P9-CMO-264

CANCER CHEMOTHERAPY AND BIOTHERAPY: PRINCIPLES AND PRACTICE

Third Edition

CANCER CHEMOTHERAPY AND BIOTHERAPY: PRINCIPLES AND PRACTICE

Third Edition

EDITED BY

Bruce A. Chabner, M.D.

Professor of Medicine
Harvard Medical School
Clinical Director
Massachusetts General Hospital Cancer Center
Boston, Massachusetts

Dan L. Longo, M.D.

Scientific Director
National Institute on Aging
National Institutes of Health
Baltimore, Maryland

with 66 contributing authors

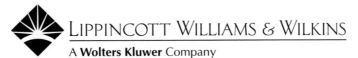

LIPPINCOTT WILLIAMS & WILKINS
A **Wolters Kluwer** Company

Philadelphia • Baltimore • New York • London
Buenos Aires • Hong Kong • Sydney • Tokyo

Acquisitions Editor: Jonathan Pine
Developmental Editor: Pamela Sutton
Supervising Editor: Mary Ann McLaughlin
Production Editor: Alyson Langlois, Silverchair Science + Communications, Inc.
Manufacturing Manager: Tim Reynolds
Cover Designer: Christine Jenny
Compositor: Silverchair Science + Communications
Printer: Edwards Brothers

© 1990, 1996, 2001 by LIPPINCOTT WILLIAMS & WILKINS
530 Walnut Street
Philadelphia, PA 19106 USA
LWW.com

All rights reserved. This book is protected by copyright. No part of this book may be reproduced in any form or by any means, including photocopying, or utilized by any information storage and retrieval system without written permission from the copyright owner, except for brief quotations embodied in critical articles and reviews. Materials appearing in this book prepared by individuals as part of their official duties as U.S. government employees are not covered by the above-mentioned copyright.

Printed in the USA

ISBN: 0-7817-2269-1

Care has been taken to confirm the accuracy of the information presented and to describe generally accepted practices. However, the authors, editors, and publisher are not responsible for errors or omissions or for any consequences from application of the information in this book and make no warranty, expressed or implied, with respect to the currency, completeness, or accuracy of the contents of the publication. Application of this information in a particular situation remains the professional responsibility of the practitioner.

The authors, editors, and publisher have exerted every effort to ensure that drug selection and dosage set forth in this text are in accordance with current recommendations and practice at the time of publication. However, in view of ongoing research, changes in government regulations, and the constant flow of information relating to drug therapy and drug reactions, the reader is urged to check the package insert for each drug for any change in indications and dosage and for added warnings and precautions. This is particularly important when the recommended agent is a new or infrequently employed drug.

Some drugs and medical devices presented in this publication have Food and Drug Administration (FDA) clearance for limited use in restricted research settings. It is the responsibility of health care providers to ascertain the FDA status of each drug or device planned for use in their clinical practice.

10 9 8 7 6 5 4 3 2 1

CONTENTS

v

CONTRIBUTING AUTHORS

Carmen J. Allegra, M.D.
Vice Deputy Director for Extramural Science
National Cancer Institute
Bethesda, Maryland

Susan G. Arbuck, M.D., M.Sc.
Head, Developmental Chemotherapy Section
Cancer Therapy Evaluation Program
Division of Cancer Treatment and Diagnosis
National Cancer Institute
Rockville, Maryland

Steven D. Averbuch, M.D.
Senior Medical Director
U.S. Drug Development
Astrazeneca Pharmaceuticals, LP
Wilmington, Delaware

Tracy T. Batchelor, M.D.
Assistant Professor of Neurology
Harvard Medical School
Director of Neuromedical Oncology
Brain Tumor Center
Massachusetts General Hospital
Boston, Massachusetts

Ernest C. Borden, M.D.
Director, Center for Cancer Drug Discovery
  and Development
Cleveland Clinic Foundation
Cleveland, Ohio

Ronald M. Bukowski, M.D.
Director of Experimental Therapeutics
Cleveland Clinic Taussig Cancer Center
Cleveland Clinic Foundation
Cleveland, Ohio

Bruce A. Chabner, M.D.
Professor of Medicine
Harvard Medical School
Clinical Director
Massachusetts General Hospital Cancer Center
Boston, Massachusetts

Jeffrey W. Clark, M.D.
Assistant Professor of Medicine
Medical Director, Clinical Protocol Office
Massachusetts General Hospital Cancer Center
Boston, Massachusetts

C. Norman Coleman, M.D.
Director, Radiation Oncology Sciences Program
Center for Cancer Research and Division of Cancer
  Treatment and Diagnosis
National Cancer Institute
Bethesda, Maryland

Jerry M. Collins, Ph.D.
Director, Laboratory of Clinical Pharmacology
U.S. Food and Drug Administration
Rockville, Maryland

O. Michael Colvin, M.D.
Director, Duke Comprehensive Cancer Center
Duke University Medical Center
Durham, North Carolina

Brendan D. Curti, M.D.
Associate Professor of Medicine
Division of Hematology/Oncology
Pennsylvania State University College
  of Medicine
Milton S. Hershey Medical Center
Hershey, Pennsylvania

Harry D. Dawson, Ph.D.
Laboratory of Immunology
Gerontology Research Center
National Institute on Aging
National Institutes of Health
Baltimore, Maryland

Robert B. Diasio, M.D.
Professor of Medicine and Pharmacology
Chairman, Department of Pharmacology
  and Toxicology
University of Alabama School of Medicine
Birmingham, Alabama

Ross C. Donehower, M.D.
Professor of Oncology and Medicine
Johns Hopkins University School of Medicine
Director, Division of Medical Oncology
Johns Hopkins Oncology Center
Baltimore, Maryland

James H. Doroshow, M.D.
Chairman, Department of Medical Oncology
    and Therapeutics Research
City of Hope Comprehensive Cancer Center
Duarte, California

Glenn Dranoff, M.D.
Associate Professor of Medicine
Department of Adult Oncology
Harvard Medical School
Dana-Farber Cancer Institute
Boston, Massachusetts

Matthew J. Ellis, M.D., Ph.D., F.R.C.P.
Associate Professor of Medicine
Department of Medicine
Division of Oncology
Duke University School of Medicine
Duke University Medical Center
Durham, North Carolina

Charles Erlichman, M.D.
Professor of Oncology
Department of Medical Oncology
Mayo Medical School
Mayo Clinic and Mayo Foundation
Rochester, Minnesota

James H. Finke, Ph.D.
Department of Immunology
Cleveland Clinic Foundation
Cleveland, Ohio

Joseph A. Fontana, M.D., Ph.D.
Professor of Medicine and Oncology
Karmanos Cancer Institute
Wayne State University School of Medicine
Chief, Hematology–Medical Oncology
John D. Dingell Veterans Administration Medical Center
Detroit, Michigan

Henry S. Friedman, M.D.
James B. Powell Jr. Professor of Neuro-Oncology
Department of Surgery
Duke University School of Medicine
Duke University Medical Center
Durham, North Carolina

Rocio Garcia-Carbonero, M.D.
Consultant in Medical Oncology
Department of Hematology-Oncology
Hospital Clinico Universitario de Valencia
Valencia, Spain

Michel P. Gatineau, M.D.
Visiting Fellow
Division of Hematology-Oncology
Massachusetts General Hospital
Boston, Massachusetts

François Goldwasser, M.D., Ph.D.
Professor of Medical Oncology
Université Paris V
Hôpital Cochin
Paris, France

William J. Gradishar, M.D.
Associate Professor of Medicine
Department of Medicine
Division of Hematology-Oncology
Northwestern University Medical School
Robert H. Lurie Comprehensive Cancer Center
Chicago, Illinois

Jean L. Grem, M.D., F.A.C.P.
Senior Investigator
Head, Cellular and Clinical Pharmacology
    Section
Medical Oncology Program
Center for Cancer Research
National Cancer Institute
Bethesda, Maryland

Kenneth R. Hande, M.D.
Professor of Medicine and Pharmacology
Department of Medicine and Pharmacology
Vanderbilt University School of Medicine
Nashville, Tennessee

Melinda G. Hollingshead, D.V.M., Ph.D.
Veterinary Medical Officer
Biological Testing Branch, Developmental
    Therapeutics Program
Division of Cancer Treatment
    and Diagnosis
National Cancer Institute
Frederick, Maryland

Jill I. Johnson, B.S.
Developmental Therapeutics Program
National Cancer Institute
Rockville, Maryland

Carl H. June, M.D.
Professor of Pathology and Laboratory Medicine
University of Pennsylvania Health System
Director, Translational Research Programs
Philadelphia, Pennsylvania

Richard P. Junghans, M.D., Ph.D.
Assistant Professor of Medicine
Director, Biotherapeutics Development Laboratory
Harvard Institute of Human Genetics
Harvard Medical School
Division of Hematology-Oncology
Beth Israel Deaconess Medical Center
Boston, Massachusetts

Dwight C. Kaufman, M.D., Ph.D.
Jackson Clinic
Jackson, Tennessee

Joanne Kurtzberg, M.D.
Professor of Pediatrics
Associate Professor of Pathology
Department of Pediatrics
Duke University Medical Center
Durham, North Carolina

John S. Lazo, Ph.D.
Professor and Chairman, Department of Pharmacology
University of Pittsburgh School of Medicine
Pittsburgh, Pennsylvania

Ann L. Mellott, M.D.
Department of Hematology-Oncology
Northwestern University Medical School
Chicago, Illinois

Richard A. Messmann, M.D., M.H.S., M.Sc.
Deputy Associate Director
National Cancer Institute
Bethesda, Maryland

James B. Mitchell, Ph.D.
Radiation Biology Branch
National Institute of Cancer
Bethesda, Maryland

Anne Monks, Ph.D.
Senior Scientist
Screening Technologies Branch
Scientific Applications International Corporation
Frederick, Maryland

Malcolm Moore, M.D.
Associate Professor
Department of Medicine and Pharmacology
Princess Margaret Hospital
University of Toronto
Toronto, Canada

Kees Nooter, Ph.D.
Senior Scientist
Department of Medical Oncology
University Hospital Rotterdam
Rotterdam, The Netherlands

Luis Paz-Ares, M.D., Ph.D.
Consultant in Medical Oncology
Division of Medical Oncology
Hospital Universitario Doce de Octubre
Madrid, Spain

William P. Petros, Pharm.D.
Associate Professor
Department of Clinical Pharmacology
West Virginia University School of Pharmacy
Morgantown, West Virginia

Yves G. Pommier, M.D., Ph.D.
Chief, Laboratory of Molecular Pharmacology
National Cancer Institute
Center for Cancer Research
National Institutes of Health
Bethesda, Maryland

Eddie Reed, M.D.
Professor of Medicine
Laurence and Jean DeLynn Chair
     of Oncology
West Virginia University School of Medicine
Director of the Mary Babb Randolph
     Cancer Center
Robert C. Byrd Health Science Center
Morgantown, West Virginia

Arun K. Rishi, Ph.D.
Associate Professor
Department of Internal Medicine
Karmanos Cancer Institute
Wayne State University School of Medicine
John D. Dingell Veterans Administration
     Medical Center
Detroit, Michigan

Eric K. Rowinsky, M.D.
Clinical Professor of Medicine
Director, Department of Clinical Research
Institute for Drug Development
University of Texas Health Sciences Center
San Antonio, Texas

David P. Ryan, M.D.
Instructor in Medicine
Division of Hematology-Oncology
Harvard Medical School
Massachusetts General Hospital
Boston, Massachusetts

Stephen E. Sallan
Professor of Pediatrics
Department of Pediatric Oncology
Dana-Farber Cancer Institute
Boston, Massachusetts

Edward A. Sausville, M.D., Ph.D.
Associate Director of Developmental Therapeutics
    Program
National Cancer Institute
Rockville, Maryland

Eric Schaffer, Ph.D.
Laboratory of Immunology
National Institute on Aging
Baltimore, Maryland

David A. Scheinberg, M.D., Ph.D.
Member, Sloan-Kettering Institute
Professor, Department of Medicine and Molecular
    Pharmacology
Weill Medical College of Cornell University
New York, New York

Richard L. Schilsky, M.D.
Professor of Medicine
Associate Dean for Clinical Research
Biological Sciences Division
University of Chicago
Chicago, Illinois

George Sgouros, Ph.D.
Associate Member, Department of Medical Physics
Memorial Sloan-Kettering Cancer Center
New York, New York

Matthew R. Smith, M.D., Ph.D.
Instructor in Medicine
Harvard Medical School
Division of Hematology-Oncology
Massachusetts General Hospital
Boston, Massachusetts

Alex Sparreboom, Ph.D.
Pharmacologist
Department of Medical Oncology
Rotterdam Cancer Institute
Rotterdam, The Netherlands

Dirk Strumberg, M.D.
Department of Internal Medicine and
    Medical Oncology
University of Essen Medical School
West German Cancer Center
Essen, Germany

Jeffrey G. Supko, Ph.D.
Assistant Professor of Medicine
Division of Hematology/Oncology
Harvard Medical School
Massachusetts General Hospital Cancer Center
Boston, Massachusetts

Sandra M. Swain, M.D.
Acting Chief of Medicine Branch
National Cancer Institute
National Institutes of Health
Bethesda, Maryland

Chris H. Takimoto, M.D., Ph.D.
Associate Professor of Medicine
Department of Medicine
Division of Medical Oncology
University of Texas Health Sciences Center
San Antonio, Texas

Charles S. Tannenbaum, Ph.D.
Project Scientist
Department of Immunology
Cleveland Clinic Foundation
Cleveland, Ohio

Dennis D. Taub, Ph.D.
Chief, Laboratory of Immunology
National Institute on Aging
National Institutes of Health
Baltimore, Maryland

Kenneth D. Tew, Ph.D., D.Sc.
Chairman of Pharmacology, Senior Member
G. Willing Pepper Chair in Cancer Research
Fox Chase Cancer Center
Philadelphia, Pennsylvania

Jaap Verweij, M.D., Ph.D.
Professor
Department of Medical Oncology
Rotterdam Cancer Institute and University Hospital
Rotterdam, The Netherlands

Deborah J. Vestal, Ph.D.
Department of Molecular Biology
Cleveland Clinic Foundation
Cleveland, Ohio

Taolin Yi, Ph.D.
Associate Staff
Department of Cancer Biology
Lerner Research Institute
Cleveland Clinic Foundation
Cleveland, Ohio

PREFACE

You know that medicines, when well used, restore health to the sick; they will be well used when the doctor together with his understanding of their nature shall understand also what man is, what life is, and what constitution and health are. Know these well and you will know their opposites; and when this is the case you will know well how to devise a remedy.

—Leonardo da Vinci, *Codex Atlantico*

The third edition of this book is an attempt to provide information that will help caregivers better understand the nature of the medicines available to treat a particularly unpleasant "opposite" in human health, cancer, and possibly better understand cancer as well. The therapeutic index of agents used to treat cancer is extraordinarily small in most cases. We do not always know why this is true, but we surmise that the root cause is that the cancer cell is more like normal cells than we have been willing to admit. The first effective chemical agents attacked DNA synthesis based on the hypothesis that cancer cells proliferate more or faster than normal cells. But this hypothesis is wrong. By the time it becomes clinically apparent, the growth fraction of acute leukemia is, if anything, similar to or lower than the growth fraction of normal bone marrow. Human solid tumors are decreasing their growth fraction and their growth rate at the point they are diagnosed. So when we use antiproliferative agents, we attack all dividing cells, including both the 2% to 5% of tumor cells that are dividing and the normal cells that are dividing. We count on the hope that the normal proliferating cells will recover the capacity to proliferate (and restore normal organ function) faster than the cancer cells do. In many cases, this hope is true.

Despite the fact that proliferation is not a feature restricted to tumor cells, new agents that appear to be effective in certain cancers continue to emerge that target proliferation, including the nucleosides (such as gemcitabine and fludarabine), the taxanes (paclitaxel and docetaxel), and the camptothecin derivatives (such as irinotecan and topotecan). Advances in our understanding of their pharmacology and metabolism are resulting in safer and more effective applications to cancer treatment. Continued efforts are underway to develop even more active and less toxic variants and analogues that bypass the cell's resistance mechanisms.

Among the many changes in the practice of oncology since the last edition of this text is the wide range of targets that are now the focus of anticancer drug development efforts. We now have approved drugs that interfere with histone deacetylase and thus alter the pattern of gene expression and the level of differentiation of malignant cells (arsenic trioxide in acute promyelocytic leukemia). Another approved drug targets an oncogenic tyrosine kinase that is a keystone of neoplastic transformation [Gleevec (imatinib mesylate) inhibiting abl in chronic myeloid leukemia]. New hormonal agents target a novel set of retinoic acid receptors (RXR; bexarotene in cutaneous T-cell lymphoma). Other new agents that interfere with the synthesis of estrogen (aromatase inhibitors) have become the estrogen antagonists of choice, supplanting the partially antagonistic and partially agonistic estrogen receptor blocker tamoxifen as first-line hormonal therapy in breast cancer. Additional agents in all of these classes that hit all of these targets, as well as additional targets (neovascularization, other steps in metastasis, protein synthesis and turnover, and many others), are well into the clinical phase of drug development, and many will be approved in the next few years.

Biologic approaches to cancer treatment are finally beginning to show clinically significant results. Humanized monoclonal antibodies have overcome many of the problems that limited the efficacy of murine antibodies in the initial trials applying this technology. Safe and effective antibodies are now readily available that target a number of tumor-associated products (for example, rituximab against CD20 and trastuzumab against the HER2/neu receptor tyrosine kinase). Adoptive cellular therapy in the form of donor lymphocyte infusions is clearly effective in patients with chronic myeloid leukemia who relapse after allogeneic bone marrow transplantation. The application of lymphocytes to cancer treatment is increasing with the growing use of the so-called minitransplant approach in which fully functional (and sometimes tumor-specific) lymphocytes are transferred to an immunosuppressed cancer-bearing host. Cancer vaccines have, for the first time, been shown to have antitumor effects; a lymphoma vaccine has been shown to eradicate polymerase chain reaction–detectable persistent tumor after a chemotherapy-induced remission. Cytokines and chemokines that are capable of regulating immune responses continue to be applied to cancer treatment in various ways. Efforts continue to try to reverse the immune defects associated with the tumor-bearing state and to restore normal immune function after the serious deleterious effects of cancer treatments on the immune system.

Supportive care tools are also burgeoning. Erythropoietin for red cells, granulocyte or granulocyte-macrophage colony-stimulating factors for granulocytes, and interleukin 11 for platelets are widely used to speed marrow recovery after myelotoxic chemotherapy. Better antiemetics (such as granisetron), better methods of pain control, and better antidepressants and sleep medications are all contributing to preserving the quality of life of cancer patients. Bisphosphonates have been shown to reduce the risk of morbidity associated with cancers that spread to bone.

Progress has also been made in the use of drugs to enhance the efficacy of radiation therapy and to protect normal tissue from radiation damage. Hypoxic cell sensitizers have not yet made a major impact on clinical management of patients, but that situation could change. Biophysical barriers to the delivery of drugs to tumors, which uniformly show increased interstitial pressure that resists penetrance of a drug to the center of a tumor, also need to be overcome. These are areas of ongoing research and development.

All the progress that is being made in the development of new and apparently more effective cancer treatments has begun to make an impact on cancer mortality rates. However, the rate of decline in cancer mortality has lagged significantly behind the development of effective treatments. Although the causes of this discordance may be multifacto-

rial, it is now emerging that at least one major contributor to the failure of treatment advances to lower mortality is that patients are not receiving life-extending therapy. Only approximately 50% of people with node-positive colorectal cancer older than the age of 65 actually receive a 5-fluorouracil–containing adjuvant chemotherapy regimen despite the confirmed result that mortality rates can be decreased by 40% to 50% by such therapy. It is our hope that we can combat this lack of penetrance of cancer treatment advances into the community practice of medicine with information about the drugs and how they can be used safely.

The skilled physicians treating patients with cancer have a daunting task in that they need to understand pharmacology, pharmacokinetics, pharmacogenetics, pharmacodynamics, drug metabolism, drug resistance, cancer cell biology, normal cell biology, and myriad drug interactions, in addition to considerations of alterations in physiology caused by the cancer or associated with concurrent disease or advanced age that influence these distinct facets that in turn influence drug action. In this book, we have attempted to incorporate relevant information that will assist the caregiver in planning the optimal treatment approach for each individual patient. It is our intention to keep the information in this text up to date through the addition of relevant information on newly approved drugs to the new online version of this book that appears at http://www.lwwoncology.com. We look forward to your feedback about how to make this book more useful to you.

Bruce A. Chabner, M.D.
Dan L. Longo, M.D.

ACKNOWLEDGMENTS

We would like to express our gratitude to our editor, Stuart Freeman, who retired at the end of 2000, but who graciously stayed on his watch to finish our third edition. Stuart was very ably assisted by Will Wiebalck, but Stuart's friendship and his great interest in the field of cancer made this working relationship special. Good rowing and smooth waters ahead, Stuart.

We would like to thank our wives, Nancy and Davi-Ellen, who have indulged us once again in this eternal project. The late nights, busy weekends, and e-mails continued unabated, but it is a project that we care about, and we hope it helps our readers understand this rapidly changing field. If we have done it correctly, this text will help to develop better drugs and make them safer and more effective in clinical practice.

Finally, to our editorial assistants, Pat Duffey and Ellen Patton, our heartfelt thanks. We could not have done this without your help in organizing the projects, preparing manuscripts, and keeping those status reports up to date.

1

CLINICAL STRATEGIES FOR CANCER TREATMENT: THE ROLE OF DRUGS

DWIGHT C. KAUFMAN
BRUCE A. CHABNER

Cancer treatment requires the cooperative efforts of multiple medical specialties. Although surgeons traditionally have been the first to treat the cancer patient, new treatment approaches have created important roles for the radiotherapist and medical oncologist in the initial management of cancer patients and have placed the responsibility for care of the majority of patients with metastatic cancer in the hands of these specialists. The array of alternatives for the treatment of cancer is constantly expanding. With the demonstration of effectiveness of new drugs and new biologics, and with the evolution of more effective strategies for integrating chemotherapy, surgery, and radiation, the development of a treatment plan becomes increasingly complex. The plan must be based on a thorough understanding of the potential for beneficial response and an awareness of the acute and late toxicities of each component of the treatment regimen.

As a general rule, the medical oncologist is urged to use standard effective regimens as described in the *Physician Data Query* (*PDQ*) system of the National Cancer Institute (NCI).* *PDQ* contains information on state-of-the-art treatments for each pathologic type of cancer, as well as a listing of experimental protocols for each disease. An important alternative to "standard" therapy is the clinical trial, which should be considered for every eligible patient. Both the patient and the physician must understand that every NCI-supported clinical trial offers the patient therapy that is thought by a panel of experts to be at least as effective as the recognized standard of care. In many randomized clinical trials (phase III trials), the current state-of-the-art standard treatment regimen is compared with a new regimen

that is hoped or even expected to be an improvement, and if the new regimen is found to be superior, it becomes the new standard. With either choice, standard therapy or a clinical trial, the medical oncologist must be fully aware of the rationale for choosing specific drugs or combinations of drugs, or combinations of drugs and biologics. All these considerations enter into the choice of a treatment plan. Steps in the treatment decision-making process are discussed in this chapter to provide the reader with an understanding of the overall role of drugs in cancer treatment.

DETERMINANTS OF TREATMENT PLANNING

The first and primary determinant of treatment is the histologic diagnosis. Malignant neoplasms occur in over 100 different pathologic forms, each with a characteristic natural history, pattern of progression, and responsiveness to treatment. Thus the *histologic diagnosis*, usually made by surgical biopsy or excision of a primary tumor, is of critical importance as a first step in treatment planning. The clinical oncologist must be alert to the possibility of atypical presentations of treatable and even curable tumors, such as germ cell tumors of the testis and breast cancer, and must ask for special histologic tests to rule in or out a potentially curable tumor type. For example, germ cell tumors on occasion may arise in the thoracic or abdominal cavity in the absence of a primary testicular tumor; still, these unusual presentations retain an excellent response to appropriate chemotherapy.[1] In certain cases—for example, lung carcinoma or the non-Hodgkin's lymphomas—accurate histologic *subtyping* of tumors is important because the subtypes of these diseases have different patterns of clinical response to treatment. Subtyping may require the characterization of cell surface immunologic markers (e.g., to distinguish T- and B-cell lymphomas) or the identification of specific intracellular secretory granules or enzymatic markers, such as dopa decarboxylase in small cell carcinoma of the lung. Molecular

---

PDQ is available to physicians at most medical libraries, at many hospitals, through the Internet, or through private computer software vendors. Access to *PDQ* is also available directly from the NCI through the NCI Information Associates Program. For information about accessing *PDQ*, call the Information Associates Program Customer Service Desk at 1-800-NCI-7890 (301-816-2083 outside the United States).

or genetic analysis may reveal important prognostic information for subtyping leukemias, lymphomas, or other cancers.[2] The essential point is that the precise histologic identity of a tumor is the single most important determinant of treatment choice and patient management. Blind treatment, in cases lacking a precise histologic diagnosis, is usually not successful,[3] although treatment for the most responsive possible diagnosis, such as testicular carcinoma in a patient with poorly differentiated carcinoma of uncertain origin, occasionally may produce durable responses.[4]

Although histologic subtyping may contribute essential information to the treatment plan, biochemical, molecular, and cytokinetic features also may provide important prognostic information and influence treatment planning. For instance, in premenopausal women with stage I breast cancer (less than 2 cm primary, node negative), certain adverse tumor features, such as a high S-phase (DNA synthetic phase) fraction, absence of estrogen or progesterone receptors, or high expression of the *c-erbB-2/HER-2-neu* oncogene, may guide the selection of drugs for adjuvant chemotherapy; in fact, high *HER-2-neu* expression in node-positive breast cancer may indicate dose-intensive adjuvant chemotherapy.[5] In the future, molecular analysis of tumors probably will be useful in identifying drug-responsive tumors and will guide the selection of therapy.

The next step in treatment planning is to determine the extent of disease, specifically to determine whether the tumor is curable by local treatment measures such as surgery or radiation therapy. The process of determining the extent of disease is termed *staging* and plays an important role in making therapeutic choices for diseases that are responsive to multiple types of treatment. For example, non-Hodgkin's lymphomas with "indolent" histology are curable with radiotherapy in a majority of cases when the tumor is confined to a single lymph node region (stage I). Because the indolent subtypes of malignant lymphoma are usually incurable, even with aggressive early chemotherapy, when more extensive lymph node involvement or dissemination to extranodal sites is present, immediate treatment of stage I disease with radiation is indicated, whereas, paradoxically, no immediate therapy may be indicated for patients with disease of stage III to IV.

The choice of specific therapies depends on histology, stage, and a third factor, the patient's probable tolerance for the side effects of the various possible treatments. Thus, although curative chemotherapy regimens exist for a substantial fraction of patients with diffuse large cell lymphoma, not all patients with this diagnosis are suitable candidates for intensive treatment.[2] Severely debilitated patients and those with underlying medical problems—for example, heart disease, diabetes, or chronic obstructive pulmonary disease—might well suffer severely disabling or fatal complications from potentially curative regimens, as indicated in Table 1-1. In such cases the physician must weigh the chances of successful treatment against the prob-

TABLE 1-1. TOXICITY OF CHOP REGIMEN FOR TREATING DIFFUSE LARGE CELL LYMPHOMA

Drugs	Toxicity[a]	Risk Factors
Cyclophosphamide	Hair loss, myelosuppression, hemorrhagic cystitis, secondary leukemia	Underlying infection
Doxorubicin hydrochloride (Adriamycin)	Cardiomyopathy, myelosuppression, hair loss	History of heart disease, prior chest irradiation
Vincristine sulfate (Oncovin)	Peripheral and autonomic neuropathy	Liver dysfunction, other neurotoxic drugs, inherited peripheral nerve disease
Prednisone	Glucose intolerance, immune suppression, bone and muscle loss	Diabetes, underlying infection

[a]In general, elderly patients are at increased risk of toxicity because of underlying medical problems and altered rates of drug elimination.

ability of serious side effects from each of the therapeutic alternatives. The ultimate decision must be based on a thorough understanding of the disease process under consideration, the *clinical* pharmacology of the drugs in question, and the potential benefits and risks of alternative forms of treatment, such as chemotherapy, radiotherapy, or surgery.

Finally, possessing the information about histology, stage, and other tumor-related variables and about the patient's age and baseline health, the oncologist must decide whether a realistic opportunity exists for curative treatment. A decision to treat with curative intent demands a high degree of adherence to drug dosing and scheduling requirements, as specified in the standard or experimental regimen, and an acceptance of treatment-related toxicity. When cure is not a realistic expectation, a decision to treat must be based on an expectation for prolongation of the patient's life or an improvement in the quality of life. In these cases, treatment-related side effects may be minimized by dosage adjustments or treatment delays when necessary, but at the cost of antitumor efficacy. When the probability for benefit is low, chemotherapy should be offered only after frank and thorough discussion of the likely outcome. In such cases, experimental phase I or phase II drugs may be a more attractive alternative in the setting of a clinical trial.

DRUGS IN CANCER TREATMENT

Drugs are now used at some time during the course of the illness of most cancer patients. Cytotoxic drugs can cure some disseminated cancers (Table 1-2) and can be effective in decreasing tumor volume, alleviating symptoms, and even prolonging life in many other types of metastatic cancer.

TABLE 1-2. CURABILITY OF DISSEMINATED CANCER WITH DRUGS

Disease	Therapy	Probable Cure Rate
Adults		
Intermediate- and high-grade non-Hodgkin's lymphomas	Combination chemotherapy	35–50%
Hodgkin's disease (stage III or IV)	Combination chemotherapy	50% or higher
Testicular carcinoma (stage III)	Combination chemotherapy followed by surgery	90% or higher
Gestational choriocarcinoma	Methotrexate sodium ± dactinomycin (actinomycin D)	90%
Ovarian carcinoma	Platinum-containing combination chemotherapy	10%
Acute myelocytic leukemia	Combination chemotherapy	20%
Hairy cell leukemia	Cladribine	80–90%
Children		
Acute lymphocytic leukemia	Combination chemotherapy plus cranial irradiation	50% or higher
Intermediate- and high-grade non-Hodgkin's lymphomas	Combination chemotherapy	50% or higher
Wilms' tumor and sarcomas	Surgery, chemotherapy, and irradiation	50%

Adjuvant chemotherapy regimens are used in patients who have had primary tumors resected and who, although possibly cured by surgery, are at significant risk of recurrence. Adjuvant therapy has been shown in randomized trials to delay tumor recurrence and prolong survival (and possibly cure) patients with breast cancer, colorectal cancer, cervical cancer (with irradiation), and osteosarcoma.[6] *Neoadjuvant* chemotherapy has been used to reduce the bulk of primary tumors before surgical resection or irradiation of locally extensive head and neck carcinomas, esophageal cancer, non–small cell lung cancer, osteosarcoma and soft tissue sarcomas, bladder cancer, and locally advanced breast cancer. This can improve the probability of total surgical resection, decrease local recurrence, and allow organ preservation. Furthermore, this strategy may eradicate micrometastatic disease, and the initial clinical response of the tumor mass can serve as an indication to continue therapy after surgery.

The design of drug treatment regimens is based on a number of considerations. These include (a) prior knowledge of the responsiveness of the pathologic category of tumor to specific drugs, (b) an understanding of the biochemical mechanisms of the drugs' cytotoxic activity as well as the mechanisms of resistance to the drugs, and (c) knowledge of the drugs' pharmacokinetic behavior and of patterns of normal organ toxicity. Some chemotherapy regimens have been designed to minimize emergence of drug resistance, based on the predictions of theoretical models of drug resistance. The biologic and pharmacokinetic features of individual drugs are considered in detail in succeeding chapters, but the impact of these and other factors such as cell kinetics on trial design is reviewed briefly at this juncture to illustrate the way in which multiple factors are integrated into a protocol.

Kinetic Basis of Drug Therapy

The objective of cancer treatment is to reduce the tumor cell population to zero cells. Chemotherapy experiments using rapidly growing transplanted tumors in mice have established the validity of the *fractional cell kill hypothesis*, which states that a given drug concentration applied for a defined time period will kill a constant fraction of the cell population, independent of the absolute number of cells. Regrowth of tumor occurs during the drug-free interval between cycles. Thus, each treatment cycle kills a specific fraction of the remaining cells. The results of treatment are a direct function of (a) the dose of drug administered and (b) the number and frequency of repetitions of treatment.

Most current chemotherapy regimens are based on cytokinetic considerations and use cycles of intensive therapy repeated as frequently as allowed by the tolerance of dose-limiting tissues such as bone marrow or gastrointestinal tract. The object of these cycles is to reduce the absolute number of remaining tumor cells to zero (or less than one) through the multiplicative effect of successive fractional cell kills. [For example, given 99% cell kill per cycle, a tumor burden of 10^{11} cells will be reduced to less than 1 cell with six cycles of treatment: $(10^{11}$ cells$) \times (0.01)^6 < 1$.]

The fractional cell kill hypothesis was defined initially in animal models of leukemia and was applied most successfully in human leukemia and lymphoma. The fundamental assumption of constant fractional cell kill per cycle with constant dosing is unlikely to be valid for the more heterogeneous, slowly growing solid tumors in humans. Most clinical neoplasms are recognized at a stage of decelerating growth, which may be due to poor tumor vascularity with resulting hypoxia or poor nutrient supply, or to other unidentified factors. These tumors contain a high fraction of slowly dividing or noncycling cells (termed G_0 cells). Because most antineoplastic agents, particularly the antimetabolites and antitumor antibiotics, are most effective against rapidly dividing cells and some are *phase specific* (i.e., most effective in killing cells in a specific phase in the cell cycle), the initial kinetic situation is unfavorable for treatment with most drugs. Exceptions to this rule are the DNA alkylators and metalators (platinum derivatives), which are equally active against nondividing cells. An initial reduction in cell numbers produced by surgery, radiotherapy, or non–cell-cycle-specific drugs (e.g., alkylating agents) may stimulate the slowly dividing cells into more rapid cell division or may recruit nondividing cells into the cell cycle, where they become increasingly susceptible to therapy with cell-cycle-specific agents (e.g., methotrexate sodium, cytosine arabinoside). Thus an initially slowly responding tumor may become more responsive to therapy after surgical debulking or with continued treatment. The fractional cell kill may actually increase with sequential courses of treatment.

Biochemical heterogeneity of human tumors introduces additional complexity to the simple hypothesis that multiple cycles of fractional cell kill translate into tumor cure. Isoenzyme typing and karyotypic analysis of tumors demonstrate that most human tumors studied thus far have evolved clonally from a single malignant cell.[7] Techniques for *in vitro* cloning of solid tumors have shown, however, that this original homogeneity does not persist during later stages of tumor growth; in fact, both experimental and human tumors are composed of cell types with differing biochemical, morphologic, and drug-response characteristics.[8] This heterogeneity results from the inherent genetic instability of malignant cells. Indeed, mutations in cell-cycle checkpoint control genes, such as *p53*, and in DNA repair genes, such as the *MSH* genes in familial colon cancer, may be the initial event in malignant transformation, establishing a fundamentally mutable clone from which myriad genetic mutations occur. Thus gene amplifications, deletions, or other alterations of genes coding for target proteins that control drug response and cell cycle lead to heterogeneity of the tumor cell population and probably account for outgrowth of resistant tumor cells during relapse of formerly sensitive tumors. When cells are subjected to the selective pressure of drug treatment, sensitive tumor cells are destroyed, but subpopulations of resistant cells survive and proliferate. This process of selecting out resistant cells has been amply demonstrated in cell culture as well as in patients.[9] Thus cell kill tends to decrease with subsequent courses of treatment as resistant cell types are selected out. With the possible exceptions of treatment of gestational choriocarcinoma with methotrexate, cyclophosphamide treatment for African Burkitt's lymphoma, and cladribine treatment for hairy cell leukemia, single-agent chemotherapy has not produced long-term survival or cure of advanced malignancies. The most successful drug treatment regimens have combined multiple agents with different mechanisms of action.

Prediction of Drug Response to Individual Agents

The selection of drugs for treating specific types of cancer is based largely on the results of previous clinical trials and is often empirical. To avoid the needless toxicity of ineffective agents, especially in diseases with only modest rates of response, predicting sensitivity for the specific tumor and patient at hand would be desirable. Various experimental systems for testing tumor cells or tumor fragments for response to panels of drugs have been studied intensively in the hope that they would accurately predict response in patients. Although some of these tests have been quite accurate in predicting resistance to various drugs in populations of highly resistant patients, none has satisfactorily predicted clinical responsiveness, and in general, prospective, randomized testing has not been done. Considering the rather formidable list of limitations (discussed later) inherent in these assays, none of the *in vitro* assay systems has become an important aid in choosing antineoplastic therapy.

Human tumor fragments grown in immunologically incompetent mice[10] (athymic, or nude, mice or thymectomized and irradiated mice) or under the renal capsule of mice[11] have been used in drug sensitivity assays; however, the *in vitro* culture of human tumors in semisolid medium[12] offers a less cumbersome means of pretreatment selection of agents. The *in vitro* tumor cell colony–forming assay allows fairly reliable culture of human ovarian cancers, renal cell carcinomas, malignant melanomas, soft tissue sarcomas, and multiple myeloma cells but less consistent growth of other forms of malignancy. The assay seems useful in predicting resistance, which potentially allows the avoidance of ineffective drugs,[13] but has some clear practical as well as theoretical disadvantages. Most significantly, the success rate in growing important solid tumors such as breast, lung, and colon carcinoma is poor (less than 25%). Consequently, the number of colonies formed is usually less than 50 per plate, which results in a test system that is able to detect cell kill only over a narrow range of 1 log cell kill or less. That the clinical behavior of a large and very heterogeneous tumor can be predicted accurately based on the *in vitro* behavior of the 1% of cells most amenable to forming soft agar colonies seems improbable. Other limitations include (a) the difficulty in completely disrupting the specimen into true single-cell suspensions, which results in difficulty in distinguishing tumor clumps from true proliferative colonies; (b) the time required to obtain results (2 to 3 weeks); (c) the problem of testing drugs that require metabolic activation in noncancer tissue, such as cyclophosphamide, procarbazine hydrochloride, and hexamethylmelamine (altretamine); and (d) the failure of testing conditions to simulate the drug concentration and duration of exposure that occur *in vivo*.

Biochemical tests based on a knowledge of the mechanism of action of specific drugs have provided helpful predictions of response in animal tumor systems, but few have been evaluated carefully in humans. Test systems have focused on one or several specific determinants, such as the concentration of a key enzyme (deoxycytidine kinase for arabinosylcytosine)[13] or the presence of a specific cytoplasmic receptor, such as the estrogen receptor for hormonal therapy of breast cancer. A few of these tests—most notably the test for estrogen receptor in breast cancer—have become cornerstones for therapeutic decision making; other tests offer considerable promise. In one retrospective study, the response of patients with ovarian cancer to platinum derivatives correlated with the level of platinum-DNA adducts in patients' peripheral white blood cells after therapy,[15] which is perhaps an indication of innate DNA reparability shared by tumor and host. Similarly, high concentrations of dihydrofolate reductase have been associated with resistance to methotrexate as is a failure to transport or polyglutamate the drug.[16,17] High levels of the DNA repair enzyme O^6-alkyl-guanine alkyl transferase predict resistance to nitrosoureas, dacarbazine, and temozolomide, which damage DNA by alkylating the O^6 position of guanine.[18] The latter test may prove useful in predicting which patients will benefit from pretreatment with O^6-benzyl guanine, an irreversible inhibitor of the alkyl transferase enzyme that is in clinical testing. Mutations in mismatch DNA repair are associated experimentally with cisplatin resistance.[19] None of these biochemical tests has been studied prospectively in a sizable patient population to prove its value in routine treatment. In each case, other potentially important changes are known to occur in experimental examples of resistance to the various drugs.

Molecularly targeted drug discovery offers the hope of identifying new drugs tailored specifically to the mutations critical for malignant transformation and tumor progression, with limited toxicity to normal tissues lacking the molecular target. Thus tumor-specific targets include the tyrosine kinase resulting from the bcr-abl translocation in chronic myelocytic leukemia.[20] A potent kinase inhibitor, STI-571, was identified by screening compounds for inhibitory activity and for selective inhibition of this kinase. The drug has striking activity in chronic and blastic phases of chronic myelocytic leukemia. Because it also inhibits the platelet-derived growth factor receptor, it will be tested against prostate cancer and primary brain tumors, which overexpress this receptor.

The epidermal growth factor receptor has also become the object of targeted drug discovery. Antibodies or small molecules that bind to and inhibit this receptor show potent tumor inhibitory activity against epithelial tumors that overexpress the epidermal growth factor receptor. In addition they show striking synergy with chemotherapy and irradiation. The synergy is believed to result from blockade of a critical growth factor signal, an event that lowers the tumor cell threshold for apoptosis. Other drug-signaling interactions, leading to synergistic cell kill, have been described for antiangiogenic drugs, protein kinase C inhibitors, the *HER-2-neu* receptor, and insulin-like growth factor I receptor. This general principle of drug-signaling interaction will undoubtedly be exploited in treating cancers that present biologic targets related to overexpressed growth factor pathways. The reader is referred to the chapter on molecularly targeted therapies for a more detailed discussion of this subject.

Pharmacokinetic Determinants of Response

Although the outcome of cancer chemotherapy depends in large part on the inherent sensitivity of the specific tumor being treated, the chances for success, even in patients with sensitive tumors, can be compromised by failure to consider important pharmacokinetic factors such as drug absorption, metabolism, and elimination in designing protocols that determine the dose, schedule, and route of drug administration.

Not only may protocol design affect pharmacokinetics and response, but even among patients with apparently normal hepatic and renal function, considerable variability is seen in peak drug concentration, area under the concentration × time curve (AUC).[21] The origin of this variability is uncertain. Clearly pharmacogenetics (inherited differences in expression of drug-metabolizing enzymes) plays an important role in the elimination of some drugs, including irinotecan hydrochloride (by glucuronidases) and 5-fluorouracil (by dihydropyrimidine dehydrogenase). In addition, differences in hepatic P-450 isoenzyme activity, protein binding of drug, and age-related changes in renal tubular function all contribute to this variability. The fact remains that most pharmacokinetic studies show at least a two- to threefold range of drug concentration and AUC for a given dose of drug.

Pharmacokinetic factors are important not only in designing general protocol but also in determining specific modifications of dosage in individual patients. Dosage may be increased or decreased based on observed patterns of toxicity or lack of same and in some cases based on direct drug concentration measurements. Renal or hepatic dysfunction leads to delayed drug elimination, which sometimes results in overwhelming toxicity. To avoid such toxicity, dosages of certain agents must be modified based on estimates of renal or hepatic function (Table 1-3). Interindividual variations are not predictable solely on the basis of renal or hepatic function, however, and direct measurement of plasma drug concentrations can provide a better guide for dosage adjustment to ensure adequate and safe drug exposure, as shown by studies of maintenance therapy in children with acute lymphocytic leukemia who receive methotrexate and 6-mercaptopurine.[22] One important source of the interindividual variability in pharmacokinetics is the variable oral absorption of a number of agents, including hexamethylmelamine, etoposide, methotrexate (in doses of more than 15 mg per m²), 6-mercaptopurine, 5-fluorouracil (5-FU), and phenylalanine mustard. This problem has been documented by pharmacokinetic studies, and this must be taken into consideration in planning the route of therapy. Drug concentration monitoring may provide a valuable guide to delayed elimination of agents such

TABLE 1-3. DRUGS REQUIRING DOSE MODIFICATION FOR ORGAN DYSFUNCTION

Agent	Organ Dysfunction	Suggested Dose Modification
Methotrexate sodium	Renal insufficiency	
Cisplatin	Renal insufficiency	In proportion to C_{cr}/100 when C_{cr} <60 mL/min
Carboplatin	Renal insufficiency	Target AUC of 5–7 mg/mL × min
		AUC = Dose/(C_{cr} + 25)
Bleomycin sulfate	Renal failure (GFR <25% normal)	50–75% decrease
m-AMSA (amsacrine)	Renal failure (GFR <25% normal)	50–75% decrease
Streptozotocin	Renal failure (GFR <25% normal)	50–75% decrease
Hydroxyurea		
Etoposide		
Deoxycoformycin	Renal insufficiency	In proportion to C_{cr}/100 when C_{cr} <60 mL/min
Fludarabine phosphate		
Chlorodeoxyadenosine		
Doxorubicin hydrochloride and daunorubicin hydrochloride	Hepatic dysfunction (no clear correlation of pharmacokinetics or toxicity proven)	Use caution with bilirubin ≥2.5; advisable to begin with reduced dose and escalate as tolerated
Paclitaxel (Taxol)	Hepatic dysfunction	50% decrease for patients with hepatic dysfunction (bilirubin >2 mg/dL)
Vincristine sulfate		Only approximate guidelines can be offered and are probably inaccurate; see text
Vinblastine sulfate		
m-AMSA	Hepatic dysfunction	
Thiotepa (thiotriethylene phosphoramide)		For bilirubin >1.5 mg/dL, reduce initial dose by 50%
Epirubicin hydrochloride		For bilirubin >3.0 mg/dL, reduce initial dose by 75%

AUC, area under the concentration × time curve; C_{cr}, creatinine clearance; GFR, glomerular filtration rate.

as methotrexate,[23] which thus allows dosage adjustment of the cytotoxic drug in later cycles and early institution or prolongation of rescue procedures. Reliable assays are available for many antineoplastic agents (Table 1-4); most assays use high-pressure liquid chromatography, a technique available in most cancer centers. A few others, such as the assays for methotrexate, have established importance as guides to the prediction of drug toxicity in high-dose therapy (Table 1-4). The utility of various assays is indicated in the discussion of individual agents in subsequent chapters.

Combination Chemotherapy

Rationale for Combination Chemotherapy

Although the first effective drugs for treating cancer were brought to clinical trial in the 1940s, initial therapeutic results were disappointing. Impressive regressions of acute lymphocytic leukemia and adult lymphomas were obtained with single agents such as nitrogen mustard, antifolates, corticosteroids, and the vinca alkaloids, but responses were only partial and of short duration. When complete remissions were obtained, as in acute lymphocytic leukemia, they lasted less than 9 months, and relapse was associated with resistance to the original drug. The introduction of cyclic combination chemotherapy for acute lymphocytic leukemia of childhood in the late 1950s marked a turning point in the effective treatment of neoplastic disease. Such combinations are now a standard component of most treatment strategies for advanced cancer. The superior results of combination chemotherapy compared with single-agent treatment derive from the following considerations. First, initial resistance to any given single agent is frequent, even in the most responsive tumors; for example, in patients with Hodgkin's disease, the complete response rates to alkylating agents or procarbazine do not exceed 20%, and virtually all patients relapse. Second, initially responsive tumors rapidly acquire resistance after drug exposure, probably owing to selection of preexisting resistant tumor cells from a hetero-

TABLE 1-4. DRUG MONITORING IN CANCER THERAPY

Agent	Assay	Use
Methotrexate (MTX) sodium	HPLC	Aids in early detection of patients at high risk of toxicity. MTX level >5 × 10^{-7} mol/L at 48 h alerts to need for increased leucovorin calcium dose for prolonged period. For toxic reactions, tailor leucovorin dosage to plasma MTX level. (See Antifolates, Chapter 6.) CSF MTX level aids in differential diagnosis of neurotoxicity. High level favors drug reaction. Predicts drug clearance in patients with renal insufficiency. Allows choice of safe dose.
5-Fluorouracil	HPLC	Confirms defect in drug elimination (dihydropyrimidine dehydrogenase deficiency).
6-Mercaptopurine	HPLC	Determines plasma levels after oral therapy to assure adequate bioavailability.

CSF, cerebrospinal fluid; HPLC, high-pressure liquid chromatography.

TABLE 1-5. CROSS-RESISTANCE PATTERNS OF DIFFERENT PROTEINS THAT MEDIATE MULTIDRUG RESISTANCE

Mediator	Resistance Patterns					
	VCR	Dox	Tax	Camp	Ara-C	MTX
MDR (P-170) ↑	+	+	+	−	−	−
MRP ↑	+	+	+	−	−	+
BCRP ↑	−	+	−	+	−	−
Deletion of topo I ↓	−	−	−	+	+	−

+, resistant; −, sensitive; Ara-C, cytosine arabinoside; BCRP, breast cancer resistance protein, also called the *mitoxantrone-resistance half-transporter* (see ref. 72); Camp, irinotecan hydrochloride (SN-38), topotecan hydrochloride; Dox, doxorubicin hydrochloride; MDR (P-170), P-170 glycoprotein; MRP, multidrug resistance protein; MTX, methotrexate sodium; Tax, paclitaxel, docetaxel; topo I, topoisomerase I (see ref. 73); VCR, vincristine sulfate.

geneous tumor cell population. Some anticancer drugs themselves increase the rate of mutation to resistance in experimental studies, as does hypoxia.[24] The use of multiple agents, each with cytotoxic activity in the disease under consideration but with different mechanisms of action, allows independent cell killing by each agent. Cells resistant to one agent might still be sensitive to the other drugs in the regimen.

Patterns of cross-resistance must be taken into consideration in formulating drug combinations. Resistance to many agents may result from unique and specific mutations, as for example may occur in the target enzymes of antimetabolites. Mutations that alter binding of inhibitors of topoisomerase II, an enzyme that promotes DNA strand breaks in the presence of anthracyclines, epipodophyllotoxins, and amsacrine, may mediate resistance to each of these agents.[25] In other cases, a single mutational change may lead to multidrug resistance. Table 1-5 describes cross-resistance patterns for some of the well-defined mechanisms of multidrug resistance. The most thoroughly studied and undoubtedly one of the more important mechanisms of multidrug resistance is increased expression of the MDR-1 gene. This gene codes for the P-170 membrane glycoprotein, which promotes the efflux of vinca alkaloids, anthracyclines, dactinomycin (actinomycin D), epipodophyllotoxins, and other natural products. This protein occurs constitutively in many normal tissues, including epithelial cells of the kidney, large bowel, and adrenal gland,[26] and has been identified in tumors derived from these tissues, as well as in posttreatment lymphomas, leukemias, non–small cell lung cancer, multiple myeloma, and other cancers.[27] P-170–mediated resistance results from decreased intracellular drug levels and can be reversed experimentally by administration of calcium-channel blockers, amiodarone, quinidine, and derivatives of cyclosporine, as well as by a variety of aprotic polar solvents. At this time, evidence suggests that P-170 contributes to clinical drug resistance in multiple myeloma, non-Hodgkin's lymphomas, pediatric sarcomas, and acute nonlymphocytic leukemia.[27a] Many clinical trials investigating the use of agents reversing multidrug resistance have been initiated, but the results of these trials are inconclusive. Many of the P-170 inhibitors also inhibit

hepatic clearance of doxorubicin hydrochloride, which significantly complicates the design and interpretation of these studies.[28] A second mechanism for multidrug resistance involves the multidrug resistance protein (MRP), which promotes drug efflux and confers resistance to anthracyclines, etoposide, and vinca alkaloids. Members of the MRP family may also mediate efflux of methotrexate.[29] Multiple members of the MRP gene family have been identified, and again their role in clinical drug resistance remains uncertain. The MRP family of genes is widely expressed in epithelial tumors,[30,31] and their potential for mediating multiagent resistance deserves further study. Finally, the fact that the classic alkylating agents (cyclophosphamide, melphalan hydrochloride, nitrogen mustard) share cross-resistance related to enhanced DNA repair mediated by nucleotide excision repair enzymes and by increased levels of intracellular nucleophilic thiols, such as glutathione, is well established. As mentioned earlier, resistance to the nitrosourea, procarbazine, and dacarbazine classes of alkylators is mediated by increased levels of a different enzyme, O^6-alkylguanine alkyl transferase. Undoubtedly, most resistant tumors have acquired a variety of mechanisms for avoiding the toxic effects of chemotherapy.

A third consideration supports combination chemotherapy. If drugs have nonoverlapping patterns of normal organ toxicity, each can be used in full dosage, and the effectiveness of each agent will be fully maintained in the combination. Drugs such as vincristine sulfate, prednisone, bleomycin sulfate, hexamethylmelamine, L-asparaginase, high-dose methotrexate/leucovorin calcium, and biologics, all lacking bone marrow toxicity, are particularly valuable in combination with traditional myelosuppressive agents. Based on these principles, curative combinations have been devised for diseases that are not curable with single-agent treatment, including acute lymphocytic leukemia (vincristine, prednisone, doxorubicin, and L-asparaginase), Hodgkin's disease [mechlorethamine, Oncovin (vincristine), procarbazine, and prednisone (MOPP) and Adriamycin (doxorubicin), bleomycin, vinblastine, and dacarbazine (ABVD)], diffuse large cell lymphoma (the combination of cyclophosphamide, doxorubicin, vincristine, and prednisone, as well as a variety of third-generation five- to eight-drug regimens), and testicular carcinoma (bleomycin, cisplatin, and vinblastine or etoposide).

Schedule Development in Combination Therapy: Kinetic and Biochemical Considerations

The detailed scheduling of drugs in multidrug regimens was based initially on both practical and theoretical considerations. Intermittent cycles of treatment were used to allow periods of recovery of host bone marrow, gastrointestinal tract, and immune function, with the expectation that recovery of the tumor cell population would be slower than that of the injured normal tissues. This strategy allowed retreatment with full therapeutic doses as frequently as possible in keeping with the fractional cell kill hypothesis. A commonly used strategy is to incorporate myelotoxic agents on day 1 of each cycle, while delivering nonmyelosuppressive agents, such as bleomycin, vincristine, prednisone, or high-dose methotrexate with leucovorin rescue, in the period of bone marrow suppression (e.g., on day 8 of a 21-day cycle) to provide continuous suppression of tumor growth while allowing maximum time for marrow recovery. High-dose methotrexate with leucovorin rescue has proved to be particularly useful in this capacity during the "off period" because of its minimal effect on white blood cell and platelet counts.

Cytokinetic considerations also influence the specific sequencing of drugs in combination regimens. S-phase–specific drugs, such as cytosine arabinoside and methotrexate, are capable of killing cells only when they are present during the period of DNA synthesis. Experimentally, these agents are most effective if administered during the period of rapid recovery of DNA synthesis that follows a period of suppression of DNA synthesis. Thus an initial phase of cytoreduction with drugs that are not cell-cycle-phase–specific, such as the bifunctional alkylating agents or nitrosoureas (if these are known to be active against the disease in question), reduces tumor bulk and recruits slowly dividing cells into active DNA synthesis. These drugs can then be followed within the same cycle of treatment by cell-cycle-phase–specific agents such as methotrexate or the fluoropyrimidines, which kill cells during periods of DNA synthesis. Monitoring cytokinetic parameters during routine clinical treatment is difficult, although positron emission tomography may provide metabolic information on solid tumors.

Although most of the common anticancer regimens use intermittent bolus delivery of drugs, in recent years advantages of constant-infusion chemotherapy have been suggested. Early clinical trials have suggested improved therapeutic ratios for several drugs, including doxorubicin, 5-FU, etoposide, ifosfamide, and cytosine arabinoside.[32,33] Constant exposure of cells to cell-cycle-phase–specific agents such as antimetabolites or cytosine arabinoside allows a greater fraction of the tumor cell population to cycle through the sensitive phase than is likely to occur with intermittent bolus therapy. An additional consideration is the experimental evidence suggesting that constant exposure of agents such as natural products, resistance to which is mediated by P-170, may overwhelm the pump, which allows the killing of otherwise resistant cells.[34] Finally, infusional regimens may change the toxicity of cancer drugs. For example, the cardiotoxicity associated with anthracyclines is more closely correlated with the peak concentration than with AUC. Liposomal preparations of doxorubicin and daunorubicin provide the same advantage of prolonged exposure to drug, low peak concentrations, and decreased cardiotoxicity as does continuous intravenous infusion of the same agents.[35]

Problem of Drug Resistance: Additional Considerations in Combination Chemotherapy

Drug resistance, either apparent with initial treatment or emerging at the time of relapse after an initial response, inevitably occurs in all but the few cancer types that are curable with chemotherapy (Table 1-2). A panoply of potential mechanisms conferring resistance to cancer cells has been described (Tables 1-5 and 1-6). As has become increasingly obvious, resistance is in most cases a complex process involving multiple mechanisms that may emerge in parallel or in series. With the appreciation of this complexity has come increasing skepticism that strategies aimed at reversal of discrete pathways conferring resistance to specific drugs or drug classes will have a major impact on the treatment of the common solid tumors. On the other hand, recent research suggests that a very common process conferring resistance to many, if not virtually all, chemotherapeutic agents is the suppression or inactivation of cell-damage–induced apoptosis, or programmed cell death, the common pathway mediating cell death in response to many cytotoxic drugs as well as to radiation. Inactivation of apoptotic mechanisms, which can occur in addition to the biochemical mechanisms associated with resistance to specific drugs or drug classes, can be mediated by inactivation of the *p53* tumor suppressor gene (also termed a *death pathway gene*) or by inappropriate expression of genes that suppress apoptosis, such as *bcl*-2. The *p53* gene is mutated in almost 50% of human cancers at diagnosis, and in an even higher percentage of tumors at the time of emergence of drug resistance.[36] Thus genes intimately involved with the fundamental processes of malignant transformation are now known to contribute directly to drug resistance.

Apoptosis is an active, energy-requiring, and protein synthesis–dependent process whereby cells, in response to specific signals, undergo an orderly, programmed series of intracellular events that lead to death. This process is a necessary component of normal development in all multicellular organisms and is required for the maintenance of normal function of many proliferating or renewable tissues. Overexpression of *bcl*-2 is linked to the pathogenesis of B-cell lymphomas.[37] Activation of the apoptotic pathway in

TABLE 1-6. MECHANISMS OF RESISTANCE

Mechanism of Resistance	Drug Involved	Pharmacologic Defect
Decreased drug uptake	Methotrexate sodium	Decreased expression of the folate transporter
Decreased drug activation	Cytosine arabinoside	Decreased deoxycytidine kinase
	Fludarabine phosphate	Decreased folylpolyglutamyl synthetase
	Cladribine	
	Methotrexate	
Increased drug target	Methotrexate	Amplified DHFR
	5-fluorouracil	Amplified TS
Altered drug target	Etoposide	Altered topo II
	Doxorubicin hydrochloride	Altered DHFR
	Methotrexate	
Increased detoxification	Alkylating agents	Increased glutathione or glutathione transferase
Enhanced DNA repair	Alkylating agents	Increased nucleotide excision repair
	Platinum derivatives	Increased O^6-alkyl-guanine alkyl transferase
	Nitrosoureas	
Defective recognition of DNA adducts	Cisplatin	Mismatch repair defect
Increased drug efflux	Doxorubicin	Increased MDR expression or MDR gene amplification
	Etoposide	
	Vinca alkaloids	
	Paclitaxel	
Defective checkpoint function and apoptosis	Most anticancer drugs	*p53* mutations

DHFR, dihydrofolate reductase; MDR, multidrug resistance; topo II, topoisomerase II; TS, thymidylate synthase.

response to DNA damage, in a *p53*-requiring process, is responsible for cytotoxicity of chemotherapy drugs and radiation.[38] Lowe et al.[39] elegantly demonstrated that, in the presence of normal *p53*, transformation of normal mouse embryo fibroblasts (MEF) with the adenovirus E1A transforming gene (functionally equivalent to loss of c-*myc* regulation) created a cell line with supersensitivity to doxorubicin, 5-FU, and etoposide, as well as x-irradiation, and that the cells died through the process of apoptosis. MEF cells lacking the *p53* gene were resistant to doxorubicin, 5-FU, and etoposide, as well as x-irradiation. This experiment may explain the selectivity of chemotherapeutic agents for malignant cells over nonmalignant cells with similar prolif-

erative rates and, reinforcing the results of other studies tying loss of cell-cycle control to resistance to chemotherapeutic agents,[40] offers an explanation for the high rate of inherent resistance of many *p53*-mutated solid tumors to chemotherapeutic agents (Fig. 1-1). Furthermore, these results suggest potential targets for effectively bypassing the elaborate defense machinery available to the cancer cell. If drugs can be found that are capable of direct activation of apoptosis (as opposed to the indirect activation of the apoptotic response by cell-damaging agents) or of reversal of suppression of the apoptotic response, perhaps the other resistance mechanisms would be moot. The search for such drugs has begun.

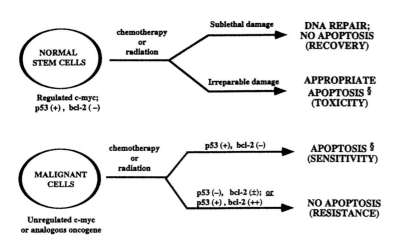

FIGURE 1-1. Effect of c-*myc* regulation, *p53*, and *bcl*-2 on sensitivity of normal and malignant cells proliferating at comparable rates. (§The dose of drug or radiation causing apoptosis of normal stem cells with regulated c-*myc* is much higher than the dose causing apoptosis of malignant cells with normal *p53*, but unregulated c-*myc* or analogous oncogene.)

The acquisition of drug resistance is widely believed to be the product of random mutations in a tumor cell population. A corollary to this hypothesis is the concept that the probability of *de novo* drug resistance in any tumor population increases with increasing number of cells and number of cell divisions. More than 20 years ago, Goldie and Coldman and colleagues[41,42] proposed a mathematical model based on the random-mutation hypothesis. It suggested several important considerations in protocol design to minimize treatment failure due to acquired drug resistance: (a) Treatment should begin as early as possible when the malignant cell population is at its smallest. (b) To avoid selection of doubly resistant mutants by sequential chemotherapy, multiple mutually non–cross-resistant drugs should be used together rather than sequentially. (c) To achieve maximal kill of both sensitive and moderately resistant cells, cytotoxic drugs should be administered as frequently as possible and in doses well above the minimally cytotoxic doses. The Goldie-Coldman model was used as the basis for the design of a number of innovative multidrug protocols for the treatment of aggressive non-Hodgkin's lymphoma and Hodgkin's disease, with the hope that these regimens would improve cure rates in these diseases in comparison with empirically designed regimens.[43] For example, regimens of methotrexate, Adriamycin (doxorubicin), cyclophosphamide, Oncovin (vincristine), prednisone, and bleomycin (MACOP-B); methotrexate, bleomycin, Adriamycin, cyclophosphamide, Oncovin, and dexamethasone (M-BACOD); moderate-dose methotrexate, bleomycin, Adriamycin, cyclophosphamide, Oncovin; and dexamethasone (m-BACOD), and ProMACE-CytaBOM [prednisone, methotrexate, doxorubicin, etoposide, cytosine arabinodise (ara-C), bleomycin, oncovin] for non-Hodgkin's lymphomas used six to eight separate cytotoxic drugs in each 3-week (or even 2-week) cycle, whereas the MOPP/dactinomycin, bleomycin, and vincristine (ABV) hybrid regimen combined all but one of the drugs from the two most effective relatively non–cross-resistant regimens for Hodgkin's disease (MOPP and ABVD). However, randomized trials comparing regimens based on the Goldie-Coldman hypothesis with the older, empirically designed four-drug regimens have failed to demonstrate any improvement in the cure rates of either non-Hodgkin's lymphoma[44–47] or Hodgkin's disease.[48,49] Although these studies do not negate the principle of random, spontaneous mutation to drug resistance followed by positive selection favoring overgrowth of the resistant clone, they do suggest that the assumptions made to allow the formal mathematical modeling were overly simplified. For instance, the Goldie-Coldman mathematical model assumes that resistance develops to individual agents, one at a time, and thus does not account for multidrug resistance patterns. Multidrug resistance and broad resistance to apoptosis as conferred by inactivation of *p53* or overexpression of *bcl-2* are not considered. That oncologists lack sophisticated understanding of this complex, multifactorial process at this point in the development of our field is now obvious.

As an alternative to classical combination chemotherapy, Norton and colleagues have proposed a scheme in which individual drugs are given sequentially at their highest possible dose. They have demonstrated outstanding clinical results with sequential cyclophosphamide, doxorubicin, and paclitaxel, each given in doses 50% to 100% above standard combination doses alone for three cycles.[50] Their initial study resulted in 80% 4-year disease-free survival in women with primary breast cancer and four or more positive lymph nodes, a group that would have a greater than 50% relapse rate at 4 years with standard cyclophosphamide plus doxorubicin chemotherapy. The advantages of the Norton scheme are (a) higher individual doses of each drug and (b) the rapid shift to a new agent to prevent selection of resistant cells. One should recognize, however, that the higher drug doses, in this twofold escalation range, are not clearly more active individually, and the higher doses do increase the risk of cardiotoxicity, leukemia, neuropathy, and other late effects on normal tissues.

Dose-Intensification Strategies

Dose intensification has received increasing emphasis in recent years as a strategy for overcoming resistance to chemotherapy. A steep dose-response effect for drug-responsive tumors has long been known, and the importance of delivering maximum tolerated doses in potentially curable diseases has been emphasized repeatedly. The concept of *dose intensity*, defined as the mg per m^2 of delivered drug per week of therapy, has been used by Levin and Hryniuk[51] in retrospective comparisons of published response rates obtained with different chemotherapeutic regimens (using the published protocol doses rather than actual delivered doses) in breast cancer, colon cancer, and ovarian cancer trials. They concluded that a dose-response correlation exists for 5-FU in colon cancer, doxorubicin in breast cancer, and cisplatin in ovarian cancer. Similarly, retrospective analyses of MOPP or MOPP derivatives in Hodgkin's disease have concluded that delivered dose of vincristine, as well as of alkylators and procarbazine, correlates with response rates and disease-free interval.[52–54] These studies have been criticized because they are retrospective (i.e., an alternative and very plausible interpretation is that tumor-related or patient-related factors that are associated with inability to tolerate full chemotherapy doses also predict for poor response) and, in addition, in the case of the Levin and Hryniuk studies, because of the rather sweeping assumptions the authors made regarding drug equivalency, which allowed numerical dose-intensity assignments to regimens containing different drugs.

A prospective, randomized cancer and leukemia group B trial[4] comparing three dosage levels of cyclophosphamide, 5-FU, and doxorubicin adjuvant chemotherapy for women with node-positive breast cancer demonstrated a highly significant dose-response effect, measured by survival and disease-free survival, but *only* for the subset of patients whose tumors had high levels of expression of the c-*erbB*-2 (*HER-2-neu*) oncogene. In their multivariate analysis, this factor, with tumor size and number of positive lymph nodes, was the only significant independent prognostic variable. No benefit was found from higher dosages in patients with absent or low levels of expression of c-*erbB*-2.

The dose-response relationships discerned from the cancer and leukemia group B study[4] are probably applicable to other diseases, despite the lack of other randomized studies. That is, in potentially curable cancers, readily tolerable ("standard") doses of effective combination chemotherapy drugs are sufficient for a subset of patients with sensitive tumors, whereas higher and, in some cases, very high doses may be necessary for the subset of patients with relative drug resistance. The challenge is to develop reliable *de novo* predictive markers (such as, potentially, *bcl*-2 overexpression or mutations in *p53* or K-*ras* genes) for each tumor to determine which patients will benefit from the higher doses. In the absence of such markers, treating every potentially curable patient with maximally tolerated doses, as established by the published or experimental protocol, is important. The following dosing principles have been used for the treatment of Hodgkin's disease,[55] but we believe they are broadly applicable to other potentially curable cancers: (a) Do not modify planned doses or schedules of chemotherapy in anticipation of toxicity that has not yet happened, nor for short-term, non–life-threatening toxicity, such as emesis or mild neuropathy. (b) Because significant individual variation may exist in the pharmacokinetics of drugs or in the sensitivity of the bone marrow (and other normal organs) to drug-related toxicity, the granulocyte count should be used as an *in vivo* biologic assay of the individual dosage limits of those agents with predominant myelotoxicity. If 100% of the planned doses do not produce a nadir granulocyte count of less than 1,000 per mm^3, the doses of the myelotoxic drugs are probably too low for that patient and should be increased in subsequent cycles to achieve a significant but tolerable level of myelotoxicity. (As a guideline, we aim for granulocyte nadirs in each cycle of between 500 and 1,000 per mm^3.) (c) Tumor response should be assessed at regular intervals throughout therapy. If evidence is seen of lack of response or of tumor regrowth, an alternative, non–cross-resistant regimen should be started.

The use of recombinant hematopoietic growth factors can mitigate the bone marrow toxicity of chemotherapy. Two recombinant agents, granulocyte colony-stimulating factor and granulocyte-macrophage colony-stimulating factor, are effective in decreasing the duration of granulocyte nadir after myelotoxic chemotherapy, although neither affects thrombocytopenia. Other factors that may have roles in ameliorating both the platelet and granulocyte toxicities are under investigation. Human thrombopoietin is available for clinical testing. No clear indications exist for its use in standard chemotherapy.[56] Studies have already demonstrated that granulocyte and granulocyte-macrophage colony-stimulating factors are capable of reducing the incidence of infectious complications and requirement

for hospitalization during chemotherapy. Whether the use of these marrow-stimulating agents, which allow significant chemotherapy dosage escalations, will improve the outcome of cancer therapy remains to be seen.

Another alternative is to use marrow-ablative dosages of chemotherapy to increase tumor cell kill and to rescue the host with either autologous bone marrow or peripheral blood stem cells, or stem cells, or marrow from a histocompatible donor. During the past 20 years, this approach has been investigated in many centers as salvage therapy for patients with relapsed leukemias, Hodgkin's and non-Hodgkin's lymphomas, as well as some solid tumors. Rescue with marrow from a human leukocyte antigen–compatible donor has the advantage of being free of malignant cells. Marrow donated by a second person contains T lymphocytes, however, which may cause graft-versus-host disease, a potentially lethal complication. On the other hand, evidence exists that a "graft-versus-tumor" effect may be beneficial in prolonging remissions, in comparison with syngeneic or autologous marrow rescue. The drugs used in these programs have myelosuppression as the primary dose-limiting toxicity and are used in doses above the lethal dose to bone marrow in the absence of marrow reinfusion but below the limits of nonhematologic toxicity. Alkylators such as busulfan, ifosfamide, and nitrosoureas are prominent in most ablative regimens because characteristically their extramyeloid toxicity occurs at two- to sevenfold higher dosages than the myeloablative dosage. Some high-dose toxicities, such as cystitis, can be prevented through the use of mesna. Total-body, total-lymphoid, or limited-field radiation has been used frequently as an adjunct to chemotherapy. Hematopoietic growth factors and peripheral blood stem cells have been used in conjunction with high-dose chemotherapy and marrow reinfusion to shorten the duration of marrow aplasia and reduce infection complications.

Randomized trials comparing high-dose regimens with best conventional therapy generally have not proven the value of dose escalation in patients with metastatic breast cancer.[57] High-dose regimens with allogeneic bone marrow transplant appear to be very effective in some younger patients with acute myeloid leukemia and in chronic myelogenous leukemia, whereas autologous bone marrow transplant or peripheral blood stem cell transplant regimens appear to be effective in drug-responsive Hodgkin's disease in first or second relapse and in intermediate- and high-grade non-Hodgkin's lymphoma in first relapse. Reported trials generally have consisted of relatively small numbers of highly selected patients, however, and follow-up in most cases is still brief. One should remember that both early and late sequelae of high-dose chemotherapy bone marrow transplant regimens, both allogeneic and autologous, may be high.[58] Acute pulmonary toxicity and vascular occlusive disease with liver failure contribute to acute mortality due to a high-dose regimen. Later, heart and lung toxicity, particularly in patients who have received radiation, also may be seen. The risk of treatment-related death from allogeneic programs may be as high as 15% to 40% depending on the age and underlying health of the patient.

Drug Interactions in Combination Chemotherapy

Specific drug interactions, both favorable and unfavorable, must be considered in developing combination regimens. These interactions may take the form of pharmacokinetic, cytokinetic, or biochemical effects of one drug that influence the effectiveness of a second component of a combination. Patterns of overlapping toxicity are a primary concern. Drugs that cause renal toxicity, such as cisplatin, must be used cautiously in combination with other agents (such as methotrexate or bleomycin) that depend on renal elimination as their primary mechanism of excretion. Regimens that use cisplatin before methotrexate, as in the treatment of head and neck cancer, must incorporate careful monitoring of renal function, pretreatment plasma volume expansion, and dose adjustment for methotrexate to ensure that altered methotrexate excretion does not lead to severe drug toxicity. The sequence of drug administration may be critical; in many experimental systems, administration of paclitaxel before cisplatin gives additive or synergistic results, whereas the opposite sequence yields antagonism and increased toxicity.[59] Extensive interactions between P-450 inducers such as phenytoin or phenobarbital and P-450 substrates such as irinotecan, paclitaxel, or vincristine lead to marked increases in drug clearance and the need for upward dosage adjustment (Chapter 22). The potential for important interactions between cancer drugs and other medications must be kept in mind during the routine care of cancer patients.

Biochemical interactions also may be important considerations in determining the choice of agents and their sequence of administration.[60] Both synergistic and antagonistic interactions have been described. A chemotherapeutic drug may be modulated by a second agent that has no antitumor activity in its own right but that enhances the intracellular activation or target binding of the primary agent or inhibits the repair of lesions produced by the primary drug. The best example of this synergy is the use of leucovorin (5-formyltetrahydrofolate), which itself has no cytotoxic effect but which enhances the affinity of the binding of 5-FU to its target enzyme, thymidylate synthase, by forming a ternary complex among the enzyme, 5-FU, and folate.[61] This combination is more effective clinically than 5-FU alone in colorectal cancer. A number of such combinations have reached the clinic and are described in greater detail in subsequent chapters.

Dose Adjustment Based on Toxicity

Finally, all drug combination regimens require dose-adjustment scales to allow increases or decreases in dosage according to toxicity. Determining which of the several agents is responsible for excessive toxicity becomes difficult if overlapping toxicity patterns are present. In this setting, arbitrary scales of dose adjustment based primarily on bone marrow toxicity are provided with protocols. Underdosing also may be a problem, particularly for drugs given by the oral route, such as 6-mercaptopurine, hexamethylmelamine, melphalan, or methotrexate, which display variable bioavailability. Drug-level monitoring could be useful in this situation but has not been used routinely to verify bioavailability of oral agents. As previously discussed, the granulocyte count can be used as an *in vivo* biologic assay of the effect of myelotoxic agents and may suggest the necessity, in regimens that are potentially curative, for dosage increases of these drugs when granulocyte nadirs are modest. In the treatment of certain curable malignancies, such as testicular carcinomas and high-grade lymphomas, chemotherapy is given on schedule and in full doses, regardless of bone marrow toxicity. In these situations the risk of toxicity is more than balanced by the need for aggressive treatment.

Combination of Chemotherapy with Radiotherapy or Biologic Agents

A further innovation in the use of antineoplastic drugs is to combine drugs with irradiation or biologic agents. Many clinical protocols have been designed to take advantage of the well-documented synergy between irradiation and drugs such as cisplatin, paclitaxel and 5-FU. In addition, drugs specifically designed as radiosensitizers or protectors, as discussed in Chapter 25, have entered clinical trial, although their value is not clear. The design of integrated chemotherapy-radiotherapy trials presents special problems because of the synergistic effects of the two therapies on both normal and malignant tissue. The normal tissue of greatest concern is the bone marrow, although the heart, lungs, and brain may also be affected by such interactions.[62] Radiation given to the pelvic or midline abdominal areas produces a decline in blood counts, myelofibrosis, and a decrease in bone marrow reserve. This can severely compromise the ability to deliver myelotoxic chemotherapy, even months or years after the radiation. The use of conformal irradiation, administered through multiple portals, can preserve a greater portion of the marrow-bearing tissue. For some toxicities, the sequence of administration may be crucial. For example, mediastinal irradiation after combination chemotherapy for massive mediastinal Hodgkin's disease has proven to be practicable and effective. Because the initial chemotherapy results in significant shrinkage of the mediastinal tumor, smaller radiation portals can be used to encompass the residual tumor completely, with proportionately less resultant radiation pneumonitis. In small cell carcinoma of the lung confined to the thorax, simultaneous administration of radiotherapy and chemotherapy has produced better results than either therapy alone or in sequence.[63] Similarly, simultaneous radiation and chemotherapy is superior to radiotherapy alone in adjuvant therapy for cervical cancer[6] and rectal cancer.[64] Thus, although considering the cumulative toxicities of chemotherapy and radiation on bone marrow and other vulnerable tissues in the radiation field is essential, the net benefits of simultaneous irradiation and chemotherapy often outweigh the disadvantages.

Many chemotherapeutic agents greatly potentiate the effects of irradiation and may lead to synergistic toxicity for organs usually resistant to radiation damage. Doxorubicin sensitizes both normal and malignant cells to radiation damage, possibly because both doxorubicin and x-rays produce free-radical damage to tissues. Doxorubicin adjuvant chemotherapy given in conjunction with irradiation to the left chest wall increases the risk of increased cardiac toxicity.[65] Similarly, bleomycin and radiation cause synergistic pulmonary toxicity. When more than one effective chemotherapy regimen is available, the choice must be informed by consideration of these possible mutually potentiating toxicities. For example, as mentioned earlier, combined-modality therapy is indicated for massive mediastinal Hodgkin's disease, generally with mantle radiation after six cycles of chemotherapy. Although ABVD has been shown to be a more effective therapy for Hodgkin's disease than is MOPP, the potential heart and lung toxicity when mediastinal radiation is added militates against this choice. Either sequential MOPP-ABVD or the hybrid MOPP-ABV regimens offer treatment efficacy equal to that of ABVD (as demonstrated in randomized trials) while decreasing by half the cumulative doses of doxorubicin and bleomycin, which thus decreases the probability of cardiac and pulmonary toxicity.[66] Corticosteroids may suppress the immediate inflammatory reaction to lung irradiation, but withdrawal of steroids may be associated with a severe, life-threatening radiation pneumonitis. When interdigitation of chemotherapy and radiation is necessary, these various toxic interactions must be anticipated and minimized by reduction of radiation dosage or chemotherapy dosage, avoidance of irradiation to specific sites during drug administration, or an alteration in drug dosage or schedule.

A final consideration in the combined use of radiotherapy and chemotherapy is the carcinogenicity of both, although in most cases little conclusive evidence exists for synergistic or even additive risk for specific secondary malignancy. The most important late side effect of cancer treatment among patients who are cured of their primary tumors is a secondary solid tumor induced by ionizing radiation. In studies of patients cured of Hodgkin's disease, the risk for secondary solid tumors begins to increase significantly after 10 years and continues to increase steadily into the second and third decades. The cumulative risk for all secondary radiation-induced (i.e., occurring within the radiation portal) solid tumors is approximately 15% at 15 years and may be as high as 20% at 25 years. On the other

hand, little evidence exists that concomitant chemotherapy increases this risk. The most important chemotherapy-related second malignancy is myeloid malignancy due to DNA alkylating or metalating agents. Among the most potently leukemogenic agents are the mustard-type alkylators, nitrosoureas, and procarbazine. The risk for leukemia increases with cumulative dose of alkylators, a fact that must be considered when long-term or high-dose alkylator use is contemplated. Leukemia has been reported after therapy for Hodgkin's disease, non-Hodgkin's lymphoma, breast cancer (adjuvant therapy), ovarian cancer, multiple myeloma, and other kinds of cancer (see Chapter 5). The most thoroughly studied group of patients consists of long-term survivors of Hodgkin's disease after MOPP chemotherapy. The cumulative risk for leukemia or myelodysplasia after MOPP is approximately 3% at 10 years. The risk for secondary myeloid malignancy decreases rapidly thereafter and approaches the age-related baseline 10 years after MOPP. Although earlier reports suggested a further increased risk for myeloid malignancy when radiation was added, either before MOPP or after MOPP, many analyses of large numbers of patients treated with both radiation and MOPP have not demonstrated any significant increased risk due to radiation.[67] One should mention that the risk for myeloid leukemia is not increased after ABVD therapy for Hodgkin's disease. A qualitatively different type of secondary nonlymphocytic leukemia is associated with topoisomerase II inhibitors, including etoposide, teniposide, and doxorubicin.[68,69] Characteristically, acute nonlymphoblastic leukemia associated with topoisomerase II inhibitor therapy has a much shorter latency period than does alkylator-induced leukemia, is frequently of the myelomonocytic or monocytic Fab subtypes (M-4 or M-5, respectively), and is frequently associated with reciprocal chromosomal translocations involving band 11q23. The risk of this type of leukemia is associated with higher total cumulative dose of the topoisomerase II inhibitor and with a weekly or twice-weekly schedule. In addition, the risk may be increased when the topoisomerase II agent is combined with high-dose alkylators or with agents that inhibit DNA repair.

The combined use of standard chemotherapeutic drugs and biologic agents also offers considerable promise based on the nonoverlapping toxicities and differing modes of action of these classes of agents. Laboratory studies demonstrate additive or synergistic interaction between interferon-γ and 5-FU, and between *HER-2-neu* antibodies and paclitaxel or cisplatin. The combination of trastuzumab (Herceptin) and paclitaxel or trastuzumab, cyclophosphamide, and doxorubicin enhances response rates and increases survival of patients with metastatic breast cancer.[70] These same trials of trastuzumab and doxorubicin/cyclophosphamide demonstrated an unacceptable rate of cardiotoxicity (28%), however, despite limitation of the anthracycline to accepted levels of total dose (less than 550 mg per m²). The reason for enhanced cardiotoxicity of the combination is unclear.

Possibilities include a drug interaction resulting in delayed doxorubicin clearance or, alternatively, a direct action of trastuzumab on the myocardium, leading to enhancement of doxorubicin toxicity. This toxic interaction illustrates the point that, until drug and biologic combinations are tested clinically, one cannot assume that patterns of toxicity of individual agents will be unaffected by their combined use.

Adjuvant Chemotherapy

Despite an apparently complete surgical resection of primary tumor, certain patients are at high risk of developing recurrent disease at distant sites. This increased risk can in some cases be predicted by the size or known local-regional extension of the primary tumor or by certain biologic markers found on the tumor. Although chemotherapeutic agents are a logical choice for treatment of patients with disseminated malignancy, drug therapy also may be used to advantage in some patients who have no evidence of metastatic disease but who are at high risk of relapse. In this setting the logical course is to consider the benefits of prophylactic or adjuvant chemotherapy after surgical removal of the tumor and lymph nodes. For patients with primary breast cancer adjuvant chemotherapy with cyclophosphamide, methotrexate, and fluorouracil; cyclophosphamide, doxorubicin, and fluorouracil; or cyclophosphamide and doxorubicin has delayed systemic recurrence and improved overall survival. Similarly, tamoxifen citrate, an antiestrogen, has extended survival in postmenopausal patients with positive lymph nodes. Adjuvant 5-FU with irradiation has improved survival in patients with rectal cancer and, in combination with leucovorin, has resulted in improved survival in patients with Dukes B2 and C colon cancer. The reader should refer to other sources for a more complete discussion of the results of adjuvant therapy in specific disease. A brief review of the theoretical basis for adjuvant treatment, however, may aid in understanding the rationale, objectives, and strategies of such therapy.

The need for adjuvant therapy arises because of (a) the high recurrence rate after surgery for apparently localized solid tumors, such as stage II breast cancer and Dukes B2 and C colon cancer, and (b) the failure of chemotherapy or combined-modality treatment to cure these patients after recurrence of disease. In addition, some experimental evidence supports the hypothesis that neoplasms are most sensitive to chemotherapy at their earliest stages of growth. This increased sensitivity of subclinical tumors may result from their high growth fraction (most cells are in active progression through the cell cycle) and shorter cell-cycle times, with resulting greater fractional cell kill for a given dose of drug. In addition, physical access of drug to tumor cells is greatest with microscopic cell collections. Perhaps most important, the probability of biochemical resistance is lowest with minimal total-body burden of tumor cells. In some tumors, *p53* mutations may occur as a later event. As the same tumors become clinically obvious, their growth fraction falls, the cell-cycle time lengthens, areas of poor perfusion increase, and the biochemical heterogeneity and probability of spontaneous resistance increase—consequently, the tumor becomes much less susceptible to treatment and cure.

The disadvantages of adjuvant therapy relate to immediate patient discomfort and to the short- and long-term risks of such treatment. A fraction of patients receiving adjuvant treatment, and in some instances, the majority, will have been cured by the primary surgical procedure and will therefore experience needless risks and toxicity if treated with adjuvant therapy. Unfortunately, at present no proven way exists of identifying these "cured" patients at the time of surgery. Factors such as S-phase fraction, *c-erbB-2/HER-2-neu* expression, or lack of estrogen receptor expression may identify high-risk subsets of patients with breast cancer, and other predictive factors may be identified for other cancers. The risks of immediate and late toxicities of chemotherapy also must be considered. When drugs are used in the adjuvant setting, late complications such as carcinogenicity and sterility assume greater importance than when the same drugs are used for patients with metastatic disease. Other late effects also must be weighed in making a decision for adjuvant chemotherapy. These include both immediate and delayed cardiotoxicity due to doxorubicin, pulmonary fibrosis due to bleomycin and the nitrosoureas, and bone marrow hypoplasia and acute leukemia due to alkylating agents, especially nitrosoureas. A telling example of late toxicity is provided by the NCI study of doxorubicin, cyclophosphamide, and methotrexate for adjuvant therapy of soft tissue sarcoma.[71] In a nonrandomized trial, 6 of the 62 treated patients developed overt congestive heart failure due to doxorubicin cardiac toxicity. Finally, one must emphasize that, irrespective of the perceived ultimate risk for relapse after initial tumor resection, use of adjuvant chemotherapy, except as part of a clinical trial, is difficult to justify unless randomized clinical trials have unequivocally demonstrated a benefit.

In summary, cancer chemotherapeutic agents have had a profound influence on the treatment and survival of patients with cancer. Because these agents have the potential for causing severe or disabling toxicity and yet must be used at maximal dosages to ensure full therapeutic benefit, the physician is literally walking a therapeutic tightrope and must constantly balance gain against likely toxicities. In this effort, every advantage afforded by a knowledge of the patient, the disease, and the therapy must be used to achieve maximum benefit. The foregoing discussion should make it apparent that an intimate knowledge of drug action, drug disposition, and drug interactions is essential to the design and application of effective cancer chemotherapy. The essential information for this task is presented in the following chapters on individual drugs and is summarized in the initial tables that describe key features of each agent. This information can only enhance the chances of success in the difficult but rewarding task of treating cancer.

REFERENCES

1. McLeod DG, Taylor HG, Skoog SJ, et al. Extragonadal germ cell tumors: clinicopathologic findings and treatment experience in 12 patients. *Cancer* 1988;61:1187.
2. Kwiatkowski DJ, Harpole DH, Godleski J, et al. Molecular-pathologic substaging in 244 stage I non-small cell lung cancer patients: clinical implications. *J Clin Oncol* 1998;16:2468.
3. Woods RL, Fox RM, Tattersal MH, et al. Metastatic adenocarcinoma of unknown primary site: a randomized study of two combination-chemotherapy regimens. *N Engl J Med* 1980;303:87.
4. Greco FA, Vaughn WK, Hainsworth JD. Advanced poorly differentiated carcinoma of unknown primary site: recognition of a treatable syndrome. *Ann Intern Med* 1986;104:547.
5. Slamon DJ, Godolphin W, Jones LA, et al. Studies of the HER-2/neu proto-oncogene in human breast and ovarian cancer. *Science* 1989;244:707.
6. Rose PG, Bundy BN, Watkins EB, et al. Concurrent cisplatin-based chemoradiation improves progression-free and overall survival in advanced cervical cancer: results of a randomized Gynecologic Oncology Group study. *N Engl J Med* 1999;340:1144.
7. Fialkow PJ. Clonal origin of human tumors. *Biochim Biophys Acta* 1976;458:283.
8. Shapiro JR, Shapiro WR. Clonal tumor cell heterogeneity. *Prog Exp Tumor Res* 1984;27:49.
9. Curt GA, Chabner BA. Gene amplification in drug resistance: of mice and men. *J Clin Oncol* 1984;2:62.
10. Giovanella BC, Stehlin JS, Williams JJ, et al. Heterotransplantation of human cancers into nude mice—a model for human cancer chemotherapy. *Cancer* 1978;42:2269.
11. Bogden AE, Haskell PM, LePage DI, et al. Growth of human tumor xenografts implanted under the renal capsule of normal immunocompetent mice. *Exp Cell Biol* 1979;47:281.
12. Hamburger AW, Salmon SE. Primary bioassay of human tumor stem cells. *Science* 1977;197:461.
13. Salmon SE, Alberts DS, Duriel GM, et al. Clinical correlations of drug sensitivity in the human tumor stem cell assay. *Recent Results Cancer Res* 1980;74:300.
14. Flasshove M, Strumberg D, Ayscue L, et al. Structural analysis of the deoxycytidine kinase gene in patients with the acute myeloid leukemia and resistance to cytosine arabinoside. *Leukemia* 1993;8:780.
15. Reed E, Parker RJ, Gill I, et al. Platinum-DNA adduct in leukocyte DNA of a cohort of 49 patients with 24 different types of malignancy. *Cancer Res* 1993;53:3694.
16. Curt GA, Carney DN, Cowan KH, et al. Unstable methotrexate resistance in human small-cell carcinoma associated with double-minute chromosomes. *N Engl J Med* 1983;308:199.
17. Gorlick R, Goker E, Trippett T, et al. Defective transport is a common mechanism of acquired methotrexate resistance in acute lymphocytic leukemia and is associated with decreased reduced folate carrier expression. *Blood* 1997;89:1013.
18. Scudiero DA, Meyer SA, Clatterbuck BE, et al. Sensitivity of human cell strains having different abilities to repair O^6-methyl guanine in DNA to inactivation by alkylating agents including chloroethyl nitrosoureas. *Cancer Res* 1984;44:2467.
19. Fink D, Aebi S, Howell SB. The role of DNA mismatch repair in drug resistance. *Clin Cancer Res* 1998;4:1.
20. Druker BJ, Lydon NB. Lessons learned from the development of an Abl tyrosine kinase inhibitor for chronic myelogenous leukemia. *J Clin Invest* 2000;105:1.
21. Hande K, Messenger M, Wagner J, et al. Inter- and intrapatient variability in etoposide kinetics with oral and intravenous drug administration. *Clin Cancer Res* 1999;5(10):2742.
22. Relling MV, Hancock ML, Rivera GK, et al. Mercaptopurine therapy intolerance and heterozygosity at the thiopurine S-methyltransferase gene locus. *J Natl Cancer Inst* 1999;91:23.
23. Stoller R, Hande KR, Jacobs SA, et al. The use of plasma pharmacokinetics to predict and prevent methotrexate toxicity. *N Engl J Med* 1977;297:630.
24. Rice GC, Hoy C, Schimke RT. Transient hypoxia enhances the frequency of DHFR gene amplification in Chinese hamster ovary cells. *Proc Natl Acad Sci U S A* 1986;83:5978.
25. Strumberg D, Nitiss JL, Dong J, et al. Molecular analysis of yeast and human type II topoisomerases. *J Biol Chem* 1999;274:40.
26. Fojo AT, Ueda K, Slamon DJ, et al. Expression of a multidrug-resistance gene in human tumors and tissues. *Proc Natl Acad Sci U S A* 1987;84:265.
27. Marie JP, Zittoun R, Sikic BI. Multidrug resistance (mdr1) gene expression in adult acute leukemias: correlation with treatment outcomes and in vitro drug sensitivity. *Blood* 1991;78:586.
27a. McKenna SL, Padua RA. Multidrug resistance in leukemia. *Br J Haematol* 1997;96:659.
28. Van der Kolk, deVries E, Loning J, et al. Activity and expression of the multidrug resistance proteins MRP1 and MRP2 in acute myeloid leukemia cells, tumor cell lines, and normal hematopoietic CD34+ peripheral blood cells. *Clin Cancer Res* 1998;4:1727.
29. Lee K, Belinsky MG, Bell DW, et al. Isolation of MOAT-B, a widely expressed multidrug resistance-associated protein/canalicular multispecific organic anion transporter-related transporter. *Cancer Res* 1998;58:2741.
30. Zhan Z, Sandor VA, Gamelin E, et al. Expression of the multidrug resistance-associated protein gene in refractory lymphoma quantitation by a validated polymerase chain reaction assay. *Blood* 1997;89:3795.
31. Doyle LA, Yang W, Abruzzo LV, et al. A multidrug resistance transporter from human MCF-7 breast cancer cells. *Proc Natl Acad Sci U S A* 1998;95:15665.
32. Anderson H, Hopwood P, Prendiville J, et al. A randomized study of bolus versus continuous pump infusion of ifosfamide and doxorubicin with oral etoposide for small cell lung cancer. *Br J Cancer* 1993;67:1385.
33. De Gramont A, Bosset JF, Milan C, et al. Randomized trial comparing monthly low-dose leucovorin and fluorouracil bolus with bimonthly high-dose leucovorin and fluorouracil bolus plus continuous infusion for advanced colorectal cancer: a French intergroup study. *J Clin Oncol* 1997;15:808.
34. Cowens JW, Creaven PJ, Greco WR, et al. Initial clinical (phase I) trial of TLC-D-99 (doxorubicin encapsulated in lyposomes). *Cancer Res* 1993;53:2796.
35. Bottini A, Bersiga A, Brizzi M. p53 but not bcl-2 immunostaining is predictive for poor clinical complete response to primary chemotherapy in breast cancer patients. *Clin Cancer Res* 2000;6(7):2751.

36. Lai GM, Chen YN, Mickley LA, et al. P-glycoprotein expression and schedule dependence of Adriamycin cytotoxicity in human colon carcinoma cell lines. *Int J Cancer* 1991;49:696.

37. Korsmeyer SJ. *Bcl-2* initiates a new category of oncogenes: regulators of cell death. *Blood* 1992;80:879.

38. Green DR, Bissonnette RP, Cotter TG. Apoptosis and cancer. *PPO Updates* 1994;8:1.

39. Lowe SW, Ruley HE, Jacks T, et al. *p53*-dependent apoptosis modulates the cytotoxicity of anticancer agents. *Cell* 1993;74:957.

40. Kohn KW, Jackman J, O'Connor PM. Cell cycle control and cancer chemotherapy. *J Cell Biochem* 1994;54:440.

41. Goldie JH, Coldman AJ. A mathematic model for relating the drug sensitivity of tumors to their spontaneous mutation rate. *Cancer Treat Rep* 1979;63:1727.

42. Goldie JH, Coldman AJ, Gudanskas GA. Rationale for the use of alternating non-cross-resistant chemotherapy. *Cancer Treat Rep* 1982;65:439.

43. DeVita VT, Hubbard SM, Longo DL. The chemotherapy of lymphomas: looking back, moving forward—The Richard and Hinda Rosenthal Foundation Award Lecture. *Cancer Res* 1987;47:5810.

44. Fisher RI, Gaynor ER, Dahlberg S, et al. Comparison of a standard regimen (CHOP) with three intensive chemotherapy regimens for advanced non-Hodgkin's lymphoma. *N Engl J Med* 1993;328:1002.

45. Fisher RI, Gaynor ER, Dahlberg S, et al. A phase III comparison of CHOP versus m-BACOD versus ProMACE-CytaBOM versus MACOP-B in patients with intermediate- or high-grade non-Hodgkin's lymphoma: results of SWOG-8516 (Intergroup 0067), the National High-Priority Lymphoma Study. *Ann Oncol* 1994;5[Suppl 2]:91.

46. Cooper IA, Wolf MM, Robertson TI, et al. Randomized comparison of MACOP-B with CHOP in patients with intermediate-grade non-Hodgkin's lymphoma: the Australian and New Zealand Lymphoma Group. *J Clin Oncol* 1994;12:769.

47. Gordon LI, Harrington D, Andersen J, et al. Comparison of a second-generation combination chemotherapeutic regimen (m-BACOD) with a standard regimen (CHOP) for advanced diffuse non-Hodgkin's lymphoma. *N Engl J Med* 1992;327:1342.

48. Canellos GP, Anderson JR, Propert KJ, et al. Chemotherapy of advanced Hodgkin's disease with MOPP, ABVD, or MOPP alternating with ABVD. *N Engl J Med* 1992;327:1478.

49. Connors JM, Klimo P, Adams G, et al. MOPP/ABV hybrid versus alternating MOPP/ABVD for advanced Hodgkin's disease. *Proc Am Soc Clin Oncol* 1992;11:317(abst 1073).

50. Hudis C, Seidman A, Baselga J, et al. Sequential dose-dense doxorubicin, paclitaxel, and cyclophosphamide for resectable high-risk breast cancer: feasibility and efficacy. *J Clin Oncol* 1999;17:1.

51. Levin L, Hryniuk WM. Dose intensity analysis of chemotherapy regimens in ovarian carcinoma. *J Clin Oncol* 1987;5:756.

52. Longo DL, Young RC, Wesley M, et al. Twenty years of MOPP therapy for Hodgkin's disease. *J Clin Oncol* 1986;4:1295.

53. van Rijswijk RE, Haanen C, Dekker AW, et al. Dose intensity of MOPP chemotherapy and survival in Hodgkin's disease. *J Clin Oncol* 1989;7:1776.

54. Bezwoda WR, Dansey R, Bezwoda MA. Treatment of Hodgkin's disease with MOPP chemotherapy: effect of dose and schedule modification on treatment outcome. *Oncology* 1990;47:29.

55. Kaufman D, Longo DL. Hodgkin's disease. *Crit Rev Oncol Hematol* 1992;13:135.

56. Kuter DJ. Megakaryocytopoiesis and thrombopoiesis. In: Beutler E, Lichtman MA, Coller BS, et al., eds. *Williams' hematology*, 6th ed. New York: McGraw-Hill, 2001:1339.

57. Stadtmauer EA, O'Neill A, Goldstein LJ, et al., and the Philadelphia Bone Marrow Transplant Group. Conventional-dose chemotherapy compared with high-dose chemotherapy plus autologous hematopoietic stem-cell transplantation for metastatic breast cancer. *N Engl J Med* 2000;342:15.

58. Socio G, Stone JV, Wingard JR, et al. Long term survival and late deaths after allogeneic bone marrow transplantation. *N Engl J Med* 1999;341:14.

59. Liebmann J, Fisher J, Teague D, et al. Sequence dependence of paclitaxel (Taxol®) combined with cisplatin or alkylators in human cancer cells. *Oncol Res* 1994;6:25.

60. Kobayashi K, Schilsky RL. Update on biochemical modulation of chemotherapeutic agents. *Oncology (Huntingt)* 1993;7:99.

61. Sotos GA, Grogan L, Allegra CJ. Preclinical and clinical aspects of biomodulation of 5-fluorouracil. *Cancer Treat Rev* 1994;20:11.

62. Pihkalan J, Saarinen UM, Lundstrom U, et al. Myocardial function in children and adolescents after therapy with anthracyclines and chest irradiation. *Eur J Cancer* 1996;32A:97.

63. Bunn PA, Lichter AS, Makuch RW, et al. Chemotherapy alone or chemotherapy plus chest radiation therapy in limited-stage small-cell lung cancer. *Ann Intern Med* 1987;106:655.

64. Fisher B, Wolmark N, Rockette H, et al. Postoperative adjuvant chemotherapy or radiation therapy for rectal cancer: results from NSABP protocol R-01. *J Natl Cancer Inst* 1988;80:21.

65. Shapiro CL, Harrigan Hardenbergh P, Gelman R, et al. Cardiac effects in adjuvant doxorubicin and radiation therapy in breast cancer patients. *J Clin Oncol* 1998;16:11.

66. Longo DL, Russo A, Duffey PL, et al. Treatment of advanced stage massive mediastinal Hodgkin's disease: the case for combined modality treatment. *J Clin Oncol* 1991;9:227.

67. Lavey RS, Eby NL, Prosnitz LR. Impact on second malignancy risk of the combined use of radiation and chemotherapy for lymphomas. *Cancer* 1990;66:80.

68. Pui CH, Ribeiro RC, Hancock ML, et al. Acute myeloid leukemia in children treated with epipodophylotoxins for acute lymphoblastic leukemia. *N Engl J Med* 1991;321:1682.

69. Winick NJ, McKenna RW, Shuster JJ, et al. Secondary acute myeloid leukemia in children with acute lymphoblastic leukemia treated with etoposide. *J Clin Oncol* 1993;11:209.

70. Slamon D, Leyland-Jones B, Shak S, et al. Addition of Herceptin (humanized anti-HER2 antibody) to first line chemotherapy for HER2 overexpressing metastatic breast cancer (HER2+/MBC) markedly increases anticancer activity: a randomized multinational controlled phase III trial. *Proc Am Soc Clin Oncol* 1998;17:98a(abstr 377).

71. Gottdiener JS, Mathisen DJ, Borer JS, et al. Doxorubicin cardiotoxicity: assessment of late left ventricular dysfunction by radionuclide cineangiography. *Ann Intern Med* 1981;94:430.

72. Brangi M, Litman T, Ciotti M, et al. Camptothecin resistance: role of the ATP-binding cassette (ABC), mitoxantrone-resistance half-transporter (MXR), and potential for glucuronidation in MXR-expressing cells. *Cancer Res* 1999;59:5938.

73. Pourquier P, Takebayashi Y, Urasaki Y, et al. Induction of topoisomerase I cleavage complexes by 1-beta-D-arabinofuranosylcytosine (ara-C) in vitro and in ara-C-treated cells. *Proc Natl Acad Sci U S A* 2000;97:2040.

2

PRECLINICAL ASPECTS OF CANCER DRUG DISCOVERY AND DEVELOPMENT

JILL I. JOHNSON
ANNE MONKS
MELINDA G. HOLLINGSHEAD
EDWARD A. SAUSVILLE

This chapter provides an overview of the preclinical phase of the development of any drug, which has two overall goals. The first is the discovery of a new molecule with therapeutic potential and demonstration of its activity in model systems leading to definition of its pharmacology and toxicology. These studies allow an assessment of how the new molecule differs from currently available therapeutic agents. The second is to conduct a series of studies directed at fulfilling regulatory requirements for entry into initial human clinical trials. This chapter also provides a demarcation of special development issues relating to anticancer drugs in light of new and continually improving information regarding cancer cell pathophysiology.

The past two decades have seen a revolution come to pass in our understanding of how cancer cells differ from normal cells. Accordingly, a shift is occurring in the methods used to discover anticancer drugs. Figure 2-1A illustrates the former or "empirical" paradigm in which the initial basis for enthusiasm about a compound was evidence of toxicity for tumor cells either growing in tissue culture (*in vitro*), or as tumors (*in vivo*) in animals. Optimization of the molecule and the schedule in an animal model in which it elicited antitumor effect then occurred. An initial assessment of toxicology allowed definition of projected dose levels that would allow inception of a human clinical trial. Note that this development path does not necessarily consider the mechanism of action of the agent as an important feature. Also, no attempt is made to relate the pharmacologic and pharmacokinetic features of the agent to pharmacodynamic measures of drug action at the tumor site in this approach. In contrast, Figure 2-1B illustrates the paradigm to which the cancer drug development community, including academic and industrial interests, is shifting. Initial selection of candidate drug molecules is made with a particular molecular target in mind. Thus, the first screen for drug activity occurs at the level of a pure target, using either a biochemical reagent or cells that have been engineered to overexpress the target or target-containing pathway. Chemical optimization relies extensively on pharmacology to assure that active concentrations of drug in terms of possibly affecting the target are achievable in animals. Then, at a relatively late stage in the molecule's development, a potentially very focused evaluation can occur *in vivo* using models that are specialized to reflect the action of the target molecule. These ideally are accompanied by documentation of effect on the biochemical target correlating with or leading to a useful effect *in vivo*.

The reason for these two potentially competing strategies in cancer drug development stems in part from the historical reality that, before the elucidation of the basis for deregulated cancer cell growth, empirical evidence of tumor shrinkage was all that could be followed, and empirical activity *in vivo* was optimistically viewed as predicting antitumor activity in humans. Because agents were cytotoxic, the only end point that mattered was tumor regression. Molecularly targeted drug discovery has now yielded drugs with a variety of actions, some of which may not lead to immediate shrinkage of tumor; verification of engagement of the target is an essential first step in drug evaluation. Even now, although reversal of the deregulation of particular oncogenes, cell-cycle regulatory mechanisms, and tumor suppressor genes is known to cause useful effects in experimental tumor models, "real" cancer cells in humans may not be affected. These tumors unfortunately have a number of molecular lesions. Therefore, even the most rationally conceived drug molecule may fail because of mutational changes downstream from its intended target or metabolic features of tumors that never allow the drug to reach its target. Thus, to view cancer drug discovery and development as ever amenable to a totally "rational" approach is naive, for empiricism must at some level enter into defining new lead structures directed against biochemical targets, or in causing promis-

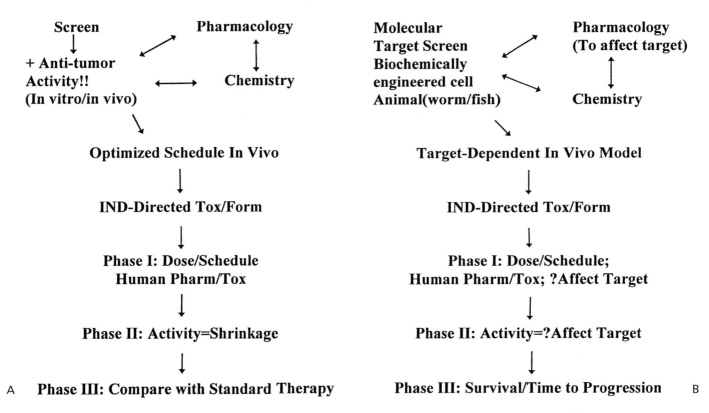

FIGURE 2-1. Comparison of the empirical (**A**) and rational (**B**) drug discovery algorithms. (IND, investigative new drug; pharm, pharmacology; tox, toxicology.)

ing leads to perform optimally in animals. On the other hand, the wealth of biochemical and genetic information defining cancer cell biology surely is leading to exciting new opportunities for clinical trials.

MAXIMIZATION OF DIVERSITY IN LEAD IDENTIFICATION

Whether the initial screen leading to a candidate drug is a mechanistically driven biochemical screen or an empirical antiproliferative screen, the greater the diversity in the types of molecules examined, the more likely a successful novel structure will be identified. Historically, natural products—defined here as extracts of plant, microbial, and animal organisms—were a source of activity in screening assays conducted as bioassays of drug effect. Examples of drugs discovered in this fashion include digitalis, the penicillins, and the antihypertensives derived from *Rauwolfia*. In cancer treatment, the vinca alkaloids, anthracyclines, camptothecins, and taxanes came to attention from these sources. Natural product extracts as a source of cancer drug discovery have been extensively reviewed[1,2] and are not discussed further except to emphasize that natural product extracts remain an important source of incredibly diverse lead structures, whose value is

most definable when used in chemically and biologically well-characterized screens.

Beginning in the 1960s, screens using pure compounds directed against enzymes or biologically well-characterized targets yielded many classes of drugs, for example, new generations of antihypertensives such as the angiotensin-converting enzyme inhibitors, the cholesterol-lowering "statins," and, in the more modern era, reverse transcriptase and protease inhibitors directed against human immunodeficiency virus. These latter examples in particular have emphasized the power of combining a knowledge of an intended target's structure at the atomic level with efforts to design useful inhibitors, and is the paradigm that will be increasingly followed in the derivation of cancer therapeutics. Thus, technologies that maximize the diversity of structures available to molecularly directed screens are of great interest.

Combinatorial Chemistry

The method of purposely synthesizing more than one compound as a result of a single reaction began approximately 15 years ago with the synthesis by Geysen[3] of multiple numbers of peptides on polyethylene rods. Accordingly, the product represented "combinations" of products deriving from a set of reactants and hence the term "combinational" chemistry. This technique of arranging solid supports in 96-well plates to allow facile addition of sequential reactants was dubbed "pin technology." The "split-pool" method (in which each individual reactant is added to equally divided solid support material for coupling, then solid supports are pooled for washing, and then supports are divided for the next reactant coupling) was an improvement on the pin technique because the resultant products exist in theoretically equimolar amounts. The next technical advance was the enclosure of the solid support resin within porous polypropylene bags—the "tea bag" method developed by Houghten.[4] The tea bag method also used split-pool synthesis, and the final product mixtures were washed from the resins. This method allowed for the synthesis of mixtures of millions of peptides in solution phase, which could be used for testing. A third variation of the split-pool approach involved the use of tagged polymeric beads as the solid support.[5] Either the beads could be used directly in assays, or the peptides could be cleaved from the beads into solution.

The synthesis of small peptide libraries, although an interesting chemical approach, was of limited use to cancer drug discovery, as small peptides do not enter cells and therefore are, in general, not suitable drug candidates. A variation of the chemistry was discovered that could produce peptide-like molecules[6] or "peptoids," which, lacking amide bonds, are less susceptible to enzymatic cleavage. The report by Bunin and Ellman[7] of the synthesis of a low-molecular-weight nonpeptidic benzodiazepine library demonstrated the utility of the combinatorial library approach for the first time as a drug discovery tool. Subsequent advances in the field included more efficient deconvolution schemes such as the positional scanning approach,[8] use of a greater number of scaffolds on which to construct libraries, and use of a wider variety of reagents and amenable reaction conditions. Virtually all pharmaceutical companies now use the methods of combinatorial chemistry in their drug discovery and development programs, particularly in the phase of lead discovery.

Computer-Based Drug Design and Computational Analysis

Medicinal chemists have traditionally used parameters such as steric bulk, hydrogen-bonding ability, hydrophobic interactions, and knowledge of active compound structure to design new test agents. Computational chemistry greatly increases the efficiency in approaching these parameters. Factors such as the structural biochemistry of the target enzyme or receptor, the nature of the substrate, the mechanism of the target-substrate interaction, and compound solubility and pharmaceutical tractability are used as modeling tools and as a selection basis for a target pharmacophore. Before a combinatorial library is actually synthesized, computer models create "virtual libraries," which are then evaluated for how thoroughly "diversity" or "multiparameter" space, as well as functional space, is covered by the selected moieties to be added to the scaffold structure.

Examples of computer models designed to synthesize virtual libraries include the Universal Library (Sphinx, Durham, NC), Icepick (Axys, South San Francisco, CA), and Matrix (ComGenex, Budapest, Hungary). Software has been designed to order the reactants and solvents in the necessary amounts and even to analyze the cost and time required for the synthesis of the library. The CombiChem drug discovery system (San Diego, CA) uses an unbiased Universal Informer Library[9] with which to screen new biologic targets. Information from the initial hits is then used to design second-generation or daughter libraries in an iterative drug discovery cycle.

Numerous algorithms exist by which the diversity of a set of compound structures can be measured and representative sublibraries selected. Little agreement is found, however, on the best approach to estimating the diversity score of a library. Libraries can be partitioned into a uniform array of blocks or cells on the basis of descriptor coordinates. The algorithm then selects one compound from each cell.[10] Atom pair fingerprints, which indicate the presence or absence of pairs of atom types separated by a defined number of bonds, can be used to describe and then differentiate each structure. The most dissimilar structures are then selected for the virtual sublibrary. Algorithms exist that then cluster structures into groups. The Jarvis-Patrick[10] clustering algorithm requires that each member of a cluster have in common a predefined number of chemical neighbors. The similar Hodes clustering model[11] is currently used by the National Cancer Institute (NCI) to assess structural novelty for primary screening candidates.

The goal of these computer algorithms is to define a library of the smallest number of compounds that covers the greatest diversity space with the greatest likelihood of being active in an assay. Detractors point out that by using these for the most part unproven tools and thus limiting the compounds screened, one runs the very real risk of decreasing the chance of finding drug leads. On the other hand, the economics of screening purified target molecules calls for efficient use of reagents.

The rapid synthesis of compounds and their evaluation in the hundreds of thousands of assays per week initially created bottlenecks in data management and analysis. Just as software has come into existence to analyze diversity space, a concomitant development of library and biologic information-handling tools has occurred, although the widespread effective use of these tools for data mining has yet to occur.[12] Examples of newly developed bioinformatics systems include Project Library[13] from MDL (San Leandro, CA), which tracks actual and virtual library synthesis, compound, and mixture registration and data, and LiBrain (Alanex Corp., San Diego, CA), which also facilitates optimization steps to produce viable drug candidates.[14]

High-Throughput Screening

Current weekly screening goals extend from hundreds to thousands, and even hundreds of thousands, of data points. Rather than limit the number of compounds to be tested, this technology promotes a much broader screening experience. The synthesis of larger combinatorial libraries in smaller sample quantities has in part driven high-throughput screening (HTS) technology, as has the availability of automated robotic work stations.

Whereas initial HTS focused on receptor-based assays, advances in fluorescence spectroscopy and fluorescence polarization have allowed the development of reliable cell-based HTS assays. Dispensing techniques such as microdrop and inkjet technologies have led to increased miniaturization. The once standard 96-well microtiter plate has been replaced by the 1,536-well plate, which may soon be supplanted by the 9,600-well plate and the 0.2-µL assay.

Advances have also been made in the types of interactions that can be studied in HTS assays. To take advantage of new targets identified by genomics consisting of aggregated proprietary and public-access sequence information, companies are developing HTSs that are more general in nature and rely on common physical characteristics of molecules such as thermal unfolding or binding affinity, using capillary electrophoresis capable of distinguishing between low-, moderate-, and high-affinity binders in collections of crude natural products, combinatorial mixtures, or pure compounds.

Key to successful HTS is the ability of the assay to properly predict drug-target interactions. In addition, such a screening program must be supported by a strong infrastructure, which includes an efficient source of samples to be assayed, a reliable robotics system, and a database system specifically designed for storing and analyzing hundreds of thousands of data points. The most astonishing advance in screening technology is the development of the biochip.[16] The chips resemble computer integrated circuits and are fabricated from sheets of thin glass, plastic, or silicon. Fluid-carrying channels and larger reaction chambers are etched into the sheets by photolithography. Reactants are pumped along the reaction pathway by miniature valves. The technology makes use of electric fields and pressure to move fluids along the channels, and tiny air bubbles maintain separation of materials.

Companies developing such "microfluidic" devices include Caliper, which is adapting conventional drug screens to biochips, and Aurora, which has created a microchip capable of assaying more than 3,400 compounds at a single time. Cadus has produced the next-generation microchip (Living Chip), a compact disc–sized device capable of holding up to 100,000 wells from which assay results can be read directly. Chips are also being created that synthesize compounds singly or in parallel. Orchid Pharmaceuticals[15] has produced a 2.5-cm square chip that contains 144 minireactors for simultaneous synthesis and has a 10,000-chamber chip in development.

Absorption, Distribution, Metabolism, and Excretion

A criticism of HTS is that such assays are designed to find the compound that is the most potent and selective against a particular target without regard to pharmaceutical or druglike factors such as solubility, toxicity, and bioavailability. Drug discovery programs historically have spent much effort defining drug leads that then fail in the development process due to toxicity, lack of *in vivo* efficacy, or poor biopharmaceutical properties. The development of predictive, inexpensive *in vitro* assays for absorption, distribution, metabolism, and excretion should alleviate the lead development bottleneck and could greatly enhance the multidisciplinary character of drug discovery. For example, *in vitro* assays like those developed by MetaXen and Xenogen use parameters such as partition coefficients, P-glycoprotein efflux, solubility, and P-450 CYP3A4 metabolism to predict absorption, P-450 induction to predict metabolism, and protein binding, drug resistance, mechanism susceptibility, and solubility information to predict distribution and excretion factors. These assays have been standardized to the greatest extent possible with the use of *in vivo* data from both animals and humans.

INITIAL ASSESSMENT OF COMPOUND ACTIVITY *IN VITRO*

The strategies described above lead to large numbers of candidate agents for assays of antiproliferative activity. Historically, pure chemical compounds and natural product extracts have initially been studied *in vivo* or *in vitro*. *In vivo* screening is discussed later. Both *in vitro* and *in vivo* approaches were primarily empirical, in that clear knowledge of a compound's target was not available. As described in the introduction to this chapter, these approaches are being supplanted by approaches in which definition of a compound's biochemical target exists before any efficacy experiment (*in vitro* or *in vivo*) is undertaken. Ultimately, whether a compound is created with a target in mind or is simply a novel chemotype, assessment of antiproliferative potential is conventionally done both *in vitro* and *in vivo*.

In the early 1980s, the NCI evaluated the *in vitro* Hamburger and Salmon colony-forming assay[16] for its potential to discover new antitumor drugs.[17] The NCI organized a cooperative effort to evaluate the human tumor colony–forming assay,[18] and this approach showed some promise. Technical limitations inherent in the methodology, however, notably limited-colony forming efficiencies, argued against its application to large-scale screening.

In Vitro Cell Line Screening

In 1985, the NCI initiated feasibility studies to develop a new *in vitro* screening model based on the use of established human tumor cell lines.[19] This screen initially focused on lung cancer, but by 1990 when it became fully operational, the screen included cell lines from most of the major human malignancies. The current model uses approximately 60 human tumor cell lines representing hematologic malignancies, melanoma, and cancers of the lung, colon, breast, brain, kidney, and prostate. The rationale for this approach[20] was that human cell lines, particularly from solid malignancies, provided an improved model for human cancer and might allow for selection of agents with activity toward a specific histologic type of cancer.[21,22] The operation of the screen began with evaluation of toxicity in multiple cell lines using tetrazolium-based assays,[23,24] but due to the variable behavior of tetrazolium dyes, the core assay was changed to a protein-based measurement, previously described.[25,26] The selection of cell lines and assay parameters has been reviewed formerly.[22]

The method uses continuous drug incubation for 48 hours with a relatively high starting cell inoculum (5,000 to 20,000 cells per well in a 96-well plate). Such an approach allows for calculation of net cell loss as a result of drug treatment and can allow cell kill to be distinguished from growth inhibition.[26] Furthermore, evidence has indicated that this approach minimized the effects of the variable doubling times of cell lines and minimizes masking of nonspecific antiproliferative effects.

Discussion of the validity of the screening parameters selected has continued over the years. In response to an overview of screening results by Weinstein et al.,[27] the 2-day incubation was criticized as not predicting clinical response as well as cell kill as measured by clonogenic survival.[28] Yet clearly short-term growth-inhibitory assays and clonogenic assays do not necessarily predict for the same cellular response. Evidence is found that therapeutic damage induced in isogenic sets of cell lines differing by one gene can lead to rapid apoptosis in one cell population but not in another *in vitro*.[29,30] When the response is measured in the clonogenic assay, however, both isogenic cell populations are equally inhibited. Thus, the *in vitro* growth inhibition assay in this case would predict for a difference in sensitivity whereas the clonogenic assay would not. In fact, the NCI *in vitro* screening assay is intended to be focused less on predicting clinical utility than on detecting previously unknown chemotypes with the potential to act as antiproliferative agents. Another study[31] illustrates an instance in which the clonogenic assay incorrectly predicted an *in vivo* outcome in a xenograft model, involving treatment with effectors of checkpoint function. Thus, clono-

genic assay behavior cannot be regarded as a gold standard on which to base decisions to pursue a compound's development. Both *in vitro* cell culture and clonogenic screens offer the potential to convey useful information about the action of novel compounds.

The NCI *in vitro* anticancer drug screen has been operational since April 1990. As of October 1998, 70,702 pure compounds have been studied in 60 cell lines; 6,452 compounds have shown evidence of *in vitro* activity; and 1,546 have been selected for *in vivo* studies. A large fraction of the data is available to the public through a web-based search system (http://dtp.nci.nih.gov). The clinical value of the compounds that have entered clinical trial has not been fully defined at this time.

A major issue in interpreting the results of *in vitro* screening studies emerging from the 60 cell line screen was the orderly display and comparison of different patterns of dose-response curves. Paull and colleagues[32] developed the "mean graph" representation of screening data (Fig. 2-2) in which the mean concentration affecting all cells to a similar degree pharmacologically is plotted in the midline of the graph, and the behavior of individual cell lines is represented as a deflection to the left, by convention, for cells more resistant than the mean, and to the right for cells more sensitive than the mean.

As is apparent from Figure 2-2, an unexpected and important application of this manner of presentation, which still forms the basis for more sophisticated pattern-recognition programs used currently, is the richly informative patterns of activity that emerge. Correlations of activity patterns could be quantified using an NCI-developed computer program named COMPARE.[33] COMPARE quantitatively estimates the similarity of the pattern of activity of a test compound in the screen to the pattern of known molecules. Use of COMPARE led to the recognition that compounds with the same or similar mechanisms of action despite different chemical structures often showed mean graph patterns that were closely correlated.[33] This approach resulted in identification of new structures with tubulin-binding activity,[34,35] topoisomerase I[36] and II activity,[37] and antimetabolites.[38,39] In addition, compounds with unique profiles of growth inhibition, which suggest modes of action not shared with known clinically active classes of chemotherapeutic agents, have also been identified.[40] As another example, the use of COMPARE linked the effects of cucurbitacin[41] and jasplakinolide[42,43] to the actin cytoskeleton. Alternatively, the COMPARE algorithm can suggest which in a series of analogs has a mechanism likely to be distinct from the lead. Thus, evaluation of cytotoxicity profiles from a variety of platinum analogs by COMPARE indicated that oxaliplatin had a different spectrum of activity than and low cross-reactivity with cisplatin. This suggested that oxaliplatin might be valuable in cisplatin-refractory disease or in combination with cisplatin, a prediction that seems to be emerging in the clinic as well.[44]

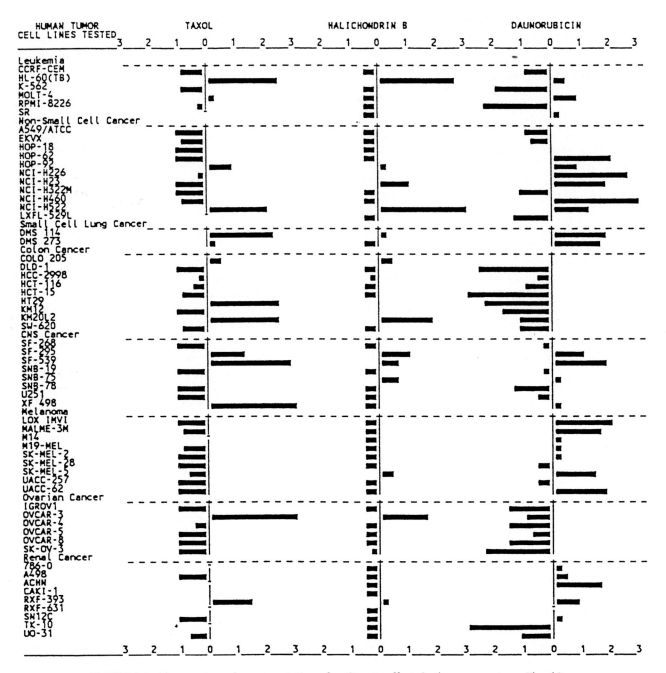

FIGURE 2-2. The mean graph representation of antitumor effects in the cancer screen. The data summarized here are modified to present a visual image consistent with the results obtained from the National Cancer Institute cancer screen. The effects of a specific agent on the tumor cell lines in the screen can be depicted by the construction of a mean graph presentation of the data. A mean of the logarithms of the concentrations of the agent that produces a particular level of response (e.g., GI_{50}, 50% growth inhibition; TGI, total growth inhibition; or LC_{50}, 50% cytotoxicity) for all the cell lines in the screen forms an anchor point for this graphic presentation. The individual response of each cell line to the agent is then depicted by a bar graph extending either to the right or to the left of the mean, depending on whether the response of the cell line was either more or less sensitive than the average response. The length of each bar is proportional to the relative sensitivity compared with the mean determination. Typical mean graphs for three agents are presented in this figure and show that a characteristic "fingerprint" of cellular responsiveness for agents can be visualized from the data. Interestingly, Taxol (paclitaxel) and halichondrin B (tubulin-interactive agents) have similar patterns in contrast to daunorubicin (a topoisomerase-interactive agent).

TABLE 2-1. PURE COMPOUNDS PRIORITIZED BY NATIONAL CANCER INSTITUTE (NCI) SCREEN FOR INCEPTION OF PHASE I CLINICAL TRIALS

Alkylphospholipid (ASTA Medica)
Proteosome inhibitor PS341 (ProScript)
Rapamycin analog CC1-779 (Wyeth-Ayerst)
17-Allylaminogeldanamycin (NCI)
Quinocarmycin DX52-1 (Kyowa Hakko Kogyo)
UCN-01 (Kyowa Hakko Kogyo)
Flavopiridol (Hoechst Marion Roussel)
KRN 5500 (Kirin Brewery Co.)
MGI-114 (MGI Pharma)
Depsipeptide (Fujisawa Research)

With the NCI *in vitro* screening data used as an empiric discovery tool, several compounds have advanced to early phase I clinical trial based in part on performance in the screening system (Table 2-1). Criteria for further advancement from *in vitro* to *in vivo* studies include demonstration of a broad range of activity against several cell lines, with differential cytotoxicity not suggesting any known mechanism of action; potency, in which the average GI_{50} (concentration causing 50% inhibition of cell growth) is less than 30 nmol per L; and selectivity or specificity for a particular histology. These compounds, as they progress through phase I and phase II trials, will provide critical information for the evaluation of whether such an empirical screening paradigm can actually generate useful initial leads.

Molecular Targets

The expression of molecular targets in the cell line panel, which allowed a distinct application of the screening data, emerged from the observation that, when function and expression of the *mdr*-1 drug resistance efflux pump was examined and the data were represented in mean graph format, one could define in the database compounds with a similar pattern of activity that were subsequently shown to interact with the *mdr*-1 gene product.[45,46] This remarkable finding suggested that quantitation of targets in the cell lines could discover previously unreported activities of unknown compounds that interact with the target. This has been borne out particularly in experience with agents interacting with the epidermal growth factor receptor.[47] Other examples include quinones, whose activities could be correlated with expression of DT-diaphorase.[48] The reduced folate carrier implicated in methotrexate resistance was measured in 40 of the 60 cell lines. The resulting pattern correlated positively with 6-day exposure data for methotrexate, but negatively with those for trimetrexate,[49] a lipid-soluble antrofolate that enters cells by diffusion. Not all molecular target estimates yield meaningful correlations with compound activity. For example, expression of *mrp*, *lrp,* and topoisomerase II has not yielded correlations with compound activity in a way that points to novel compounds affecting those targets.

To address the increasing complexity of the emerging data, other computational tools have been used in addition to COMPARE. Weinstein and colleagues explored the use of neural networks[50] to group drugs by mechanism of action and biologic response profile in the screen. The Kohonen self-organizing map was also used to suggest the mechanism of action of compounds identified by the screen as potentially useful chemotherapeutic agents and to probe the biology of the cell lines in the cancer screen.[51] More recent database analyses used cluster algorithms (Discovery) in an effort to allow patterns of compound response to "self-assemble" into coherent patterns of activity.[27]

The cells in the screen have also been characterized in part for pathways relevant to chemotherapy response. For example, the *p53* tumor suppressor pathway was characterized in the cell lines,[52] including *p53* complementary DNA sequence, measurement of basal *p53* protein levels, and functional assessment of (a) transcriptional activity, (b) G_1 cell-cycle arrest, and (c) gamma-ray–induced expression of *CIP1/WAF1*, *GADD-45*, and *MDM2* messenger RNA. COMPARE and Discovery analyses revealed that most commonly used clinical agents tended to be less effective against cells expressing the *p53* mutant sequence, with the exception of antimitotic agents, notably paclitaxel (Taxol).[27] Moreover, mining of the database to discover other *p53*-independent compounds led to the finding that ellipticiniums, but not ellipticines, were more potent against *p53* mutant cells than *p53* wild-type cells.[53]

That the fingerprint patterns of activity from the screening program encode incisive information on mechanisms of action, and potential interaction with a particular protein target, was also illustrated in an analysis of a two-dimensional gel electrophoresis protein expression database of the 60 cell lines.[54]

Other important pathways measured in the cell lines include that of the *ras* oncogene, a mutated version of which clustered in the leukemias and non–small cell lung and colon carcinoma subpanels.[55] A striking similarity in cytosine arabinoside sensitivity was observed in cell lines harboring *ras* mutations that was not present in tumor lines with wild-type alleles. Similar correlations with mutations were also observed for certain topoisomerase II inhibitors. The results suggested that the *ras* oncogene might play an important role in rendering tumor cells sensitive to these agents. More recent data indicate that the enhanced sensitivity of cells harboring a *ras* mutation is due to a potentiation of the apoptotic response in these cells.[56] This hypothesis is concordant with a clinical study in which the presence of *ras* oncogene was associated with improved survival of patients in response to treatment primarily with cytosine arabinoside and a topoisomerase II inhibitor.[57] It also correlates with the sensitivity of pancreatic cancer and bladder cancer to the closely related cytidine analog, gemcitabine hydrochloride.

Nm23 expression as a marker of metastatic potential was measured in the cells of the screen, and in conjunction with

COMPARE, at least one compound was identified that gave initial evidence of *in vivo* activity in a hollow fiber model against a variety of human tumor cells.[58]

Evolution of the National Cancer Institute Screen

In response to the Developmental Therapeutics Program Review of 1998, the initial NCI screening paradigm has been altered to screen for antiproliferative activity using three cell lines chosen to be sensitive enough to cytotoxic agents so that at least one of the triad would have detected more than 95% of the compounds scored as active using the assay containing all 60 cell lines. Compounds scoring as active in the three cell line prescreen are then studied in the full 60 cell line assay to allow COMPARE assessment of pattern uniqueness and development of hypotheses relating to the mechanism of action.

ASSESSMENT OF COMPOUND ACTIVITY *IN VIVO*

A variety of animal models for evaluating anticancer therapies have been described. Although each model has its advocates, no single model is ideal for all applications. Thus, one must determine what information is desired from the *in vivo* study to make an informed choice regarding which model or models to use. Compound availability, assay costs, assay time requirements, statistical validity of the assay, behavior of clinical agents in the model, technical difficulty of the assay system, rate and frequency with which tumor appears, and reproducibility of the results are some of the factors to consider when selecting an animal model. Perhaps without exception, however, experimental agents derived from molecular or cellular screens, or other *in vitro* sources, require verification of activity, and, if possible, of molecular action, in an *in vivo* system before clinical trial. Table 2-2 lists the types of critical information needed from efficacy studies.

Initial Detection of Antitumor Activity

The history of *in vivo* screening at NCI was reviewed by Plowman et al.[59] The initial screens, introduced in 1955, consisted of several tumor panels with varying rodent and human tumor cell line content, which were introduced as

TABLE 2-2. QUESTIONS ANSWERED BY *IN VIVO* EFFICACY TESTING

Does the compound show antiproliferative activity?
Is efficacy observed at sublethal doses?
How do metabolism and excretion impact efficacy?
What administration route(s) is(are) effective?
What dose and schedule are optimal?
Are toxic phenomena associated with an efficacious dose?
How do analogs and prodrugs compare in efficacy?
Which physiologic compartment does the compound reach?

opportunity arose and as science evolved. The first 20 years of screening relied largely on testing with the murine L1210 leukemia model. Compound leads were further evaluated against various rodent tumors, particularly sarcoma 180, carcinoma 755, Walker 256 carcinosarcoma, P388 leukemia, B16 melanoma, and Lewis lung carcinoma.

In 1975, the NCI selected intraperitoneally implanted murine P388 leukemia as its first-line model, with active agents studied in additional tumor systems.[60] During this period, human tumor models began playing a role in the drug discovery and development process. The discovery of the athymic mouse in the late 1960s[61] allowed researchers to develop transplantable human tumor xenografts.[62,63] Thus, in 1976 a panel of three human tumors, consisting of a colon line (CX-1), a lung line (LX-1), and a breast line (MX-1), was introduced for efficacy studies. The early xenograft models were often conducted as subrenal capsule assays in which small tumor fragments were implanted under the renal capsule and monitored for growth by sequential sacrifice.[64] These assays were labor intensive and were subsequently replaced by assays of subcutaneous xenografts.

An analysis of the results obtained between 1976 and 1982 found a broad range of sensitivity and compound yield among the various tumor models.[61] This conclusion led the NCI to implement a strategy that involved sequential testing of compounds against a smaller panel of tumors (MX-1, B16, and L1210). These lines were very sensitive to test agents, and they were thought to have the highest probability of identifying active agents.

The development of primary *in vitro* screening approaches, described earlier, promoted the development of human tumor xenografts using the 60 cell lines represented in the *in vitro* screen. This approach allowed the mouse efficacy studies to be designed based on the activity of a compound in the *in vitro* assay. The methods used, as well as the resulting tumor xenograft panel, have been well described.[59,65,66] A significant problem which rapidly emerged was that the number of lead compounds generated by the *in vitro* screen led to increased time and costs associated with the need to conduct hundreds of xenograft studies annually. The desire to implement a high-throughput, low-cost *in vivo* prescreen so that lead compounds could be prioritized for efficacy testing in the xenograft models led to development of the hollow fiber assay.[67] This assay has emerged as the initial *in vivo* screen by the NCI for lead compounds with cytostatic or cytotoxic potential. Compounds with activity in the hollow fiber assay are considered for testing in human tumor xenografts after compound mechanism of action, formulation, and pharmacokinetic issues are considered.

Hollow Fiber Assay

The selection criteria for an *in vivo* efficacy prescreen included a high volume capacity, a short assay time, a limited need for compound, a low false-negative rate, and a minimal challenge for the test agent to overcome. The hollow fiber assay[65,67] allows screening of 50+ compounds per

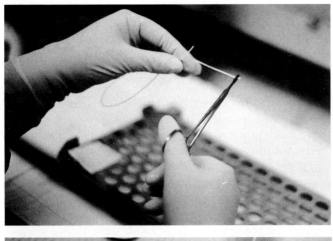

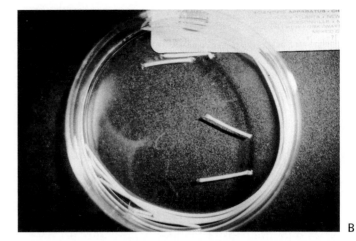

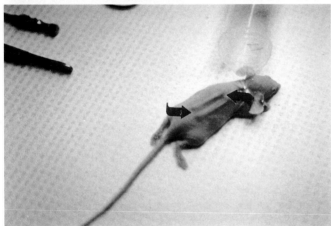

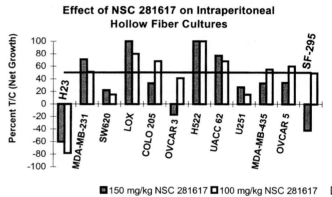

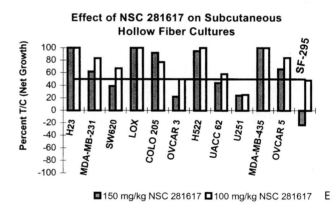

FIGURE 2-3. Hollow fiber *in vivo* model. **A:** Preparation of fibers loaded with tumor cells. **B:** Fibers before injection. **C:** Fibers (*arrows*) in the subcutaneous compartment of a mouse. **D,E:** Intraperitoneal and subcutaneous activity of test agent NSC 281617 in cells grown in hollow fibers. Activity is suggested in SW620, COLO 205, OVCAR 3, U251, MDA-MB-435, and OVCAR 5, with evidence of cell kill in H23 and SF295 in the peritoneal compartment. (T/C, <50% net growth.)

week in a 10-day assay that uses less than 500 mg of compound while testing for growth suppression of less than 10^6 tumor cells. The assay evaluates the activity of a test agent against a standard panel of 12 cell lines consisting of two lines each from the breast, colon, lung, melanoma, brain, and ovarian tumor histology subpanels. The cell lines used were selected by ranking the sensitivity of the *in vitro* cell lines to 3,500 compounds potentially suitable for *in vivo* testing and selecting the two most sensitive cell lines from each histologic subpanel. The prostate and renal lines are not represented in the standard panel, because separate assays are conducted for compounds active against cells of

these two histologic types. For the standard assay, compounds are evaluated at two dose levels based on the maximum tolerated dose (MTD) determined in mouse toxicity assays. A convenient extrapolation from the single-dose MTD to a multiple-day dosing scheme is afforded by setting the high test dose at [(1.5) (MTD)]/4, and the low dose at 67% of the high test dose. Hollow fiber cultures of each cell line are prepared *in vitro* and implanted subcutaneously and intraperitoneally into mice (Fig. 2-3). Because compound delivery is accomplished through intraperitoneal injection, the anticellular activity can be assessed in a same site (intraperitoneal/intraperitoneal) and a distant site (subcutaneous/intraperitoneal) in the same mouse. The mice are treated with a vehicle or test agent for 4 days, and the fibers are retrieved for evaluation of viable cell mass using a formazan dye conversion assay. The percent net growth of each cell line is calculated by comparison to a set of control fibers assessed for viable cell mass on the day of implantation.

For a compound to be selected for additional testing, it must meet one of three referral criteria. These criteria are (a) percent net growth must be reduced by 50% or more in 10 of the 48 combinations tested; (b) the percent net growth of cells in the subcutaneous compartment must be reduced by 50% or more in 4 of the 24 combinations; and (c) a negative net cell growth (cell kill) must occur in one or more combinations. Each compound is evaluated in a total of 24 mice (four sets of cell lines × three mice per dose × two doses) with six data points generated in each mouse (three intraperitoneal and three subcutaneous fibers). This produces 144 data points for each compound tested in the hollow fiber assay. Thus, this system allows a compound to demonstrate activity in a simple pharmacologic assay that merely asks whether the compound can or cannot reach the target cells in therapeutic concentrations under the conditions tested. The basis for this scoring system is that its application to the selected cell lines would have resulted in detection of 95% of the currently available cytotoxic agents used in "standard" oncologic practice.

Rodent Tumor Models: Additional Consideration

A variety of tumor models have been described in rodents, those of greatest interest using rats or mice. This results in part from their relatively low body weights, which minimize the amount of chemotherapeutic agent needed, and in part from the fact that their physiology is the best understood of the rodent species. Many inbred strains are available. Murine leukemias, grown in the peritoneal cavity and producing mortality as an end point, have been used for many years. Use of the L1210 and P388 leukemias in drug screening efforts was reviewed by Waud.[68] In addition to the leukemias, a variety of solid tumors are available for modeling antitumor activity. These include tumors of varying histologic types and implant sites. These tumor systems have been thoroughly reviewed by Corbett et al.[69]

Human Tumor Xenograft Models

The literature is rich with human tumor xenograft models that rely on immunocompromised mice as hosts for tumors of various histologies.[59,63,65,70,71] These models can be divided into subgroups based on the site at which the tumor cells are inoculated as well as the end point measured by the assay. Tumors have been successfully generated after tumor cell inoculation into the peritoneal cavity, the subcu-

taneous tissues, and the vascular network via cardiac or tail vein puncture, or under the renal capsule as well as into various other organ sites.

Intraperitoneal Tumors

One of the simplest xenograft models involves direct injection of tumor cells into the peritoneal cavity with subsequent administration of the test agent by one of several routes. In most cases, the end point for these intraperitoneal xenograft assays is host morbidity or mortality. This results from ascites and intraperitoneal tumor formation as well as dissemination to distant organs, for example, brain, for some tumor cell lines. Because daily tumor measurements are not required, these assays are less labor intensive and, thus, less cost prohibitive than with other xenograft models. Unfortunately, not all cells are amenable to growth in the peritoneal cavity, so the desired cell line must be assessed for its growth potential. Because the tumor is difficult to observe until ascites is present, standardization of the assay is important so that all of the inoculated mice produce viable tumor growth. Determining the minimum inoculum required to give the desired end point in all of the test mice, such as time to ascites development, is also valuable. The NCI *in vivo* screening program has found that the HL-60 promyelocytic leukemia, U251 glioblastoma, LOX melanoma, and several other ovarian, leukemic, and lymphoma cell lines provide evaluable growth as intraperitoneal tumor models (M. Hollingshead, *unpublished results*). With these models, direct administration of the test agent into the peritoneal cavity offers the greatest potential for activity for most compounds because they do not have to achieve effective plasma concentrations or distribute to the target tissues. This approach is often referred to as a "same-site" model because the target (tumor cells) and the test agent are placed in close proximity. Although this does not address issues such as agent uptake, distribution, metabolism, and excretion, it does allow an initial assessment of the *in vivo* potential of the test article. The occurrence of protein binding, local cellular uptake, rapid systemic absorption and distribution, metabolism, and host toxicity can be preliminarily assessed in these same-site models. Nonetheless, activity only in a same-site model is less valuable than activity that occurs after traversal of several pharmacologic compartments.

Subcutaneous Tumors

The subcutaneous xenograft model is commonly used for chemotherapeutic assessment, as the tumor growth can be monitored visually throughout the experiment. For these assays, tumor cells are placed under the skin of immunocompromised mice (e.g., SCID, nu/nu, NIH-III, SCID/bg, SCID/NOD), and the cells are monitored for growth by

TABLE 2-3. SUBCUTANEOUS XENOGRAFT EFFICACY PARAMETERS

Number of tumor-free mice at end of experiment
Optimal percent of treated/control based on median tumor weight
Median days until tumor reaches specified weight or doubling of volume
Growth delay at a specified tumor weight or doubling volume
Net log cell kill
Number of partial/complete tumor regressions
Number of toxicity-related deaths
Number of treatment-related weight loss

daily observation. When tumors are detected at the inoculation site, daily measurement of the tumor volume can be accomplished by means of calipers. Generally, the tumor length and width are measured, and the tumor volume is calculated using one of several formulas.[72] The NCI assumes the tumor to be a prolate ellipsoid, so the volume equals [(tumor length in mm) × (tumor width in mm)²]/2. Assuming a unit volume of 1, then the volume in mm³ is equal to the tumor weight in mg. The tumor weights versus time can be plotted to produce tumor growth curves that are compared for control and experimentally treated mice to ascertain whether treatment has an impact on tumor growth. Parameters for measuring compound efficacy in these subcutaneous xenograft models have been described elsewhere. The parameters used in the NCI drug screening program are given in Table 2-3.

Although the subcutaneous models have contributed to anticancer drug development by allowing detection of activity and schedule optimization, concern continues as to the ability of these models to predict response of a specific tumor type in the clinic. For example, little correlation was found between the results of xenograft studies and those of phase II clinical trials for 39 agents studied (E. Sausville and L. Rubinstein, *unpublished results*). Numerous factors can account for the lack of correspondence between murine models and experience in the clinic. Notable differences can exist in murine compared with human pharmacology. Tumors "trained" to grow as murine xenografts over a short period may not be representative of human tumors in a host. Murine xenografts frequently use athymic or otherwise immunocompromised animals, and therefore misrepresent important contributions by the immune system. Finally, different end points may be more easily achieved in mice than in humans (e.g., regression in mice versus inhibition or stasis, rather than regression, in humans). Clearly, improvements are needed in the application of these models to clinical practice. Murray[73] supported this concept by comparing the outcome of animal studies to those of clinical trials for small cell lung cancer patients. He concluded that the applicability of the animal data is dependent on what clinical goal is desired: cure, symptom relief, or survival gain. Houghton and colleagues[74] also conclude that

murine xenograft models may have greater predictability if dosing schedules are based on total drug exposure rather than on simple MTD calculations.

Factors to consider in improving predictability of xenograft models for the clinic include species differences in protein binding, metabolism, organ-specific toxicity, total dose tolerated, biologic half-life, dose and route effects, length of treatment required, tumor site, tumor biology, and tumor sensitivity. Although several of these are amenable to *in vitro* testing or pharmacologic/pharmacokinetic studies, the issues of tumor site, biology, and sensitivity are not readily resolved in the absence of animal tumor models. These issues have led researchers to develop tumor models that more closely mimic the clinical setting.

Orthotopic Implants

One of the deficiencies of the subcutaneous xenograft model is its failure to produce the metastatic lesions that ultimately kill many cancer patients.[75,76] Although a few subcutaneous xenograft models do produce metastatic lesions (e.g., LOX melanoma, SK-MEL-28 melanoma, MDA-MB-435 breast, and DU-145 prostate), they are the exception rather than the rule. Fidler and colleagues[77,78] demonstrated that the occurrence of metastatic lesions is not the result of a random event. Rather, it is selective, and the metastatic event consists of a series of steps that are dependent on the tumor cell injection site. Their studies have in general confirmed the concept of Paget[79] that tumor cell "seeds" need the appropriate growth environment provided by certain organs ("soil") to produce metastatic lesions. Fidler demonstrated that a tumor implanted "orthotopically," that is, into the organ of origin, behaved more like the clinical disease and was thus a better model for human cancer than subcutaneous models. This concept has proven useful for studying tumor biology and therapies, as orthotopic implantation generates tumors that produce metastatic lesions similar to those seen in humans.[80–82] To further extend the importance of orthotopic xenografts, Fidler's group[83] demonstrated differences in drug sensitivity between orthotopically and subcutaneously implanted tumor tissue. Although tissues of any origin can be implanted orthotopically, those most commonly used are breast, colon, brain, melanoma, and lung tumors. Building on the concept of orthotopic implantation, Hoffman[84] developed and patented the MetaMouse. This model differs from other orthotopic models in that the implanted tumor material consists of surgically attached pieces of tumor rather than cell suspensions or simple trocar-implanted tumor fragments. The tumor fragments used in the MetaMouse are obtained directly from human patients or from human tumor xenografts grown subcutaneously in immunocompromised mice. Giavazzi[85] and Hoffman[76] have reviewed orthotopic models and the resulting metastatic lesions.

Metastatic Models

Metastasis, the process by which tumor cells leave their tissue of origin and colonize in distant tissues, has become a target for new antineoplastic therapies. The metastatic process consists of multiple events that result from invasion of the tissue, and vascular and lymphatic components adjacent to the primary tumor. This process is initiated by basement membrane invasion resulting from proteolysis and cell motility. After tumor cell intravasation into the circulation, tumor cell emboli are trapped in distant capillary beds where extravasation can occur.[86] A small percentage of these embolic tumor cells may survive to produce tumors.[87] Another critical component in these events is the tumor vasculature, as it supplies the tumor with nutrients for growth as well as provides a pathway by which tumor cells gain entry to distant tissues. Each step in the metastatic process is being evaluated as a potential target for interruption of tumor spread.[88] Unfortunately, the *in vivo* tumor models currently available do not assess the individual targets but rely on demonstration of an effect downstream of these targets, for example, an antitumor effect. This can be measured with standard subcutaneous xenograft models if the target is applicable, for instance, for antiangiogenic agents. If the target is not relevant in the subcutaneous models, as, for example, basement membrane proteolysis, then the orthotopic models are an option. These models are generally metastatic, so an effect on one or more steps in the metastasis process should reduce the number of detectable tumor nodules at the metastatic site(s).

Intravenous Tumor (Disseminated Tumor)

Disseminated tumor models in which intravenously injected tumor cells colonize the lungs and other tissues offer another method for evaluating agents effective in the later stages of metastasis. Perhaps the best known of the disseminated tumor models is the murine melanoma B16-BL6.[89] The B16-BL6 melanoma is able to metastasize from a primary subcutaneous site as well as after intravenous injection. Thus, the same tumor cell can be used to assess both upstream and downstream events in the metastatic process.[89] This model has been used successfully to evaluate a matrix metalloproteinase inhibitor designed to inhibit basement membrane degradation.[90] Although not as well characterized as B16-BL6, human xenograft models exist in which intravenously administered cells produce disseminated disease in immunodeficient mice, particularly SCID mice. Examples of human tumor cell lines producing this effect are LOX melanoma, SK-MEL-28 melanoma, K562 chronic myelogenous leukemia, AS-283 AIDS-related lymphoma, and A549 lung tumor.[91] The problem with the disseminated models is the need for reproducible intravenous inoculations in rodents and the inability to identify the exact cause for reductions in numbers of metastases in lung or other organs.

Antiangiogenic Agents

The impact of inhibiting angiogenesis on tumor growth and metastasis has led to the development of specific antiangiogenic assays in addition to the standard tumor growth inhibition assays. Various *in vitro* assays can assess the impact of a therapeutic agent on endothelial cell proliferation, migration, and cord formation.[92] Although these assays help delineate the mechanism of action for a potential therapeutic agent, they may not show activity with all agents. Compounds whose effects are mediated through a secondary mechanism, for example, cytokine induction, would not demonstrate effects in these *in vitro* assays. For *in vivo* studies, many laboratories use the chicken chorioallantoic membrane as a substrate to assess antiangiogenic agents.[93] Although this is a more complex assay than the *in vitro* assays, it does lack several features of human neoplasia. These differences include the following: (a) it is not mammalian; (b) it is embryonic; (c) it does not simulate the tumor angiogenesis microenvironment; (d) it is only semiquantitative; and (e) some workers feel that it may not measure clinically relevant activity.

Various *in vivo* models are described that measure the growth of blood vessels into an exogenously administered substrate. Although various substrates have been described,[92] the most commonly used is Matrigel, to which various angiogenic agents, such as vascular endothelial growth factor (VEGF) or basic fibroblast growth factor (bFGF), have been added.[94] Matrigel is a basement membrane extract in which new blood vessels develop after injection into the subcutaneous tissue of rodents. By quantitating the number of vessels or the hemoglobin content, the angiogenesis response can be defined. Of note, Matrigel can be used to support xenogeneic tumor cells for injection into mice because it protects the tumor cells, provides a physiologic support, and may provide a medium into which vascular components can migrate.

The corneal angiogenesis assay[95] provides another tumor-independent assay. For this, controlled-release pellets containing angiogenic agents, for example, bFGF or VEGF, are placed into corneal micropockets, and vessel growth is quantified in the presence or absence of treatment with putative antiangiogenic agents. This approach has been used to assess the antiangiogenic potential of TNP-470 and thalidomide, two compounds currently in clinical trials.[96]

Molecular Targets and Transgenic Animals

One current interest in cancer therapeutics involves modulation of various molecular targets in neoplastic cells. These targets include oncogenes that promote unregulated cell growth (e.g., *ras, fos, myc, sis,* and *erb*) and tumor suppressor genes that suppress tumor growth (e.g., *p16, pRB,* and *p53*). Although a large number of targets have been defined, the importance of each of them in determining the causes of human disease is uncertain. Interest in these targets has led to a two-pronged strategy to develop animal models and validate them both as important tumorigenicity targets and as chemotherapeutic targets. One approach is to transfect cells with oncogenes so that the effect of the oncogene on cellular activity can be assessed both *in vitro* and *in vivo*. If the nontransfected cell line is tumorigenic, then the *in vivo* activity of a compound against the transfected and nontransfected cells can be compared using methodologies described earlier. Examples of this approach include ultimately successful efforts to derive inhibitors of the bcr-abl tyrosine kinase[97] and several farnesyl transferase inhibitors.[98]

Another approach is the generation of transgenic mice bearing one or more mutations. In many instances these transgenic mice develop spontaneous tumors at a defined age. The impact of chemotherapeutic agents on tumor development and growth may be assessed after treatment at various times relative to the predicted tumor occurrence. Barrington and colleagues,[99] using transgenic mice expressing one or more oncogenes in the presence or absence of *p53*, reported that L-744,832, a farnesyl transferase inhibitor, is *p53* independent. These transgenic mice offer an exciting method of manipulating potential treatment targets; however, their use for routine *in vivo* screening is often limited by the time required for tumor development and the amount of compound necessary to treat the animal for a protracted period of time. In addition, the number of mice developing tumors may be less than 50%, so extremely large treatment groups are necessary to obtain statistically relevant results.

Tumor Model Application

Although each of these models has value for chemotherapeutic evaluations, the models also have limitations. In applying any efficacy model to drug screening, one must consider whether the model can answer the desired question and whether a simpler means exists to get the same answer. Table 2-4 compares several characteristics of the models described here. Choosing the correct model with regard to both the immune status of the host and the tumor

selected for treatment is important. If the therapeutic protocol being evaluated depends on the host's immune system, a syngeneic model would be appropriate. Conversely, if the role of the immune response is to be minimized, then an immunocompromised host may be necessary. Host immune compromise can be either genetic, as in the SCID mouse, or induced, for example by irradiation. Another important consideration is which tumor line to use, because the target sensitivity is dependent on various parameters, such as molecular target expression, tumor doubling time, hormonal sensitivity, tumor growth fraction, and implant site.[72] If subcutaneous models are selected, the importance of the tumor implant site must not be overlooked. Differences in the site of implantation can have a significant impact on the tumor growth rate; therefore, a uniform technique must be applied to all experimental mice.[100] Another important consideration is whether the tumor is passed from mouse to mouse or initiated from tissue culture–derived cells. Both approaches are valid and each offers advantages. For tumors in which phenotypic shift can occur, for example, MDR expression, it may be important to initiate tumors from tissue culture–derived cells so that phenotypic shift is less likely. On the other hand, tumors passed from mouse to mouse tend to have higher tumor take rates and more homogeneous growth curves. To avoid undesirable phenotypic and genotypic shifts, the recommendation is that a tumor line undergo only approximately ten *in vivo* passages before new tumors are initiated from frozen cell and tumor stocks.

Once a tumor model is selected, the experimental design must be developed in light of the information available about the test agent. One of the first determinations made must be the scheduling of treatment relative to the time of tumor inoculation or, for transgenic mice, their age and onset of spontaneous tumors. Treatment can be initiated the day after tumor implantation or it can be withheld until the tumor reaches a predetermined size or stage (e.g., staged tumor). Generally, the sooner treatment is started relative to tumor inoculation, the more likely one is to see an effect, because the treatment must overcome or suppress a smaller tumor burden. Similarly, treatment of transgenic mice can be initiated early in life, for example, at weaning, or treat-

TABLE 2-4. COMPARISON OF TUMOR MODELS

Host Model	Immune Status	Assay Length	Relative Cost	Difficulty	End Point
Murine leukemia	Competent	10–15 d	Low	Low	Morbidity/mortality
Murine solid tumor	Competent	10–30 d	Low	Moderate	Tumor mass
Human i.p. xenograft	Deficient	15–90 d	Moderate	Low	Morbidity/mortality
Human s.c. xenograft	Deficient	15–90 d	Moderate	Moderate	Tumor mass
Orthotopic model	Either	Weeks to months	Low to moderate	Moderate to high	Morbidity/mortality/tumor metastases
Disseminated tumor	Either	14–90 d	Low to moderate	Moderate to high	Morbidity/mortality/tumor metastases
Transgenic mice	Either	Weeks to months	Moderate to high	Moderate to high	Morbidity/mortality/tumor metastases

ment can be delayed until signs of tumor development occur. These treatment approaches should be tailored to the expected use of a compound. The regression of large, well-established tumors more closely mimics the expected clinical use of an agent in patients with metastatic disease, whereas "early-stage" tumors may be more relevant to use of an agent as an adjuvant or "cytostatic" treatment.

Consideration must be given to the dose, route, and treatment schedule for compound administration. If no data exist regarding the compound's MTD, then determining the MTD before initiating efficacy trials may be desirable. If this is not done, then an empiric dose must be selected based on the solubility of the agent, the level of activity of similar compounds, the availability of material for testing (e.g., natural product extracts), pharmacokinetic parameters, or other factors, for the initial trials. Corbett and colleagues[101] recommend use of a flexible dose and schedule so that the MTD can be achieved in the initial tests. Venditti[102] demonstrated early that the treatment schedule for a compound could be critical to showing activity. The NCI program generally uses repeated doses administered either once daily for 5 days or once every fourth day for a total of three doses. The decision as to which protocol is used depends, at least in part, on the tumor doubling time. If a tumor has a doubling time in excess of 2.5 days, then the intermittent treatment protocol is generally selected unless the compound is known to require continuous exposure to achieve an effect.

Along with choice of the dose and schedule, a route of administration must be selected for initial studies. The intraperitoneal route has been used in many screening programs because of the ease of administering test agents by this route to large numbers of animals bearing intraperitoneally inoculated leukemias. This route may not offer the best outcome against tumors inoculated into tissues other than the peritoneum, however, because of agent uptake, distribution, and rapid loss due to liver metabolism. The intravenous route of administration has perhaps the greatest correlation with the clinical situation. Unfortunately, this route requires the greatest expertise, restricts the number of injections given because of the limited availability of vessels, and requires a compound with adequate solubility to allow administration. The subcutaneous, intramuscular, and oral routes offer acceptable alternatives. The issue of oral bioavailability must be considered before selecting this administration route, as administering the test article by the oral route is of no value if the agent is not available systemically because of absorption or metabolism effects. With some agents the need for continuous exposure is an important consideration in treatment strategies. Although human patients can receive multihour intravenous infusions, limitations exist when modeling these treatment protocols in rodent systems. Options for sustained-release delivery include osmotic pumps (Alza Scientific, Palo Alto, CA), slow-release pellets (Innovative Research of America,

Sarasota, FL), and emulsions or liposomal formulations. The body weights of the mice must be monitored during treatment so that significant weight loss is noted, both to determine the MTD and to assess its impact on the growth of the tumors, as noted by Giovanella and colleagues.[63] The use of multiple dose levels for a given compound provides for a margin of error regarding MTD and also allows development of a dose-response curve. The NCI program routinely uses three dose levels in its preliminary evaluation of a new chemotherapeutic agent. The difference between doses represents a 33% reduction from the high to intermediate and intermediate to low doses, for example, 100, 67, and 45 mg per kg per injection. Another common stepdown between doses is 50%, which allows a broader range of doses to be covered. Care must be exercised in selecting the test doses, because a decrease in test sensitivity can occur as the distance between doses increases. This is because the range between toxic and ineffective doses is often narrow for cytotoxic agents.

Finally, the treatment group size must be given adequate attention if meaningful data are to be generated. The importance of this consideration cannot be overstated, nor does a single right answer exist. If the selected model has extremely high reproducibility, then a smaller number of mice are required to achieve meaningful reductions in tumor growth rates or burdens. For example, the murine leukemias grow as intraperitoneal tumors with very narrow death patterns. For these tumors, a control group of 15 to 20 mice with treatment groups of six mice per dose often provides reproducible evidence of efficacy. At the other extreme, a transgenic model in which only 30% of mice develop tumors may require hundreds of test animals to achieve statistical validity. The NCI program generally uses 20 mice in each control or vehicle-treated group and six to ten mice per dose for the treated groups. Consulting a statistician to aid in determining the appropriate treatment group size for a given tumor model is recommended before one embarks on a chemotherapy trial.

What Tumor Models Ultimately Tell Us

As noted above, despite great efforts, little direct correspondence is found between effects of clinically tested agents and clinical outcome, if one compares the preclinical models in which an agent is active with the outcome of studies in tumors with the same histology in humans. Nonetheless, the larger the number of preclinical models in which an agent does show activity, the greater the likelihood that activity will be seen in some human neoplasm.

As cancer drug discovery and development transitions from an actively empirical to a more rationally driven enterprise, a more refined use of tumor models will have the following general outline. Agents will be selected for detailed study based on their ability to affect a molecule important to a tumor's pathophysiology. The *in vivo* model used to further develop the agent will be known beforehand to depend on the activity of the drug's target. The drug will be studied in the model using a formulation and schedule known to give drug concentrations adequate to engage and affect functions of its target. The object of the *in vivo* model then becomes a demonstration that the drug molecule is performing as expected. Critical to this pathway of development is the actual demonstration that the drug is affecting its target in the tumor model. The exceedingly useful outcome of this type of development scheme will be the potential to transfer the assay of target effect from the *in vivo* model to patient specimens from early clinical trials.

Molecular Targets in Cancer Drug Discovery

The extraordinary number of potential drug targets for cancer treatments is beginning to yield useful drug molecules. Included are numerous targets related to growth factor–induced signal transduction. The licensing of the monoclonal antibody Herceptin (trastuzumab) directed at the *erbB-2*[proto-oncogene product presages intense efforts to define "small molecules" with analogous effects. Promising early results have been obtained with a bcr-abl–directed tyrosine kinase antagonist.[103] Broad programs directed at inhibitors of epidermal growth factor,[104] platelet-derived growth factor,[105] and VEGF[106] action are under way. Other kinase targets are directed at normalizing aberrant cell-cycle control and include modulators of cyclin-dependent kinases, such as flavopiridol[107] and UCN-01.[108] Farnesyl transferase inhibitors may allow *ras*-stimulated signals to be modulated,[109,110] and matrix metalloproteinase inhibitors broadly target the metastatic ability of tumors.[111] Although the fact that the majority of these molecules are advancing to the clinic along the rational pathway described above is gratifying, virtually all have some level of activity in classical xenograft tumor model systems. What remains unclear is the level of activity in such target-directed systems that will ultimately result in a useful clinical effect.

PRECLINICAL PHARMACOLOGY AND TOXICOLOGY STUDIES

After demonstration of activity in an animal model, the next phase of a drug's preclinical development addresses its effects on the host organism. The goal of preclinical toxicology studies for anticancer drugs is to determine in appropriate animal models the MTD and the nature of dose-limiting toxicity, and to demonstrate schedule-dependent toxicity and the reversibility of that toxicity.[112–114] This allows estimation of a "safe" starting dose for initial clinical trials, which for small molecules is one-tenth of the MTD or one-third of the toxic dose low in nonrodents.[113] The toxic dose low is defined as the highest toxic dose that, when doubled, corresponds to a nonlethal dose. In no case

is a dose that just begins to elicit reversible toxicity used to define the starting dose.

Toxicologic evaluations are typically divided into preliminary or "range-finding" studies, and "investigational new drug (IND)–directed" studies. Range-finding studies assess clinical characteristics of drugs administered at a range of dosages to bracket those that are effective and those that are toxic. More detailed IND–directed toxicology evaluations focus on the actual proposed clinical use schedule and seek to define a nontoxic, minimally toxic, and overtly toxic series of dosages. During these evaluations, animals are followed for the appearance and reversibility of clinical signs, and studies of clinical chemistry, hematology, and histopathology of all organs are performed.[113] These studies are currently required by the Food and Drug Administration (FDA) to use two species, at least one nonrodent, both of which are treated with the proposed clinical dose and schedule.[114] In contrast, evaluation of "biologics," including antibodies, immunotoxins, vaccines, and so forth, generally uses only the most relevant animal species, which is exposed to the agent administered using the clinical route and schedule.[115]

Previously, toxicology evaluations used standard protocols. For example, the standard NCI toxicology protocols from 1980 to 1988 included determination of the LD_{10} (dose lethal to 10% of test subjects) on day 1 and days 1 through 5 of the dosing schedule, followed by assessment of safety and dose-limiting toxicities when administered at the LD_{10} on day 1 and days 1 through 5 of the schedule.[116] The current development paradigm targets the most effective route and schedule of administration. For example, twice weekly dosing for the proteasome inhibitor PS341,[117] and continuous infusion for phenylacetate[118] for periods as long as 14 days, have been used in initial phase I schedules.

Preclinical pharmacology studies routinely define a suitable assay for study of bulk and formulated drug stability, and a separate assay for the drug in biologic fluids. Pharmacology studies are conducted to determine pharmacokinetics of the agents in rats and dogs after single intravenous doses and by the route and schedule that mimics that which was efficacious in animal models. Toxicokinetic studies are conducted as part of the toxicology studies. Additional studies that increase confidence that the drug will perform well in clinical trials include demonstration that one can obtain efficacious drug levels *in vivo*, with correlation of drug plasma levels and AUC, or both, with toxicity.

One should note that the toxicology studies described above are required for all drugs, whereas the development of assays to measure drug levels in plasma is always pursued, but in some cases a useful assay is not ready at the time toxicology studies are completed. Not all antineoplastic agents have been amenable to assay at the time of entry into clinical trial (especially highly potent natural products), so pharmacology information is desirable but not required by the FDA. Nonetheless, a focused effort to develop a suitable assay should be routinely considered part of the normal drug development process to allow an informed interpretation of toxicity and early clinical data.

INITIATION OF CLINICAL STUDIES

The regulatory requirements for use of an agent vary with the type of use. To permit entry into early clinical trials (e.g., phase I or II), documentation that the proposed schedule may be safely given is the goal of FDA review. To allow marketing of the agent, FDA must determine that the agent is safe and effective. The latter is customarily defined by behavior in phase III trials, in which the test agent is compared to standard or no therapy. An increasingly popular strategy is to attempt to gain "accelerated approval" for an agent to treat a dire or life-threatening disease. Phase II data could be used to obtain such accelerated approval if the following end points were obtained: unequivocal evidence of tumor diminution or clear documentation of preserved performance status in the absence of a response, including favorable outcome on quality of life indicators. When accelerated approval is given, postmarketing stipulations to assure continued judgment of likely benefits are defined. A series of discussions by the Oncology Drug Advisory Committee of the FDA[119] reaffirmed survival benefit as the most important criterion for recommendation of full approval for cytotoxic agents. Surrogate end points for survival, such as response or time to progression, were seen as more able to support accelerated approval, with monitoring to detect subsequent evidence of survival benefit in postmarketing studies. An important issue in further discussion of these policies is the influence of relative toxicity and quality of life. Especially for nontoxic agents, a basis exists for further debate and consideration of these issues.

The drug is ready for entry into the clinic provided that a reliable and workable formulation of the agent has been defined, and reversible toxicity (as opposed to poorly predictable and irreversible toxicity) is demonstrated to be likely after the first manifestation of a drug's adverse effects. Before beginning the clinical trial, an IND application must be approved by the FDA. The components of an IND application include: cover sheet (Form 1571); Table of Contents; Introductory Statement; General Investigative Plan; Investigator's Brochure; Initial Clinical Protocol; Chemistry, Manufacturing, and Control (this extremely important section provides for the precise description and chemical characteristics of the drug under study, how it was made, and how it is to be labeled); Toxicology Data; Pharmacology Data (if available); Previous Human Experience; and Miscellaneous (including potential for abuse and results of radiotracer experiments).

Responsibility of the sponsor for phase I studies includes submitting the IND application, assuring qualifications of investigators, writing and securing local institutional review board approval of protocols, shipping investigational agents and maintaining detailed shipping records corresponding to lots sent, assessing adverse drug reactions and submitting reports on them in a timely fashion to FDA, preparing an annual report of the IND's activities to the FDA, monitoring quality of the data through periodic audits, assuring that the use and disposition of the investigational agent is properly accounted for at the study sites, assuring that informed consent is obtained for each patient entering the study, tracking amendments made to protocols after inception of clinical studies, and informing investigators of new information pertinent to the trial. These regulations are contained in 21 C.F.R. 312.50.

REFERENCES

1. Cragg GM, Newman DJ. Discovery and development of antineoplastic agents from natural product sources. *Cancer Invest* 1999;17:153–163.
2. Cragg G, Newman DJ, Weiss RB. Coral reefs, forests and thermal vents: the worldwide exploration of nature for novel antitumor agents. *Semin Oncol* 1997;24:156–163.
3. Geysen HM, Meleon RH, Barteling SJ. Use of peptides synthesis to prove viral antigens for epitopes to a resolution of a single amino acid. *Proc Natl Acad Sci U S A* 1984; 81:3998–4002.
4. Houghten RA, Pinella C, Blondelle SE, et al. Generation and use of synthetic peptide combinatorial libraries for basic research and drug discovery. *Nature* 1991;354:84–86.
5. Lam KS, Salmon SE, Hersh EM, et al. A new type of synthetic peptide library for identifying ligand-binding activity. *Nature* 1991;354:82–84.
6. Zuckermann RN, Martin EJ, Spellmeyer DC, et al. Discovery of nanomolar ligands for 7-transmembrane G-protein-coupled receptors from a diverse N-(substituted)glycine peptoid library. *J Med Chem* 1994;37:2678–2685.
7. Bunin BA, Ellman J. A general and expedient method for the solid-phase synthesis of 1,4-benzodiazepine derivatives. *J Am Chem Soc* 1992;114:10997–10998.
8. Dooley CT, Houghten RA. The use of positional scanning synthetic peptide combinatorial libraries for the rapid determination of opioid receptor ligands. *Life Sci* 1993;52(18):1509–1517.
9. Myers P. A rapid and reliable methodology for drug discovery using informative compound libraries. Paper presented at: The 1997 Charleston Conference Advancing New Lead Discovery; March 3–5, 1997; Isle of Palms, SC.
10. Clark RD, Cramer RD. Taming the combinatorial centipede. *Chemtech* 1997;27(5):24–31.
11. Hodes L. Clustering a large number of compounds. 1. Establishing the method on an initial sample. *J Chem Info and Comp Sci* 1988;29:66–71.
12. DeWitt SH, Zaborowski M. Data management for combinatorial chemistry. *Network Science.* Available at http://www.netsci.org.
13. MDL. Combinatorial chemistry: a strategy for the future. *Network Science.* Available at http://www.netsci.org.

14. Polinsky A. Integration of combinatorial chemistry into the drug discovery process. Paper presented at: The 1997 Charleston Conference Advancing New Lead Discovery; March 3–5, 1997; Isle of Palms, SC.

15. Service RF. Coming soon: the pocket DNA sequencer. *Science* 1998;282:399–401.

16. Hamburger AW, Salmon SE. Primary bioassay of human tumor stem cells. *Science* 1977;197:461–463.

17. Shoemaker RH, Wolpert-DeFilippes MK, Kern DH, et al. Application of a human tumor colony-forming assay to new drug screening. *Cancer Res* 1985;45(5):2145–2153.

18. Shoemaker RH. New approaches to antitumor drug screening: the human tumor colony-forming assay. *Cancer Treat Rep* 1986;70(1):9–12.

19. Boyd MR. National Cancer Institute drug discovery and development. In: Frei E II, Freireich E, eds. *Accomplishments in oncology*. Philadelphia: JB Lippincott, 1986:68–76.

20. Boyd MR. Status of the NCI preclinical antitumor drug discovery screen. In: DeVita VT Jr, Hellman S, Rosenberg SA, eds. *Cancer: principles and practice of oncology updates.* 3(10). Philadelphia: JB Lippincott, 1989:1–12.

21. Grever ME, Schepartz SA, Chabner BA. The National Cancer Institute: cancer drug discovery and development program. *Semin Oncol* 1992;19(6):622–638.

22. Boyd MR. The NCI *in vitro* anticancer drug discovery screen. In: Teicher B, ed. *Anticancer drug development guide: preclinical screening, clinical trials, and approval.* Totowa, NJ: Humana Press, 1996:23–42.

23. Alley M, Scudiero DA, Monks A, et al. Feasibility of drug screening with panels of human tumor cell lines using a microculture tetrazolium assay. *Cancer Res* 1988;48(3):589–601.

24. Scudiero DA, Shoemaker RH, Paull KD, et al. Evaluation of a soluble tetrazolium/formazan assay for cell growth and drug sensitivity in culture using human and other tumor cell lines. *Cancer Res* 1988;48(17):4827–4833.

25. Skehan P, Storeng R, Scudiero D, et al. New colorimetric cytotoxicity assay for anticancer-drug screening. *J Natl Cancer Inst* 1990;82(13):1107–1112.

26. Monks A, Scudiero D, Skehan P, et al. Feasibility of a high-flux anticancer drug screen using a diverse panel of cultured human tumor cell lines. *J Natl Cancer Inst* 1991;83(11):757–766.

27. Weinstein JN, Myers TG, O'Conner PM, et al. An information-intensive approach to the molecular pharmacology of cancer. *Science* 1997;275(5298):343–349.

28. Brown JM. NCI's anticancer drug screening program may not be selecting for clinically active compounds. *Oncol Res* 1997;9(5):213–215.

29. Lock RB, Stribinskiene L. Dual modes of death induced by etoposide in human epithelial tumor cells allow Bcl-2 to inhibit apoptosis without affecting clonogenic survival. *Cancer Res* 1996;56(17):4006–4012.

30. Han JW, Dionne CA, Kedersha NL, et al. P53 status affects the rate of the onset but not the overall extent of doxorubicin-induced cell death in rat-1 fibroblasts constitutively expressing c-Myc. *Cancer Res* 1997;57(1):176–182.

31. Waldman T, Zhang Y, Dillehapy L, et al. Cell-cycle arrest versus cell death in cancer therapy. *Nat Med* 1997;3(9):1034–1036.

32. Paull KD, Shoemaker RH, Hodes L, et al. Display and analysis of patterns of differential activity of drugs against human tumor cell lines: development of mean graph and COMPARE algorithm. *J Natl Cancer Inst* 1989;81(14):1088–1092.

33. Paull KD, Hamel E, Malspeis L. Prediction of biochemical mechanisms of action from the *in vitro* antitumor screen of the National Cancer Institute. In: Foye W, ed. *Cancer chemotherapeutic agents.* Washington: ACS Professional Reference Book 9, 1995.

34. Bai R, Paull KD, Herald CL, et al. Halichondrin B and homohalichondrin B, marine natural products binding in the vinca domain of tubulin. Discovery of tubulin-based mechanism of action by analysis of differential cytotoxicity data. *J Biol Chem* 1991;266(24):15882–15889.

35. Paull KD, Lin CM, Malspeis L, et al. Identification of novel antimitotic agents acting at the tubulin level by computer-assisted evaluation of differential cytotoxicity data. *Cancer Res* 1992;52(14):3892–3900.

36. Kohlhagen G, Paull KD, Cushman M, et al. Protein-linked DNA strand breaks induced by NSC 314622, a novel non-camptothecin topoisomerase I poison. *Mol Pharmacol* 1998;54(1):50–58.

37. Leteurtre F, Kohlhagen G, Paull KD, et al. Topoisomerase II inhibition and cytotoxicity of the anthrapyrazoles DuP 937 and DuP 941 (Losoxantrone) in the National Cancer Institute preclinical antitumor drug discovery screen. *J Natl Cancer Inst* 1994;86(16):239–244.

38. Jayaram HN, Gharehbaghi K, Jayaram NH, et al. Cytotoxicity of a new IMP dehydrogenase inhibitor, benzamide riboside, to human myelogenous leukemia K562 cells. *Biochem Biophys Res Commun* 1992;186(3):1600–1606.

39. Cleaveland ES, Monks A, Vaigro-Wolff A, et al. Site of action of two novel pyrimidine biosynthesis inhibitors accurately predicted by the COMPARE program. *Biochem Pharmacol* 1995;49(7):947–954.

40. Bradshaw TD, Wrigley S, Shi DF, et al. 2-(4-amino-phenyl) benzothiazoles: novel agents with selective profiles of in vitro antitumor activity. *Br J Cancer* 1998;77(5):745–752.

41. Duncan KKK, Duncan MD, Alley MC, et al. Cucurbitacin E–induced disruption of the actin and vimentin cytoskeleton in prostate carcinoma cells. *Biochem Pharmacol* 1996;52:1553–1560.

42. Bubb MR, Senderowicz AMJ, Sausville EA, et al. Jasplakinolide, a cytotoxic natural product, induces actin polymerization and competitively inhibits the binding of phalloidin to F-actin. *J Biol Chem* 1994;269:14869–14871.

43. Senderowicz AMJ, Kaur G, Sainz E, et al. Jasplankinolide's inhibition of the growth of prostate carcinoma cells in vitro with disruption of the actin cytoskeleton. *J Natl Cancer Inst* 1995;87:46–51.

44. Rixe O, Ortuzar W, Alvarez M, et al. Oxaliplatin, tetraplatin, cisplatin, and carboplatin: spectrum of activity in drug-resistant cell lines and in the cell lines of the National Cancer Institute's anticancer drug screen panel. *Biochem Pharmacol* 1996;52(12):1855–1865.

45. Alvarez M, Paull K, Monks A, et al. Generation of a drug resistance profile by quantitation of mdr-1/P-glycoprotein in the cell lines of the National Cancer Institute anticancer drug screen. *J Clin Invest* 1995;95(5):2205–2214.

46. Lee JS, Paull K, Alvarez M, et al. Rhodamine efflux patterns predict P-glycoprotein substrates in the National Cancer Institute drug screen. *Mol Pharmacol* 1994;46(4):627–638.

47. Wosikowski K, Schuurhuis D, Johnson K, et al. Identification of epidermal growth factor receptor and c-erbB2 pathway inhibitors by correlation with gene expression patterns. *J Natl Cancer Inst* 1997;89(20):1505–1515.

48. Fitzsimmon SA, Workman P, Grever M, et al. Reductase enzyme expression across the National Cancer Institute tumor cell line panel: correlation with sensitivity to mitomycin C and E09. *J Natl Cancer Inst* 1996;88(5):259–269.

49. Moscow JA, Connolly T, Myers TG, et al. Reduced folate carrier gene (RFC1) expression and anti-folate resistance in transfected and non-selected cell lines. *Int J Cancer* 1997;72(1):184–190.

50. Weinstein JN, Kohn KW, Grever MR, et al. Neural computing in cancer drug development: predicting mechanism of action. *Science* 1992;258(5081):447–451.

51. Van Osdol WW, Myers TG, Paull KD, et al. Use of the Kohonen self-organizing map to study the mechanisms of action to chemotherapeutic agents. *J Natl Cancer Inst* 1994;86(24):1853–1859.

52. O'Connor PM, Jackman J, Bae I, et al. Characterization of the p53 tumor suppressor pathway in cell lines of the National Cancer Institute anticancer drug screen and correlations with the growth-inhibitory potency of 123 anticancer agents. *Cancer Res* 1997;7(19):4285–4300.

53. Shi LM, Myers TG, Fan Y, et al. Mining the National Cancer Institute anticancer drug discovery database: cluster analysis of ellipticine analogs with p53-inverse and central nervous system-selective patterns of activity. *Mol Pharmacol* 1998;53(2):241–251.

54. Myers TG, Anderson NL, Waltham M, et al. A protein expression database for the molecular pharmacology of cancer. *Electrophoresis* 1997;18(3–4):647–653.

55. Koo HM, Monks A, Mikheev A, et al. Enhanced sensitivity to 1-beta-D-arabinofuranosylcytosine and topoisomerase II inhibitors in tumor cell lines harboring activated ras oncogenes. *Cancer Res* 1996;56(22):5211–5216.

56. Koo HM, Gray-Goodrich M, Kohlhagen G, et al. The ras oncogene-mediated sensitization of human cells to topoisomerase II inhibitor-induced apoptosis. *J Natl Cancer Inst* 1999;91(3):236–244.

57. Neubauer A, Dodge RK, George SL, et al. Prognostic importance of mutations in the ras proto-oncogenes in de novo acute myeloid leukemia. *Blood* 1994;83(6):1603–1611.

58. Freije JM, Lawrence JA, Hollingshead MG, et al. Identification of compounds with preferential inhibitory activity against low-Nm23-expressing human breast carcinoma and melanoma cell lines. *Nat Med* 1997;3(4):395–401.

59. Plowman J, Dykes DJ, Hollingshead M, et al. Human tumor xenograft models in NCI drug development. In: Teicher BA, ed. *Anticancer drug development guide: preclinical screening, clinical trials, and approval.* Totowa, NJ: Humana Press, 1997:101–125.

60. Venditti JM, Wesley RA, Plowman J. Current NCI preclinical antitumor screening *in vivo*: results of tumor panel screening, 1976-1982, and future directions. In: Garrattini S, Golden A, Hawking F, eds. *Advances in pharmacology and chemotherapy*, vol. 20. Orlando, FL: Academic, 1984:1–20.

61. Flanagan SP. "Nude," a new hairless gene with pleiotropic effects in the mouse. *Genet Res* 1966;8:295–309.

62. Rygaard J, Povlsen CO. Heterotransplantation of a human malignant tumor to "nude" mice. *Acta Pathol Microbiol Scand* 1969;77:758–760.

63. Giovanella BC, Stehlin JS. Heterotransplantation of human malignant tumors in "nude" thymusless mice. I. Breeding and maintenance of "nude" mice. *J Natl Cancer Inst* 1973;51:615–619.

64. Bogden A, Kelton D, Cobb W, et al. A rapid screening method for testing chemotherapeutic agents against human tumor xenografts. In: Houchens D, Ovejera A, eds. *Proceeding of the Symposium on the Use of Athymic (Nude) Mice in Cancer Research.* New York: Gustav Fischer, 1987:231–250.

65. Dykes DJ, Abbott BJ, Mayo JG, et al. Development of human tumor xenograft models for *in vivo* evaluation of new antitumor drugs. In: Feibig HH, Berger DP, eds. *Contributions to oncology*, vol 42. *Immunodeficient mice in oncology.* Basel: S. Karger, 1992:1–22.

66. Stinson SF, Alley MC, Kopp WC, et al. Morphological and immunocytochemical characteristics of human tumor cell lines for use in a disease-oriented anticancer drug screen. *Anticancer Res* 1992;12:1035–1054.

67. Hollingshead MG, Alley MC, Camalier RF, et al. In vivo cultivation of tumor cells in hollow fibers. *Life Sci* 1995;57:131–141.

68. Waud WR. Murine L1210 and P388 leukemias. In: Teicher BA, ed. *Anticancer drug development guide: preclinical screening, clinical trials, and approval.* Totowa, NJ: Humana Press, 1997:59–74.

69. Corbett T, Valeriote F, LoRusso P, et al. *In vivo* methods for screening and preclinical testing: use of rodent solid tumors for drug discovery. In: Teicher BA, ed. *Anticancer drug development guide: preclinical screening, clinical trials, and approval.* Totowa, NJ: Humana Press, 1997:75–99.

70. Leonessa F, Green D, Licht T, et al. MDA435/LCC6 and MDA435/LCC6^MDR1: ascites models of human breast cancer. *Br J Cancer* 1996;73:154–161.

71. McLemore TL, Abbott BJ, Mayo JG, et al. Development and application of new orthotopic *in vivo* models for use in the US National Cancer Institute's drug screening program. In: Wu BQ, Zheng J, eds. *Immune-deficient animals in experimental medicine. Sixth International Workshop of Immune-Deficient Animals, Beijing, 1988.* Basel: S. Karger, 1989:334–343.

72. Clarke R. Issues in experimental design and endpoint analysis in the study of experimental cytotoxic agents in vivo in breast cancer and other models. *Breast Cancer Res Treat* 1997;46:255–278.

73. Murray N. Importance of dose and dose intensity in the treatment of small-cell lung cancer. *Cancer Chemother Pharmacol* 1997;40[Suppl]:S58–S63.

74. Houghton PJ, Steward CF, Thompson J, et al. Preclinical and clinical results with irinotecan extending principles learned in model systems to clinical trials design. *Oncol* 1998;12([Suppl 6]:84–93.

75. Fine DL, Fodstad O, Shoemaker R, et al. Metastasis models tumors in athymic mice: useful models for drug development. *Cancer Detect Prev* 1987;1[Suppl]:291–299.

76. Hoffman RM. Patient-like models of human cancer in mice. *Curr Perspect Mol Cell Oncol* 1992;1:311–326.

77. Fidler IJ, Wilmanns C, Staroselsky A, et al. Modulation of tumor cell response to chemotherapy by the organ environment. *Cancer Metastasis Rev* 1994;13:209–222.

78. Fidler IJ. Rationale and methods for the use of nude mice to study the biology and therapy of human cancer metastasis. *Cancer Metastasis Rev* 1986;5:29–49.

79. Paget S. The distribution of secondary growths in cancer of the breast. *Lancet* 1989;1:571–573.

80. Giavazzi R, Jessup JM, Campbell DE, et al. Experimental nude mouse model of human colorectal cancer liver metastases. *J Natl Cancer Inst* 1986;77:1303–1308.

81. Mohammad RM, Al-Katib A, Pettit GR, et al. An orthotopic model of human pancreatic cancer in severe combined immunodeficient mice: potential application for preclinical studies. *Clin Cancer Res* 1998;4:887–894.

82. Berry KK, Siegal GP, Boyd JA, et al. Development of a metastatic model for human endometrial carcinoma using orthotopic implantation in nude mice. *Int J Oncol* 1994;4: 1163–1171.

83. Wilmanns C, Fan D, O'Brian CA, et al. Modulation of doxorubicin sensitivity and level of P-glycoprotein expression in human colon carcinoma cells by ectopic and orthotopic environments in nude mice. *Int J Oncol* 1993;3:413–422.

84. Hoffman M. Fertile seed and rich soil. In: Teicher BA, ed. *Anticancer drug development guide: preclinical screening, clinical trials, and approval.* Totowa, NJ: Humana Press, 1997:127–144.

85. Giavazzi R. Metastatic models. In: Boven E, Winograd B, eds. *The nude mouse in oncology research.* Boca Raton, FL: CRC Press, 1991:117–132.

86. Dickson RB, Johnson MD, Maemura M, et al. Anti-invasion drugs. *Breast Cancer Res Treat* 1996;38:121–132.

87. Fidler IL. Selection of successive tumor lines for metastasis. *Nat New Biol* 1973;242:148–149.

88. Zetter BR. Angiogenesis and tumor metastasis. *Ann Rev Med* 1998;49:407–424.

89. Talmadge JE, Fidler IJ. Cancer metastasis is selective or random dependent on the parent tumor population. *Nature* 1982;297:593–594.

90. Chirivi RGS, Garofalo A, Crimmis MJ, et al. Inhibition of the metastatic spread and growth of B16-BL6 murine melanoma by a synthetic matrix metalloproteinase inhibitor. *Int J Cancer* 1994;58:460–464.

91. Guilbaud N, Kraus-Berthier L, Saint-Dizier D, et al. Antitumor activity of S 16020-0 in two orthotopic models of lung cancer. *Anticancer Drugs* 1997;8:276–282.

92. O'Reilly MS. The preclinical evaluation of angiogenesis inhibitors. *Invest New Drugs* 1997;15:5–13.

93. Schlatter P, Konig MF, Karlsson LM, et al. Quantitative study of intussusceptive capillary growth in the chorioallantoic membrane (CAM) of the chicken embryo. *Microvasc Res* 1997;54:65–73.

94. Passaniti A, Taylor RM, Pili R, et al. A simple, quantitative method for assessing angiogenesis and antiangiogenic agents using reconstituted basement membrane, heparin, and fibroblast growth factor. *Lab Invest* 1992;67:519–528.

95. Muthukkaruppan V, Auerbach R. Angiogenesis in the mouse cornea. *Science* 1979;28:1416–1418.

96. Kenyon BM, Voest EE, Chen CC, et al. A model of angiogenesis in the mouse cornea. *Invest Ophthalmol Vis Sci* 1996; 37:1625–1632.

97. Druker BJ, Tamura S, Buchdunger E, et al. Effects of a selective inhibitor of the Abl tyrosine kinase on the growth of Bcr-Abl positive cells. *Nat Med* 1996;2(5):561–566.

98. Mangues R, Corral T, Kohl NE, et al. Antitumor effect of a farnesyl protein transferase inhibitor in mammary and lymphoid tumors overexpressing –ras in transgenic mice. *Cancer Res* 1998;58(6):1253–1259.

99. Barrington RE, Subler MA, Rands E, et al. A farnesyltransferase inhibitor induces tumor regression in transgenic mice harboring multiple oncogenic mutations by mediating alterations in both cell cycle control and apoptosis. *Mol Cell Biol* 1998;18(1):85–92.

100. Auerbach R, Auerbach W. Regional differences in the growth of normal and neoplastic cells. *Science* 1982;215: 127–134.

101. Corbett TH, Valeriote FA, Demchik L, et al. Discovery of cryptophycin-1 and BCN-183577: examples of strategies and problems in the detection of antitumor activity in mice. *Invest New Drugs* 1997;5:207–218.

102. Venditti J. Treatment schedule dependency of experimentally active antileukemic (L1210) drugs. *Cancer Chemother Rep* 1972;2:35–59.

103. Druker BJ, Sawyers CL, Talpaz M, et al. Phase I trial of a specific Abl tyrosine kinase inhibitor CGP 57148 in interferon refractory chronic myelogenous leukemia. *Proc Am Soc Clin Oncol* 1999;18(24):7a.

104. Fry DW, Kraker AJ, Connors RC, et al. Strategies for the discovery of novel tyrosine kinase inhibitors with anticancer activity. *Anticancer Drug Des* 1994;9(4):331–351.

105. Maguire MP, Sheets KR, McVety K, et al. A new series of PDGF receptor tyrosine kinase inhibitors: 3-substituted quinoline derivatives. *J Med Chem* 1994;37(14):2129–2137.

106. Fong TA, Shawver LK, Sun L, et al. SU5416 is a potent and selective inhibitor of the vascular endothelial growth factor receptor (Flk-1/KDR) that inhibits tyrosine kinase catalysis, tumor vascularization, and growth of multiple tumor types. *Cancer Res* 1999;59(1):99–106.

107. Patel V, Senderowicz AM, Pinto D Jr, et al. Flavopiridol, a novel cyclin-dependent kinase inhibitor, suppresses the growth of head and neck squamous cell carcinomas by inducing apoptosis. *J Clin Invest* 1998;102(9):1674–1681.

108. Wang Q, Fan S, Eastman A, et al. UCN-01: a potent abrogator of G2 checkpoint function in cancer cells with disrupted p53. *J Natl Cancer Inst* 1996;88(14):956–965.

109. Oliff A. Farnesyltransferase inhibitors: targeting the molecular basis of cancer. *Biochem Biophys Acta* 1999;1423(3): C19–30.

110. Sebti S, Hamilton AD. Inhibitors of prenyl transferases. *Curr Opin Oncol* 1997;9(6):557–561.

111. Kleiner DE, Stetler-Stevenson WG. Matrix metalloproteinases and metastasis. *Cancer Chemother Pharmacol* 1999;43[Suppl]:S42–51.

112. Grieshaber CK. Agent-directed preclinical toxicology for new antineoplastic drugs. In: Valeriote FA, Corbett H, eds. *Cytotoxic anticancer drugs: models and concepts for drug dis-*

covery and development. Boston: Kluwer Academic Publishers, 1992:247–260.

113. Tomaszewski JE, Smith AC. Safety testing of antitumor agents. In: Williams PD, Hottendorf GH, eds. *Comprehensive toxicology, toxicity testing and evaluation.* Oxford: Elsevier Science, 1997:299–309.

114. DeGeorge JJ, Ahn C, Andrews PA, et al. Regulatory considerations for preclinical development of anticancer drugs. *Cancer Chemother Pharmacol* 1998;41:173–185.

115. Food and Drug Administration. International Conference on Harmonization. Preclinical safety evaluation of biotechnology-derived pharmaceuticals. *Federal Register* 1997;62:61515.

116. Lowe MC, Davis RD. The current toxicology protocol of the National Cancer Institute. In: Hellman D, Carter S, eds. *Fundamentals of cancer chemotherapy.* New York: McGraw-Hill, 1987:228–235.

117. Adams J, Palombella VJ, Sausville EA, et al. Proteasome inhibitors: a novel class of potent and effective antitumor agents. *Cancer Res* 1999;59(11):2615–2622.

118. Thibault A, Cooper MR, Figg WD, et al. A phase I and pharmacokinetic study of intravenous phenylacetate in patients with cancer. *Cancer Res* 1994;54(7):1690–1694.

119. Goldberg KB, Goldberg P. Advisors reaffirm survival as standard for full FDA approval of cancer drugs. *Cancer Lett* 1999;25:6–8.

3

PHARMACOKINETICS AND CLINICAL MONITORING

JERRY M. COLLINS

Pharmacokinetic studies of anticancer drugs are used routinely in many clinical trials. One group[1] has even suggested that "it is now inconceivable to perform clinical research in cancer chemotherapy without obtaining adequate pharmacokinetic data." Before describing the technical details of this discipline, we need to step back and evaluate the potential benefits of pharmacokinetic studies both at the population level (i.e., the "average" patient) and at the level of the individual patient.

First, a clear distinction needs to be made between the *effects* of a drug (dynamics) and its concentration-time history (kinetics). The role of *pharmacodynamics* is to define the therapeutic goals, which are attained using kinetics to formulate an administration strategy to achieve these goals. For infectious diseases, the goal is prolonged maintenance of plasma concentration above a minimal inhibitory concentration or minimal bactericidal concentration but below a level toxic to the host. In anticancer chemotherapy, although the general goal of killing tumor cells is clearly defined, in most cases we are severely limited by an inability to select concentration-time parameters that separate antitumor effects from normal tissue toxicity. Much remains to be learned about the differences between normal and tumor tissues that can be exploited therapeutically. Thus, although pharmacokinetics is a tool that can be used to evaluate the feasibility of a strategy based on pharmacodynamics, it is not a replacement for knowledge of exploitable differences between host and tumor.

BENEFITS FOR THE AVERAGE PATIENT: ROUTE, SCHEDULING, AND DOSAGE

For the average patient, pharmacokinetics can help answer the fundamental questions in delivery of drugs: (a) What route of administration? (b) How often (schedule)? and (c) How much (dose)? These questions are answered using empiric observation (what works best in an experimental or clinical setting) and biochemical, cell kinetic, and pharmacokinetic considerations.

The choice of drug administration *route* is based primarily on pharmacokinetic assessment of bioavailability (the ability of drug to reach its target site in an active form) and the ability to formulate an acceptable dose preparation for oral, intravenous (IV), intramuscular, intrathecal, or subcutaneous use. The IV route, although it necessitates a venipuncture, is the preferred route for water-soluble compounds because complete absorption is guaranteed if the IV infusion is performed correctly. Bioavailability is judged by comparison of plasma, or urine concentrations, or both, produced by the oral (or intramuscular or subcutaneous) dose versus an IV dose.

Many factors influence oral bioavailability. Absorption through the lipid-bilayer cell membrane of the intestinal mucosa is determined by molecular size, lipid solubility, and the presence of specific transport systems such as the folate transport mechanism for antifolates. Absorption is also affected by drug stability in gastric acid and breakdown by intestinal enzymes such as cytidine deaminase (which hydrolyses cytosine arabinoside). The physiologic state of the intestinal tract may be affected adversely by disease or by previous drug therapy. Vomiting induced by chemotherapeutic drugs may lead to loss of a major portion of an oral dose. Thus, highly emetic agents such as cisplatin cannot be used in combination with orally administered drugs. In addition to intestinal absorption, hepatic metabolism or uptake and biliary excretion may prevent orally administered drugs from reaching the systemic circulation in an active form. Mercaptopurine is an example of a drug with very low and erratic bioavailability,[2] whereas azidothymidine is a drug with consistently high bioavailability.[3]

On occasion, a tumor may grow in a body compartment, such as the central nervous system or peritoneal cavity, that is not penetrated readily by systemically administered drugs. The rate of penetration into these compartments is influenced by the same factors that determine intestinal absorption (size, lipid solubility, and specific transport processes). Direct intrathecal, intraperitoneal, intravesical, or topical administration may be advantageous in these cases, but the relative advantage as compared to that of systemic therapy will be determined by pharmacokinetic factors, such as relative rates of clearance from the central and peripheral compartments. These considerations are dealt with in detail later in this chapter (see Regional Administration).

In addition to route, the *schedule* of drug administration is highly dependent on pharmacokinetic considerations and requires a choice of the duration of administration (bolus versus prolonged infusion), frequency of repetition of the dose, and the sequencing of multiple drugs or drugs and other modalities such as radiation. Bolus dosing provides maximal peak drug levels in plasma but a rapid decline thereafter as drug is eliminated from the plasma compartment by metabolism or excretion. This form of dosing is convenient for drugs that are non–cell-cycle-phase-dependent and therefore do not have to be present during a specific phase of the cell cycle. Examples are the nitrosoureas, alkylating agents, procarbazine, and other drugs that chemically interact with DNA.

For agents that act preferentially in specific phases of the cell cycle, such as S-phase–specific drugs (e.g., cytosine arabinoside or methotrexate), prolonged IV infusions (6 to 120 hours) have advantages, particularly if the drug has a short plasma half-life. Prolonged infusions have the additional advantage of providing a specific and constant plasma concentration of the drug, a desirable feature if one has information regarding the sensitivity of the tumor, as provided by various *in vitro* tests. Intermediate-length infusions (1 to 4 hours) may provide a means to overcome the acute toxicities that are produced by the delivery of high peak drug levels to target organs. Particularly for neurotoxic or cardiotoxic compounds, rapid IV infusions may present unacceptable dangers, but intermediate-length infusions may reduce peak drug levels adequately while retaining some of the convenience of bolus dosing.

The final consideration in drug administration is the choice of *dose*. Dose is usually determined by an empiric phase I trial using a set schedule, with stepwise evaluation of toxicity at progressively higher doses. This procedure is called *modified Fibonacci escalation*.[4] In certain circumstances, dose also may be determined by setting pharmacologic objectives, such as a target drug concentration in a specific body compartment such as plasma, cerebrospinal fluid (CSF), or ascites. This type of regimen planning requires pharmacokinetic design and verification by drug level monitoring and has been used in only a few clinical oncologic settings, such as intrathecal chemotherapy with methotrexate (MTX) and intraperitoneal therapy with MTX and 5-fluorouracil (5-FU). Additional information on the relationship of drug concentration to tumor cell kill, as provided by *in vitro* assays, may provide a basis for more precise pharmacokinetic adjustment of dosage.

Pharmacologically guided dose escalation was developed as an alternative to the predetermined escalation proce-

dure.[5] After the first set of patients has been treated in a phase I setting, the rate of dose escalation is determined by the plasma levels of drug relative to target plasma levels measured in mice at the maximum tolerated dose or mouse lethal dose$_{10}$ (dose that kills 10% of mice). With this approach, investigators can estimate the difference between the target concentration and plasma levels produced by the current dose level. Such information is desirable in itself for planning a short or long trial. But the greatest value derives from the opportunity to intervene at an early stage in the phase I trial. If it is determined that the current plasma levels are close to the target, a cautious escalation may be indicated. If the current plasma levels are far from the target values, then a rapid escalation could generate considerable savings in time and clinical resources, and fewer patients will be exposed to doses that are not biologically active. Although this procedure is still not widely used, it has found support in Europe and Japan, as well as the United States.[6–8]

CLINICAL MONITORING

For the individual, clinical monitoring and pharmacokinetics offer the possibility of tailoring drug delivery to the particular patient's needs. The standard doses derived from group studies do not allow for interindividual variability. However, doses may be adjusted on the basis of direct measurements of drug concentration in the individual patient, indicators of renal or hepatic dysfunction, or interactions of the anticancer drug with concomitant medications (see Chapter 1).

Drug concentration measurements are the heart of clinical monitoring and pharmacokinetic studies. Many anticancer drugs are difficult to measure because of inherent instability, either spontaneously degrading or being degraded by enzymes in blood or tissues. Although the study of many anticancer drugs has been facilitated by the use of radiolabeled material, separation methods are required because the majority are extensively metabolized. Advances in separation methodology, such as high-performance liquid chromatography, coupled with mass spectrometry and with improvements in the sensitivity of detectors and the development of highly sensitive and specific competitive protein binding assays, have provided an improved basis for drug concentration measurement.

For some purposes, a model is necessary to interpret data, but often questions may be answered without a formal model construction. Simple concentration-time measurements of drug levels in plasma or other body fluids may be used to determine the basis of a population's therapeutic or toxic response. This is a process of determining target levels. Once target levels are established, measurements in problematic patients may be used to directly adjust an individual patient's dose when levels outside the target range are

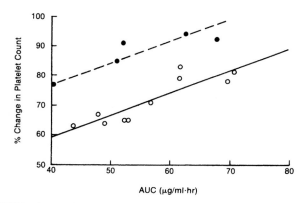

FIGURE 3-1. Relationship between thrombocytopenia and plasma levels of carboplatin. (AUC, area under the concentration × time curve.) (From Egorin MJ, Van Echo DA, Olman EA, et al. Prospective validation of a pharmacologically based dosing scheme for the *cis*-diamminedichloroplatinum(II) analog diamminecyclobutanedicarboxylatoplatinum. *Cancer Res* 46:6502, 1985, with permission.)

encountered. This principle was demonstrated by Bleyer[9] in studies of the toxicity of intrathecal MTX. Stoller et al.[10] used this approach to identify patients who required intensive leucovorin rescue after high-dose MTX. It has been demonstrated that monitoring plasma levels of menogaril,[11] medroxyprogesterone,[12] and fluorouracil[13] can be used to titrate toxicity in patients. In addition to these examples of toxicity avoidance, a similar monitoring strategy could be useful for improving response to therapy with MTX[14] or teniposide.[15]

If one knows the pharmacokinetics of a given agent, specifically the route of elimination, adjustments in dose can be made for altered renal or hepatic function to accommodate abnormalities in individual patients. In general, these adjustments would be expected to be less precise than adjustments based on drug-level measurements. Occasionally, there is a close relationship between a renal function indicator (e.g., serum creatinine) and plasma pharmacokinetics. Egorin et al.[16] have elegantly applied such correlations for dose adjustments of carboplatin (Fig. 3-1) and hexamethylene bisacetamide.[17] Other groups have reported a close relationship between etoposide pharmacokinetics and renal function.[18,19] Powis[20] reviewed the effects of both renal and hepatic dysfunction for anticancer drugs.

Another important but relatively unexplored area of clinical monitoring and pharmacokinetics is drug-drug interaction. Essentially all treatment protocols include combinations of drugs, encompassing two or more anticancer drugs, as well as various other drugs related to general symptomatic and supportive therapy of the patient. Several types of interaction among these agents may occur, but perhaps the most important are alterations of clearance. Changes in clearance might result in unexpected toxicity, due to increased levels, or lessened effectiveness due to decreased levels. Although many of these interactions can be determined by straightforward observational stud-

ies, the work by Zimm et al.[21] on 6-mercaptopurine and allopurinol demonstrates the utility of modeling in assessing the components of drug interactions. Measurements of plasma levels and pharmacokinetic modeling were required to explain the interference of allopurinol with the catabolism of mercaptopurine via the oral route but not via the IV route.

The serious adverse reactions caused by administration of ketoconazole to patients taking terfenadine,[22] the widely used and relatively safe antihistamine, provide a cautionary note for potential interactions with anticancer drugs because of their much narrower therapeutic index. Another common drug, cimetidine, is reported to inhibit the metabolism of cyclophosphamide[23] and hexamethylmelamine.[24] On the other hand, anticancer drugs are reported to interfere with the absorption of noncancer drugs, such as digoxin.[25] Balis[26] reviewed the literature of drug interactions related to anticancer drugs. When evaluating drug-drug interactions, recent findings with paclitaxel illustrate the difficulties generated by interspecies differences in metabolic pathways.[27]

The fundamental obstacle to greater success in application of pharmacokinetics and clinical monitoring to anticancer therapy is our limited knowledge of pharmacodynamics. We need to develop pharmacologic goals based on measurements of drugs in body fluids or other end points.

The intensive effort to establish *in vitro* biochemical and clonogenic screening tests offers the potential for more efficacious use of pharmacokinetics. In the test situation, drug concentration and exposure duration required for cell kill can be defined, and these conditions can be used to select specific drugs and schedules of administration. In acute myelogenous leukemia, efforts have focused on the ability of cells *in vitro* to form the active triphosphate nucleotide 1-β-D-arabinofuranosylcytosine triphosphate (ara-CTP) from cytosine arabinoside (ara-C), the formation of which appears to correlate with *in vivo* responses. This approach has been extended to determination of ara-CTP levels in leukemic cells harvested from patients on therapy.[28,29] Finally, the drug delivery rate and schedule are being adjusted in a prospective fashion to determine the utility of this monitoring.[30]

An alternative to direct measurement of drug metabolism is the assessment of tumor tissue parameters, such as rates of DNA synthesis or other intracellular biochemical processes after treatment.[31] Serial studies might determine the optimal timing for the next treatment, although the invasive nature of such sampling must be considered.

PHARMACOKINETIC MODELING

Anticancer drugs have become prime modeling targets, because the therapeutic index of these drugs is so low that the modeling effort is thought to be worthwhile. A pharmacokinetic model is a mathematic model (i.e., an equation or set of equations) that can be used to describe the concentration versus time history of a drug. By convention, pharmacokinetic models are often presented in terms of box diagrams. Each box is called a *compartment* and corresponds to a region in the body with specific kinetic properties. The compartments may or may not represent real, identifiable anatomic regions.

Even for those models that are empirically constructed from concentration-time data, the model may provide insight that is not obvious from an examination of the raw data. For data that exhibit great variation, a model may suggest which variables (e.g., binding or elimination) are probable sources of this variation and may lead to adjustments of drug delivery based on clinical laboratory tests, such as glomerular filtration rate or plasma protein analysis. For cases in which routine drug level measurement is not feasible, a high-risk population might be identified for selective monitoring. This approach was used for test-dose studies with MTX.[32] Models also can improve the dosage-adjustment process when there is nonlinear pharmacokinetic behavior or for situations in which a change must be made in the drug delivery pattern.

Generally, a model or application of a model is no better than the data on which it is built. However, one special use of a model is in those cases for which no data are available, such as when drug levels are too low to measure or no reliable assay method exists. This type of predictive modeling requires tremendous confidence in the modeling process, as well as a keen understanding of the limitations of modeling. Above all, the modeling process forces us to make judgments about a drug's kinetic behavior, and this process clarifies the importance of what is unknown and the uncertainty of what is "known."

Mass-Balance Concepts

Once the structure for the model has been established, the next step is formulation of mass balances (i.e., equations to describe the transfer processes between the compartments and the reaction or excretory processes within the compartments). A mass balance for a compartment is simply an overall accounting of the rate processes that influence the amount of drug in the compartment:

$$\text{Net change} = \text{input(s)} - \text{output(s)} \pm \text{reaction(s)} \quad \text{[3-1]}$$

$$[\text{Rate of change of drug in compartment}] \quad \text{[3-2]}$$
$$= [\text{rate of absorption or injection}]$$
$$+ [\text{rate of inflow with blood}] + [\text{rate of diffusion in}]$$
$$- [\text{rate of outflow with blood}] - [\text{rate of diffusion out}]$$
$$- [\text{rate of conversion by reaction}]$$
$$- [\text{rate of excretion}]$$

The mass balances constitute a set of differential equations that form the basis of the model. Details of the various

rate processes may be well understood (e.g., in terms of active or passive transport), empirically observed, or inferred to account for conservation of mass. A complete mass balance considers all species: free (ionized), free (un-ionized), and bound forms. Because such equations can be quite complex structurally, and since only total drug concentration is normally measured, the balances are usually expressed in terms of total drug. If the free concentration is desired, it may be calculated from the binding relationships.

After the differential mass balances have been formulated and initial conditions specified, these equations are integrated to yield mass as a function of time. For those cases without an analytic solution, numeric integration procedures are used.

The major advantage of the mass-balance approach is flexibility, because once the derivation is understood, the equation can be modified readily. For example, the volume of distribution may not be constant, the delivery schedule may be novel, or other changes in assumptions may present the kineticist with a previously undescribed solution.

An especially useful conceptual approach invokes the steady state, a situation in which there is constant input of drug balanced by constant removal by the elimination processes. Practically, this is achieved by a constant IV infusion. The set of differential equations simplifies to a set of algebraic equations, which are far easier to use.

For linear pharmacokinetic models, all transfer and elimination processes are first order, meaning proportional to drug concentration. The most commonly used inputs are short bolus injection, constant infusion, and exponentially declining absorption. The steady-state concentration during constant infusion represents the time-averaged concentration for intermittent administration.

One-Compartment Model

The one-compartment model, in which the whole body is assumed to be kinetically homogeneous, is the most commonly used clinical model. There are some situations in which the one-compartment model is an adequate system. For example, large molecules, such as the enzyme carboxypeptidase, do not enter cells.[33] Also, some drugs have slow elimination phases compared with the time scale for distribution to body tissues. Suramin is an example of this class of compounds.[34] Although any drug departs from single-compartment behavior if samples are taken early or late enough, one phase may dominate to the extent that the one-compartment model is a useful approximation. For suramin, the extraordinarily slow elimination phase (half-life of 50 days) dominates even the slowest distribution processes and therefore renders the drug suitable for one-compartment modeling. Additionally, the concepts learned in the analysis of one-compartment kinetics can be transferred to more complex models.

The mass balance for the linear one-compartment model is simplified by the absence of intercompartmental transfer terms, so that the rate of change in drug mass equals the drug infusion rate minus the drug elimination rate:

$$V_d\left(\frac{dC_p}{dt}\right) = G - k_{el}V_d C_p \qquad [3\text{-}3]$$

Concentration measured in plasma, C_p, has units of mass per volume. The apparent volume of distribution, V_d, is simply the mass in the compartment divided by concentration in the compartment. As presented in Equation 3-3, V_d is assumed to be constant for the time scale of interest. All excretory and reaction terms are considered to be parallel elimination pathways, with the overall elimination rate constant k_{el} (time^{-1}) representing the sum of these individual processes:

$$k_{el} = k_{renal} + k_{mile} + k_{enzymatic} + \dots \qquad [3\text{-}4]$$

In Equation 3-3, the product of the elimination rate constant and the volume of distribution is identical to total-body clearance, CL_{TB}. Input is defined by the function G (units: mass per time), which may represent intermittent or continuous drug delivery. Figure 3-2 is a representation of the kinds of concentration-time curves that are observed for different input forms of a drug that behaves according to a one-compartment model.

When drug input is by bolus injection, the dose is assumed to be instantly mixed throughout the compartment volume, providing the initial condition for the differential equation: $C_0 = $ dose$/V_d$, and $G = 0$. Integration of the differential model Equation 3-3 yields

$$C_p(t) = C_0 \exp(-k_{el}t) \qquad [3\text{-}5]$$

When plotted on semilogarithmic paper (see Fig. 3-2A), this equation is a straight line with a slope of $-k_{el}$.

One of the more popular features of the one-compartment model is the *half-life* or *half-time*, $t_{1/2}$, which is the time required for the concentration (at any point on the concentration-time curve) to achieve half its value (see Fig. 3-2A). This formula may be applied repetitively so that in two half-times 25% of drug is present, and so forth. This half-time is inversely related to the elimination rate constant:

$$t_{1/2} = \frac{(\ln 2)}{k_{el}} = \frac{0.693}{k_{el}} \qquad [3\text{-}6]$$

Constant infusion may be preferred to bolus injection. Although it requires more support services, this route provides constant levels of drug, especially in cases in which the drug half-time is short. The same mass balance shown in Equation 3-3 applies, except that $G = G_0$ (constant). When therapy is initiated, $C_p = 0$, and the integration yields

$$C_p(t) = C_{ss}[1 - \exp(-k_{el}t)] \qquad [3\text{-}7]$$

The steady-state concentration C_{ss} is $G/(k_{el}V_d)$ or G/CL_{TB}.

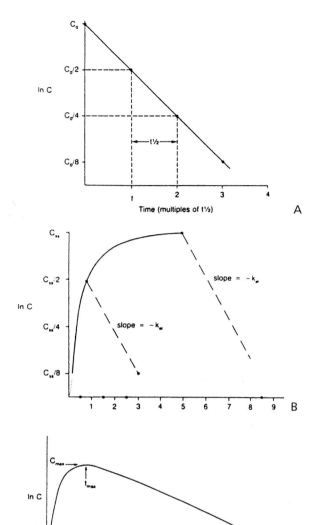

FIGURE 3-2. Concentration × time profiles observed after various inputs to one-compartment model: bolus **(A)**; constant infusion **(B)**; first-order input **(C)**. (C, concentration; k_{el}, elimination rate constant.)

As shown in Figure 3-2B, there is a rapid increase in drug concentration that levels off toward a plateau concentration, C_{ss}, and is then maintained for the duration of the infusion. Regardless of when the infusion is terminated, first-order decay of drug concentration is observed with the same rate constant k_{el} exhibited after bolus administration. The time to achieve plateau level depends on k_{el} only and is independent of the infusion rate. The time required to reach one-half the plateau level, $t_{1/2}$, is identical to the time required for a concentration decrease of 50% after bolus injection. Also, 75% of the plateau level is reached in two half-times, and so forth. For practical purposes, the plateau level is said to be reached in three to five half-times.

Many combinations of drug injection schedules might be used. For all linear kinetic models, each injection can be analyzed independently and the analyses combined to yield the resulting concentration-time profile. For example, if it is desirable to achieve the steady-state concentration rapidly, a *loading dose* may be given as a bolus at the same time the infusion is started. The bolus dose is usually selected to achieve an initial concentration $C_0 = C_{ss}$ by administering a dose calculated as follows: dose = $V_d C_{ss}$. In this way, the time lag to plateau is eliminated.

As an alternative to continuous drug infusion, periodic bolus injections may be given to maintain reasonably constant plasma levels. As with the infusion, there is an approach to steady-state values (peaks and valleys), or the steady state can be reached immediately with the proper choice of loading dose. The most common such schedule targets the peak concentration to be twice the valley concentration. This design requires dosing once each half-time. An initial dose of twice the successive (maintenance) doses abolishes the time lag. As the dosing frequency increases, the ratio of peak-to-valley concentrations approaches 1, and the concentration-time curve looks more like a constant infusion.

Oral, subcutaneous, intramuscular, intrathecal, and intraperitoneal routes of delivery are not used as commonly for anticancer drugs as are the IV modes, but they deserve some mention. All these routes are thought to give an exponentially decreasing rate of drug delivery after initial dosing. This process is referred to as *first-order absorption*, and the mass balance is

$$V_d = \frac{dC_p}{dt} = k_a F X_0 \exp(-k_a t) - k_{el} V_d C_p \quad [3\text{-}8]$$

X_0 is the dose administered, k_a is the first-order absorption rate constant (time^{-1}), and F is the fractional bioavailability. For subcutaneous or intramuscular administration, F is usually 1. For oral and intraperitoneal routes, absorption may be erratic or subject to first-pass elimination by the liver before reaching the systemic circulation, or both. This differential model may be integrated subject to an initial condition of zero concentration:

$$C_p(t) = \frac{k_a F X_0 / V_d}{(k_a - k_{el})} = [\exp(-k_{el}t) - \exp(-k_a t)] \quad [3\text{-}9]$$

As shown in Figure 3-2C, the concentration rises to a peak value and then declines. It is useful to know what this peak concentration is and when it occurs. The time of maximal concentration, t_{max}, is found when $dC_p/dt = 0$, which is

$$t_{max} = \frac{\ln(k_a / k_{el})}{k_a - k_{el}} \quad [3\text{-}10]$$

The maximal concentration C_{max} is found by substituting t_{max} for t in Equation 3-9:

$$C_{max} = C_p(t_{max}) = \frac{F X_0}{V_d} = \exp(-k_{el} t_{max}) \quad [3\text{-}11]$$

Nonlinear One-Compartment Model

Linear models are quite useful for studying concentrations in certain ranges and also for concept formation. However, anticancer drugs are given to maximally tolerated doses, and some exhibit deviations from linear behavior, especially during high-dose chemotherapy. After bolus administration, deviations due to nonlinearities are expressed as convex curves on semilogarithmic plots (i.e., slower rates of drug elimination at high concentrations compared to low concentrations). In contrast, linear multicompartment effects are expressed as concave curvature.

There are three types of nonlinearities that may be encountered, all of which are saturation effects that may be approximated by linear models below saturation levels: (a) excretion (e.g., limited capacity for renal tubular secretion), (b) metabolism (e.g., limited capacity for biochemical conversion), and (c) protein binding in plasma or tissue (e.g., a fixed number of binding sites). The mass balance for nonlinear elimination is a straightforward modification of Equation 3-3:

$$V_d = \frac{dC_p}{dt} = G - v_{max}\left(\frac{C_p}{K_M + C_p}\right) \quad [3\text{-}12]$$

The maximal capacity of the body to eliminate drug (mass per time) is v_{max}, and K_M is the concentration (mass per volume) at which the mass rate of elimination is half-maximal.

For continuous infusions, Equation 3-12 can be solved for steady-state concentration:

$$C_{ss} = \frac{G K_M}{v_{max} - G} \quad [3\text{-}13]$$

As the rate of infusion approaches the body's maximal elimination capacity, small changes in the infusion rate produce disproportionately large increases in C_{ss}. A clear example of this phenomenon was reported recently for high-dose ara-C infusions.[35]

For bolus administration ($G = 0$), the differential model (see Equation 3-12) plus the initial condition ($C_0 = $ dose/V_d) cannot be integrated and solved explicitly for C_p as a function of time. Implicit analytic solutions or numerically integrated solutions are available and can be used to generate simulations such as Figure 3-3, which illustrates the convex curvature characteristic of a saturable enzymatic elimination process. At concentrations below K_M, the reaction rate in typical enzymatic conversions is roughly proportional to substrate (drug) concentrations. Above K_M, the rate of reaction does not increase in proportion to drug concentration and reaches a maximal value. Increasingly longer times are required to decrease concentration by a factor of two. Half-time now depends on concentration and is a less useful concept than for linear models. If the therapeutic or toxic effect of a drug depends on either $C \times T$ or time above some inhib-

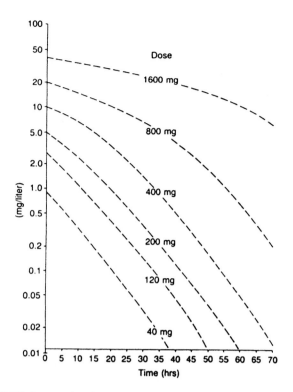

FIGURE 3-3. Dose dependency in one-compartment model with Michaelis-Menten elimination after bolus input. ($K_M = 5$ mg/L; $v_{max} = 25$ mg/h; $V_d = 40$ L.)

itory concentration, disproportionate increases in effect are produced by dose increases.

Two-Compartment Linear Model

Although the one-compartment model has provided an important introduction to kinetic analysis, most drugs require two compartments for satisfactory analysis.[36] The two-compartment model has become the most widely published research model. Figure 3-4 illustrates the concentration-time profile for doxorubicin after bolus administration.

In general, input of administered drug and elimination from the body can occur in either compartment in a two-compartment model. The most common situation is illustrated in Figure 3-5; input and elimination are located only in compartment one, which includes plasma and is also called the *central* compartment. The second compartment is often referred to as the *peripheral* compartment. Conceptually, the biphasic behavior arises from the initial process of distribution, in which transfer of drug from compartment one to compartment two dominates, and elimination, during which the two compartments have equilibrated, and elimination of drug dominates.

For a bolus injection ($G = 0$), the initial concentration in the first compartment $C_1(0)$ is dose/V_1, where V_1 is the volume of the first compartment. The initial concentration in

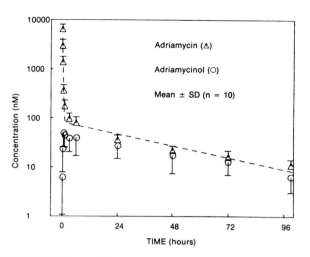

FIGURE 3-4. Plasma disappearance curve for doxorubicin after a bolus dose of 75 mg/m². (SD, standard deviation.) (From Greene RF, Collins JM, Jenkins JF, et al. Plasma pharmacokinetics of Adriamycin and Adriamycinol: implications for the design of in vitro experiments and treatment protocols. *Cancer Res* 43:3417, 1983, with permission.)

the second compartment $C_2(0)$ is 0. Differential mass balances can be written for each compartment and solved simultaneously to yield

$$C_1(t) = A \exp(-\alpha t) + B \exp(-\beta t) \qquad [3\text{-}14]$$

$$C_2(t) = H[\exp(-\beta t) - \exp(-\alpha t)] \qquad [3\text{-}15]$$

where A, B, H, α, and β are algebraic functions of rate constants, volumes, and dose.[37]

Only $C_1(t)$ is usually measurable. The zero-time concentration for C_1 is $A + B$. B is the zero-time intercept for C_1 extrapolated from the elimination phase, α is the initial dis-

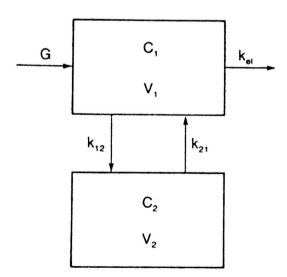

FIGURE 3-5. Two-compartment model (box diagram). (C, concentration; G, input; k_{el}, elimination rate constant; V, volume.)

appearance rate, and β is the terminal disappearance rate. $C_2(t)$ reaches a peak value at $t = t_{max}$:

$$t_{max} = \ln\left(\frac{\alpha/\beta}{\alpha - \beta}\right) \qquad [3\text{-}16]$$

The half-time for C_1 is continuously increasing and is bounded by the terminal slope (elimination phase). After the distribution phase is essentially complete, curves for C_1 and C_2 are nearly parallel, and the system becomes a pseudo–one-compartment model.

When a drug is given by constant infusion, there is an accumulation of drug until steady state is reached, and the plateau concentration is the same as for the one-compartment model:

$$C_{ss} = \ln\left(\frac{G_0}{CL_{TB}}\right) \qquad [3\text{-}17]$$

However, the behavior after the infusion has stopped is no longer independent of the infusion time. Frequently, an α phase that is clearly seen postbolus is barely perceptible postinfusion.

As with one-compartment linear analysis, each injection in a multidose regimen behaves independently of other doses. However, rapid achievement of a plateau is not possible with a single loading dose.

Three or More Compartments

In reality, there is a continuous spectrum of blood-tissue exchange rates in the body. Any separation of tissues into various boxes is somewhat arbitrary. The complexity (number of compartments) of the model is dictated by the application for the model. It is difficult to justify more than two or at most three compartments on statistical grounds; therefore, a pharmacologic or physiologic rationale is needed. Any compartment large enough to influence the drug's distribution must be included. Additionally, a compartment that may not be important in terms of overall distribution may be required if it functions as a target organ.

Physiologic Pharmacokinetic Models

For pharmacologists interested in developing an understanding of drug disposition in individual tissue compartments, models that incorporate physiologic compartments are of considerable interest. These models require measurements of actual physiologic parameters, such as volumes and blood flow rates, as well as drug concentrations in various compartments, and therefore are based primarily on data from experimental animals. Entry into specific areas such as the central nervous system may be of critical importance in the use of drugs, and physiologic models can allow

comparisons of $C \times T$ profiles for various schedules and routes of administration.

In the most general form, physiologic pharmacokinetic models are overly complex and require too large a database for routine clinical use. However, they provide a basis for understanding a drug's kinetic behavior that can be incorporated into simpler models, either physiologic or hybrid, assimilating both empiric observations and physiologic information. Physiologic modeling goes beyond the usual goals of empiric pharmacokinetic modeling to allow for incorporation of data into the model that has been obtained in other species or *in vitro*.

Several model systems have been used to study *in vitro* metabolism: subcellular (e.g., microsomes[38]), cellular (e.g., hepatocytes), tissue homogenates,[39] and whole organs (e.g., isolated perfused liver[35]). In each case, a determination of the drug metabolism parameters v_{max} and K_M can be made, and these values are incorporated into the model.

The compartments comprising a physiologic pharmacokinetic model have an anatomic basis, and the transfer processes in the model have a physiologic or pharmacologic identity. Each organ is modeled separately; then, the model connections are provided by blood flow. For any organ that does not receive input of drug from an external source or does not have diffusional contact with another compartment, the change in drug mass is determined by the arteriovenous concentration difference and any local clearance:

$$V_i \frac{dC_i}{dt} = Q_i C_{art} - Q_i C_{vein} - CL_i C_i \qquad [3\text{-}18]$$

where C_i, V_i, and Q_i are the compartment parameters for concentration, volume, and flow; C_{art} is the concentration of drug in arterial blood supplying the organ; C_{vein} is the mixed-venous blood draining the organ, and CL_i is the intrinsic drug clearance of the organ, a measure of its maximal capacity to remove the drug by all routes.

If the transcapillary and transcellular exchange rates are assumed to be rapid compared to perfusion, the organ concentration is said to be *blood flow–limited*. In this case, the organ concentration is in equilibrium with the venous blood exiting the tissue. These are identical when the partition coefficient is unity:

$$V_i \frac{dC_i}{dt} = Q_i C_{art} - Q_i C_i - CL_i C_i \qquad [3\text{-}19]$$

Because each term except CL_i can be measured, if tissue can be biopsied, a CL_i characteristic of each compartment can be determined.

Simple exercises with physiologic mass balances are often adequate to describe the most important features of a drug's kinetics in the body. It is important to realize that compartments such as muscle and fat, which may have no drug receptors and usually have no role in drug elimination, profoundly influence the time course of drug concentrations (and, potentially, response) throughout the body by acting as reservoirs for redistribution of drugs. Therefore, the most demanding test of physiologic modeling is whole-body simulation.

Ara-C is a drug with considerable usefulness in the treatment of leukemias. Its mechanism of action and other pharmacologic properties are summarized in Chapter 8. It requires intracellular conversion to the triphosphate nucleotide ara-CTP, but much of the drug is deactivated instead by deaminating enzymes [ara-C → arabinosyluracil (ara-U)] in various body tissues. The distribution of these enzymes is a source of considerable variation in mammalian species. The structure for the physiologic model for ara-C is presented in Figure 3-6.[36]

In this model, the mass balances are simplified; the drug is assumed to be freely transported across cell membranes, and thus is flow limited (valid until saturation occurs above 100 μm). There is no binding or partitioning of ara-C between blood and other tissues. The mass balance for blood *B* is

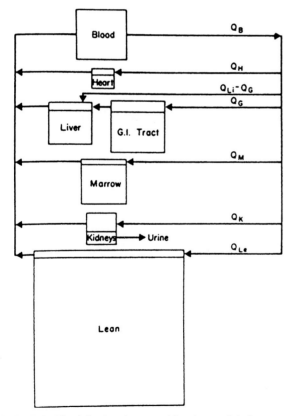

FIGURE 3-6. Physiologic pharmacokinetic model for cytosine arabinoside. (GI, gastrointestinal.) [From Dedrick RL, Forrester DD, Cannon JN, et al. Pharmacokinetics of 1-β-D-arabinofuranosylcytosine (ara-C) deamination in several species. *Biochem Pharmacol* 22:2405, 1973, with permission.]

$$V_{\mathrm{B}}\frac{dC_{\mathrm{B}}}{dt} = \sum(Q_i C_i) - C_{\mathrm{B}}\sum Q_i - \frac{v_{\mathrm{max,B}} C_{\mathrm{B}}}{K_{\mathrm{M}} + C_{\mathrm{B}}} + G \qquad [3\text{-}20]$$

Because drug clearance depends on enzymatic degradation, clearance is expressed as a saturable enzymatic (Michaelis-Menten) process. The maximal rate of enzymatic conversion within the blood is $v_{\mathrm{max,B}}$, and K_{M} is the drug concentration that produces a half-maximal rate of conversion.

Mass balances for the heart, gastrointestinal tract, bone marrow, and lean compartments have identical form:

$$V_i\frac{dC_i}{dt} = Q_i(C_{\mathrm{B}} - C_i) - \frac{v_{\mathrm{max,i}} C_i}{K_{\mathrm{M}} + C_i} \qquad [3\text{-}21]$$

The mass balance for the kidney is similar, with an additional elimination term for urinary removal. The liver mass balance incorporates input from the hepatic artery and portal vein. Simulations compared favorably with data for mouse, monkey, dog, and human parameters, despite considerable variation in elimination rates in these four species.[39]

MTX was the first anticancer drug for which a physiologic pharmacokinetic model was developed.[40] The original model incorporated two features not required in the ara-C model but essential to MTX distribution: strong nonlinear intracellular binding to dihydrofolate reductase and biliary secretion with possible enterohepatic circulation of the drug. An impressive presentation comparing simulations with experimental data required four cycles of semilogarithmic paper to illustrate all tissues simultaneously. Several subsequent modifications have been published. A complete presentation of the currently used model is available.[41] Additional changes could be implemented now that studies of MTX metabolism in tumor cells have demonstrated that conversion to polyglutamylation does occur.[42]

Physiologic models have been constructed for many other anticancer drugs. Among those for the most important drugs in clinical practice, models have been published for 5-FU,[43] cisplatin,[44] and doxorubicin.[45]

REGIONAL ADMINISTRATION

Due to the low therapeutic index of most anticancer drugs, several unusual routes of administration have been implemented to maximize delivery of drugs to the site of the tumor and to reduce the deleterious effects associated with ordinary systemic administration. Examples of these routes are given in Table 3-1. At least two of these routes have become accepted therapeutic practice: intrathecal delivery for meningeal leukemia and intravesical delivery for transitional-stage bladder carcinoma. As reviewed in a later section, the intraperitoneal route has been the subject of many pilot studies and formal phase I and phase II trials by our

TABLE 3-1. MODES OF REGIONAL DRUG DELIVERY

Intracavitary
    Intrathecal
    Intravesical
    Intraperitoneal
    Intrapleural
Intravascular
    Intraarterial:
        First-pass effects
        Device removal
    Intraportal vein

group and others. Some promising pharmacologic results have been obtained, and more definitive therapeutic trials are in progress. Similarly, the intraarterial (IA) route (especially studies of hepatic arterial delivery) has been actively investigated and is reviewed in more detail below. Other intravascular maneuvers include intraportal drug delivery, studied by Taylor,[46] and the recovery of drug from venous drainage before it reaches the systemic circulation.[47]

Pharmacokinetic analysis can help to evaluate the potential usefulness of these approaches; the functional form of the equations is quite similar. The conceptual basis for this functional similarity has been described.[48]

Intraarterial

IA infusion is a delivery mode almost unique to anticancer chemotherapy. It has been applied to a number of arteries in the body, most commonly in patients with liver metastases, brain tumors, and head and neck cancer, or in conjunction with limb-isolation procedures. Fenstermacher and Cowles[49] have used a physiologic pharmacokinetic model to simulate drug concentration in tumor and various body tissues as a result of a carotid artery infusion. Eckman et al.[50] have developed equations that quantitate the potential concentration advantage expected from IA infusion compared with IV administration. They also have discussed the possible impact on pharmacodynamics (drug effects), with emphasis on our lack of understanding in that area.

The quantitative advantage of IA infusion is most easily expressed in terms of the area under the concentration versus time curve (AUC), although this may not be the most appropriate measure for some drugs, such as antimetabolites.[51] As long as all transfer processes are linear, this area is independent of the particular time course of delivery. To examine the selective advantage of IA versus IV infusion, the key index is the ratio of drug concentration in the tumor (AUC_T) being perfused (i.e., the circulation exiting the tissue) to drug concentration in the systemic circulation (AUC_S) supplying potential sites of toxicity (e.g., bone marrow). The therapeutic advantage for drug delivery R_d can be expressed as the ratio of the index value for IA versus the ratio of the index value for IV delivery:

$$R_d = \frac{(AUC_T/AUC_S)_{IA}}{(AUC_T/AUC_S)_{IV}} \qquad [3\text{-}22]$$

For a region that does not eliminate drug from the body, R_d is a function only of the local artery flow rate Q_i and the total-body clearance, CL_{TB}, observed after IV administration:

$$R_d = \frac{CL_{TB}}{Q_i} + 1 \qquad [3\text{-}23]$$

This equation suggests that the smaller the blood flow in the artery being infused, the greater is the advantage for IA delivery. Also, for a given artery, the advantage can be increased by selection of a drug with a high total-body clearance. For example, MTX infusion (assume $CL_{TB} = 200$ mL/min) into a carotid artery (assume $Q_i = 300$ mL/min) yields an R_d of 1.67, whereas doxorubicin infusion (assume $CL_{TB} = 900$ mL/min) yields an R_d of 4. Naturally, tumor sensitivity to the drug also must be considered. Because there is no elimination by the perfused tissue, the AUC in all other body tissues is unchanged (same for IA or IV). Thus tumor exposure can be increased, whereas systemic exposure is not. R_d for this case is simply the ratio of $AUC_T(IA)/AUC_T(IV)$.

For a tissue that does eliminate drug (e.g., the liver), there is an additional advantage. R_d is now related to the fraction of drug E eliminated on a single pass through the tissue:

$$R_d = \frac{CL_{TB}}{Q(1-E)} + 1 \qquad [3\text{-}24]$$

For the particular case of elimination only in the perfused region (e.g., hepatic artery infusion of certain drugs),

$$R_d = \frac{1}{(1-E)} \qquad [3\text{-}25]$$

because $E = CL_{TB}/Q_i$.

The experimental demonstration of the pharmacokinetic advantage of IA delivery has lagged behind the development of the theory. Two approaches can be used: (a) comparison of plasma levels in the same patient who is given matched IA and IV infusions on separate occasions or (b) comparison of ipsilateral versus contralateral tissue levels for a unilateral infusion. Speth et al.[52] have reported results for both of these techniques. In most patients, iododeoxyuridine (IdUrd) was infused into the common hepatic artery, and plasma levels were compared. In one patient, IdUrd was selectively infused into the right branch of the hepatic artery, and biopsies were obtained from both the left and right lobes. A two- to sevenfold advantage was found for IA delivery. The demonstration of a pharmacokinetic advantage is encouraging, but the ultimate value of IA therapy depends on improved response rates and efficacy. For

IdUrd, the initial therapeutic responses (50% objective responses) certainly warrant further investigation.[53]

Intrathecal

Intrathecal administration has been used primarily to obtain adequate drug levels in the cerebrospinal fluid (CSF) to eradicate cancer cells that are otherwise protected from effective therapy. Intrathecal delivery generates high levels of the drug in meningeal areas but does not provide effective drug delivery to parenchymal brain tumors due to a sharp gradient in drug concentration from the meningeal surface inward.[54] A mass balance for the CSF space can be written:

$$V_{CSF} = \frac{dC_{CSF}}{dt} \qquad [3\text{-}26]$$
$$= K(C_p - C_{CSF}) - Q_{CSF}C_{CSF} + P + G_{it}$$

where K is the blood–brain barrier permeability, Q_{CSF} is the rate of CSF formation and removal from the brain, and P represents any active transport of drug into the CSF (assume negligible for this analysis). G_{it} is the intrathecal input function. G_{it} is included in the CSF mass balance for intrathecal delivery but is zero for IV input. The advantage for intrathecal administration R_d is the ratio of C_{CSF} achieved via the intrathecal versus IV routes. When all transfer processes are linear, this advantage is determined only by the permeability and total-body clearance:

$$R_d = \frac{CL_{TB}}{K} + 1 \qquad [3\text{-}27]$$

Although Q_{CSF} strongly affects the concentration in CSF regardless of administration route, its effects are equally felt by all routes. MTX has been most often studied by this route.[9] A comparative study of several anticancer drugs has also been published.[55]

Intraperitoneal

Peritoneal dialysis is currently being evaluated as an intraperitoneal delivery vehicle for anticancer drugs when disease is localized to the abdomen.[56] The pharmacokinetic rationale suggests that tumor tissue may be exposed to high local concentrations, whereas systemic levels are no greater than normally encountered with IV therapy. In an analogous fashion to intrathecal delivery, only cells in close contact with the peritoneal fluid will benefit from this mode of drug delivery.

For a drug that is not subject to "first pass" elimination by the liver, the therapeutic advantage R_d for intraperitoneal versus IV delivery is the ratio of peritoneal fluid concentrations that are achievable:

$$R_d = \frac{CL_{TB}}{PA} + 1 \qquad [3\text{-}28]$$

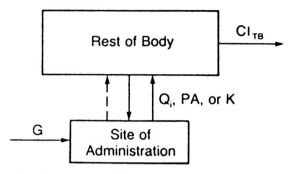

FIGURE 3-7. Regional drug administration. Solid arrows illustrate symmetric intercompartmental transfer, designated in text as Q_i for intraarterial administration, *PA* for intraperitoneal administration, and *K* for intrathecal administration. Asymmetric routes of transfer, such as lymph or cerebrospinal fluid flow, are shown as a dashed arrow. (Cl_{TB}, total-body clearance.)

assuming all transfer processes are linear. *PA* is the permeability-area product for peritoneal drug administration. It is determined by multiplying the volume of intraperitoneal fluid by the slope obtained from a semilogarithmic plot of peritoneal concentration versus time. For most hydrophilic anticancer drugs, PA ranges from 5 to 20 mL per minute, and CL_{TB} ranges from approximately 100 to several thousand mL per minute. R_d of approximately 25 was found for MTX,[57] and R_d of approximately 300 was found for 5-FU.[58,59] Howell and colleagues[60] have studied the intraperitoneal pharmacology of a number of additional drugs. R_d was 12 for cisplatin, which has a very steep dose-response curve.[60] After correction for protein binding, R_d was 65 for etoposide.[61] Gyves and co-workers[62] have pioneered the use of implantable devices for peritoneal access.

Similarities

The structural similarity of Equations 3-23, 3-27, and 3-28 emphasizes the conceptual similarity (Fig. 3-7) of these three modes of regional administration. Furthermore, the same concepts apply to the oral route, which is occasionally used for anticancer drugs. Presumably, higher local levels in the gastrointestinal tract and portal vein can be achieved than with IV dosing, but incomplete or erratic absorption, or both, often make the oral route unacceptable. Furthermore, delivery of the drug to the liver via the portal vein for "first pass" metabolism can be a disadvantage for treatment of systemic disease.

CONCLUDING REMARKS

The ultimate goal of pharmacokinetics is to assist in the optimization of therapy. Before pharmacokinetics can make substantial contributions to the treatment process, several preliminary steps are required. A substantial database made up of measurement of concentration-time profiles after drug administration is needed. Another important step is the development of kinetic models, both physiologic and empiric. There is a continuing need for these steps in the progression toward our ultimate goal, but sufficient headway has been made to justify more emphasis being placed on studies designed to provide fundamental information.

Although progress has been made in pharmacokinetic areas, the limiting step for optimization of therapy is inadequate knowledge of the relationship between drug concentration-time profiles and drug effects. Pharmacokinetics can serve as a useful tool to help elucidate pharmacodynamic relationships by determining which profiles are feasible and by helping design administration strategies. Also, because overall drug effect results from both kinetic and dynamic variables, studies can be designed to adjust doses individually so kinetic differences between patients can be minimized and attention can be focused solely on drug dynamics.

Finally, pharmacokinetics can serve a useful role in the process of drug development by assisting the overall integration of data between preclinical testing and early clinical trials.[63] Initial human studies rely heavily on toxicologic and pharmacologic data obtained in mice and dogs, and pharmacokinetics provides a convenient approach to comparative analysis.

REFERENCES

1. Donelli MG, D'Incalci M, Garattini S. Pharmacokinetic studies of anticancer drugs in tumor-bearing animals. *Cancer Treat Rep* 1984;68:381.
2. Zimm S, Collins JM, Riccardi R, et al. Variable bioavailability of oral mercaptopurine: Is maintenance chemotherapy in acute lymphoblastic leukemia being optimally delivered? *N Engl J Med* 1983;308:1005.
3. Klecker RW, Collins JM, Yarchoan R, et al. Plasma and cerebrospinal fluid pharmacokinetics of 3'-azido-3'-deoxythymidine: a novel pyrimidine analog with potential application for the treatment of patients with AIDS and related diseases. *Clin Pharmacol Ther* 1987;41:407.
4. Goldsmith MA, Slavik M, Carter SK. Quantitative prediction of drug toxicity in humans from toxicology in small and large animals. *Cancer Res* 1975;35:1354.
5. Collins JM, Zaharko DS, Dedrick RL, et al. Potential roles for preclinical pharmacology in phase I trials. *Cancer Treat Rep* 1986;70:73.
6. EORTC Pharmacokinetics and Metabolism Group. Pharmacokinetically guided dose escalation in phase I clinical trials. *Eur J Cancer Clin Oncol* 1987;23:1083.
7. Fuse E, Kobayashi S, Inaba M, et al. Application of pharmacokinetically guided dose escalation with respect to cell cycle phase specificity. *J Natl Cancer Inst* 1994;86(13):989.
8. Collins JM, Grieshaber CK, Chabner BA. Pharmacologically guided phase I trials based upon preclinical development. *J Natl Cancer Inst* 1990;82:1321.
9. Bleyer WA. The clinical pharmacology of intrathecal methotrexate: II. An improved dosage regimen derived from age-related pharmacokinetics. *Cancer Treat Rep* 1977;61:1419.
10. Stoller RG, Hande KR, Jacobs SA, et al. Use of plasma pharmacokinetics to predict and prevent methotrexate toxicity. *N Engl J Med* 1977;297:630.
11. Egorin MJ, Van Echo DA, Whitacre MY, et al. Human pharmacokinetics, excretion, and metabolism of the anthracycline antibiotic menogaril (7-OMEN, NSC 269148) and their correlation with clinical toxicities. *Cancer Res* 1986;46:1513.
12. Beex L, Burghouts J, van Turnhout J, et al. Oral vs. IM administration of high-dose medroxyprogesterone acetate in pretreated patients with advanced breast cancer. *Cancer Treat Rep* 1987;71:1151.
13. Thyss A, Milano G, Renee N, et al. Clinical pharmacokinetic study of 5-FU in continuous 5-day infusions for head and neck cancer. *Cancer Chemother Pharmacol* 1986;6:64.
14. Evans WE, Crom WR, Abromowitch M, et al. Clinical pharmacodynamics of high-dose methotrexate in acute lymphocytic leukemia: identification of a relation between concentration and effect. *N Engl J Med* 1986;314:471.
15. Rodman JH, Abromowitch M, Sinkule JA, et al. Clinical pharmacodynamics of continuous infusion teniposide: systemic exposure as a determinant of response in a phase I trial. *J Clin Oncol* 1987;5:1007.
16. Egorin MJ, Van Echo DA, Olman EA, et al. Prospective validation of a pharmacologically based dosing scheme for the cis-diamminedichloroplatinum(II) analogue diamminecyclobutanedicarboxylatoplatinum. *Cancer Res* 1985;45:6502.
17. Egorin MJ, Sigman LM, Van Echo DA, et al. Phase I clinical and pharmacokinetic study of hexamethylene bisacetamide (NSC95580) administered as a five-day continuous infusion. *Cancer Res* 1987;47:617.
18. Arbuck SG, Douglass HO, Crom WR, et al. Etoposide pharmacokinetics in patients with normal and abnormal organ function. *J Clin Oncol* 1986;4:1690.
19. D'Incalci M, Rossi C, Zucchetti M, et al. Pharmacokinetics of etoposide in patients with abnormal renal and hepatic function. *Cancer Res* 1986;46:2566.
20. Powis G. Effect of human renal and hepatic disease on the pharmacokinetics of anticancer drugs. *Cancer Treat Rev* 1982;9:85.
21. Zimm S, Collins JM, O'Neill D, et al. Inhibition of first-pass metabolism in cancer chemotherapy: the interaction of 6-mercaptopurine and allopurinol. *Clin Pharmacol Ther* 1983;34:810.
22. Peck CC, Temple R, Collins JM. Understanding consequences of concurrent therapies. *JAMA* 1993;269:1550.
23. Dorr RT, Soble MJ, Alberts DS. Interaction of cimetidine but not ranitidine with cyclophosphamide in mice. *Cancer Res* 1986;46:1795.
24. Hande K, Combs G, Swingle R, et al. Effect of cimetidine and ranitidine on the metabolism and toxicity of hexamethylmelamine. *Cancer Treat Rep* 1986;70:1443.
25. Bjornsson TD, Huang AT, Roth P, et al. Effects of high-dose cancer chemotherapy on the absorption of digoxin in two different formulations. *Clin Pharmacol Ther* 1986;39:25.
26. Balis FM. Pharmacokinetic drug interactions of commonly used anticancer drugs. *Clin Pharmacokinet* 1986;11:223.

27. Jamis-Dow CA, Klecker RW, Katki AG, et al. Metabolism of Taxol by human and rat liver in vitro: a screen for drug interactions and interspecies differences. *Cancer Chemother Pharmacol* 1995;36:107.

28. Rustum YM, Preisler HD. Correlation between leukemic cell retention of 1-β-D-arabinofuranosylcytosine-5'-triphosphate and response to therapy. *Cancer Res* 1979;39:42.

29. Liliemark JO, Plunkett W, Dixon DO. Relationship of 1-β-D-arabinofuranosylcytosine-5'-triphosphate levels in leukemic cells during treatment with high-dose 1-β-D-arabinofuranosylcytosine. *Cancer Res* 1985;45:5952.

30. Plunkett W, Liliemark JO, Adams TM, et al. Saturation of 1-β-D-arabinofuranosylcytosine-5'-triphosphate accumulation in leukemia cells during high-dose 1-β-D'-arabinofuranosylcytosine therapy. *Cancer Res* 1987;47:3005.

31. Young RC. Kinetic aids to proper chemotherapeutic scheduling: labeled nucleoside incorporation studies in vivo. *Cancer Treat Rep* 1976;60:1947.

32. Kerr IG, Jolivet J, Collins JM, et al. Test dose for predicting high-dose methotrexate infusions. *Clin Pharmacol Ther* 1983;33:44.

33. Howell SB, Blair HE, Uren J, et al. Haemodialysis and enzymatic cleavage of methotrexate in man. *Eur J Cancer* 1978;14:787.

34. Collins JM, Klecker RW, Yarchoan R, et al. Clinical pharmacokinetics of suramin in patients with HTLV-III/LAV infection. *J Clin Pharmacol* 1986;26:22.

35. Donehower RC, Karp JE, Burke PJ. Pharmacology and toxicity of high-dose cytarabine by 72-hour continuous infusion. *Cancer Treat Rep* 1986;70:1059.

36. Oates J, Wilkinson G. Principles of drug therapy. In: Thorn GW, et al., eds. *Harrison's principles of internal medicine*, 8th ed. New York: McGraw-Hill, 1977:334–346.

37. Gibaldi M, Perrier D. *Pharmacokinetics*, 2nd ed. New York: Marcel Dekker, 1982.

38. McManus ME, Monks A, Collins JM, et al. Nonlinear pharmacokinetics of misonidazole and desmethylmisonidazole in the isolated perfused rat liver. *J Pharmacol Exp Ther* 1981;219:669.

39. Dedrick RL, Forrester DD, Cannon JN, et al. Pharmacokinetics of 1-β-D-arabinofuranosylcytosine (ara-C) deamination in several species. *Biochem Pharmacol* 1973;22:2405.

40. Bischoff KB, Dedrick RL, Zaharko DS, et al. Methotrexate pharmacokinetics. *J Pharm Sci* 1971;60:1128.

41. Dedrick RL, Myers CE, Bungay PM, et al. Pharmacokinetic rationale for peritoneal drug administration in the treatment of ovarian cancer. *Cancer Treat Rep* 1978;62:1.

42. Jacobs SA, Stoller RG, Chabner BA, et al. Dose-dependent metabolism of methotrexate in man and rhesus monkeys. *Cancer Treat Rep* 1977;61:651.

43. Collins JM, Dedrick RL, King FG, et al. Nonlinear pharmacokinetic models for 5-fluorouracil in man: intravenous and intraperitoneal routes. *Clin Pharmacol Ther* 1980; 28:235.

44. Farris FF, King FG, Dedrick RL, et al. Physiologic model for the pharmacokinetics of cis-dichlorodiammineplatinum(II)(DDP) in the tumored rat. *J Pharmacokinet Biopharm* 1985;13:13.

45. Chan KK, Cohen JL, Gross JF, et al. Prediction of Adriamycin disposition in cancer patients using a physiologic, pharmacokinetic model. *Cancer Treat Rep* 1978;62:1161.

46. Taylor I. Cytotoxic perfusion for colorectal liver metastases. *Br J Surg* 1978;65:109.

47. Oldfield EH, Dedrick RL, Chatterji DC, et al. Reduced systemic drug exposure by combining intracarotid chemotherapy with hemoperfusion of jugular drainage. *Surg Forum* 1983;34:535.

48. Collins JM. Pharmacologic rationale for regional drug delivery. *J Clin Oncol* 1984;2:498.

49. Fenstermacher JD, Cowles AL. Theoretic limitations of intracarotid infusions in brain tumor chemotherapy. *Cancer Treat Rep* 1977;61:519.

50. Eckman WW, Patlak CS, Fenstermacher JD. A critical evaluation of the principles governing the advantages of intraarterial infusions. *J Pharmacokinet Biopharm* 1974;2:257.

51. Collins JM. Pharmacokinetic rationale for intraarterial therapy. In: Howell SB, ed. *Intra-arterial and intracavitary cancer chemotherapy*. Boston: Martinus Nijhoff, 1985:1.

52. Speth PAJ, Kinsella TJ, Chang AE, et al. Selective incorporation of iododeoxyuridine into DNA of hepatic metastases versus normal human liver. *Clin Pharmacol Ther* 1988; 44:369.

53. Chang AE, Collins JM, Speth PAJ, et al. Phase I study of intraarterial iododeoxyuridine in patients with colorectal liver metastases. *J Clin Oncol* 1989;7:662.

54. Blasberg R, Patlak CS, Fenstermacher JD. Intrathecal chemotherapy: brain tissue profiles after ventriculocisternal perfusion. *J Pharmacol Exp Ther* 1975;195:73.

55. Collins JM. Pharmacokinetics of intraventricular administration. *J Neurooncol* 1983;1:283.

56. Myers CE, Collins JM. Pharmacology of intraperitoneal chemotherapy. *Cancer Invest* 1983;1:395.

57. Jones RB, Collins JM, Myers CE, et al. High-volume intraperitoneal chemotherapy with methotrexate in patients with cancer. *Cancer Res* 1981;41:55.

58. Speyer JL, Collins JM, Dedrick RL, et al. Phase I and pharmacologic studies of intraperitoneal 5-fluorouracil. *Cancer Res* 1980;40:567.

59. Speyer JL, Sugarbaker PH, Collins JM, et al. Portal levels and hepatic clearance of 5-fluorouracil after intraperitoneal administration in man. *Cancer Res* 1981;41:1916.

60. Howell SB, Pfeifle CE, Wung WE, et al. Intraperitoneal cis-diamminedichloroplatinum with systemic thiosulfate protection. *Cancer Res* 1983;43:426.

61. Zimm S, Cleary SM, Lucas WE, et al. Phase I/pharmacokinetic study of intraperitoneal cisplatin and etoposide. *Cancer Res* 1987;47:1712.

62. Gyves JW, Ensminger WD, Stetson P, et al. Constant intraperitoneal infusion of 5-fluorouracil via a totally implanted system. *Clin Pharmacol Ther* 1984;35:83.

63. Collins JM. Pharmacology and drug development. *J Natl Cancer Inst* 1988;80:790.

4

INFERTILITY AFTER CANCER CHEMOTHERAPY

RICHARD L. SCHILSKY

Cytotoxic chemotherapy has produced sustained clinical remissions and cures for many patients with Hodgkin's disease,[1] acute lymphoblastic leukemia,[2] choriocarcinoma,[3] testicular carcinoma,[4] and other malignant and nonmalignant disorders. As detailed in subsequent chapters most of the commonly used antineoplastic drugs produce immediate toxicities in organs composed of self-renewing cell populations such as bone marrow, skin, and gastrointestinal tract epithelium. Pancytopenia, stomatitis, alopecia, nausea, and vomiting occur frequently but generally are not prolonged or irreversible once chemotherapy is completed. Some antitumor agents are associated with more delayed toxic effects, such as the cardiomyopathy of doxorubicin (Adriamycin) or the pulmonary fibrosis associated with bleomycin, which may become clinically apparent even after chemotherapy is completed. However, as patients continue to survive longer after chemotherapy, previously unrecognized toxic effects are becoming manifest. Important among these late effects is infertility, which is of particular concern for successfully treated patients hoping to return to a normal lifestyle. In this chapter, we consider this late effect of cancer chemotherapy.

GONADAL DYSFUNCTION AFTER CANCER CHEMOTHERAPY

Neoplastic disease and its treatment can interfere with any of the cellular, anatomic, physiologic, or behavioral processes that make up normal sexual and reproductive function. Indeed, many drugs used in the treatment of cancer have profound and, often, lasting effects on the testis and the ovary. Germ cell production and endocrine function may be altered. These effects are generally related to the age, pubertal status, and menstrual status of the patient as well as to the particular drug class, dosage, or combination administered.

Chemotherapy Effects in Men

The adult testis functions as an exocrine and endocrine gland, producing spermatozoa and testosterone. Spermatogenesis proceeds in the seminiferous tubules, which constitute more than 75% of the mass of the testis, although the interstitial cells of Leydig carry on the endocrine functions of the gland. The remainder of the testis consists of supporting and vascular tissues necessary for the protection and nourishment of the developing spermatozoa.

The seminiferous tubules are lined by a stratified epithelium composed of two cell types: spermatogenic cells and Sertoli cells. The spermatogenic cells are arranged in an orderly fashion; spermatogonia lie directly on the basement membrane, and primary and secondary spermatocytes, spermatids, and maturing spermatozoa progress centrally toward the tubular lumen. Sertoli cells also lie on the basement membrane. These specialized cells help to maintain the blood–testis barrier and to regulate the release of mature spermatozoa from the germinal epithelium.[5]

In any area of the seminiferous tubule, five to six generations of germ cells can be identified. These generations are not randomly distributed but occur in fixed cell associations. Thus spermatids at a particular stage in their development are always associated with the same types of spermatocytes and spermatogonia. Six typical cell associations in the human testis synchronously evolve in the process of sperm maturation. A complete series of cell associations constitutes a cycle of the germinal epithelium, and each cell association may be considered a stage of the cycle. The entire process of spermatogenesis proceeds continuously throughout the tubule, and it has been estimated that 64 to 90 days elapse from spermatogonial stem cell mitosis to release of mature spermatozoa from the seminiferous epithelium.[6]

Spermatogenesis is a dynamic and complex process divided into three phases: (a) proliferation of spermatogonia to produce spermatocytes and to renew the stem cell pool, (b) meiotic division of spermatocytes to reduce the

TABLE 4-1. SITE OF TOXICITY OF ANTINEOPLASTIC DRUGS IN THE GERMINAL EPITHELIUM

Drug	Cell Type Affected	Reference
Actinomycin D	Stem cells, early spermatogonia	9
Bischloroethyl-nitrosourea (carmustine)	Stem cells, intermediate spermatogonia	9
Bleomycin	Intermediate spermatogonia	8
Busulfan	Type A spermatogonia	11, 12
Chloroethylcyclo-hexylnitrosourea (lomustine)	Intermediate spermatogonia, spermatocytes	9
Cisplatin	Spermatogonia, spermatocytes, spermatids	9, 10
Arabinosylcytosine	Late spermatogonia, spermatocytes	8
Cyclophosphamide	Early and late spermatogonia, spermatocytes	8, 10
Doxorubicin	Stem cells, spermatocytes	8, 10
5-Fluorouracil	Spermatids	10
Methotrexate	Early spermatogonia	9, 10
Mitomycin C	Stem cells, spermatogonia	9
Mechlorethamine hydrochloride	Intermediate and late spermatogonia	9
Procarbazine	Stem cells, early spermatogonia	9

chromosome number in the germ cells by half, and (c) maturation of the spermatids to become spermatozoa.[7] Cytotoxic agents could affect this process in a number of ways: (a) A specific cell type within the germinal epithelium might be selectively damaged or destroyed; (b) the proliferative and meiotic phases of spermatogenesis might proceed normally, but sperm maturation might be abnormal, leading to functionally incompetent mature spermatozoa; or (c) chemotherapy might damage Sertoli cells, Leydig cells, or other supportive or nutritive constituents of the testis in such a way as to alter the particular microenvironment necessary for normal germ cell production.

With knowledge of the normal histology of the germinal epithelium and of the kinetics of spermatogenesis, it is possible to estimate the specific site of a drug's effect, either by examining the testis microscopically or by performing sperm counts or mating studies at some interval after administration of the drug. The morphology of the spermatids can be used to define the stage of the germinal epithelial cycle at the time of biopsy, and the presence or absence of cells supposed to be found at that stage can be noted. Flow cytometry can also be used to examine the DNA content and cell-cycle progression of spermatogenic cells obtained from animals injected with bromodeoxyuridine. Known kinetic parameters can then be used to determine precisely which spermatogenic cell was destroyed by drug administration. For example, examination of mouse testes 11 days after doxorubicin administration revealed an absence of pachytene primary spermatocytes, indicating that type A2 (primitive) spermatogonia are most sensitive to injury by this drug.[8] Similar analysis after cisplatin administration demonstrated that intermediate spermatogonia are most sensitive to cisplatin and that, at high doses (10 mg per kg), even late-stage spermatids may be affected, suggesting the occurrence of Sertoli cell damage at this dose level.[9] Following administration of 5-fluorouracil (5-FU), spermatogonial damage is not seen; rather, arrest of spermatid development is noted.[10] Failure of sperm release from the germinal epithelium has been observed after the administration of 5-FU, cisplatin, doxorubicin, or methotrexate (MTX), suggesting Sertoli cell damage by all these agents.[10]

Serial mating studies, whereby animals are mated at varying intervals after drug administration and the onset of infertility is noted, can provide similar, although less precise, information. In the rat, an infertile mating occurring 6 to 7 weeks after drug treatment implies that spermatocytes were affected primarily by the drug in question, whereas infertility occurring 10 weeks after drug treatment reflects spermatogonial destruction.[11,12] As long as the dynamics of the germinal epithelium of the species under study have been delineated, some insight into the effects of cytotoxic agents on spermatogenesis can be obtained. Table 4-1 summarizes the results of both biopsy and mating studies in rats and mice for several commonly used antineoplastic agents.

Clearly, such studies cannot be performed in men, and one must rely primarily on reproductive history, clinical examination, and specific laboratory tests in the evaluation of testicular function. Table 4-2 provides a summary of this type of evaluation. Because the seminiferous tubules comprise a large proportion of the testicular mass, damage to the germinal epithelium frequently results in testicular atrophy, which is readily detectable on physical examination. Impaired spermatogenesis is also manifest as a decrease in the number, morphology, or motility of sperm in the ejaculate and as an increase in the serum level of follicle-stimu-

TABLE 4-2. EVALUATION OF THE PATIENT WITH SUSPECTED GERMINAL APLASIA

	Normal	Germinal Aplasia
Testicular size (mL)	20–30	8–15
Follicle-stimulating hormone (mIU/mL)	4–25	25–90
Luteinizing hormone (mIU/mL)	4–18	8–25
Testosterone (ng/dL)	250–1,200	200–700
Sperm count (10^6/mL)	>20	0

lating hormone (FSH). More recently, detection of chromosomal abnormalities in human sperm has been accomplished. Human sperm are fused with hamster oocytes, and human pronuclear sperm chromosomes are identified by banding techniques.[13] Using this technique, the reported frequency of chromosomal structural abnormalities in normal sperm is 7% to 9%.[13,14] The frequency of structural abnormalities has been examined in only a few patients after chemotherapy but is reported to be 9% to 40%, with more damage seen in patients who received multiple chemotherapeutic agents.[14,15] In addition, flow cytometry has been used to determine ploidy in human sperm after radiation and chemotherapy. One year after radiation therapy, the percentage of condensed haploid cells was markedly reduced compared to a cohort who received chemotherapy, but this difference was no longer present at 3 years.[16] In chemotherapy and radiation-treated patients, a low pretreatment percentage of condensed haploid cells correlated with a lack of recovery of sperm cell production at 1 year. Sperm chromatin structure can also be assessed using acridine orange staining of spermatozoa. Although the presence of abnormal chromatin does not seem to be related to pretreatment sperm count, it may predict for resumption of spermatogenesis after cytotoxic chemotherapy.[17] Leydig cell dysfunction also may occur after cancer treatment and is detected by an increase in serum luteinizing hormone (LH) and, if uncompensated, a fall in serum testosterone level. Indeed, decreased daily testosterone production and low free testosterone levels have been noted in men with germinal aplasia despite normal plasma LH levels.[18] Leydig cell dysfunction has been detected in up to 30% of men treated with alkylating-agent based combination chemotherapy although clinically overt testosterone deficiency is rare.[19]

There seem to be common pathophysiologic changes that occur in the testis independent of the type of drug administered but related to the total dose used. The primary testicular lesion caused by all antitumor agents studied thus far is depletion of the germinal epithelium lining the seminiferous tubules.[20–24] Testicular biopsy in most patients reveals complete germinal aplasia, with only Sertoli cells left lining the tubular lumen. Occasionally, scattered spermatogonia, spermatocytes, or spermatids may be seen, or there may be evidence for maturation arrest at the spermatocyte stage.[25] The tubules appear atrophic, and peritubular fibrosis is sometimes seen, although the interstitial cells of Leydig and the Sertoli cells remain normal in appearance.

Clinically, there is a marked decrease in testicular volume noted on physical examination, in association with severe oligospermia or azoospermia and infertility.[26,27] Depletion of the germinal epithelium is accompanied by a marked increase in serum FSH levels.[28] This finding suggests that the seminiferous tubule may be the site of production of a feedback inhibitor of gonadotropin secretion.

Abnormalities of serum testosterone or changes in secondary sexual characteristics after chemotherapy are infrequent. However, subtle abnormalities of Leydig cell function may be present. Administration of LH-releasing hormone (LHRH) to men after combination chemotherapy for Hodgkin's disease produces excessively high serum LH and FSH levels consistent with compensated Leydig cell failure.[29–31] This abnormality has not been correlated with any specific clinical changes in sexual function.

Among the anticancer drugs, alkylating agents have most consistently caused male infertility. In particular, chlorambucil and cyclophosphamide (Cytoxan) deplete the testicular germinal epithelium in a dose-related fashion. Progressive oligospermia occurs in men with lymphoma who are treated with up to 400 mg of chlorambucil.[23] Those patients receiving cumulative doses in excess of 400 mg are uniformly azoospermic. Similarly, decreased sperm counts may occur in men treated with 50 to 100 mg of cyclophosphamide daily for courses as brief as 2 months, although azoospermia and germinal aplasia are infrequent until 6 to 10 g of the drug has been administered.[20] Both sperm count and motility are markedly reduced during treatment with a cyclophosphamide-containing regimen in patients with bone and soft tissue sarcomas.[21] Antimetabolites in conventional doses seem to have relatively few effects on spermatogenesis, although one study suggested that high-dose MTX (250 mg per kg) may produce transient oligospermia in some patients.[32] This modest effect of MTX on spermatogenesis may be due to the presence of a significant barrier to MTX passage from blood to seminiferous tubule.[33] These data suggest the presence of a threshold dose for the development of testicular germinal aplasia for each particular drug. However, prospective studies of testicular function in large numbers of men receiving a variety of antitumor agents are needed to provide more reliable information concerning the threshold drug dose above which severe or irreversible testicular injury occurs.

Little information is presently available concerning the impact of other classes of antineoplastic agents on the testis. Several reports have suggested that doxorubicin may be less toxic to the human testis than expected based on animal studies. In both the mouse[8] and the rat,[10,34] doxorubicin produces severe germinal epithelial injury, yet recent clinical studies of the effects of doxorubicin-containing regimens on testicular function in men have revealed reversible testicular injury in the majority of patients under age 40.[35–38]

Amsacrine, a recently introduced acridine derivative with activity in acute leukemia, causes rapidly reversible azoospermia, suggesting that this drug produces little toxicity to stem cells in the human testis.[39] Recombinant interferon-α-2b, an active agent in the treatment of some chronic leukemias and solid tumors, seems to have no adverse effects on testicular function in men treated chronically for hairy cell leukemia.[40]

The effects of cisplatin alone on testicular function are difficult to discern from available information. Patients with testicular cancer treated with cisplatin-based combination chemotherapy uniformly become severely oligospermic or azoospermic soon after chemotherapy is initiated.[41–47] It is apparent that higher doses of cisplatin or more cycles of chemotherapy are associated with more profound and persistent decreases in sperm counts.[48,49] Although the specific contribution of cisplatin to the gonadal toxicity of cisplatin (Platinol), vinblastine sulfate hydrate (Velban), and bleomycin (PVB) or the vinblastine, actinomycin D, bleomycin, cisplatin, cyclophosphamide regimen[44] is difficult to sort out, these regimens have been used routinely in the treatment of testicular cancer, and their effects on fertility in a patient population likely to be cured deserve particular emphasis. Unfortunately, many of these individuals are azoospermic at the time of diagnosis, and others will be infertile due to retrograde ejaculation that may occur after retroperitoneal lymph node dissection.

As might be expected, other combination chemotherapy regimens that include alkylating agents have profound effects on spermatogenesis. Sherins and DeVita[50] reported the effects of combination chemotherapy on the fertility of 16 men with lymphoma in complete remission 2 months to 7 years after mechlorethamine, vincristine (Oncovin), procarbazine, prednisone (MOPP); cyclophosphamide, vincristine, prednisone (CVP); or cyclophosphamide alone.[50] Testicular biopsy in 15 patients revealed germinal aplasia in ten, scattered spermatogonia with arrest of spermatogenesis in two, and normal spermatogenesis in three. All except the three patients with normal biopsies had azoospermia or severe oligospermia on semen analysis. Those patients with normal ejaculates and biopsies, of whom two received MOPP and one received CVP, had been off therapy for 2 to 7 years. Subsequent studies have confirmed that at least 80% of men treated with MOPP combination chemotherapy become azoospermic or severely oligospermic.[51–54] Chapman et al.[52] found that all 74 men receiving cyclic combination chemotherapy for Hodgkin's disease were azoospermic after treatment, and only four of 74 recovered spermatogenesis after a median follow-up of 27 months. A decline in libido and decreased sexual activity also occurred during therapy and only partially recovered after treatment. At least 50% of men with advanced Hodgkin's disease are azoospermic *before* the initiation of treatment, complicating the interpretation of posttreatment status.[55,56]

The gonadal effects of cyclophosphamide-containing regimens for the treatment of aggressive non-Hodgkin's lymphoma have only recently been studied. Unlike patients with Hodgkin's disease, those with non-Hodgkin's lymphoma often have normal pretreatment sperm counts and motility.[57] Regimens containing modest doses of cyclophosphamide such as MTX-leucovorin, doxorubicin hydrocloride (Adriamycin), cyclophosphamide, vincristine sulfate (Oncovin), prednisone, bleomycin (MACOP-B) or vinblastine, doxoru-bicin hydrocloride (Adriamycin), cyclophosphamide, vincristine sulfate (Oncovin), prednisone, bleomycin (VACOP-B) have produced only transient azoospermia with total recovery of spermatogenesis in 100% of patients at a median of 28 months after completion of therapy.[57] However, with the standard cyclophosphamide, doxorubicin, vincristine, and prednisone regimen, sperm counts recovered in only two-thirds of patients at 7 years.[58] Those receiving more than 9.5 g per m^2 of cyclophosphamide and those who also received pelvic irradiation had more profound and longer-lasting damage.[58]

Leydig cell dysfunction also may occur more often than previously recognized. Although Leydig cells remain morphologically intact after chemotherapy and basal serum LH levels tend to remain normal, many patients have hypersecretion of LH in response to the administration of LHRH, an indication of Leydig cell dysfunction.[52,53] Evidence of Sertoli cell dysfunction has been observed as well. Plasma levels of immunoreactive inhibin, a product of Sertoli cells, may be reduced after chemotherapy, but the decrease is not necessarily correlated with abnormal LH, FSH, testosterone, or sperm counts.[59] These biochemical abnormalities also have not been associated with specific clinical changes in sexual desire or function.

With the completion of chemotherapy, the recovery of spermatogenesis is unpredictable for the individual patient but is probably related to the age of the patient, the total dose of drug administered, the type of drug, and the duration of time off therapy. Complete recovery of spermatogenesis was reported in three of five previously azoospermic patients after therapy with chlorambucil in doses ranging from 410 to 2,600 mg.[27] In these patients, sperm counts were normal at 33, 34, and 42 months after completion of chemotherapy. Two additional patients, who received the highest cumulative drug doses, demonstrated a partial return of spermatogenesis at 38 and 58 months after discontinuing treatment. In a similar study, 26 men treated for 5 to 34 months with 50 to 100 mg of cyclophosphamide daily all became azoospermic within 6 months of starting therapy.[60] However, serial sperm counts demonstrated a return of spermatogenesis in 12 patients a mean period of 31 months after discontinuation of cyclophosphamide. Those patients demonstrating a recovery of spermatogenesis tended to receive lower initial drug doses. These studies, along with numerous anecdotal reports,[61,62] clearly demonstrate that the germinal epithelium can regenerate and spermatogenesis can resume after single-agent chemotherapy. Furthermore, the evidence suggests that the rapidity with which spermatogenesis resumes may be related to the total dose of chemotherapy administered.

Treatment with combination chemotherapy may produce longer-lasting azoospermia than therapy with single agents. Sherins and DeVita[50] observed azoospermia and testicular germinal aplasia in patients for as long as 4 years after completion of MOPP combination chemotherapy, and Chapman et al.[31] observed a return of spermatogenesis in only four of 64 men followed as long as 51 months after the completion of mechlorethamine, vinblastine, procarbazine, and prednisone (MVPP) chemotherapy. Other recent studies[63] have confirmed these findings, and it now appears that only approximately 10% of patients receiving MOPP or MVPP will ultimately have a return of spermatogenesis. Permanent infertility is most likely to occur when more than three cycles of such chemotherapy have been administered.[64]

Several studies have suggested that the use of procarbazine in these regimens is particularly damaging to the germinal epithelium.[65,66] In one report, 32 patients receiving combination chemotherapy for lymphoma were studied. Thirty-one of 32 developed increased serum FSH levels during their initial therapy, and of 15 studied, all had azoospermia. Sixteen patients were evaluated for recovery of testicular function. In seven of ten patients treated with CVP or a related regimen, plasma FSH levels returned to normal during 34 months of follow-up. Of four patients studied, three had normal sperm counts, and the fourth was oligospermic. In contrast, only one of six patients treated with a procarbazine-containing regimen demonstrated a decrease of serum FSH or an increase in sperm count during 52 months of follow-up. In another study, patients treated with combination chemotherapy for non-Hodgkin's lymphoma appeared to have a lower incidence of gonadal dysfunction than those treated for Hodgkin's disease, despite receiving similar cumulative doses of cyclophosphamide and vincristine. However, most of the Hodgkin's disease patients also received procarbazine whereas those treated for non-Hodgkin's lymphoma did not.[66] Although the patient numbers are small, these data suggest that the use of procarbazine, in combination chemotherapy regimens may be associated with longer-lasting testicular damage than seen with the use of alkylating agents alone. Indeed, Sieber et al.[67] demonstrated that procarbazine by itself is toxic to the germinal epithelium in adult male monkeys. An aggressive eight-drug regimen that did not contain procarbazine was used in the treatment of adult acute lymphocytic leukemia and was associated with preservation of fertility in the majority of patients.[68]

In recent years, a number of alternative combination chemotherapy regimens to MOPP have been proposed for treatment of advanced Hodgkin's disease. Among these, the doxorubicin hydrochloride [Adriamycin, bleomycin, vinblastine, and dacarbazine (ABVD)] seems to be equally efficacious and generally less toxic than the MOPP regimen. A recent comparison of the treatment regimens revealed that azoospermia occurs in 100% of MOPP-treated patients but in only 35% of patients receiving ABVD and that recovery of spermatogenesis occurs rarely in MOPP-treated patients but nearly always in those treated with ABVD.[69,70] Similarly, 90% of patients with Hodgkin's disease treated with three cycles of mitoxantrone, vincristine, vinblastine, and prednisone fol-

lowed by radiation therapy developed severe oligospermia or azoospermia within 1 month of beginning chemotherapy, but sperm counts returned to normal in 63% of patients between 2.6 and 4.5 months after the completion of chemotherapy.[71] A hybrid regimen of MOPP and ABVD produced persistent testicular dysfunction in approximately 60% of patients at 27 months posttreatment; pretreatment sperm quality did not have an impact on posttreatment recovery.[56] This information may play an important role in treatment planning for young men with Hodgkin's disease who are concerned about preservation of fertility during and after treatment.

Similar concerns face patients with testicular cancer who are about to begin chemotherapy. Although most commonly used regimens for testis cancer produce gonadal injury, there seems to be a high degree of reversibility of testicular dysfunction, with as many as 50% of patients demonstrating resumption of spermatogenesis within 2 years of completing chemotherapy. Among 98 patients with testicular germ cell cancers, 28 were treated with cisplatin-based chemotherapy and had profound decreases in sperm counts 1 year later; their median sperm counts had returned to pretreatment levels 3 years after chemotherapy.[72] This was paralleled by a normalization of FSH values. Compared with stage I patients who were treated with orchiectomy alone, patients with metastatic disease receiving PVB had similar sperm counts 1.5 years after treatment.[73] However, in both groups, these counts were considered subnormal in 55% of patients. Recovery of spermatogenesis and fertility may occur even longer after treatment. A patient with malignant teratoma who underwent orchiectomy, chemotherapy, and pelvic irradiation was found to be azoospermic 8 years after completing treatment but recovered fertility 6 years later, 14 years after completing treatment.[74] Higher doses of chemotherapy generally induce longer-lasting oligospermia.[48] Patients with pretreatment oligo- or azoospermia seem least likely to resume spermatogenesis after treatment. However, recovery of spermatogenesis 2 years after cisplatin-based chemotherapy may occur in up to 50% of patients who had pretreatment azoospermia or oligospermia.[75] In patients whose FSH level does not normalize within 2 years of chemotherapy, recovery of fertility is very unlikely.[76] Similar rates of recovery of spermatogenesis (approximately 40% at 5 years) have been noted in osteosarcoma patients receiving doxorubicin or cyclophosphamide-based chemotherapy, or a combination of the two.[21,38,77]

Little information is available about fertility after high-dose chemotherapy with autologous or allogeneic bone marrow transplantation. In men receiving a preparative regimen of high-dose cyclophosphamide alone, potential for recovery of spermatogenesis is reasonably high. In 72 men who received this treatment in Seattle, 65% had normal FSH and normal sperm counts, and 94% had normal serum LH and testosterone levels.[78] Recovery of spermatogenesis is not age-related in this population. After total-body irradiation, however, spermatogenesis is permanently absent in most patients.[79]

The recognition that some chemotherapy regimens produce irreversible gonadal injury has prompted a search for means to protect the testis from the toxic effects of these drugs. Reducing the rate of spermatogenesis by interrupting the pituitary-gonadal axis has been proposed as a means of rendering the germinal epithelium relatively resistant to cytotoxic agents.

Gonadotropin-releasing hormone (GnRH) analogs, both agonists and antagonists, have been shown to inhibit spermatogenesis in the rat,[80] dog,[81] monkey,[82] and man.[83] Glode et al.[84] originally reported that treatment of mice with a GnRH analog resulted in protection of the testis from the damaging effects of cyclophosphamide. More recent studies have failed to confirm these observations,[85] but other reports have indicated that GnRH analogs seem to protect the rat testis from the effects of x-irradiation[86] and procarbazine.[87] Notably, complete suppression of spermatogenesis during treatment does not appear to be necessary for the protective benefit.[87] Indeed, one recent report suggests that hormone pretreatment does not protect the rat testis from the damaging effects of procarbazine through arrest of spermatogonial proliferation.[88] The primate testis also may be protected from alkylating agents with the use of these agents.[89] These experimental findings have stimulated the initiation of clinical trials to evaluate this approach in patients receiving cancer chemotherapy. In one study,[90] six men receiving combination chemotherapy for lymphoma were treated with D-Trp[6]-Pro[9]-*N*-ethylamide–LHRH before and during chemotherapy administration. All patients had a fall in serum testosterone, LH, and FSH levels during treatment, and all patients became oligospermic or azoospermic. Nevertheless, after completion of chemotherapy, there was a rapid rise in serum FSH in all patients, and five of six patients developed persistent azoospermia with a median follow-up of 52 weeks. A prospective comparative study of the LHRH agonist D-Ser-(TBU)[6]LHRH ethylamide versus control has recently been completed in 14 patients with germ cell tumors receiving PVB.[91] Six patients received the LHRH agonist and demonstrated suppressed FSH, LH, and testosterone levels during treatment. However, all patients (six "protected" and eight controls) demonstrated posttreatment azoospermia that normalized within 24 months after therapy. A larger study of 30 men with Hodgkin's disease treated with MVPP or a related regimen also failed to demonstrate a protective effect of the LHRH analog buserelin.[92] In a similar study involving 20 men with Hodgkin's disease and other solid tumors who received MOPP, ABVD, radiotherapy, or a combination of the three, buserelin again failed to protect spermatogenesis.[93]

Testosterone administration also has the potential to inhibit spermatogenesis reversibly and has shown some ability to protect the rat testis from the damaging effects of procarbazine.[94–96] The protective effect of testosterone along with 17β-estradiol in rats is selective for the survival and recovery of early stem spermatogonia.[95] At present, it seems that hormonal manipulation of spermatogenesis is a promising experimental approach to protection of the testis from cytotoxic chemotherapy, but many more studies are required to determine the optimal method of applying this intervention in the clinic. The problem simply may be related to duration of therapy. In the successful mouse experiments, mice were pretreated for up to 6 weeks with GnRH agonists before being exposed to chemotherapy. In the human studies, hormone treatment either preceded chemotherapy by a short interval or was coincident with chemotherapy. From knowledge of the kinetics of spermatogenesis in mice and humans, it seems likely that a much longer period of hormone suppression is necessary to achieve a beneficial effect in men. However, it may not be appropriate to delay initiation of potentially curative therapy for the time necessary to test this approach.

Testicular circulatory isolation, a method for diminishing blood flow to the testis resulting in regional drug exclusion, has been tested in rats and resulted in preservation of fertility after doxorubicin administration.[97] A phase I study has been conducted in humans demonstrating the safety of transscrotal placement of an aortic clamp for up to 1 hour.[98] However, this method has not yet been tested in humans during chemotherapy administration.

Chemotherapy Effects in Women

The evaluation of chemotherapy effects on ovarian function is hampered by the relative inaccessibility of the ovary to biopsy. There is no readily available direct measurement of the female germ cell population analogous to semen analysis in men. Only recently have animal models been developed to assess the effects of cytotoxic drugs on ovarian function. Thus, one must rely primarily on menstrual and reproductive history and on determinations of serum hormone levels to assess the functional status of the ovary.

Oogenesis is the process of maturation of the primitive female germ cell to the mature ovum. This process occurs primarily during intrauterine life and involves multiple mitotic divisions to increase the number of germ cells, followed by the beginning of the first meiotic division, which will eventually reduce the diploid chromosome number to half before fertilization. At the time of birth, the oocytes are in the long prophase of their first meiotic division, and they remain in that state until the formation of a mature follicle before ovulation.[99]

In the postnatal ovary, most of the ongoing cellular growth and replication is related to the growth and development of follicles. Primordial follicles develop during gestation and consist of a primary oocyte covered by a layer of mesenchymal cells called *granulosa cells*. At the time of birth, the ovary may contain 150,000 to 500,000 primordial follicles, many of which subsequently become atretic. From childhood to menopause, follicular growth occurs as a continuous process, with ovulation occurring in a cyclic fashion.[100] The granulosa cells surrounding the primary oocyte proliferate, follicular fluid accumulates, and the ovum completes its first meiotic division to become a secondary oocyte. At this time, the follicle is known as a *secondary* or *graafian follicle*. The follicle continues to enlarge until the time of ovulation. Those follicles not undergoing ovulation become atretic and regress. During the reproductive life of a woman, only 300 to 400 oocytes mature and are extruded in the process of ovulation; the remainder undergo some form of atresia.

It is the process of follicular growth and maturation that is most likely to be affected by cytotoxic chemotherapy. In rats, cyclophosphamide causes destruction of ovarian follicles in a dose-dependent fashion.[101] Incubation of mouse oocytes with doxorubicin results in a series of morphologic and biochemical events resembling apoptosis. Indeed, functional bax protein appears to be necessary for doxorubicin-induced cell death to occur.[102] Knowledge of the molecular events surrounding chemotherapy-induced ovarian failure might permit the development of strategies to prevent this complication of treatment.

The primary histologic lesion noted in the ovaries of women receiving antineoplastic chemotherapy is ovarian fibrosis and follicle destruction.[103–105] Clinically, amenorrhea ensues and is accompanied by elevation of serum FSH and LH levels and by a fall in serum estradiol. Vaginal epithelial atrophy and endometrial hypoplasia occur, and patients may complain of menopausal symptoms such as "hot flashes" or of symptoms of estrogen deficiency such as vaginal dryness and dyspareunia.

The onset and duration of amenorrhea seem to be both dose and age-related. Generally, younger patients are able to tolerate larger cumulative drug doses before amenorrhea occurs and have a greater likelihood of resumption of menses when therapy is discontinued.

Among the anticancer drugs, alkylating agents are the most frequent cause of ovarian dysfunction. During the early clinical trials of busulfan, amenorrhea was a common side effect. Several investigators noted the onset of permanent amenorrhea among patients receiving busulfan in doses varying from 0.5 to 14.0 mg per day for at least 3 months.[106,107]

Cyclophosphamide has been noted to cause a dose-related depletion of antral follicles, a decrease in follicle diameter, and a fall in serum estradiol and progesterone levels in rats receiving the drug.[108] The effects of cyclophosphamide on ovarian function in humans were first noted in the rheumatology literature, as early cessation of menses and menopausal symptoms developed in six of 33 patients treated for rheumatoid arthritis with daily cyclophosphamide for 6 to 40 months.[109] One of these patients had elevated serum FSH levels consistent with primary ovarian

failure. Subsequently, several investigators documented the occurrence of amenorrhea, decreased urinary estrogens, and increased urinary gonadotropins in at least 50% of premenopausal women receiving 40 to 120 mg of cyclophosphamide daily for an average of 18 months.[110,111] Ovarian biopsy in some patients has demonstrated arrest of follicular maturation and absence of ova.

Studies of the use of adjuvant chemotherapy for the prevention of recurrence of breast cancer suggest that the onset of amenorrhea and the resumption of menses are related to the age of the patient during chemotherapy and to the total dose administered.[112–114] Amenorrhea developed in 17 of 18 women treated with adjuvant cyclophosphamide for 13 to 14 months postoperatively.[115] Permanent cessation of menses occurred after a mean total dose of 5.2 g in all patients 40 years of age and older. Amenorrhea also developed in four of five women younger than age 40, but only after a mean cyclophosphamide dose of 9.3 g had been administered. Menses subsequently returned in two of these patients within 6 months of discontinuing therapy. Furthermore, a prospective study of ovarian function in premenopausal women receiving melphalan alone or in combination with 5-FU demonstrated the occurrence of amenorrhea in 22% of patients younger than age 39 but in 73% of patients older than age 40.[116] Time to the development of amenorrhea also appears to be age-related after adjuvant treatment with cyclophosphamide, MTX, and 5-FU (CMF).[117] In women younger than age 35, mean time to the onset of amenorrhea is 5.54 months; for women aged 35 to 45 years, the mean time is 2.31 months, and in women older than age 45, amenorrhea develops very quickly, with a mean onset of 1.01 months. It seems, then, that alkylating agent chemotherapy accelerates the onset of menopause, particularly in older patients, whereas younger patients may tolerate higher total doses before amenorrhea becomes irreversible. Other large studies examining the effects of CMF also have documented this dramatic age-related effect.[118–121]

Among the antimetabolites, only high-dose MTX has been evaluated and seems to have no immediate ovarian toxicity.[32] The effects of oral etoposide on ovarian function were evaluated in one study of 22 patients receiving this agent. Age-related oligo- or amenorrhea occurred in 41% of patients after a mean cumulative etoposide dose of 5 g.[122] Doxorubicin administration does not appear to have profound ovarian ablative effects. In women younger than age 35 who received adjuvant cyclophosphamide, doxorubicin, and 5-FU, 32% had temporary amenorrhea during treatment, and only 9% had permanent amenorrhea.[123]

Studies of adjuvant chemotherapy for breast cancer have yielded other important information regarding the effects of dose and treatment duration on menstrual cycles. Evaluation of 95 premenopausal women who received cyclophosphamide, MTX, 5-FU, vincristine, and prednisone documented permanent amenorrhea in 70.5% of patients.[124] Women receiving chemotherapy for 12 weeks had a 55% incidence of amenorrhea, whereas 83% of women receiving a 36-week regimen were rendered amenorrheic. Breast cancer recurrence and mortality rates in women who experienced amenorrhea were lower than in those who continued to menstruate, even within each treatment group, suggesting a potential therapeutic benefit of ovarian ablation. However, the contribution of treatment-induced amenorrhea to the beneficial effects of adjuvant chemotherapy remains uncertain and controversial.

The risk of ovarian failure after other combination chemotherapy is also clearly related to the age of the patient at the time of treatment. Overall, at least 50% of women treated with MOPP or related regimens become amenorrheic.[125–132] The cessation of menses is accompanied by elevations of serum FSH and LH consistent with primary ovarian failure. Apart from age, no clear differences have been noted between those women who become amenorrheic during therapy and those who do not. In one study, follow-up of MOPP-treated patients for a median of 9 years after the completion of chemotherapy revealed that 46% had developed permanent amenorrhea.[128] Of these women, 89% were older than 25 years at the time of treatment. Moreover, the time of onset of amenorrhea seemed to be age-related; ovarian failure occurred within 1 year of discontinuing therapy in all patients 39 years of age or older, whereas in younger patients there was a gradual decrease in frequency of menses occurring more than several years after therapy. At present, it seems unlikely that those patients treated when younger than age 25 will experience any significant therapy-related ovarian dysfunction during the initial 5 to 10 years after the completion of therapy.

Data suggest that ABVD chemotherapy may be less likely to produce premature menopause, although longer follow-up is required to be certain. Other chemotherapy programs, particularly those used for treatment of germ cell tumors of the ovary, cause relatively little ovarian toxicity.[133] In one study, 70% of women maintained regular menses after treatment with a variety of regimens containing drugs such as actinomycin D, vincristine, and cyclophosphamide. Combination chemotherapy regimens for aggressive non-Hodgkin's lymphoma also do not consistently cause premature ovarian failure, perhaps because procarbazine is rarely included in such regimens.[66] Among seven women aged 35 to 43 treated with MACOP-B or VACOP-B, only one developed amenorrhea.[57] From the same series, two young women who underwent high-dose cyclophosphamide, BCNU, and etoposide followed by autologous bone marrow reinfusion had normal ovarian function 2 years after treatment. From the Seattle experience, cyclophosphamide-containing preparative regimens for allogeneic bone marrow transplantation induced reversible amenorrhea in women younger than 26 years of age but permanent amenorrhea in 67% of women older than

age 26.[78] Regimens using total-body irradiation caused premature menopause in nearly all patients.

Efforts to protect the ovary from the toxic effects of chemotherapy have focused on the use of oral contraceptives to induce ovarian suppression. Preliminary data reported by Chapman and Sutcliffe[134] suggested that ovarian follicles could be protected and normal menses could be preserved by the administration of oral contraceptives during chemotherapy. Only a small number of young women were studied, and follow-up was brief. More recent studies with longer follow-up failed to demonstrate a protective effect of oral contraceptives.[131,132] GnRH analogs may partially protect ovarian follicles and fertility in rats from the damaging effects of cyclophosphamide,[101,135,136] with variable protective effects from x-irradiation.[137,138] However, preliminary clinical observations have failed to demonstrate a protective effect of the LHRH analog buserelin on ovarian function in women undergoing chemotherapy for Hodgkin's disease.[92] In contrast, GnRH agonists may have a protective effect in young women receiving chemotherapy for lymphoma.[139] Buserelin, administered with cyclophosphamide, doxorubicin, and 5-FU for metastatic breast cancer, has been shown to induce ovarian ablation during therapy, but long-term effects on ovarian function have not been reported.[140] Continued long-term, prospective follow-up of women maintaining normal menses during chemotherapy is necessary to determine the degree of risk of premature ovarian failure and early menopause in these individuals.

Chemotherapy Effects in Children

Any study of the effects of cytotoxic chemotherapy on gonadal function in children is particularly complex because of the variables introduced by the continuum of sexual development in this patient population. Thus, the effects of chemotherapy can be expected to vary according to when drugs are given and when their effects are evaluated relative to puberty. The available reports suggest differences in the sensitivity of the prepubertal, pubertal, and adult testis to alkylating-agent chemotherapy. For example, one investigator reported that 15 boys treated with cyclophosphamide when prepubertal or in early puberty had normal serum FSH, LH, and testosterone levels for their age when studied.[141] All had been off therapy for 1.5 to 5.5 years when evaluated, but most were still prepubertal or in early puberty. Testicular biopsy in one patient who received 5.7 g of cyclophosphamide was normal, and biopsies in four other patients receiving 7.5 to 21.5 g showed only focal tubular atrophy.

A prospective evaluation of gonadal function in 14 boys undergoing combination chemotherapy (prednisone, vincristine, MTX, and 6-mercaptopurine) for acute lymphoblastic leukemia showed that these particular agents do not cause irreversible damage to the germinal epithelium.[142] Nine patients were prepubertal, four were intrapubertal, and one was sexually mature at the start of treatment. After a median follow-up of 5.5 years, all patients had normal testicular size and normal serum gonadotropin and testosterone levels. Five of six patients tested had normal semen analyses; one had a low-normal sperm count. Shalet et al.,[143] in a study of 44 patients undergoing chemotherapy for acute lymphoblastic leukemia, found a median decrease of 51% in the number of seminiferous tubules containing spermatogonia as compared with normal age-matched controls. Follow-up of similar patients indicates that testicular function may improve gradually over many years; five of 11 patients who had less than 50% of their tubules containing spermatozoa immediately after chemotherapy for leukemia recovered normal germ cell function (normal testicular volume, FSH level, sperm counts, or a combination of the three) more than 10 years later.[144] These findings suggest that leukemia therapy has definite, although at least partially reversible, effects on the germinal epithelium of the prepubertal and intrapubertal boy.

Although these data suggest that the prepubertal testis may be more resistant to the effects of alkylating agents than the adult gonad, in some patients the time elapsed from cessation of therapy to evaluation may have been sufficient to allow recovery of a previously damaged testis. Etteldorf et al.[145] demonstrated that even for the prepubertal patient, a dose-toxicity relationship may exist. These investigators evaluated eight boys treated with cyclophosphamide at ages 7.5 to 13.0 years. All had been off therapy for 6.5 to 10.0 years when studied. All patients receiving total cyclophosphamide doses of 6.2 to 10.5 g, as well as one patient receiving 14.3 g, had normal sperm counts, testicular histology, and serum gonadotropins, whereas those patients receiving 11.8 to 39.3 g of the drug were uniformly azoospermic with germinal aplasia on biopsy. Clearly, the prepubertal state cannot always protect the germinal epithelium from high doses of alkylating agents. Among 19 prepubertal boys receiving MOPP or more than 9 g per m^2 of cyclophosphamide, 12 were sterile at a mean follow-up of 9 years.[146] Other studies have confirmed that MOPP is toxic to prepubertal testes.[147] From these and other data,[148,149] one can conclude that the prepubertal testis may be more tolerant of moderate doses of alkylating agents than is the adult testis, yet a threshold dose does seem to exist above which germinal epithelial injury will result.[150,151] Malnutrition may further enhance the susceptibility of the prepubertal testis to cytotoxic chemotherapy.[152]

Chemotherapy delivered to male patients during puberty may have profound effects on both germ cell production and endocrine function. Sherins et al.[153] reported studies of testicular function in boys treated with MOPP combination chemotherapy for Hodgkin's disease. Gynecomastia developed in nine of 13 pubertal patients a mean of 28 months after initiation of treatment. This was accompanied by elevated serum FSH and LH levels and by low to normal serum testosterone levels. Testicular biopsy in six patients with gynecomastia

revealed germinal aplasia. Among 12 prepubertal and pubertal boys who received at least six cycles of MOPP for Hodgkin's disease at Stanford, all patients who provided semen for analysis had complete azoospermia as long as 11 years after treatment.[148] Two of these boys (ages 8 and 12 at diagnosis) had recovery of fertility and subsequently fathered children 12 and 15 years after therapy. None of the boys treated during puberty recovered spermatogenesis. However, all boys attained normal sexual maturation, and androgen replacement was not necessary in any patient. These and other data[154] suggest that the germinal epithelium may be permanently damaged by combination chemotherapy in pubertal patients. Leydig cell dysfunction also occurs in some patients and may be manifest as gynecomastia.

Testicular relapse of childhood acute lymphoblastic leukemia occurs in 10% to 15% of patients, usually within 1 year of completion of therapy.[155,156] Treatment of this condition ordinarily involves bilateral testicular irradiation to 2,400 rads along with additional systemic chemotherapy. It has been assumed that although the germinal epithelium may be destroyed by such radiation, Leydig cell function is not adversely affected. Several studies have now appeared, however, that clearly indicate that Leydig cell function and testosterone production may be severely impaired by testicular irradiation.[157–159] In some patients, progression through puberty may be delayed, and testosterone replacement therapy may be required.

Less information is available concerning the effects of cytotoxic chemotherapy on ovarian function in children. There seems to be no delay in menarche and no interruption of menses in girls treated with single-agent cyclophosphamide.[141,151,160,161] Furthermore, Arneil[149] reported normal ovarian histology at postmortem examination in six girls treated with cyclophosphamide for malignancy. However, the drug dosages were not clearly specified. Ovarian biopsy in girls treated for acute lymphoblastic leukemia showed a reduction in the number of follicles and cortical stromal fibrosis, with more severe changes noted in postmenarchal girls.[162] Other investigators have noted absence or inhibition of follicle development after cytotoxic chemotherapy in girls dying from leukemia[163] and solid tumors.[164]

A careful study of ovarian function in girls treated with combination chemotherapy for acute leukemia yielded more encouraging results. Treatment included intermittent cycles of prednisone, vincristine, MTX, and 6-mercaptopurine, with some receiving cyclophosphamide also. Seventeen patients were prepubertal at the time of treatment, 11 were aged 10.5 to 15.5 years but were premenarchal, and seven were postmenarchal.[165] Overall, 80% of the patients demonstrated normal ovarian function when studied. Sixteen of 17 prepubertal patients either had achieved spontaneous menarche or were progressing normally through puberty. Seven of 11 patients of pubertal age at the time of treatment achieved spontaneous menarche, five while receiving chemotherapy. Three patients developed secondary amenorrhea and elevated gonadotropins consistent with ovarian failure, but menses subsequently returned in two. Although ovarian dysfunction was not prominent in this series, it is difficult to draw generally applicable conclusions, because the chemotherapy administered consisted primarily of antimetabolites. It seems that these drugs do not cause ovarian dysfunction in young girls. However, with long-term follow-up, some patients may later experience premature menopause.[166] The effects of combination chemotherapy, including alkylating agents on the prepubertal and pubertal ovary, have been studied in girls receiving treatment for Hodgkin's disease. Preliminary data suggest that ovarian function is likely to be preserved in the majority of patients.[147,167] Preservation of fertility has also been noted in a high proportion of long-term survivors of childhood non-Hodgkin's lymphoma treated with regimens containing cyclophosphamide, vincristine, doxorubicin, and high-dose MTX.[168] However, in one study of 13 prepubertal girls receiving nitrosoureas or procarbazine, or both, for brain tumors, nine showed biochemical evidence of primary ovarian failure (elevated basal FSH level or abnormal peak FSH response to GnRH stimulation), and only three had normal pubertal development and menarche.[169] Longer follow-up is required to determine whether these patients will experience premature menopause.

With the introduction of antineoplastic chemotherapy, lasting clinical remissions have been obtained for many patients who otherwise would have died. The long-term effects of such therapy are only now being recognized. Among them, infertility must be considered an unfortunate but acceptable side effect for many patients. Although alkylating agents seem to be primarily responsible for gonadal injury, doxorubicin,[34] arabinosylcytosine,[170] procarbazine,[67] and vinblastine[171] also have been implicated. A listing of the drugs with cytotoxic effects on fertility is shown in Table 4-3. As new effective antitumor agents are introduced into clinical practice, further screening for gonadal toxicity will become necessary. In addition, long-term prospective studies of reproductive function in patients receiving cancer chemotherapy are necessary to determine the magnitude and duration of gonadal dysfunction resulting from any therapeutic regimen.

TABLE 4-3. DRUG-RELATED INFERTILITY

Definite	Probable	Unlikely
Chlorambucil	Doxorubicin (Adriamycin)	Methotrexate
Cyclophosphamide	Vinblastine	5-Fluorouracil
L-Phenylalanine mustard	Arabinosylcytosine	6-Mercapto-
	Cisplatin	purine
Mechlorethamine hydrochloride	Nitrosoureas	Vincristine
	Amsacrine	Interferon
Busulfan	Etoposide	
Procarbazine	Mitoxantrone	
	Bleomycin	

COUNSELING

For patients facing the problem of chemotherapy-induced sterility, sperm banking before therapy remains a consideration. Although the technology of freezing, preserving, and thawing human semen has advanced considerably, ultimate conception rates using preserved semen remain at only 50% to 60%.[172–175] However, conception rates as high as 80% have been reported for patients who cryopreserved sperm before treatment for Hodgkin's disease.[176] In 1973, Sherman[172] summarized the results of artificial insemination with frozen human semen. Of 621 reported pregnancies, the spontaneous abortion rate was 8% and the congenital abnormality rate was only 1%, both less than expected for the general population. Most physicians practicing artificial insemination, however, prefer fresh donor semen. Among those using frozen semen, the great majority do not store it for longer than 24 months.[174]

For patients with cancer, sperm banking and successful insemination may be even less likely because of poor quality semen. As many as 50% of male patients with Hodgkin's disease and testicular cancer are severely oligospermic or azoospermic before receiving any therapy.[55,56,177–181] The cause of impaired spermatogenesis is unknown. In previously untreated patients with Hodgkin's disease, oligospermia does not correlate with age, stage, presence of systemic symptoms, or fever.[182] Minimal standards of sperm quality for cryopreservation have been proposed to maximize the chances of successful insemination. These include sperm concentration of at least 20×10^6 per mL, postthaw motility greater than 40%, and postthaw progression greater than 2+. Two studies demonstrated that fewer than 20% of lymphoma patients meet these criteria. These findings indicate a low probability of successful semen preservation and, ultimately, of conception. Nevertheless, for some patients, successful artificial insemination or *in vitro* fertilization is possible even when cryopreserved sperm quality is poor.[175,183–185] Thus sperm banking at a reliable institution should be offered to patients if they are properly informed of the cost-benefit ratio of the procedure. Other strategies that have been explored recently include *in vitro* fertilization[186] and gamete micromanipulation. Intracytoplasmic sperm injection is a type of gamete micromanipulation that holds particular promise for azoospermic and oligospermic cancer survivors. Intracytoplasmic sperm injection is the direct injection of a single sperm into the cytoplasm of an oocyte in the context of *in vitro* fertilization. Patients with semen samples devoid of sperm are still candidates for the procedure, because sperm may be obtained through epididymal aspiration or testicular sperm extraction (TESE). Through TESE, testicular biopsy tissue is macerated, centrifuged, and examined for the presence of sperm. TESE is an important method of sperm recovery for patients who have undergone cytotoxic chemotherapy and have apparent germinal aplasia. One group showed that 76% of patients with either complete germinal aplasia or maturation arrest on biopsy had recoverable sperm after TESE, presumably because of adjacent areas of intact spermatogenesis.[187] The reported pregnancy rates range from 30% to 40% and do not appear to be significantly altered by the source of sperm or the testicular history.[187–190]

Until recently, no reliable techniques existed for women who wished to retain the ability to bear children following ovarian ablative chemotherapy. Oocyte freezing and storage have been partially successful. However, embryos may now be cryopreserved for later intrafallopian or intrauterine transfer.[191] Before initiation of chemotherapy, women may have oocytes harvested and fertilized *in vitro* with husband or donor sperm. The embryos can be stored in liquid nitrogen and thawed for implantation at a later date when the patient's endometrium has been hormonally prepared. This option has been associated with pregnancy and take-home baby rates of 30% to 35% and 29%, respectively.[192] In women who did not have frozen zygotes or embryos stored before chemotherapy, donor ova are available for fertilization and implantation at specialized fertility centers.

A technique that holds great promise for women anticipating treatment with potentially sterilizing chemotherapy is ovarian autografting. Already in clinical trials in England, the technique relies on the removal of oocyte-rich ovarian cortical tissue that is then slowly cooled and stored in a cryopreservative. At a later date, the tissue may be thawed and reimplanted near the fallopian tubes for potentially natural ovulation and fertilization. Gosden's group, which pioneered this technique, reported successful pregnancies in sheep and is now applying the technique to humans.[193–196]

Patients in whom reproductive capacity returns after chemotherapy frequently have questions concerning the risks of spontaneous abortion and fetal abnormalities. The incidence of spontaneous abortions was significantly higher among nurses who handled chemotherapeutic agents during pregnancy than among women who were not exposed (26% versus 15%).[197] Cytotoxic chemotherapy administered during pregnancy, particularly the first trimester, is teratogenic. However, the magnitude of the risk is difficult to estimate from anecdotal reports in the literature. A recent review of pregnancy outcome in 58 women treated for acute leukemia during pregnancy revealed a higher incidence of spontaneous abortion and premature delivery when leukemia was diagnosed and treated during the first or second trimester.[198] However, congenital malformations were rare, and long-term follow-up of a small number of children has shown normal growth and development thus far. Another study examined pregnancy outcome among 21 women who were treated with chemotherapy during pregnancy for a variety of malignancies.[199] Thirteen women received chemotherapy during the first trimester. There were four spontaneous

abortions and four elective abortions. Only five were carried to term, and of those, two had major congenital malformations. Among four women who were treated during the second trimester, there was one stillbirth, one elective abortion, and two normal live births. All infants exposed to chemotherapy *in utero* during the third trimester were normal at birth. The children born alive had lower birth weights, lower gestational age at birth, and significant intrauterine growth retardation compared with a control group matched for maternal age. This study suggested a serious teratogenic effect of chemotherapy during the first trimester and lesser effects when chemotherapy was administered during the third trimester. Few studies report long-term follow-up of the children exposed to chemotherapy *in utero*, but available reports suggest that there are no adverse effects detected in childhood or adolescence in children who are born alive and well.[200]

The mutagenic potential of cancer chemotherapy remains largely undefined. Some anecdotal reports suggest that there is no increased incidence of spontaneous abortion or fetal abnormalities in those women treated with chemotherapy in comparison with the general population.[123,201–204] Several larger series and reviews have generally confirmed this.[205–209] However, one study indicated that structural congenital cardiac defects are more prevalent among children of women previously treated with dactinomycin.[205] Another study has suggested that women previously treated with both chemotherapy and irradiation have a greater chance of pregnancy ending in abortion or with delivery of an abnormal child than do sibling controls.[210] When male rats are exposed to chemotherapy before mating with nonexposed females, there is reduced litter size[211,212] and increased incidence of fetal losses[213] in the resulting pregnancies. In the subsequent progeny, there is also a slight increase in congenital malformations,[212,213] abnormal karyotypes,[212] and tumors.[211] At present, it is impossible to define the risk of fetal wastage or abnormality in patients previously treated with cytotoxic drugs. Whether a specific fetal abnormality may occur more commonly than others or whether a specific drug class, dose, or combination is more mutagenic than others remains unknown. Additional studies carried out over many years are required before the true risks to subsequent generations are known.

Women who develop premature ovarian failure due to cytotoxic chemotherapy and those taking tamoxifen also may be subject to the physical and emotional disorders that accompany estrogen deficiency. Depressed libido, irritability, sleep disturbances, and poor self-image all occur commonly in women with treatment-related amenorrhea.[127,214] Hormone replacement therapy may be of considerable benefit to patients with chemotherapy-induced amenorrhea, frequently producing dramatic relief of hot flashes, dyspareunia, and irritability. Another potential benefit of estrogen replacement therapy may be prevention of postmenopausal osteoporosis and diminished risk of premature atherosclerosis.

The long-term consequences of cancer treatment will take many more years to define. The effects of the disease and its treatment may become increasingly difficult to separate as cancer survivors become older. A recent follow-up of 2,283 long-term survivors of childhood cancer reveals that the extent of fertility impairment depends on the gender of the patient and the diagnosis, as well as on the type of therapy received.[215] Evaluation of the late effects of cancer treatment is an ongoing responsibility of the oncology community. Clearly, continued long-term follow-up of cancer survivors is necessary to define fully the spectrum of delayed toxicities of cancer treatment.

REFERENCES

1. Longo DL, Young RC, Wesley M, et al. Twenty years of MOPP therapy for Hodgkin's disease. *J Clin Oncol* 1986; 4:1295.
2. George SL, Aur RJA, Mauer AM, et al. A reappraisal of the results of stopping therapy in childhood leukemia. *N Engl J Med* 1979;300:269.
3. Lewis JL. Current status of treatment of gestational trophoblastic disease. *Cancer* 1976;38:620.
4. Einhorn LH, Donohue J. cis-Diamminedichloroplatinum, vinblastine, and bleomycin combination chemotherapy in disseminated testicular cancer. *Ann Intern Med* 1977;87:293.
5. Walsh PC, Amelar RD. Embryology, anatomy and physiology of the male reproductive system. In: Amelar RD, Dubin L, Walsh PC, eds. *Male infertility*. Philadelphia: WB Saunders, 1977:3.
6. Helen CG, Clermont Y. Kinetics of the germinal epithelium in man. *Recent Prog Horm Res* 1964;20:545.
7. Clermont Y. Kinetics of spermatogenesis in mammals: seminiferous epithelium cycle and spermatogonial renewal. *Physiol Rev* 1972;52:198.
8. Lu CC, Meistrich ML. Cytotoxic effects of chemotherapeutic drugs on mouse testis cells. *Cancer Res* 1979;39:3575.
9. Meistrich ML, Finch M, da Cunha MF, et al. Damaging effects of fourteen chemotherapeutic drugs on mouse testis cells. *Cancer Res* 1982;42:122.
10. Russell LD, Russell JA. Short-term morphologic response of the rat testis to administration of five chemotherapeutic agents. *Am J Anat* 1991;192:142.
11. Jackson H. The effects of alkylating agents on fertility. *Br Med Bull* 1964;20:107.
12. Jackson H, Fox BW, Craig AW. Antifertility substances and their assessment in the male rodent. *J Reprod Fertil* 1961; 2:447.
13. Martin RH. Detection of genetic damage in human sperm. *Reprod Toxicol* 1993;7:47.
14. Genesca A, Miro R, Caballin MR, et al. Sperm chromosome studies in individuals treated for testicular cancer. *Hum Reprod* 1990;5:286.
15. Jenderny J, Jacobi ML, Ruger A, et al. Chromosome aberrations in 450 sperm complements from eight controls and lack of increase after chemotherapy in two patients. *Hum Genet* 1992;90:151.
16. Fossa SD, Melvik JE, Juul NO, et al. DNA flow cytometry in sperm cells from testicular cancer patients: impact of different treatment modalities on spermatogenesis. *Eur Urol* 1991;19:125.
17. Fossa SD, DeAngelis P, Kraggerud SM, et al. Prediction of posttreatment spermatogenesis in patients with testicular cancer by flow cytometric sperm chromatin structure assay. *Cytometry* 1997;30:192–196.
18. Booth JD, Loriaux DL. Selective control of follicle stimulating hormone secretion: new perspectives. In: D'Aguta R, Lipsett MB, Polosa P, et al., eds. *Recent advances in male reproduction: molecular basis and clinical implications.* New York: Raven Press, 1983:269.
19. Howell SJ, Radford JA, Ryder WDJ, et al. Testicular function after cytotoxic chemotherapy: evidence of Leydig cell insufficiency. *J Clin Oncol* 1999;17(5):1493–1498.
20. Fairley KF, Barrie JU, Johnson W. Sterility and testicular atrophy related to cyclophosphamide therapy. *Lancet* 1972;1:568.
21. Meistrich ML, Wilson G, Brown BW, et al. Impact of cyclophosphamide on long-term reduction in sperm count in men treated with combination chemotherapy for Ewing and soft tissue sarcomas. *Cancer* 1992;70:2703.
22. Kumar R, Biggart JD, McEvoy J, et al. Cyclophosphamide and reproductive function. *Lancet* 1972;1:1212.
23. Richter P, Calamera JC, Morgenfeld MC, et al. Effect of chlorambucil on spermatogenesis in the human with malignant lymphoma. *Cancer* 1970;25:1026.
24. Miller DG. Alkylating agents and human spermatogenesis. *JAMA* 1971;217:1662.
25. Maguire LC, Dick FR, Sherman BM. The effects of antileukemia therapy on gonadal histology in adult males. *Cancer* 1981;48:1967.
26. Qureshi MJA, Goldsmith HJ, Pennington HJ, et al. Cyclophosphamide therapy and sterility. *Lancet* 1972;2:1290.
27. Cheviakoff J, Calamera JC, Morgenfeld M, et al. Recovery of spermatogenesis in patients with lymphoma after treatment with chlorambucil. *J Reprod Fertil* 1973;33:155.
28. Van Thiel DH, Sherins RJ, Myers GH, et al. Evidence for a specific seminiferous tubular factor affecting follicle-stimulating hormone secretion in man. *J Clin Invest* 1972; 51:1009.
29. Mecklenberg RS, Sherins RJ. Gonadotropin response to luteinizing hormone releasing hormone in men with germinal aplasia. *J Clin Endocrinol Metab* 1974;38:1005.
30. Jacobson RJ, Sagel J, Distiller LA, et al. Leydig cell dysfunction in male patients with Hodgkin's disease receiving chemotherapy. *Clin Res* 1978;26:437A.
31. Chapman RM, Sutcliffe SB, Rees LH, et al. Cyclical combination chemotherapy and gonadal function. *Lancet* 1979; 1:285.
32. Shamberger RC, Rosenberg SA, Seipp CA, et al. Effects of high dose methotrexate and vincristine on ovarian and testicular functions in patients undergoing postoperative adjuvant treatment of osteosarcoma. *Cancer Treat Rep* 1981;65:739.
33. Riccardi R, Vigersky R, Bleyer WA, et al. Studies of the blood-testis barrier to methotrexate in rats. *Proc Am Soc Clin Oncol* 1981;22:365.

34. Lui R, LaRegina M, Johnson F. Testicular cytotoxicity of doxorubicin in rats. *Proc Am Assoc Cancer Res* 1985;26:371.

35. Shamberger RC, Sherins RJ, Rosenberg SA. The effect of postoperative adjuvant chemotherapy and radiotherapy on testicular function in men undergoing treatment for soft tissue sarcoma. *Cancer* 1981;47:2368.

36. Meistrich ML, da Cunha MF, Chawla SP, et al. Sperm production following chemotherapy for sarcomas. *Proc Am Assoc Cancer Res* 1985;26:170.

37. Bonadonna G, Santoro A. Chemotherapy in the treatment of Hodgkin's disease. *Cancer Treat Rep* 1982;9:21.

38. Meistrich ML, Chawla SP, da Cunha MF, et al. Recovery of sperm production after chemotherapy for osteosarcoma. *Cancer* 1989;63:2115.

39. da Cunha MF, Meistrich MF, Haq MM, et al. Temporary effects of AMSA chemotherapy on spermatogenesis. *Cancer* 1982;49:2459.

40. Schilsky RL, Davidson HS, Magid D, et al. Gonadal and sexual function in male patients with hairy cell leukemia: lack of adverse effects of recombinant alpha-2 interferon treatment. *Cancer Treat Rep* 1987;71:179.

41. Drasga RE, Einhorn LH, Williams SD, et al. Fertility after chemotherapy for testicular cancer. *J Clin Oncol* 1983;1:179.

42. Tseng A, Kessler R, Freiha F, et al. Male fertility before and after treatment of testicular cancer. *Proc Am Soc Clin Oncol* 1984;3:161.

43. Nijman JM, Koops HS, Kremer J, et al. Gonadal function after surgery and chemotherapy in men with stage II and III nonseminomatous testicular tumors. *J Clin Oncol* 1987;5:651.

44. Leitner SP, Bosl GJ, Bajorunas D. Gonadal dysfunction in patients treated for metastatic germ cell tumors. *J Clin Oncol* 1986;4:1500.

45. Hansen SW, Berthelsen JG, von der Maase H. Long-term fertility and Leydig cell function in patients treated for germ cell cancer with cisplatin, vinblastine, and bleomycin versus surveillance. *J Clin Oncol* 1990;8:1695.

46. Stephenson WT, Poirier SM, Rubin L, Einhorn LH. Evaluation of reproductive capacity in germ cell tumor patients following treatment with cisplatin, etoposide and bleomycin. *J Clin Oncol* 1995;13(9):2278–2280.

47. Grossfeld GD, Small EJ. Long-term side effects of treatment for testis cancer. *Urol Clin North Am* 1998;25(3):503–515.

48. Stuart NSA, Woodroffe CM, Grundy R, et al. Long-term toxicity of chemotherapy for testicular cancer—the cost of cure. *Br J Cancer* 1989;61:479.

49. Pont J, Albrecht W. Fertility after chemotherapy for testicular germ cell cancer. *Fertil Steril* 1997;68(1):1–5.

50. Sherins RJ, DeVita VT. Effects of drug treatment for lymphoma on male reproductive capacity. *Ann Intern Med* 1973;79:216.

51. Asbjornsen G, Molne K, Klepp O, et al. Testicular function after combination chemotherapy for Hodgkin's disease. *Scand J Haematol* 1976;16:66.

52. Chapman R, Sutcliffe SB, Rees L, et al. Cyclical combination chemotherapy and gonadal function: retrospective study in males. *Lancet* 1979;1:265.

53. Whitehead E, Shalet SM, Blackledge G, et al. The effects of Hodgkin's disease and combination chemotherapy on gonadal function in the adult male. *Cancer* 1982;49:418.

54. Wang C, Ng RP, Chan TK, et al. Effect of combination chemotherapy on pituitary gonadal function in patients with lymphoma and leukemia. *Cancer* 1980;45:2030.

55. Chapman RM, Sutcliffe SB, Malpas JS. Male gonadal dysfunction in Hodgkin's disease: a prospective study. *JAMA* 1981;245:1323.

56. Viviani S, Ragni G, Santoro A, et al. Testicular dysfunction in Hodgkin's disease before and after treatment. *Eur J Cancer* 1991;27:1389.

57. Muller U, Stahel RA. Gonadal function after MACOP-B or VACOP-B with or without dose intensification and ABMT in young patients with aggressive non-Hodgkin's lymphoma. *Ann Oncol* 1993;4:399.

58. Pryzant RM, Meistrich ML, Wilson G, et al. Long-term reduction in sperm count after chemotherapy with and without radiation therapy for non-Hodgkin's lymphomas. *J Clin Oncol* 1993;11:239.

59. Brennemann W, Stoffel-Wagner B, Bidlingmaier F, et al. Immunoreactive plasma inhibin levels in men after polyvalent chemotherapy of germinal cell cancer. *Acta Endocrinol* 1992;126:224.

60. Buchanan JD, Fairley KF, Barrie JU. Return of spermatogenesis after stopping cyclophosphamide therapy. *Lancet* 1975;2:156.

61. Hinkes E, Plotkin D. Reversible drug-induced sterility in a patient with acute leukemia. *JAMA* 1973;223:1490.

62. Blake DA, Heller RH, Hsu SH, et al. Return of fertility in a patient with cyclophosphamide-induced azoospermia. *Johns Hopkins Med J* 1976;139:20.

63. Waxman JHX, Terry YA, Wrigley PFM, et al. Gonadal function in Hodgkin's disease: long-term follow-up of chemotherapy. *Br Med J* 1982;285:1612.

64. da Cunha MF, Meistrich ML, Fuller LM, et al. Recovery of spermatogenesis after treatment for Hodgkin's disease: limiting dose of MOPP chemotherapy. *J Clin Oncol* 1984;2:571.

65. Roeser HP, Stocks AE, Smith AJ. Testicular damage due to cytotoxic drugs and recovery after cessation of therapy. *Aust N Z J Med* 1978;8:250.

66. Bokemeyer C, Schmoll H-J, van Rhee J, et al. Long-term gonadal toxicity after therapy for Hodgkin's and non-Hodgkin's lymphoma. *Ann Hematol* 1994;68:105–110.

67. Sieber SM, Correa P, Dalgard DW, et al. Carcinogenic and other adverse effects of procarbazine in nonhuman primates. *Cancer Res* 1978;38:2125.

68. Evenson DP, Arlin Z, Welt S, et al. Male reproductive capacity may recover following drug treatment with the L-10 protocol for acute lymphocytic leukemia. *Cancer* 1984;53:30.

69. Santoro A, Bonadonna G, Valagussa P, et al. Long-term results of combined chemotherapy-radiotherapy approach in Hodgkin's disease: superiority of ABVD plus radiotherapy versus MOPP plus radiotherapy. *J Clin Oncol* 1987;5:27.

70. Kulkarni SS, Sastry PS, Saikia TK, et al. Gonadal function following ABVD therapy for Hodgkin's disease. *Am J Clin Oncol* 1997;20(4):354–357.

71. Meistrich ML, Wilson G, Mathur K, et al. Rapid recovery of spermatogenesis after mitoxantrone, vincristine, vinblastine, and prednisone chemotherapy for Hodgkin's disease. *J Clin Oncol* 1997;15(12):3488–3495.

72. Fossa SD, Aabyholm T, Vepestad S, et al. Semen quality after treatment for testicular cancer. *Eur Urol* 1993;23:172.

73. Hansen PV, Trykker H, Helkjaer PE, et al. Testicular function in patients with testicular cancer treated with orchiectomy alone or orchiectomy with cisplatin-based chemotherapy. *J Natl Cancer Inst* 1989;81:1246.

74. Chakraborty PR, Neave F. Recovery of fertility 14 years following radiotherapy and chemotherapy for testicular tumor. *Clin Oncol* 1993;5:253.

75. Fosse SD, Theodorsen L, Norman N, et al. Recovery of impaired pretreatment spermatogenesis in testicular cancer. *Fertil Steril* 1990;54:493.

76. Kader HA, Rostom AY. Follicle-stimulating hormone levels as a predictor of recovery of spermatogenesis following cancer therapy. *Clin Oncol* 1991;3:37.

77. Siimes MA, Elomaa I, Koskimies A. Testicular function after chemotherapy for osteosarcoma. *Eur J Cancer* 1990;26:973.

78. Sanders J, Sullivan K, Witherspoon R, et al. Long-term effects and quality of life in children and adults after bone marrow transplantation. *Bone Marrow Transplant* 1989;4:27.

79. Keilholz U, Max R, Scheibenbogen C, et al. Endocrine function and bone metabolism 5 years after autologous bone marrow/blood-derived progenitor cell transplantation. *Cancer* 1997;79:1617–1622.

80. Heber D, Dodson R, Peterson M, et al. Counteractive effects of agonistic and antagonistic gonadotropin-releasing hormone analogs on spermatogenesis: sites of action. *Fertil Steril* 1984;41:309.

81. Vickery BH, McRae GI, Briones W, et al. Effects of an LHRH agonist analog upon sexual function in male dogs: suppression, reversibility and effect of testosterone replacement. *J Androl* 1984;5:28.

82. Bint Akhtar F, Marshall GR, Wickings EJ, et al. Reversible induction of azoospermia in rhesus monkeys by constant infusion of a GnRH agonist using osmotic minipumps. *J Clin Endocrinol Metab* 1983;56:534.

83. Linde R, Doelle GC, Alexander N, et al. Reversible inhibition of testicular steroidogenesis and spermatogenesis by a potent gonadotropin-releasing hormone agonist in normal men. *N Engl J Med* 1981;305:663.

84. Glode LM, Robinson J, Gould SF. Protection from cyclophosphamide-induced testicular damage with an analog of gonadotropin-releasing hormone. *Lancet* 1981;1:1132.

85. da Cunha MF, Meistrich ML, Nader S. Absence of testicular protection by a gonadotropin-releasing hormone analog against cyclophosphamide-induced testicular cytotoxicity in the mouse. *Cancer Res* 1987;47:1093.

86. Schally AV, Paz-Bouza JL, Schlosser JV, et al. Protective effects of analogs of luteinizing hormone-releasing hormone against x-irradiation-induced testicular damage in rats. *Proc Natl Acad Sci U S A* 1987;84:851.

87. Ward JA, Robinson J, Furr BJA. Protection of spermatogenesis in rats from the cytotoxic procarbazine by the depot formulation of Zoladex, a gonadotropin-releasing hormone agonist. *Cancer Res* 1990;50:568.

88. Meistrich ML, Wilson G, Zhang Y, et al. Protection from procarbazine-induced testicular damage by hormonal pretreatment does not involve arrest of spermatogonial proliferation. *Cancer Res* 1997;57:1091–1097.

89. Lewis RW, Dowling KJ, Schally AV. D-Tryptophan-6 analog of luteinizing hormone-releasing hormone as a protective agent against testicular damage caused by cyclophosphamide in baboons. *Proc Natl Acad Sci U S A* 1985;82:2975.

90. Johnson DH, Linde R, Hainsworth JD, et al. Effect of a luteinizing hormone releasing hormone agonist given during combination chemotherapy on posttherapy fertility in male patients with lymphoma: preliminary observations. *Blood* 1985;65:832.

91. Kreuser ED, Hetzel WD, Hautmann R, et al. Reproductive toxicity with and without LHRHA administration during adjuvant chemotherapy in patients with germ cell tumors. *Horm Metab Res* 1990;22:494.

92. Waxman JH, Ahmed R, Smith D, et al. Failure to preserve fertility in patients with Hodgkin's disease. *Cancer Chemother Pharmacol* 1987;19:159.

93. Krause W, Pfluger KH. Treatment with the gonadotropin-releasing hormone agonist buserelin to protect spermatogenesis against cytotoxic treatment in young men. *Andrologia* 1989;21:265.

94. Dehe JI, Bush C, Peckham MJ. Protection from procarbazine-induced damage of spermatogenesis in the rat by androgen. *Cancer Res* 1986;46:1909.

95. Meistrich ML, Wilson G, Ye W-S, et al. Hormonal protection from procarbazine-induced testicular damage is selective for survival and recovery of stem spermatogonia. *Cancer Res* 1994;54:1027.

96. Parchuri N, Wilson G, Meistrich ML. Protection by gonadal steroid hormones against procarbazine-induced damage to spermatogenic function in LBNF$_1$ hybrid rats. *J Androl* 1993;14:257.

97. Johnson FE, Liebscher GJ, LaRegina MC, et al. Preservation of fertility following doxorubicin administration in the rat. *Surg Oncol* 1992;1:145.

98. Gibbons JJ, Parra RO, Andriole GL, et al. Testicular circulatory isolation: a phase I study. *Surg Oncol* 1992;1:413.

99. Mayer DL, Odell WD. *Physiology of reproduction*. St Louis: CV Mosby, 1971:20.

100. Peters H, Byskov AG, Himelstein-Braw R, et al. Follicular growth: the basic event in the mouse and human ovary. *J Reprod Fertil* 1975;4:559.

101. Montz FJ, Wolff AJ, Gambone JC, et al. Gonadal protection and fecundity in cyclophosphamide-treated rats. *Cancer Res* 1991;51:2124.

102. Tilly JL. Molecular and genetic basis of normal and toxicant-induced apoptosis in female germ cells. *Toxicol Lett* 1998;102–103:497–501.

103. Belohorsky B, Siracky J, Sandor L, et al. Comments on the development of amenorrhea caused by Myleran in cases of chronic myelosis. *Neoplasma* 1960;4:397.

104. Sobrinho LG, Levine RA, DeConti RC. Amenorrhea in patients with Hodgkin's disease treated with antineoplastic agents. *Am J Obstet Gynecol* 1971;109:135.

105. Miller JJ, Williams GF, Leissring JC. Multiple late complications of therapy with cyclophosphamide including ovarian destruction. *Am J Med* 1971;50:530.

106. Louis J, Limarzi LR, Best WR. Treatment of chronic granulocytic leukemia and Myleran. *Arch Intern Med* 1957;97:299.

107. Galton DAG, Till M, Wiltshaw E. Busulfan: summary of clinical results. *Ann N Y Acad Sci* 1958;68:967.

108. Janell J, Young Lai EV, Bau R, et al. Ovarian toxicity of cyclophosphamide alone and in combination with ovarian irradiation in the rat. *Cancer Res* 1987;47:2340.

109. Fosdick WM, Parsons JL, Hill DF. Long-term cyclophosphamide therapy in rheumatoid arthritis. *Arthritis Rheum* 1968;11:151.

110. Warne GL, Fairley KF, Hobbs JB, et al. Cyclophosphamide-induced ovarian failure. *N Engl J Med* 1973;289:1159.

111. Uldall PR, Kerr DNS, Tacchi D. Sterility and cyclophosphamide. *Lancet* 1972;1:693.

112. Dnistrian AM, Schwartz MK, Fracchia AA, et al. Endocrine consequences of CMF adjuvant therapy in premenopausal and postmenopausal breast cancer patients. *Cancer* 1983;51:803.

113. Samaan NA, DeAsis DN, Buzdar AU, et al. Pituitary-ovarian function in breast cancer patients on adjuvant chemoimmunotherapy. *Cancer* 1978;41:2084.

114. Ravdin PM, Fritz NF, Tormey DC, et al. Endocrine status of premenopausal node-positive breast cancer patients following adjuvant chemotherapy and long term tamoxifen. *Cancer Res* 1988;48:1026.

115. Koyama H, Wada T, Nishizawa Y, et al. Cyclophosphamide-induced ovarian failure and its therapeutic significance in patients with breast cancer. *Cancer* 1977;39:1403.

116. Fisher B, Sherman B, Rockette H, et al. L-Phenylalanine mustard in the management of premenopausal patients with primary breast cancer. *Cancer* 1979;44:847.

117. Mehta RR, Beattie CW, Das Gupta TK. Endocrine profile in breast cancer patients receiving chemotherapy. *Breast Cancer Res Treat* 1991;20:125.

118. Goldhirsch A, Gelber RD, Castiglione M. The magnitude of endocrine effects of adjuvant chemotherapy for premenopausal breast cancer patients. *Ann Oncol* 1990;1:183.

119. Reichman BS, Green KB. Breast cancer in young women: effect of chemotherapy on ovarian function, fertility and birth defects. *J Natl Cancer Inst Mono* 1994;16:125–129.

120. Bines J, Oleske DM, Cobleigh MA. Ovarian function in premenopausal women treated with adjuvant chemotherapy for breast cancer. *J Clin Oncol* 1996;14(5):1718–1729.

121. Hensley ML, Reichman BS. Fertility and pregnancy after adjuvant chemotherapy for breast cancer. *Crit Rev in Oncl/Hema* 1998;28:121–128.

122. Choo YC, Chan SYW, Wong LC, et al. Ovarian dysfunction in patients with gestational trophoblastic neoplasia treated with short intensive courses of etoposide. *Cancer* 1985;55:2348.

123. Sutton R, Buzdar AU, Hortobagyi GN. Pregnancy and offspring after adjuvant chemotherapy in breast cancer patients. *Cancer* 1990;65:847.

124. Reyno LM, Levine MN, Skingley P, et al. Chemotherapy induced amenorrhea in a randomized trial of adjuvant chemotherapy duration in breast cancer. *Eur J Cancer* 1993;29A:21.

125. Morgenfeld MC, Goldberg V, Parisier H, et al. Ovarian lesions due to cytostatic agents during the treatment of Hodgkin's disease. *Surg Gynecol Obstet* 1972;134:826.

126. Sherins R, Winokur S, DeVita VT, et al. Surprisingly high risk of functional castration in women receiving chemotherapy for lymphoma. *Clin Res* 1975;23:343.

127. Chapman RM, Sutcliffe SB, Malpas JS. Cytotoxic-induced ovarian failure in women with Hodgkin's disease: I. Hormone function. *JAMA* 1979;242:1877.

128. Schilsky RL, Sherins RJ, Hubbard SM, et al. Long-term follow-up of ovarian function in women treated with MOPP chemotherapy for Hodgkin's disease. *Am J Med* 1981;71:552.

129. Horning SJ, Hoppe RT, Kaplan HS, et al. Female reproductive potential after treatment for Hodgkin's disease. *N Engl J Med* 1981;304:1377.

130. Andrieu JM, Ochoa-Molina ME. Menstrual cycle, pregnancies and offspring before and after MOPP therapy for Hodgkin's disease. *Cancer* 1983;52:435.

131. Whitehead E, Shalet SM, Blackledge G, et al. The effect of combination chemotherapy on ovarian function in women treated for Hodgkin's disease. *Cancer* 1993;52:988.

132. Specht L, Hansen MM, Geisler C. Ovarian function in young women in long-term remission after treatment for Hodgkin's disease stage I or II. *Scand J Haematol* 1984;32:265.

133. Gershenson DM. Menstrual and reproductive function after treatment with combination chemotherapy for malignant ovarian germ cell tumors. *J Clin Oncol* 1988;6:270.

134. Chapman RM, Sutcliffe SB. Protection of ovarian function by oral contraceptives in women receiving chemotherapy for Hodgkin's disease. *Blood* 1981;58:849.

135. Ataya KM, McKanna JA, Neintraub AM, et al. A luteinizing hormone–releasing hormone agonist for the prevention of chemotherapy-induced ovarian failure in rats. *Cancer Res* 1985;45:3651.

136. Ataya K, Ramahi-Ataya A. Reproductive performance of female rats treated with cyclophosphamide and/or LHRH agonist. *Reprod Toxicol* 1993;7:229.

137. Janell J, Younglai EV, McMahon A, et al. Effects of ionizing radiation and pretreatment with [D-Leu(6), des-Gly(10)]luteinizing hormone-releasing hormone ethylamide on developing rat ovarian follicles. *Cancer Res* 1987;47:5005.

138. Jarrell JF, McMahon A, Barr RD, et al. The agonist (D-leu-6, des-gly-10)-LHRH-ethylamide does not protect the fecundity of rats exposed to high dose unilateral ovarian irradiation. *Reprod Toxicol* 1991;5:385.

139. Blumenfeld Z, Haim N. Prevention of gonadal damage during cytotoxic therapy. *Ann Med* 1997;29:199–206.

140. Falkson G, Falkson HC. CAF and nasal buserelin in the treatment of premenopausal women with metastatic breast cancer. *Eur J Clin Oncol* 1989;25:737.

141. Pennisi AJ, Grushkin CM, Lieberman E. Gonadal function in children with nephrosis treated with cyclophosphamide. *Am J Dis Child* 1975;129:315.

142. Blatt J, Poplack DG, Sherins RJ. Testicular function in boys after chemotherapy for acute lymphoblastic leukemia. *N Engl J Med* 1981;304:1121.

143. Shalet SM, Hann IM, Lendon M, et al. Testicular function after combination chemotherapy in childhood for acute lymphoblastic leukemia. *Arch Dis Child* 1981;56:275.

144. Wallace WHB, Shalet SM, Lendon M, et al. Male fertility in long-term survivors of childhood acute lymphoblastic leukaemia. *Int J Androl* 1991;14:312.

145. Etteldorf JN, West CD, Pitcock JA, et al. Gonadal function, testicular histology, and meiosis following cyclophosphamide therapy in patients with nephrotic syndrome. *J Pediatr* 1976;88:206.

146. Aubier F, Flamant F, Brauner R, et al. Male gonadal function after chemotherapy for solid tumors in childhood. *J Clin Oncol* 1989;7:304.

147. Ortin TT, Shostak CA, Donaldson SS. Gonadal status and reproductive function following treatment for Hodgkin's disease in childhood: the Stanford experience. *Int J Radiat Oncol Biol Phys* 1990;19:873.

148. Kirkland RT, Bongiovanni AM, Cornfeld D, et al. Gonadotropin responses to luteinizing releasing factor in boys treated with cyclophosphamide for nephrotic syndrome. *J Pediatr* 1976;89:941.

149. Arneil GC. Cyclophosphamide and the prepubertal testis. *Lancet* 1972;2:1259.

150. Rapola J, Koskimies O, Hutternen NP, et al. Cyclophosphamide and the pubertal testis. *Lancet* 1973;1:98.

151. Lentz RD, Bergstein J, Steffes MW, et al. Post-pubertal evaluation of gonadal function following cyclophosphamide therapy before and during puberty. *J Pediatr* 1977;91:385.

152. Matus-Ridley M, Nicosia SV, Meadows AT. Gonadal effects of cancer therapy in boys. *Cancer* 1985;55:2353.

153. Sherins RJ, Olweny CLM, Ziegler JL. Gynecomastia and gonadal dysfunction in adolescent boys treated with combination chemotherapy for Hodgkin's disease. *N Engl J Med* 1978;299:12.

154. Whitehead E, Shalet SM, Morris-Jones PH, et al. Gonadal function after combination chemotherapy for Hodgkin's disease in childhood. *Arch Dis Child* 1982;47:287.

155. Askin FB, Land VJ, Sullivan MP, et al. Occult testicular leukemia: testicular biopsy at three years continuous complete remission of childhood leukemia: a Southwest Oncology Group Study. *Cancer* 1981;47:470.

156. Hensle TW, Burbige KA, Shepard BR, et al. Chemotherapy and its effect on testicular morphology in children. *J Urol* 1984;131:1142.

157. Brauner R, Czernichow P, Cramer P, et al. Leydig cell function in children after direct testicular irradiation for acute lymphoblastic leukemia. *N Engl J Med* 1983;309:25.

158. Leiper AD, Grant DB, Chessells JM. The effect of testicular irradiation on Leydig cell function in prepubertal boys with acute lymphoblastic leukemia. *Arch Dis Child* 1983;58:906.

159. Blatt J, Sherins RJ, Niebrugge D, et al. Leydig cell function in boys following treatment for testicular relapse of acute lymphoblastic leukemia. *J Clin Oncol* 1985;3:1227.

160. Chiu J, Drummond KN. Long-term follow-up of cyclophosphamide therapy in frequent relapsing minimal lesion nephrotic syndrome. *J Pediatr* 1974;84:825.

161. DeGroot GW, Faiman C, Winter JSD. Cyclophosphamide and the prepubertal gonad: a negative report. *J Pediatr* 1974;84:123.

162. Marcello MF, Nuciforo G, Romeo R, et al. Structural and ultrastructural study of the ovary in childhood leukemia after successful treatment. *Cancer* 1990;66:2099.

163. Himelstein-Braw R, Peters H, Faber M. Morphological study of the ovaries of leukemic children. *Br J Cancer* 1978;38:82.

164. Nicosia SV, Matus-Ridley M, Meadows AT. Gonadal effects of cancer therapy in girls. *Cancer* 1985;55:2364.

165. Siris EJ, Leventhal BG, Vaitukaitis JL. Effects of childhood leukemia and chemotherapy on puberty and reproductive function in girls. *N Engl J Med* 1976;294:1143.

166. Byrne J, Fears TR, Gail MH, et al. Early menopause of long-term survivors of cancer during adolescence. *Am J Obstet Gynecol* 1992;66:788.

167. Green DM, Brecher ML, Lindsay AN, et al. Gonadal function in pediatric patients following treatment for Hodgkin's disease. *Med Pediatr Oncol* 1981;9:235.

168. Haddy TB, Adde MA, McCalla J, et al. Late effects in long-term survivors of high-grade non-Hodgkin's lymphomas. *J Clin Oncol* 1998;16(6):2070–2079.

169. Clayton PE, Shalet SM, Price DA, et al. Ovarian function following chemotherapy for childhood brain tumors. *Med Pediatr Oncol* 1979;17:92.

170. Lendon M, Hann IM, Palmer MK, et al. Testicular histology after combination chemotherapy in childhood for acute lymphoblastic leukaemia. *Lancet* 1978;2:439.

171. Vilar O. Effect of cytostatic drugs on human testicular function. In: Mancini RE, Martini L, eds. *Male fertility and sterility*. New York: Academic Press, 1974:423.

172. Sherman JK. Synopsis of the use of frozen human semen since 1964: state-of-the-art human semen banking. *Fertil Steril* 1973;24:397.

173. Ansbacher R. Artificial insemination with frozen spermatozoa. *Fertil Steril* 1978;29:375.

174. Curie-Cohen M, Luttrell L, Shapiro J. Current practice of artificial insemination by donor in the United States. *N Engl J Med* 1979;300:585.

175. Sanger WG, Olson JH, Sherman JK. Semen cryobanking for men with cancer—criteria change. *Fertil Steril* 1992;58:1024.

176. Tournaye H, Camus M, Bollen N, et al. In vitro fertilization techniques with frozen-thawed sperm: a method for preserving the progenitive potential of Hodgkin patients. *Fertil Steril* 1991;55:443.

177. Brachen RB, Smith KD. Is semen cryopreservation helped in testicular cancer? *Urology* 1980;15:581.

178. Chlebowski RT, Heber D. Hypogonadism in male patients with metastatic cancer prior to chemotherapy. *Cancer Res* 1982;42:2495.

179. Sanger WG, Armitage JO, Schmidt MA. Feasibility of semen cryopreservation in patients with malignant disease. *JAMA* 1980;244:789.

180. Thachil JV, Jewett MAS, Rider WD. The effects of cancer and cancer therapy on male fertility. *J Urol* 1981;126:141.

181. Berthelsen JG, Skakkebaek NE. Gonadal function in men with testis cancer. *Fertil Steril* 1983;39:68.

182. Redman JR, Bajorunas DR, Goldstein MC, et al. Semen cryopreservation and artificial insemination for Hodgkin's disease. *J Clin Oncol* 1987;5:233.

183. Milligan DW, Hughes R, Linday KS. Semen cryopreservation in men undergoing cancer chemotherapy—a UK survey. *Br J Cancer* 1989;60:966–967.

184. Rhodes EA, Hoffman DJ, Kaempfer SH. Ten years of experience with semen cryopreservation by cancer patients: follow-up and clinical considerations. *Fertil Steril* 1985;44:512–516.

185. Scammell GE, White N, Stedronska J, et al. Cryopreservation of semen in men with testicular tumour or Hodgkin's disease: results of artificial insemination of their partners. *Lancet* 1985;2:31–32.

186. Hakim LS, Lobel SM, Oates RD. The achievement of pregnancies using assisted reproductive technologies for male factor infertility after retroperitoneal lymph node dissection for testicular carcinoma. *Fertil Steril* 1995;64(6):1141–1146.

187. Tournaye H, Liu J, Nagy PZ, et al. Correlation between testicular histology and outcome after intracytoplasmic sperm injection using testicular spermatozoa. *Hum Reprod* 1996; 11:127–132.

188. Palmero GD, Cohen J, Alikani M, et al. Intracytoplasmic sperm injection: a novel treatment for all forms of male factor infertility. *Fertil Steril* 1995;63:1231–1240.

189. Oehninger S, Veeck L, Lanzendorf S, et al. Intracytoplasmic sperm injection achievement of high pregnancy rates in couples with severe male factor infertility is dependent primarily upon female not male factors. *Fertil Steril* 1995;64:977–981.

190. Harari O, Bourne H, McDonald M, et al. Intracytoplasmic sperm injection: a major advance in the management of severe male subfertility. *Fertil Steril* 1995;64:360–368.

191. Abdalla HI, Baber RJ, Kirkland A, et al. Pregnancy in women with premature ovarian failure using tubal and intrauterine transfer of cryopreserved zygotes. *Br J Obstet Gynaecol* 1989;96:1071.

192. Pados G, Camus M, Van Waesberghe L, et al. Oocyte and embryo donation: evaluation of 412 consecutive trials. *Hum Reprod* 1992;7:1111.

193. Gosden RG, Baird DT, Wade JC, et al. Restoration of fertility to oophorectomized sheep by ovarian autografts stored at −196°C. *Hum Reprod* 1994;9:597–603.

194. Newton H, Aubard Y, Rutherford A, et al. Low temperature storage and grafting of human ovarian tissue. *Hum Reprod* 1996;11:1487–1491.

195. Law C. Freezing ovary tissue may help cancer patients preserve fertility. *J Natl Cancer Inst* 1996;88:1184–1185.

196. Newton H. The cryopreservation of ovarian tissue as a strategy for preserving the fertility of cancer patients. *Hum Reprod Update* 1998;4(3):237–247.

197. Stucker I, Caillard JF, Collin R, et al. Risk of spontaneous abortion among nurses handling antineoplastic drugs. *Scand J Work Environ Health* 1990;16:102.

198. Reynosa EE, Shepherd FA, Messner HA, et al. Acute leukemia during pregnancy: the Toronto leukemia study group experience with long term followup of children exposed in vitro to chemotherapeutic agents. *J Clin Oncol* 1987;5:1098.

199. Zemlickis D, Lishner M, Degendorfer P, et al. Fetal outcome after in utero exposure to cancer chemotherapy. *Arch Intern Med* 1992;152:573.

200. Aviles A, Diaz-Maqueo JC, Talavera A, et al. Growth and development of children of mothers treated with chemotherapy during pregnancy: current status of 43 children. *Am J Hematol* 1991;36:243.

201. Johnson SA, Goldman JM, Hawkins DF. Pregnancy after chemotherapy for Hodgkin's disease. *Lancet* 1979;2:93.

202. Li FP, Fine W, Jaffee N, et al. Offspring of patients treated for cancer in childhood. *J Natl Cancer Inst* 1979;62:1193.

203. Van Tiel DH, Ross GT, Lipsett MB. Pregnancies after chemotherapy of trophoblastic neoplasms. *Science* 1970; 169:1326.

204. Kung F-T, Chang S-Y, Tsae Y-C, et al. Subsequent reproduction and obstetric outcome after methotrexate treatment of cervical pregnancy: a review of original literature and international collaborative follow-up. *Human Rep* 1997; 12(3):591–595.

205. Green DM, Zevon MA, Lowrie G, et al. Congenital anomalies in children of patients who received chemotherapy for cancer in childhood and adolescence. *N Engl J Med* 1991; 325:141.

206. Aisner J, Wiernik PH, Pearl P. Pregnancy outcome in patients treated for Hodgkin's disease. *J Clin Oncol* 1993; 3:507.

207. Dodds L, Marrett LD, Tomkins DJ, et al. Case-control study of congenital anomalies in children of cancer patients. *Br Med J* 1993;307:164.

208. Doll DC, Ringenberg QS, Yarbro JW. Antineoplastic agents and pregnancy. *Semin Oncol* 1989;16:337–346.

209. Garber JE. Long-term follow-up of children exposed in utero to antineoplastic agents. *Semin Oncol* 1989;16: 437–444.

210. Holmes GE, Holmes FF. Pregnancy outcome of patients treated for Hodgkin's disease. *Cancer* 1978;41:1317.

211. Tomatis L, Turusov VS, Cardis E, et al. Tumor incidence in the progeny of male rats exposed to ethylnitrosourea before mating. *Mutat Res* 1990;229:231.

212. Francis AJ, Anderson D, Evans JG, et al. Tumours and malformations in the adult offspring of cyclophosphamide-treated and control male rats—preliminary communication. *Mutat Res* 1990;229:239.

213. Seethalakshmi L, Flores C, Kinkead T, et al. Effects of subchronic treatment with cis-platinum on testicular function, fertility, pregnancy outcome, and progeny. *J Androl* 1992; 13:65.

214. Mortimer JE, Boucher L, Baty J, Knapp DL, Ryan E, Rowland JH. Effect of tamoxifen on sexual functioning in patients with breast cancer. *J Clin Oncol* 1999;17(5):1488–1492.

215. Byrne J, Mulvihill JS, Myers MH, et al. Effects of treatment on fertility in long-term survivors of childhood or adolescent cancer. *N Engl J Med* 1987;317:1315.

5

CARCINOGENESIS: A LATE COMPLICATION OF CANCER CHEMOTHERAPY

CHARLES ERLICHMAN
MALCOLM MOORE

Although the potential of antineoplastic agents to induce new malignancies was suggested by Haddow[1] in 1947 on the basis of the ability of chemical carcinogens to cause growth inhibition, convincing evidence for carcinogenic effects of these agents in humans has been reported only in the past 30 years. The major reasons for this belated recognition of the problem are the long latency periods seen for expression of carcinogenicity in humans (3 to 4 years) and the brief survival of most patients treated with chemotherapy. Only in the past three decades have a sizable number of patients with advanced malignancy been cured by chemotherapy or been treated with adjuvant chemotherapy; thus, sufficient time has elapsed and sufficient numbers of individuals are now at risk for second tumors to be seen in clinically significant numbers. Although survival benefits will undoubtedly continue to accrue from the use of these agents and will probably outweigh the risks of second neoplasms, greater concern for this complication is necessary in the use of antineoplastic drugs in adjuvant programs and in nonneoplastic conditions such as renal transplantation or autoimmune disease, in which long-term survival of a large fraction of the treated population is ensured. In these instances, the benefits and risks of alternative therapies must be weighed carefully against those of the antineoplastic agents, and carcinogenicity must be included in the equation.

Definition of the risk of carcinogenesis due to chemotherapy is a difficult task. Prediction of carcinogenicity at the experimental level depends on test systems that examine the ability of chemicals to cause mutation of bacteria or mammalian cells, malignant transformation of mammalian cells, chromosomal aberrations, or tumors in mice or rats. Such tests are subject to interspecies variability in drug metabolism and target-tissue kinetics, and to other host factors that influence tumor development. These factors make extrapolation of the quantitative risk to humans a difficult, if not impossible, task. Second, the immune status of the patient is believed to play an important role in determining carcinogenicity, as indicated by the increased risk of lymphoid and cutaneous neoplasms in patients receiving immunosuppressive therapy; in cancer patients, the immune system is suppressed both as a result of the neoplastic process and as a consequence of therapy. This immunosuppression undoubtedly influences the risk of carcinogenesis but is not duplicated in test systems. Finally, the assessment of risk in humans at present is based in part on analyses of retrospective series, which often give incomplete information regarding key parameters of treatment (dose, duration) and which lack a control or untreated population. Such a control population is particularly important in risk assessment, because an increased incidence of second tumors, such as acute myelocytic leukemia in patients with Hodgkin's disease, may exist in the absence of treatment. More recently, analyses of randomized trials that compare adjuvant chemotherapy regimens with no additional treatment have been undertaken with respect to incidence of second malignancies. The information derived from these studies clarifies some of the confounding variables mentioned.

With these limitations in mind, this chapter considers available information concerning the carcinogenic potential of antitumor agents. This discussion examines the common pharmacologic properties shared by antineoplastic agents and classic carcinogens, specific predictions of carcinogenicity based on nonhuman test systems, and clinical evidence for an increased risk of second neoplasms in patients receiving these agents.

RELATIONSHIP OF ANTINEOPLASTIC AGENTS TO CHEMICAL CARCINOGENS

The chemical induction of cancer in animals is thought to involve a multistage process with a long latency period. This

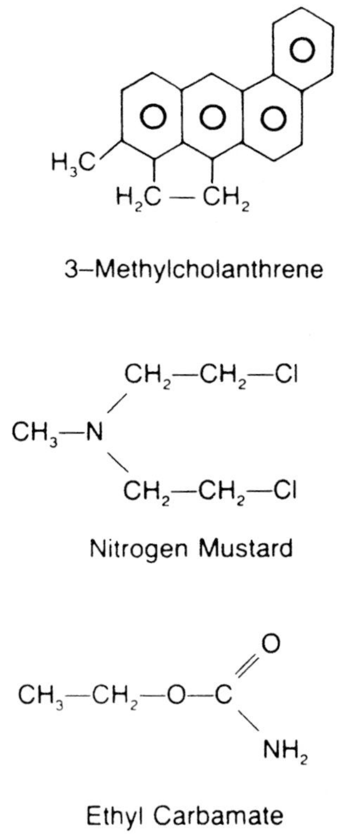

3–Methylcholanthrene

Nitrogen Mustard

Ethyl Carbamate

FIGURE 5-1. Chemical structures of three carcinogenic agents.

process can be initiated by a variety of chemical structures that have at least one common thread in their mode of action—an interaction with DNA.[2-4] Initiation results from irreversible genetic alterations, such as mutations or deletions in DNA.[5] One of the most carefully studied systems of tumor induction is the induction of skin cancer in mice and rabbits by alkylating agents, polycyclic hydrocarbons, and ethyl carbamate (Fig. 5-1). Repeated applications of these agents over long periods result in the development of benign or malignant tumors. Exposure to these compounds in limited doses, however, causes morphologic changes in the epithelium but does not result in tumors unless this stage of initiation is followed by the introduction of a promoter, such as a phorbol ester, an ingredient of croton oil. Promoters are not carcinogenic by themselves but lead to tumor production if applied after the initiating agent. Treatment with a specific promoter before exposure to the initiating agent does not result in tumor formation. This stage of promotion occurs over weeks and months and is reversible in its early stages. Promotion involves changes not in DNA structure but in the expression of the genome mediated through promoter-receptor interaction. The binding of promoter to receptor alters the expression of genes downstream. For example, estrogens and androgens may act as promoters by binding to the estrogen and androgen receptors, respectively, in liver or mammary tissue. Promoters such as phorbol-12-myristate-13-acetate have a variety of biologic actions; they alter differentiation, cause changes in cell surface glycopep-

tides, alter various metabolic activities, and suppress immune surveillance of tumors by cytotoxic macrophages and natural killer cells.[6] The final stage of progression is irreversible and is characterized by karyotypic instability and malignant growth. Thus, carcinogenesis is a multistep process that may be arrested at intermediate stages, that requires a long latency period for induction, and that can be influenced by, if it does not require, a promoting agent.

The existence or identity of an associated promoter has not been established for well-documented carcinogens in humans. For cancer patients, induction of second tumors may require not only an initiator but also a promoter, a function that may be fulfilled by a second chemotherapeutic agent, by radiotherapy, or by a disease-related abnormality in metabolism or immune function. This consideration could explain the higher risk of second tumors in patients receiving a combination of drugs and irradiation.

Chemical carcinogens show a diversity of structures but share important metabolic features. Most are inert and require microsomal metabolic activation to positively charged (or electrophilic) intermediates that react with DNA bases. The primary sites for attack of DNA are relatively negatively charged (or nucleophilic) sites, such as the 7 position of guanine[7,8] (see Chapter 12). This characteristic of carcinogens—namely, microsomal metabolism to an electrophilic intermediate that attacks DNA—is shared by certain antineoplastic agents such as cyclophosphamide and mitomycin C and is essential in the antineoplastic action of these drugs. Other agents, such as L-phenylalanine mustard and nitrogen mustard, do not require metabolic activation to form alkylating species. Carcinogenicity has also been ascribed to ionizing irradiation, which produces free radicals, such as superoxide or hydroxyl radicals. A number of antitumor drugs have the same ability to promote formation of reactive oxygen intermediates; such agents include those that possess quinone functional groups [doxorubicin hydrochloride and plicamycin (mithramycin)] and those that bind electron-donating heavy metals (such as bleomycin sulfate and its analogs). Four antineoplastic agents suspected as carcinogens and their probable carcinogenic intermediates are given in Figure 5-2; the varied chemical features of their reactive intermediates are illustrated.

The identification of oncogenes and suppressor genes recently has added another variable to the equation. Their role in carcinogenesis is being pursued aggressively, and several possible mechanisms of actions have been proposed. The loss of one allele in a tumor suppressor gene such as *p53* can potentially increase the risk of a drug-induced mutation in the other allele and development of the malignant phenotype. Oncogenes can be activated by a variety of mechanisms summarized in Table 5-1. Point mutations, chromosomal translocations, and gene amplification can alter expression of these genes. Just as altered oncogene expression and mutation occur with exposure to potential carcinogens, exposure to carcinogenic antitumor drugs likely alters oncogene expres-

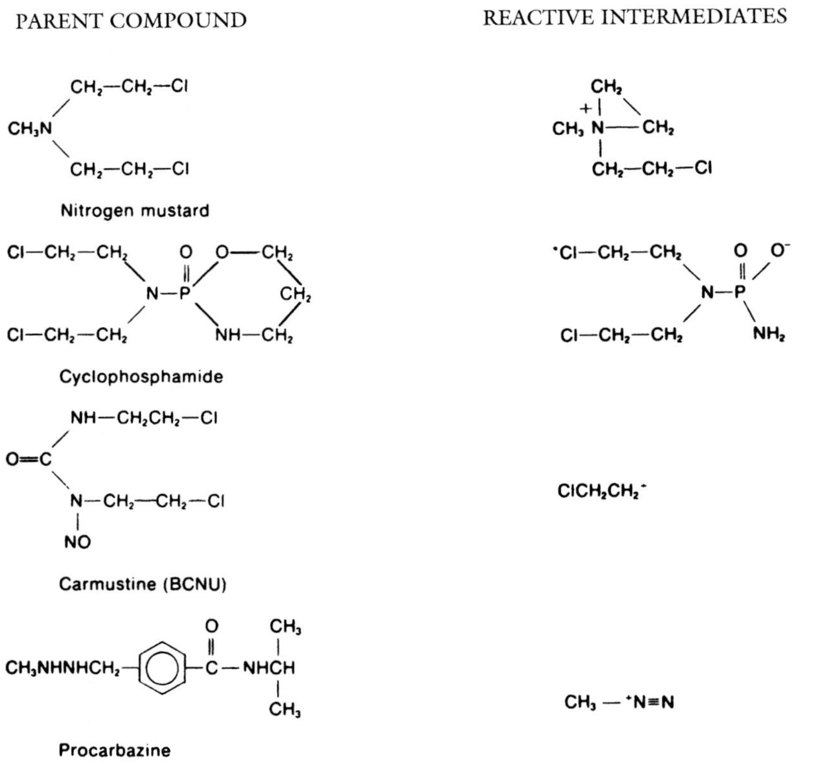

PARENT COMPOUND

REACTIVE INTERMEDIATES

Nitrogen mustard

Cyclophosphamide

Carmustine (BCNU)

$CH_3 - ^+N \equiv N$

Procarbazine

FIGURE 5-2. Antineoplastic agents with reactive intermediates.

sion and increases the risk of second malignancies. Studies using nitrosomethylurea-induced mammary tumors have identified an activated *ras* oncogene in the majority of the tumors, which contained a substitution of adenine for guanine in the twelfth codon. This change is consistent with methylation of the oxygen in the 6 position of guanine, which would result in the replacement of guanine by adenine on DNA replication.[9] Such studies bring together environmental and genetic factors in cancer causation.

TESTING OF ANTINEOPLASTIC AGENTS FOR CARCINOGENIC POTENTIAL

In view of the damaging effects of many antineoplastic agents on DNA and the suggestive clinical evidence of their

TABLE 5-1. ONCOGENE ACTIVATION

Alteration	Effect
Base mutation in coding sequence	New gene product with altered activity
Base deletion in noncoding sequence	Altered regulation of normal gene product
Chromosomal translocation	Altered message and level of expression
Gene amplification	Increased gene expression

Adapted from Pitot HC. The molecular biology of carcinogenesis. *Cancer* 1993;72:962, with permission.

carcinogenicity, application of methods for determining carcinogenic potential before widespread use of new agents in humans has become imperative. An ideal test system would be simple, rapid, inexpensive, and yet specific for carcinogens and sensitive to modestly potent agents. Unfortunately, the various methods available, ranging from *in vitro* bacterial mutagenesis assays to long-term studies in rodents, all have recognized drawbacks.[10]

Five types of test systems for carcinogen exposure are available. Mutagenesis assays attempt to quantify the frequency with which a chemical induces mutational events based on the assumption that mutagenicity correlates with the likelihood of causing cancer in animals. The underlying premise is that carcinogenesis is the product of a mutational event that can be expressed in the short term as a change in biochemical features of a test organism. Cytogenetic studies attempt to correlate drug-induced chromosomal aberrations such as sister chromatid exchanges (SCEs) with carcinogenicity. Although certain characteristic karyotypic changes are associated with specific malignancies, such as the Ph[1] chromosome with chronic granulocytic leukemia, cytogenetic abnormalities are not proven either necessary or sufficient causes of neoplastic transformation. Tests of oncogenesis in tissue culture are based on the hypothesis that agents that produce neoplastic transformation in culture are likely to be carcinogenic in the whole animal. Like the Ames assay of bacterial mutagenesis, this system entails the assumption that the drug concentration, duration of exposure, and metabolism of the suspected carcinogen are relevant to the *in vivo* situation, but this assumption is of uncertain validity, and metabolic information is not available for many of the compounds tested. *In vivo* mammalian studies are conducted usually in rodents over extended periods and at great expense. The primary drawbacks of this system are the known species, sex, and age dependencies of drug metabolism in rodents and the lack of pharmacologic information that would allow an extrapolation of results from rodents to humans. The fifth approach, a measure of carcinogen exposure, uses detection of carcinogen-macromolecular adducts or somatic gene mutation in either target tissue or peripheral blood elements.

Mutagenesis Assays

Among the many mutagen-testing systems, the Ames test satisfies the requirements of simplicity and rapid return of results and in addition appears to possess high specificity for carcinogens, although certain exceptions have been identified. This test[11] uses specific strains of *Salmonella typhimurium* that are histidine-requiring mutants. Exposure of these strains to the suspected mutagen in a histidine-free medium leads to growth of revertant mutants if the appropriate mutation is induced. Small amounts of chemicals (less than 1 mg) can be used, and results are obtained in approximately 2 days. For agents that require metabolic activation (as do many carcinogens), rat or human liver microsomes can be added to the test plates.

In extensive testing of a wide variety of agents previously documented to be carcinogens and noncarcinogens, 90% of the known carcinogens gave positive results in the Ames assay, and 87% of the noncarcinogens were inactive.[12,13] These findings suggest that the system has a high degree of specificity. Many of the antineoplastic agents in use today have been examined in the Ames system,[14–17] and some of the results are incorporated in Table 5-2. Most antimetabolites and the vinca alkaloids give negative results in both the Ames test and *in vivo* systems, whereas alkylating agents and many antitumor antibiotics give positive results in both assay systems. Both procarbazine hydrochloride and dactinomycin (actinomycin D), however, are carcinogenic in animals but give negative results in the Ames test. In the case of procarbazine, this discrepancy may be due to the failure of the test system to simulate the metabolism of procarbazine as it occurs *in vivo*. The agent 6-mercaptopurine, which has been reported to be carcinogenic in animals, shows weakly mutagenic results in the *Salmonella* system.

From the foregoing analysis, the Ames test would appear to be an excellent screening procedure but one with obvious false-negative results. An analysis of the Ames test results by Rinkus and Legator[18] indicates that the false-negative rate is particularly high for specific chemical classes. At least seven classes of agents known to contain carcinogenic compounds are poorly detected in the Ames system, including azo compounds, carbonyl, hydrazine,

TABLE 5-2. RESULTS OF TESTING ANTINEOPLASTIC AGENTS IN THREE SYSTEMS FOR CARCINOGENICITY

Agent	Ames Test	Sister Chromatid Exchanges	Animal Studies
Mechlorethamine hydrochloride	+	+	+
Cyclophosphamide	+	+[a]	+
Melphalan	+	+	+
Thiotriethylene phosphoramide (thiotepa)	+	+	+
Chlorambucil	NR	+	+
Procarbazine hydrochloride	–	+[a]	–
Lomustine (CCNU)	NR	+[b]	–
Doxorubicin hydrochloride	+	+	+
Streptozotocin	+	NR	+
Bleomycin sulfate	–	+[c]	–
Dactinomycin (actinomycin D)	–	±	+
Mitomycin C	+	+	+
Dacarbazine (DTIC)	NR	–[b]	+
Cisplatin	+	+	NR
5-Fluorouracil	–	NR	NR
6-Mercaptopurine	+	–	+
Cytosine arabinoside (ara-C)	–	NR	–
Vincristine sulfate	–	±	–
Vinblastine sulfate	–	NR	+
Methotrexate sodium	–	+	–

+, positive result reported in at least one study; –, no positive result reported; ±, slight decrease over control (which is of unknown significance); NR, no result reported.
[a]Drug must be activated.
[b]Test done on patient lymphocytes after treatment with agent.
[c]Concentration giving positive results also causes significant numbers of other chromosomal aberrations.

chloroethylene, steroid, and antimetabolite structures. In some cases, known carcinogens such as urethane probably cannot be metabolized to their carcinogenic form in the test system.

Another assay approach based on mutations measures the mutation frequency in the hypoxanthine-guanine phosphoribosyltransferase (*HGPRT*) gene.[19] This technique can be used *in vitro* in mammalian cells and *in vivo* in patient samples. Assessment of mutation frequency at baseline and after treatment, and comparison between control groups and populations treated with chemotherapy have been carried out.[20,21] Whether these assays are predictive of increased malignant risk is yet to be determined.

In vivo mutational assays have been developed using transgenic rodent models.[22] These models are comprised of an altered genomic sequence that is inheritable—often the *Escherichia coli lacI* (lac repressor) or *lacZ* (β-galactosidase) genes. Animals are treated with the potentially carcinogenic agent and after sufficient time has passed to fix DNA adducts as mutations, genomic DNA is extracted, and the target gene is isolated by such methods as magnetic affinity capture. The transgenic model allows for rapid assessment of tissue-specific mutation after chemical treatment. This may focus subsequent clinical monitoring on specific organs. As with other *in vivo* studies, factors such as drug pharmacokinetics, DNA repair, animal age, diet, strain, sex, drug dose, and dosing duration influence the results.

Assay of Sister Chromatid Exchanges

Chromosomal damage resulting from exposure to chemical substances *in vitro* or *in vivo* has been used as an index of mutagenic or carcinogenic potential for many years but has required significant skill in recognizing the many different possible aberrations. Assay of sister chromatid exchange (SCE), a type of chromosomal study that detects the exchange of small DNA fragments between sister chromatid pairs, has considerable appeal because relatively few cells need to be examined, exchanges can be visualized easily, and the system is quite sensitive to small amounts of chemicals. The exchange is symmetric and does not alter the overall chromosomal morphology.[23]

The ability of various chemotherapeutic agents to induce SCE indicates that this technique might be useful as an assay for mutagenesis and ultimately carcinogenesis, but limitations of its potential also have become clear.[23,24] Ionizing radiation, known to be a potent mutagen and carcinogen, causes only slight increments in SCE; these changes are minimal in comparison with other chromosomal damage, including breaks, deletions, and other aberrations induced at the same dose level. On the other hand, ultraviolet light evokes dramatic increases in SCE frequency. Alkylating agents and some DNA intercalators induce a high frequency of SCE in addition to other chromosomal damage. Cyclophosphamide induces SCEs only after

microsomal activation.[25] Among the antimetabolites, methotrexate sodium, which is not carcinogenic in laboratory animals, has been reported to induce SCE, but 6-mercaptopurine, a suspected carcinogen, does not cause these chromosomal abnormalities.[26]

The use of SCE has particular appeal because the effects of chemotherapeutic agents can be assessed *in vivo* by performing this test on peripheral lymphocytes from patients receiving antineoplastic therapy. Studies of lymphocytes from patients before and at intervals after chemotherapy have shown a marked increase in SCEs after the administration of lomustine (CCNU), dacarbazine (DTIC), and mitomycin.[27–29] Whether such increases in SCE frequency reflect the likelihood of carcinogenicity is still unclear.

Cell Culture Systems

Cell culture systems also have been advocated for the testing of carcinogenicity. Morphologic transformation of cells in culture and the ability of these cells to produce tumors when implanted in animals have been the primary criteria used for carcinogenicity. Three major test systems, which use hamster embryo cells, fibroblasts from the ventral prostate, or 3T3-like cells, have been applied to the screening of environmental carcinogens.[30,31] Using all three lines, investigators have shown a good quantitative correlation between transformation *in vitro* and *in vivo* carcinogenesis, although the number of antineoplastic agents tested has been limited. Mammalian cell culture systems, however, are subject to many of the same problems as those of bacterial mutagenesis assays discussed previously, including the need to activate compounds to reactive intermediates. An additional problem pertinent to these three systems is the use of cells of nonhuman and nonepithelial origin. Finally, tumors resulting from the implantation of transformed cells are sarcomas and, thus, may not reflect the potential of the tested agent to cause tumors in epithelial cells or in humans.

The results of testing antineoplastic drugs in cell transformation systems have not correlated well with tests of carcinogenicity in experimental animals.[32,33] Carcinogenic alkylating agents [melphalan and thiotriethylene phosphoramide (thiotepa)] increased the transformation frequency of C3H/10T1/2 cells, and dactinomycin and bleomycin showed a concentration-dependent increase in transformation frequency. These results are consistent with the known carcinogenicity of these agents. However, methotrexate also caused a concentration-dependent increase in transformation but at a relatively low frequency, whereas two other antimetabolites, 5-fluorodeoxyuridine and arabinosylcytosine, produced transformation in synchronized cells exposed during the S phase of the cell cycle. None of these antimetabolites has proved to be carcinogenic in animals or humans.

More recently, the use of cultured human tissue and cells for carcinogenesis studies has become possible.[34] Studies in these systems overcome some of the drawbacks of using nonhuman systems. Drug metabolism to the ultimate carcinogen, uptake of drug into human cells, the identification of specific DNA adducts, and the presence of DNA repair systems more closely approach the *in vivo* situation.

Animal Studies

The classic yardstick for assessing carcinogenicity has been the ability of the suspected agent to induce tumors in laboratory animals. These studies, although the most direct and reliable source of experimental information, are fraught with difficulties, including high cost, interspecies variability in susceptibility to carcinogens, and the long time required to obtain results. In addition, efforts must be made to design protocols of drug administration that mimic the intensity and duration of exposure found in humans, a problem compounded by differences in drug metabolism and pharmacokinetics in humans and rodents. A definite advantage of the bioassay system in intact animals is the preservation of the role of the immune system in determining the outcome. This factor is obviously missing in any of the *in vitro* assays.

The results of various bioassays of antineoplastic agents are recorded in Table 5-2.[35–38] Some results are conflicting and seem to depend on the age, sex, and species of animal used in the test. In general, however, most alkylating agents and antitumor antibiotics are carcinogenic in animals, whereas antimetabolites, including methotrexate, cytosine arabinoside (ara-C), and hydroxyurea, give negative results. Drug combinations have received only limited testing in bioassay systems.[39] Tests of the combination of prednisone and azathioprine, commonly used in organ transplantation, showed a decrease in time before tumor appearance compared with azathioprine alone. With other combinations (e.g., prednisone plus CCNU, ara-C plus CCNU, and prednisone, vincristine sulfate, and cyclophosphamide), the median time before tumor appearance was longer than with the alkylating agent alone. Of the ten combinations studied, four resulted in slightly higher tumor incidence than controls, whereas six caused fewer tumors than did the individual drugs.

Molecular and Biochemical Assays

Advances in the detection of carcinogen-molecular adducts and somatic gene mutations have opened the opportunity to study carcinogen exposure in humans.[40,41] The polymerase chain reaction and DNA sequencing enable rapid assessment of oncogene and tumor suppressor gene mutations in small patient samples. The use of ^{32}P-postlabeling thin-layer chromatography and autoradiography assays, enzyme-linked immunosorbent assays, synchronous fluorescence spectroscopy, and gas chromatography/mass spectroscopy has made it feasible to detect low levels of adducts in human samples. Carcinogen-DNA adducts, exposure to chemicals, and carcinogenicity have been correlated with each other; but in the past, the low levels of adducts present in human samples limited the conventional assay systems. The use of enzyme immunoassays combined with synchronous fluorescence spectroscopy has increased sensitivity and specificity for polycyclic aromatic hydrocarbon–DNA adducts. The use of high-pressure liquid chromatography or immunoaffinity chromatography in combination with ^{32}P-postlabeling assay or immunoassay can be used to detect alkyl adducts in the human tissue with assay detection limits ranging from 1 to 600 adducts per 10^8 nucleotides depending on assay and tissue examined. Such assays make it feasible to perform epidemiologic studies in patients receiving chemotherapy.

CLINICAL STUDIES IMPLICATING ANTINEOPLASTIC AGENTS IN CARCINOGENESIS

Although experimental evidence demonstrating the carcinogenic potential of many antineoplastic agents was abundant, the clinical evidence of this problem was slower to appear. The fact that the rate of development of "secondary" cancers in patients with malignant lymphoma, pediatric cancers, ovarian cancer, and breast cancer is higher than that seen in an age-matched normal population has become clear. Many good reviews of this topic are now available in the medical literature.[42–44] The reporting of second tumors in patients with prior histories of cancer comes from a variety of sources. Initial reports were mainly anecdotal and thus did not allow an analysis of factors that might be important. Data reported more recently have come from hospital-based, national, and international tumor registries and from longer follow-up of chemotherapy and hormonal therapy studies. The use of longer-term clinical trial data has the advantage that the initial cohort and treatment are tightly controlled. This provides a better analysis of how different drugs and treatments would impact the risk of second cancers. The use of clinical trial data for this purpose is somewhat limited by patient numbers, which rarely exceed 1,000. Registries, on the other hand, can have several thousand or tens of thousands of patients and thus allow a better assessment regarding less common second cancers such as acute leukemia or sarcoma. Determining treatment and outcome from registries can be quite labor intensive, however. One method that is used to identify treatment factors involved in the development of new cancers from a registry is referred to as a "nested" case-control study. In this approach, patients in the registry who develop a second cancer are compared with others who did not. These comparisons have provided a better estimate of the risks and the factors that influence the development of second cancers. Clinical information about the total dosages of drugs, concomitant therapy, and the duration of treatment is important in estimating risk. For some drugs such as the alkylating agents or etoposide, a threshold exists above which the risk of neoplasia rises sharply. Such thresholds have been previously identified in experimental carcinogenesis and in the induction of SCEs. Duration of treatment also may have a bearing, because a brief but intense exposure to a cytotoxic agent may be less carcinogenic than long-term low-dose exposure.

Another issue in assessing the true risk of second cancers from cytotoxic agents is the existence of other factors that may also influence their development. An underlying increased incidence of second malignancy is found independent of therapy in patients with retinoblastoma, Wilms' tumor, multiple myeloma, Hodgkin's disease, and other tumors such as those associated with the hereditary nonpolyposis colorectal cancer syndrome. Other therapies used to treat the cancer, particularly radiation therapy, also impact the development of secondary cancers. Recently evidence is accumulating of an increase in solid tumors after therapy for Hodgkin's disease and testicular cancer that is most likely related to radiation rather than chemotherapy. In many reports, combination treatment regimens or regimens using irradiation and chemotherapy were used. Thus, the carcinogenic effects cannot necessarily be ascribed to one compound of the regimen with certainty, although the used of the nested case-control method may allow conclusions to be drawn regarding the carcinogenicity of different components of the regimen.

Interpretation of studies in this area must also take into consideration the statistical methods used to assess relative risk.[45] The use of a person-years-of-risk analysis assumes that the yearly incidence of second malignancies is constant for the entire follow-up period and does not allow for the fact that a patient must live a certain time through the latency period for the occurrence of a second malignancy. Such an analysis allows a reasonable estimate of the carcinogenic effects of a single therapy, but its use when comparing two treatments biases results against the treatment that leads to a longer survival. Many studies compare the risk of cancer in the treated group with that of an age-matched cohort in the normal population to determine a relative risk. For a tumor that is uncommon in this age-matched population, an increase in the relative risk of fivefold to tenfold sounds impressive but may only translate into a problem for less than 1% of patients who received therapy. On the other hand, small increases in relative risk for the more common solid tumors such as lung or breast cancer translate into a much greater problem in terms of absolute risk. This is the case with treatments for Hodgkin's disease as described later. One method that is useful in determining the overall impact of a secondary cancer in a population is to describe it in terms of the number of new cancers that occur per 10,000 patients treated.

Based on information currently available, one can attempt to categorize antineoplastic agents into high, moderate, low, and unknown risk groups on the basis of their oncogenic potential in humans (Table 5-3). The primary basis for this classification is reports of second malignancy in patients treated for both hematologic and solid tumors, with additional information coming from trials of cytotoxic agents in patients with immune diseases or after organ transplantation. Given that the latency period for the development of secondary cancers can range from 2 to 3 years (e.g., for etoposide-induced leukemias) to 10 to 20 years for solid tumors, the risk for many newer agents such as paclitaxel, docetaxel, irinotecan hydrochloride, and gemcitabine hydrochloride cannot yet be properly determined. A true assessment of agents primarily used in palliative therapy is also difficult, because most patients may not survive long enough for problems such as second cancers to manifest.

The development of a new cancer can occur many years after treatment of the initial cancer. This means that large numbers of patients and long follow-up are required to define the risk of carcinogenesis and to understand which drugs and schedules are the probable cause. Some investigators have used preneoplastic lesions as markers of carcinogenicity to provide an earlier estimate of the risk. For example, a small group of patients with breast cancer who had been randomized previously to receive adjuvant chemotherapy or oophorectomy underwent cytologic and colposcopic screening of the uterine cervix.[46] The results were compared with those for 79 controls with no known breast malignancy. Significantly more breast cancer patients who had received chemotherapy had cervical intraepithelial neo-

TABLE 5-3. CATEGORIZATION OF ANTINEOPLASTIC AGENTS ACCORDING TO CARCINOGENIC RISK IN HUMANS

High Risk	Moderate Risk	Low Risk	Unknown
Melphalan	Doxorubicin hydrochloride	Vinca alkaloids	Bleomycin sulfate
Mechlorethamine hydrochloride	Thiotriethylene phosphoramide	Methotrexate sodium	Taxanes
Nitrosoureas	(thiotepa)	Cytosine arabinoside (ara-C)	Busulfan
Etoposide	Cyclophosphamide	5-Fluorouracil	Gemcitabine hydrochloride
Teniposide	Procarbazine hydrochloride	L-Asparaginase	Irinotecan hydrochloride
Azathioprine	Dacarbazine (DTIC)	Carboplatin	Mitoxantrone hydrochloride
	Cisplatin		

plasia (p <.01) than did controls; the proportion of breast cancer patients in the oophorectomy group who had cervical intraepithelial neoplasia did not differ significantly from the proportion in the control group. The incidence of chromosome abnormalities and structural chromosome changes in ovarian cancer patients treated with melphalan was higher than in a control group.[47] For patients receiving both melphalan and radiation therapy, the frequency of chromosomal aberrations was even higher. Whether these chromosomal changes act as a marker for subsequent development of secondary leukemia is not yet known. In children with hematologic cancer who had previously received chemotherapy and cranial irradiation, the total-body mole counts were compared with those of their siblings. The median number of moles was 20.0 in the patient group (n = 79) and 11.0 in the healthy siblings (n = 88).[48] In another study, a total-body count of melanocytic nevi in children receiving treatment for hematologic cancer was carried out before therapy and repeated 3 years later. Total-body nevus counts were significantly increased 3 years after treatment.[49] To what degree these results predict subsequent cancer development is yet unknown. With increasing knowledge of progression from benign to neoplastic growth in diseases like colorectal and pancreatic cancer, however, assessment of precursor lesions may be a useful way to evaluate risk.

SECOND MALIGNANCIES IN SPECIFIC POPULATIONS OF CANCER PATIENTS

Pediatric Patients

Long-term survival is now possible for many patients with pediatric malignancies. This group of patients is being followed closely for the development of late complications of treatment. Some pediatric tumors such as retinoblastoma are known to be associated with genetic abnormalities that may predispose to other cancers.[50] Overall, the risk of development of a second cancer 20 years after childhood cancer has been estimated to be 8% to 20%.[51,52] One consistent finding has been an association between treatment with the epipodophyllotoxins, etoposide, or teniposide, and secondary acute nonlymphocytic leukemia (ANLL), often with monocytic features. One series examined 205 children with acute lymphoblastic leukemia (ALL) who were treated with a four-drug induction with prednisone, L-asparaginase, vincristine, and daunorubicin hydrochloride followed by maintenance therapy with oral 6-mercaptopurine, methotrexate, L-asparaginase, etoposide, and cytarabine. The etoposide was given twice weekly. The risk of secondary ANLL at 4 years was 5.9% ± 3.2%. Because none of these children received alkylating agent therapy or irradiation, etoposide was most likely responsible for these secondary leukemias.[53] Risk factors for secondary ANLL

in 734 consecutively treated children with ALL who attained complete remission and received maintenance treatment with epipodophyllotoxins were reported by Pui et al.[54] Secondary ANLL was diagnosed in 21 of the 734 patients, and the overall cumulative risk at 6 years was 3.8% (2.3% to 6.1%). For the subgroups treated twice weekly or weekly with etoposide or teniposide, the risk of ANLL at 6 years was 12.3%, whereas for the subgroups treated with these drugs only during remission induction, or every 2 weeks during maintenance treatment, the risk was 1.6%. In their analysis, the schedule of the epipodophyllotoxin administration was important, whereas the cumulative dose of drug did not appear to influence the risk of secondary leukemia. At the Dana-Farber Cancer Institute, no epipodophyllotoxin was used in their regimens. They reviewed 752 children with ALL who entered complete remission after induction therapy. Only two had developed ANLL after a median follow-up of 4 years.[55] Clinical and cytologic findings in epipodophyllotoxin-induced leukemia are a short latency period (mean 24 to 36 months) between the completion of treatment and the development of ANLL, a Fab M-4 or M-5 subtype, a translocation of the *MLL* gene at chromosome band 11q23, and a poor response to treatment.[56] Studies have shown an association between the breakpoints in the *MLL* gene and DNA topoisomerase II cleavage sites that are stimulated by etoposide. Secondary leukemia due to alkylating agents is characterized by a different phenotype with a longer latency period, antecedent myelodysplasia, and deletions of chromosomes 5 or 7.[42]

In view of this apparent increased risk of leukemia with epipodophyllotoxins, the National Cancer Institute Cancer Therapy Evaluation Program has instituted a monitoring plan for secondary leukemias after treatment with these agents. In one report[57] from this program, they examined 12 cooperative group clinical trials, 11 in the pediatric population, that used cumulative doses of etoposide ranging from less than 1.5 g per m² to more than 3.0 g per m².[58] Risk of development of secondary leukemia at 6 years was 3.3%, 0.7%, and 2.2% in the dose ranges of less than 1.5 g per m², 1.5 to 2.99 g per m², and more than 3.0 g per m², respectively. Their overall conclusions were that, at doses of less than 5 g per m², only a minor risk of secondary leukemia is found. The risk of leukemia in patients receiving etoposide probably is influenced by other agents used in the regimens, particularly alkylating agents and other topoisomerase inhibitors. Relatively high rates of secondary leukemia have been reported in small series after the use of intensive treatments for pediatric tumors with poor prognosis that included both topoisomerase II inhibitors and alkylating agents.[59]

The development of secondary solid tumors in pediatric cancer patients is an issue of growing concern. Roswell Park Cancer Institute reviewed the courses of 1,406 patients younger than 20 years of age who were treated over a 30-year period.[60] The actuarial risk of a second malignant tumor 25 years after diagnosis was 5.6%. Prior therapy with carmustine (BCNU) and doxorubicin were the only factors that were significantly associated with the risk of a second malignant tumor. In Italy, a registry of all patients with childhood cancer who achieved complete remission was followed for a median time of 52 months after treatment. Twenty second malignancies occurred, which included nine hematologic malignancies (four ANLL, two chronic myelocytic leukemia, three non-Hodgkin's lymphoma), eight central nervous system tumors (all in patients given central nervous system radiation), and three other solid tumors.[61] Others have reported the occurrence of unusual tumors such as squamous cell cancers of the skin occurring in teenagers who have previously received therapy for ANLL.[62] In a follow-up of 674 patients treated in the German Ewing's sarcoma studies, the cumulative risk of a second malignancy was 0.7%, 2.9%, and 4.7% after 5, 10, and 15 years, respectively. The interval until the development of myelodysplasia/leukemia was 17 to 96 months and until development of solid tumors was 82 to 136 months.[63] The importance of the development of second malignancy must be interpreted in relation to the risks of failure of therapy of the primary cancer. In the analysis of the German Ewing's sarcoma trials, second malignancies accounted for only 3 of the 328 deaths in this population; the remainder were due to Ewing's sarcoma. Similarly, a review of all ALL patients treated at Dana-Farber Cancer Institute demonstrated a risk of second malignancy of 2.7%, but the risk of other adverse events, including relapse, death, or induction failure, was 31%.[64] A review from Stanford of 694 children with Hodgkin's disease showed a risk of both solid tumors and hematologic malignancies similar to that reported for adults with this disease (discussed later). Of note, the actuarial risk at 20 years in men was 10.6% and in women was 15.4% due to the additional risk of breast cancers occurring within the radiation field.[65] Similar observations were made by the Late Effects Study Group, which found the relative risk for second tumors in children treated for Hodgkin's disease to be 18.1, with approximately a 35% risk of breast cancer by the age of 40.[66] Risk of breast cancer was increased when the patient was of pubertal age at the time of radiation, and when the dose of radiation was higher. Risk of leukemia was associated with use of alkylating agents and advanced stage at diagnosis.

Overall, the risk of ANLL peaks a few years after therapy, whereas the risk of a solid tumor increases with the length of follow-up. It is still too early to assess what additional risk this population will experience when they enter an age group in which the development of cancer is more common. In this setting, a modest increase in relative risk could translate into a substantial increase in the overall absolute risk of cancer. This has already been observed to some degree in the population treated for Hodgkin's disease.

Patients with Ovarian Cancer

Advanced ovarian cancer was treated initially with alkylating agents such as melphalan.[67] Several reports have implicated alkylating agents (particularly melphalan and cyclophosphamide used as single agents) as a causative factor in the high incidence of ANLL in this group of patients.[68–71] A review of 5,455 cases of ovarian cancer revealed a 36.1-fold increased risk of acute leukemia compared with an age-matched control group. For patients surviving at least 2 years after the institution of therapy, the risk was 174.4-fold higher than that in the controls.[72] Many patients with acute leukemia identified in this series also received radiotherapy alone or in combination with alkylating agents. Thus, determining which agent was responsible for the leukemia was impossible. An analysis of a large cohort of patients with ovarian cancer treated with melphalan or cyclophosphamide revealed a 93-fold increased risk of ANLL in women treated with chemotherapy.[73] The risk was highest 5 to 6 years after the initiation of therapy and decreased thereafter. A dose-response relationship was apparent for melphalan and was suggested for cyclophosphamide. Melphalan was more likely to induce secondary leukemia than was cyclophosphamide. In an international collaborative group of cancer registries and hospitals, 114 cases of leukemia were identified after ovarian cancer.[74] Chemotherapy alone was associated with a relative risk for leukemia of 12 compared with surgery alone, whereas radiotherapy alone did not produce a significant increase in risk. The risk of leukemia was greatest 4 to 5 years after chemotherapy and was increased for at least 8 years. Cyclophosphamide, chlorambucil, melphalan, thiotepa, and treosulfan were independently associated with significantly increased risks of leukemia. Chlorambucil and melphalan were the most leukemogenic. These studies support the clinical impression that a dose-response effect may exist, that the carcinogenic potential of all alkylating agents is not necessarily the same, and that the latency period is approximately 5 years. They also suggest that the risk for secondary leukemia does decrease after a period. The largest analysis of second tumors in ovarian cancer was done on nine population registries of the National Cancer Institute and Connecticut Tumor Registry.[75] Researchers examined 32,251 women with ovarian cancer and found a relative risk of second cancers of 1.28 [95% confidence interval (CI), 1.21 to 1.35], with an excess of leukemia [relative risk (RR) = 4.1] and colorectal (RR = 1.4), bladder (RR = 2.1), and breast (RR = 1.2) cancers. The association with rectal and breast cancer was probably related to genetic predisposition; the risk of leukemia, to alkylating agents; and the risk of sarcomas and abdominal tumors, to previous radiation.

Ovarian cancer is now treated primarily with platinum-based regimens, and melphalan and chlorambucil are rarely used. The leukemogenic potential of cisplatin is assumed to be less than for other alkylating agents. Anecdotal reports exist of patients developing ANLL after cisplatin therapy, but the relative risk of developing ANLL after cisplatin is not yet well known.[76,77] The newest agents for the treatment of ovarian cancer are paclitaxel and topotecan hydrochloride. It is too early to assess the carcinogenic potential of the topoisomerase I inhibitors and taxanes.

Patients with Breast Cancer

Breast cancer is another malignancy responsive to various cytotoxic and hormonal agents that are associated with an increased risk of secondary malignancies.[78] Among patients receiving adjuvant chemotherapy for breast cancer, no increased risk of leukemia was identified in a group of 1,265 who received postoperative thiotepa (with or without radiotherapy), compared with untreated controls.[79] The ongoing prospective adjuvant studies in breast cancer have addressed this question more definitively.[80–82] The results of the National Surgical Adjuvant Breast and Bowel Program database analysis indicate that risk of leukemia in patients receiving melphalan-based adjuvant chemotherapy increases fivefold. An initial analysis of the Milan studies of cyclophosphamide, methotrexate, and 5-fluorouracil (CMF) adjuvant chemotherapy revealed no increased incidence of leukemia or other second malignancies.[83] A more recent analysis of 2,465 patients with localized breast cancer treated in Milan from 1973 to 1990 revealed a 15-year cumulative risk of second cancers of 8.4% after local treatment only, 6.4% after CMF therapy, and 5.1% after doxorubicin-based chemotherapy. The relative risk for women receiving CMF treatment was 1.29.[84] An analysis of 1,113 patients in Sweden treated with adjuvant CMF or radiation therapy did not demonstrate any increase in second cancers in the first 10 years of follow-up.[85] Patients receiving chemotherapy actually had a lower rate of such cancers than those receiving radiation therapy.

The typical features of ANLL secondary to alkylating agent exposure include a latency period of 3 to 5 years, during which dysplasia of the myeloid lineage often becomes apparent; deletions of part or all of chromosome 5 or chromosome 7; and an unfavorable response to chemotherapy. Case reports have described the occurrence of a different type of ANLL with monocytic features associated with a translocation at 11q23 (the locus of the *MLL* gene) in patients who have received epirubicin hydrochloride–containing combination therapy for breast cancer.[86] These cases occur after a brief latency period of 1 to 3 years rather than the more prolonged interval preceding ANLL induced by alkylating agents and are similar, if not identical, to the cases of leukemia associated with etoposide, another topoisomerase II inhibitor.[57]

The M. D. Anderson Cancer Center reviewed data on 1,474 patients treated on six adjuvant or neoadjuvant trials that included 5-fluorouracil, doxorubicin, and cyclophosphamide.[87] The median follow-up was only 8 years, which is too short to evaluate risk of solid tumors. The 10-year estimated acute leukemia rate was 2.5% in patients who received both chemotherapy and radiation and 0.5% in the chemotherapy-only group. This suggests that any leukemogenic risk from the use of anthracycline therapy is modest. Curtis et al.[88] reviewed the Surveillance, Epidemiology, and End Results database of 21,708 patients with breast cancer and found an 11.5 relative risk of developing secondary leukemias in patients treated with alkylating agents with or without radiation therapy as an adjuvant after a median follow-up of 4.2 years. In an attempt to assess the contributions of adjuvant radiotherapy, melphalan, or cyclophosphamide, Curtis and colleagues also reported a case-control study in a cohort of 82,700 women diagnosed with breast cancer.[89] Results indicate a 2.4-fold increase in relative risk of leukemia after radiotherapy alone, a 10-fold increase after chemotherapy alone, and a 17.4-fold increase after a combination of the two. Melphalan was tenfold more leukemogenic than cyclophosphamide, with little increase seen in the risk of leukemia after cumulative doses of cyclophosphamide of less than 20 g. The results from these analyses are consistent with data from the treatment of other malignancies. They do not rule out the possibility that second solid tumors that have a much longer latency period than leukemias may still develop.[90]

Adjuvant therapy with tamoxifen citrate is now well established to improve relapse-free survival and overall survival in selected patients with breast cancer. A number of large studies randomizing women to receive tamoxifen or placebo after surgery have been completed. Longer follow-up on these patients has provided evidence about the influence of tamoxifen on the subsequent development of other malignancies. The short- and long-term adverse effects of tamoxifen have been thought to be due to its estrogenic effects. In postmenopausal women, tamoxifen treatment leads to endometrial hyperplasia and polyps.[91] Tamoxifen also stimulates the growth of endometrial cancer *in vitro*.[92] An association is found between tamoxifen and the development of endometrial cancer. A relative risk of 6.4 was seen in a Scandinavian study in which 40 mg per day was used and was continued for 5 years.[93] Other studies using lower tamoxifen dosages and a shorter duration of treatment have reported lower relative risks.[94] Some have not reported any increased risk of endometrial cancer. Not all studies, however, prospectively collected information on second primaries.[95] The National Surgical Adjuvant Breast and Bowel Program reviewed 2,843 patients randomized to receive tamoxifen or placebo in their B-14 study.[96] The relative risk of endometrial cancer in the tamoxifen-treated group was 7.5, and the overall annual hazard rate for the development of endometrial cancer was 1.6 per 1,000. If the estrogenic effects of tamoxifen cause endometrial cancer, those tumors that develop should be of low grade and have a relatively good prognosis. This assumption has been confirmed in some of the studies reported.[97] Others have shown a distribution of grade and stage similar to that seen in non–hormonally induced cancers.[98] In an analysis of 3,457 women with breast cancer, 53 subsequently developed endometrial cancer.[99] Of these women, 15 had received tamoxifen and 38 had not. The number of high-grade cancers increased significantly in the tamoxifen-treated women, who also were more likely to die of their endometrial cancer. In a Japanese study, however, 825 women with primary breast cancer were followed prospectively with annual gynecologic examinations.[100] Thirteen cases of endometrial cancer were discovered, but the incidence was no different in women who were and who were not taking tamoxifen. In a review of the Stockholm randomized trial of 2 years of adjuvant tamoxifen in postmenopausal women (n = 4,914; median follow-up of 9 years), an increased risk of endometrial cancer (RR = 4.1) and a decreased risk of contralateral breast cancers were noted.[101] In addition, an increase in colorectal (RR = 1.9) and gastric (RR = 3.2) cancers was associated with the use of tamoxifen. In summary, most studies have demonstrated that adjuvant tamoxifen leads to a higher rate of endometrial cancer. The highest relative risks are associated with higher dosages and a longer duration of therapy. The histopathologic features of tamoxifen-associated endometrial cancer are less clear, because each reported series had only small numbers of such cancers. Tamoxifen can induce liver cancer in laboratory animals, but no increased incidence of primary liver cancer has been seen in the adjuvant breast studies. These tumors could well be missed, because any tumor developing in the liver probably would be presumed to be a recurrence of the previous breast cancer.

Several studies have reported a reduction in the development of cancers in the contralateral breast with tamoxifen use.[101–105] This either could represent a reduction in the incidence of other breast cancers or could just be a manifestation of a reduction in the incidence of recurrence of the initial cancer within the contralateral breast. Reports have also appeared of reductions in cardiovascular mortality and increases in thromboembolic events when women take tamoxifen. An analysis of the impact of adjuvant tamoxifen on mortality was undertaken using published risks of endometrial cancers and thromboembolic events as well as reductions in contralateral breast cancer and cardiovascular mortality.[106] This analysis concluded that the overall impact of tamoxifen was favorable with between 3 and 41 deaths avoided per 1,000 patients treated, depending on the age of the women being treated. The importance of breast cancer as a source of morbidity and mortality in women and the observations of reductions in contralateral breast cancers with adjuvant tamoxifen have led to two breast cancer prevention trials in which healthy women were randomized to receive tamoxifen or placebo. In a prevention trial, the increased risks of adverse events such as second malignancies are more of a concern. This was all taken into account when these trials were developed; however, some reservations have been expressed about exposing women to an increased risk of endometrial cancer.[107] No intervention is without risk; whether long-term tamoxifen usage leads to an overall health benefit to women can only be truly answered by these prevention trials.

Patients with Multiple Myeloma

Multiple myeloma, a disease commonly treated with single-agent alkylators such as melphalan, also has been associated with a high incidence of ANLL.[108–110] Because myeloma itself involves a bone marrow element, the possibility exists that a common process may be responsible for both diseases. However, the reported incidence of leukemia in patients with myeloma who do not receive alkylating therapy is no greater than expected for an age-matched population.[111] This suggests that the alkylating agents have contributed to the high incidence of leukemia. This contention is supported by a prospective trial of alkylating therapy for myeloma, which found that the actuarial risk of developing acute leukemia was 17.4% at 50 months—214 times that expected.

Patients with Malignant Lymphoma

The incidence of second malignancies among patients with malignant lymphoma was no higher than expected during the era before intensive therapy.[112] The use of combination chemotherapy and combined radiotherapy and chemotherapy has been associated with a high incidence of second malignancies, specifically ANLL and solid tumors.[113–117] Many of these patients, however, would not have survived long enough to be exposed to the risk of a second malignancy before the introduction of intensive therapy. Many lymphoma patients have defective immune function, which may predispose to a higher risk of cancer on exposure to an inciting agent. Mechlorethamine hydrochloride and procarbazine, components of MOPP combination chemotherapy for Hodgkin's disease, are potent carcinogens in animals.[37] A case-control study of 1,939 patients treated for Hodgkin's disease in the Netherlands assessed factors influencing the development of acute leukemia.[118] The cumulative dose of mechlorethamine was the most important factor. The use of lomustine was also associated with secondary leukemia, as was a requirement for a second course of chemotherapy. Overall, patients receiving chemotherapy had a 40-fold greater risk of leukemia than those receiving radiation therapy alone, whereas the use of combined-modality therapy did not increase the risk of leukemia beyond that seen with chemotherapy. Other analyses have similarly confirmed the importance of mechlorethamine, procarbazine, and nitrosoureas in the risk of second leukemia after treatment for lymphoma.[119,120] These studies also demonstrated that chemotherapy that did not include these three agents had a negligible risk of secondary leukemia.

Although many reports have been concerned with an increased risk of acute leukemia, solid tumors also occur more frequently in patients with malignant lymphoma after intensive therapy.[121–124] Approximately one out of five patients with Hodgkin's disease develops a second cancer within 15 years of primary treatment.[122,125] Three-fourths of these are solid tumors, and the remainder are equally divided between leukemia and lymphoma. One hundred and thirteen second cancers were seen in 2,846 British patients treated for Hodgkin's disease from 1970 to 1987.[126] The relative risk compared with that of the general population for leukemia and non-Hodgkin's lymphoma was 16, but the chance of developing colon, lung, and thyroid cancer, as well as osteogenic sarcoma, was also higher. In a German series of over 1,500 patients with Hodgkin's disease treated with radiation therapy, with or without chemotherapy, from 1940 to 1991, the cumulative risk for malignancy was 1.5%, 4.2%, 9.4%, and 21% at 5, 10, 15, and 20 years, respectively.[127] At the 20-year period, the risk for solid tumors, lymphoma, and leukemia was 19%, 1.9%, and 0.6%, respectively. Three-fourths of the solid tumors occurred within the radiation field. In patients receiving both chemotherapy and radiation therapy, the regimen of doxorubicin, bleomycin, vinblastine sulfate, and dacarbazine (ABVD) was associated with the highest risk. In a case-control study of patients who developed lung cancer, the use of chemotherapy led to a higher risk than the use of radiation therapy.[128] Arseneau et al.[116] reported a 23-fold increased risk of sarcoma after combined-modality therapy in Hodgkin's disease patients. The overall risk of second malignancies increased 2.8-fold with intensive chemotherapy. In 885 women treated for Hodgkin's disease from 1961 to 1990, the relative risk of developing and dying from breast cancer was increased fourfold to fivefold.[121] Although this is due primarily to upper mantle irradiation, the concurrent use of chemotherapy further increased the relative risk. Because combined-modality therapy exposes patients to a higher risk of neoplasm, a long-term assessment of its benefits and risks continues to be necessary. One interesting analysis examined 313 patients with early-stage Hodgkin's disease who received either full-dose radiation therapy or chemotherapy followed by a lower dose of involved-field radiation.[129] The relative risk of a second cancer was 1.5 (95% CI, 0.6 to 3.5; p value not significant) in the combined-modality group but was 3.3 (95% CI, 2.2 to 5.3; p <.001) in the group receiving full-dose radiation.

Longer follow-up of patients receiving combination chemotherapy and radiotherapy for Hodgkin's disease has suggested that the increased risk of leukemia in this patient population may peak at between 3 and 9 years, followed by a decline thereafter.[51,113,130–132] The risks for the development of solid tumors appear to continue to increase over time.[132] Although the relative risk is highest for the development of leukemia and lymphoma, the twofold to threefold increase seen in the more common solid tumors accounts for most of the absolute increase in cancer cases in these patients.

Patients with Gastrointestinal Cancer

Analysis of randomized trials of adjuvant methyl-CCNU in the management of patients with gastrointestinal cancers performed by Boice et al.[133] has added more information regarding the leukemogenic potential of this treatment. The results of this analysis indicated that a 12.4 relative risk of leukemia exists in patients treated with methyl-CCNU. This risk seems to be dose dependent when cumulative dose is considered. The latency period varies from 6 to 69 months and may continue to rise beyond that. Because the current data do not suggest a benefit in survival with such therapy, the leukemogenic risk has led to the removal of methyl-CCNU from adjuvant treatment regimens. The most important drug in adjuvant regimens for colorectal cancer is 5-fluorouracil, and it has not been associated with an increased risk of second cancers.

Patients with Testicular Cancer

More than 15 years have now passed since cisplatin-based chemotherapy was first used for the treatment of advanced testicular cancer. This treatment has led to a large increase in the number of patients cured with chemotherapy, and reports about the long-term consequences of this therapy are only beginning to appear. In a group of 1,909 patients in the Netherlands diagnosed between 1971 and 1985, 78 second cancers occurred, or 1.6 times the number expected.[134] Significant increases were seen in gastrointestinal cancers (RR = 2.6) and leukemia (RR = 5.1). In this analysis, radiation therapy was the main contributing factor; patients treated with chemotherapy did not have an increased rate of second malignancies and actually had a decrease in the incidence of cancer in the contralateral testis. In a Norwegian series, the use of chemotherapy plus infradiaphragmatic radiation did increase the relative risk of second cancers over that seen with infradiaphragmatic radiation alone (RR = 1.3 versus 2.4).[135] The highest risk was seen in patients who received both infradiaphragmatic and supradiaphragmatic radiation. An update of the Norwegian experience confirmed a modest increase in relative risk from the use of combined-modality therapy.[136] The use of modern cisplatin-containing chemotherapy alone did not appear to increase the risk of a second cancer. In a cohort of 1,025 German patients treated between 1970 and 1990, 224 received surgery only, 332 had radiation therapy, and

413 received chemotherapy, which in 293 cases included etoposide.[137] The incidence of secondary neoplasm increased in patients receiving radiation therapy but not in those who received chemotherapy. The median follow-up in this review was relatively short (61 months). In a more recent review from France of 131 patients with seminoma, the relative risk of second tumors was not increased by infradiaphragmatic radiation. It was increased threefold, however, in patients receiving both infradiaphragmatic and supradiaphragmatic radiation and was increased 26-fold in the small number of patients who received chemotherapy plus radiation.[138]

No increases in second cancers have been reported after the use of cisplatin, vinblastine, and bleomycin (PVB) for testicular cancer.[139] Etoposide is now used rather than vinblastine because a randomized trial demonstrated the improved effectiveness of cisplatin, etoposide, and bleomycin over PVB.[140] The association between etoposide and secondary leukemia in the pediatric population led to a more detailed scrutiny of this relationship in testicular cancer patients. Among 315 patients at Indiana University receiving etoposide, two cases of acute leukemia (0.63%) occurred.[141] Of 340 patients treated with etoposide at Memorial Sloan-Kettering Cancer Center, two cases of acute leukemia also were seen.[142] The overall conclusion of these and other reviews of etoposide use is that the dosages used in most germ cell cancer protocols are associated with a slightly increased risk of acute leukemia that is acceptable, given the benefits of etoposide-based therapy in treating this disease.[143]

The largest review of second neoplasms in patients with testicular cancer includes data for almost 29,000 men in 16 different tumor registries.[144] Overall, 1,406 second cancers were identified yielding a relative risk of 1.43. Increased tumors found included leukemias (RR = 3.07 to 5.20), melanoma (RR = 1.69), lymphoma (RR = 1.88), and a variety of gastrointestinal tumors (RR = 1.27 to 2.21). An analysis of the relationship between treatment and these new tumors revealed that the gastrointestinal tumors were associated with radiation therapy, whereas the secondary leukemia was associated with both radiation and chemotherapy.

Patients Receiving High-Dose Therapies

High-dose chemotherapy with autologous bone marrow transplantation (ABMT) or peripheral blood stem cell transplantation is being used with increased frequency in patients with hematologic malignancies and breast cancer. In this setting, very high doses of drugs are given over a short period of time, in contrast to the more conventional method of giving lower doses over a period of 4 to 12 months. The agents used differ slightly depending on the institution and tumor being treated, but commonly the oxazaphosphorine nitrogen mustards (cyclophosphamide

and ifosfamide), carboplatin, and etoposide are used. The doses delivered with marrow rescue are threefold to sixfold higher than can be given with such support; thus, the total dose of drug delivered is similar to that given when such drugs are used in conventional regimens. Myelodysplastic syndrome (MDS) and ANLL have been reported in patients who receive allogeneic, autologous, or peripheral blood transplantation for a variety of malignancies.[145,146] Most patients who have an ABMT, however, also receive other chemotherapy before this procedure, which confounds estimation of risk. A review of all 649 patients who received ABMT or peripheral blood stem cell transplantation at the University of Chicago from 1985 to 1997 revealed 7 cases (1%) of MDS, ALL, or ANLL that were felt to be therapy related.[147] These occurred in patients with Hodgkin's disease (5), non-Hodgkin's lymphoma (1), and breast cancer (1). The median latency period between initial standard-dose treatment of the cancer and development of leukemia/MDS was approximately 5 years, whereas the interval was less than 2 years from the high-dose therapy. This suggests that conventional chemotherapy before the high-dose therapy was the more likely cause. In a situation in which high-dose therapy is given repeatedly, however, the risk of secondary leukemia may become prohibitive. In a series of 86 patients with poor-risk solid tumors treated with repeated high doses of cyclophosphamide/ifosfamide, etoposide, and doxorubicin, the risk of ANLL at 24 months increased 5,000-fold.[148] Cytogenetic analysis was consistent with leukemias induced both by alkylators and by etoposide.

Patients who receive allogeneic transplants are also demonstrated to have an increased risk of solid tumors.[146] One advantage in analyzing this population is the existence of good registries for many of the patients. In an analysis of 19,229 patients at 235 centers, the relative risk of solid tumors at 10 years was 8.3; the cumulative incidence was 2.2% at 10 years and 6.7% at 15 years. Solid tumors with a notable increase in risk included tumors of the skin, oral cavity, central nervous system, connective tissue, and liver. A younger age and higher dose of total-body irradiation predicted for a higher relative risk. The increased risk of skin and oral cavity tumors was primarily related to the presence of graft-versus-host disease.

Patients Receiving Cyclophosphamide Therapy

Bladder toxicity associated with the use of the oxazaphosphorine nitrogen mustards cyclophosphamide and ifosfamide has been long recognized.[149] The acute cystitis is likely related to toxic metabolites and can be limited by the concomitant use of mesna. An increased number of reports have now been published of bladder cancer in patients who received long-term cyclophosphamide therapy.[150,151] The most common situations in which this occurs are in some pediatric protocols, in low-grade lymphomas, and in immunosuppressive therapy. A review of a cohort of 6,171 medium- or long-term survivors of non-Hodgkin's lymphoma revealed 48 cases of urothelial cancer.[151] Overall, a 4.5-fold increase in risk of bladder cancer was estimated from the use of cyclophosphamide; however, the cumulative dose was critical in determining risk. In patients who received more than 50 g of cyclophosphamide, the risk increased 15-fold, which translated to an absolute risk of 7% within 15 years of treatment. The long-term use of cyclophosphamide is now less common in treating pediatric and adult cancers; however, the risk of secondary urothelial cancer may be an important consideration in decisions about therapy in immunologic diseases.

Patients Receiving Immunosuppressive Agents

Cytotoxic agents such as azathioprine and cyclophosphamide are also immunosuppressive agents and have been used in the treatment of rheumatoid arthritis, scleroderma, Wegener's granulomatosis, nephrotic syndrome, and glomerulonephritis, as well as in the control of rejection in renal transplantation.[152–154]

Accumulated experience with these and other immunosuppressive agents suggests a different mechanism of tumor induction from that observed in patients treated for neoplastic conditions. Patients treated with immunosuppressive agents have a high incidence of malignant lymphomas, often with evidence of the presence of Epstein-Barr virus, which show a predilection for primary sites in the brain; this may be due to long-term immunosuppression resulting in decreased immune surveillance. This state resembles the chronic immunodeficiency of certain inherited disorders, such as Wiskott-Aldrich syndrome, which is also associated with a high incidence of lymphomas.[155]

Further evidence supporting the contention that long-term immunosuppression contributes to neoplastic induction is found in the experience of inadvertent engraftment of human tumors in donor kidneys. In one case, immunosuppression led to the development of a tumor of donor origin, but tumor rejection occurred rapidly after cytotoxic therapy ceased. Immunosuppression is not an entirely satisfactory explanation for the high incidence of lymphomas in transplant patients because long-term alkylating-agent therapy leads to nonlymphocytic leukemia in patients with multiple myeloma or ovarian carcinoma. Continued investigations into the role of immune surveillance in carcinogenesis are necessary to define the mechanisms responsible for the development of neoplasms in immunosuppressed patients. The complex interaction of various factors (such as the interleukins and interferons) is being defined. How antineoplastic drugs interact with these factors must be defined before the impact of antineoplastic agents on immune surveillance is known.

CONCLUSION

Both clinical and laboratory studies have implicated alkylating agents and epipodophyllotoxins as potent carcinogens. Strong evidence exists for carcinogenicity in laboratory systems for the antitumor antibiotics and procarbazine; the clinical evidence suggests less of a risk. Antimetabolites as a group are much less hazardous, likely due to fewer interactions with DNA. Newer agents such as the topoisomerase I inhibitors and the taxanes have not been used for a sufficient duration to allow estimation of any carcinogenic risk. Long-term immunosuppression with azathioprine has led to an increased incidence of lymphoid malignancies, perhaps by an entirely different mechanism than those producing mutagenic effects. The combined use of chemotherapy and radiotherapy definitely increases the risk of tumor induction. All of this, however, must be interpreted in the context of the need successfully to treat a potentially lethal primary cancer.

The available data suggest that certain guidelines should be followed in the design, use, and follow-up of chemotherapy (and radiation therapy) for patients with potentially curable disease. A careful surveillance must be conducted for secondary neoplasms during long-term follow-up of these patients. An attempt should be made to establish the quantitative risk of neoplasia for any regimen that proves curative, and efforts should be made to limit the use of the more highly carcinogenic agents. On the basis of present information, caution is required when using alkylating agents or epipodophyllotoxins. Careful prospective and retrospective studies should be aimed at establishing whether a total-dose threshold exists for carcinogenicity of suspected carcinogens in humans and whether modification of the schedule of administration affects this risk. Finally, further attention should be directed to the development of new agents that do not have mutagenic or cytotoxic actions but that exert regulatory actions on cell growth and differentiation.

REFERENCES

1. Haddow A. Mode of action of chemical carcinogens. *Br Med Bull* 1947;4:331–342.
2. Miller A. Carcinogenesis by chemicals: an overview—G.H.A. Clowes Memorial Lecture. *Cancer Res* 1970;30:559–576.
3. Farber E. Carcinogenesis—cellular evolution as a unifying thread: presidential address. *Cancer Res* 1973;33:2537–2550.
4. Miller EC. Some current perspectives on chemical carcinogenesis in humans and experimental animals: presidential address. *Cancer Res* 1978;38:1479–1496.
5. Pitot HC. The molecular biology of carcinogenesis. *Cancer* 1993;72:962–970.
6. Keller R. Suppression of natural antitumor defense mechanisms by phorbol esters. *Nature* 1979;282:729–731.
7. Price CC, Gaucher GM, Koneru P, et al. Mechanism of

action of alkylating agents. *Ann N Y Acad Sci* 1969; 163:593–600.

8. Singer B. Sites in nucleic acids reacting with alkylating agents of differing carcinogenicity or mutagenicity. *J Toxicol Environ Health* 1977;2:1279–1295.

9. Zarbl H, Sukumar S, Arthur AV, et al. Direct mutagenesis of *ha-ras*-1 oncogenes by *N*-nitroso-*N*-methylurea during initiation of mammary carcinogenesis in rats. *Nature* 1985;315:382–385.

10. Nath J, Krichna G. Fundamental and applied genetic toxicology. In: Craig E, Stitzel RE, eds. *Modern pharmacology with clinical applications.* Boston: Little, Brown and Company, 1997:69–77.

11. McCann J, Ames BN. A simple method of detecting environmental carcinogens as mutagens. *Ann N Y Acad Sci* 1976;271:5–13.

12. McCann J, Choi E, Yamasaki E, et al. Detection of carcinogens as mutagens in the *Salmonella*/microsome test: assay of 300 chemicals. *Proc Natl Acad Sci U S A* 1975;72:5135–5139.

13. McCann J, Ames BN. Detection of carcinogens as mutagens in the *Salmonella*/microsome test: assay of 300 chemicals [Discussion]. *Proc Natl Acad Sci U S A* 1975;73: 950–954.

14. Seino Y, Nagao M, Yahagi T, et al. Mutagenicity of several classes of antitumor agents to *Salmonella typhimurium* TA98, TA100, and TA92. *Cancer Res* 1978;38:2148–2156.

15. Brundrett RB, Colvin M, White EH. Comparison of mutagenicity, antitumor activity, and chemical properties of selected nitrosoureas and nitrosoamides. *Cancer Res* 1979; 39:1328–1333.

16. Genther CS, Schoeny RS, Loper JC. Mutagenic studies of folic acid antagonists. *Antimicrob Agents Chemother* 1977;12:84–92.

17. Benedict WF, Baker MS, Haroun L, et al. Mutagenicity of cancer chemotherapeutic agents in the *Salmonella*/microsome test. *Cancer Res* 1977;37:2209–2213.

18. Rinkus SJ, Legator MS. Chemical characterization of 465 known or suspected carcinogens and their correlation with mutagenic activity in the *Salmonella typhimurium* system. *Cancer Res* 1979;39:3289–3318.

19. Albertini RJ, Castle KL, Borcherding WR. T-cell cloning to detect the mutation 6-thioguanine-resistant lymphocytes present in human peripheral blood. *Proc Natl Acad Sci U S A* 1982;79:6617–6621.

20. Hirota H, Kubota M, Hashimoto H, et al. Analysis of hprt gene mutation following anti-cancer treatment in pediatric patients with acute leukemia. *Mutat Res* 1993;319:113–120.

21. Hirota H, Kirota M, Adachi A, et al. Somatic mutation at T-cell antigen receptor and glycophorin A loci in pediatric leukemia patients following chemotherapy: comparison with HPRT locus mutation. *Mutat Res* 1994;315:95–103.

22. Musalis JC, Monteforte JA, Winegar RA. Transgenic animal models for detection of in vivo mutations. *Annu Rev Pharmacol Toxicol* 1995;35:145–164.

23. Kato H. Spontaneous and induced sister chromatid exchanges as revealed by the BUdr-labeling method. *Int Rev Cytol* 1977;49:55–97.

24. Perry P, Evans HJ. Cytological detection of mutagen-carcinogen exposure by sister chromatid exchange. *Nature* 1977; 258:121–125.

25. Guerrero PR, Rounds DE, Hall TC. Bioassay procedure for the detection of mutagenic metabolites in human urine with the use of sister chromatid exchange analysis. *J Natl Cancer Inst* 1979;62:805–809.

26. Banerjee A, Benedict WF. Production of sister chromatid exchanges by various cancer chemotherapeutic agents. *Cancer Res* 1979;39:797–799.

27. Lambert B, Ringborg U, Harper E, et al. Sister chromatid exchanges in lymphocyte cultures of patients receiving chemotherapy for malignant disorders. *Cancer Treat Rep* 1979;62:1413–1419.

28. Lambert B, Ringborn U, Linblad A, et al. The effects of DTIC, melphalan, actinomycin D and CCNU on the frequency of sister chromatid exchanges in peripheral lymphocytes of melanoma patients. In: Jones, Salmon SE, eds. *Adjuvant therapy of cancer II.* New York: Grune & Stratton, 1979:55–62.

29. Ohtsuru M, Ishi Y, Takai S, et al. Sister chromatid exchanges in lymphoctyes of cancer patients receiving mitomycin C treatment. *Cancer Res* 1980;40:477–480.

30. Heidelberger C. Chemical oncogenesis in culture. *Cancer Res* 1973;18:317–366.

31. Heidelberger C. Chemical carcinogenesis. *Cancer* 1977;40: 430–433.

32. Benedict WF, Banerjee A, Gardner A. Induction of morphological transformation in mouse C3H/10T1/2 clone 8 cells and chromosomal damage in hamster A(T1)C1-3 cells by cancer chemotherapeutic agents. *Cancer Res* 1977;37: 2202–2208.

33. Jones PA, Benedict WF, Baker MS. Oncogenic transformation of C3H/10T1/2 clone 8 mouse embryo cells by halogenated pyrimidine nucleosides. *Cancer Res* 1976;36:101–107.

34. Gabrielson EW, Harris CC. Use of cultured human tissues and cells in carcinogenesis research. *J Cancer Res Clin Oncol* 1985;110:1–10.

35. Schamhl D, Habs M. Experimental carcinogenesis of antitumor drugs. *Cancer Treat Rev* 1978;5:175–184.

36. Weisburger JH, Griswald DP, Prejean JD, et al. The carcinogenic properties of some of the principal drugs used in clinical cancer chemotherapy: recent results. *Cancer Res* 1975;52:1–17.

37. Weisburger EK. Bioassay program for carcinogenic hazards of cancer chemotherapeutic agents. *Cancer* 1977;40:1935–1949.

38. Solcia E, Ballerini L, Bellini O, et al. Mammary tumors induced in rats by Adriamycin and daunomycin. *Cancer Res* 1978;38:1444–1446.

39. Sieber SM, Adamson RH. Toxicity of antineoplastic agents in man: chromosomal aberrations, antifertility effects, congenital malformations and carcinogenic potential. *Cancer Res* 1978;22:57–155.

40. Harris C. Chemical and physical carcinogenesis: advances and perspectives for the 1990s. *Cancer Res* 1991;151: 5023S–5044S.

41. Sugamiua H, Weston A, Caporaso NE. Biochemical and molecular epidemiology of cancer. *Biomed Environ Sci* 1991;4:73–92.

42. Smith MA, McCaffrey RP, Karp JE. The secondary leukemias: challenges and research directions. *J Natl Cancer Inst* 1996;88:407–418.

43. Bokemeyer C, Schmoll HJ. Treatment of testicular cancer and the development of secondary malignancies. *J Clin Oncol* 1995;13:283–292.

44. Van Leeuwen F. Second cancers. In: DeVita VT Jr, Hellman S, Rosenberg SA, eds. *Cancer: principles and practice of oncology*, 5th ed. Philadelphia: Lippincott, 1997:2773–2796.

45. Makuch R, Simon R. Recommendations for the analysis of the effect of treatment on the development of second malignancies. *Cancer* 1979;44:250–253.

46. Hughes RG, Colquhoun M, Alloub M, et al. Cervical intraepithelial neoplasia in patients with breast cancer: a cytological and colposcopic study. *Br J Cancer* 1993;67:1082–1085.

47. Islam MQ, Kopf I, Levan A, et al. Cytogenetic findings in 111 ovarian cancer patients: therapy-related chromosome aberrations and heterochromatic variants. *Cancer Genet Cytogenet* 1993;65:35–46.

48. De Wit PE, de Vaan GA, de Boo TM, et al. Prevalence of naevocytic naevi after chemotherapy for childhood cancer. *Med Pediatr Oncol* 1990;18:336–338.

49. Baird EA, McHenry PM, MacKie RM. Effect of maintenance chemotherapy in childhood on numbers of melanocytc naevi. *Br J Med* 1992;305:799–801.

50. Li FP, Abramson DH, Tarone RE, et al. Hereditary retinoblastoma, lipoma and second primary cancer. *J Natl Cancer Inst* 1997;89:83–84.

51. Tucker MA, D'Angi GJ, Boice JD, et al. Bone sarcomas linked to radiotherapy and chemotherapy in children. *N Engl J Med* 1987;317:588–593.

52. Tucker MA, Meadows AT, Boice JD, et al. Leukemia after therapy with alkylating agents for childhood cancer. *J Natl Cancer Inst* 1987;78:459–464.

53. Winick NJ, McKenna RW, Shuster JJ, et al. Secondary acute myeloid leukemia in children with acute lymphoblastic leukemia treated with etoposide. *J Clin Oncol* 1993;11:209–217.

54. Pui CH, Ribeiro RC, Hancock ML, et al. Acute myeloid leukemia in children treated with epipodophyllotoxins for acute lymphoblastic leukemia. *N Engl J Med* 1991;325:1682–1687.

55. Kreissman SG, Gelber RD, Cohen HJ, et al. Incidence of secondary acute myelogenous leukemia after treatment of childhood acute lymphoblastic leukemia. *Cancer* 1992;70:2208–2213.

56. Felix CA. Secondary leukemias induced by topoisomerase-targeted drugs. *Biochim Biophys Acta* 1998;1400:233–255.

57. Smith MC, Rubinstein L, Ungerleider RS. Therapy-related acute myeloid leukemia following treatment with epipodophyllotoxins: estimating the risk. *Med Pediatr Oncol* 1994;23:86–98.

58. Smith MA, Rubinstein L, Anderson JR, et al. Secondary leukemia or myelodysplastic syndrome after treatment with epipodophyllotoxins. *J Clin Oncol* 1999;17:569–577.

59. Kushner BH, Cheung NKV, Kramer K, et al. Neuroblastoma and treatment related myelodysplasia/leukemia: the MSKCC experience. *J Clin Oncol* 1998;16:3880–3889.

60. Green DM, Zevon MA, Reese PA, et al. Second malignant tumors following treatment during childhood and adolescence for cancer. *Med Pediatr Oncol* 1994;22:1–10.

61. Jankovic M, Fraschini D, Amici A, et al. Outcome after cessation of therapy in childhood acute lymphoblastic leukaemia. *Eur J Cancer* 1993;29a:1839–1843.

62. Morland BJ, Radford M. Cutaneous squamous cell carcinoma following treatment for acute lymphoblastic leukaemia. *Med Pediatr Oncol* 1993;21:150–152.

63. Dunst J, Ahrens S, Paulussen M, et al. Second malignancies after treatment for Ewing's sarcoma: a report of the CESS-studies. *Int J Radiat Oncol Biol Phys* 1998;42:379–384.

64. Kimball Dalton VM, Gelber RD, Li F, et al. Second malignancies in patients treated for childhood acute lymphoblastic leukemia. *J Clin Oncol* 1998;16:2848–2853.

65. Wolden SL, Lamborn KR, Cleary SF, et al. Second cancers following pediatric Hodgkin's disease. *J Clin Oncol* 1998;16:536–544.

66. Bhatia S, Robison LL, Oberlin O, et al. Breast cancer and other second neoplasms after childhood Hodgkin's disease. *N Engl J Med* 1996;334:745–751.

67. Bagley CM, Young RC, Canellos GP, et al. Treatment of ovarian carcinoma: possibilities for progress. *N Engl J Med* 1972;287:856–862.

68. Einhorn N. Acute leukemia after chemotherapy (melphalan). *Cancer* 1978;41:444–447.

69. Sotrel G, Jafari K, Lash AF, et al. Acute leukemia in advanced ovarian carcinoma after treatment with alkylating agents. *Obstet Gynecol* 1976;47:67S–71S.

70. Morrison J, Yon JL. Acute leukemia following chlorambucil therapy of advanced ovarian and fallopian tube carcinoma. *Gynecol Oncol* 1978;6:115–120.

71. Casciato DA, Scott JL. Acute leukemia following prolonged cytotoxic agent therapy. *Medicine* 1979;53:32–47.

72. Reimer PR, Hoover R, Fraumeni J, et al. Acute leukemia after alkylating-agent therapy of ovarian cancer. *N Engl J Med* 1977;297:177–181.

73. Greene MH, Harris EL, Gershenson DM, et al. Melphalan may be a more potent leukemogen than cyclophosphamide. *Ann Intern Med* 1986;105:360–367.

74. Kaldor JM, Day NE, Pettersson F, et al. Leukemia following chemotherapy for ovarian cancer. *N Engl J Med* 1990;322:1–6.

75. Travis LB, Curtis RE, Boice JD, et al. Second malignant neoplasms among long-term survivors of ovarian cancer. *Cancer Res* 1996;56:1564–1570.

76. Sprance HE, Hempling RE, Piver MS. Leukemia following cisplatin-based chemotherapy for ovarian carcinoma. *Eur J Gynecol Oncol* 1992;13:131–137.

77. Reed E, Evans MK. Acute leukemia following cisplatin-based chemotherapy in a patient with ovarian cancer. *J Natl Cancer Inst* 1990;82:431–432.

78. Carbone PP, Bauer M, Baud P, et al. Chemotherapy of disseminated breast cancer: current status and prospects. *Cancer* 1977;39:2916–2922.

79. Chan PYM, Sadoff L, Winkley JH. Second malignancies following first breast cancer in prolonged thio-TEPA adjuvant chemotherapy. In: Salmon SE, Jones SE, eds. *Adjuvant therapy of cancer*. Amsterdam: North-Holland, 1977:597–607.

80. Lerner HJ. Acute myelogenous leukemia in patients receiving chlorambucil as long-term adjuvant chemotherapy for stage II breast cancer. *Cancer Treat Rep* 1978;62:1135–1138.

81. Fisher B, Glass A, Redmond C, et al. L-phenylalanine mustard (L-PAM) in the management of primary breast cancer: an update of earlier findings and a comparison with those utilizing L-PAM plus 5-fluorouracil (5-FU). *Cancer* 1977;39:2883–2903.

82. Fisher B, Rockette H, Fisher ER, et al. Leukemia in breast cancer patients following adjuvant chemotherapy or postoperative radiation: the NSABP experience. *J Clin Oncol* 1985;3:1640–1658.

83. Valagussa P, Tancini G, Bonadonna G. Second malignancies after CMF for resectable breast cancer. *J Clin Oncol* 1987;5:1138–1142.

84. Valagussa P, Moliterni A, Terenziani M, et al. Second malignancies following CMF-based adjuvant chemotherapy in resectable breast cancer. *Ann Oncol* 1994;5:803–808.

85. Arriagada R, Rutqvist LE. Adjuvant chemotherapy in early breast cancer and incidence of new primary malignancies. *Lancet* 1991;338:535–538.

86. Pederson-Bjergaard J, Siqsgaard T, Nielsen D, et al. Acute monocytic or myelomonocytic leukemia with balanced chromosome translocations to band 11q23 after therapy with 4 epidoxorubicin and cisplatin or cyclophosphamide for breast cancer. *J Clin Oncol* 1992;10:1444–1451.

87. Diamandidou E, Buzdar AU, Smith TL, et al. Treatment-related leukemia in breast cancer patients treated with fluorouracil-doxorubicin-cyclophosphamide combination adjuvant chemotherapy: the University of Texas M.D. Anderson Cancer Center experience. *J Clin Oncol* 1996;14:2722–2730.

88. Curtis RE, Boice JD, Moloney WC, et al. Leukemia following chemotherapy for breast cancer. *Cancer Res* 1990;50:2741–2746.

89. Curtis RE, Boice JD, Stovall M, et al. Risk of leukemia after chemotherapy and radiation treatment for breast cancer. *N Engl J Med* 1990;326:1745–1751.

90. Henne T, Schmahl D. Occurrence of second primary malignancies in man—a second look. *Cancer Treat Rev* 1985;12:77–94.

91. Rutqvist LE. Long-term toxicity of tamoxifen. *Cancer Res* 1993;127:257–266.

92. Satyaswaroop PG, Zaino RJ, Marbel R. Estrogen-like effects of tamoxifen on human endometrial carcinoma transplanted into nude mice. *Cancer Res* 1984;44:4006–4010.

93. Fornander T, Rutqvist LE, Cedermark B, et al. Adjuvant tamoxifen in early breast cancer: occurrence of new primary cancers. *Lancet* 1989;1:117–120.

94. Andersson M, Storm HH, Mouridsen HT. Incidence of new primary cancers after adjuvant tamoxifen therapy and radiotherapy for early breast cancer. *J Natl Cancer Inst* 1991;83:1013–1017.

95. Ribeiro G, Swindell R. The Christie Hospital adjuvant tamoxifen trial. *Monogr Natl Cancer Inst* 1992;11:121–125.

96. Fisher B, Costantino JP, Redmond CK, et al. Endometrial cancer in tamoxifen-treated breast cancer patients: findings from the National Surgical Adjuvant Breast and Bowel Project (NSABP) B-14. *J Natl Cancer Inst* 1994;86:527–537.

97. Seoud MA, Johnson J, Weed JC. Gynecological tumors in tamoxifen-treated women with breast cancer [Review]. *Obstet Gynecol* 1993;82:165–169.

98. Fornander T, Hellstrom AC, Moberger B. Descriptive clinicopathologic study of 17 patients with endometrial cancer during or after adjuvant tamoxifen in early breast cancer. *J Natl Cancer Inst* 1993;85:1850–1855.

99. Magriples U, Naftolin F, Schwartz PE, et al. High-grade endometrial carcinoma in tamoxifen-treated breast cancer patients. *J Clin Oncol* 1993;11:485–490.

100. Katase K, Sugiyama Y, Hasumi K, et al. The incidence of subsequent endometrial carcinoma with tamoxifen use in patients with primary breast cancer. *Cancer* 1998;82:1698–1703.

101. Rutqvist LE, Johansson H, Signomklao T, et al. Adjuvant tamoxifen therapy for early stage breast cancer and second primary malignancies. *J Natl Cancer Inst* 1995;87:645–651.

102. Fisher B, Costantino J, Redmond C, et al. A randomized clinical trial evaluating tamoxifen in the treatment of patients with node negative breast cancer. *N Engl J Med* 1989;320:479–484.

103. Stewart HJ. The Scottish trial of adjuvant tamoxifen in node-negative breast cancer: Scottish Cancer Trials Breast Group. *Monogr Natl Cancer Inst* 1992;11:117–120.

104. Rutqvist LE, Cedermark B, Glas U, et al. Contralateral primary tumors in breast cancer patients in a randomized trial of adjuvant tamoxifen therapy. *J Natl Cancer Inst* 1991;83:1299–1306.

105. Rubagotti A, Perrotta A, Casella C, et al. Risk of new primaries after chemotherapy and/or tamoxifen treatment for early breast cancer. *Ann Oncol* 1996;7:239–244.

106. Ragaz J, Coldman A. Survival impact of adjuvant tamoxifen on competing causes of mortality in breast cancer survivors. *J Clin Oncol* 1998;16:2018–2024.

107. Friedman MA, Trimble EL, Abrams JS. Tamoxifen: trials, tribulations, and tradeoffs. *J Natl Cancer Inst* 1994;86:478–479.

108. Rosner F, Grunwald H. Multiple myeloma terminating in acute leukemia. *Am J Med* 1974;57:927–939.

109. Kyle RA, Pierre RV, Bayard ED. Multiple myeloma and acute leukemia associated with alkylating agents. *Arch Intern Med* 1975;135:185–192.

110. Bergsagel DE, Bailey AJ, Langley GR, et al. The chemotherapy of plasma-cell myeloma and the incidence of acute leukemia. *N Engl J Med* 1979;301:743–748.

111. Sieber SM. Cancer chemotherapeutic agents and carcinogenesis. *Cancer Chemother Rep* 1975;59:915–918.

112. Moertel CG, Hagedorn AB. Leukemia or lymphoma and coexistent primary malignant lesions: a review of the literature and study of 120 cases. *Blood* 1957;12:788.

113. Tucker MA, Coleman CN, Cox RS, et al. Risk of second cancers after treatment for Hodgkin's disease. *N Engl J Med* 1988;318:76–81.

114. Krikorian JG, Burke JS, Rosenberg SA, et al. Occurrence of non-Hodgkin's lymphoma after therapy for Hodgkin's disease. *N Engl J Med* 1979;300:452–458.

115. Canellos GP, Arseneau JC, De Vita VT, et al. Second malignancies complicating Hodgkin's disease in remission. *Lancet* 1975;1:947–949.

116. Arseneau JC, Canellos GP, Johnson R, et al. Risk of new cancers in patients with Hodgkin's disease. *Cancer* 1977;40:1912–1916.

117. Rodriguez MA, Fuller LM, Zimmerman SO, et al. Hodgkin's disease: study of treatment intensities and incidences of second malignancies. *Ann Oncol* 1993;4:125–131.

118. Van Leeuwen FE, Chorus AM, van den Belt-Dusebout AW, et al. Leukemia risk following Hodgkin's disease: relation to cumulative dose of alkylating agents, treatment with teniposide combinations, number of episodes of chemotherapy, and bone marrow damage. *J Clin Oncol* 1994;12:1063–1073.

119. Brusamolini E, Anselm AP, Klersy C, et al. The risk of acute leukemia in patients treated for Hodgkin's disease is signifi-

cantly higher after combined modality programs than after chemotherapy alone and is correlated with the extent of radiotherapy and type and duration of chemotherapy: a case-control study. *Haematologica* 1998;83:812–823.

120. Travis LB, Curtis RE, Stovall M, et al. Risk of leukemia following treatment for non-Hodgkin's lymphoma. *J Natl Cancer Inst* 1994;86:1450–1457.

121. Hancock SL, Tucker MA, Hoppe RT. Breast cancer after treatment of Hodgkin's disease. *J Natl Cancer Inst* 1993;85:25–31.

122. Sont JK, van Stiphout WA, Noordijk EM, et al. Increased risk of second cancers in managing Hodgkin's disease: the 20-year Leiden experience. *Ann Hematol* 1992;65:213–218.

123. Henry-Amar M. Second cancers after treatment of Hodgkin's disease: experience at the International Database on Hodgkin's disease (IDHD). *Bull Cancer* 1992;79:389–391.

124. Abrahamsen JF, Andersen A, Hannisdal E, et al. Second malignancies after treatment of Hodgkin's disease: the influence of treatment, follow-up time, and age. *J Clin Oncol* 1993;11:255–261.

125. Boice JD. Second cancer after Hodgkin's disease—the price of success? *J Natl Cancer Inst* 1993;85:4–5.

126. Swerdlow AJ, Douglas AM, Vaughn Hudson G, et al. Risk of second primary cancers after Hodgkin's disease by type of treatment. *Br J Med* 1992;304:1137–1143.

127. Slanina J, Heinemann F, Henne K, et al. Second malignancies after the therapy of Hodgkin's disease: the Freiburg collective 1940 to 1991. *Strahlenther Onkol* 1999;175:154–161.

128. Kaldor JM, Day NE, Pettersson F, et al. Lung cancer following Hodgkin's disease. *Int J Cancer* 1992;52:677–681.

129. Salloum E, Doria R, Schubert W, et al. Second solid tumors in patients with Hodgkin's disease cured after radiation or chemotherapy plus adjuvant low-dose radiation. *J Clin Oncol* 1996;14:2435–2443.

130. Blayney DW, Longo DL, Young RC, et al. Decreasing risk of leukemia with prolonged follow-up after chemotherapy and radiotherapy for Hodgkin's disease. *N Engl J Med* 1987;316:710–714.

131. Meadows AT, Baum E, Fossati-Bellani F, et al. Second malignant neoplasms in children: an update from the Late Effects Study Group. *J Clin Oncol* 1985;3:532–538.

132. Glanzmann C, Veraguth A, Lutolf UM. Incidence of second solid cancer in patients after treatment of Hodgkin's disease. *Strahlenther Onkol* 1994;170:140–146.

133. Boice JD, Greene MH, Killen JY, et al. Leukemia after adjuvant chemotherapy with semustine (methyl-CCNU). *N Engl J Med* 1986;314:119–120.

134. Van Leeuwen FE, Stiggelbout AM, van den Belt AW, et al. Second cancer risk following testicular cancer. *J Clin Oncol* 1993;11:415–424.

135. Fossa SD, Langmark F, Aass N, et al. Second non-germ cell malignancies after radiotherapy of testicular cancer with or without chemotherapy. *Br J Cancer* 1990;61:639–643.

136. Wanderas EJ, Fossa SD, Tretli S. Risk of subsequent non–germ cell cancer after treatment of germ cell cancer in 2006 Norwegian male patients. *Eur J Cancer* 1997;33:253–262.

137. Bokemeyer C, Schmoll HJ. Secondary neoplasms following treatment of malignant germ cell tumors. *J Clin Oncol* 1993;11:1703–1709.

138. Bachaud JM, Berthier F, Souile M, et al. Second non-germ cell malignancies in patients treated for state I–II testicular seminoma. *Radiother Oncol* 1999;50:191–197.

139. Nichols CR, Hoffman R, Einhorn LJ, et al. Hematologic malignancies associated with primary mediastinal germ cell tumors. *Ann Intern Med* 1985;102:603–609.

140. Williams SD, Birch R, Einhorn LH, et al. Treatment of disseminated germ-cell tumors with cisplatin, bleomycin and either vinblastine or etoposide. *N Engl J Med* 1987;316:1435–1440.

141. Nichols CR, Breeden ES, Loehrer PJ, et al. Secondary leukemia associated with a conventional dose of etoposide: review of serial germ cell tumor protocols. *J Natl Cancer Inst* 1993;85:36–40.

142. Bajorin DF, Motzer RJ, Rodriguez E, et al. Acute nonlymphocytic leukemia in germ cell tumor patients treated with etoposide-containing chemotherapy. *J Natl Cancer Inst* 1993;85:60–62.

143. Kollmannsberger C, Beyer J, Droz JP, et al. Secondary leukemia following high cumulative doses of etoposide in patients treated for advanced germ cell tumors. *J Clin Oncol* 1998;16:3386–3391.

144. Travis LB, Curtis RE, Storm H, et al. Risk of second malignant neoplasms among long-term survivors of testicular cancer. *J Natl Cancer Inst* 1997;89:1429–1439.

145. Oddou S, Vey N, Viens P, et al. Second neoplasms following high-dose chemotherapy and autologous transplantation for malignant lymphomas. *Leuk Lymphoma* 1998;31:187–194.

146. Curtis RE, Rowlings PA, Deeg HJ, et al. Solid cancers after bone marrow transplantation. *N Engl J Med* 1997;336:897–904.

147. Sobecks RM, Le Beau MM, Anastasi J, et al. Myelodysplasia and acute leukemia following high-dose chemotherapy and autologous bone marrow or peripheral blood stem cell transplantation. *Bone Marrow Transplant* 1999;23:1161–1165.

148. Kushner BH, Heller G, Cheung N, et al. High risk of leukemia after short-term dose-intensive chemotherapy in young patients with solid tumors. *J Clin Oncol* 1998;16:3016–3020.

149. Siu LL, Moore MJ. Evidence based guidelines: use of mesna in the prevention of ifosfamide induced urotoxicity. *Support Care Cancer* 1998;6:144–152.

150. Inagaki T, Ebisuno S. Cyclophosphamide induced urinary bladder and renal pelvic tumor: a case report. *Nippon Hinyokika Gakkai Zasshi* 1998;89:674–677.

151. Travis LB, Curtis RE, Glimelius B, et al. Bladder and kidney cancer following cyclophosphamide therapy for non-Hodgkin's lymphoma. *J Natl Cancer Inst* 1995;87:524–530.

152. Roberts MM, Bell R. Acute leukemia after immunosuppressive therapy. *Lancet* 1976;2:768–770.

153. Penn I. Second malignant neoplasms associated with immunosuppressive medication. *Cancer* 1976;37:1024–1032.

154. Steinberg AD, Plotz PH, Wolff SM, et al. Cytotoxic drugs in treatment of nonmalignant disease. *Ann Intern Med* 1972;76:619–642.

155. Penn I. Occurrence of cancer in immune deficiencies. *Cancer* 1974;34:858–866.

6

STEROID HORMONE THERAPIES FOR CANCER

MATTHEW J. ELLIS
SANDRA M. SWAIN

A detailed understanding of drug action and clinical pharmacology are prerequisites for the rational application of chemotherapy. This principle is well illustrated by the treatment of cancer with therapies that target steroid hormones and steroid hormone receptors. A century of progress in safety and efficacy in this field has inspired generations of cancer researchers. Investigators have documented that cancer can be treated with steroid deprivation, steroid receptor blockade, or administration of potent synthetic steroids. The correct application of steroid hormone therapy requires an appreciation of (a) steroid synthesis and metabolism, (b) the endocrine regulation of these processes, (c) the molecular basis of steroid signaling through nuclear hormone receptors, and (d) the response of cancer cells to modulation of steroid receptor signaling. This chapter aims to provide a reference source on this basis, focusing on "classic" steroid therapies that signal through glucocorticoid, androgen, estrogen, and progesterone nuclear hormone receptors to achieve control of tumor growth.

HISTORICAL PERSPECTIVE

In 1849, Berthold demonstrated that the effects of castration on the cockerel cockscomb could be prevented by testis transplantation. The field of endocrinology therefore began with androgen deprivation and restoration. Sex steroid deprivation was arguably the first successful therapy for metastatic cancer in Western medicine, established by the description of breast cancer regression[1] and, later, prostate cancer regression after surgical castration.[2] With the successful synthesis of steroids in the 1930s and 1940s, further progress in cancer treatment was achieved with potent glucocorticoids, androgens, estrogens, and progestins.

The next step was to achieve sex hormone deprivation through medical rather than surgical means. First, only aminoglutethimide, a nonspecific inhibitor of steroid biosynthesis, was available.[3] Subsequently, estrogen deprivation has been achieved in a selective manner with luteinizing hormone–releasing hormone (LHRH) antagonists[4] and aromatase inhibitors.[5] Androgen deprivation can also be induced medically with LHRH antagonists, 5α-reductase inhibitors,[6] and high dosages of the antifungal drug, ketoconazole.[7]

Another phase of development in steroid hormone–based therapies was initiated when the estrogen receptor (ER) antagonist tamoxifen was shown to induce breast cancer regression in the early 1970s.[8] Tamoxifen is not a steroid and is associated with a better side effect profile than high-potency estrogen treatment, the contemporary treatment for advanced breast cancer at the time when tamoxifen was introduced.[9,10] Because long-term tamoxifen administration is safe and well tolerated, clinical trials of adjuvant therapy are possible. The aim is to prevent relapse after initial surgical treatment, rather than to treat established metastatic disease. These studies eventually established that 5 years of tamoxifen is a safe and effective adjuvant therapy for the treatment of ER positive breast cancer, reducing systemic relapse by approximately 50%.[11] Indeed, the introduction of tamoxifen likely contributed to the recent decline in breast cancer mortality observed in high-incidence Western countries.[12]

A series of alternative ER antagonists is the latest focus in the effort to improve the safety and efficacy of endocrine therapy for breast cancer. A number of these agents are in clinical trial.[13] Nonsteroidal androgen receptor (AR) antagonists have been developed for prostate cancer, and they have made a significant impact on the control of advanced disease.[14] Furthermore, studies of adjuvant endocrine therapy in prostate cancer have begun to show improved survival with the early institution of androgen deprivation.[15] Recently, it has been established that tamoxifen can reduce the incidence of breast cancer when given to women at high risk for the disease.[16]

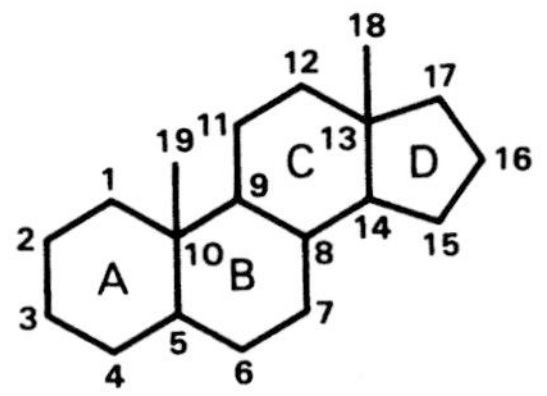

FIGURE 6-1. The structure and numbering of the cyclopentane-perhydrophenanthrene nucleus.

STEROID STRUCTURE, BIOSYNTHESIS, AND TRANSPORT

Structure

Physiologically important steroids include adrenocortical steroids (glucocorticoids and mineralocorticoids), steroids required for sexual function (androgens, estrogens, and progestins), bile acids, and sterols. All steroids have the same hydrated four-ring structure (cyclopentane-perhydro-phenanthrene), in which a five-sided cyclopentane ring (designated the D ring) is attached to three six-sided phenan-threne rings (designated A, B, and C rings) (Fig. 6-1). The carbon atoms that form these rings are numbered 1 to 17. Additional side chain carbons in sex steroids are attached to either carbon atom 10 or 13, designated carbon atom 19 for androgens and carbon atom 18 for estrogens. Corticoids and progestins are characterized by a two carbon–side chain, car-bons (21 and 22), attached to carbon atom 17. The trivial (or common) and systematic names of the steroid hormones used for cancer therapy are shown in Figure 6-2, together with their structures. Table 6-1 provides a list of the deriva-tive names for most approved steroidal and nonsteroidal compounds available to manipulate steroid action for thera-peutic effect. Detailed chemical descriptions and steroid nomenclature are available from a number of sources.[17–20]

Biosynthesis

The ultimate source of all endogenous steroid molecules is cholesterol, which derives directly from the diet or via

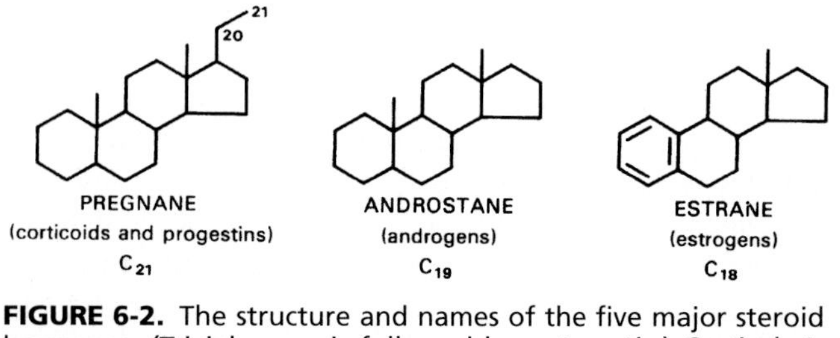

FIGURE 6-2. The structure and names of the five major steroid hormones. (Trivial name is followed by systematic.) Cortisol, 4-pregnen-11β,17α, 21-triol-3,20-dione; aldosterone, 4-pregnen-11β,21-diol-18-al-3,20-dione; progesterone, 4-pregnen-3,20-dione; testosterone, 4-androsten-17β-ol-3-one; estradiol, 1,3,5(10)-estratrien-3,17β-diol.

endogenous synthesis. All tissues, except possibly the adult brain, can synthesize cholesterol, although quantitatively the liver is the most important source.[21] The adrenal glands synthesize and secrete variable amounts of all five classes of the steroid hormones: glucocorticoids, mineralocorticoids, androgens, estrogens, and progestins. The testes and ovaries synthesize and secrete androgens and estrogens in differing amounts. Progesterone, the most significant endogenous progestin, is generated in a cyclic manner by the corpus luteum. However, the placenta is responsible for the increased amounts of progesterone and estrogens synthe-sized during pregnancy. Figure 6-3 summarizes the enzy-matic steps required for the formation of these compounds.

Transport

Steroids circulate in the bloodstream predominantly bound to albumin and steroid-binding globulins. Cortisol and progesterone circulate bound primarily to corticosteroid-binding globulin (CBG), and the androgens and estrogens are transported via testosterone and estradiol-binding globulin (TEBG) or sex steroid–binding globulin. The unbound, or free, hormone enters the cell by a non–energy-dependent process, the cell membrane providing a favorable lipid-rich environment for passage of the hor-mone by diffusion. Once inside the cell, steroid hormones and their synthetic competitors bind to hormone-specific nuclear receptors.

Nuclear Steroid Hormone Receptors

The effects of steroid hormones are mediated through a family of nuclear hormone receptors that include the ER, progesterone receptor (PgR), AR, glucocorticoid receptor (GR), and mineralocorticoid receptor. This receptor family also includes receptors for nonsteroidal nuclear hormones, the retinoids (retinoid alpha receptor and retinoid X recep-tor), vitamin D or deltanoids, and thyroid hormone. The amino acid homologies that define this receptor family are illustrated in Figure 6-4. Nuclear hormone receptors oper-ate as ligand-dependent transcription factors that bind to DNA to direct changes in gene expression in response to hormone binding.[22,23] These receptors share certain struc-tural features or functional "domains." This can be illus-trated by considering structure and function relationships in an ER. An ER has six domains, designated A to E (Fig. 6-4). Estradiol binds to the ligand-binding site in the E domain. The E domain also mediates ER dimerization, with assistance from residues in domain C. The sequence-specific DNA binding function resides in domain C. Domain D contains a nuclear localization signal required for transfer of the ER from the cytoplasm to the nucleus. Domains that promote transcription, or activation func-tions (AF), are present in domains A and B (AF1) and domain E (AF2). The basic structure and function relation-ships for all steroid hormones follow the same pattern, with

TABLE 6-1. TRIVIAL AND SYSTEMATIC NAMES FOR CLINICALLY RELEVANT STEROIDS AND ANALOGS

Trivial	Systematic
Adrenal steroids and antagonists	
Androstenedione	Androst-4-ene-3,17-dione
Betamethasone	9-Fluoro-11β,17,21-trihydroxy-16β-methylpregna-1,4-diene-3,20-dione valerate
Cortisone	17α,21-Dihydroxy-pregna-4-ene-3,11,20-trione
Dehydroepiandrosterone	3β-Hydroxyandrost-5-en-17-one
Dexamethasone	9α-Fluoro-16α-methyl-11β,17α,20-trihydroxypregna-1,4-diene-3,20-dione
Fluorocortisone	9α-Fluoro-11β,17α,21-trihydroxy-pregna-4-ene-3,20-dione
Methylprednisolone	16α-Methyl-11β,17α,21-trihydroxypregna-1,4-diene-3,20-dione
Prednisolone	11β,17α,21-Trihydroxypregna-1,4-diene-3,20-dione
Prednisone	17α,21-Dihydroxypregna-1,4-diene-3,11,20-trione
Spironolactone	17-Hydroxy-7-mercapto-3-oxo-17α-pregna-4-ene-21-carboxylic acid flactone, 7-acetate
Triamcinolone	9α-Fluoro-11β,16α,21-tetrahydroxypregna-1,4-diene-3,20-dione
Androgens and antiandrogens	
Steroidal	
Cyproterone	6-Chloro-1α,2α-methylene-4,6-pregnadien-17-ol-3,20-dione acetate
Fluoxymesterone	9α-Fluoro-17α-methyl-4-androsten-4β,17-diol-3-one
Methyltestosterone	17α-Methyl-4-androstan-17-ol-3-one
Testosterone propionate	4-Androsten-17β-ol-3-one-propionate
Finasteride (MK906)	*N*-(2-methyl-2-propyl)-3-oxo-4-aza-5α-androst-1-ene-17β-carboxamide
Nonsteroidal	
Flutamide	4'-Nitro-3'-trifluoromethylisobutyranilide
Anadron (RU 23908)	5,5-Dimethyl-3-[4-nitro-3-(trifluoromethyl-19-nor-1,3,5(10)-pregnatrien-20-yne-3,17-diol
Bicalutamide	± -4'-Cyano-α,α,α-trifluoro-3-[(?fluorophenyl)sulfonyl]-2-methyl-m-lactoto-luidide
Ketoconazole	*cis*-1-Acetyl-4-[4{[2-(2,4-dichlorophenyl)-2-(1*H*-imidazol-1-ylmethyl)-1,3-dioxolan-4-yl]methoxyl}phenyl]piperazine
Estrogens and antiestrogens	
Steroidal	
Estradiol	1,3,5-Estratriene-3,17β-diol
Estradiol benzoate	1,3,5-Estratriene-3,17β-diol-3 benzoate
Estriol	1,3,5-Estratriene-3,16α,17β-triol
Estrone	1,3,5-Estratriene-3-ol-17-one
Ethinyl estradiol	17α-Ethinyl-1,3,5-estratriene-3,17β-diol
Faslodex (ICI 182,780)	7α-[9-(4,4,5,5,5-Pentafluoropentylsulfinyl)nonyl]estra-1,3,5,(10)-triene-3,17β-diol
Nonsteroidal	
Diethylstilbestrol	3,4-Di-*p*-hydroxyphenylhex-3-ene
Tamoxifen	*trans*-1-(*p*-β-Dimethylaminoethoxyphenyl)-1,2-diphenylbut-1-ene
Toremifene	4-Chloro-1,2-diphenyl-1-{4-[2-*N,N*-dimethylamino)ethoxy]-phenyl}-1-butane
Droloxifene (or 3-hydroxytamoxifen)	Σ-1-[4'-(2-Dimethylaminoethoxy)phenyl]-1-(3'-hydroxyphenyl)-2-phenyl-but-1-ene citrate
Raloxifene	[6-Hydroxy-2(4-hydroxyphenyl)benzo[*b*]thien-3-yl]{4-[2-(1-piperidinyl)ethoxy]phenyl}methanone-hydrochloride
Progesterones	
Medoxyprogesterone acetate	6α-Methyl-4-pregnon-17-ol-3,20-dione acetate
Megestrol acetate	6-Methyl-4,6-pregnadien-17-ol-3,20-dione acetate
Anti-progestins	
Mifepristone (RU-486)	11β-(4-Dimethylaminophenyl)-17β-hydroxy-17α-propenyl-4,9-estradiene-3-one
Onapristone	11β-[(4-Dimethylamino)phenyl]-17α-hydroxy-17β-(3-hydroxypropyl)-13α-methyl-4,9-gonadien-3-on(e)
Aromatase inhibitors	
Aminoglutethimide	3-(4-Aminophenyl)-3-ethylpiperidine-2,6-dione
Letrozole	[4,4'-(1*H*-1,2,4-Triazol-1-yl-methylene)-bis-benzonitrile]
Anastrozole	2,2'-[5-(1*H*-1,2,4-Triazol-1-ylmethyl)-1,3-phenylene]bis(2-methyl-propiononitrile)
4-Hydroxyandrostenedione (4OHA) (Formestane)	4-Hydroxyandrost-4-ene-3,17-dione
Exemestane	6-Methylenandrosta-1,4-diene-3,17-dione

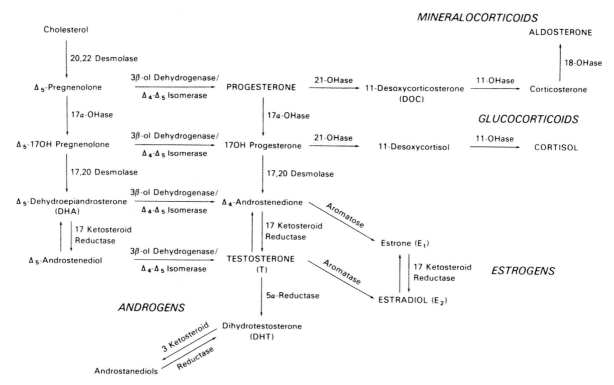

FIGURE 6-3. Enzymatic steps in the biosynthesis of the steroid hormone.

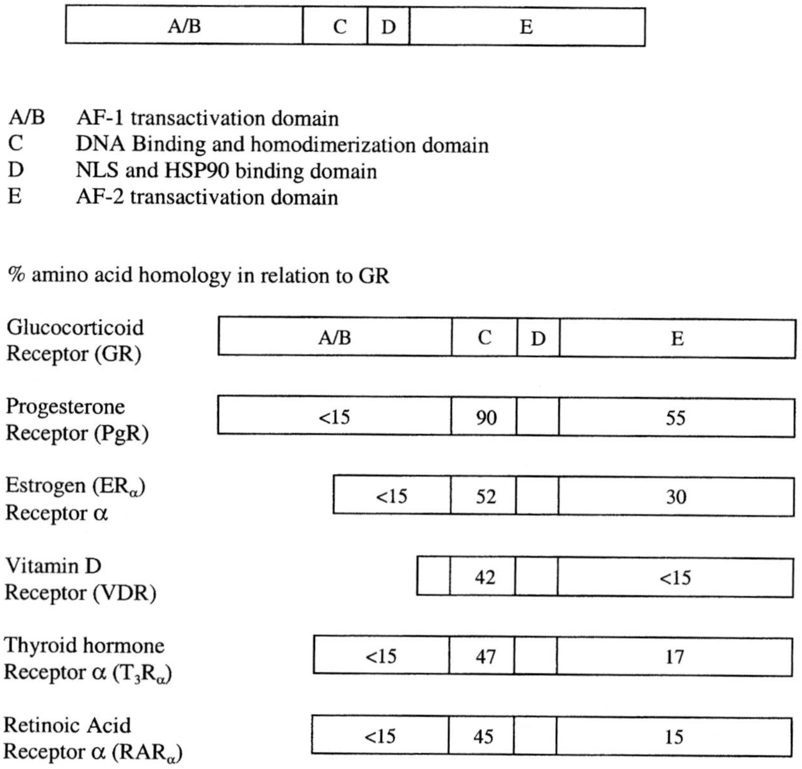

A/B		C	D	E	

A/B   AF-1 transactivation domain
C   DNA Binding and homodimerization domain
D   NLS and HSP90 binding domain
E   AF-2 transactivation domain

% amino acid homology in relation to GR

Glucocorticoid
Receptor (GR)

A/B	C	D	E

Progesterone
Receptor (PgR)

<15	90		55

Estrogen (ER$_\alpha$)
Receptor α

<15	52		30

Vitamin D
Receptor (VDR)

42		<15

Thyroid hormone
Receptor α (T$_3$R$_\alpha$)

<15	47		17

Retinoic Acid
Receptor α (RAR$_\alpha$)

<15	45		15

FIGURE 6-4. Examples of amino acid homology between nuclear hormone receptors. (A/B, activation function 1 transactivation domain; C, DNA-binding and homodimerization domain; D, nuclear localization signal and heat-shock protein 90–binding domain; E, activation function 2 transaction domain.)

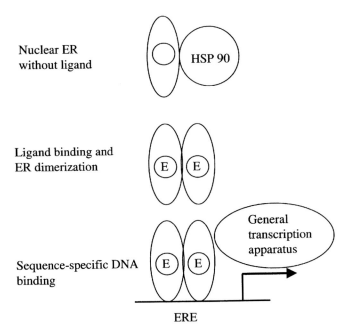

Nuclear ER
without ligand

HSP 90

Ligand binding and
ER dimerization

E E

Sequence-specific DNA
binding

E E

General
transcription
apparatus

ERE

FIGURE 6-5. Simplified operational details of nuclear hormone action, using the estrogen receptor as an example. (E, estrogen-occupied ligand-binding site; ER, estrogen receptor; ERE, estrogen response element; HSP, heat-shock protein.)

a hormone-binding site, dimerization domain, transactivation domain(s), and a nuclear localization signal.

Estrogen Receptor as an Example of Steroid Receptor Function

Simplified operational details of nuclear hormone action are illustrated in Figure 6-5, using ER as an example. Estrogens bind to the ligand-binding domain (LBD), ER is released from heat-shock protein (HSP) 90, and dimerization occurs. Sequence-specific DNA binding to a sequence referred to as an estrogen response element (ERE) follows. In the presence of estrogen, messenger RNA (mRNA) transcription is promoted though AF2. Residues in AF1 also promote transcription, although the function of AF1 does not require the presence of estrogen.[24] Each nuclear hormone operates in a similar manner, activating different patterns of gene expression through receptor-specific response elements. The DNA sequences of these elements have a common structure, consisting of a palindromic sequence separated by a spacer sequence, which varies in length according to the cognate receptor. The consensus DNA binding sites for each of the nuclear hormones are illustrated in Figure 6-6.

Coactivators and Corepressors

"Liganded" (or ligand-bound) receptors interact with a family of "coactivator" and "corepressor" proteins that are sensitive to the conformational changes that occur in the LBD of each receptor. Coactivators promote interactions between the nuclear hormone receptor and the basic transcriptional

machinery to activate gene transcription. An increasing number of proteins have been described with coactivator properties. For ER, the list includes CREB-binding protein,[25] transcriptional mediators/intermediary factors 2,[26] glucocorticoid receptor-interacting protein-1,[27] estrogen receptor associated p160,[28] and steroid receptor coactivator-1.[29] Corepressors have the opposite function and hold the DNA bound receptor in an inactive state.[30,31] The list of corepressors is shorter but is also growing and includes nuclear receptor corepressor (N-CoR)[32] and silencing mediator for retinoid and thyroid receptors (SMRT).[33,34] A general mechanism for the coactivator and corepressor-mediated switch of nuclear receptors from an inactive to active state has recently been proposed. On ligand binding, a histone deacetylase–containing corepressor complex is displaced from the nuclear receptor in exchange for a histone acetyltransferase–containing coactivator complex. These enzymes cause the

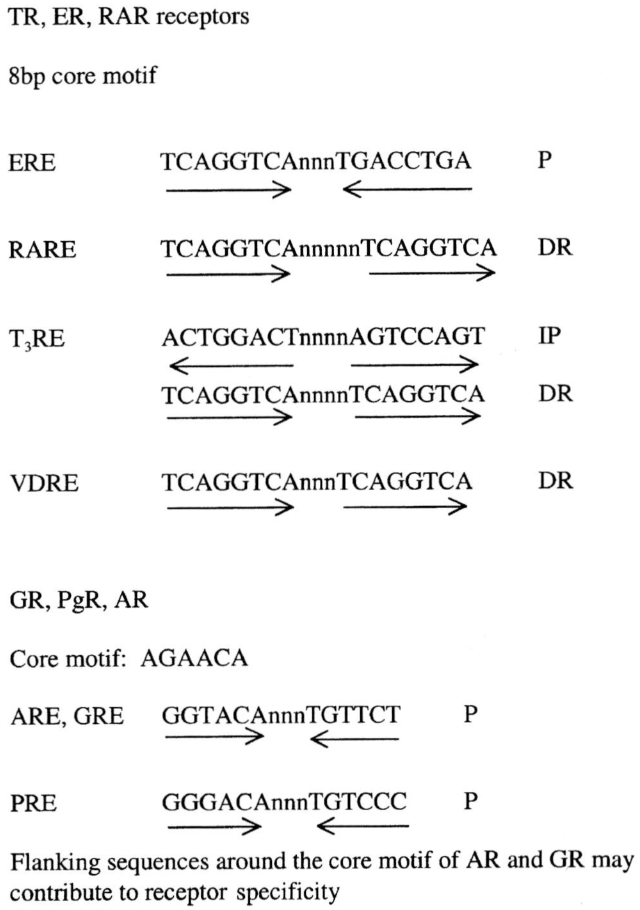

TR, ER, RAR receptors

8bp core motif

ERE	TCAGGTCAnnnTGACCTGA	P
RARE	TCAGGTCAnnnnnTCAGGTCA	DR
T_3RE	ACTGGACTnnnnAGTCCAGT	IP
	TCAGGTCAnnnnTCAGGTCA	DR
VDRE	TCAGGTCAnnnTCAGGTCA	DR

GR, PgR, AR

Core motif: AGAACA

| ARE, GRE | GGTACAnnnTGTTCT | P |
| PRE | GGGACAnnnTGTCCC | P |

Flanking sequences around the core motif of AR and GR may contribute to receptor specificity

FIGURE 6-6. Consensus core response element motifs for nuclear hormone receptors. (AR, androgen receptor; ARE, androgen receptor response element; DR, direct repeat; ER, estrogen receptor; ERE, estrogen response element; GR, glucocorticoid receptor; GRE, glucocorticoid response element; IP, inverted palindrome; n, any nucleotide; P, palindrome; PgR, progesterone receptor; PRE, progesterone receptor response element; RAR, retinoic acid receptor; RARE, retinoic acid receptor response element; T_3RE, triiodothyronine receptor response element; VDRE, vitamin D receptor response element.)

acetylation of histones, a structure responsible for organizing DNA into chromosomes. When histones become acetylated in the vicinity of the liganded nuclear receptor, DNA becomes unwound, or open, allowing access to the RNA polymerase complex, and transcription is initiated.[35]

Steroid Hormone Receptors as Targets for Signal Transduction Pathways

It is important to emphasize that nuclear hormones are not simply receptors for lipid-soluble hormones, but they are also critical signaling targets for protein phosphorylation–dependent second messenger pathways. For example, ER can be activated by the mitogen-activated protein (MAP) kinase cascade though epidermal growth factor receptor (EGFR) family members, including EGFR and ErbB2[36–38] and the insulin-like growth factor I (IGF-I) receptor.[39–41] Furthermore, the neurotransmitter dopamine[42] and the second messenger cyclic adenosine monophosphate (cAMP)[43–45] also influence ER function through phosphorylation. AR function is also modulated by growth factors. For example, nerve growth factor, IGF, epidermal growth factor, and cAMP all influence AR function and androgen-dependent prostate cancer cell growth.[46–48] These functional relationships, or cross-talk, with growth factor pathways suggest that nuclear hormone receptors have an integration function which ultimately determines the cellular response to a complex set of extracellular signals.

GLUCOCORTICOIDS

Historical Perspective

Glucocorticoids are required for the normal function of essentially all tissues. The major physiologic effects are summarized in Table 6-2. Historical insights into the role

TABLE 6-2. MAJOR PHYSIOLOGIC EFFECTS OF GLUCOCORTICOIDS

Metabolic effects
  Carbohydrate
    Increased blood sugar
    Increased hepatic glycogenolysis and gluconeogenesis
    Decreased peripheral uptake of glucose by the adipose, lymphoid, and connective tissue
  Protein: increased protein degradation and decreased protein synthesis in muscle, adipose, lymphoid, and connective tissue, providing increased amino acids for hepatic protein synthesis and gluconeogenesis
  Lipid: increased mobilization of free fatty acids from triglyceride
Circulatory effects
  Increased cardiac output
  Increased sensitivity to the pressor effects of catecholamines
  Sodium retention by the kidney
Musculoskeletal effects
  Increased capacity for work
Immune modulation

of glucocorticoid hormones were gained through the description of the clinical consequences of glucocorticoid deficiency and excess. In 1855, Addison provided the classic description of a wasting disease associated with the destruction of the "suprarenal" glands,[49] and shortly thereafter, Brown-Sequard demonstrated the essential role of the adrenal gland in sustaining life in dogs.[50] A syndrome of glucocorticoid excess was first characterized in 1932 by Cushing.[51] The role of the pituitary gland in regulating adrenal function was established in 1926, when Foster and Smith observed that hypophysectomy caused adrenal atrophy,[52] which, in 1932, was shown to be reversed by treatment with pituitary extract.[53] The active agent in pituitary extracts, adrenocorticotropic hormone (ACTH), was purified by 1943,[54] chemically and structurally identified by 1956,[55] and synthesized by 1963.[56]

Synthesis Regulation

Under the negative feedback mechanisms governing the release of ACTH, glucocorticoids are synthesized in the fasciculata zone of the adrenal cortex from cholesterol after stimulation of the ACTH receptor on the surface of steroid synthesizing cells (Fig. 6-3). The ACTH receptor is most closely related to the melanocyte stimulating hormone receptor and signals via G proteins to adenyl cyclase.[57] Stimulation of the ACTH receptor elevates cAMP and protein kinase A (PKA) activity.[58] Increased cAMP activates the steroidogenic acute regulatory protein by serine phosphorylation. Steroidogenic acute regulatory protein acts to promote cholesterol translocation to the inner mitochondrial membrane, where conversion to 5-pregnenolone, the major rate-limiting step for glucocorticoid synthesis, occurs.[59] Through this mechanism, the adrenal gland can up-regulate steroidogenesis within minutes, achieving up to a tenfold elevation in circulating levels during periods of stress.[60]

Serum-Binding Proteins

Once synthesized in the adrenal gland, cortisol enters the circulation and reaches target organs mostly bound to albumin, CBG, or transcortin orosomucoid (α-acidic glycoprotein).[61] At physiologic concentrations of cortisol in human plasma (approximately 10 μg per dL), 76% of cortisol is bound to CBG, 13.5% is bound to albumin, 10.5% is unbound, and negligible amounts are bound to orosomucoid. Steroid binding to plasma proteins serves a storage or buffer function. Large quantities of hormone circulate in a biologically inert reservoir, from which the active agent is readily available by dissociation.

Serum protein binding also protects steroids from degradation and excretion, decreasing the metabolic clearance rate. Furthermore, protein binding decreases the accumulation of highly lipophilic steroids in adipose tissue, where they would otherwise be relatively inaccessible for transport to target organs. Changes in endocrine status can alter CBG levels and the total blood levels of the steroids (although the amount of free hormone does not change markedly because of negative feedback on pituitary ACTH secretion). For example, estrogens stimulate CBG synthesis in the liver, and, as a result, total cortisol levels are markedly elevated during pregnancy.[62] Corticosteroids also affect CBG levels. Adrenalectomy causes a decrease in plasma CBG that is reversible with cortisol replacement.

Effects of Pharmacologic Dosages of Corticosteroids

On dissociation from the plasma binding proteins, cortisol enters the cell nucleus, binds to the GR, and activates expression from glucocorticoid responsive genes. The pharmacologic effects of glucocorticoids are listed in Table 6-3. Many of the actions on the list are the basis for the side effect profile associated with the therapeutic use of corticosteroids, including immunosuppression and nosocomial infections, Cushing's syndrome, diabetes mellitus, poor wound healing, posterior subcapsular cataracts, osteoporosis, euphoria, and psychosis. From a therapeutic standpoint, the effects of glucocorticoids on the immune cell

TABLE 6-3. MAJOR PHARMACOLOGIC EFFECTS OF GLUCOCORTICOIDS

Antiinflammatory and immunosuppressive effects
  Decreased vascular permeability
  Decreased polymorphonuclear leukocyte diapedesis, chemotaxis, and phagocytosis
  Decreased mast cell histamine reaccumulation and release
  Decreased antibody formation, especially the primary response
  Decreased thymocyte and lymphocyte mass and impaired delayed hypersensitivity
  Decreased resistance to bacterial, viral, fungal, and parasitic infections
  Decreased Fc receptor concentration
  Decreased response to T-cell mitogen
  Decreased synthesis of lymphokines
Connective tissue effects
  Decreased collagen formation
  Decreased mucopolysaccharide formation
  Impaired granulation tissue formation and wound healing
  Osteoporosis
Musculoskeletal effects
  Proximal muscular weakness (steroid myopathy)
Central nervous system effects
  Euphoria, mood lability, psychosis
  Sleeplessness
Eye effects
  Posterior subcapsular cataracts
Developmental effects
  Induction of surfactant, myelin, retinal proteins, pancreatic and breast proteins, etc.
  Inhibition of skeletal growth
Miscellaneous effects
  Decreased intestinal calcium absorption
  Decreased pituitary thyroid-stimulating hormone secretion

function and inflammatory processes are the basis for the value of corticosteroids in cancer treatment. In epithelial malignancies, glucocorticoids are not generally thought to be directly cytotoxic but are used to control the effects of malignancy on normal tissues. For example, corticosteroids are used to reduce tissue edema in the treatment of cerebral and spinal cord metastasis and to provide an adjunct to opiate analgesia to control the pain and aesthenia associated with advanced malignancy. In addition, corticosteroids are frequently used in antiemetic regimens for the treatment of chemotherapy-induced nausea.

Anticancer Effects

In treatment of lymphoid malignancies, leukemia and myeloma corticosteroids are critical antineoplastic agents with a direct cytotoxic action on malignant cells. Glucocorticoids at pharmacologic concentrations induce marked lymphocytopenia and thymic atrophy in experimental animals[63] and are cytotoxic for leukemic lymphoblasts in humans.[64] These actions are mediated through the GR, which is present in normal peripheral blood lymphocytes and monocytes,[65,66] as well as leukemia, myeloma, and lymphoma cells.[67–69] The cytotoxic action of glucocorticoids depends on the ability of these hormones to induce apoptosis in sensitive cells.[70] The level of apoptosis in the presence of corticosteroids depends on the expression of pro- and antiapoptotic proteins and signal transduction pathways.[70–73]

Pharmacokinetics

Many protocols use suprapharmacologic concentrations of glucocorticoid. Plasma concentrations as high as 1 g of prednisolone per m^2 of body surface area approach 1,000 times those required to saturate receptor and induce killing of sensitive cells *in vitro*. However, on a once-daily dosage, 20 or more half-lives may elapse before the next dose of drug is administered, so there is a rationale for using such large dosages. Glucocorticoid effects at normal physiologic levels are short lived, with a rapid metabolic clearance of cortisol (plasma half-life of approximately 60 minutes). Other steroids are cleared from the plasma at rates of approximately 2,000 L per day, which correspond to a plasma half-life of 20 minutes.[74] The half-lives of several synthetic steroids in dog plasma are as follows: prednisone, 33 minutes; dexamethasone, 60 minutes; prednisolone, 60 to 71 minutes; 6 α-methylprednisolone, 81 minutes; and triamcinolone, 116 minutes.[75]

Cortisol is extensively metabolized to inactive glucuronides, sulfates, and other forms in a number of tissues such that only 1% to 2% of the unaltered steroid ends up in the urine.[76] By far the most important organ for metabolism is the liver. The liver also plays a crucial role in activating certain synthetic 11-keto glucocorticoids, such as cortisone and prednisone, which must be converted to 11-hydroxy

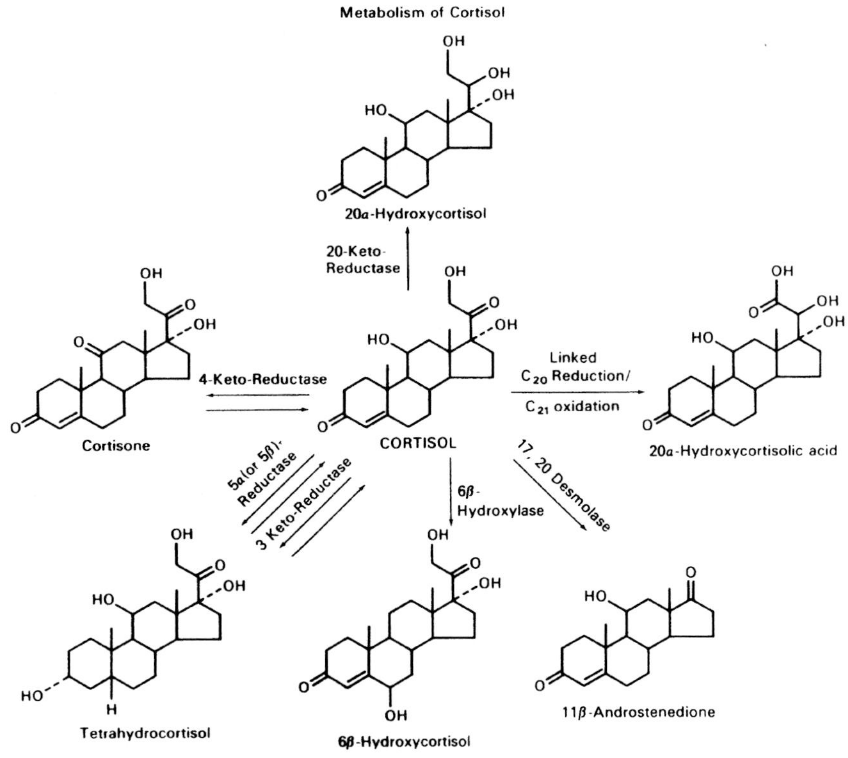

FIGURE 6-7. A summary of the enzymatic transformations of cortisol.

metabolites to exert activity. Thus, patients with compromised hepatic function may not respond to these agents because of decreased ability to convert to the 11β-OH steroid by 11-keto reductase enzymes. Hyperthyroidism markedly shifts the equilibrium of this reaction in favor of the inactive oxidized forms, whereas hypothyroidism does the reverse.[77] Anorexia nervosa and other malnourished states favor the 11β-OH steroids in a manner similar to the effect of hypothyroidism.[78] Drugs that induce hepatic enzymes may increase metabolism of glucocorticoids. These include barbiturates, phenytoin, and rifampin.[79]

Metabolism

At least seven enzymatic reactions that occur predominantly in the liver contribute to the metabolism of cortisol (Fig. 6-7). Of the seven, tetrahydroreduction of the steroid A ring provides nearly half the total urinary metabolites.[80] Synthetic 11-keto glucocorticoids (cortisone, prednisone, prednisolone) must be reduced to their hydroxy analogs to become active. An example is prednisone, which is rapidly converted to prednisolone.[79] In children, a considerable proportion of the urinary steroids are excreted unconjugated or free, whereas in adults, most of the steroids are conjugated to form inactive glucuronides and a smaller amount of sulfates.[81] Conjugated metabolites and unmetabolized drugs are subject to renal excretion. Only negligible amounts are excreted in the bile, with no enterohepatic circulation.[79] Because the metabolic clearance rate of cortisol is quite uniform, the replacement dosage of hydrocorti-

sone (12 to 15 mg per m² per day) is fairly uniform. There is systemic absorption from the skin and mucous membranes; therefore, topical preparations containing triamcinolone or other potent fluorinated glucocorticoid analogs have systemic effects if used in sufficient quantities.

The dosages of drugs used can be described as physiologic or that which is normally secreted by the adrenal gland (equivalent to 20 mg daily of hydrocortisone). Pharmacologic dosages are greater than physiologic dosages. Table 6-4 provides a reference for approximate equivalent oral dosages of commonly used corticosteroids. Use of glucocorticoids with no mineralocorticoid activity may reduce toxicity. Synthetic steroids with little mineralocorticoid activity include dexamethasone, methylprednisone, prednisolone, prednisone, and triamcinolone.

ANDROGENS

Historical Perspective

Although the first androgenic effect (growth of the capon comb) was demonstrated by Berthold in 1849, it was not until 1931 that Butenandt isolated a crystalline androgen that he called "testicular hormone."[82] Active testicular extracts were first prepared in 1927 by Loewe and Voss,[83] but the identification and synthesis of testosterone was not accomplished until 1935.[84] Many steroids with androgenic activity were subsequently identified. Naturally occurring androgens were isolated from ovarian, adrenal, and testicular tissue, and numerous analogs and derivatives were syn-

TABLE 6-4. APPROXIMATE EQUIVALENT ORAL DOSAGES OF COMMONLY USED CORTICOSTEROIDS

Drug	Antiinflammatory Potency	Dose (mg)	Sodium Retention Capacity	Half-life (h)
Cortisone	0.8	25	0.8	8–12
Hydrocortisone	1	20	1.0	8–12
Prednisone	4	5	0.8	12–36
Prednisolone	4	5	0.8	12–36
Methylprednisolone	5	4	0.5	12–36
Triamcinolone	5	4	0	12–36
Betamethasone	25	0.8	0	36–72
Dexamethasone	30	0.8	0	36–72

Adapted from Dujovne CA, Azarnoff DL. Clinical complications of corticosteroid therapy. A selected review. *Med Clin North Am* 1973;57:1331–1342; Gums JG, Wilt VM. Disorders of the adrenal gland. In: DiPiro JT, Talbert RL, Yee GC, et al., eds. *Pharmacotherapy—a pathophysiologic approach*, 3rd ed. Stamford, CT: Appleton & Lange, 1997; Melby JC. Drug spotlight program: systemic corticosteroid therapy: pharmacology and endocrinologic considerations. *Ann Intern Med* 1974;81:505–512; Schimmer BP, Parker KL. Adrenocorticotropic hormone—adrenocortical steroids and their synthetic analogs: inhibitors of the synthesis and actions of adrenocortical hormones. In: Hardman JG, Limbird LE, Molinoff PB, et al. *Goodman & Gilman's The pharmacological basis of therapeutics*, 9th ed. New York: McGraw-Hill, 1996; Gelman CR, Rumack BH, Hess AJ, eds. *Drugdex system*. Englewood, CO: Micromedex, Inc, 1999, with permission.

thesized. A summary of the effects of androgens in humans is presented in Table 6-5.

Synthesis

The synthesis and secretion of testosterone from the testes is under the regulation of the pituitary gland via a trophic hormone, luteinizing hormone (LH) (Fig. 6-3). A small amount of testosterone (approximately 0.1 mg per day) is also secreted from the adrenal glands in men and women via synthesis along the Δ5 pathway, involving Δ5 pregnenolone, 17-hydroxypregnenolone, and dehydroepiandrosterone. As with ACTH, LH regulates the first step of the five-step pathway: conversion of cholesterol to Δ5 pregnenolone by 20α-hydroxylation (Fig. 6-3). The LH effect is mediated by the LH receptor, a seven-membrane spanning G protein–linked receptor that activates cAMP-dependent PKA in response to LH binding.[85,86] Testosterone is secreted at a steady rate throughout the day in amounts totaling approximately 7 mg per day, reaching blood levels of approximately 500 ng per dL. Circulating hormone is more than 95% bound to test TEBG and albumin.[87] Free testosterone has a plasma half-life of approximately 15 minutes, but little is excreted unchanged in urine.

TABLE 6-5. PHYSIOLOGIC EFFECTS OF ANDROGENS

Male sexual differentiation *in utero*
Enlargement of male internal and external genitalia
Pubertal expression of male secondary sex characteristics
    Growth of pubic and axillary hair
    Deepening of voice
    Beard growth
    Increase in muscle mass
Onset and maintenance of spermatogenesis (with follicle-stimulating hormone)
Increased growth velocity and epiphyseal closure
Awakening and maintenance of libido
Suppression of breast development and growth
Increase in red cell mass

The three major metabolic pathways for clearance of testosterone are (a) conversion of testosterone back to androstenedione via the reversible 17-keto reductase step, (b) reduction of the double bond at the five position to form the potent androgen dihydrotestosterone (DHT), and (c) reduction of the 3-ketone to an alcohol. The products of the latter reaction are the weakly androgenic 5α-androsterone (20%) and its inactive 5β-isomer, etiocholanolone (26%), which are excreted in the urine largely as sulfates and glucuronides. Hydroxylations also occur at the 6β, 11β, 16, and 18 positions.[19] When androstenedione or testosterone tagged with carbon 14 is given to humans, approximately 90% of the dose is excreted in the urine within two days, and approximately 6% is excreted in the feces.[19] The extent to which testosterone is bound influences its metabolic clearance rate.[88] Small amounts of testosterone are converted to estradiol by aromatase in peripheral tissues, including muscle and adipose tissue. Although the percentage of conversion is small, the contribution to the total urinary estrogen is substantial, and this pathway is highly significant in the pathogenesis of postmenopausal breast cancer (see Estrogens).

Androgen Therapy for Breast Cancer

Historical Perspective

Although historically important, the current role of potent androgens in the treatment of breast cancer is in question. It is unclear whether AR is a true therapeutic target for breast cancer, because synthetic androgens reduce estrogen levels. Estrogen levels are suppressed by synthetic androgens (e.g., testololactone and fluoxymesterone),[89] because these drugs bind to the aromatase substrate binding site without subsequent conversion to estrogens.[90] This prevents endogenous androgenic substrates for aromatase being converted to estrogen (see Steroidal

Aromatase Inhibitors). This insight led to the development of attenuated androgens (exemestane and formestane) for breast cancer therapy that exhibit reduced androgenic side effects but enhanced binding to the aromatase enzyme. Synthetic androgens are occasionally used as third- or fourth-line treatment for patients still considered candidates for endocrine therapy (slowly progressing bone, soft tissue disease, or both). However, the response rate to androgen therapy after estrogen deprivation therapy with a potent aromatase inhibitor is uncertain and probably low. Any benefit of instituting androgen therapy needs to be balanced against risks associated with these relatively toxic compounds. On this basis, the authors consider potent synthetic androgen therapy for breast cancer obsolete and superceded by the steroidal aromatase inhibitor and attenuated androgen, exemestane.

Side Effects

Virilizing effects occur in essentially all female patients treated with androgens. In addition, nonvirilizing effects may also occur, including water retention, weight gain, edema, and jaundice.[91] Cholestatic jaundice occurs with a 10% to 20% incidence and is a problem for all patients receiving steroids with a 17α-methyl substitution, such as fluoxymesterone.[92] Hepatic adenocarcinomas have been reported in patients with aplastic anemia receiving 17-alkyl derivatives for 1 to 7 years.[93] The most typical schedule of androgen administration is 10 mg of fluoxymesterone orally twice a day.[94] No schedule-dependent differences in response have been reported. The major side effects of virilization (nearly universal) and cholestatic jaundice (up to 20%) may require discontinuation of the drug. As with other endocrine therapies, hypercalcemia may occasionally occur and should be treated with bisphosphonates before gradual reinstitution of therapy.

Other Synthetic Androgens for Breast Cancer Therapy

Danazol, a synthetic derivative of ethisterone (ethinyl testosterone), has activity in metastatic breast cancer[95,96] and should also be mentioned for historical correctness, but this drug is generally considered to be an obsolete treatment. However, danazol has been used for severely symptomatic fibrocystic breast disease with some success.[97,98] Danazol is a weak impeded androgen that decreases levels of plasma estradiol and sex steroids by inhibiting 3β-hydroxysteroid dehydrogenase, 17α-hydroxylase, and 17,20-lyase.[99] Danazol also suppresses ovulation by preventing the mid-cycle LH and follicle-stimulating hormone (FSH) surge.[100] Oral administration of 200 mg of danazol twice daily results in plasma concentrations ranging from 80 to 293 ng per mL and requires 14 days to achieve a steady state. Side effects include androgenic effects, decreased breast size, amenorrhea, and menopausal symptoms.

Androgen Deprivation Therapy for Prostate Cancer

Historical Perspective

Huggins[101,102] established that the prostate gland is dependent on testicular androgens, and his finding that castration caused regression of prostate cancer initiated the era of endocrine therapy for this disease.[2] Subsequently, investigators confirmed that androgen therapy, achieved surgically by orchiectomy or by treatment with LHRH antagonists, is the mainstay medical therapy for prostate cancer. Eighty percent to 90% of men with metastatic disease experience regression or disease stabilization on androgen ablation, with a median time to progression of 18 to 36 months. Progestins are weak AR antagonists and provide a second-line approach after the development of hormone refractory disease. However, a series of potent AR antagonists was subsequently developed for use as second-line therapy or in combination with androgen ablation as an initial treatment approach. High-dose estrogen with diethylstilbestrol (DES) to suppress androgen levels, although of historical importance, is now only used occasionally. A fourth approach involves suppression of adrenal androgen synthesis. The production of androgens by the adrenal glands is small compared to production by the testis. However, this source provides an important stimulus for prostate cancer growth in the absence of functioning testes.[103] Interference with adrenal androstenedione production with ketoconazole and hydrocortisone has recently demonstrated a valuable salvage therapy for hormone refractory prostate cancer.[104] Corticosteroids can also be used as monotherapy to reduce endogenous steroid production. Finally, in humans and many other species, the active intracellular androgen is DHT, a metabolite of testosterone.[105] Studies of prostate in organ culture suggest that a metabolite of DHT, 5α-androstane-3, 17β-diol, specifically stimulates prostatic secretion, whereas DHT induces prostatic growth.[106] This view is best supported by male human pseudohermaphrodites with 5α-reductase deficiency.[107] These patients have normal plasma testosterone levels, spermatogenesis, erections, and ejaculations but vestigial prostate development. When given DHT, prostate growth ensues. These observations led to the development of a competitive inhibitor of 5α-reductase (e.g., finasteride) for treatment of benign prostatic hypertrophy. A 5-mg daily dose of finasteride improves obstructive symptoms, increases urinary flow, and decreases prostate volume.[108] Data from experimental tumor models[109] suggest prostate cancer may be prevented by 5α-reductase inhibitor treatment, and a large prevention trial is under way.[110]

Androgen Receptors and Prostate Cancer

Unlike the measurement of ERs in breast cancer, there is little value in measuring ARs in prostate cancer. A biochemical methodology, requiring tissue extracts, is inaccurate because stromal cells in the normal or hypertrophied prostate express high levels of AR. Furthermore, plasma contains a high-affinity binding protein that interferes with competitive binding assays, and prostate tissue is capable of rapid metabolism of radiolabeled androgen into nonbinding metabolites.[111,112] More recently, quantitative AR immunohistochemistry has shown promise as a means to predict response to prostate cancer endocrine therapy.[113] However, the clinical utility of AR analysis is principally limited by the lack of an effective alternative to endocrine therapy for prostate cancer treatment. Clinicians are therefore unlikely to forgo a clinical trial of androgen ablation on the basis of a negative test result for AR.

Medical Suppression of Testicular Function

Historical Perspective

To this day, orchiectomy remains a standard approach to androgen deprivation for advanced prostate cancer. Alternatives to surgery were initially explored with synthetic estrogens or progestins. Estrogens, natural androgen antagonists, resulted in some success in the treatment of prostate carcinoma. Estrogens block LH and the production of testosterone in the testis. Progestins have also been used because they suppress LH and compete directly with testosterone for prostatic ARs.[114] However, treatment with high-dose synthetic steroids has been replaced with LHRH antagonists as the major medical alternative to surgery. These agents are considered equivalent to surgery or high-dose estrogen in terms of a response rate, but they have a low incidence of side effects and avoid the adverse psychologic effects of orchiectomy.[115]

Luteinizing Hormone–Releasing Hormone Agonists

More than 1,600 LHRH agonists and antagonists have been synthesized and the actions of these drugs have been extensively reviewed elsewhere.[115,116] The hypothalamic hormone that controls release of FSH and LH from the pituitary gland is called *LHRH* or *gonadotropin-releasing hormone (GnRH)*.[117] Expression of LHRH is limited to the hypothalamus, where it is released in a pulsatile manner and delivered to the pituitary by the portal veins.[118,119] LHRH binds to the LHRH receptor on pituitary cells with activation of LH gene expression and release through a cAMP-dependent mechanism. LHRH release is controlled by neurotransmitters (neuropeptide Y) and negative feedback by estrogen and testosterone.[120,121]

The ten amino acid sequence of endogenous LHRH is provided in Figure 6-8.[122] When it was appreciated that the major site of enzymatic degradation of LHRH was the glycine at position six, a series of six-substituted analogs were synthesized that were resistant to degradation and had a longer duration of action. Overriding the normal pulsatile pattern of endogenous LHRH activity with long-acting analogs increased the duration of LHRH receptor occupancy and caused profound receptor down-regulation and degradation. After a transient increase in FSH and LH levels, these agents inhibited testicular and ovarian function due to loss of gonadotrophin signaling.[4,123] Further increases in potency of six substituted LHRH analogs were possible through N-terminal substitutions to increase receptor affinity, and, after a series of initial clinical trials, several LHRH analogs became available for routine clinical practice (Fig. 6-8).[4]

In addition to effects on LH and FSH release, some investigators concluded that LHRH agonists had a direct anti-tumor effect on breast cancer cells *in vitro*.[124–126] However, Wilding et al. found that a high concentration of peptide was needed and that there was low affinity of LHRH binding to tumor cell receptors. This suggested that LHRH agonists have little direct inhibitory effects on breast cancer cells *in vivo*.[127] Similarly, direct inhibitory actions of LHRH agonists on prostate cancer cells have been proposed.[128,129] In these experiments, a LHRH agonist was found to inhibit epidermal growth factor–dependent prostate cancer cell proliferation. The contribution of direct antitumor effects to the clinical activity of LHRH agonist therapy for prostate cancer is unclear but deserves further investigation.

Endocrine Effects in Men. Continuous treatment with an LHRH agonist causes an initial LH and FSH surge followed by an inhibition of gonadotropin release and a castration-like effect on circulating sex hormone levels.[130] Animals treated with LHRH agonists develop a decrease in testis, ventral prostate, and seminal vesicle weight.[123] Chronic treatment of men with LHRH agonists results in decreased basal testosterone, DHT, estradiol, and progesterone levels and a decline in sperm density and mobility.[131,132] A fall in serum levels of 17α-hydroxyprogesterone suggests that gonadal steroidogenesis is blocked early in the steroid synthetic pathway. Santen et al. noted that men treated with daily leuprolide subcutane-

GnRH

pyro Glu-His-Trp-Ser-Tyr-Gly-Leu-Arg-Pro-Gly-NH$_2$

    1   2   3   4   5   6   7   8   9   10

Leuprolide

pyro Glu-His-Trp-Ser-Tyr-D-Leu-Leu-Arg-Pro-ethylamide

    1   2   3   4   5   6   7   8   9   10

Goserelin

pyro Glu-His-Trp-Ser-Tyr-D-Ser (tert Butyl)-Leu-Arg-Pro-Azgly

    1   2   3   4   5   6   7   8   9   10

FIGURE 6-8. Gonadotropin-releasing hormone (GnRH) and analogs. (Arg, arginine; Glu, glucose; Gly, glycerol; His, histidine; Leu, leucine; Pro, proline; Ser, serine; Trp, tryptophan; Tyr, tyrosine.)

ously (s.c.) experienced an initial fourfold rise in LH and twofold increase in testosterone 8 hours after the first dose. The initial rise in testosterone resolved after 1 week, and levels declined rapidly thereafter. Gonadotropins became fully suppressed after 2 to 4 weeks of continuous therapy. Therapy for 1 or 2 years revealed no escape from the androgen suppression. Similar results were reported when men were treated with buserelin s.c., followed by intranasal (i.n.) chronic administration. After a 2- to 3-day period of testosterone stimulation to levels of 122% to 158% of baseline, a decrease in testosterone levels was documented at 3 to 9 weeks and a decrease in LH and FSH at 5 to 8 weeks.[133] Through these mechanisms, LHRH agonists suppress the function of sexual organs and induce the regression of hormone-dependent prostate cancer.

Pharmacokinetics. The oral bioavailability of LHRH agonists is low because proteolysis occurs in the gastrointestinal tract. Rectal administration also has low potency. Vaginal administration reveals higher potency than other mucosal routes but less than the s.c. route. With intravenous (i.v.) administration, native LHRH has a half-life of 2 to 8 minutes in the initial phase and 15 to 60 minutes in the slower phase. The i.v. route of administration is not used for the treatment of cancer in clinical trials. The i.n. route is convenient, and lipophilic analogs are more effectively absorbed through this route than the native LHRH.[119] However, it proved difficult to administer sufficient LHRH analog to achieve castrate estradiol levels by the i.n. route.[133] Therefore, the most widely used route of administration is s.c. injection. The plasma pharmacokinetics of this route are limited by absorption, which depends on formulation, injection volume, local blood flow, injection trauma, site of injection, and proteolytic degradation at the injection site. The bioavailability of unmodified LHRH is 75% to 90% by the s.c. route. Injection in the deltoid area gives higher levels than do injections into the abdominal wall. Once-monthly biodegradable depot formulations have been synthesized to improve efficacy and convenience of s.c. administration. The formulation used for one of these preparations, goserelin, is a rod of D,L-lactide-glycolide copolymer that releases drug for 28 days. The polymer degrades to lactic and glycolic acids. Depot dosages of goserelin, 3.6, 1.8, and 0.9 mg, release 120, 60, or 30 μg of drug daily for at least 28 days, respectively. These three dosages decreased testosterone to castration levels in men by 2 to 3 weeks. The 3.6-mg monthly dosage was equivalent to 250 μg per day s.c. Subcutaneous implantation of a 3.6-mg dose of goserelin sustained amenorrhea in premenopausal women for 61 to 71 days.[134] At 5 weeks, a rise in LH concentration is noted. This drug demonstrated a potency 100 to 200 times that of native GnRH.[134–137] Pharmacokinetic information on LHRH agonists is provided in Table 6-6.

TABLE 6-6. PHARMACOLOGY OF LUTEINIZING HORMONE–RELEASING HORMONE AGONISTS

Mechanisms of action	Inhibition of gonadotropin secretion with resultant castration levels of testosterone in men and estrogens in women
	Direct inhibitory effects on steroidogenesis through blockade of 17,20-desmolase and 17α-hydroxylase enzymes
	Direct antitumor effect on human mammary cancer *in vitro*
Metabolites of buserelin	5–9 pentapeptide, C-terminal fragments, 6–9 tetrapeptide, and 7–9 tripeptide
Pharmacokinetics	Gonadotropin-releasing hormone $t_{1/2\alpha}$, 2–8 min $t_{1/2\beta}$, 15–60 min
	Goserelin s.c. 4.9 h
	Buserelin s.c. 60–80 min
	Decapeptyl s.c. 51.7 min
	Nafarelin 2.5–3.5 h
	Leuprolide s.c. 3 h
Elimination	Enzymatic degradation by pyroglutamate aminopeptidase, endopeptidase, and post-proline-cleaving enzymes and renal excretion
Drug interactions	None known
Toxicity	Hot flashes
	Reduced libido
	Impotence
	Local irritation at the injection site
	Polyuria and polydipsia
	Gastrointestinal problems, such as indigestion, nausea and vomiting, and constipation
	Taste sensations
	Peripheral edema
	Rash
	Gynecomastia and mastodynia
	Disease flare
	General allergic reaction
Precautions	Because there is an initial surge of luteinizing hormone, follicle-stimulating hormone, and testosterone, an acute exacerbation of disease may be seen

$t_{1/2}$, half-life.

Clinical Activity in Prostate Cancer. Initial experience with LHRH agonists in men with prostate cancer is equivalent to orchiectomy or DES.[138] Approximately 40% of patients have objective regression of tumor, and the majority of patients experience relief of bone pain. Androgen deprivation with a LHRH agonist is currently the standard initial approach to advanced prostate cancer. More recently, adjuvant therapy with LHRH agonists has been explored. When LHRH agonists was administered concurrently or toward the end of a course of radiotherapy for locally advanced prostate cancer, gains in relapse-free and overall survival were noted.[15] LHRH agonists have also been successfully administered before radiotherapy to reduce cancer volume and, thereby, the long-term complications of radical radiation to the prostate.[139]

Side Effects. Side effects from the administration of LHRH agonists in men include loss of libido in many and impotence in all patients.[140,141] Impotence is reversible after discontinuation in previously potent men. One study evaluated the testicular histology of men treated with LHRH agonists before orchiectomy. Histologic examination revealed marked peritubular thickening, a decreased number of Leydig cells, and fibrosis. The authors suggested that suppression of spermatogenesis may not be reversible after long-term treatment.[142] Other side effects included hot flashes in a majority of men; gastrointestinal disturbances, such as diarrhea, constipation, and indigestion; peripheral edema; weight gain; rash; gynecomastia; mastodynia; general allergic reactions; and exacerbation of tumor-related symptoms or disease flare, thought to be due to the initial gonadotropin stimulation.[143] Symptoms such as an acute exacerbation of bone pain (with spinal cord compression), urinary retention, and an increase in soft tissue tumor deposits are particularly noted during the initial month of treatment and can be ablated by the concurrent use of the antiandrogen flutamide.[138] Also, local reactions and hematoma at the injection site can occur.

ANTIANDROGENS

Historical Perspective

The first antiandrogen used in prostate cancer was the steroid cyproterone acetate. Cyproterone acetate binds to the AR, but does so with relatively low affinity with respect to testosterone. The clinical activity of cyproterone acetate against prostate cancer may be due to inhibition of LH secretion with subsequent androgen deprivation.[144] Cyproterone acetate has been rendered obsolete by the nonsteroidal antiandrogens flutamide, bicalutamide, and nilutamide. Interest in steroidal antiandrogens persists, however, with several new agents in preclinical development.[145] Currently, only flutamide and bicalutamide are in routine clinical use, as nilutamide is associated with ocular (light and dark adaption), lung, and liver toxicities.[146,147]

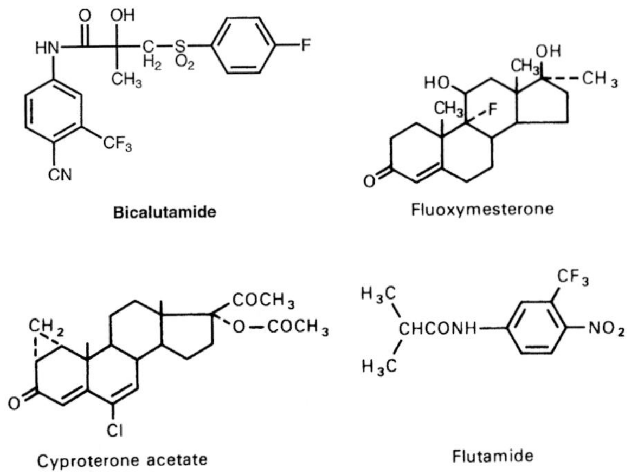

FIGURE 6-9. Synthetic androgens and antiandrogens.

Flutamide

Flutamide is a nonsteroidal antiandrogen (Fig. 6-9). The parent compound and its hydroxy metabolite are pure antiandrogens that competitively block binding of androgens to the AR. Flutamide reduces DNA synthesis and organ weight in the prostate in rats. Plasma levels of testosterone rise because of a compensatory increase in LH. However, the cellular levels of testosterone and DHT are reduced in androgen target tissues, probably because of competition of the drug and its metabolite for receptor binding. The effect of flutamide on gonadotropin release has been studied. Flutamide increases FSH and LH pulse frequency with increases in plasma concentrations of testosterone and estradiol.[148] Other studies showed that flutamide increases the formation of the adrenal C-19 steroids and their metabolism to conjugated compounds.[149]

Pharmacokinetics

Flutamide itself is metabolized to the more potent antiandrogen α-hydroxyflutamide. Flutamide itself has a weak binding affinity for the AR. The relative binding affinity (RBA) of flutamide compared with testosterone (RBA = 100) for the AR at 30 minutes is 0.3 and at 24 hours is less than 0.1. The RBA of hydroxyflutamide for the AR is 4.5 at 30 minutes and 0.5 at 24 hours. These results suggest that the metabolite is the active compound.[150] One hour after a 200-mg oral dose, only 2.5% of the parent compound is found in the plasma.[151] However, metabolite D, hydroxyflutamide, constitutes 23% of the administered drug at 1 hour. At least six other metabolites have been tentatively identified (Table 6-7). Four additional metabolites are known but have not been precisely identified. The plasma half-life of the α-hydroxy metabolite is 5 to 6 hours.[152] The mean trough plasma concentration of hydroxyflutamide during chronic treatment with 250 mg of flutamide three times daily is approximately 3.4 μm and remains unchanged after 6 to 18 months of treatment.

TABLE 6-7. FLUTAMIDE PHARMACOLOGY

Mechanism of action	Pure antiandrogen, interferes with the activated androgen-receptor complex formation in target cells
	Inhibits DNA synthesis in the prostate
Metabolism	A—α,α,α-trifluoro-4'-amino-*m*-acetotoluidide
	B—α,α,α-trifluoro-4'-amino-2-methyl-*m*-lactotoluidide
	C—α,α,α-trifluoro-4'-nitro-*m*-acetotoluidide
	D—α,α,α-trifluoro-2-methyl-4'-nitro-*m*-lactoluidide (hydroxyflutamide)
	E—α,α,α-trifluoro-4'-amino-2-methyl-*m*-propionotoluidide
	F—α,α,α-trifluoro-6-nitro-*m*-toluidine
	G—α,α,α-trifluoro-2-amino-5-nitro-*p*-cresol
Pharmacokinetics	Plasma half-life of D (major metabolite), 5–6 h
Elimination	51.1% excreted in the urine in 5 d, 4.7% in feces, remaining through skin and lungs
Toxicity	Mastodynia, gynecomastia, hot flashes, diminished libido, hepatotoxicity

Peak plasma levels occur at 2 to 4 hours after the dose. The maximum concentration reaches a mean of approximately 8.5 µm.

Clinical Activity in Prostate Cancer

The treatment of prostate cancer patients without prior endocrine therapy with flutamide resulted in subjective, objective responses, or both, in 63 of 72 (87.5%) patients.[14] However, most patients receive combined therapy with a LHRH agonist and an antiandrogen. For patients who received an LHRH agonist or orchiectomy alone as initial therapy, and the disease is progressing, adding therapy with an antiandrogen is also appropriate.

Toxicity

Side effects of flutamide include mastodynia, gynecomastia (36%), secretion of colostrum in men, hot flashes, decreased libido, loss of facial hair, loss of male escutcheon, elevation of liver function test results, and abdominal discomfort.[152,153] Sexual potency was maintained in 32 of 37 (86%) of previously potent patients in one study, but in nine of the 32 potency eventually decreased.

Bicalutamide

Bicalutamide is a potent AR antagonist and an analog of an active metabolite of flutamide. The relative potencies of the two drugs have been controversial,[154] however, a single daily dose of bicalutamide 50 mg is thought to be the clinical equivalent of 250 mg of flutamide three times a day.[155] As with flutamide, central inhibition of ARs by bicalutamide causes an increase in LH and testosterone levels during monotherapy.[156]

Pharmacokinetics

Bicalutamide is a racemate with an R-enantiomer and an S-enantiomer. The R-enantiomer provides most of the antiandrogenic effect, because the plasma concentrations of the R-enantiomer (or – enantiomer) in serum are approximately nine times higher than those of the S-enantiomer (or + enantiomer). These differences in plasma concentrations reflect the long half-life of the R-enantiomer (5.8 days) compared with the S-enantiomer (1.2 days).[157,158] There is no significant effect of food on area under the plasma concentration × time curve (AUC) or half-life.[157] The peak maximum concentration of R-bicalutamide after a single 50-mg dose is 559 to 970 ng per mL and occurs between 19 and 48 hours after dosing.[159] During daily administration bicalutamide accumulates approximately tenfold in plasma, consistent with the long half-life. The mean plasma levels are approximately 9 µg per mL for a once-a-day 50-mg dose.[158] Bicalutamide is subjected to glucuronidation, and approximately half of an oral dose is excreted in the urine and half in the feces.[159]

Clinical Activity in Prostate Cancer

A recently reported comparison between bicalutamide, 150 mg, and surgical castration for patients with metastatic disease favored surgery in terms of median survival,[160] although this difference was not replicated in a second study.[161] However, the clinical development of bicalutamide has generally emphasized combination therapy with LHRH agonists. The lower dosage of 50 mg is generally recommended in combination with androgen deprivation, as this dosage is well tolerated and effective when testosterone levels are suppressed. Combinations of the LHRH agonists goserelin and leuprolide and either flutamide or bicalutamide were compared in a randomized study.[162] Leuprolide and flutamide appeared to be the least effective of the four regimens studied.

Toxicity

Flutamide and bicalutamide are equivalently well tolerated, with diarrhea more common with flutamide and hematuria more common with bicalutamide.[162] Rare cases of eosinophilic pneumonitis with bicalutamide have been described,[163,164] but this side effect is much less frequent than with nilutamide.

Antiandrogen Withdrawal

For patients whose disease has progressed on antiandrogen therapy, withdrawal of the antiandrogen is an appropriate therapeutic maneuver that can lead to a decrease in prostate-specific antigen (PSA) and clinical improvement in 30% to 50% of patients. A response can be expected within 2 to 4 weeks of stopping flutamide and nilutamide, as the elimination half-lives are short for these compounds (7.8 to 9.6 hours and 38 to 59 hours, respectively). A withdrawal response may be delayed up to 4 to 6 weeks for bicalutamide because the half-life is longer (4.9 to 6.7 days). Median duration of a withdrawal response is 4 months. A withdrawal response in some cases is associated with mutations in AR.[165] Mutated AR has been shown to recognize flutamide as an agonist, leading to the stimulation of prostate cancer growth. A switch from flutamide to high-dose bicalutamide on disease progression stabilizes disease in approximately 20% of patients, suggesting these two drugs are not completely cross resistant.[166] In fact, clinical benefit for the switch to bicalutamide is most frequent for patients with AR mutations.[165] AR mutation does not explain all cases of antiandrogen withdrawal, and in model systems a switch from antagonist to agonist actions after long-term bicalutamide exposure can occur without AR mutation or gene amplification.[167]

INHIBITORS OF STEROID SYNTHESIS PATHWAYS AND PROSTATE CANCER

Ketoconazole

The antifungal agent ketoconazole inhibits the cleavage reaction converting 17α-hydroxyprogesterone to androstenedione, the direct precursor of testosterone.[168] For patients with metastatic prostate carcinoma given 400 mg of ketoconazole every 8 hours, plasma testosterone, androstenedione, and dehydroepiandrosterone levels decrease, whereas 17α-hydroxyprogesterone and progesterone levels increase.[169] There is no change in cortisol or aldosterone, whereas 11-deoxycorticosterone and 11-deoxycortisol increase. These data suggest that ketoconazole blocks the 17,20-lyase step in the adrenal gland and testes in humans with little effect on 20,22-desmolase.[170] As expected, the response to ACTH stimulation is impaired by the administration of high-dose ketoconazole.[171] Therefore, ketoconazole is usually administered with 20 mg of prednisone. Adding a corticosteroid has the additional advantage of suppressing the ACTH-dependent release of androgens.

Ketoconazole has been used in limited studies of prostate cancer with response rates of 20% to 30%. The most common dosage is 400 mg orally every 8 hours.[7] The combination of ketoconazole and prednisone has produced declines in PSA in up to 60% of patients with disease progression after treatment with androgen deprivation and an antiandrogen. Tumor regression and an improvement in pain have been documented, and the median duration of response is 4 months.[172] Ketoconazole requires an acid environment for dissolution and absorption and therefore should not be administered with H_2-receptor antagonists. It is primarily eliminated by hepatic metabolism and should be used with caution for patients with compromised hepatic function. The serum half-life is 1.4 to 3.3 hours,

and the terminal half-life is 8 hours. The only serious toxicity is hepatocellular necrosis, and careful monitoring of liver function is mandatory, although recent data on the safety of ketoconazole has been reassuring.[173] Side effects associated with androgen deprivation are commonly observed. New, more potent and selective inhibitors of 17α-hydroxylase-C17, 20-lyase are under development and may be available for clinical trial soon.[174,175]

Finasteride

Another approach to androgen deprivation therapy is blockade of the 5α-reductase reaction required for conversion of testosterone to DHT, the active intracellular androgen in the prostate. 5α-Reductase is expressed by the prostate gland, liver, genital skin, and frontal scalp. Synthetic inhibitors of 5α-reductase inhibit growth of animal models of prostate carcinoma.[176,177]

Finasteride, a synthetic 4-azasteroid compound,[6] is a competitive inhibitor of 5α-reductase that does not affect the binding of testosterone or DHT to the AR (Fig. 6-10). In addition to controlling the growth of the prostate, DHT production causes male-pattern baldness. The decrease in DHT is associated with a decrease in PSA, an increase in testosterone, and an increase in LH serum levels.[108] Dosages of 10 and 100 mg suppressed DHT by 70% and 82%, respectively.[178] The K_i (inhibition constant) of finasteride for human prostatic 5α-reductases is 26 nM.[179] When finasteride is given, the major 5α-reduced metabolite of cortisol, 5α-pregnane-3α,11β,17α,21-tetrol-20-one, is decreased in the urine, indicating inhibition of hepatic 5α-reductase.[180] The mean bioavailability of oral finasteride was found to be 63%, with a maximum plasma concentration averaging 37 ng per mL at 1 to 2 hours after dosing. Ninety percent of finasteride is bound to plasma proteins. Finasteride does cross the blood–brain barrier. The drug accumulates after multiple dosing with plasma concentrations 47% to 54% higher than after the first dosage.[181] The mean plasma half-life of elimination of a 5-mg dose is 6 hours and is increased to 8 hours in men 70 years of age or older.[182] Five metabolites have been described, including a monohydroxylated and monocarboxylic acid metabolites.[6] Thirty-nine percent of finasteride is excreted as metabolites in the urine, and 57% in the feces.[183] For patients with renal impairment, urinary metabolites were decreased and fecal excretion increased. Also, plasma metabolites are increased with renal impairment.[181]

Side effects include decreased libido, decreased ejaculate volume, and impotence.[108] Also, headache[183]; breast tenderness and enlargement; hypersensitivity reactions, including lip swelling and skin rash[181]; deep vein thrombosis[184]; and dizziness[185] have been reported. Finasteride is currently approved for treatment of benign prostate hyperplasia and is being prospectively tested in a large national prostate cancer prevention trial.[110] Finasteride has been used in one

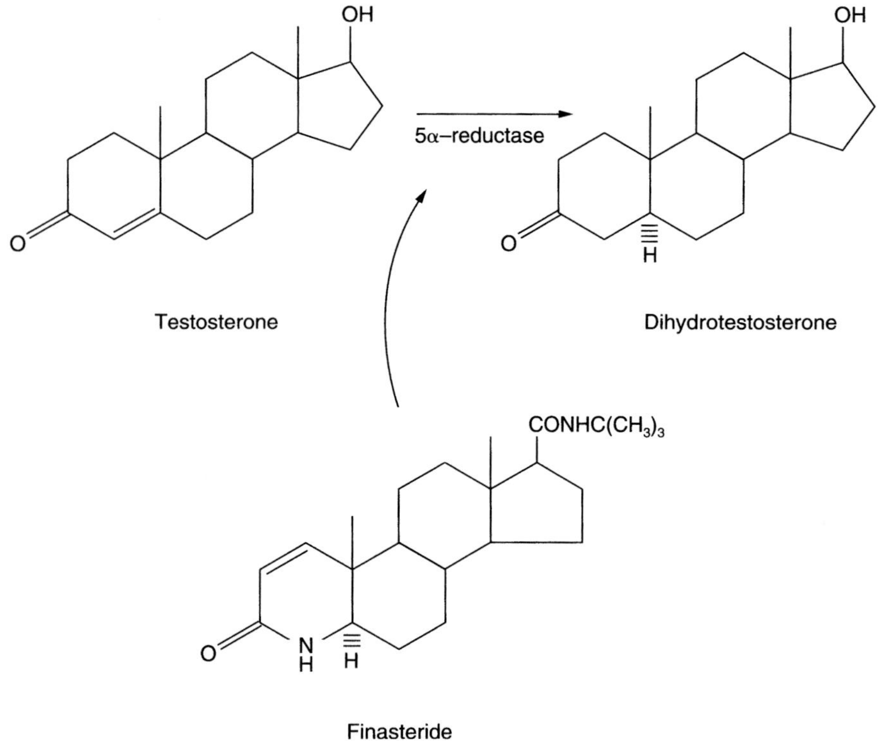

FIGURE 6-10. Finasteride inhibition of 5α-reductase.

study of prostate cancer with limited responses.[186] There are several other 5α-reductase inhibitors for which various preclinical studies are in progress, including epristeride,[187] turosteride,[188] and LY191704.[189]

ESTROGENS

Historical Perspective

The demonstration by Knauer in 1900 that ovarian transplants prevented uterine atrophy and loss of sexual function accompanying ovariectomy established the hormonal nature of ovarian function in regulating reproductive function.[190] With the development by Allen and Doisy in 1923 of a rat bioassay for assessing changes in the vaginal smear induced by ovarian extracts, Frank et al. in 1925 were able to demonstrate a female sex hormone in the blood of various species.[191] In 1926, Loewe and Lange discovered a hormone in the urine of menstruating women that varied in concentration with the phase of the menstrual cycle.[192] In 1928, Zondek reported the presence of large amounts of estrogen in the urine during pregnancy.[193] This finding led to the isolation and crystallization of an active substance, later identified and synthesized as estradiol.[194]

Estrogens are synthesized by the adrenal glands, testes, and ovarian follicles. However, ovarian steroidogenesis is cyclic in response to the cyclic secretory patterns of FSH and LH established by GnRH (LHRH) release from the arcuate

nucleus of the hypothalamus. Steroidogenesis in the ovary is initiated by the binding of LH to LH receptors on theca interna cells with activation of adenylate cyclase, the formation of cAMP, and activation of PKA. Uniquely, ovarian estrogens are synthesized by the cooperative action of two cell types. Androgens (either androstenedione or testosterone) are synthesized by ovarian thecal cells and converted to estrogens in the neighboring granulosa cells by aromatase.

Aromatase is an enzyme complex consisting of the P-450 cytochrome, P-450arom, and a flavoprotein, nicotinamide adenine dinucleotide phosphate cytochrome P-450 reductase, that regenerates active aromatase after completion of the aromatization reaction. The active site of aromatase contains a heme complex responsible for the nucleophilic attack on the androgenic precursor C19 methyl group that generates formic acid and an aromatized A ring characteristic of estrogenic steroids (Fig. 6-11).[195,196] The gene encoding the cytochrome component of aromatase, cytochrome P-450 (CYP) 19, has low homology with other members of the CYP family and has been mapped to chromosome 15.[197] Aromatase is regulated by LH during the menstrual cycle,[198] and expression is directly regulated by cAMP.[199]

Estradiol is readily formed from estrone, and can also be formed directly by aromatization of testosterone. Hydroxylation of estrone at the 16 position results in the formation of estriol, the other biologically important estrogen in humans. These compounds are shown in Figure 6-12. Estrogen metabolism occurs primarily in the liver, where there is free interconversion between estrone and estra-

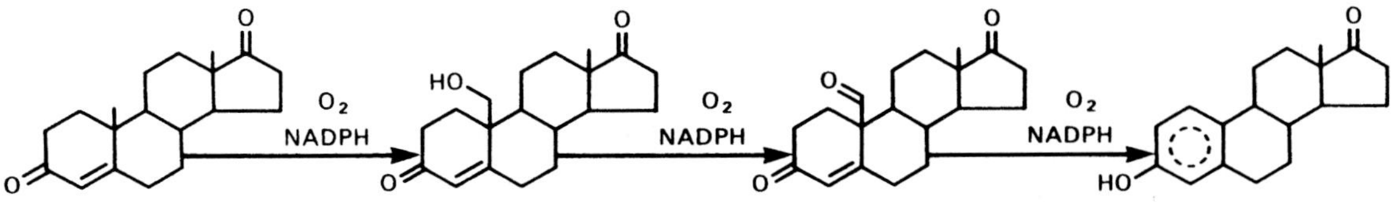

FIGURE 6-11. Aromatase reaction. (NADPH, nicotinamide adenine dinucleotide phosphate.)

diol.[200] Equilibrium slightly favors estrone, which probably serves as the main precursor for the hydroxylated estrogen metabolites in urine.[201]

Serum Levels during Menstrual Cycling

As with the androgens, circulating estrogens are bound to TEBG, although the extent of binding is uncertain.[202,203] Total blood concentrations of estradiol range from a low of approximately 10 pg per mL in the early follicular phase to as high as 500 pg per mL during mid cycle. This peak is quite sharp and usually precedes the ovulatory gonadotropin surge.[204] A second rise in serum estrogen occurs during the luteal phase and is lower but more prolonged. The estrogens are responsible, in concert with other hormones, for the development and maintenance of female sexual organs and secondary sexual characteristics and for the maintenance of the menstrual cycle and pregnancy (Table 6-8).

Metabolism

All three endogenous estrogens are excreted in the urine predominantly as glucuronides and sulfates, although numerous other water-soluble metabolites have been identified.[205] Estrogens undergo enterohepatic recirculation. More than half of the estrogen metabolites and one-third of the progesterone metabolites are excreted in the bile shortly after the administration of radioactive hormone. Eventu-

ally, 50% to 80% of an administered dose is excreted as metabolites in the urine within 4 to 6 days, and up to 18% may be found in the feces. In the liver, two systems for sulfation exist, one for the estrogens and the other for 3β-hydroxy steroids. Glucuronides are formed from diphosphoglucuronic acid by the microsomal enzyme glucuronyl transferase. Detailed reviews of metabolism and physiology are available.[206,207]

Estrogen Therapy

Historical Perspective

High-dose estrogen therapy was the first medical treatment for metastatic prostate and breast carcinoma. The antiandrogenic actions of estrogen explain the activity of estrogen against prostate cancer, but why high-dose estrogen causes remissions in metastatic breast cancer remains an unresolved paradox. Physiologic dosages of estradiol stimulate receptor-positive tumor cell growth *in vitro*[208–210] and *in vivo*.[211] However, high dosages inhibit breast cancer growth *in vitro*[212] and *in vivo*.[213] One study suggested that estrogens promote chromosomal nondisjunction, which could cause loss of cellular viability.[214]

Endocrine Effects of High-Dose Estrogen

Men treated for prostate carcinoma with high-dose estrogens exhibit a marked decrease in plasma testosterone con-

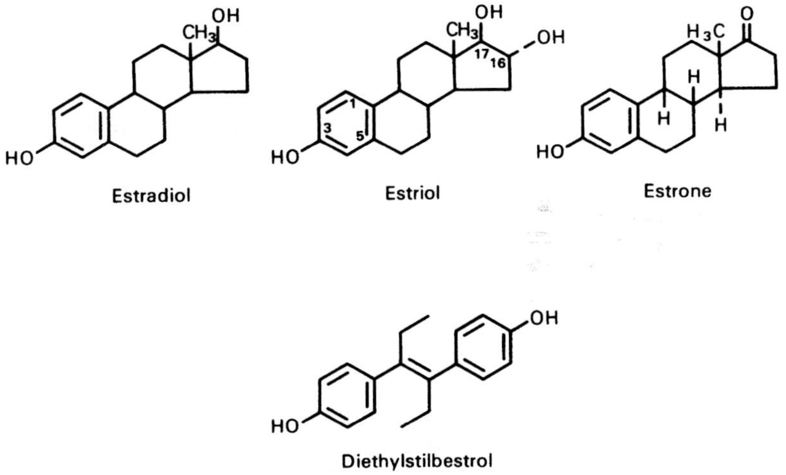

FIGURE 6-12. Endogenous and synthetic estrogens.

TABLE 6-8. PHYSIOLOGIC EFFECTS OF ESTROGENS

Growth and maintenance of female genitalia
Pubertal expression of female secondary sex characteristics
    Breast enlargement
    Increase in size and pigmentation of nipple and areolae
    Molding of body contour with alteration in subcutaneous fat
      deposition
    Promotion of female psyche formation
    Alteration in skin texture
Maintenance of pregnancy (in concert with progestins)
Sodium retention

centrations.[215,216] Suppression of testosterone is probably due to inhibition of Leydig cell function, because estrogen blunts the increase in testosterone normally associated with exposure to human chorionic gonadotropin.[217] Most studies also reveal decreases in plasma LH and FSH in women and men.[215,218] Estrogen treatment has a broad range of additional effects of uncertain importance. The long-term effects of estrogens on testicular function may be irreversible with long-term suppression of testosterone production by the Leydig cells, even after high-dose estrogen therapy has been stopped.[219]

Estrogen Preparations

Several different estrogens have been used in clinical trials in the treatment of prostate and breast carcinoma. These include polyestradiol phosphate, micronized 17β-estradiol, ethinyl estradiol, conjugated equine estrogenic hormones, DES diphosphate, estradiol undecylate, stilbestrol, and DES. The most widely used agent was DES, a nonsteroidal synthetic estrogen; however, this agent is now not freely available in the United States. Nonetheless, these agents are briefly discussed, as the therapeutic value of high-dose estrogen continues to be explored in the third-line endocrine therapy setting in breast and prostate cancer.

The relative potency of several estrogens has been assayed by determination of effects on plasma FSH, a measure of the systemic effect, and by increases in SHBG, CBG, and angiotensinogen, all of which indicate the hepatic effect. Piperazine estrone sulfate and micronized estradiol were equipotent with respect to increases in SHBG, whereas conjugated estrogens were 3.2-fold more potent, DES was 28.4-fold more potent, and ethinyl estradiol was 600-fold more potent. With respect to decreased FSH, conjugated estrogens were 1.4-fold, DES was 3.8-fold, and ethinyl estradiol was 80 to 200-fold more potent than was piperazine estrone sulfate. The dose equivalents for ethinyl estradiol (50 µg) and DES (1 mg) reflect these relative potencies.[220] Intravaginal administration of creams containing either conjugated estrogens or 17β-estradiol results in substantial pharmacologic levels of estradiol and estrone with subsequent decreases in LH and FSH.[221] Therefore, vaginal creams containing estrogens should be used with caution for patients who are at high risk of developing breast cancer or who have a history of early breast cancer.

Diethylstilbestrol

DES, a potent synthetic estrogen (Fig. 6-12), is absorbed well after an oral dosage. Patients given 1 mg of DES daily had plasma concentrations at 20 hours ranging from 0.9 to 1.9 ng per mL. The initial half-life of DES is 80 minutes, with a secondary half-life of 24 hours.[222] The principal pathways of metabolism are conversion to the glucuronide and oxidation. The oxidative pathways include aromatic hydroxylation of the ethyl side chains and dehydrogenation to (Z,Z)-dienestrol, producing transient quinone-like intermediates that react with cellular macromolecules and cause genetic damage in eukaryotic cells.[223] Metabolic activation of DES may explain its well-established carcinogenic properties.[224]

Ethinyl Estradiol

Ethinyl estradiol, a more potent estrogen than DES, has a biologic half-life in plasma of approximately 28 hours. It is excreted in urine as a glucuronide and as unchanged drug. It is 600-fold more potent than piperazine estrone sulfate and 22-fold more effective than DES in increasing sex hormone–binding globulin (SHBG), a parameter of estrogen potency.[220] The usual dosage is 1 mg three times a day for female breast cancer and 150 µg per day for prostate cancer.

Toxicity

Estrogens have substantial response rates in untreated prostate[225] and breast[9] cancer. However, serious complications, including exacerbation of ischemic heart disease, hypertension, congestive heart failure, venous thromboembolic disease, and cerebral ischemia, have limited the value of this treatment approach.[9,226,227] These side effects are dose dependent and most troublesome with DES doses of 5 mg daily. In addition, estrogens induce increased platelet aggregation and increases in factor VII and plasminogen, with decreased antithrombin III.[228,229] Hypertension is believed to result from estrogen-related fluid retention. Other side effects of exogenous estrogens include nausea and vomiting, diarrhea, abdominal cramps, anorexia, and glucose intolerance. Chloasma, erythema multiforme, erythema nodosum, hirsutism, and alopecia have been reported.[230,231] Estrogens cause various central nervous system side effects, including dizziness, headache, and depression. Keratoconus, or change in the corneal curvature, has been noted, with resultant intolerance to contact lenses for patients treated with estrogens. Hypercalcemia and increased bone pain are associated with a greater likelihood of subsequent antitumor response. Women may develop pigmentation of the nipples, vaginal bleeding, urinary urgency, and incontinence. Premenopausal women report mastodynia, venous dilatation of the breast, amenorrhea, and dysmenorrhea. Men develop gynecomastia and masto-dynia. The risk of gallbladder disease is higher in post-menopausal women taking conjugated estrogens.[232] Elevated liver function tests and cholestatic jaundice have been seen. Hepatocellular adenomas have been reported in oral contraceptive users.[233] The use of conjugated estrogens without a progestational agent is associated with an increased risk of endometrial carcinoma.[234] Estrogens are rarely used to treat premenopausal breast cancer, but they should never be administered to pregnant patients. Vaginal adenosis is found in 66.8%, and vaginal or cervical ridges are found in 40% of DES-exposed offspring.[235] Also, the occurrence of clear cell adenocarcinoma of the vagina has been correlated to DES exposure *in utero*.[236] A recent analysis of DES-exposed offspring reveals a risk through age 34 of one case per 1,000 women.

Drug Interactions

Inducers of the hepatic microsomal enzymes, such as rifampin, barbiturates, carbamazepine, phenylbutazone, phenytoin, and primidone, enhance the metabolism of estrogen and decrease estrogenic activity. Estrogens have been reported to decrease the activity of oral anticoagulants because of the induction of the synthesis of clotting factors. Estrogens increase the half-life and pharmacologic effects of glucocorticoids but induce the metabolism and anticonvulsant activity of phenytoin and other hydantoin anticonvulsants.

Antiestrogen Therapy

Historical Perspective

The recent decline in breast cancer mortality in Western countries is considered to be in part due to the introduction of the antiestrogen tamoxifen,[12] and tamoxifen remains arguably the single most useful drug in the treatment of early and advanced stage disease.[237] Tamoxifen is a nonsteroidal triphenylethylene first synthesized in 1966. The drug was initially developed as an oral contraceptive, but instead of blocking ovarian function, tamoxifen was found to induce ovulation. Activity in metastatic breast cancer was first described in the early 1970s, and tamoxifen rapidly became the drug of choice for advanced disease, with response rates ranging from 16% to 56%.[238–241] The preference for tamoxifen is not because it proved better than contemporary alternatives, but because it was found to be safe and easy to tolerate.[9,242,243] In fact, the tolerability of tamoxifen was one of the chief reasons for the success of tamoxifen adjuvant trials, as patients are able to take the drug for prolonged periods of time with acceptable levels of toxicity. A recent metaanalysis indicated that 5 years of tamoxifen therapy almost halves the 10-year recurrence risk for patients with ER-positive tumors and reduces the ten-year risk of death by 26%.[11] These data

contrast with the metastatic setting, in which tamoxifen is not associated with permanent remission. Nonetheless, patients with metastatic disease may achieve excellent disease control with tamoxifen. Although the overall time to disease progression is approximately 6 months,[243,244] the median time to progression for patients with a response is 12 to 18 months, with disease control in some patients lasting for years.

Tamoxifen Is a Mixed Estrogen Receptor Agonist and Antagonist

Tamoxifen affects organ systems besides the breast. Organs affected by tamoxifen administration include endometrium (endometrial cancer and hypertrophy),[245–247] coagulation system (thrombosis),[248,249] bone (modulation of mineral density),[250–252] and liver (alterations of blood lipid profile).[253,254] In the organ systems listed above, tamoxifen generally acts as an agonist, mimicking the effect of estrogen, in contrast to the action on breast epithelial cells where tamoxifen generally acts as an antagonist. Therefore, tamoxifen is correctly described as an organ site–specific mixed agonist and antagonist. The agonist properties of tamoxifen also manifest in the treatment of advanced breast cancer. Flare reactions, withdrawal responses, and the experimental demonstration of breast tumor growth stimulated by tamoxifen (see next section) are evidence that tamoxifen operates as an agonist in breast tissue under certain circumstances. The simple model of ER function presented in Figure 6-5 does not provide any insights concerning these complex effects of tamoxifen. Figure 6-12 is an attempt to summarize some recent observations at the molecular level that may explain the mixed agonist and antagonist properties of tamoxifen and related compounds.

Corepressors and Coactivators

Figure 6-13A focuses on the identification of nuclear proteins that interpret the difference between estrogen-bound ER and tamoxifen-bound ER. These proteins are termed *coactivators* and *corepressors* and are discussed in more detail in an earlier section. Tamoxifen distorts the LBD, generating an abnormal conformation that disrupts coactivator binding.[255] Subsequently, corepressor molecules are recruited to ER, holding ER in an inactive state.[256] Because tamoxifen induces dimerization and DNA binding, inactivation of ER depends on the net effect of tamoxifen on coactivator and corepressor interactions, which may differ between cell types and tumors. In some cells, AF2 inhibition may be bypassed when enough coactivator function is recruited to the N-terminal, ligand-independent domain, AF1.[257] Other cells may express a coactivator protein that can bind and activate AF2 despite the presence of tamoxifen.[32] Coactivator and corepressor proteins are therefore consid-

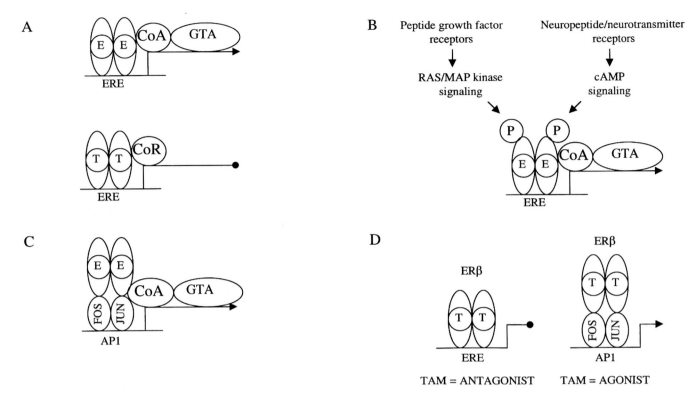

FIGURE 6-13. More complex models of estrogen receptor (ER) models. **A:** Estrogen (E) promotes coactivator (CoA) interactions that activate the general transcription apparatus (GTA). Tamoxifen (T) promotes corepressor (CoR) interactions that prevent activation of the general transcription apparatus. **B:** Estrogen receptor is phosphorylated by protein kinases activated by growth factors and neurotransmitters. **C:** ER interacts with other DNA-binding transcription factors to modulate the transcription of genes that do not possess an ERE. **D:** ERβ, a second ER, interacts with classic EREs and forms complexes with AP1 transcription factors. Activities in the presence of estrogens and antiestrogens (T) differ from ERα. (cAMP, cyclic adenosine monophosphate; ERE, estrogen response element; MAP, mitogen-activated protein kinase; P, phosphate.)

ered key to the molecular basis for the tissue-specific mixed agonist and antagonist profile of tamoxifen. Differences in coactivator and corepressor status between tumors may help to explain the variable response to tamoxifen in ER-positive breast cancer.[258]

Modulation of Estrogen Receptor Function through Second Messenger Pathways

ER expression and function are strongly influenced by growth factor signaling (Fig. 6-13B). As a result, ER expression levels correlate with distinct patterns of growth factor receptor overexpression. For example, ER-negative tumors overexpress EGFR family members, in particular EGFR[259,260] and ErbB2.[261,262] When ErbB2 or EGFR is activated in experimental systems, ER expression is suppressed. For example, chronic activation with heregulin, a ligand for the ErbB family of receptors, leads to ER down-regulation and the acquisition of an ER-negative phenotype.[36,37] These data suggest that EGFR and ErbB2 signaling bypass the requirement for estrogen for breast cancer cell growth and drive breast

cancer cells into an ER-negative, endocrine therapy–resistant state.[38]

In contrast, signaling through the IGF-I receptor provides an example of a positive interaction between growth factors signaling and ER function. Several key components of the IGF system (e.g., the IGF-I receptor and the signaling intermediate insulin receptor substrate-I) are regulated by estrogen. As a result, IGF-I and estrogen synergistically promote the growth of breast cancer cells.[40,263,264] The angiogenic fibroblast growth factor family also regulates ER function, with induction of tamoxifen resistance, in an animal model.[265] Finally, the neurotransmitter dopamine[42] and the second messenger cAMP[43–45] also influence ER function through phosphorylation. Interestingly, activation of cAMP leads to phosphorylation in the AF2 domain, altering the agonist and antagonist response to tamoxifen.[266] This suggests a role for cAMP in modulating the tissue-specific effects of tamoxifen. In conclusion, ER is at the center of a complex web of signaling interactions that become deregulated as breast cancer cells evolve towards an estrogen-independent (and tamoxifen-resistant) phenotype. Insights into the cross-talk between ER and other signal transduction pathways provide a rationale for novel therapeutic approaches, as well as suggest new predictive tests for endocrine therapy sensitivity.

Estrogen Receptor Function through "Nonclassic" Estrogen Response Elements

The classic estrogen response element consists of two palindromic DNA sequences separated by a three–base pair spacer sequence (Fig. 6-6). ER binds most strongly to this sequence; however, it is also capable of promoting transcription through sequences that have only partial homology to a classic ERE. In these cases, nearby response elements for other transcription factors (e.g., SP-1) contribute to ER activity.[267,268] Clearly, the activity of any ERE is dependent on overall promoter context. In perhaps the most surprising departure from the "standard model," ER can induce transcription without direct contact with DNA (Fig. 6-13C). In these instances, ER operates in conjunction with a second transcription factor that provides the sequence-specific DNA binding function. Through this indirect mechanism, ER can influence transcription through a greater variety of promoter sequences. Examples include the AP1 site (a target for many signals involved in cellular proliferation)[269,270] and a polypurine tract in the transforming growth factor beta promoter referred to as a *raloxifene response element*.[271,272] Because AP1 transcription factors, such as c-fos and c-jun, are key regulators of cell growth, ER-dependent AP1 activation may be critical to estrogen-dependent cell-cycle progression. Furthermore, new classes of antiestrogen do not have the same profile of activities at AP1 sites as tamoxifen, which may help to explain differences in the clinical activity between compounds.[270]

Estrogen Receptor β, a Second Estrogen Receptor Gene

The identification of a second ER gene, ERβ,[273,274] has provided a further layer of complexity to our understanding of estrogen regulated gene expression (Fig. 6-13D). ERβ is similar in structure to ER (now designated *ERα*) but is less important than ERα for normal reproductive organ development and function (at least in the mouse).[275] Nonetheless, ERβ mRNA is expressed by breast cancer cells and has a potential role in breast cancer pathogenesis and endocrine therapy sensitivity.[276] ERα and ERβ are highly homologous in the DNA binding domain (96%), with ERα and ERβ heterodimers readily forming on an ERE.[277] The homology in the LBD between the two receptors is also high (58%); however, affinities for estrogens and antiestrogens vary between ERα and ERβ.[278] Consequently, responses to different ligands may be more distinct than anticipated from primary sequence analysis.[279]

In contrast to the hormone and DNA binding domains, ERα and ERβ are not homologous in the N-terminal A and B (transactivation) domains, and, as a result, the transcriptional properties of ERα and ERβ are dissimilar. When the activity of an ERβ homodimer through an ERE is examined, tamoxifen is a potent antagonist with no partial agonist actions (due to a lack of an AF1 ligand independent activation function).[280] In contrast, tamoxifen is an agonist through ERβ when signaling is through an AP1 site. This suggests that an increase in ERβ activity through AP1 might be an additional explanation for the agonist effects of tamoxifen, as well as for tamoxifen resistance.[270] Information on the clinical significance of ERβ expression in breast cancer is limited at this time. However, Speirs et al. have observed that breast cancers that coexpress ERα and ERβ tend to be node positive and higher grade than tumors that express ERα alone,[281] and Dotzlaw et al. noted a tendency for ERβ-expressing tumors to be PgR negative.[282] These correlations suggest an adverse effect of ERβ expression on prognosis.

Tamoxifen Metabolism

The metabolism of tamoxifen is complex and has been extensively studied by thin-layer chromatography, high-pressure liquid chromatography, and gas chromatography.[283] Ten major metabolites have been identified in patient sera (Fig. 6-14 and Table 6-9).[284,285] An excellent review of tamoxifen and its metabolism is available that presents in schematic form the proposed metabolic pathways of tamoxifen.[286] Originally, it was believed that 4-hydroxytamoxifen was the major metabolite,[283] but Adam et al. found by using a different solvent system the major plasma metabolite was *N*-desmethyltamoxifen.[287] Metabolism of tamoxifen is mediated in the liver by cytochrome P-450–dependent oxidases. The metabolites are excreted largely in the bile as conjugates with little tamoxifen eliminated in the unchanged form. In two subjects given 14C-labeled tamoxifen, Fromson et al. found that 74% to 78% of the radioactivity was recovered in the feces, and 9% to 14% was recovered in the urine.[288] Sutherland et al. reported that impaired renal function does not result in elevated blood levels of tamoxifen.[289] Also, metabolite BX, or 4-hydroxy-*N*-demethyl-tamoxifen, has been detected in serum from patients receiving tamoxifen; its biologic significance is unknown at the present time.[290]

The estrogen agonist and antagonist effects of the metabolites of tamoxifen have been tested in the rat and mouse systems.[284,291,292] Agonist effects are seen as positive uterotropic effects and antagonist actions as blocking of the uterotropic effects of estrogen.[284] It must be mentioned, however, that tamoxifen acts as an estrogen agonist in mice but as a partial agonist in rats, and that metabolite effects differ in these species. Metabolite B, or 4-hydroxytamoxifen, is an estrogen agonist in mice but a mixed agonist and antagonist in rat uteri. Metabolite D is an estrogen antago-

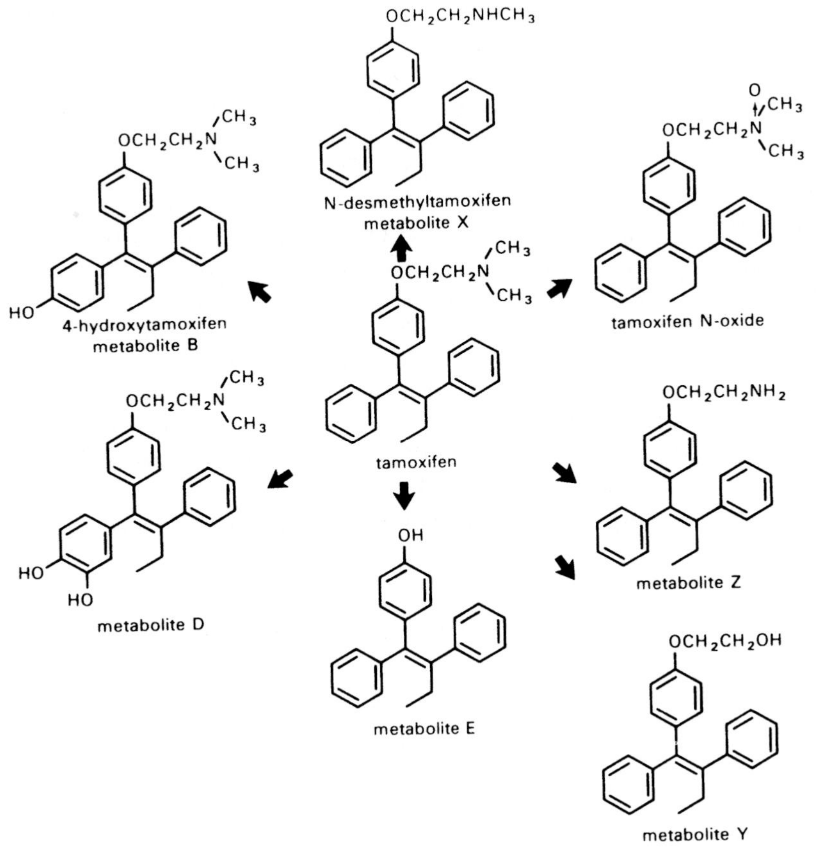

FIGURE 6-14. Tamoxifen and metabolites. (Adapted from Lyman SD, Jordan VC. Metabolism of nonsteroidal antiestrogens. In: Jordan VC, ed. *Estrogen/antiestrogen action and breast cancer therapy.* Madison: University of Wisconsin Press, 1986:191, with permission.)

nist in rat uteri and a mixed agonist and antagonist in mice. Metabolite E is the only metabolite that has no antagonist properties in any system but acts as a pure agonist. Metabolites X and Y are mixed estrogen agonists and antagonists. Metabolite A has antiuterotropic effects in rats. Finally, tamoxifen-*N*-oxide acts as a pure estrogen antagonist for MCF-7 cell proliferation.[292]

Tamoxifen Pharmacokinetics

Data concerning steady-state plasma levels and relative potency of binding to the ER suggest that the biologic actions of tamoxifen are exerted by the parent compound and its 4-hydroxy metabolite.[293–298] Estradiol is present in plasma in the range of 15 to 48 pg per mL. Tamoxifen equilibrates at levels of 300 ng per mL, its *N*-desmethyl metabolite at 470 ng per mL, and 4-hydroxytamoxifen at 7 ng per mL.[291,298] Because 4-hydroxytamoxifen binds to the ER with 25 to 50 times the affinity of tamoxifen and with an affinity equal to that of estradiol, tamoxifen and 4-hydroxytamoxifen may exert an equal biologic action. *N*-desmethyltamoxifen is probably a minor contributor to the therapeutic effect of tamoxifen, because, despite a higher plasma concentration in plasma, the binding affinity for ER is 1,250 less than 4-hydroxytamoxifen. The plasma levels of tamoxifen and metabolites remain roughly proportional to

dosage over the therapeutic dosage range, indicating no saturation of metabolic pathways.[8,297,299]

The initial plasma half-life of tamoxifen ranges from 4 to 14 hours, depending on the study, with a secondary half-life of approximately 7 days.[288,294,300,301] Steady-state concentrations of tamoxifen are achieved after 4 to 16 weeks of treatment.[294] The biologic half-life of the metabolite *N*-desmethyltamoxifen is 14 days, with a steady-state concentration reached at 8 weeks. These long half-lives reflect the high level of plasma binding to protein (greater than 99%) and enterohepatic recirculation.[284] Only free tamoxifen or metabolites can bind to ERs. Tamoxifen persists in the plasma of patients for at least 6 weeks after discontinuation of treatment.[300] Because of the long plasma half-life of tamoxifen, at least 4 weeks are required to reach steady-state levels in plasma, leading several investigators to explore the use of loading doses. In general, these investigators aimed at achieving plasma levels of 150 ng per mL, the lowest steady-state concentration observed for patients responding to the drug. Loading doses of 80 mg per m² twice daily yielded levels of 225 ng per mL at 3 hours after the first dose, whereas 50 mg per m² twice daily yielded proportionately lower levels, barely exceeding 150 ng per mL. Another study using 100 mg per m² over 24 hours on day 1 confirmed that peak concentrations of tamoxifen exceeded 150 ng per mL by the end of day 1 and could be

TABLE 6-9. TAMOXIFEN PHARMACOLOGY

Mechanism of action	Changes folding of the steroid-binding domain, preventing gene activation of estrogen receptor
	Blocks cells in mid-G_1, may be mediated by cyclin D1
	Blocks estrogen-stimulated progesterone receptor synthesis, 52-K protein synthesis, DNA polymerase activity, and tritiated thymidine incorporation
	Stimulates production of T-cell growth factor β, decreases insulin-like growth factor-I
Metabolism	Metabolite B: 4-hydroxytamoxifen
	Metabolite E: (loss of basic side chain)-phenol
	Tamoxifen *N*-oxide
	Metabolite X: *N*-desmethyltamoxifen
	Metabolite Y: primary alcohol
	Metabolite Z: desdimethyltamoxifen
	Metabolite BX: 4-hydroxy-*N*-demethyl-tamoxifen
	Metabolites A, C, D, F: (tentative)
Relative binding affinity for estrogen receptor	17β-Estradiol =100
	Tamoxifen = 6
	Metabolite B = 280
	Metabolite E = 3
	Tamoxifen *N*-oxide = 6
	Metabolite X = 4
	Metabolite Y = 0.5
Pharmacokinetics	Tamoxifen
	$t_{1/2\alpha}$ 4–14 h
	$t_{1/2\beta}$ >7 d
	Steady state, 4–16 wk
	N-Desmethyltamoxifen
	$t_{1/2}$ 9.8–14 d
	Steady state, 8 wk
Elimination	Conjugation with biliary excretion
Drug interactions	Potentiates mild hepatotoxicity induced by chronic allopurinol treatment
	Medroxyprogesterone acetate and aminoglutethimide affect metabolism
	? Inhibition of warfarin metabolism
Toxicity	Rat oncogenicity study—hepatocellular carcinoma at doses of 5–35 mg/kg/d and increased incidence of cataracts
	Intraretinal opacities, primarily paramacular, and optic neuritis
	Venous thrombosis and pulmonary embolism
	Hepatitis, fatty liver, two cases of hepatic carcinoma
	Thrombocytopenia (2%–5%)
	Increased incidence of endometrial carcinoma
	Severe lipemia on patient with prior history of hypertriglyceridemia
	Anovulation

$t_{1/2}$, half-life.

maintained above that level by a daily dose of 20 mg.[300,302] Although studies of loading doses are of theoretical interest, their clinical relevance is uncertain. It is likely that tamoxifen and its 4-hydroxy metabolite are present in excess at all dosage levels used clinically. A thorough analysis indicates that a single dose of 20 mg a day is the most appropriate approach to tamoxifen administration.[300,303] Because most tamoxifen is bound to serum proteins, tamoxifen is present in low concentrations in the cerebrospinal fluid,[304] suggesting the response to tamoxifen is likely to be poor in leptomeningeal disease and central nervous system metastasis.

Drug Interactions

The CYP3A family is responsible for *N*-demethylation of tamoxifen. Many other drugs are substrates for this enzyme family, such as erythromycin, nifedipine, cyclosporine, testosterone, diltiazem, and cortisol. The combination of tamoxifen with any of these drugs could potentially interfere with tamoxifen metabolism.[305] Mani et al.[306] have found tamoxifen *N*-demethylation is catalyzed in humans by CYP3A enzymes, whereas 4-hydroxylation is catalyzed by CYP2D6. None of the inducers of P-450 tested was able to elevate the rate of 4-hydroxylation. Inducers of P-450 enzymes do enhance *N*-demethylation but the clinical relevance of this information is unknown at this time. CYP2D6 is commonly involved in drug hydroxylation. There is an absence of hepatic CYP2D6 in 8% of whites, defining a group in which 4-hydroxytamoxifen would not be produced efficiently. The activity of CYP2D6 is also reduced by serotonin selective reuptake inhibitor antidepressants.[307] The clinical significance of a low rate of hydroxylation to 4-hydroxy tamoxifen is currently subject to investigation, in view of the widespread use of serotonin selective reuptake inhibitor antidepressants in patients with a history of breast cancer. Tamoxifen lowers plasma levels of the aromatase inhibitor letrozole, indicating these two agents should not be administered together.[308] Medroxyprogesterone acetate has been found to alter metabolism of tamoxifen.[309] Also, serum concentrations of tamoxifen and the metabolites Y, B, BX, X, and Z are reduced with the use of aminoglutethimide combined with tamoxifen. Finally, there have been reports of life-threatening interactions between warfarin and tamoxifen, but a clear interaction is not certain.[310] Careful monitoring of coagulation indices are necessary when warfarin and tamoxifen are prescribed together.

Intratumoral Tamoxifen Metabolism

Osborne et al.[311] measured tamoxifen metabolites in 14 breast tumors. The metabolite 4-hydroxy tamoxifen exists in the trans (potent antiestrogen) and cis (weak antiestrogen) forms. In nonresponding patients, all except one had reduced tumor tamoxifen levels or a high cis/trans ratio of the metabolite. It was suggested that these metabolic abnormalities might contribute to tamoxifen resistance. Another group investigated this hypothesis in an animal system; it concluded that the metabolism and isomerization of tamoxifen to more estrogenic compounds were not mechanisms of tamoxifen resistance.[312] Levels have been measured in tumor biopsy specimens after a daily dose of 40 mg.[298] The mean concentration of tamoxifen was 25.1 ng; of *N*-desmethyltamoxifen, 52 ng; and of 4-hydroxytamoxifen, 0.53 ng per mg of protein. These concentrations are sufficient to prevent specific binding of estradiol to ER in human tumors *in vitro*.

Tamoxifen Side Effects

Although tamoxifen remains the first-line endocrine therapy for early-stage and advanced breast cancer, important side effects should be considered. The tamoxifen chemoprevention trial, National Surgical Adjuvant Breast Project (NSABP) P01, established one of the most accurate sources of information on tamoxifen toxicity, because the true incidence of tamoxifen side effects was not obscured by tumor-related medical problems.[16] In NSABP P01, the excess incidence of serious adverse events (pulmonary embolus, deep venous thrombosis, cerebrovascular accident, cataract, and endometrial cancer) for patients receiving tamoxifen therapy was five to six events per 1,000 patient years of treatment. Less serious but troublesome side effects of tamoxifen included hot flashes, nausea, and vaginal discharge. Depression is also considered a side effect of tamoxifen, although there was no clear evidence of this association for women who received tamoxifen or placebo in NSABP P01. In summary, tamoxifen therapy is usually well tolerated and safe, and serious side effects occur in approximately 1 in 200 patients annually.

Ophthalmologic Side Effects

Tamoxifen retinopathy, with macular edema and loss of visual acuity, was first reported in patients receiving 120 to 160 mg per day. Three of the four originally reported patients also had corneal opacities.[313] The retinal lesions are superficial, white, refractile bodies 3 to 10 μm in diameter in the macula and 30 to 35 μm in diameter in the paramacular tissues and occur in the nerve fiber layer, suggesting that they are the product of axonal degeneration.[314] Additional cases have been described with patients receiving 30 to 180 mg per day.[315] Other ophthalmologic findings reported include optic neuritis, macular edema, crystalline macular deposits with reduced visual acuity, intraretinal crystals with noncystoid macular edema, refractile deposits in the paramacular areas with progressive retinal pigment atrophy, bilateral optic disc edema with visual impairment and retinal hemorrhages, tapetoretinal degeneration, and two cases of superior ophthalmic vein thrombosis.[316–319] It is worth emphasizing that, in the chemoprevention study, the only significant optic toxicity at increased incidence compared to placebo was cataract.[16]

Thrombosis

The increased risk of thrombosis associated with tamoxifen therapy may be associated with decreased levels of antithrombin III levels. Enck and Rios found a decreased functional activity of antithrombin III in 42% of tamoxifen-treated patients.[248] Pemberton et al. found reduced antithrombin III and protein C levels in women taking tamoxifen.[320] The incidence of venous thrombosis in this study was 5.62% compared with 0% in controls. The generally accepted rate is lower. The NASBP B-14 study reported thromboembolic events in 12 patients (0.9%) with one fatal pulmonary embolus compared with two thromboemboli (0.2%) in controls,[321] a rate similar to the P01 prevention trial.[16]

Hematologic Side Effects

Thrombocytopenia occurs in 5% of patients and is usually transient, resolving after the first week of treatment. Leukopenia is less frequent and is also transient.[94]

Lipoproteins

Changes in serum lipoproteins have been noted for patients taking tamoxifen. Changes occur that are indicative of an estrogenic effect of tamoxifen: an increase in total triglycerides, a decrease in total cholesterol, an increase in low-density lipoproteins (LDL) triglycerides, and a decrease in LDL cholesterol. Many other studies substantiate the effect of tamoxifen on lowering total cholesterol and, in most cases, LDL cholesterol and apolipoprotein B.[322–324] Despite these potentially favorable effects, there was no evidence of an improvement in the rate of cardiovascular mortality in either the Oxford metaanalysis[11] or the NSABP P01 prevention trial.[16]

Hepatic Toxicity

Tamoxifen has been associated with various hepatic abnormalities, including cholestasis, jaundice, peliosis hepatitis, and hepatitis. Carcinogenicity studies in rats reveal hepatocellular carcinoma in dosages ranging from 5 to 35 mg per kg per day.[325] The dose given to humans of 20 to 40 mg is 5 to 10 times less than the 5 mg per kg dose, and an increase in hepatocellular carcinoma in humans taking tamoxifen has not been reported. This is significant because tamoxifen forms adducts with DNA and could be mutagenic and carcinogenic.[326,327]

Bone Side Effects

The effect of tamoxifen on bone mineral content in postmenopausal women can be considered an advantageous side effect, with substantial data supporting an estrogen agonistic activity of tamoxifen on bone.[250,251,328] In the P01 study, a nonsignificant decrease in fracture rate was documented; further follow-up of this study should clarify this issue.[16] In premenopausal women, bone mineral density is decreased. Presumably in a high estrogen environment, tamoxifen operates predominantly as an antagonist.[329]

Gynecologic Side Effects

Many premenopausal patients notice a change in the duration of menses or heaviness of flow, and there have been suggestions of an increased incidence of ovarian cysts in these patients.[330] In postmenopausal women, endometrial cancer is increased, but screening for endometrial cancer is complicated by tamoxifen-induced benign endometrial hyperplasia and polyp formation. Data from the pilot British Breast Cancer Prevention Trial found that 39% of women taking tamoxifen had histologic endometrial changes, 16% with atypical hyperplasia and 8% with endometrial polyps. These results compared with 10% abnormalities in placebo-treated patients with no atypical hyperplasia and 2% with polyps. Transvaginal ultrasonography was used, with an endometrial thickness of 8 mm or more predictive for atypical hyperplasia or polyps.[331] The risk of endometrial cancer relates to age and duration of tamoxifen treatment. In the original Swedish report, 13 endometrial cancers were diagnosed in 695 tamoxifen patients at a frequency of 0.9% for patients receiving 2 years of drug versus 3% for those receiving 5 years of treatment. The frequency in the controls was similar to that of patients receiving 2 years of treatment, whereas the highest frequency was in those treated for 5 years. The increased frequency appeared in the third and fourth years of follow-up. It should be noted that the Swedish patients received the high dose of 40 mg daily. The same investigators later described the histology of 17 cases of tamoxifen-linked endometrial cancer, 16 of which were grade 1 or 2, although three patients from the group died of the uterine malignancy.[332] These frequencies are similar to those reported for the P01 study, with an increase in endometrial cancer but, overall, a low rate of death from the disease. Recently a case-control study found that exposure to tamoxifen interacts with other risk factors for endometrial cancer, namely, a history of hormone replacement therapy and higher body mass index.[333]

Recommendations for gynecologic follow-up of patients taking tamoxifen have varied from observation, to yearly vaginal ultrasound, to yearly endometrial biopsy, with no solid data for any of these approaches. Current recommendations are yearly pelvic examinations and rapid investigation of postmenopausal bleeding, but not radiologic or biopsy screening. Particular attention should be given to patients at higher risk.[333] Cyclic progestins have been considered to obviate the estrogenic effect of tamoxifen on the endometrium. Preclinical data suggest that progesterone may reverse the antitumor effect of tamoxifen in the dimethylbenzanthracene-induced rat mammary tumor model.[334] There continues to be concern about the safety of cyclic progestins. Furthermore, many postmenopausal women find regular "withdrawal" bleeding inconvenient.

Endocrine Effects

The effects of tamoxifen on circulating hormones through feedback effects on the pituitary-hypothalamus axis, through effects on plasma steroid-binding proteins, or through end-organ effects vary according to gender and menopausal status. In postmenopausal women, most investigators have found a decrease in prolactin, LH, and FSH, although all three remain within the normal range.[335–339] Thyrotropin-releasing hormone induction of prolactin secretion is suppressed.[340] Plasma estrone and estradiol remain unchanged in most studies, although one reported a minor decrease in plasma estrogens and an increased urinary excretion of glucuronide conjugates, suggesting an increase in metabolism or renal clearance of endogenous estrogens.[341] In premenopausal women, estradiol, estrogen, and progesterone have been reported to be increased after tamoxifen.[338,342] Many women continue to ovulate while taking tamoxifen, and in those who do, supraphysiologic levels of estradiol have been seen.[342] Tamoxifen causes an elevation of serum cortisol due to an increase in transcortin,[343] as well as increases in sex hormone–binding globulin, thyroxine-binding globulin, and apolipoprotein AI.[344–346] Because tamoxifen is a weak estrogen, it binds to ER and has estrogenic effects on normal hormone-responsive organs. In postmenopausal women, it causes an increase in cornification of the vaginal epithelium[347,348] and induces PgR in endometrium[349] and in breast tumors.[350] In men, the only consistent finding seems to be an increase in progesterone in plasma,[296] whereas levels of LH, estradiol, and other hormones remain unchanged in most studies.[296,298] IGF-I or somatomedin C levels have been shown to be decreased with the use of tamoxifen.[328,351,352] Because exogenous estrogens are known to decrease IGF-I levels in postmenopausal women, it is possible that the effect seen with tamoxifen is an estrogen agonist effect.[353]

Pregnancy

The effect of tamoxifen on offspring is unknown. There was one case report of a mother on tamoxifen giving birth to a baby with Goldenhar's syndrome, an oculoauriculovertebral syndrome.[354] This woman also had smoked marijuana and ingested cocaine, so the effect of tamoxifen is unclear. In the same case report, there is a discussion of 50 pregnancies on file at AstraZeneca Pharmaceuticals in women taking tamoxifen. These resulted in 19 normal births, eight terminated pregnancies, 13 unknown outcomes, and ten with a fetal and neonatal disorder, two of which had craniofacial defects. Although the teratogenicity of tamoxifen is unknown, women should be told to use mechanical contraception while on this drug.

Male Breast Cancer

There have been case reports of impotence[355] and of nocturnal priapism[356] in male breast cancer patients receiving tamoxifen. Another series reported a decrease in libido in 29.2% of male breast cancer patients.[357] The issue of impotence in men treated with tamoxifen has been studied in men treated with tamoxifen for male infertility. One paper reports a loss of libido in four cases (9%),[358] whereas studies that reported an increase in testosterone levels with tamoxifen did not report an increase in impotence.[359] These data suggest that the effect of tamoxifen on sexual function is minimal and is probably not the cause of impotence.

Flare Reactions

A transient exacerbation of symptoms or "flare reaction" was first observed during the treatment of postmenopausal women with high-dose estrogen. A clinical flare reaction is characterized by a dramatic increase in bone pain and an increase in size and number of metastatic skin nodules with erythema.[360–362] Typically, symptoms occur from 2 days to 3 weeks after starting treatment and can be accompanied by hypercalcemia, which occurs in approximately 5% of patients.[363] In clinical trials that compared endocrine therapies, an increase in bone pain or increase in skin lesions was observed in 4% to 7% of patients receiving high-dose estrogen and 3% to 13% of patients receiving tamoxifen.[10,363] Flare has also been observed with fluoxymesterone[364] and megestrol acetate.[365] Interestingly, flare has not been frequently documented with aromatase inhibitor treatment (aminoglutethimide, letrozole, and anastrozole). These data suggest flare is mainly associated with endocrine therapies with agonist properties. Tumor regression may occur as the reaction subsides. Patients should not be considered resistant to tamoxifen therapy within the first month of starting treatment if a patient has a flarelike syndrome. Pain and hypercalcemia should be treated aggressively. If symptoms are mild, tamoxifen therapy can continue to determine whether the patient will respond. In more severe cases, tamoxifen can be stopped and then reintroduced once symptoms have improved. Because tamoxifen flare is a transient phenomenon, clinicians should look for objective evidence of disease progression if the patient's symptoms are not resolving after 4 to 6 weeks.

In this context, two further manifestations of flare need to be taken into consideration, tumor marker flare and bone scintigraphic flare. Tumor marker analysis should be interpreted with caution in the first months after starting tamoxifen, because up to 75% of patients beginning a new therapy for metastatic disease will exhibit a rise in tumor marker levels that subsequently return to baseline levels or below. These tumor marker "spikes" may last as long as 30 to 60 days. Bone scans can also show flare, with an increase in uptake 2 to 4 months after initiating systemic therapy, which may confuse a radiographic evaluation of flarelike symptoms.[366–368] Plain film radiography is helpful here, as the presence of sclerosis, suggesting healing, may be documented in previously purely lytic lesions. Flare reactions can be also detected by fluorodeoxyglucose positron emission tomography.[369] In a small study, seven tamoxifen responders (none of whom had a clinical flare reaction) had a significant increase in glucose uptake seven to ten days after starting tamoxifen, whereas the four nonresponders did not. These data suggest that metabolic flare detected by positron emission tomography might predict responsiveness to tamoxifen.

Withdrawal Response

Between 25% and 35% of patients treated with estrogens have a secondary response if estrogen is stopped when disease progression is diagnosed.[9,370] The same phenomena can be observed on withdrawal of tamoxifen and progestins.[371] Convincing withdrawal responses only occur for patients who have experienced tumor regression followed by subsequent recurrence of tumor. Although frequently short lived, some patients may experience disease stability for more than 6 months.[371] Seeking a withdrawal response may be a way of increasing the total time a patient receives benefit from endocrine therapy. Tamoxifen withdrawal therapy is appropriate for patients who responded well to prior tamoxifen therapy and whose symptoms are minimal at the time of progression.[372]

Tamoxifen Resistance Mechanisms

Resistance to tamoxifen is easy to explain in the absence of ER expression. However, many ER-positive tumors are intrinsically resistant and almost all patients with ER-positive metastatic disease ultimately become refractory to tamoxifen. From a clinical standpoint, ER-positive tamoxifen-resistant breast cancer can be considered to exhibit either primary resistance (no response to tamoxifen) or secondary resistance (progression after disease regression or stability). Approximately one-third of patients with secondary tamoxifen resistance obtain clinical benefit from subsequent endocrine therapy. The following sections summarize data on this subject.

Estrogen Receptor Mutation and Alternative Messenger RNA Splicing

One hypothesis to explain the variable clinical response to tamoxifen in ER-positive breast cancer invokes ER gene mutation.[373] However, unlike AR, recent publications have established somatic mutations in ER are rare, occurring in fewer than 1% of either ER-positive or ER-negative breast cancers.[374] Mutations in ER also do not explain the majority of instances of tamoxifen resistance.[375] However, alternatively spliced ER mRNA variants have been commonly identified in normal and malignant breast tissues.[376] These mRNA variants lack one or more exons due to exon "skipping." A transcript that has received particular attention lacks exon 5, where exon 4 directly splices into exon 6 with preservation of the reading frame.[377] The exon 5–deleted variant binds to DNA, but not estrogen, and activates transcription in an estrogen-independent manner (a dominant positive receptor). These properties imply a role in estrogen independent growth.[378] However, coexpression of the exon 5–deleted variant with an intact ER did not alter the transcriptional response to estrogen, arguing against a critical role in breast cancer pathogenesis.[379,380] On the other hand, ERβ transcripts have not been fully examined, and a thorough investigation of both ER transcripts in breast cancer could still provide important information relevant to predicting tamoxifen sensitivity.

ErbB2 and Tamoxifen Resistance

As discussed in an earlier section, ER function is strongly influenced by peptide growth factor signaling. Tumors unresponsive to endocrine therapy might be identified through analysis of the expression of these growth factors and their receptors. ErbB2 expression has been extensively examined in this regard. The presence of ErbB2 tumor immunostaining was first shown to correlate with resistance to hormone therapy in a small group of patients with metastatic disease. Among patients with ER-positive tumors, ErbB2 expression was associated with a tamoxifen response rate of only 20%, and for patients with ER-negative tumors, 0%. This was in contrast to patients with ErbB2-negative tumors, in whom the response rates were 41% for ER-positive and 27% for ER-negative tumors.[381] Since this early report, several groups evaluated patients on endocrine therapy trials with a convenient immunoassay for the extracellular domain of ErbB2 (ErbB2-extracellular domain), shed by ErbB2-positive tumor cells into the circulation. A study by Leitzel et al. studied 300 patients enrolled in a trial of megestrol acetate or fadrozole as second-line endocrine therapy for advanced breast cancer. Patients with elevated serum ErbB2 levels (19% of the total) had a response rate to endocrine therapy of 20.7%, compared with 41% for patients with low serum ErbB2 levels. Duration of response and survival were significantly shorter in the ErbB2-positive group.[382] A study with a similar design reported a comparable result for patients receiving the antiestrogen droloxifene. Elevated pretreatment plasma ErbB2 levels (two standard deviations above the mean for normal subjects) were associated with a response probability of only 10%, a level generally associated with ER-negative tumors.[383]

However, the relationship between endocrine therapy response and ErbB2 expression was not observed in all studies. In a retrospective study of tissues collected from patients with metastatic breast cancer in the 1980s by the South West Oncology Group to study the effects of ER on endocrine therapy response, Elledge et al. performed immunohistochemistry for ErbB2. No difference in response rate, time to progression, or overall survival between ErbB2-positive and ErbB2-negative patients was demonstrated.[384] A potential explanation for these differences is the possibility that the ErbB2-ECD studies in particular did not rigorously exclude patients with ER-negative, ErbB2-positive tumors for whom the endocrine therapy response rates are understandably low. Given the uncertainty of the clinical evidence on the relationship between endocrine therapy resistance

and ErbB2 expression, ErbB2-positive and ER-positive patients should not be denied the potential benefits of tamoxifen or other endocrine therapies in the metastatic or early disease settings.

Coactivators and Corepressors and Tamoxifen Resistance

There is only limited information on coactivator and corepressor function in human breast cancer. However, several recent observations raise the possibility that these molecules may be critical determinants of the efficacy of endocrine therapy. For example, ER-positive MCF-7 breast cancer cells form tumors in nude mice that regress with tamoxifen treatment. If tamoxifen is continued, tumor growth resumes in a tamoxifen-dependent manner, because withdrawal of tamoxifen causes a second, temporary regression.[385] This animal model is reminiscent of clinical tumor regressions that may occur after tamoxifen is stopped for disease progression (withdrawal response) discussed above.[371] Interestingly, levels of the corepressor N-CoR are suppressed in the tamoxifen-stimulated tumors when compared with their tamoxifen-sensitive counterparts.[258] This finding suggests that prolonged tamoxifen exposure alters the coactivators and corepressor balance in favor of the agonist, growth-promoting properties of tamoxifen. Another potential player in the coactivator and corepressor profile in breast cancer cells is the gene called *amplified in breast cancer 1* (AIB1).[386] AIB1 is located in 20q12, a region amplified in breast and ovarian cancer. The encoded protein is an ER coactivator, and a recent study demonstrated that AIB1 is associated with ER expression in breast cancer samples.[387] More data can be expected on the relationship between tamoxifen resistance and coactivator and corepressor status in human breast cancer samples in the near future.

Other Antiestrogens

The structures of recently approved antiestrogens or antiestrogens currently under investigation are provided in Figure 6-15. Toremifene is the first new antiestrogen since tamoxifen to be approved in the United States and provides an alternative to tamoxifen for first-line treatment of advanced breast cancer.[388,389] It is under investigation as adjuvant therapy for breast cancer. Toremifene acts as almost a pure antiestrogen in rats and is partially agonistic in mice.[390] This drug has no hepatocarcinogenicity or DNA adduct-forming ability in rats.[391] Toremifene is reported to have antiestrogenic activity similar to tamoxifen.[392] The major metabolites are *N*-demethyl-toremifene and 4-hydroxy-toremifene. The mean terminal half-life values of toremifene and these metabolites are from 5 to 6 days.[393] Side effects were similar to those of tamoxifen, with hot flashes being the most common. Five patients developed leukopenia, with the lowest white blood cell count being 2,500. One patient had to discontinue therapy because of

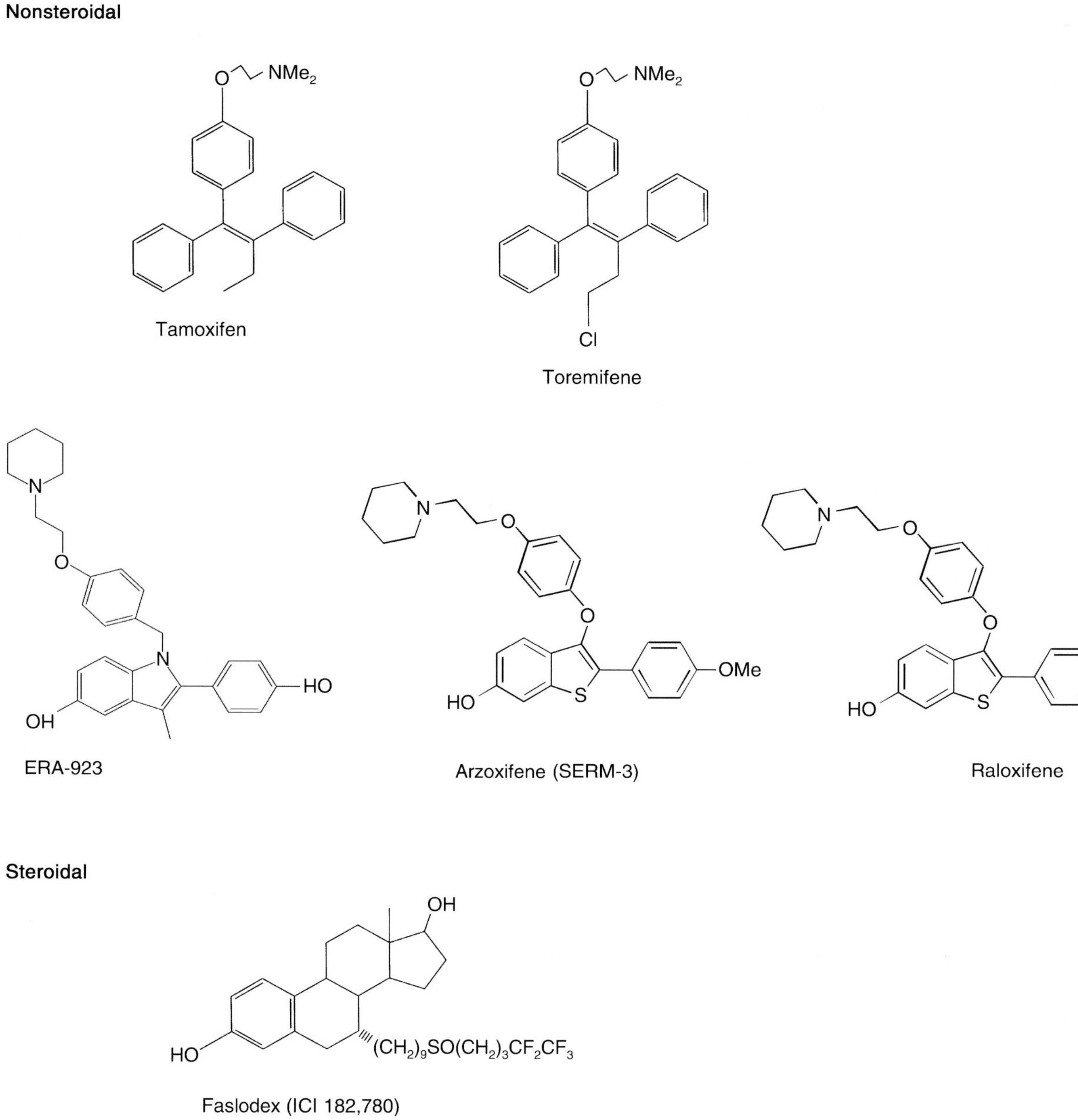

Nonsteroidal

Tamoxifen

Toremifene

ERA-923

Arzoxifene (SERM-3)

Raloxifene

Steroidal

Faslodex (ICI 182,780)

FIGURE 6-15. Antiestrogens. (SERM, selective estrogen receptor modulator.)

tremor. Toremifene is cross resistant with tamoxifen and should not be used in tamoxifen-resistant disease.[394]

Pure Antiestrogens

Because resistance to tamoxifen may be due to partial agonist effects, pure antiestrogens without agonist activity may be more effective. ICI 182,780, or Faslodex, is at an advanced stage of clinical development (Fig. 6-15). ICI 182,780 is distinct from other antiestrogens because it has a steroid structure that blocks ER dimerization, inhibits DNA binding, increases ER turnover, and suppresses ER levels.[395–397] As a result, ICI 182,780 blocks ER function before coactivator binding, theoretically overcoming resistance driven by the agonist properties of tamoxifen. Interestingly, ICI 182,780 also has activity as an aromatase inhibitor, although it is not known how much this property contributes to the clinical activity of the drug.[398] Preclinical studies in models of tamoxifen-resistant disease have been promising,[399] and clinical trials for patients with tamoxifen-resistant advanced disease are under way. ICI 182,780 is administered as a monthly intramuscular (i.m.) injection as the oral route is unreliable. Data from a small phase II trial confirmed activity in tamoxifen-resistant advanced disease, with 7 of 19 patients receiving 250 mg a month experiencing partial responses and a further 6 of 19 patients achieving stable disease for at least 24 weeks.[400] Two large clinical trials are under way: For patients with tamoxifen-resistant disease, ICI 182,780 is being compared with anastrozole (a selective aromatase inhibitor); for patients with advanced disease, who have never received tamoxifen or have not received the drug for at least one year, ICI 182,780 is being compared to tamoxifen.

ICI 182,780 is not reliably absorbed orally and is formulated as a monthly depot i.m. injection. With this preparation, peak levels of ICI 182,780 occur at a median of 8 to 9 days after dosing and decline thereafter, but remain above the projected therapeutic threshold at day 28. In careful pharmacokinetic studies, the AUC was 140 ng per day in the first month and 208 ng per day after 6 months, suggesting some drug accumulation. No clear effect on FSH levels and LH levels has been documented, indicating that ICI 182,780 has no impact on pituitary function. There were also no changes in sex hormone–binding globulin, prolactin, or lipids.[401] The effects of ICI 182,780 on ER, PgR, proliferation, and apoptosis have been examined in benign endometrial tissue and malignant breast tissue. When ICI 182,780 was given for a week before hysterectomy, it was found to decrease a Ki67-based proliferation assay, however, ER and PgR levels were not affected. In contrast, short-term exposure to ICI 182,780 before breast surgery decreased ER and PgR expression and proliferation and increased apoptosis.[397,402] These data suggest that, like other antiestrogens, there may be differences in the action of ICI 182,780 at different organ sites. Clinical development programs have recently activated for other "pure" antiestrogens. EM 652 has a nonsteroidal structure and is theoretically interesting because of an inhibitory action against ERα and ERβ, whether these receptors are operating through a classic ERE or an AP1 site (Fig. 6-12D).[403]

ERA923 is another nonsteroidal antiestrogen in early clinical trials. No preclinical information on this compound has been released.

New Selective Estrogen Receptor Modulators

Although pure antiestrogen therapy is a logical new approach to the treatment of advanced breast cancer, drugs devoid of all estrogenic activities might be problematic in the adjuvant and prevention settings, because secondary hormone replacement therapy–like benefits of tamoxifen are considered worthwhile for postmenopausal women. This concern stimulated the development of alternative antiestrogens with a modified mixed agonist and antagonist profile. Ideally, these drugs are antiestrogenic in the breast but retain beneficial effects on bone mineralization and blood lipid profile without adverse estrogenic effects on the endometrium. Drugs with a mixed agonist and antagonist profile have recently been referred to as *selective estrogen receptor modulators* (SERM), to reflect these remarkable properties (Fig. 6-15). Raloxifene is the first approved drug to exhibit a "modified" SERM profile; however, the indication for raloxifene is osteoporosis not breast cancer.[404,405] An early evaluation of activity in tamoxifen-resistant breast

cancer (when the drug was referred to as *keoxifene* or *LY156758*), was disappointing.[406] Consequently, raloxifene should not be used for the treatment of either early stage or advanced breast cancer. However, there is continued interest in this drug in the prevention setting, because a decrease in breast cancer incidence was seen in raloxifene osteoporosis trials.[407] The current NSABP prevention study compares raloxifene to tamoxifen in women at high risk of the disease.[408] A raloxifene-related drug, currently referred to as *arzoxifene*, has a similar profile as raloxifene, but with greater ER antagonist activity in breast cancer models. Arzoxifene has been subjected to phase I testing in breast cancer,[409] and information about phase II trials, as well as plans for phase III development, should be available soon. It is important to emphasize that although ideal SERMs may represent a small advance in terms of safety, they are not necessarily more efficacious.

Activity in advanced tamoxifen-resistant disease is considered by many clinicians to provide critical evidence that a new endocrine therapy may be more active than tamoxifen. Of the new antiestrogens tested thus far, where there is information, they have failed this test. The group includes idoxifene (which at best has minor activity in tamoxifen-resistant disease),[410] droloxifene,[411,412] and toremifine.[394] In general, antiestrogens that exhibit a mixed agonist and antagonist profile, even if modified in a way that improves tissue-specific toxicities, are likely to exhibit overlapping resistance and toxicity profiles with tamoxifen.[13,413] This may be because any antiestrogen that triggers ER dimerization and DNA binding is prone to the same coactivator-based resistance mechanisms that may limit the activity of tamoxifen.

Progestins

Historical Perspective

In 1897, Beard postulated that the corpus luteum was essential for pregnancy.[414] Support for this concept was provided by Fraenkel in 1905, who demonstrated that destruction of the corpora lutea in pregnant rabbits caused abortion, an event that could be prevented by the injection of luteal extracts.[415] Although progesterone, the active principle in corpus lutea extracts, was isolated in 1929 from the corpora lutea of sows by Corner and Allen,[416] the limited amounts of available hormone hampered further studies until the 1950s, when progesterones with prolonged activity were synthesized. Since that time, progestins have been widely used as oral contraceptives. High-dose progestin therapy is the last synthetic sex steroid routinely used in the treatment of advanced breast cancer. Until recently, megestrol acetate was a favored second-line therapy for patients with tamoxifen-resistant disease. However, megestrol acetate was recently relegated to third-line therapy, because phase III studies have shown that selective aromatase inhibitors provide a better side effect and efficacy profile.[5,417]

Progesterone Physiology

Progesterone is secreted mainly by the corpus luteum of the ovary during the second half of the menstrual cycle. The principal physiologic target organ for progesterone is the uterine endometrium. Progesterone secretion begins just before ovulation, coincident with the LH surge, and derives from the follicle that becomes the corpus luteum once the ovum is released.[418] Progesterone is synthesized from cholesterol and pregnenolone in all steroid-producing tissues: the ovary, testis, adrenal cortex, and placenta. Although the luteotroph varies with the species, in humans LH is the primary stimulator of progesterone synthesis.[419] The production rate of progesterone varies from a few milligrams per day during the follicular phase to 10 to 20 mg per day during the luteal phase (reaching blood levels of 10 ng per mL), increasing to several hundred milligrams daily during the latter parts of pregnancy. Rates of 1 to 5 mg per day have been measured in men and are comparable to the values in women during the follicular phase of the cycle.[420] Once secreted into the bloodstream, progesterone is either bound to CBG (with an affinity roughly equal to that of cortisol) or rapidly cleared from the circulation within a few minutes, predominantly by the liver, where glucuronidation or sulfation occurs before excretion in the urine. The isomers of pregnanediol are the principal metabolites.[75,205] In total, 50% to 60% of the progesterone C-14 given is excreted in the urine. A small and probably physiologically insignificant proportion is stored in body fat, from which it is slowly released. The enhanced biologic potency of such synthetic progestins as medroxyprogesterone acetate (6α-methyl 17α-hydroxyprogesterone acetate) may be explained by a lower metabolic clearance rate than progesterone[421] and by the greater affinity for the PgR.[422] The biologic roles of progesterone are listed in Table 6-10. Although progestins act principally through the PgR, these agents have some antiandrogenic (sometimes weakly androgenic) and antimineralocorticoid-like properties on the basis of low affinities for androgen and mineralocorticoid receptors.

TABLE 6-10. PHYSIOLOGIC EFFECTS OF PROGESTINS

Establishment and maintenance of pregnancy
Promotion of development of secretory epithelium of uterine endometrium after estrogen priming
Alterations in vaginal epithelium, causing change from abundant watery secretions to scant viscid material
Proliferation and engorgement of mammary acini (in concert with estrogens)
Thermogenesis
Weakly antiandrogenic
Weakly antimineralocorticoid

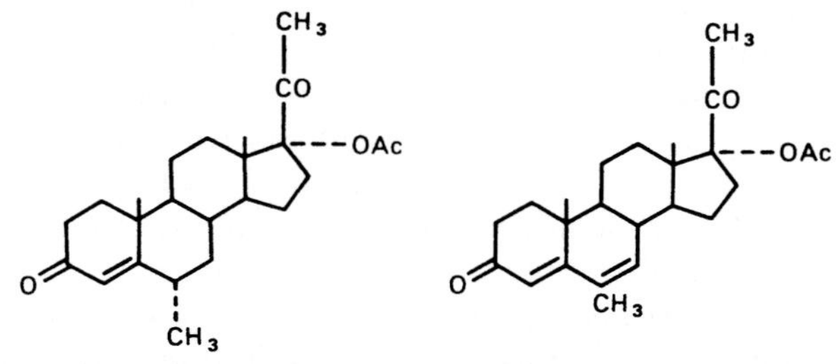

FIGURE 6-16. Progestins.

Progestins and Breast Cancer Therapy

A variety of progestins have been used for patients with hormone-dependent cancer. These include the C-21, 17-acetoxysteroids, such as medroxyprogesterone acetate and megestrol acetate, and the 19-carbon steroids, such as norethisterone (Fig. 6-16). Historically, the response rate to progestins was quoted as approximately 27% to 35% and positively correlated with estrogen and PgR expression.[94] This has been confirmed in large phase III studies in comparison with selective aromatase inhibitors, if patients who experience disease stabilization (lack of progression at 24 weeks) are included.[423,424]

The mechanism of the anticancer action of the progestins is not established, in part because these agents do not simply act through the PgR, but also through the AR and ER. Although progestins may have a direct antitumor action,[425,426] progestins also suppress basal and GnRH-simulated gonadotropin secretion, cortisol, dehydroepiandrosterone, and estradiol in a dose-dependent manner.[427] In the normal menstrual cycle, breast epithelial cell proliferation is maximal during the luteal phase (days 20 to 28), when progesterone levels are highest.[428,429] These data suggest that progestins stimulate the growth of normal mammary epithelium. Antiprogestins induce apoptosis in mammary tumor models,[430,431] suggesting that progesterone is an important stimulatory factor during mammary tumorigenesis. Also, progestins regulate metastasis-related cell surface receptors, such as the laminin receptor for adhesion molecules,[432] which may result in increased metastases. A direct antitumor action is supported by data, suggesting that progestins alter signaling through peptide growth factor receptors. Vignon et al.[426] showed that R5020, a progestin, decreases the production of a mitogenic 52-K glycoprotein.

Endocrine Effects

Progestin treatment results in a decrease in FSH and LH levels.[433–435] Also, cortisol and ACTH levels are depressed,[434–437] and the ACTH response to metyrapone is blunted.[436] The cortisol decrease is ACTH-dependent. Estrone levels are decreased in postmenopausal women by

82% compared to pretreatment,[435] as are levels of dehydroepiandrosterenedione sulfate and androstenedione.[438] Suppression of postmenopausal estrogen is therefore likely to be a predominant mode of action of progestins. This being the case, the activity of these drugs after disease progression on more potent estrogen deprivation therapies is likely to be low. Progestin therapy continues to be offered as a benign third-line endocrine therapy option, post selective aromatase inhibitor treatment, despite lack of evidence for activity in this setting. Men treated with medroxyprogesterone acetate have decreased levels of testosterone, which presumably explains the activity of progestins against prostate cancer.[434]

Medroxyprogesterone Acetate

Medroxyprogesterone acetate (MPA) was once commonly used for treating breast and endometrial cancer. The usual route of administration was i.m. As a result, when oral progestins such as megestrol acetate became available, the use of MPA declined. MPA is extensively metabolized and less than 1% of an i.v. dosage is recovered intact in the urine.[75,439] However, there were no clear correlations between plasma MPA and efficacy or between dosage and efficacy. There has been at least one study in which MPA was administered orally at a dose of 400 mg per day, with a 53% response rate in 30 patients.[94,440]

Megestrol Acetate

Megestrol acetate (MA) is the synthetic progestin most commonly prescribed for advanced breast cancer. The pharmacokinetics differ from MPA, because MA has a more rapid half-life (4 hours), greater renal excretion (56% to 78%, with 12% excreted as parent compound), and higher plasma levels.[75,433] The metabolites of MA are shown in Table 6-11. With oral dosages of 400 mg per day, plasma concentrations reach 400 ng per mL, with considerable interpatient variation. The recommended dosage is 40 mg four times each day or a single daily dose of 160 mg. MPA and MA probably have equivalent activities in

TABLE 6-11. MEGESTROL ACETATE PHARMACOLOGY

Mechanism of action	Unknown
Metabolism	17α-Acetoxy-6-hydroxymethyl-pregna-4,6-diene-3,20-dione
	2α-Hydroxy-6-hydroxymethyl-pregna-4,6-diene-3,20-dione
	17α-Acetoxy-6-hydroxymethyl-pregna-4,6-diene-3,20-dione
	2α-Hydroxy-6-hydroxymethyl-pregna-4,6-diene-3,20-dione
	17α-Acetoxy-21-hydroxy-6α-methyl-pregna-4,6-diene-3,20-dione
Pharmacokinetics	Half-life = 4 h
Elimination	Renal excretion, 56%–78%, fecal excretion, 7.7%–30.0%

breast cancer, but patients on MPA have a higher incidence of side effects.[441]

Toxicity

Pannuti et al. noted increased toxicity with high i.m. dosages of MPA, with little increase in efficacy.[442] These side effects include gluteal abscesses in 15% of patients receiving 1,500 mg i.m. daily, moon-shaped facies in 11%, fine tremors in 19%, and leg cramps in 19%; there is a much lower incidence of each of these effects with the 500-mg i.m. dose. Other side effects with MPA include sweating, vaginal discharge, and amenorrhea.[94] Another significant side effect is weight gain largely due to increased adipose tissue in the abdominal and cervicodorsal regions.[443] Weight gain ranged from 3 to 10 kg in 56% of patients treated with 1,000 to 1,500 mg i.m. daily. Because there is no difference in efficacy with different dosages or routes of administration, 400 to 500 mg orally daily is probably an adequate dosage. Crona et al.[444] reported decreases in high-density lipoprotein (HDL) cholesterol and apolipoprotein A1 with an increase in triglycerides in patients receiving 1,000 mg i.m. weekly. These results suggest that the risk of cardiovascular disease could be increased in patients taking MPA. Side effects with MA include increased appetite, weight gain of 5 to 20 kg, elevated liver function tests, thromboembolism, vaginal bleeding, hot flashes, fluid retention, nausea and vomiting, hypercalcemia and flare, and rash.[433] Most recently, megestrol acetate showed activity in cancer patients as treatment for anorexia and weight loss, rather than for antitumor activity.[445] This activity appears to result from suppression of cytokines that induce tumor cachexia.[446] Megestrol acetate in low dosages (20 mg per day) is active in the treatment of postmenopausal hot flashes in breast cancer patients.[447]

Antiprogestins

Mifepristone

The structures of antiprogestins under investigation are provided in Figure 6-17. Horwitz et al.[448] showed that progestin treatment of a cell line that lacks ER but contains the PgR (a T47D variant) inhibits proliferation. This suggests that PgR is a valid therapeutic target for breast cancer. This hypothesis was addressed through clinical trials of progesterone antagonists for treatment of advanced breast cancer. The first tested, mifepristone or RU 38486 [17 β-hydroxy-11β-(4-dimethylaminophenyl)-17α-(prop-1-ynyl) estra-4, 9-dien-3-one] (Fig. 6-17), has antiprogestational and antiglucocorticoid effects.[449] It has antiproliferative activity against ER-positive and negative cell lines[426] and inhibits 7,12-dimethylbenz[a]anthracene (DMBA)– induced mammary carcinomas in rats.[450] Pretreatment of an ER-

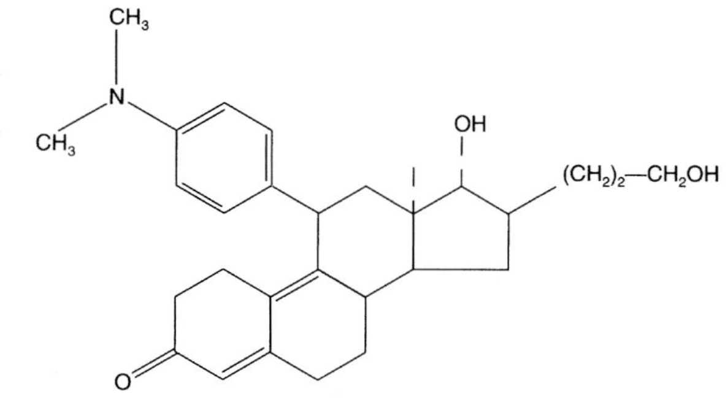

Onapristone (ZK 98299)

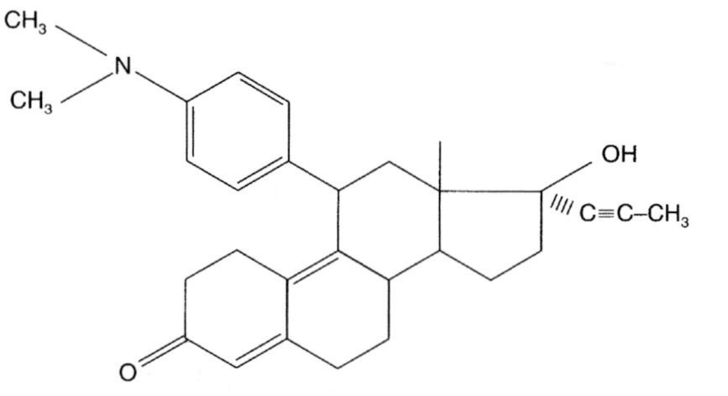

Mifepristone (RU 486)

FIGURE 6-17. Antiprogestins.

positive line with estradiol increases the effect of mifepristone, possibly through induction of PgR. The compound seems to require the presence of PgR, but not estrogen, androgen, or corticosteroid receptors, for activity. Patients who received prior estrogens develop secretory endometrial changes when receiving mifepristone, suggesting the compound has partial progestin agonist properties.[451] A clinical trial using mifepristone in metastatic breast cancer patients, 200 mg orally daily, reported a response rate of 18%.[452] The toxic effect reported was a 10% decrease in serum potassium. Plasma concentrations of FSH, LH, and prolactin were unchanged with treatment. Plasma cortisol concentrations showed a statistically significant increase from 235 ± 94 ng per mL baseline to 473 ± 141 ng per mL after 3 months of treatment. Another study tested mifepristone in 11 postmenopausal patients with an objective response in one patient.[453] Patients were treated with 200 or 400 mg per day. Endocrine parameters revealed a significant increase in cortisol, which could not be suppressed with dexamethasone. Also, plasma androstenedione and estradiol were increased. The plasma steroid hormone–binding globulin decreased with no change in gonadotropins or prolactin. Eosinophils and serum creatinine increased. Side effects reported include anorexia, nausea, tiredness, dizziness, somnolence, decrease in body weight, and a grand mal seizure suspected to be related to antiglucocorticoid activity. Although this compound is

interesting, newer drugs with less antiglucocorticoid activity are needed.

Onapristone

Onapristone is another progesterone antagonist that has also been studied in breast cancer patients with advanced disease. The drug is a synthetic steroid, 11β-[(4-dimethylamino)phenyl]-17α-hydroxy-17β-(3-hydroxypropyl)-13α-estra-4, 9(10)-dien-3-one (ZK98299) (Fig. 6-17). Onapristone binds to the PgR with an infinity ranging from 16% to 25% of that of progesterone.[454–456] Onapristone-PgR complexes do not induce progesterone response genes, indicating a lack of PgR agonist effect.[457,458] Preclinical data reveal onapristone inhibits hormone-dependent mammary tumors by blocking cells at the G0 and G1 phase of the cell cycle and inducing apoptosis.[459] Onapristone interrupts pregnancy in animal models due to PgR antagonism.[460] Also, onapristone displaces dexamethasone bound to the GR, with a relative binding affinity of 53% compared with dexamethasone.[461] The progesterone antagonistic properties are mediated through blocking of progesterone binding to the receptor.[454,456,458,462] In a small trial of onapristone as a first-line therapy in 19 elderly patients with locally advanced disease, ten experienced partial responses.[463] Clinical development is currently halted because of the development of liver function test abnormalities.

Estrogen Deprivation Therapy

Premenopausal Women

Oophorectomy versus Luteinizing Hormone–Releasing Hormone Agonists

Oophorectomy has been standard therapy for breast cancer for more than 100 years. As adjuvant therapy for premenopausal women, oophorectomy is associated with a marked reduction in relapse and death from breast cancer.[464] Because premenopausal women treated with LHRH agonists have plasma estradiol concentrations typical for postmenopausal women, surgical oophorectomy and treatment with LHRH agonists are generally held to be equivalent.[133,465–467] In premenopausal women treated with the LHRH agonist leuprolide, serum FSH and LH rise during the first few days of treatment.[466] Subsequently, FSH and LH levels fall and remain persistently suppressed. A similar pattern is seen with buserelin[133] and goserelin.[468] Plasma progesterone, estrone, estrone sulfate, and estradiol levels decrease to postmenopausal levels after 6 weeks of treatment. There is no change in androstenedione, prolactin, or cortisol levels. Unlike prostate cancer patients, in whom there is a transient rise in androgens with a risk of disease exacerbation, no rises in estrogen levels have been detected when women with advanced breast cancer are treated with LHRH agonists.[469–471]

Clinical Activity in Breast Cancer

Premenopausal women with breast cancer treated with LHRH agonists have objective response rates of between 36% and 44%.[466,468,472] The only randomized comparison between ovariectomy and LHRH agonist therapy was underpowered but did not reveal significant differences between these two approaches to estrogen deprivation.[467] Recent data have suggested the combination of an LHRH agonist and tamoxifen is superior to medical castration alone in the treatment of metastatic breast cancer, although the gains in response rate, disease-free, and overall survival were modest.[473,474] In the adjuvant setting, LHRH agonists were examined and the results released on a preliminary basis at the time of writing. Intergroup study 0101 examined the value of goserelin adjuvant therapy after chemotherapy treatment for premenopausal women with node-positive, ER-positive early stage breast cancer. The treatment of patients was randomized into three groups: no further systemic therapy after the chemotherapy was completed, monthly goserelin for a maximum of 5 years, or the combination of goserelin and tamoxifen. After a median follow-up period of 4 years, a significant increase in disease-free survival was detected for combination therapy of goserelin and tamoxifen therapy, but not for goserelin therapy alone. The lack of benefit for goserelin treatment alone could be explained on the basis that chemotherapy induced menopause in a significant proportion of women. In these women, goserelin would not be expected to provide any clinical benefit. This hypothesis was supported by several planned subgroup analyses. A benefit for goserelin therapy (in terms of disease-free survival) was detected in women less likely to have become menopausal with therapy (i.e., those aged 40 or younger), or those with premenopausal estradiol levels after chemotherapy.[475] A second larger European study was also completed in which the treatment of premenopausal women was randomly assigned to no endocrine treatment, goserelin, tamoxifen, or a combination. Chemotherapy could be administered at the discretion of the treating oncologist. A benefit for goserelin therapy was detected in all patient subgroups, including those who received chemotherapy and tamoxifen.[476] At the time of writing, information on these trials was available only as meeting abstracts. Further follow-up of the patients in these studies will be required to determine whether LHRH agonist therapy is associated with an increase in overall survival.

Toxicity

Side effects in women[466,468,472] include hot flashes, nausea and vomiting, headache, dizziness, vaginitis, sweating, emotional lability, breast atrophy, tumor flare, diarrhea, local reaction, irritability, hives, and severe polydipsia and polyuria in one patient. Also, amenorrhea is induced in all women. Bone mineral density is reduced in the lumbar spine and femur after 4 months of treatment with goserelin and does not normalize after discontinuation of treatment.[477] In the adjuvant breast cancer setting, this may be of concern and treatment with bisphosphonates may be appropriate. Total serum cholesterol, LDL cholesterol, and LDL to HDL cholesterol ratios were higher, whereas HDL cholesterol was lower in polycystic ovary patients treated with 6 months of goserelin.[478] Measurement of antithrombin III concentrations after treatment with goserelin reveals no change.[479] This suggests there may be no increased risk of thromboembolic episodes with this therapy.

Postmenopausal Women

Postmenopausal Estrogen

The therapeutic effect of reducing estrogen levels for patients with breast cancer was originally restricted to patients with functioning ovaries. However, postmenopausal women still produce significant amounts of estrogen through aromatization of circulating adrenal androgens in peripheral normal tissues, such as fat, muscle, liver, and the epithelial and stromal components of the breast.[480–482] Peripheral aromatization is increased in certain medical conditions, including obesity, hepatic disease, and hyperthyroidism, but is independent of pituitary hormone secretion. Although menopausal women continue to secrete some ovarian testosterone and androstenedione after menstrual cycling ceases, androstenedione from the adrenal gland is the major substrate for peripheral aromatization. The relative proportion of estrogens synthesized in extragonadal sites increases with age, and eventually nonovarian estrogens predominate in the circulation.[483,484]

Intratumoral Aromatase

Expression of aromatase in the breast led to the proposition that local synthesis of estrogens contributes to breast cancer growth in postmenopausal women.[485,486] In support of this theory, the decline in estrogen concentrations after menopause is less marked in breast tissue than in plasma[487] due to a combination of aromatase activity[488,489] and preferential estrogen uptake from the circulation.[490] Furthermore, aromatase activity has been shown to correlate with a marker of breast cancer cell proliferation[491] and quadrants of the breast bearing a breast cancer have more aromatase expression than those not bearing tumors. It is unclear whether an increase in aromatase expression precedes breast cancer development or is a direct consequence of the presence of a tumor.[492,493] However, aromatase activity in the breast is an attractive resolution to the paradox that breast cancer increases with age, although overall estrogen levels decline.

Regulation of Aromatase Activity

Investigations into the regulation of aromatase activity in the breast and other tissues have revealed a complex picture. The aromatase gene has a complex promoter structure, with regulatory elements targeted by gonadotrophins, glucocorticoids, growth factors, cytokines, and the intracellular signaling molecule cAMP.[481,494–496] Examples of peptide growth factors that may increase local estrogen production are the insulin-like growth factors (IGF-I and IGF-II), key players in breast cancer pathogenesis and ER function.[41] IGF-I and IGF-II promote aromatase activity in stromal cells[497,498] and the conversion of estrone to the more active molecule estradiol.[499] To develop a model of autocrine estrogen stimulation of breast cancer growth, several groups generated MCF7 breast cancer cells that overexpress aromatase by gene transfection.[500,501] Aromatase overexpressing MCF7 cells are androgen-dependent in nude mice, and growth can be efficiently inhibited by aromatase inhibitors and tamoxifen, but not antiandrogens.[502–505] Taken together, these observations suggest a model for postmenopausal breast cancer development that focuses on the interaction among locally synthesized estrogens, growth factors, and cytokines.

Aromatase Inhibitor Development

The pivotal role of aromatase in the development of breast cancer in older women defines this enzyme as a key therapeutic target. Two distinct solutions evolved to the problem of designing potent, specific, and safe aromatase inhibitors.[196] One strategy is to develop "steroidal" aromatase inhibitors, resistant to aromatase action, that bind aromatase and block conversion of androgenic substrates (Type 1 inhibitors). An alternative was to develop a family of "nonsteroidal" inhibitors that disrupt the aromatase active site by coordinating within the heme complex without affecting the active sites of other steroidogenic enzymes (Type 2 inhibitors). Both approaches led to the successful introduction into clinical practice of potent and specific aromatase inhibitors.

Aminoglutethimide

In 1973, Griffiths et al. first demonstrated the activity of aminoglutethimide, an inhibitor of cholesterol conversion to pregnenolone in the treatment of metastatic breast cancer.[3] Subsequently, it became appreciated that inhibition of aromatase, rather than suppression of general steroidogenesis, was key to the therapeutic action of aminoglutethimide.[506–508] Unfortunately, even at the lowest dosages effective against breast cancer, aminoglutethimide inhibited the formation of corticosteroids by blocking P-450 enzymes involved in cholesterol side-chain cleavage.[509] This lack of specificity exposes patients to the risk of glucocorticoid deficiency. Furthermore, the clinical utility of aminoglutethimide was limited by troublesome side effects including rash, nausea, somnolence (aminoglutethimide was originally developed as a sedative),[510] and blood dyscrasias.[511]

Clinical Activity

Clinical trials demonstrated that the clinical activity of aminoglutethimide was similar to tamoxifen as first-line treatment for advanced disease.[512,513] However, the single trial that assessed the efficacy of aminoglutethimide in the adjuvant setting did not demonstrate any clear long-term benefit with 8 years of follow-up.[514] For advanced disease patients with a history of tamoxifen responsive disease, the response to aminoglutethimide was estimated to be approximately 50%, with an overall response rate of approximately 30%.[515] Furthermore, approximately 20% of patients whose disease was initially refractory to tamoxifen therapy (primary tamoxifen resistance) remained responsive to aminoglutethimide.[512,513] These observations provided a strong rationale for the development of more potent and selective aromatase inhibitors. These newer aromatase inhibitors have now rendered aminoglutethimide an obsolete breast cancer therapy.

Steroidal Aromatase Inhibitors

A large number of androstenedione derivatives were screened in aromatase inhibition assays and two compounds, formestane (4-hydroxyandrostenedione) and exemestane, emerged as drugs suitable for clinical development.[516] As shown in the structures in Figure 6-18, both compounds retain androgenic properties but have side-chain substitutions that prevent conversion to estrogenic metabolites. Although not intrinsically reactive, formestane and exemestane (or modified forms of these drugs) exhibit tight or even irreversible binding to the aromatase active site.[517] Formestane and exemestane are therefore considered "mechanism-based" or "suicide" inhibitors because they permanently inactivate aromatase.[518] Recovery of aromatase activity after treatment with a suicide inhibitor therefore requires the synthesis of new aromatase protein. *In vivo*, the pharmacokinetics of suicide inhibition is characterized by persistently low aromatase activity despite complete drug clearance. Because suicide inhibition prolongs drug action, intermittent dosing should be possible, potentially improving the side effect to benefit ratio. However, in clinical practice this benefit remains largely theoretic because exemestane must be administered daily to maintain estrogen suppresion.

Formestane (4-Hydroxyandrostenedione). Formestane was the first alternative aromatase inhibitor to aminoglutethimide available, although it was never licensed in the United States. The drug continues to be used in several countries, but is being rapidly replaced by the nonsteroidal inhibitors anastrozole and letrozole. Formestane is 30- to 60-fold more potent than aminoglutethimide and suppresses 65% of estrogen production with, on average, a 40% decrease in serum estrone levels. Estradiol levels were suppressed by 32% to 40% within 24 hours and maximally suppressed by up to 78% seven days after treatment with 250 to 500 mg i.m. of 4-hydroxyandrostenedione.[519–521] 4-Hydroxytestosterone, a metabolite of formestane, has 65% of the aromatase inhibitory activity of 4OHA and

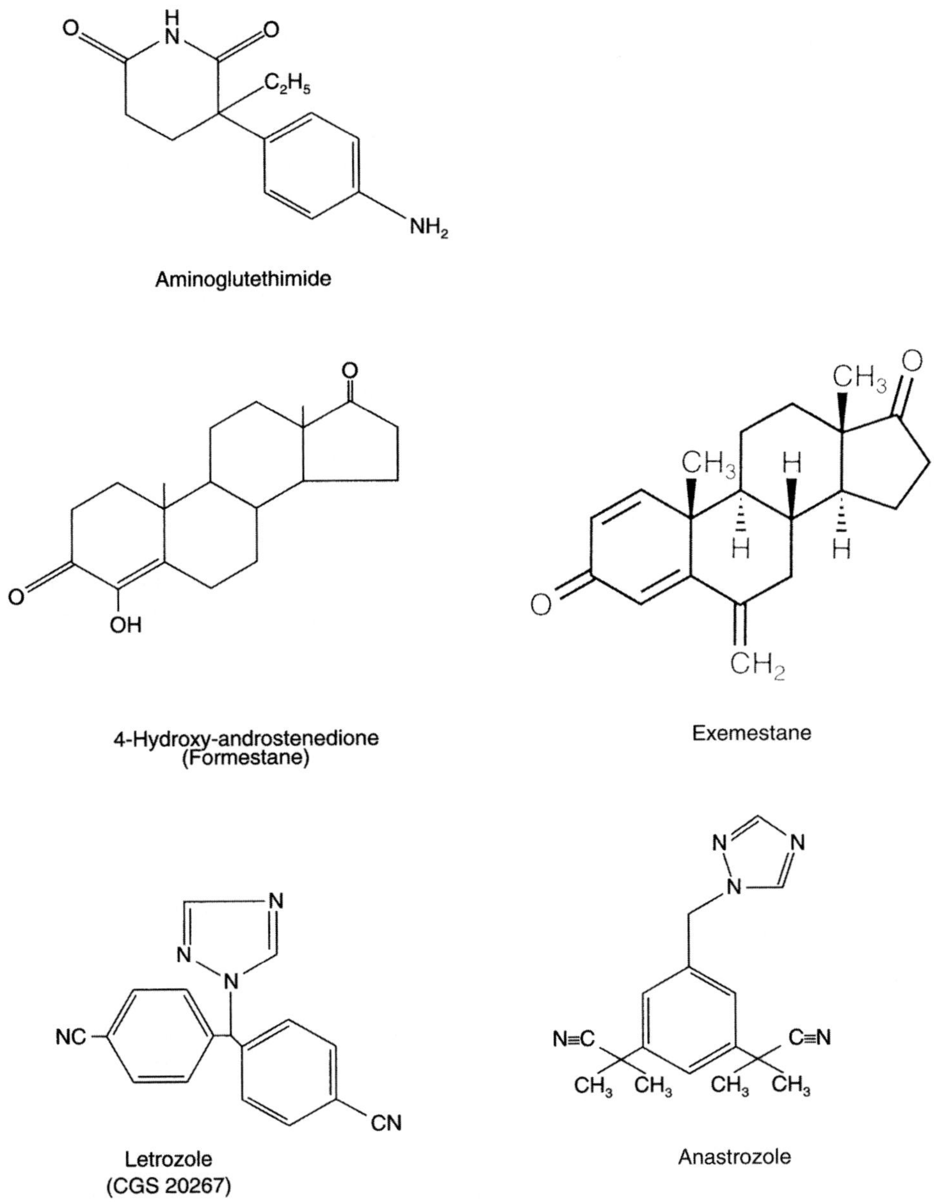

Aminoglutethimide

4-Hydroxy-androstenedione
(Formestane)

Exemestane

Letrozole
(CGS 20267)

Anastrozole

FIGURE 6-18. Aromatase inhibitors.

may contribute to the biologic activity of formestane.[522] Formestane is a highly specific aromatase inhibitor with no effects in postmenopausal women on thyroid-stimulating hormone, testosterone, androstenedione, 5α-DHT, or cortisol levels.[520]

Administration and Metabolism. Formestane is formulated as an i.m. injection, and this is considered to be one of the drawbacks of this drug. After i.m. injection, the drug is absorbed slowly and has a plasma half-life of between 5 and 10 days, with detectable levels as late as 28 days after injection.[519] Peak levels are reached at 1 to 2 days after injection.[520] A steady-state concentration, approximately 4.5 µg per mL after 250 mg, is achieved after the third or fourth fortnightly dosage.[523] After oral administration, 4OHA is

rapidly and extensively metabolized in the liver, the major product being a series of glucuronides.[520,524] The serum half-life of the drug is 2 to 3 hours. Fifty percent of an oral dose is excreted in the form of glucuronides in the first 4 hours after administration.[520] The main metabolites are the glucuronides of 4-hydroxytestosterone and 3α-hydroxy-5β-androsterone-4,17-dione. 4-Hydroxytestosterone and another metabolite, 4-hydroxyandrosta-4, 6-diene-3,17-dione, have aromatase activity, but less than the parent compound. Although the orally administered compound is active, its formulation is difficult, and it is not available for general clinical use.[519]

Clinical Activity. Phase II trials of 250 mg of formestane given every 2 weeks established response rates of 23% to

39%, with stabilization of disease for a further 14% to 29% of patients.[525-527] Predictably, responses were more frequent for patients with ER-positive tumors and a history of a response to tamoxifen. As first-line therapy, formestane produced response rates equivalent to tamoxifen (33% versus 37%); however, responses to formestane were less durable.[528] In the second-line setting, formestane proved to have antineoplastic activity similar to megestrol acetate.[529] Side effects with the use of i.m. formestane include sterile abscesses at the injection site, itching, and irritation. Lethargy, perioral edema, anaphylactoid reactions, hot flashes, vaginal spotting, emotional lability, nausea, dizziness, indigestion, ataxia, cramps, rash, arthralgia, alopecia, exacerbation of existing exanthema, increased facial hair, and, in one patient, neutropenia also have been reported. Toxicity with oral administration includes hot flashes, rash, facial swelling, and leukopenia.[530] Five percent of patients require discontinuation of treatment due to adverse effects.

Exemestane. Exemestane (6-methylenandrosta-1, 4-diene-3, 17-dione) is a synthetic steroidal irreversible aromatase inhibitor (Fig. 6-18). It has potent aromatase activity with a K_i of 26 nM and no cholesterol side-chain cleavage (desmolase) or 5α-reductase activity. It does not bind to the ER but weakly binds to the AR with an affinity 0.28% relative to DHT.[531] The binding affinity of the 17-dihydrometabolite is, however, 100 times that of the parent compound. As a result, there is slight androgenic activity in the rat with this drug.[531] The smallest dosage found to have maximal suppression of plasma estrone, estradiol, and estrone sulfate and urinary estrone and estradiol was 25 mg. This dosage inactivates peripheral aromatase by 98% and reduces basal plasma estrone, estradiol, and estrone sulphate levels by 85% to 95%.[532] Other endocrine parameters, such as cortisol, aldosterone, dehydroepiandrosterones, 17-OH-progesterone, FSH, and LH, were not significantly affected by 25 mg of exemestane.[533,534]

Administration and Metabolism. Exemestane is extensively metabolized with rapid oxidation of the methylene group at position 6 and reduction of the 17-keto group with subsequent formation of many secondary metabolites. A screen of potential metabolites for aromatase activity did not reveal any compounds with inhibitory activity greater than exemestane.[535] The drug is excreted in the urine and feces. As a consequence, clearance is affected by renal and hepatic insufficiency, with threefold elevations in the AUC under either conditions. Metabolism occurs through CYP3A4 and aldoketoreductases, and the activity of the major CYP enzymes is unaffected. The absorption of exemestane is enhanced by high fat foods, and it is recommended that the drug be taken after eating. Peak plasma concentrations are reached within 2 hours of administration and fall below the limit of detection 4 hours later (for the approved 25-mg dose).[533]

Clinical Activity. In one phase II trial of exemestane, 25 mg, involving 134 women with tamoxifen-resistant disease, the overall response rate was 22%. In addition, a further 31% had no change in disease for 24 weeks. Median duration of objective response was 68 weeks, and time to progression was 29 weeks (meeting abstract only).[536] In a second trial for patients with disease resistant to tamoxifen and megestrol acetate, the response rate was 13%, with an overall success rate (PR, CR, and stable disease for 24 weeks) of 30%.[537] Interestingly, responses were seen in visceral disease and for patients who never responded to tamoxifen (the overall response rate in this category was 25%).[536] Similar data were observed with formestane.[538] These results challenge the established dogma that further endocrine therapy should not be offered to patients who do not show an initial response to tamoxifen and have visceral disease. A recent phase III study demonstrated that exemestane achieves a similar objective response rate to megestrol acetate as second-line therapy. However, exemestane had an advantage with respect to median time to progression (4.7 months versus 3.8 months, $p = .037$).[539] Exemestane was as well tolerated as megestrol acetate and was associated with less weight gain. Common adverse events include hot flashes, nausea, and fatigue.[532]

Nonsteroidal Aromatase Inhibitors

Research has focused on a series of imidazole and triazole derivatives with "molecular shapes" that efficiently coordinate within the aromatase heme complex. Progress was assisted by new systems for rapid drug screening, and out of these screens came three drugs with the desired profile: vorozole, letrozole, and anastrozole (Fig. 6-18). Because vorozole is not available for further clinical trials despite good clinical activity,[540] our discussion focuses on letrozole and anastrozole.

Anastrozole. Anastrozole (2,2 [5-(1H-1, 2, 4-triazol-1-ylmethyl)-1, 3-phenylene] bis (2-methylpropiononitrile) is a competitive aromatase inhibitor with high potency. It inhibits human placental aromatase with an IC50 (concentration inhibiting enzyme activity by 50%) of 15 nM.[541,542] Pharmacodynamic studies reveal that subjects receiving 1 mg per day orally achieved maximal estradiol suppression and a decrease of estradiol ranging from 78% to 86% from baseline. There was no effect on glucocorticoid or mineralocorticoid secretion as tested by ACTH stimulation.[541] Anastrozole was the first selective aromatase inhibitor approved in North America and Europe. One mg of anastrozole daily rapidly suppresses estradiol, estrone, and estrone sulfate levels to close to assay detection limits and is more effective than formestane in this regard.[543] Suppression is maintained long term with no compensatory rise in androstenedione levels. Importantly, even at higher doses (5 to 10 mg), anastrozole administration does not affect basal or ACTH-stimulated cortisol and aldosterone levels.[541]

Administration and Metabolism. Anastrozole is rapidly absorbed with maximum level occurring within 2 hours after administration. Less than 10% of the drug is cleared as unchanged drug due to extensive metabolism. Degradation occurs through *N*-dealkylation, and metabolites are excreted predominantly in the urine. The half-life is approximately 50 hours, justifying a once-a-day dosing schedule. Steady-state concentrations were achieved by the tenth dose. The mean peak plasma concentration at the 1-mg dose was 13.1 ng per mL. The plasma elimination half-life with the 0.5- and 1.0-mg multiple doses ranged from 38 to 61 hours.[541]

Clinical Activity. Two international phase III clinical trials conducted in postmenopausal women with tamoxifen-resistant disease compared the activity of anastrozole with megestrol acetate (40 mg four times daily). Two doses of anastrozole were examined in these trials, 1 mg and 10 mg. Both doses suppress circulating estrogens to the limit of assay detection; however, the 10-mg dose was included to address the possibility that efficient inhibition of intratumoral aromatase might require a higher dose. An overview of both trials, incorporating data from 764 patients has recently been published.[544] Both trials were restricted to postmenopausal patients with ER-positive tumors, unless a response to tamoxifen treatment was previously documented in the case of an ER-negative and unknown tumor. Approximately half the patients developed progressive disease during or after adjuvant tamoxifen treatment; the rest developed tamoxifen resistance during treatment for metastatic disease. Few patients with advanced disease entered the trial without a history of a response to tamoxifen. Patient and tumor characteristics were evenly distributed in the three arms of the trials. Objective response rates were low: 10.3% in the 1-mg anastrozole group; 8.9% in the 10-mg anastrozole group, and 7.9% in the megestrol acetate group had either a complete or partial response. However 25.1%, 22.6%, and 26.1% of patients had stable disease equal to or greater than 6 months. Overall approximately one-third of patients benefited from therapy, with no difference emerging between the three treatment arms. With a median follow-up of 6 months, no differences in survival were detected. However, in an updated analysis, a longer median survival for 1 mg anastrozole versus megestrol acetate emerged (26.7 months versus 22.5 months, *p* = .02). There was also a higher 2-year survival in the 1-mg anastrozole group (56.1% versus 46.3%, respectively). A trend for significant improvement in median survival was also seen with the 10-mg dose (25.5 months, *p* = .10 against megestrol acetate); however, a difference in 2-year survival was not observed in the 10-mg group.[545] In both trials, anastrozole proved to be remarkably well tolerated. Anastrozole was associated with less weight gain than megestrol acetate, which will be considered a major advantage over progestins by many physicians and patients. In contrast, nausea and vomiting were more common with anastrozole. However, gastrointestinal toxicities were less troublesome with the 1-mg dose, and gastrointestinal problems rarely led to interruption of therapy.

Letrozole. Letrozole (4,4'-[(1H-1,2,4-triazol-1-yl)methylene]bisbenzonitrile) was the second nonsteroidal selective aromatase inhibitor approved for the treatment of advanced breast cancer. The IC50 for placental aromatase is 11.5 nM, marginally more potent than anastrozole or exemestane. For comparison, the IC50 for aminoglutethimide is 1,900 nM. In a preclinical model of aromatase-dependent breast cancer growth, letrozole had greater antitumor activity than did anastrozole and tamoxifen.[504,505] Letrozole has a profile similar to anastrozole, combining high potency, selectivity, and promising activity against advanced breast cancer in phase I and II trials.[546–549] Both letrozole doses examined in phase III trials, 0.5 mg and 2.5 mg, suppress estrogen levels over 90% (less than 0.5 pmol per L).[550] Clinical studies in postmenopausal women have confirmed the highly selective action of letrozole with no alteration of serum levels of the other classes of steroids.[546]

Administration and Metabolism. Oral absorption is rapid and not significantly affected by food. Like anastrozole, metabolic clearance through the liver is the major elimination pathway, and the half-life of 50 hours allows a once-a-day dosing schedule. CYP3A4 and CYP2A6 catalyze letrozole to its major metabolite that is then subjected to glucuronidation. Letrozole can be safely prescribed for patients with renal insufficiency, because only 5% of the drug is cleared in the urine. However, the drug should be used with caution for patients with severe liver impairment. There are no known drug interactions with erythromycin, warfarin, or cimetidine. As mentioned earlier, coadministration of tamoxifen reduces letrozole levels by 37%, probably due to the induction of CYP3A4.[308] Letrozole is extremely well tolerated, as only 2% of patients discontinued the drug due to adverse events in the comparison with megestrol acetate, which had an 8% discontinuation rate.[423]

Clinical Activity. A nonblinded comparison was made between aminoglutethimide, 250 mg, twice a day and two doses of letrozole, 0.5 mg and 2.5 mg. Blinding was not thought to be ethical because of the adrenal suppression associated with aminoglutethimide therapy. The dose of aminoglutethimide in this trial was predicted to achieve a 50% to 60% decrease in estrogen levels, against 85% to 95% with letrozole (the actual levels in the trial have not been reported). Five hundred and fifty-five women with tamoxifen-resistant breast cancer were entered. Response rates were highest for 2.5 mg letrozole (17.8%), compared with 0.5 mg letrozole (16.7%) and aminoglutethimide (11.2%). Both doses of letrozole were significantly superior to aminoglutethimide in time to disease progression, although the differences were small. In addition, a small but significant survival benefit emerged in favor of letrozole 2.5 mg (median survival 30 months) against aminoglutethimide (median survival 19 months; $p = .02$).[551] As a result of this trial aminoglutethimide can be considered an obsolete breast cancer treatment. In a second phase III trial, letrozole was compared to megestrol acetate.[423] Patients were allowed to enter the trial with unknown estrogen and PgR status, without a requirement for a prior response to tamoxifen. As a result, 40% of the letrozole patients had unknown ER and PgR status against 25% in the anastrozole trials. Five hundred and fifty-one patients were randomized between megestrol acetate, 160 mg a day, and letrozole, 0.5 mg and 2.5 mg. Data were analyzed for response and safety for 33 months and for survival for 45 months. Two and one-half mg of letrozole produced a significantly higher overall response rate (24%) compared with megestrol acetate (16%) and letrozole, 0.5 mg (13%). Letrozole, 2.5 mg, was also superior to letrozole 0.5 mg and megestrol acetate for time to treatment failure, although the differences were small (median duration, 5.1 months, 3.2 months, and 3.9 months, respectively), and a survival benefit has not been observed. Once again, the safety and tolerability of selective aromatase inhibitors were demonstrated. Letrozole was significantly better tolerated than megestrol acetate with respect to serious adverse experiences, discontinuation due to poor tolerability, cardiovascular side effects, and weight gain.

Future Development Plans for Aromatase Inhibitors

Three programs are being executed to assess the value of selective aromatase inhibitors as adjuvant therapy for breast cancer. In the ATAC trial [anastrozole (*A*rimidex), *ta*moxifen, and *c*ombination] approximately 10,000 patients are randomized to three arms: 5 years of anastrozole 1 mg, 5 years of tamoxifen 20 mg, or 5 years of the combination. The acronym for the letrozole adjuvant trial design is FEMTA [letrozole (*Fem*ara), *t*amoxifen *a*djuvant trial]. The FEMTA trial is a four-way randomization between 5 years of letrozole, 2.5 mg, 5 years of tamoxifen, 20 mg, and two sequential therapy arms, with either tamoxifen first (2 years), then letrozole (3 years), or the reverse.[552] An exemestane adjuvant trial is being executed that also has a sequential design examining 3 years of tamoxifen versus exemestane after an initial 2 years of tamoxifen treatment. A fourth design is currently open as a United States Intergroup study in which treatment is randomized between aromatase inhibitor and placebo after completing 5 years of tamoxifen therapy. In addition to breast cancer end points, these investigations have substudies focused on the long-term effects of extreme estrogen deprivation, including osteoporosis, cardiovascular disease, and quality of life.

Aromatase Inhibitors for the Treatment of Premenopausal Women

Hereditary aromatase deficiency, due to inherited loss-of-function mutations in the aromatase gene, is associated with a syndrome of hypergonadotrophic hypogonadism, multicystic ovaries, virilism, and bone demineralization in childhood. These problems are reversible with low-dose estrogens.[553,554] Polycystic ovary syndrome in adult women has a less well-defined etiology, although low aromatase activity is believed to play a part.[555] Treatment of premenopausal women with aromatase inhibitors is therefore likely to be complicated by polycystic ovaries and virilization. To circumvent these problems, the treatment of premenopausal women with advanced breast cancer with an LHRH analog and selective aromatase inhibitor combination is under investigation. Aminoglutethimide treatment of premenopausal women does not suppress estrogen levels, so the indication for this drug was restricted to patients without ovarian function.[556] However, more potent aromatase inhibitors are able to suppress ovarian aromatase activity. For example, in a small pharmacokinetic study, a combination of formestane and an LHRH agonist produced more effective inhibition of premenopausal estradiol levels than with the LHRH agonist alone.[557] This is also the case for the nonsteroidal aromatase vorozole, because the combination of vorozole and goserelin was markedly more effective in reducing estrogen levels when compared to goserelin alone.[558] Further investigations will be required to determine whether the extremely low estrogen levels achieved with an LHRH-A and a third-generation aromatase inhibitor will translate into increased clinical benefit. Outside of a clinical trial, the use of selective aromatase inhibitors continues to be restricted to postmenopausal women with advanced breast cancer.

SUMMARY

There has been remarkable growth in the number of steroid hormone therapies available for the treatment of breast cancer. The last 4 years have seen U.S. Food and Drug Administration approval for toremifene, anastrozole, letrozole, and exemestane. In the near future, we may see approval of the first pure antiestrogen and an increasing emphasis on the use of SERM agents in the prevention of breast cancer. In the adjuvant and advanced disease setting, aromatase inhibitors could displace tamoxifen as first-line agents. For prostate cancer, the adjuvant use of combination of an LHRH agonist and antiandrogen is likely to increase as gains in overall survival are confirmed. Prevention with 5α-reductase inhibitors may be introduced. Finally, new signal transduction inhibitors with endocrine therapy–like profiles of safety and efficacy will be introduced and combinations with classic steroid hormone therapies explored.

Despite the fast pace of these changes, the framework outlined in this chapter should stand the reader in good stead when making rational decisions concerning the clinical use of endocrine therapy for cancer.

REFERENCES

1. Beatson GW. On the treatment of inoperable carcinoma of the mamma: suggestions for a new method of treatment with illustrative cases. *Lancet* 1896;2:104–107.

2. Huggins C, Hodges CV. Studies of prostatic cancer: the effect of castration, of estrogen and of androgen injection on serum phosphatases in metastatic carcinoma of the prostate. *Cancer Res* 1941;1:293–297.

3. Griffiths CT, Hall TC, Saba Z. Preliminary trial of aminoglutethimide in breast cancer. *Cancer* 1973;32:31–37.

4. Santen RJ, Manni A, Harvey H. Gonadotropin releasing hormone (GnRH) analogs for the treatment of breast and prostatic carcinoma. *Breast Cancer Res Treat* 1986; 7(3):129–145.

5. Ellis M. Selective aromatase inhibitors: current indication and future perspectives. In: Lippman ME, Harris J, eds. *Diseases of the breast update*, vol 2. Baltimore: Lippincott–Raven, 1998.

6. Sudduth SL, Koronkowski MJ. Finasteride: the first 5 alpha-reductase inhibitor. *Pharmacotherapy* 1993;13(4): 309–325; discussion 325–329.

7. Williams G, et al. Objective responses to ketoconazole therapy in patients with relapsed progressive prostatic cancer. *Br J Urol* 1986;58(1):45–51.

8. Furr BJ, Jordan VC. The pharmacology and clinical uses of tamoxifen. *Pharmacol Ther* 1984;25(2):127–205.

9. Ingle JN, et al. Randomized clinical trial of diethylstilbestrol versus tamoxifen in postmenopausal women with advanced breast cancer. *N Engl J Med* 1981;304(1):16–21.

10. Stewart HJ, et al. The tamoxifen trial—a double-blind comparison with stilboestrol in postmenopausal women with advanced breast cancer. *Eur J Cancer* 1980;Suppl(1):83–88.

11. Tamoxifen for early breast cancer: an overview of the randomised trials. Early Breast Cancer Trialists' Collaborative Group. *Lancet* 1998;351(9114):1451–1467.

12. Hermon C, Beral V. Breast cancer mortality rates are levelling off or beginning to decline in many western countries: analysis of time trends, age-cohort and age-period models of breast cancer mortality in 20 countries. *Br J Cancer* 1996;73(7):955–960.

13. Gradishar WJ, Jordan VC. Clinical potential of new antiestrogens. *J Clin Oncol* 1997;15(2):840–852.

14. Sogani CP, Vagaiwala MR, Whitmore WF Jr. Experience with flutamide in patients with advanced prostatic cancer without prior endocrine therapy. *Cancer* 1984;54(4):744–750.

15. Bolla M. Adjuvant hormonal treatment with radiotherapy for locally advanced prostate cancer. *Eur Urol* 1999;35 (Suppl 1):23–25; discussion 26.

16. Fisher B, et al. Tamoxifen for prevention of breast cancer: report of the National Surgical Adjuvant Breast and Bowel Project P-1 Study. *J Natl Cancer Inst* 1998;90(18):1371–1388.

17. IUPAC Commission on the Nomenclature of Organic Chemistry and IUPAC-IUB Commission on Biochemical Nomenclature. Revised tentative rules for nomenclature of steroids. *Biochem J* 1969;113(1):5–28.

18. Briggs MJ, Brotherton J. *Steroid biochemistry and pharmacology*. London: Academic Press, 1970.

19. Brotherton J. *Sex hormone pharmacology*. London: Academic Press, 1976.

20. Briggs MH, Christie GA. *Advances in steroid biochemistry and pharmacology*. London: Academic Press, 1977.

21. Danielsson H, Tchen TT. Steroid metabolism. In: Greenbert DM, ed. *Metabolic pathways*. New York: Academic Press, 1968:117.

22. Evans RM. The steroid and thyroid hormone receptor superfamily. *Science* 1988;240(4854):889–895.

23. Beato M. Gene regulation by steroid hormones. *Cell* 1989;56(3):335–344.

24. Parker MG. Transcriptional activation by oestrogen receptors. *Biochem Soc Symp* 1998;63:45–50.

25. Kamei Y, et al. A CBP integrator complex mediates transcriptional activation and AP-1 inhibition by nuclear receptors. *Cell* 1996;85(3):403–414.

26. Voegel JJ, et al. TIF2, a 160 kDa transcriptional mediator for the ligand-dependent activation function AF-2 of nuclear receptors. *EMBO J* 1996;15(14):3667–3675.

27. Hong H, et al. GRIP1, a transcriptional coactivator for the AF-2 transactivation domain of steroid, thyroid, retinoid, and vitamin D receptors. *Mol Cell Biol* 1997;17(5):2735–2744.

28. Halachmi S, et al. Estrogen receptor-associated proteins: possible mediators of hormone-induced transcription. *Science* 1994;264(5164):1455–1458.

29. Onate SA, et al. Sequence and characterization of a coactivator for the steroid hormone receptor superfamily. *Science* 1995;270(5240):1354–1357.

30. Beato M, Sanchez-Pacheco A. Interaction of steroid hormone receptors with the transcription initiation complex. *Endocr Rev* 1996;17(6):587–609.

31. Beato M, et al. Interaction of steroid hormone receptors with transcription factors involves chromatin remodelling. *J Steroid Biochem* 1996;56(1–6 Spec No):47–59.

32. Jackson TA, et al. The partial agonist activity of antagonist-occupied steroid receptors is controlled by a novel hinge domain-binding coactivator L7/SPA and the corepressors N-CoR or SMRT. *Mol Endocrinol* 1997;11(6):693–705.

33. Chen JD, Evans RM. A transcriptional co-repressor that interacts with nuclear hormone receptors [see comments]. *Nature* 1995;377(6548):454–457.

34. Horlein AJ, et al. Ligand-independent repression by the thyroid hormone receptor mediated by a nuclear receptor co-repressor. *Nature* 1995;377(6548):397–404.

35. Xu L, Glass CK, Rosenfeld MG. Coactivator and corepressor complexes in nuclear receptor function. *Curr Opin Genet Dev* 1999;9(2):140–147.

36. Mueller H, et al. Selective regulation of steroid receptor expression in MCF-7 breast cancer cells by a novel member of the heregulin family. *Biochem Biophys Res Commun* 1995;217(3):1271–1278.

37. Pietras RJ, et al. HER-2 tyrosine kinase pathway targets estrogen receptor and promotes hormone-independent growth in human breast cancer cells. *Oncogene* 1995;10 (12):2435–2446.

38. El-Ashry D, et al. Constitutive raf-1 kinase activity in breast cancer cells induces both estrogen-independent growth and apoptosis. *Oncogene* 1997;15(4):423–435.

39. Ellis MJ, et al. Affinity for the insulin-like growth factor-II (IGF-II) receptor inhibits autocrine IGF-II activity in MCF-7 breast cancer cells. *Mol Endocrinol* 1996;10(3): 286–297.

40. Ellis MJ. The insulin-like growth factor network and breast cancer. In: Bowcock AM, ed. *Breast cancer: molecular genetics, pathogenesis, and therapeutics.* Totowa, NJ: Humana Press, 1999.

41. Ellis MJ, et al. Insulin-like growth factors in human breast cancer. *Breast Cancer Res Treat* 1998;52(1–3):175–184.

42. Smith CL, Conneely OM, O'Malley BW. Modulation of the ligand-independent activation of the human estrogen receptor by hormone and antihormone. *Proc Natl Acad Sci U S A* 1993;90(13):6120–6124.

43. Aronica SM, Katzenellenbogen BS. Stimulation of estrogen receptor-mediated transcription and alteration in the phosphorylation state of the rat uterine estrogen receptor by estrogen, cyclic adenosine monophosphate, and insulin-like growth factor-I. *Mol Endocrinol* 1993;7(6):743–752.

44. Le Goff P, et al. Phosphorylation of the human estrogen receptor. Identification of hormone-regulated sites and examination of their influence on transcriptional activity. *J Biol Chem* 1994;269(6):4458–4466.

45. El-Tanani MK, Green CD. Two separate mechanisms for ligand-independent activation of the estrogen receptor. *Mol Endocrinol* 1997;11(7):928–937.

46. Sortino MA, et al. Mitogenic effect of nerve growth factor (NGF) in LNCaP prostate adenocarcinoma cells: role of the high- and low-affinity NGF receptors. *Mol Endocrinol* 2000;14(1):124–136.

47. Reinikainen P, Palvimo JJ, Janne OA. Effects of mitogens on androgen receptor-mediated transactivation. *Endocrinology* 1996;137(10):4351–4357.

48. Nazareth LV, Weigel NL. Activation of the human androgen receptor through a protein kinase A signaling pathway. *J Biol Chem* 1996;271(33):19900–19907.

49. Addison T. *On the constitutional and local effects of disease of the suprarenal capsules.* London: Samuel Highley, 1855.

50. Brown-Sequard GG. Researches experimentals sur la physiologie et la pathologie des capsule surrenele. *CR Acad Sci* 1856;3:422.

51. Cushing H. The basophil adenomas of the pituitary body and their clinical manifestations. *Bull Johns Hopkins Hosp* 1932;50:137.

52. Foster GL, Smith PE. Hypophysectomy and replacement therapy in relation to basal metabolism and specific dynamic action in the rat. *JAMA* 1926;87:2151.

53. Collip JB, Anderson EM, Thompson DL. The adrenotropic hormone of the anterior pituitary lobe. *Lancet* 1933;2:347.

54. Li CH, Evans HM, Simpson ME. Adrenocorticotrophic hormone. *J Biol Chem* 1943;149:413.

55. Bell PH, Howard KS, Shepherd RG. Studies with corticotropin: II. Pepsin degradation of corticotropin. *J Am Chem Soc* 1956;78:5059.

56. Schwyzer R, Sieber P. Total synthesis of adrenocorticotropic hormone. *Nature* 1963;199:172.

57. Mountjoy KG, et al. The cloning of a family of genes that encode the melanocortin receptors. *Science* 1992;257(5074):1248–1251.

58. De Souza EB. Corticotropin-releasing factor receptors: physiology, pharmacology, biochemistry and role in central nervous system and immune disorders. *Psychoneuroendocrinology* 1995;20(8):789–819.

59. Kallen CB, et al. Unveiling the mechanism of action and regulation of the steroidogenic acute regulatory protein. *Mol Cell Endocrinol* 1998;145(1–2):39–45.

60. Ontjes DA. The pharmacologic control of adrenal steroidogenesis. *Life Sci* 1980;26(24):2023–2035.

61. Westphal U. Binding of corticosteroids by plasma proteins. In: Greep RO, Astwood EB, Blaschko H, eds. *Handbook of physiology section I: endocrinology.* Washington, DC: American Physiological Society, 1975:117.

62. Sandberg AA, Slaunwhite WRJ. Transcortin: a corticosteroid-binding protein of plasma: II. Levels in various conditions and the effects of estrogens. *J Clin Invest* 1959;38:1290.

63. Claman HN. Corticosteroids and lymphoid cells. *N Engl J Med* 1972;287(8):388–397.

64. Goldin A, et al. The chemotherapy of human and animal acute leukemia. *Cancer Chemother Rep* 1971;55(4):309–505.

65. Neifeld JP, Lippman ME, Tormey DC. Steroid hormone receptors in normal human lymphocytes. Induction of glucocorticoid receptor activity by phytohemagglutinin stimulation. *J Biol Chem* 1977;252(9):2972–2977.

66. Lippman M, Barr R. Glucocorticoid receptors in purified subpopulations of human peripheral blood lymphocytes. *J Immunol* 1977;118(6):1977–1981.

67. Lippman ME, Yarbro GK, Leventhal BG. Clinical implications of glucocorticoid receptors in human leukemia. *Cancer Res* 1978;38(11 Pt 2):4251–4256.

68. Crabtree GR, Smith KA, Munck A. Glucocorticoid receptors and sensitivity of isolated human leukemia and lymphoma cells. *Cancer Res* 1978;38(11 Pt 2):4268–4272.

69. Lippman ME, et al. Glucocorticoid-binding proteins in human acute lymphoblastic leukemic blast cells. *J Clin Invest* 1973;52(7):1715–1725.

70. Smets LA, van den Berg JD. Bcl-2 expression and glucocorticoid-induced apoptosis of leukemic and lymphoma cells. *Leuk Lymphoma* 1996;20(3–4):199–205.

71. Feinman R, et al. Role of NF-kappaB in the rescue of multiple myeloma cells from glucocorticoid-induced apoptosis by bcl-2. *Blood* 1999;93(9):3044–3052.

72. Krett NL, et al. Cyclic adenosine-3',5'-monophosphate-mediated cytotoxicity in steroid sensitive and resistant myeloma. *Clin Cancer Res* 1997;3(10):781–787.

73. McColl KS, et al. Apoptosis induction by the glucocorticoid hormone dexamethasone and the calcium-ATPase inhibitor thapsigargin involves Bcl-2 regulated caspase activation. *Mol Cell Endocrinol* 1998;39(1-2):229–238.

74. Loriaux DL, Cutler GBJ. Diseases of the adrenal glands. In: Po K, ed. *Basic clinical endocrinology.* New York: Wiley-Liss, 1981.

75. Fotherby K, James F. Metabolism of synthetic steroids. *Adv Steroid Biochem Pharmacol* 1972;3:67.

76. Peterson RE. Metabolism of adrenal corticol steroids. In: Christy NP, ed. *The human adrenal cortex.* New York: Harper & Row, 1971:87.

77. Gordon GG, Southren AL. Thyroid hormone effects on steroid hormone metabolism. *Bull N Y Acad Med* 1977;53:241–259.

78. Boyar RM, et al. Cortisol secretion and metabolism in anorexia nervosa. *N Engl J Med* 1977;296(4):190–193.

79. McEvoy GK. Adrenals. In: *Drug information 88.* Bethesda, MD: American Society of Hospital Pharmacists, 1986:1706.

80. Bradlow HL, et al. Isolation and identification of four new carboxylic acid metabolites of cortisol in man. *J Clin Endocrinol Metab* 1973;37(5):811–818.

81. Hakin HLJ, Trafford DJH. The chemistry of the steroids. *Clin Endocrinol Metab* 1972;1:333–360.

82. Butenandt A. Uber die chemische untersuchung der sexual-hormons. *Angew Chem* 1931;44:905–916.

83. Loewe S, Voss HE. Der tand der erfassung des mannlichen sexual hormons (androkinins). *Klin Wochenschr* 1930;9:481–487.

84. Ruzicka I, Wettstein A. Synthetische darstellung des testishormons. Testosteron (Androst-3-17-ol). *Helv Chim Acad* 1935;18:1264–1275.

85. Puett D, et al. hCG-receptor binding and transmembrane signaling. *Mol Cell Endocrinol* 1996;25(1–2):55–64.

86. Alvarez CA, et al. Characterization of a region of the lutropin receptor extracellular domain near transmembrane helix 1 that is important in ligand-mediated signaling. *Endocrinology* 1999;140(4):1775–1782.

87. Nisula BC, Dunn JF. Measurement of the testosterone binding parameters for both testosterone-estradiol binding globulin and albumin in individual serum samples. *Steroids* 1979;34(7):771–791.

88. Vermeulen A, Ando S. Metabolic clearance rate and interconversion of androgens and the influence of the free androgen fraction. *J Clin Endocrinol Metab* 1979;48(2):320–326.

89. Goldenberg IS. Clinical trial of delta-1-testololactone (NSC 23759), medroxy progesterone acetate (NSC 26386) and oxylone acetate (NSC 47438) in advanced female mammary cancer. A report of the cooperative breast cancer group. *Cancer* 1969;23(1):109–112.

90. Bhatnagar AS, Nadjafi C, Steiner R. Aromatase inhibitors in cancer treatment. In: Stall BA, ed. *Endocrine management of cancer 2: contemporary therapy.* Basel: Karger, 1988:30.

91. Wilson JD. Androgens. In: Goodman Gilman A, et al., eds. *The pharmacologic basis of therapeutics*, 8th ed. New York: Pergamon Press, 1990:1413.

92. Feldman EE, Carter AC. Endocrinologic and metabolic effects of 17 α-methyl-19-nortestosterone in women. *J Clin Endocrinol Metab* 1960;20:842–857.

93. Johnson FL, et al. Association of androgenic-anabolic steroid therapy with development of hepatocellular carcinoma. *Lancet* 1972;2(7790):1273–1276.

94. Henderson IC. Endocrine therapy in metastatic breast cancer. In: Harris JR, et al., eds. *Breast diseases.* Philadelphia: JB Lippincott Co, 1991:559.

95. Brodovsky HS, et al. Danazol in the treatment of women with metastatic breast cancer. *Cancer Treat Rep* 1987;71(9):875–876.

96. Coombes RC, et al. Danazol treatment of advanced breast cancer. *Cancer Treat Rep* 1980;64(10–11):1073–1076.

97. Madanes AE, Farber M. Danazol. *Ann Intern Med* 1982;96(5):625–630.

98. Tobiassen T, et al. Danazol treatment of severely symptomatic fibrocystic breast disease and long-term follow-up—the Hjorring project. *Acta Obstet Gynecol Scand Suppl* 1984;123:159–176.

99. Barbieri RL, Canick JA, Makris A. Danazol inhibits steroidogenesis. *Fertil Steril* 1977;28:809–813.

100. Greenblatt RB, et al. Clinical studies with an antigonadotropin—Danazol. *Fertil Steril* 1971;22(2):102–112.

101. Huggins C, Clark PJ. Quantitative studies of prostatic secretion. *J Exp Med* 1940;72:747.

102. Huggins C. Quantitative studies of prostatic secretion: characterization of normal section and testis extirpation and androgen substitution on the prostatic output. *J Exp Med* 1939;70:543–556.

103. Blankenstein MA, Bakker GH. Rationale for suppression of adrenal steroidogenesis in advance prostate cancer. In: Back N, Brevier GJ, Eijsvogel V, eds. *EORTC genitourinary group monograph 2.* New York: Wiley-Liss, 1985:161.

104. Small EJ, Baron A, Bok R. Simultaneous antiandrogen withdrawal and treatment with ketoconazole and hydrocortisone in patients with advanced prostate carcinoma. *Cancer* 1997;80(9):1755–1759.

105. Wilson JD. Recent studies on the mechanism of action of testosterone. *N Engl J Med* 1972;287(25):1284–1291.

106. Baulieu EE, Lasnizki I, Robel P. Metabolism of testosterone and action of metabolites on prostate glands grown in organ culture. *Nature* 1968;219(159):1155–1156.

107. Imperato-McGinley J, et al. Steroid 5alpha-reductase deficiency in man: an inherited form of male pseudohermaphroditism. *Science* 1974;86(4170):1213–1215.

108. Gormley GJ, et al. The effect of finasteride in men with benign prostatic hyperplasia. The Finasteride Study Group [see comments]. *N Engl J Med* 1992;327(17):1185–1191.

109. Petrow V. The dihydrotestosterone (DHT) hypothesis of prostate cancer and its therapeutic implications. *Prostate* 1986;9(4):343–361.

110. Coltman CA Jr, Thompson IM Jr, Feigl P. Prostate Cancer Prevention Trial (PCPT) update. *Eur Urol* 1999;35(5–6):544–547.

111. Hammond GL, et al. Serum steroids in normal males and patients with prostatic diseases. *Clin Endocrinol (Oxf)* 1978;9(2):113–121.

112. Mainwaring WIP. Androgen receptors in the future management of carcinoma of the prostate. In: Thompson EB, Lippman ME, eds. *Steroid receptor and the management of cancer.* Boca Raton, FL: CRC Press, 1979.

113. Prins GS, Sklarew RJ, Pertschuk LP. Image analysis of androgen receptor immunostaining in prostate cancer accurately predicts response to hormonal therapy. *J Urol* 1998;159(3):641–649.

114. Geller J, Albert JD. Comparison of various hormonal therapies for prostatic carcinoma. *Semin Oncol* 1983;10(4 Suppl 4):34–41.

115. Chrisp P, Goa KL. Goserelin. A review of its pharmacodynamic and pharmacokinetic properties, and clinical use in sex hormone-related conditions. *Drugs* 1991;41(2):254–288.

116. Jackson IM, Matthews MJ, Diver JM. LHRH analogues in the treatment of cancer. *Cancer Treat Rev* 1989;16(3):161–175.

117. Glode LM. The biology of gonadotropin-releasing hormone and its analogs. *Urology* 1986;27(1 Suppl):16–20.

118. Garcia A, Schiff M, Marshall JC. Regulation of pituitary gonadotropin-releasing hormone receptors by pulsatile gonadotropin-releasing hormone injections in male rats. Modulation by testosterone. *J Clin Invest* 1984;74(3):920–928.

119. Handelsman DJ, Swerdloff RS. Pharmacokinetics of gonadotropin-releasing hormone and its analogs. *Endocr Rev* 1986;7(1):95–105.

120. Veldhuis JD, Urban RJ, Dufau ML. Evidence that androgen negative feedback regulates hypothalamic gonadotropin-releasing hormone impulse strength and the burst-like secretion of biologically active luteinizing hormone in men. *J Clin Endocrinol Metab* 1992;74(6):1227–1235.

121. Urban JH, Das I, Levine JE. Steroid modulation of neuropeptide Y-induced luteinizing hormone releasing hormone release from median eminence fragments from male rats. *Neuroendocrinology* 1996;63(2):112–119.

122. Dutta AS, Furr BJA. Luteinizing hormone releasing hormone (LHRH) analogues. *Ann Rep Med Chem* 1985;20: 203–214.

123. Sandow J, von Rechenberg W, Engelbart K. Pharmacological studies on androgen suppression in therapy of prostate carcinoma. *Am J Clin Oncol* 1988;11(Suppl 1):S6–S10.

124. Foekens JA, et al. Combined effects of buserelin, estradiol and tamoxifen on the growth of MCF-7 human breast cancer cells in vitro. *Biochem Biophys Res Commun* 1986; 140(2):550–556.

125. Miller WR, et al. Growth of human breast cancer cells inhibited by a luteinizing hormone- releasing hormone agonist. *Nature* 1985;313(5999):231–233.

126. Eidne KA, Flanagan CA, Millar RP. Gonadotropin-releasing hormone binding sites in human breast carcinoma. *Science* 1985;229(4717):989–991.

127. Wilding G, Chen M, Gelmann EP. LHRH agonists and human breast cancer cells [letter]. *Nature* 1987;329 (6142):770.

128. Montagnani Marelli M, et al. Effects of LHRH agonists on the growth of human prostatic tumor cells: "in vitro" and "in vivo" studies. *Arch Ital Urol Androl* 1997;69(4):257–263.

129. Moretti RM, et al. Luteinizing hormone-releasing hormone agonists interfere with the stimulatory actions of epidermal growth factor in human prostatic cancer cell lines, LNCaP and DU 145. *J Clin Endocrinol Metab* 1996;81(11):3930–3937.

130. Nicholson RI, et al. Endocrinological and clinical aspects of LHRH action (ICI 118630) in hormone dependent breast cancer. *J Steroid Biochem* 1985;23(5B):843–847.

131. Faure N, et al. Inhibition of serum androgen levels by chronic intranasal and subcutaneous administration of a potent luteinizing hormone-releasing hormone (LH-RH) agonist in adult men. *Fertil Steril* 1982;37(3):416–424.

132. Linde R, et al. Reversible inhibition of testicular steroidogenesis and spermatogenesis by a potent gonadotropin-releasing hormone agonist in normal men: an approach toward the development of a male contraceptive. *N Engl J Med* 1981;305(12):663–667.

133. Klijn JG, et al. LHRH-agonist treatment in clinical and experimental human breast cancer. *J Steroid Biochem* 1985;23(5B):867–873.

134. Thomas EJ, et al. Endocrine effects of goserelin, a new depot luteinising hormone releasing hormone agonist. *Br Med J (Clin Res Ed)* 1986;293(6559):1407–1408.

135. Furr BJ, Nicholson RI. Use of analogues of luteinizing hormone-releasing hormone for the treatment of cancer. *J Reprod Fertil* 1982;64(2):529–539.

136. Beacock CJ, et al. The treatment of metastatic prostatic cancer with the slow release LH-RH analogue Zoladex ICI 118630. *Br J Urol* 1987;59(5):436–442.

137. Robinson MR, et al. An LH-RH analogue (Zoladex) in the management of carcinoma of the prostate: a preliminary report comparing daily subcutaneous injections with monthly depot injections. *Eur J Surg Oncol* 1985;11(2): 159–165.

138. Leuprolide versus diethylstilbestrol for metastatic prostate cancer. The Leuprolide Study Group. *N Engl J Med* 1984;311(20):1281–1286.

139. Blank KR, et al. Neoadjuvant androgen deprivation prior to transperineal prostate brachytherapy: smaller volumes, less morbidity. *Cancer J Sci Am* 1999;5(6):370–373.

140. Mathe G, et al. Phase II trial with D-Trp-6-LH-RH in prostatic carcinoma: comparison with other hormonal agents. *Prostate* 1986;9(4):327–342.

141. Peters CA, Walsh PC. The effect of nafarelin acetate, a luteinizing-hormone-releasing hormone agonist, on benign prostatic hyperplasia [published erratum appears in N Engl J Med 1988 Mar 3;318(9):580]. *N Engl J Med* 1987;317 (10):599–604.

142. Smith JA Jr, Urry RL. Testicular histology after prolonged treatment with a gonadotropin-releasing hormone analogue. *J Urol* 1985;133(4):612–614.

143. Kahan A, et al. Disease flare induced by D-Trp6-LHRH analogue in patients with metastatic prostatic cancer [letter]. *Lancet* 1984;1(8383):971–972.

144. Neumann F, Graf K. Discovery, development, mode of action and clinical use of cyproterone acetate. *J Int Med Res* 1975;3:1–9.

145. Bratoeff E, et al. Steroidal antiandrogens and 5alpha-reductase inhibitors. *Curr Med Chem* 1999;6(12):1107–1123.

146. Seigneur J, et al. Pulmonary complications of hormone treatment in prostate carcinoma. *Chest* 1988;93(5):1106.

147. Gomez JL, et al. Simultaneous liver and lung toxicity related to the nonsteroidal antiandrogen nilutamide (Anandron): a case report. *Am J Med* 1992;92(5):563–566.

148. Migliari R, et al. Short term effects of flutamide administration on hypothalamic-pituitary-testicular axis in man. *J Urol* 1988;139(3):637–639.

149. Brochu M, et al. Effects of flutamide and aminoglutethimide on plasma 5 alpha-reduced steroid glucuronide concentrations in castrated patients with cancer of the prostate. *J Steroid Biochem* 1987;28(6):619–622.

150. Belanger A, et al. Plasma levels of hydroxy-flutamide in patients with prostatic cancer receiving the combined hormonal therapy: an LHRH agonist and flutamide. *Prostate* 1988;12(1):79–84.

151. Katchen B, Buxbaum S. Disposition of a new, nonsteroid, antiandrogen, alpha,alpha,alpha-trifluoro-2-methyl-4'-nitro-m-propionotoluidide (Flutamide), in men following a single oral 200 mg dose. *J Clin Endocrinol Metab* 1975;41(2):373–379.

152. Neri R, Kassem N. Biological and clinical properties of antiandrogens. In: Breciani F, ed. *Progress in cancer research and therapy.* New York: Raven Press, 1984:507.

153. Stoliar B, Albert DJ. SCH 13521 in the treatment of advanced carcinoma of the prostate. *J Urol* 1974;111(6): 803–807.

154. Simard J, Singh SM, Labrie F. Comparison of in vitro effects of the pure antiandrogens OH-flutamide, Casodex, and nilutamide on androgen-sensitive parameters [see comments]. *Urology* 1997;49(4):580–586; discussion 586–589.

155. Kolvenbag GJ, Nash A. Bicalutamide dosages used in the treatment of prostate cancer. *Prostate* 1999;39(1):47–53.

156. Eri LM, Haug E, Tveter KJ. Effects on the endocrine system of long-term treatment with the non-steroidal anti-androgen Casodex in patients with benign prostatic hyperplasia. *Br J Urol* 1995;75(3):335–340.

157. Cockshott ID, et al. The effect of food on the pharmacokinetics of the bicalutamide ("Casodex") enantiomers. *Biopharm Drug Dispos* 1997;18(6):499–507.

158. Cockshott ID, et al. The pharmacokinetics of Casodex in prostate cancer patients after single and during multiple dosing. *Eur Urol* 1990;18(Suppl 3):10–17.

159. McKillop D, et al. Metabolism and enantioselective pharmacokinetics of Casodex in man. *Xenobiotica* 1993;23(11):1241–1253.

160. Tyrrell CJ, et al. A randomised comparison of 'Casodex' (bicalutamide) 150 mg monotherapy versus castration in the treatment of metastatic and locally advanced prostate cancer. *Eur Urol* 1998;33(5):447–456.

161. Goa KL, Spencer CM. Bicalutamide in advanced prostate cancer. A review [published erratum appears in Drugs Aging 1998;Jul;13(1):41]. *Drugs Aging* 1998;12(5):401–422.

162. Sarosdy MF, et al. Comparison of goserelin and leuprolide in combined androgen blockade therapy. *Urology* 1998;52(1):82–88.

163. Wong PW, et al. Eosinophilic lung disease induced by bicalutamide: a case report and review of the medical literature. *Chest* 1998;113(2):548–550.

164. McCaffrey JA, Scher HI. Interstitial pneumonitis following bicalutamide treatment for prostate cancer. *J Urol* 1998;160(1):131.

165. Taplin ME, et al. Selection for androgen receptor mutations in prostate cancers treated with androgen antagonist. *Cancer Res* 1999;59(11):2511–2515.

166. Joyce R, et al. High dose bicalutamide for androgen independent prostate cancer: effect of prior hormonal therapy. *J Urol* 1998;159(1):149–153.

167. Culig Z, et al. Switch from antagonist to agonist of the androgen receptor bicalutamide is associated with prostate tumour progression in a new model system. *Br J Cancer* 1999;81(2):242–251.

168. Rassmussen GH. Chemical control of androgen action. *Ann Rep Med Chem* 1986;21:179–188.

169. Trachtenberg J. Ketoconazole therapy in advanced prostatic cancer. *J Urol* 1984;132(1):61–63.

170. De Coster R, et al. Effects of high dose ketoconazole therapy on the main plasma testicular and adrenal steroids in previously untreated prostatic cancer patients. *Clin Endocrinol (Oxf)* 1986;24(6):657–664.

171. De Coster R, et al. Effects of high-dose ketoconazole and dexamethasone on ACTH-stimulated adrenal steroidogenesis in orchiectomized prostatic cancer patients. *Acta Endocrinol (Copenh)* 1987;115(2):265–271.

172. Reese DM, Small EJ. Secondary hormonal manipulations in hormone refractory prostate cancer. *Urol Clin North Am* 1999;26(2):311–321.

173. Bok RA, Small EJ. The treatment of advanced prostate cancer with ketoconazole: safety issues. *Drug Saf* 1999;20(5):451–458.

174. Wachall BG, et al. Imidazole substituted biphenyls: a new class of highly potent and in vivo active inhibitors of P450 17 as potential therapeutics for treatment of prostate cancer. *Bioorg Med Chem* 1999;7(9):1913–1924.

175. Grigoryev DN, et al. Effects of new 17alpha-hydroxylase/C(17,20)-lyase inhibitors on LNCaP prostate cancer cell growth in vitro and in vivo. *Br J Cancer* 1999;81(4):622–630.

176. Homma Y, et al. Inhibition of rat prostate carcinogenesis by a 5alpha-reductase inhibitor, FK143. *J Natl Cancer Inst* 1997;89(11):803–807.

177. Zaccheo T, Giudici D, di Salle E. Effect of the dual 5alpha-reductase inhibitor PNU 157706 on the growth of dunning R3327 prostatic carcinoma in the rat. *J Steroid Biochem Mol Biol* 1998;64(3–4):193–198.

178. Rittmaster RS, et al. Effect of MK-906, a specific 5 alpha-reductase inhibitor, on serum androgens and androgen conjugates in normal men. *J Androl* 1989;10(4):259–262.

179. Liang T, et al. Species differences in prostatic steroid 5 alpha-reductases of rat, dog, and human. *Endocrinology* 1985;117(2):571–579.

180. Vermeulen A, et al. Hormonal effects of an orally active 4-azasteroid inhibitor of 5 alpha-reductase in humans. *Prostate* 1989;14(1):45–53.

181. Finasteride formulary information monograph. Raritan, NJ: Merck & Co, 1992.

182. Gregoire S, Winchell GA, Costanzer M. Multiple dose pharmacokinetics of finasteride, a 5 alpha-reductase inhibitor, in men 45 to 60 and greater than or equal to 70 years old. *Pharmacol Res* 1990;7:553.

183. Carlin JR, et al. Disposition and pharmacokinetics of [14C]finasteride after oral administration in humans. *Drug Metab Dispos* 1992;20(2):148–155.

184. Beisland HO, et al. Scandinavian clinical study of finasteride in the treatment of benign prostatic hyperplasia. *Eur Urol* 1992;22(4):271–277.

185. Kirby RS, et al. Long-term urodynamic effects of finasteride in benign prostatic hyperplasia: a pilot study. *Eur Urol* 1993;24(1):20–26.

186. Presti JC Jr, et al. Multicenter, randomized, double-blind, placebo controlled study to investigate the effect of finasteride (MK-906) on stage D prostate cancer. *J Urol* 1992;148(4):1201–1204.

187. Levy MA, et al. Epristeride is a selective and specific uncompetitive inhibitor of human steroid 5 alpha-reductase isoform 2. *J Steroid Biochem Mol Biol* 1994;48(2–3):197–206.

188. Di Salle E, et al. Hormonal effects of turosteride, a 5 alpha-reductase inhibitor, in the rat. *J Steroid Biochem Mol Biol* 1993;46(5):549–555.

189. Hirsch KS, et al. LY191704: a selective nonsteroidal inhibitor of human steroid 5 alpha-reductase type 1. *Proc Natl Acad Sci U S A* 1993;90(11):5277–5281.

190. Knauer E. Die ovarien-transplantation. *Arch Gynaekol* 1900;60:322.

191. Frank RT, Frank ML, Gustavosn RG. Demonstration of the female sex hormone in the circulating blood: I. Preliminary report. *JAMA* 1925;85:510.

192. Loewe S, Lange F. Der gehalt des frauenharns an brur sterzengenden stoffen in abhangigkeit von ovariellen zylkus. *Klin Wochenschr* 1926;5:1038–1039.

193. Zondek B. Darstellung des weiblichen sexualhormon aus dem harn. *Klin Wochenschr* 1928;7(485).

194. Butenandt A. Uber "progynon" ein crystallisiertes, weibliches sexualhormon. *Naturwissenschaften* 1929;7(879).

195. Bagget B, Engel LL, Savard K. The conversion of testosterone 3-C14 to C14-estradiol-17β by human ovarian tissue. *J Biol Chem* 1956;221:931–941.

196. Brodie A, Njar V. Aromatase inhibitors and breast cancer. *Semin Oncol* 1996;23(4 Suppl 9):10–20.

197. Chen SA, et al. Human aromatase: cDNA cloning, Southern blot analysis, and assignment of the gene to chromosome 15. *DNA* 1988;7(1):27–38.

198. Fitzpatrick SL, et al. Expression of aromatase in the ovary: down-regulation of mRNA by the ovulatory luteinizing hormone surge. *Steroids* 1997;62(1):197–206.

199. Michael MD, Michael LF, Simpson ER. A CRE-like sequence that binds CREB and contributes to cAMP-dependent regulation of the proximal promoter of the human aromatase P450 (CYP19) gene. *Mol Cell Endocrinol* 1997;134(2):147–156.

200. Ryan KJ, Engel LL. The interconversion of estrone and estradiol by human tissue slices. *Endocrinology* 1953;52:287–291.

201. Pundel JP. Die androgen abstrichbilder. *Arch Gynaekol* 1957;188:577.

202. Vigersky RA, et al. Relative binding of testosterone and estradiol to testosterone-estradiol-binding globulin. *J Clin Endocrinol Metab* 1979;49(6):899–904.

203. Dunn JF, Nisula BC, Rodbard D. Transport of steroid hormones: binding of 21 endogenous steroids to both testosterone-binding globulin and corticosteroid-binding globulin in human plasma. *J Clin Endocrinol Metab* 1981;53(1):58–68.

204. Speroff L, Vande Wiele RL. Regulation of the human menstrual cycle. *Am J Obstet Gynecol* 1971;109(2):234–247.

205. Murad F, Kuret JA. Estrogens and progestins. In: Goodman Gilman A, et al., eds. *The pharmacological basis of therapeutics*, 8th ed. New York: Pergamon Press, 1990:1384.

206. Deghenghi R, Givner ML. The female sex hormones and analogs. In: Wolff ME, ed. *Burger's medicinal chemistry, vol. II*. New York: Wiley-Liss, 1979:917.

207. Kutsky RJ. Estradiol. In: *Handbook of vitamins, minerals, and hormones*. New York: Van Nostrand Reinhold, 1981:415.

208. Lippman M, Bolan G, Huff K. The effects of estrogens and antiestrogens on hormone-responsive human breast cancer in long-term tissue culture. *Cancer Res* 1976;36(12):4595–4601.

209. Page MJ, et al. Serum regulation of the estrogen responsiveness of the human breast cancer cell line MCF-7. *Cancer Res* 1983;43(3):1244–1250.

210. Darbre P, et al. Effect of estradiol on human breast cancer cells in culture. *Cancer Res* 1983;43(1):349–354.

211. Soule HD, McGrath CM. Estrogen responsive proliferation of clonal human breast carcinoma cells in athymic mice. *Cancer Lett* 1980;10(2):177–189.

212. Reddel RR, Sutherland RL. Effects of pharmacological concentrations of estrogens on proliferation and cell cycle kinetics of human breast cancer cell lines in vitro. *Cancer Res* 1987;47(20):5323–5329.

213. Brunner N, Spang-Thomsen M, Cullen K. The T61 human breast cancer xenograft: an experimental model of estrogen therapy of breast cancer. *Breast Cancer Res Treat* 1996;39(1):87–92.

214. Tsutsui T, et al. Aneuploidy induction and cell transformation by diethylstilbestrol: a possible chromosomal mechanism in carcinogenesis. *Cancer Res* 1983;43(8):3814–3821.

215. Bishop MC, Selby C, Taylor M. Plasma hormone levels in patients with prostatic carcinoma treated with diethylstilboestrol and estramustine. *Br J Urol* 1985;57(5):542–547.

216. Stege R, et al. Steroid-sensitive proteins, growth hormone and somatomedin C in prostatic cancer: effects of parenteral and oral estrogen therapy. *Prostate* 1987;10(4):333–338.

217. Jones TM, et al. Direct inhibition of Leydig cell function by estradiol. *J Clin Endocrinol Metab* 1978;47(6):1368–1373.

218. Franchimont P, Legros JJ, Meurice J. Effect of several estrogens on serum gonadotropin levels in postmenopausal women. *Horm Metab Res* 1972;4(4):288–292.

219. Tomic R. Pituitary function after orchiectomy in patients with or without earlier estrogen treatment for prostatic carcinoma. *J Endocrinol Invest* 1987;10(5):479–482.

220. Mashchak CA, et al. Comparison of pharmacodynamic properties of various estrogen formulations. *Am J Obstet Gynecol* 1982;144(5):511–518.

221. Rigg LA, Hermann H, Yen SS. Absorption of estrogens from vaginal creams. *N Engl J Med* 1978;298(4):195–197.

222. Abramson FP, Miller HC Jr. Bioavailability, distribution and pharmacokinetics of diethylstilbestrol produced from stilphostrol. *J Urol* 1982;128(6):1336–1339.

223. Liehr JG, et al. Diethylstilbestrol (DES) quinone: a reactive intermediate in DES metabolism. *Biochem Pharmacol* 1983;32(24):3711–3718.

224. Herbst AL, Ulfelder H, Poskanzer DC. Adenocarcinoma of the vagina. Association of maternal stilbestrol therapy with tumor appearance in young women. *N Engl J Med* 1971;284(15):878–881.

225. Denis L. Prostate cancer. Primary hormonal treatment. *Cancer* 1993;71(3 Suppl):1050–1058.

226. Lundgren R, et al. Cardiovascular complications of estrogen therapy for nondisseminated prostatic carcinoma. A preliminary report from a randomized multicenter study. *Scand J Urol Nephrol* 1986;20(2):101–105.

227. Henriksson P, Johansson SE. Prediction of cardiovascular complications in patients with prostatic cancer treated with estrogen. *Am J Epidemiol* 1987;125(6):970–978.

228. Henriksson P, et al. Activators and inhibitors of coagulation and fibrinolysis in patients with prostatic cancer treated with oestrogen or orchidectomy. *Thromb Res* 1986;44(6):783–791.

229. Agardh CD, et al. The influence of treatment with estrogens and estramustine phosphate on platelet aggregation and plasma lipoproteins in non-disseminated prostatic carcinoma. *J Urol* 1984;132(5):1021–1024.

230. Carter AC, et al. Diethylstilbestrol: recommended dosages for different categories of breast cancer patients. Report of the Cooperative Breast Cancer Group. *JAMA* 1977;237(19):2079–2080.

231. Kennedy BJ. Massive estrogen administration in premeno-

pausal women with metastatic breast cancer. *Cancer* 1962;15:641.

232. Surgically confirmed gallbladder disease, venous thromboembolism, and breast tumors in relation to postmenopausal estrogen therapy. A report from the Boston Collaborative Drug Surveillance Program, Boston University Medical Center. *N Engl J Med* 1974;290(1):15–19.

233. Ameriks JA, et al. Hepatic cell adenomas, spontaneous liver rupture, and oral contraceptives. *Arch Surg* 1975;110(5): 548–557.

234. Ziel HK, Finkle WD. Increased risk of endometrial carcinoma among users of conjugated estrogens. *N Engl J Med* 1975;293(23):1167–1170.

235. Bibbo M, et al. Follow-up study of male and female offspring of DES-exposed mothers. *Obstet Gynecol* 1977; 49(1):1–8.

236. Melnick S, et al. Rates and risks of diethylstilbestrol-related clear-cell adenocarcinoma of the vagina and cervix. An update. *N Engl J Med* 1987;316(9):514–516.

237. Osborne CK. Tamoxifen in the treatment of breast cancer. *N Engl J Med* 1998;339(22):1609–1618.

238. Westerberg H, et al. Anti-oestrogen therapy of advanced mammary carcinoma. *Acta Radiol Ther Phys Biol* 1976; 15(6):513–518.

239. Morgan LR Jr, et al. Therapeutic use of tamoxifen in advanced breast cancer: correlation with biochemical parameters. *Cancer Treat Rep* 1976;60(10):1437–1443.

240. Manni A, et al. Antihormone treatment of stage IV breast cancer. *Cancer* 1979;43(2):444–450.

241. Rose C, Mouridsen HT. Treatment of advanced breast cancer with tamoxifen. *Recent Results Cancer Res* 1984;91:230–242.

242. Ingle JN, et al. Randomized trial of bilateral oophorectomy versus tamoxifen in premenopausal women with metastatic breast cancer. *J Clin Oncol* 1986;4(2):178–185.

243. Muss HB, et al. Tamoxifen versus high-dose oral medroxyprogesterone acetate as initial endocrine therapy for patients with metastatic breast cancer: a Piedmont Oncology Association study. *J Clin Oncol* 1994;12(8):1630–1638.

244. Sawka CA, et al. A randomized crossover trial of tamoxifen versus ovarian ablation for metastatic breast cancer in premenopausal women: a report of the National Cancer Institute of Canada Clinical Trials Group (NCIC CTG) trial MA.1. *Breast Cancer Res Treat* 1997;44(3):211–215.

245. Jordan VC, Assikis VJ. Endometrial carcinoma and tamoxifen: clearing up a controversy. *Clin Cancer Res* 1995;1(5): 467–472.

246. Gorodeski GI, et al. Tamoxifen increases plasma estrogen-binding equivalents and has an estradiol agonistic effect on histologically normal premenopausal and postmenopausal endometrium. *Fertil Steril* 1992;57(2):320–327.

247. Uziely B, et al. The effect of tamoxifen on the endometrium. *Breast Cancer Res Treat* 1993;26(1):101–105.

248. Enck RE, Rios CN. Tamoxifen treatment of metastatic breast cancer and antithrombin III levels. *Cancer* 1984; 53(12):2607–2609.

249. Love RR, Surawicz TS, Williams EC. Antithrombin III level, fibrinogen level, and platelet count changes with adjuvant tamoxifen therapy. *Arch Intern Med* 1992;52(2): 317–320.

250. Turken S, et al. Effects of tamoxifen on spinal bone density in women with breast cancer. *J Natl Cancer Inst* 1989;81 (14):1086–1088.

251. Fornander T, et al. Long-term adjuvant tamoxifen in early breast cancer: effect on bone mineral density in postmenopausal women. *J Clin Oncol* 1990;8(6):1019–1024.

252. Love RR, et al. Effects of tamoxifen on bone mineral density in postmenopausal women with breast cancer. *N Engl J Med* 1992;326(13):852–856.

253. Schapira DV, Kumar NB, Lyman GH. Serum cholesterol reduction with tamoxifen. *Breast Cancer Res Treat* 1990;17(1):3–7.

254. Love RR, et al. Effects of tamoxifen therapy on lipid and lipoprotein levels in postmenopausal patients with node-negative breast cancer. *J Natl Cancer Inst* 1990;82(16): 1327–1332.

255. Shiau AK, et al. The structural basis of estrogen receptor/coactivator recognition and the antagonism of this interaction by tamoxifen. *Cell* 1998;95(7):927–937.

256. Shibata H, et al. Role of co-activators and co-repressors in the mechanism of steroid/thyroid receptor action. *Recent Prog Horm Res* 1997;52:141–164.

257. McInerney EM, Katzenellenbogen BS. Different regions in activation function-1 of the human estrogen receptor required for antiestrogen- and estradiol-dependent transcription activation. *J Biol Chem* 1996;271(39):24172–24178.

258. Lavinsky RM, et al. Diverse signaling pathways modulate nuclear receptor recruitment of N-CoR and SMRT complexes. *Proc Natl Acad Sci U S A* 1998;95(6):2920–2925.

259. Harris AL, et al. Epidermal growth factor receptor and other oncogenes as prognostic markers. *J Natl Cancer Inst Monogr* 1992;11:181–187.

260. Nicholson S, et al. Epidermal growth factor receptor (EGFr); results of a 6 year follow-up study in operable breast cancer with emphasis on the node negative subgroup. *Br J Cancer* 1991;63(1):146–150.

261. Zeillinger R, et al. HER-2 amplification, steroid receptors and epidermal growth factor receptor in primary breast cancer. *Oncogene* 1989;4(1):109–114.

262. Tetu B, Brisson J. Prognostic significance of HER-2/neu oncoprotein expression in node-positive breast cancer. The influence of the pattern of immunostaining and adjuvant therapy. *Cancer* 1994;73(9):2359–2365.

263. Lee AV, et al. Enhancement of insulin-like growth factor signaling in human breast cancer: estrogen regulation of insulin receptor substrate-1 expression in vitro and in vivo. *Mol Endocrinol* 1999;13(5):787–796.

264. Ellis MJ, et al. Insulin-like growth factors and breast cancer prognosis. *Breast Cancer Res Treatment* 1998;52:175–184.

265. McLeskey SW, et al. Tamoxifen-resistant fibroblast growth factor-transfected MCF-7 cells are cross-resistant in vivo to the antiestrogen ICI 182,780 and two aromatase inhibitors. *Clin Cancer Res* 1998;4(3):697–711.

266. Katzenellenbogen BC, et al. Antiestrogens: mechanisms of action and resistance in breast cancer. *Breast Cancer Res Treatment* 1997;44:23–38.

267. Porter W, et al. Role of estrogen receptor/Sp1 complexes in estrogen-induced heat shock protein 27 gene expression. *Mol Endocrinol* 1996;10(11):1371–1378.

268. Porter W, et al. Functional synergy between the transcription factor Sp1 and the estrogen receptor. *Mol Endocrinol* 1997;11(11):1569–1580.

269. Barsalou A, et al. Estrogen response elements can mediate agonist activity of anti-estrogens in human endometrial Ishikawa cells. *J Biol Chem* 1998;273(27):17138–17146.

270. Paech K, et al. Differential ligand activation of estrogen receptors ERalpha and ERbeta at AP1 sites. *Science* 1997;277(5331):1508–1510.

271. Yang NN, et al. Identification of an estrogen response element activated by metabolites of 17beta-estradiol and raloxifene. *Science* 1996;273(5279):1222–1225.

272. Yang NN, et al. Correction: raloxifene response needs more than an element [letter]. *Science* 1997;275(5304):1249.

273. Kuiper GG, et al. Cloning of a novel receptor expressed in rat prostate and ovary. *Proc Natl Acad Sci U S A* 1996;93(12):5925–5930.

274. Mosselman S, Polman J, Dijkema R. ER beta: identification and characterization of a novel human estrogen receptor. *FEBS Lett* 1996;392(1):49–53.

275. Krege JH, et al. Generation and reproductive phenotypes of mice lacking estrogen receptor beta. *Proc Natl Acad Sci U S A* 1998;95(26):15677–15682.

276. Dotzlaw H, et al. Expression of estrogen receptor-beta in human breast tumors. *J Clin Endocrinol Metab* 1997;82(7):2371–2374.

277. Pace P, et al. Human estrogen receptor beta binds DNA in a manner similar to and dimerizes with estrogen receptor alpha. *J Biol Chem* 1997;272(41):25832–25838.

278. Kuiper GG, et al. Comparison of the ligand binding specificity and transcript tissue distribution of estrogen receptors alpha and beta. *Endocrinology* 1997;138(3):863–870.

279. Barkhem T, et al. Differential response of estrogen receptor alpha and estrogen receptor beta to partial estrogen agonists/antagonists. *Mol Pharmacol* 1998;54(1):105–112.

280. McInerney EM, et al. Transcription activation by the human estrogen receptor subtype beta (ER beta) studied with ER beta and ER alpha receptor chimeras. *Endocrinology* 1998;139(11):4513–4522.

281. Speirs V, et al. Coexpression of estrogen receptor alpha and beta: poor prognostic factors in human breast cancer? *Cancer Res* 1999;59:525–528.

282. Dotzlaw H, et al. Estrogen receptor beta messenger RNA expression in human breast tumor biopsies: relationship to steroid receptor status and regulation by progestins. *Cancer Res* 1999;59:529–532.

283. Fromson JM, Pearson S, Bramah S. The metabolism of tamoxifen (I.C.I. 46,474) in laboratory animals. *Xenobiotica* 1973;3(11):693–709.

284. Lyman SD, Jordan VC. Metabolism of nonsteroidal antiestrogens. In: Jordan VC, ed. *Estrogen/antiestrogen action and breast cancer therapy*. Madison, WI: University of Wisconsin Press, 1986:191.

285. Bain RR, Jordan VC. Identification of a new metabolite of tamoxifen in patient serum during breast cancer therapy. *Biochem Pharmacol* 1983;32(2):373–375.

286. Lonning PE, et al. Clinical pharmacokinetics of endocrine agents used in advanced breast cancer. *Clin Pharmacokinet* 1992;22(5):327–358.

287. Adam HK, Douglas EJ, Kemp JV. The metabolism of tamoxifen in human. *Biochem Pharmacol* 1979;28(1):145–147.

288. Fromson JM, Pearson S, Bramah S. The metabolism of tamoxifen (I.C.I. 46,474). II. In female patients. *Xenobiotica* 1973;3(11):711–714.

289. Sutherland CM, et al. Effect of impaired renal function on tamoxifen. *J Surg Oncol* 1984;27(4):222–223.

290. Langan-Fahey SM, Tormey DC, Jordan VC. Tamoxifen metabolites in patients on long-term adjuvant therapy for breast cancer. *Eur J Cancer* 1990;26(8):883–888.

291. Kemp JV, et al. Identification and biological activity of tamoxifen metabolites in human serum. *Biochem Pharmacol* 1983;32(13):2045–2052.

292. Bates DJ, et al. Metabolism of tamoxifen by isolated rat hepatocytes: anti-estrogenic activity of tamoxifen N-oxide. *Biochem Pharmacol* 1982;31(17):2823–2827.

293. Fabian C, Tilzer L, Sternson L. Comparative binding affinities of tamoxifen, 4-hydroxytamoxifen, and desmethyltamoxifen for estrogen receptors isolated from human breast carcinoma: correlation with blood levels in patients with metastatic breast cancer. *Biopharm Drug Dispos* 1981;2(4):381–390.

294. Fabian C, et al. Clinical pharmacology of tamoxifen in patients with breast cancer: correlation with clinical data. *Cancer* 1981;48(4):876–882.

295. Nicholson RI, et al. The binding of tamoxifen to oestrogen receptor proteins under equilibrium and non-equilibrium conditions. *Eur J Cancer* 1979;15(3):317–329.

296. Wakeling AE, Slater SR. Estrogen-receptor binding and biologic activity of tamoxifen and its metabolites. *Cancer Treat Rep* 1980;64(6–7):741–744.

297. Daniel CP, et al. Determination of tamoxifen and an hydroxylated metabolite in plasma from patients with advanced breast cancer using gas chromatography-mass spectrometry. *J Endocrinol* 1979;83(3):401–408.

298. Daniel P, et al. Determination of tamoxifen and biologically active metabolites in human breast tumours and plasma. *Eur J Cancer Clin Oncol* 1981;17(11):1183–1189.

299. Wilkinson PM, et al. Tamoxifen (Nolvadex) therapy—rationale for loading dose followed by maintenance dose for patients with metastatic breast cancer. *Cancer Chemother Pharmacol* 1982;10(1):33–35.

300. Fabian C, Sternson L, Barnett M. Clinical pharmacology of tamoxifen in patients with breast cancer: comparison of traditional and loading dose schedules. *Cancer Treat Rep* 1980;64(6–7):765–773.

301. Adam HK, Patterson JS, Kemp JV. Studies on the metabolism and pharmacokinetics of tamoxifen in normal volunteers. *Cancer Treat Rep* 1980;64(6–7):761–764.

302. Ribeiro GG, Wilkinson PM. A clinical assessment of loading dose tamoxifen for advanced breast carcinoma. *Clin Oncol* 1984;10(4):363–367.

303. Buzdar AU, et al. Bioequivalence of 20-mg once-daily tamoxifen relative to 10-mg twice-daily tamoxifen regimens for breast cancer [published erratum appears in J Clin Oncol 1994 Jun;12(6):1337] [see comments]. *J Clin Oncol* 1994;12(1):50–54.

304. Noguchi S, et al. Inability of tamoxifen to penetrate into cerebrospinal fluid [letter]. *Breast Cancer Res Treat* 1988;12(3):317–318.

305. Jacolot F, et al. Identification of the cytochrome P450 IIIA family as the enzymes involved in the N-demethylation of tamoxifen in human liver microsomes. *Biochem Pharmacol* 1991;41(12):1911–1919.

306. Mani C, et al. Metabolism of the antimammary cancer antiestrogenic agent tamoxifen. I. Cytochrome P-450-catalyzed N-demethylation and 4-hydroxylation [published erratum appears in Drug Metab Dispos Biol Fate Chem 1993;21(6):1174]. *Drug Metab Dispos* 1993;21(4):645–656.

307. Crewe HK, et al. The effect of selective serotonin re-uptake inhibitors on cytochrome P4502D6 (CYP2D6) activity in human liver microsomes. *Br J Clin Pharmacol* 1992;34(3): 262–265.

308. Dowsett M, et al. Impact of tamoxifen on the pharmacokinetics and endocrine effects of the aromatase inhibitor letrozole in postmenopausal women with breast cancer. *Clin Cancer Res* 1999;5(9):2338–2343.

309. Reid AD, et al. Tamoxifen metabolism is altered by simultaneous administration of medroxyprogesterone acetate in breast cancer patients. *Breast Cancer Res Treat* 1992;22(2): 153–156.

310. Tenni P, Lalich DL, Byrne MJ. Life threatening interaction between tamoxifen and warfarin. *BMJ* 1989;298(6666):93.

311. Osborne CK, et al. Tamoxifen and the isomers of 4-hydroxytamoxifen in tamoxifen-resistant tumors from breast cancer patients. *J Clin Oncol* 1992;10(2):304–310.

312. Wolf DM, et al. Investigation of the mechanism of tamoxifen-stimulated breast tumor growth with nonisomerizable analogues of tamoxifen and metabolites. *J Natl Cancer Inst* 1993;85(10):806–812.

313. Kaiser-Kupfer MI, Lippman ME. Tamoxifen retinopathy. *Cancer Treat Rep* 1978;62(3):315–320.

314. Kaiser-Kupfer MI, Kupfer C, Rodrigues MM. Tamoxifen retinopathy. A clinicopathologic report. *Ophthalmology* 1981;88(1):89–93.

315. McKeown CA, et al. Tamoxifen retinopathy. *Br J Ophthalmol* 1981;65(3):177–179.

316. Pugesgaard T, Von Eyben FE. Bilateral optic neuritis evolved during tamoxifen treatment. *Cancer* 1986;58(2): 383–386.

317. Griffiths MF. Tamoxifen retinopathy at low dosage. *Am J Ophthalmol* 1987;104(2):185–186.

318. Bentley CR, Davies G, Aclimandos WA. Tamoxifen retinopathy: a rare but serious complication. *BMJ* 1992;304 (6825):495–496.

319. Chang T, Gonder JR, Ventresca MR. Low-dose tamoxifen retinopathy. *Can J Ophthalmol* 1992;27(3):148–149.

320. Pemberton KD, Melissari E, Kakkar VV. The influence of tamoxifen in vivo on the main natural anticoagulants and fibrinolysis. *Blood Coagul Fibrinolysis* 1993;4(6):935–942.

321. Fisher B, et al. A randomized clinical trial evaluating tamoxifen in the treatment of patients with node-negative breast cancer who have estrogen-receptor-positive tumors. *N Engl J Med* 1989;320(8):479–484.

322. Bruning PF, et al. Tamoxifen, serum lipoproteins and cardiovascular risk. *Br J Cancer* 1988;58(4):497–499.

323. Ingram D. Tamoxifen use, oestrogen binding and serum lipids in postmenopausal women with breast cancer. *Aust N Z J Surg* 1990;60(9):673–675.

324. Jones AL, et al. Haemostatic changes and thromboembolic risk during tamoxifen therapy in normal women. *Br J Cancer* 1992;66(4):744–747.

325. Gau TC. Letter to physicians. Stuart Pharmaceuticals, 1987.

326. Potter GA, McCague R, Jarman M. A mechanistic hypothesis for DNA adduct formation by tamoxifen following hepatic oxidative metabolism. *Carcinogenesis* 1994;15(3): 439–442.

327. Pathak DN, Bodell WJ. DNA adduct formation by tamoxifen with rat and human liver microsomal activation systems. *Carcinogenesis* 1994;15(3):529–532.

328. Fornander T, et al. Oestrogenic effects of adjuvant tamoxifen in postmenopausal breast cancer. *Eur J Cancer* 1993;4:497–500.

329. Gotfredsen A, Christiansen C, Palshof T. The effect of tamoxifen on bone mineral content in premenopausal women with breast cancer. *Cancer* 1984;53(4):853–857.

330. Planting AS, et al. Tamoxifen therapy in premenopausal women with metastatic breast cancer. *Cancer Treat Rep* 1985;69(4):363–368.

331. Kedar RP, et al. Effects of tamoxifen on uterus and ovaries of postmenopausal women in a randomised breast cancer prevention trial [see comments]. *Lancet* 1994;343(8909): 1318–1321.

332. Fornander T, Hellstrom AC, Moberger B. Descriptive clinicopathologic study of 17 patients with endometrial cancer during or after adjuvant tamoxifen in early breast cancer. *J Natl Cancer Inst* 1993;85(22):1850–1855.

333. Bernstein L, et al. Tamoxifen therapy for breast cancer and endometrial cancer risk. *J Natl Cancer Inst* 1999;91(19): 1654–1662.

334. Robinson SP, Jordan VC. Reversal of the antitumor effects of tamoxifen by progesterone in the 7,12-dimethylbenzanthracene-induced rat mammary carcinoma model. *Cancer Res* 1987;47(20):5386–5390.

335. Sherman BM, et al. Endocrine consequences of continuous antiestrogen therapy with tamoxifen in premenopausal women. *J Clin Invest* 1979;64(2):398–404.

336. Manni A, Pearson OH. Antiestrogen-induced remissions in premenopausal women with stage IV breast cancer: effects on ovarian function. *Cancer Treat Rep* 1980;64(6–7):779–785.

337. Paterson AG, et al. The effect of tamoxifen on plasma growth hormone and prolactin in postmenopausal women with advanced breast cancer. *Eur J Cancer Clin Oncol* 1983;19(7):919–922.

338. Jordan VC, et al. Alteration of endocrine parameters in premenopausal women with breast cancer during long-term adjuvant therapy with tamoxifen as the single agent. *J Natl Cancer Inst* 1991;83(20):1488–1491.

339. Golder MP, et al. Plasma hormones in patients with advanced breast cancer treated with tamoxifen. *Eur J Cancer* 1976;12(9):719–723.

340. Szamel I, et al. Hormonal changes during a prolonged tamoxifen treatment in patients with advanced breast cancer. *Oncology* 1986;43(1):7–11.

341. Levin J, et al. Effect of tamoxifen treatment on estrogen metabolism in postmenopausal women with advanced breast cancer. *Anticancer Res* 1982;2(6):377–380.

342. Ravdin PM, et al. Endocrine status of premenopausal node-positive breast cancer patients following adjuvant chemo-

therapy and long-term tamoxifen. *Cancer Res* 1988;48(4): 1026–1029.

343. Wilking N, et al. Effects of tamoxifen on the serum levels of oestrogens and adrenocortical steroids in postmenopausal breast cancer patients. *Acta Chir Scand* 1982;148 (4):345–349.

344. Sakai F, et al. Increases in steroid binding globulins induced by tamoxifen in patients with carcinoma of the breast. *J Endocrinol* 1978;76(2):219–226.

345. Fex G, Adielsson G, Mattson W. Oestrogen-like effects of tamoxifen on the concentration of proteins in plasma. *Acta Endocrinol (Copenh)* 1981;97(1):109–113.

346. Gordon D, et al. The effect of tamoxifen therapy on thyroid function tests. *Cancer* 1986;58(7):1422–1425.

347. Boccardo F, et al. Estrogen-like action of tamoxifen on vaginal epithelium in breast cancer patients. *Oncology* 1981; 38(5):281–285.

348. Ferrazzi E, et al. Oestrogen-like effect of tamoxifen on vaginal epithelium [letter]. *Br Med J* 1977;1(6072):1351–1352.

349. Luciani L, et al. Hormonal and receptor status in postmenopausal women with endometrial carcinoma before and after treatment with tamoxifen. *Tumori* 1984;70(2): 189–192.

350. Namer M, Lalanne C, Baulieu EE. Increase of progesterone receptor by tamoxifen as a hormonal challenge test in breast cancer. *Cancer Res* 1980;40(5):1750–1752.

351. Lien EA, et al. Influence of tamoxifen, aminoglutethimide and goserelin on human plasma IGF-I levels in breast cancer patients. *J Steroid Biochem Mol Biol* 1992;41(3–8): 541–543.

352. Pollak M, et al. Effect of tamoxifen on serum insulinlike growth factor I levels in stage I breast cancer patients. *J Natl Cancer Inst* 1990;82(21):1693–1697.

353. Dawson-Hughes B, et al. Regulation of growth hormone and somatomedin-C secretion in postmenopausal women: effect of physiological estrogen replacement. *J Clin Endocrinol Metab* 1986;63(2):424–432.

354. Cullins SL, Pridjian G, Sutherland CM. Goldenhar's syndrome associated with tamoxifen given to the mother during gestation [letter]. *JAMA* 1994;271(24):1905–1906.

355. Collinson MP, Hamilton DA, Tyrrell CJ. Two case reports of tamoxifen as a cause of impotence in male subjects with carcinoma of the breast. *Breast* 1998;2:48.

356. Fernando IN, Tobias JS. Priapism in patient on tamoxifen [letter]. *Lancet* 1989;1(8635):436.

357. Anelli TF, et al. Tamoxifen administration is associated with a high rate of treatment-limiting symptoms in male breast cancer patients. *Cancer* 1994;74(1):74–77.

358. Traub AI, Thompson W. The effect of tamoxifen on spermatogenesis in subfertile men. *Andrologia* 1981;13(5): 486–490.

359. Gooren LJ. Androgen levels and sex functions in testosterone-treated hypogonadal men. *Arch Sex Behav* 1987;16(6): 463–473.

360. McIntosh IH, Thynne GS. Tumour stimulation by antioestrogens. *Br J Surg* 1977;64:900.

361. Clarysse A. Hormone induced tumor flare. *Eur J Cancer Clin Oncol* 1985;21:585.

362. Plotkin D, et al. Tamoxifen flare in advanced breast cancer. *JAMA* 1978;240(24):2644–2646.

363. Beex L, et al. Tamoxifen versus ethinyl estradiol in the treatment of postmenopausal women with advanced breast cancer. *Cancer Treat Rep* 1981;65(3–4):179–185.

364. Tormey DC, Simon RM, Lippman ME. Evaluation of tamoxifen dose in advanced breast cancer: a progress report. *Cancer Treat Rep* 1976;60:1451.

365. Ettinger DS, et al. Megestrol acetate v tamoxifen in advanced breast cancer: correlation of hormone receptors and response. *Semin Oncol* 1986;13(4 Suppl 4):9–14.

366. Rossleigh MA, et al. Serial bone scans in the assessment of response to therapy in advanced breast carcinoma. *Clin Nucl Med* 1982;7(9):397–402.

367. Coleman RE, et al. Bone scan flare predicts successful systemic therapy for bone metastases. *J Nucl Med* 1988; 29(8):1354–1359.

368. Vogel CL, et al. Worsening bone scan in the evaluation of antitumor response during hormonal therapy of breast cancer. *J Clin Oncol* 1995;13(5):1123–1128.

369. Dehdashti F, et al. Positron emission tomographic assessment of "metabolic flare" to predict response of metastatic breast cancer to antiestrogen therapy. *Eur J Nucl Med* 1999;26:51–56.

370. Kaufman RJ, Escher GC. Rebound regression in advanced mammary carcinoma. *Surg Gynecol Obstet* 1961;113:635.

371. Howell A, et al. Response after withdrawal of tamoxifen and progestogens in advanced breast cancer. *Ann Oncol* 1992;3(8):611–617.

372. Hayes DF, Henderson IC, Shapiro CL. Treatment of metastatic breast cancer: present and future prospects. *Semin Oncol* 1995;22(Suppl 5):5–21.

373. Fuqua SA, Chamness GC, McGuire WL. Estrogen receptor mutations in breast cancer. *J Cell Biochem* 1993;51(2): 135–139.

374. Roodi N, et al. Estrogen receptor gene analysis in estrogen receptor-positive and receptor-negative primary breast cancer. *J Natl Cancer Inst* 1995;87(6):446–451.

375. Karnik PS, et al. Estrogen receptor mutations in tamoxifen-resistant breast cancer. *Cancer Res* 1994;54(2):349–353.

376. Pfeffer U, et al. Alternative splicing of the estrogen receptor primary transcript normally occurs in estrogen receptor positive tissues and cell lines. *J Steroid Biochem Mol Biol* 1996;56(1–6 Spec No):99–105.

377. Zhang QX, Borg A, Fuqua FA. An exon 5 deletion variant of the estrogen receptor frequently coexpressed with wild-type estrogen receptor in human breast cancer. *Cancer Res* 1993;53(24):5882–5884.

378. Gallacchi P, et al. Increased expression of estrogen-receptor exon-5-deletion variant in relapse tissues of human breast cancer. *Int J Cancer* 1998;79(1):44–48.

379. Rea D, Parker MG. Effects of an exon 5 variant of the estrogen receptor in MCF-7 breast cancer cells. *Cancer Res* 1996;56(7):1556–1563.

380. Pfeffer U, Fecarotta E, Vidali G. Coexpression of multiple estrogen receptor variant messenger RNAs in normal and neoplastic breast tissues and in MCF-7 cells. *Cancer Res* 1995;55(10):2158–2165.

381. Wright C, et al. Relationship between c-erbB-2 protein product expression and response to endocrine therapy in advanced breast cancer. *Br J Cancer* 1992;65(1):118–121.

382. Leitzel K, et al. Elevated serum c-erbB-2 antigen levels and

decreased response to hormone therapy of breast cancer. *J Clin Oncol* 1995;13(5):1129–1135.

383. Yamauchi H, et al. Prediction of response to antiestrogen therapy in advanced breast cancer patients by pretreatment circulating levels of extracellular domain of the HER-2/c-neu protein. *J Clin Oncol* 1997;15(7):2518–2525.

384. Elledge RM, et al. HER-2 expression and response to tamoxifen in estrogen receptor-positive breast cancer: a Southwest Oncology Group Study. *Clin Cancer Res* 1998; 4(1):7–12.

385. Gottardis MM, Jordan VC. Development of tamoxifen-stimulated growth of MCF-7 tumors in athymic mice after long-term antiestrogen administration. *Cancer Res* 1988;48 (18):5183–5187.

386. Anzick SL, et al. AIB1, a steroid receptor coactivator amplified in breast and ovarian cancer. *Science* 1997;277(5328): 965–968.

387. Bautista S, et al. In breast cancer, amplification of the steroid receptor coactivator gene AIB1 is correlated with estrogen and progesterone receptor positivity. *Clin Cancer Res* 1998;4(12):2925–2929.

388. Hayes DF, et al. Randomized comparison of tamoxifen and two separate doses of toremifene in postmenopausal patients with metastatic breast cancer. *J Clin Oncol* 1995;13(10):2556–2566.

389. Vogel CL. Phase II and III clinical trials of toremifene for metastatic breast cancer. *Oncology (Huntingt)* 1998;12(3 Suppl 5):9–13.

390. Kangas L, et al. A new triphenylethylene compound, Fc-1157a. II. Antitumor effects. *Cancer Chemother Pharmacol* 1986;17(2):109–113.

391. Hard GC, et al. Major difference in the hepatocarcinogenicity and DNA adduct forming ability between toremifene and tamoxifen in female Crl:CD(BR) rats. *Cancer Res* 1993;53(19):4534–4541.

392. Kangas L. Review of the pharmacological properties of toremifene. *J Steroid Biochem* 1990;36(3):191–195.

393. Wiebe VJ, et al. Pharmacokinetics of toremifene and its metabolites in patients with advanced breast cancer. *Cancer Chemother Pharmacol* 1990;25(4):247–251.

394. Buzdar AU, Hortobagyi GN. Tamoxifen and toremifene in breast cancer: comparison of safety and efficacy. *J Clin Oncol* 1998;16(1):348–353.

395. Dauvois S, et al. Antiestrogen ICI 164,384 reduces cellular estrogen receptor content by increasing its turnover. *Proc Natl Acad Sci U S A* 1992;89(9):4037–4041.

396. Dauvois S, White R, Parker MG. The antiestrogen ICI 182780 disrupts estrogen receptor nucleocytoplasmic shuttling. *J Cell Sci* 1993;106(Pt 4):1377–1388.

397. DeFriend DJ, et al. Investigation of a new pure antiestrogen (ICI 182780) in women with primary breast cancer. *Cancer Res* 1994;54(2):408–414.

398. Long BJ, et al. The steroidal antiestrogen ICI 182,780 is an inhibitor of cellular aromatase activity. *J Steroid Biochem Mol Biol* 1998;67(4):293–304.

399. Osborne CK, et al. Comparison of the effects of a pure steroidal antiestrogen with those of tamoxifen in a model of human breast cancer. *J Natl Cancer Inst* 1995;87(10): 746–750.

400. Howell A, et al. Response to a specific antioestrogen (ICI 182780) in tamoxifen-resistant breast cancer. *Lancet* 1995; 345(8941):29–30.

401. Howell A, et al. Pharmacokinetics, pharmacological and anti-tumour effects of the specific anti-oestrogen ICI 182780 in women with advanced breast cancer. *Br J Cancer* 1996;74(2):300–308.

402. Ellis PA, et al. Induction of apoptosis by tamoxifen and ICI 182780 in primary breast cancer. *Int J Cancer* 1997;72(4): 608–613.

403. Labrie F, et al. EM-652 (SCH 57068), a third generation SERM acting as pure antiestrogen in the mammary gland and endometrium. *J Steroid Biochem Mol Biol* 1999;69(1–6):51–84.

404. Lufkin EG, et al. Treatment of established postmenopausal osteoporosis with raloxifene: a randomized trial. *J Bone Miner Res* 1998;13(11):1747–1754.

405. Balfour JA, Goa KL. Raloxifene. *Drugs Aging* 1998;12(4): 335–41; discussion 342.

406. Buzdar AU, et al. Phase II evaluation of Ly156758 in metastatic breast cancer. *Oncology* 1988;45(5):344–345.

407. Ettinger B, et al. Reduction of vertebral fracture risk in postmenopausal women with osteoporosis treated with raloxifene: results from a 3-year randomized clinical trial. Multiple Outcomes of Raloxifene Evaluation (MORE) Investigators [see comments]. *JAMA* 1999;282(7):637–645.

408. Jordan VC. Targeted antiestrogens to prevent breast cancer. *Trends Endocrinol Metab* 1999;10(8):312–317.

409. Hudis C, et al. Phase 1 study of a third-generation selective estrogen receptor modulator (SERM3, LY353381, HCL) in refractory, metastatic breast cancer (abstract). *Breast Cancer Res Treat* 1998;50:306.

410. Coombes RC, et al. Idoxifene: report of a phase I study in patients with metastatic breast cancer. *Cancer Res* 1995; 55(5):1070–1074.

411. Grasser WA, et al. Common mechanism for the estrogen agonist and antagonist activities of droloxifene. *J Cell Biochem* 1997;65(2):159–171.

412. Haarstad H, et al. Influence of droloxifene on metastatic breast cancer as first-line endocrine treatment. *Acta Oncol* 1998;37(4):365–368.

413. O'Regan RM, et al. Effects of the antiestrogens tamoxifen, toremifene, and ICI 182,780 on endometrial cancer growth. *J Natl Cancer Inst* 1998;90(20):1552–1558.

414. Beard J. The span of gestation and the cause of birth. Fisher G, ed. Jena:1897.

415. Fraenkel L. Die funktion des corpus luteum. *Arch Gynaekol* 1905;68:483–545.

416. Corner GW, Allen WM. Physiology of the corpus luteum. II. Production of a special uterine reaction (progestational proliferation) by extracts of the corpus luteum. *Am J Physiol* 1929;88:326–339.

417. Buzdar A, Plourde P, Hortobagyi G. Aromatase inhibitors in metastatic breast cancer. *Semin Oncol* 1996;23(4 Suppl 9):28–32.

418. Saunders FJ, Elton RL. Effects of ethynodiol diacetate and mestranol in rats and rabbits, on conception, on the outcome of pregnancy and on the offspring. *Toxicol Appl Pharmacol* 1967;11:229–244.

419. Williams MT, Clark MR, Ling WY. Role of cyclic AMP in the action of luteinizing hormone on steroidogenesis in the

corpus luteum. In: George WJ, Ignarro L, eds. *Advances in cyclic nucleotide research,* vol 9. New York: Raven Press, 1978:573.

420. Van de Wiele RL, Gurpide E, Kelly WG. The secretory rate of progesterone and aldosterone in normal and abnormal late pregnancy. *Acta Endocrinol Suppl (Copenh)* 1960; 51:159.

421. Gupta C, et al. In vivo metabolism of progestins. V. The effect of protocol design on the estimated metabolic clearance rate and volume of distribution of medroxyprogesterone acetate in women. *J Clin Endocrinol Metab* 1979;48(5):816–820.

422. Janne O, et al. Oestrogen-induced progesterone receptor in human uterus. *J Steroid Biochem* 1975;6(3–4):501–509.

423. Dombernowsky P, et al. Letrozole, a new oral aromatase inhibitor for advanced breast cancer: double-blind randomized trial showing a dose effect and improved efficacy and tolerability compared with megestrol acetate. *J Clin Oncol* 1998;16(2):453–461.

424. Buzdar AU, et al. Anastrozole versus megestrol acetate in the treatment of postmenopausal women with advanced breast carcinoma: results of a survival update based on a combined analysis of data from two mature phase III trials. *Arimidex Study Group Cancer* 1998;83(6):1142–1152.

425. Allegra JC, Kiefer SM. Mechanisms of action of progestational agents. *Semin Oncol* 1985;12(1 Suppl 1):3–5.

426. Vignon F, Bardon S, Chalbos D. Antiproliferative effect of progestins and antiprogestins in human breast cancer cells. In: Klijn JGM, Paridaens R, Foekens JA, eds. *Hormonal manipulation of cancer: peptides, growth factors, and new (anti) steroidal agents.* New York: Raven Press, 1987:47.

427. Blossey HC, et al. Pharmacokinetic and pharmacodynamic basis for the treatment of metastatic breast cancer with high-dose medroxyprogesterone acetate. *Cancer* 1984;54(6 Suppl):1208–1215.

428. Going JJ, et al. Proliferative and secretory activity in human breast during natural and artificial menstrual cycles. *Am J Pathol* 1988;130(1):193–204.

429. Potten CS, et al. The effect of age and menstrual cycle upon proliferative activity of the normal human breast. *Br J Cancer* 1988;58(2):163–170.

430. Michna H, et al. The antitumor mechanism of progesterone antagonists is a receptor mediated antiproliferative effect by induction of terminal cell death. *J Steroid Biochem* 1989;34(1–6):447–453.

431. Michna H, et al. Progesterone antagonists block the growth of experimental mammary tumors in G0/G1 [letter]. *Breast Cancer Res Treat* 1990;17(2):155–156.

432. Shi YE, et al. Expression of 67 kDa laminin receptor in human breast cancer cells: regulation by progestins. *Clin Exp Metastasis* 1993;11(3):251–261.

433. Sikic BI, et al. High-dose megestrol acetate therapy of ovarian carcinoma: a phase II study by the Northern California Oncology Group. *Semin Oncol* 1986;13(4 Suppl 4):26–32.

434. Sadoff L, Lusk W. The effect of large doses of medroxyprogesterone acetate (MPA) on urinary estrogen levels and serum levels of cortisol T4 LH and testosterone in patients with advanced cancer. *Obstet Gynecol* 1974;43(2):262–267.

435. Vesterinen E, et al. Effect of medroxyprogesterone acetate on serum levels of LH, FSH, cortisol, and estrone in patients with endometrial carcinoma. *Arch Gynecol* 1981;230(3):205–211.

436. Hellman L, et al. The effect of medroxyprogesterone acetate on the pituitary-adrenal axis. *J Clin Endocrinol Metab* 1976;42(5):912–917.

437. Papaleo C, et al. ACTH and cortisol plasma levels in cancer patients treated with medroxyprogesterone acetate at high dosages. *Chemioterapia* 1984;3(4):220–222.

438. van Veelen H, et al. Endocrine effects of medroxyprogesterone acetate: relation between plasma levels and suppression of adrenal steroids in patients with breast cancer. *Cancer Treat Rep* 1985;69(9):977–983.

439. Antal EJ, Gillespie WR, Albert KS. The bioavailability of an orally administered medroxyprogesterone acetate suspension. *Int J Clin Pharmacol Ther Toxicol* 1983;21(5): 257–259.

440. Neomto T, Patel J, Rosner D. Oral medroxyprogesterone acetate (NSC-26386) in metastatic breast cancer. *Proc Am Assoc Cancer Res* 1983;24:320.

441. Willemse PH, et al. A randomized comparison of megestrol acetate (MA) and medroxyprogesterone acetate (MPA) in patients with advanced breast cancer. *Eur J Cancer* 1990;26(3):337–343.

442. Pannuti F, et al. Prospective, randomized clinical trial of two different high dosages of medroxyprogesterone acetate (MAP) in the treatment of metastatic breast cancer. *Eur J Cancer* 1979;15(4):593–601.

443. De Lena M, Brambilla C, Valagussa P. High-dose medroxyprogesterone acetate in breast cancer resistant to endocrine and cytotoxic therapy. *Cancer Chemother Pharmacol* 1979;2:175–180.

444. Crona N, Enk L, Samsioe G. Medroxyprogesterone acetate (MPA) in adjuvant treatment of endometrial carcinoma—changes in serum lipoproteins. *Steroid Biochem* 1983;195:198.

445. De Conno F, et al. Megestrol acetate for anorexia in patients with far-advanced cancer: a double-blind controlled clinical trial. *Eur J Cancer* 1998;34(11):1705–1709.

446. Mantovani G, et al. Cytokine involvement in cancer anorexia/cachexia: role of megestrol acetate and medroxyprogesterone acetate on cytokine downregulation and improvement of clinical symptoms. *Crit Rev Oncog* 1998;9(2):99–106.

447. Quella SK, et al. Long term use of megestrol acetate by cancer survivors for the treatment of hot flashes. *Cancer* 1998;82(9):1784–1788.

448. Horwitz KB, et al. Progestin action and progesterone receptor structure in human breast cancer: a review. *Recent Prog Horm Res* 1985;41:249–316.

449. Henderson D. Antiprogestational and antiglucocorticoid activities of some novel 11 β-aryl substituted steroids. In: Furr BJA, Wakeling AE, eds. *Pharmacological and clinical uses of inhibitors of hormone secretion and action.* London: Bailliere Tindall, 1987:184.

450. Bakker GH, Setyono-Han B, de Jong FH. Mifepristone in treatment of experimental breast cancer in rats. In: Klijn JGM, Paridaens R, Foekens JA, eds. *Hormonal manipulation of cancer: peptides, growth factors, and new (anti) steroidal agents.* New York: Raven Press, 1987:39.

451. Bell MR, Batzold FH, Winneker RC. Chemical control of fertility. *Ann Rep Med Chem* 1986;21:169–177.

452. Maudelonde T, Romieu G, Ulmann A. First clinical trial on the use of the anti progestin RU486 in advanced breast cancer. In: Klijn JGM, Paridaens R, Foekens JA, eds. *Hormonal manipulation of cancer: peptides, growth factors, and new (anti) steroidal agents.* New York: Raven Press, 1987:55.

453. Klijn JG, et al. Antiprogestins, a new form of endocrine therapy for human breast cancer. *Cancer Res* 1989; 49(11):2851–2856.

454. Pongubala JM, Elger WA, Puri CP. Relative binding affinity of antiprogestins ZK 98.299 and ZK 98.734 for progesterone receptors in the endometrium and myometrium of bonnet monkeys. *J Recept Res* 1987;7(6):903–920.

455. D'Souza A, Hinduja IN, Puri CP. Antiprogestin ZK-98.299 and progesterone display differential binding characteristics in the human myometrial cytosol. *Biochim Biophys Acta* 1992;1175(1):73–80.

456. Puri CP, et al. Binding characteristics of progesterone and antiprogestin ZK 98.299 in human endometrial and myometrial cytosol. *Biochim Biophys Acta* 1989;1011(2–3):176–182.

457. Klein-Hitpass L, et al. Two types of antiprogestins identified by their differential action in transcriptionally active extracts from T47D cells. *Nucleic Acids Res* 1991;19(6):1227–1234.

458. Takimoto GS, et al. Hormone-induced progesterone receptor phosphorylation consists of sequential DNA-independent and DNA-dependent stages: analysis with zinc finger mutants and the progesterone antagonist ZK98299. *Proc Natl Acad Sci U S A* 1992;89(7):3050–3054.

459. Schneider MR, et al. Antitumor activity of the progesterone antagonists ZK 98.299 and RU 38.486 in the hormone-dependent MXT mammary tumor model of the mouse and the DMBA- and the MNU-induced mammary tumor models of the rat. *Eur J Cancer Clin Oncol* 1989;25(4):691–701.

460. Elger W, et al. Studies on the mechanisms of action of progesterone antagonists. *J Steroid Biochem* 1986;25(5B):835–845.

461. Zakula Z, Moudgil VK. Interaction of rat liver glucocorticoid receptor with a newly synthesized antisteroid ZK98299. *Biochim Biophys Acta* 1991;1092(2):188–195.

462. van den Berg HW, Lynch M, Martin JH. The relationship between affinity of progestins and antiprogestins for the progesterone receptor in breast cancer cells (ZR-PR-LT) and ability to down-regulate the receptor: evidence for heterospecific receptor modulation via the glucocorticoid receptor. *Eur J Cancer* 1993;12(5):1771–1775.

463. Robertson JF, et al. Onapristone, a progesterone receptor antagonist, as first-line therapy in primary breast cancer. *Eur J Cancer* 1999;35(2):214–218.

464. Ovarian ablation in early breast cancer: overview of the randomised trials. Early Breast Cancer Trialists' Collaborative Group [see comments]. *Lancet* 1996;348(9036):1189–1196.

465. Walker KJ, et al. Preliminary endocrinological evaluation of a sustained-release formulation of the LH-releasing hormone agonist D-Ser(But)6Azgly10LHRH in premenopausal women with advanced breast cancer. *J Endocrinol* 1986;111(2):349–353.

466. Harvey HA, et al. Medical castration produced by the GnRH analogue leuprolide to treat metastatic breast cancer. *J Clin Oncol* 1985;3(8):1068–1072.

467. Taylor CW, et al. Multicenter randomized clinical trial of goserelin versus surgical ovariectomy in premenopausal patients with receptor-positive metastatic breast cancer: an intergroup study. *J Clin Oncol* 1998;16(3):994–999.

468. Nicholson RI, Walker KJ, Turkes A. The British experience with LH-RH agonist Zoladex (ICI 118630) in the treatment of breast cancer. In: Klijn JGM, Paridaens R, Foekens JA, eds. *Hormonal manipulation of cancer: peptides, growth factors, and new (anti) steroidal agents.* New York: Raven Press, 1987:331.

469. Dowsett M, et al. Clinical and endocrine effects of leuprorelin acetate in pre- and postmenopausal patients with advanced breast cancer. *Clin Ther* 1992;14(Suppl A):97–103.

470. Robertson JF, et al. Combined endocrine effects of LHRH agonist (Zoladex) and tamoxifen (Nolvadex) therapy in premenopausal women with breast cancer. *Br J Surg* 1989;76(12):1262–1265.

471. Lissoni P, et al. Endocrine and clinical effects of an LHRH analogue in pretreated advanced breast cancer. *Tumori* 1988;74(3):303–308.

472. Blamey RW, et al. Goserelin depot in the treatment of premenopausal advanced breast cancer. *Eur J Cancer* 1992: 810–814.

473. Jonat W, et al. A randomised study to compare the effect of the luteinising hormone releasing hormone (LHRH) analogue goserelin with or without tamoxifen in pre- and perimenopausal patients with advanced breast cancer. *Eur J Cancer* 1995;2:137–142.

474. Klijn JGM, et al. Combination LHRH–agonist plus tamoxifen treatment is superior to medical castration alone in premenopausal metastatic breast cancer (abstract). *Breast Cancer Res Treat* 1998;50:227.

475. Davidson N, et al. Effect of chemohormonal therapy in premenopausal, node (+), receptor (+) breast cancer: an Eastern Cooperative Oncology Group phase III intergroup trial (E5188, INT-0101). Abstract 249. *Proc ASCO* 1999;18:67a.

476. Rutqvist LE. Zoladex and tamoxifen as adjuvant therapy in premenopausal breast cancer: a randomized trial by the Cancer Research Campaign (C.R.C.) Breast Cancer Trials Group, the Stockholm Breast Cancer Study Group, the South-East Sweden Breast Cancer Group and the Gruppo Interdisiplinare Valutazione Interveni in Oncologica (G.I.V.I.O.). Abstract 251. *Proc ASCO* 1999;18:67a.

477. Devogelaer JP, Nagant DE, Deuxchaisnes C. Effect of goserelin implants, an LH-RH analogue, on lumbar and hip BMD as studied by deka technique [abstract 207]. *Gynecol Endocrinol* 1990;4(Suppl 2):114.

478. Obhrai H, Samra JS, Brown P. Effects of medical oophorectomy on fasting lipids and lipoproteins in women with polycystic ovarian syndrome (PCOS) [abstract 123]. *Gynecol Endocrinol* 1990;4(Suppl 2):72.

479. Varenhorst E, et al. Antithrombin III concentration, thrombosis, and treatment with luteinising hormone releasing hormone agonist in prostatic carcinoma. *Br Med J (Clin Res Ed)* 1986;292(6525):935–936.

480. Santner SJ, et al. Estrone sulfate: a potential source of estradiol in human breast cancer tissues. *Breast Cancer Res Treat* 1986;7(1):35–44.

481. Santner SJ, et al. Aromatase activity and expression in breast cancer and benign breast tissue stromal cells. *J Clin Endocrinol Metab* 1997;82(1):200–208.

482. Santen R, et al. Estrogen production via the aromatase enzyme in breast carcinoma: which cell type is responsible? *J Steroid Biochem Mol Biol* 1997;61:267–271.

483. MacDonald P, Rombaut R, Siiteri P. Plasma percursors of estrogen. I. Extent of conversion of plasma alpha-4 androstenedione to estrone in normal males and nonpregnant normal, castrate and adrenalectomized females. *J Clin Endocrinol Metab* 1967;27:1103–1111.

484. Longcope C. Metabolic clearance and blood production rates of estrogens in postmenopausal women. *Am J Obstet Gynecol* 1971;111:778–781.

485. Abul-Hajj Y, Iverson R, Kiang D. Aromatization of androgens by human breast cancer. *Steroids* 1979;33:205–222.

486. Dowsett M, et al. The control and biological importance of intratumoral aromatase in breast cancer. *J Steroid Biochem Mol Biol* 1996;56(1–6):145–150.

487. Pasqualini JR, et al. Concentrations of estrone, estradiol, and estronesulfate and evaluation of sulfatase and aromatase activities in pre- and postmenopausal breast cancer patients. *J Clin Endocrinol Metab* 1996;81(4):1460–1464.

488. de Jong P, et al. Inhibition of breast cancer tissue aromatase activity and estrogen concentrations by the third-generation aromatase inhibitor vorozole. *Cancer Res* 1997;57(11):2109–2111.

489. Thorsen T, Tangen M, Stoa K. Concentrations of endogenous estradiol as related to estradiol receptor sites in breast tumor cytosol. *Eur J Cancer Clin Oncol* 1982;18:333–337.

490. Masamura S, et al. Mechanism for maintenance of high breast tumor estradiol concentrations in the absence of ovarian function: role of very high affinity tissue uptake. *Breast Cancer Res Treat* 1997;42:215–216.

491. Lu Q, et al. Expression of aromatase protein and messenger ribonucleic acid in tumor epithelial cells and evidence of functional significance of locally produced estrogen in human breast cancers. *Endocrinology* 1996;137(7):3061–3068.

492. Bulun S, et al. A link between breast cancer and local estrogen biosynthesis suggested by quantification of breast adipose tissue aromatase cytochrome P450 transcripts using competitive polymerase chain reaction after reverse transcription. *J Clin Endocrinol Metab* 1993;77:1622–1628.

493. Bulun S, Mahendroo M, Simpson E. Aromatase gene expression in adipose tissue: relationship to breast cancer. *J Steroid Biochem Mol Biol* 1994;49:319–326.

494. Hseuh A, Adashi E, Jones P. Hormonal regulation of the differentiation of cultured ovarian granulosa cells. *Endocr Rev* 1984;5:76–127.

495. Simpson ER, Zhao Y. Estrogen biosynthesis in adipose. Significance in breast cancer development. *Ann N Y Acad Sci* 1996;784:18–26.

496. Zhou D, et al. Identification of a promoter that controls aromatase expression in human breast cancer and adipose stromal cells. *J Biol Chem* 1996;271(25):15194–15202.

497. Emoto N, Ling N, Baird A. Growth factor-mediated regulation of aromatase activity in human skin fibroblasts. *Proc Soc Exp Biol Med* 1991;196:351–358.

498. Schmidt M, Loffler G. Induction of aromatase in stromal vascular cells from human breast adipose tissue depends on cortisol and growth factors. *FEBS Lett* 1994;341:177–181.

499. Singh A, Reed M. Insulin-like growth factor type I and insulin-like growth factor type II stimulate oestradiol-17

beta hydroxysteroid dehydrogenase (reductive) activity in breast cancer cells. *J Endocrinol* 1991;129:45–48.

500. Macaulay VM, et al. Biological effects of stable overexpression of aromatase in human hormone-dependent breast cancer cells. *Br J Cancer* 1994;69(1):77–83.

501. Yue W, et al. A new nude mouse model for postmenopausal breast cancer using MCF-7 cells transfected with the human aromatase gene. *Cancer Res* 1994;54(19):5092–5095.

502. Lee K, et al. An in vivo model of intratumoral aromatase using aromatase-transfected MCF7 human breast cancer cells. *Int J Cancer* 1995;62(3):297–302.

503. Yeu W, et al. In situ aromatization enhances breast tumor estradiol levels and cellular proliferation. *Cancer Res* 1998;58:927–932.

504. Brodie A, et al. Preclinical studies using the intratumoral aromatase model for postmenopausal breast cancer. *Oncology (Huntingt)* 1998;12(3 Suppl 5):36–40.

505. Brodie A, et al. Intratumoral aromatase model: the effects of letrozole (CGS 20267). *Breast Cancer Res Treat* 1998;49(Suppl 1):S23–S26, discussion S33–S37.

506. Samojlik E, Santen R, Wells S. Adrenal suppression with aminoglutethimide II. Differential effects of aminoglutethimide on plasma androstendione and estrogen levels. *J Clin Endocrinol Metab* 1977;45:480–487.

507. Bonneterre J, Coppens H, Mauriac L. Aminoglutethimide (AG) in advanced breast cancer (BC). Low dose vs. standard dose. *Eur J Cancer Clin Oncol* 1985;21:1153–1158.

508. Santen RJ, et al. Aminoglutethimide inhibits extraglandular estrogen production in postmenopausal women with breast carcinoma. *J Clin Endocrinol Metab* 1978;47(6):257–265.

509. Carella MJ, et al. Adrenal effects of low-dose aminoglutethimide when used alone in postmenopausal women with advanced breast cancer. *Metabolism* 1994;43(6):723–727.

510. Goldhirsch A, Gelber RD. Endocrine therapies of breast cancer. *Semin Oncol* 1996;23(4):494–505.

511. Lawrence B, et al. Pancytopenia induced by aminoglutethimide in the treatment of breast cancer. *Cancer Treat Rep* 1978;62(10):1581–1583.

512. Smith I, et al. Tamoxifen versus aminoglutethimide in advanced breast carcinoma: a randomized cross-over trial. *Br Med J (Clin Res Ed)* 1981;283:1432–1434.

513. Smith I, et al. Tamoxifen versus aminoglutethimide versus combined tamoxifen and aminoglutethimide in the treatment of advanced breast carcinoma. *Cancer Res* 1982;42:3430s–3433s.

514. Jones A, et al. Adjuvant aminoglutethimide for postmenopausal patients with primary breast cancer: analysis at 8 years. *J Clin Oncol* 1992;10:1547–1552.

515. Harris A, et al. Aminoglutethimide for the treatment of advanced postmenopausal breast cancer. *Eur J Cancer Clin Oncol* 1983;19:11–17.

516. Banting L. Inhibition of aromatase. *Prog Med Chem* 1996;33:147–184.

517. Sjoerdsma A. Suicide enzyme inhibitors as potential drugs. *Clin Pharmacol Ther* 1981;30(1):3–22.

518. Brodie A, Hendrickson J, Tsai-Morris C. Inactivation of aromatase in vitro by 4-OHA and 4-acetoxyandrostenedione and sustain effects in vivo. *Steroids* 1981;38:696–702.

519. Dowsett M, et al. Dose-related endocrine effects and pharmacokinetics of oral and intramuscular 4-hydroxyandro-

stenedione in postmenopausal breast cancer patients. *Cancer Res* 1989;49:1306–1312.

520. Dowsett M, Coombes R. Second generation aromatase inhibitor—4-hyroxyandrostenedione. *Breast Cancer Res Treat* 1994;30:81–87.

521. Santner SJ, et al. Additive effects of aminoglutethimide, testololactone, and 4-hydroxyandrostenedione as inhibitors of aromatase. *J Steroid Biochem* 1984;20(6A):1239–1242.

522. Brodie AM, Romanoff LP, Williams KI. Metabolism of the aromatase inhibitor 4-hydroxy-4-androstene-3,17-dione by male rhesus monkeys. *J Steroid Biochem* 1981;14(8): 693–696.

523. Wiseman LR, McTavish D. Formestane. A review of its pharmacodynamic and pharmacokinetic properties and therapeutic potential in the management of breast cancer and prostatic cancer. *Drugs* 1993;45(1):66–84.

524. Poon GK, et al. Determination of 4-hydroxyandrost-4-ene-3,17-dione metabolism in breast cancer patients using high-performance liquid chromatography-mass spectrometry. *J Chromatogr* 1991;565(1–2):75–88.

525. Brodie AM, Santen RJ. Aromatase and its inhibitors in breast cancer treatment—overview and perspective. *Breast Cancer Res Treat* 1994;30(1):1–6.

526. Goss PE, Gwyn KM. Current perspectives on aromatase inhibitors in breast cancer. *J Clin Oncol* 1994;12(11): 2460–2470.

527. Bajetta E, et al. A multicentre, randomized, pharmacokinetic, endocrine and clinical study to evaluate formestane in breast cancer patients at first relapse: endocrine and clinical results. The Italian Trials in Medical Oncology (I.T.M.O.) group. *Ann Oncol* 1997;8:649–654.

528. Perez Carrion R, et al. Comparison of the selective aromatase inhibitor formestane with tamoxifen as first-line hormonal therapy in postmenopausal women with advanced breast cancer. *Ann Oncol* 1994;5(Suppl 7):S19–S24.

529. Thurlimann B, et al. Formestane versus megestrol acetate in postmenopausal breast cancer patients after failure of tamoxifen: a phase III prospective randomised cross over trial of second-line hormonal treatment (SAKK 20/90). Swiss Group for Clinical Cancer Research (SAKK). *Eur J Cancer* 1997;33:989–990.

530. Cunningham D, Powles T, Dowsett M. Oral 4-hydroxyandrostenedione, a new endocrine treatment for disseminated breast cancer. *Cancer Chemother Pharmacol* 1987; 20:253–255.

531. Di Salle E, et al. 4-Aminoandrostenedione derivatives: a novel class of irreversible aromatase inhibitors. Comparison with FCE 24304 and 4-hydroxyandrostenedione. *J Steroid Biochem Mol Biol* 1990;37(3):369–374.

532. Scott LJ, Wiseman LR. Exemestane. *Drugs* 1999;58(4): 675–680, discussion 681–682.

533. Evans T, et al. Phase I and endocrine study of exemestane (FCE 24304), a new aromatase inhibitor, in postmenopausal women. *Cancer Res* 1992;52:5933–5939.

534. Zilembo N, et al. Endocrinological and clinical evaluation of exemestane, a new steroidal aromatase inhibitor. *Br J Cancer* 1995;72:1007–1012.

535. Buzzetti F, et al. Synthesis and aromatase inhibition by potential metabolites of exemestane (6-methylenandrosta-1,4-diene-3,17-dione). *Steroids* 1993;58(11):527–532.

536. Kvinnsland S, et al. Antitumor efficacy of exemestane, a novel, irreversible, oral, aromatase inhibitor in postmenopausal patients with metastatic breast cancer failing tamoxifen. *Breast Cancer Res Treat* 1997;46:Abstract 217.

537. Jones S, et al. Multicenter, phase II trial of exemestane as third-line hormonal therapy of postmenopausal women with metastatic breast cancer. Aromasin Study Group. *J Clin Oncol* 1999;17(11):3418–3425.

538. Noberasco C, et al. Activity of formestane in de novo tamoxifen-resistant patients with metastatic breast cancer. *Oncology* 1995;52:454–457.

539. Kaufmann M, et al. Survival Advantage of Exemestane (EXE, Aromasin) over megestrol acetate (MA) in postmenopausal women with advanced breast cancer (ABC) refractory to tamoxifen (TAM): results of a phase III randomized double blind study. Abstract 412. *Proc ASCO* 1999;18:109a.

540. Boccardo F, et al. Clinical efficacy and endocrine activity of vorozole in postmenopausal breast cancer patients. Results of a multicentric phase II study. *Ann Oncol* 1997; 8(8):745–750.

541. Plourde PV, Dyroff M, Dukes M. Arimidex: a potent and selective fourth–generation aromatase inhibitor. *Breast Cancer Res Treat* 1994;30(1):103–111.

542. Plourde PV, et al. Arimidex: a new, oral once-a-day aromatase inhibitor. *J Steroid Biochem Mol Biol* 1995;53(1–6): 175–179.

543. Dowsett M, et al. A randomized comparison assessing oestrogen suppression with arimadex (anastrozole) and formestane in postmenopausal advanced breast cancer patients. *Eur J Cancer* 1996;32A(Suppl 2):49.

544. Buzdar A, et al. Anastrozole, a potent and selective aromatase inhibitor, versus megestrol acetate in postmenopausal women with advanced breast cancer: results of overview analysis of two phase III trials. Arimidex Study Group. *J Clin Oncol* 1996;14(7):2000–2011.

545. Howell A, et al. Significantly improved survival with Arimadex (anastrozole) compared with megestrol acetate in postmenopausal women with advanced breast cancer: updated results of two randomized trials (abstract). *Breast Cancer Res Treat* 1997;46:18.

546. Iveson T, et al. Phase I study of the oral nonsteroidal aromatase inhibitor CGS 20267 in postmenopausal patients with advanced breast cancer. *Cancer Res* 1993;53:266–270.

547. Bisagni G, et al. Letrozole, a new oral non-steroidal aromatase inhibitor in treating postmenopausal patients with advanced breast cancer. A pilot study. *Ann Oncol* 1996; 7:99–102.

548. Tominaga T, Ohashi Y, Abe R. Phase II trial of letrozole (a novel oral nonsteroidal aromatase inhibitor) in postmenopausal patients with advanced or recurrent breast cancer (abstract). *Eur J Cancer* 1995;31A(Suppl 5):S81.

549. Lipton A, et al. Letrozole (CGS 20267). A phase I study of a new potent oral aromatase inhibitor of breast cancer. *Cancer* 1995;75(8):2132–2138.

550. Klein KO, et al. Use of ultrasensitive recombinant cell bioassay to measure estrogen levels in women with breast cancer receiving the aromatase inhibitor, letrozole. *J Clin Endocrinol Metab* 1995;80(9):2658–2660.

551. Gershanovich M, et al. Letrozole, a new oral aromatase inhibitor: randomised trial comparing 2.5 mg daily, 0.5 mg

daily and aminoglutethimide in postmenopausal women with advanced breast cancer. Letrozole International Trial Group (AR/BC3). *Ann Oncol* 1998;9(6):639–645.

552. Goldhirsch A, Coates A. New trial with Letrozole. *International Breast Cancer Study Group News Letter* 1997; 3(3):2.

553. Ito Y, et al. Molecular basis of aromatase deficiency in an adult female with sexual infantilism and polycystic ovaries. *Proc Natl Acad Sci U S A* 1993;90:11673–11677.

554. Conte F, et al. A syndrome of female pseudohermaphrodism, hypergonadotropic hypogonadism, and multicystic ovaries associated with missense mutations in the gene encoding aromatase (P450arom). *J Clin Endocrinol Metab* 1994;78:1287–1292.

555. Agarwal S, Judd H, Magoffin D. A mechanism for the suppression of estrogen production in polycystic ovary syndrome. *J Clin Endocrinol Metab* 1996;81:3686–3691.

556. Santen RJ, Samojlik E, Wells SA. Resistance of the ovary to blockade of aromatization with aminoglutethimide. *J Clin Endocrinol Metab* 1980;51(3):473–477.

557. Celio L, et al. Premenopausal breast cancer patients treated with a gonadotropin-releasing hormone analog alone or in combination with an aromatase inhibitor: a comparative endocrine study. *Anticancer Res* 1999;19(3B):2261–2268.

558. Dowsett M, et al. Vorozole results in greater oestrogen suppression than formestane in postmenopausal women and when added to goserelin in premenopausal women with advanced breast cancer. *Breast Cancer Res Treat* 1999;56(1):25–34.

7

ANTIFOLATES

RICHARD A. MESSMANN
CARMEN J. ALLEGRA

The folate-dependent enzymes represent attractive targets for antitumor chemotherapy because of their critical role in the synthesis of the nucleotide precursors of DNA (Fig. 7-1). In 1948, Farber and associates were the first to show that aminopterin, a four-amino analog of folic acid, could inhibit the proliferation of leukemic cells and produce remissions in acute leukemia cases.[1] Their findings ushered in the era of antimetabolite chemotherapy and generated great interest in the antifolate class of agents. Since then, the clinical value of antifolate compounds has been proven in the treatment of the leukemias; head and neck, breast, and bladder cancers; lymphomas; and choriocarcinoma.[2] Their clinical application has also extended to the treatment of nonneoplastic disorders, including rheumatoid arthritis,[3] graft-versus-host disease after bone marrow transplantation,[4] psoriasis,[5] bacterial and plasmodial infections,[6] and opportunistic infections associated with the acquired immunodeficiency syndrome.[7] It is fair to state that this class of agents is one of the best understood and most versatile of all the cancer chemotherapeutic drugs (Table 7-1).

MECHANISM OF ACTION

Substitution of an amino group for the hydroxyl at position 4 of the pteridine ring is the critical change in the structure of antifolate compounds that leads to their antitumor activity (Fig. 7-2). This change transforms the molecule from a substrate to a tight-binding inhibitor of dihydrofolate reductase (DHFR), a key enzyme in intracellular folate homeostasis. The critical importance of DHFR stems from the fact that folic acid compounds are active as coenzymes only in their fully reduced tetrahydrofolate form. Two specific tetrahydrofolates play essential roles as one-carbon carriers in the synthesis of DNA precursors. The cofactor 10-formyltetrahydrofolate provides its one-carbon group for the *de novo* synthesis of purines in reactions mediated by glycineamide ribonucleotide (GAR) transformylase and aminoimidazole carboxamide ribonucleotide (AICAR) trans-

formylase. A second cofactor, 5,10-methylenetetrahydrofolate (CH_2-FH_4), donates its one-carbon group to the reductive methylation reaction, converting deoxyuridylate to thymidylate (Fig. 7-1). In addition to contributing a one-carbon group, 5,10-methylenetetrahydrofolate is oxidized to dihydrofolate, which must then be reduced to tetrahydrofolate by the enzyme DHFR for it to rejoin the pool of active reduced-folate cofactors. In actively proliferating tumor cells, inhibition of DHFR by methotrexate (MTX) (Fig. 7-2) or other 2,4-diamino antifolates leads to an accumulation of folates in the inactive dihydrofolate form, with variable depletion of reduced folates.[8-14] Folate depletion, however, does not fully account for the metabolic inhibition associated with antifolate treatment because the critical reduced-folate pools may be relatively preserved even in the presence of cytotoxic concentrations of MTX. Additional factors may contribute to MTX-associated cytotoxicity, including metabolism of the parent compound to polyglutamated derivatives and the accumulation of dihydrofolate and 10-formyldihydrofolate polyglutamates as a consequence of DHFR inhibition.[8,9,15-17] MTX polyglutamates, dihydrofolate polyglutamates, and 10-formyldihydrofolate metabolites represent potent direct inhibitors of the folate-dependent enzymes of thymidylate and purine biosynthesis.[18-23] Thus, inhibition of DNA biosynthesis by 2,4-diamino folates is a multifactorial process consisting of both partial depletion of reduced-folate substrates and direct inhibition of folate-dependent enzymes. The relative roles of each of these mechanisms in determining antifolate-associated metabolic inhibition may depend on specific cellular factors that vary among different cancer cell lines and tumors.

CHEMICAL STRUCTURE

Various heterocyclic compounds with the 2,4-diamino configuration have antifolate activity and include pyrimidine analogs such as pyrimethamine and trimethoprim[20-29] (Fig. 7-2); classical pteridines such as aminopterin and MTX[2];

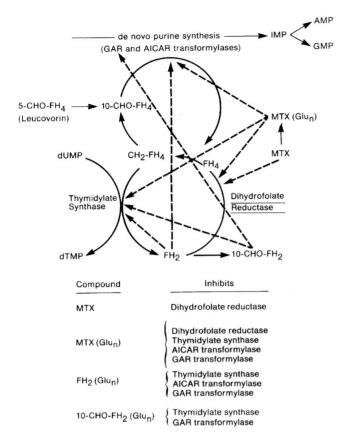

FIGURE 7-1. Sites of action of methotrexate (MTX), its poly-glutamated metabolites [MTX(Glu_n)], and folate by-products of the inhibition of dihydrofolate reductase, including dihydrofolate (FH_2) and 10-formyldihydrofolate (10-CHO-FH_2). Also shown are 5,10-methylenetetrahydrofolate (CH_2-FH_4), the folate cofactor required for thymidylate synthesis, and 10-formyltetrahydrofolate (10-CHO-FH_4), the required intermediate in the synthesis of purine precursors. (AICAR; aminoimidazole carboxamide ribonucleotide; AMP, adenosine monophosphate; dUMP, deoxyuridylate; dTMP, thymidylate; GAR; glycineamide ribonucleotide; GMP, guanosine monophosphate; IMP, inosine monophosphate.) (From DeVita VT, Hellman S, Rosenberg SA, eds. *Cancer: principles and practice of oncology*. Philadelphia: JB Lippincott, 1989:349–397.)

and compounds with replacement of the nitrogen at either the 5 or 8 position or both with a carbon atom, such as the quinazolines (trimetrexate; piritrexim)[24–26] and 10-ethyl-10-deazaaminopterin (10-EDAM, Edatrexate).[27] Compounds with preservation of the benzoylglutamate terminal group are transported by a folate-specific system in the cell membrane, whereas those lacking a terminal glutamate do not require active transmembrane transport and have activity against MTX-resistant cells that lack the folate transporter.[28] Investigators have designed antifolate analogs directed at targets other than DHFR, including those folate-dependent enzymes required for the *de novo* synthesis of purines and thymidylate. A host of potent thymidylate synthase (TS) inhibitors such as 10-propargyl-5,8-dideazafolate (PDDF, CB3717)[30] and closely related compounds ZD1694 [raltitrexed (Tomudex)] and ZD9331,[31]

TABLE 7-1. KEY FEATURES OF METHOTREXATE SODIUM (MTX)

Mechanism of action	Inhibition of dihydrofolate reductase leads to partial depletion of reduced folates
	Polyglutamates of MTX and dihydrofolate inhibit purine and thymidylate biosynthesis
Metabolism	Converted to polyglutamates in normal and malignant tissues
	7-Hydoxylation in liver
Pharmacokinetics	$t_{1/2\alpha}$ = 2–3 h; $t_{1/2\beta}$ = 8–10 h
Elimination	Primarily as interact drug in urine
Drug interactions	High-dose toxicity to normal tissues rescued by leucovorin calcium
	L-Asparaginase blocks toxicity and antitumor activity
	Pretreatment with MTX increases 5-fluorouracil and cytosine arabinoside nucleotide formation
	Nonsteroidal antiinflammatory agents decrease renal clearance and increase toxicity
Toxicity	Myelosuppression
	Mucositis, gastrointestinal epithelial denudation
	Renal tubular obstruction and injury
	Hepatotoxicity
	Pneumonitis
	Hypersensitivity
	Neurotoxicity
Precaution	Reduce dose in proportion to creatinine clearance
	Do not administer high-dose MTX to patients with abnormal renal function
	Monitor plasma concentrations of drug, hydrate patients during high-dose therapy (see Tables 7-2 and 7-4)

$t_{1/2}$, half-life.

LY231514 (multitargeted antifolate, MTA),[32] 1843U89,[33] and 5,8-dideazatetrahydrofolic acid (DDATHF, lometrexol) and LY231514,[34] both inhibitors of GAR transformylase, have been developed. Although the analogs with DHFR as the primary target have unique structural features distinct from MTX and have equal or greater potency for inhibiting DHFR and other folate-dependent enzymes, none has yet replaced MTX in the clinic. This is primarily because of the greater familiarity with both the cytotoxic activity and host toxicity patterns of MTX and the current lack of evidence that these analog compounds have therapeutic efficacy greater than that of MTX or other available standard agents.

CELLULAR PHARMACOLOGY AND MECHANISMS OF RESISTANCE

In this section, the sequence of events that leads to the cytotoxic action of MTX is considered, beginning with drug movement across the cell membrane, followed by its

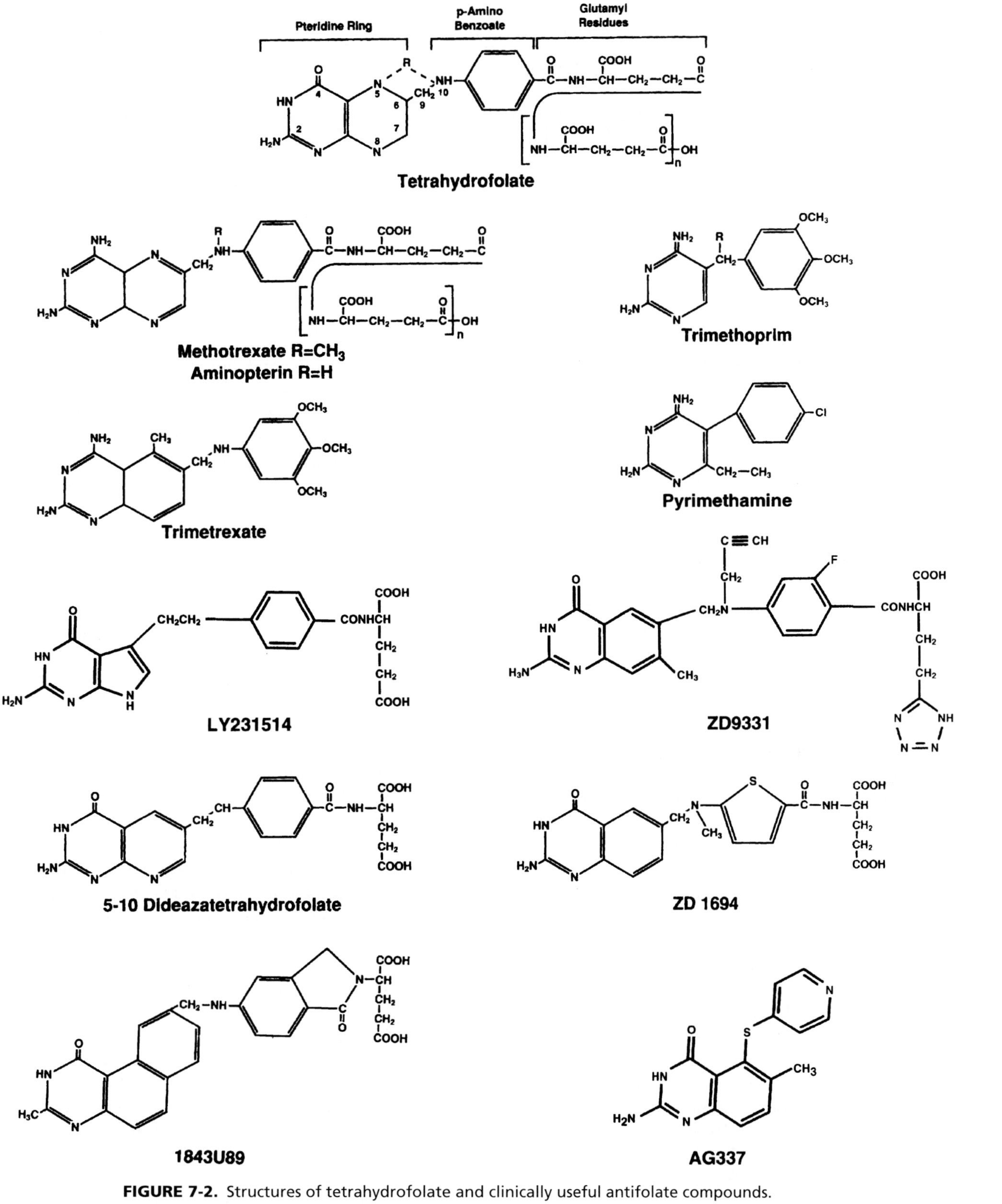

FIGURE 7-2. Structures of tetrahydrofolate and clinically useful antifolate compounds.

intracellular metabolism to the polyglutamate derivatives, binding to DHFR and other folate-dependent enzymes, effects on intracellular folates, and, finally, inhibition of DNA synthesis. Each of these steps plays an essential role in determining the ultimate clinical efficacy and toxicity of MTX and other antifolate compounds.

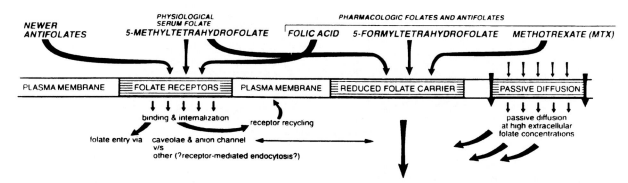

FIGURE 7-3. Transport systems identified for the physiologic folates and various antifolates. (Adapted from Antony AC. The biological chemistry of folate receptors. *Blood* 1992;79:2807–2820.)

Transmembrane Transport

Folate influx into mammalian cells proceeds via two distinct transport systems: (a) the reduced-folate carrier (RFC) system and (b) the folate receptor (FR) system (Fig. 7-3).[35–38] The proliferative or kinetic state of tumor cells influences the rate of folate and MTX transport. In general, rapidly dividing cells have a greater rate of MTX uptake and a lower rate of drug efflux[39] than cells that are either in the stationary phase or that are slowly growing.[40] In some experiments, induction of differentiation of tumor cells, independent of effects on growth rate, markedly decreased MTX transport.[41] The RFC system, with its large transport capacity, transports folic acid inefficiently [K_t (transport coefficient) = 200 μmol per L] and is a primary transport mechanism of the reduced folates and antifolates like MTX (K_t = 0.7 to 6.0 μmol per L), at pharmacologic drug concentrations.[42–48] The RFC system also transports the naturally occurring reduced folates, including the rescue agent 5-formyltetrahydrofolate (leucovorin).[36,37,49–52] Studies have mapped the RFC gene to the long arm of chromosome 21, and this site encodes a protein with predicted molecular size of 58 to 68 kd.[53–57]

In the second folate transport mechanism, FRs mediate the internalization of folates via a high-affinity membrane-bound 38-kd glycoprotein. The FR gene family encodes three homologous glycoproteins that share a similar folate-binding site. The α and β FRs are anchored to the plasma membrane by a carboxyl-terminal glycosylphosphatidylinositol tail and transport the reduced folates and MTX at a lower capacity than the RFC system. The function of the FR, which is inefficiently anchored to plasma membranes by a glycosylphosphatidylinositol tail and is primarily secreted into the media, is unknown. FRs are expressed in normal tissues and, at high levels, on the surface of some epithelial tumors such as ovarian cancer.[58,59] The FR system has a 10- to 30-fold higher affinity for folic acid and the reduced folates [K_a (dissociation constant) = 1 to 10 μmol per L] than for MTX. In addition, MTX polyglutamates demonstrate a 75-fold increased affinity for FR compared with the monoglutamate form of MTX.[60] Variation in exogenous folate concentrations and normal physiologic conditions, such as pregnancy, can alter the tissue expression of FR.

The FR isoforms (α, β, γ) are independently expressed in mammalian cells[61] and normal human tissues.[62] FR-α is expressed in human epithelial neoplasms (ovarian cancer and nasopharyngeal KB carcinoma cells) where it is upregulated by folate depletion and down-regulated in folate-replete medium.[35,44] Elwood et al. have shown that FR-α is expressed in a complex manner involving promoters upstream from exons 1 and 4 and differential messenger RNA (mRNA) splicing of 5′ exons, all of which may play a role in transcriptional and translational regulation.[63–65] FR-β is expressed in human placenta and nonepithelial tumors. FR-γ, found in hematopoietic and lymphatic cells and tissues, lacks a glycosylphosphatidylinositol membrane anchor and is secreted.[57] Although human FR-α, FR-β, and FR-γ share 70% amino acid sequence homology, they differ in binding affinities for stereoisomers of folates.[66]

Although the precise mechanism of FR-mediated folate uptake remains controversial,[67] two separate pathways for FR-mediated folate uptake have been reported: (a) the classic receptor-mediated internalization of the ligand-receptor complex through clathrin-coated pits with subsequent formation of secondary lysosomes and (b) a mechanism of small molecule uptake, termed potocytosis,[68–70] in which receptor complexes accumulate within distinct subdomains of the plasma membrane known as caveolae that internalize to form intracellular vesicles.[71] Once internalization has occurred, acidification within the vesicle causes the folate-receptor complex to dissociate and translocate across the cell membrane. Studies suggest that the depletion of membrane cholesterol and the blockage of sphingolipid synthesis inhibit human FR-mediated transport[63] and that disruption of the cytoskeletal elements (e.g., actin) decreases receptor-mediated uptake.[72]

Although questions remain as to the relative importance of the FR and RFC transport systems in the uptake of antifolates during chemotherapy, studies[73,74] suggest that the RFC system is the more relevant transporter of MTX in mammalian cells, even in cells expressing high levels of FR.

Both *in vitro* and *in vivo* experimental systems have identified defective transport as a common mechanism of intrinsic or acquired resistance to MTX.[75–78] Other factors, however, including intracellular levels of DHFR, affinity of DHFR for MTX, polyglutamation, and levels of TS, may also influence the cytotoxic action of MTX, and their effects may not be easily separable from drug transport. A number of MTX-resistant cell lines with functional defects in the RFC have now been described, with the majority being established by single step selection in the presence of MTX.[79–83] The conditions used to generate these mutant cell lines *in vitro* often involve a higher folate concentration (1 to 5 μmol per L) than that normally found *in vivo* (5 to 50 nmol per L). Therefore, neoplastic cells with a markedly reduced capacity to transport folates may not be able to survive *in vivo* in a low-folate environment.[84] An MTX-resistant human lymphoblastic CCRF-CEM/MTX cell line was established and maintained in physiologic concentrations of folate (2 nmol per L).[85] These cells lacked the RFC protein and, for this reason, were resistant to MTX. These cells retained the folate binding protein, however, and were able to use this transport process to maintain growth even in nanomolar concentrations of folic acid. This study is of particular interest because the concentration of folate used was in the physiologic range, and thus this mechanism of transport-mediated resistance may have direct clinical relevance.

Using L1210 cells exposed to low pH conditions, Sierra et al. reported altered MTX uptake kinetics, which suggests an additional and separate MTX transport system, but further studies are required to define its importance as related to cytotoxicity.[86] Zhao et al. have characterized a mutated murine RFC (RFC1) with increased affinity for folic acid and decreased affinity for MTX, which suggests that amino acids in the first predicted transmembrane domain play an important role in determining the spectrum of affinities for, and mobility of, RFC1. This domain is also a cluster region for mutations that occur when cells are placed under selective pressure with antifolates that use RFC1 as the major route of entry into mammalian cells.[87,88] Using transport-defective L1210 leukemia cell lines, Zhao and colleagues found that the large intracellular loop between the sixth and seventh transmembrane domains of the RFC1 protein also plays a key role in RFC1 inactivation resulting from single point mutations.[89]

To identify clinical MTX resistance on the basis of impaired transport, a sensitive competitive displacement assay using the fluorescent analog of MTX, *N*-(4-amino-4-deoxy-*N*10-methylpteroyl)-*N*-(4'-fluoresceinthiocarbamyl)-L-lysine (PT430) was developed.[90] An analysis of 17 patients with acute lymphoblastic leukemia (ALL) revealed that blast cells from 2 of 4 patients in relapse after initial treatment with MTX-based combination chemotherapy demonstrated defective MTX transport. This study offers suggestive evidence that impaired transport may play a role in the development of clinical MTX resistance. Using semi-

quantitative reverse-transcription polymerase chain reaction techniques, Guo et al.[91] investigated MTX resistance in tumors obtained from patients with high-grade osteosarcoma. In this study 13 of 20 osteosarcoma samples (65%) were found to have decreased RFC expression at the time of initial biopsy and 17 of 26 tumor samples (65%) derived from patients with poor response to chemotherapy had decreased RFC expression. The authors concluded that the relatively high frequency of decreased RFC expression suggested that impaired transport of MTX is a common mechanism of intrinsic resistance in osteosarcoma. For an in-depth analysis of RFC activity as it relates to transport-mediated MTX resistance, the reader is referred to the review by Moscow.[92]

Significant differences in the characteristics of antifolate drug transport have prompted interest in the development of new analogs. The nonglutamated antifolates such as trimetrexate and piritrexim, as well as the glutamyl esters of MTX, do not require active cellular transport and demonstrate activity against transport-resistant mutants.[93–95] The quinazoline antifolates have a higher rate of influx and a lower rate of efflux than does MTX, whereas aminopterin has a faster influx rate; these differences correlate with the greater intracellular accumulation of the quinazolines and aminopterin, compared with MTX, after equimolar doses *in vivo*.[96] The compound 10-EDAM is more avidly accumulated in tumor cells than in normal bone marrow or intestinal epithelium and has broader therapeutic activity and less marrow toxicity than MTX in experimental systems.[28,97] Although the parent compound 10-EDAM has essentially no inhibitory activity against TS, its polyglutamated forms have significant inhibitory activity.[98] This effect of polyglutamation is similar to that noted for MTX.[99,100]

In contrast to MTX, which has a relatively poor affinity for the folate binding proteins, several of the more recently synthesized antifolate inhibitors such as CB3717, raltitrexed, DDATHF, LY231514, and BW1843U89 rely heavily on the high-affinity folate binding proteins for cellular transport.[101,102] Because several of these compounds are efficiently transported by either folate transport system, however, they may be less susceptible to the emergence of clinical resistance resulting from alterations in membrane transport. The clinical importance of human FR in transport of these newer antifolates was examined by Pinard et al., who concluded that, in RFC nonfunctional cells, the amount of FR activity may be an important determinant of cellular sensitivity to the newer high-affinity FR antifolates.[103] Homofolate is a DHFR inhibitor that is primarily transported by the folate binding proteins and has extremely potent activity against malignant cells overexpressing this protein.[104] This antifolate analog and the TS inhibitors may prove to be particularly interesting agents for the treatment of human solid tumors that have developed MTX resistance due to either downregulation or alterations of the RFC system. Sen et al.

reviewed the relationship between FR expression and the toxicity of lometrexol, which inhibits purine synthesis through inhibition of GAR transformylase. These investigators found that *de novo* resistance to lometrexol was mediated by the extent of its polyglutamylation and intracellular half-life, in addition to changes in FR-mediated transport.[105] In addition, low-folate conditions that up-regulate FR expression may have clinical relevance. Research has demonstrated that mice maintained on a low-folate diet had higher FR expression on their normal tissues and experienced significantly greater lometrexol toxicity, which suggests the potential for a human corollary in cancer patients with poor nutritional intake.[106]

Trimetrexate and piritrexim have demonstrated only modest activity against human solid tumors.[107–109] Trimetrexate combined with leucovorin calcium has significant activity against the pulmonary pathogen *Pneumocystis carinii*, whose DHFR enzyme is highly sensitive to this combination; in contrast, it has limited sensitivity to the commonly used antiinfectious agent trimethoprim.[7,110] Hum and colleagues[111] have applied the same pharmacologic principles used to develop trimetrexate and leucovorin for the treatment of *P. carinii* and have suggested using high-dose trimetrexate and minimal-dose leucovorin rescue to treat cancers resistant to MTX because of decreased transport of MTX and folate.

The compound 10-EDAM has clinical activity against a variety of human solid tumors. Its dose-limiting toxicity is mucositis rather than the myelosuppression normally associated with MTX therapy.[100,112] Phase II testing has shown this agent to be active in the treatment of non–small cell lung cancers, soft tissue sarcomas, and breast cancers, with overall response rates of 17%, 14%, and 41%, respectively.[100,113,114]

Using L1210 cells, Saxena has characterized two functionally distinct MTX efflux transporters that are sensitive to chemical inhibition.[115] One pathway is inhibited by bromosulfophthalein, probenecid, prostaglandin A, and high concentrations of potassium chloride and is shared by cyclic nucleotides.[116–119] Assaraf et al. demonstrated the potential importance of these transporters in Chinese hamster ovary cells, in which the decreased activity of the efflux pump conferred selective resistance to lipophilic antifolates.[120] Although the efflux pathways for MTX in human leukemic lymphoblasts (CCRF-CEM cells) are identical to those described for the murine cells, the bromosulfophthalein-sensitive route is quantitatively insignificant.[121]

The potential interaction between the P-glycoprotein efflux pump and MTX is an area of research interest. The *MDR* gene encodes a P-glycoprotein drug efflux pump, and cells expressing the *MDR-1* phenotype, although not cross-resistant to MTX, are cross-resistant to lipophilic antifolates such as trimetrexate.[122] In addition, *MDR* expression may confer resistance to MTX in cells, such as human leukemic CCRF-CEM cells, that do not express functional human FR or FRC systems.[123] Additional studies are required to define the clinical relevance of MTX-based chemotherapy as related to the expression of *MDR*.

Using a tetracycline-inducible expression system in an osteosarcoma cell line (SaOs-2), Li et al.[124] found that p21/waf1-induced cells exhibited greater sensitivity to doxorubicin hydrochloride, raltitrexed, and MTX than noninduced cells and that this condition was associated with increased apoptosis. The SaOs-2 cells lack both p53 and a functional retinoblastoma protein. Overexpression of p21/waf1 protein was associated with diminished E2F-1 phosphorylation, which resulted in an increase in E2F-1 binding activity and enhanced expression of E2F-responsive genes (DHFR and TS). The authors suggested that this mechanism may mediate sensitivity to anticancer drugs by contributing to increased S–G_2 cell-cycle arrest or delay and increased cell susceptibility to apoptosis.

Intracellular Transformation

Naturally occurring folates exist within cells in a polyglutamated form. The polyglutamation of folate substrates is facilitated by folylpolyglutamyl synthetase (FPGS), an enzyme that adds up to four to six glutamyl groups in γ peptide linkage. This reaction serves three main purposes for folates: (a) it facilitates the accumulation of intracellular folates in vast excess of the monoglutamate pool that is freely transportable into and out of cells, (b) it allows selective intracellular retention of these relatively large anionic molecules and thus prolongs intracellular half-life, and (c) it enhances folate cofactor affinity for several folate-dependent enzymes. MTX polyglutamates are more potent inhibitors of DHFR, TS, AICAR transformylase, and GAR transformylase than is MTX-Glu_1.[16,17] MTX and the other glutamyl-terminal analogs also undergo polyglutamation (Fig. 7-2) in normal liver cells,[75] bone marrow myeloid precursors,[125,126] human fibroblasts,[127] and a variety of leukemic and carcinoma cell lines.[126,128–133] FPGS activity is especially high in MTX-sensitive leukemic cell lines and in human lymphoblastic leukemia cells.[133]

The efficiency of the polyglutamation reaction is dependent on the particular folate substrate and may vary widely among the antifolate compounds. The polyglutamation of MTX occurs over 12 to 24 hours of exposure, at which time most intracellular drug exists in the polyglutamate form.[129,134] In the few studies of polyglutamate formation *in vivo*, 80% or more of MTX in both normal and malignant tissues exists in the form of polyglutamates.[133,135–137] Human liver retains MTX polyglutamates for several months after drug administration.[138] Thus, the selective retention and depot formation in excess of free monoglutamate, as seen with physiologic folates, appears to characterize MTX polyglutamates as well.

FPGS is a 62-kd magnesium-, adenosine triphosphate–, and potassium-dependent protein.[139–147] The most avid substrate for this enzyme is dihydrofolate [K_m (binding affinity) = 2 μmol per L] > tetrahydrofolate (K_m = 6 μmol per L) > 10-formyltetrahydrofolate or 5-methyltetrahydrofolate > aminopterin > leucovorin > MTX. Because of the relatively slow rate of formation of MTX polyglutamates compared with the naturally occurring folates, reductions in FPGS activity or cellular glutamate levels that have little effect on folate polyglutamate pools may have critical effects on the level of MTX polyglutamates and on the ultimate cytotoxicity of MTX. Some have postulated that the relatively inefficient metabolism of 5-methyltetrahydrofolate (the predominant folate present in human serum) to its polyglutamate form may be responsible for the folate depletion that occurs in vitamin B_{12} deficiency. Lack of B_{12} would inhibit methionine synthetase, which is responsible for the demethylation of 5-methyltetrahydrofolate to tetrahydrofolate, an excellent substrate for FPGS.[144] The accumulation of MTX polyglutamates in liver reduces the polyglutamation of natural folates in that tissue[147] and may, in part, account for the chronic hepatotoxicity associated with MTX. Potent inhibitors of FPGS have been synthesized, such as the ornithine analog of aminopterin [K_i (inhibition constant) = 0.15 μmol per L]; this compound also inhibits DHFR, but, unfortunately, has little cytotoxicity, presumably due to its poor transmembrane transport. The intracellular content of polyglutamate derivatives represents a balance between the activity of two different enzymes, FPGS and γ-glutamyl hydrolase (GGH, conjugase).[148] The latter, a γ-glutamyl-specific peptidase, removes terminal glutamyl groups and returns MTX polyglutamates to their parent monoglutamate form. Hydrolase activity is induced by MTX exposure,[148] and this induction of enzyme has been implicated as a possible mechanism of folate depletion with resultant neurotoxicity.[136]

Yao et al.[149] isolated and cloned the complementary DNA (cDNA) for GGH, which codes for an enzyme of 318 amino acids and has a molecular weight of 36 kd. Human GGH acts as an exopeptidase, yielding MTX polyglutamate forms ranging in size from Glu_4 to Glu_1. Rhee[150] further characterized human cellular GGH and found that the enzyme cleaved both the ultimate and penultimate γ-linkages of MTX polyglutamates. Using human HT-1080 fibrosarcoma cells, Waltham et al.[151] characterized the native form of secreted GGH, which is derived from a lysosomal compartment within the cell, and the enzyme displayed a marked preference for long-chain polyglutamate forms. Several glutamine antagonists including azaserine, acivicin, and 6-diazo-5-oxo-L-norleucine are potent inhibitors of partially purified GGH in cell-free systems.

MTX polyglutamates exist essentially only within cells and enter or exit cells sparingly.[130,152–154] The diglutamate form has an uptake velocity of one-fifteenth that of MTX,[155] whereas higher glutamates have even slower transport rates.[130,152–154] Thus, MTX polyglutamates are selectively retained in preference to parent drug as extracellular

levels of MTX fall after drug exposure. The assumption has widely been made that the enhanced cellular retention of MTX polyglutamates relative to MTX was determined at the level of transmembrane transport as it relates specifically to efflux. Studies using an inside-out plasma membrane vesicle system, however, revealed that MTX and MTX polyglutamates are equal as permeants for efflux of MTX through the plasma membrane.[156] These results suggest that intracellular compartmentalization of MTX polyglutamates may play a more critical role in determining their final intracellular accumulation.

Several parameters influence a cell's ability to polyglutamate MTX. Paramount among these factors is the rate of cell growth[131,157–159] and the level of intracellular folates.[157–162] Enhancement of cell proliferation with growth factors such as insulin,[132,161] dexamethasone, tocopherol,[132] and estrogen in hormone-responsive cells increases polyglutamation, whereas deprivation of essential amino acids[163] results in inhibition of polyglutamation. Methionine appeared to decrease polyglutamation in normal rat hepatocytes, whereas it increased or had little effect on this process in hepatoma cells.[161] MTX and L-asparaginase are frequently used in combination for the treatment of acute leukemia. Conversion of MTX to polyglutamate forms can be markedly inhibited by preexposure to L-asparaginase, presumably through amino acid deprivation with resultant growth arrest.[164] Increasing intracellular folate pools through exposure of cells to high concentrations of leucovorin or 5-methyltetrahydrofolate results in a decrease in MTX polyglutamation.[127,160,162] Conversely, the process is enhanced in human hepatoma cells either by incubating cells with MTX in folate-free medium or by first depleting the intracellular folates by "permeabilizing" cell membranes with lysolecithin in a folate-free environment.[157–159]

An important factor in the selective nature of MTX cytotoxicity may derive from diminished polyglutamate formation in normal tissues relative to that in malignant tissues. Although little metabolism to polyglutamates is observed in normal murine intestinal cells *in vivo*, most murine leukemias and Ehrlich ascites tumor cells efficiently convert MTX to higher polyglutamate forms in tumor-bearing animals.[45,165] Normal human and murine myeloid progenitor cells form relatively small amounts of MTX polyglutamates compared with leukemic cells.[125,126] Human myeloid precursor cells polyglutamated MTX to levels that were insufficient to saturate DHFR after a 24-hour exposure to a concentration of 1 μmol per L and resulted in no cytotoxicity.[125,126] DHFR saturation by MTX polyglutamates was generated with a drug exposure of 10 μmol per L, a finding that correlated with cytotoxicity.

In addition to increasing its retention within cells, polyglutamation of MTX enhances its inhibitory effects on specific folate-dependent enzymes. The pentaglutamates have a slower dissociation rate from DHFR than does MTX[128,166] and a markedly enhanced inhibitory potency for TS (K_i = 50 nmol per L), AICAR transformylase (K_i = 57 nmol per L),[167] and, to a lesser extent, GAR transformylase (K_i = 2 μmol per L) in the presence of monoglutamated folate substrates.[14,167] The well-described incomplete depletion of physiologic folate cofactors by MTX suggests that direct enzymatic inhibition of purine and TS by MTX polyglutamates may contribute to MTX cytotoxicity. These effects may also explain the competitive nature of leucovorin rescue and the selective rescue of normal versus malignant tissues, in that rescue may depend on the ability of leucovorin and its derived tetrahydrofolates to compete with MTX polyglutamates at sites other than DHFR.

The ability of antifolate analogs to undergo polyglutamation is one of several properties that influences cytotoxicity. Aminopterin is a better substrate for FPGS than is MTX and is a more potent cytotoxic agent. A fluorinated MTX analog, PT430, is a weak substrate for FPGS and has little cytotoxic activity.[168] The ability to generate MTX polyglutamates has been correlated with sensitivity to MTX in studies of both human and murine tumor cells,[168,169] and several cancer cell lines have been isolated that are highly resistant to MTX on the basis of decreased polyglutamate formation.[169,170]

Although defective polyglutamation may coexist with other metabolic alterations, examples of pure polyglutamation defects have been described in human leukemia cell lines (CCRF-CEM)[171] and in human squamous cancer cell lines derived from head and neck tumors.[172] In an attempt to simulate the clinical use of MTX, a resistant subline was established after short-term (24-hour) exposure to moderately high MTX concentrations. Resistance to MTX was due solely to an impaired ability to polyglutamate MTX, which was the result of a decreased level of FPGS enzyme activity.[173] Faessel et al.[174] evaluated the combined action among polyglutamylatable and nonpolyglutamylatable antifolates directed against DHFR, TS, glycinamide ribonucleotide formyltransferase, and 5-aminoimidazole-4-carboxamide ribonucleotide formyltransferase in human ileocecal HCT-8 cells *in vitro*. The authors determined that polyglutamation played a critical role in fostering synergy between inhibitors of DHFR and inhibitors of other folate-requiring enzymes. Further evidence for the role of polyglutamation as a determinant of drug sensitivity stems from investigations using other antifolates such as the GAR transformylase inhibitor DDATHF. Polyglutamates of DDATHF were readily formed in cultured human leukemia cell lines and were found to be retained for prolonged periods in drug-free conditions. The FPGS-deficient CCRF-CEM cell line generated few DDATHF polyglutamates and was insensitive to drug exposure.[175] An MTX-resistant rat hepatoma H35 cell line was established that demonstrated cross-resistance to the antifolate analog CB3717, an inhibitor of TS.[176] In this resistant cell line, the level of CB3717 polyglutamates was significantly less than that in the parental rat hepatoma H35 cell line, and

this impaired level of polyglutamation was due to an enhanced level of GGH enzyme activity. Jackman et al.[176a] described the cellular pharmacology and *in vivo* activity of ZD9331, a nonpolyglutamylatable, water-soluble TS inhibitor. Using the mouse cell line L1210:RD1694, which is characterized by an acquired resistance to ZD1694 due to reduced folylpolyglutamate synthetase, the authors noted that antitumor activity was not significantly cross-resistant to ZD9331.

Polyglutamation has been investigated as a determinant of response to MTX in clinical chemotherapy. In a study of six human small cell carcinoma cell lines that had demonstrated resistance *in vitro* after clinical treatment with MTX, two were resistant on the basis of a low capacity to form MTX polyglutamates.[177] One of seven samples from MTX-resistant leukemic patients demonstrated a decreased ability to form MTX polyglutamates as the sole explanation for resistance.[82] Investigating the reduced accumulation of long-chain MTX polyglutamates in ALL patients, Longo found a decrease in the binding affinity (K_m) of MTX to FPGS from blast cells of patients with acute myelogenous leukemia (AML) as opposed to ALL.[152] This difference in affinity resulted in a predominance of MTX-Glu$_1$ species in AML cells, and MTX Glu$_{3-5}$ in ALL cells. No corresponding disparity in binding affinity was found when the equivalently cytotoxic antifolate TS inhibitors raltitrexed and BW1843U89, which exhibited similar levels of accumulation of the higher polyglutamate forms, were examined. A more recent study by Longo et al.[178] suggests that the evaluation of GGH and folylpolyglutamate synthetase activity at the time of clinical diagnosis may be used as a predictor of the extent of MTX polyglutamation and, therefore, of response to MTX therapy and outcome in patients with acute leukemias. Hyperdiploid status in childhood ALL is a good prognostic feature, and patients exhibiting hyperdiploid lymphoblasts show higher levels of synthesis of cytotoxic MTX polyglutamates than patients exhibiting aneuploid or diploid lymphoblasts. Galpin et al.[179] found a higher concentration of MTX long-chain polyglutamates in T than in B lymphoblasts and an increased level of expression of FPGS mRNA in B-lineage cells. These findings suggest that the higher response rates observed in patients with B-cell ALL may result from increased levels of FPGS activity that, in turn, facilitate enhanced intracellular formation of more cytotoxic MTX polyglutamates. A 3-day *in situ* assay for TS was established to characterize antifolate resistance in previously untreated patients with soft tissue sarcomas.[180,181] When fresh tumor specimens were used, 12 of 15 human sarcomas were determined to be naturally resistant to MTX as a result of impaired polyglutamation.[180]

Binding to Dihydrofolate Reductase

The physical characteristics of binding of NADPH [reduced form of nicotinamide adenine dinucleotide phosphate (NADP)] and MTX to DHFR have been established by x-ray crystallographic studies, nuclear magnetic resonance spectroscopy, amino acid sequencing of native and chemically modified enzyme, and site-directed mutagenesis. Enzyme from microbial, chicken, and mammalian sources have been studied[182–194]; strong amino acid sequence homology is found at positions involved in substrate cofactor and inhibitor binding.[195] In general, a long hydrophobic pocket binds MTX and is formed in part by the isoleucine-5, alanine-7, aspartate-27, phenylalanine-31 (Phe-31), phenylalanine-34 (Phe-34), and other amino acid residues. Several particularly important interactions contribute to the binding potency of the 4-amino antifolates: (a) hydrogen bonding of the carbonyl oxygen of isoleucine-5 to the 4-amino group of the inhibitor; (b) a salt bridge between aspartate and the N-1 position of MTX, which is not involved in binding to the physiologic substrates; (c) hydrophobic interactions of the inhibitor with DHFR, particularly with Phe-31 and Phe-34; (d) hydrogen bonding of the 2-amino group to aspartate-27 and to a structurally consistent bound water molecule; and (e) hydrogen binding of the terminal glutamate to an invariant arginine-70 residue. Investigations have identified the importance of the interactions of MTX with Phe-31 and Phe-34 because mutations in these positions result in a 100-fold and 80,000-fold decrease in MTX affinity for the enzyme, respectively.[196,197] Mutation of arginine-70 results in a decrease in MTX affinity by greater than 22,000-fold but does not alter the binding affinity of trimetrexate, which lacks the terminal glutamate moiety. This finding supports the essential role of arginine-70 in the binding of inhibitors that preserve the terminal glutamate structure.[198] Mutations outside the enzyme active site also may result in marked reductions in folate and antifolate affinities.[199] In addition, the physiologic substrate dihydrofolate is bound to the enzyme in an inverted, or "upside down," configuration compared with the inhibitor MTX[186,193,196,200] The reader is referred to more detailed reviews of this subject for consideration of substrate and cofactor binding characteristics and mutated DHFR cDNA studies.[188–194,201–211]

Optimal binding of MTX to DHFR is dependent on the concentration of NADPH. NADH (reduced form of nicotinamide adenine dinucleotide) may also act as a cosubstrate for DHFR but, unlike NADPH, it does not promote binding of MTX to the enzyme.[212] Thus, the intracellular ratios of NADPH/NADP and NADPH/NADH may play an important role in the selective action of MTX to the extent that the cosubstrate ratios may differ in malignant and in normal tissues.[165,212] In the presence of excess NADPH, the binding affinity of MTX for DHFR has been estimated to lie between 10 and 200 pmol per L,[211,213,214] although this affinity is significantly affected by pH, salt concentration, and the status of enzyme sulfhydryl groups. Under conditions of low pH and with a low ratio

of inhibitor to enzyme, binding is essentially stoichiometric,[215] that is, one molecule of MTX is bound to one molecule of DHFR.

Binding of MTX to DHFR isolated from bacterial and mammalian sources in the presence of NADPH generates a slowly formed ternary complex. The overall process has been termed slow, tight-binding inhibition and involves an initial rapid but weak enzyme-inhibitor interaction followed by a slow but extremely tight-binding isomerization to the final complex.[190,209,216–220] The final isomerization step probably involves a conformational change of the enzyme with subsequent binding of the para-aminobenzoyl moiety to the enzyme.[191,220] Other folate analogs, such as aminopterin, follow the same slow, tight-binding kinetic process, in contrast to the pteridines and pyrimethamine, which behave as classic inhibitors of the bacterial enzymes.[211] Trimethoprim is considered to be a classical, albeit weak, inhibitor of mammalian DHFR. Of note, it does not undergo an isomerization process to the ternary complex form.[209]

In the therapeutic setting, MTX acts as a tight-binding but reversible inhibitor. Under conditions of high concentrations of competitive substrate (dihydrofolate) and at neutral intracellular pH, a considerable excess of free drug is required to fully inhibit the enzyme. Both in tissue culture and in cell-free systems, tritium-labeled MTX bound to intracellular enzyme can be displaced by exposure of cells to unlabeled drug, dihydrofolate,[9,221–223] or reduced folates such as leucovorin and 5-methyltetrahydrofolate,[165] which indicates a slow but definite "off rate" or dissociation of MTX from the enzyme.[165,224,225] Thus, an excess of free, or unbound, drug is required to maintain total inhibition of DHFR.[226]

The polyglutamates of MTX have similar potency in their tight-binding inhibition of mammalian DHFR[129,209,227] and possess a slower rate of dissociation from the enzyme than the parent compound. In pulse-chase experiments using intact human breast cancer cells, MTX pentaglutamate was found to have a dissociation half-life of 120 minutes compared to 12 minutes for the parent compound. Cell-free experiments using purified preparations of mammalian enzyme indicate that MTX polyglutamation has a modest effect in enhancing binding and catalytic inhibition (twofold to sixfold) of DHFR.[14,209,214,228] Like MTX, enzyme-bound MTX polyglutamates may also be displaced by reduced folates[165] and high concentrations of dihydrofolate,[229,230] albeit at a slower rate than MTX.

These observations indicate that, in the absence of free drug, a small fraction of intracellular DHFR, either through new synthesis or through dissociation from the inhibitor, becomes available for catalytic activity and is adequate to allow for continued intracellular metabolism. The requirement for excess free drug to inhibit enzyme activity completely is important in understanding the clinical effects and toxicity of this agent, and is fundamental to the relationship between pharmacokinetics and pharmacodynamics. Jackson et al. have reported a close correlation between cytotoxicity and the affinity of drug binding to DHFR for a series of murine leukemias with differing sensitivity to MTX.[213] Resistance to MTX as a result of decreased DHFR binding affinity for MTX has been described in murine leukemic cells,[199,231–234] Chinese hamster ovary[235] and lung[236] cells, and murine and hamster lung fibroblast cells.[237–239] These mutant enzymes may have several thousand–fold reduced binding affinity for MTX and, in general, are less efficient in catalyzing the reduction of dihydrofolate than is wild-type DHFR. Analysis of a DHFR cDNA isolated from a DHFR-amplified and MTX-resistant human colon cancer cell revealed a single base mutation that resulted in an amino acid substitution at position 31 (phenylalanine → serine).[69] Binding studies further demonstrated that the DHFR enzyme had an eightfold decrease in binding affinity for MTX compared with DHFR isolated from the parent cell line. A similar finding of DHFR gene amplification with altered MTX affinity has been observed in an MTX-resistant Chinese hamster ovary cell line.[240]

Drug-sensitive Chinese hamster lung cells have been found to express two different forms of DHFR encoded by distinct alleles.[236,241,242] The two species differ in molecular weight and isoelectric point (21,000 versus 20,000 and 6.7 versus 6.5) and result from a single amino acid substitution of asparagine for aspartic acid at position 95. Either allele may be predominantly expressed in various subclones of the parent cell line. This observation raises the possibility that distinct naturally occurring DHFR alleles may exist in a variety of tissues and, to the extent that they may confer differential sensitivity to MTX, this DHFR genetic polymorphism of the host may serve as a mechanism by which cells may become clinically MTX resistant.

DHFR with reduced affinity for MTX may represent a clinically important mechanism of MTX resistance, as this phenomenon was observed in the leukemic cells of 4 of 12 patients with resistant AML.[243]

A common finding in MTX-resistant cells is an increase in the expression of DHFR protein with no associated change in the enzyme's affinity for MTX.[244] Elevated levels of DHFR enzyme may be detected by assaying tumor cell homogenates or by labeling the enzyme with a fluorescent MTX derivative. The latter compound has been used for the identification and recovery of resistant clones with as little as twofold increases in DHFR gene copy.[245–247] Elevations in DHFR may persist for many generations of cell renewal in tumor cells from resistant patients.[248] In resistant murine leukemic cells, the increased DHFR activity results from reduplication of the DHFR gene (Fig. 7-4), a process that has been shown to occur by exposing murine and

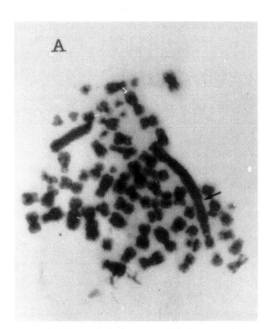 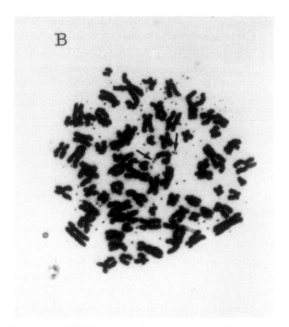

FIGURE 7-4. A: Marker chromosomes found in methotrexate (MTX)-resistant breast cancer cells. A human breast cancer cell line, MCF-7, resistant to MTX was isolated by growing cells in gradually increasing drug concentrations. These cells are resistant to drug concentrations more than 200-fold higher than those that kill wild-type cells and contain more than 30-fold increases in dihydrofolate reductase (DHFR). The arrow indicates a marker chromosome with a greatly expanded homogenously staining region. (Courtesy of Cowan K, Lippman M, and Douglas P, National Cancer Institute, Bethesda, MD 20892.) **B:** Metaphase plate of a small cell lung cancer carcinoma cell line taken from a patient with clinical MTX resistance. The prominent double-minute chromosomes (*arrows*) were associated with amplification of the drug target enzyme, DHFR. (From Curt GA, Carney DN, Cowan KH, et al. Unstable methotrexate resistance in human small-cell carcinoma associated with double minute chromosomes. *N Engl J Med* 1983;308:199–202.)

human leukemia and carcinoma cells in culture to stepwise increases in the concentration of MTX.[239,241,245,249–259] Gene reduplication may take the form of a homogeneously staining region (HSR) on chromosomes or nonintegrated pieces of DNA known as double-minute chromosomes (Fig. 7-4B). Although HSRs appear to confer stable resistance to the cell, double-minute chromosomes are unequally distributed during cell division,[239,253,254] and in the absence of the continued selective pressure of drug exposure, the cells revert to the original low-DHFR genotype. Evidence exists that gene amplification occurs initially in the form of double-minute chromosomes, because this is the predominant abnormality in low-level drug-resistant cells, whereas HSRs occur in highly resistant cells that contain multiple gene copies.[239,253,254,259] A third mechanism of gene amplification has been identified in an MTX-resistant HeLA 10B3 cell line in which were found submicroscopic extrachromosomal elements (amplisomes) containing amplified DHFR genes. These amplisomes appeared early in the development of MTX resistance and were not found to be integrated into the chromosome nor were they associated with double-minute chromosomes. Although these amplisomes were lost in the absence of the selective pressure of MTX, they disappeared at a much slower rate than would be predicted from simple dilution of nonreplicating elements.

Although MTX resistance through DHFR gene amplification becomes apparent only after the prolonged selective pressure of drug exposure, studies[260,261] indicate that highly MTX-resistant cells may be generated by gene amplification within a single cell cycle. Early S-phase cells exposed transiently to agents that block DNA synthesis (e.g., hydroxyurea) may undergo reduplication of multiple genes synthesized during early S phase, including DHFR, after removal of the DNA synthetic inhibitor. This finding has broad implications for the rapid development of drug resistance in patients treated with MTX and other inhibitors of DNA synthesis. Exposure of cells to a variety of chemical and physical agents unrelated to MTX—including hypoxia, alkylating agents,[262,263] ultraviolet irradiation,[263,264] phorbol esters,[263–266] *cis*-diamminedichloro-platinum,[267,268] doxorubicin,[269,270] and 5-fluorodeoxyuridine[271]—may induce MTX resistance through DHFR gene amplification, with subsequent increases in DHFR protein. The induction of MTX resistance by a variety of chemical and physical agents may explain *de novo* MTX resistance in certain human tumors, given the constant presence of a host of environmental carcinogens.

To begin to identify the underlying molecular basis for the process of gene amplification, studies have investigated the interaction between overexpression of oncogenes and DHFR gene amplification and the subsequent development of MTX resistance.[272] Of note, the induced expression of *c-myc* mRNA in rat embryo fibroblasts was associated with DHFR gene amplification and MTX resistance.

Unlike in malignant cells, amplification of DNA has not been reported in normal cells of patients undergoing therapy with cytotoxic agents. To further address this issue, drug-resistant colonies of either normal mammary epithelial cells or normal diploid fibroblast cells were established after selection in MTX.[273] Although some MTX-resistant colonies were observed when normal fibroblast cells were treated with MTX, no evidence was found of DHFR gene amplification. Thus, the process of DHFR gene amplification appears to be rare in normal human cell lines compared with human cancers and cancer cell lines.

In addition to gene amplification, more subtle mechanisms exist for increasing DHFR expression. Molecular analysis of the DHFR gene encoding for overexpressed DHFR protein has occasionally revealed significant differences in non–protein coding regions that may impact mRNA expression.[241] Exposure of human breast cancer cells to MTX results in an acute increase (up to fourfold) in the cellular DHFR content that is dependent on both duration of exposure to drug and drug concentration.[257,274,275] The expression of DHFR protein appears to be controlled at the level of mRNA translation, as no acute associated change occurs in the amount of DHFR mRNA or DHFR gene copy number after MTX exposure nor are alterations seen in DHFR enzyme stability. When an RNA gel mobility shift assay was used, human recombinant DHFR protein was shown specifically to bind to its corresponding DHFR mRNA.[276] Incubation of DHFR protein either with the normal substrates dihydrofolate or NADPH, or with MTX completely represses its binding to the target DHFR mRNA. In an *in vitro* translation system, this specific interaction between DHFR and its message is associated with inhibition of translation. These studies provide evidence for a translational autoregulatory mechanism underlying the control of DHFR expression (Fig. 7-5). The presence of either excess MTX or dihydrofolate prevent DHFR protein from performing its normal autoregulatory function, thereby allowing for increased DHFR protein synthesis. Thus, the ability to regulate DHFR expression at the translational level allows normal cellular function to be maintained in the setting of an acute cellular stress and represents a unique mechanism whereby cells can react to and overcome the inhibitory effects of MTX and antifolate analogs. In further attempts to characterize DHFR autoregulation, Bertino et al.[277] used a series of truncated DHFR mRNA probes to investigate whether the enzyme directly contacts its cognate mRNA. A resultant DHFR protein/RNA interaction was found in an approximately 100–base-pair portion in the protein coding region that contains two putative stem-loop structures (Fig. 7-5). In addition, the DHFR/RNA interaction was prevented by the binding of MTX to DHFR, which thereby relieved translational autoregulation.

Although various *in vitro* and *in vivo* model systems have clearly demonstrated an association between DHFR gene amplification and MTX resistance, the clinical significance of gene amplification remains uncertain. Tumor samples from patients resistant to MTX have been evaluated, and several clinical specimens have been found to possess elevated levels of DHFR enzyme in association with DHFR gene amplification.[278–281] A small cell lung carcinoma cell line isolated from

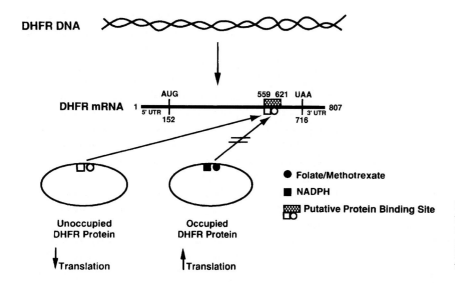

FIGURE 7-5. Proposed model for autoregulatory control of dihydrofolate reductase (DHFR) messenger RNA (mRNA) translation by DHFR protein. Numbers correspond to nucleic acid base location. (NADPH, reduced form of nicotinamide adenine dinucleotide phosphate.)

a patient clinically resistant to high-dose MTX was found to have amplification of the DHFR gene and increased expression of DHFR protein.[278,282] This amplification was associated with the presence of double-minute chromosomes (Fig. 7-4B). After serial passage in drug-free media, cells lost the double-minute chromosomes on which the amplified genes resided and regained drug sensitivity. Clinical MTX resistance attributable to DHFR amplification was also investigated in two patients with acute leukemia and in one patient with ovarian cancer. In all three cases, amplification of DHFR gene copies (twofold to threefold) with increased DHFR protein (threefold to sixfold) was observed, and the increase in DHFR gene copy number was postulated to be directly associated with the development of MTX resistance.[279–281] Matherly et al. found a markedly greater frequency of DHFR overexpression in T-cell ALL than in B-precursor ALL in children. The authors speculated that this difference in DHFR expression was associated with the poorer prognosis of T-cell ALL treated with standard doses of antimetabolites, implying that higher-dose MTX consolidation therapy may be better used in this population.[283,284]

Pharmacologic approaches directed toward circumventing MTX resistance due to altered or amplified DHFR have included the use of lipophilic MTX analogs such as trimetrexate and piritrexim. These agents achieve intracellular concentrations 30- to 60-fold higher than MTX at comparable extracellular drug concentrations[30,285] and are only partially cross-resistant with MTX in DHFR-amplified cell lines.[95]

Consequences of Dihydrofolate Reductase Enzyme Inhibition

The critical cellular events associated with MTX inhibition of DHFR are illustrated in Figure 7-1. Thymidylate synthase catalyzes the sole biochemical reaction resulting in the oxidation of tetrahydrofolates.

The compound 5,10-methylenetetrahydrofolate is oxidized to dihydrofolate and a methylene group is transferred to deoxyuridylate, which leads to the formation of thymidylate. Continued activity of this enzymatic reaction in the presence of DHFR inhibition results in rapid accumulation of intracellular levels of dihydrofolate in the polyglutamated form. This accumulation is temporally associated with a depletion of several critical reduced-folate pools, most notably 5-methyltetrahydrofolate. In several *in vitro* cell systems studied to date, however, the reduced-folate cofactors required for *de novo* purine and thymidylate synthesis (10-formyltetrahydrofolate and 5,10-methylenetetrahydrofolate) are relatively preserved in the presence of cytotoxic concentrations of MTX.[9–12,14,286] In studies using human breast cancer cells, purified normal human myeloid precursor cells, and murine leukemia cells, exposure to lethal concentrations of MTX resulted in a 70% to 80% preservation of 10-formyltetrahydrofolate pools compared with untreated controls (Fig. 7-6). Additional studies using human breast cancer cells, promyelocytic leukemia cells, normal human myeloid progenitor cells, and Krebs ascites cells and L1210 murine leukemia cells grown in the peritoneal cavity of mice confirm a partial preservation of 5,10-methylenetetrahydrofolate pools (50% to 70%) during MTX exposures that produce profound TS inhibition and cytotoxicity.[13,14] Subsequent computer modeling of the intracellular human folate pools based on experimental data confirm the importance of direct inhibition of the various folate-dependent enzymes in the metabolic inhibition associated with MTX exposure.[22] To determine the importance of the inhibitory effects of MTX polyglutamates as distinct from the effects of folate depletion and direct dihydrofolate inhibition, several investigators have examined the change in folate pools associated with exposure to trimetrexate, an antifolate that is not polyglutamated but remains a potent inhibitor of DHFR.[22,287–289] Results of

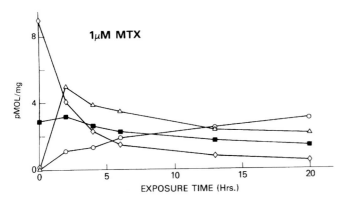

FIGURE 7-6. Effects of 1 μmol/L methotrexate (MTX) on intracellular folate pools in human breast cancer cells (MCF-7). (Δ, dihydrofolate; o, 10-formyldihydrofolate; ■, 10-formyltetrahydrofolate; ◊, 5-methyltetrahydrofolate.) (From Allegra CJ, Fine RL, Drake JC, et al. The effect of methotrexate on intracellular folate pools in human MCF-7 breast cancer cells. Evidence for direct inhibition of purine synthesis. *J Biol Chem* 1986;261:6478–6485.)

various studies are conflicting. In murine leukemia cells, folate pools were relatively preserved and dihydrofolate polyglutamates seemed to serve an essential role in metabolic inhibition. In contrast, folate depletion appeared to be the more critical event in rat hepatoma cells. Presumably, intrinsic differences between these cell lines with regard to the levels of TS, folate pools, and intracellular folate regulation may determine the relative roles of direct enzyme inhibition versus substrate depletion in the metabolic inhibitory effects of MTX. Although partial depletion of reduced-folate cofactors undoubtedly contributes to the inhibition of metabolic pathways, the accumulated dihydrofolate and MTX polyglutamates appear also to play a critical role as direct inhibitors of folate-dependent enzymes in both *de novo* purine and thymidylate synthesis. As mentioned previously, these metabolites are potent inhibitors of TS, AICAR transformylase, and GAR transformylase, and of enzymes responsible for the interconversion of the various folate forms, including 5,10-methylenetetrahydrofolate reductase. The inhibition constants (K_is) for these enzymes are generally in the 0.05 to 5 μmol per L range, depending on the specific reaction and the polyglutamated form of the competing folate substrates. In addition to the finding of partial depletion of reduced folates, the importance of direct metabolic inhibition, particularly by dihydrofolate polyglutamates, is suggested by the strong correlation between the accumulation of these inhibitory metabolites and the profound inhibition of the *de novo* purine synthetic pathway. A novel intracellular folate, 10-formyldihydrofolate, has also been described in MTX-treated human myeloid and breast cancer cells. This folate appears to arise from enzymatic formylation of the accumulated dihydrofolate, and it is a potent inhibitor of GAR transformylase and TS. Interestingly, the compound is a substrate for AICAR transformylase with an

affinity equivalent to that of the natural substrate (10-formyltetrahydrofolate), which provides further evidence that substrate depletion is not the sole mechanism for the metabolic inhibition produced by MTX. Studies have suggested that the primary site of inhibition of *de novo* purine synthesis induced by MTX may be either at or before the reaction catalyzed by GAR transformylase, specifically involving the enzyme amidophosphoribosyltransferase.[23] Isolated enzyme kinetic studies revealed that the polyglutamated forms of dihydrofolate and MTX were potent noncompetitive inhibitor of the enzyme, with apparent K_i values of 3.4 μmol per L and 6 μmol per L, respectively.[290] Thus, MTX-induced metabolic inhibition is a multifactorial process involving various biochemical pathways.

Reduced-folate (leucovorin) rescue of MTX-treated cells may be anticipated to result in an accumulation of reduced folates that would compete with and overcome direct enzymatic inhibition rather than simply replete tetrahydrofolate levels (*vide infra*). This feature may, in large part, explain the competitive nature of leucovorin rescue observed *in vitro* and clinically. Also, selectivity of the cytotoxic effects of MTX and selectivity of leucovorin rescue may depend on the extent to which various normal and malignant cells generate dihydrofolate and MTX polyglutamates.

Relative Importance of Thymidylate and Purine Synthesis Inhibition

Although metabolic inhibition of DNA precursor synthesis is the most obvious effect of antifolates, the relative importance of purine depletion compared with thymidylate depletion is unclear. Zaharko and colleagues have shown that in murine bone marrow cells a block in thymidylate synthesis was established by MTX concentrations of 10 nmol per L or greater, whereas inhibition of purine synthesis occurred only at drug levels of 100 nmol per L or higher.[291] These findings imply that purine synthesis may be relatively conserved at the expense of thymidylate synthesis. Further work with human breast cancer cells in culture has confirmed this difference in sensitivity to MTX between the two folate-dependent pathways.[292] Investigations have demonstrated that DDATHF, by inhibiting purine synthesis, protects cells in a dose-dependent manner from the cytotoxic effects of TS inhibition. These results are consistent with the concept that unbalanced inhibitory effects of MTX on purine and thymidylate synthesis are critical for the cytotoxic efficacy of MTX.[293]

Studies by Taylor and Tattersall using human leukemia cells found that cytotoxicity is best correlated with inhibition of DNA synthesis.[294,295] In general, sources of both purines and thymidine are required to rescue fully from the toxicity of MTX. The relative importance of MTX effects on purine synthesis and on thymidylate synthesis, however, appears to vary with the particular cell line under investigation. Both the antipurine and antithymidylate effects of MTX are a function of the growth rate of cells. TS activity increases during S phase, as does cell sensitivity to MTX.[296] In an examination of four hepatoma cell lines, each with a different growth rate, the most rapidly proliferating cells were most sensitive to the combination of MTX and thymidine, a combination that should allow isolated inhibition of purine synthesis. The slowest growing cells were least sensitive to this combination.[297] In addition, differences in sensitivity to antipurine effects are found even among rapidly growing tumor cells. Tattersall et al. noted that the antipurine effect correlated with the relative cellular activities of 5,10-methylenetetrahydrofolate dehydrogenase and TS.[298] Cells with higher 5,10-methylenetetrahydrofolate dehydrogenase activity, and presumably greater rates of purine synthesis, showed greater sensitivity to the antipurine effects of MTX. The activities of both 5,10-methylenetetrahydrofolate[299,300] and TS[82,177,301,302] influence sensitivity to MTX. Inhibition of TS by 5-fluorodeoxyuridylate or by depletion of its substrate deoxyuridylate diminishes sensitivity to MTX. TS activity in human leukemia, lung carcinoma, and colon carcinoma influences MTX sensitivity; specifically, low levels of TS activity are usually associated with MTX resistance.[82,177,301] In cells with low levels of TS, the slow rate of oxidation of 5,10-methylenetetrahydrofolate creates less dependence on DHFR to regenerate tetrahydrofolates. A block in DHFR produces minimal accumulation of the toxic dihydrofolate and minimal depletion of tetrahydrofolates.

Mechanisms of Cell Death

As a consequence of the multiple effects of antifolates on nucleotide biosynthesis, several mechanisms of cell death are possible. Deoxythymidine triphosphate thymidine 5'-triphosphate and deoxypurine nucleotides are required for both the synthesis of DNA and its repair. Inhibition of thymidylate and purine synthesis leads to a cessation of DNA synthesis, but whether this inhibition, alone, kills cells is unclear. A close correlation is found between DNA strand breaks and cell death in Ehrlich ascites tumor cell exposed to MTX[303]; because the breaks occurred in mature DNA, the authors attributed them to ineffective repair mechanisms due to lack of nucleotides. This work was supported by similar experimental findings in a mutant murine cell line lacking TS activity and grown in thymidine-deplete media[304] and in a Chinese hamster ovary cell line in which DNA damage was prevented by the use of thymidine and hypoxanthine.[305] Another hypothesis that attempts to explain MTX cytotoxicity concerns the increase in intracellular dUMP pools that occurs as a consequence of inhibition of *de novo* thymidylate synthesis. Clearly the high concentrations of dUMP may ultimately lead to misincorporation of dUMP and deoxyuridine triphosphate into cellular DNA; in the presence of 10 μmol per L MTX, human lymphoblasts incorporate approximately 1 pmol of dUMP

per 1 μmol DNA.[306,307] An enzyme, uracil-DNA-glycosylase, specifically excises uracil bases from DNA, a process that may be responsible for the fragments of DNA observed in antifolate-treated cells with high levels of uracil incorporation.[308–311] These studies implicate the presence of lesions expected in DNA undergoing excision repair of misincorporated uracil nucleotides. Further evidence for the importance of uracil misincorporation derives from a study of seven cell lines that varied widely in deoxyuridine triphosphatase activity.[312] An inverse correlation between deoxyuridine triphosphatase activity and MTX toxicity was found, which suggests that the level of deoxyuridine triphosphate misincorporation into DNA is an important factor in MTX cytotoxicity. Although these studies offer insights into the consequences of uracil misincorporation into DNA, they do not explain the marked toxicity of MTX-thymidine combinations, which must act through an antipurine effect. Probably both uracil nucleotide misincorporation (with subsequent excision repair) and the combined effects of purine and pyrimidine depletion result in the formation of DNA strand breaks. Although the induction of DNA strand breaks is central to the activity of MTX, it is the cellular response to these breaks that ultimately determines whether a cell incurring a given level of DNA damage dies.[313–315] The identification of the critical cell death effectors will enable the development of more potent and hopefully more selective therapeutic strategies.

Pharmacokinetic and Cytokinetic Determinants of Cytotoxicity

At least two pharmacokinetic factors—drug concentration and duration of cell exposure—are critical determinants of cytotoxicity. In tissue culture and in intact animals, extracellular drug concentrations of 10 nmol per L are required to inhibit thymidylate synthesis in normal bone marrow. This same drug concentration is associated with depletion of bone marrow cellularity when maintained for 24 hours or longer. The rate of cell loss from murine bone marrow increases with increasing drug concentrations up to 10 μmol per L[316] (Fig. 7-7). Similar findings have been reported in studies with murine tumor cells. Compared with drug concentration, the duration of exposure to MTX is a more critical factor in determining cell death, provided the minimal threshold concentration for cytotoxicity is exceeded. For a given dose of drug, cell loss is directly proportional to the time period of exposure but doubles only with a tenfold increase in drug concentration.[317] This relationship is likely the result of the S-phase specificity of MTX. With longer duration of exposure, more cells are allowed to enter the vulnerable DNA-synthetic phase of the cell cycle.

Time and concentration correlates of cytotoxicity for human tumor cells have also been studied. Hryniuk and Bertino found variable inhibition of thymidine incorporation into DNA of human leukemic cells in short-term cul-

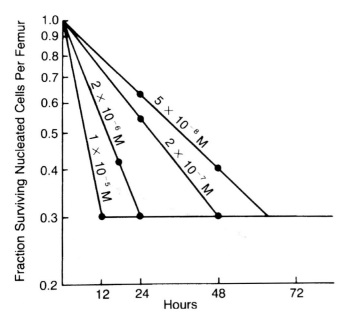

FIGURE 7-7. Nucleated cells per femur remaining after constant infusion of methotrexate sodium into mice to achieve indicated drug concentration for various periods. (From Pinedo HM, Zaharko DS, Bull J, et al. The relative contribution of drug concentration and duration of exposure to mouse bone marrow toxicity during continuous methotrexate infusion. *Cancer Res* 1977;37:445–450.)

ture when these cells were exposed to 1 μmol per L MTX for 1 hour or less.[318] In leukemia cell lines, the duration of exposure appears to play a far more important role than absolute drug concentration. A marked increase in toxicity (30-fold) was appreciated only when the duration rather than drug concentration was increased,[317] provided both parameters were changed by similar increments.

In addition to pharmacokinetic and cytokinetic factors, physiologic compounds in the cellular environment may profoundly affect the cytotoxicity of MTX. Most prominent among these factors are the naturally occurring purine bases, purine nucleosides, and thymidine. In bone marrow and intestinal epithelium, the *de novo* synthesis of both thymidylate and purines is inhibited by concentrations of MTX above 100 nmol per L, but cells can survive this block when bone marrow is supplied with 10 μmol per L thymidine and a purine source (adenosine, inosine, or hypoxanthine) at similar concentrations. Thymidine alone is incapable of completely reversing the cytotoxic effect of MTX.[299] The purine salvage pathways in normal bone marrow appear to be highly efficient, however, and the endogenous concentrations of purines in this tissue are high, albeit variable.[319] Plasma thymidine levels in humans have been reported to be approximately 0.2 μmol per L,[320] whereas the concentration of the purine bases and nucleosides is somewhat higher (0.5 μmol per L).[321] Thus, under basal conditions, the concentrations of purines and thymidine would appear inadequate to rescue cells. Clinical investigations using the nucleoside transport inhibitor

dipyridamole, however, have demonstrated an increase in toxicity when combined with MTX, which suggests that physiologic concentrations of nucleosides may affect the toxicity and potentially the antitumor activity of MTX.[322] Pharmacologic interventions, such as allopurinol treatment (which elevates circulating hypoxanthine concentrations) and chemotherapy, with subsequent tumor lysis, may further raise levels of the circulating nucleosides and ameliorate toxicity to tumor or host tissues.

In an effort to improve MTX antitumor activity and reduce host toxicity in normal tissue, investigators have tested combinations of MTX and thymidine in animals and humans. This combination is based on the rationale that normal tissues might be less sensitive to the antipurine effects of MTX (see Consequences of Dihydrofolate Reductase Enzyme Inhibition) and might have greater ability to use thymidine than tumor cells. When MTX is administered first, an antipurine effect is established, and subsequent exposure to thymidine reverses only the antithymidylate action of MTX.[225] In non–tumor-bearing animals, thymidine is ineffective in reversing or preventing toxicity to normal tissues, probably due to the low concentrations of circulating purines.[323] In tumor-bearing animals, thymidine rescue does ameliorate host toxicity, and the combination produces results superior to those of MTX alone in selected test systems.[324,325] Clearly, however, therapeutic gains observed in a given model system may not be extrapolated to other model systems,[326] and caution should be used in attempting to apply nucleoside rescue to humans, based on animal models. These concerns are rooted in the lack of predictability in a given tumor and the ability of normal tissues to salvage exogenous nucleosides. Although exogenous nucleosides can rescue normal cells, they can also prevent toxicity to malignant cells, and in some systems these effects occur in parallel and result in little therapeutic gain.[326] The toxic and therapeutic results of clinical trials of this combination clearly indicate that antifolate toxicity is lessened in humans by thymidine, but the therapeutic value of the combination is doubtful. Augmentation of the cytotoxicity of MTX has also been achieved in human colon cancer cell lines by inhibiting thymidine salvage with the use of the nucleoside transport inhibitor dipyridamole.[327] Although of potential importance, the selectivity of this approach with respect to normal tissues has not been fully investigated.

A third determinant of antifolate cytotoxic action is the concentration of reduced folate in the circulation. The compound 5-methyltetrahydrofolate (the predominant circulating folate cofactor), when present in sufficient concentration, can readily reverse MTX toxicity,[328] as can leucovorin.[329] Circulating levels of 5-methyltetrahydrofolate are approximately 0.01 μmol per L and of little pharmacologic relevance. Exogenous administration of reduced folates, however, is able to reverse MTX toxicity in a competitive manner. Leucovorin is commonly used after MTX administration to reduce or prevent toxicity and is effective when

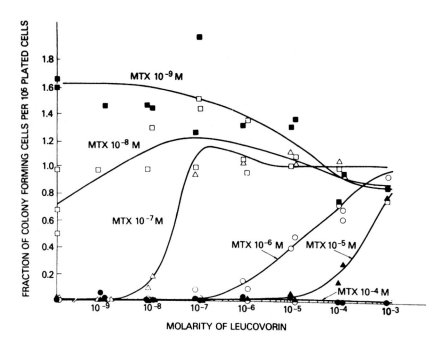

FIGURE 7-8. Effect of various combinations of leucovorin calcium and methotrexate sodium (MTX) on formation of granulocyte colonies *in vitro* by mouse bone marrow. Values are normalized to control value for marrow incubated without either drug. (MTX concentrations: ■, 10^{-9} mol/L; □, 10^{-8} mol/L; △, 10^{-7} mol/L; ○, 10^{-6} mol/L; ▲, 10^{-5} mol/L; ●, 10^{-4} mol/L.) (From Pinedo HM, Zaharko DS, Bull JM, et al. The reversal of methotrexate cytotoxicity to mouse bone marrow cells by leucovorin and nucleosides. *Cancer Res* 1976;36:4418–4424.)

given within 24 to 36 hours after MTX treatment. The concentration of leucovorin required to prevent MTX toxicity increases as the drug concentration increases (Fig. 7-8).[299] The reasons for this competitive relationship are only partly understood. However, given the current knowledge of direct enzymatic inhibition of the folate-dependent enzymes in *de novo* purine and thymidylate synthesis by intracellular metabolites formed after MTX treatment, several possibilities exist. Competition may occur at the level of membrane transport because both MTX and the reduced folates share a common transmembrane transport system. When given concurrently with MTX, leucovorin decreases the rate of MTX polyglutamation. An important consideration in leucovorin rescue is its effect on intracellular reduced-folate pools. Competitive concentrations of reduced folate are required to overcome inhibition by dihydrofolate and MTX polyglutamates at folate-dependent enzymes such as TS and AICAR transformylase. In addition, by raising intracellular concentrations of dihydrofolate, leucovorin indirectly increases substrate competition with MTX for the inhibited DHFR enzyme and leads to repletion of the tetrahydrofolate pools. In support of this latter mechanism as the basis for leucovorin rescue are studies that show nearly quantitative conversion of leucovorin to dihydrofolate and the ability of dihydrofolate to (a) compete with MTX and MTX polyglutamates for DHFR binding in intact human cancer cells, (b) reactivate DHFR, and (c) rescue cells from MTX cytotoxicity.[9,222,223,230,330] Furthermore, an important factor in the clinical efficacy of leucovorin rescue relates to the timing and dose of leucovorin.[331] Because leucovorin is capable of reversing the cytotoxic effects of MTX on host and malignant cells, the minimum dose of leucovorin needed to rescue host cells should be used. In patients with head and

neck cancer randomized to receive standard-dose MTX and either leucovorin or placebo rescue starting 24 hours later,[332] both overall toxicity and response rate were significantly lower in patients treated with MTX and leucovorin. This study emphasizes that careful consideration must be given to the dose and timing of leucovorin when used in combination with MTX to avoid rescue of both cancerous and normal tissues.

METHOTREXATE ASSAY

Two methods are commonly used for the rapid assay of MTX and include one that is based on tight binding of drug to DHFR and another that depends on antibody-drug interactions. Both methods provide extremely sensitive measurement of MTX levels greater than 10 nmol per L in biologic fluids. Significant differences are seen, however, in the time required to perform them and in their specificity for parent compound as opposed to metabolites (Table 7-2). The first widely used method,[333] the enzyme inhibition assay, measures MTX concentration by determining the ability of a clinical sample to inhibit DHFR activity. This assay requires the availability of DHFR enzyme and a recording spectrophotometer; samples are assayed in sequence, and serial dilutions of the sample must be tested to find a dilution that inhibits enzyme in the linear range of 25% to 75% inhibition. Thus, the enzyme inhibition assay is time-consuming. Automation and microcomputer technology, however, may allow for a more efficient use of this very sensitive and specific assay.[334]

A competitive binding assay that uses DHFR as the binding protein is available and preserves the specificity

TABLE 7-2. METHOTREXATE ASSAY METHODS

Assay	Advantages	Disadvantages
Dihydrofolate reductase (DHFR) inhibition	Sensitive, no cross-reaction with metabolites	Time consuming
Competitive DHFR binding	Sensitive, no cross-reaction with metabolites, rapid	Not automated
Immunoassay		
Fluorescence polarization	Sensitive, rapid, automated	Cross-reacts with metabolites
Enzyme multiplied	Rapid, automated	Relatively insensitive, cross-reacts with metabolites
High-pressure liquid chromatography	Methotrexate and metabolites individually quantitated	Time consuming, expensive

for parent compound that is observed in the enzyme inhibition assay. In the binding assay, MTX in a biologic sample competes for DHFR binding sites with a known quantity of radiolabeled drug. Enzyme-bound tritium-labeled MTX is separated from free drug by albumin-coated charcoal adsorption of the unbound material, and the bound fraction remaining in the supernatant is assayed for radioactivity. Multiple samples can be run simultaneously and results can be reported on the same day.[335] Trimethoprim, which is commonly used in the oncologic population in combination with sulfonamides for the treatment and prophylaxis of *P. carinii* pneumonia and bacterial infections, cross-reacts with MTX in this assay and may lead to spuriously elevated results when the bacterial enzyme is used.[336] This cross-reaction may be avoided by using a mammalian source of DHFR (e.g., bovine) that does not bind trimethoprim at clinically achievable serum concentrations.

Radioimmunoassays and fluorescence-polarization immunoassays for MTX are also available for routine clinical use,

and employ antibodies generated by an MTX-bovine serum albumin complex.[337,338] These assays are as sensitive (0.01 to 800 μmol per L) and as rapid as the competitive DHFR binding procedure but have somewhat different specificity. The immunoassay antibodies cross-react with one MTX metabolite, 2,4-diamino-N_{10}-methyl pteroic acid (DAMPA) (40%), but not with 7-hydroxymethotrexate (7-OH-MTX) (1%) (Fig. 7-9). At later time points after drug administration, DAMPA is found in plasma in relatively high concentrations (equal to or greater than that of MTX) and thus produces values for the parent compound[339] that are on an average twofold to fourfold higher than the DHFR binding method. A variant of the radioimmunoassay (enzyme-multiplied immunoassay), based on antibody inhibition of an enzyme-MTX complex, is the most rapid assay available but also cross-reacts with DAMPA[340] and has a sensitivity limit of approximately 0.2 μmol per L. This limitation is critical when evaluating patient samples beyond 48 hours, when MTX concentrations may be at the limit of the assay's sensitivity. Prudent

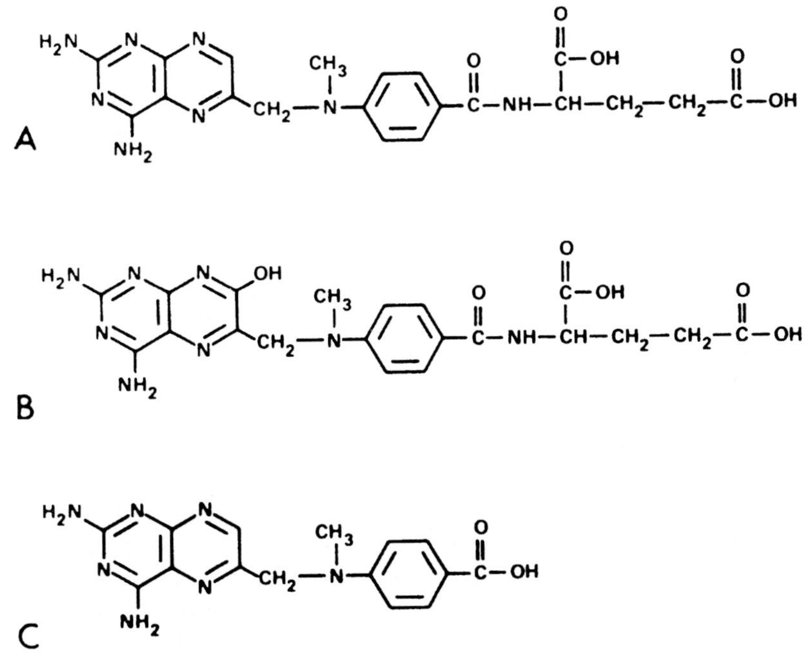

FIGURE 7-9. Methotrexate (MTX) metabolites in humans. **A** is the parent compound; **B** is 7-hydroxymethotrexate (7-OH-MTX); and **C** is 2,4-diamino-N_{10}-methyl pteroic acid (DAMPA).

use of hydration and continued leucovorin can be guided only by accurate measurements of MTX concentrations down to the nontoxic level (approximately 10 nmol per L).[341]

High-pressure liquid chromatography (HPLC) can be used to separate and quantitate MTX and its various metabolites.[339,342] Although the sensitivity of HPLC is primarily limited by the ultraviolet detection systems commonly used (0.2 μmol per L), its sensitivity may be markedly enhanced by serum concentration methods,[342,343] electrochemical detection,[344] or postcolumn derivatization and fluorescence detection.[345] Although HPLC technology is generally too cumbersome for routine clinical monitoring, its use is required when high sensitivity and specificity along with an ability to measure individual MTX metabolites are required. Reports have compared the two more commonly used assay techniques, enzyme-multiplied immunoassay and fluorescence-polarization immunoassay, with HPLC and in over 100 patient plasma samples tested found a high concordance among all three methods.[346,347] Thus, several assays are available for the accurate and rapid measurement of MTX levels in patient samples. The final selection of an assay to be used in the clinical setting may ultimately depend on the requirements for sensitivity, specificity, identification of specific MTX metabolites, and cost and time constraints.

PHARMACOKINETICS

Although the pharmacologic properties of MTX are now better understood at the biochemical and molecular levels, clinical exploitation of this knowledge depends on a detailed understanding of the time profile of drug concentration in extracellular and intracellular spaces and the complex relationship of drug levels to effects on specific tissues. Although antifolate pharmacokinetics is well understood, the important second step—that is, definition of the relationship between drug concentration and effect (pharmacodynamics)—requires continued investigation.

The first attempts to define the distribution and disposition of MTX in a comprehensive manner were reported by Zaharko et al.[348] These authors developed a detailed model for MTX pharmacokinetics that accurately predicted drug-derived radioactivity in various tissue compartments for a 4-hour period after drug administration. The primary elements of that model were (a) elimination of MTX by renal excretion, (b) an active enterohepatic circulation, (c) metabolism of at least a small fraction of drug within the gastrointestinal tract by intestinal flora, and (d) multiple drug half-lives in plasma, the longest of which was found to be approximately 3 hours. Each of these elements has been observed in humans, although a longer terminal half-life is now appreciated, estimated to be between 8 and 27 hours,

depending on the assay method used.[348] HPLC has also disclosed extensive metabolism of MTX in both mice and humans.

Absorption

MTX is absorbed from the gastrointestinal tract by a saturable active transport system.[349] Although small doses are well absorbed, absorption is incomplete at higher doses. Bioavailability for doses of 50 mg per m^2 or greater may be enhanced by subdividing the dose rather than delivering as a single large dose.[349–352] An investigation of the oral bioavailability of MTX given to 15 patients with acute leukemia (6 to 28 mg per m^2) revealed a longer absorptive phase and a lower fractional absorption of the drug for doses greater than 12 mg per m^2 (2.5 hours and 51%, respectively) than for doses less than 12 mg per m^2 (1.5 hours and 87%, respectively).[353]

Drug absorbed in the intestine enters the portal circulation and thus must pass through the liver, where hepatocellular uptake, polyglutamation, and storage all occur; orally administered drug is further subject to degradation (deglutamylation) by intestinal flora to DAMPA, a metabolite that is inactive pharmacologically but that cross-reacts in commonly used radioimmunoassay systems for MTX. Drugs taken orally are also subject to the variability of intestinal absorption created by drug-induced epithelial damage, motility changes, and alterations in flora. One or all of these factors may be responsible for the highly variable nature of MTX pharmacokinetics observed in children receiving small doses of MTX (20 mg per m^2) by mouth.[354] For these reasons, MTX is usually given by systemic routes.

Distribution

The volume of distribution of MTX approximates that of total body water. The drug is loosely bound to serum albumin, with approximately 60% binding at concentrations at or above 1 μmol per L in plasma.[355] Weak organic acids such as aspirin[356] can displace MTX from plasma proteins, but the clinical significance of this displacement process has not been proven.

MTX penetrates slowly into third-space fluid collection, such as pleural effusions[357] or ascites,[358] reaching steady-state plasma concentrations in approximately 6 hours. It also exits slowly from these compartments, producing a concentration gradient of severalfold in favor of the loculated fluid at later time points. The clearance of MTX from peritoneal fluid is approximately 5 mL per minute, substantially less than its clearance from the plasma compartment, which equals or exceeds glomerular filtration (120 mL per minute). The accumulation of drug in closed spaces forms the basis for clinical trials of intraperitoneal chemotherapy with MTX and other antineoplastic agents.[358] In brief, the mechanism responsible for drug accumulation in closed fluid spaces relates to the limited permeability of the peritoneal surface to both charged and high-molecular-weight compounds[359]; thus, only small amounts of drug are able to cross the peritoneal membrane and enter the portal circulation. Drug either not retained or metabolized in the liver passes into the systemic circulation and is then excreted rapidly in the urine. Intraperitoneal installation of MTX produces intraperitoneal drug levels 18- to 36-fold higher than that in plasma, thus providing a large increase in the therapeutic index for the treatment of intraperitoneal disease.[360]

Third-space retention of intravenously administered drug is associated with a prolongation of the terminal drug half-life in plasma, owing presumably to the slow reentry of sequestered drug into the bloodstream.[358] This effect must be considered when treating patients with ascites or pleural effusions. Although no strict guidelines exist for dose adjustment in patients with third-space accumulations, evacuation of this fluid before treatment and close monitoring of plasma drug concentrations in such patients is strongly advisable.

Fossa et al.[361] have described unexpectedly high levels of MTX in bladder cancer patients receiving MTX-based combination chemotherapy who had previously undergone cystectomy and ileal conduit diversion. Plasma levels of MTX greater than 80 nmol per L were observed in 73% of patients who had undergone this surgical procedure but in only 22% of patients with an intact bladder, presumably due to drug resorption from the ileal conduit. Moreover, these patients experienced greater host toxicity in the form of mucositis and diarrhea. Thus, special care must be given to patients with ileal conduit diversions, who are at increased risk for delayed MTX elimination and subsequent MTX toxicity.

Plasma Pharmacokinetics

After the initial distribution phase, which lasts a relatively few minutes, at least two phases of drug disappearance from plasma are observed in laboratory animals and humans. Conventional doses of 25 to 100 mg per m^2 produce peak plasma concentrations of 1 to 10 µmol per L, whereas high-dose infusion regimens using 1.5 g per m^2 or more yield peak levels of 0.1 to 1 mmol per L.[347,353] Whether plasma concentrations are strictly proportional to dose is unclear. Lawrence et al. found a 50% decrease in MTX clearance and disproportionately higher plasma levels after 100 mg intravenous MTX compared with 25 mg doses in the same patient.[362] This nonlinearity was ascribed to saturation of the renal tubular secretory mechanism for MTX, although no direct evidence for this hypothesis was presented. The initial phase of drug disappearance from plasma has a half-life of 2 to 3 hours, with no apparent variation as doses are increased to the high-dose range. This phase extends for the first 12 to 24 hours after drug administration and is largely determined by the rate of renal

excretion of MTX. Prolongation of this phase, as well as of the terminal phase of drug disappearance from plasma, is observed in patients with renal dysfunction, in whom half-life is approximately proportional to the serum creatinine.[363] Bressolle[364] and colleagues studied the effects of moderate renal insufficiency on pharmacokinetics of MTX in patients with rheumatoid arthritis. Intramuscular MTX was administered to four separate groups of patients segregated according to creatinine clearance: less than 45, 45 to 60, 61 to 80, and more than 80 mL per minute. Noting an increased elimination half-life and reduced total clearance that correlated with the degree of renal impairment, the authors concluded that individual renal function testing was preferred over a general decrease of the MTX dose based only on observed serum creatinine. In patients with normal creatinine clearance, the half-life of the initial phase of drug disappearance increases with advancing age of the patient, which lends additional variability to plasma levels, disappearance kinetics, and toxicity.

The final phase of drug disappearance has a considerably longer half-life of 8 to 10 hours[358,361,365,366]; this half-life may further lengthen in patients with renal dysfunction or with third-space fluid such as ascites. After conventional doses of 25 to 200 mg per m^2, this terminal phase begins at drug concentrations above the threshold for toxicity to bone marrow and gastrointestinal epithelium. Thus, any prolongation of the terminal half-life is likely to be associated with significant toxicity.

The use of constant-infusion MTX has received increasing consideration, because it offers the advantage of providing predictable blood and cerebrospinal fluid (CSF) concentrations for a specific period of time. Bleyer[367] has used the following formulas for achieving a desired plasma concentration in patients with normal renal function:

(a) Priming dose (in mg/m^2) = 15 × plasma MTX (in µmol/L) concentration

(b) Infusion dose (in mg/m^2/hour) = 3 × plasma MTX (in µmol/L) concentration

An approximate correction for renal function may be made by reducing the infusion doses in proportion to the reduction in creatinine clearance, based on a normal creatinine clearance of 60 mL per minute per m^2. The terminal elimination phase of MTX increases from 3 to 5 hours in proportion to the duration of the constant infusion over the range of 24 to 72 hours.[368] This variation probably represents slow tissue release of poorly effluxable MTX polyglutamates that form in cells in a time- and dose-dependent manner.

The plasma pharmacokinetics of MTX may independently predict relapse in children treated during the maintenance phase of ALL with intermediate drug doses (1 g per m^2). In a study of 108 children, a rapid drug clearance (84 to 132 mL per minute per m^2) was associated with a 40% risk of relapse, whereas those children with relatively slow drug clearance (45 to 72 mL per minute per m²) had a significantly decreased (p_2 = .01) risk of relapse (25%).[369] Steady-state MTX concentrations of less than 16 µmol per L were also associated with a lower probability of remaining in remission (p <.05) than in patients with concentrations in excess of 16 µmol per L.[370] These associations were further supported by the finding of a systemic clearance of 123 mL per minute per m² in 25 children who relapsed with ALL versus 72 mL per minute per m² in 33 children who remained in continuous remission.[371] These results suggest that dose should be increased in children with rapid drug clearance and low steady-state MTX levels.[372]

Renal Excretion

The bulk of drug is excreted in the urine in the first 12 hours after administration, with renal excretion varying from 44% to virtually 100% of the administered dose.[361,365,366,373] The higher figure is likely to be true for patients with normal renal function. MTX clearance by the kidney has exceeded creatinine clearance in some patients studied. Hande et al. calculated MTX renal clearance to be 194 mL per minute in a patient recovering from drug-induced renal failure,[374] and Monjanel et al. consistently found MTX clearance to exceed creatinine clearance.[375] Other studies, however, have determined

TABLE 7-3. AQUEOUS SOLUBILITY OF METHOTREXATE AND METABOLITES

	Solubility (mg/mL)		
	pH 5.0	pH 6.0	pH 7.0
Methotrexate	0.39	1.55	9.04
7-Hydroxy methotrexate	0.13	0.37	1.55
2,4-diamino-N_{10}-methyl pteroic acid	0.05	0.10	0.85

MTX clearance to be at a level somewhat lower than creatinine clearance.[376]

During high-dose infusion, rapid drug excretion may lead to high MTX concentrations in the urine. These concentrations, approaching 10 mmol per L, exceed the solubility of the drug below pH 7.0 (Table 7-3) and are believed to be responsible for intrarenal precipitation of drug and renal failure. Thus, in high-dose regimens, hydration and alkalinization of the urine are recommended to avoid renal toxicity (Table 7-4). To ensure adequate intrarenal dissolution of MTX during high-dose therapy (0.7 to 8.4 g per m²), a 20-fold greater urine flow is required at pH 5.0 (2 to 42 mL per minute per m²) than at pH 7.0 (0.1 to 1.2 mL per minute per m²).[376] Intensive hydration does not affect the clearance of MTX or the plasma pharmacokinetics, aside from its effects on the prevention of renal damage.[377]

TABLE 7-4. HIGH-DOSE METHOTREXATE SODIUM (MTX) THERAPY

Hydration and urinary alkalinization

Administer 2.5–3.5 L/m²/d of i.v. fluids starting 12 h before and for 24–48 h after administration of MTX drug infusion. Sodium bicarbonate 45–50 mEq/L i.v. fluid to ensure that urine pH is >7.0 at the time of drug infusion.

Commonly used drug infusion regimens

MTX Dose	Duration (h)	Fluid (L/24 h)	Bicarbonate (mEq/24 h)	Leucovorin Calcium Rescue	Onset of Rescue (h after start of MTX)
1.5–7.5 g/m²	6.0	3/m²	NS	15 mg i.v. q3h, then 15 mg p.o. q6h × 7	18
8–12 g/m²	4.0	1.5–2.0/m²	2–3/kg	10 mg p.o. q6h × 10	20
3.0–7.5 g/m²	0.3	3/m²	288/kg	10 mg/m² i.v. × 1, then 10 mg/m² p.o. q6h × 12	24
1 g/m²	24.0	2.4/m²	48/m²	15 mg/m² i.v. q6h × 2, then 3 mg/m² p.o. q12h × 3	36
1.0–7.5 g/m²	0.5	3/m²	288/kg	10 mg/m² i.v. × 1, then 10 mg/m² p.o. q6h × 11	24

NS, not specified.
Adapted from Ackland SP, Schilsky RL. High-dose methotrexate: a critical reappraisal. *J Clin Oncol* 1987;5:2017–2031.

Monitor points

MTX drug levels above 5×10^{-7} mol/L at 48 h after the start of MTX infusion require continued leucovorin rescue. A general guideline for leucovorin rescue is as follows:

MTX Level	Leucovorin Dosage
5×10^{-7} mol/L	15 mg/m² q6h × 8
1×10^{-6} mol/L	100 mg/m² q6h × 8
2×10^{-6} mol/L	200 mg/m² q6h × 8

MTX drug levels should be measured every 24 h and the dosage of leucovorin adjusted until the MTX level is $<5 \times 10^{-8}$ mol/L.

The exact mechanism of MTX excretion in the human kidney has not been fully elucidated. In dog and monkey, active secretion of MTX takes place in the proximal renal tubule, with reabsorption in the distal tubule.[378] As noted earlier, the high clearance values in excess of creatinine clearance suggest that active tubular secretion of MTX occurs in humans. MTX excretion is inhibited by weak organic acids such as aspirin,[307] piperacillin,[379,380] penicillin G,[381] and probenecid, an inhibitor of organic acid secretion.[310] The cephalosporins, including ceftriaxone, ceftriazone, ceftazidime, and sulfamethoxazole, enhance the renal elimination of MTX, probably through competition for tubular reabsorption.[380,381] Simultaneous folic acid administration blocks MTX reabsorption, which suggests that leucovorin might accelerate MTX excretion in high-dose rescue regimens.

Although MTX is primarily excreted via the kidneys, the pharmacokinetic pattern of MTX cannot entirely be predicted based on knowledge of the renal function in an individual patient.[375] In one study of 20 patients with normal serum creatinine, the total body clearance of MTX varied from 40 to 400 mL per minute. Decreased renal tubular function, not reflected in creatinine clearance, may be responsible for this variability.

In high-dose MTX therapy, despite interindividual variation in pharmacokinetics, blood levels of drug may be accurately predicted by a preliminary determination of drug clearance using a small test dose (10 to 50 mg per m^2).[375,382] Pharmacokinetic measurements made after delivery of this test dose provide a basis for calculating high-dose infusion rates according to the following formula (units of conversion must be carefully considered):

$$\text{Clearance (mL/minute)} = \text{dose (50 mg/}m^2)/\frac{\text{area under concentration}}{} \times \frac{\text{time}}{\text{curve}}$$

$$\text{Infusion rate} = \frac{\text{plasma MTX concentration (in μmol/L)}}{} \times \text{MTX clearance}$$

Thus, the desired infusion rate is the product of the target steady-state concentration multiplied by the MTX clearance rate, as determined from the test dose.[375]

Extrapolation from the test dose of 50 mg per m^2 to a high-dose infusion schedule has proven to be reliable as long as renal function remains normal during the infusion period. The test dose technique has also been used to identify the subset of patients with impaired MTX elimination who are at increased risk for toxicity.[383]

Hepatic Uptake and Biliary Excretion

MTX undergoes uptake, storage, and metabolism in the liver, but the relative contribution of each of these processes to drug pharmacokinetics is unclear.

MTX is actively transported into hepatocytes by an uptake system that appears to have several components, as previously discussed.[384,385] In the hepatocyte, MTX is converted to polyglutamate forms that persist for several months after drug administration.[386] The parent drug also undergoes excretion into the biliary tract and is reabsorbed into the systemic circulation from the small intestine. Strum et al.[387] found that other chemotherapeutic agents affect the hepatic uptake and biliary secretion of MTX. Vincristine sulfate and cyclophosphamide inhibit both hepatic uptake and biliary excretion, but the net effect of these actions is to produce a fall in intrahepatic drug concentration. Dactinomycin (actinomycin D) strongly inhibits biliary secretion of MTX, with little effect on hepatic uptake, and causes a marked increase in intrahepatic levels of the drug. The pharmacokinetic effects of these drug interactions have not been examined in detail in humans; the possibility exists that the combination of MTX and dactinomycin may increase MTX levels in liver and enhance its hepatic toxicity.

The effects of conjugated and unconjugated bile salts on the enterohepatic circulation of MTX have been investigated *in vivo* in perfused rat intestinal preparations.[388] This study demonstrated a saturable intestinal transport mechanism (K_t = 0.98 μmol per L). The unconjugated bile salt deoxycholate and the conjugated salt taurocholate significantly diminished MTX absorption. Folic acid, 5-methyltetrahydrofolate, and the organic anions rose bengal and sulfobromophthalein also inhibited transport. These compounds might be useful in altering both systemic and specific hepatic toxicities associated with MTX by promoting MTX excretion in the stool.

Widely divergent estimates have been made of the relative importance of biliary excretion of MTX in humans. Lerne et al.,[389] using tritium-labeled MTX, found only 0.41% of an administered dose in the bile of a patient with a biliary fistula. Subsequent studies have variously estimated that 6.7% to 9%[390] or 20%[373] of an administered dose enters the biliary tract. Calvert and co-workers used the highly specific DHFR inhibition assay to measure biliary concentrations of MTX and found that biliary levels were 2,500-fold to 10,000-fold higher than simultaneous concentrations in the plasma.[373] Despite these high concentrations in bile, less than 10% of an intravenous dose of MTX is eliminated in the feces. In the presence of diminished renal function, the enterohepatic circulation may become an important determinant of drug elimination.[391] Under these conditions, intestinal binding of the drug with activated charcoal[392] or the anion-exchange resin cholestyramine,[393] which has a 5.4-fold greater binding capacity than charcoal, may be used to enhance the nonrenal excretion of MTX. Most MTX excreted in bile is reabsorbed as intact drug, whereas an undefined fraction is metabolized by intestinal flora to the inactive derivative DAMPA (Fig. 7-9).[394] The intraluminal metabolism of MTX by intestinal flora can be reduced by nonabsorbable antibiotics. Shen and Azarnoff[390] have observed that patients pretreated with kanamycin sulfate have higher levels of intact MTX and lower concentrations of metabolites in their plasma, presumably owing to decreased metabolism in the gastrointestinal tract.

METHOTREXATE METABOLISM

The introduction of high-dose MTX regimens has led to the identification of at least two MTX metabolites in humans. Jacobs et al. identified 7-OH-MTX in the urine of patients receiving high-dose infusions[395]; 7-OH-MTX constituted 20% to 46% of material excreted in the urine in the interval between 12 and 24 hours after the start of the infusion. The fraction of drug in the form of this metabolite was estimated to be as high as 86% in the period from 24 to 48 hours. A second metabolite, DAMPA, has also been identified in plasma and urine, and, at later times, this metabolite makes up an important fraction of drug-derived material, comprising a mean of 25% of material excreted in the interval from 24 to 48 hours.[339] Both of these metabolites are known to accumulate in plasma, and at 24 to 48 hours after high-dose MTX administration, they account for most of the MTX-derived material found in plasma.

Both metabolites can be completely separated and quantitated by HPLC.[339] As previously discussed, DAMPA cross-reacts strongly with antibodies to MTX prepared by conjugating the glutamate end of the MTX molecule to serum albumin. These antibodies, which are used in radioimmunoassays of MTX, distinguish poorly between the parent compound and metabolite, and in the presence of high circulating concentrations of the metabolite yield plasma MTX values twofold to fourfold higher than values obtained by either the DHFR inhibition or competitive binding assays.

The pharmacokinetics of 7-OH-MTX has been studied after bolus or infusion doses of MTX. The kinetics of 7-OH-MTX was studied after high-dose MTX (12 g per m^2) in 93 cycles from 19 patients with osteosarcoma. A monophasic serum elimination with a half-life of 5.5 hours was noted, and by 12 hours after the 4-hour MTX infusions, 7-OH-MTX levels exceeded MTX levels by an average of 16-fold.[396] In eight patients, 7-OH-MTX levels were found to be up to 30-fold higher than parent MTX levels at 24 hours after MTX administration.[397] Marked interpatient variations in 7-OH-MTX concentrations were noted in 37 patients with head and neck cancer treated with intermediate doses (100 mg per m^2) of MTX.[398] Concentrations in excess of 1 μmol per L of 7-OH-MTX were achieved after 6 to 8 hours, and the median elimination half-life was 13 hours. In both this and a separate study of 29 children with ALL,[399] no association was found between the levels of 7-OH-MTX and either tumor response, duration of response, or toxicity. Concentrations of 7-OH-MTX may exceed those of MTX in tissue as well as in serum. The level of this metabolite in bone marrow was found to be threefold greater than that of MTX[399]; tumor samples taken from patients with osteogenic sarcoma 24 to 48 hours after MTX administration contained up to 60% of the drug as the 7-OH metabolite.[135] CSF concentrations of the 7-OH-MTX metabolite are one-hundredth that of serum levels.[399] To the extent that 7-OH-MTX competes with MTX for cellular transport, polyglutamation, and enzyme binding (see later in this section), it may alter MTX responsiveness and the durability of MTX-induced remissions in certain tumor types.

Regarding the sites of MTX metabolism, 7-OH-MTX is probably formed through the action of the liver enzyme aldehyde oxidase. Levels of the 7-OH-MTX metabolite have been found to be 700-fold higher in bile than in serum.[400] This reaction has been characterized in rabbits and rats, and it appears to be saturable.[400] MTX, aminopterin, and dichloromethotrexate are all substrates for rabbit liver aldehyde oxidase. Although MTX polyglutamates may also be hydroxylated, they are poor substrates for aldehyde oxidase compared with MTX.[401,402] Thus, in addition to prolonging intracellular retention, polyglutamation retards the degradation of MTX to the less-potent 7-OH-MTX. Differences in the relative rates of 7-hydroxylation and polyglutamation have been observed in normal and neoplastic tissues. For example, normal rat hepatocytes readily hydroxylate MTX but only poorly polyglutamate the 7-OH product. In contrast, hepatoma cells have a limited ability to hydroxylate MTX but can efficiently polyglutamylate the 7-OH derivative.[403] In a study by Chladek et al.,[404] the authors examined *in vitro* MTX hydroxylation in both rat and human liver; they concluded that MTX is oxidized by a soluble enzymatic system in both species and suggested that aldehyde oxidase and xanthine oxidase may play an important role in MTX metabolism. In examining the role of human liver aldehyde oxidase in the metabolism of MTX to the 7-OH product, however, Jordan et al.[405] found minimal involvement of the enzyme with regard to MTX oxidation.

The extent to which polyglutamated 7-OH-MTX is formed in malignant but not in normal cells may be important in the selective action of MTX, because the 7-OH polyglutamates have measurable effects on several critical intracellular pathways. The polyglutamates of 7-OH-MTX are inhibitors of the folate-dependent enzymes AICAR transformylase and TS, with potency similar to that of MTX polyglutamates (K_i = 3 and 0.4 μmol per L, respectively).[406] These metabolites can bind to DHFR[126,190] but are relatively weak inhibitors (K_i = 9 nmol per L) of this enzyme compared with MTX.[209,228,407] Unlike with the inhibition of certain folate-dependent enzymes, polyglutamation has relatively minor effects on the potency of DHFR inhibition by 7-OH-MTX.[209,407] Exposure of murine leukemia cells to high concentrations of 7-OH-MTX (100 μmol per L) resulted in only mild inhibition of cell growth.[286] Despite primary metabolism of MTX to the 7-OH-MTX metabolite by the liver, no dosage adjustment of MTX appears to be necessary for patients with hepatic dysfunction.

The pteroic acid metabolite DAMPA is probably formed by the action of bacterial carboxypeptidases in the gastrointestinal tract. Enzymes specific for glutamate terminal peptide bonds have been characterized.[408] DAMPA is also produced by the enzymatic cleavage of MTX in a rescue regimen initially tested in the treatment of brain tumors.[409] In this protocol, high-dose systemic MTX is followed by the infusion of the bacterial enzyme carboxypeptidase G1, which degrades MTX in the systemic circulation but leaves drug intact in the brain and CSF.

The role of these metabolites in producing MTX toxicity or influencing therapeutic activity is uncertain. Both 7-OH-MTX and the pteroic acid metabolite are less soluble than the parent drug (Table 7-3). Jacobs and colleagues demonstrated that 7-OH-MTX constituted more than 50% of precipitated intrarenal material in their study of MTX-induced renal failure in monkeys,[395] but the role of either metabolite in the clinical syndrome of MTX-associated nephrotoxicity in humans is unproved.

TOXICITY

Primary Toxic Effects

The primary toxic effects of folate antagonists are myelosuppression and gastrointestinal mucositis. The incidence of these and other toxicities depends on the specific dose, schedule, and route of drug administration and is summarized in Table 7-5. The intestinal and oral epithelia are somewhat more sensitive than granulocyte and platelet precursors, in that drug schedules that produce intense mucositis (particularly those with prolonged, low drug concentrations) may cause little marrow suppression. The threshold plasma concentration of MTX required to

inhibit DNA synthesis in bone marrow has been estimated to be 10 nmol per L, whereas gastrointestinal epithelium is inhibited at 5 nmol per L plasma concentrations.[410] This greater sensitivity of gastrointestinal epithelium is believed to result from greater accumulation and persistence of MTX in intestinal epithelium than in bone marrow.[411] Mucositis usually appears 3 to 7 days after drug administration and precedes the onset of a fall in white blood count or platelet count by several days. The duration and intensity of these acute toxicities are, in general, determined by drug dose and individual pharmacokinetics. In patients with compromised renal function, small doses on the order of 25 mg may provide cytotoxic blood levels for up to 3 to 5 days and may result in serious bone marrow toxicity. Myelosuppression and mucositis usually are completely reversed within 2 weeks, unless drug excretion mechanisms are severely impaired.

The introduction of high-dose MTX regimens with leucovorin rescue[412,413] has been associated with a new spectrum of clinical toxicities and has required more careful monitoring of drug pharmacokinetics in individual patients. These regimens use otherwise lethal doses in a 6- to 36-hour infusion, followed by a 24- to 48-hour period of multiple leucovorin doses to terminate the toxic effect of MTX. Several of the more commonly used high-dose regimens and their related pharmacokinetics are presented in Table 7-4. For each regimen, successful rescue by leucovorin depends on the rapid elimination of MTX by the kidneys. Early experience with high-dose regimens, however, indicated that MTX itself may have acute toxic effects on renal function during the period of drug infusion,[413] which can lead to delayed drug clearance, ineffective rescue by leucovorin, and a host of secondary toxicities, including severe myelosuppression, mucositis, and epithelial desquamation.[361,365] During the early clinical trials of high-dose MTX, a number of toxic deaths were recorded.[414]

TABLE 7-5. TOXICITIES ASSOCIATED WITH VARIOUS DOSES/ROUTES OF METHOTREXATE SODIUM ADMINISTRATION

	Myelotoxicity	Nephrotoxicity	Hepatotoxicity	Mucositis	Pulmonary Toxicity	Neurotoxicity
Intermediate i.v. (50–100 mg/m²)	+++	+	+ (transaminasemia)	++	±	−
High-dose i.v. with leucovorin calcium (100–12,000 mg/m²)	+	+++ (requires urinary alkalinization and hydration)	++ (transaminasemia)	++	±	++ (acute and chronic)
Low-dose p.o., daily dose (5–25 mg/m²)	−	−	+++ (up to 25% cirrhosis)	−	±	−
Low-dose p.o., pulse therapy (5–25 mg/m²)	−	−	++ (rarely cirrhosis)	−	+	−
Intrathecal	−	−	−	−	−	++ (acute, subacute, and chronic)

+, some toxicity; ++, moderate toxicity; +++, high toxicity; −, no toxicity; ±, possible toxicity.

The cause of drug-induced renal dysfunction, which is usually manifested as an abrupt rise in serum blood urea nitrogen and creatinine with a corresponding fall in urine output, is thought to arise from the precipitation of MTX and possibly its less soluble metabolites, 7-OH-MTX and DAMPA, in acidic urine.[395,397] A direct toxic effect of antifolates on the renal tubule, however, has been suggested by the observation that aminopterin, an equally soluble compound that is used at one-tenth the dose of MTX, is also associated with renal toxicity.[415] Jacobs et al.[395] were able to reproduce the syndrome of MTX-induced renal failure in a monkey model system and demonstrated precipitation of both MTX and 7-OH-MTX in the renal tubules. Both of these compounds have limited solubility under acid pH conditions. To prevent precipitation, most centers now use vigorous hydration (2.5 to 3.5 L of fluid per m^2 per 24 hours, beginning 12 hours before MTX infusion and continuing for 24 to 48 hours), with alkalinization of the urine (45 to 50 mEq of sodium bicarbonate per liter of intravenous fluid). The MTX infusion should not begin until urine flow exceeds 100 mL per hour and urine pH is 7.0 or higher, and these parameters should be carefully monitored during the course of drug infusion (Table 7-4).

With this regimen, the incidence of renal failure and myelosuppression has been markedly reduced. No change in the rate of MTX excretion or alteration of plasma pharmacokinetics results from the intense hydration used in the preparatory regimen described above[377]; thus, these safety measures should have no deleterious effect on the therapeutic efficacy of the regimen.

Despite careful attention to the details of hydration and alkalinization, occasional patients can develop serious or even fatal toxicity.[414] Almost all of these toxic episodes are associated with delayed MTX clearance from plasma and can be predicted by routine monitoring of drug concentration in plasma at appropriate times after drug infusion.[416] The specific time for monitoring, and the guidelines for distinguishing between normal and dangerously elevated levels, must be determined for each regimen and for each assay procedure. In general, a time point well into the final phase of drug disappearance, such as 24 or 48 hours after the start of infusion, should be chosen (Table 7-4). The value of monitoring has been established by numerous studies. The National Cancer Institute (NCI) experience in administering adjuvant therapy for osteosarcoma is typical. The investigators used a 6-hour infusion of 50 to 250 mg per kg MTX, followed 2 hours after infusion by 15 mg per m^2 leucovorin repeated every 6 hours for eight doses.[413] They observed that in each of seven patients with moderate to severe myelosuppression, plasma MTX concentrations were 0.9 µmol per L or higher at 48 hours after drug administration; this finding alerted physicians to the high risk of toxicity. Of note, in three of these seven patients, renal function remained normal; this finding confirmed that determination of serum creatinine was unreliable as a

sole predictor of toxicity.[365] Earlier time points may be used for monitoring drug disappearance and for guiding patient management. After a 6-hour high-dose infusion regimen, plasma concentrations of less than 5 µmol per L at 24 hours are associated with a low incidence of toxicity.[417] Pretreatment elevations of urinary *N*-acetyl-α-D-glucosaminidase (more than 1.5 U per mmol creatinine) have been found to predict prolonged MTX clearance and subsequent enhanced toxicity,[418] but the utility of this marker has not been tested in large prospective trials.

The use of ketoprofen, a nonsteroidal antiinflammatory drug (NSAID), has been associated with severe MTX toxicity.[419] A review of 118 cases of single-agent high-dose MTX therapy revealed four cases of fatal toxicity associated with the use of NSAIDs. Patients treated with ketoprofen demonstrated a marked prolongation of serum MTX half-life that was postulated to be due to decreased renal elimination secondary to inhibition of renal prostaglandin synthesis or competitive secretion of the two drugs. This specific drug interaction is of particular clinical importance, given the widespread use of NSAIDs and MTX in the management of patients with cancer and rheumatoid arthritis.

Early detection of elevated concentrations of MTX allows institution of specific clinical measures. Continuous medical supervision is warranted until the severity and duration of myelosuppression can be determined. Leucovorin in increased doses is required and must be continued until plasma MTX concentration falls below 50 nmol per L. Because of the competitive relationship between MTX and leucovorin, the leucovorin dose must be increased in proportion to the plasma concentration of MTX. Small doses of leucovorin are unable to prevent toxicity in patients with elevated drug levels, even when leucovorin is continued beyond 48 hours.[365,416] In the NCI osteosarcoma study,[416] leucovorin dosages of 50 to 100 mg per m^2 every 6 hours successfully rescued four of four patients with MTX levels above 0.9 µmol per L at 48 hours, whereas five of five patients with similarly high levels who received 12 to 30 mg per m^2 of leucovorin experienced severe myelosuppression. As a general rule, a reasonable course is to treat with leucovorin at a dosage of 100 mg per m^2 every 6 hours for patients with MTX levels of 1 µmol per L and to increase this dosage in proportion to the MTX level up to a maximum of 500 mg per m^2 (Table 7-4). Subsequent leucovorin dosage adjustments should be based on repeated plasma MTX levels taken at 24-hour intervals. The results of *in vitro* studies indicate that leucovorin may not be able to rescue patients with plasma MTX concentrations above 10 µmol per L. In these patients, supportive care, including antibiotics, platelet transfusion, and hydration, must be relied on to carry them through the prolonged period of myelosuppression.

The absorption of oral leucovorin is saturable such that the bioavailability of the compound is limited above total doses of 40 mg. The fractional absorption of a 40-mg dose is 0.78, whereas that of 60- and 100-mg doses is 0.62 and

0.42, respectively.[139] For this reason, leucovorin is usually administered intravenously to assure its absorption.

The persistence of high concentrations of MTX in plasma presents a serious danger to patients who have received high-dose MTX. Because of the variable effectiveness of leucovorin in preventing toxicity in patients with levels of 10 μmol per L or greater at 48 hours, alternative methods of rescue have been proposed. Both hemodialysis and peritoneal dialysis are ineffective in removing significant quantities of MTX; clearance was estimated to be 40 mL per minute by hemodialysis[374] but only 5 mL per minute by peritoneal dialysis. In one carefully studied patient, despite the presence of moderate renal failure, renal clearance of MTX exceeded hemodialysis clearance by greater than twofold.[374] Although hemodialysis produced a transient decrease in plasma concentration of MTX, a rapid rebound to predialysis levels was observed on cessation of the procedure. This rebound was likely the result of entry of drug into the plasma space from deeper compartments. The use of charcoal hemoperfusion columns is capable of removing MTX and other antineoplastic drugs from whole blood and has been applied successfully in a few patients; however, platelet adherence to these columns may lead to thrombocytopenia. Relling et al.[420] documented a case in which a patient developed severe renal failure immediately after receiving high-dose MTX and was effectively treated with repeated hemodialysis and charcoal hemoperfusion with subsequent leucovorin and thymidine rescue. Gastrointestinal and hematologic toxicities were completely prevented in the patient, and serum creatinine normalized within 24 days after onset of therapy. Abelson and co-workers have used a bacterial enzyme, carboxypeptidase G1,[409] which inactivates MTX by removal of its terminal glutamate, to destroy circulating MTX. The regimen of high-dose MTX followed by intravenous carboxypeptidase was well tolerated, but this form of enzymatic rescue carries a risk of hypersensitivity to the bacterial enzyme. Bertino et al. have demonstrated the feasibility of attaching the enzyme to hollow fiber tubing, which can then be used in an extracorporeal shunt for drug removal[421] and thus avoid immune sensitization. One potential disadvantage of carboxypeptidase G1, however, is its relatively high affinity for natural folates as well as MTX. An alternative enzyme that cleaves MTX but not reduced folates has been isolated by Albrecht and co-workers.[422] DeAngelis[423] and colleagues conducted a pilot study to determine the efficacy of carboxypeptidase G2 (CPG2) rescue after high-dose MTX in patients with recurrent cerebral lymphoma. All patients had at least a 2-log decline in plasma MTX levels within 5 minutes of CPG2 administration, whereas CSF MTX concentrations remained elevated for 4 hours after CPG2. No MTX or CPG2 toxicity was observed and anti-CPG2 activity antibodies were not detected in any patient. The authors concluded that CPG2 rescue was a safe and effec-

tive alternative to leucovorin rescue after high-dose MTX chemotherapy. Additional utility of CPG2 was suggested in patients with MTX-sensitive central nervous system tumors, as no affect was seen on CSF MTX levels. In an NCI study on the use of CPG2 in pediatric patients who developed nephrotoxicity while receiving high-dose MTX, Widemann et al.[424] found that CPG2 and thymidine rescue was well tolerated and resulted in a rapid and effective reduction in the plasma MTX concentration with only mild to moderate MTX-related toxicity.

Physicians worldwide (except in Europe) may request CPG2 by calling the Cancer Therapy Evaluation Program (CTEP) of the National Cancer Institute at 301-496-6138 (Internet address: http://ctep.info.nih.gov/). The contact for physicians requesting CPG2 in Germany, Austria, and Switzerland is Professor Udo Bode at phone ++49 (0) 228 287 3215. All other callers from Europe should contact Professor Tony Atkinson at ++44 (0) 123 582 0555.

The rationale for rescue of MTX with thymidine has been discussed previously. Preliminary reports have described the successful prevention of MTX toxicity in humans using 6- to 40-hour infusions of the antifolate followed by a 72-hour infusion of thymidine at a rate of 8 g per m^2 per day.[320,425] Patients receiving a bolus dose of MTX, 3 g per m^2, were successfully rescued by thymidine infusion (1 g per m^2 per day); the infusion was begun 24 hours after MTX administration and continued until MTX concentration in the plasma reached 50 nmol per L.[426] Thymidine infusions of 1 g per m^2 per day produced only a twofold rise in serum thymidine concentration, which indicates a very steep dose-response relationship for thymidine rescue. The serum concentration of thymidine is proportional to thymidine dose up to infusion rates of 3 g per m^2 per day. Above that rate, little further increase occurs in serum thymidine concentration.[426] Few antitumor responses were noted in these initial trials, but the number of treated patients was small, and the therapeutic value of this approach remains unproved.

In the experimental setting, MTX toxicity can also be blocked by drugs that prevent cell progression into the S phase of the cell cycle. The antagonistic effect of L-asparaginase on MTX toxicity is a representative example; through depletion of the amino acid asparagine, L-asparaginase inhibits protein synthesis and prevents entry of cells into the DNA-synthetic phase of the cell cycle.[427] Rescue regimens[428] that use high doses of MTX (up to 400 mg per m^2), followed within 24 hours by 20,000 to 40,000 U per m^2 of L-asparaginase, produce minimal bone marrow toxicity and mucositis, and appear to have some effectiveness in patients refractory to low-dose MTX alone. Yap et al.[428] reported a complete remission rate of 62% (13 of 21 cases) in adult patients with ALL who had failed initial therapy with conventional induction regimens (vincristine, prednisone, daunomycin). The regimen is less effective in previously treated patients with AML, producing a remission rate of only 18%. Lobel et al. have concluded[429] that continued responsiveness to L-asparaginase is a requirement for achievement of complete remission with this regimen.

MTX toxicity is also prevented by drugs that inhibit the TS reaction, thereby preventing alterations in the composition of the intracellular folate pools and negating the effect of DHFR enzyme inhibition. This effect has been studied in detail and seems to explain the antagonism of fluoropyrimidine pretreatment followed by MTX.[430]

Poor nutritional status has been associated with an increased risk of toxicity from MTX.[431–433] Poorly nourished patients appear to have an approximately twofold decrease in their clearance of MTX. Animals fed a chemically defined, elemental liquid diet also demonstrated decreased clearance of MTX resulting in an enhancement of toxicity.[434–437] The reason for this delayed drug clearance appears to be a protracted enterohepatic circulation. Providing dietary protein in the form of polypeptides (rather than amino acids) either alone or in combination with cholestyramine treatment to bind intestinal MTX may be useful in avoiding excess toxicity associated with nutritional deficiencies.

Other Toxicities

Hepatotoxicity

In addition to its inhibitory effects on rapidly dividing tissues, MTX has toxic effects on nondividing tissues not easily explained by its primary action on DNA synthesis. Long-term MTX therapy is associated with portal fibrosis, which may, on occasion, progress to frank cirrhosis. Chronic liver disease has occurred most frequently in patients with psoriasis or rheumatoid arthritis or in children with acute leukemia who have received maintenance therapy over a period of several years. The incidence of cirrhosis has been estimated to be 10% in MTX-treated patients with psoriasis but may reach as high as 25% to 30% in those patients treated for 5 years or longer with continuous daily therapy.[438] A high underlying incidence of chronic hepatic disease related to alcohol or to arsenicals used for psoriasis treatment found in this patient population may have a contributory role.[439] Cirrhosis does not always progress with continued antifolate treatment. Of 11 patients with psoriasis who showed cirrhotic changes on liver biopsy and continued to receive treatment, only 3 showed progression on subsequent biopsy, and 3 had no pathologic findings on a follow-up biopsy.[438] The association of cirrhosis with long-term oral therapy has led to the hypothesis that MTX hepatotoxicity is due to a high "first-pass" drug exposure. One study in rats, however, found no difference in hepatic drug exposure when the animals were treated with subcutaneous administration or with intraperitoneal administration (to simulate oral use).[440]

The use of "pulsed" weekly therapy rather than continuous daily treatment appears to lessen the incidence of MTX-associated hepatotoxicity.[441,442] Several studies suggest that the incidence of hepatic cirrhosis is no different in patients with rheumatoid arthritis treated with MTX pulse therapy than in untreated patients despite long-term therapy (longer than 5 years).[443,444] Evidence of hepatic toxicity was detected on liver biopsy in 76% of 29 patients receiving weekly (7.5-mg) pulse therapy with MTX for rheumatoid arthritis; however, only one patient had severe fibrosis.[443] These patients had been treated for an average of approximately 2.5 years (1,500 mg total dose). Abnormal elevations in serum transaminases have been found in up to 70% of patients treated with long-term weekly MTX; however, the enzyme elevations were poor predictors of liver damage.[445] In a series of 45 patients who underwent liver biopsy while being treated with long-term weekly MTX, 22% had fibrotic changes but less than 3% demonstrated cirrhosis.[446] Interestingly, the authors found that the occurrence of hepatic fibrosis was associated with pulmonary fibrosis and obesity. Finally, Scully and colleagues reported a 30% incidence of hepatic fibrosis in patients treated with weekly MTX with a mean MTX dose of 1,300 mg over 2.7 years.[445] None of these patients were found to have evidence of cirrhosis. An analysis of 859 patients treated with weekly MTX revealed an overall incidence of hepatic fibrosis of 17% with no patient demonstrating evidence of cirrhosis.[445] Thus, the use of pulse therapy appears to mitigate the development of chronic hepatotoxicity associated with low-dose continuous therapy.

Acute elevations of liver enzymes (alanine transaminase, aspartate transaminase, L-lactate dehydrogenase) are commonly observed after high-dose MTX administration and usually return to normal within 10 days. The frequency and severity of liver enzyme elevations appear to be directly related to the number of MTX doses received.[447] Liver biopsy in such patients has revealed fatty infiltration but no evidence of hepatocellular necrosis or periportal fibrosis. The late occurrence of cirrhosis in patients treated with high-dose MTX has not been reported.

The biochemical basis for MTX hepatotoxicity is not known. MTX causes increased lipid deposition in liver, possibly through interference with synthesis of choline (which requires a one-carbon transfer).[448] Acute MTX hepatotoxicity in rats can be reversed by choline administration. Cholestasis has been reported in rats treated with high doses of MTX (1,000 mg per kg) due to the formation of biliary precipitates comprised almost entirely of 7-OH-MTX.[449]

Interestingly, Bergasa et al.[450] conducted a pilot study of low-dose oral MTX treatment for primary biliary cirrhosis in which 10 symptomatic patients were treated with MTX at a dosage of 15 mg per week. Although all patients experienced transient mucositis and intermittent dyspepsia, the authors concluded that patients with early disease may have benefited from MTX administration manifested as decreased symptomatology (pruritus, fatigue), improved serum biochemical indices, and decreased hepatic inflammation.

Pneumonitis

Treatment with MTX is associated with a poorly characterized, self-limited pneumonitis, with fever, cough, and an interstitial pulmonary infiltrate.[449,451] Eosinophilia has not been a consistent finding, either in the peripheral blood or in open lung biopsy specimens. Lung biopsies have revealed a variety of findings, from simple interstitial edema and a mononuclear infiltrate to noncaseating granulomas. The possibility that MTX pneumonitis may not represent a hypersensitivity phenomenon has been raised because of the failure of some patients to react to reinstitution of MTX therapy. However, bronchoalveolar lavage in three patients with presumptive MTX-induced lung damage revealed a predominance of T8 suppressor lymphocytes. In contrast to peripheral lymphocytes obtained from MTX-treated patients with no lung damage, lymphocytes from the study patients elaborated leukocyte inhibitory factor in response to MTX exposure.[452] This study supports an immunologic basis for MTX-related lung damage. The possibility exists, however, that many case reports of "MTX lung" in fact represent unrecognized viral infections or allergic reactions to unsuspected allergens. This is supported by the lack of significant effects on pulmonary function in 38 adolescents treated with high-dose MTX.[453] With the increasing use of long-term weekly low-dose MTX therapy for rheumatoid arthritis, however, a number of cases of MTX-associated lung damage have been reported.[454,455] A review of 168 patients treated with MTX for rheumatoid arthritis uncovered 9 cases (5%) of probable MTX-associated lung toxicity.[456] Using a retrospective combined-cohort review and abstraction from the medical literature, Kremer, Alarcon, and colleagues[457] characterized the clinical features of MTX-associated lung injury in patients with rheumatoid arthritis. Clinical symptoms of MTX toxicity in the cohort included the subacute development of shortness of breath (93%), cough (82%), and fever (69%) with resultant death in 5 of 27 patients. The authors concluded that early symptom recognition and the cessation of MTX administration could avoid the serious and sometimes fatal outcome of this MTX-associated toxicity in rheumatoid arthritis patients. Corticosteroids have been used in a small number of patients who ultimately recovered,[458] but the utility of this approach has yet to be established. Alarcon et al.[459] found that the strongest predictors of MTX-induced lung injury in rheumatoid arthritis patients included older age, presence of diabetes, rheumatoid pleuropulmonary involvement, presence of hypoalbuminemia, and prior use of disease-modifying antirheumatic drugs.

Hypersensitivity

True anaphylactic reactions to MTX are rare. Two cases of acute hypersensitivity reaction to MTX have been described.[460] The first patient experienced acute cardiovascular collapse, which was reproduced on rechallenge of the patient with MTX. In the second case, the acute reaction consisted of facial edema, rash, and generalized pruritus, and again was elicited on rechallenge. Both patients were receiving bacille Calmette-Guérin in conjunction with MTX at the time of these reactions, and thus may have developed a heightened sensitivity to MTX. Three cases of toxic erythema and desquamation of the hands were reported in patients receiving high doses (1.5 g per m^2) of MTX for the treatment of non-Hodgkin's lymphoma.[461] This toxic reaction was associated with severe mucositis and was ameliorated by MTX dose reductions on subsequent treatment.

Reversible oligospermia with testicular failure has been reported in men treated with high-dose MTX.[462] No alterations in follicle-stimulating hormone, luteinizing hormone, estradiol, or progesterone have been observed in women exposed to MTX.

PHARMACOKINETICS AND TOXICITY OF METHOTREXATE IN THE CENTRAL NERVOUS SYSTEM

Because of its high degree of ionization at physiologic pH, MTX penetrates into the CSF with difficulty. During a constant intravenous drug infusion,[463] the ratio of venous MTX concentration to CSF concentration is approximately 30:1 at equilibrium. Thus, plasma levels in excess of 30 µmol per L would be required to achieve the concentration of 1 µmol per L that is thought to be necessary for killing of leukemic cells. Protocols for prophylaxis against meningeal leukemia and lymphoma using systemic high-dose infusions of MTX have demonstrated that high-dose MTX infusions are a reasonable treatment alternative to intrathecal prophylaxis. Overt meningeal leukemia increases the CSF to plasma ratio by approximately tenfold.[464] In children with ALL, a diminished CSF to plasma ratio has been found to be a useful predictor of CNS relapse.[465,466]

Direct intrathecal injection of MTX has been used for the treatment and prophylaxis of meningeal malignancy. The readers are referred to a comprehensive review on this topic.[467] Drug injected into the intrathecal space distributes in a total volume of approximately 120 mL for patients over 3 years of age. Thus, a maximal total dose of 12 mg is advised for all patients over 3 years, with lower doses indicated for younger children. Bleyer[367] has recommended a dose of 6 mg for age 1 or younger, 8 mg for ages 1 to 2, and 10 mg for ages 2 to 3. The peak CSF concentration achieved by this schedule is approximately 100 µmol per L. Lumbar CSF drug concentrations decline in a biphasic pattern with a terminal half-life of 7 to 16 hours.[465] This terminal phase of disappearance may be considerably prolonged in patients with active meningeal disease and in older age patients.[467,468] Injection of radiolabeled MTX into the ventricular space of rabbits demonstrated rapid but variable distribution of MTX in the gray matter adjacent to the CSF, which suggests a mechanism for the various syndromes associated with MTX neurotoxicity.[469] MTX is cleared from spinal fluid by bulk resorption of spinal fluid (i.e., "bulk flow"), a process that may be prolonged by increases in intracranial pressure and the administration of acetazolamide.[465] A second component of resorption involves the active transport of this organic anion by the choroid plexus. Probenecid is an inhibitor of the active transport process and may be used to prolong CSF MTX exposure.[465] A prolongation of the terminal half-life is also found in patients who develop drug-related neurotoxicity, although a causal relationship between abnormal pharmacokinetics and neurotoxicity has not been firmly established.

MTX administered into the lumbar space distributes poorly over the cerebral convexities and into the ventricular spaces.[463] The concentration gradient between lumbar and ventricular CSF may exceed 10:1. Although this uneven distribution has no documented role in determining clinical relapse of patients treated for meningeal leukemia, awareness of this potential problem has led to clinical trials using direct intraventricular injection of MTX via an Ommaya reservoir. Bleyer and colleagues[470] have demonstrated that a concentration × time regimen in which 1 mg MTX was injected into the Ommaya reservoir every 12 hours for 3 days yielded continuous CSF levels above 0.5 μmol per L and achieved therapeutic results equivalent to those with the conventional intralumbar injection of 12 mg every 4 days. Moreover, this concentration × time regimen was associated with a considerable reduction in neurotoxic side effects, presumably owing to the avoidance of high peak levels of drug associated with higher MTX doses. Glantz et al.[471] reported on the use of high-dose intravenous MTX as the sole treatment for nonleukemic meningitis. Sixteen patients with solid tumor neoplastic meningitis received high-dose intravenous MTX (8 g per m² over 4 hours) with leucovorin rescue. Compared with a reference group of patients receiving standard intrathecal MTX, the high-dose intravenous group exhibited cytotoxic CSF and serum MTX concentrations that were maintained much longer than with intrathecal dosing. In addition, median survival in the high-dose intravenous MTX group was 13.8 months versus 2.3 months for the intrathecal reference group (p = .003).

Three different neurotoxic syndromes have been observed after treatment with intrathecal MTX.[470] The most common and most immediate neurotoxic side effect is an acute chemical arachnoiditis manifested as severe headache, nuchal rigidity, vomiting, fever, and inflammatory cell pleocytosis of the spinal fluid. This constellation of symptoms appears to be a function of the frequency and dose of drug administered, and may be ameliorated either by reduction in dose or by a change in therapy to intrathecal cytosine arabinoside. A less acute but more serious neurotoxic syndrome has been observed in approximately 10% of patients treated with intrathecal MTX. This subacute

toxicity appears during the second or third week of treatment, usually in adult patients with active meningeal leukemia, and is manifested as motor paralysis of the extremities, cranial nerve palsy, seizures, or coma. Because MTX pharmacokinetics is abnormal in these patients, the suspicion is that this subacute neurotoxicity may be the result of extended exposure to toxic drug concentrations.[467] Finally, a more chronic demyelinating encephalopathy has been observed in children months or years after intrathecal MTX therapy. The primary symptoms of this toxicity are dementia, limb spasticity, and, in more advanced cases, coma. Computerized axial tomography (CT) has revealed ventricular enlargement, white matter changes, cortical thinning, and diffuse intracerebral calcification in children who have received prophylactic intrathecal MTX.[472,473] Most of these patients had also received cranial irradiation (greater than 2,000 rads) and all had received systemic chemotherapy.

Treatment with repeated courses of high-dose intravenous MTX may also result in encephalopathy.[474] In these patients, symptoms of dementia and paresis may develop in the second or third month after treatment and may also be associated with diffuse cortical hypodensities on CT scan. A second form of cerebral dysfunction associated with high-dose MTX is an acute transient dysfunction described in 4% to 15% of treated patients.[475–477] The syndrome consists of any combination of paresis, aphasia, behavioral abnormalities, and seizures. The neurologic events occur an average of 6 days after the MTX dose and completely resolve, usually within 48 to 72 hours. Patients may have received any number of MTX doses before the onset of this neurotoxic event, and some patients may have repeat episodes with subsequent MTX doses. In general, CSF and head CT scans are normal, but low-density lesions have been noted in some cases.[478] The electroencephalogram may represent the only abnormal study and shows a diffuse or focal slowing. No clinical evidence exists to support the use of leucovorin, either acutely after intrathecal MTX or over the long term in patients who develop neurotoxic symptoms. Although leucovorin can enter the CSF, its penetration appears to be poor.[479,480] In a study of ten patients with osteosarcoma treated with high-dose MTX and leucovorin rescue, little or no increase in CSF folates was observed during rescue.[479] When positron emission tomography scanning was used in a rat model, however, high-dose leucovorin infusions (1,000 mg per kg) given over 24 hours reversed the global decrease in glucose metabolism associated with MTX exposure.[481] A comparison of neurologic toxicities was undertaken in a randomized trial involving 49 children with acute leukemia treated with either intrathecal MTX plus radiation or high-dose systemic MTX for central nervous system prophylaxis.[482] Long-term toxicities were similar with either treatment option, and overall decreases in intelligence quotients were found to be clinically significant in 61% of the children. In addition, 58% of the patients treated with systemic therapy had abnormal electroencephalograms and 57% of those treated with intrathecal MTX and radiation experienced somnolence syndrome. Mahoney and colleagues[483] described the incidence of acute neurotoxicity in 1,304 children with lower risk B-precursor lymphoid leukemia treated as part of the Pediatric Oncology Group 9005 trial. After remission induction, patients were randomized into one of three 24-week intensification schedules (intermediate-dose MTX or divided-dose oral MTX with or without intravenous mercaptopurine and extended intrathecal therapy). Overall, acute neurotoxicity occurred in 7.8% (95 of 1,218) of eligible patients, and the authors found that intensification with repeated intravenous MTX and low-dose leucovorin rescue was associated with a higher risk of acute neurotoxicity and leukoencephalopathy, especially in patients who received concomitant triple intrathecal therapy (MTX, dexamethasone, cytosine arabinoside).

The etiology of the MTX-associated neurotoxicity is unknown. Vascular events in the form of vasospasm or emboli have been proposed to explain these neurologic abnormalities, and studies have suggested alterations in brain glucose metabolism after MTX treatment.[481,484] Long-term exposure of rat cerebellar explants to 1 μmol per L MTX resulted in axonal death 2 weeks after drug exposure and loss of myelin sheaths in 5 weeks, which suggests a direct toxic effect of MTX on axonal cells.[485] DHFR is present in brain tissue, but its biochemical role in the cerebral cortex, the primary site of MTX neurotoxicity, is uncertain. Several studies have demonstrated the ability of cranial radiation to increase blood–brain barrier permeability to serum proteins and MTX.[486,487] Because radiation and MTX are frequently used together, this interaction may be an important mechanism for enhanced toxicity. Blood–brain barrier disruption has also been used in an attempt to increase drug delivery to central nervous system disease. Barrier disruption with internal carotid artery infusions of 25% mannitol solutions and 6% polysorbate-80 intravenous infusions have resulted in markedly higher levels of MTX in the brain.[488,489] Whether or not a similar degree of enhanced uptake occurs in brain tumors that probably do not have an intact blood–brain barrier is not known. Inadvertent overdose of intrathecal MTX generally has a fatal outcome. Immediate lumbar puncture with CSF removal along with ventriculolumbar perfusion has been successfully used to avert catastrophe in such situations.[490]

CLINICAL DOSAGE SCHEDULES

A variety of dosage schedules and routes of administration are used clinically, including high-dose therapy with the addition of leucovorin rescue. The selection of an appropriate schedule depends largely on the specific disease being treated, on other antineoplastic agents or radiation to be used in combination regimens, on the patient's tolerance for host toxicity, and on other factors that might alter pharmacokinetics. Parenteral schedules are preferred for induction therapy regimens in which maximal concentrations and duration of exposure are desirable in an effort to achieve complete remission. High-dose MTX regimens and leucovorin rescue offer the advantage of minimal bone marrow toxicity, a particularly attractive feature in combination chemotherapy. This regimen, however, can safely be used only in patients with normal renal and hepatic function and under conditions in which no large extracellular accumulations of fluid are present. As emphasized earlier, high-dose regimens should be instituted only when plasma monitoring is available to determine the adequacy of drug clearance and the risk of serious toxicity. Furthermore, because leucovorin may rescue tumor cells as well as normal cells, the optimal dose, schedule, and clinical utility of high-dose MTX with leucovorin in rescue needs to be more carefully defined through continued clinical investigation.

OTHER ANTIFOLATES

LY231514

TS represents a logical target for new drug development using folate analogs, and LY231514 (MTA), a pyrrolo(2,3-d)pyrimidine-based multitargeting antifolate analog, is a potent inhibitor of TS. LY231514 is mainly transported into cells via the RFC system before being metabolized to the polyglutamated forms, which are potent inhibitors of several folate-dependent enzymatic reactions. The multitargeting effect of LY231514 was seen in studies by Shih et al., who suggested that, at higher concentrations, LY231514 and its polyglutamates not only act as TS inhibitors but also inhibit other key folate-requiring enzymes, including DHFR, glycinamide ribonucleotide formyltransferase, and to a lesser extent 5-aminoimidazole-4-carboxamide ribonucleotide formyltransferase and C1-tetrahydrofolate synthase.[491] The combined inhibitory effects of LY231514 give rise to a cellular level end-product reversal pattern that is different from those of other inhibitors such as MTX and the quinazoline antifolates. In addition, the metabolic effects exerted by LY231514 on the folate and nucleotide pools are also quite distinct from those of MTX.[492] Chen et al. compared LY231514 with MTX, raltitrexed, and a glycinamide ribonucleotide formyltransferase inhibitor (LY309887) for their effects on intracellular folate and on nucleoside triphosphate pools in CCRF-CEM cells.[493] Although LY231514 was found to have minimal effects on folate pools, it caused rapid depletion of deoxythymidine triphosphate thymidine 5'-triphosphate, deoxycytidine triphosphate, and deoxyguanosine triphosphate. The authors concluded that the inhibitory effects of LY231514, in CCRF-CEM cells, was exerted primarily against the thymidylate cycle and secondarily against *de novo* purine biosynthesis. In studies evaluating the effects of folic acid on modulating the toxicity and antitumor efficacy of LY231514 in human tumor cell lines adapted to growth in low-folate medium, folic acid was shown to be 100- to 1,000-fold less active than folinic acid at protecting cells from LY231514-induced cytotoxicity.[494] Further, folic acid supplementation was demonstrated to preserve the antitumor activity of LY231514 while reducing toxicity in mice. The study suggested that a combination of folic acid and LY231514 may provide a mechanism for enhanced clinical antitumor selectivity. Although completed phase I trials have determined that the clinical toxicities of LY231514 include neutropenia and minor gastrointestinal disturbances, larger ongoing clinical trials will determine the benefit and utility of this multitargeting agent.[495,496]

AG337

AG337 (nolatrexed dihydrochloride, THYMITAQ) is a nonclassic inhibitor of TS specifically designed to avoid potential resistance mechanisms that can limit the activity of the classic antifolate antimetabolites.[497] AG337 is a lipophilic molecule designed using x-ray structure–based methodologies to interact at the folate cofactor binding site of the TS enzyme. TS was suggested as the locus of action of AG337 by the ability of thymidine to antagonize cell growth inhibition and the direct demonstration of TS inhibition in whole cells using a tritium-release assay.[498] AG337 is characterized as a non–glutamate-containing molecule that does not require facilitated transport for uptake and does not undergo, nor require, intracellular polyglutamylation for activity. L1210 cells treated with AG337 exhibited S-phase cell-cycle arrest and a pattern of nucleotide pool modulations, including a reduction in thymidine triphosphate levels, consistent with inhibition of TS.[498] Rafi et al. measured plasma concentrations of deoxyuridine (dUrd) in patients receiving doses of AG337 at levels of more than 600 mg per m^2 and found elevation in plasma dUrd levels (60% to 290%), which implied that TS inhibition was being achieved in patients.[497] In all cases dUrd concentrations quickly returned to pretreatment levels after the end of the infusion; this suggested that TS inhibition was not maintained, presumably due to the brief intracellular half-life of the nonpolyglutamated parent compound. A phase I trial evaluating intravenous administration of AG337 found dose-limiting myelosuppression and a high incidence of thrombotic phenomena.[499] A second trial evaluating 5-day oral administration of nolatrexed showed rapid absorption with a median bioavailability of 89%; dose-limiting toxicities were gastrointestinal. The authors concluded that nolatrexed could be safely administered as an oral preparation at a dosage of 800 mg per m^2 per day for 5 days.[500] A phase I study of 10-day oral administration found nausea, vomiting, stomatitis, and liver function test abnormalities as dose-limiting toxicities.[501]

Raltitrexed

Raltitrexed (ZD1694, Tomudex) is a water-soluble TS inhibitor that appears to have an acceptable toxicity profile, convenient dosing schedule, and antitumor activity in colorectal, breast, and pancreatic cancers.[502–504] This drug is a second-generation agent designed to overcome the major toxicity associated with its predecessor, CB3717—namely, poorly predictable nephrotoxicity. CB3717, also a TS inhibitor, blocked DNA replication through depletion of deoxythymidine triphosphate thymidine 5'-triphosphate pools and without exhibiting an antipurine effect, while retaining antitumor activity against transport-defective MTX-resistant as well as DHFR-overproducing cells.[505] Yin and colleagues[506] conducted *in vitro* studies on the human A253 head and neck squamous carcinoma cell line to evaluate the downstream molecular alterations induced by the potent and sustained inhibition of TS by raltitrexed. TS inhibition by raltitrexed resulted in a time-dependent induction of megabase DNA fragmentation followed by a secondary 50- to 300-kilobase DNA fragmentation, which may correlate with reduced expression of *p27* and increase in cyclin E and cdk2 kinase activity. Sotelo-Mundo et al.[507] evaluated the crystal structures of mammalian TS bound to dUMP and raltitrexed with findings that suggest a ligand-induced conformational change similar to that of *Escherichia coli* protein but without induction of the "closed" conformation. Cunningham[504] reviewed the results of three large controlled studies which suggest that raltitrexed is an effective alternative to 5-fluorouracil–based therapy in patients with advanced colorectal cancer and that raltitrexed has the advantage of a predictable toxicity profile, minimization or avoidance of mucositis, and convenient dosing schedule. The data concerning progression-free survival and survival are not consistent, however, with at least one large study demonstrating inferiority with respect to therapy with 5-fluorouracil and leucovorin.

ZD9331

ZD9331 is a potent quinazoline antifolate inhibitor of TS that does not require polyglutamation by folylpolyglutamate synthetase for activity. The lack of required polyglutamation of ZD9331, which is in contrast to raltitrexed, may allow for antitumor activity in cells with low FPGS activity. ZD9331 is transported into cells predominantly by the RFC system and competes with both MTX and folinic acid for cellular uptake. Jackman and colleagues found that ZD9331 had reduced activity against two cell lines (L1210:1565 and CEM/MTX) that were low expressers of RFC.[176a] Using a mouse model, the authors observed both gastrointestinal toxicity and myelosuppression in the form of weight loss and neutropenia/thrombocytopenia, respectively. Walton et al.[508] reviewed the effects of bolus dosing and route of administration in mice, and found ZD9331 to be nonnephrotoxic at active antitumor doses (50 mg per kg via intraperitoneal administration). Intravenous doses of 200 mg per kg resulted in peak kidney drug concentrations that were 20-fold greater than after intraperitoneal administration and resulted in a significant reduction in glomerular filtration, which also was not found with intraperitoneal administration of drug.

1843U89

1843U89 (U89, GW1843) is an antifolate inhibitor of TS that retains a terminal glutamate moiety and therefore requires transportation into the cell by the RFC. It undergoes metabolism to the polyglutamate state but only up to the addition of a single glutamic acid moiety to the parent compound, that is, to a diglutamate.[509] In addition to being a potent inhibitor of TS (K_i = 0.09 nmol per L), 1843U89 differs from other folate-based inhibitors of TS in that the parent compound (monoglutamate) is as potent an enzyme inhibitor as the diglutamated metabolite.[509,510] Studies examining the 1.95 Å crystal structure of *E. coli* TS bound to 1843U89 and dUMP found that the 1843U89 binding site included a normally buried hydrophobic patch accessible to the drug only after insertion of 1843U89 into the wall of the TS active site and resultant local distortion of the protein.[511] Smith and colleagues[512] used canine and murine models to investigate whether the antitumor selectivity of 1843U89 could be enhanced by combining the drug with folic acid. They found that oral folic acid administered 30 minutes before intravenous administration of 1843U89 increased the maximally tolerated and lethal doses of 1843U89 in dogs and thymidine-depleted mice. Further, folic acid administration blocked mouse and dog intestinal toxicity without decreasing efficacy of 1843U89.

Antibody-Directed Enzyme Therapy

Antibody-directed enzyme therapy (ADEPT) systems separate cytotoxic and targeting functions by binding to cell surface markers expressed specifically on malignant cells and activating molecules, including antifolate compounds like MTX at the target cell. This targeted binding and activation theoretically minimizes generalized toxicity secondary to nonspecific delivery of cytotoxic drug. Studies done by Springer et al. delivered an antibody-CPG2 enzyme before the nontoxic prodrug CMDA. Once delivered, CMDA was converted to a cytotoxic drug by the action of the localized conjugate at the tumor site.[513] In addition, prodrugs of quinazoline antifolate TS inhibitors (ZD1694 and ICI198583) have been designed and synthesized for use in ADEPT systems. The α-linked L-dipeptide prodrugs were designed to be activated to their corresponding TS inhibitors at the tumor site by prior administration of a monoclonal antibody conjugated to the enzyme carboxypeptidase A. Activation of the α-linked L-alanine dipeptides with carboxypeptidase A led to a cytotoxicity enhancement of ten- to 100-fold.[514] ADEPT holds the potential of providing an effective and relatively nontoxic treatment of cancer.[515]

REFERENCES

1. Farber S, Diamond LK, Mercer RD, et al. Temporary remission in acute leukemia in children produced by folic acid antagonist 4-amethopteroylglutamic acid (aminopterin). *N Engl J Med* 1948;238:787.
2. DeVita VT. *Cancer: principles and practice of oncology*, 4th ed. Philadelphia, JB Lippincott, 1993.
3. Hoffmeister RT. Methotrexate therapy in rheumatoid arthritis: 15 years' experience. *Am J Med* 1983;75:69–73.
4. Storb R, Deeg HJ, Fisher L, et al. Cyclosporine v methotrexate for graft-v-host disease prevention in patients given marrow grafts for leukemia: long-term follow-up of three controlled trials. *Blood* 1988;71:293–298.
5. Rees RB, Bennett JH, Maibach HI, et al. Methotrexate for psoriasis. *Arch Dermatol* 1967;95:2–11.
6. Calabresi P, Chabner BA. Chemotherapy of neoplastic diseases. In: Gilman AG, Rall TW, Dies DS, et al., eds. *The pharmacologic basis of therapeutics*, 8th ed. New York: Pergamon Press, 1990:1202.
7. Allegra CJ, Chabner BA, Tuazon CU, et al. Trimetrexate for the treatment of Pneumocystis carinii pneumonia in patients with the acquired immunodeficiency syndrome. *N Engl J Med* 1987;317:978–985.
8. Allegra CJ, Fine RL, Drake JC, et al. The effect of methotrexate on intracellular folate pools in human MCF-7 breast cancer cells. Evidence for direct inhibition of purine synthesis. *J Biol Chem* 1986;261:6478–6485.
9. Matherly LH, Barlowe CK, Phillips VM, et al. The effects of 4-amino-antifolates on 5-formyltetrahydrofolate metabolism in L1210 cells. *J Biol Chem* 1987;262:710–717.
10. Baram J, Allegra CJ, Fine RL, et al. Effect of methotrexate on intracellular folate pools in purified myeloid precursor cells from normal human bone marrow. *J Clin Invest* 1987;79:692–697.
11. Kesavan V, Sur P, Doig MT, et al. Effects of methotrexate on folates in Krebs ascites and L1210 murine leukemia cells. *Cancer Lett* 1986;30:55–59.
12. Bunni M, Doig MT, Donato H, et al. Role of methylenetetrahydrofolate depletion in methotrexate-mediated intracellular thymidylate synthesis inhibition in cultured L1210 cells. *Cancer Res* 1988;48:3398–3404.
13. Seither RL, Trent DF, Mikulecky DC, et al. Folate-pool interconversions and inhibition of biosynthetic processes after exposure of L1210 leukemia cells to antifolates. Experimental and network thermodynamic analyses of the role of dihydrofolate polyglutamylates in antifolate action in cells. *J Biol Chem* 1989;264:17016–17023.
14. Priest DG, Bunni M, Sirotnak FM. Relationship of reduced folate changes to inhibition of DNA synthesis induced by

methotrexate in L1210 cells in vivo. *Cancer Res* 1989; 49:4204–4209.

15. Allegra CJ, Hoang K, Yeh GC, et al. Evidence for direct inhibition of de novo purine synthesis in human MCF-7 breast cells as a principal mode of metabolic inhibition by methotrexate. *J Biol Chem* 1987;262:13520–13526.

16. Baram J, Chabner BA, Drake JC, et al. Identification and biochemical properties of 10-formyldihydrofolate, a novel folate found in methotrexate-treated cells. *J Biol Chem* 1988;263:7105–7111.

17. Kumar P, Kisliuk RL, Gaumont Y, et al. Inhibition of human dihydrofolate reductase by antifolyl polyglutamates. *Biochem Pharmacol* 1989;38:541–543.

18. Allegra CJ, Chabner BA, Drake JC, et al. Enhanced inhibition of thymidylate synthase by methotrexate polyglutamates. *J Biol Chem* 1985;260:9720–9726.

19. Allegra CJ, Drake JC, Jolivet J, et al. Inhibition of phosphoribosylaminoimidazolecarboxamide transformylase by methotrexate and dihydrofolic acid polyglutamates. *Proc Natl Acad Sci U S A* 1985;82:4881–4885.

20. Baggott JE, Vaughn WH, Hudson BB. Inhibition of 5-aminoimidazole-4-carboxamide ribotide transformylase, adenosine deaminase and 5'-adenylate deaminase by polyglutamates of methotrexate and oxidized folates and by 5-aminoimidazole-4-carboxamide riboside and ribotide. *Biochem J* 1986;236:193–200.

21. Chu E, Drake JC, Boarman D, et al. Mechanism of thymidylate synthase inhibition by methotrexate in human neoplastic cell lines and normal human myeloid progenitor cells. *J Biol Chem* 1990;265:8470–8478.

22. Morrison PF, Allegra CJ. Folate cycle kinetics in human breast cancer cells. *J Biol Chem* 1989;264:10552–10566.

23. Lyons SD, Sant ME, Christopherson RI. Cytotoxic mechanisms of glutamine antagonists in mouse L1210 leukemia. *J Biol Chem* 1990;265:11377–11381.

24. Bertino JR, Sawicki WL, Moroson BA, et al. 2,4-diamino-5-methyl-6-[(3,4,5-trimethoxyanilino)methyl]quinazoline (tmq), a potent non-classical folate antagonist inhibitor—I effect on dihydrofolate reductase and growth of rodent tumors in vitro and in vivo. *Biochem Pharmacol* 1979;28: 1983–1987.

25. O'Dwyer PJ, Shoemaker DD, Plowman J, et al. Trimetrexate: a new antifol entering clinical trials. *Invest New Drugs* 1985;3:71–75.

26. Sigel CW, Macklin AW, Woolley JL Jr, et al. Preclinical biochemical pharmacology and toxicology of piritrexim, a lipophilic inhibitor of dihydrofolate reductase. *J Natl Cancer Inst Monogr* 1987;5:111–120.

27. Sirotnak FM, DeGraw JI, Schmid FA, et al. New folate analogs of the 10-deaza-aminopterin series. Further evidence for markedly increased antitumor efficacy compared with methotrexate in ascitic and solid murine tumor models. *Cancer Chemother Pharmacol* 1984;12:26–30.

28. Kamen BA, Eibl B, Cashmore A, et al. Uptake and efficacy of trimetrexate (TMQ, 2,4-diamino-5-methyl-6-[(3,4,5-trimethoxyanilino)methyl] quinazoline), a non-classical antifolate in methotrexate-resistant leukemia cells in vitro. *Biochem Pharmacol* 1984;33:1697–1699.

29. Jones TR, Calvert AH, Jackman AL, et al. A potent antitumour quinazoline inhibitor of thymidylate synthetase: synthesis, biological properties and therapeutic results in mice. *Eur J Cancer* 1981;17:11–19.

30. Jones TR, Calvert AH, Jackman AL, et al. A potent antitumor quinazoline inhibitor of thymidylate synthetase, biological properties and therapeutic results in mice. *Eur J Cancer* 1981;17:11–19.

31. Cheng YC, Dutschman GE, Starnes MC, et al. Activity of the new antifolate N10-propargyl-5,8-dideazafolate and its polyglutamates against human dihydrofolate reductase, human thymidylate synthetase, and KB cells containing different levels of dihydrofolate reductase. *Cancer Res* 1985;45:598–600.

32. Grindey GB, Shih C, Bernett CJ, et al. A novel pyrrolopyrimidine antifolate that inhibits thymidylate synthase (TS). *Am Assoc Cancer Res* 1992:2451.

33. Humphreys J, Smith G, Waters K, et al. Antitumor activity of the novel thymidylate synthase inhibitor 1843U89 in cells resistant to antifolates by multiple mechanisms. *Am Assoc Cancer Res* 1993:1625.

34. Beardsley GP, Taylor EC, Grindley GB, et al. Deaza derivatives of tetrahydrofolic acid: a new class of folate antimetabolite. In: Cooper BA, Whitehead VM, eds. *Chemistry and biology of pteridines*. Berlin: Walter deGruyter, 1986:953.

35. Antony AC, Kane MA, Portillo RM, et al. Studies of the role of a particulate folate-binding protein in the uptake of 5-methyltetrahydrofolate by cultured human KB cells. *J Biol Chem* 1985;260:14911–14917.

36. Kamen BA, Capdevila A. Receptor-mediated folate accumulation is regulated by the cellular folate content. *Proc Natl Acad Sci U S A* 1986;83:5983–5987.

37. Fan J, Vitols KS, Huennekens FM. Biotin derivatives of methotrexate and folate. Synthesis and utilization for affinity purification of two membrane-associated folate transporters from L1210 cells. *J Biol Chem* 1991;266:14862–14865.

38. Brigle KE, Westin EH, Houghton MT, et al. Characterization of two cDNAs encoding folate-binding proteins from L1210 murine leukemia cells. Increased expression associated with a genomic rearrangement. *J Biol Chem* 1991;266: 17243–17249.

39. Kamen BA, Bertino JR. Folate and anti-folate transport in mammalian cells. *Antibiot Chemother* 1980;28:62–67.

40. Chello PL, Sirotnak FM, Dorick DM. Alterations in the kinetics of methotrexate transport during growth of L1210 murine leukemia cells in culture. *Mol Pharmacol* 1980;18: 274–280.

41. Corin RE, Haspel HC, Sonenberg M. Transport of the folate compound methotrexate decreases during differentiation of murine erythroleukemia cells. *J Biol Chem* 1984; 259:206–211.

42. Knight CB, Elwood PC, Chabner BA. Future directions for antifolate drug development. *Adv Enzyme Regul* 1989; 29:3–12.

43. Henderson GB, Zevely EM. Affinity labeling of the 5-methyltetrahydrofolate/methotrexate transport protein of L1210 cells by treatment with an N-hydroxysuccinimide ester of [3H]methotrexate. *J Biol Chem* 1984;259:4558–4562.

44. Kane MA, Portillo RM, Elwood PC, et al. The influence of extracellular folate concentration on methotrexate uptake by human KB cells. Partial characterization of a membrane-

associated methotrexate binding protein. *J Biol Chem* 1986; 261:44–49.

45. Price EM, Freisheim JH. Photoaffinity analogues of methotrexate as folate antagonist binding probes. 2. Transport studies, photoaffinity labeling, and identification of the membrane carrier protein for methotrexate from murine L1210 cells. *Biochemistry* 1987;26:4757–4763.

46. Goldman ID, Lichtenstein NS, Oliverio VT. Carrier-mediated transport of the folic acid analogue, methotrexate, in the L1210 leukemia cell. *J Biol Chem* 1968;243:5007–5017.

47. Sirotnak FM, Donsbach RC. Kinetic correlates of methotrexate transport and therapeutic responsiveness in murine tumors. *Cancer Res* 1976;36:1151–1158.

48. Warren RD, Nichols AP, Bender RA. Membrane transport of methotrexate in human lymphoblastoid cells. *Cancer Res* 1978;38:668–671.

49. Henderson GB, Tsuji JM, Kumar HP. Transport of folate compounds by leukemic cells. Evidence for a single influx carrier for methotrexate, 5-methyltetrahydrofolate, and folate in CCRF-CEM human lymphoblasts. *Biochem Pharmacol* 1987;36:3007–3014.

50. Antony AC. The biological chemistry of folate receptors. *Blood* 1992;79:2807–2820.

51. Sirotnak FM, Goutas LJ, Jacobsen DM, et al. Carrier-mediated transport of folate compounds in L1210 cells. Initial rate kinetics and extent of duality of entry routes for folic acid and diastereomers of 5-methyltetrahydrohomofolate in the presence of physiological anions. *Biochem Pharmacol* 1987;36:1659–1667.

52. Matherly LH, Czajkowski CA, Angeles SM. Identification of a highly glycosylated methotrexate membrane carrier in K562 human erythroleukemia cells up-regulated for tetrahydrofolate cofactor and methotrexate transport. *Cancer Res* 1991;51:3420–3426.

53. Wong SC, Proefke SA, Bhushan A, et al. Isolation of human cDNAs that restore methotrexate sensitivity and reduced folate carrier activity in methotrexate transport-defective Chinese hamster ovary cells. *J Biol Chem* 1995;270:17468–17475.

54. Moscow JA, Gong M, He R, et al. Isolation of a gene encoding a human reduced folate carrier (RFC1) and analysis of its expression in transport-deficient, methotrexate-resistant human breast cancer cells. *Cancer Res* 1995;55:3790–3794.

55. Prasad PD, Ramamoorthy S, Leibach FH, et al. Molecular cloning of the human placental folate transporter. *Biochem Biophys Res Commun* 1995;206:681–687.

56. Williams FM, Flintoff WF. Isolation of a human cDNA that complements a mutant hamster cell defective in methotrexate uptake. *J Biol Chem* 1995;270:2987–2992.

57. Ratnam M, Marquardt H, Duhring JL, et al. Homologous membrane folate binding proteins in human placenta: cloning and sequence of a cDNA. *Biochemistry* 1989;28:8249–8254.

58. Campbell IG, Jones TA, Foulkes WD, et al. Folate-binding protein is a marker for ovarian cancer. *Cancer Res* 1991; 51:5329–5338.

59. Coney LR, Tomassetti A, Carayannopoulos L, et al. Cloning of a tumor-associated antigen: MOv18 and MOv19 antibodies recognize a folate-binding protein. *Cancer Res* 1991;51:6125–6132.

60. Elwood PC, Kane MA, Portillo RM, et al. The isolation, characterization, and comparison of the membrane-associated and soluble folate-binding proteins from human KB cells. *J Biol Chem* 1986;261:15416–15423.

61. Shen F, Ross JF, Wang X, et al. Identification of a novel folate receptor, a truncated receptor, and receptor type beta in hematopoietic cells: cDNA cloning, expression, immunoreactivity, and tissue specificity. *Biochemistry* 1994;33: 1209–1215.

62. Roberts SJ, Petropavlovskaja M, Chung KN, et al. Role of individual N-linked glycosylation sites in the function and intracellular transport of the human alpha folate receptor. *Arch Biochem Biophys* 1998;351:227–235.

63. Roberts SJ, Chung KN, Nachmanoff K, et al. Tissue-specific promoters of the alpha human folate receptor gene yield transcripts with divergent 5' leader sequences and different translational efficiencies. *Biochem J* 1997;326:439–447.

64. Elwood PC, Nachmanoff K, Saikawa Y, et al. The divergent 5' termini of the alpha human folate receptor (hFR) mRNAs originate from two tissue-specific promoters and alternative splicing: characterization of the alpha hFR gene structure. *Biochemistry* 1997;36:1467–1478.

65. Sun XL, Murphy BR, Li QJ, et al. Transduction of folate receptor cDNA into cervical carcinoma cells using recombinant adeno-associated virions delays cell proliferation in vitro and in vivo. *J Clin Invest* 1995;96:1535–1547.

66. Shen F, Zheng X, Wang J, et al. Identification of amino acid residues that determine the differential ligand specificities of folate receptors alpha and beta. *Biochemistry* 1997;36:6157–6163.

67. Wu M, Fan J, Gunning W, et al. Clustering of GPI-anchored folate receptor independent of both cross-linking and association with caveolin. *J Membr Biol* 1997;159:137–147.

68. Anderson RG, Kamen BA, Rothberg KG, et al. Potocytosis: sequestration and transport of small molecules by caveolae. *Science* 1992;255:410–411.

69. Kamen BA, Smith AK, Anderson RG. The folate receptor works in tandem with a probenecid-sensitive carrier in MA104 cells in vitro. *J Clin Invest* 1991;87:1442–1449.

70. Chang WJ, Rothberg KG, Kamen BA, et al. Lowering the cholesterol content of MA104 cells inhibits receptor-mediated transport of folate. *J Cell Biol* 1992;118:63–69.

71. Smart EJ, Mineo C, Anderson RG. Clustered folate receptors deliver 5-methyltetrahydrofolate to cytoplasm of MA104 cells. *J Cell Biol* 1996;134:1169–1177.

72. Lewis CM, Smith AK, Kamen BA. Receptor-mediated folate uptake is positively regulated by disruption of the actin cytoskeleton. *Cancer Res* 1998;58:2952–2956.

73. Spinella MJ, Brigle KE, Sierra EE, et al. Distinguishing between folate receptor-alpha-mediated transport and reduced folate carrier-mediated transport in L1210 leukemia cells. *J Biol Chem* 1995;270:7842–7849.

74. Westerhof GR, Rijnboutt S, Schornagel JH, et al. Functional activity of the reduced folate carrier in KB, MA104, and IGROV-I cells expressing folate-binding protein. *Cancer Res* 1995;55:3795–3802.

75. Kessel D, Hall TC, Roberts D, et al. Uptake as a determinant of methotrexate response in mouse leukemias. *Science* 1965;150:752–754.

76. Fisher GA. Defective transport of amethopterin (methotrexate) as a mechanism of resistance to the antimetabolite in L5178 leukemia cells. *Biochem Pharmacol* 1962;11:1233–1234.

77. Galivan J. Transport and metabolism of methotrexate in

normal and resistant cultured rat hepatoma cells. *Cancer Res* 1979;39:735–743.

78. Sirotnak FM, Moccio DM, Kelleher LE, et al. Relative frequency and kinetic properties of transport-defective phenotypes among methotrexate-resistant L1210 clonal cell lines derived in vivo. *Cancer Res* 1981;41:4447–4452.

79. Browman GP, Gorka C, Mehta C, et al. Studies with a 2,4-diamino-5-(3',4'-dichlorophenyl)-6-methylpyrimidine (DDMP)-resistant L1210 leukemia cell line without cross-resistance to methotrexate. *Biochem Pharmacol* 1980;29:2241–2245.

80. Schuetz JD, Matherly LH, Westin EH, et al. Evidence for a functional defect in the translocation of the methotrexate transport carrier in a methotrexate-resistant murine L1210 leukemia cell line. *J Biol Chem* 1988;263:9840–9847.

81. Assaraf YG, Schimke RT. Identification of methotrexate transport deficiency in mammalian cells using fluoresceinated methotrexate and flow cytometry. *Proc Natl Acad Sci U S A* 1987;84:7154–7158.

82. Rodenhuis S, McGuire JJ, Narayanan R, et al. Development of an assay system for the detection and classification of methotrexate resistance in fresh human leukemic cells. *Cancer Res* 1986;46:6513–6519.

83. Schuetz JD, Westin EH, Matherly LH, et al. Membrane protein changes in an L1210 leukemia cell line with a translocation defect in the methotrexate-tetrahydrofolate cofactor transport carrier. *J Biol Chem* 1989;264:16261–16267.

84. Kano Y, Ohnuma T, Holland JF. Folate requirements of methotrexate-resistant human acute lymphoblastic leukemia cell lines. *Blood* 1986;68:586–591.

85. Jansen G, Westerhof GR, Kathmann I, et al. Identification of a membrane-associated folate-binding protein in human leukemic CCRF-CEM cells with transport-related methotrexate resistance [published erratum appears in Cancer Res 1995;55(18):4203]. *Cancer Res* 1989;49:2455–2459.

86. Sierra EE, Brigle KE, Spinella MJ, et al. pH dependence of methotrexate transport by the reduced folate carrier and the folate receptor in L1210 leukemia cells. Further evidence for a third route mediated at low pH. *Biochem Pharmacol* 1997;53:223–231.

87. Zhao R, Assaraf YG, Goldman ID. A mutated murine reduced folate carrier (RFC1) with increased affinity for folic acid, decreased affinity for methotrexate, and an obligatory anion requirement for transport function. *J Biol Chem* 1998;273:19065–19071.

88. Zhao R, Assaraf YG, Goldman ID. A reduced folate carrier mutation produces substrate-dependent alterations in carrier mobility in murine leukemia cells and methotrexate resistance with conservation of growth in 5-formyltetrahydrofolate. *J Biol Chem* 1998;273:7873–7879.

89. Zhao R, Sharina IG, Goldman ID. Pattern of mutations that results in loss of reduced folate carrier function under antifolate selective pressure augmented by chemical mutagenesis. *Mol Pharmacol* 1999;56:68–76.

90. Trippett T, Schlemmer S, Elisseyeff Y, et al. Defective transport as a mechanism of acquired resistance to methotrexate in patients with acute lymphocytic leukemia. *Blood* 1992;80:1158–1162.

91. Guo W, Healey JH, Meyers PA, et al. Mechanisms of methotrexate resistance in osteosarcoma. *Clin Cancer Res* 1999;5:621–627.

92. Moscow JA. Methotrexate transport and resistance. *Leuk Lymphoma* 1998;30:215–224.

93. Taylor IW, Slowiaczek P, Friedlander ML, et al. Selective toxicity of a new lipophilic antifolate, BW301U, for methotrexate-resistant cells with reduced drug uptake. *Cancer Res* 1985;45:978–982.

94. Rosowsky A, Lazarus H, Yuan GC, et al. Effects of methotrexate esters and other lipophilic antifolates on methotrexate-resistant human leukemic lymphoblasts. *Biochem Pharmacol* 1980;29:648–652.

95. Mini E, Moroson BA, Franco CT, et al. Cytotoxic effects of folate antagonists against methotrexate-resistant human leukemic lymphoblast CCRF-CEM cell lines. *Cancer Res* 1985;45:325–330.

96. Sirotnak FM, Donsbach RC. Comparative studies on the transport of aminopterin, methotrexate, and methasquin by the L1210 leukemia cell. *Cancer Res* 1972;32:2120–2126.

97. Schmid FA, Sirotnak FM, Otter GM, et al. Combination chemotherapy with a new folate analog: activity of 10-ethyl-10-deaza-aminopterin compared to methotrexate with 5-fluorouracil and alkylating agents against advanced metastatic disease in murine tumor models. *Cancer Treat Rep* 1987;71:727–732.

98. Nair MG, Nanavati NT, Kumar P, et al. Synthesis and biological evaluation of poly-gamma-glutamyl metabolites of 10-deazaaminopterin and 10-ethyl-10-deazaaminopterin. *J Med Chem* 1988;31:181–185.

99. Van der Laan BF, Jansen G, Kathmann GA, et al. In vitro activity of novel antifolates against human squamous carcinoma cell lines of the head and neck with inherent resistance to methotrexate. *Int J Cancer* 1992;51:909–914.

100. Grant SC, Kris MG, Young CW, et al. Edatrexate, an antifolate with antitumor activity: a review. *Cancer Invest* 1993;11:36–45.

101. Jansen G, Schornagel JH, Westerhof GR, et al. Multiple membrane transport systems for the uptake of folate-based thymidylate synthase inhibitors. *Cancer Res* 1990;50:7544–7548.

102. Westerhof GR, Jansen G, van Emmerik N, et al. Membrane transport of natural folates and antifolate compounds in murine L1210 leukemia cells: role of carrier- and receptor-mediated transport systems. *Cancer Res* 1991;51:5507–5513.

103. Pinard MF, Jolivet J, Ratnam M, et al. Functional aspects of membrane folate receptors in human breast cancer cells with transport-related resistance to methotrexate. *Cancer Chemother Pharmacol* 1996;38:281–288.

104. Henderson GB, Strauss BP. Growth inhibition by homofolate in tumor cells utilizing a high-affinity folate binding protein as a means for folate internalization. *Biochem Pharmacol* 1990;39:2019–2025.

105. Sen S, Erba E, D'Incalci M, et al. Role of membrane folate-binding protein in the cytotoxicity of 5,10-dideazatetrahydrofolic acid in human ovarian carcinoma cell lines in vitro. *Br J Cancer* 1996;73:525–530.

106. Mendelsohn LG, Gates SB, Habeck LL, et al. The role of dietary folate in modulation of folate receptor expression, folylpolyglutamate synthetase activity and the efficacy and toxicity of lometrexol. *Adv Enzyme Regul* 1996;36:365–381.

107. Lin JT, Cashmore AR, Baker M, et al. Phase I studies with trimetrexate: clinical pharmacology, analytical methodology, and pharmacokinetics. *Cancer Res* 1987;47:609–616.

108. Stewart JA, McCormack JJ, Tong W, et al. Phase I clinical and pharmacokinetic study of trimetrexate using a daily ×5 schedule. *Cancer Res* 1988;48:5029–5035.

109. Laszlo J, Brenckman WD Jr, Morgan E, et al. Initial clinical studies of piritrexim. *J Natl Cancer Inst Monogr* 1987;5:121–125.

110. Allegra CJ, Kovacs JA, Drake JC, et al. Activity of antifolates against Pneumocystis carinii dihydrofolate reductase and identification of a potent new agent. *J Exp Med* 1987;165:926–931.

111. Hum M, Holcenberg JS, Tkaczewski I, et al. High-dose trimetrexate and minimal-dose leucovorin: a case for selective protection? *Clin Cancer Res* 1998;4:2981–2984.

112. Currie VE, Warrell RP Jr, Arlin Z, et al. Phase I trial of 10-deaza-aminopterin in patients with advanced cancer. *Cancer Treat Rep* 1983;67:149–154.

113. Casper ES, Christman KL, Schwartz GK, et al. Edatrexate in patients with soft tissue sarcoma. Activity in malignant fibrous histiocytoma. *Cancer* 1993;72:766–770.

114. Vandenberg TA, Pritchard KI, Eisenhauer EA, et al. Phase II study of weekly edatrexate as first-line chemotherapy for metastatic breast cancer: a National Cancer Institute of Canada Clinical Trials Group study. *J Clin Oncol* 1993;11:1241–1244.

115. Saxena M, Henderson GB. Identification of efflux systems for large anions and anionic conjugates as the mediators of methotrexate efflux in L1210 cells. *Biochem Pharmacol* 1996;51:974–982.

116. Sirotnak FM, Moccio DM, Young CW. Increased accumulation of methotrexate by murine tumor cells in vitro in the presence of probenecid which is mediated by a preferential inhibition of efflux. *Cancer Res* 1981;41:966–970.

117. Sirotnak FM, Moccio DM, Hancock CH, et al. Improved methotrexate therapy of murine tumors obtained by probenecid-mediated pharmacological modulation at the level of membrane transport. *Cancer Res* 1981;41:3944–3949.

118. Henderson GB, Zevely EM. Inhibitory effects of probenecid on the individual transport routes which mediate the influx and efflux of methotrexate in L1210 cells. *Biochem Pharmacol* 1985;34:1725–1729.

119. Henderson GB, Tsuji JM. Methotrexate efflux in L1210 cells. Kinetic and specificity properties of the efflux system sensitive to bromosulfophthalein and its possible identity with a system which mediates the efflux of 3′,5′-cyclic AMP. *J Biol Chem* 1987;262:13571–13578.

120. Assaraf YG, Goldman ID. Loss of folic acid exporter function with markedly augmented folate accumulation in lipophilic antifolate-resistant mammalian cells. *J Biol Chem* 1997;272:17460–17466.

121. Henderson GB, Tsuji JM, Kumar HP. Characterization of the individual transport routes that mediate the influx and efflux of methotrexate in CCRF-CEM human lymphoblastic cells. *Cancer Res* 1986;46:1633–1638.

122. Norris MD, De Graaf D, Haber M, et al. Involvement of MDR1 P-glycoprotein in multifactorial resistance to methotrexate. *Int J Cancer* 1996;65:613–619.

123. De Graaf D, Sharma RC, Mechetner EB, et al. P-glycoprotein confers methotrexate resistance in 3T6 cells with deficient carrier-mediated methotrexate uptake. *Proc Natl Acad Sci U S A* 1996;93:1238–1242.

124. Li WW, Fan J, Hochhauser D, et al. Overexpression of p21waf1 leads to increased inhibition of E2F-1 phosphorylation and sensitivity to anticancer drugs in retinoblastoma-negative human sarcoma cells. *Cancer Res* 1997;57:2193–2139.

125. Koizumi S, Curt GA, Fine RL, et al. Formation of methotrexate polyglutamates in purified myeloid precursor cells from normal human bone marrow. *J Clin Invest* 1985;75:1008–1014.

126. Fabre I, Fabre G, Goldman ID. Polyglutamylation, an important element in methotrexate cytotoxicity and selectivity in tumor versus murine granulocytic progenitor cells in vitro. *Cancer Res* 1984;44:3190–3195.

127. Rosenblatt DS, Whitehead VM, Dupont MM, et al. Synthesis of methotrexate polyglutamates in cultured human cells. *Mol Pharmacol* 1978;14:210–214.

128. Whitehead VM. Synthesis of methotrexate polyglutamates in L1210 murine leukemia cells. *Cancer Res* 1977;37:408–412.

129. Schilsky RL, Bailey BD, Chabner BA. Methotrexate polyglutamate synthesis by cultured human breast cancer cells. *Proc Natl Acad Sci U S A* 1980;77:2919–2922.

130. Jolivet J, Schilsky RL, Bailey BD, et al. Synthesis, retention, and biological activity of methotrexate polyglutamates in cultured human breast cancer cells. *J Clin Invest* 1982;70:351–360.

131. Kennedy DG, Van den Berg HW, Clarke R, et al. The effect of the rate of cell proliferation on the synthesis of methotrexate poly-gamma-glutamates in two human breast cancer cell lines. *Biochem Pharmacol* 1985;34:3087–3090.

132. Galivan J, Nimec Z, Rhee M. Synergistic growth inhibition of rat hepatoma cells exposed in vitro to N10-propargyl-5,8-dideazafolate with methotrexate or the lipophilic antifolates trimetrexate or metoprine. *Cancer Res* 1987;47:5256–5260.

133. Whitehead VM, Rosenblatt DS, Vuchich MJ, et al. Methotrexate polyglutamate synthesis in lymphoblasts from children with acute lymphoblastic leukemia. *Dev Pharmacol Ther* 1987;10:443–448.

134. Jolivet J, Chabner BA. Intracellular pharmacokinetics of methotrexate polyglutamates in human breast cancer cells. Selective retention and less dissociable binding of 4-NH2-10-CH3-pteroylglutamate4 and 4-NH2-10-CH3-pteroylglutamate5 to dihydrofolate reductase. *J Clin Invest* 1983;72:773–778.

135. Samuels LL, Feinberg A, Moccio DM, et al. Detection by high-performance liquid chromatography of methotrexate and its metabolites in tumor tissue from osteosarcoma patients treated with high-dose methotrexate/leucovorin rescue. *Biochem Pharmacol* 1984;33:2711–2714.

136. Winick NJ, Kamen BA, Balis FM, et al. Folate and methotrexate polyglutamate tissue levels in rhesus monkeys following chronic low-dose methotrexate. *Cancer Drug Deliv* 1987;4:25–31.

137. Shane B. Folylpolyglutamate synthesis and role in the regulation of one-carbon metabolism. *Vitam Horm* 1989;45:263–335.

138. Gewirtz DA, White JC, Randolph JK, et al. Formation of methotrexate polyglutamates in rat hepatocytes. *Cancer Res* 1979;39:2914–2918.

139. McGuire J, Kitamoto Y, Hsieh P, et al. Characterization of mammalian folyl polyglutamate synthetase. In: Kisliuk RL, Brown GM, eds. *Chemistry and biology of pteridines*. New York: Elsevier/North Holland, 1978:471–476.

140. Clarke L, Waxman DJ. Human liver folylpolyglutamate synthetase: biochemical characterization and interactions

with folates and folate antagonists. *Arch Biochem Biophys* 1987;256:585–596.

141. Cichowicz DJ, Shane B. Mammalian folylpoly-gamma-glutamate synthetase. 1. Purification and general properties of the hog liver enzyme. *Biochemistry* 1987;26:504–512.

142. Cichowicz DJ, Shane B. Mammalian folylpoly-gamma-glutamate synthetase. 2. Substrate specificity and kinetic properties. *Biochemistry* 1987;26:513–521.

143. George S, Cichowicz DJ, Shane B. Mammalian folylpoly-gamma-glutamate synthetase. 3. Specificity for folate analogues. *Biochemistry* 1987;26:522–529.

144. Cook JD, Cichowicz DJ, George S, et al. Mammalian folylpoly-gamma-glutamate synthetase. 4. In vitro and in vivo metabolism of folates and analogues and regulation of folate homeostasis. *Biochemistry* 1987;26:530–539.

145. McGuire JJ, Hsieh P, Coward JK, et al. Enzymatic synthesis of folylpolyglutamates. Characterization of the reaction and its products. *J Biol Chem* 1980;255:5776–5788.

146. McGuire JJ, Hsieh P, Franco CT, et al. Folylpolyglutamate synthetase inhibition and cytotoxic effects of methotrexate analogs containing 2,omega-diaminoalkanoic acids. *Biochem Pharmacol* 1986;35:2607–2613.

147. Shin YS, Buehring KU, Stokstad EL. The metabolism of methotrexate in Lactobacillus casei and rat liver and the influence of methotrexate on metabolism of folic acid. *J Biol Chem* 1974;249:5772–5777.

148. Galivan J, Johnson T, Rhee M, et al. The role of folylpolyglutamate synthetase and gamma-glutamyl hydrolase in altering cellular folyl- and antifolylpolyglutamates. *Adv Enzyme Regul* 1987;26:147–155.

149. Yao R, Schneider E, Ryan TJ, et al. Human gamma-glutamyl hydrolase: cloning and characterization of the enzyme expressed in vitro. *Proc Natl Acad Sci U S A* 1996;93:10134–10138.

150. Rhee MS, Lindau-Shepard B, Chave KJ, et al. Characterization of human cellular gamma-glutamyl hydrolase. *Mol Pharmacol* 1998;53:1040–1046.

151. Waltham MC, Li WW, Gritsman H, et al. Gamma-glutamyl hydrolase from human sarcoma HT-1080 cells: characterization and inhibition by glutamine antagonists. *Mol Pharmacol* 1997;51:825–832.

152. Longo GS, Gorlick R, Tong WP, et al. Disparate affinities of antifolates for folylpolyglutamate synthetase from human leukemia cells. *Blood* 1997;90:1241–1245.

153. Fry DW, Yalowich JC, Goldman ID. Rapid formation of poly-gamma-glutamyl derivatives of methotrexate and their association with dihydrofolate reductase as assessed by high pressure liquid chromatography in the Ehrlich ascites tumor cell in vitro. *J Biol Chem* 1982;257:1890–1896.

154. Fry DW, Yalowich JC, Goldman ID. Augmentation of the intracellular levels of polyglutamyl derivatives of methotrexate by vincristine and probenecid in Ehrlich ascites tumor cells. *Cancer Res* 1982;42:2532–2536.

155. Sirotnak FM, Chello PL, Piper JR, et al. Growth inhibitory, transport and biochemical properties of the gamma-glutamyl and gamma-aspartyl peptides of methotrexate in L1210 leukemia cells in vitro. *Biochem Pharmacol* 1978;27:1821–1825.

156. Schlemmer SR, Sirotnak FM. Retentiveness of methotrexate polyglutamates in cultured L1210 cells. Evidence against

157. Galivan J, Nimec Z. Effects of folinic acid on hepatoma cells containing methotrexate polyglutamates. *Cancer Res* 1983;43:551–555.

158. Galivan J, Nimec Z, Balinska M. Regulation of methotrexate polyglutamate accumulation in vitro: effects of cellular folate content. *Biochem Pharmacol* 1983;32:3244–3247.

159. Nimec Z, Galivan J. Regulatory aspects of the glutamylation of methotrexate in cultured hepatoma cells. *Arch Biochem Biophys* 1983;226:671–680.

160. Kennedy DG, Van den Berg HW, Clarke R, et al. The effect of leucovorin on the synthesis of methotrexate poly-gamma-glutamates in the MCF-7 human breast cancer cell line. *Biochem Pharmacol* 1985;34:2897–2903.

161. Galivan J, Pupons A, Rhee MS. Hepatic parenchymal cell glutamylation of methotrexate studied in monolayer culture. *Cancer Res* 1986;46:670–675.

162. Jolivet J, Faucher F, Pinard MF. Influence of intracellular folates on methotrexate metabolism and cytotoxicity. *Biochem Pharmacol* 1987;36:3310–3312.

163. Jolivet J, Cole DE, Holcenberg JS, et al. Prevention of methotrexate cytotoxicity by asparaginase inhibition of methotrexate polyglutamate formation. *Cancer Res* 1985;45:217–220.

164. Sur P, Fernandes DJ, Kute TE, et al. L-asparaginase-induced modulation of methotrexate polyglutamylation in murine leukemia L5178Y. *Cancer Res* 1987;47:1313–1318.

165. Matherly LH, Fry DW, Goldman ID. Role of methotrexate polyglutamylation and cellular energy metabolism in inhibition of methotrexate binding to dihydrofolate reductase by 5-formyltetrahydrofolate in Ehrlich ascites tumor cells in vitro. *Cancer Res* 1983;43:2694–2699.

166. Allegra CJ, Drake JC, Jolivet J, et al. Inhibition of folate-dependent enzymes by methotrexate polyglutamates. In: Goldman ID, ed. *Proceedings of the Second Workshop on Folyl and Antifolyl Polyglutamates.* New York: Praeger, 1985:348–359.

167. Galivan J, Inglese J, McGuire JJ, et al. Gamma-fluoromethotrexate: synthesis and biological activity of a potent inhibitor of dihydrofolate reductase with greatly diminished ability to form poly-gamma-glutamates. *Proc Natl Acad Sci U S A* 1985;82:2598–2602.

168. Samuels LL, Moccio DM, Sirotnak FM. Similar differential for total polyglutamylation and cytotoxicity among various folate analogues in human and murine tumor cells in vitro. *Cancer Res* 1985;45:1488–1495.

169. Matherly LH, Voss MK, Anderson LA, et al. Enhanced polyglutamylation of aminopterin relative to methotrexate in the Ehrlich ascites tumor cell in vitro. *Cancer Res* 1985;45:1073–1078.

170. Cowan KH, Jolivet J. A methotrexate-resistant human breast cancer cell line with multiple defects, including diminished formation of methotrexate polyglutamates. *J Biol Chem* 1984;259:10793–10800.

171. Pizzorno G, Mini E, Coronnello M, et al. Impaired polyglutamylation of methotrexate as a cause of resistance in CCRF-CEM cells after short-term, high-dose treatment with this drug. *Cancer Res* 1988;48:2149–2155.

172. Pizzorno G, Chang YM, McGuire JJ, et al. Inherent resistance of human squamous carcinoma cell lines to metho-

trexate as a result of decreased polyglutamylation of this drug. *Cancer Res* 1989;49:5275–5280.

173. McCloskey DE, McGuire JJ, Russell CA, et al. Decreased folylpolyglutamate synthetase activity as a mechanism of methotrexate resistance in CCRF-CEM human leukemia sublines. *J Biol Chem* 1991;266:6181–6187.

174. Faessel HM, Slocum HK, Jackson RC, et al. Super in vitro synergy between inhibitors of dihydrofolate reductase and inhibitors of other folate-requiring enzymes: the critical role of polyglutamylation. *Cancer Res* 1998;58:3036–3050.

175. Pizzorno G, Sokoloski JA, Cashmore AR, et al. Intracellular metabolism of 5,10-dideazatetrahydrofolic acid in human leukemia cell lines. *Mol Pharmacol* 1991;39:85–89.

176. Rhee MS, Wang Y, Nair MG, et al. Acquisition of resistance to antifolates caused by enhanced gamma-glutamyl hydrolase activity. *Cancer Res* 1993;53:2227–2230.

176a. Jackman AL, Kimbell R, Aherne GW, et al. Cellular pharmacology and in vivo activity of a new anticancer agent, ZD9331: a water-soluble, nonpolyglutamatable, quinazoline-based inhibitor of thymidylate synthase. *Clin Cancer Res* 1997;3:911–921.

177. Curt GA, Jolivet J, Carney DN, et al. Determinants of the sensitivity of human small-cell lung cancer cell lines to methotrexate. *J Clin Invest* 1985;76:1323–1329.

178. Longo GS, Gorlick R, Tong WP, et al. Gamma-glutamyl hydrolase and folylpolyglutamate synthetase activities predict polyglutamylation of methotrexate in acute leukemias. *Oncol Res* 1997;9:259–263.

179. Galpin AJ, Schuetz JD, Masson E, et al. Differences in folylpolyglutamate synthetase and dihydrofolate reductase expression in human B-lineage versus T-lineage leukemic lymphoblasts: mechanisms for lineage differences in methotrexate polyglutamylation and cytotoxicity. *Mol Pharmacol* 1997;52:155–163.

180. Li WW, Lin JT, Tong WP, et al. Mechanisms of natural resistance to antifolates in human soft tissue sarcomas. *Cancer Res* 1992;52:1434–1438.

181. Li WW, Lin JT, Schweitzer BI, et al. Intrinsic resistance to methotrexate in human soft tissue sarcoma cell lines. *Cancer Res* 1992;52:3908–3913.

182. Gupta SV, Greenfield NJ, Poe M, et al. Dihydrofolate reductase from a resistant subline of the L1210 lymphoma. Purification by affinity chromatography and ultraviolet difference spectrophotometric and circular dichroic studies. *Biochemistry* 1977;16:3073–3079.

183. Nakamura H, Littlefield JW. Purification, properties, and synthesis of dihydrofolate reductase from wild type and methotrexate-resistant hamster cells. *J Biol Chem* 1972;247:179–187.

184. Gready JE. Dihydrofolate reductase: the current story [News]. *Nature* 1979;282:674–675.

185. Matthews DA, Alden RA, Bolin JT, et al. X-ray structural studies of dihydrofolate reductase. In: Kisliuk RL, Brown GM, eds. *Chemistry and biology of pteridines.* New York: Elsevier/North Holland, 1979:465.

186. Charlton PA, Young DW, Birdsall B, et al. Steriochemistry of reduction of folic acid using dihydrofolate reductase. *Chem Commun* 1979;20:922.

187. Matthews DA, Alden RA, Bolin JT, et al. Dihydrofolate reductase: x-ray structure of the binary complex with methotrexate. *Science* 1977;197:452–455.

188. Matthews DA, Bolin JT, Burridge JM, et al. Refined crystal structures of Escherichia coli and chicken liver dihydrofolate reductase containing bound trimethoprim. *J Biol Chem* 1985;260:381–391.

189. Matthews DA, Bolin JT, Burridge JM, et al. Dihydrofolate reductase. The stereochemistry of inhibitor selectivity. *J Biol Chem* 1985;260:392–399.

190. Appleman JR, Howell EE, Kraut J, et al. Role of aspartate 27 in the binding of methotrexate to dihydrofolate reductase from Escherichia coli. *J Biol Chem* 1988;263:9187–9198.

191. Taira K, Benkovic SJ. Evaluation of the importance of hydrophobic interactions in drug binding to dihydrofolate reductase. *J Med Chem* 1988;31:129–137.

192. Thillet J, Absil J, Stone SR, et al. Site-directed mutagenesis of mouse dihydrofolate reductase. Mutants with increased resistance to methotrexate and trimethoprim. *J Biol Chem* 1988;263:12500–12508.

193. Oefner C, D'Arcy A, Winkler FK. Crystal structure of human dihydrofolate reductase complexed with folate. *Eur J Biochem* 1988;174:377–385.

194. Cody V, Ciszak E. Computer graphic modeling in drug design—conformational analysis of antifolate binding to avian dihydrofolate reductase: crystal and molecular structures of 2,4-diamino-5-cyclohexyl-6-methylpyrimidine and 5-cyclohexyl-6-methyluracil. *Anticancer Drug Des* 1991;6:83–93.

195. Freisheim JH, Kumar AA, Blankenship D. Structure-function relationships of dihydrofolate reductases: sequence homology considerations and active center residues. In: Kislink RL, Brown GM, eds. *Chemistry and biology of pteridines.* New York: Elsevier/North Holland, 1979:419.

196. Blakely RL, Freisheim JH. Effects of conversion of phenylalanine-31 to leucine on the function of dihydrofolate reductase. *Biochemistry* 1989;28:4645–4650.

197. Schweitzer BI, Srimatkandada S, Gritsman H, et al. Probing the role of two hydrophobic active site residues in the human dihydrofolate reductase by site-directed mutagenesis. *J Biol Chem* 1989;264:20786–20795.

198. Thompson PD, Freisheim JH. Conversion of arginine to lysine at position 70 of human dihydrofolate reductase: generation of a methotrexate-insensitive mutant enzyme. *Biochemistry* 1991;30:8124–8130.

199. Dicker AP, Waltham MC, Volkenandt M, et al. Methotrexate resistance in an in vivo mouse tumor due to a non-active-site dihydrofolate reductase mutation. *Proc Natl Acad Sci U S A* 1993;90:11797–11801.

200. Bystroff C, Kraut J. Crystal structure of unliganded Escherichia coli dihydrofolate reductase. Ligand-induced conformational changes and cooperativity in binding. *Biochemistry* 1991;30:2227–2239.

201. Zhao SC, Banerjee D, Mineishi S, et al. Post-transplant methotrexate administration leads to improved curability of mice bearing a mammary tumor transplanted with marrow transduced with a mutant human dihydrofolate reductase cDNA. *Hum Gene Ther* 1997;8:903–909.

202. Flasshove M, Banerjee D, Leonard JP, et al. Retroviral transduction of human CD34+ umbilical cord blood progenitor cells with a mutated dihydrofolate reductase cDNA. *Hum Gene Ther* 1998;9:63–71.

203. Patel M, Sleep SE, Lewis WS, et al. Comparison of the protec-

tion of cells from antifolates by transduced human dihydro-folate reductase mutants. *Hum Gene Ther* 1997;8:2069–2077.

204. Blakley RL, Sorrentino BP. In vitro mutations in dihydro-folate reductase that confer resistance to methotrexate: potential for clinical application. *Hum Mutat* 1998;11:259–263.

205. Mareya SM, Sorrentino BP, Blakley RL. Protection of CCRF-CEM human lymphoid cells from antifolates by retroviral gene transfer of variants of murine dihydrofolate reductase. *Cancer Gene Ther* 1998;5:225–235.

206. May C, James RI, Gunther R, et al. Methotrexate dose-escalation studies in transgenic mice and marrow transplant recipients expressing drug-resistant dihydrofolate reductase activity. *J Pharmacol Exp Ther* 1996;278:1444–1451.

207. Braun SE, McIvor RS, Davidson AS, et al. Retrovirally mediated gene transfer of Arg22 and Tyr22 forms of dihydrofolate reductase into the hematopoietic cell line K562: a comparison of methotrexate resistance. *Cancer Gene Ther* 1997;4:26–32.

208. Lewis WS, Cody V, Galitsky N, et al. Methotrexate-resistant variants of human dihydrofolate reductase with substitutions of leucine 22. Kinetics, crystallography, and potential as selectable markers. *J Biol Chem* 1995;270:5057–5064.

209. Appleman JR, Prendergast N, Delcamp TJ, et al. Kinetics of the formation and isomerization of methotrexate complexes of recombinant human dihydrofolate reductase. *J Biol Chem* 1988;263:10304–10313.

210. Morrison JF. The slow-binding and slow, right binding inhibition of enzyme-catalyzed reactions. *Trends Biochem Sci* 1982;7:102.

211. Stone SR, Morrison JF. Mechanisms of inhibition of DHFRs from bacterial and vertebrate sources by various classes of folate analogues. *Biochim Biophys Acta* 1986;869:275–285.

212. Kamen BA, Whyte-Bauer W, Bertino JR. A mechanism of resistance to methotrexate. NADPH but not NADH stimulation of methotrexate binding to dihydrofolate reductase. *Biochem Pharmacol* 1983;32:1837–1841.

213. Jackson RC, Hart LI, Harrap KR. Intrinsic resistance to methotrexate of cultured mammalian cells in relation to the inhibition kinetics of their dihydrofolate reductases. *Cancer Res* 1976;36:1991–1997.

214. Kumar P, Kisliuk RL, Gaumont Y, et al. Interaction of poly-glutamyl derivatives of methotrexate, 10-deazaaminopterin, and dihydrofolate with dihydrofolate reductase. *Cancer Res* 1986;46:5020–5023.

215. Werkheiser WC. The biochemical, cellular and pharmacological action and effects of the folic acid antagonists. *Cancer Res* 1963;23:1277.

216. Cha S. Tight-binding inhibitors—III. A new approach for the determination of competition between tight-binding inhibitors and substrates—inhibition of adenosine deaminase by coformycin. *Biochem Pharmacol* 1976;25:2695–2702.

217. Williams JW, Morrison JF, Duggleby RG. Methotrexate, a high-affinity pseudosubstrate of dihydrofolate reductase. *Biochemistry* 1979;18:2567–2573.

218. Williams JW, Duggleby RG, Cutler R, et al. The inhibition of dihydrofolate reductase by folate analogues: structural requirements for slow- and tight-binding inhibition. *Biochem Pharmacol* 1980;29:589–595.

219. Blakley RL, Cocco L. Role of isomerization of initial complexes in the binding of inhibitors to dihydrofolate reductase. *Biochemistry* 1985;24:4772–4777.

220. Taira K, Fierke CA, Chen JT, et al. On interpreting the inhibition of and catalysis by DHFR. *Trends Biochem Sci* 1987;12:213.

221. White JC. Reversal of methotrexate binding to dihydrofolate reductase by dihydrofolate. Studies with pure enzyme and computer modeling using network thermodynamics. *J Biol Chem* 1979;254:10889–10895.

222. Mead JR, Venditti JM, Schrecker AW, et al. The effect of reduced derivatives of folic acid on toxicity and antileukemic effect of methotrexate in mice. *Biochem Pharmacol* 1963;12:371.

223. Allegra CJ, Boarman D. Interaction of methotrexate polyglutamates and dihydrofolate during leucovorin rescue in a human breast cancer cell line (MCF-7). *Cancer Res* 1990;50:3574–3578.

224. Cohen M, Bender RA, Donehower R, et al. Reversibility of high-affinity binding of methotrexate in L1210 murine leukemia cells. *Cancer Res* 1978;38:2866–2870.

225. Jackson RC, Niethammer D, Hart LI. Reactivation of dihydrofolate reductase inhibited by methotrexate or aminopterin. *Arch Biochem Biophys* 1977;182:646–656.

226. White JC, Loftfield S, Goldman ID. The mechanism of action of methotrexate. III. Requirement of free intracellular methotrexate for maximal suppression of (14C)formate incorporation into nucleic acids and protein. *Mol Pharmacol* 1975;11:287–297.

227. Galivan J. Evidence for the cytotoxic activity of polyglutamate derivatives of methotrexate. *Mol Pharmacol* 1980;17:105–110.

228. Drake JC, Allegra CJ, Baram J, et al. Effects on dihydrofolate reductase of methotrexate metabolites and intracellular folates formed following methotrexate exposure of human breast cancer cells. *Biochem Pharmacol* 1987;36:2416–2418.

229. Boarman DM, Baram J, Allegra CJ. Mechanism of leucovorin reversal of methotrexate cytotoxicity in human MCF-7 breast cancer cells. *Biochem Pharmacol* 1990;40:2651–2660.

230. Kruger-McDermott C, Balinska M, Galivan J. Dihydrofolate-mediated reversal of methotrexate toxicity to hepatoma cells in vitro. *Cancer Lett* 1986;30:79–84.

231. Goldie JH, Krystal J, Hartley D, et al. A methotrexate-insensitive variant of folate reductase present in two lines of methotrexate-resistant L5178Y cells. *Eur J Cancer* 1980;16:1539–1546.

232. Goldie JH, Dedhar S, Krystal G. Properties of a methotrexate-insensitive variant of dihydrofolate reductase derived from methotrexate-resistant L5178Y cells. *J Biol Chem* 1981;256:11629–11635.

233. Dedhar S, Goldie JH. Overproduction of two antigenically distinct forms of dihydrofolate reductase in a highly methotrexate-resistant mouse leukemia cell line. *Cancer Res* 1983;43:4863–4871.

234. McIvor RS, Simonsen CC. Isolation and characterization of a variant dihydrofolate reductase cDNA from methotrexate-resistant murine L5178Y cells. *Nucleic Acids Res* 1990;18:7025–7032.

235. Flintoff WF, Essani K. Methotrexate-resistant Chinese hamster ovary cells contain a dihydrofolate reductase with an altered affinity for methotrexate. *Biochemistry* 1980;19:4321–4327.

236. Melera PW, Davide JP, Hession CA, et al. Phenotypic expression in Escherichia coli and nucleotide sequence of two Chinese hamster lung cell cDNAs encoding different dihydrofolate reductases. *Mol Cell Biol* 1984;4:38–48.

237. Melera PW, Wolgemuth D, Biedler JL, et al. Antifolate-resistant Chinese hamster cells. Evidence from independently derived sublines for the overproduction of two dihydrofolate reductases encoded by different mRNAs. *J Biol Chem* 1980;255:319–322.

238. Melera PW, Lewis JA, Biedler JL, et al. Antifolate-resistant Chinese hamster cells. Evidence for dihydrofolate reductase gene amplification among independently derived sublines overproducing different dihydrofolate reductases. *J Biol Chem* 1980;255:7024–7028.

239. Haber DA, Schimke RT. Unstable amplification of an altered dihydrofolate reductase gene associated with double-minute chromosomes. *Cell* 1981;26:355–362.

240. Dicker AP, Volkenandt M, Schweitzer BI, et al. Identification and characterization of a mutation in the dihydrofolate reductase gene from the methotrexate-resistant Chinese hamster ovary cell line Pro-3 MtxRIII. *J Biol Chem* 1990;265:8317–8321.

241. Cowan KH, Goldsmith ME, Levine RM, et al. Dihydrofolate reductase gene amplification and possible rearrangement in estrogen-responsive methotrexate-resistant human breast cancer cells. *J Biol Chem* 1982;257:15079–15086.

242. Melera PW, Davide JP, Oen H. Antifolate-resistant Chinese hamster cells. Molecular basis for the biochemical and structural heterogeneity among dihydrofolate reductases produced by drug-sensitive and drug-resistant cell lines. *J Biol Chem* 1988;263:1978–1990.

243. Dedhar S, Hartley D, Fitz-Gibbons D, et al. Heterogeneity in the specific activity and methotrexate sensitivity of dihydrofolate reductase from blast cells of acute myelogenous leukemia patients. *J Clin Oncol* 1985;3:1545–1552.

244. Friedkin M, Crawford E, Humphreys SR, et al. The association of dihydrofolate reductase with amethopterin resistance in mouse leukemia. *Cancer Res* 1962;22:600.

245. Kaufman RJ, Bertino JR, Schimke RT. Quantitation of dihydrofolate reductase in individual parental and methotrexate-resistant murine cells. Use of a fluorescence activated cell sorter. *J Biol Chem* 1978;253:5852–5860.

246. Rosowsky A, Wright JE, Cucchi CA, et al. Transport of a fluorescent antifolate by methotrexate-sensitive and methotrexate-resistant human leukemic lymphoblasts. *Biochem Pharmacol* 1986;35:356–360.

247. Johnston RN, Beverley SM, Schimke RT. Rapid spontaneous dihydrofolate reductase gene amplification shown by fluorescence-activated cell sorting. *Proc Natl Acad Sci U S A* 1983;80:3711–3715.

248. Bertino JR, Donohue DR, Simmons B, et al. Induction of dihydrofolate reductase activity in leukocytes and erythrocytes of patients treated with amethopterin. *J Clin Invest* 1963;42:466.

249. Alt FW, Kellems RE, Schimke RT. Synthesis and degradation of folate reductase in sensitive and methotrexate-resistant lines of S-180 cells. *J Biol Chem* 1976;251:3063–3074.

250. Berenson RJ, Francke U, Dolnick BJ, et al. Karyotypic analysis of methotrexate-resistant and sensitive mouse L5178Y cells. *Cytogenet Cell Genet* 1981;29:145–152.

251. Hamlin JL, Biedler JL. Replication pattern of a large homogenously staining chromosome region in antifolate-resistant Chinese hamster cell lines. *J Cell Physiol* 1981;107:101–114.

252. Milbrandt JD, Heintz NH, White WC, et al. Methotrexate-resistant Chinese hamster ovary cells have amplified a 135-kilobase-pair region that includes the dihydrofolate reductase gene. *Proc Natl Acad Sci U S A* 1981;78:6043–6047.

253. Brown PC, Beverley SM, Schimke RT. Relationship of amplified dihydrofolate reductase genes to double minute chromosomes in unstably resistant mouse fibroblast cell lines. *Mol Cell Biol* 1981;1:1077–1083.

254. Kaufman RJ, Brown PC, Schimke RT. Loss and stabilization of amplified dihydrofolate reductase genes in mouse sarcoma S-180 cell lines. *Mol Cell Biol* 1981;1:1084–1093.

255. Tyler-Smith C, Alderson T. Gene amplification in methotrexate-resistant mouse cells. I. DNA rearrangement accompanies dihydrofolate reductase gene amplification in a T-cell lymphoma. *J Mol Biol* 1981;153:203–218.

256. Flintoff WF, Weber MK, Nagainis CR, et al. Overproduction of dihydrofolate reductase and gene amplification in methotrexate-resistant Chinese hamster ovary cells. *Mol Cell Biol* 1982;2:275–285.

257. Domin BA, Grill SP, Bastow KF, et al. Effect of methotrexate on dihydrofolate reductase activity in methotrexate-resistant human KB cells. *Mol Pharmacol* 1982;21:478–482.

258. Domin BA, Grill SP, Cheng Y. Establishment of dihydrofolate reductase-increased human cell lines and relationship between dihydrofolate reductase levels and gene copy. *Cancer Res* 1983;43:2155–2158.

259. Meltzer PS, Cheng YC, Trent JM. Analysis of dihydrofolate reductase gene amplification in a methotrexate-resistant human tumor cell line. *Cancer Genet Cytogenet* 1985;17:289–300.

260. Hoy CA, Rice GC, Kovacs M, et al. Over-replication of DNA in S phase Chinese hamster ovary cells after DNA synthesis inhibition. *J Biol Chem* 1987;262:11927–11934.

261. Mariani BD, Schimke RT. Gene amplification in a single cell cycle in Chinese hamster ovary cells. *J Biol Chem* 1984;259:1901–1910.

262. Fanin R, Banerjee D, Volkenandt M, et al. Mutations leading to antifolate resistance in Chinese hamster ovary cells after exposure to the alkylating agent ethylmethanesulfonate. *Mol Pharmacol* 1993;44:13–21.

263. Kleinberger T, Etkin S, Lavi S. Carcinogen-mediated methotrexate resistance and dihydrofolate reductase amplification in Chinese hamster cells. *Mol Cell Biol* 1986;6:1958–1964.

264. Sharma RC, Schimke RT. Enhancement of the frequency of methotrexate resistance by gamma-radiation in Chinese hamster ovary and mouse 3T6 cells. *Cancer Res* 1989;49:3861–3866.

265. Barsoum J, Varshavsky A. Mitogenic hormones and tumor promoters greatly increase the incidence of colony-forming cells bearing amplified dihydrofolate reductase genes. *Proc Natl Acad Sci U S A* 1983;80:5330–5334.

266. Bojan F, Kinsella AR, Fox M. Effect of tumor promoter 12-O-tetradecanoylphorbol-13-acetate on recovery of methotrexate-, N-(phosphonoacetyl)-L-aspartate-, and cadmium-resistant colony-forming mouse and hamster cells. *Cancer Res* 1983;43:5217–5221.

267. Newman EM, Lu Y, Kashani-Sabet M, et al. Mechanisms of cross-resistance to methotrexate and 5-fluorouracil in an A2780 human ovarian carcinoma cell subline resistant to cisplatin. *Biochem Pharmacol* 1988;37:443–447.

268. Rosowsky A, Wright JE, Cucchi CA, et al. Collateral methotrexate resistance in cultured human head and neck carcinoma cells selected for resistance to cis-diaminedichloroplatinum(II). *Cancer Res* 1987;47:5913–5918.

269. Rice GC, Ling V, Schimke RT. Frequencies of independent

and simultaneous selection of Chinese hamster cells for methotrexate and doxorubicin (Adriamycin) resistance. *Proc Natl Acad Sci U S A* 1987;84:9261–9264.

270. Mandelbaum-Shavit F, Ramu A. Dihydrofolate reductase activity in Adriamycin and methotrexate sensitive and resistant P388 leukemia cells. *Cell Biol Int Rep* 1987;11:389–396.

271. Schuetz JD, Gorse KM, Goldman ID, et al. Transient inhibition of DNA synthesis by 5-fluorodeoxyuridine leads to overexpression of dihydrofolate reductase with increased frequency of methotrexate resistance. *J Biol Chem* 1988;263:7708–7712.

272. Denis N, Kitzis A, Kruh J, et al. Stimulation of methotrexate resistance and dihydrofolate reductase gene amplification by c-myc. *Oncogene* 1991;6:1453–1457.

273. Wright JA, Smith HS, Watt FM, et al. DNA amplification is rare in normal human cells. *Proc Natl Acad Sci U S A* 1990;87:1791–1795.

274. Cowan KH, Goldsmith ME, Ricciardone MD, et al. Regulation of dihydrofolate reductase in human breast cancer cells and in mutant hamster cells transfected with a human dihydrofolate reductase minigene. *Mol Pharmacol* 1986;30:69–76.

275. Bastow KF, Prabhu R, Cheng YC. The intracellular content of dihydrofolate reductase: possibilities for control and implications for chemotherapy. *Adv Enzyme Regul* 1984;22:15–26.

276. Chu E, Takimoto CH, Voeller D, et al. Specific binding of human dihydrofolate reductase protein to dihydrofolate reductase messenger RNA in vitro. *Biochemistry* 1993;32:4756–4760.

277. Ercikan-Abali EA, Banerjee D, Waltham MC, et al. Dihydrofolate reductase protein inhibits its own translation by binding to dihydrofolate reductase mRNA sequences within the coding region. *Biochemistry* 1997;36:12317–12322.

278. Curt GA, Carney DN, Cowan KH, et al. Unstable methotrexate resistance in human small-cell carcinoma associated with double minute chromosomes. *N Engl J Med* 1983;308:199–202.

279. Horns RC Jr, Dower WJ, Schimke RT. Gene amplification in a leukemic patient treated with methotrexate. *J Clin Oncol* 1984;2:2–7.

280. Trent JM, Buick RN, Olson S, et al. Cytologic evidence for gene amplification in methotrexate-resistant cells obtained from a patient with ovarian adenocarcinoma. *J Clin Oncol* 1984;2:8–15.

281. Carman MD, Schornagel JH, Rivest RS, et al. Resistance to methotrexate due to gene amplification in a patient with acute leukemia. *J Clin Oncol* 1984;2:16–20.

282. Curt GA, Jolivet J, Bailey BD, et al. Synthesis and retention of methotrexate polyglutamates by human small cell lung cancer. *Biochem Pharmacol* 1984;33:1682–1685.

283. Matherly LH, Taub JW, Wong SC, et al. Increased frequency of expression of elevated dihydrofolate reductase in T-cell versus B-precursor acute lymphoblastic leukemia in children. *Blood* 1997;90:578–589.

284. Matherly LH, Taub JW, Ravindranath Y, et al. Elevated dihydrofolate reductase and impaired methotrexate transport as elements in methotrexate resistance in childhood acute lymphoblastic leukemia. *Blood* 1995;85:500–509.

285. Rodenhuis S, McGuire JJ, Sawicki WL, et al. Effects of methotrexate and of the "nonclassical" folate antagonist trimetrexate on human leukemia cells. *Leukemia* 1987;1:116–120.

286. Seither RL, Rape TJ, Goldman ID. Further studies on the pharmacologic effects of the 7-hydroxy catabolite of meth-

otrexate in the L1210 murine leukemia cell. *Biochem Pharmacol* 1989;38:815–822.

287. Rhee MS, Balinska M, Bunni M, et al. Role of substrate depletion in the inhibition of thymidylate biosynthesis by the dihydrofolate reductase inhibitor trimetrexate in cultured hepatoma cells. *Cancer Res* 1990;50:3979–3984.

288. Rhee MS, Coward JK, Galivan J. Depletion of 5,10-methylenetetrahydrofolate and 10-formyltetrahydrofolate by methotrexate in cultured hepatoma cells. *Mol Pharmacol* 1992;42:909–916.

289. Trent DF, Seither RL, Goldman ID. Compartmentation of intracellular folates. Failure to interconvert tetrahydrofolate cofactors to dihydrofolate in mitochondria of L1210 leukemia cells treated with trimetrexate [published erratum appears in Biochem Pharmacol 1991;42(12):2405]. *Biochem Pharmacol* 1991;42:1015–1019.

290. Sant ME, Lyons SD, Phillips L, et al. Antifolates induce inhibition of amido phosphoribosyltransferase in leukemia cells. *J Biol Chem* 1992;267:11038–11045.

291. Zaharko DS, Fung WP, Yang KH. Relative biochemical aspects of low and high doses of methotrexate in mice. *Cancer Res* 1977;37:1602–1607.

292. Donehower RC, Allegra JC, Lippman ME, et al. Combined effects of methotrexate and 5-fluoropyrimidine on human breast cancer cells in serum-free culture. *Eur J Cancer* 1980;16:655–661.

293. Kwok JB, Tattersall MH. Inhibition of 2-desamino-2-methyl-10-propagyl-5,8-dideazafolic acid cytotoxicity by 5,10-dideazatetrahydrofolate in L1210 cells with decrease in DNA fragmentation and deoxyadenosine triphosphate pools. *Biochem Pharmacol* 1991;42:507–513.

294. Taylor IW, Tattersall MH. Methotrexate cytotoxicity in cultured human leukemic cells studied by flow cytometry. *Cancer Res* 1981;41:1549–1558.

295. Taylor IW, Slowiaczek P, Francis PR, et al. Biochemical and cell cycle perturbations in methotrexate-treated cells. *Mol Pharmacol* 1982;21:204–210.

296. Fernandes DJ, Sur P, Kute TE, et al. Proliferation-dependent cytotoxicity of methotrexate in murine L5178Y leukemia. *Cancer Res* 1988;48:5638–5644.

297. Jackson RC, Weber G. Enzyme pattern directed chemotherapy. The effects of combinations of methotrexate, 5-fluorodeoxyuridine and thymidine on rat hepatoma cells in vitro. *Biochem Pharmacol* 1976;25:2613–2618.

298. Tattersall MH, Jackson RC, Jackson ST, et al. Factors determining cell sensitivity to methotrexate: studies of folate and deoxyribonucleoside triphosphate pools in five mammalian cell lines. *Eur J Cancer* 1974;10:819–826.

299. Pinedo HM, Zaharko DS, Bull JM, et al. The reversal of methotrexate cytotoxicity to mouse bone marrow cells by leucovorin and nucleosides. *Cancer Res* 1976;36:4418–4424.

300. Jackson RC. Modulation of methotrexate toxicity by thymidine: sequence-dependent biochemical effects. *Mol Pharmacol* 1980;18:281–286.

301. White JC, Goldman ID. Methotrexate resistance in al L1210 cell line resulting from increased dihydrofolate reductase, decreased thymidylate synthetase activity, and normal membrane transport. Computer simulations based on network thermodynamics. *J Biol Chem* 1981;256:5722–5727.

302. Ayusawa D, Koyama H, Seno T. Resistance to methotrexate in

thymidylate synthetase-deficient mutants of cultured mouse mammary tumor FM3A cells. *Cancer Res* 1981;41:1497–1501.

303. Li JC, Kaminskas E. Accumulation of DNA strand breaks and methotrexate cytotoxicity. *Proc Natl Acad Sci U S A* 1984;81:5694–5698.

304. Hori T, Ayusawa D, Shimizu K, et al. Chromosome breakage induced by thymidylate stress in thymidylate synthase-negative mutants of mouse FM3A cells. *Cancer Res* 1984;44:703–709.

305. Borchers AH, Kennedy KA, Straw JA. Inhibition of DNA excision repair by methotrexate in Chinese hamster ovary cells following exposure to ultraviolet irradiation or ethylmethanesulfonate. *Cancer Res* 1990;50:1786–1789.

306. Fridland A. Effect of methotrexate on deoxyribonucleotide pools and DNA synthesis in human lymphocytic cells. *Cancer Res* 1974;34:1883–1888.

307. Goulian M, Bleile B, Tseng BY. Methotrexate-induced misincorporation of uracil into DNA. *Proc Natl Acad Sci U S A* 1980;77:1956–1960.

308. Grafstrom RH, Tseng BY, Goulian M. The incorporation of uracil into animal cell DNA in vitro. *Cell* 1978;15:131–140.

309. Golos B, Malec J. Enhancement of methotrexate-induced growth inhibition, cell killing and DNA lesions in cultured L5178Y cells by the reduction of DNA repair efficiency. *Biochem Pharmacol* 1989;38:1743–1748.

310. Richards RG, Brown OE, Gillison ML, et al. Drug concentration-dependent DNA lesions are induced by the lipid-soluble antifolate, piritrexim (BW301U). *Mol Pharmacol* 1986;30:651–658.

311. Curtin NJ, Harris AL, Aherne GW. Mechanism of cell death following thymidylate synthase inhibition: 2'-deoxyuridine-5'-triphosphate accumulation, DNA damage, and growth inhibition following exposure to CB3717 and dipyridamole. *Cancer Res* 1991;51:2346–2352.

312. Beck WR, Wright GE, Nusbaum NJ, et al. Enhancement of methotrexate cytotoxicity by uracil analogues that inhibit deoxyuridine triphosphate nucleotidohydrolase (dUTPase) activity. *Adv Exp Med Biol* 1986;195:97–104.

313. Bertino JR, Goker E, Gorlick R, et al. Resistance mechanisms to methotrexate in tumors. *Oncologist* 1996;1:223–226.

314. Li W, Fan J, Hochhauser D, et al. Lack of functional retinoblastoma protein mediates increased resistance to antimetabolites in human sarcoma cell lines. *Proc Natl Acad Sci U S A* 1995;92:10436–10440.

315. Goker E, Waltham M, Kheradpour A, et al. Amplification of the dihydrofolate reductase gene is a mechanism of acquired resistance to methotrexate in patients with acute lymphoblastic leukemia and is correlated with p53 gene mutations. *Blood* 1995;86:677–684.

316. Pinedo HM, Zaharko DS, Bull J, et al. The relative contribution of drug concentration and duration of exposure to mouse bone marrow toxicity during continuous methotrexate infusion. *Cancer Res* 1977;37:445–450.

317. Cherry LM, Hsu TC. Restitution of chromatid and isochromatid breaks induced in the G2 phase by actinomycin D. *Environ Mutagen* 1982;4:259–265.

318. Hryniuk WM, Bertino JR. Treatment of leukemia with large doses of methotrexate and folinic acid: clinical-biochemical correlates. *J Clin Invest* 1969;48:2140–2155.

319. Howell SB, Mansfield SJ, Taetle R. Thymidine and hypoxanthine requirements of normal and malignant human cells for protection against methotrexate cytotoxicity. *Cancer Res* 1981;41:945–950.

320. Howell SB, Ensminger WD, Krishan A, et al. Thymidine rescue of high-dose methotrexate in humans. *Cancer Res* 1978;38:325–330.

321. Rustum YM. High-pressure liquid chromatography. I. Quantitative separation of purine and pyrimidine nucleosides and bases. *Anal Biochem* 1978;90:289–299.

322. Willson JK, Fischer PH, Remick SC, et al. Methotrexate and dipyridamole combination chemotherapy based upon inhibition of nucleoside salvage in humans. *Cancer Res* 1989;49:1866–1870.

323. Straw JA, Talbot DC, Taylor GA, et al. Some observations on the reversibility of methotrexate toxicity in normal proliferating tissues. *J Natl Cancer Inst* 1977;58:91–97.

324. Tattersall MH, Brown B, Frei Ed. The reversal of methotrexate toxicity by thymidine with maintenance of antitumour effects. *Nature* 1975;253:198–200.

325. Semon JH, Grindey GB. Potentiation of the antitumor activity of methotrexate by concurrent infusion of thymidine. *Cancer Res* 1978;38:2905–2911.

326. Uitendaal MP, Schornagel JH, Leyva A, et al. Influence of concomitant infusion of thymidine and inosine on methotrexate activity in normal and P388-bearing mice. *Eur J Cancer Clin Oncol* 1984;20:1527–1532.

327. Van Mouwerik TJ, Pangallo CA, Willson JK, et al. Augmentation of methotrexate cytotoxicity in human colon cancer cells achieved through inhibition of thymidine salvage by dipyridamole. *Biochem Pharmacol* 1987;36:809–814.

328. Novelli A, Mini E, Liuffi M, et al. Clinical data on rescue of high-dose methotrexate with N^5-methyltetrahydrofolate in human solid tumors. In: Periti P, ed. *High-dose methotrexate pharmacology, toxicology and chemotherapy.* Firenze, Italy: Giuntina, 1978:299.

329. Goldin A, Mantel N, Greenhouse SW, et al. Effect of delayed administration of citrovorum factor on antileukemic effectiveness of amethopterin in mice. *Cancer Res* 1954;14:43.

330. Matherly LH, Barlowe CK, Goldman ID. Antifolate polyglutamylation and competitive drug displacement at dihydrofolate reductase as important elements in leucovorin rescue in L1210 cells. *Cancer Res* 1986;46:588–593.

331. Bernard S, Etienne MC, Fischel JL, et al. Critical factors for the reversal of methotrexate cytotoxicity by folinic acid. *Br J Cancer* 1991;63:303–307.

332. Browman GP, Goodyear MD, Levine MN, et al. Modulation of the antitumor effect of methotrexate by low-dose leucovorin in squamous cell head and neck cancer: a randomized placebo-controlled clinical trial. *J Clin Oncol* 1990;8:203–208.

333. Bertino JR, Fischer GA. Techniques for study of resistance to folic acid antagonists. *Methods Med Res* 1964;10:297.

334. Yap AK, Luscombe DK. Rapid and inexpensive enzyme inhibition assay of methotrexate. *J Pharmacol Methods* 1986;16:139–150.

335. Myers CE, Lippman ME, Elliot HM, et al. Competitive protein binding assay for methotrexate. *Proc Natl Acad Sci U S A* 1975;72:3683–3686.

336. Hande K, Gober J, Fletcher R. Trimethoprim interferes with serum methotrexate assay by the competitive protein binding technique. *Clin Chem* 1980;26:1617–1619.

337. Pesce MA, Bodourian SH. Evaluation of a fluorescence polarization immunoassay procedure for quantitation of methotrexate. *Ther Drug Monit* 1986;8:115–121.

338. Bertino JR, Isacoff WH. Methods of measuring methotrexate in body fluids. In: Pinedo HM, ed. *Clinical pharmacology of antineoplastic drugs*. Amsterdam: Elsevier/North Holland, 1978:3.

339. Donehower RC, Hande KR, Drake JC, et al. Presence of 2,4-diamino-N10-methylpteroic acid after high-dose methotrexate. *Clin Pharmacol Ther* 1979;26:63–72.

340. Oellerich M, Engelhardt P, Schaadt M, et al. Determination of methotrexate in serum by a rapid, fully mechanized enzyme immunoassay (EMIT). *J Clin Chem Clin Biochem* 1980;18:169–174.

341. Allegra CJ, Drake JC, Bell BA, et al. Measuring levels of methotrexate [Letter]. *N Engl J Med* 1985;313:184.

342. So N, Chandra DP, Alexander IS, et al. Determination of serum methotrexate and 7-hydroxymethotrexate concentrations. Method evaluation showing advantages of high-performance liquid chromatography. *J Chromatogr* 1985;337:81–90.

343. Stout M, Ravindranath Y, Kauffman R. High-performance liquid chromatographic assay for methotrexate utilizing a cold acetonitrile purification and separation of plasma or cerebrospinal fluid. *J Chromatogr* 1985;342:424–430.

344. Palmisano F, Cataldi TR, Zambonin PG. Determination of the antineoplastic agent methotrexate in body fluids by high-performance liquid chromatography with electrochemical detection. *J Chromatogr* 1985;344:249–258.

345. Salamoun J, Smrz M, Kiss F, et al. Column liquid chromatography of methotrexate and its metabolites using a postcolumn photochemical reactor and fluorescence detection. *J Chromatogr* 1987;419:213–223.

346. Slordal L, Prytz PS, Pettersen I, et al. Methotrexate measurements in plasma: comparison of enzyme multiplied immunoassay technique, TDx fluorescence polarization immunoassay, and high pressure liquid chromatography. *Ther Drug Monit* 1986;8:368–372.

347. Najjar TA, Matar KM, Alfawaz IM. Comparison of a new high-performance liquid chromatography method with fluorescence polarization immunoassay for analysis of methotrexate. *Ther Drug Monit* 1992;14:142–146.

348. Zaharko DS, Dedrick RL, Bischoff KB, et al. Methotrexate tissue distribution: prediction by a mathematical model. *J Natl Cancer Inst* 1971;46:775–784.

349. Chungi VS, Bourne DW, Dittert LW. Drug absorption VIII: kinetics of GI absorption of methotrexate. *J Pharm Sci* 1978;67:560–561.

350. Henderson ES, Adamson RH, Denham C, et al. The metabolic fate of tritiated methotrexate. I. Absorption, excretion, and distribution in mice, rats, dogs and monkeys. *Cancer Res* 1965;25:1008–1017.

351. Henderson ES, Adamson RH, Oliverio VT. The metabolic fate of tritiated methotrexate. II. Absorption and excretion in man. *Cancer Res* 1965;25:1018–1024.

352. Stuart JF, Calman KC, Watters J, et al. Bioavailability of methotrexate: implications for clinical use. *Cancer Chemother Pharmacol* 1979;3:239–241.

353. Balis FM, Savitch JL, Bleyer WA. Pharmacokinetics of oral methotrexate in children. *Cancer Res* 1983;43:2342–2345.

354. Balis FM, Holcenberg JS, Poplack DG, et al. Pharmacokinetics and pharmacodynamics of oral methotrexate and mercaptopurine in children with lower risk acute lymphoblastic leukemia: a joint children's cancer group and pediatric oncology branch study. *Blood* 1998;92:3569–3577.

355. Steele WH, Lawrence JR, Stuart JF, et al. The protein binding of methotrexate by the serum of normal subjects. *Eur J Clin Pharmacol* 1979;15:363–366.

356. Liegler DG, Henderson ES, Hahn MA, et al. The effect of organic acids on renal clearance of methotrexate in man. *Clin Pharmacol Ther* 1969;10:849–857.

357. Wan SH, Huffman DH, Azarnoff DL, et al. Effect of route of administration and effusions on methotrexate pharmacokinetics. *Cancer Res* 1974;4:3487–3491.

358. Chabner BA, Stoller RG, Hande K, et al. Methotrexate disposition in humans: case studies in ovarian cancer and following high-dose infusion. *Drug Metab Rev* 1978;8:107–117.

359. Torres IJ, Litterst CL, Guarino AM. Transport of model compounds across the peritoneal membrane in the rat. *Pharmacology* 1978;17:330–340.

360. Jones RB, Collins JM, Myers CE, et al. High-volume intraperitoneal chemotherapy with methotrexate in patients with cancer. *Cancer Res* 1981;41:55–59.

361. Fossa SD, Heilo A, Bormer O. Unexpectedly high serum methotrexate levels in cystectomized bladder cancer patients with an ileal conduit treated with intermediate doses of the drug. *J Urol* 1990;143:498–501.

362. Stoller RG, Jacobs SA, Drake JC, et al. Pharmacokinetics of high-dose methotrexate. *Cancer Chemother Rep* 1975;6:19.

363. Kristenson L, Weismann K, Hutters L. Renal function and the rate of disappearance of methotrexate from serum. *Eur J Clin Pharmacol* 1975;8:439–444.

364. Bressolle F, Bologna C, Kinowski JM, et al. Effects of moderate renal insufficiency on pharmacokinetics of methotrexate in rheumatoid arthritis patients. *Ann Rheum Dis* 1998;57:110–113.

365. Nirenberg A, Mosende C, Mehta BM, et al. High-dose methotrexate with citrovorum factor rescue: predictive value of serum methotrexate concentrations and corrective measures to avert toxicity. *Cancer Treat Rep* 1977;61:779–783.

366. Isacoff WH, Morrison PF, Aroesty J, et al. Pharmacokinetics of high-dose methotrexate with citrovorum factor rescue. *Cancer Treat Rep* 1977;61:1665–1674.

367. Bleyer WA. The clinical pharmacology of methotrexate: new applications of an old drug. *Cancer* 1978;41:36–51.

368. Howell SB, Tamerius RK. Achievement of long duration methotrexate exposure with concurrent low dose thymidine protection: influence of methotrexate pharmacokinetics. *Eur J Cancer* 1980;16:1427–1432.

369. Evans WE, Crom WR, Stewart CF, et al. Methotrexate systemic clearance influences probability of relapse in children with standard-risk acute lymphocytic leukaemia. *Lancet* 1984;1:359–362.

370. Evans WE, Crom WR, Abromowitch M, et al. Clinical pharmacodynamics of high-dose methotrexate in acute lymphocytic leukemia. Identification of a relation between concentration and effect. *N Engl J Med* 1986;314:471–477.

371. Borsi JD, Moe PJ. Systemic clearance of methotrexate in the prognosis of acute lymphoblastic leukemia in children. *Cancer* 1987;60:3020–3024.

372. Pearson AD, Amineddine HA, Yule M, et al. The influence of serum methotrexate concentrations and drug dosage on outcome in childhood acute lymphoblastic leukaemia [see comments]. *Br J Cancer* 1991;64:169–173.

373. Calvert AH, Bondy PK, Harrap KR. Some observations on the human pharmacology of methotrexate. *Cancer Treat Rep* 1977;61:1647–1656.

374. Hande KR, Balow JE, Drake JC, et al. Methotrexate and hemodialysis [Letter]. *Ann Intern Med* 1977;87:495–496.

375. Monjanel S, Rigault JP, Cano JP, et al. High-dose methotrexate: preliminary evaluation of a pharmacokinetic approach. *Cancer Chemother Pharmacol* 1979;3:189–196.

376. Sasaki K, Tanaka J, Fujimoto T. Theoretically required urinary flow during high-dose methotrexate infusion. *Cancer Chemother Pharmacol* 1984;13:9–13.

377. Romolo JL, Goldberg NH, Hande KR, et al. Effect of hydration on plasma-methotrexate levels. *Cancer Treat Rep* 1977;61:1393–1396.

378. Huang KC, Wenczak BA, Liu YK. Renal tubular transport of methotrexate in the rhesus monkey and dog. *Cancer Res* 1979;39:4843–4848.

379. Iven H, Brasch H. Influence of the antibiotics piperacillin, doxycycline, and tobramycin on the pharmacokinetics of methotrexate in rabbits. *Cancer Chemother Pharmacol* 1986;17:218–222.

380. Iven H, Brasch H. The effects of antibiotics and uricosuric drugs on the renal elimination of methotrexate and 7-hydroxymethotrexate in rabbits. *Cancer Chemother Pharmacol* 1988;21:337–342.

381. Iven H, Brasch H. Cephalosporins increase the renal clearance of methotrexate and 7-hydroxymethotrexate in rabbits. *Cancer Chemother Pharmacol* 1990;26:139–143.

382. Kerr IG, Jolivet J, Collins JM, et al. Test dose for predicting high-dose methotrexate infusions. *Clin Pharmacol Ther* 1983;33:44–51.

383. Favre R, Monjanel S, Alfonsi M, et al. High-dose methotrexate: a clinical and pharmacokinetic evaluation. Treatment of advanced squamous cell carcinoma of the head and neck using a prospective mathematical model and pharmacokinetic surveillance. *Cancer Chemother Pharmacol* 1982;9:156–160.

384. Gewirt DA, White JC, Goldman ID. Transport, binding and polyglutamation of methotrexate (MTX) in freshly isolated hepatocytes. *Am Assoc Cancer Res* 1979:147.

385. Strum WB, Liem HH. Hepatic uptake, intracellular protein binding and biliary excretion of amethopterin. *Biochem Pharmacol* 1977;26:1235–1240.

386. Jacobs SA, Derr CJ, Johns DG. Accumulation of methotrexate diglutamate in human liver during methotrexate therapy. *Biochem Pharmacol* 1977;26:2310–2313.

387. Strum WB, Liem HH, Muller-Eberhard U. Effect of chemotherapeutic agents on the uptake and excretion of amethopterin by the isolated perfused rat liver. *Cancer Res* 1978;38:4734–4736.

388. Said HM, Hollander D. Inhibitory effect of bile salts on the enterohepatic circulation of methotrexate in the unanesthetized rat: inhibition of methotrexate intestinal absorption. *Cancer Chemother Pharmacol* 1986;16:121–124.

389. Lerne PR, Creaven PJ, Allen LM, et al. Kinetic model for the disposition and metabolism of moderate and high-dose methotrexate in man. *Cancer Chemother Rep* 1975;59:811–817.

390. Shen DD, Azarnoff DL. Clinical pharmacokinetics of methotrexate. *Clin Pharmacokinet* 1978;3:1–13.

391. Steinberg SE, Campbell CL, Bleyer WA, et al. Enterohepatic circulation of methotrexate in rats in vivo. *Cancer Res* 1982;42:1279–1282.

392. Breithaupt H, Kuenzlen E. Pharmacokinetics of methotrexate and 7-hydroxymethotrexate following infusions of high-dose methotrexate. *Cancer Treat Rep* 1982;66:1733–1741.

393. Erttmann R, Landbeck G. Effect of oral cholestyramine on the elimination of high-dose methotrexate. *J Cancer Res Clin Oncol* 1985;110:48–50.

394. Valerino DM, Johns DG, Zaharko DS, et al. Studies of the metabolism of methotrexate by intestinal flora. I. Identification and study of biological properties of the metabolite 4-amino-4-deoxy-N10-methylpteroic acid. *Biochem Pharmacol* 1972;21:821–831.

395. Jacobs SA, Stoller RG, Chabner BA, et al. 7-Hydroxymethotrexate as a urinary metabolite in human subjects and rhesus monkeys receiving high dose methotrexate. *J Clin Invest* 1976;57:534–538.

396. Erttmann R, Bielack S, Landbeck G. Kinetics of 7-hydroxymethotrexate after high-dose methotrexate therapy. *Cancer Chemother Pharmacol* 1985;15:101–104.

397. Lankelma J, van der Klein E, Ramaekers F. The role of 7-hydroxymethotrexate during methotrexate anti-cancer therapy. *Cancer Lett* 1980;9:133–142.

398. Stewart AL, Margison JM, Wilkinson PM, et al. The pharmacokinetics of 7-hydroxymethotrexate following medium-dose methotrexate therapy. *Cancer Chemother Pharmacol* 1985;14:165–167.

399. Sonneveld P, Schultz FW, Nooter K, et al. Pharmacokinetics of methotrexate and 7-hydroxy-methotrexate in plasma and bone marrow of children receiving low-dose oral methotrexate. *Cancer Chemother Pharmacol* 1986;18:111–116.

400. Bremnes RM, Slordal L, Wist E, et al. Formation and elimination of 7-hydroxymethotrexate in the rat in vivo after methotrexate administration. *Cancer Res* 1989;49:2460–2464.

401. Fabre G, Seither R, Goldman ID. Hydroxylation of 4-amino-antifolates by partially purified aldehyde oxidase from rabbit liver. *Biochem Pharmacol* 1986;35:1325–1330.

402. Rosowsky A, Wright JE, Holden SA, et al. Influence of lipophilicity and carboxyl group content on the rate of hydroxylation of methotrexate derivatives by aldehyde oxidase. *Biochem Pharmacol* 1990;40:851–857.

403. Rhee MS, Galivan J. Conversion of methotrexate to 7-hydroxymethotrexate and 7-hydroxymethotrexate polyglutamates in cultured rat hepatic cells. *Cancer Res* 1986; 46:3793–3797.

404. Chladek J, Martinkova J, Sispera L. An in vitro study on methotrexate hydroxylation in rat and human liver. *Physiol Res* 1997;46:371–379.

405. Jordan CG, Rashidi MR, Laljee H, et al. Aldehyde oxidase-catalysed oxidation of methotrexate in the liver of guinea-pig, rabbit and man. *J Pharm Pharmacol* 1999;51:411–418.

406. Sholar PW, Baram J, Seither R, et al. Inhibition of folate-dependent enzymes by 7-OH-methotrexate. *Biochem Pharmacol* 1988;37:3531–3534.

407. Clendeninn NJ, Drake JC, Allegra CJ, et al. Methotrexate polyglutamates have a greater affinity and more rapid on-rate for purified human dihydrofolate reductase than MTX. *Proc Am Assoc Cancer Res* 1985:232.

408. McCullough JL, Chabner BA, Bertino JR. Purification and properties of carboxypeptidase G1. *J Biol Chem* 1971;246:7207–7213.

409. Abelson HT, Ensminger W, Rosowsky A, et al. Comparative effects of citrovorum factor and carboxypeptidase G1 on

cerebrospinal fluid-methotrexate pharmacokinetics. *Cancer Treat Rep* 1978;62:1549–1552.

410. Chabner BA, Young RC. Threshold methotrexate concentration for in vivo inhibition of DNA synthesis in normal and tumorous target tissues. *J Clin Invest* 1973;52:1804–1811.

411. Sirotnak FM, Moccio DM. Pharmacokinetic basis for differences in methotrexate sensitivity of normal proliferating tissues in the mouse. *Cancer Res* 1980;40:1230–1234.

412. Ackland SP, Schilsky RL. High-dose methotrexate: a critical reappraisal. *J Clin Oncol* 1987;5:2017–2031.

413. Jaffe N. Recent advances in the chemotherapy of metastatic osteogenic sarcoma. *Cancer* 1972;30:1627–1631.

414. Von Hoff DD, Penta JS, Helman LJ, et al. Incidence of drug-related deaths secondary to high-dose methotrexate and citrovorum factor administration. *Cancer Treat Rep* 1977;61:745–748.

415. Glode LM, Pitman SW, Ensminger WD, et al. A phase 1 study of high doses of aminopterin with leucovorin rescue in patients with advanced metastatic tumors. *Cancer Res* 1979;39:3707–3714.

416. Stoller RG, Hande KR, Jacobs SA, et al. Use of plasma pharmacokinetics to predict and prevent methotrexate toxicity. *N Engl J Med* 1977;297:630–634.

417. Evans WE, Pratt CB, Taylor RH, et al. Pharmacokinetic monitoring of high-dose methotrexate. Early recognition of high-risk patients. *Cancer Chemother Pharmacol* 1979;3:161–166.

418. Goren MP, Wright RK, Horowitz ME, et al. Urinary N-acetyl-beta-D-glucosaminidase and serum creatinine concentrations predict impaired excretion of methotrexate. *J Clin Oncol* 1987;5:804–810.

419. Thyss A, Milano G, Kubar J, et al. Clinical and pharmacokinetic evidence of a life-threatening interaction between methotrexate and ketoprofen. *Lancet* 1986;1:256–258.

420. Relling MV, Stapleton FB, Ochs J, et al. Removal of methotrexate, leucovorin, and their metabolites by combined hemodialysis and hemoperfusion. *Cancer* 1988;62:884–888.

421. Bertino JR, Condos S, Horvath C, et al. Immobilized carboxypeptidase G1 in methotrexate removal. *Cancer Res* 1978;38:1936–1941.

422. Albrecht AM, Boldizsar E, Hutchison DJ. Carboxypeptidase displaying differential velocity in hydrolysis of methotrexate, 5-methyltetrahydrofolic acid, and leucovorin. *J Bacteriol* 1978;134:506–513.

423. DeAngelis LM, Tong WP, Lin S, et al. Carboxypeptidase G2 rescue after high-dose methotrexate. *J Clin Oncol* 1996;14:2145–2149.

424. Widemann BC, Balis FM, Murphy RF, et al. Carboxypeptidase-G2, thymidine, and leucovorin rescue in cancer patients with methotrexate-induced renal dysfunction. *J Clin Oncol* 1997;15:2125–2134.

425. Schornagel JH, Leyva A, Bucsa JM, et al. Thymidine prevention of methotrexate toxicity in head-and-neck cancer. In Pinedo HM, ed. *Clinical pharmacology of antineoplastic drugs.* Amsterdam: Elsevier/North Holland, 1978:83.

426. Howell SB, Herbst K, Boss GR, et al. Thymidine requirements for the rescue of patients treated with high-dose methotrexate. *Cancer Res* 1980;40:1824–1829.

427. Capizzi RL. Schedule-dependent synergism and antagonism between methotrexate and L-asparaginase. *Biochem Pharmacol* 1974;23:151.

428. Yap BS, McCredie KB, Benjamin RS, et al. Refractory acute leukaemia in adults treated with sequential colaspase and high-dose methotrexate. *BMJ* 1978;2:791–793.

429. Lobel JS, O'Brien RT, McIntosh S, et al. Methotrexate and asparaginase combination chemotherapy in refractory acute lymphoblastic leukemia of childhood. *Cancer* 1979;43:1089–1094.

430. Moran RG, Mulkins M, Heidelberger C. Role of thymidylate synthetase activity in development of methotrexate cytotoxicity. *Proc Natl Acad Sci U S A* 1979;76:5924–5928.

431. Rajeswari R, Shetty PA, Gothoskar BP, et al. Pharmacokinetics of methotrexate in adult Indian patients and its relationship to nutritional status. *Cancer Treat Rep* 1984;68:727–732.

432. Mihranian MH, Wang YM, Daly JM. Effects of nutritional depletion and repletion on plasma methotrexate pharmacokinetics. *Cancer* 1984;54:2268–2271.

433. Torosian MH, Mullen JL, Miller EE, et al. Reduction of methotrexate toxicity with improved nutritional status in tumor-bearing animals. *Cancer* 1988;61:1731–1735.

434. Kehoe JE, Harvey LP, Daly JM. Alteration of chemotherapy toxicity using a chemically defined liquid diet in rats. *Cancer Res* 1986;46:4047–4052.

435. McAnena OJ, Ridge JA, Daly JM. Alteration of methotrexate metabolism in rats by administration of an elemental liquid diet. II. Reduced toxicity and improved survival using cholestyramine. *Cancer* 1987;59:1091–1097.

436. McAnena OJ, Harvey LP, Bonau RA, et al. Alteration of methotrexate toxicity in rats by manipulation of dietary components. *Gastroenterology* 1987;92:354–360.

437. McAnena OJ, Rossi M, Mehta BM, et al. Alteration of methotrexate metabolism in rats by administration of an elemental liquid diet. I. Changes in drug enterohepatic circulation. *Cancer* 1987;59:31–37.

438. Zachariae H, Kragballe K, Sogaard H. Methotrexate induced liver cirrhosis. Studies including serial liver biopsies during continued treatment. *Br J Dermatol* 1980;102:407–412.

439. Dahl MG, Gregory MM, Scheuer PJ. Liver damage due to methotrexate in patients with psoriasis. *BMJ* 1971;1:625–630.

440. Balis FM, Murphy RF, Lester CM, et al. The influence of route of administration on the hepatic uptake of methotrexate. *Cancer Drug Deliv* 1986;3:239–242.

441. Dahl MG, Gregory MM, Scheuer PJ. Methotrexate hepatotoxicity in psoriasis—comparison of different dose regimens. *BMJ* 1972;1:654–656.

442. Podurgiel BJ, McGill DB, Ludwig J, et al. Liver injury associated with methotrexate therapy for psoriasis. *Mayo Clin Proc* 1973;48:787–792.

443. Willkens RF, Clegg DO, Ward JR, et al. Liver biopsies in patients on low-dose pulse methotrexate for the treatment of rheumatoid arthritis. In: *Sixteenth International Congress on Rheumatology.* Sydney, Australia: 1985:88(abst).

444. Mackenzie AH. Hepatotoxicity of prolonged methotrexate therapy for rheumatoid arthritis. *Cleve Clin Q* 1985;52:129–135.

445. Scully CJ, Anderson CJ, Cannon GW. Long-term methotrexate therapy for rheumatoid arthritis. *Semin Arthritis Rheum* 1991;20:317–331.

446. Phillips CA, Cera PJ, Mangan TF, et al. Clinical liver disease in patients with rheumatoid arthritis taking methotrexate. *J Rheumatol* 1992;19:229–233.

447. Weber BL, Tanyer G, Poplack DG, et al. Transient acute hepatotoxicity of high-dose methotrexate therapy during childhood. *J Natl Cancer Inst Monogr* 1987;5:207–212.

448. Tuma DJ, Barak AJ, Sorrell MF. Interaction of methotrexate with lipotropic factors in rat liver. *Biochem Pharmacol* 1975;24:1327–1331.

449. Clarysse AM, Cathey WJ, Cartwright GE, et al. Pulmonary disease complicating intermittent therapy with methotrexate. *JAMA* 1969;209:1861–1868.

450. Bergasa NV, Jones A, Kleiner DE, et al. Pilot study of low dose oral methotrexate treatment for primary biliary cirrhosis. *Am J Gastroenterol* 1996;91:295–299.

451. Sostman HD, Matthay RA, Putman CE, et al. Methotrexate-induced pneumonitis. *Medicine* (Baltimore) 1976;55:371–388.

452. Akoun GM, Mayaud CM, Touboul JL, et al. Use of bronchoalveolar lavage in the evaluation of methotrexate lung disease. *Thorax* 1987;42:652–655.

453. Wall MA, Wohl ME, Jaffe N, et al. Lung function in adolescents receiving high-dose methotrexate. *Pediatrics* 1979;63:741–746.

454. Kremer JM, Phelps CT. Long-term prospective study of the use of methotrexate in the treatment of rheumatoid arthritis. Update after a mean of 90 months. *Arthritis Rheum* 1992;35:138–145.

455. Searles G, McKendry RJ. Methotrexate pneumonitis in rheumatoid arthritis: potential risk factors. Four case reports and a review of the literature. *J Rheumatol* 1987;14:1164–1171.

456. Carson CW, Cannon GW, Egger MJ, et al. Pulmonary disease during the treatment of rheumatoid arthritis with low dose pulse methotrexate. *Semin Arthritis Rheum* 1987;16:186–195.

457. Kremer JM, Alarcon GS, Weinblatt ME, et al. Clinical, laboratory, radiographic, and histopathologic features of methotrexate-associated lung injury in patients with rheumatoid arthritis: a multicenter study with literature review [see comments]. *Arthritis Rheum* 1997;40:1829–1837.

458. Hargreaves MR, Mowat AG, Benson MK. Acute pneumonitis associated with low dose methotrexate treatment for rheumatoid arthritis: report of five cases and review of published reports. *Thorax* 1992;47:628–633.

459. Alarcon GS, Kremer JM, Macaluso M, et al. Risk factors for methotrexate-induced lung injury in patients with rheumatoid arthritis. A multicenter, case-control study. Methotrexate Lung Study Group. *Ann Intern Med* 1997;127:356–364.

460. Goldberg NH, Romolo JL, Austin EH, et al. Anaphylactoid type reactions in two patients receiving high dose intravenous methotrexate. *Cancer* 1978;41:52–55.

461. Doyle LA, Berg C, Bottino G, et al. Erythema and desquamation after high-dose methotrexate. *Ann Intern Med* 1983;98:611–612.

462. Shamberger RC, Rosenberg SA, Seipp CA, et al. Effects of high-dose methotrexate and vincristine on ovarian and testicular functions in patients undergoing postoperative adjuvant treatment of osteosarcoma. *Cancer Treat Rep* 1981;65:739–746.

463. Shapiro WR, Young DF, Mehta BM. Methotrexate: distribution in cerebrospinal fluid after intravenous, ventricular and lumbar injections. *N Engl J Med* 1975;293:161–166.

464. Bleyer WA, Drake JC, Chabner BA. Neurotoxicity and elevated cerebrospinal-fluid methotrexate concentration in meningeal leukemia. *N Engl J Med* 1973;289:770–773.

465. Bode U, Magrath IT, Bleyer WA, et al. Active transport of methotrexate from cerebrospinal fluid in humans. *Cancer Res* 1980;40:2184–2187.

466. Morse M, Savitch J, Balis F, et al. Altered central nervous system pharmacology of methotrexate in childhood leukemia: another sign of meningeal relapse. *J Clin Oncol* 1985;3:19–24.

467. Blaney SM, Balis FM, Poplack DG. Current pharmacological treatment approaches to central nervous system leukaemia. *Drugs* 1991;41:702–716.

468. Ettinger LJ, Chervinsky DS, Freeman AI, et al. Pharmacokinetics of methotrexate following intravenous and intraventricular administration in acute lymphocytic leukemia and non-Hodgkin's lymphoma. *Cancer* 1982;50:1676–1682.

469. Grossman SA, Reinhard CS, Loats HL. The intracerebral penetration of intraventricularly administered methotrexate: a quantitative autoradiographic study. *J Neurooncol* 1989;7:319–328.

470. Bleyer WA, Poplack DG, Simon RM. "Concentration × time" methotrexate via a subcutaneous reservoir: a less toxic regimen for intraventricular chemotherapy of central nervous system neoplasms. *Blood* 1978;51:835–842.

471. Glantz MJ, Cole BF, Recht L, et al. High-dose intravenous methotrexate for patients with nonleukemic leptomeningeal cancer: is intrathecal chemotherapy necessary? *J Clin Oncol* 1998;16:1561–1567.

472. Peylan-Ramu N, Poplack DG, Blei CL, et al. Computer assisted tomography in methotrexate encephalopathy. *J Comput Assist Tomogr* 1977;1:216–221.

473. Paakko E, Vainionpaa L, Lanning M, et al. White matter changes in children treated for acute lymphoblastic leukemia. *Cancer* 1992;70:2728–2733.

474. Shapiro WR, Allen JC, Horten BC. Chronic methotrexate toxicity to the central nervous system. *Clin Bull* 1980;10:49–52.

475. Jaffe N, Takaue Y, Anzai T, et al. Transient neurologic disturbances induced by high-dose methotrexate treatment. *Cancer* 1985;56:1356–1360.

476. Fritsch G, Urban C. Transient encephalopathy during the late course of treatment with high-dose methotrexate. *Cancer* 1984;53:1849–1851.

477. Walker RW, Allen JC, Rosen G, et al. Transient cerebral dysfunction secondary to high-dose methotrexate. *J Clin Oncol* 1986;4:1845–1850.

478. Kubo M, Azuma E, Arai S, et al. Transient encephalopathy following a single exposure of high-dose methotrexate in a child with acute lymphoblastic leukemia. *Pediatr Hematol Oncol* 1992;9:157–165.

479. Allen J, Rosen G, Juergens H, et al. The inability of oral leucovorin to elevate CSF 5-methyl-tetrahydrofolate following high dose intravenous methotrexate therapy. *J Neurooncol* 1983;1:39–44.

480. Mehta BM, Glass JP, Shapiro WR. Serum and cerebrospinal fluid distribution of 5-methyltetrahydrofolate after intravenous calcium leucovorin and intra-Ommaya methotrexate administration in patients with meningeal carcinomatosis. *Cancer Res* 1983;43:435–438.

481. Phillips PC, Thaler HT, Allen JC, et al. High-dose leucovorin reverses acute high-dose methotrexate neurotoxicity in the rat. *Ann Neurol* 1989;25:365–372.

482. Ochs J, Mulhern R, Fairclough D, et al. Comparison of neuropsychologic functioning and clinical indicators of neurotoxicity in long-term survivors of childhood leukemia given cranial radiation or parenteral methotrexate: a prospective study. *J Clin Oncol* 1991;9:145–151.

483. Mahoney DH Jr, Shuster JJ, Nitschke R, et al. Acute neurotoxicity in children with B-precursor acute lymphoid leukemia: an association with intermediate-dose intravenous methotrexate and intrathecal triple therapy—a Pediatric Oncology Group study. *J Clin Oncol* 1998;16:1712–1722.

484. Phillips PC, Dhawan V, Strother SC, et al. Reduced cerebral glucose metabolism and increased brain capillary permeability following high-dose methotrexate chemotherapy: a positron emission tomographic study. *Ann Neurol* 1987;21:59–63.

485. Gilbert MR, Harding BL, Grossman SA. Methotrexate neurotoxicity: in vitro studies using cerebellar explants from rats. *Cancer Res* 1989;49:2502–2505.

486. Livrea P, Trojano M, Simone IL, et al. Acute changes in blood-CSF barrier permselectivity to serum proteins after intrathecal methotrexate and CNS irradiation. *J Neurol* 1985;231:336–339.

487. Storm AJ, van der Kogel AJ, Nooter K. Effect of X-irradiation on the pharmacokinetics of methotrexate in rats: alteration of the blood-brain barrier. *Eur J Cancer Clin Oncol* 1985;21:759–764.

488. Azmin MN, Stuart JF, Florence AT. The distribution and elimination of methotrexate in mouse blood and brain after concurrent administration of polysorbate 80. *Cancer Chemother Pharmacol* 1985;14:238–242.

489. Neuwelt EA, Frenkel EP, Rapoport S, et al. Effect of osmotic blood-brain barrier disruption on methotrexate pharmacokinetics in the dog. *Neurosurgery* 1980;7:36–43.

490. Spiegel RJ, Cooper PR, Blum RH, et al. Treatment of massive intrathecal methotrexate overdose by ventriculolumbar perfusion. *N Engl J Med* 1984;311:386–388.

491. Shih C, Chen VJ, Gossett LS, et al. LY231514, a pyrrolo[2,3-d]pyrimidine-based antifolate that inhibits multiple folate-requiring enzymes. *Cancer Res* 1997;57:1116–1123.

492. Shih C, Habeck LL, Mendelsohn LG, et al. Multiple folate enzyme inhibition: mechanism of a novel pyrrolopyrimidine-based antifolate LY231514 (MTA). *Adv Enzyme Regul* 1998;38:135–152.

493. Chen VJ, Bewley JR, Andis SL, et al. Preclinical cellular pharmacology of LY231514 (MTA): a comparison with methotrexate, LY309887 and raltitrexed for their effects on intracellular folate and nucleoside triphosphate pools in CCRF-CEM cells. *Br J Cancer* 1998;78:27–34.

494. Worzalla JF, Shih C, Schultz RM. Role of folic acid in modulating the toxicity and efficacy of the multitargeted antifolate, LY231514. *Anticancer Res* 1998;18:3235–3239.

495. McDonald AC, Vasey PA, Adams L, et al. A phase I and pharmacokinetic study of LY231514, the multitargeted antifolate. *Clin Cancer Res* 1998;4:605–610.

496. Rinaldi DA, Burris HA, Dorr FA, et al. Initial phase I evaluation of the novel thymidylate synthase inhibitor, LY231514, using the modified continual reassessment method for dose escalation. *J Clin Oncol* 1995;13:2842–2850.

497. Rafi I, Taylor GA, Calvete JA, et al. Clinical pharmacokinetic and pharmacodynamic studies with the nonclassical antifolate thymidylate synthase inhibitor 3, 4-dihydro-2-amino-6-methyl-4-oxo-5-(4-pyridylthio)-quinazoline dihydrochloride (AG337) given by 24-hour continuous intravenous infusion. *Clin Cancer Res* 1995;1:1275–1284.

498. Webber S, Bartlett CA, Boritzki TJ, et al. AG337, a novel lipophilic thymidylate synthase inhibitor: in vitro and in vivo preclinical studies. *Cancer Chemother Pharmacol* 1996;37:509–517.

499. Creaven PJ, Pendyala L, Meropol NJ, et al. Initial clinical trial and pharmacokinetics of Thymitaq (AG337) by 10-day continuous infusion in patients with advanced solid tumors. *Cancer Chemother Pharmacol* 1998;41:167–170.

500. Hughes AN, Rafi I, Griffin MJ, et al. Phase I studies with the nonclassical antifolate nolatrexed dihydrochloride (AG337, THYMITAQ) administered orally for 5 days. *Clin Cancer Res* 1999;5:111–118.

501. Jodrell DI, Bowman A, Rye R, et al. A phase I study of the lipophilic thymidylate synthase inhibitor Thymitaq (nolatrexed dihydrochloride) given by 10-day oral administration. *Br J Cancer* 1999;79:915–920.

502. Zalcberg JR, Cunningham D, Van Cutsem E, et al. ZD1694: a novel thymidylate synthase inhibitor with substantial activity in the treatment of patients with advanced colorectal cancer. Tomudex Colorectal Study Group. *J Clin Oncol* 1996;14:716–721.

503. Cunningham D, Zalcberg J, Smith I, et al. "Tomudex" (ZD1694): a novel thymidylate synthase inhibitor with clinical antitumour activity in a range of solid tumours. "Tomudex" International Study Group. *Ann Oncol* 1996;7:179–182.

504. Cunningham D. Mature results from three large controlled studies with raltitrexed ("Tomudex"). *Br J Cancer* 1998;77:15–21.

505. Fry DW, Jackson RC. Biological and biochemical properties of new anticancer folate antagonists. *Cancer Metastasis Rev* 1987;5:251–270.

506. Yin MB, Guo B, Panadero A, et al. Cyclin E-cdk2 activation is associated with cell cycle arrest and inhibition of DNA replication induced by the thymidylate synthase inhibitor Tomudex. *Exp Cell Res* 1999;247:189–199.

507. Sotelo-Mundo RR, Ciesla J, Dzik JM, et al. Crystal structures of rat thymidylate synthase inhibited by Tomudex, a potent anticancer drug. *Biochemistry* 1999;38:1087–1094.

508. Walton MI, Mitchell F, Aherne GW, et al. The renal effects of the water-soluble, non-folylpolyglutamate synthetase-dependent thymidylate synthase inhibitor ZD9331 in mice. *Br J Cancer* 1998;78:1457–1463.

509. Duch DS, Banks S, Dev IK, et al. Biochemical and cellular pharmacology of 1843U89, a novel benzoquinazoline inhibitor of thymidylate synthase. *Cancer Res* 1993;53:810–818.

510. Hanlon MH, Ferone R. In vitro uptake, anabolism, and cellular retention of 1843U89 and other benzoquinazoline inhibitors of thymidylate synthase. *Cancer Res* 1996;56:3301–3306.

511. Weichsel A, Montfort WR. Ligand-induced distortion of an active site in thymidylate synthase upon binding anticancer drug 1843U89. *Nat Struct Biol* 1995;2:1095–1101.

512. Smith GK, Amyx H, Boytos CM, et al. Enhanced antitumor activity for the thymidylate synthase inhibitor 1843U89 through decreased host toxicity with oral folic acid. *Cancer Res* 1995;55:6117–6125.

513. Springer CJ, Poon GK, Sharma SK, et al. Analysis of antibody-enzyme conjugate clearance by investigation of prodrug and active drug in an ADEPT clinical study. *Cell Biophys* 1994;25:193–207.

514. Springer CJ, Bavetsias V, Jackman AL, et al. Prodrugs of thymidylate synthase inhibitors: potential for antibody directed enzyme prodrug therapy (ADEPT). *Anticancer Drug Des* 1996;11:625–636.

515. Syrigos KN, Epenetos AA. Antibody directed enzyme prodrug therapy (ADEPT): a review of the experimental and clinical considerations. *Anticancer Res* 1999;19:605–613.

8

5-FLUOROPYRIMIDINES

JEAN L. GREM

Despite many efforts to synthesize antineoplastic drugs on a rational basis, few agents have fulfilled the expectations of biochemical, pharmacologic, and clinical activity. The 5-fluorinated pyrimidines, synthesized by Heidelberger et al., represent an exception.[1] The impetus for synthesis of fluorinated pyrimidines came from the observation that rat hepatomas use radiolabeled uracil more avidly than nonmalignant tissues.[2] This implied that the enzymatic pathways for use of uracil, and possibly analogs of uracil, differ between malignant and normal cells and represent a possible target for antimetabolite chemotherapy. These drugs have shown the predicted biochemical action and have become useful in the treatment of human solid tumors, including breast cancer, gastrointestinal (GI) adenocarcinomas, and squamous cell carcinomas arising in the head and neck. They have invoked interest not only because of their inherent *antitumor* activity, but also because of their synergistic interaction with other antitumor agents, irradiation, physiologic nucleosides, and leucovorin (LV).

STRUCTURE AND CELLULAR PHARMACOLOGY

The chemical structures of the initial two 5-fluoropyrimidines to enter clinical trials are shown in Figure 8-1. The simplest derivative, 5-fluorouracil [5-FU, molecular weight (MW) = 130], is an analog of uracil with a fluorine atom substituted at the carbon-5 position of the pyrimidine ring in place of hydrogen. The key features of 5-FU are outlined in Table 8-1. The fluorine atom is slightly bulkier than hydrogen but does not impede the anabolism of 5-FU. Activation to the nucleotide level is essential to the antitumor activity of this class of compounds. The ribonucleoside derivative 5-fluorouridine (FUrd) has been used extensively in preclinical studies but is not used in the clinic. The deoxyribonucleoside derivative 5-fluoro-2'-deoxyuridine (FdUrd, MW = 246) is commercially available (floxuridine, FUDR) and is used primarily for regional administration.

Transport

In human erythrocytes, 5-FU and uracil exhibited similar saturable [K_m (binding affinity) approximately equal to 4 mmol per L; v_{max} 500 pmol per second per 5 μL cells] and nonsaturable (rate constant approximately equal to 80 pmol per second per 5 μL cells) components of influx. Competitive-inhibition experiments and countertransport studies suggest that 5-FU shares the same facilitated-transport system as uracil, adenine, and hypoxanthine. The system is neither temperature nor energy-dependent.[3–5] 5-FU permeation is quite pH-dependent. Ionization of the hydroxyl group attached to the fourth carbon [pK (ionization constant of acid) = 8.0] markedly depresses the transmembrane passage of drug. 5-FU entry into erythrocytes via nonfacilitated diffusion and a facilitated nucleobase transport system clearly differs from that used by pyrimidine nucleosides.[4–5] In a rat hepatoma cell line, maximal accumulation of free intracellular 5-FU occurs within 200 seconds.[3] Total intracellular 5-FU continues to increase thereafter due to the formation of nucleotides and RNA incorporation.

FdUrd uses the facilitated nucleoside transport system and rapidly gains entry into cells.[6] In Ehrlich ascites cells, intracellular FdUrd reaches equilibrium with extracellular drug within 15 seconds. Total intracellular drug continues to accumulate thereafter due to formation of fluorodeoxyuridylate (5-fluoro-2'-deoxyuridine-5'monophosphate) (FdUMP) and other nucleotides. The phosphorylation process, rather than membrane transport, is rate-limiting in the continued formation of intracellular nucleotides.

Metabolic Activation

Activation of 5-FU to the ribonucleotide level may occur through one of two pathways, as outlined in Figure 8-2.[7–18] These involve direct transfer of a ribose phosphate to 5-FU from 5'-phospho-α-D-ribosyl 1-pyrophosphate (PRPP) as catalyzed by orotic acid phosphoribosyl transferase (OPRTase, also called pyrimidine PRTase) or a two-step sequence involving the addition of a ribose moiety by uridine (Urd) phosphorylase as the initial step; phosphorylation is then

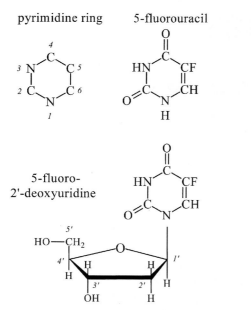

FIGURE 8-1. Structures of pyrimidine ring, 5-fluorouracil, and 5-fluoro-2'-deoxyuridine.

accomplished by Urd kinase. Sequential action of pyrimidine monophosphate kinase and pyrimidine diphosphate kinase result in the formation of fluorouridine diphosphate (FUDP) and fluorouridine triphosphate (FUTP). The fraudulent nucleotide FUTP is incorporated into RNA by the action of RNA polymerase.

The first pathway, catalyzed by OPRT, appears to be of primary importance for 5-FU activation in normal tissues, because its inhibition by a nucleotide metabolite of allopurinol diminishes toxicity to bone marrow and GI mucosa.[9,12,14] The OPRT pathway is the dominant route of 5-FU activation in many murine leukemias[7,8]; other cancer cell lines, such as Novikoff hepatoma, Walker 256, continuously cultured carcinoma cell line used for tissue cultures HeLA), and some human colon carcinoma xenografts, activate the drug by the action of Urd phosphorylase and Urd kinase.[9,10,12–14] These conclusions are in part derived indirectly from drug interactions affecting the availability of ribose-1-phosphate and PRPP (substrates for the various activation pathways) and do not represent direct measurement of enzyme activities.[10,11] Although one activation pathway may appear to predominate in a given cancer cell under certain conditions, many cancer cells can use both pathways.

In the presence of a deoxyribose-1-phosphate (dR-1-P) donor, 5-FU is converted to FdUrd by thymidine (dThd) phosphorylase. dThd kinase transforms FdUrd to FdUMP, a potent inhibitor of thymidylate synthase (TS). FdUMP can be formed indirectly on conversion of FUDP to fluorodeoxyuridine diphosphate (FdUDP) by ribonucleotide reductase, followed by dephosphorylation to FdUMP. FdUMP and FdUDP are substrates for pyrimidine monophosphate and diphosphate kinase, respectively, resulting

in the formation of fluorodeoxyuridine triphosphate (FdUTP). FdUTP can be incorporated into DNA by DNA polymerase.

Physiologic Urd metabolites are largely present *in vivo* as nucleotide sugars that are necessary for the glycosylation of proteins and lipids; this process plays an important role in cytoplasmic and cell membrane metabolism. 5-FU nucleotide sugars, such as FUDP-glucose, FUDP-hexose, FUDP-*N*-acetylglucosamine, and FdUDP-*N*-acetylglucosamine, also have been detected in mammalian cells.[19–21] The extent to which 5-FU nucleotide sugars are incorporated into proteins and lipids and the possible metabolic consequences are unclear.

In terms of catabolic pathways, acid and alkaline phosphatases convert the various nucleotide derivatives of 5-FU to the nucleoside level, and 5'-nucleotidases convert FdUMP to FdUrd. The pyrimidine phosphorylases catalyze the reversible conversion of pyrimidine base to nucleoside. FdUrd serves as a substrate for Urd and dThd phosphorylases, depending on the tissue, yielding 5-FU.[17,18] The further metabolic degradation of 5-FU *in vivo* is discussed later. dThd phosphorylase is now known to be homologous to platelet-derived endothelial growth factor, which is involved in angiogenesis.

MECHANISM OF ACTION

Inhibition of Thymidylate Synthase

At least two primary mechanisms of action appear capable of causing cell injury: (a) inhibition of TS and (b) incorporation into RNA. The first occurs through the generation of FdUMP, which binds tightly to TS and prevents formation of thymidylate (thymidine 5'-monophosphate, dTMP Thymidylate is the essential precursor of thymidine 5'-triphosphate (dTTP), one of four deoxyribonucleotides required for DNA synthesis and repair. The second mechanism results from the incorporation of FUTP into RNA and the subsequent effects on RNA function. The functional TS enzyme comprises a dimer of two identical subunits, each of molecular weight approximately 30 kd (bacterial) to 36 kd (human). Each subunit has a nucleotide-binding site and at least two distinct folate binding sites, one for $5,10\text{-}CH_2FH_4$ mono- or polyglutamate and one for polyglutamates of dihydrofolate. FdUMP competes with the natural substrate deoxyuridine monophosphate (dUMP) for the catalytic site on TS.[22,23] In the methylation of dUMP, transfer of the folate methyl group to dUMP is made possible by elimination of the hydrogen attached to the carbon-5 position of uracil. This elimination cannot occur with the more tightly bound fluorine atom of FdUMP, and the enzyme is trapped in a slowly reversible ternary complex (Fig. 8-3). The "thymineless state" that ensues is toxic to actively dividing cells. Toxicity can be circumvented by salvage of dThd in cells that contain dThd

TABLE 8-1. KEY FEATURES OF 5-FLUOROURACIL

Mechanism of action	Incorporation of fluorouridine triphosphate into RNA interferes with RNA synthesis and function.
	Inhibition of thymidylate synthase by fluorodeoxyuridylate (FdUMP) leads to depletion of thymidine 5' monophosphate and thymidine 5' triphosphate, and accumulation of deoxyuridine monophosphate and deoxyuridine triphosphate.
	Incorporation of fluorodeoxyuridine triphosphate and deoxyuridine triphosphate into DNA may affect DNA stability.
	Genotoxic stress triggers programmed cell death pathways.
Metabolism	Converted enzymatically to active nucleotide forms intracellularly.
	DPD catalyzes the initial, rate-limiting step in 5-fluorouracil (5-FU) catabolism.
Pharmacokinetics	Primary half-life is 8–14 min after i.v. bolus.
	Nonlinear pharmacokinetics due to saturable catabolism: Total body clearance decreases with increasing doses; clearance is faster with infusional schedules.
	Volume of distribution slightly exceeds extracellular fluid space.
Elimination	Approximately 90% is eliminated by metabolism (catabolism→anabolism).
	<10% unchanged drug excreted by kidneys.
	Reduction of 5-FU to dihydrofluorouracil by DPD is rate limiting. Thereafter: dihydrofluorouracil→fluoroureidopropionic acid→fluoro-β-alanine.
	5-FU and its catabolites undergo biliary excretion.
Pharmacokinetic drug interactions	Interference with 5-FU catabolism markedly prolongs its half-life.
	Inhibitors of DPD:
	Thymidine and thymine
	Uracil (component of uracil and ftorafur)
	5-chloro-2,4-dihydroxypyridine (component of ftorafur, 5-chloro-2,4-dihydroxypyridine, and potassium oxonate)
	3-cyano-2,6-dihydroxypyridine (component of emitefur, 3-{3-[6-benzoyloxy-3-cyano-2-pyridyloxycarbonyl]benzoyl}-1-ethoxymethyl-5-fluorouracil)
	(E)-5-(2-bromovinyl)uracil (metabolite of sorivudine)
	Eniluracil
	Chronic administration of cimetidine (but not ranitidine) may decrease the clearance of 5-FU.
	Dipyridamole increases 5-FU clearance during continuous i.v. infusion.
	Interferon-α may decrease 5-FU clearance in some individuals in a dose- and schedule-dependent manner.
Biochemical drug interactions	Thymidine salvage via thymidine kinase repletes thymidine 5' triphosphate pools, decreases FdUMP formation, and antagonizes the DNA-directed toxicity of 5-FU and 5-fluoro-2'deoxyuridine; thymidine may increase fluorouridine triphosphate formation and its incorporation into RNA.
	Sequential methotrexate→5-FU increases 5-FU toxicity and increases fluorouridine triphosphate (FUTP) incorporation into RNA; may antagonize DNA-directed toxicity of 5-FU.
	Leucovorin increases intracellular pools of reduced folates; 5,10-methylenetetrahydrofolate polyglutamates enhance the stability of reduced folate-FdUMP–thymidylate synthase ternary complex; the magnitude and duration of thymidylate synthase inhibition is increased.
	Inhibitors of de novo pyrimidine synthesis (N-phosphonoacetyl-L-aspartic acid, brequinar) increase 5-FU anabolism to the ribonucleotide level and 5-FU–RNA incorporation; uridine triphosphate, cytidine triphosphate, deoxycytidine triphosphate, and deoxyuridine monophosphate depletion may enhance RNA- and DNA-directed toxicity of 5-FU.
Toxicity	Gastrointestinal epithelial ulceration
	Myelosuppression
	Dermatologic
	Ocular
	Neurotoxicity (cognitive dysfunction and cerebellar ataxia)
	Cardiac (coronary spasm)
	Biliary sclerosis (hepatic arterial infusion of FdUrd)
Precautions	Nonlinear pharmacokinetics: difficulty in predicting plasma concentrations and toxicity at high doses.
	Patients with deficiency of DPD may have life-threatening or fatal toxicity if treated with 5-fluoropyrimidines.
	Duration of DPD inhibition with eniluracil may be prolonged (8-wk washout period recommended).
	Patients receiving sorivudine should not receive concurrent 5-fluoropyrimidines (4-wk washout period recommended).
	Elderly, female, and poor performance status patients have greater risk of toxicity.

DPD, dihydropyrimidine dehydrogenase.

kinase. The circulating concentrations of dThd in humans are not thought to be sufficient (approximately 0.1 μmol per L) to afford protection.[24] In contrast, the plasma levels of dThd are approximately tenfold higher in rodents, which complicates preclinical evaluation of the antitumor activity of various TS inhibitors.

The presence of the reduced-folate cofactor is required for tight binding of the inhibitor to TS. The natural cofactor for the TS reaction, 5,10-CH$_2$FH$_4$, in its mono- and polyglutamate forms, binds through its methylene group to the carbon-5 position of FdUMP. The polyglutamates of 5,10-CH$_2$FH$_4$ are much more effective in stabilizing the ternary complex.[25,26] Other naturally occurring folates also promote FdUMP binding to the enzyme but result in a more readily dissociable complex. Exceptions are the polyglutamates of dihydrofolic acid (FH$_2$), which promote extremely tight

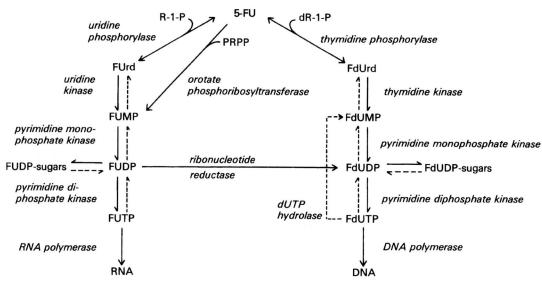

FIGURE 8-2. Intracellular activation of 5-fluorouracil (5-FU). (dUTP, deoxyuridine triphosphate; FdUDP, fluorodeoxyuridine diphosphate; FdUMP, fluorodeoxyuridylate; FdUrd, 5-fluoro-2'-deoxyuridine; FdUTP, fluorodeoxyuridine triphosphate; FUDP, fluorouridine diphosphate; FUMP, fluorouridine monophosphate; FUrd, 5-fluorouridine; FUTP, fluorouridine triphosphate; PPRP, phosphoribosyl phosphate.)

binding of FdUMP to the enzyme.[26,27] Dihydrofolate accumulates in cells exposed to methotrexate (MTX). Although MTX is a relatively weak inhibitor of TS in cell-free experiments, MTX polyglutamates are more potent inhibitors.[28] MTX polyglutamates decrease the rate of formation of ternary complex among FdUMP, folate cofactor, and enzyme. The ability of MTX polyglutamates to inhibit ternary-complex formation is highly influenced by the glutamation state of the reduced-folate cofactor and is substantially reduced in the presence of 5,10-CH$_2$FH$_4$ pentaglutamate.[28] Similarly, in tissue culture, MTX-induced depletion of intracellular reduced folates causes a marked reduction in the rate of formation of ternary complex.[27,29]

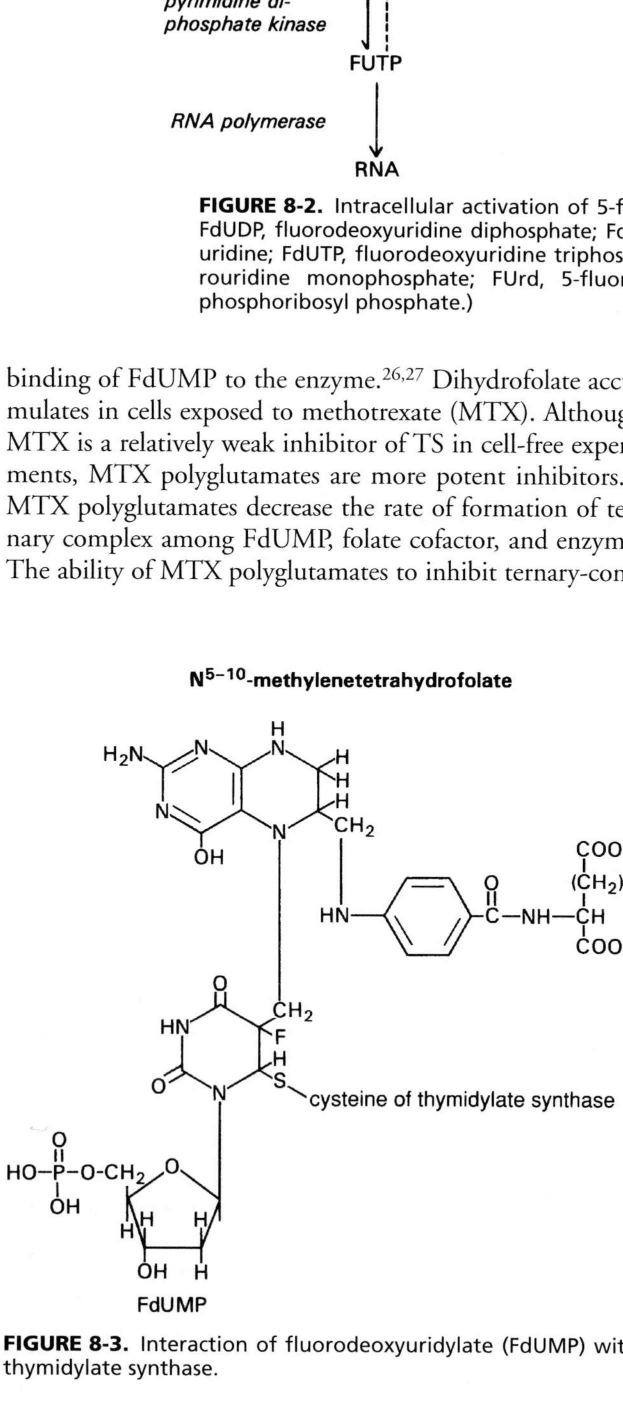

The kinetics of formation and dissociation of the ternary complex have been studied using the enzyme from *Lactobacillus casei*.[30] Only one site in the free enzyme is accessible for binding to FdUMP; the second site becomes exposed after occupancy of the first site by inhibitor and 5,10-CH$_2$FH$_4$. The two binding sites seem to be nonequivalent in terms of their dissociation constants, with K_d values of 1.1×10^{-11} and 2×10^{-10} mol per L.[31] FdUMP binds less avidly to the mammalian enzyme, with a dissociation half-life ($t_{1/2}$) of 6.2 hours, indicating that inhibition of the mammalian enzyme is slowly reversible.[32]

Elucidation of the crystal structure of TS has permitted a complex kinetic and thermodynamic description of the association between TS, FdUMP, and 5,10-CH$_2$FH$_4$.[33,34] The interaction proceeds by an ordered mechanism with initial nucleotide binding followed by 5,10-CH$_2$FH$_4$ binding to form a rapidly reversible noncovalent ternary complex. Enzyme-catalyzed conversions result in the formation of a covalent bond between carbon-5 of FdUMP and the one-carbon unit of the cofactor. The equilibrium constant between the noncovalent and covalent ternary complexes is approximately 2×10^4; the overall dissociation constant of 5,10-CH$_2$FH$_4$ from the covalent complex is approximately 10^{-11} mol per L.

The three-dimensional conformation of free and bound TS has been characterized through molecular modeling and

N$^{5-10}$-methylenetetrahydrofolate

FIGURE 8-3. Interaction of fluorodeoxyuridylate (FdUMP) with thymidylate synthase.

iterative crystallographic analysis.[33,35,36] The crystal structures of the enzymes from *Escherichia coli* and *L. casei* have been more accurately resolved than the human form. Although the molecular weight and amino acid composition of the bacterial and mammalian enzymes differ, the primary sequence and the active site residues that form the folate binding site of the bacterial enzymes show high homology with the human sequence. The bacterial ternary complex serves as an appropriate surrogate for the design of inhibitors of human TS, including the antifolate TS inhibitors, which bind to the folate-binding active site rather than to the dUMP-binding site.

Despite the high specificity and potency of TS inhibition by FdUMP and the well-established lethality of dTMP and dTTP depletion, inhibition of TS is not the sole cause of 5-FU toxicity. If 5-FU toxicity results from dTTP depletion, then dThd should reverse the toxic effects. Examples of complete protection from 5-FU cytotoxicity by dThd have been reported, but dThd shows variable effectiveness in rescuing cells exposed to 5-FU.[37–40] Murine lymphoma cells experience two phases of drug toxicity when exposed to 5-FU.[39] The early phase of toxicity during the initial 24 hours of drug exposure has the characteristics of S-phase specificity, including S-phase accumulation. Addition of dThd prevents the S-phase block induced by dTTP depletion and abolishes the early phase of growth inhibition. The later phase of 5-FU inhibition of growth has different characteristics. After 24 hours (approximately one cell-cycle length) of incubation with 5-FU, dThd no longer prevents lethality; instead, toxicity is maximal for cells exposed during the G_1 phase of the cell cycle. This second phase of inhibition is attributed to progressive incorporation of 5-FU into RNA with subsequent deleterious effects on RNA processing and function. In another model, a 3-hour incubation with 5-FU at low concentrations (5 to 20 µmol per L) produces a dThd-reversible toxicity, although dThd could not reverse toxicity associated with high 5-FU concentrations.[40]

Additional experimental evidence from *in vivo* studies supports the contention that 5-FU toxicity is at least partially independent of its effect on TS. Coadministration of 5-FU and dThd prevents the early inhibition of DNA synthesis but markedly increases 5-FU toxicity to normal tissues in the whole animal, increases the antitumor effect of 5-FU against various animal tumors, and increases [³H]FUrd incorporation into the RNA of normal and malignant cells.[41–44] Other pharmacologic measures that increase FUTP formation and its RNA incorporation also increase its toxicity.[42–45]

RNA-Directed Effects

Mammalian cells have several different classes of RNA. The majority of cellular RNA is ribosomal RNA (rRNA), which forms the major component of ribosomes. Ribosomes are large ribonucleoprotein particles consisting of a small and

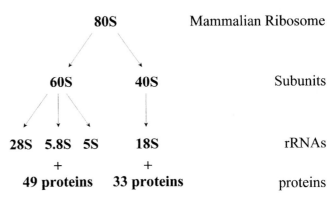

FIGURE 8-4. Organization of mammalian ribosomes. (rRNAs, ribosomal RNAs; S, sedimentation behavior.)

large subunit, each of which has distinct proteins and RNAs (Fig. 8-4). The ribosomes are molecular machines that coordinate the interplay of transfer RNA (tRNA), messenger RNA (mRNA), and proteins in the complex process of protein synthesis. tRNA carries amino acids in activated form to the ribosome for peptide bond formation. Mature tRNA, designated 4S based on its sedimentation behavior, is 75 nucleotides in length and accounts for approximately 15% of cellular RNA. After initial transcription, mature tRNA and rRNA are generated by cleavage and modification of nascent RNA chains. Additional processing may include the addition of nucleotides to the termini of the RNA chain and enzymatic modification of bases and ribose moieties. mRNA serves as the template for protein synthesis and comprises approximately 5% of cellular RNA. mRNA expression entails a complex series of events (Table 8-2). The initial transcription product, designated *pre-mRNA* or *heterogeneous nuclear RNA*, has modifications of the 5'-end and 3'-end and contains both exons (the coding sequences) and introns (the intervening untranslated sequences). The introns are removed by a process called *splicing*. Small nuclear RNA molecules (snRNAs), designated as U1–U6, associate with specific proteins to form small nuclear ribonucleoproteins (snRNPs). Spliceosomes are large (60S) complexes that contain specific snRNPs that recognize the 5'- and 3'-splice sites and the branch site of precursor mRNA; the spliceosome holds the exons of the precursor mRNA during the excision of the noncoding sequences until the exons are joined. The mRNA with the intact coding sequence is then transported into the cytoplasm, whereas the introns are rapidly degraded in the nucleus. Translation proceeds in the cytoplasm in three steps: initiation, elongation, and termination.

The contribution of RNA-directed toxicity to ultimate lethality *in vitro* and *in vivo* varies greatly depending on the type of cancer cell line and the experimental conditions. 5-FU is extensively incorporated into nuclear and cytoplasmic RNA fractions, which may result in alterations in RNA processing and function (Table 8-3).[46–49] Incorporation of 5-FU into RNA inhibits the processing of the initial pre-rRNA transcripts to the cytoplasmic rRNA species in a

TABLE 8-2. EXPRESSION OF MESSENGER RNA (MRNA) IN MAMMALIAN CELLS

1. Transcription begins; 5'-end of mRNA is modified.
2. 3'-end of mRNA is released and is then polyadenylated.
3. RNA splicing by spliceosome (60S complex).
   a. Small nuclear RNAs that exist as ribonucleoprotein particles:
      i. U1
      ii. U2
      iii. U5
      iv. U4/U6
   b. Consensus sequences are recognized; spliceosome complex forms.
   c. Exon-intron junctions are broken, and intron is removed.
   d. Exons are joined.
4. mRNA with intact coding sequence is transported to the cytoplasm.
5. mRNA is translated in the ribosomes.
   a. mRNA associates with the small subunit.
   b. Two transfer RNAs (tRNAs) span both the large and small subunit.
   c. Incoming aminoacyl-tRNA binds to the A site (or acceptor site): codon "n + 1."
   d. Peptidyl-tRNA occupies the P site (or donor site): codon "n."
   e. Peptide bond formation: Peptide carried by peptidyl-tRNA is transferred to the aminoacyl-tRNA.
   f. Translocation moves ribosome by one codon.
   g. Deacylated tRNA leaves via the E site.
   h. Incoming aminoacyl-tRNA binds to the A site.
   i. Elongation proceeds.
   j. Termination:
      i. Release of polypeptide chain from tRNA
      ii. Ribosome dissociates from mRNA

S, sedimentation behavior.

dose- and time-dependent manner.[46–53] Lethality in erythroleukemia cells correlates with incorporation of 5-FU into pre-rRNA in the nucleus and inhibition of maturation to cytoplasmic 28S and 18S rRNA species.[49]

Net RNA synthesis may be inhibited during and after fluoropyrimidine exposure in a concentration and time-dependent fashion. In human breast and colon cancer cell lines, a highly significant relationship exists between 5-FU incorporation into total cellular RNA and the loss of clonogenic survival.[11,54,55] The incorporation into RNA and

TABLE 8-3. RNA-DIRECTED CYTOTOXIC EFFECTS OF 5-FLUOROURACIL (5-FU)

Decrease in net RNA synthesis.
Inhibition with RNA processing.
Inhibition of messenger RNA polyadenylation.
Alteration of the secondary structure of RNA.
5-FU residues in transfer RNA form covalent complex with enzymes involved in posttranslational modification of uracil residues.
Incorporation into uracil-rich small nuclear RNA species interferes with normal splicing.
Quantitative changes in protein synthesis.
Qualitative changes in protein synthesis.
Up-regulation of thymidylate synthase (TS) protein synthesis.
   TS bound in ternary complex cannot bind to TS messenger RNA.
   TS protein translation no longer repressed.

decrease in viability are a function of 5-FU concentration and time of exposure. 5-FU is incorporated into all species of RNA; substantial amounts of [³H]5-FU accumulate in low-molecular-weight (4S) RNA at lethal drug concentrations.[55] Even under conditions of exposure to high concentrations of 5-FU, the analog replaces only a small percentage of uracil residues in RNA in intact cells; nonetheless, the incorporated 5-FU residues appear to be stable and to persist in RNA for many days after drug administration.[40,56,57]

5-FU exposure also affects mRNA processing and translation. Polyadenylation of mRNA, a process thought to confer stability, is inhibited at relatively low concentrations of 5-FU.[58] The functional significance of the effect on polyadenylation and 5-FU-mRNA incorporation is unclear.[59] Polyadenylated mRNA containing 5-FU is associated with an increased rate of protein synthesis in one cell-free system, but the proteins show no qualitative differences in their electrophoretic profile.[60] In permeabilized K-562 erythroleukemia cells, preexposure to α-amanitin, an inhibitor of RNA polymerase II, decreases [³H]FUrd incorporation into polyadenylated mRNA and antagonizes its cytotoxicity.[61]

Altered metabolism of dihydrofolate reductase (DHFR) precursor mRNA or processing intermediates, or both, is seen in some fluoropyrimidine-treated cells. Nuclear and cytoplasmic labeling experiments demonstrated a decreased rate of nuclear DHFR precursor mRNA conversion to cytoplasmic DHFR mRNA.[62,63] Incorporation of 5-FU into RNA may affect quantitative and qualitative aspects of protein synthesis.[64–69] 5-FU exposure leads to a dose-dependent increase in the mRNA coding for DHFR in MTX-resistant KB cells. Furthermore, the DHFR protein product has alterations in MTX binding affinity and reactivity with polyclonal anti-DHFR antiserum, suggesting possible translational miscoding.[64,65] In other studies, the processing of nuclear precursor mRNA coding for DHFR and polyadenylation of the mRNA species are both decreased.[67,70] 5-FU decreases globin gene transcription and translation in erythroleukemia cells.[66] In the MCF-7 human breast cancer cell line, 5-FU exposure has different effects on various mRNAs, causing increases and decreases in total mRNA levels of specific species.[68]

In vitro transcribed TS mRNA with 100% substitution of 5-FU has an altered pattern of migration in nondenaturing gels and of denaturation in RNA melting-temperature studies, consistent with changes in the secondary structure of mRNA.[71] However, no differences in the translational efficiency of 5-FU–substituted TS mRNA are seen. Analysis of the *in vitro* translated protein product by Western immunoblotting, isoelectric focusing, FdUMP-binding, and TS catalytic activity experiments showed no difference compared with control mRNA containing only uracil.[71] In this cell-free system, therefore, 5-FU substitution in mRNA does not result in miscoding during translation. In another system, 100% substitution of uracil residues in human-TS complementary DNA (cDNA) with either FUTP or 5-bromouridine 5'-triphosphate (BrUTP) indicated that the translational rate is inhibited in the presence of BrUTP-substituted cDNA, but not with FUTP substitution.[70] The stability of the transcribed mRNA in a rabbit reticulocyte lysate system is increased by three- and tenfold with FUTP and BrUTP, respectively. Finally, nondenaturing gel electrophoresis shows different conformations for each of the substituted mRNA species.

Changes in the structure and levels of snRNAs and snRNPs may result from fluoropyrimidine treatment.[71–76] With 8% replacement of Urd residues with 5-FU in HeLA cells, the levels of U2-snRNA and -snRNPs decrease in nuclear extracts.[73] The substitution of FUTP for uridine triphosphate (UTP) in a cell-free system (84% replacement of uracil residues by 5-FU) leads to pH-dependent *mis*splicing of ^{32}P-labeled human β-globin precursor mRNA, and pH values favoring 5-FU ionization promote missplicing.[74]

The splicing reaction of precursor RNA exposed to either 1 mmol per L UTP or 1 mmol per L FUTP has been compared in *Tetrahymena* rRNA, an autocatalytic, self-splicing system with one intron and two exons.[75] Polyacrylamide and urea gel electrophoresis indicates that the rate and extent of formation of all RNA product species is decreased with 100% FUTP substitution. Furthermore, 5-FU substitution greatly increases the pH and temperature sensitivity of the process. Partial ionization of 5-FU residues at physiologic pH (pK 5-FU = 7.8 vs. pK uracil = 10.1) may therefore destabilize the active conformation of RNA.[75]

Another potential locus of 5-FU action is inhibition of enzymes involved in posttranscriptional modification of RNA.[53,77–80] 5-FU exposure inhibits tRNA uracil 5-methyltransferase, which may explain the decreased formation of modified Urd (pseudouridine) bases in tRNA.[77] In the presence of S-adenosylmethionine, 5-FU–substituted tRNA forms a stable covalent complex containing uracil 5-methyltransferase, 5-FU–tRNA, and the methyl group of S-adenosylmethionine.[78] Thus, irreversible inhibition of RNA methylation may contribute to RNA-directed cytotoxicity of 5-FU. 5-FU–substituted yeast glycine tRNAs form highly stable covalent complexes with pseudouridine synthase.[79] Many nucleotide positions in tRNA, rRNA, and snRNA are posttranscriptionally modified from Urd to pseudouridine, although the precise physiologic role of the modified residue is unclear. In an *in vitro* assembly and modification system, 5-FU incorporation alters the biosynthesis of U2 snRNA with subsequent effects on snRNA-protein interactions.[80] Even low levels of 5-FU incorporation (5% replacement) inhibit the formation of the pseudouridine modification.[80] Subtle changes in the structures of these essential splicing cofactors may thus have profound effects on snRNP–precursor mRNA interactions and interfere with precursor mRNA splicing.

5-FU–associated cytotoxicity in cancer cells exposed in the presence of sufficient concentrations of dThd to circumvent TS inhibition is presumed to result from RNA-directed effects of 5-FU. A paradox is that significant incorporation of 5-FU into RNA may occur in some cancer cell lines in the absence of toxicity. The factors that influence whether 5-FU–RNA incorporation results in cytotoxicity are not clear. In murine S-180 cells, the cytotoxicity of several different radiolabeled fluoropyrimidines given at equal concentrations was correlated to the extent of RNA incorporation. FUrd has the highest rate of RNA incorporation and the greatest cytotoxicity, whereas 5'-deoxy-5-fluorouridine (5'-dFUrd) has the lowest rate of RNA incorporation and is minimally toxic.[66] At cytotoxic concentrations, [^{3}H]FUrd is preferentially incorporated into nucleolar RNA (composed predominantly of pre-rRNA) with little incorporation into nucleoplasmic RNA (composed mainly of heterogeneous nuclear RNA but also containing tRNA and 5S rRNA).[68] The observation that only 10% of the [^{3}H]RNA is present in mature 28S and 18S cytoplasmic rRNA species is consistent with a block in the processing of rRNA.[68] Exposure to [^{3}H]5'-dFUrd at a nontoxic concentration produces slightly greater total RNA incorporation, but the distribution into nuclear and nucleoplasmic RNA is similar. Furthermore, a time-dependent increase in [^{3}H]5'-dFUrd accumulation into mature 28S and 18S cytoplasmic rRNA species is noted, suggesting that [^{3}H]5'-dFUrd incorporation does not impair pre-rRNA processing. The rate of RNA incorporation and the species into which the fluoropyrimidine is incorporated appear to be more important determinants of cytotoxicity than is the total amount incorporated. These findings and those from other studies suggest that 5-FU and FUrd may be channeled into different ribonucleotide compartments and, ultimately, into distinct classes of RNA.[81]

In summary, the changes that result in altered pre-RNA processing and mRNA metabolism are not uniform for all RNA species after 5-FU exposure. Effects on precursor and mature rRNA, precursor and mature mRNA, tRNA, and snRNA species suggest inhibition of processing; incorporated 5-FU residues also inhibit enzymes involved in posttranscriptional modification of uracil. Many of the RNA-directed effects of fluoropyrimidines undoubtedly occur as a consequence of their fraudulent incorporation into various RNA species. However, rapid changes in mRNA levels suggest that at least some of these alterations may be mediated by other 5-FU–associated alterations in cellular metabolism or posttranslational modification.[82] The changes in certain key mRNAs resulting from 5-FU exposure may be relevant as a mechanism of cytotoxicity. 5-FU–mediated interference with the production of enzymes involved in DNA repair may have cytotoxic consequences, such as 5-FU–mediated inhibition of ERCC-1 mRNA expression in cisplatin-resistant cancer cells.[83] 5-FU and FUrd produce structural and functional alterations in uracil-rich snRNAs and consequently in snRNPs with potential repercussions on cellular growth and metabolism. The RNA-directed effects of 5-FU are even more complex than previously appreciated, and some RNA effects may be independent of 5-FU incorporation into RNA.

TABLE 8-4. DNA-DIRECTED CYTOTOXIC EFFECTS OF 5-FLUOROURACIL

Biochemical consequences of thymidylate synthase inhibition
Deoxyribonucleotide imbalance
Depletion of thymidine monophosphate and thymidine triphosphate
Accumulation of deoxyuridine monophosphate
   Elevation of extracellular deoxyuridine
   Formation of deoxyuridine triphosphate
Accumulation of deoxyadenosine triphosphate
Direct and indirect effects on DNA synthesis and integrity
Inhibition of net DNA synthesis
"Uracil" misincorporation into DNA (fluoro- and deoxyuridine triphosphate)
Interference with nascent DNA chain elongation
Altered stability of nascent DNA
Induction of single-strand breaks in nascent DNA
Interference with DNA repair
Induction of single- and double-strand breaks in parental DNA

DNA-Directed Cytotoxic Mechanisms

The biochemical consequences of TS inhibition and the potential effects on DNA integrity are summarized in Table 8-4. Inhibition of TS results in depletion of dTMP and dTTP, thus leading to inhibition of DNA synthesis and interference with DNA repair. Accumulation of dUMP occurs behind the blockade of TS, and further metabolism to the deoxyuridine triphosphate (dUTP) level may occur.[84–86] Inhibition of TS is accompanied by elevated concentrations of deoxyuridine in the extracellular media in cell culture models and in plasma of rodents; monitoring changes in plasma deoxyuridine levels may, therefore, serve as an indirect reflection of TS inhibition.

FdUTP and dUTP are substrates for DNA polymerase, and their incorporation into DNA is a possible mechanism of cytotoxicity.[87–99] 5-FU cytotoxicity in some models correlates with the level of 5-FU–DNA.[93,95,99] Two mechanisms tend to prevent incorporation of FdUTP and dUTP into DNA. The enzyme dUTP pyrophosphatase or dUTP hydrolase catalyses the hydrolysis of FdUTP to FdUMP and inorganic pyrophosphate.[100–101] The DNA repair enzyme uracil-DNA-glycosylase hydrolyzes the fluorouracil-deoxyribose glycosyl bond of the FdUMP residues in DNA, thereby creating an apyrimidinic site.[98,102] Endonucleolytic cleavage of the base-free deoxyribose site results in a single-strand break, which is subsequently repaired. In the face of thymidine triphosphate depletion, however, the efficiency of the repair process is substantially weakened. Uracil-DNA-glycosylase is a cell-cycle–dependent enzyme with maximal levels of activity at the G1 and S interface, such that excision of the fraudulent bases occurs before DNA replication. The activity of uracil-DNA-glycosylase inversely correlates with the level of FdUrd incorporation into DNA in human lymphoblastic cells.[92] Because the affinity of human uracil-DNA-glycosylase is much lower for 5-FU than for uracil, it is removed more slowly from DNA by this mechanism.[102] Furthermore, recent studies suggest that FdUTP inhibits the activity of uracil-DNA-glycosylase.[103] Accumula-

tion of deoxyadenosine triphosphate (dATP) accompanies TS inhibition.[104–106] Thus, the combined effects of deoxyribonucleotide imbalance (high dATP, low dTTP, high dUTP) and misincorporation of FdUTP into DNA may have several deleterious consequences affecting DNA synthesis and the integrity of nascent DNA.

A variety of DNA-directed effects has been described.[107–118] 5-FU treatment inhibits DNA elongation and decreases the average DNA chain length.[91,107,108,109] DNA strand breaks accumulate in 5-FU–treated cells and correlate with excision of [³H]5-FU from DNA.[108] In human ileocecal and colon carcinoma cells, 5-FU and FdUrd result in single and double-stranded DNA breaks in a concentration and time-dependent fashion.[110,111] LV seems to enhance DNA damage, whereas dThd exposure limits it.[110,112] FdUrd exposure may result in the formation of large (one to five-megabase) DNA fragments as a result of double-strand DNA breaks; the time course and extent of DNA megabase fragmentation correlates with loss of clonogenicity in HT29 cells (Fig. 8-5).[113] The pattern of

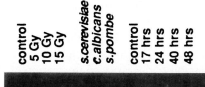

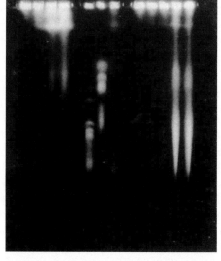

2.2 Mb -

1.0 Mb -

FIGURE 8-5. Induction of megabase DNA fragments by 5-fluoro-2'-deoxyuridine (FdUrd): After treatment with 100 nmol/L FdUrd for the indicated time periods, agarose cell blocks containing either DNA treated with various doses of γ-radiation or intact HT29 cells were digested in a solution to remove RNA and protein, then subjected to pulsed-field gel electrophoresis. The size standards shown in the middle lanes represent yeast chromosomes. DNA-megabase fragmentation was seen after 40- and 48-hour FdUrd exposure and produced a pattern distinct from that seen with γ-radiation. [Reproduced from Dusenbery CE, Davis MA, Lawrence TS, et al. Induction of megabase DNA fragment by 5-fluorodeoxyuridine in human colorectal tumor (HT29) cells. *Mol Pharmacol* 1991;39:285–289, with permission from the American Society for Pharmacology and Experimental Therapeutics.]

DNA fragmentation is distinct from that associated with gamma radiation, which produces random breaks. The pattern of high-molecular-weight DNA damage differs during FdUrd exposure in two colon cancer cell lines; although both are equally sensitive to FdUrd-induced inhibition of TS, higher drug concentrations and longer exposure times are necessary to achieve a comparable degree of DNA fragmentation and cytotoxicity in SW620 cells.[101,114] The basis for the resistance of SW620 cells to FdUrd-induced DNA damage correlates with higher activity of dUTP and failure to accumulate dUTP, findings that implicate dUTP (and perhaps its incorporation into DNA) in 5-FU–induced DNA damage.[101] In contrast to the DNA megabase fragmentation seen in the two colon cancer cell lines, dThd starvation of a TS-deficient murine cell line produces much smaller DNA fragments, 50 to 200 kb in length.[115]

Fibroblast cells isolated from patients with Bloom's syndrome (associated with altered regulation of uracil-DNA-glycosylase) have increased DNA fragmentation after 5-FU treatment compared with normal fibroblast cells. In this model, DNA damage is prevented by aphidicolin, an inhibitor of DNA polymerase-α that stops the movement of replication forks and, therefore, decreases the incorporation of FdUTP into DNA.[116] Inhibition of protein synthesis by cycloheximide within 8 hours of FdUrd exposure dramatically reduces DNA double-strand breakage and lethality in murine FM3A cells, suggesting that FdUrd exposure triggers the synthesis of an endonuclease capable of inducing DNA strand breaks.[104] In rat prostate cancer cells with intact programmed cell-death pathways, FdUrd induces oligonucleosomal fragmentation of genomic DNA.[118]

Factors that regulate recognition of DNA damage and apoptosis contribute to 5-FU lethality. The oncogene *p53* plays a pivotal role in the regulation of cell-cycle progression and apoptosis and influences the sensitivity of murine embryonic fibroblasts to 5-FU.[119] Transfection and expression of the *bcl*-2 oncogene in a human-lymphoma cell line renders it resistant to FdUrd. TS inhibition, dTTP depletion, and induction of single-strand breaks in nascent DNA are similar in vector control cells and *bcl*-2–expressing cells.[120] In vector control cells, in contrast, induction of double-stranded DNA fragmentation in parental DNA coincides with onset of apoptosis.[120] These studies indicate that factors operating downstream from TS influence drug sensitivity. The contribution of DNA damage to cell lethality varies among different malignant lines, and DNA fragmentation does not appear to contribute to 5-FU–mediated cytotoxicity in some cancer cell lines.[121,122]

In summary, TS inhibition, as seen in "pure" form with FdUrd treatment in the absence of dThd salvage, and 5-FU incorporation into RNA are capable of producing lethal effects on cells. DNA damage also contributes to cytotoxicity and can occur in the absence of detectable FdUTP incorporation into DNA. The combined effects of deoxyribonucleotide imbalance (high dATP, low dTTP, high dUTP) and misincorporation of FdUTP and dUTP into DNA result in a number of deleterious consequences affecting DNA synthesis and the integrity of nascent DNA. The pattern and extent of DNA damage induced by fluoropyrimidines in human colorectal cancer cells varies and may be affected by the activity of enzymes involved in DNA repair and by downstream pathways that are required to implement cellular destruction. It is now recognized that the genotoxic stress resulting from TS inhibition activates programmed cell-death pathways, resulting in induction of parental DNA fragmentation. Depending on the cell line in question, two different patterns of parental DNA damage may be noted: internucleosomal DNA laddering, the hallmark of classical apoptosis, and high-MW DNA fragmentation with segments ranging from approximately 50 kb to 1 to 3 megabases (mb). Differences in the type and activity of endonucleases and DNA-degradative enzymes triggered in a given cell line most likely explain these disparate patterns of parental DNA fragmentation. In "apoptosis-competent" cancer cell lines, such as HL60 promyelocytic leukemia cells, genotoxic stress results in rapid (within hours) induction of programmed cell death, with classic DNA laddering. In contrast, many cancer cell lines derived from epithelial tumors, including colon cancer, appear to undergo delayed programmed cell death. This phenomenon may reflect a "postmitotic" cell death, in which one or more rounds of mitosis are needed before cell death occurs.[123] In such cell lines, the duration of the genotoxic insult may determine whether induction of cytostasis or programmed cell death occurs. One possible explanation for delayed apoptosis is that originally sublethal damage to genes, which are essential for cell survival, may ultimately lead to cell death with subsequent rounds of DNA replication.

Factors operating downstream from TS clearly influence the cellular response to genotoxic stress, such as overexpression of the cellular oncoproteins bcl-2 and mutant p53. Disruption of the signal pathways that sense genotoxic stress or lead to induction of programmed cell death, or both, may render a cancer cell inherently resistant to 5-FU. In some cancer cell lines, thymineless death may be mediated by Fas and Fas-ligand interactions.[124,125] Fas is a cell surface receptor that belongs to the tumor necrosis factor–receptor superfamily; Fas and Fas-ligand are known to regulate apoptosis. Modulation of Fas expression may thus represent a strategy to enhance the sensitivity of cancer cells to TS inhibitors, including 5-FU and LV. A final point is that although induction of programmed cell death is generally thought to be a consequence of DNA-directed events, 5-FU–mediated induction of apoptosis in intestinal crypt cells with an intact p53 pathway appears to be a consequence of RNA-directed effects.[126] Although induction of apoptosis is the final common pathway for cell death, DNA and RNA-directed effects of 5-FU may provide the triggering stimulus.

Relative Importance of RNA versus DNA-Directed Effects

The relative contributions of DNA and RNA-directed mechanisms to the cytotoxicity of 5-FU are influenced by the specific patterns of intracellular metabolism, which vary among different normal and tumor tissues. 5-FU concentration and duration of exposure play pivotal roles in determining the basis of cytotoxicity. The improved response rates observed with LV-modulation of bolus 5-FU therapy, the correlation between high TS expression in tumor tissue and insensitivity to 5-FU–based therapy, and the clinical activity of the antifolate-based TS inhibitors provide strong evidence that TS is an important therapeutic target. In some models, RNA-directed effects have been predominant with prolonged duration of exposure and are not necessarily cell-cycle dependent, whereas DNA-directed effects have been important during short-term exposure of cells in S phase. In different models, contrary results have been observed. The mechanism of insensitivity differs in human colon cancer cells selected for resistance to either short-term, high-concentration 5-FU exposure (1,000 μmol per L for 4 hours, simulating bolus administration) or more prolonged, lower-concentration exposure (15 μmol per L for 7 days).[127] A subline resistant to short-term 5-FU exposure has decreased 5-FU–RNA incorporation, whereas the subline insensitive to protracted 5-FU exposure displays more rapid recovery from TS inhibition after drug exposure. Of interest, the subline with RNA-directed resistance retains sensitivity to protracted exposure.[128]

In two human colon carcinoma cell lines, the determinants of cytotoxicity with prolonged (120-hour) exposure to 5-FU at pharmacologically relevant concentrations (0.1–1.0 μmol per L) have been assessed.[129] In this model, DNA-directed effects (inhibition of TS and induction of single-strand breaks in nascent DNA) and the gradual and stable accumulation of 5-FU into RNA contribute to 5-FU toxicity. Thus, the primary mechanism of 5-FU cytotoxicity varies among cancer cell lines and can change within a given cell line by alterations in the schedule of administration or the circumstances of drug exposure (the presence or absence of potential modulators of toxicity). Furthermore, more than one mechanism of action may be operative, and each may contribute to cytotoxicity.

DETERMINANTS OF SENSITIVITY TO FLUOROPYRIMIDINES

Because of the complexity of fluoropyrimidine metabolism and the multiple sites of biochemical action, it has not been possible to specify one unique feature that distinguishes sensitive from resistant tumor cells. Rather, multiple factors may be associated with responsiveness to this class of antimetabolites (Table 8-5).

TABLE 8-5. DETERMINANTS OF SENSITIVITY TO 5-FLUOROURACIL

Extent of 5-fluorouracil anabolism
  Cellular uptake FUrd and FdUrd require facilitated nucleoside transport)
  Activity of anabolic enzymes
  Availability of (deoxy)ribose-1-phosphate donors and phosphoribosyl phosphate
Activity of catabolic pathways
  Alkaline and acid phosphatases
  Dihydropyrimidine dehydrogenase
Thymidylate synthase (TS)
  Baseline activity of enzyme
  Affinity of TS for fluorodeoxyuridine monophosphate
  Stability of the ternary complex
  Intracellular reduced-folate content
  Transport across cell membranes
  Polyglutamation
    Folylpolyglutamate synthetase activity
    Folylpolyglutamate hydrolase activity
  Concentration of deoxyuridine monophosphate
  Up-regulation of TS protein expression with TS inhibition
Extent of fluorouridine triphosphate incorporation into RNA: concentration of competing normal substrates (uridine triphosphate, cytidine 5' triphosphate)
Salvage pathways
  Thymidine rescue
  Uridine rescue
Extent of deoxyuridine triphosphate (dUTP) and dUTP incorporation into DNA
  Ability to accumulate dUTP (dUTP hydrolase activity)
  Uracil-DNA-glycosylase activity
Extent and type of DNA damage
  Single-strand breaks
  Double-strand breaks
  Newly synthesized DNA vs. parental DNA
  Activity of DNA repair enzymes
Cellular response to genotoxic stress
  Cytostasis vs. cell death
  Intact DNA damage recognition pathways
  Intact programmed cell death signaling pathways
  Duration of genotoxic stress

FdUrd, 5-fluoro-2'-deoxyuridine; FUrd, 5-fluoro-uridine.

Deletion of or diminished activity of the various activating enzymes may result in resistance to 5-fluoropyrimidines.[130–143] Conversely, elevated levels of certain activating enzymes have been associated with increased fluoropyrimidine sensitivity. A series of clones derived from murine leukemia selected for stable resistance to either 5-FU, FUrd, or FdUrd is each deficient in one enzyme involved in pyrimidine metabolism: Decreased OPRT was associated with 5-FU resistance, whereas FdUrd and FUrd resistance was associated with deletion of dThd and Urd kinase, respectively.[136,137] Because the subclones retained sensitivity to alternate fluoropyrimidines, resistance to 5-FU may not preclude sensitivity to FdUrd, or vice versa.

In addition to the importance of these activating enzymes, the availability of ribose-1-phosphate, dR-1-P, and PRPP may influence activation and response.[10,11,144–147]

For example, inosine and deoxyinosine augment 5-FU activation to the ribonucleotide and deoxyribonucleotide levels *in vitro* by serving as a source of ribose-1-phosphate and dR-1-P, respectively.

The formation of 5-fluoropyrimidine nucleotides within target cells and the size of the competitive physiologic pools of UTP and dTTP also influence 5-FU cytotoxicity.[148–156] The extent of 5-FU incorporation into RNA depends on FUTP formation and the size of the competing pool of UTP. Strategies that increase FUTP formation generally increase incorporation of FUTP into RNA and enhance 5-FU toxicity. Modulators including 6-methylmercaptopurine riboside (MMPR), *N*-phosphonoacetyl-L-aspartic acid (PALA), pyrazofurin, MTX, and dThd may increase FUTP formation by virtue of inhibiting *de novo* purine or pyrimidine synthesis, thereby increasing PPRP levels. Through feedback inhibition, expansion of dTTP pools decreases FdUMP formation by two means: blocking phosphorylation of FdUrd by dThd kinase, and inhibiting the reduction of FUDP to FdUDP. In contrast, expansion of UTP or cytidine triphosphate (CTP) pools inhibits formation of FUMP by Urd kinase. Changes in nucleotide pool size have been implicated in 5-FU resistance in Chinese hamster fibroblast and in murine S49 lymphoma sublines, which have altered CTP synthase activity, increased CTP pools, and decreased UTP pools.[157,158]

Because RNA and DNA-directed effects of 5-FU may differ in importance among different malignant cell lines, any single manipulation of 5-FU metabolism may produce conflicting results if different tumor models are compared. The development and application of sensitive assays that permit reliable measurement of FUTP, 5-FU–RNA levels, and TS inhibition in patient samples will hopefully answer questions concerning clinical determinants of sensitivity to fluorinated pyrimidines given by various schedules.

Determinants of Thymidylate Synthase Inhibition

The ability of FdUMP to inhibit TS is influenced by several variables, including the concentration of enzyme; the amount of FdUMP formed and its rate of breakdown; the levels of dUMP, the competing normal substrate; and $5,10\text{-}CH_2FH_4$ cofactor and its extent of polyglutamation. The degree and persistence of TS inhibition is a crucial determinant of cytotoxicity in *in vitro* and *in vivo* models. In one model, blockade of TS leads to a gradual expansion of the intracellular dUMP pool; resumption of DNA synthesis is a function of two factors: (a) the rate of decrease of intracellular FdUMP and (b) the rate of increase in dUMP, which competes with FdUMP for newly synthesized TS and for an enzyme that has dissociated from the ternary complex.[149] In bone marrow, recovery is related to 20-fold expansion of the dUMP pool, whereas recovery of DNA synthesis in the intestine correlates with a more rapid fall in FdUMP. In

5-FU–sensitive P1534 leukemia cells, free intracellular FdUMP persists for up to 7 days and is opposed by only a modest increase in free dUMP concentration.[150]

FdUMP accumulates rapidly in responsive L1210 leukemia and resistant Walker 256 carcinoma, but the rapid recovery of DNA synthesis in the insensitive carcinoma correlates to an accelerated decline in intracellular free FdUMP concentration.[151] Other studies have confirmed that a more rapid decline in FdUMP concentration may be characteristic of resistant neoplasms, perhaps due to increased phosphatase activity.[127,132,152] The basis for resistance in some cells may be explained by the rate of nucleotide inactivation rather than slower formation of the active product.

Determination of TS content in tumor tissue may help to clarify the relationship between pretreatment TS levels and prognosis, response, or both, to 5-FU therapy. Biochemical assays permit measurement of dUMP, TS, the ternary complex, and free FdUMP.[153–156,159,160] The total content of TS is estimated by the [³H]FdUMP-binding assay. TS catalytic activity is determined by a tritium release assay (using either [5-³H]dUrd in intact cells or [5-³H]dUMP in cytosolic preparations); during dTMP formation, the addition of a methyl group displaces the [³H] from the carbon-5 of dUMP. Although these assays are extremely useful for preclinical studies, their application to clinical tumor samples has been limited by the requirement for relatively large quantities of tissue (greater than or equal to 50 mg); the assay requires functional TS and must be performed on fresh or frozen tumor tissue. Despite the limitations, these biochemical assays have yielded important information. In biopsies of solid tumor and normal liver obtained 20 to 240 minutes after administration of 500 mg per m² 5-FU to 21 patients undergoing elective surgery, maximal TS inhibition occurred within 90 minutes and averaged 70% to 80% in tumor tissue compared with approximately 50% inhibition in histologically normal tissue.[161] Patients whose tumors were responsive to 5-FU had greater inhibition of TS.[161,162] In malignant tumor and adjacent normal tissue specimens from ten patients with previously untreated colorectal cancer, a large variation in TS binding and catalytic activity was observed in primary colon tumors, and the overall enzyme levels were significantly higher than in adjacent normal colonic tissue.[163]

Measurement of TS gene expression provides an alternative to directly assaying intracellular TS enzyme. A polymerase chain reaction (PCR)–based method can quantitate the expression of TS in clinical tumor samples, and TS gene expression correlates with the intracellular level of TS protein.[164,165] Overexpression of TS in tumor biopsies correlates to insensitivity to 5-FU–based regimens in several studies.[164–167] Because of the exquisite sensitivity, such PCR-based techniques may provide the means for predicting response to fluoropyrimidine-based regimens and encourage the development of individualized therapy for patients.

Monoclonal antibodies have been developed that are capable of detecting human TS in immunoprecipitation and enzyme-linked immunosorbent assays (ELISA) and by Western immunoblot analysis.[168] Johnston et al. demonstrated that the antibodies had high specificity and tight binding affinities (K_d range, 0.3 to 11.0 nmol per L), and immunologic detection was sensitive and quantitative. Two antibodies reacted with TS on immunohistochemical staining of human colon cancer cell lines and tissue. Immunologic quantitation of TS in ten 5-FU–sensitive and resistant human cancer cell lines showed a good correlation with biochemical assays, and the limit of sensitivity was 0.3 fmol protein in cellular lysates.[169] Increasing TS levels correlated with higher 5-FU concentrations required for 50% growth inhibition. TS protein content in 1-mg tumor biopsy specimens can be measured with an ultrasensitive ELISA and chemiluminescent technique with a lower limit of detection of 30 amol (10^{-18} mol per L).[170] The immunohistochemical methodology was applied in a retrospective analysis of the relationship between TS content in tumor tissue at the time of surgery and clinical outcome in patients with rectal cancer entered in the National Surgical Adjuvant Breast and Bowel Project Protocol R-01.[171,172] The expression of TS in tumor tissue at the time of surgery provides additional prognostic information beyond that conferred by Dukes stage.[171] Patients whose tumors had high expression of TS had a significantly inferior disease-free and overall survival compared to patients with tumors with low expression. This methodology may permit elucidation of the importance of TS as a chemotherapeutic target.

Quantitative and qualitative changes in TS have been identified in cells with innate or acquired resistance to fluoropyrimidines.[173–183] Amplification of the TS gene, with corresponding elevation of enzyme content, has been found in lines resistant to 5-FU or FdUrd.[173–178] Resistant cell lines may have an altered TS protein with decreased binding affinity for FdUMP.[179,180] A colon cancer cell line with intrinsic insensitivity to FdUrd has an altered structural form of TS with decreased affinity for FdUMP and 5,10-CH_2FH_4.[182,183] Two point mutations were identified: one in the 3'-untranslated region, and a substitution of histidine for tyrosine in codon 33 of the protein-coding region. Fluoropyrimidine exposure may be accompanied by acute changes in TS content; the potential contribution of this phenomenon to drug resistance is discussed in the following section.

Adequate reduced-folate pools are required to form and maintain a stable ternary complex. Administration of exogenous reduced folates enhanced the cytotoxicity of 5-FU and FdUrd in several preclinical models.[155,156] Clinical administration of LV is intended to elevate the reduced-folate content in the cancer cell.[184] However, tumor cells must be able to transport LV into the cell and convert the reduced folates to the more potent and stable polyglutamated state.[185–188] Deficiency of the low-affinity, high-capacity folate transport system (impaired membrane transport) and reduced folylpolyglutamate synthetase activity (impaired polyglutamation) impair the ability of LV to expand the reduced-folate pools. Decreased stability of the ternary complex has been described in HCT 8 ileocecal cancer cells with acquired resistance to 5-FU and LV.[189] The rate of LV uptake, expansion of the reduced-folate pool, and polyglutamate chain length distribution of 5,10-methylenetetrahydrofolate are similar in the resistant and parental cells, suggesting that a mutation in TS may account for the reduced formation and stability of the ternary complex.

dTTP depletion after fluoropyrimidine exposure influences sensitivity; salvage of preformed dThd by dThd kinase can bypass FdUMP-mediated TS inhibition and represents a potential mechanism of resistance.[190,191] Coadministration of 5-FU with an inhibitor of nucleoside transport would theoretically prevent cellular entry of preformed dThd. In a human colon parental line (GC_3C_1) and a subline selected for dThd kinase deficiency, the cytotoxicity and cellular pharmacology of 5-FU were similar, although only the parental line could be rescued by exogenous dThd.[192] Studies comparing the efficacy of 5-FU against parental and dThd kinase–deficient mutants *in vivo* may be used to clarify the role of dThd salvage as a resistance mechanism.

In summary, to inhibit TS, 5-FU must reach the tumor and then be metabolized to FdUMP. Cell lines lacking the capacity for nucleoside transport are unresponsive to FdUrd but retain sensitivity to 5-FU.[193,194] Additional factors influence the ability of FdUMP to inhibit TS. The tumor cell must enter the vulnerable synthetic phase of the cell cycle during drug exposure. The intracellular reduced-folate content must be adequate to promote stable inhibition of TS. The ratio of endogenous dUMP to FdUMP pools can affect the duration of TS inhibition. In certain cell lines, however, dUMP accumulation is associated with increased formation of dUTP; incorporation of dUTP into DNA may subsequently contribute to cytotoxicity by enhancing DNA damage.

Regulation of Thymidylate Synthase

Given the relevance of TS in determining response to fluoropyrimidines, characterization of the molecular mechanisms controlling TS gene expression has been the focus of intense research. TS belongs to a class of enzymes required for DNA replication; its activity is higher in rapidly proliferating cells than in noncycling cells. When nonproliferating cells are synchronized and stimulated to enter the synthetic phase of the cell cycle, TS content may increase up to 20-fold.[195–197] In continuously proliferating cancer cells, TS activity varies by approximately four- to eightfold from resting to synthetic phase.[198,199] Increased expression of the TS gene at the G1-S boundary appears to be controlled by posttranscriptional regulation, although functional elements in the promoter region of the human TS gene may also be involved in the regulation of gene expression.[200,201]

Fluoropyrimidine exposure may be accompanied by an acute increase in TS content in malignant and nonmalignant cells, which may in turn permit recovery of enzymatic activity.[202–205] The increase in total TS content is a function of fluoropyrimidine concentration and time of exposure.[203,205] A phenomenon of similar magnitude also occurs in patients.[206] Serial tumor biopsies obtained before treatment and 24 hours after intravenous (i.v.) bolus 5-FU and LV in patients with refractory breast cancer indicated that total TS content increased approximately 2.6-fold 24 hours after 5-FU.[206] In NCI-H630 colorectal cancer cells, TS content increases up to 5.5-fold during 5-FU exposure and is regulated at the translational level.[207] In a reticulocyte lysate system, human TS–mRNA translation is specifically inhibited in the presence of exogenous human recombinant TS protein. Incubation of TS protein with FdUMP, dUMP, or $5,10\text{-}CH_2FH_4$ abrogates the inhibitory effect of TS protein on new TS protein synthesis.[208] The ability of TS protein to specifically interact with radiolabeled full-length TS-mRNA can be demonstrated by RNA–gel retardation assays. A decrease in the level of free unbound TS leads to an increase in TS-mRNA translation. Two *cis*-acting elements of the full-length TS-mRNA to which human recombinant TS protein binds have been identified; the first site includes the translational start site contained within a putative stem-loop structure, and the second site corresponds to a 200-nucleotide sequence within the protein coding region.[209] Variant TS-RNA sequences with either a deletion or mutation at the translational start site are unable to bind TS protein. These findings indicate that TS protein binds to specific regions in its corresponding TS-mRNA and that TS-mRNA protein binding contributes to the regulation of TS-mRNA translation. These findings have suggested new strategies to down-regulate TS-mRNA expression. For example, antisense oligodeoxynucleotides targeted at the AUG translational start site of TS-mRNA inhibits translation in rabbit reticulocyte lysate, and transfection of KB31 nasopharyngeal cancer cells with a plasmid construct containing the TS antisense fragment decreases the expression of TS protein and enhances the sensitivity to FdUrd by eightfold.[210]

Other cellular factors, such as the reduced-folate content, influence TS expression. A functionally TS-negative mutant (TS-C1) has been described that has normal levels of TS-mRNA transcripts and immunologically reactive TS protein.[211,212] High concentrations of folate in medium substitutes for dThd and supports clonogenic growth, suggesting that the TS-C1 mutant is folate responsive. The mutant TS protein has greatly reduced affinity for the reduced-folate cofactor, and the endogenous total reduced-folate pools are only 6% of the level in the parental line. Exposure of TS-C1 cells to 20 µmol per L LV stimulated *de novo*

dTMP synthesis within 6 hours, whereas more than 80% of the TS activity was lost within 24 hours after LV removal.[212] Certain human breast and colon cancer cell lines selected for resistance to doxorubicin are cross-resistant to 5-FU on the basis of enhanced expression of TS protein.[213]

Importance of Schedule of Administration in Preclinical Models

Drug concentration and duration of exposure *in vitro* are important determinants of response to fluoropyrimidines.[40,49,214–217] High drug concentrations (greater than or equal to 100 µmol per L) are generally required for cytotoxicity if the duration of exposure is brief (less than 6 hours), whereas prolonged exposure (greater than or equal to 72 hours) to concentrations between 1 and 10 µmol per L results in relatively uniform sensitivity to 5-FU among a variety of tumor types. *In vivo* studies have shown that infusional 5-FU is superior to bolus administration in some, but not all, tumor models.[216] The clinical evidence concerning schedule dependency is discussed later in this chapter.

CLINICAL PHARMACOLOGY OF 5-FLUOROURACIL

The pharmacokinetics of 5-FU are important because of the wide choice of routes and schedules of administration available for this drug, each of which have slightly different toxicity profiles. Regional approaches permit the selective exposure of specific tumor-bearing sites to high local concentrations of drug. Pharmacokinetic studies have played an important role in assessing these therapeutic alternatives.

Clinical Pharmacology Assay Methods

The most widely used methods for quantitating 5-FU in biologic fluids are high-performance liquid chromatography (HPLC) and gas chromatography–mass spectrometry (GC-MS). Various methods are used to extract 5-FU from biologic fluids. In general, an initial deproteination step is performed by chemical or filtration techniques. Subsequent steps separate 5-FU from other constituents in biologic fluids that might interfere with 5-FU detection.

A number of different HPLC assays have been described for the analysis of 5-FU, including reversed-phase, reversed-phase ion-pairing, and normal-phase chromatography.[218–229] HPLC methods using ultraviolet detection of 5-FU are typically associated with limits of detection in the range of 25 to 100 ng per mL (0.2 to 1.0 µmol per L). Column or valve-switching techniques and the use of microbore-HPLC columns can improve the limits of detection to 5 to 10 ng per mL (40 to 80 nmol per L).[224,227]

The nucleoside metabolites of 5-FU can be separated from parent drug on reversed-phase and ion-exchange columns, whereas separation of the nucleotide metabolites is obtained with either anion-exchange or reversed-phase ion-pairing methods. Preclinical studies describing the intracellular metabolism of 5-FU generally use radiolabeled 5-FU, and HPLC with inline liquid scintillation detection is used to quantify the metabolites.

Derivitization of 5-FU is required for GC-MS. Mass spectrometry generally provides much greater sensitivity than that achievable with HPLC, with limits of detection as low as 0.5 ng per mL (4 nmol per L) for a 1-mL plasma sample.[230–231] Recent advances in fluorine-19 magnetic resonance imaging (MRI) have permitted monitoring of the pharmacokinetics and *in vivo* cellular pharmacology of 5-FU, thus providing a potential means of noninvasive determination of 5-FU content in tissues.[232]

5-FU is unstable in whole blood and plasma at room temperature, and catabolism is much more rapid in whole blood than in plasma.[233,234] Blood samples should be placed on ice immediately, and plasma should be separated as quickly as possible. 5-FU is stable in plasma at 4°C for up to 24 hours and is stable for prolonged periods when stored at –20°C or –70°C.

Absorption and Distribution

5-FU is usually administered by the i.v. route. Bioavailability by the oral route is erratic, and usually less than 75% of a dose reaches the systemic circulation.[234–236] When 5-FU is administered by i.v. bolus or infusion, it readily penetrates the extracellular space, as well as cerebrospinal fluid (CSF) and extracellular "third-space" accumulations, such as ascites or pleural effusions. Conventional doses of i.v. 5-FU yield CSF concentrations above 0.01 μmol per L for 12 hours.[237] In primates, CSF exposure to 5-FU varies depending on the schedule of administration, with a higher

CSF area under the concentration × time curve (AUC) provided by bolus delivery than by slow infusion.[238] The volume of distribution (V_d) ranges from 13 to 18 L (8 to 11 L per m²) after i.v. bolus doses of 370 to 720 mg per m², which slightly exceeds extracellular fluid space.[230,239]

Plasma Pharmacokinetics

The pharmacokinetic profile of 5-FU varies according to dose and schedule of administration. After i.v. bolus injection of conventional doses of 370 to 720 mg per m², peak concentrations of 5-FU in plasma levels reach 300 to 1,000 μmol per L (Table 8-6).[218,225,230,239,240] Thereafter, rapid metabolic elimination leads to a fall in plasma levels, with a primary $t_{1/2}$ of 8 to 14 minutes. The 5-FU plasma level falls below 1 μmol per L within 2 hours.

Several pharmacokinetic models have been proposed that describe the observed plasma levels and disappearance of 5-FU after i.v. bolus doses or continuous infusion (CI). McDermott et al. reported triexponential elimination of i.v. bolus 5-FU with $t_{1/2}$ values of 2, 12, and 124 minutes.[241] Using more sensitive GC-MS methodology, a prolonged third elimination phase of 5-FU was noted after bolus administration with a $t_{1/2}$ of approximately 5 hours.[231] 5-FU plasma levels ranged from 36 to 136 nmol per L 4 to 8 hours after i.v. bolus doses of 500 to 720 mg per m² and possibly reflect release of 5-FU from tissues.

The clearance of 5-FU is much faster with CI than with bolus administration and increases as the dose rate decreases (Table 8-7).[221,226,232,236,242–245] As the duration of 5-FU infusion increases, the tolerated daily dose decreases. A recommended starting dose of single-agent 5-FU given by protracted CI is 300 mg per m²; the achieved steady-state plasma levels (C_{ss}) are in the submicromolar range. With CI over 96 to 120 hours, a daily dose of 1,000 mg per

TABLE 8-6. PHARMACOKINETICS OF 5-FLUOROURACIL GIVEN BY INTRAVENOUS BOLUS

Investigator	Dose mg/m²/d	No.	Half-Life (min)	Clearance (mL/min/m²)	Plasma Concentration (μmol/L)	AUC per Dose (μmol/L/min)
Grem[239]	370	16	8.1 ± 0.4	862 ± 24	C_0: 332 ± 27 15 min: 82 ± 6 60 min: 4 ± 1	3,761 ± 286
Macmillan[218]	400	8	11.4 ± 1.5	744 ± 145	5 min: 469 ± 85 20 min: 100 ± 20 60 min: 13 ± 6	9,885 ± 1,569
Heggie[225]	500	10	12.9 ± 7.3	594 ± 7.3	5 min: 420 ± 102 20 min: 114 ± 52 60 min: 10 ± 11	7,125 ± 2,371
Van Gröeningen[230]	500	15	9.8 ± 2.4	558	Not stated	7,338 ± 1,708
	600	18		404		12,000 ± 2,446
	720	7	14.4 ± 2.5	349		16,200 ± 2,446
Grem[240]	425	11	9.8 ± 0.5 (all doses)	743 ± 81	C_0: 378 ± 46	4,401 ± 363
	490	13		713 ± 28	393 ± 24	5,304 ± 227

AUC, area under the concentration × time curve; C_0, estimated initial concentration.
Note: If either AUC or clearance was not provided, it was calculated from the following equation: intravenous dose/AUC = clearance. The molecular weight of 5-fluorouracil = 130.

TABLE 8-7. PHARMACOKINETICS OF 5-FLUOROURACIL GIVEN BY CONTINUOUS INTRAVENOUS INFUSION

Investigator	Duration of Infusion	Daily Dose (mg/m²)	No.	C_{ss} (μmol/L)	Clearance (mL/min/m²)
Grem[243]	Protracted	64–200	24	0.30 ± 0.04 (0.14–1.04)	3,050 ± 330
Anderson[231]	Protracted	176–300	3	0.32 (0.05–0.57)	Not provided
Harris[253]	Protracted	300	7	0.13 ± 0.01	Not provided
Yoshida[226]	Protracted	190–600	19	1.15 ± 0.15 (0.08–2.40)	2,033
Petit[243]	120 h	450–966	7	2.6 ± 0.2	Not provided
Fleming[244]	120 h	1,000	57	2.1	2,523 ± 684
Fraile[236]	96 h	1,000–1,100	6	24–48 h, 1.3 ± 0.1	Not provided
				72–96 h, 1.8 ± 0.3	
Benz[221]	24 h	1,500	7	4 (1.94–5.63)	2,118 (1,235–3,471)
Erlichman[245]	120 h	1,250	15	3.4 ± 0.4	2,410
		1,500	6	5.1 ± 1.0	1,790
		1,750	14	6.4 ± 0.9	1,990
		2,000	25	7.2 ± 0.7	1,910
		2,250	17	7.5 ± 1.0	2,000
Remick[246]	72 h	1,655	6	5.4 ± 0.3	1,750 ± 105
		2,875	8	13.9 ± 0.5	1,117 ± 37
Grem[247]	72 h	1,150–1,525	19	3.4 ± 0.5	3,011 ± 356
		1,750	31	5.0 ± 0.5	2,671 ± 563
		2,000	53	6.5 ± 0.9	2,651 ± 324
		2,300	14	8.8 ± 1.3	2,116 ± 572
		2,645–3,500	10	10.0 ± 2.1	2,247 ± 443

C_{ss}, plasma concentration at steady state.
Note: Plasma clearance converted from mL/min assuming an average body surface area of 1.7 m² and from mL/kg assuming a conversion factor of 37 from kg to m².

m² 5-FU produces a C_{ss} in the 1- to 3-μmol per L range, and an intermittent schedule is necessary. The 5-FU content of whole bone marrow sonicates relative to simultaneous 5-FU plasma levels is much lower after CI than after bolus dosing, which is consistent with decreased myelotoxicity of CI schedules.[201] CI of 2,000 to 2,600 mg per m² 5-FU daily given either for 72 hours every 3 weeks or for 24 hours weekly yields an average C_{ss} of 5 to 10 μmol per L.

In addition to dose- and schedule-dependent variations in 5-FU pharmacokinetics, 5-FU clearance varies considerably between individuals on a given schedule. A number of studies indicate that the elimination kinetics of 5-FU are nonlinear.[230,234,235,241,248-252] The following are noted with increasing doses: (a) a decrease in hepatic extraction ratio, (b) an increase in bioavailability, (c) an increase in plasma $t_{1/2}$, (d) a decrease in total-body clearance, and (e) an increase in 5-FU AUC. Although the change in 5-FU clearance or AUC with increasing 5-FU dosage on a given schedule may be linear over a certain dose range, with higher dosages the decrease in clearance and increase in AUC may change disproportionately. This nonlinear behavior represents saturation of metabolic processes at higher drug concentrations, leading to difficulty in predicting plasma levels or toxicity at higher dosages.

Variation in 5-FU pharmacokinetics has been reported according to time of day. Petit et al. reported a 2.2-fold difference in 5-FU C_{ss} during a 5-day infusion of 1,000 mg per m² per day (with i.v. cisplatin on day 1); the peak value averaged 4.5 μmol per L and occurred at 1:00 a.m., whereas the minimum value averaged 2 μmol per L and occurred at 1:00

p.m.[243] With protracted CI of 300 mg per m² per day 5-FU, Harris et al. reported that the maximum 5-FU C_{ss} was 0.22 μmol per L around noon; the trough 5-FU value, 0.04 μmol per L, occurred around midnight.[253] The discrepancy between the times of day at which peak and trough 5-FU levels occurred in these two studies suggests that other factors, perhaps geographic, seasonal, individual sleep and wake habits, administration of other drugs, or a combination of the four, may influence 5-FU clearance.

The diurnal and interindividual variations in 5-FU pharmacokinetics suggest that to compare and assess pharmacokinetic parameters with clinical outcome (e.g., toxicity) or the impact of another drug on 5-FU clearance, it is important for clinical investigators to (a) state the time of day at which samples were drawn; (b) for consecutive daily schedules, state the day of therapy on which samples were drawn; (c) have each patient serve as his or her own control whenever possible; (d) obtain samples for pharmacokinetic studies at the same time of day and, for consecutive daily schedules, on the same day of treatment; and (e) collect pharmacokinetic samples for all subjects within as narrow a time window as possible.

In the past several years, a number of investigators have described correlations between 5-FU pharmacokinetic parameters and clinical toxicity with i.v. bolus and infusion schedules (Table 8-8).[227,231,239,242,247,254-256] Serious clinical toxicity tends to increase with higher systemic exposure, reflected by total AUC with bolus injection and C_{ss} with 5-FU infusion. These findings suggest that pharmacokinetic monitoring might be used to adjust 5-FU doses to

TABLE 8-8. CORRELATION OF 5-FLUOROURACIL PHARMACOKINETIC PARAMETERS WITH CLINICAL TOXICITY

Reference	Dose (mg/m²/d)	Intra-venous Schedule	Parameter AUC, μmol/L/min; C_{ss}, μmol/L	Toxicity Grade	Incidence (%)	No. Patients	p Value (Test)
231	500–720	Bolus	AUC: ≤8,300	≥1	11	11	Not stated
			>8,300		71	28	
239	370	Bolus	AUC: <4,000	≥3	0	15	.03 (Wilcoxon rank sum)
			4,000–5,000		21	14	
			>5,000		43	7	
227	190–360	Protracted CI	C_{ss}: 0.8 ± 0.4[a]	≤2	100	9	<.05 (Bonferroni)
			1.5 ± 0.7[a]	≥3	100	10	
242	64–200	Protracted CI	C_{ss}: 0.24 ± 0.02[a]	≤1	100	19	.02 (Mann-Whitney)
			0.53 ± 0.14[a]	≥2	100	5	
254	1,000	120 h CI	AUC: <1,800	≥1	3	31	<.01 (not stated)
			≥1,800		78	32	
247	1,150–3,500	72 h CI		≥3	Gastrointestinal toxicity / absolute granulocyte count / platelet:		
			C_{ss}: ≤8.9		1/14/0	91	.02, .01, .007 (Fisher's exact)
			≥9.0		14/41/14	11	
255	185–3,600	72 h CI	C_{ss}: ≤2.0	≥1	6	32	% Mucositis = 100(1 – $e^{-0.114C_{ss}}$)
			2.1–4.0		28	32	
			>4.0		70	50	r^2 = 0.88
256	~1,000	96 h CI	AUC[b] 27,622 ± 962[a]	0–2 heme toxicity		65	.035 (t-test)
			31,451 ± 1,358[a]	3–4		26	

AUC, area under the concentration × time curve; CI, continuous infusion; C_{ss}, plasma concentration at steady state.
[a]Mean ± SE.
[b]AUC units are ng•h/mL over 96 h.

avoid or minimize serious clinical toxicity. This approach has been used successfully in patients receiving infusional 5-FU in several clinical trials.[256,257] However, not all patients with relatively high 5-FU systemic exposure experience serious toxicity, and some patients have toxicity despite relatively low 5-FU systemic exposure, suggesting that other factors also contribute to clinical toxicity.

The relationship between antitumor activity and 5-FU pharmacokinetics is less clear. Although two nonrandomized trials have suggested an association between clinical response and higher 5-FU–plasma exposure during 96- or 120-hour infusions given with cisplatin on day 1 in head and neck cancer patients,[258,259] other studies have shown no such correlation.[226,239,242,247] A randomized trial in head and neck cancer, in which standard dosing was compared to pharmacokinetically guided dose adaptation of 5-FU, showed that although the AUC and certain clinical toxicities were appreciably greater in the standard arm, the objective response rate was comparable in the two arms.[256]

When given systemically, FdUrd is generally given by continuous infusion. The achieved C_{ss} with protracted schedules have not been well defined. The plasma concentrations anticipated with a low-dose CI are well below the detection limits of HPLC assays, and analysis by GC-MS has been hampered by the difficulty in preparing stable, volatile derivatives of FdUrd. With i.v. bolus administration of FdUrd on a weekly schedule, in contrast, the AUC of 5-FU is two- to threefold greater than FdUrd, suggesting

that FdUrd is acting in part as a precursor to 5-FU (Fig. 8-6).[260] At the recommended dose of 1,650 mg per m² given at the midpoint of a 2-hour infusion of 500 mg per m² LV, the median clearance was 3,500 mL per min.

Regional Administration of 5-Fluorouracil

The administration of 5-FU and FdUrd by intrahepatic arterial infusion (HAI) is a strategy to maximize the regional exposure while limiting systemic toxicity. Ensminger et al. found that 19% to 51% of infused 5-FU is cleared in its first pass through the liver.[248] In contrast, FdUrd clearance by the liver exceeds 94% in the first pass. In patients receiving 6 successive 2-hour infusions of escalating dose rates of 5-FU either i.v. or by HAI, the systemic and hepatic metabolic clearances and extraction ratios decrease progressively with increasing 5-FU dose rates. Systemic exposure to 5-FU after HAI ranges from 12% to 52% of that after i.v. administration of dose rates equivalent to 0.37 to 10.00 g per m²; the regional advantage relative to systemic exposure varies from sixfold at the lowest 5-FU doses to twofold at the highest doses.[252] With 1 g 5-FU given over 2 hours by HAI, systemic drug exposure is 0.7-fold lower, and the clearance is 1.5-fold higher compared to the i.v. route.[261] Increasing the duration of HAI to 24 hours increases the clearance by 2.3-fold versus i.v. infusion, and systemic drug exposure is decreased. Thus, drug dose, blood flow, and the rate of

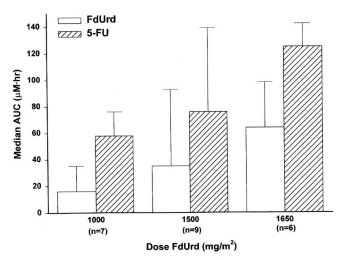

FIGURE 8-6. Area under the plasma concentration × time curve (AUC) values after intravenous bolus 5-fluoro-2'-deoxyuridine (FdUrd): FdUrd was given by bolus administration weekly for 6 of 8 weeks at the midpoint of a 2-hour infusion of 500 mg per m² leucovorin. The median AUC and upper limit of the range for FdUrd and 5-fluorouracil (5-FU) are shown for three different FdUrd doses. The number of patients is shown in parentheses. (Adapted from Creaven PJ, Rustum YM, Petrelli NJ, et al. Phase I and pharmacokinetic evaluation of floxuridine/leucovorin given on the Roswell Park weekly regimen. *Cancer Chemother Pharmacol* 1994;34:261–265, with permission from Springer-Verlag New York.)

administration influence the extent of hepatic removal and systemic exposure.

5-FU has also been given by hepatic portal venous perfusion, based on the premise that although most large metastases obtain their blood supply predominantly from the arterial circulation, small metastases may be fed by the portal circulation. After intraoperative bolus administration of [³H]FdUrd into either the hepatic artery or the portal vein, mean tumor uptake of FdUrd in patients with established metastases is 15.5-fold greater with HAI, whereas the uptake into normal liver is similar.[262] HAI is clearly the logical alternative in patients with clinically detectable metastases. However, portal perfusion may be effective in the setting of micrometastatic disease, an approach that has been used in the adjuvant setting in patients with Dukes B and C colon cancer.

5-FU and FdUrd also may be administered by the intraperitoneal (i.p.) route. Low-molecular-weight compounds injected into the peritoneal cavity are absorbed primarily through the portal circulation, passing through the liver before reaching the systemic circulation. The rates of absorption and clearance from the peritoneal cavity depend on the drug's lipid solubility and MW, as well as the surface area of the peritoneum (which may be altered by tumor, adhesions, or other pathologic changes).

Intraperitoneal dialysate concentrations of 5 mmol per L 5-FU or less maintained by intermittent exchanges of fluid can be tolerated for up to 5 days.[263,264] The mean 5-FU clearance from the peritoneal cavity was 840 mL per

minute in one trial, approximately fivefold slower than the systemic clearance, and the ratio of i.p. to systemic 5-FU concentrations was approximately 300.[263] Higher i.p. drug concentrations (greater than 5 mmol per L) saturate hepatic clearance mechanisms, with increased systemic levels and significant myelosuppression. Mild to moderate local intolerance (abdominal pain, chemical peritonitis) is sometimes observed, particularly with repeated administration. A more recent phase I trial evaluated 5-FU given i.p. in escalating concentrations for 4 hours along with a fixed dose of cisplatin (90 mg per m²) every 28 days.[265] Dose-limiting granulocytopenia was observed with 5-FU concentrations of 20 mmol per L or more, and other toxicities included nausea and vomiting and diarrhea. Peak-plasma concentrations of 5-FU occurred 1 hour after i.p. instillation and increased in proportion to dose. Between dialysate concentrations of 5 and 24 mmol per L, the mean peritoneal fluid levels of 5-FU ranged from 2.2 to 12.5 mmol per L, and peak plasma levels ranged from 6 to 60 μmol per L. At the recommended dose of 3,900 mg 5-FU, the average 5-FU concentration in the dialysate was 15 mmol per L, and the peritoneal to plasma AUC ratio was 212.

Muggia et al. evaluated i.p. FdUrd given in 2 L of 1.5% dialysate with a dwell time of up to 3 days (Fig. 8-7).[266] At the recommended dose of 3 g FdUrd, local tolerance was excellent; the major systemic toxicity was nausea and vomiting, which was well controlled with antiemetics. Pharmacokinetic sampling of peritoneal fluid and peripheral blood

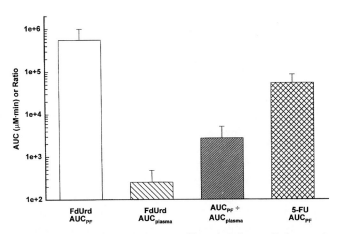

FIGURE 8-7. Pharmacokinetic profile of 5-fluoro-2'-deoxyuridine (FdUrd) given by intraperitoneal instillation. Peritoneal fluid and peripheral blood samples were obtained at 0.5, 10, 15, and 30 minutes and at 1, 2, and 4 hours after initial intraperitoneal installation and treated with 3,000 mg FdUrd in 2 L 1.5% dialysate for 3 days. The data are shown as the mean ± standard deviation (n = ten patients). The area under the concentration × time curve (AUC) values have been converted from μg × min/mL to μmol/L × min. (AUC_PF, AUC in peritoneal fluid; AUC_plasma, AUC in plasma extrapolated to infinity; 5-FU, 5-fluorouracil.) (Adapted from Muggia FM, Chan KK, Russell C, et al. Phase I and pharmacologic evaluation of intraperitoneal 5-fluoro-2'-deoxyuridine. *Cancer Chemother Pharmacol* 1991;28:241–250, with permission from Springer-Verlag New York.)

was performed over the initial 4 hours. The peritoneal FdUrd levels were above 1,000 μg per mL (greater than 4 mmol per L), and the peritoneal 5-FU levels were also high (100 to 200 μg per mL, or approximately 0.75 to 1.50 mmol per L). With i.p. FdUrd, the plasma levels of FdUrd were generally below 0.5 μg per mL (approximately 2 μmol per L), whereas the plasma levels of 5-FU were much higher: 20 to 40 μg per mL (approximately 150 to 300 μmol per L). The AUC values extrapolated to infinity for patients treated with the recommended dose indicate a pharmacologic advantage for FdUrd in peritoneal fluid versus plasma of approximately 2,700.[7] The $t_{1/2}$ and clearance of FdUrd in peritoneal fluid averaged 97 minutes and 31 mL per minute, respectively. In two patients who received a 30-minute i.v. infusion of 2 g FdUrd, in contrast, these values were 7.5 minutes and 7,000 mL per minute, respectively.[266] The addition of LV 640 mg to the dialysate did not alter the tolerance of i.p. FdUrd, and the regional pharmacologic advantage for LV was approximately sixfold.[267]

Topical 5-FU, 2% to 5% in a hydrophilic cream base or propylene glycol, is used by dermatologists for the treatment of multiple actinic keratoses of the face, intraepidermal carcinomas, superficial basal cell carcinoma, vaginal intraepithelial neoplasia, and genital condylomas. Local application of 5-FU has also been used by ophthalmologists after trabeculectomy in patients with uncontrolled glaucoma to improve intraocular pressure control.

Mechanisms of Drug Elimination

Approximately 90% of a dosage of 5-FU is eliminated by metabolism (catabolism > anabolism), although less than 10% undergoes renal excretion.[225,268] The initial rate-limiting step in the degradation of 5-FU involves reduction of the pyrimidine ring by dihydropyrimidine dehydrogenase (DPD) (Fig. 8-8). In the presence of the reduced form of nicotinamide adenine dinucleotide phosphate (NADPH), DPD converts pyrimidines, such as uracil and 5-FU, to the dihydropyrimidine form [dihydrouracil and dihydrofluorouracil (DHFU)]. Kinetic studies of purified DPD from a number of mammalian tissues, including human liver, have shown that the affinity of uracil and 5-FU are similar (apparent K_m values range from 1.8 to 5.5 μmol per L in cell-free assays).[269–273] Saturation of DPD at drug concentrations severalfold above the K_m likely accounts for the

dose-dependent pharmacokinetics. DPD is widely distributed in tissues throughout the body, including the liver, GI mucosa, and peripheral blood mononuclear cells (PBMCs).[274,275] Because of the size of the organ, the liver has the highest total content of DPD in the body and is a major site of 5-FU catabolism.

The clearance of 5-FU during CI exceeds hepatic blood flow (1,000 mL per minute or approximately 600 mL per minute per m²) by severalfold, suggesting that a substantial portion of 5-FU metabolism occurs in extrahepatic tissue. In clinical practice, the dosage of 5-FU is not usually reduced in the presence of hepatic dysfunction. There is only limited information about 5-FU pharmacokinetics in patients with severe hepatic dysfunction. Ansfield et al. reported that patients with liver metastases associated with jaundice experienced severe toxicity when treated with full-dose i.v. 5-FU.[276] However, full-dose 5-FU has been given by HAI to patients with extensive liver replacement and jaundice; improvement or resolution of jaundice may occur in some of these patients without undue systemic toxicity.[277] Patients with severe hepatic dysfunction in general have been excluded from randomized trials of HAI FdUrd. 5-FU clearance does not seem to correlate with hepatic chemistry tests in patients with relatively normal liver function.[278] Preliminary results from a phase I study of 5-FU administered as a weekly 24-hour infusion with LV in patients with either hepatic (bilirubin greater than or equal to 1.5 mg per dL) or renal dysfunction indicated no consistent changes in clearance with increasing bilirubin.[279] Thus, the dosage of 5-FU need not be reduced automatically for hepatic dysfunction; however, a more conservative approach may be prudent in jaundiced patients with a poor performance status.

DHFU appears rapidly after i.v. bolus 5-FU. The pyrimidine ring is subsequently opened by dihydropyrimidinase-forming α-fluoroureido-propionic acid (FUPA); FUPA is then irreversibly converted by β-alanine synthase to fluoro-β-alanine (FBAL), with the release of ammonia from the nitrogen-3 position and CO_2 from the carbon-2 position of the pyrimidine ring. In ten patients receiving 500 to 700 mg per m² [³H]5-FU, peak DHFU levels of 10 to 30 μmol per L were seen 30 to 90 minutes after dosing. FUPA reached maximum plasma levels of approximately 13 μmol per L at 90 minutes, and maximum levels of FBAL occurred between 60 to 90 minutes (approximately 60 μmol per L). The excretion

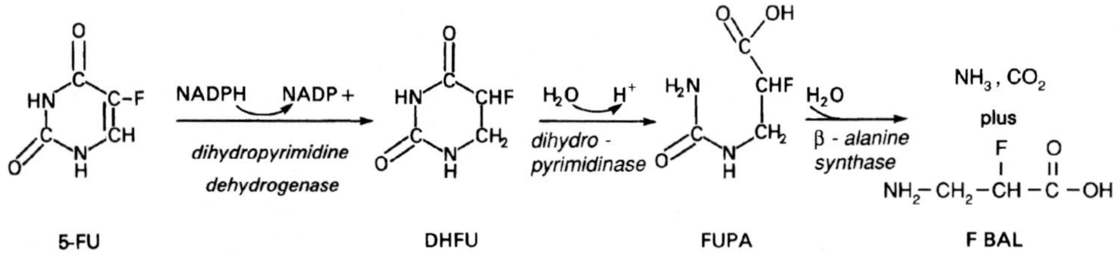

FIGURE 8-8. Catabolism of 5-fluorouracil (5-FU). (DHFU, dihydrofluorouracil; FBAL, fluoro-β-alanine; FUPA, α-fluoroureido-propionic acid; NADP, nicotinamide adenine dinucleotide; NADPH, nicotinamide adenine dinucleotide phosphate.)

of unchanged drug, FBAL, and FUPA in the urine occurred within the initial 6 hours, and FBAL was the major urinary metabolite.[225]

Significant biliary concentrations of 5-FU (11 to 259 μmol per L) have been detected during the first hour after an i.v. bolus dose.[225] A conjugate of FBAL and cholic acid was seen within 30 minutes, and peak values of approximately 1 mmol per L were seen within 2 to 4 hours.[225,280] Other metabolites identified in an isolated rat liver perfusion model include glucuronides and conjugates with α-muricolic acid, cholic acid, and chenodeoxycholic acid.[281]

After i.v. bolus administration of [³H]FBAL in rats, urinary excretion of free FBAL was the primary route of elimination.[282] The tissue levels of FBAL were at least five- to tenfold higher than the corresponding plasma levels for up to 8 days; the radioactivity was present as free FBAL in all tissues except liver, where FBAL undergoes enterohepatic circulation as FBAL-bile acid conjugates. FBAL accumulated in tissues that correspond to sites of 5-FU toxicity in humans, suggesting that FBAL might contribute to host toxicity.

Correlation between Dihydropyrimidine Dehydrogenase Activity and 5-Fluoropyrimidine–Associated Toxicity

In humans, the clearance of 5-FU is governed by the activity of DPD, an enzyme that indirectly influences the amount of 5-FU available for anabolism to the active nucleotide metabolites. Human DPD protein has been purified and characterized.[272,273] DPD enzymatic activity has often been measured by incubating cellular lysates at 37°C with excess NADPH and radiolabeled 5-FU, with separation of 5-FU and DHFU by HPLC with inline scintillation detection. This is a labor-intensive assay that has generally limited its availability to research laboratories. Although there appears to be a relationship between DPD activity and 5-FU clearance, the correlation is not tight in general study populations of cancer patients that have not been preselected for insensitivity to 5-FU–based therapy.[242,244,283] In contrast, profound DPD deficiency is more likely to be identified in patients who have experienced excessive toxicity with a 5-FU–based therapy.[284–290] DPD activity in human PBMCs serves as a surrogate marker for total-body enzyme activity, and population studies suggest the activity is described by a Gaussian distribution.[283,288,291–296] Although total DPD deficiency is relatively rare, a cutoff value of 100 pmol per minute per mg may designate patients with partial DPD deficiency at increased risk of toxicity with 5-FU–based therapy.[288,291] The wide interpatient variability noted for DPD activity in these population-based clinical studies is consistent with the broad interpatient variations in 5-FU clearance mentioned previously.

The human cDNA for DPD has been cloned, and the gene is localized to the centromeric region of human chromosome 1 between 1p22 and q21.[296,297] The structural organization of the human DPD gene indicates that it is approximately 150 kb in length and consists of 23 exons ranging in size from 69 to 1,404 base pairs.[298] Given the large size of the DPD protein, several different molecular defects have been described in different populations of DPD-deficient kindreds, including point mutations and deletions due to exon skipping.[299–305]

Familial studies suggest that total DPD deficiency is associated with an autosomal-recessive pattern of inheritance.[284–289,299–305] However, childhood familial thymine-uraciluria in homozygous-deficient patients has been associated with a variable clinical phenotype; not all subjects with the DPD-deficient genotype exhibit the abnormal phenotype.[304,305]

Pharmacokinetic interactions between 5-FU and several compounds are related to interference with 5-FU catabolism by DPD. Clinical studies using pharmacologic doses of dThd with 5-FU demonstrated marked slowing of 5-FU clearance.[306–308] The clearance of 5-FU was inversely related to the plasma level of thymine, which competitively inhibits the catabolism of 5-FU by DPD.[307] Pyrimidine nucleosides and bases competitively interfere with the catabolism of various substrates by DPD.[309] Chronic cimetidine therapy (1,000 mg daily in divided doses for 4 weeks) has been reported to decrease the clearance of 5-FU (555 mg per m² i.v. bolus) by 28%.[310] Preclinical studies in rats and monkeys confirm that chronic cimetidine treatment decreases the clearance of 5-FU, apparently as a result of inhibition of DPD activity.[311] Cimetidine is an H₂-receptor antagonist; of note, ranitidine is chemically distinct and does not affect 5-FU clearance.

In Japan, shortly after the commercial release of 1-β-D-arabinofuranosyl-(E)-5-(2-bromovinyl)uracil or sorivudine, an oral antiviral agent with activity against herpes zoster, 15 patients died, and other patients experienced severe clinical toxicity while taking oral 5-FU prodrugs at the same time as sorivudine.[312–314] The basis for this interaction was shown to be production of (E)-5-(2-bromovinyl)uracil (BVU) by gut flora.[312] In the presence of NADPH, BVU forms a covalent complex with DPD, thereby inhibiting its activity. Japanese investigators documented that rats treated with the combination of oral ftorafur and sorivudine had markedly elevated levels of 5-FU in plasma and in tissues, including bone marrow and intestine, and all animals died within 10 days. Marked myelosuppression, prominent atrophy of intestinal membrane mucosa, bloody diarrhea, and severe anorexia occurred in the terminal phase, similar to the clinical picture of the Japanese patients. In contrast, rats treated with either sorivudine or ftorafur alone had no noticeable toxicity.

Studies of patients taking sorivudine have documented prolonged inhibition of DPD. In 19 patients with herpes zoster taking sorivudine orally (40 mg once daily) for 10 consecutive days, serum sorivudine, BVU, and circulating uracil and DPD activity in PBMCs were determined before, during, and after administration of sorivudine.[313] BVU was eliminated from the circulation within 7 days after the last sorivudine dose. DPD activity was completely suppressed in 18 of the 19 subjects and markedly suppressed in the remaining subject during the 10-day course of sorivudine. DPD activity reached baseline levels within 19 days after the last dose of sorivudine in all subjects. Sorivudine is currently an investigational antiviral agent in North America and Europe. The tragic experience in Japan highlights the potential for unexpected life-threatening drug interactions when promising new drugs are introduced into clinical practice, particularly when different specialists might be responsible for prescribing agents used for diverse medical problems. The previous pharmacodynamic study suggests that patients receiving sorivudine should not receive other fluoropyrimidines for at least 4 weeks after

completing sorivudine therapy and should be monitored carefully thereafter.[314]

Impact of Schedule of Administration on Clinical Toxicities

The main toxic effects of 5-FU and FdUrd are exerted on rapidly dividing tissues, primarily the GI mucosa and bone marrow. The spectrum of toxicity associated with 5-FU (Table 8-9) and FdUrd (Table 8-10) varies according to dose, schedule, and route of administration.[315–349] A general observation is considerable variation in the incidence and severity of these toxicities among patients.

An early regimen consisted of a 5-day loading course (10 to 15 mg per kg per day) of i.v. bolus 5-FU followed by half dosages every other day for 11 dosages or until toxicity supervened.[315,316] This regimen was associated with a 3% mortality rate and was subsequently modified to a 5-day loading course followed on recovery by single weekly dos-

TABLE 8-9. RELATIONSHIP OF ROUTE AND SCHEDULE TO TOXICITY OF 5-FLUOROURACIL

Reference	Route/Schedule	Daily Dose: mg/m² (Exceptions Noted)	Toxicities
317–320	i.v. bolus daily for 5 d q 4 wk	500 425 (+LV 20) 370–400 (+LV 200)	Myelosuppression, mucositis, diarrhea[a] Ocular, dermatitis
321, 322	i.v. bolus weekly (for 6 of 8 wk)	750 500–600 (+LV 500/2-h)	Myelosuppression, diarrhea[a] Mucositis, ocular
323–327	i.v. CI 24 h q wk	2,600 2,300–2,600 (+LV 50–500/24 h)	Neurologic, diarrhea[a] Mucositis, skin (hand-foot), myelosuppression
328, 329	i.v. CI 48 h q wk	1,750/24 h (3,500 total)	Diarrhea, mucositis,[a] skin (hand-foot), myelosuppression, neurologic
246, 247	i.v. CI 72 h q 3 wk	2,300/24 h (6,900 total) 2,000 (+LV 500/24 h)	Mucositis[a] Diarrhea, myelosuppression
236, 244, 330	i.v. CI over 96–120 h q 3 wk	1,000/24 h (4,000–5,000 total)	Mucositis, diarrhea,[a] myelosuppression, dermatitis
330a	i.v. CI over 144 h q 3 wk	750/24 h	Mucositis, skin (hand-foot),[a] diarrhea
326, 331	i.v. CI over 24 h daily × 4 wk q 5 wk	300 200 (+LV 20 q wk)	Skin (hand-foot), mucositis[a] Diarrhea, myelosuppression
332	i.v. bolus →CI over 22-h d 1,2 q 2-wk	400 →600/22 h (+LV 200/2 h)	Myelosuppression, diarrhea[a] Mucositis, conjunctivitis
333, 334	i.v. bolus →CI over 48 h q 2 wk	400 →3,600/48 h (+LV 400/2-h d 1)	Myelosuppression, diarrhea, mucositis[a]
335	i.v. CI over 48 h q 2 wk	1,500–2,000 (+LV 500/2 h d 1, 2)	Diarrhea, mucositis,[a] myelosuppression, skin (hand-foot), neurologic
336	HAI CI over 24 h daily for 14–21 d	750–1,100	Mucositis, diarrhea,[a] upper gastrointestinal ulceration, myelosuppression, chemical hepatitis
337	HAI i.v. over 15 min → CI over 22 h d 1,2 q 2 wk	400 →1,600 (+LV 200/2 h d 1, 2)	Diarrhea, cardiac, neurotoxicity[a]
263, 264	i.p. installation for 32–120 h q 28 d	5 mmol/L	Mucositis, diarrhea,[a] peritonitis, myelosuppression
266, 267	i.p. installation over 4 h q 28 d	3,900 mg (15 mmol/L) (+ cisplatin 90 mg/m²)	Myelosuppression, nausea and vomiting,[a] diarrhea, abdominal pain
338, 339	Topical daily	5% cream	Local inflammation,[a] systemic toxicity rare unless patient is dihydropyrimidine dehydrogenase deficient

CI, continuous infusion; HAI, hepatic arterial infusion; LV, leucovorin.
[a]Dose-limiting.

TABLE 8-10. TOXICITY ASSOCIATED WITH VARIOUS CLINICAL SCHEDULES OF 5-FLUORO-2'-DEOXYURIDINE

| Reference | Route/Schedule | Leucovorin | Maximum Daily Dose | | Toxicities |
			mg/kg	mg/m²	
315	i.v. bolus × 5 d q 4 wk	No	30	1,110	Diarrhea, mucositis[a]
340		Yes (high)	22	800	Myelosuppression, dermatitis
341	i.v. bolus q wk × 6 q 8 wk	Yes (high)	45	1,650	Diarrhea[a]
342	i.v. CI × 3 d	No	30	1,100	Diarrhea, mucositis, and myelosuppression[a]
342–344	i.v. CI × 5–7 d q 3–4 wk	No	0.75–1.00	28–37	Mucositis, diarrhea[a]
	i.v. CI × 5 d q 3 wk	Yes (high)	0.3	11.1	Myelosuppression
345–347	i.v. CI × 14 d q 4 wk	No	0.15	5.6	Diarrhea[a]
		Yes (low)	0.075	2.8	
348	i.v. CI × 24 h q wk × 3–4 wk	No	125–150	4,400–5,500	Diarrhea, fatigue[a] Mucositis, (skin) hand-foot
345, 346, 349	HAI × 14 d q 28 d	No	0.125–0.150	7.4–11.0	Chemical hepatitis, cholestatic jaundice, and biliary sclerosis,[a] upper gastrointestinal ulceration
266	i.p. × 4 h d × 3 q 3 wk	No		3,000	Nausea and vomiting

CI, continuous infusion; HAI, hepatic arterial infusion.
[a]Dose-limiting.

ages. Side effects included leukopenia, mucositis, nausea and vomiting, diarrhea, and dermatitis. FdUrd also has been given as a rapid i.v. injection daily for 5 days (30 mg per kg per day) followed by half dosages every other day for 11 dosages or until toxicity supervened. The toxicity profile was similar, except that the incidence of nausea and vomiting and dermatitis appears to be higher with i.v. bolus FdUrd, whereas alopecia is more common with 5-FU.[315] Another commonly used schedule is i.v. bolus 5-FU given daily for 5 days every 4 weeks.[317–320] Mucositis and diarrhea are dose limiting, although significant granulocytopenia also may occur. A single i.v. bolus dose given weekly is also used commonly, with myelosuppression, diarrhea, and mucositis as the most frequent toxicities.[321,322]

5-FU has been administered as a CI, with the duration ranging from 24 hours to several weeks. With infusion durations of 72 to 120 hours, 5-FU is generally given at 3-week intervals. In general, the tolerated daily dosage is lower as the duration of infusion increases. For a CI of 4 or 5 days' duration, a common daily dosage is 1,000 mg per m² per day.[236,244,330] Mucositis is usually dose limiting, although diarrhea and dermatitis occur. Myelosuppression is generally of mild to moderate severity. With a 72-hour CI, 2,300 mg per m² per day is tolerated in the absence of LV modulation. Mucositis (18% grade 3 to 4) is dose limiting with CI of 750 mg per m² 5-FU daily for 7 days every 3 weeks, and 14% of patients experience grade 2 or worse palmar-plantar erythrodysesthesia (hand-foot syndrome).[330a] Intermittent doses up to 14 g (8 g per m²) over a 24-hour period have been tolerated, but this latter schedule is not currently in clinical use.[342]

Several high-dose infusion regimens that are repeated on a weekly basis are also popular. With a weekly 24-hour CI schedule, the recommended dosage is 2,600 mg per m², with dose-limiting neurotoxicity and GI toxicity.[323–327] When given by weekly 48-hour infusion, the daily 5-FU dosage is 1,750 mg per m²; diarrhea and mucositis are generally dose limiting.

With protracted CI of single-agent 5-FU, the recommended dosage is 300 mg per m² per day.[326,331] When initially developed, the intention was to continue the infusion indefinitely until toxicity supervened.[331] However, a daily-for-28-days schedule followed by a 1-week break is now more frequently used. Mucositis and hand-foot syndrome are dose limiting, whereas diarrhea is less common.

In colorectal cancer patients who have progressed after bolus 5-FU therapy, salvage therapy with 5-FU given either by protracted infusion or high-dose weekly 24-hour infusion is associated with response rates of 11% to 23%.[350,351] An every-2-week schedule of LV-modulated 5-FU given by combined bolus and CI has been evaluated primarily in Europe.[332–335] The premise for these combined schedules is the potential for different mechanisms of action with bolus versus infusional 5-FU. It is hoped that combining bolus and high-dose infusional schedules may result in a better antitumor effect. A large French Intergroup study compared the monthly schedule of low-dose LV and bolus 5-FU with a high-dose LV and 5-FU bolus plus CI every 2 weeks as first-line therapy of patients with metastatic colorectal cancer. The response rate (32.6% vs. 14.4%, $p = .0004$) and median progression-free survival (27.6 vs. 22 weeks, $p = .0012$) were significantly higher with the every-2-week regimen.[332]

The highest tolerated dose of FdUrd administered as a 14-day CI is 0.125 to 0.150 mg per kg per day (4.6 to 5.6 mg per m² per day). Diarrhea is the predominant toxicity, whereas mucositis is less common. Severe myelosuppression is distinctly uncommon with prolonged CI of either 5-FU or FdUrd. When considering comparable schedules of 5-FU and FdUrd (Tables 8-8 and 8-9), the tolerated doses of bolus FdUrd with weekly 24-hour CI FdUrd are approximately twofold higher than 5-FU. In contrast, with more prolonged CI of FdUrd for either 5 or 14 days, the tolerated daily doses are approximately 90- and 50-fold lower, respectively, than those recommended for 5-FU. The pharmacokinetics and pharmacodynamics associated with these prolonged infusional schedules of FdUrd have not been well characterized, and the basis for the discrepancy between tolerated doses of 5-FU and FdUrd is unclear.

Myelosuppression

Myelosuppression is more common with i.v. bolus schedules of 5-FU and FdUrd. The greatest impact is on leukocytes and granulocytes, although anemia may also be problematic in some patients. Serious thrombocytopenia occurred with the loading schedules but is uncommon with the currently used clinical schedules. In one study using a daily-for-5-days schedule of bolus 5-FU with LV, the median onset of the leukocyte nadir was day 19 (range, 15 to 27 days).[239] Serial bone marrow aspirates examined in patients undergoing loading courses of 5-FU revealed alterations in metamyelocytes as early as 24 hours after the first dose of 5-FU; megaloblastic erythropoiesis was the dominant process in the bone marrow between days 5 and 7, and recovery of the marrow to normoblastic hematopoiesis was apparent within 3 to 5 days after discontinuing 5-FU.[352] Interference with conversion of dUMP to dTMP as a consequence of decreased activity of TS or DHFR formed the basis of the deoxyuridine suppression test, which was previously used to confirm the basis of the megaloblastic anemia. The acute megaloblastic changes seen with the loading schedule might, therefore, be explained by inhibition of TS with this bolus 5-FU schedule. Pharmacodynamic studies are needed to clarify the cytotoxic mechanisms that result in 5-FU–associated myelosuppression with various clinical schedules.

Gastrointestinal Toxicity

5-FU–associated GI toxicity can be severe and life threatening. Mucositis may be preceded by a sensation of dryness that is followed by erythema; formation of a white, patchy membrane; ulceration; and necrosis. Similar lesions have been observed throughout the GI tract and in the stoma of colostomies. Enteric lesions may occur at any level, resulting in clinical symptoms of dysphagia, retrosternal burning, watery diarrhea, abdominal pain, and proctitis. The diarrhea can be bloody, and nausea, vomiting, and profuse diarrhea can lead to marked dehydration and even hypotension. Disruption of the integrity of the gut lining may permit access of enteric organisms into the bloodstream, with the potential for overwhelming sepsis, particularly if the granulocyte nadir coincides with diarrhea. Radiographic changes on small bowel series have shown extensive or segmental narrowing of the ileum and thickening or effacement of the mucosal folds in the distal ileum.[353]

Before each dose, it is essential to question whether the patient has experienced mouth soreness, watery stools, or both. 5-FU should be withheld in the face of ongoing mucositis or diarrhea, even if mild, and subsequent dosages should be reduced when the patient has fully recovered. If diarrhea occurs, supportive care and vigorous hydration should be given as dictated by the severity of the toxic reaction. Antidiarrheal agents may provide symptomatic relief from mild diarrhea, but they have been less effective in the setting of moderate to severe diarrhea. In a randomized trial comparing octreotide [somatostatin analog, 0.1 mg subcutaneously (s.c.) twice daily × 3] to oral loperamide (4 mg initially then 2 mg every 6 hours daily × 3) in patients with 5-FU–induced diarrhea, resolution of diarrhea occurred more quickly (within 3 days) in patients receiving octreotide than in those receiving loperamide.[354] On complete recovery, 5-FU should be resumed at a reduced dose.

An oral hygiene program is often used to help reduce the severity of mucositis, and topical anesthetics can provide local pain relief. Although initial experience suggested a potential benefit of allopurinol mouthwash, a randomized, double-blind crossover study in patients receiving 5-FU with LV daily for 5 days showed no amelioration of mucositis.[355,356] Mouth cooling (oral cryotherapy) with oral ice chips for 30 minutes starting immediately before bolus 5-FU substantially reduces the severity of mucositis.[356]

Skin Toxicity

Dermatologic toxicity occurs with bolus and CI schedules.[357–359] Loss of hair, occasionally progressing to total alopecia; nail changes (onycholysis and pigmentation); dermatitis; and increased pigmentation and atrophy of the skin may occur. Manifestations vary from erythema alone to a maculopapular erythematous rash. 5-FU enhances the cutaneous toxicity of radiation, and reactions typically occur within 7 days of radiation. Erythema followed by dry desquamation occurs, with vesicle formation in severe cases. Photosensitivity reactions may occur and can result in exaggerated sunburn reactions, residual tanning, or both, in the distribution of sunlight exposure. Hyperpigmentation over the veins into which 5-FU has been administered also occurs. Allergic contact dermatitis may occur with topical 5-FU. Actinic keratoses may develop an erythematous inflammatory reaction after systemic administration of 5-FU. Hand-foot syndrome is particularly common with CI schedules. It has been suggested that oral pyridoxine may ameliorate this toxicity, but definitive data are lacking.[360,361]

Neurotoxicity

5-FU may produce acute neurologic symptoms. A cerebellar syndrome has been most frequently reported and may be accompanied by ataxia, global motor weakness, bulbar palsy, bilateral oculomotor nerve palsy, and upper motor neuron signs.[352–368] Serious cognitive impairment, such as somnolence, coma, organic brain syndrome, and dementia, have also been seen. These symptoms are usually reversible on discontinuation of the drug. Neurologic toxicity has been seen on several 5-FU schedules but is more prominent on schedules that feature high daily doses (bolus and 24- to 48-hour infusions) or with intensive daily schedules. Neurotoxicity also has been prominent in some clinical studies of 5-FU given in combination with modulators, such as dThd, PALA, and allopurinol.[323,326,369–371] Anecdotal reports suggest a potential benefit for thiamine supplementation.[365]

Severe neurotoxic reactions, including coma, have been reported in patients with previously unrecognized complete deficiency of DPD after receiving conventional doses of 5-FU, and the time to recovery may be longer than in non–DPD-deficient patients.[285,286,289] Pharmacokinetic analysis of one such patient confirmed a markedly prolonged $t_{1/2}$ of 5-FU; no catabolites were identified in serum, urine, or CSF, and the neurotoxic reactions correlated with prolonged exposure to elevated 5-FU plasma levels.[285] A patient who was subsequently found to be DPD deficient developed severe neurotoxicity and remained in a comatose state for 4 days; dramatic improvement in the neurologic status occurred after CI of dThd at 8 g per m² per day.[289]

An uncommon complication of 5-FU and levamisole therapy is a cerebral demyelinating process reminiscent of multifocal leukoencephalopathy.[372,373] Although most reports of 5-FU–associated neurotoxicity indicate a relatively acute onset, the symptoms occurred in the latter patients after several months of adjuvant therapy with 5-FU and levamisole and included a decline in mental status, ataxia, and loss of consciousness. MRI scans with gadolinium enhancement showed prominent multifocal-enhancing white matter lesions.[372] Cerebral biopsy performed in two patients showed morphologic features of an active, demyelinating disease.[372] The myelin loss was associated with numerous dispersed, as well as vasocentric, macrophages; sparing of axons; and perivascular lymphocytic inflammation. Three patients improved after cessation of therapy and a short course of corticosteroids, but recovery was incomplete in two other patients.[372,373] Because a similar phenomenon has not been reported in adjuvant studies involving 5-FU and LV or single-agent levamisole, the leukoencephalopathy may be unique to the combination of 5-FU and levamisole.

A possible role for 5-FU catabolites has been raised in preclinical models. Prolonged accumulation of [³H]FBAL is noted in brain tissue of rats.[282] In a canine model, 5-FU administration with osmotic blood–brain barrier disruption produces neurotoxicity accompanied by foci of hemorrhagic necrosis and edema in brain tissue.[374] The administration of eniluracil, an inhibitor of DPD, protects dogs from neurotoxicity associated with a 72-hour CI of 5-FU.[375] Cats receiving either orally administered 5-FU or direct instillation of FBAL into the left ventricle have similar neuropathologic changes.[376] In this feline model, FBAL is more toxic than fluoroacetic acid, a potential metabolite of FBAL. Because neurotoxicity is a prominent feature of 5-FU toxicity in DPD-deficient patients who do not produce 5-FU catabolites, it seems likely that the basis of 5-FU–associated neurotoxicity may be direct effects of the parent compound or its anabolites, at least in these patients.

In rhesus monkeys, after a 10-mg intraventricular dose, 5-FU disappears from ventricular CSF in a monoexponential fashion with a $t_{1/2}$ of 51 minutes.[377] The peak ventricular 5-FU concentration is 10 to 15 mmol per L, and the AUC is greater than 18 mmol per L per hour, but without evident toxicity. After intralumbar administration, however, delayed onset of bilateral hind limb paralysis was seen. Necropsy revealed abnormalities ranging from demyelination of the lumbar and sacral cords to severe necrosis of the ventral horn of the sacral spinal cord.[377] This catastrophic complication indicates that intralumbar administration of 5-FU is unsafe and provides further evidence of direct 5-FU neurotoxicity. *In vitro,* FdUrd is much more toxic to glial cancer cells than is 5-FU, but it is far less toxic to cultured neurons than either 5-FU or FUrd.[378] CSF does not contain dThd phosphorylase, suggesting a potential role for intrathecal administration of FdUrd, but the safety of such an approach in preclinical models has not yet been established.[378]

Cardiotoxicity

5-FU therapy may be complicated by cardiac toxicity characterized by chest pain, arrhythmia, and changes in electrocardiograms (ECGs) with bolus and infusional schedules.[379–382] Chest pain generally occurs in temporal association with 5-FU administration. The chest discomfort is often accompanied by ECG and serum enzyme changes indicative of myocardial ischemia. Some of these episodes have occurred in patients with a prior history of chest irradiation or cardiac disease, but coronary angiography performed subsequent to the acute ischemic event in other patients demonstrated no evidence of atherosclerotic disease, suggesting that coronary vasospasm might be involved. Cardiac shock and sudden death have also been reported. A prospective study of 16 patients receiving a monthly schedule of 5-FU and LV revealed transient decreases in left ventricular systolic and diastolic function during therapy by echocardiogram, unassociated with clinical symptoms. Estimates of the overall incidence of fluorouracil cardiotoxicity have varied widely from 1.2% to 18.0% of patients, and some information has been derived from retrospective studies and from trials in which 5-FU was given in combination with other cytotoxic agents, including cisplatin.[379] In a prospective multicenter cohort study of 483 patients receiving CI 5-FU, the incidence of suspected or documented cardiotoxic events was 1.9%, and preexisting cardiac disease appeared to be a risk factor.[380] There is no unequivocally effective prophylaxis or treatment for this syndrome. Once

5-FU administration is discontinued, symptoms are usually reversible, although fatal events have been described. There is a high risk of recurrent cardiac symptoms' relapse when patients are reexposed to this drug after previous cardiac incidents, and, therefore, it seems prudent to discontinue 5-FU. Raltitrexed has been safely given to patients with prior 5-FU–associated cardiac toxicity.[383]

The pathophysiology of fluorouracil-associated cardiac adverse events is controversial. 5-FU metabolites have been suggested to contribute to cardiotoxicity. [³H]FBAL accumulates in cardiac tissue of rats for up to 8 days after a single dose.[282] Using fluorine-19 MRI, fluoroacetic acid was detected in the perfusates of isolated rabbit hearts; accumulation of citrate was also noted, presumably reflecting inhibition of citrate metabolism.[384] Interestingly, these abnormalities were seen only with the commercial formulations of 5-FU (available as an aqueous solution of 50 mg per mL buffered with either Tris, pH 8.5, or sodium hydroxide), but not with 5-FU freshly prepared from reagent-grade powder.[384] Impurities in the commercial formulation were detected and are thought to result from degradation of 5-FU in the basic medium used to dissolve the drug. One of these impurities, fluoroacetaldehyde, is metabolized into fluoroacetate by the isolated perfused rabbit heart. Fluoroacetate was detected in the urine of 15 patients treated with CI 5-FU alone, or in combination with LV, mitomycin C, or cisplatin; six of these patients developed signs or symptoms of cardiac toxicity.[384] This study suggests that preparation of 5-FU immediately before clinical administration might avoid its chemical degradation to potentially toxic products. Two patients who developed 5-FU–associated cardiac toxicity were reported to have high venous levels of endothelin-1, a potent naturally occurring vasoconstrictor, but whether this is cause or effect is unclear.[385]

The effects of 5-FU on the vasoreactivity of vascular smooth muscle were studied in rings of aorta freshly isolated from rabbits.[386] Concentration-dependent vasoconstriction was noted, occurring in 23% and 54% of rings within minutes of exposure to 70 and 700 µmol per L 5-FU, respectively. FdUrd did not produce vasoconstriction in this model. Pretreatment with an inhibitor of protein kinase C reduced 5-FU–induced vasoconstriction, whereas activators of protein kinase C increased it. Nitroglycerin abolished 5-FU–associated vasoconstriction *in vitro*, suggesting that nitrates might be effective therapy.

Ocular Toxicity

5-FU may cause significant ocular toxicity, such as epiphora, blepharitis, conjunctivitis, cicatricial ectropion, tear duct stenosis, and sclerosing canaliculitis.[387–391] Excessive lacrimation is usually the most frequent ocular symptom, but ocular pruritus and burning also occur. Conjunctivitis is reversible with discontinuation of 5-FU at an early point in the patient's course, but progression of the inflammatory response may require surgical correction of dacryostenosis and ectropion. In one study, 5-FU was detected in the tears of 12 patients within several minutes after i.v. 5-FU (peak concentrations exceeding 400 µmol per L), but tear concentrations did not correlate with the presence or absence of ocular toxicity. There is no established antidote. In a randomized, crossover trial in 62 patients with 5-FU–associated ocular toxicity, ocular ice pack therapy lessened 5-FU–induced ocular toxicity to a clinically moderate degree.[392] Ocular toxicity often improves with dose reduction. Early ophthalmologic evaluation should be considered to avoid potentially permanent damage from fibrosis.

Pulmonary Toxicity

Three patients with renal cell cancer receiving FdUrd as a 14-day continuous systemic i.v. infusion every 4 weeks developed nonproductive cough, dyspnea, and fever after a median of 15 months of therapy (range, 8 to 27 months).[393] Chest radiographs showed interstitial disease, and pulmonary function tests revealed a restrictive pattern. Lung biopsies in two patients showed a pattern of interstitial inflammation. The patients improved after discontinuation of FdUrd and institution of oral prednisone therapy (40 to 80 mg per day) but required maintenance low-dose steroids to preserve their pulmonary function. One patient developed recurrent symptoms when rechallenged with i.v. FdUrd. Although pneumonitis has been reported as a rare complication of other antimetabolites, such as methotrexate and fludarabine phosphate, pulmonary toxicity has not previously been attributed to 5-FU or FdUrd therapy.

Toxicity of Hepatic Arterial Infusion Regimens

In patients with metastases confined to the liver, HAI of 5-FU or FdUrd is often used to provide high local drug concentrations. Systemic toxicities are usually dose limiting with HAI of 5-FU, presumably because more drug reaches the systemic circulation, and include oral mucositis, nausea, vomiting, and diarrhea.[336,337] Chemical hepatitis is usually mild in severity. A strategy to limit systemic toxicity is to use continuous low-dose HAI of 5-FU.[394]

In contrast, systemic toxicities are uncommon with FdUrd, whereas local-regional toxicities predominate.[345,346,349,394–401] Hepatic toxicity is dose limiting. Peptic ulcers, gastritis, and duodenitis occurred in up to 25% of patients in older studies, but the incidence is lower in more recent studies, owing to improved surgical technique, including ligation of distal vessels that supply the superior border of the distal stomach and proximal duodenum and verification of catheter position. Chemical hepatitis, evidenced by elevations of alkaline phosphatase, transaminases, bilirubin, or a combination of the four, not attributable to disease progression, occurs commonly with HAI FdUrd. Cholestatic jaundice is a serious complication of HAI of FdUrd and may progress to biliary sclerosis. This complication is believed to result from perfusion of the blood supply of the gallbladder and upper bile duct, via the hepatic artery, with high local drug concentrations. In more severely affected patients, cholangiograms reveal characteristic radiographic changes; narrowing of the common hepatic duct and the lobar ducts, with varying degrees of intrahepatic ductal stricture; and sparing of the common bile duct. Liver biopsy specimens reveal canalicular cholestasis and focal pericholangitis. The hepatocytes appear normal, although reactive changes of Kupffer's cells (hyperplasia, intracellular bile staining, and small clusters of neutrophils in association with aggregates of Kupffer's cells) are present. Some patients may require cholecystectomy for acalculous cholecystitis; at surgery, the gallbladders appear shrunken, hypovascular, and densely fibrotic. The onset of biliary sclerosis can be delayed by decreasing the initial dose (the median time to toxicity at 0.2 or 0.3 mg per kg per day is five or three cycles, respectively). Although FdUrd may be reinstituted at a lower dose after normalization of liver enzymes, most patients became progressively intolerant. In some cases, the clinical picture does not improve after interruption of therapy.

A lower starting dose (0.2 mg per kg per day) of FdUrd given by HAI may be associated with less hepatotoxicity. Liver enzymes should be monitored carefully, and therapy should be interrupted if elevations of alkaline phosphatase, transaminases, or both, occur. Imaging studies are indicated to rule out tumor progression. In a randomized trial comparing HAI of FdUrd (0.3 mg per kg per day for 14 of 28 days) with or without dexamethasone (20 mg total), the incidence of patients experiencing greater than or equal to twofold increase in bilirubin was decreased from 30% to 9%.[397] The incidence of biliary sclerosis, 12%, seemed to be higher when low-dose LV was given concurrently with HAI FdUrd.[398] In a subsequent phase II study in which

Decadron (dexamethasone, 20 mg total dose) was added to FdUrd (0.30 mg per kg per day) and LV (15 mg per m² per day) as a 14-day HAI, the incidence of biliary sclerosis was only 3%.[399] Thus, concurrent use of regional Decadron seems to decrease the incidence of biliary sclerosis.

Catheter-related complications may result from long-term infusion and include thrombosis of the artery used for catheterization, hemorrhage or infection at the arterial puncture site, and accidental slippage of the catheter into the arterial supply of the duodenum or stomach, with necrosis of the intestinal epithelium, hemorrhage, and perforation.[396] This latter catastrophe is usually heralded by epigastric pain or vomiting; these symptoms should alert the clinician to reassess the catheter position promptly. In some patients, it may not be possible to use HAI because of difficulties in catheter placement, thrombosis of the portal vein, or variations in vascular anatomy.

Age and Gender as Prognostic Factors for Clinical Toxicity Associated with 5-Fluorouracil

A number of clinical studies have reported significantly greater clinical toxicity in female and elderly patients treated with 5-FU–based therapy.[402–405] Among 334 patients treated in a Gastrointestinal Tumor Study Group trial comparing monthly bolus 5-FU with weekly bolus 5-FU and LV, the incidence of clinical toxicities of grade 3 to 4 severity was significantly higher in patients older than 70 years compared to younger patients, and in women compared to men (Fig. 8-9).[402] Similar results were observed in another trial involving 212 patients who received a monthly schedule of 5-FU and low-dose LV.[403] With patients categorized as younger than 60 years, between 60 and 69 years, and 70 years or older, the incidence of grade 3 to 4 leukopenia (21% vs. 32% vs. 40%) and mucositis (11% vs. 26% vs. 36%) increased with

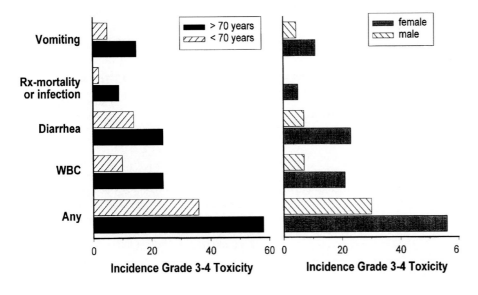

FIGURE 8-9. Influence of age and gender on 5-fluorouracil (5-FU) toxicity: The incidence of severe clinical toxicity according to age and gender was determined in 331 patients participating in a multiinstitutional phase III trial comparing 5-FU alone (500 mg/m²/d × i.v. bolus every 28 days), with 5-FU 600 mg per m² given with either high-dose leucovorin (500 mg per m² over 2 hours) or low-dose leucovorin (25 mg per m² leucovorin over 10 minutes) weekly for 6 of 8 weeks. The top bar reflects treatment-related mortality for age, but infection for gender. The incidence of each toxicity was significantly higher in patients 70 years or older (*p* ≤.01) and in females (vomiting, *p* = .03; others, *p* ≤.01). (WBC, white blood cell count.) (Adapted from Stein BJ, Petrelli NJ, Douglass HO, et al. Age and sex are independent predictors of 5-fluorouracil toxicity. *Cancer* 1995;75:11–17, with permission from Lippincott Williams & Wilkins.)

advancing age. Women also had a higher incidence of grade 3 to 4 leukopenia than did men (39% vs. 23%).[403] Women experienced more severe granulocytopenia, diarrhea, and stomatitis than men in an intergroup adjuvant study in rectal cancer comparing two cycles of either 5-FU, 5-FU and LV, 5-FU and levamisole, or 5-FU, LV, and levamisole before and after chemoradiation with 5-FU ± LV.[404] The largest experience has been reported by the Meta-Analysis Group in Cancer.[405] Using individual data from six randomized trials comparing infusional with bolus 5-FU, the incidence of toxicities associated with the two schedules was evaluated to identify predictive factors for toxicity. Female patients, older patients, and those with poorer performance had a significantly higher risk of nonhematologic toxicity (diarrhea, mucositis, nausea, and vomiting). Hand-foot syndrome was 2.6-fold more common in patients receiving infusional 5-FU (34% vs. 13% with bolus 5-FU, $p < .0001$); female patients and older patients also had a substantially higher risk of hand-foot syndrome. Grade 3 to 4 hematologic toxicity, mainly neutropenia, was approximately sevenfold more common with bolus 5-FU therapy (31% vs. 4%, $p < .0001$); poor performance status was also a significant prognostic factor for serious hematologic toxicity.

The possible influence of age and gender on 5-FU clearance and DPD activity (in PBMCs or liver tissue) has yielded inconsistent results in different clinical studies.[244,283,288,291,406–409] Even in trials that report a difference according to gender, there is considerable overlap in the values between men and women. Furthermore, the correlation between either age and gender and 5-FU clearance or DPD activity is not tight. For example, in a study of 104 patients receiving a 5-day infusion of 5-FU (1,000 mg per m² in conjunction with cisplatin, 100 mg per m² on day 1) univariate analysis indicated that age had the greatest impact on 5-FU clearance compared to several other covariables; the p value was less than .001, indicating that the slope of the regression line was significantly different from zero.[409] However, the r² value was only 0.14, suggesting a weak correlation with considerable scatter and distance of the data points from the regression line. In a preclinical model, a study of DPD activity in liver tissue obtained

from rats at ages 3, 8, 40, and over 60 weeks found no gender or age-related changes in DPD activity.[410]

Other factors may also account for the increased toxicity in female and elderly patients. For example, age-related physiologic changes in the liver and kidneys, perhaps involving organ mass and function, and alterations in regional blood flow might account for the reduced elimination of metabolized drugs, such as 5-FU, in the elderly population.[411] i.v. bolus 5-FU causes greater toxicity and higher mortality in female mice. Although the basis for this phenomenon is not clearly understood, administration of testosterone enanthate to female mice for 2 days before 5-FU (130 mg per kg) significantly reduced myelosuppression and decreased mortality from 50% to 20% but did not diminish antitumor activity.[412]

It is possible that combined information from large numbers of patients might clarify these issues, but the present literature suggests that interindividual differences in DPD activity may contribute more to the interindividual variability observed in different studies than do potential gender or age differences. Because of the reports of increased clinical toxicity, it seems prudent to monitor blood counts and symptoms in elderly and female patients closely during 5-FU–based therapy with appropriate dose adjustments. However, it is not currently recommended that the dose of 5-FU be lowered *a priori* in these patient subsets. It will be of interest to determine whether any apparent influence of age or gender on clinical toxicity is seen with oral 5-FU combined with DPD inhibitors.

Comparison of Various Fluoropyrimidine Routes and Schedules in Randomized Trials

Numerous randomized studies have been conducted to compare various routes and schedules of 5-FU given either as a single agent or with putative modulators. Metaanalysis of primary data from randomized clinical trials is a powerful tool to convincingly establish or refute the benefit of a clinical strategy. A series of such metaanalyses has been performed by the Advanced Colorectal Cancer Meta-Analysis Group, and the results are summarized in Table 8-11.[413–417] Continuous infu-

TABLE 8-11. METAANALYSES COMPARING ROUTES AND SCHEDULES OF 5-FLUOROPYRIMIDINE THERAPY

Reference	Comparison	No. of Patients	% Responding (p value)	Median Survival (mo) (p value)
413	Bolus 5-FU	578	11.1	11
	Bolus 5-FU + leucovorin	803	22.5 ($<1 \times 10^{-7}$)	11.5
414	5-FU	570	10	9.1
	5-FU + methotrexate	608	19 (<.0001)	10.7 (.024)
416	± i.v. 5-FU or 5-fluoro-2'-deoxyuridine	655 (391 + chemotherapy)	14	11 (12 mo + chemotherapy)
	HAI 5-fluoro-2'-deoxyuridine	654	41 ($<1 \times 10^{-10}$)	16 (.0009 vs. all controls) (0.14 vs. + i.v. chemotherapy)
417	Bolus 5-FU	41% ($<1 \times 10^{-10}$)	13.6	11.3
	CI 5-FU	552	22.5 (.0002)	12.1 (.04)

CI, continuous infusion; 5-FU, 5-fluorouracil; HAI, hepatic arterial infusion.

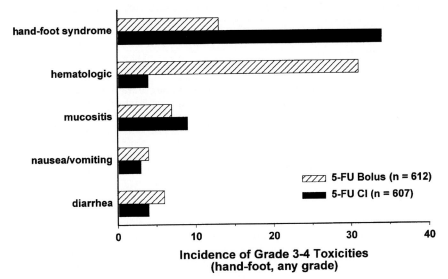

FIGURE 8-10. Comparison of fluorouracil toxicity given by intravenous bolus or continuous infusion (CI) in patients with metastatic colorectal cancer: The clinical toxicity associated with single-agent 5-fluorouracil (5-FU) was determined in a metaanalysis based on 1,219 individual patients from six randomized trials that compared 5-FU given by either intravenous bolus or continuous infusion. Hand-foot syndrome was significantly more common with infusional 5-FU (adjusted relative risk 1.87 vs. bolus, *p* <.0001), whereas the incidence of hematologic toxicity was significantly lower (adjusted relative risk 0.14, *p* <.0001). (Adapted from Toxicity of fluorouracil in patients with advanced colorectal cancer: effect of administration schedule and prognostic factors. The meta-analysis group in cancer. *J Clin Oncol* 1998;16:3537–3541, with permission from the American Society of Clinical Oncology.)

sion is superior to i.v. bolus 5-FU when given as a single agent. In addition, striking differences in toxicity are seen (Fig. 8-10). HAI of 5-FU or FdUrd consistently produced higher response rates in patients with liver metastases compared to systemic infusion of 5-FU or FdUrd. Improvement in survival was significant only when data from two trials in which patients randomized to the control arm may have remained untreated. Current strategies for patients with metastasis confined to the liver include administration of regional and systemic therapy in various sequences, and the use of dexamethasone to decrease the biliary toxicity of HAI FdUrd. For patients who undergo complete resection of hepatic metastases, the benefit of postoperative therapy is not clear. A recently reported trial demonstrated that after resection of liver metastases from colorectal cancer, a combination of HAI FdUrd and dexamethasone, plus systemic chemotherapy (5-FU and LV or infusional 5-FU), led to improved survival at 2 years compared to systemic chemotherapy alone.[417a] The use of LV and MTX as modulators of 5-FU is addressed in subsequent sections.

PROTECTION STRATEGIES

A number of approaches have been explored in an effort to ameliorate toxic reactions of 5-FU in the experimental host (Table 8-12).

Allopurinol Protection

Allopurinol is converted to oxypurinol ribonucleotide, which inhibits orotidylate decarboxylase and causes a buildup in the pools of orotidylate and orotic acid (orotate), which blocks 5-FU activation by OPRT.[9,11] Because host tissues, but not all tumors, may depend on this activation pathway, coadministration of allopurinol diminishes host toxicity in some *in vivo* models. Antitumor responses are maintained in tumors that use Urd phosphorylase and Urd kinase to acti-

vate 5-FU to FUMP. Patients receiving CI 5-FU were able to tolerate twice the daily dose of 5-FU if given with allopurinol (2.2 vs. 1.1 g per m^2 per day).[418] The granulocyte nadir in 20 patients who received a single dose of 5-FU 1,200 mg per m^2 alone the first cycle (mean, 577 per µL) was 75% lower than that observed during the second cycle, in which allopurinol was given with the same dose of 5-FU. Allopurinol appeared to increase the maximally tolerated dose of 5-FU by 1.5-fold.[370] However, reduction of 5-FU toxicity by allopurinol has not been consistently seen. The combination of high-dose allopurinol with bolus 5-FU on biweekly and daily-for-5-days schedules was associated with unacceptable neurotoxicity manifested by encephalopathy and cerebellar signs.[419,420] Although allopurinol did not affect the clearance of 5-FU given by CI over 5 days, it appeared to increase the $t_{1/2}$ of 5-FU by 67% on a weekly i.v. bolus schedule.[245,420] An initial report suggested amelioration of 5-FU–associated mucositis by allopurinol mouthwash, but this was not confirmed in a randomized trial.[355,356] A concern is the potential for allopurinol to interfere with 5-FU activation in tumors that rely on the OPRT pathway. In a rat model, allopurinol decreased FdUMP formation in colon carcinoma tissue by more than twofold but did not affect FdUMP levels in regenerating liver tissue.[197]

By consuming PRPP, purine bases (e.g., hypoxanthine and adenine) can reduce 5-FU toxicity in some cell lines that use the OPRT pathway. Coadministration of hypoxanthine or adenine with 5-FU promptly reduced PRPP levels to less than 20% of baseline and reversed 5-FU toxicity in L5178Y cells.[421,422] There is currently no clinical role for allopurinol or purine bases as modulators of 5-FU.

Uridine Rescue

Several preclinical studies demonstrate a selective rescue of normal tissue from 5-FU toxicity by delayed Urd.[423–427] Delayed administration of pharmacologic doses of Urd

TABLE 8-12. STRATEGIES TO REDUCE THE TOXICITY OF 5-FLUOROURACIL (5-FU) IN NORMAL TISSUES

| Modulator | Evidence for Protection in Preclinical Models | | Reduction in Clinical Toxicity | Mechanism(s) |
	In vitro	In vivo		
Allopurinol	Yes	Yes	Mixed results	Oxypurinol ribonucleotide inhibits orotate decarboxylase; orotate buildup inhibits 5-FU activation by orotate phosphoribosyl transferase; decreased leukopenia observed in some trials.
Purine bases	Yes	Yes	Unknown	Depletion of phosphoribosyl phosphate decreases 5-FU activation via orotate phosphoribosyl transferase.
Uridine rescue	Yes	Yes	Yes	Delayed administration of pharmacologic doses of uridine increases the clearance of 5-FU from RNA and DNA and allows faster recovery from RNA and DNA synthetic inhibition (host effect > tumor effect in tumors with limited capacity to salvage uridine).
Hematopoietic growth factors	NA	Yes	Mixed results	Amelioration of 5-FU–associated myelosuppression; in clinical trials with sequential 5-FU → granulocyte- or granulocyte-macrophage colony-stimulating factor or interleukin-1, granulocytopenia may be diminished but gastrointestinal toxicity is dose-limiting; concurrent administration of granulocyte- or granulocyte-macrophage colony-stimulating factor + 5-FU/leucovorin increases granulocytopenia.
Variable-rate CI "chronomodulation"	NA	Yes	Yes	In preclinical models, toxicity of 5-FU and 5-fluoro-2'-deoxyuridine influenced by time of administration; circadian-modulated CI regimens may reduce clinical toxicity of 5-fluoro-2'-deoxyuridine given systemically or by HAI.
Thymidine	Yes	No	No	Thymidine used *in vitro* to replete deoxythymidine triphosphate pools via thymidine kinase salvage, thus antagonizing DNA-directed toxicity of 5-FU.

CI, continuous infusion; HAI, hepatic arterial infusion; NA, not applicable.

(800 mg per kg every 2 hours for 3 doses followed 18 hours later by 4 additional doses every 2 hours) in tumor-bearing mice reduces 5-FU toxicity to the host without affecting its antitumor activity.[423] Urd administration expands UTP pools and increases the clearance of [³H]5-FU from RNA and DNA in tumor and normal tissues.[424] Delayed administration of Urd doubles the tolerated dose of 5-FU given i.p. once weekly, increases [³H]5-FU incorporation into RNA by 2.2-fold, and improves the antitumor effect.[427]

Delayed administration of Urd by CI (5 g per kg daily for 5 days s.c.) allows a threefold increase in 5-FU dose from 200 to 600 mg per kg and resulted in an improved therapeutic index in mice bearing B16 melanoma but not L1210 leukemia.[425] An improved therapeutic index with 5-FU and delayed Urd rescue also occurs in mice bearing either murine colon carcinoma 26 or 38, with less severe hematologic toxicity and more rapid recovery.[426] The biochemical mechanism allowing selective Urd rescue of normal tissues with retention of antitumor activity in these murine models is uncertain but is suspected to involve differences in Urd uptake and UTP-pool expansion in normal versus tumor cells, resulting in inhibition of further 5-FU–RNA formation and faster clearance of 5-FU from RNA. Tumors with limited capacity to salvage Urd represent the most logical model for selective protection.

Parenteral Urd as a modulator of 5-FU toxicity has been evaluated in clinical trials.[374–376] Dosages of Urd less than or equal to 12 g per m² as a 1-hour i.v. infusion were well tolerated and increased plasma Urd above 100 μmol per L for up to 8 hours, but delayed administration of 5 to 6 g per m² 24- and 48-hours after bolus 5-FU did not prevent myelosuppression.[428] CI of Urd produced dose-limiting febrile reactions.[429] An intermittent schedule of 3 g per m² over 3 hours, alternating with a 3-hour rest, over 72 hours was tolerable and resulted in peak and trough Urd levels in the 1-mmol per L and approximately 100- to 300-μmol per L range, respectively.[429] This intermittent Urd schedule starting 3 hours after weekly bolus 5-FU ameliorated the leukopenia but did not affect platelet toxicity.[430] Phlebitis of peripheral veins necessitates administration of Urd via a central venous catheter.

Preclinical studies suggested that adequate plasma levels of Urd could be achieved by oral administration.[431,432] A phase I trial of oral Urd indicated that the bioavailability was only 6% to 10% for single-dose levels of 8 to 12 g per m².[433] When given orally every 6 hours for 3 days, diarrhea was dose limiting, and 5 g per m² Urd was the recommended dose.[434] This multiple-dose oral schedule reversed leukopenia, but not thrombocytopenia associated with weekly bolus 5-FU therapy.[434] Oral Urd, 8 g per m² given every 6 hours for 12 doses starting 24 hours after bolus 5-FU, allowed escalation of the 5-FU dosage in a combination regimen that also included high-dose MTX, LV, and doxorubicin.[435] Because of the poor bioavailability with oral Urd, PN401, an investigational Urd ester prodrug with high bioavailability, is currently being evaluated as a modulator of 5-FU toxicity. A 6-g tablet of PN401 given every 6 hours for 10 doses starting 24 hours after bolus 5-FU given weekly for 6 of 8 weeks results in sustained plasma-Urd levels greater than or equal to 50 µmol per L; the recommended dosage of 5-FU with PN401 rescue is 800 mg per m².[436] In a different trial, PN401 (6 g) was given every 2 hours for 4 doses, then every 6 hours for 15 doses starting 8 hours after a bolus dose of 5-FU, and led to sustained Urd concentrations greater than or equal to 100 µmol per L for 12 hours.[437] At the recommended 5-FU dosage of 1,250 mg per m² given weekly for 3 of 4 weeks with PN401 rescue, the 5-FU AUC was 18,540 µmol per L per minute.[437] Whether this strategy will translate into improved antitumor activity remains to be determined. Protection might be afforded to tumors with high levels of Urd kinase, and the timing of Urd rescue after 5-FU therapy might affect the rescue of normal tissues versus tumor tissue.

Hematopoietic Growth Factors

In mice, daily administration of recombinant human granulocyte colony-stimulating factor (G-CSF) and granulocyte-macrophage colony-stimulating factor (GM-CSF) permits accelerated recovery from granulocytopenia induced by intermittent bolus 5-FU therapy.[438,439]

The use of G-CSF and GM-CSF as modulators of the toxicity associated with 5-FU and LV has produced mixed results. No reduction in the incidence and severity of mucositis was observed with the combination of G-CSF starting on either day 1 or day 6 with bolus 5-FU and low-dose LV given daily for 5 days, whereas severe myelosuppression occurred with the concurrent schedule.[440] A different trial evaluated GM-CSF (*E. coli*) starting on either day 1 or day 6 in conjunction with escalating doses of 5-FU and high-dose LV given daily for 5 days.[441] The absolute granulocyte nadirs for all cycles at 5-FU dosages of 425, 490, and 560 mg per m² per day were significantly lower when GM-CSF was initiated on day 1 versus day 6, supporting the premise that concurrent administration of hematopoietic growth factors with chemotherapy increases granulocyte toxicity. The dosage of 5-FU was escalated according to individual tolerance, and 35% and 6% of patients ultimately experienced grade 3 to 4 mucositis and diarrhea. GM-CSF had no apparent effect on the clearance of 5-FU, and an appropriate increase in 5-FU AUC was noted with increasing 5-FU dosage.[441] The incidence of diarrhea was potentially lower than may have been anticipated in view of the higher 5-FU doses and the more frequent treatment interval. 5-FU dose escalation was not possible in a separate trial using 5-FU and LV on days 1 to 5 and GM-CSF on days 6 to 15 because of mucositis.[442]

The effect of colony-stimulating factors on the toxicity associated with 5-FU modulated by interferon (IFN) alone or with LV has also been evaluated. G-CSF, 5 µg per kg, given s.c. for 5 days beginning 6 hours after a weekly 24-hour infusion of 5-FU with 9 MU IFN-α s.c. 3 times weekly allowed an increase in the tolerated 5-FU dose from 2,600 to 3,400 mg per m².[443] In contrast, G-CSF given daily for 4 days starting the day after a bolus dose of 5-FU on a weekly schedule with 9 MU IFN-α s.c. 3 times a week did not permit dose escalation above 750 mg per m².[443] The toxicities and 5-FU dose intensity in patients receiving IFN-α 5 MU per m² s.c. days 1 through 7, 5-FU 370 mg per m² plus LV 500 mg per m² on days 2 through 6, and GM-CSF (*Saccharomyces cerevisiae*) 250 µg per m² s.c. days 7 through 18 every 3 weeks was compared to that observed in an earlier phase II study using the identical regimen of 5-FU, LV, and IFN-α without GM-CSF.[444] The addition of GM-CSF appeared to allow greater 5-FU dosage intensity and decreased the severity of granulocytopenia, mucositis, and skin rash when compared to the earlier trial, at the cost of greater nausea, vomiting, and fatigue. The potential impact of increased 5-FU dosage intensity on clinical response is unclear. Further studies may clarify whether the use of colony-stimulating factors with 5-FU–based therapy is a cost-effective strategy.

Circadian-Dependent Toxicity of Fluoropyrimidines

In several preclinical models, the time of administration of 5-FU and FdUrd influences host toxicity.[445–450] In a murine model, drug administration during the active phase produces greater hematologic toxicity, whereas treatment during the rest phase results in longer tumor growth delay and smaller tumor volume in a 5-FU–sensitive tumor.[447] The toxicity of an i.p. bolus dose of FdUrd (1,200 mg per kg) administered at six different times (4-hour intervals) was compared in rats.[450] FdUrd was not lethal when administered at 12:00 p.m. (midpoint of the resting phase) but killed 40% of rats when given at 4:00 a.m. (late active phase).[450] In rats bearing a s.c.-implanted adenocarcinoma, a variable-rate infusion pattern of FdUrd that gave maximum drug flow during the late activity and early rest phase of the recipient was less toxic and provided the most effective tumor control than other patterns or constant-rate infusion.[448]

These observations may be explained by circadian-dependent changes in the rates of DNA and RNA synthesis and activities of enzymes involved with 5-FU anabolism and catabolism.[450–454] Peak DNA synthetic activity in normal tissues of the mouse occurs during the mid-dark (active) phase.[451] Several studies in humans have also shown that DNA synthesis in bone marrow and intestinal mucosa follows a circadian pattern.[455–457] The highest DNA synthetic rate in human bone marrow occurs during the waking hours, with lowest DNA synthesis during the sleep span (12:00 a.m. to 4:00 a.m.).[455,456]

Circadian variations of DPD activity and dThd kinase activity in rat liver and spleen have been noted.[450,453,454] When measured simultaneously, an inverse circadian relationship is seen between the activities of dThd kinase and DPD in several tissues in rats.[454] One study indicated that peak dThd kinase activity in bone marrow and intestine was at 4:00 a.m. (end of the active phase), whereas trough activity was 12 hours later (end of the inactive phase). Peak and trough dThd kinase activity in liver cytoplasm occurred 2 hours sooner. The ratio between peak and trough enzyme activity in the different tissues varied from 1.6- to 10-fold. The higher the activity of dThd kinase, the lower was the survival due to increased host toxicity.[454] In contrast, peak DPD activity occurred at mid-resting phase in bone marrow and liver, whereas trough activity was seen in the mid-active phase and varied approximately twofold.[453]

As mentioned before, 5-FU pharmacokinetics during constant rate CI may vary in a diurnal fashion,[243,253] and one study showed an inverse correlation between 5-FU plasma levels and DPD activity.[253] In other studies in which either 5-FU–plasma levels or DPD activity was monitored on several occasions, however, marked inter- and intraindividual variations have been noted.[458–460] It is possible, however, to impose a circadian profile on 5-FU pharmacokinetics through the use of programmable infusion pumps (Fig. 8-11).[459,461]

Several variable-rate infusion schedules have been explored in an effort to minimize host activity. In a clinical trial evaluating FdUrd administered as either a fixed-rate infusion (0.15 mg per kg per day for 14 days) or a variable-rate infusion (15% of the total dose from 9:00 a.m. to 3:00 p.m., 68% from 3:00 p.m. to 9:00 p.m., 15% from 9:00 p.m. to 3:00 a.m., 2% from 3:00 a.m. to 9:00 a.m.), the incidence and severity of diarrhea was significantly lower with the variable-rate infusion program.[462] In a subsequent dose-escalation study, patients tolerated an average of 1.5-fold more FdUrd with minimal toxicity with variable-rate infusion.[463] Variable-rate HAI of FdUrd appears to be less toxic than does fixed-rate infusion.[464]

Levi and colleagues have developed a 5-day chronomodulated CI regimen, in which 5-FU and LV (600 and 300 mg per m² per day) are given between 10:15 p.m. and 9:45 a.m., with peak delivery at 4:00 a.m., and oxaliplatin (20 mg per m² per day) is given between 10:15 a.m. and 9:45 p.m., with a peak at 4:00 p.m., repeated every 21 days. A randomized trial comparing this regimen versus fixed-rate infusion of all three drugs concurrently over 24 hours daily in patients with metastatic colorectal cancer indicated superiority of the chronomodulated arm; a lower incidence of severe mucositis (18% vs. 89%), higher median tolerated 5-FU dose (700 vs. 500 mg per m²), and higher response rate (53% vs. 32%).[465] A second trial of identical design confirmed these results.[466] Multicenter evaluation of an intensified chronotherapy regimen has been reported in which 5-FU and LV (600 and 300 mg per m² per day) are given over 11.5 hours with peak delivery rate at 4:00 a.m.), with oxaliplatin (25 mg per m² per day) given over 11.5 hours with a peak delivery rate at 4:00 p.m. daily for 4 days every 14 days, and the dose of 5-FU was escalated per individual tolerance.[467] Among 90 patients, 66% had an objective response, and 38% of patients were alive at 2 years. The apparent improvement in activity was associated with increased toxicity; greater than or equal to grade 3 mucositis and diarrhea occurred in 30% and 41% of patients, respectively. The worth of this intensified ambulatory chronotherapy regimen is currently being evaluated in a multicenter randomized study conducted by the European Organization for Research and Treatment of Cancer Chronotherapy Study Group.

It is not clear whether the reduction in clinical toxicity with the Levi regimen is due to having an intermittent 11.5-hour exposure to drug with a 12.5-hour drug-free interval each day as opposed to specific timing of peak drug infusion. Other investigators have recommended a variable-rate schedule in which two-thirds of the total daily dose of 5-FU would be administered during the evening hours.[468] A mechanistic basis for the recommendation of different optimal times of peak drug infusion in different trials is not clear. However, a general finding in the clinical trials evaluating variable-rate infusion schedules is that higher doses of 5-FU or FdUrd are tolerated, with reduced host toxicity.

Several key issues are unresolved. It is not yet known whether the major enzymes involved in 5-FU anabolism and catabolism in tumor tissue display circadian variation

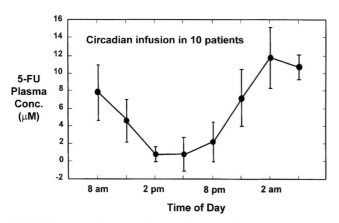

FIGURE 8-11. 5-Fluorouracil (5-FU) plasma levels during variable-rate infusion. 5-FU plasma levels were measured at 3-hour intervals over the second day of a 72-hour infusion of 5-FU 1,750 mg per m² per day using a programmable infusion pump that delivered a smooth continuous sinusoidal variable infusion rate with a peak at 4 a.m. and a trough rate of 0 at 4 p.m. The data, from ten patients, are shown as the mean and the standard deviation. (Conc, concentration.) (Reproduced from Takimoto CH, Yee LK, Venzon D, et al. High inter- and intrapatient variation in 5-fluorouracil plasma concentrations during a prolonged drug infusion. *Clin Cancer Res* 1999;5:1347–1352, with permission from the American Association for Cancer Research.)

and whether the pattern differs from that of the normal tissues of the host. A theoretical concern is that if the pattern of enzyme activity in tumor tissues parallels that of normal tissues, then drug administration at a time intended to reduce host toxicity also may lead to decreased activation in tumor. This concern does not seem to be born out, considering the clinical activity of the variable-rate infusion regimens. Given human genetic diversity; heterogeneity of lifestyles with different sleep and wake cycles; the geographic and seasonal changes that influence the duration of sunlight; and the possible influences of other drugs, hormones, feeding and fasting, and rate of cell proliferation on circadian rhythms, it is perhaps not surprising that there is wide inter- and intrapatient variability in diurnal profiles of 5-FU–plasma levels and DPD activity.

BIOCHEMICAL STRATEGIES TO INCREASE THE CYTOTOXICITY OF 5-FLUOROURACIL

A number of important interactions have been demonstrated between 5-FU and other antineoplastic drugs or normal metabolites in experimental and clinical investigations (Table 8-13). These strategies include attempts to increase the conversion of 5-FU to its active metabolites, modulate its binding to TS, increase its incorporation into

TABLE 8-13. STRATEGIES TO ENHANCE THE CYTOTOXICITY OF 5-FLUOROURACIL (5-FU) IN CANCER CELLS

Modulator	Evidence for Increased Cytotoxicity in Preclinical Models		Enhancement of Clinical Activity	Putative Mechanism(s)
	In Vitro	*In Vivo*		
Methotrexate	Yes	Yes	Yes: phase III trials	Sequential methotrexate → 5-FU inhibits *de novo* purine synthesis, causing expansion of phosphoribosyl phosphate pools, increased formation of FUTP, and increased incorporation of FUTP into RNA.
Leucovorin	Yes	Yes	Yes: phase III trials	Expansion of 5,10-CH$_2$FH$_4$ mono- and polyglutamate pools increases the stability of the reduced folate-fluorodeoxyuridylate-TS ternary complex; enhances DNA-directed effects of 5-FU.
Thymidine	Yes	Yes	No: phase I, II trials	Thymidine antagonizes the DNA-directed effects of 5-FU, but pharmacologic doses may increase 5-FU anabolism to FUTP and increase FUTP-RNA incorporation; thymidine and thymine competitively decrease 5-FU catabolism by dihydropyrimidine dehydrogenase, markedly prolonging the $t_{1/2}$ of 5-FU and increasing toxicity to the host.
N-(phosphonoacetyl)-L-aspartic acid, brequinar	Yes	Yes	*N*-(phosphonoacetyl)-L-aspartic acid: No: randomized phase II and III trials	Inhibition of *de novo* pyrimidine synthesis leads to depletion of uridine triphosphate and cytidine triphosphate pools, which compete with FUTP for RNA incorporation; less feedback inhibition of uridine kinase; decreased uridine triphosphate and cytidine triphosphate pools in turn result in decreased formation of deoxyuridine monophosphate and deoxycytidine triphosphate; increased phosphoribosyl phosphate pools and decreased production of orotic acid favor formation of fluorouridine monophosphate; increased FUTP incorporation into RNA; may increase RNA and DNA-directed toxicities of 5-FU.
IFN α, β, γ	Yes	Yes	IFN-α: No: phase III trials	Mechanism of interaction may differ in various cancer cell lines; IFN-α may increase fluorodeoxyuridylate formation, enhance DNA-damage, and potentiate natural killer cell–mediated cytotoxicity; IFN-γ may abrogate acute increase in TS content during 5-FU exposure, thus extending the extent and duration of TS inhibition; *in vivo*, IFN-α may affect 5-FU clearance in a dose and schedule-dependent manner in some individuals.
Cisplatin and analogs	Yes	Yes	Cisplatin: Yes: phase III trials, squamous cell cancers Oxaliplatin: Yes: phase III trials in colorectal cancer	Cisplatin may indirectly increase the FH$_4$ and 5,10-CH$_2$FH$_4$ pools; 5-FU may interfere with the repair of cisplatin-associated DNA damage. Oxaliplatin is active against DNA mismatch repair deficient cancer cells; clinical evidence of synergy between oxaliplatin and 5-FU in colorectal cancer; underlying mechanism uncertain.
Ionizing radiation	Yes	Yes	Yes: phase III trials: various squamous cell cancers and rectal cancer	Augmentation of DNA-directed cytotoxicity.

FUTP, fluorouridine triphosphate; IFN, interferon; TS, thymidylate synthase.

RNA or DNA, decrease the competing pools of normal nucleotides by blocking the *de novo* and salvage pathways of pyrimidine synthesis, decrease the catabolism of 5-FU and its metabolites, and combine 5-FU with other agents with complementary mechanisms of cytotoxicity. Several of these strategies have yielded convincing evidence of clinical benefit, whereas others have failed to improve the therapeutic index.

Sequential Methotrexate-Fluorouracil

The interaction of 5-FU with MTX has particular importance because of the frequent clinical use of these drugs in the combination chemotherapy regimens. Both inhibit the synthesis of dTMP and dTTP, 5-FU through the binding of FdUMP to TS and MTX through the depletion of intracellular reduced folates and the generation of toxic polyglutamates (Fig. 8-12). Several biochemical interactions are possible.[469] The reduced folate 5,10-CH_2FH_4, which is required for binding of FdUMP to TS, is oxidized to FH_2 in the TS reaction and cannot be resynthesized in the presence of MTX. Pretreatment of cells with MTX would be expected to deplete the 5,10-

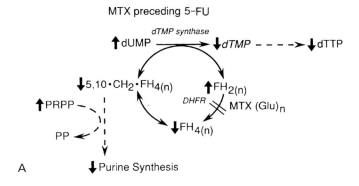

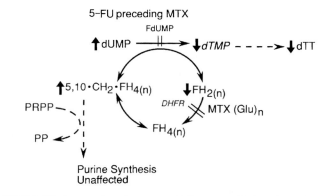

FIGURE 8-12. Interaction between 5-fluorouracil (5-FU) and methotrexate (MTX). **A:** MTX preceding 5-FU. (DHFR, dihydrofolate reductase; dTMP, thymidine 5'-monophosphate; dTTP, thymidine 5'-triphosphate; dUMP, deoxyuridine monophosphate; FdUMP, fluorodeoxyuridylate; PP, pyrophosphate; PRPP, phosphoribosyl phosphate.)

CH_2FH_4 cofactor and thereby diminish FdUMP's binding to TS.[28] Because depletion of reduced folates by MTX is only partial, however, this may be insufficient to affect FdUMP's binding to TS. In addition, FH_2 polyglutamates, which accumulate in the presence of antifolates, may substitute for 5,10-CH_2FH_4 in the ternary complex with FdUMP and TS.[25] MTX pretreatment also results in accumulation of dUMP, which may compete with FdUMP for binding to TS.

MTX pretreatment, however, augments FUTP formation.[11] Above threshold concentrations of 0.1 to 1.0 µmol per L, MTX inhibits *de novo* purine synthesis, thus causing an expansion of the intracellular pool of PRPP. PRPP is then available for the conversion of 5-FU to FUMP by OPRT; FUTP formation, 5-FU–RNA incorporation, and cytotoxicity are thereby increased. This sequence of events has been demonstrated in L1210 cells, and cytotoxic synergism is seen with MTX preceding 5-FU.[11] 5-FU activation is promoted in a similar manner by MTX in human tumors in culture, although longer periods of incubation with MTX may be required to produce expansion of the PPRP pools. Enhancement of 5-FU toxicity in some human cell lines is greatest when exposure to greater than or equal to 1 µmol per L MTX is maintained for 24 hours before 5-FU administration.[13,469,470] In MCF-7 human breast cancer cells, in contrast, pretreatment with MTX did not enhance 5-FU activation.[471] The synergistic cytotoxicity of sequential MTX → 5-FU *in vitro* requires medium containing serum with low concentrations of hypoxanthine, dThd (i.e., dialyzed fetal bovine serum), or both, because the addition of physiologic concentrations of hypoxanthine (1 to 10 µmol per L) and dThd (0.5 µmol per L) diminishes the synergism of sequential MTX → 5-FU.[472] Several *in vivo* models have shown improved antitumor activity when MTX was given 22 to 24 hours before bolus 5-FU and confirmed that this strategy increases formation of 5-FU ribonucleotides and 5-FU–RNA incorporation.[473–475]

The reverse sequence of drug administration (5-FU → MTX) produces the least favorable antitumor effects in cell culture and *in vivo* models.[11,469,474–477] The sequence-dependent antagonism is thought to be a consequence of 5-FU–mediated antagonism of MTX's antipurine effects. The antipurine action of MTX is believed to result from two factors (Fig. 8-12): (a) partial depletion of 10-formyl FH_4, and (b) buildup of FH_2, an inhibitor of *de novo* purine synthesis. Ongoing dTMP synthesis is required to deplete the cellular reduced-folate pool. Pretreatment with 5-FU inhibits TS and thereby blocks the conversion of reduced folates to FH_2. As a result, the reduced-folate pool is spared for purine synthesis; furthermore, the FH_2 pool does not expand.[477] When MTX precedes 5-FU, in contrast, ongoing dTMP synthesis leads to depletion of reduced folates and accumulation of FH_2 pools, thus allowing establishment of the block in purine biosynthesis. Pretreatment of a DHFR gene-amplified KB cell line with 5-FU results in increased levels of DHFR-mRNA; the newly expressed DHFR enzyme has decreased affinity for MTX, suggesting another possible factor's contributing to the sequence-dependent antagonism.[71,72]

In summary, despite potential interference with the formation of the ternary complex involving FdUMP, TS, and reduced folate, experimental sequences using MTX before 5-FU have produced more favorable results than have regimens using 5-FU first, presumably through enhancement of the RNA-directed toxicities of 5-FU. The disparate results of randomized clinical trials suggest that the dosage and scheduling of these two agents may be of crucial importance. The dosage of MTX and the interval before 5-FU administration must be sufficient to allow the biochemical effects of MTX to become established. Pharmacodynamic studies suggest that PRPP levels are significantly increased 24 hours after MTX.[478] One randomized trial in colorectal cancer demonstrated that a 24-hour interval between MTX and 5-FU was superior to a 1-hour interval.[479] In contrast, a trial involving MTX, 5-FU, and LV in head and neck cancer patients showed no advantage for an 18-hour interval compared to concurrent administration in terms of response rate, but host toxicity was greater with sequential MTX → 5-FU and LV.[480] These results suggest that the ability of MTX to modulate 5-FU toxicity and the optimal time of administration may depend on the tissue type. A metaanalysis of eight randomized trials comparing MTX modulation of 5-FU with bolus 5-FU alone in patients with metastatic colorectal cancer documents a doubling of the response rate with MTX modulation (Table 8-11).[414]

When higher-than-standard doses of MTX are used, LV rescue is used to protect the patient, which may contribute to the improved activity of MTX, 5-FU, and LV regimens. The strategy of LV rescue is based on the assumption that delayed administration of LV will be more likely to rescue normal tissues than tumor tissues, although the potential for protection of the tumor remains a concern. Substitution of the lipophilic-antifolate trimetrexate for MTX in regimens involving sequential antifolate → 5-FU with LV rescue may be advantageous, because trimetrexate and LV do not compete for transport or polyglutamation. Sequence-dependent synergism is seen with trimetrexate given before 5-FU in several preclinical models.[481,482] A phase I trial of sequential trimetrexate, LV, and bolus 5-FU recommended trimetrexate, 110 mg per m² over 30 minutes, followed 24 hours later by LV, 500 mg per m² i.v.; 5-FU, 600 mg per m² i.v.; and oral LV, 10 mg per m² every 6 hours for 7 doses weekly for 6 of 8 weeks.[483] Phase II studies with this regimen in patients with colorectal cancer used the same dosage and schedule of trimetrexate, but with slightly lower doses of 5-FU and LV, and showed promising results.[484] The benefit of this three-drug combination versus 5-FU and LV alone is being tested in randomized clinical trials in previously untreated colorectal cancer.[485]

Modulation of Fluorinated Pyrimidines by Folinic Acid

The ability to form and maintain a stable ternary complex is a critical determinant of sensitivity to 5-FU and FdUrd. The concentration of reduced folate in equilibrium with the ternary complex inversely correlates with its rate of dissociation.[34,486–489] High levels of intracellular reduced folates are, therefore, necessary for the optimal binding and inhibition of TS by FdUMP. Enhanced inhibition of TS over a sustained period results in further depletion of dTTP pools, greater inhibition of DNA synthesis, increased DNA damage, and, finally, enhanced cytotoxicity. In preclinical models, the endogenous reduced-folate levels are insufficient to promote maximal inhibition of TS in many tumors; in 5-FU-sensitive tumors, in contrast, maximal FdUMP binding into the ternary complex may occur without exogenous LV.[487–492] Exogenous LV (folinic acid, citrovorum factor, 5-formyltetrahydrofolate, 5-CHO-FH$_4$) has been used in an effort to expand intracellular reduced-folate pools and thereby permit maximal ternary-complex formation.[184] LV increases the *in vitro* and *in vivo* cytotoxicity of 5-FU in many, but not all, cancer cell types in a concentration and time-dependent manner.[29,110,112,185–187,212,492–508] In general, concentrations of LV below 1 μmol per L have been insufficient to expand intracellular folate pools, and 10 μmol per L is often cited as the target concentration. As the duration of exposure increases, the concentration of LV required to optimally modulate total intracellular levels of 5,10-CH$_2$FH$_4$ and enhance fluoropyrimidine toxicity decreases. With brief exposures to 5-FU or FdUrd, several preclinical studies suggest that it is important to administer LV before or at least concurrently with the fluoropyrimidine to permit metabolism of LV to 5,10-CH$_2$FH$_4$ polyglutamates, which are more effective in promoting ternary-complex formation.[489,493,500,503] Other investigators have argued that 5-FU should be given 30 to 40 minutes before LV to achieve peak concentrations of FdUMP and 5,10-CH$_2$FH$_4$ simultaneously.[490,505] These differences suggest that the optimal concentration of LV and time of administration relative to fluoropyrimidine exposure may vary depending on the tumor model used. For example, in two different human cancer cell lines, maximum ternary complex formation occurred when 5-FU exposure was delayed for either 4 hours or 18 hours after exposure to LV; the time of peak folate-polyglutamate formation coincided with the time of peak TS complex formation and total TS protein in each cell line.[495] The ability of LV to modulate cytotoxicity is also influenced by the duration of exposure to 5-FU.[496]

LV is chemically synthesized and consists of equal amounts of the diastereoisomers *R*- (or *D*-) and *S*- (or *L*-)

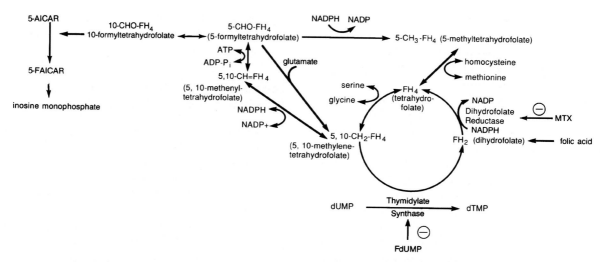

FIGURE 8-13. Interconversions of reduced folates. (ADP, adenosine 5'-diphosphate; 5-AICAR, 5-aminoimidazole-4-carboxamide ribonucleotide; ATP, adenosine 5'-triphosphate; dTMP, thymidine 5'-monophosphate; dUMP, deoxyuridine monophosphate; 5-FAICAR, 5-formamidoimidazole-4-carboxamide ribonucleotide; FdUMP, fluorodeoxyuridylate; MTX, methotrexate; NADP, nicotinamide adenine dinucleotide; NADPH, nicotinamide adenine dinucleotide phosphate; –, inhibition.)

5-CHO-FH$_4$. The natural diastereoisomer is *S*-5-CHO-FH$_4$ which must be metabolized to exert its modulatory effects on 5-FU (Fig. 8-13). After i.v. administration, *S*-5-CHO-FH$_4$ is rapidly cleared from plasma by conversion to its metabolite *S*-5-methyl-tetrahydrofolate (5-CH$_3$-FH$_4$) and by urinary excretion.[184] 5-CHO-FH and 5-CH$_3$-FH$_4$ are transported across the cell membrane by a common saturable reduced-folate carrier and subsequently undergo complex intracellular metabolism, including polyglutamation. An important determinant of sensitivity to LV modulation is the variation in the intracellular metabolism of 5-CHO-FH$_4$ and 5-CH$_3$-FH$_4$ to 5,10-CH$_2$FH$_4$ and its conversion to polyglutamates. In cell-free systems, 5,10-CH$_2$FH$_4$ with a 5-chain length polyglutamate binds more tightly to TS than the monoglutamate (apparent K_m, 0.6 vs. 23 µmol per L for Glu-5 and Glu-1, respectively) and is 40-fold more potent in promoting ternary-complex formation.[26] In addition, the intracellular $t_{1/2}$ increases as the number of glutamate residues increases. Using TS purified from a human colon cancer xenograft, 5,10-CH$_2$FH$_4$ with 3 or 6 glutamate residues was 18-fold and 200-fold more effective in stabilizing the ternary complex than the monoglutamate form.[501] The increase in total reduced folate cofactor content is concentration dependent; prolonged exposure is necessary to permit accumulation of the more potent longer chain length polyglutamates.[185–187,501,506] Cell lines with impaired ability to transport, metabolize, and polyglutamate reduced folates are relatively insensitive to attempted LV modulation of fluoropyrimidine toxicity in proportion to the severity of the metabolic defect in folate metabolism.[188,189,494,506] Although exposure to higher doses of LV may not be necessary to promote optimal formation and stabilization of ternary complex in all cancer cell types, increasing the dosage and duration of LV expo-

sure may sensitize certain tumors that might otherwise be unaffected by low-dose or short-term exposure to LV. A 20- to 200-fold excess of the inactive *R*-stereoisomer did not affect the uptake, metabolism, or polyglutamation of *S*-LV in several human cancer cell lines.[185,186,509]

The combination of 5-FU and LV has been extensively tested in the clinic. Dose, route, and schedule of LV administration have varied. Pharmacokinetic studies have been performed for several LV regimens. With i.v. bolus injection of 50 mg racemic LV, plasma levels of bioactive reduced folates (*S*-5-CHO-FH$_4$ and 5-CH$_3$-FH$_4$) remain above 1 µmol per L for approximately 1 hour.[510] When the i.v. bolus dose is increased to 200 mg per m,^{2} and with a 2-hour infusion of 500 mg per m^2 LV, peak plasma levels of bioactive reduced folates exceed 40 µmol per L.[511,512] With CI of 500 mg per m^2 LV, the C_{ss} values of *S*-5-CHO-FH$_4$ and 5-CH$_3$-FH$_4$ are 4 to 5 µmol per L each.[513] Priest et al. compared the bioavailability and metabolism of LV after i.v. or oral administration of five different dosages, ranging from 10 to 500 mg per m^2.[514] LV absorption after oral administration was saturable. Accumulation of several metabolites was greater after i.v. than oral administration, and peak plasma levels of FH$_4$ and 5,10-CH$_2$-FH$_4$ exceeded 2 µmol per L after an i.v. dose of 500 mg per m^2.[514] The observation that host-mediated biotransformation of LV to the active metabolite occurs before tumor uptake may provide additional rationale for high-dose i.v. LV.

Numerous randomized phase III trials have evaluated the worth of LV-modulation of i.v. bolus 5-FU. In general, the highest tolerated dose of 5-FU when given in combination with LV is lower than that for single-agent 5-FU, and a qualitative alteration in the toxicity pattern has been noted with increased GI epithelial toxicity with 5-FU and LV (Table 8-9). A metaanalysis of nine randomized trials of

5-FU and LV compared with 5-FU alone in patients with advanced colorectal cancer indicated that 5-FU and LV therapy showed a highly significant benefit over single-agent 5-FU in terms of tumor response rate (Table 8-11), although this did not translate into a survival advantage.[413]

No apparent differences were noted between weekly and monthly (daily for 5 days) schedules in the metaanalysis of 5-FU and LV trials.[413] Furthermore, randomized trials comparing the monthly 5-FU and low-dose LV with weekly 5-FU high-dose LV schedules in advanced colorectal cancer and as adjuvant therapy reveal similar efficacy, although the toxicity profile differs.[322,515]

Interferon with 5-Fluorouracil

IFNs are a group of proteins that regulate a wide spectrum of cell functions and modulate responses to infection and malignancy. The binding of type I (α and β) and type II (γ) IFNs to high-affinity cell surface receptors activates a post-receptor signaling mechanism that leads to functional changes in gene expression; effects on gene transcription, protein expression, enzyme activities, nucleotide pools, and cell-cycle distribution have been described. *In vivo*, IFN therapy affects the function of natural killer (NK) cells, T cells, and macrophages, and induces other cytokines.

Numerous *in vitro* studies have demonstrated that each of the interferons (α, β, and γ) may interact with 5-FU or FdUrd in a greater than additive fashion to produce cytotoxicity in a variety of human cancer cell lines.[203,516-533] The type of IFN that maximally enhances fluoropyrimidine cytotoxicity differs among cell lines. Because of the ability of dThd to rescue cells from the additive effects of IFN-α and -γ, several investigators have concluded that IFN enhances the DNA-directed actions of 5-FU.[106,125,203,207,516,523,524] In several models, pretreatment with IFN for 24 to 48 hours followed by concurrent exposure to 5-FU and IFN produced optimal effects; other studies gave IFN concurrently with 5-FU for 24 to 72 hours. New protein synthesis appears to be a requirement for IFN-mediated augmentation of fluoropyrimidine toxicity in some studies.[125,519,520,522,526,530] In some leukemia and colon cancer cell lines, IFN-α and IFN-γ increase FdUMP formation and enhance TS inhibition, apparently due to an IFN-mediated increase in the activities of dThd phosphorylase.[517,519,520]

In other models, enhancement of 5-FU cytotoxicity by IFN-α is noted in the absence of an effect on 5-FU metabolism or the extent of TS inhibition, and the locus of interaction appears to be at the level of DNA damage.[523,524,531] Houghton et al. found that DNA single and double-strand breaks were significantly enhanced by IFN-α, and the addition of LV to 5-FU and IFN-α further potentiated DNA damage.[524] In H630 colon cancer cells, IFN-γ abrogates the increase in TS content induced by 5-FU; enhanced inhibition of TS is the basis for potentiation of 5-FU toxicity.[203]

This effect on TS protein appeared to be at the level of TS-mRNA translation.[203,207] In HT29 colon cancer cells, the combination of IFN-α, IFN-γ, and 5-FU led to more than additive cytotoxic effects.[532] More profound dTTP depletion occurred with the triple combination compared to 5-FU alone, and this was not due to enhanced TS inhibition. The exaggerated dTTP depletion was accompanied by greater imbalance in the ratio of dATP to dTTP pools and more pronounced inhibition of DNA synthesis and damage to nascent and parental DNA.[532]

Other investigators have shown that combination treatment with 5-FU and IFN-α results in enhanced NK-cell–mediated cytotoxicity.[526,527] The various IFNs have also improved the activity of 5-FU in some murine tumor and xenograft models. The underlying basis for the apparent enhancement of 5-FU cytotoxicity by IFN in preclinical studies includes several mechanisms and appears to be highly dependent on the specific cancer cell line or tumor model studied. In addition to biochemical and molecular mechanisms, immunomodulatory effects may be operative *in vivo*. Increasing attention is now being directed toward the use of IFNs as up-regulators of cellular proteins or cell surface receptor ligands.[125,520,533]

The potential impact of IFN-α on the activity of 5-FU plus or minus LV has been extensively evaluated in clinical trials using a variety of dosages and schedules.[534-547] Wadler et al. introduced a regimen involving continuous administration of 9 MU s.c. 3 times weekly beginning on day 1, in conjunction with an initial 5-day CI of 5-FU (750 mg per m² per day) followed, upon recovery, by weekly bolus 5-FU 750 mg per m².[534] These investigators documented induction of dThd phosphorylase in PBMCs isolated from patients receiving this IFN regimen.[535] The response rates in phase II studies seemed much higher than expected with 5-FU or 5-FU and LV alone.[534,536] Unfortunately, the overall experience from randomized clinical trials comparing 5-FU and IFN with either 5-FU alone (bolus and infusional regimens) or with LV modulation in patients with advanced colorectal cancer has failed to identify a clear benefit for IFN in terms of response rate, although IFN definitely increases host toxicity, particularly with higher dosages.[537-543] The National Surgical Adjuvant Breast and Bowel Project compared 5-FU and LV given on a daily-for-5-days monthly schedule with or without IFN-α 5 MU per m² s.c. days 1 through 7 as adjuvant therapy for 2,176 patients with colon cancer.[544] Unfortunately, IFN-α conferred no benefit in this large, randomized trial; clinical toxicity was higher, and a greater proportion of patients failed to complete the six cycles of therapy.

The increased toxicity with IFN-α and 5-FU with or without LV suggests that IFN is modulating host toxicity, with no selective preference for tumor. The basis for the enhanced clinical toxicity may, in part, be explained by alterations in dThd phosphorylase expression in host tissues and by a pharmacologic interaction between IFN-α and

5-FU. Several investigators have reported a decrease in 5-FU clearance by IFN-α.[239,545–547] In one study, patients received 5-FU and LV daily for 5 days during the initial cycle. If tolerated, the same dose of 5-FU and LV was given in the second cycle, with the addition of IFN-α-2a s.c. at either 3, 5, or 10 MU per m² per day, starting 24 hours before the first dose of 5-FU and then continued daily for 7 or 14 days. Plasma samples were obtained on day 4 or 5 of therapy in 18 matched cycles. With each patient serving as his or her own control, a dose-dependent decrease in 5-FU clearance with an increase in the 5-FU AUC by 1.3- and 1.5-fold was observed in patients receiving 5 or 10 MU per m² per day; no such effect was apparent in patients receiving 3 MU per m² per day.[239] The catabolism of [³H]5-FU in intact PBMCs obtained from patients receiving this same IFN, 5-FU, and LV regimen was then measured with samples obtained at the same time on days 1, 2, and 4 before the daily doses of chemotherapy.[548] In 47 matched patient cycles, [³H]5-FU catabolism in mononuclear cells was significantly decreased compared with baseline by 20% and 41% on days 2 and 4 of therapy. These observations suggest that changes in 5-FU catabolism during therapy with IFN-α, 5-FU, and LV may account for the decreased clearance. With a 5-day CI of 5-FU (750 mg per m² per day) with IFN-α-2b s.c. 0.1 to 15.0 MU per m² per day, the mean 5-FU C_{ss} was significantly higher after IFN administration (1.3 vs. 1.0 μmol per L), but there was no apparent relationship between IFN dosage and change in 5-FU clearance.[545] Schuller et al. compared the influence of IFN-α (3 to 5 MU per m² s.c. three times a week) on 5-FU pharmacokinetics in patients receiving weekly i.v. bolus 5-FU (750 per m²) with or without 200 mg per m² LV.[547] Dose-dependent effects of IFN-α on 5-FU clearance were noted; of interest, the magnitude of the decrease in 5-FU clearance by IFN-α was greater in the absence of LV. The correlation noted between higher 5-FU AUC or C_{ss} and increased GI toxicity in several of these studies suggests that the pharmacokinetic interaction of IFN-α with 5-FU contributes to the toxicity of the combination.[239,545]

Fluorouracil and Thymidine

Although dThd is known to reverse the cytotoxicity of low concentrations of 5-FU *in vitro*, high concentrations of 5-FU (above 10 μmol per L) may not be countered effectively by dThd in all cancer cells. Furthermore, enhancement of 5-FU potency by pharmacologic doses of dThd has been observed *in vivo*.[41–44] Figure 8-14 summarizes the potential pharmacologic and biochemical interactions between dThd and 5-FU. Thymine, produced from the catabolism of dThd by dThd phosphorylase, competes with 5-FU for degradation by DPD, thus prolonging the plasma $t_{1/2}$ of 5-FU. dThd is anabolized to dTMP via dThd kinase, which has several consequences. First, dThd can compete with FdUrd for dThd kinase,

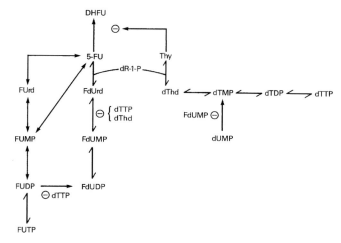

FIGURE 8-14. Interaction between 5-fluorouracil (5-FU) and thymidine (dThd). (DHFU, dihydrofluorouracil; dR-1-P, deoxyribose-1-phosphate; dTDP, thymidine 5'-diphosphate; dThd, thymidine; dTMP, thymidine 5'-monophosphate; dTTP, thymidine 5'-triphosphate; dUMP, deoxyuridine monophosphate; FdUDP, fluorodeoxyuridine diphosphate; FdUMP, fluorodeoxyuridylate; FdUrd, 5-fluoro-2'-deoxyuridine; FUDP, fluorouridine diphosphate; FUMP, fluorouridine monophosphate; FUrd, 5-fluorouridine; FUTP, fluorouridine triphosphate; Thy, thymine; –, inhibition.)

thereby decreasing FdUMP formation. Subsequent metabolism of dThd monophosphate to dTTP will expand the dTTP pools; dTTP, in turn, acts as a feedback inhibitor of dThd kinase and ribonucleotide reductase. Inhibition of the latter enzyme prevents FUDP conversion to FdUDP and consequently FdUMP, thus allowing enhanced FUTP formation and its incorporation into RNA. dThd acts as a donor of the deoxyribose moiety to promote the direct conversion of 5-FU to FdUrd by dThd phosphorylase; in some models, low concentrations of dThd may promote 5-FU incorporation into DNA.[92] In general, pharmacologic concentrations of dThd are intended to increase the RNA-directed effects of 5-FU while negating the DNA-directed toxicity.[41–44,549]

Clinical trials of the 5-FU and dThd combination have confirmed enhancement of 5-FU toxicity.[306–308,549,550] CI of dThd 8 g per day produces a C_{ss} of approximately 1 μmol per L; when given with 5-FU doses of 370 to 555 mg per m² daily for 5 days, severe myelosuppression and mucositis occurred.[550] Pretreatment of patients with dThd (7.5 to 45.0 g) 1 hour before 5-FU produced severe thrombocytopenia, leukopenia, mucositis, and diarrhea.[307] dThd markedly alters 5-FU plasma pharmacokinetics.[306–308] A bolus dose of 15 g of dThd produces peak plasma levels of 1 mmol per L; when given 1 hour before i.v. bolus of 5-FU, the $t_{1/2}$ of 5-FU increased to approximately 3 hours.[307] Patients receiving [2-¹⁴C]5-FU with dThd had marked reduction in the excretion of respiratory [¹⁴C]CO₂, which is released from the pyrimidine ring during 5-FU catabolism, and renal excretion became the primary route of 5-FU clearance. FdUrd was detected in plasma at levels of 10 to 50 μmol per

L in patients receiving 7.5 to 45.0 g dThd. A loading dose of dThd (15 g per m²) followed by a 5-day concurrent infusion of 5-FU (278 mg per m² per day) and dThd (8 g per m²) produced plasma dThd levels of 30 to 600 µmol per L during the initial 24 hours, whereas C_{ss} levels of 2 to 3 µmol per L dThd were maintained by the infusion.[308] 5-FU clearance was sevenfold lower than that measured in a separate cohort of patients receiving 5-FU alone, and median FdUrd levels were 0.7 to 1.3 µmol per L in the first 24 hours.

The clinical results do not indicate a differential effect on tumor cells as opposed to the host. Severe hematologic, GI, and CNS toxicity has been a feature of virtually all 5-FU/dThd regimens irrespective of dose or schedule. The increase in clinical toxicity with the combination of dThd and 5-FU required a more than 50% 5-FU dose reduction from conventional regimens, with no improvement in antitumor activity.

5-Fluorouracil and Inhibitors of *De Novo* Pyrimidine Biosynthesis

A number of inhibitors of the *de novo* synthesis of pyrimidines have received extensive preclinical evaluation, including pyrazofurin and 6-azauridine, inhibitors of orotidylate decarboxylase; acivicin, an inhibitor of carbamoylphos-

phate synthetase and CTP synthase; PALA, an inhibitor of aspartate carbamoyltransferase; and brequinar, an inhibitor of the mitochondrial enzyme dihydroorotate dehydrogenase (Fig. 8-15).[551–561] Inhibition of specific steps in the *de novo* pathway by these compounds causes reductions in pyrimidine nucleotide pools and promotes use of preformed pyrimidines, such as 5-FU. Inhibitors of orotate decarboxylase also elevate intracellular levels of orotic acid, which competitively inhibits the conversion of 5-FU to FUMP by OPRT.

PALA inhibits the second step in the *de novo* pathway of pyrimidine biosynthesis and has been tested extensively as a modulator of 5-FU.[554–564] Pretreatment with PALA may enhance the RNA-directed and DNA-directed cytotoxicity of 5-FU through several mechanisms.[562] Depletion of UTP and CTP results in diminished feedback inhibition of Urd-cytidine kinase activity, thereby favoring formation of FUMP through the salvage pathway and decreased competition with FUTP for RNA polymerase. Inhibition of the *de novo* pathway increases the availability of PRPP and decreases formation of orotic acid, thus favoring the formation of FUMP via OPRT. Depletion of pyrimidine nucleotide pools decreases dUMP formation through the ribonucleotide reductase pathway, with less competition with FdUMP for TS binding. Finally, decreased deoxycyti-

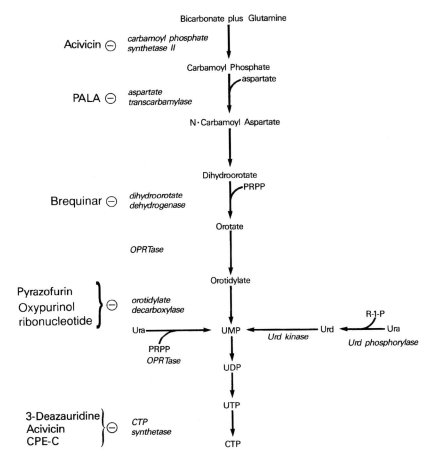

FIGURE 8-15. Sites of action of inhibitors of *de novo* pyrimidine biosynthesis. (CPE-C, cyclopentenyl cytosine; CTP, cytidine triphosphate; OPRTase, orotate phosphoribosyl transferase; PALA, *N*-phosphonoacetyl-L-aspartic acid; PRPP, phosphoribosyl phosphate; R-1-P, ribose-1-phosphate; UDP, uridine diphosphate; UMP, uridine monophosphate; Ura, uracil; Urd, uridine; UTP, uridine triphosphate; –, inhibition.)

dine triphosphate pools might enhance the DNA-directed toxicity of 5-FU. A number of these biochemical effects have been noted in preclinical *in vitro* and *in vivo* models, and a common feature of PALA modulation is increased 5-FU incorporation into RNA.

Preclinical studies indicate that initial biochemical effects of PALA are evident within a few hours; with persistent enzyme inhibition, the magnitude of pyrimidine nucleotide depletion becomes more profound during the initial 24 hours.[554,555,558,562,563] Pretreatment with PALA at intervals ranging from 3 to 24 hours modulates 5-FU metabolism.[556,558,559,561] The duration of the biochemical effects varies according to the type of host and tumor tissue. In general, sensitive tissues show persistent enzyme inhibition for many days after PALA administration, whereas more rapid recovery is noted in less sensitive tissues. Some preclinical studies in mice bearing PALA-sensitive murine solid tumors, such as Lewis lung carcinoma and spontaneous breast tumor, suggested that subtherapeutic doses of PALA may selectively produce depletion of Urd and cytidine nucleotide pools in tumor tissue.[555,561] Other studies, however, suggest great heterogeneity in the sensitivity of various cancer cell lines to PALA.[562–564] Aspartate carbamoyltransferase (ACTase) activity in some tumor tissues is much higher compared to normal tissues.[565] ACTase activity appears to correlate with the proliferative rate of the tumor and host tissue. Less sensitive tumors tended to have higher ACTase levels, and higher concentrations of PALA are required for biochemical effects to be evident.

The combination of PALA and 5-FU has been tested extensively in the clinic.[562] In the majority of the early studies, PALA was administered at close to its highest tolerated dose, and consequently, the dose of 5-FU had to be reduced. Diarrhea and mucositis were dose limiting in the majority of clinical trials using a daily-for-5-days bolus or CI schedule of PALA and 5-FU, although myelosuppression and skin rash also were prominent. In phase II studies conducted primarily in patients with colorectal cancer, the combination produced results consistent with that expected from 5-FU alone.[562] One randomized trial failed to show an advantage of PALA and 5-FU over 5-FU alone.[566]

Based on preclinical studies that showed enhancement of 5-FU activity with low-dose PALA, clinical interest resurfaced in exploring lower, but biochemically active, dosages of PALA in conjunction with 5-FU given at its maximally tolerated dose. Pharmacodynamic studies have led to different recommendations regarding the PALA dosage, depending on the biochemical indicator used. The biochemical effects of PALA have been monitored by either direct measurement of ACTase activity in tumor or a surrogate host tissue or by indirect assessment of ACTase activity (changes in plasma or urinary levels of pyrimidines).

A number of investigators have reported decreases in plasma Urd as early as 4 hours after administration of PALA.[247,567,568] Preclinical studies using the isolated rat liver perfusion model have documented the pivotal role of the liver in regulating the concentration of circulating Urd.[569,570] The liver appears to degrade essentially all incoming Urd; the hepatic pools of uracil nucleotides, formed predominantly by *de novo* synthesis, are responsible for the plasma-Urd concentrations leaving the liver.[569,570] The pharmacologic basis of the decrease in plasma-Urd levels during PALA treatment, therefore, may largely reflect decreased synthesis and export of Urd by the liver, although increased salvage of preformed Urd by various tissues also contributes.

In a phase I study of PALA given 24 hours before i.v. bolus 5-FU, the biochemical effects of PALA were monitored using a surrogate normal tissue end point: the effect on pyrazofurin-mediated urinary excretion of orotic acid and orotidine.[571] Because PALA (250 mg per m²) was associated with a biochemical effect and allowed administration of full-dose bolus 5-FU, this dose was selected for subsequent clinical studies. The biochemical assay used in this trial may largely reflect inhibition of *de novo* pyrimidine synthesis in the liver. Preclinical studies suggest that the liver is an especially sensitive target organ to PALA-mediated inhibition of ACTase.[563,572,573] More profound and persistent inhibition has been noted in liver tissue compared with other normal tissues, including bone marrow, spleen, and intestine, and, in some cases, tumor tissue.[563,572,573] The occurrence of dose-limiting hepatic toxicity (characterized by ascites, hyperbilirubinemia, and hypoalbuminemia) with PALA (250 mg per m²), given in conjunction with weekly i.v. bolus 5-FU, provides clinical evidence that low-dose PALA is capable of enhancing the toxicity of 5-FU in hepatic tissue on this particular schedule.[574]

In contrast, other clinical studies that directly monitored ACTase activity have concluded that the enzyme is incompletely and transiently inhibited by PALA, 250 mg per m² or higher. In one study, PALA was given 24 hours before a loading dose of high-dose LV, followed by a concurrent 72-hour CI of 5-FU and LV.[247] Patients were treated at seven PALA dosages ranging from 250 to 2,848 mg per m²; biochemical assessment was performed at each dosage using two surrogate end points: target enzyme activity in PBMCs and plasma-Urd levels. The delivered 5-FU dosage intensity across all cycles of therapy for patients treated with 1,750 mg per m² per day, or more, of 5-FU was not significantly different with PALA dosages of less than or equal to 1,266 mg per m², but it was much lower with PALA dosages of 1,899 mg per m² or more. Compared with each patient's own baseline, PALA at or below 844 mg per m² failed to appreciably inhibit ACTase activity at 24 hours in most patients. More consistent inhibition was seen at or above 1,266 mg per m² of PALA. Even with the highest PALA dosages, however, ACTase activity had returned toward baseline by 96 hours in most patients. In contrast, a modest decrease in plasma-Urd levels was evident at all PALA dosage levels, which persisted for at least 96 hours.[247] A different trial monitored leukocyte ACTase activity; with 250, 500, and 1,000 mg per m² PALA, ACTase activity was inhibited by 13%, 17%, and 49%, respectively.[575]

Moore et al. reported the change in ACTase activity in serial tumor biopsies taken from 16 patients at baseline and again after PALA (administered on one of several schedules). Baseline ACTase activity varied by fourfold among tumor specimens.[576] Sixteen to 24 hours after an initial dose of either 1,000, 3,600, or 6,000 mg per m² of PALA, ACTase was inhibited by 17%, 47%, and 75%, respectively. Inhibition of ACTase was accompanied by changes in UTP pools; after either 1,000 or 5,000 to 6,000 mg per m² of PALA, UTP pools were decreased by 16% and 43%, respectively. The only specimens that showed more than a 60% decrease were from patients having low initial ACTase activity who were treated with 3,600 mg per m² or more of PALA. Inhibition of ACTase by PALA and the ensuing depletion of pyrimidine nucleotides in human tumors thus occurred in a dose-dependent manner.[576]

Ardalan et al. combined a fixed dose of PALA, 250 mg per m², given 24 hours before a 24-hour CI of 5-FU on a weekly schedule, and recommended a 5-FU dose of 2,600 mg per m² per week, with or without PALA per week.[323] Based on promising phase II response rates in patients with colorectal cancer, this weekly schedule has been compared with the same schedule of 5-FU alone and with other 5-FU–modulated regimens in randomized trials.[326,577,578] Unfortunately, on this schedule, PALA did not improve the activity of 5-FU.

MTX and MMPR are also associated with expansion of PRPP pools; the addition of either modulator with PALA and 5-FU has led to improved antitumor activity in preclinical models compared to any of the individual combinations alone.[558,579] The combination of PALA, MTX, and 5-FU or PALA, MMPR, and 5-FU has been explored in preliminary clinical studies.[580,581] PRPP levels were measured in tumor specimens before treatment, and 12 and 24 hours after PALA and MMPR, in a phase I trial of weekly low-dose PALA given in conjunction with escalating dosages of MMPR 24 hours before the start of a 24-hour CI of 5-FU (1,300 mg per m²).[581] A twofold increase in PRPP at 12 hours was seen in two of four patients treated with 75 mg per m² MMPR, whereas more consistent increases in PRPP were evident with 150 and 225 mg per m² MMPR, although the PRPP levels returned toward baseline by 24 hours.[581] Further clinical evaluation will be required to determine whether PALA administered as part of a multimodulatory regimen including 5-FU will result in enhancement of the therapeutic index.

Brequinar enhances 5-FU cytotoxicity in *in vitro* and *in vivo* tumor models.[582–585] The cytotoxicity of brequinar can be reversed by Urd and cytidine in a concentration-dependent manner, depending on the capacity of the tumor to salvage pyrimidine nucleosides.[582–585] In the murine colon tumor 38, which has minimal capacity to salvage Urd, low

dosages of brequinar that were nontherapeutic when given alone resulted in a selective decrease in Urd nucleotide pools in tumor tissue compared with normal tissues.[582] Pretreatment with brequinar 4 and 24 hours before 5-FU significantly increased the incorporation of [³H]5-FU into tumor RNA, but the 4-hour interval was associated with the best therapeutic index. These preclinical studies provide a rationale for the clinical evaluation of brequinar as a biochemical modulator of 5-FU.[586]

Hydroxyurea

Hydroxyurea, an inhibitor of ribonucleotide reductase, has been combined with fluoropyrimidines as a strategy to decrease dUMP formation. In mice bearing L1210 leukemia, the combination of hydroxyurea (100 mg per kg daily i.p.) and FdUrd (75 mg per day i.p. on days 1 to 5, 8, 11, and 14) resulted in significantly longer survival compared with either drug alone at optimal dosages.[587] The combination of hydroxyurea and 5-FU has been explored clinically in the treatment of colorectal carcinoma, but several randomized trials have shown no apparent advantage.[588–590]

Combination with Purines and Pyrimidines

In cell lines that possess Urd phosphorylase, dThd phosphorylase, Urd kinase, and dThd kinase, simultaneous exposure of cancer cells to 5-FU and purines, such as inosine and deoxyinosine, or low concentrations (10 to 25 μmol per L) of pyrimidines, such as Urd and dUrd, may enhance 5-FU toxicity.[84,142,591–596] Donation of ribose-1-phosphate and dR-1-P moieties increases the formation of FUrd and FdUrd. In a human colon cancer cell line, the addition of 25 μmol per L dUrd to 5-FU enhanced FdUMP and dUMP formation, the extent of DNA damage, and cytotoxicity.[84] Urd functions as a potent inhibitor of DPD [K_i (inhibition constant) is 0.7 μmol per L for DPD isolated from hepatic tissue], and at 10 μmol per L, Urd can totally inhibit 5-FU catabolism by this enzyme.[595] Such observations highlight the importance of sequence of administration and the drug concentration to the outcome.

Normal tissues can catabolize FdUrd by either Urd phosphorylase or dThd phosphorylase. Some malignant cells are known to be deficient in dThd phosphorylase while retaining Urd phosphorylase. In such tumors, the combination of FdUrd with an inhibitor of Urd phosphorylase is predicted to prevent its catabolism to 5-FU and increase anabolism to FdUMP. In contrast, host tissues that contain dThd and Urd phosphorylases would retain the ability to catabolize FdUrd, despite inhibition of the latter enzyme. This hypothesis has been confirmed with two investigational inhibitors of Urd phosphorylase: benzylacyclouridine (BAU) and 5-(benzyloxybenzyl)barbituric acid (BBBAU).[597–599] BAU potentiates the cytotoxicity of FdUrd against human carcinoma cell lines *in vitro* and *in vivo*.[597] Furthermore, delayed administration of BAU in combination with Urd reduces host toxicity from 5-FU, and the combination of 5-FU and BAU, with or without Urd, was more effective than 5-FU alone against murine colon tumor 38 *in vivo*.[598] Coadministration of 20 nmol per L BBBAU enhances the cytotoxicity of FdUrd in DLD human colon cancer cells *in vitro*, and administration of BBBAU at 30 mg per kg per day with FdUrd 4,000 mg per kg per day (daily for 4 days) increased tumor growth inhibition of DLD cells growing s.c. by approximately three-fold in immunosuppressed mice.[599]

5-Fluoropyrimidines as Biochemical Modulators of Other Halogenated Pyrimidines

The halogenated pyrimidines iododeoxyuridine (IdUrd) and bromodeoxyuridine have attracted considerable attention as radiosensitizers by virtue of incorporation of their 5'-triphosphate metabolites into DNA.[600] IdUrd also has cytotoxic properties as a single agent. Iododeoxyuridine triphosphate (IdUTP) and bromodeoxyuridine triphosphate (BrdUTP) compete with dTTP for incorporation into DNA. Iododeoxyuridine monophosphate and bromodeoxyuridine monophosphate can serve as substrates for TS; this interaction results in cleavage of the iodine or bromine from the carbon-5 position.[601] Coadministration of an inhibitor of TS is expected to diminish the inactivation of iododeoxyuridine monophosphate and bromodeoxyuridine monophosphate, whereas depletion of dTTP should stimulate incorporation of IdUTP and BrdUTP into DNA. The success of this approach depends on duration of exposure and substrate competition for phosphorylation by dThd kinase. The activity of dThd kinase is dependent on feedback inhibitors, such as dTTP and IdUTP. 5-FU may be converted to FdUMP by alternate pathways not involving dThd kinase, thus avoiding potential competition with IdUrd or bromodeoxyuridine. In several models, 5-FU and FdUrd increase the DNA incorporation of IdUTP or BrdUTP, resulting in increased cytotoxicity, radiosensitization, or both, in several human cancer cell lines *in vitro* and *in vivo*.[602–607] In a human bladder cancer cell line, enhancement of IdUrd-DNA incorporation and cytotoxicity requires exposure times of 4 to 24 hours or more.[604] In contrast, a concurrent 1-hour exposure to 3 μmol per L each of IdUrd and FdUrd is antagonistic, with decreased formation of FdUMP.[608] In HT 29 colon cancer cells, the increased radiosensitization associated with IdUrd and FdUrd appeared to result from at least two effects: decreased dTTP pools accompanied by increased incorporation of IdUrd into DNA, and cell-cycle redistribution with an accumulation of cells in the G_1 and S phases.

In early clinical trials, IdUrd was generally given by short i.v. infusions of 2 hours or less. The combination of FdUrd and IdUrd was associated with some tumor regressions, but toxicity was severe.[609–611] With a prolonged infusional schedule, up to 1,000 mg per m² per day IdUrd for 14 days can be administered safely; at this dose, IdUrd C_{ss} values of approximately 3 μmol per L were achieved, and up to 11% substitution of dThd by IdUrd was observed in the DNA of peripheral granulocytes.[612–614] Selective incorporation of IdUrd into DNA of hepatic tumor was seen compared with normal liver when IdUrd was given by either systemic infusion or HAI.[615] IdUrd (200 to 675 mg per m² per day) and FdUrd (0.6 to 3.5 mg per m² per day, 15% to 78% of the single-agent highest tolerated dose) were subsequently combined as a concurrent 14-day CI.[616] At a fixed dosage of IdUrd, increasing dosages of FdUrd did not appear to increase IdUrd C_{ss} or percent IdUrd substitution. With escalating doses of IdUrd and fixed doses of FdUrd, the C_{ss} for IdUrd rose proportionally, as did the percent IdUrd substitution. However, no clinically relevant enhancement of IdUrd incorporation into DNA by FdUrd was evident. Dose-limiting toxicities included thrombocytopenia, diarrhea, mucositis, and elevation of serum transaminases.[616] The addition of LV 200 mg per m² to a 14-day infusion of IdUrd reduced the highest tolerated dose to 400 mg per m² (C_{ss} 0.7 μmol per L) but did not enhance IdUrd-DNA incorporation in peripheral blood granulocytes.[617]

A 4-day HAI of 5-FU, 300 mg per day (approximately 180 mg per m² per day), was studied with escalating doses of IdUrd given as a 3-hour HAI on days 8 to 14.[618] With IdUrd infusions of 37 to 81 mg per m² per day, the systemic peak plasma levels of IdUrd (0.2 to 0.8 μmol per L) and iodouracil (0.4 to 1.8 μmol per L) increased. Of interest, although 5-FU was undetectable during infusion of 5-FU alone, plasma levels of approximately 0.5 μmol per L were seen during infusion of IdUrd doses of 37 mg per m² per day or more.[618] Hepatic toxicity was dose limiting, and biliary sclerosis was documented in one patient. Although tumor regression occurred in some cases, the use of this regimen is limited by hepatic toxicity, reminiscent of that seen with HAI of FdUrd.

Combination with Nucleoside Transport Inhibitors

Human colon carcinomas possess high levels of the enzymes necessary for nucleoside salvage, and dThd salvage represents a potential mechanism of resistance to 5-FU or FdUrd.[619] Dipyridamole, nitrobenzylthioinosine, and dilazep inhibit the uptake and efflux of nucleosides, such as dThd, FdUrd, and dUrd, in a dose-dependent manner.[620–622] In some *in vitro* models, dipyridamole-mediated interference with nucleoside salvage increases the toxicity of several antimetabolites, including PALA, MTX, and acivicin.[623–625] Because the effects of dipyridamole on nucleoside transport are rapidly reversible on drug removal, continuous exposure is necessary to modulate 5-FU toxicity. In HCT 116 colon cancer cells, dipyridamole and NBMPR increase FdUMP formation and the cytotoxicity of 5-FU.[622,626,627] The augmentation of 5-FU toxicity is concentration dependent; free dipyridamole concentrations as low as 50 nmol per L modulated 5-FU toxicity, but optimal effects required 500 nmol per L.[626] The increase in FdUMP levels results in part from blockade of the efflux of FdUrd and other deoxyribonucleosides, such as dUrd, which serve as donors of dR-1-P.[84,627] The expansion of dUMP pools with 5-FU is accompanied by increased production of alkaline-labile sites in newly synthesized DNA.[84] Other investigators have confirmed enhanced DNA damage with 5-FU and dipyridamole.[628] A direct correlation is noted between increased accumulation of dUTP and increased DNA fragility in cells treated with the antifolate TS inhibitor CB3717 and dipyridamole.[85] The interaction between nucleoside transport inhibitors and 5-FU and FdUrd is complex, and more than one mechanism resulting in augmentation of toxicity may exist.

The combination of 5-FU with or without LV and dipyridamole has been explored in clinical trials using either intermittent oral dosing or CI of dipyridamole.[246,629,630] With 175 mg per m^2 dipyridamole by mouth (p.o.) every 6 hours, mean peak and trough free drug concentrations are 38 and 23 nmol per L, respectively, which are considerably lower than the optimal concentrations in cell culture models.[629] With CI of 285 mg per m^2 per day of dipyridamole for 3 days (the highest tolerated dose), the mean C_{ss} of total and free dipyridamole is 6.7 μmol per L and 24 nmol per L, respectively.[631] In paired patient courses of CI 5-FU, with or without dipyridamole, dipyridamole administration was associated with significantly lower 5-FU C_{ss} and a faster clearance.[246,255] Thus, the relatively high concentrations of free dipyridamole needed to optimally modulate 5-FU toxicity, metabolism, and DNA damage in tissue culture systems are not clinically achievable with systemic administration. The achievable C_{ss} of free dipyridamole with infusional or high-dose oral therapy may be sufficient to modulate the transport of dThd and other nucleosides in normal tissues and some tumor tissues.[631,632] However, orally administered dipyridamole failed to improve the activity of a 5-FU and LV regimen in a randomized trial in patients with advanced colorectal cancer.[633]

Interaction of 5-Fluorouracil with Platinum Analogs

Synergism between cisplatin and 5-FU has been demonstrated in preclinical models *in vitro* and *in vivo*.[634–643] The precise mechanism(s) for the synergism has not been completely defined, but preclinical studies point to enhancement of DNA-directed toxicity. In some models, the toxicity of 5-FU and cisplatin is abrogated by dThd but potentiated by LV.[637,642,643] In an ovarian cancer cell line, a 1-hour incubation with cisplatin (10 μmol per L) increased FH_4 and CH_2FH_4 pools by 2.5-fold and increased ternary

complex formation by the same magnitude.[637] The apparent basis is cisplatin-mediated inhibition of methionine uptake, which stimulates the endogenous synthesis of methionine from homocysteine and increases the conversion of $5\text{-}CH_3FH_4$ to FH_4, which is a precursor of 5,10-CH_2FH_4 (Fig. 8-13).[637] Other effects of cisplatin on DNA integrity or interactions with cell surface nucleic acids and plasma membrane also may be important. Enhanced DNA damage and inhibition of the repair of cisplatin-induced DNA interstrand cross-links have been noted with the combination.[640,643]

In some preclinical models, concurrent exposure to both drugs was efficacious.[637,642] In other models, however, preexposure to 5-FU before cisplatin administration was superior to the opposite sequence.[638–641,643] With dosages that were only minimally effective when given alone, the sequence 5-FU (35 mg per kg) followed 24 hours later by cisplatin (3 mg per kg) given weekly for 5 doses significantly reduced the tumor burden in a murine colon cancer model.[638] In contrast, the opposite sequence was more toxic in terms of treatment-related deaths and was less efficacious in reducing tumor burden. In a human squamous cancer cell line, optimal cytotoxicity was seen with a 24-hour preexposure to 5-FU, followed by cisplatin after a 24- to 48-hour drug-free interval; the removal of cisplatin-induced DNA interstrand cross-links was significantly reduced compared with cells exposed to cisplatin alone or to 5-FU followed immediately by cisplatin.[640] The lag time for 5-FU effects and the inability of dThd to reverse the interaction raised the possibility that RNA-directed effects might be involved. 5-FU inhibits ERCC1 and γ-glutamyl-cysteine synthetase mRNA expression in a cisplatin-resistant human squamous carcinoma cell line, suggesting that 5-FU mediated interference with the expression of DNA repair enzymes might enhance DNA damage associated with cisplatin exposure.[83] In NCI H548 colon cancer cells, preexposure to 5-FU for 24 hours followed by cisplatin for 2 hours produced more than additive cytotoxicity and a greater degree of single-stranded–DNA fragmentation in parental and nascent DNA compared to the opposite sequence.[643]

Although phase II studies suggested a beneficial effect of 5-FU plus cisplatin in colorectal carcinoma, in randomized studies comparing bolus or infusional 5-FU with or without bolus cisplatin, the clinical toxicity was increased without a corresponding improvement in overall disease control.[644–648] Cisplatin is inactive as a single agent in colorectal cancer, so perhaps the necessary cellular events allowing a positive interaction were not present in this tumor type. In contrast, the combination of 5-FU and cisplatin has shown promising results in diseases in which both agents have single-agent activity, including squamous cell cancers arising in the anus, head and neck, esophagus, and cervix. The influence of sequence and timing of cisplatin and 5-FU administration in determining the extent of therapeutic effect, toxicity, or both, has not been carefully studied in clinical trials.

Oxaliplatin has also shown additive or synergistic cytotoxic properties with 5-FU in *in vitro* and *in vivo* studies.[648,649] More impressive is the evidence of clinical synergy between oxaliplatin and 5-FU in metastatic colorectal cancer. Objective responses have been seen when oxaliplatin is added to a 5-FU–based regimen on which patients have had documented disease progression.[650–653] Results from an initial randomized trial in advanced colorectal cancer suggest a substantial improvement in the response rate when oxaliplatin is added to 5-FU and LV as first-line therapy.[654] Additional phase III trials evaluating the worth of oxaliplatin with 5-FU and LV as adjuvant therapy for colon cancer and for patients with advanced disease are ongoing. The basis of the interaction between oxaliplatin and cisplatin and how it might differ from that between cisplatin and 5-FU is the subject of ongoing investigation.

5-Fluorouracil and Levamisole

Several adjuvant therapy trials in colon cancer have indicated a benefit for node-positive patients treated with the combination of 5-FU (450 mg per m² i.v. bolus daily for 5 days, followed in 28 days by weekly injection of 450 mg per m² for 48 weeks) and the immunomodulator levamisole (50 mg p.o. three times daily for 3 days, repeated every 2 weeks for 1 year) compared with patients receiving no additional therapy or levamisole alone.[655–657] In contrast, 5-FU and levamisole have not shown improved results compared with 5-FU alone in advanced colorectal cancer.[658,659] Although levamisole is associated with a variety of immunorestorative and cellular effects in preclinical and clinical studies, the basis for the apparent clinical benefit derived from 5-FU and levamisole in the adjuvant setting is not clear.[659,660]

In three human-colon cancer cell lines, 24- to 72-hour exposures to levamisole at concentrations of 100 μmol per L or less were not cytotoxic and did not appear to potentiate the cytotoxicity of 5-FU.[66] More than additive toxicity with 5-FU was only evident with 500 and 1,000 μmol per L levamisole, concentrations that exceed the peak-plasma concentrations achieved with standard oral dosing (1 to 5 μmol per L) by several orders of magnitude.[659,661] Another study indicated that continuous exposure to 125 μmol per L or greater levamisole enhanced the cytotoxicity of 5-FU, but not FdUrd, against a panel of human solid tumor cell lines. dThd was not protective in this model.[662] The metabolite p-hydroxytetramisole potentiated 5-FU–mediated cytotoxicity at equimolar concentrations as the parent compound. 5-FU cytotoxicity was also enhanced by 1-p-bromotetramisole, an analog with tenfold greater inhibitory activity against the enzyme alkaline phosphatase, and orthovanadate, an inhibitor of tyrosine phosphatase, but not by okadaic acid, an inhibitor of serine-threonine phosphatases. These results sug-

gest that the antiphosphatase activity of levamisole may contribute to the potentiation of 5-FU cytotoxicity.[662]

Adjuvant therapy with 5-FU and levamisole has been accompanied by neurotoxicity and hepatic toxicity, which are not generally seen with either agent given alone at the same dosages and schedules. Neurotoxicity occurs in approximately 5% of patients, manifest by headache, dizziness, vertigo, anxiety, irritability, and ataxia.[373,374,655,656,663–666] MRI studies with gadolinium enhancement have shown prominent multifocal enhancing white matter lesions in affected patients, suggesting an inflammatory leukoencephalopathy. Stereotactic cerebral biopsy in two patients revealed features of active demyelination.[373] The neurologic symptoms may improve on cessation of therapy and institution of a short course of corticosteroids, but recovery may be incomplete.

Approximately 40% of patients receiving 5-FU and levamisole develop laboratory abnormalities consistent with hepatic toxicity, occurring a median of 2.5 months after starting therapy.[667,668] Elevation of alkaline phosphatase is the most common abnormality and is frequently accompanied by elevations of transaminases and serum bilirubin. These changes are usually mild, not associated with symptoms, and resolve when therapy is stopped. In some instances, elevated carcinoembryonic-antigen levels increase in the absence of disease progression; fatty liver was noted on CT scan or liver biopsy in some patients.

A major criticism of the 5-FU and levamisole data is that the definitive trials showing benefit of the combination did not include an arm containing 5-FU alone, and many oncologists remained skeptical of the contribution of levamisole to the therapeutic benefit. For these reasons, an Italian trial compared one year of therapy with 5-FU and levamisole with 5-FU alone as adjuvant therapy for colon cancer. Preliminary results suggest a similar outcome on both arms, casting doubt on the worth of levamisole to the therapeutic effect.[669] Recent results from adjuvant phase III trials in colon cancer indicate that bolus 5-FU modulated by LV, given on either a monthly schedule for six cycles or a schedule consisting of weekly dosages for 6 of 8 weeks for a four-cycle schedule, is as effective as one year of 5-FU and levamisole therapy, and both are superior to 6 months of 5-FU and levamisole.[515] In view of the toxicity considerations and the more recent clinical results, the use of levamisole plus 5-FU is likely to be supplanted by 5-FU and LV.

5-Fluorouracil and Azidothymidine

Zidovudine (AZT, Azidothymidine) is an important component of multi-agent therapy for acquired immunodeficiency syndrome (AIDS) and AIDS-related complex. The potential role of AZT as an antineoplastic agent is a subject of investigation. Preclinical models suggest that the antiproliferative activity of AZT in cancer cell lines correlates with incorporation of AZT triphosphate into DNA and the induction of DNA damage. Enhanced cytotoxicity has been seen with the combination of 5-FU and AZT *in vitro* and *in vivo*; this effect is dThd-reversible.[670–675] In some models, AZT does not affect the metabolism of 5-FU, FdUMP-mediated TS inhibition, or 5-FU–RNA incorporation, and the basis for the synergism appears to be 5-FU–mediated potentiation of AZT incorporation into DNA, presumably by decreasing the competing pools of dTTP. In other models, AZT-mediated inhibition of dThd kinase and interference with dThd salvage seems important. Although the basis for the interaction may be complex, a common final pathway with combined AZT and 5-FU may be increased DNA damage. Based on the preclinical data, the combination of 5-FU and AZT, with or without LV, is currently being investigated in the clinical setting.[676–679]

5-Fluorouracil and Paclitaxel

Paclitaxel is a taxane derivative that binds to the β-subunit of tubulin in the microtubule and promotes the formation of extremely stable microtubules. The impaired ability of paclitaxel-stabilized microtubules to disassemble in turn interferes with their normal functions, including formation of the mitotic spindle apparatus during cell division, maintenance of cell shape, motility, anchorage, mediation of signals between surface receptors and the nucleus, and intracellular transport. Prominent sequence-dependent interactions have been described in patients for paclitaxel combined with several anticancer agents, including cisplatin, doxorubicin, and cyclophosphamide.

Several preclinical studies describe antagonism between paclitaxel and 5-FU *in vitro*. Sequential 24-hour exposures to paclitaxel followed by 5-FU led to additive effects in four different human cancer cell lines using the MTT assay, whereas the opposite sequence, 5-FU followed by paclitaxel, led to subadditive effects in three of the four cell

lines.[680] Concurrent continuous exposure of BCap37 breast cancer cells and KB cells to 100 nmol per L paclitaxel and 10 μmol per L 5-FU inhibited the customary oligonucleosomal-DNA fragmentation seen with paclitaxel alone at 48 and 72 hours.[681] In this model, although 5-FU given alone did not produce noticeable changes in the cell-cycle profile, it diminished the ability of paclitaxel to produce G_2-M blockade and prevented apoptosis.

In MCF-7 breast cancer cells, 24-hour exposures to 5-FU and paclitaxel in various sequences suggested that pre-exposure to 5-FU, followed by paclitaxel, resulted in marked antagonism, whereas sequential paclitaxel followed by 5-FU was optimal.[682] Concurrent or preexposure to paclitaxel did not affect [³H]5-FU metabolism, [³H]5-FU–RNA incorporation, or the extent of 5-FU–mediated TS inhibition. Paclitaxel led to G_2-M phase accumulation that persisted for up to 24 hours after drug exposure, whereas a 24-hour 5-FU exposure produced S-phase accumulation. 5-FU preexposure diminished paclitaxel-associated G_2-M phase block, whereas subsequent exposure to 5-FU after paclitaxel did not. 5-FU exposure resulted in transient induction of p53 and p21, which returned to basal levels 24 hours after drug removal. p53 and p21 protein content also markedly increased during paclitaxel exposure, accompanied by phosphorylation of Bcl-2. Pronounced DNA fragmentation was seen at 48 hours when cells were exposed to paclitaxel for an initial 24-hour period. Paclitaxel-associated DNA fragmentation was not prevented by concurrent or subsequent exposure to 5-FU (Fig. 8-16). In this model, paclitaxel-mediated G_2-M phase arrest appeared to be a crucial step in induction of DNA fragmentation. Because an initial 24-hour paclitaxel exposure did not interfere with subsequent 5-FU metabolism, or TS inhibition, and delayed exposure to 5-FU did not impede either paclitaxel-mediated induction of mitotic blockade or DNA fragmentation, this sequence seems logical for clinical trials. Clinical trials often use empirically

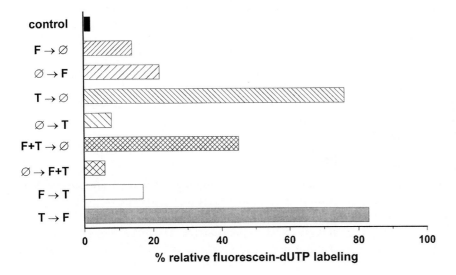

% relative fluorescein-dUTP labeling

FIGURE 8-16. 5-Fluorouracil preexposure antagonizes paclitaxel-mediated DNA damage in MCF-7 breast cancer cells. MCF-7 cells were treated with various 24-hour sequences of either no drug (ø), 4 μmol/L 5-fluorouracil (F), or 40 nmol/L paclitaxel (T) as indicated. After 48 hours, DNA strand breakage was determined by fluorescein–deoxyuridine triphosphate (dUTP) labeling of 3'-OH DNA ends by terminal deoxynucleotidyl transferase as assessed by flow cytometry. A boundary for fluorescein intensity was established for control cells, and intensity beyond this level is presented as percent of the total fluorescent distribution. (Reprinted from Grem JL, Nguyen D, Monahan BP, et al. Sequence-dependent antagonism between fluorouracil and paclitaxel in human breast cancer cells. *Biochem Pharmacol* 1999;58:477–486, with permission from Elsevier Science.)

derived schedules for drug combinations. Additional clinical studies will be needed to determine whether the sequence of paclitaxel and 5-FU administration influences toxicity and response to therapy.

Interaction of 5-Fluorouracil with Ionizing Radiation

Heidelberger et al. discovered that growth-inhibitory doses of radiotherapy in rodent tumors were made curative by the addition of 5-FU.[683] Conversely, ineffective regimens of 5-FU became active by the addition of a single dose of radiotherapy. The synergistic interaction has been confirmed by other investigators using *in vitro* and *in vivo* models.[684–695] Combined treatment with 5-FU and radiotherapy leads to dosage and time-dependent enhancement of cell killing in HeLA and HT-29 cells.[685–687] Enhanced radiosensitization depends on 5-FU exposure for a period longer than the cell-doubling time; thus, the optimal effects for these two cancer cell lines are observed when 5-FU continues for at least 48 hours after irradiation, with little or no synergy if 5-FU is given either before or for only 3 hours after irradiation. However, the optimal schedule for 5-FU radiosensitization in preclinical models varies depending on the model system used. In DU-145 prostate cancer cells, 5-FU modulation of radiosensitivity is apparent with either a 1-hour pulse of 100 μmol per L 5-FU plus irradiation at 30 minutes or with continuous exposure to 4 μmol per L 5-FU and irradiation given either immediately before or 17 hours after 5-FU.[688]

In *p53* mutant HT-29 cells, time-dependent radiosensitization occurs after a 2-hour exposure to 0.5 μmol per L FdUrd.[691] TS is maximally inhibited at the end of FdUrd exposure, but TS inhibition persists for up to 32 hours after drug removal, accompanied by dTTP pool depletion. An increase in radiosensitivity, however, is not apparent until 16 hours after drug removal. The increase in radiation sensitivity parallels the gradual accumulation of cells in early S phase, a relatively radiosensitive phase of the cell cycle. In another model, 8- or 24-hour preexposures to low concentrations of FdUrd enhance DNA damage, apparently by inhibiting repair of double-stranded breaks; the addition of LV and dipyridamole enhances FdUrd-mediated radiosensitization and the interference with DNA repair.[689,690] Although HT-29 and SW-620 colon cancer cells have the same *p53* mutation, the response to FdUrd-mediated radiosensitization is different.[693] Exposure to 100 nmol per L FdUrd for 14 hours produces comparable inhibition of TS activity by 75% to 80%, yet the radiosensitive HT-29 cell line progresses into S phase, whereas the insensitive cell line arrests at the G_1-S boundary. Although cyclin D protein levels do not change with FdUrd treatment in either cell line, cyclin E protein content increases by seven- to ninefold in both lines. Cyclin E–dependent kinase activity increases appreciably only in HT-29 cells, and this may account for the ability of this cell line to progress into S phase and become radiosensitized.[693] These interesting findings suggest that a G_1-S checkpoint that influences radiosensitization produced by FdUrd is not dependent on normal *p53* function.

In vivo, the combination of 5-FU, with or without LV, with radiation on several schedules has proven effective in increasing the delay in tumor regrowth.[683,684,686,687] In general, however, the bulk of the experimental evidence supports the notion that more prolonged exposure to fluoropyrimidines is optimal. The underlying mechanism(s) for this synergistic interaction may be influenced by schedule and duration of exposure. FdUMP-mediated inhibition of TS with resulting dTTP pool depletion, deoxyribonucleotide imbalance, increased DNA damage, inhibition of DNA repair, and accumulation of cells in S phase appear to be important features of radiosensitization. The RNA-directed effects of 5-FU might conceivably play a role, but they have not been clearly implicated.

5-FU given alone or in combination with other agents (including cisplatin or mitomycin C) during radiotherapy has demonstrated efficacy in patients with either squamous cell cancers arising in the anal canal, cervix, head and neck, and esophagus, or adenocarcinomas arising in the rectum.[695–701] Diverse schedules of 5-FU have been used—for example, bolus administration of 5-FU only during the first and final 3 days of radiation, 96- to 120-hour CI for the first and last week of radiation, and prolonged CI throughout the entire radiation treatment. A randomized trial in high-risk rectal cancer patients comparing 5-FU given by intermittent bolus injections with protracted CI during postoperative radiation therapy to the pelvis demonstrated significant improvements in time to relapse and survival in favor of the infusional 5-FU arm.[701]

ORALLY BIOAVAILABLE 5'-FLUOROPYRIMIDINES

There is keen interest in developing 5-FU–based therapy that can be administered orally, and the structures of agents that are either commercially available or in clinical trials are shown in Figure 8-17. Two of the drugs, ftorafur and doxifluridine, were initially tested with i.v. administration, whereas the other drugs were developed as a strategy to permit oral administration. Features of the oral 5-fluoropyrimidine drugs are shown in Table 8-14.

Ftorafur

Ftorafur [1-(2-tetrahydrofuranyl)-5-fluorouracil, tegafur, MW = 200] is a furan nucleoside that was originally synthesized and tested in the Soviet Union. Ftorafur has clinical activity against adenocarcinomas and is less myelosuppressive but more neurotoxic than 5-FU. Ftorafur is a prodrug

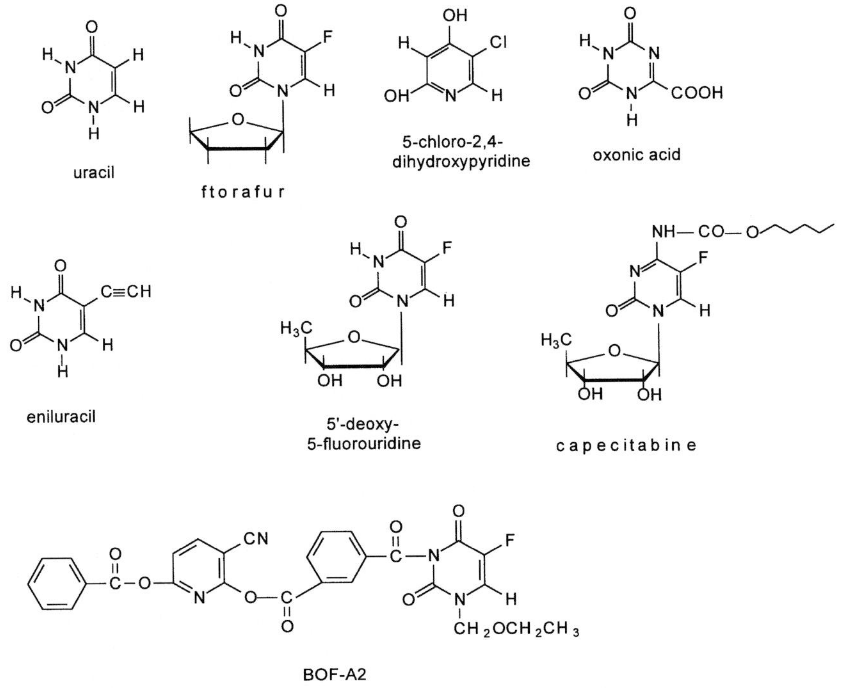

FIGURE 8-17. Structures of orally administered 5-fluoropyrimidine analogs. (BOF-A2, emitefur, 3-{3-[6-benzoyloxy-3-cyano-2-pyridyloxycarbonyl]benzoyl}-1-ethoxymethyl-5-fluorouracil.)

TABLE 8-14. ORALLY ADMINISTERED 5-FLUOROPYRIMIDINES

Agents	Pharmacologic Effect	Common Clinical Schedules

UFT, 2-drug combination: uracil and ftorafur (4:1 molar ratio)
Orzel = UFT + calcium leucovorin
	Prodrug containing
	  Uracil is a competitive inhibitor of DPD.
	  Ftorafur is an oral fluorouracil prodrug.
		UFT 300 mg/m^2 + LV 75–150 mg p.o. daily in 3 divided doses for 28 of 35 d
		or
		LV 500 mg/m^2 i.v. + UFT 195 mg/m^2 p.o. d 1 then oral LV 15 mg + UFT 195 mg/m^2 q 12 h for 14 of 28 d

Eniluracil with oral 5-FU	Eniluracil is a mechanism-based inhibitor of DPD; It renders 5-FU bioavailability near 100%; It prevents formation of 5-FU catabolites.	Eniluracil 20 mg p.o. + 1 mg/m^2 5-FU p.o. twice daily for 28 of 35 d

S-1, 3-drug combination:
  Ftorafur
  5-chloro-2,4-dihydroxypyridine
 	
  Potassium oxonate 1:0.4:1 molar ratio
	
	Ftorafur is an oral fluorouracil prodrug.
	5-chloro-2,4-dihydroxypyridine is a potent, competitive inhibitor of DPD.
	Potassium oxonate is a competitive inhibitor of orotate phosphoribosyl transferase (decreases 5-FU anabolism and gastrointestinal toxicity).
		40 mg/m^2 (40–60 mg) p.o. twice daily for 28 of 42 d
		or
		30 mg/m^2 p.o. twice daily for 28 of 35 d

Capecitabine (Xeloda)	Oral 5-FU prodrug. Parent drug absorbed intact. Converted sequentially to 5'-deoxy-5-fluorocytidine, 5'-deoxy-5-fluorouridine, and 5-FU. 5-FU liberated by thymidine phosphorylase.	2,500 mg/m^2 p.o. daily in 2 divided doses for 14 of 21 d

BOF-A2 (emitefur)
  1-ethoxymethyl-5-fluorouracil
  3-cyano-2,6-dihydroxypyridine
	
	Masked oral 5-FU prodrug.
	Parental drug absorbed intact.
	5-FU liberated by hepatic microsomal enzymes.
	3-cyano-2,6-dihydroxypyridine is a potent competitive inhibitor of DPD.
		200 mg p.o. twice daily for 14 of 28 d
		or
		200 mg/m^2 p.o. + LV 60 mg p.o. in 2 divided doses daily for 14 of 21 d

BOF-A2, emitefur, 3-{3-[6-benzoyloxy-3-cyano-2-pyridyloxycarbonyl]benzoyl}-1-ethoxymethyl-5-fluorouracil; DPD, dihydropyrimidine dehydrogenase; 5-FU, 5-fluorouracil; LV, leucovorin; UFT, uracil and ftorafur.

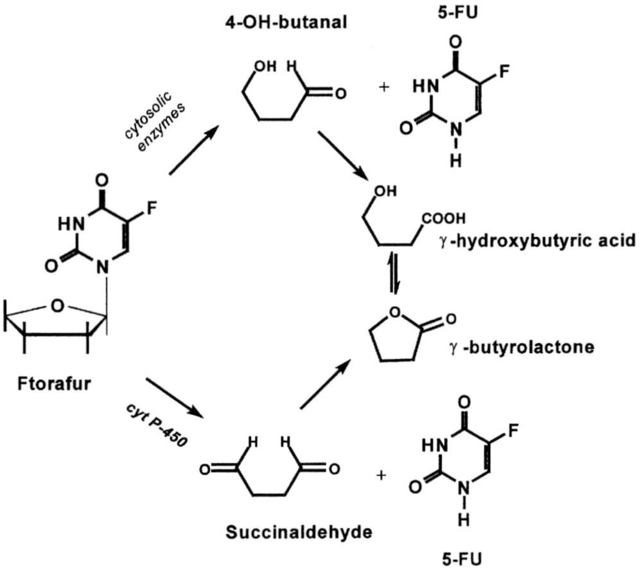

FIGURE 8-18. Metabolism of ftorafur. (5-FU, 5-fluorouracil.)

and is slowly metabolized to 5-FU by two major metabolic pathways.[702–709] One pathway is mediated by microsomal cytochrome P-450 oxidation at the 5'-carbon of the tetrahydrofuran moiety, resulting in the formation of a labile intermediate (5'-hydroxyftorafur) that spontaneously cleaves to produce succinaldehyde and 5-FU (Fig. 8-18). The second pathway, mediated by soluble enzymes, proceeds via enzymatic cleavage of the N-1-C-2' bond to yield 5-FU and 4-hydroxybutanal; the latter undergoes further enzymatic conversion to form γ-butyrolactone (γ-BL) or γ-hydroxybutyric acid (γ-HB); succinaldehyde is at least partially converted to these latter two compounds. *In vivo*, the liver is the major source of cytochrome P-450, with lower levels in the GI tract and much lower levels in the brain. *In vitro* studies with tissue homogenates from liver, GI tract, and the brain containing the soluble enzyme pathway have documented metabolism of ftorafur to 5-FU. Small amounts of 3'- and 4'-hydroxyl derivatives have been isolated from urine.[702,703] After i.v. bolus injection of 1 g per m², ftorafur and a major metabolite, dehydroftorafur, were detected in serum, whereas 5-FU was not.[707] Other investigators have confirmed that 5-FU plasma concentrations are low.[708,709] These findings raise the possibility that metabolic conversion of ftorafur to 5-FU occurs intracellularly, without subsequent redistribution via the systemic circulation. Plasma levels of 5-FU may not accurately reflect the extent of this intracellular conversion.

The pharmacokinetic behavior of ftorafur has been described for i.v. and oral routes of administration. After i.v. bolus injection, ftorafur undergoes an initial distribution phase, followed by a prolonged $t_{1/2}$ ranging from 6 to 16 hours.[702,703,707–710] The clearance is approximately 31 mL per minute per m², and the V_d (15 to 30 L per m²) approximates that of total-body water.[707–710] After oral administration, absorption is virtually 100%. After 2 g per m² p.o., ftorafur appears in plasma by 11 minutes, and peak plasma levels occur at 3.2 hours.[710] Simultaneous sampling of blood from portal and peripheral veins indicates that ftorafur appears sooner in the portal vein; peak levels in the peripheral vein occur 1.7 hours later, consistent with rapid absorption and hepatic retention.

Pretreatment of tumor-bearing mice with an inhibitor of microsomal enzymes enhances the acute neurotoxic effects of ftorafur and interferes with the antitumor activity, whereas induction of microsomal enzyme activity produces the opposite effects.[711,712] Administration of phenobarbital and glutathione to patients receiving mitomycin C and ftorafur leads to significantly lower plasma levels of ftorafur, suggesting that stimulation of hepatic microsomal enzymes accelerates ftorafur metabolism.[712] These studies suggest that the liver is the major site of metabolism, although other enzyme pathways may be responsible for the formation of various metabolites.

Ftorafur has been administered intravenously in doses of 1.50 to 2.25 g per m² daily for 4 or 5 days or single doses of 4 g per m² weekly.[713–718] The primary clinical toxicities with these schedules are GI symptoms (diarrhea, cramps, vomiting, and mucositis) and neurologic side effects (altered mental status, cerebellar ataxia, and, rarely, coma). The neurotoxic side effects resemble those of intracarotid infusion of 5-FU and have been attributed to the high concentrations of parent drug found in the CSF.[702,708,709] The ftorafur metabolite γ-hydroxybutyrate occurs physiologically in brain and CSF, has anesthetic properties, and produces concentration-dependent CNS depression; thus, it may contribute to neurotoxicity. A recommended oral dose is 1.5 g per m² daily for 14 to 21 days, although some investigators suggest that a less-intensive regimen of 0.8 to 1.0 g per m² daily (in divided doses) for 14 of 28 days is better tolerated.[719,720] GI side effects are predominant with the oral route; neurotoxicity in the form of dizziness and lethargy occurs infrequently.

Phase II trials in a variety of solid tumors indicate that ftorafur has comparable activity with that of 5-FU.[713–721] Some patients failing 5-FU–containing regimens have responded to a protracted oral schedule of ftorafur.[720,721] A randomized trial indicated similar antitumor activity for single-agent ftorafur and 5-FU, whereas toxicity profiles differed.[722] Ftorafur-containing combination chemotherapy regimens yielded results similar to historic control 5-FU–containing regimens.[723,724] Randomized trials using a substitution design with either ftorafur or 5-FU showed superiority of the 5-FU–containing arms in two studies, although both arms were equivalent in another trial.[725–727]

The option for oral administration has maintained interest in the use of ftorafur. Oral ftorafur has been combined with oral LV on a 21-day schedule and appears to be active; the recommended dose is 1,600 mg (approximately

900 mg per m²) in 3 divided doses with 500 mg LV in 5 divided doses.[728]

UFT

UFT, a combination of uracil and ftorafur (molar ratio of 4:1), entered into clinical trials in Japan in the early 1980s. Preclinical studies indicate that UFT results in significantly higher tumor to serum 5-FU ratios than observed with ftorafur alone.[729–730] UFT is usually given orally in divided doses daily for either 5 or 28 days. With oral doses ranging from 50 to 300 mg per m², maximum plasma levels of ftorafur and 5-FU occur between 0.6 and 2.1 hours; ftorafur levels (2.7 to 20.0 µg per mL, 13.5 to 100.0 µmol per L) exceed 5-FU levels by 10- to 15-fold (0.025 to 0.900 µg per mL, 0.2 to 7.0 µmol per L), and ftorafur clearance is approximately 70 mL per minute per m².[731] In patients undergoing nephrectomy for renal cell carcinoma 1 day after a 5-day course of twice-daily ftorafur (1 capsule: 100 mg ftorafur, 224 mg uracil), intratumoral 5-FU levels were significantly higher (2.3-fold) than in normal kidney tissue.[732] In another study, the maximum 5-FU concentration in bladder cancer tissue was four- and tenfold higher than in normal bladder epithelium and peripheral blood, respectively.[733]

Combined phase II data from 438 patients revealed that UFT had activity in cancers arising in the stomach (28%), pancreas (25%), gallbladder and bile duct (25%), liver (19%), colon and rectum (25%), breast (32%), and lung (7%).[734] In this series, hematologic toxicity was mild; GI toxicity included anorexia (24%), nausea and vomiting (12.5%), and diarrhea (12%). Another summary article indicated phase II response rates of more than 30% in patients with head and neck, bladder, or breast cancer.[735] A randomized trial of prophylactic oral UFT (300 to 400 mg per day starting within 14 days of surgery for 2 years) for patients with superficial bladder cancer showed a significantly lower recurrence rate in the UFT group (26% vs. 43% for control); with this low-dose schedule, GI symptoms occurred in fewer than 10% of patients.[736]

UFT subsequently entered clinical evaluation on an international basis. Comparison of 5-FU pharmacokinetics with equimolar total daily doses of UFT and CI 5-FU indicated that during the first day, the C_{ss} and AUC_{0-8h} were 1.8- and 1.7-fold higher with infusional 5-FU, respectively (Fig. 8-19).[737] By day 5, however, no appreciable differences were noted between these parameters. With a 28-day schedule followed by a 2-week break, administration of UFT in 3 divided doses every 8 hours was much better tolerated than single-daily or twice-daily dosing.[738] Pharmacokinetic analysis suggested saturation of ftorafur kinetics, resulting in disproportionate increases in the AUC and toxicities with increasing dose levels. A daily dose of 400 mg per m² given in 3 divided doses was recommended on this schedule.[738] A phase II study of UFT (300 to 350 mg per m²) p.o. plus LV (150 mg p.o.) in 3 divided doses daily for

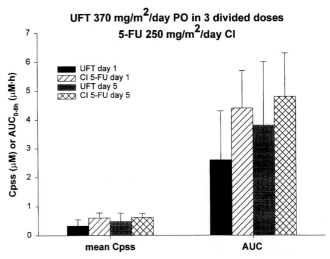

FIGURE 8-19. Comparison of 5-fluorouracil (5-FU) pharmacokinetics in patients receiving continuous infusion 5-FU and uracil and ftorafur (UFT). 5-FU plasma levels were compared in ten patients who received 5-FU 250 mg per m² per day by continuous infusion (CI) for 5 days, followed by a 1-week washout period by UFT 370 mg per m² per day in 3 divided doses for 28 consecutive days. The mean and standard deviation are shown. (AUC, area under the curve; Cpss, concentration of plasma at the steady state.) [Adapted from Ho DH, Pazdur R, Covington W, et al. Comparison of 5-fluorouracil pharmacokinetics in patients receiving continuous 5-fluorouracil infusion and oral uracil plus N_1-(2'-tetrahydrofuryl)-5-fluorouracil. *Clin Cancer Res* 1998;4:2085–2088, with permission from The American Association for Cancer Research.]

28 days revealed a 42% response rate in 45 patients with previously untreated colorectal cancer.[739] With this schedule, GI toxicity is generally mild to moderate in severity and includes anorexia, nausea, vomiting, and diarrhea. Hematologic toxicity is mild, and symptomatic hand-foot syndrome is uncommon. A different schedule tested by the Oncopaz Cooperative Group used a single i.v. dose of LV (500 mg per m²) followed by oral UFT (195 mg per m²) on day 1, followed by oral LV (15 mg) and UFT (195 mg per m²) every 12 hours on days 2 through 14, followed by a 2-week rest.[740] The response rate as first-line therapy in 75 patients with advanced colorectal cancer was 39%. The primary toxicity was GI but was of grade 3 to 4 severity in only 3.5%; hematologic toxicity was minimal, and the regimen was safe even in elderly patients.

The extent of TS inhibition was determined in tumor tissue taken from gastric cancer patients assigned treatment with UFT alone (400 mg ftorafur per day) or with LV (30 mg per day) in divided doses every 12 hours for 3 days before gastrectomy, with the last dose approximately 6 hours before surgery.[741] TS inhibition, estimated by comparing free versus total TS with a ligand-binding assay, was significantly greater in eight patients treated with UFT and LV compared to that measured in nine patients receiving UFT alone (61% vs. 32% inhibition, respectively).[741] A bioavailability study compared the pharmacokinetics of UFT and LV in 18 patients after UFT alone, LV alone, or a combination of the two.[742] When LV was coadministered with UFT, there were no significant effects on tegafur, uracil, or 5-FU C_{max} or AUC; no significant differences were seen in LV and 5-methyltetrahydrofolate plasma levels after LV alone or with UFT. As might be expected, however, great interpatient variability in UFT and LV pharmacology was noted.[742] Although no randomized trials have directly evaluated the benefit of combining LV with UFT versus UFT alone, Bristol-Myers Squibb elected to pursue clinical development in Western countries with a proprietary combination of UFT and oral calcium LV (Orzel) based on the activity seen in phase II studies.[743] The monthly schedule was selected for randomized trials owing to the higher projected dose intensity (2,100 vs. 1,365 mg per m² per week) and excellent safety profile.

The results of two large phase III trials comparing UFT plus LV with the monthly schedule of bolus 5-FU plus LV in patients with metastatic colorectal cancer suggest comparable efficacy (response rates, 12% vs. 15% and 11% vs. 9%) but a more favorable safety profile with significantly fewer episodes of febrile neutropenia and infection (Fig. 8-20).[744,745] The National Surgical Breast and Bowel Project protocol C-06 has compared the 28-day schedule of UFT plus LV with weekly bolus 5-FU and high-dose LV as adjuvant therapy for stage II and III colon cancer.[746] Accrual was completed in mid-1999, and the data are maturing.

5'-Deoxy-5-Fluorouridine

The synthetic fluoropyrimidine 5'-deoxy-5-fluorouridine (5'-dFUrd, doxifluridine, Furtulon, MW = 246) has shown promising antitumor activity and increased specificity for tumor cells as compared with normal tissues in some preclinical models.[747–760] Because the 5'-carbon of the ribose moiety lacks a hydroxyl group, 5'-dFUrd cannot serve as a

substrate for Urd kinase. Urd and dThd phosphorylase are potentially capable of liberating 5-FU by cleaving the glycosidic bond. 5-FU is thus released intracellularly and can undergo further metabolic activation.[747,748,751–754,756–761] Urd phosphorylase primarily cleaves pyrimidine ribonucleosides but also cleaves pyrimidine 2'- and 5'-deoxyribonucleosides. In contrast, dThd phosphorylase is thought to be relatively specific for pyrimidine 2'- and 5'-deoxyribonucleosides.[17,18,752,753,761–765] Urd phosphorylase is present in virtually all normal and tumor tissues studied, whereas the activity of dThd phosphorylase is much more variable in human and rodent tumors.[17,18,597,753,756,763–765] Distinct differences exist between the enzymes isolated from human and mouse tissues in terms of biologic properties, substrate specificities, and their roles in the metabolism of natural-pyrimidine nucleosides and their 5-fluorinated analogs.[761] Substrate specificity also varies between enzymes from different human tissues, suggesting the presence of isoenzymes. In human liver, dThd phosphorylase contributes from 99% to 100% of the phosphorolysis of 5'-dFUrd and FdUrd, whereas the contribution from dThd phosphorylase isolated from mouse liver (73% and 83%, respectively) or human placenta (86% and 93%, respectively) is lower.[761] The inter- and intraspecies differences in substrate specificities and activities between human and murine pyrimidine nucleoside phosphorylases suggest problems in extrapolating information from murine studies involving modulators of these enzymes, in combination with fluoropyrimidines, to the clinical setting.

A number of preclinical studies suggest that 5'-dFUrd shows selective cytotoxicity against tumor tissues and relatively low toxicity against normal tissues, presumably because of greater enzymatic activation in neoplastic tissues than in normal tissues.[751–756,758] When 5'-dFUrd is used as the substrate, human and rodent tumor tissue (including esophagus,

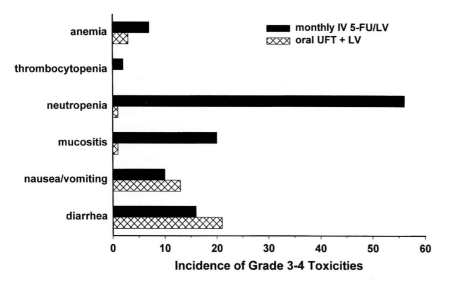

FIGURE 8-20. Toxicity profile of uracil and ftorafur (UFT) plus leucovorin (LV) versus a monthly schedule of 5-fluorouracil (5-FU) plus LV. The incidence of grades 3 and 4 toxicities are shown for patients treated in a phase III trial comparing oral UFT (300 mg per m² per day) and LV (75 or 90 mg per day) on a 28-day schedule every 5 weeks or intravenous 5-FU (425 mg per m² per day) plus LV (25 mg per m² per day) on a daily-for-5-days schedule every 4 weeks. The incidence of severe mucositis, neutropenia, thrombocytopenia, and anemia was significantly lower with UFT and LV. (Adapted from Pazdur R, Douillard J-Y, Skillings JR, et al. Multicenter phase III study of 5-fluorouracil or UFT in combination with leucovorin in patients with metastatic colorectal cancer. *Proc Am Soc Clin Oncol* 1999;18:263a, with permission from the American Society of Clinical Oncology.)

stomach, intestine, pancreas, breast, urinary bladder, and lung) usually contains higher specific activity of pyrimidine phosphorylase(s) than do normal tissues from the same organs, suggesting potentially selective cytotoxicity.[753,756,760] In contrast, nonmalignant human liver tissue has much higher activity than do normal tissues of other digestive organs, but its activity is either comparable to or higher than that in malignant tissues from various origins.[760]

The cytotoxicity of 5'-dFUrd *in vitro* correlates with activity of the pyrimidine phosphorylases.[747,748,751,754,758,759] 5'-dFUrd has selective action in culture against human B cells, which have high levels of Urd phosphorylase.[751] In contrast, human T cells and murine L1210 leukemia cells lack Urd phosphorylase and are resistant to 5'-dFUrd. Comparison of the toxicity of 5'-dFUrd in human tumor cells and human bone marrow *in vitro* indicates that 5'-dFUrd, but not 5-FU or FdUrd, has selective tumor toxicity.[754] Cytokine-mediated increases in Urd and dThd phosphorylase activity have been associated with enhanced *in vitro* sensitivity of human and murine cancer cells to 5'-dFUrd.[747,748,759]

Several investigators have reported that the antitumor activity of 5'-dFUrd against human tumor xenografts, however, does not correlate with the ability of tumor homogenates to convert [^{3}H]5'-dFUrd to 5-FU.[757,760] A possible explanation is that the liver may be the major site of metabolic activation of this prodrug *in vivo*.

Clinical trials have been carried out in Europe and Japan using several schedules. Pharmacokinetic studies after i.v. administration by either rapid 30- or 60-minute infusions reveals nonlinear elimination: 5'-dFUrd metabolism is saturable at plasma levels above 40 to 50 µmol per L; a fall in clearance of the drug occurs with increasing dose.[766–768] With low doses (1 to 2 g per m^2 over 30 minutes), the disappearance of 5'-dFUrd follows first-order kinetics.[766–768] With higher dosages (15 g per m^2), the peak plasma levels are approximately 175 µmol per L, with a primary $t_{1/2}$ of 25 minutes.[768] With rapid i.v. injection of 2 or 4 g per m^2, the clearance falls from 330 to 200 mL per minute per m^2. The peak plasma levels of 5-FU are much lower than 5'-dFUrd levels, and the ratio is influenced by the infusion rate.[769–773] Urinary excretion is virtually 100%; unchanged drug and FBAL account for the majority of the compounds.[770,771] After i.v. bolus, the renal clearance of 5'-dFUrd (166 mL per minute per m^2) exceeds the expected glomerular filtration rate, suggesting that 5'-dFUrd undergoes renal tubular secretion; however, there is no evidence that renal clearance is saturable.[768] The cumulative biliary excretion has been estimated to be 0.8% of the injected dosage.[771] FBAL accounts for approximately 10% of the biliary metabolites, whereas a FBAL–bile acid conjugate is the major metabolite.[771] When 5'-dFUrd is administered by CI over 5 days (0.75 to 4 g per m^2 per day), nonrenal clearance does not appear saturable; C_{ss} levels range from 167 to 6,519 ng per mL (0.7 to 26.5 µmol per L) and increase linearly with dose.[772] Nonrenal clearance averages 728 mL per minute per m^2 and is approximately seven times higher than renal clearance (109 mL per minute per m^2).[772]

Initial phase I testing indicated that myelosuppression and stomatitis were dose limiting at 4,000 mg per m^2 per day for 5 days i.v.; CNS toxicity and ECG changes were also noted.[772,773] With a 6-hour i.v. infusion weekly-for-3-weeks schedule of 5'-dFUrd, neurotoxicity is dose limiting with 10 to 12.5 g per m^2 per week.[772,774] Nausea and vomiting, diarrhea, and cutaneous reactions occur with both schedules.

In phase II studies using the weekly 6-hour infusion schedule, clinical activity was seen in breast cancer (36% response rate) and colorectal cancer (22% response rate).[774] Neurologic toxicity (dizziness, ataxia, and alterations of consciousness) was prominent, however, occurring in 42% of the patients, with four lethal events. 5'-dFUrd is active in colorectal, breast, ovarian, and head and neck cancer when given by rapid i.v. infusion on a daily for 5-days schedule.[775–777] Unfortunately, a high incidence of dose-related neurotoxicity occurred, and the symptoms were reminiscent of Wernicke-Korsakoff syndrome: unsteadiness and diplopia occurred during the second week; ataxia, confusion, and abnormal electroencephalograms were noted by the fourth week.[778] A randomized trial comparing 5-FU (450 mg per m^2 per day × 5) with 5'-dFUrd (4,000 mg per m^2 per day × 5) was interrupted because of cardiac toxicity (chest pain, arrhythmias, and ventricular fibrillation) on the 5'-dFUrd arm; furthermore, 48% of the patients receiving 5'-dFUrd experienced neurotoxicity.[776] The response rate favored the 5'-dFUrd arm (20% of 25 patients vs. 7% of 27 patients with 5-FU). Cardiac toxicity was also observed sporadically in other clinical trials.

Lengthening the infusion of 5'-dFUrd (4 g per m^2 per day × 5) to 1 hour reduces the incidence and severity of neurotoxicity to 16% to 23%.[779,780] A 5-day CI of 5'-dFUrd is well tolerated at daily doses less than or equal to 3.5 g per m^2 except for mild nausea; dose-limiting toxicities at 4 g per m^2 per day include granulocytopenia, thrombocytopenia, mucositis, and rash.[772] Protracted CI of 5'-dFUrd 0.75 g per m^2 daily for 3 months is well tolerated, but hand-foot syndrome is dose limiting.[781]

Two randomized trials compared a 1-hour infusion of either 5'-dFUrd (4 g per m^2 per day) or 5-FU (450 or 500 mg per m^2 per day) daily for 5 days in advanced colorectal cancer.[779,780] The response rate was higher with 5'-dFUrd on both trials (23% of 31 and 5% of 112 patients, respectively) compared with 5-FU (7% of 30 and 1% of 110 patients, respectively), and the time to disease progression favored the 5'-dFUrd arm in one study (48 vs. 39 weeks, $p = .02$); survival was not improved on either trial. A potential criticism of these trials is that the arms were not equitoxic: The 1-hour infusion of 5-FU was relatively nontoxic, but dose escalation was not allowed.

Unlike 5-FU, 5'-dFUrd is well absorbed by the oral route. An oral regimen of 5'-dFUrd 1,200 mg daily for 28 days is well tolerated, with mild to moderate diarrhea, nausea and vomiting as the principal side effects; higher doses were complicated by a higher incidence of diarrhea.[781] Another commonly used oral regimen is *l*-LV 25 mg p.o. followed 2 hours later by 5'-dFUrd 1,200 mg per m² daily for 5 days followed by 5 days rest. With this schedule, C_{max} values for 5'-FdUrd and 5-FU average approximately 67 and 6 µmol per L, respectively.[782] Among 62 previously untreated patients with colorectal cancer, 32% responded, as did 13% of patients with prior systemic–5-FU therapy.[782]

Capecitabine

Capecitabine (N^4-pentoxycarbonyl-5'-deoxy-5-fluorocytidine, Xeloda) is the first oral 5-FU prodrug to be approved in the United States, based on its activity in metastatic breast cancer patients refractory to two earlier regimens.[783] This agent is absorbed intact as the parent drug through the GI mucosa. It then undergoes a three step enzymatic conversion to 5-FU: Hepatic carboxylesterase yields 5'-deoxy-5-fluorocytidine; cytidine deaminase, a widely distributed enzyme, produces 5'-dFUrd; and dThd phosphorylase then generates 5-FU (Fig. 8-21). Clinical studies have documented rapid GI absorption of the parent drug with efficient conversion to doxifluridine, whereas systemic levels of 5-FU have been low.[784,785]

Preclinical studies comparing intracellular accumulation of 5-FU in four human-cancer xenografts (3 sensitive, 1 insensitive to capecitabine), after administration of either oral capecitabine or i.p. 5-FU at their maximum tolerated doses (MTD) on a daily for a 7-day schedule.[786] With 1.5 mmol per kg capecitabine, the median AUC of 5-FU in tumor tissue was 250 nmol per hour per g, which was 120-fold higher than the AUC in plasma. After 0.15 mmol per kg 5-FU, in contrast, the median 5-FU AUC in tumor tissue was 12.2 nmol per hour per g, representing only a two-fold increase over the plasma AUC. Despite the tenfold higher dose of capecitabine, the 5-FU AUC in plasma was approximately one-third of that observed with i.p. injection

of 5-FU. This study provides strong evidence that 5-FU is preferentially formed in tumor tissue versus plasma after capecitabine administration.

In an *in vivo* model, 18 (75%) of 24 human cancer xenografts were sensitive to capecitabine.[787] Among 15 tumors with dThd-phosphorylase activity greater than 50 µg per mg per hr, 87% were sensitive, but 56% of tumors with lower enzyme activity were also sensitive.[787] The authors found that the ratio of dThd phosphorylase to DPD activity, however, provided additional information: Tumors with relatively low ratios were more likely to be resistant, whereas tumors with higher ratios were uniformly sensitive. This information suggests that tumors with low dThd-phosphorylase activity may still retain sensitivity to capecitabine provided the activity of DPD is also low. Conversely, capecitabine might not be effective in tumors with higher dThd phosphorylase if the DPD activity is also high.

The activities of carboxylesterase, cytidine deaminase, and dThd phosphorylase were measured in human tumor and adjacent normal tissue surgically resected from patients with a variety of cancers.[788] Using capecitabine as the substrate, carboxylesterase activity was almost exclusively localized in human-liver and hepatocellular carcinoma, with minimal activity in other tumors and organs, including the intestinal tract and plasma. Homogenates prepared from most normal and tumor tissues were able to deaminate 5'-dFCyd, although normal liver had the highest activity. With 5'-dFUrd as substrate, dThd-phosphorylase activity was detected in all normal tissues, with the highest activity in liver tissue. dThd-phosphorylase activities showed much greater variability in tumor tissue, but with few exceptions, the activity was higher in tumor tissue obtained from 11 different sites of origin than that of the corresponding normal tissues.

Two schedules have been evaluated in the clinic: a continuous schedule for 28 days (MTD 1,600 mg per m² p.o. daily), and a daily for 14 days every 3-weeks schedule (MTD 3,200 mg per m² p.o. daily).[784,785] Capecitabine is given as two equal doses approximately 12 hours apart,

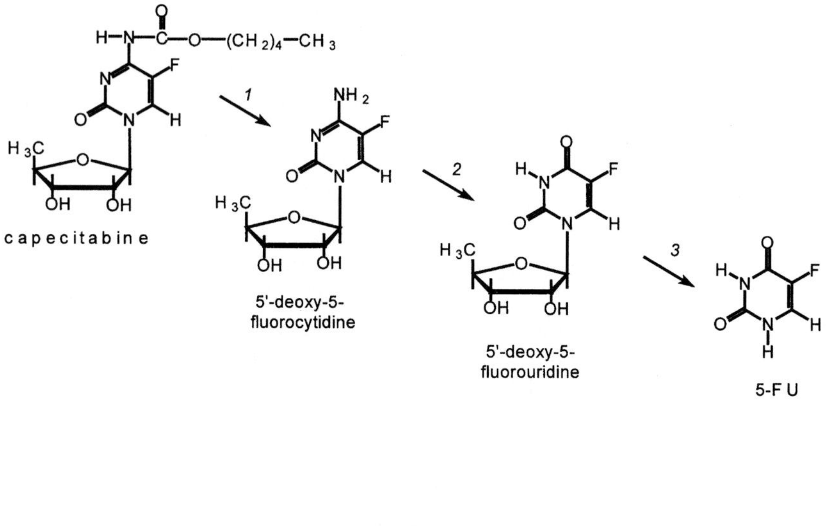

FIGURE 8-21. Activation of capecitabine: The enzymes are 1, carboxylesterase; 2, cytidine deaminase; 3, thymidine phosphorylase. (5-FU, 5-fluorouracil.)

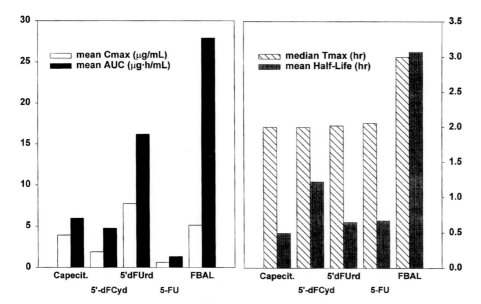

FIGURE 8-22. Pharmacokinetic parameters of capecitabine (Capecit.) on a twice-daily schedule for 14 consecutive days. Pharmacokinetic data of capecitabine and its metabolites from eight patients on day 1 of oral capecitabine, 2,510 mg per m^2 in two equal divided doses. The maximum plasma concentration (Cmax) and area under the plasma concentration-time curve (AUC) are shown as the geometric mean, the time of maximum plasma concentration (Tmax) is shown as the arithmetic median, and the half-life is shown as the arithmetic mean. (5'-DFUR, 5'-deoxy-5-fluorouridine; FBAL, fluoro-β-alanine; 5-FU, 5-fluorouracil; 5'-dFCyd, 5'-deoxy-5-fluorocytidine.) (Adapted from Mackean M, Planting A, Twelves C, et al. Phase I and pharmacologic study of intermittent twice-daily oral therapy with capecitabine in patients with advanced and/or metastatic cancer. *J Clin Oncol* 1998;16:2977-2985, with permission from the American Society of Clinical Oncology.)

taken within 30 minutes after a meal. The toxicity profile favors the daily for 14- of 21-days schedule, with a recommended total daily dose of 2,510 mg per m^2 p.o. When given with low-dose oral LV (60 mg p.o. daily), the recommended total daily dose is 1,650 mg per m^2 for 14 of 21 days.[789] Dose-limiting toxicities include diarrhea, nausea, vomiting, and hand-foot syndrome, whereas myelosuppression is uncommon.

The pharmacokinetics of capecitabine and its metabolites have been measured using a validated liquid chromatography mass spectrometry technique.[785] Representative pharmacokinetic parameters from eight patients after an initial dose of 1,255 mg per m^2 (total daily dose 2,510 mg per m^2) are shown in Figure 8-22. Peak-plasma concentrations are reached approximately 2 hours after oral dosing. The $t_{1/2}$ are approximately 1 hour for all metabolites except for FBAL, which has an initial $t_{1/2}$ of 3 hours. The AUC of 5'-dFUrd is the greatest and exceeds the AUC of 5-FU by approximately 12-fold. Over the dosage range used clinically, there is no evidence of dose dependency in the pharmacokinetic parameters. No appreciable accumulation of either parent drug or metabolites is noted when comparing pharmacokinetic values from days 1 and 14, other than a 22% higher 5-FU AUC on day 14, suggesting a change in 5-FU clearance with time. The relatively low circulating concentrations of 5-FU support the notion that its formation occurs primarily within cells.

Comparison of capecitabine pharmacokinetics before and after food intake indicates a profound effect on the C_{max} of capecitabine and most of its metabolites.[790] The AUC of capecitabine is 1.5-fold higher when taken before food; a moderate effect is also noted for 5'-dFCyd, with a 1.26-fold higher AUC before food. Food ingestion has only a minor influence on the AUC of the other metabolites. The elimination $t_{1/2}$ are not affected. Because the clinical

safety of capecitabine has been determined exclusively with capecitabine taken within 30 minutes after a meal, it is currently recommended that capecitabine be administered with food. The pharmacokinetics of capecitabine have been evaluated in patients with hepatic dysfunction.[791] Although plasma concentrations of capecitabine, 5'-dFUrd, 5-FU, DHFU, and FBAL were, in general, higher in patients with liver dysfunction, the opposite was found for 5'-dFCyd. These effects did not appear to be clinically significant. Twelves et al. concluded that caution should be used when treating patients with moderately impaired hepatic function, but there is no *a priori* need for dose reduction.[791]

Two large randomized phase III trials comparing capecitabine with the monthly schedule of 5-FU and LV (425 mg per m^2 and 20 mg per m^2 daily for 5 days, respectively) in patients with advanced colorectal cancer have been conducted.[792,793] A multiinstitutional trial done in North and South America, involving 605 patients, demonstrated a response rate in favor of capecitabine (23% vs. 16%).[792] Grade 3 to 4 toxicities included hand-foot syndrome (18%) and diarrhea (15%) for capecitabine and neutropenia (26%), mucositis (16%), and diarrhea (14%) for 5-FU and LV. A second international trial using the identical design involved 602 patients. The response rate again favored capecitabine (27% vs. 18%).[793] Hand-foot syndrome and diarrhea of grade 3 to 4 severity occurred in 16% and 10% of capecitabine patients, whereas severe or worse neutropenia, mucositis, and diarrhea occurred in 20%, 13%, and 10% of patients receiving 5-FU and LV.

Eniluracil

The uracil analog eniluracil (776C85, 5-ethynyluracil) is an extremely potent mechanism-based inactivator of DPD and is approximately ninefold more potent than bromvinyl-

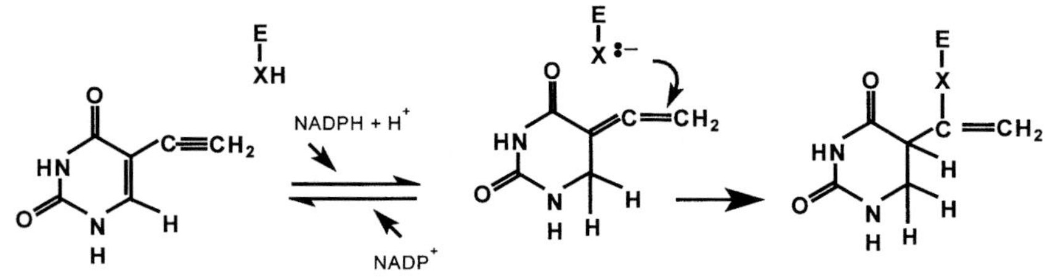

FIGURE 8-23. Interaction between eniluracil and dihydropyrimidine dehydrogenase. (E, dihydropyrimidine dehydrogenase; NADP, nicotinamide adenine dinucleotide; NADPH, nicotinamide adenine dinucleotide phosphate.)

uracil.[794] On binding of eniluracil to DPD (apparent K_m, approximately 1.6 µmol per L), an unstable intermediate is formed, after which the drug becomes covalently linked to the enzyme through modification of an amino acid residue (Fig. 8-23).[794] Administration of eniluracil to animals and humans results in complete inhibition of DPD throughout the body, as evidenced directly by enzyme assays and indirectly by up to 100-fold elevations of plasma-uracil levels.[795–797] When given with eniluracil, renal excretion of 5-FU becomes the predominant route of elimination. Oral administration of 5-FU with eniluracil renders 5-FU completely bioavailable.

Although eniluracil appears to be nontoxic when given alone, it shifts the 5-FU dose toxicity–response curves to lower doses. When 5-FU is given alone at the MTD on a daily-for-4-days schedule, 75% of rats bearing advanced colon cancers have partial responses.[797] In contrast, when eniluracil (1 mg per kg per day) is combined with 5-FU at one-tenth the single-agent dose, 100% of the rats have complete tumor regressions that are sustained for at least 90 days posttherapy.[197] Moreover, the results with eniluracil plus 5-FU are superior to those obtained with 5-FU given by continuous infusion for 4 days, suggesting that the improved antitumor activity is not simply due to prolonged 5-FU plasma exposure. Additional studies in rats bearing s.c. colon cancer compared treatment with either ftorafur, UFT, eniluracil plus ftorafur, or eniluracil plus UFT.[798] The combination of ftorafur plus eniluracil had the greatest antitumor activity and was superior to UFT and ftorafur alone; eniluracil did not improve the activity of UFT. The total 5-FU AUC did not correlate with the rank order of antitumor efficacy. Endogenous plasma-uracil levels (1 to 3 µmol per L) were not affected by ftorafur but increased to approximately 100 µmol per L after 5-FU and eniluracil and to approximately 800 µmol per L after UFT.[798] These findings suggest that although moderately elevated levels of uracil may be beneficial, high uracil levels seen with UFT may counteract the antitumor effects. To test the hypothesis that 5-FU catabolites may attenuate the antitumor activity of 5-FU, the antitumor activity of three regimens was compared in the rat model: 5-FU alone (100 mg per kg), eniluracil (1 mg per kg) followed by 5-FU (10 mg per kg), and eniluracil (10 mg per kg) followed by 5-FU (10 mg per kg) and DHFU (90 mg per kg). The regimen was repeated

weekly for 3 weeks on all arms. The complete response rate was 13% with 5-FU alone, 94% with eniluracil plus 5-FU, and 38% with the three-drug combination, indicating that administration of DHFU interfered with the efficacy of eniluracil plus 5-FU.[799]

5-FU metabolism was monitored in an isolated rat liver perfusion model with fluorine-19 nuclear magnetic resonance spectroscopy during perfusion with 5-FU alone (15 mg per kg) or 5-FU preceded by eniluracil (0.5 mg per kg). Eniluracil produced a striking 27-fold decrease in the formation of catabolites and a sevenfold increase in anabolite formation.[800] Specifically, eniluracil prevented the formation of the toxic catabolites FBAL, fluoroacetate, and 2-fluoro-3-hydroxypropionic acid, which have been implicated in 5-FU–associated neurotoxicity and cardiac toxicity. This methodology has also been used to study the effect of eniluracil on the metabolism of 5-FU in mice bearing murine colon 38 tumors.[801] *Ex vivo* measurements of tissue extracts from liver, kidney, and tumor indicate a greater than 95% elimination of FUPA and FBAL signals in the tissues of mice that received 2 mg per kg of EU before administration of 5-FU. Furthermore, a prolonged presence of 5-FU and increased formation of fluoronucleotides was noted in normal and tumor tissues.[801] In a canine model, a 26-hour CI of 5-FU (40 mg per kg), which produces C_{ss} of 1.3 µmol per L, is associated with severe neurotoxicity manifest by seizures, muscle tremors, and ataxia. Administration of eniluracil (1 mg per kg s.c.) 30 minutes before the start of 5-FU infusion, then repeated every 6 hours during a CI of 5-FU (at 1.6 and 4.0 mg per kg), was associated with much higher mean C_{ss} plasma levels (2.4 and 5.3 µmol per L, respectively); neurotoxicity was not observed, although mild GI toxicity occurred with the higher dosage of 5-FU.[375] The preclinical data clearly indicate that eniluracil-mediated inhibition of DPD prevents the formation of potentially toxic catabolites but also increases 5-FU anabolism within tissues.

Interspecies allometric scaling of 5-FU pharmacokinetic data obtained from mice, rats, and dogs treated with eniluracil followed by 5-FU predicted that the MTD of 5-FU given as a single i.v. bolus, or by CI for 5 or 12 days, would be 110, 50, and 30 mg per m², respectively.[802] Initial studies of oral eniluracil given once daily for 7 days at 0.74, 3.7, or 18.5 mg per m² indicated that DPD activity in PBMCs was inactivated within 1 hour and remained inhibited by 93%

to 98% 24 hours after dosing.[803] Fourteen days post eniluracil, mean-DPD activity was approximately 60% (0.74 mg per m^2), 70% (3.7 mg per m^2), and 125% (18.5 mg per m^2) relative to baseline values. Because lower dosages of eniluracil would be expected to produce faster recovery, the observations from this early study perhaps suggest variability in the duration of DPD inhibition among patients.

Pharmacokinetic comparison of 5-FU (10 mg per m^2) given either i.v. or p.o. on day 2 with oral eniluracil (3.7 mg per m^2 p.o.) on days 1 and 2 (24 hours and 30 minutes before the 5-FU dose) indicated complete oral bioavailability of 5-FU.[804] The terminal $t_{1/2}$ of 5-FU was prolonged to approximately 4.5 hours, and the systemic clearance was reduced to approximately 60 mL per minute per m^2. Patients later received escalating doses of oral 5-FU on days 2 through 6 with eniluracil (3.7 mg per m^2 p.o.) on days 1 through 7. The MTD of 5-FU was 25 mg per m^2. In a second phase I trial, no toxicity was observed after the administration of eniluracil at doses of 0.74, 3.7, and 18.5 mg per m^2 p.o. daily for 7 days.[803] After a 14-day washout period, the assigned dose of eniluracil was given daily for 3 days with 5-FU (10 mg per m^2 i.v.) on day 2. No toxicity was seen during this second period. With 50 mg of eniluracil on days 1 through 3 and either 10 mg per m^2 i.v. or 20 mg p.o. 5-FU on day 2, the $t_{1/2}$ of 5-FU averaged 4.9 and 6.1 hours, respectively. After another 14-day washout, patients received eniluracil p.o. on days 1 through 7 with escalating doses of either oral or i.v. 5-FU. Neutropenia and thrombocytopenia were dose limiting; nonhematologic toxicities occurred less frequently but included nausea, vomiting, diarrhea, anorexia, mucositis, and fatigue. When 5-FU was given on days 2 through 6 with 50 mg each of eniluracil and LV on days 1 through 7, the recommended dose of oral 5-FU was 15 mg per m^2, which is 28-fold lower than the customary dose of 5-FU and LV on a monthly schedule.

A 28-day schedule has also been explored in which eniluracil and 5-FU were administered orally twice a day. The currently recommended doses of eniluracil and 5-FU are 10 and 1 mg per m^2 twice daily for 28 of 35 days. For the majority of the subsequent phase II and III trials, a combination tablet that incorporates eniluracil and 5-FU in a dose ratio of 10 to 1 is being used. Preliminary results of phase II trials using the oral 28-day regimen of eniluracil indicate the regimen is active as first-line therapy in breast cancer (52% of 29 patients responded) and colorectal cancer (24% of 45 patients responded).[805,806] In the phase II trial in breast cancer, using the 10 and 1 mg per m^2 twice daily for 28 of 35 days schedule, diarrhea and mucositis of mild to moderate severity occurred in 36% and 12% of patients.[805] Other common grade 1 to 2 toxicities included fatigue and lethargy (27%), nausea (24%), and headache (9%). In the colorectal cancer trial, patients received either 1 or 1.15 mg per m^2 5-FU with a tenfold excess of eniluracil twice daily for 28 of 35 days. Toxicity was slightly greater in this trial, and grade 3 to 4 toxicities of the following types were seen: diarrhea, 13%; mucositis, 3%; granulocytopenia, 3%.[806] In contrast to protracted infusional 5-FU, hand-foot syndrome was not a problem. Phase III trials are under way that are comparing the oral 28-day schedule of eniluracil and 5-FU as first-line therapy for colorectal cancer with either i.v. bolus 5-FU plus LV or protracted infusional 5-FU.

A weekly schedule intended to simulate a high-dose 24-hour CI of 5-FU used 20 mg eniluracil and 15 mg LV orally twice daily for 3 days, with oral 5-FU given twice daily on day 2, repeated weekly for 3 of 4 weeks. GI toxicity was dose limiting, and the recommended dose of 5-FU was 10 mg per m^2 p.o. twice daily.[807] The tolerated daily doses of 5-FU plus eniluracil on the schedules intended to mimic CI 5-FU are more than 100-fold lower than the comparable i.v. dose of 5-FU without eniluracil (Table 8-15), whereas the recommended 5-FU dose with eniluracil on schedules, intended to reflect a monthly i.v. bolus schedule, are 20- to 30-fold lower. The explanation may be that twice-daily dosing of 5-FU and eniluracil results in more sustained exposure of normal tissues to 5-FU metabolites.

Because some patients receiving a subsequent 5-FU–type regimen 3 to 5 weeks after completing protocol ther-

TABLE 8-15. COMPARISON OF RECOMMENDED 5-FLUOROURACIL DOSAGES ± CONCURRENT ENILURACIL

Cycle	Oral Eniluracil	5-Fluorouracil (mg/m^2)	Leucovorin (mg)	Difference in Total Daily 5-Fluorouracil Dose
q 4 wk	0	425 i.v. d 1–5	20/m^2 d 1–5	—
q 4 wk	50 mg d 1–7	15 p.o. d 2–6	50 p.o. d 2–6	28-fold
q 4 wk	10 mg d 1–7	20 i.v. d 2–6	50 i.v. d 2–6	21-fold
q 4 wk	0	500 i.v. d 1–5	0	—
q 4 wk	10 mg d 1–7	25 i.v. d 2–6	0	20-fold
q 4 wk	3.7 mg/m^2 or 10 mg d 1–7	25 p.o. d 2–6	0	20-fold
q 5 wk	0	300 i.v. d 1–28	0	—
q 5 wk	10 mg/m^2 b.i.d. d 1–28	1.0 p.o. b.i.d. d 1–28	0	150-fold
q wk	0	2,600	±500 mg/m^2	—
q wk	20 mg b.i.d. d 1–3 q wk × 3 of 4 wk	10 p.o. b.i.d. d 2 q wk × 3 of 4 wk	15 mg p.o. b.i.d. d 1–3 q wk × 3 of 4 wk	130-fold

apy with eniluracil and 5-FU have experienced life-threatening or fatal toxicity, it is currently recommended that a minimum of 8 weeks elapse between the last dose of eniluracil and subsequent therapy with another 5-fluoropyrimidine. In the phase I trial simulating the weekly high-dose CI schedule, pharmacodynamic studies suggested prolonged inhibition of DPD for up to 19 days after the last dose of eniluracil as reflected by DPD-catalytic activity in PBMCs and elevated uracil levels compared to baseline values.[807] Additional pharmacodynamic studies are planned by Glaxo-Wellcome to define more precisely the duration of DPD inhibition in a population-based study of patients treated with the 28-day twice-daily schedule.

S-1

S-1 is a three-drug preparation containing ftorafur, 5-chloro-2,4-dihydroxypyridine, and potassium oxonate in a 1.0 to 0.4 to 1.0 molar ratio.[808] 5-Chloro-2,4-dihydroxypyridine is a competitive, reversible inhibitor of DPD and is approximately 180-fold more potent than uracil *in vitro*. Oxonic acid (5-aza-orotic acid) strongly inhibits the anabolism of 5-FU to FUMP by OPRT *in vitro* and *in vivo*. Preclinical studies evaluating oral administration of 5-FU and oxonic acid have documented reduced formation of FUMP and 5-FU–RNA incorporation in GI tissues, but not in tumor or bone marrow.[809–816] The GI toxicity is greatly reduced compared to 5-FU alone, without loss of antitumor activity.[809]

The antitumor activity of S-1 and UFT was compared against human colon carcinoma orthotopically transplanted in nude rats.[810] After implantation of a single-cell suspension of KMC12 cells into the subserosal layer of the colon, extensive local tumor growth and invasion to the mucosa and serosa occurred, followed by metastatic foci in lymph nodes and lung. Equitoxic doses of S-1 (15 mg per kg per day) and UFT (30 mg per kg per day) were given by mouth for 14 consecutive days starting 7 days after tumor implantation. Tumor weight, measured on day 21, indicated that S-1 inhibited tumor growth to a much greater extent than did UFT (57% vs. 18%).[810] Pharmacokinetic studies revealed that the 5-FU AUC over a 24-hour period was 3.5-fold higher after a single dose of S-1 compared to that achieved with UFT; this translated into 1.3-fold higher 5-FU–RNA levels in colonic tumor tissue. Maximal TS inhibition, seen 4 hours after dosing, was 55% after S-1 and 35% with UFT.

The antitumor activity, toxicity, and achieved plasma concentrations of 5-FU with MTD of S-1, ftorafur, and 5-FU were compared in rats bearing advanced colorectal cancer.[815] When given on a 7- or 28-day schedule, S-1 produced less stomatitis, diarrhea, and alopecia than either ftorafur or 5-FU. Furthermore, the therapeutic index (the ratio of the MTD vs. the minimum effective dose) was 5.3 (7 day) and 3.8 (28 day), compared to ratios less than or equal to 1.0 to

1.25 for ftorafur and 5-FU on both schedules. 5-FU plasma levels were comparable 4 and 8 hours post S-1 dosing compared to infusional 5-FU, but were approximately 60% lower by 24 hours. S-1 therapy resulted in more sustained inhibition of TS and induction of apoptosis in tumor cells and produced superior antitumor activity.[815]

A daily-for-7-days schedule of either oral S-1 (30 mg per kg per day) or CI 5-FU (40 mg per kg per day) resulted in almost complete inhibition of the tumor growth in Yoshida sarcoma–bearing rats.[816] Rats given infusional 5-FU had significantly more toxicity, however, manifest by marked weight loss and severe diarrhea. The ratio of the 5-fluoronucleotide concentrations in normal GI versus tumor tissue was lower in rats treated with S-1. Thus, although both regimens produced equal antitumor effects, S-1 had a markedly superior therapeutic index compared to infusional 5-FU.

Phase II testing in Japan used a twice-daily oral administration for 28 days followed by a 2-week rest, with a total daily dosage equivalent to 50 mg to 80 mg per m² of ftorafur. In the late phase II trials, patients tended to receive a fixed daily dose depending on their body surface area (total daily dosage given in two divided doses): less than 1.25 m², 80 mg; 1.25 to 1.50 m², 100 mg; greater than or equal to 1.5 m², 120 mg. S-1 appears to have activity in a number of tumor types. Two trials in gastric cancer revealed response rates of 49% (n = 51) and 40% (n = 50).[817,818] The same schedule of S-1 was associated with response rates of 36% in colorectal cancer (n = 62), 29% in head and neck cancer (n = 59), and 41% in breast cancer (n = 27).[819–821] Clinical toxicity tended to be mild. In four trials, the incidence of grade 3 to 4 granulocytopenia ranged from 5% to 13%, whereas grade 3 to 4 diarrhea was observed in fewer than 2% of patients.[817–820]

An HPLC and gas chromatography–negative ion chemical ionization mass spectrometry method has been developed to analyze the constituents of S-1 and 5-FU in plasma and urine.[822] In four patients receiving a 50-mg dose of S-1, the C_{max} of ftorafur and 5-FU were 1,693 ng per mL (8.5 μmol per L) at approximately 3 hours and 83 ng per mL (0.64 μmol per L) at 4 hours, respectively. Similar results were seen in another trial: The C_{max} of ftorafur and 5-FU occurred at approximately 2.4 hours and 3.5 hours after dosing; the C_{max} of ftorafur was approximately tenfold higher than that of 5-FU (9.9 μmol per L vs. 0.99 μmol per L), whereas the AUC_{0-48h} was 25-fold higher (141 μmol per L per hour vs. 5.6 μmol per L per hour).[823] The plasma $t_{1/2}$ are approximately 13 (ftorafur) and 2 (5-FU) hours.

Two trials done in the Netherlands and North America also evaluated the twice daily for 28 days schedule followed by a 7-day rest.[824,825] In one trial, diarrhea was dose limiting at doses greater than or equal to 40 mg per m², whereas 25 or 35 mg per m² doses were better tolerated.[824] The $t_{1/2}$ of 5-FU was approximately 3 hours, and the occurrence of diarrhea correlated with the AUC, but not with the C_{max}. In the other trial, dose-limiting diarrhea and neutropenia occurred at greater than or equal to 35 mg per m^2; 30 mg per m^2 was the recommended dose.[825] Additional clinical trials are planned on an international basis.

BOF-A2

BOF-A2 (emitefur, 3-{3-[6-benzoyloxy-3-cyano-2-pyridyl-oxycarbonyl]benzoyl}-1-ethoxymethyl-5-fluorouracil; MW, approximately 558) is composed of 1-ethoxymethyl-5-fluorouracil, a masked 5-FU prodrug, and 3-cyano-2,6-dihydroxypyridine (CNDP), a potent inhibitor of DPD.[826–828] CNDP is an approximately 2,000-fold more potent inhibitor of 5-FU catabolism by DPD than uracil, but does not affect the enzymes involved in 5-FU activation. *In vivo*, BOF-A2 is degraded to 1-ethoxymethyl–5-FU and CNDP; the former is gradually converted to 5-FU in hepatic microsomes. When given on a daily schedule, BOF-A2 has antitumor activity against various experimental tumors and human lung cancer xenografts.[826–833]

Using a rat model of lung tumors established from i.v.-injected Yoshida sarcoma cells, the concentration of 5-FU in tumor tissue was determined at 2, 6, and 12 hours after oral administration of either BOF-A2 (36 μmol per kg) or UFT (50 μmol per kg); these doses were selected to achieve similar 5-FU plasma concentrations 1 hour after dosing.[829] The highest 5-FU level in tumor tissue (90 ng per g) occurred 6 hours after UFT dosing, at which time it was 14- and 1.4-fold higher than that in the plasma and normal lung tissue; by 12 hours, the intratumoral 5-FU level had decreased almost fivefold to 19 ng per g.[829] After BOF-A2, the highest 5-FU level in tumor tissue (217 ng per g) also was noted at 6 hours and was 7- and 2.4-fold higher than that in the plasma and normal lung tissue. By 12 hours, the intratumoral–5-FU level had decreased by less than twofold to 130 ng per g.

There is, as yet, only limited information from clinical trials of this novel oral 5-FU prodrug. A multicenter phase II trial of BOF-A2, 200 mg p.o. twice daily for 14 days, followed by a 2-week rest period, was reported in Japanese patients with non–small cell lung cancer; approximately half the patients had received prior chemotherapy.[834] The response rate in 62 evaluable patients was 18%, and responses were noted in squamous cell and adenocarcinoma histologies. This regimen was well tolerated, with grade 2 or worse myelosuppression occurring in fewer than 10% of patients. The incidence of grade 2 or worse GI toxicity was similarly low (anorexia, 19%; diarrhea, mucositis, and nausea and vomiting, approximately 10% each).

A North American phase I trial evaluated BOF-A2 and LV, 90 mg p.o., given in 3 divided doses daily for 14 days, followed by a 1-week rest.[835] Dose-limiting mucositis and diarrhea were seen at the initial dose level with a total daily dose of 200 mg per m^2 BOF-A2. The same total daily dose of BOF-A2 given with 60 mg LV in 2 divided doses with was better tolerated. Preliminary information suggests

some activity in colorectal cancer patients resistant to prior 5-FU–based therapy. However, ongoing trials will define suitable dosages for phase II trials.

REFERENCES

1. Heidelberger C, Chaudhuari NK, Daneberg P, et al. Fluorinated pyrimidines. A new class of tumor inhibitory compounds. *Nature* 1957;179:663–666.
2. Rutman RJ, Cantarow A, Paschkis KE. Studies on 2-acetylaminofluorene carcinogenesis: III. The utilization of uracil-2-C^{14} by pre-neoplastic rat liver. *Cancer Res* 1954;14:119–126.
3. Wohlhueter RM, McIvor RS, Plagemann PGW. Facilitated transport of uracil and 5-fluorouracil, and permeation of orotic acid into cultured mammalian cells. *J Cell Physiol* 1980;104:309–319.
4. Walliser S, Redmann K. Effect of 5-fluorouracil and thymidine on the transmembrane potential of HeLa cells. *Cancer Res* 1978;40:3555–3559.
5. Domin BA, Mahony WB, Zimmerman TP. Transport of 5-fluorouracil and uracil into human erythrocytes. *Biochem Pharmacol* 1993;46:503–510.
6. Bowen D, Diasio RB, Goldman ID. Distinguishing between membrane transport and intracellular metabolism of fluorodeoxyuridine in Ehrlich ascites tumor cells by application of kinetic and high-performance liquid chromatographic techniques. *J Biol Chem* 1979;254:5333–5339.
7. Reyes P, Hall TC. Synthesis of 5-fluorouridine 5'-phosphate by a pyrimidine phosphoribosyltransferase of mammalian origin: I. Some properties of the enzyme from P-1534J mouse leukemia cells. *Biochemistry* 1969;8:2057–2062.
8. Kessel D, Deacon J, Coffey B, et al. Some properties of a pyrimidine phosphoribosyltransferase from murine leukemia cells. *Mol Pharmacol* 1972;8:731–739.
9. Schwartz PM, Handschumacher RE. Selective antagonism of 5-fluorouracil cytotoxicity by 4-hydroxypyrazolopyrimidine (allopurinol) in vitro. *Cancer Res* 1979;39:3095–3101.
10. Cory J, Breland JB, Carter GL. Effect of 5-fluorouracil on RNA metabolism in Novikoff hepatoma cells. *Cancer Res* 1979;39:4905–4913.
11. Cadman E, Davis L, Heimer R. Enhanced 5-fluorouracil nucleotide formation following methotrexate: biochemical explanation for drug synergism. *Science* 1979;205:1135–1137.
12. Houghton JA, Houghton RJ. 5-Fluorouracil in combination with hypoxanthine and allopurinol: toxicity and metabolism in xenografts of human colonic carcinomas in mice. *Biochem Pharmacol* 1980;29:2077–2080.
13. Benz C, Cadman E. Modulation of 5-fluorouracil metabolism and cytotoxicity by antimetabolite pretreatment in human colorectal adenocarcinoma HCT-8. *Cancer Res* 1981;41:994–999.
14. Houghton JA, Houghton PJ. Elucidation of pathways of 5-fluorouracil metabolism in xenografts of human colorectal adenocarcinoma. *Eur J Cancer Clin Oncol* 1983;19:807–815.
15. Finan PJ, Kiklitis PA, Chisholm EM, et al. Comparative levels of tissue enzymes concerned in the early metabolism of 5-fluorouracil in normal and malignant human colorectal tissue. *Br J Cancer* 1984;50:711–715.

16. Schwartz PM, Moir RD, Hyde CM, et al. Role of uridine phosphorylase in the anabolism of 5-fluorouracil. *Biochem Pharmacol* 1987;34:3585–3589.

17. Woodman PW, Sarrif AM, Heidelberger C. Specificity of pyrimidine nucleoside phosphorylases and the phosphorolysis of 5-fluoro-2' deoxyuridine. *Cancer Res* 1980;40:507–511.

18. Niedzwicki JG, El Kouni MH, Chu SH, et al. Structure activity relationship of ligands of the pyrimidine nucleoside phosphorylases. *Biochem Pharmacol* 1983;32:399–415.

19. Pogolotti AL, Nolan PA, Santi DV. Methods for the complete analysis of 5-fluorouracil metabolites in cell extracts. *Anal Biochem* 1981;117:178–186.

20. Peterson MS, Ingraham HA, Goulian M. 2'-Deoxyribosyl analogues of UDP-N-acetylglucosamine in cells treated with methotrexate or 5-fluorodeoxyuridine. *J Biol Chem* 1983;258:10831–10834.

21. Peters GJ, Laurensse E, Lankelma J, et al. Separation of several 5-fluorouracil metabolites in various melanoma cell lines: evidence for the synthesis of 5-fluorouracil-nucleotide sugars. *Eur J Cancer Clin Oncol* 1984;20:1425–1431.

22. Santi DV, McHenry CS, Sommer A. Mechanisms of interactions of thymidylate synthetase with 5-fluorodeoxyuridylate. *Biochemistry* 1974;13:471–480.

23. Sommer A, Santi DV. Purification and amino acid analysis of an active site peptide from thymidylate synthetase containing covalently bound 5'-fluoro-2'-deoxyuridylate and methylene tetrachloride. *Biochem Biophys Res Commun* 1974;57:689–696.

24. Howell SB, Mansfield SJ, Taetle R. Significance of variation in serum thymidine concentration for the marrow toxicity of methotrexate. *Cancer Chemother Pharmacol* 1981;5:221–226.

25. Dolnick BJ, Cheng Y-C. Human thymidylate synthetase derived from blast cells of patients with acute myelocytic leukemia. *J Biol Chem* 1977;252:7697–7703.

26. Dolnick BJ, Cheng Y-C. Human thymidylate synthase: II. Derivatives of pteroylmono- and polyglutamates as substrates and inhibitors. *J Biol Chem* 1978;253:3563–3567.

27. Fernandes DJ, Bertino JR. 5-Fluorouracil-methotrexate synergy: enhancement of 5-fluorodeoxyuridylate binding to thymidylate synthetase by dihydropteroylpolyglutamates. *Proc Natl Acad Sci U S A* 1980;77:5663–5667.

28. Allegra CJ, Chabner BA, Jolivet J. Enhanced inhibition of thymidylate synthase by methotrexate polyglutamates. *J Biol Chem* 1986;230:9720–9726.

29. Ullman B, Lee M, Martin DW Jr, et al. Cytotoxicity of 5-fluoro-2'-deoxyuridine: requirement for reduced folate cofactors and antagonism by methotrexate. *Proc Natl Acad U S A* 1978;75:980–983.

30. Danenberg KD, Danenberg PV. Evidence for sequential interaction of the subunits of thymidylate synthetase. *J Biol Chem* 1979;254:4345–4348.

31. Murinson DS, Anderson T, Schwartz HS, et al. Competitive radioassay for 5-fluorodeoxyuridine 5'-monophosphate in tissues. *Cancer Res* 1979;39:2471–2479.

32. Washtien WL, Santi DV. Assay of intracellular free and macromolecular-bound metabolites of 5-fluorodeoxyuridine and 5-fluorouracil. *Cancer Res* 1979;39:3397–3404.

33. Hardy LW, Finer-Moore JS, Montfort WR, et al. Atomic structure of thymidylate synthase: target for rational drug design. *Science* 1987;235:448–455.

34. Santi DV, McHenry CS, Raines RT, et al. Kinetics and thermodynamics of the interaction of 5-fluoro-2'-deoxyuridylate. *Biochemistry* 1987;26:8606–8613.

35. Appelt K, Bacquet RJ, Bartlett CA, et al. Design of enzyme inhibitors using iterative protein crystallographic analysis. *J Med Chem* 1991;34:1925–1934.

36. Schoichet BK, Stroud RM, Santi DV, et al. Structure-based discovery of inhibitors of thymidylate synthase. *Science* 1993;259:1445–1450.

37. Madoc-Jones J, Bruce WR. On the mechanism of the lethal action of 5-fluorouracil in mouse L-cells. *Cancer Res* 1968;28:1976–1981.

38. Murgo AJ, Fried J, Burchenal D, et al. Effects of thymidine and thymidine plus 5-fluorouracil on the growth kinetics of a human lymphoid cell line. *Cancer Res* 1980;40:1543–1549.

39. Maybaum J, Ullman B, Mandel HG, et al. Regulation of RNA- and DNA-directed actions of 5-fluoropyrimidines in mouse T-lymphoma (S-49) cells. *Cancer Res* 1980;40:4209–4215.

40. Evans RM, Laskin JD, Hakala MT. Assessment of growth-limiting events caused by 5-fluorouracil in mouse cells and in human cells. *Cancer Res* 1980;40:4113–4122.

41. Spiegelman S, Nayak R, Sawyer R, et al. Potentiation of the antitumor activity of 5-FU by thymidine and its correlation with the formation of (5-FU) RNA. *Cancer* 1980;45:1129–1134.

42. Spiegelman S, Sawyer R, Nayak R, et al. Improving the antitumor activity of 5-fluorouracil by increasing its incorporation into RNA via metabolic modulation. *Proc Natl Acad Sci U S A* 1980;77:4996–4970.

43. Santelli G, Valeriote F. In vivo enhancement of 5-fluorouracil cytotoxicity to AKR leukemia cells by thymidine in mice. *J Natl Cancer Inst* 1978;61:843–847.

44. Carrico CK, Glazer RI. Augmentation by thymidine of the incorporation and distribution of 5-fluorouracil into ribosomal RNA. *Biochem Biophys Res Commun* 1979;87:664–670.

45. Kufe DW, Egan EM. Enhancement of 5-fluorouracil incorporation into human lymphoblast ribonucleic acid. *Biochem Pharmacol* 1981;30:129–133.

46. Wilkinson DS, Tisty TD, Hanas RJ. The inhibition of ribosomal RNA synthesis and maturation in Novikoff hepatoma cells by 5-fluorouridine. *Cancer Res* 1975;35:3014–3020.

47. Chaudhuri NK, Montag BJ, Heidelberger C. Studies on fluorinated pyrimidines: III. The metabolism of 5-fluorouracil-2-^{14}C and 5-fluoroorotic-2-^{14}C acid in vivo. *Cancer Res* 1958;18:318–328.

48. Harbers E, Chaudhuri NK, Heidelberger C. Studies on fluorinated pyrimidines: VIII. Further biochemical and metabolic investigations. *J Biol Chem* 1959;234:1255–1262.

49. Herrick D, Kufe DW. Lethality associated with incorporation of 5-fluorouracil into preribosomal RNA. *Mol Pharmacol* 1984;26:135–140.

50. Kanamaru R, Kakuta H, Sato T, et al. The inhibitory effects of 5-fluorouracil on the metabolism of preribosomal and ribosomal RNA in L-1210 cells in vitro. *Cancer Chemother Pharmacol* 1986;17:43–46.

51. Greenhalgh DA, Parish JH. Effect of 5-fluorouracil combination therapy on RNA processing in human colonic carcinoma cells. *Br J Cancer* 1990;61:415–419.

52. Ghoshal K, Jacob ST. Specific inhibition of pre-ribosomal RNA processing in extracts from the lymphosarcoma cells treated with 5-fluorouracil. *Cancer Res* 1994;54:632–636.

53. Ghoshal K, Jacob ST. An alternative molecular mechanism of action of 5-fluorouracil, a potent anticancer drug. *Biochem Pharmacol* 1997;53:1569–1575.

54. Kufe DW, Major PP. 5-Fluorouracil incorporation into human breast carcinoma RNA correlates with cytotoxicity. *J Biol Chem* 1981;256:9802–9805.

55. Glazer RI, Lloyd LS. Association of cell lethality with incorporation of 5-fluorouracil and 5-fluorouridine into nuclear RNA in human colon carcinoma cells in culture. *Mol Pharmacol* 1982;21:468–473.

56. Laskin JD, Evans RM, Slocum HK, et al. Basis for natural variation in sensitivity to 5-fluorouracil in mouse and human cells in culture. *Cancer Res* 1979;39:383–390.

57. Spears CP, Shani J, Shahinian AH, et al. Assay and time course of 5-fluorouracil incorporation into RNA of L1210/0 ascites cells in vivo. *Mol Pharmacol* 1985;27:302–307.

58. Carrico CK, Glazer RI. The effect of 5-fluorouracil on the synthesis and translation of poly(A) RNA from regenerating liver. *Cancer Res* 1979;39:3694–3701.

59. Tseng W-C, Medina D, Randerath K. Specific inhibition of transfer RNA methylation and modification in tissue of mice treated with 5-fluorouracil. *Cancer Res* 1978;38:1250–1257.

60. Glazer RI, Legraverend M. The effect of 5-fluorouridine 5'-triphosphate on RNA transcribed in isolated nuclei in vitro. *Mol Pharmacol* 1980;17:279–282.

61. Heimer R, Sartorelli AC. RNA polymerase II transcripts as targets for 5-fluorouridine cytotoxicity: antagonism of 5-fluorouridine actions by α-amanitin. *Cancer Chemother Pharmacol* 1989;24:80–86.

62. Will CL, Dolnick BJ. 5-Fluorouracil augmentation of dihydrofolate reductase RNA containing contiguous exon and intron sequences in KB7B cells. *J Biol Chem* 1987;262:5433–5436.

63. Will CL, Dolnick BJ. 5-Fluorouracil inhibits dihydrofolate reductase precursor mRNA processing and/or nuclear mRNA stability in methotrexate-resistant KB cells. *J Biol Chem* 1989;264:21413–21421.

64. Dolnick BJ, Pink JJ. 5-Fluorouracil modulation of dihydrofolate reductase RNA levels in methotrexate-resistant KB cells. *J Biol Chem* 1983;258:13299–13306.

65. Dolnick BJ, Pink JJ. Effects of 5-fluorouracil on dihydrofolate reductase mRNA from methotrexate-resistant KB cells. *J Biol Chem* 1985;260:3006–3014.

66. Iwata T, Watanabe T, Kufe DW. Effects of 5-fluorouracil on globin mRNA synthesis in murine erythroleukemia cells. *Biochemistry* 1986;25:2703–2707.

67. Armstrong RD, Lewis M, Stern SG, et al. Acute effect of 5-fluorouracil on cytoplasmic and nuclear dihydrofolate reductase messenger RNA metabolism. *J Biol Chem* 1986;261:7366–7371.

68. Armstrong RD. RNA as a target for antimetabolites. In: Glazer RI, ed. *Developments in cancer chemotherapy*, vol 2. Boca Raton, FL: CRC Press, 1989:154–174.

69. Takimoto CH, Voeller DB, Strong JM, et al. Effects of 5-fluorouracil substitution on the RNA conformation and in vitro translation of thymidylate synthase messenger RNA. *J Biol Chem* 1993;28:21438–21442.

70. Schmittgen TD, Danenberg KD, Horikoshi T, et al. Effect of 5-fluoro- and 5-bromouracil substitution on the translation of human thymidylate synthase mRNA. *J Biol Chem* 1994;269:16269–16275.

71. Armstrong RD, Takimoto CH, Cadman EC. Fluoropyrimidine-mediated changes in small nuclear RNA. *J Biol Chem* 1986;261:21–24.

72. Takimoto CH, Cadman EC, Armstrong RD. Precursor-dependent differences in the incorporation of fluorouracil in RNA. *Mol Pharmacol* 1986;29:637–642.

73. Sierakowska H, Shukla RR, Dominsksi A, et al. Inhibition of pre-mRNA splicing by 5-fluoro-, 5-chloro- and 5-bromouridine. *J Biol Chem* 1989;264:19185–19191.

74. Doong SL, Dolnick BJ. 5-Fluorouracil substitution alters pre-mRNA splicing in vitro. *J Biol Chem* 1988;263:4467–4473.

75. Danenberg PV, Shea LCC, Danenberg K. Effect of 5-fluorouracil substitution on the self-splicing activity of Tetrahymena ribosomal RNA. *Cancer Res* 1990;50:1757–1763.

76. Lenz H-J, Manno DJ, Danenberg KD, et al. Incorporation of 5-fluorouracil into U2 and U6 snRNA inhibits mRNA precursor splicing. *J Biol Chem* 1994;269:31962–31968.

77. Randerath K, Tseng W-C, Harris JS, et al. Specific effects of fluoropyrimidines and 5-azapyrimidines on modification of the 5 position of pyrimidines, in particular the synthesis of 5-methyluracil and 5-methylcytosine in nucleic acids. *Cancer Res* 1983;84:283–297.

78. Santi DV, Hardy LW. Catalytic mechanism and inhibition of tRNA (uracil-5-)methyltransferase: evidence for covalent catalysis. *Biochemistry* 1987;26:8599–8606.

79. Samuelsson T. Interactions of transfer RNA pseudouridine synthases with RNAs substituted with fluorouracil. *Nucleic Acids Res* 1991;19:6139–6144.

80. Patton JR. Ribonucleoprotein particle assembly and modification of U2 small nuclear RNA containing 5-fluorouridine. *Biochemistry* 1993;32:8939–9844.

81. Shani J, Danenberg PV. Evidence that intracellular synthesis of 5-fluorouridine-5'-phosphate from 5-fluorouracil and 5-fluorouridine is compartmentalized. *Biochem Biophys Res Commun* 1984;122:439–445.

82. Jin Y, Heck DE, DeGeorge G, et al. 5-Fluorouracil suppresses nitric oxide biosynthesis in colon carcinoma cells. *Cancer Res* 1996;56:1978–1982.

83. Fujishima H, Niho Y, Kondo T, et al. Inhibition by 5-fluorouracil of ERCC1 and gamma-glutamylcysteine synthetase messenger RNA expression in a cisplatin-resistant HST-1 human squamous carcinoma cell line. *Oncol Res* 1997;9:167–172.

84. Grem JL, Mulcahy RT, Miller EM, et al. Interaction of deoxyuridine with fluorouracil and dipyridamole in a human colon cancer cell line. *Biochem Pharmacol* 1989;38:51–59.

85. Curtin NJ, Harris AL, Aherne GW. Mechanism of cell death following thymidylate synthase inhibition: 2'-deoxy-5'-triphosphate accumulation, DNA damage, and growth inhibition following exposure to CB3717 and dipyridamole. *Cancer Res* 1991;51:2346–2352.

86. Aherne GW, Hardcastle A, Raynaud F, et al. Immunoreactive dUMP and TTP pools as an index of thymidylate synthase inhibition; effect of tomudex (ZD1694) and a nonpolyglutamated quinazoline antifolate (CB30900) in L1210 mouse leukaemia cells. *Biochem Pharmacol* 1996;51:1293–1301.

87. Tanaka M, Yoshida S, Saneyoshi M, et al. Utilization of 5-fluoro-2'-deoxyuridine triphosphate and 5-fluoro-2'-deoxycytidine triphosphate in DNA synthesis by DNA polymerases alpha and beta from calf thymus. *Cancer Res* 1981;41:4132–4135.

88. Ingraham HA, Tseng BY, Goulian M. Mechanism for exclusion of 5-fluorouracil from DNA. *Cancer Res* 1980; 40:998–1001.

89. Tanaka M, Kimura K, Yoshida S. Increased incorporation of 5-fluorodeoxyuridine into DNA of human T-lymphoblastic cell lines. *Gann* 1984;75:986–992.

90. Herrick D, Major PP, Kufe DW. Effect of methotrexate on incorporation and excision of 5-fluorouracil residues in human breast carcinoma DNA. *Cancer Res* 1982;42:5015–5017.

91. Cheng Y-C, Nakayama K. Effects of 5-fluoro-2'-deoxyuridine on DNA metabolism in HeLa cells. *Mol Pharmacol* 1983;23:171–174.

92. Tanaka M, Kimura K, Yoshida S. Enhancement of the incorporation of 5-fluorodeoxyuridylate into DNA of HL-60 cells by metabolic modulations. *Cancer Res* 1983;43:5145–5150.

93. Kufe DW, Scott P, Fram R, et al. Biologic effect of 5-fluoro-2'-deoxyuridine incorporation in L1210 deoxyribonucleic acid. *Biochem Pharmacol* 1983;32:1337–1340.

94. Major PP, Egan E, Herrick D, et al. 5-Fluorouracil incorporation in DNA of human breast carcinoma cells. *Cancer Res* 1982;42:3005–3009.

95. Schuetz JD, Wallace HJ, Diasio RB. 5-Fluorouracil incorporation into DNA of CF-1 mouse bone marrow cells as a possible mechanism of toxicity. *Cancer Res* 1984;44:1358–1363.

96. Lonn U, Lonn S. Interaction between 5-fluorouracil and DNA of human colon adenocarcinoma. *Cancer Res* 1984; 44:3414–3418.

97. Sawyer RC, Stolfi RL, Martin DS, et al. Incorporation of 5-fluorouracil into murine bone marrow DNA in vivo. *Cancer Res* 1984;44:1847–1851.

98. Caradonna DJ, Cheng YC. The role of deoxyuridine triphosphate nucleotidohydrolase, uracil-DNA glycosylase, and DNA polymerase alpha in the metabolism of FUdR in human tumor cells. *Mol Pharmacol* 1980;18:513–520.

99. Chu E, Lai GM, Zinn S, et al. Resistance of a human ovarian cancer line to 5-fluorouracil associated with decreased levels of 5-fluorouracil in DNA. *Mol Pharmacol* 1990;38:410–417.

100. Harris JM, McIntosh EM, Muscat GE. Structure/function analysis of a dUTPase: catalytic mechanism of a potential chemotherapeutic target. *J Mol Biol* 1999;2:275–287.

101. Canman CE, Lawrence TS, Shewach DS, et al. Resistance to fluorodeoxyuridine-induced DNA damage and cytotoxicity correlates with an elevation of deoxyuridine triphosphatase activity and failure to accumulate deoxyuridine triphosphate. *Cancer Res* 1993;53:5219–5224.

102. Mauro DJ, De Riel JK, Tallarida RJ, et al. Mechanisms of excision of 5-fluorouracil by uracil DNA glycosylase in normal human cells. *Mol Pharmacol* 1993;43:854–857.

103. Wurzer JC, Tallarida RJ, Sirover MA. New mechanism of action of the cancer chemotherapeutic agent 5-fluorouracil in human cells. *J Pharmacol Exp Ther* 1994;269:39–43.

104. Yoshioka A, Tanaka S, Hiraoka O, et al. Deoxyribonucleoside triphosphate imbalance—fluorodeoxyuridine-induced DNA double strand breaks in mouse FM3A cells and the mechanism of cell death. *J Biol Chem* 1987;262:8235–8241.

105. Houghton JA, Tillman DM, Harwood FG. Ratio of 2'-deoxyadenosine-5'-triphosphate/thymidine-5'-triphosphate influences the commitment of human colon carcinoma cells to thymineless death. *Clin Cancer Res* 1995;1:723–730.

106. Wadler S, Horowitz R, Mao X, et al. Effect of interferon of 5-fluorouracil-induced perturbations in pools of deoxynucleotide triphosphates and DNA strand breaks. *Cancer Chemother Pharmacol* 1996;38:529–535.

107. Schuetz JD, Diasio RB. The effect of 5-fluorouracil on DNA chain elongation in intact bone marrow cells. *Biochem Biophys Res Commun* 1985;133:361–367.

108. Schuetz JD, Collins JM, Wallace HJ, et al. Alteration of the secondary structure of newly synthesized DNA from murine bone marrow cells by 5-fluorouracil. *Cancer Res* 1986;46:119–123.

109. Jones S, Willmore E, Durkacz BW. The effects of 5-fluoropyrimidines on nascent DNA synthesis in Chinese hamster ovary cells monitored by pH-step alkaline and neutral elution. *Carcinogenesis* 1994;15:2435–2438.

110. Yin M, Rustum YM. Comparative DNA strand breakage induced by FUra and FdUrd in human ileocecal adenocarcinoma (HCT-8) cells: relevance to cell growth inhibition. *Cancer Commun* 1991;3:45–51.

111. Lonn U, Lonn S. DNA lesions in human neoplastic cells and cytotoxicity of 5-fluoropyrimidines. *Cancer Res* 1986; 46:3866–3870.

112. Lonn U, Lonn S. Increased levels of DNA lesions induced by leucovorin-5-fluoropyrimidine in human colon adenocarcinoma. *Cancer Res* 1988;48:4153–4157.

113. Dusenbury CE, Davis MA, Lawrence TS, et al. Induction of megabase DNA fragments by 5-fluorodeoxyuridine in human colorectal tumor (HT29) cells. *Mol Pharmacol* 1991;39:285–289.

114. Canman CE, Tang H-Y, Normolle DP, et al. Variations in patterns of DNA damage induced in human colorectal tumor cells by 5-fluorodeoxyuridine. Implications for mechanisms of resistance and cytotoxicity. *Proc Natl Acad U S A* 1992;89:10474–10478.

115. Ayusawa D, Arai H, Wataya Y, et al. A specialized form of chromosomal DNA degradation induced by thymidylate stress in mouse FM3A cells. *Mutat Res* 1988;200:221–230.

116. Lonn U, Lonn SB, Nylen U. Increased levels of 5-fluorouracil-induced DNA lesions in Bloom's syndrome. *Int J Cancer* 1990;45:494–499.

117. Li Z-R, Yin M-B, Arredendo MA, et al. Down-regulation of c-myc gene expression with induction of high molecular weight DNA fragments by fluorodeoxyuridine. *Biochem Pharmacol* 1994;48:327–334.

118. Kyprianou N, Isaacs JT. "Thymineless" death in androgen-independent prostatic cancer cells. *Biochem Biophys Res Commun* 1989;165:73–81.

119. Lowe SW, Ruley HE, Jacks T, et al. p53-Dependent apoptosis modulates the cytotoxicity of anticancer agents. *Cell* 1993;74:957–967.

120. Fisher TC, Milner AE, Gregory CD, et al. Bcl-2 modulation of apoptosis induced by anticancer drugs: resistance to thymidylate stress is independent of classical resistance pathways. *Cancer Res* 1993;53:3321–3326.

121. Lonn U, Lonn S. The increased cytotoxicity in colon adenocarcinoma of methotrexate-5-fluorouracil is not associated

with increased induction of lesions in DNA by 5-fluorouracil. *Biochem Pharmacol* 1986;35:177–181.

122. Parker WB, Kennedy KA, Klubes P. Dissociation of 5-fluorouracil-induced DNA fragmentation from either its incorporation into DNA or its cytotoxicity in murine T-lymphoma (S-49). *Cancer Res* 1987;47:979–982.

123. Darzynkiewicz Z. Methods in analysis of apoptosis and cell necrosis. In: Parker J, Stewart C, eds. The Purdue cytometry CD-ROM, vol 3. West Lafayette, IN: Purdue University, 1997.

124. Houghton JA, Harwood FG, Tillman DM. Thymineless death in colon carcinoma cells is mediated via Fas signaling. *Proc Natl Acad U S A* 1997;94:8144–8149.

125. Tillman DM, Petak I, Houghton JA. A fas-dependent component in 5-fluorouracil/leucovorin-induced cytotoxicity in colon carcinoma cells. *Clin Cancer Res* 1999;5:425–430.

126. Pritchard DM, Watson AJM, Potten CS, et al. Inhibition of uridine but not thymidine of p53-dependent intestinal apoptosis initiated by 5-fluorouracil: evidence for the involvement of RNA perturbation. *Proc Natl Acad U S A* 1997;94:1795–1799.

127. Aschele C, Sobrero A, Faderan MA, et al. Novel mechanisms of resistance to 5-fluorouracil in human colon cancer (HCT-8) sublines following exposure to two different clinically relevant dose schedules. *Cancer Res* 1992;52:1855–1964.

128. Sobrero AF, Aschele C, Guglielmi AP, et al. Synergism and lack of cross-resistance between short-term and continuous exposure to fluorouracil in human colon adenocarcinoma cells. *J Natl Cancer Inst* 1993;85:1937–1944.

129. Ren Q-F, Van Groeningen CJ, Geoffroy F, et al. Determinants of cytotoxicity with prolonged exposure to fluorouracil in human colon cancer cells. *Oncol Res* 1997;9:77–88.

130. Reyes P, Hall TC. Synthesis of 5-fluorouridine 5'-phosphate by a pyrimidine phosphoribosyltransferase of mammalian origin: II. Correlation between the tumor levels of the enzyme and 5-fluorouracil-promoting increase in survival of tumor-bearing mice. *Biochem Pharmacol* 1969;18:2587–2590.

131. Nahas A, Savlov ED, Hall TC. Phosphoribosyl transferase in colon tumor and normal mucosa as an aid in adjuvant chemotherapy with 5-fluorouracil (NSC-19893). *Cancer Chemother Rep* 1974;58:909–912.

132. Reichard P, Skold O, Klein G, et al. Studies on resistance against 5-fluorouracil: I. Enzymes of the uracil pathway during development of resistance. *Cancer Res* 1962;22:235–243.

133. Bresnick E, Thompson UB. Properties of deoxythymidine kinase partially purified from animal tumors. *J Biol Chem* 1965;240:3967–3974.

134. Hande KR, Chabner BA. Pyrimidine nucleoside monophosphate kinase from human leukemic blast cells. *Cancer Res* 1978;38:579–585.

135. Ardalan B, Cooney DA, Jayaram HN, et al. Mechanisms of sensitivity and resistance of murine tumors to 5-fluorouracil. *Cancer Res* 1980;40:1431–1437.

136. Mulkins MA, Heidelberger C. Isolation of fluoropyrimidine-resistant murine leukemic cell lines by one-step mutation and selection. *Cancer Res* 1982;42:956–964.

137. Mulkins MA, Heidelberger C. Biochemical characterization of fluoropyrimidine-resistant murine leukemic cell lines. *Cancer Res* 1982;42:965–973.

138. Piper AA, Fox RM. Biochemical basis for the differential sensitivity of human T- and B-lymphocyte lines to 5-fluorouracil. *Cancer Res* 1982;42:3753–3760.

139. Ardalan B, Villacorte D, Heck D, et al. Phosphoribosyl pyrophosphate pool size and tissue levels as a determinant of 5-fluorouracil response in murine colonic adenocarcinomas. *Biochem Pharmacol* 1982;31:1989–1992.

140. Au J L-S, Rustum YM, Minowad J, et al. Differential selectivity of 5-fluorouracil and 5'-deoxy-5-fluorouridine in cultured human B lymphocytes and mouse L1210 leukemia. *Biochem Pharmacol* 1983;32:541–546.

141. Yoshida M, Hoshi A. Mechanism of inhibition of phosphoribosylation of 5-fluorouracil by purines. *Biochem Pharmacol* 1984;33:2863–2867.

142. El-Assouli SM. The molecular basis for the differential sensitivity of B and T lymphocytes to growth inhibition by thymidine and 5-fluorouracil. *Leuk Res* 1985;9:391–398.

143. Peters GJ, Laurensse E, Leyva A, et al. Sensitivity of human, murine and rat cells to 5-fluorouracil and 5'-deoxy-5-fluorouridine in relation to drug-metabolizing enzymes. *Cancer Res* 1986;46:20–28.

144. Tamemasa O, Tezuka M. Additive formation of antineoplastic 5-fluorouracil nucleosides from 5-fluorouracil by Ehrlich ascites tumor extracts in the presence of ribose 1-phosphate/uridine or deoxyribose 1-phosphate/deoxyuridine. *J Pharmacobiodyn* 1982;5:720–726.

145. Beltz RE, Waters RN, Hegarty TJ. Enhancement and depression by inosine of the growth inhibitory action of 5-fluorouracil on cultured Jensen tumor cells. *Biochem Biophys Res Commun* 1983;112:235–241.

146. Washtien WL. Comparison of 5-fluorouracil metabolism in two human gastrointestinal tumor cell lines. *Cancer Res* 1984;44:909–914.

147. Iigo M, Yamaizumi Z, Nishimura S, et al. Mechanism of potentiation of antitumor activity of 5-fluorouracil by guanine ribonucleotides against adenocarcinoma 755. *Eur J Cancer Clin Oncol* 1987;23:1059–1065.

148. Kessel D, Hall TC, Wodinsky I. Nucleotide formation as a determinant of 5-fluorouracil response in mouse leukemia. *Science* 1966;154:911–913.

149. Myers CE, Young RC, Chabner BA. Biochemical determinants of 5-fluorouracil response in vivo: the role of deoxyuridylate pool expansion. *J Clin Invest* 1975;56:1231–1238.

150. Ardalan B, Buscaglia MD, Schein PS. Tumor 5-fluorodeoxyuridylate concentrations as a determinant of 5-fluorouracil response. *Biochem Pharmacol* 1977;27:2009–2013.

151. Klubes P, Connelly K, Cerna I, et al. Effects of 5-fluorouracil on 5-fluorodeoxyuridine 5-monophosphate and 2-deoxyuridine 5'-monophosphate pools and DNA synthesis in solid mouse L1210 and rat Walker 256 tumors. *Cancer Res* 1978;38:2325–2331.

152. Fernandes DJ, Cranford SK. Resistance of CCRF-CEM cloned sublines to 5-fluorodeoxyuridine associated with enhanced phosphatase activities. *Biochem Pharmacol* 1985;34:125–132.

153. Moran RG, Spears CP, Heidelberger C. Biochemical determinants of tumor sensitivity to 5-fluorouracil: ultrasensitive methods for determination of 5-fluoro-2'-deoxyuridylate, 2'-deoxyuridylate, and thymidylate synthetase. *Proc Natl Acad Sci U S A* 1979;76:1456–1460.

154. Rustum YM, Danhauser L, Luccioni C, et al. Determinants of response to antimetabolites and their modulation by normal purine and pyrimidine metabolites. *Cancer Treat Rep* 1981;65(suppl 3):73–82.

155. Berger SH, Hakala MT. Relationship of dUMP and free FdUMP pools to inhibition to thymidylate synthase by 5-fluorouracil. *Mol Pharmacol* 1984;25:303–309.

156. Houghton JA, Weiss KD, Williams LG, et al. Relationship between 5-fluoro-2'-deoxyuridylate, 2'-deoxyuridylate, and thymidylate synthase activity subsequent to 5-fluorouracil administration, in xenografts of human colon adenocarcinomas. *Biochem Pharmacol* 1986;35:1351–1358.

157. Kaufman ER. Resistance to 5-fluorouracil associated with increased cytidine triphosphate levels in V79 Chinese hamster cells. *Cancer Res* 1984;44:3371–3376.

158. Aronow B, Watts T, Lassetter J, et al. Biochemical phenotype of 5-fluorouracil-resistant murine T-lymphoblasts with genetically altered CTP synthetase activity. *J Biol Chem* 1984;259:9035–9043.

159. Fernandes DJ, Cranford SK. A method for the determination of total, free, and 5-fluorodeoxyuridylate-bound thymidylate synthase in cell extracts. *Anal Biochem* 1984;142:378–385.

160. Yalowich JC, Kalman TI. Rapid determinations of thymidylate synthase activity and its inhibition in intact L1210 leukemia cells in vitro. *Biochem Pharmacol* 1985;34:2319–2324.

161. Spears CP, Gustavsson BG, Mitchell MS, et al. Thymidylate synthetase inhibition in malignant tumors and normal liver of patients given intravenous 5-fluorouracil. *Cancer Res* 1984;44:4144–4150.

162. Spears CP, Gustavsson BG, Berne M, et al. Mechanisms of innate resistance to thymidylate synthase inhibition after 5-fluorouracil. *Cancer Res* 1988;48:5894–5900.

163. Peters GJ, van Groeningen CJ, Leurensse EJ, et al. Thymidylate synthase from untreated human colorectal cancer and colonic mucosa: enzyme activity and inhibition by 5-fluoro-2-deoxyuridine-5-monophosphate. *Eur J Cancer* 1991;27:263–267.

164. Horikoshi T, Danenberg KD, Staglbauer THW, et al. Quantitation of thymidylate synthase, dihydrofolate reductase, and DT-diaphorase gene expression in human tumors using the polymerase chain reaction. *Cancer Res* 1992;52:108–116.

165. Johnston PG, Lenz H-J, Leichman CG, et al. Thymidylate gene and protein expression correlate and are associated with response to 5-fluorouracil in human colorectal and gastric tumors. *Cancer Res* 1995;55:1407–1412.

166. Lenz H-J, Leichman CG, Danenberg KD, et al. Thymidylate synthase mRNA level in adenocarcinoma of the stomach: a predictor for primary tumor response and overall survival. *J Clin Oncol* 1985;14:176–182.

167. Leichman CG, Lenz H-J, Leichman L, et al. Quantitation of intratumoral thymidylate synthase expression predicts for disseminated colorectal cancer response and resistance to protracted-infusion fluorouracil and weekly leucovorin. *J Clin Oncol* 1997;15:3223–3229.

168. Johnston PG, Liang C-M, Henry S, et al. Production and characterization of monoclonal antibodies that localize human thymidylate synthase in the cytoplasm of human cells and tissue. *Cancer Res* 1991;51:6668–6676.

169. Johnston PG, Drake JC, Trepel J, et al. Immunological quantitation of thymidylate synthase using the monoclonal antibody TS 106 in 5-fluorouracil-sensitive and -resistant human cancer cell lines. *Cancer Res* 1992;52:4306–4312.

170. Johnston PG, Drake JC, Steinberg SM, et al. The quantitation of thymidylate synthase in human tumors using an ultrasensitive enzyme-linked immunoassay. *Biochem Pharmacol* 1993;12:2483–2486.

171. Johnston PG, Fisher E, Rockette HE, et al. The role of thymidylate synthase expression in prognosis and outcome to adjuvant therapy in rectal cancer. *J Clin Oncol* 1994;12:2640–2647.

172. Fisher B, Wolmark N, Rockette H, et al. Postoperative adjuvant chemotherapy or radiation therapy for rectal cancer: results from NSABP protocol R-01. *J Natl Cancer Inst* 1988;80:21–29.

173. Washtien WL. Thymidylate synthase levels as a factor in 5-fluorodeoxyuridine and methotrexate cytotoxicity in gastrointestinal tumor cell lines. *Mol Pharmacol* 1982;21:723–728.

174. Priest DG, Ledford BE, Doig MT. Increased thymidylate synthetase in 5-fluorodeoxyuridine-resistant cultured hepatoma cells. *Biochem Pharmacol* 1980;29:1549–1553.

175. Jenh C-H, Geyer PK, Baskin F, et al. Thymidylate synthase gene amplification in fluorodeoxyuridine-resistant mouse cell lines. *Mol Pharmacol* 1985;28:80–85.

176. Berger SH, Jenh C-H, Johnson LF, et al. Thymidylate synthase overproduction and gene amplification in fluorodeoxyuridine-resistant human cells. *Mol Pharmacol* 1985;28:461–467.

177. Clark JL, Berger SH, Mittelman A, et al. Thymidylate synthase gene amplification in a colon tumor resistant to fluoropyrimidine chemotherapy. *Cancer Treat Rep* 1987;71:261–265.

178. Copur S, Aiba K, Drake JC, et al. Thymidylate synthase gene amplification in human colon cancer cell lines resistant to 5-fluorouracil. *Biochem Pharmacol* 1995;49:1419–1426.

179. Jastreboff MM, Kedzierska B, Rode W. Altered thymidylate synthetase in 5-fluorodeoxyuridine-resistant Ehrlich ascites carcinoma cells. *Biochem Pharmacol* 1985;32:2259–2267.

180. Bapat AR, Zarow C, Danenberg PV. Human leukemic cells resistant to 5-fluoro-2'deoxyuridine contain a thymidylate synthase with a lower affinity for nucleotides. *J Biol Chem* 1983;258:4130–4136.

181. Newman EM, Lu Y, Kashani-Sabet M, et al. Mechanisms of cross-resistance to methotrexate and 5-fluorouracil in an A2780 human ovarian carcinoma cell subline resistant to cisplatin. *Biochem Pharmacol* 1988;37:443–447.

182. Berger SH, Barbour KW, Berger FG. A naturally occurring variation in thymidylate synthase structure is associated with a reduced response to 5-fluoro-2'-deoxyuridine in a human colon tumor cell line. *Mol Pharmacol* 1988;34:480–484.

183. Barbour KW, Berger SH, Berger SG. Single amino acid substitution defines a naturally occurring genetic variant of human thymidylate synthase. *Mol Pharmacol* 1990;37:515–518.

184. Grem JL, Hoth DF, Hamilton JM, et al. Overview of current status and future direction of clinical trials with 5-fluorouracil in combination with folinic acid. *Cancer Treat Rep* 1987;71:1249–1264.

185. Zhang Z-G, Rustum YM. Effects of diastereoisomers of 5-formyl-tetrahydrofolate on cellular growth, sensitivity to 5-fluoro-2'-deoxyuridine, and methylenetetrahydrofolate polyglutamate levels in HCT-8 cells. *Cancer Res* 1991;51:3476–3481.

186. Boarman DM, Allegra CJ. Intracellular metabolism of 5-formyltetrahydrofolate in human breast and colon cell lines. *Cancer Res* 1992;52:36–44.

187. Romanini A, Lin JT, Niedzwiecki D, et al. Role of folylpolyglutamates in biochemical modulation of fluoropyrimidines by leucovorin. *Cancer Res* 1991;51:789–793.

188. Wang F-S, Aschele C, Sobrero A, et al. Decreased folylpolyglutamate synthetase expression: a novel mechanism of fluorouracil resistance. *Cancer Res* 1993;53:3677–3680.

189. Lu K, McGuire JJ, Slocum HK, et al. Mechanisms of acquired resistance to modulation of 5-fluorouracil by leucovorin in HCT-8 human ileocecal carcinoma cells. *Biochem Pharmacol* 1997;53:689–696.

190. Cohen A, Ullman B. Role of intracellular dTTP levels in fluorodeoxyuridine toxicity. *Biochem Pharmacol* 1984;33:3298–3301.

191. Grem JL, Fischer PH. Enhancement of 5-fluorouracil's anticancer activity by dipyridamole. *Pharmacol Ther* 1989;40:349–371.

192. Radparvar S, Houghton PJ, Germain G, et al. Cellular pharmacology of 5-fluorouracil in a human colon adenocarcinoma cell line selected for thymidine kinase deficiency. *Biochem Pharmacol* 1990;39:1759–1765.

193. Sobrero AF, Moir RD, Bertino JR, et al. Defective facilitated diffusion of nucleosides, a primary mechanism of resistance to 5-fluoro-2'-deoxyuridine in the HCT-8 human carcinoma. *Cancer Res* 1985;45:3155–3160.

194. Sobrero AF, Handschumacher RE, Bertino JR. Highly selective drug combinations for human colon cancer cells resistant in vitro to 5-fluoro-2'-deoxyuridine. *Cancer Res* 1985;45:3161–3163.

195. Navalgund LG, Rossana C, Muench AJ, et al. Cell cycle regulation of thymidylate synthetase gene expression in cultured mouse fibroblasts. *J Biol Chem* 1980;255:7386–7390.

196. Rode W, Scanlon KJ, Moroson BA, et al. Regulation of thymidylate synthetase in mouse leukemia cells (L1210). *J Biol Chem* 1980;255:1305–1311.

197. Jenh C-H, Rao LG, Johnson LF. Regulation of thymidylate synthase enzyme synthesis in 5-fluorodeoxyuridine-resistant mouse fibroblasts during the transition from the resting to growing state. *J Cell Physiol* 1985;122:149–154.

198. Conrad AH. Thymidylate synthetase activity in cultured mammalian cells. *J Biol Chem* 1971;246:1318.

199. Cadman E, Heimer R. Levels of thymidylate synthetase during normal culture growth of L1210 cells. *Cancer Res* 1986;46:1195–1198.

200. Johnson LF. Post transcriptional regulation of thymidylate synthase gene expression. *J Cell Biochem* 1994;54:378–392.

201. Horie N, Takeishi K. Identification of functional elements in the promoter region of the human gene for thymidylate synthase and nuclear factors that regulate the expression of the gene. *J Biol Chem* 1997;272:18375–18381.

202. Berne M, Gustavsson B, Almersjo O, et al. Concurrent allopurinol and 5-fluorouracil: 5-fluoro-2'-deoxyuridylate formation and thymidylate synthase inhibition in rat colon carcinoma in regenerating rat liver. *Cancer Chemother Pharmacol* 1987;20:193–197.

203. Chu E, Zinn S, Boarman D, et al. Interaction of interferon and 5-fluorouracil in the H630 human colon carcinoma cell line. *Cancer Res* 1990;50:5834–5840.

204. Van der Wilt CL, Pinedo HM, Smid K, et al. Elevation of thymidylate synthase following 5-fluorouracil treatment is prevented by the addition of leucovorin in murine colon tumors. *Cancer Res* 1992;52:4922–4928.

205. Parr AL, Drake JC, Gress RE, et al. 5-Fluorouracil-mediated thymidylate synthase induction in malignant and nonmalignant human cells. *Biochem Pharmacol* 1998;56:231–235.

206. Swain SM, Lippman ME, Chabner BA, et al. Fluorouracil and high-dose leucovorin in previously treated patients with metastatic breast cancer. *J Clin Oncol* 1989;7:890–899.

207. Chu E, Voeller DM, Johnston PG, et al. Regulation of thymidylate synthase in human colon cancer cells treated with 5-fluorouracil and interferon-gamma. *Mol Pharmacol* 1993;43:527–533.

208. Chu E, Koeller DM, Casey JL, et al. Autoregulation of human thymidylate synthase messenger RNA translation by thymidylate synthase. *Proc Natl Acad U S A* 1991;88:8977–8981.

209. Chu E, Voeller D, Koeller DM, et al. Identification of an RNA binding site for human thymidylate synthase. *Proc Natl Acad U S A* 1993;90:517–521.

210. Ju J, Kane SE, Lenz HJ, et al. Desensitization and sensitization of cells to fluoropyrimidines with different antisenses directed against thymidylate synthase messenger RNA. *Clin Cancer Res* 1998;4:2229–2236.

211. Houghton PJ, Germain GS, Hazelton VJ, et al. Mutant of human colon adenocarcinoma selected for thymidylate synthase deficiency. *Proc Natl Acad Sci U S A* 1989;86:1377–1381.

212. Houghton PJ, Rahman A, Will CL, et al. Mutations of the thymidylate synthase gene of human adenocarcinoma cells causes a thymidylate synthase-negative phenotype that can be attenuated by exogenous folates. *Cancer Res* 1992;52:558–565.

213. Chu E, Drake JC, Koeller DM, et al. Induction of thymidylate synthase associated with multidrug resistance in human breast and colon cancer cell lines. *Mol Pharmacol* 1991;39:136–143.

214. Calabro-Jones PM, Byfield JE, Ward JF, et al. Time-dose relationships for 5-fluorouracil cytotoxicity against human epithelial cancer cells in vitro. *Cancer Res* 1982;42:4413–4420.

215. Drewinko B, Yang L-Y. Cellular basis for the inefficacy of 5-FU in human colon carcinoma. *Cancer Treat Rep* 1985;69:1391–1398.

216. Santelli G, Valeriote F. Schedule-dependent cytotoxicity of 5-fluorouracil in mice. *J Natl Cancer Inst* 1986;76:159–164.

217. Moran RG, Scanlon KL. Schedule-dependent enhancement of the cytotoxicity of fluoropyrimidines to human carcinoma cells in the presence of folinic acid. *Cancer Res* 1991;51:4618–4623.

218. MacMillan WE, Wolberg WH, Welling PG. Pharmacokinetics of fluorouracil in humans. *Cancer Res* 1978;38:3479–3482.

219. Buckpitt AR, Boyd MR. A sensitive method for determination of 5-fluorouracil and 5-fluoro-2'-deoxyuridine in human plasma by high-pressure liquid chromatography. *Anal Biochem* 1980;106:432–437.

220. Stetson PL, Shukla US, Ensminger WD. Sensitive high-performance liquid chromatographic method for the determination of 5-fluorouracil in plasma. *J Chromatogr* 1985;344:385–390.

221. Benz C, DeGregorio M, Saks S, et al. Sequential infusions of methotrexate and 5-fluorouracil in advanced cancer: pharmacology, toxicity, and response. *Cancer Res* 1985;45:3354–3358.

222. Klecker RW Jr, Jenkins JF, Kinsella TJ, et al. Clinical pharmacology of 5-iodo-2'-deoxyuridine and 5-iodouracil and endogenous pyrimidine modulation. *Clin Pharmacol Ther* 1985;38:45–51.

223. Michaelis HC, Foth H, Kahl FG. Determination of 5-fluoro-2'-deoxyuridine in human plasma by high-performance liquid chromatography with pre-column fluorimetric derivatization. *J Chromatogr* 1987;416:176–182.

224. LaCreta FP, Williams WM. High-performance liquid chromatographic analysis of fluoropyrimidine nucleosides and fluorouracil in plasma. *J Chromatogr* 1987;414:197–201.

225. Heggie GD, Sommadossi J-P, Cross DS, et al. Clinical pharmacokinetics of 5-fluorouracil and its metabolites in plasma, urine, and bile. *Cancer Res* 1987;47:2203–2206.

226. Yoshida T, Araki E, Iigo M, et al. Clinical significance of monitoring serum levels of 5-fluorouracil by continuous infusion in patients with advanced colonic cancer. *Cancer Chemother Pharmacol* 1990;26:352–354.

227. Barberi-Heyob M, Merlin JL, Weber B. Analysis of 5-fluorouracil in plasma and urine by high-performance liquid chromatography. *J Chromatogr* 1992;581:281–286.

228. Gamelin E, Boisdron-Celle M, Turcant A, et al. Rapid and sensitive high-performance liquid chromatographic analysis of halogenopyrimidines in plasma. *J Chromatogr B Biomed Sci Appl* 1997;695:409–416.

229. Jung M, Berger G, Pohlen U, et al. Simultaneous determination of 5-fluorouracil and its active metabolites in serum and tissue by high-performance liquid chromatography. *J Chromatogr B Biomed Sci Appl* 1997;702:193–202.

230. van Gröeningen CJ, Pinedo HM, Heddes J, et al. Pharmacokinetics of 5-fluorouracil assessed with a sensitive mass spectrometric method in patients on a dose escalation schedule. *Cancer Res* 1988;48:6956–6961.

231. Anderson LW, Parker RJ, Collins JM, et al. Gas chromatographic-mass spectrometric method for routine monitoring of 5-fluorouracil in plasma of patients receiving low-level protracted infusions. *J Chromatogr* 1992;581:195–201.

232. Wolf W, Waluch V, Presant CA. Non-invasive ¹⁹F-NMRS of 5-fluorouracil in pharmacokinetic and pharmacodynamic studies. *NMR Biomed* 1998;11:380–387.

233. Murphy RF, Balis FM, Poplack DG. Stability of 5-fluorouracil in whole blood and plasma. *Clin Chem* 1987;33:2299–2300.

234. Almersjo OE, Gustavsson BG, Regardh CG, et al. Pharmacokinetic studies of 5-fluorouracil after oral and intravenous administration in man. *Acta Pharmacol Toxicol* 1980;46:329–336.

235. Christophidis N, Vajda FJE, Lucas I, et al. Fluorouracil therapy in patients with carcinoma of the large bowel: a pharmacokinetic comparison of various rates and routes of administration. *Clin Pharmacokinet* 1978;3:330–336.

236. Fraile RJ, Baker LH, Buroker TR, et al. Pharmacokinetics of 5-fluorouracil administered orally by rapid intravenous and by slow infusion. *Cancer Res* 1980;40:2223–2228.

237. Clarkson B, O'Connor A, Winston L, et al. The physiologic disposition of 5-fluorouracil and 5-fluoro-2'-deoxyuridine in man. *Clin Pharmacol Ther* 1964;5:581–610.

238. Kerr IG, Zimm S, Collins JM, et al. Effect of intravenous dose and schedule on cerebrospinal fluid pharmacokinetics of 5-fluorouracil in the monkey. *Cancer Res* 1984;44:4929–4932.

239. Grem JL, McAtee N, Murphy RF, et al. A pilot study of interferon alfa-2a in combination with fluorouracil plus high-dose leucovorin in metastatic gastrointestinal carcinoma. *J Clin Oncol* 1991;9:1811–1820.

240. Grem JL, McAtee N, Murphy RF, et al. Phase I and pharmacokinetic study of recombinant human granulocyte-macrophage colony-stimulating factor given in combination with fluorouracil plus calcium leucovorin in metastatic gastrointestinal adenocarcinoma. *J Clin Oncol* 1994;12:560–568.

241. McDermott BJ, van der Berg HW, Murphy RF. Nonlinear pharmacokinetics for the elimination of 5-fluorouracil after intravenous administration in cancer patients. *Cancer Chemother Pharmacol* 1982;9:173–178.

242. Grem JL, McAtee N, Balis F, et al. A phase II study of continuous infusion 5-fluorouracil and leucovorin with weekly cisplatin in metastatic colorectal carcinoma. *Cancer* 1993;72:663–668.

243. Petit E, Milano G, Levi F, et al. Circadian rhythm-varying plasma concentration of 5-fluorouracil during a five-day continuous venous infusion at a constant rate in cancer patients. *Cancer Res* 1988;48:1676–1680.

244. Fleming RF, Milano G, Thyss A, et al. Correlation between dihydropyrimidine dehydrogenase activity in peripheral mononuclear cells and systemic clearance of fluorouracil in cancer patients. *Cancer Res* 1982;52:2899–2902.

245. Erlichman C, Fine S, Elhakim T. Plasma pharmacokinetics of 5-FU given by continuous infusion with allopurinol. *Cancer Treat Rep* 1986;70:903–904.

246. Remick SC, Grem JL, Fischer PH, et al. Phase I trial of 5-fluorouracil and dipyridamole administered by 72-hour concurrent continuous infusion. *Cancer Res* 1990;50:2667–2672.

247. Grem JL, McAtee N, Steinberg SM, et al. A phase I study of continuous infusion 5-fluorouracil plus calcium leucovorin in combination with n-(phosphonacetyl)-L-aspartate in metastatic gastrointestinal adenocarcinoma. *Cancer Res* 1993;53:4828–4836.

248. Ensminger WD, Rosowsky A, Raso VO, et al. A clinical pharmacological evaluation of hepatic arterial infusion of 5-fluoro-2'-deoxyuridine and 5-fluorouracil. *Cancer Res* 1978;38:3784–3792.

249. Collins JM, Dedrick RL, King FG, et al. Nonlinear pharmacokinetic models for 5-fluorouracil in man: intravenous and intraperitoneal routes. *Clin Pharmacol Ther* 1980;28:235–246.

250. Schwartz PM, Turek PJ, Hyde CM, et al. Altered plasma kinetics of 5-FU at high dosage in rat and man. *Cancer Treat Rep* 1985;69:133–136.

251. Collins JM. Pharmacokinetics of 5-fluorouracil infusions in the rat: comparison with man and other species. *Cancer Chemother Pharmacol* 1985;14:108–111.

252. Wagner JG, Gyves JW, Stetson PL, et al. Steady-state nonlinear pharmacokinetics of 5-fluorouracil during hepatic arterial and intravenous infusions in cancer patients. *Cancer Res* 1986;46:1499–1506.

253. Harris BE, Song R, Soong SJ, et al. Relationship between dihydropyrimidine dehydrogenase activity and plasma 5-fluorouracil levels with evidence for circadian variation of enzyme activity and plasma drug levels in cancer patients receiving 5-fluorouracil by protracted continuous infusion. *Cancer Res* 1990;50:197–201.

254. Thyss A, Milano G, Renee N, et al. Clinical pharmacokinetic study of 5-FU in continuous 5-day infusions for head and neck cancer. *Cancer Chemother Pharmacol* 1986;16:64–66.

255. Trump DL, Egorin MJ, Forrest A, et al. Pharmacokinetic and pharmacodynamic analysis of fluorouracil during 72-hour continuous infusion with and without dipyridamole. *J Clin Oncol* 1991;9:2027–2035.

256. Fety R, Rolland F, Barberi-Heyob M. Clinical impact of pharmacokinetically-guided dose adaptation of 5-fluorouracil: results from a multicentric randomized trial in patients

with locally advanced head and neck carcinomas. *Clin Cancer Res* 1998;4:2039–2045.

257. Santini J, Milano G, Thyss A, et al. 5-FU therapeutic monitoring with dose adjustment leads to an improved therapeutic index in head and neck cancer. *Br J Cancer* 1989;59:287–290.

258. Milano G, Etienne MC, Renee N. Relationship between fluorouracil systemic exposure and tumor response and patient survival. *J Clin Oncol* 1994;12:1291–1295.

259. Vokes EE, Mick R, Kies MS, et al. Pharmacodynamics of fluorouracil-based induction chemotherapy in advanced head and neck cancer. *J Clin Oncol* 1996;14:1663–1671.

260. Creaven PJ, Rustum YM, Petrelli NJ, et al. Phase I and pharmacokinetic evaluation of floxuridine/leucovorin given on the Roswell Park weekly regimen. *Cancer Chemother Pharmacol* 1994;34:261–265.

261. Goldberg JA, Kerr DJ, Watson DG, et al. The pharmacokinetics of 5-fluorouracil administered by arterial infusion in advanced colorectal hepatic metastases. *Br J Cancer* 1990;61:913–915.

262. Sigurdson ER, Ridge JA, Kemeny N. Tumor and liver drug uptake following hepatic artery and portal vein infusion. *J Clin Oncol* 1987;5:1836–1840.

263. Speyer JL, Collins JM, Dedrick RL, et al. Phase I and pharmacologic studies of 5-fluorouracil administered intraperitoneally. *Cancer Res* 1980;40:567–572.

264. Sugarbaker PH, Gianola FJ, Speyer JC, et al. Prospective, randomized trial of intravenous versus intraperitoneal 5-fluorouracil in patients with advanced primary colon or rectal cancer. *Surgery* 1985;98:414–422.

265. Schilsky RL, Choi KE, Grayhack J, et al. Phase I clinical and pharmacologic study of intraperitoneal cisplatin and fluorouracil in patients with advanced intra-abdominal cancer. *J Clin Oncol* 1990;8:2054–2061.

266. Muggia FM, Chan KK, Russell C, et al. Phase I and pharmacologic evaluation of intraperitoneal 5-fluoro-2'-deoxyuridine. *Cancer Chemother Pharmacol* 1991;28:241–250.

267. Israel VK, Jiang C, Muggia FM, et al. Intraperitoneal 5-fluoro-2'-deoxyuridine (FUDR) and (S)-leucovorin for disease predominantly confined to the peritoneal cavity: a pharmacokinetic and toxicity study. *Cancer Chemother Pharmacol* 1995;37:32–38.

268. Coustere C, Mentre F, Sommadossi J-P, et al. A mathematical model of the kinetics of 5-fluorouracil and its metabolites in cancer patients. *Cancer Chemother Pharmacol* 1991;28:123–129.

269. Shiotani T, Weber T. Purification and properties of dihydrothymine dehydrogenase from rat liver. *J Biol Chem* 1981;256:219–224.

270. Podschun B, Wahler G, Schnackerz KD. Purification and characterization of dihydropyrimidine dehydrogenase from pig liver. *Eur J Biochem* 1989;185:219–224.

271. Podschun B, Cook PF, Schnackerz KD. Kinetic mechanism of dihydropyrimidine dehydrogenase in pig liver. *J Biol Chem* 1990;265:12966–12972.

272. Lu Z, Zhang R, Diasio RB. Purification and characterization of dihydropyrimidine dehydrogenase from human liver. *J Biol Chem* 1992;267:17102–17109.

273. Lu Z, Zhang R, Diasio RB. Comparison of dihydropyrimidine dehydrogenase from human, rat, pig, and cow liver: biochemical and immunological properties. *Biochem Pharmacol* 1993;46:945–952.

274. Naguib FN, El Kouni MH, Cha S. Enzymes of uracil catabolism in normal and neoplastic tissues. *Cancer Res* 1985;45:5405–5412.

275. Ho DH, Townsend L, Luna MA, et al. Distribution and inhibition of dihydrouracil dehydrogenase activities in human tissues using 5-fluorouracil as a substrate. *Anticancer Res* 1986;6:781–784.

276. Ansfield FJ, Schroeder JM, Curreri AR. Five years clinical experience with 5-fluorouracil. *JAMA* 1962;181:295–299.

277. Ansfield FJ, Ramirez G, Davis HL, et al. Further clinical studies with intrahepatic arterial infusion with 5-fluorouracil. *Cancer* 1975;36:2413–2417.

278. Fleming RA, Milano GA, Etienne MC, et al. No effect of dose, hepatic function, or nutritional status on 5-FU clearance following continuous (5-day), 5-FU infusion. *Br J Cancer* 1992;66:668–672.

279. Fleming FG, Schilsky RL, O'Brien SM, et al. Phase I and pharmacologic study of 5-fluorouracil in patients with hepatic or renal dysfunction. *Proc Am Assoc Cancer Res* 1993;34:396.

280. Sweeny DJ, Barnes S, Heggie GD, et al. Metabolism of 5-fluorouracil to an n-cholyl-2-fluoro-β-alanine conjugate: previously unrecognized role for bile acids in drug conjugation. *Proc Natl Acad Sci U S A* 1987;84:5439–5443.

281. Sweeny FJ, Barnes S, Diasio RG. Formation of conjugates of 2-fluoro-beta-alanine and bile acids during the metabolism of 5-fluorouracil and 5-fluoro-2-deoxyuridine in the isolated perfused rat liver. *Cancer Res* 1988;48:2010–2014.

282. Zhang R, Soong S-J, Liu T, et al. Pharmacokinetics and tissue distribution of 2-fluoro-β-alanine in rats: potential relevance to toxicity pattern of 5-fluorouracil. *Drug Metab Dispos* 1992;20:113–119.

283. Etienne MC, Lagrange JL, Dassonville O, et al. Population study of dihydropyrimidine dehydrogenase in cancer patients. *J Clin Oncol* 1994;12:2248–2253.

284. Tuchman M, Stoeckeler JS, Kiang DT, et al. Familial pyrimidinemia and pyrimidinuria associated with severe fluorouracil toxicity. *N Engl J Med* 1985;313:245–249.

285. Diasio RB, Beavers TL, Carpenter T. Familial deficiency of dihydropyrimidine dehydrogenase: biochemical basis for familial pyrimidinemia and severe 5-fluorouracil-induced toxicity. *J Clin Invest* 1988;81:47–51.

286. Harris BE, Carpenter JT, Diasio RB. Severe 5-fluorouracil toxicity secondary to dihydropyrimidine dehydrogenase deficiency. *Cancer Res* 1991;68:499–501.

287. Lyss AP, Lilenbaum RC, Harris BE, et al. Severe 5-fluorouracil toxicity in a patient with decreased dihydropyrimidine dehydrogenase activity. *Cancer Invest* 1993;11:239–240.

288. Lu A, Zhang R, Diasio RB. Dihydropyrimidine dehydrogenase activity in human peripheral blood mononuclear cells and liver: population characteristics, newly identified deficient patients, and clinical implication in 5-fluorouracil chemotherapy. *Cancer Res* 1993;53:5433–5438.

289. Takimoto CH, Lu Z-H, Zhang R, et al. Severe neurotoxicity following 5-fluorouracil-based chemotherapy in a patient with dihydropyrimidine dehydrogenase deficiency. *Clin Cancer Res* 1996;2:477–481.

290. Milano G, Etienne MC, Pierrefite V, et al. Dihydropyrimidine dehydrogenase deficiency and fluorouracil-related toxicity. *Br J Cancer* 1999;79:627–630.

291. Lu Z, Zhang R, Diasio RB. Population characteristics of hepatic dihydropyrimidine dehydrogenase activity, a key metabolic enzyme in 5-fluorouracil chemotherapy. *Clin Pharmacol Ther* 1995;58:512–522.

292. Lu Z, Zhang R, Carpenter JT, et al. Decreased dihydropyrimidine dehydrogenase activity in a population of patients with breast cancer: implication for 5-fluorouracil-based chemotherapy. *Clin Cancer Res* 1998;4:325–329.

293. McLeod HL, Sludden J, Murray GI, et al. Characterization of dihydropyrimidine dehydrogenase in human colorectal tumours. *Br J Cancer* 1998;77:461–465.

294. McMurrough J, McLeod HL. Analysis of the dihydropyrimidine dehydrogenase polymorphism in a British population. *Br J Clin Pharmacol* 1996;41:425–427.

295. Chazal M, Etienne MC, Renee N, et al. Link between dihydropyrimidine dehydrogenase activity in peripheral blood mononuclear cells and liver. *Clin Cancer Res* 1996;2:507–510.

296. Yokota H, Fernandez-Salguero P, Furuya H, et al. cDNA cloning and chromosome mapping of human dihydropyrimidine dehydrogenase, an enzyme associated with 5-fluorouracil toxicity and congenital thymine uraciluria. *J Biol Chem* 1994;269:23192–23196.

297. Takai S, Fernandez-Salguero P, Kimura S, et al. Assignment of the human dihydropyrimidine dehydrogenase gene (DPYD) to chromosome region 1p22 by fluorescence in situ hybridization. *Genomics* 1994;24:613–614.

298. Johnson MR, Diasio RB, Albin N, et al. Structural organization of the human dihydropyrimidine dehydrogenase gene. *Cancer Res* 1997;57:1660–1663.

299. Meinsma R, Fernandez-Salguero P, Van Kuilenburg AB, et al. Human polymorphism in drug metabolism: mutation in the dihydropyrimidine dehydrogenase gene results in exon skipping and thymine uracilurea. *DNA Cell Biol* 1995;14:1–6.

300. Kouwaki M, Hamajima N, Sumi S, et al. Identification of novel mutations in the dihydropyrimidine dehydrogenase gene in a Japanese patient with 5-fluorouracil toxicity. *Clin Cancer Res* 1998;4:2999–3004.

301. Ridge SA, Sludden J, Brown O, et al. Dihydropyrimidine dehydrogenase pharmacogenetics in Caucasian subjects. *Br J Clin Pharmacol* 1998;46:151–156.

302. Ridge SA, Sludden J, Wei X, et al. Dihydropyrimidine dehydrogenase pharmacogenetics in patients with colorectal cancer. *Br J Cancer* 1998;77:497–500.

303. Sohn DR, Cho MS, Chung PJ. Dihydropyrimidine dehydrogenase activity in a Korean population. *Ther Drug Monit* 1999;21:152–154.

304. Fernandez-Salguero PM, Gonzalez FJ, Idle JR, et al. Lack of correlation between phenotype and genotype for the polymorphically expressed dihydropyrimidine dehydrogenase in a family of Pakistani origin. *Pharmacogenetics* 1997;7:161–163.

305. Van Kuilenburg AB, Vreken P, Abeling NG, et al. Genotype and phenotype in patients with dihydropyrimidine dehydrogenase deficiency. *Hum Genet* 1999;104:1–9.

306. Kirkwood JM, Ensminger W, Rosowsky A, et al. Comparison of pharmacokinetics of 5-fluorouracil and 5-fluorouracil with concurrent thymidine infusions in a phase I trial. *Cancer Res* 1980;40:107–113.

307. Woodcock TM, Martin DS, Damin LEM, et al. Clinical trials with thymidine and fluorouracil: a phase I and clinical pharmacologic evaluation. *Cancer* 1980;45:1135–1143.

308. Au JL-S, Rustum YM, Ledesma EJ, et al. Clinical pharmacological studies of concurrent infusion of 5-fluorouracil and thymidine in treatment of colorectal carcinomas. *Cancer Res* 1982;42:2930–2937.

309. Tuchman M, O'Dea RF, Ramnaraine MLR, et al. Pyrimidine base degradation in cultured murine C-130 neuroblastoma cells and in situ tumors. *J Clin Invest* 1988;81:425–430.

310. Harvey VJ, Slevin ML, Dilloway MR, et al. The influence of cimetidine on the pharmacokinetics of 5-fluorouracil. *Br J Clin Pharmacol* 1984;18:421–430.

311. Dilloway MR, Lant AF. Effect of H_2-receptor antagonists on the pharmacokinetics of 5-fluorouracil in the rat and monkey. *Biopharm Drug Dispos* 1991;12:17–28.

312. Okuda H, Watabe T, Kawaguchi Y, et al. Lethal drug interactions of sorivudine, a new antiviral drug, with oral 5-fluorouracil prodrugs. *Drug Metab Dispos* 1997;25:270–273.

313. Yan J, Tyring SK, McCrary MM, et al. The effect of sorivudine on dihydropyrimidine dehydrogenase activity in patients with acute herpes zoster. *Clin Pharmacol Ther* 1997;61:563–573.

314. Diasio RB. Sorivudine and 5-fluorouracil; a clinically significant drug-drug interaction due to inhibition of dihydropyrimidine dehydrogenase. *Br J Clin Pharmacol* 1998;46:1–4.

315. Curreri AR, Ansfield FJ, McIvor FA, et al. Clinical studies with 5-fluorouracil. *Cancer Res* 1958;18:478–484.

316. Ansfield R, Klotz J, Nealon T, et al. A phase III study comparing the clinical utility of four regimens of 5-fluorouracil. *Cancer* 1977;39:34–40.

317. Erlichman C, Fine S, Wong A, et al. A randomized trial of fluorouracil and folinic acid in patients with metastatic colorectal carcinoma. *J Clin Oncol* 1988;6:469–475.

318. Poon MA, O'Connell MJ, Moertel CG, et al. Biochemical modulation of fluorouracil: evidence of significant improvement of survival and quality of life in patients with advanced colorectal carcinoma. *J Clin Oncol* 1989;7:1407–1418.

319. Cocconi G, Cunningham D, van Cutsem E, et al. Open, randomized multicenter trial of raltitrexed versus fluorouracil plus high-dose leucovorin in patients with advanced colorectal cancer. *J Clin Oncol* 1998;16:2943–2952.

320. Cunningham D, Zalcberg JR, Rath U, et al. Final results of a randomised trial comparing "Tomudex" (raltitrexed) with 5-fluorouracil plus leucovorin in advanced colorectal cancer. *Ann Oncol* 1996;7:961–965.

321. Petrelli N, Douglass HD, Herrera L, et al. The modulation of fluorouracil with leucovorin in metastatic colorectal carcinoma: a prospective randomized phase III trial. *J Clin Oncol* 1991;7:1419–1426.

322. Buroker TR, O'Connell MJ, Wieand HS, et al. Randomized comparison of two schedules of fluorouracil and leucovorin in the treatment of advanced colorectal cancer. *J Clin Oncol* 1994;12:14–20.

323. Ardalan B, Singh G, Silberman HA. Randomized phase I and phase II study of short-term infusion of high-dose fluorouracil with or without n-(phosphonacetyl)-L-aspartic acid in patients with advanced pancreatic and colorectal cancer. *J Clin Oncol* 1988;6:1053–1058.

324. O'Dwyer PJ, Paul AR, Walczak J, et al. Phase II study of biochemical modulation of fluorouracil by low-dose PALA in patients with colorectal cancer. *J Clin Oncol* 1990;8:1497–1503.

325. Haas NB, Hines JB, Hudes GR, et al. Phase I trial of 5-flu-orouracil by 24-hour infusion weekly. *Invest New Drugs* 1993;11:181–185.

326. Leichman CG, Fleming TR, Muggia FM, et al. Phase II study of fluorouracil and its modulation in advanced colorectal cancer: a Southwest Oncology Group study. *J Clin Oncol* 1995;13:1303–1311.

327. Kohne CH, Schoffski P, Wilke H, et al. Effective biomodulation by leucovorin of high-dose infusion fluorouracil given as a weekly 24-hour infusion: results of a randomized trial in patients with advanced colorectal cancer. *J Clin Oncol* 1998;16:418–426.

328. Díaz-Rubio E, Aranda E, Camps C, et al. A phase II study of weekly 48-hour infusion with high-dose 5-fluorouracil in advanced colorectal cancer: an alternative to biochemical modulation. *J Infus Chemother* 1994;4:58–61.

329. Aranda E, Diaz-Rubio E, Cervantes A, et al. Randomized trial comparing monthly low-dose leucovorin and fluorouracil bolus with weekly high-dose 48-hour continuous-infusion fluorouracil for advanced colorectal cancer: a Spanish Cooperative Group for Gastrointestinal Tumor Therapy (TTD) study. *Ann Oncol* 1998;9:727–731.

330. Seifert P, Baker L, Reed ML, et al. Comparison of continuously infused 5-fluorouracil with bolus injection in treatment of patients with colorectal adenocarcinoma. *Cancer* 1975;36:123–128.

330a. Rougier P, Paillot B, LaPlanche A, et al. 5-Fluorouracil (5-FU) continuous intravenous infusion compared with bolus administration. Final results of a randomised trial in metastatic colorectal cancer. *Eur J Cancer* 1997;33:1789–1793.

331. Lokich JJ, Ahlgren JD, Gullo JJ, et al. A prospective randomized comparison of continuous infusion fluorouracil with a conventional bolus schedule in metastatic colorectal carcinoma: a Mid-Atlantic Oncology Program Study. *J Clin Oncol* 1989;7:425–432.

332. de Gramont A, Bosset JF, Milan C, et al. Randomized trial comparing monthly low-dose leucovorin and fluorouracil bolus with bimonthly high-dose leucovorin and fluorouracil bolus plus continuous infusion for advanced colorectal cancer: a French intergroup study. *J Clin Oncol* 1997;15:808–815.

333. de Gramont A, Louvet C, Andre T, et al. A simplified bimonthly regimen with leucovorin and 5-fluorouracil for metastatic colorectal cancer. Feasibility study. *Proc Am Soc Clin Oncol* 1997;16:287a.

334. de Gramont A, Louvet C, Andre T, et al. A review of GERCOD trials of bimonthly leucovorin plus 5-fluorouracil 48-h continuous infusion in advanced colorectal cancer: evolution of a regimen. Groupe d'Etude et de Recherche sur les Cancers de l'Ovaire et Digestifs (GERCOD). *Eur J Cancer* 1998;34:619–626.

335. Beerblock K, Rinaldi Y, Andre T, et al. Bimonthly high dose leucovorin and 5-fluorouracil 48-hour continuous infusion in patients with advanced colorectal carcinoma. Groupe d'Etude et de Recherche sur les Cancers de l'Ovaire et Digestifs (GERCOD). *Cancer* 1997;79:1100–1105.

336. Ansfield F, Ramirez G, Skibba JL, et al. Intrahepatic arterial infusion with 5-fluorouracil. *Cancer* 1971;28:1147–1151.

337. Kerr DJ, Ledermann JA, McArdle CS, et al. Phase I clinical and pharmacokinetic study of leucovorin and infusional hepatic arterial fluorouracil. *J Clin Oncol* 1995;13:2968–2972.

338. Goette DK. Topical chemotherapy with 5-fluorouracil. A review. *J Am Acad Dermatol* 1981;4:633–649.

339. Johnson MR, Hageboutros A, Wang K, et al. Life-threatening toxicity in a dihydropyrimidine dehydrogenase-deficient patient after treatment with topical 5-fluorouracil. *Clin Cancer Res* 1999;5:2006–2011.

340. Levin RD, Gordon JH. Fluorodeoxyuridine with continuous leucovorin infusion. A phase II clinical trial in patients with metastatic colorectal cancer. *Cancer* 1993;72:2895–2901.

341. Creaven PJ, Rustum YM, Petrelli NJ, et al. Phase I and pharmacokinetic evaluation of floxuridine/leucovorin given on the Roswell Park weekly regimen. *Cancer Chemother Pharmacol* 1994;34:261–265.

342. Sullivan RD, Young CW, Miller E, et al. The clinical effects of the continuous administration of fluorinated pyrimidines (5-fluorouracil and 5-fluoro-2'-deoxyuridine). *Cancer Chemother Rep* 1960;8:77–83.

343. Sullivan RD, Miller E. The clinical effects of prolonged intravenous infusion of 5-fluoro-2'-deoxyuridine. *Cancer Res* 1965;25:1025–1030.

344. Vokes EE, Raschko JW, Vogelzang NJ, et al. Five day infusion of fluorodeoxyuridine with high-dose oral leucovorin: a phase I study. *Cancer Chemother Pharmacol* 1991;28:69–73.

345. Kemeny N, Daly J, Reichman B, et al. Intrahepatic or systemic infusion of fluorodeoxyuridine in patients with liver metastases from colorectal carcinoma. *Ann Intern Med* 1987;107:459–465.

346. Hohn D, Stagg R, Friedman M, et al. A randomized trial of continuous intravenous versus hepatic intraarterial floxuridine in patients with colorectal cancer metastatic to the liver: the Northern California Oncology Group trial. *J Clin Oncol* 1989;7:1646–1654.

347. Anderson N, Lokich J, Bern M, et al. A phase I clinical trial of combined fluoropyrimidines with leucovorin in a 14-day infusion. Demonstration of biochemical modulation. *Cancer* 1989;63:233–237.

348. Ardalan B, Sparling L, Sridhar KS, et al. Phase II trial of high dose 24-hour infusion of fluorodeoxyuridine in patients with metastatic colorectal cancers (previously failed multiple chemotherapeutic modalities). *Proc Am Soc Clin Oncol* 1999;18:249a.

349. Martin JK, O'Connell MJ, Wieand HS, et al. Intra-arterial floxuridine vs systemic fluorouracil for hepatic metastases from colorectal cancer. *Arch Surgery* 1990;125:1022–1027.

350. Thirion P, Cunningham D, Findlay M, et al. Pooled analysis of phase II trials with low-dose 5-fluorouracil continuous infusion as a second line chemotherapy in advanced colorectal cancer. *Proc Am Soc Clin Oncol* 1998;17:272a.

351. Nobile MT, Chiara S, Barzacchi MC, et al. Pretreated advanced colorectal cancer: phase II study with high-dose 24 hours 5-fluorouracil infusion plus 1-leucovorin. *Proc Am Soc Clin Oncol* 1998;17:275a.

352. Brennan MJ, Waitkevicius VK, Rebuck JW. Megaloblastic anemia associated with inhibition of thymine synthesis (observations during 5-fluorouracil treatment). *Blood* 1960;14:1535–1545.

353. Kelvin FM, Gramm HF, Gluck WL, et al. Radiologic manifestations of small-bowel toxicity due to floxuridine therapy. *AJR Am J Roentgenol* 1986;146:39–43.

354. Cascinu S, Fedeli A, Fedeli SL, et al. Octreotide versus

loperamide in the treatment of fluorouracil-induced diarrhea: a randomized trial. *J Clin Oncol* 1993;11:148–151.

355. Mahood DJ, Kose AM, Loprinzi CL, et al. Inhibition of fluorouracil-induced stomatitis by oral cryotherapy. *J Clin Oncol* 1991;9:449–452.

356. Loprinzi CL, Cianflone SG, Dose AM, et al. A controlled evaluation of an allopurinol mouthwash as prophylaxis against 5-fluorouracil induced stomatis. *Cancer* 1990;65:1879–1882.

357. Donagin WG. Clinical toxicity of chemotherapeutic agents: dermatologic toxicity. *Semin Oncol* 1982;9:14–22.

358. Vukelja SJ, Bonner MW, McCollough M, et al. Unusual serpentine hyperpigmentation associated with 5-fluorouracil. Case report and review of cutaneous manifestations associated with systemic 5-fluorouracil. *J Am Acad Dermatol* 1991;25:905–908.

359. Pujol RM, Rocamora V, Lopez-Pousa A, et al. Persistent supravenous erythematous eruption. A rare local complication of intravenous 5-fluorouracil therapy. *J Am Acad Dermatol* 1998;39:839–842.

360. Fabian CJ, Molina R, Slavik M, et al. Pyridoxine therapy for palmar-plantar erythrodysesthesia associated with continuous 5-fluorouracil infusion. *Invest New Drugs* 1990;8:57–63.

361. Mortimer JE, Anderson I. Weekly fluorouracil and high-dose leucovorin. Efficacy and treatment of cutaneous toxicity. *Cancer Chemother Pharmacol* 1990;26:449–452.

362. Riehl JL, Brown WJ. Acute cerebellar syndrome secondary to 5-fluorouracil therapy. *Neurology* 1964;14:961–967.

363. Moertel CG, Reitemeier RJ, Bolton CF, et al. Cerebellar ataxia associated with fluorinated pyrimidine therapy. *Cancer Chemother Rep* 1964;41:15–18.

364. Lynch HT, Droszcz CP, Albano WA, et al. "Organic brain syndrome" secondary to 5-fluorouracil toxicity. *Dis Colon Rectum* 1981;24:130–131.

365. Moore DH, Fowler WC Jr, Crumpler LS. 5-Fluorouracil neurotoxicity. *Gynecol Oncol* 1990;36:152–154.

366. Macdonald DR. Neurologic complications of chemotherapy. *Neurol Clin* 9:955–967, 1991.

367. Tuxen MK, Hansen SW. Neurotoxicity secondary to antineoplastic drugs. *Cancer Treat Rev* 1994;20:191–214.

368. Bygrave HA, Geh JI, Jani Y, et al. Neurological complications of 5-fluorouracil chemotherapy. Case report and review of the literature. *Clin Oncol* 1998;10:334–336.

369. O'Connell MJ, Powis G, Rubin J, et al. Pilot study of PALA and 5-FU in patients with advanced cancer. *Cancer Treat Rep* 1982;66:77–80.

370. Wooley PV, Ayoob MJ, Smith FP, et al. A controlled trial of the effect of 4-hydroxypyrazolopyrimidine (Allopurinol) on the toxicity of a single bolus dose of 5-fluorouracil. *J Clin Oncol* 1985;3:103–109.

371. Muggia FM, Camacho FJ, Kaplan BH, et al. Weekly 5-fluorouracil combined with PALA. Toxic and therapeutic effects in colorectal cancer. *Cancer Treat Rep* 1987;71:253–256.

372. Hook CC, Kimmel DW, Kvols LK, et al. Multifocal inflammatory leukoencephalopathy with 5-fluorouracil and levamisole. *Ann Neurol* 1992;31:262–267.

373. Figueredo AT, Fawcet SE, Molloy DW, et al. Disabling encephalopathy during 5-fluorouracil and levamisole adjuvant therapy for resected colorectal cancer. A report of two cases. *Cancer Invest* 1995;13:608–611.

374. Neuwelt EA, Barnet PA, Glasberg M, et al. Neurotoxicity of chemotherapeutic agents after blood-brain barrier modification neuropathological studies. *Ann Neurol* 1983;14:316–324.

375. Davis ST, Joyner SS, Baccanari DP, et al. 5-Ethynyluracil (776C85). Protection from 5-fluorouracil-induced neurotoxicity in dogs. *Biochem Pharmacol* 1994;48:233–236.

376. Okada R, Shibutani M, Matsuo T, et al. Experimental neurotoxicity of 5-fluorouracil and its derivatives is due to poisoning by the monofluorinated organic metabolites, monofluoroacetic acid and α-fluoro-β-alanine. *Acta Neuropathol* 1990;81:66–73.

377. Berg SL, Balis FM, McCully CL, et al. Intrathecal 5-fluorouracil in the rhesus monkey. *Cancer Chemother Pharmacol* 1992;31:127–130.

378. Yamada M, Nakagawa H, Fukushima M, et al. In vitro study on intrathecal use of 5-fluoro-2'-deoxyuridine (FdUrd) for meningeal dissemination of malignant brain tumors. *J Neurooncol* 1998;37:115–121.

379. Becker K, Erckenbrecht JF, Haussinger D, et al. Cardiotoxicity of the antiproliferative compound fluorouracil. *Drugs* 1999;57:475–484.

380. Meyer CC, Calis KA, Burke LB, et al. Symptomatic cardiotoxicity associated with 5-fluorouracil. *Pharmacotherapy* 1997;17:729–736.

381. Grandi AM, Pinotti G, Morandi E, et al. Noninvasive evaluation of cardiotoxicity of 5-fluorouracil and low doses of folinic acid. A one-year follow-up study. *Ann Oncol* 1997;8:705–708.

382. Wang WS, Hsieh RK, Chiou TJ, et al. Toxic cardiogenic shock in a patient receiving weekly 24-h infusion of high-dose 5-fluorouracil and leucovorin. *Jpn J Clin Oncol* 1998;28:551–554.

383. Köhne C-H, Thuss-Patience P, Friedrich M, et al. Raltitrexed (Tomudex). An alternative drug for patients with colorectal cancer and 5-fluorouracil associated cardiotoxicity. *Br J Cancer* 1998;77:973–977.

384. Lemaire L, Malet-Martino MC, de Forni M, et al. Cardiotoxicity of commercial 5-fluorouracil stems from the alkaline hydrolysis of this drug. *Br J Cancer* 1992;66:119–127.

385. Porta C, Moroni M, Ferrari S, et al. Endothelin-1 and 5-fluorouracil-induced cardiotoxicity. *Neoplasma* 1998;45:81–82.

386. Mosseri M, Fingert HJ, Varticovoski L, et al. In vitro evidence that myocardial ischemia resulting from 5-fluorouracil chemotherapy is due to protein kinase C-mediated vasoconstriction of vascular smooth muscle. *Cancer Res* 1993;53:3028–3033.

387. Haidak DJ, Hurwitz BS, Yeung KY. Tear-duct fibrosis (dacrostenosis) due to 5-fluorouracil. *Ann Intern Med* 1978;88:657.

388. Fraunfelder FT, Meyer SM. Ocular toxicity of antineoplastic agents. *Ophthalmology* 1984;90:1–3.

389. al-Tweigeri T, Nabholtz JM, Mackey JR. Ocular toxicity and cancer chemotherapy. A review. *Cancer* 1996;78:1359–1373.

390. Lee V, Bentley CR, Olver JM. Sclerosing canaliculitis after 5-fluorouracil breast cancer chemotherapy. *Eye* 1998;12:343–349.

391. Loprinzi CL, Love RR, Garrity JA, et al. Cyclophosphamide, methotrexate, and 5-fluorouracil (CMF)-induced ocular toxicity. *Cancer Invest* 1990;8:459–465.

392. Loprinzi CL, Wender DB, Veeder MH, et al. Inhibition of 5-fluorouracil-induced ocular irritation by ocular ice packs. *Cancer* 1994;74:945–948.

393. Wong MK, Bjarnason GA, Hrushesky WJ, et al. Steroid-responsive interstitial lung disease in patients receiving 2'-deoxy-5-fluorouridine infusion chemotherapy. *Cancer* 1995;75:2558–2564.

394. Boyle FM, Smith RC, Levi JA. Continuous hepatic artery infusion of 5-fluorouracil for metastatic colorectal cancer localised to the liver. *Aust N Z J Med* 1993;23:32–34.

395. Kemeny MM, Battifora H, Blayney DW, et al. Sclerosing cholangitis after continuous hepatic artery infusion of FUDR. *Ann Surg* 1985;202:176–181.

396. Hohn DC, Rayner AA, Economou JS, et al. Toxicities and complications of implanted pump hepatic arterial and intravenous floxuridine infusion. *Cancer* 1986;57:465–470.

397. Kemeny N, Seiter K, Niedzwiecki D, et al. A randomized trial of intrahepatic infusion of fluorodeoxyuridine with dexamethasone versus fluorodeoxyuridine alone in the treatment of metastatic colorectal cancer. *Cancer* 1992;69:327–334.

398. Kemeny N, Seiter K, Conti JA, et al. Hepatic arterial floxuridine and leucovorin for unresectable liver metastases from colorectal carcinoma. New dose schedules and survival update. *Cancer* 1994;73:1134–1142.

399. Kemeny N, Conti JA, Cohen A, et al. Phase II study of hepatic arterial floxuridine, leucovorin, and dexamethasone for unresectable liver metastases from colorectal carcinoma. *J Clin Oncol* 1994;12:2288–2295.

400. Chang AE, Schneider PD, Sugarbaker PH, et al. A prospective randomized trial of regional versus systemic continuous 5-fluorodeoxyuridine chemotherapy in the treatment of colorectal liver metastases. *Ann Surg* 1987;206:685–693.

401. Rougier P, Laplanche A, Huguier M, et al. Hepatic arterial infusion of floxuridine in patients with liver metastases from colorectal carcinoma: long-term results of a prospective randomized trial. *J Clin Oncol* 1992;10:1112–1118.

402. Stein BN, Petrelli NJ, Douglass HO, et al. Age and sex are independent predictors of 5-fluorouracil toxicity. *Cancer* 1995;75:11–17.

403. Zalcberg J, Kerr D, Seymour L, et al. Haematological and non-haematological toxicity after 5-fluorouracil and leucovorin in patients with advanced colorectal cancer is significantly associated with gender, increasing age and cycle number. Tomudex International Study Group. *Eur J Cancer* 1998;34:1871–1875.

404. Tepper JE, O'Connell MJ, Petroni GR, et al. Adjuvant postoperative fluorouracil-modulated chemotherapy combined with pelvic radiation therapy for rectal cancer. Initial results of intergroup 0114. *J Clin Oncol* 1997;15:2030–2039.

405. Toxicity of fluorouracil in patients with advanced colorectal cancer. Effect of administration schedule and prognostic factors. Meta-analysis group in cancer. *J Clin Oncol* 1988;16:3537–3541.

406. Tuchman M, Roemeling RV, Hrushesky WA, et al. Dihydropyrimidine dehydrogenase activity in human blood mononuclear cells. *Enzyme* 1989;42:15–24.

407. Port RE, Daniel B, Ding RW, et al. Relative importance of dose, body surface area, sex and age for 5-fluorouracil clearance. *Oncology* 1991;48:277–281.

408. Milano G, Etienne MC, Cassuto-Viguier E, et al. Influence of sex and age on fluorouracil clearance. *J Clin Oncol* 1992;10:1171–1175.

409. Etienne MC, Chatelut E, Pivot X, et al. Co-variables influencing 5-fluorouracil clearance during continuous venous infusion. A NONMEM analysis. *Eur J Cancer* 1998;34:92–97.

410. Tateishi T, Watanabe M, Nakura H, et al. Sex- or age-related differences were not detected in the activity of dihydropyrimidine dehydrogenase from rat liver. *Pharmacol Res* 1997;35:103–106.

411. Durnas C, Loi CM, Cusack BJ. Hepatic drug metabolism and aging. *Clin Pharmacokinet* 1990;19:359–389.

412. Stolfi RL, Sawyer RC, Rabandranath N, et al. Protection by testosterone from fluorouracil-induced toxicity without loss of anticancer activity against autochthonous murine breast tumors. *Cancer Res* 1980;40:2730–2735.

413. Modulation of fluorouracil by leucovorin in patients with advanced colorectal cancer. Evidence in terms of response rate. The advanced colorectal cancer meta-analysis project. *J Clin Oncol* 1992;10:896–903.

414. Meta-analysis of randomized trials testing the biochemical modulation of fluorouracil by methotrexate in metastatic colorectal cancer. The advanced colorectal cancer meta-analysis project. *J Clin Oncol* 1994;12:960–969.

415. Efficacy of intravenous continuous infusion of fluorouracil compared with bolus administration in advanced colorectal cancer. Meta-analysis group in cancer. *J Clin Oncol* 1998;16:301–308.

416. Reappraisal of hepatic arterial infusion in the treatment of nonresectable liver metastases from colorectal cancer. Meta-analysis group in cancer. *J Natl Cancer Inst* 1996;88:252–258.

417. Toxicity of fluorouracil in patients with advanced colorectal cancer. Effect of administration schedule and prognostic factors. Meta-analysis group in cancer. *J Clin Oncol* 1998; 16:3537–3541.

417a. Kemeny N, Huang Y, Cohen A, et al. Hepatic arterial infusion of chemotherapy after resection of hepatic metastases from colorectal cancer. *N Engl J Med* 1999;341:2039–2048.

418. Fox RM, Woods RL, Tattersall MHN. Allopurinol modulation of high-dose fluorouracil toxicity. *Cancer Treat Rev* 1979;6(suppl):143–147.

419. Campbell TN, Howell SB, Pfeifle C, et al. High-dose allopurinol modulation of 5-FU toxicity. Phase I trial of an outpatient dose schedule. *Cancer Treat Rep* 1982;66:1723–1727.

420. Howell SB, Pfeifle CE, Wung WE. Effect of allopurinol on the toxicity of high-dose 5-fluorouracil administered by intermittent bolus injection. *Cancer* 1983;51:220–225.

421. Yoshida M, Hoshi A, Kuretani K. Prevention of antitumor effect of 5-fluorouracil by hypoxanthine. *Biochem Pharmacol* 1978;27:2979–2982.

422. Yoshida M, Hoshi A. Mechanism of inhibition of phosphoribosylation of 5-fluorouracil by purines. *Biochem Pharmacol* 1984;33:2863–2867.

423. Martin DS, Stolfi RL, Sawyer RC, et al. High-dose 5-fluorouracil with delayed uridine "rescue" in mice. *Cancer Res* 1982;42:3864–3970.

424. Sawyer RC, Stolfi RL, Spiegelman S, et al. Effect of uridine on the metabolism of 5-fluorouracil in the CD8F1 murine mammary carcinoma system. *Pharm Res* 1984;2:69–75.

425. Klubes P, Cerna I. Use of uridine rescue to enhance the antitumor selectivity of 5-fluorouracil. *Cancer Res* 1983;43: 3182–3186.

426. Peters GJ, van Dijk J, Laurensse E, et al. In vitro biochemical and in vivo biological studies of the uridine "rescue" of 5-fluorouracil. *Br J Cancer* 1988;57:259–265.

427. Nord LK, Stolfi RL, Martin DS. Biochemical modulation of 5-fluorouracil with leucovorin or delayed uridine rescue. *Biochem Pharmacol* 1992;43:2543–2549.

428. Leyva A, van Groeningen CJ, Kraal I, et al. Phase I and pharmacokinetic studies of high-dose uridine intended for rescue from 5-fluorouracil toxicity. *Cancer Res* 1984;44:5928–5933.

429. van Groeningen CJ, Leyva A, Kraal I, et al. Clinical and pharmacokinetic studies of prolonged administration of high-dose uridine intended for rescue from 5-FU toxicity. *Cancer Treat Rep* 1986;70:745–750.

430. van Groeningen CJ, Peters GJ, Leyva A, et al. Reversal of 5-fluorouracil-induced myelosuppression by prolonged administration of high-dose uridine. *J Natl Cancer Inst* 1989;81:157–162.

431. Martin DS, Stolfi RL, Sawyer RC. Utility of oral uridine to substitute for parenteral uridine rescue of 5-fluorouracil therapy, with and without a uridine phosphorylase inhibitor (5-benzylacyclouridine). *Cancer Chemother Pharmacol* 1989;24:9–14.

432. Klubes P, Geffen DB, Cysyk RL. Comparison of the bioavailability of uridine in mice after either oral or parenteral administration. *Cancer Chemother Pharmacol* 1986;17:236–240.

433. van Groeningen CJ, Peters GJ, Nadal JC, et al. Clinical and pharmacological study of orally administered uridine. *J Natl Cancer Inst* 1991;83:437–441.

434. van Groeningen CJ, Peters GJ, Pinedo HM. Reversal of 5-fluorouracil-induced toxicity by oral administration of uridine. *Ann Oncol* 1993;4:317–320.

435. Schwartz GK, Christman K, Saltz L, et al. A phase I trial of a modified, dose intensive FAMTX regimen (high dose 5-fluorouracil + doxorubicin + high dose methotrexate + leucovorin) with oral uridine rescue. *Cancer* 1996;78:1988–1995.

436. Kelsen DP, Martin D, O'Neil J, et al. Phase I trial of PN401, an oral prodrug of 5-FU, to prevent toxicity from fluorouracil in patients with advanced cancer. *J Clin Oncol* 1997;15:1511–1517.

437. Hidalgo MA, Villalona-Calero R, Drengler L, et al. A phase I and pharmacokinetic study of the oral uridine prodrug PN401 as a rescue agent for escalating doses of 5-fluorouracil in patients with advanced cancer. *Proc Am Soc Clin Oncol* 1998;17:233a.

438. Shimamura M, Kobayashi Y, Yuo A, et al. Effect of human recombinant granulocyte colony-stimulating factor on hematopoietic injury in mice induced by 5-fluorouracil. *Blood* 1987;69:353–355.

439. O'Reilly M, Gamelli RL. Recombinant granulocyte-macrophage colony-stimulating factor improves hematopoietic recovery after 5-fluorouracil. *J Surg Res* 1988;45:104–111.

440. Meropol NJ, Miller LL, Korn DL, et al. Severe myelosuppression resulting from concurrent administration of granulocyte colony-stimulating factor and cytotoxic therapy. *J Natl Cancer Inst* 1992;84:1201–1203.

441. Grem JL, McAtee N, Murphy RF, et al. Phase I and pharmacokinetic study of recombinant human granulocyte-macrophage colony-stimulating factor given in combination with fluorouracil plus calcium leucovorin in metastatic gastrointestinal adenocarcinoma. *J Clin Oncol* 1994;12:560–568.

442. Moore DF Jr, Pazdur R. Phase I study of 5-fluorouracil with folinic acid combined with recombinant human granulocyte-macrophage colony-stimulating factor. *Am J Clin Oncol* 1992;15:464–466.

443. Wadler S, Atkins M, Karp D, et al. Clinical trial of weekly intensive therapy with 5-fluorouracil on two different schedules combined with interferon alpha-2a and filgrastim in patients with advanced solid tumors. Eastern cooperative oncology group study P-Z991. *Cancer J Sci Am* 1998;4:261–268.

444. Shapiro JD, Harold N, Takimoto C, et al. A pilot study of interferon α-2a, fluorouracil and leucovorin given with granulocyte-macrophage colony stimulating factor in advanced gastrointestinal adenocarcinoma. *Clin Cancer Res* 1999;5:2399–2408.

445. Gardner MLG, Plumb JA. Diurnal variation in the intestinal toxicity of 5-fluorouracil in the rat. *Clin Sci* 1981;61:717–722.

446. Burns ER, Beland SS. Effect of biological time on the determination of the LD50 of 5-fluorouracil in mice. *Pharmacology* 1984;28:296–300.

447. Peters GJ, van Dijk J, Nadal JC, et al. Diurnal variation in the therapeutic efficacy of 5-fluorouracil against murine colon cancer. *In Vivo* 187;1:113–118.

448. van Roemeling R, Hrushesky WJM. Determination of the therapeutic index of floxuridine by its circadian infusion pattern. *J Natl Cancer Inst* 1990;82:386–393.

449. Minshull M, Gardner MLG. The effects of time of administration of 5-fluorouracil on leucopenia in the rat. *Eur J Cancer Clin Oncol* 1984;20:857–858.

450. Zhang R, Lu Z, Liu T, et al. Relationship between circadian-dependent toxicity of 5-fluorodeoxyuridine and circadian rhythms of pyrimidine enzymes. Possible relevance to fluoropyrimidine therapy. *Cancer Res* 1993;53:2816–2822.

451. Burns ER. Circadian rhythmicity in DNA synthesis in untreated and saline-treated mice as a basis for improved chemotherapy. *Cancer Res* 1981;41:2795–2802.

452. Burns ER, Beland SS. Induction by 5-fluorouracil of a major phase difference in the circadian profiles of DNA synthesis between the Ehrlich ascites carcinoma and five normal organs. *Cancer Lett* 1983;20:235–239.

453. Harris BE, Song R, He YJ, et al. Circadian rhythm of rat liver dihydropyrimidine dehydrogenase. *Biochem Pharmacol* 1988;37:4759–4762.

454. Zhang R, Lu Z, Liu T, et al. Circadian rhythm of rat spleen cytoplasmic thymidine kinase. *Biochem Pharmacol* 1993;45:1115–1119.

455. Smaaland R, Laerum OD, Lote K, et al. DNA synthesis in human bone marrow is circadian stage dependent. *Blood* 1991;77:2603–2611.

456. Smaaland R, Svardal AM, Lote K, et al. Glutathione content in human bone marrow and circadian stage relation to DNA synthesis. *J Natl Cancer Inst* 1991;83:1092–1098.

457. Buchi KN, Moore JG, Hrushesky WJM, et al. Circadian rhythm of cellular proliferation in human rectal mucosa. *Gastroenterology* 1991;101:410–415.

458. Takimoto CH, Yee LK, Venzon D, et al. High inter- and intrapatient variation in 5-fluorouracil plasma concentrations during a prolonged drug infusion. *Clin Cancer Res* 1999;5:1347–1352.

459. Grem JL, Yee LK, Venzon DJ, et al. Inter- and intraindividual variation in dihydropyrimidine dehydrogenase activity in peripheral blood mononuclear cells. *Cancer Chemother Pharmacol* 1997;40:117–125.

460. Fleming GH, Schilsky RL, Mick R, et al. Circadian variation of 5-fluorouracil plasma levels during continuous infu-

sion 5-FU and leucovorin inpatients with hepatic or renal dysfunction. *Ann Oncol* 1995;5(suppl 5):236.

461. Metzger G, Massari C, Etienne MC, et al. Spontaneous or imposed circadian changes in plasma concentrations of 5-fluorouracil coadministered with folinic acid and oxaliplatin. Relationship with mucosal toxicity in patients with cancer. *Clin Pharmacol Ther* 1994;56:190–201.

462. von Roemeling R, Hrushesky WJM. Circadian patterning of continuous floxuridine infusion reduces toxicity and allows higher dose intensity in patients with widespread cancer. *J Clin Oncol* 1989;7:1710–1719.

463. Hrushesky WJM, von Roemeling R, Lanning TM, et al. Circadian-shaped infusions of floxuridine for progressive metastatic renal cell carcinoma. *J Clin Oncol* 1990;8:1504–1513.

464. Wesen C, Hrushesky WJM, van Roemeling R. Circadian modification of intra-arterial 5-fluoro-2'-deoxyuridine infusion rate reduces its toxicity and permits higher dose-intensity. *J Infus Chemother* 1992;2:69–75.

465. Levi FA, Zidani R, Vannetzel JM, et al. Chronomodulated versus fixed-infusion-rate delivery of ambulatory chemotherapy with oxaliplatin, fluorouracil, and folinic acid (leucovorin) in patients with colorectal cancer metastases. A randomized multi-institutional trial. *J Natl Cancer Inst* 1994;86:1608–1617.

466. Levi F, Zidani R, Misset JL. Randomised multicentre trial of chronotherapy with oxaliplatin, fluorouracil, and folinic acid in metastatic colorectal cancer. International organization for cancer chronotherapy. *Lancet* 1997;350:681–686.

467. Levi F, Zidani R, Brienza S, et al. A multicenter evaluation of intensified, ambulatory, chronomodulated chemotherapy with oxaliplatin, 5-fluorouracil, and leucovorin as initial treatment of patients with metastatic colorectal carcinoma. International organization for cancer chronotherapy. *Cancer* 1999;85:2532–2540.

468. Bjarnason GA, Kerr IG, Doyle N, et al. Phase I study of 5-fluorouracil by a 14-day circadian infusion in metastatic adenocarcinoma patients. *Cancer Chemother Pharmacol* 1993; 33:221–228.

469. Bertino JR. Biomodulation of 5-fluorouracil with antifolates. *Semin Oncol* 1997;24(suppl 18):52–56.

470. Benz C, Tillis T, Tattelman E, et al. Optimal scheduling of methotrexate and 5-fluorouracil in human breast cancer. *Cancer Res* 1982;42:2081–2086.

471. Donehower RC, Allegra JC, Lippman ME, et al. Combined effects of methotrexate and 5-fluoropyrimidines on human breast cancer cells in serum-free tissue culture. *Eur J Cancer* 1980;16:655–661.

472. Piper AA, Nott SE, Mackinnon WB, et al. Critical modulation by thymidine and hypoxanthine of sequential methotrexate-5-fluorouracil synergism in murine L1210 cells. *Cancer Res* 1983;43:5101–5105.

473. Sawyer RC, Stolfi RL, Martin DS, et al. Inhibition by methotrexate of the stable incorporation of 5-fluorouracil into murine bone marrow DNA. *Biochem Pharmacol* 1989;38:2305–2311.

474. El-Tahtawy A, Wolf W. In vivo measurements of intratumoral metabolism, modulation, and pharmacokinetics of 5-fluorouracil, using 19F nuclear magnetic resonance spectroscopy. *Cancer Res* 1991;51:5806–5812.

475. McSheehy PMJ, Prior MJW, Griffiths JR. Enhanced 5-fluorouracil cytotoxicity and elevated 5-fluoronucleotides in the rat walker carcinosarcoma following methotrexate pre-treatment. A 19 F-MRS study in vivo. *Br J Cancer* 1992;65:369–375.

476. Tattersall MHN, Jackson RC, Connors TA, et al. Combination chemotherapy. The interaction of methotrexate and 5-fluorouracil. *Eur J Cancer* 1973;9:733–739.

477. Bertino JR, Sawicki WL, Linquist CA, et al. Schedule-dependent antitumor effects of methotrexate and 5-fluorouracil. *Cancer Res* 1977;37:327–328.

478. Kemeny N, Ahmed T, Michaelson R, et al. Activity of sequential low-dose methotrexate and fluorouracil in advanced colorectal carcinoma. Attempt at correlation with tissue and blood levels of phosphoribosylpyrophosphate. *J Clin Oncol* 1984;2:311–315.

479. Marsh JC, Bertino JR, Katz KH, et al. The influence of drug interval on the effect of methotrexate and fluorouracil in the treatment of advanced colorectal cancer. *J Clin Oncol* 1991;9:371–380.

480. Browman GP, Levine MN, Goodyear MD, et al. Methotrexate/fluorouracil scheduling influences normal tissue toxicity but not antitumor effects in patients with squamous cell head and neck cancer. Results from a randomized trial. *J Clin Oncol* 1988;6:963–968.

481. Elliot WL, Howeard CT, Kykes DJ, et al. Sequence and schedule-dependent synergy of trimetrexate in combination with 5-fluorouracil in vitro and in mice. *Cancer Res* 1989;15:5586–5590.

482. Romanini A, Li WW, Colofiore JR, et al. Leucovorin enhances cytotoxicity of trimetrexate/fluorouracil, but not methotrexate/fluorouracil, in CCRF-CEM cells. *J Natl Cancer Inst* 1992;84:1033–1038.

483. Conti JA, Kemeny N, Seiter K, et al. Trial of sequential trimetrexate, fluorouracil, and high-dose leucovorin in previously treated patients with gastrointestinal carcinoma. *J Clin Oncol* 1994;12:695–700.

484. Blanke CD, Kasimis B, Schein P, et al. Phase II study of trimetrexate, fluorouracil, and leucovorin for advanced colorectal cancer. *J Clin Oncol* 1997;15:915–920.

485. Punt CJA, Keizer HJ, Douma J, et al. Multicenter randomized trial of 5-fluorouracil and leucovorin with or without trimetrexate as first line treatment in patients with advanced colorectal cancer. *Proc Am Soc Clin Oncol* 1999;18:262.

486. Danenberg PV, Danenberg KD. Effect of 5,10-methylenetetrahydrofolate and the dissociation of 5-fluorodeoxyuridylate binding of human thymidylate synthetase. Evidence for an ordered mechanism. *Biochemistry* 1978;17:4018–4024.

487. Houghton JA, Maroda SJ, Phillips JO, et al. Biochemical determinants of responsiveness to 5-fluorouracil and its derivatives in xenografts of human colorectal adenocarcinomas in mice. *Cancer Res* 1981;41:144–149.

488. Houghton JA, Schmidt C, Houghton PF. The effect of derivatives of folic acid on the fluorodeoxyuridylate-thymidylate synthetase covalent complex in human colon xenografts. *Eur J Cancer Clin Oncol* 1982;18:347–354.

489. Houghton JA, Torrance PM, Radparvar S, et al. Binding of 5-fluorodeoxyuridylate to thymidylate synthase in human colon adenocarcinoma xenografts. *Eur J Cancer Clin Oncol* 1986;22:505–510.

490. Spears CP, Gustavsson BG, Fiosing R. Folinic acid modulation of fluorouracil. Tissue kinetics of bolus administration. *Invest New Drugs* 1989;7:27–36.

491. Evans RM, Laskin JD, Hakala MT. Effects of excess folates and deoxyinosine on the activity and site of action of 5-fluorouracil. *Cancer Res* 1981;41:3288–3295.

492. Yin M-B, Zakrzewski SF, Hakala MT. Relationship of cellular folate cofactor pools to the activity of 5-fluorouracil. *Mol Pharmacol* 1983;23:190–197.

493. Cao S, Frank C, Rustum YM. Role of fluoropyrimidine Schedule and (6R,S)leucovorin dose in a preclinical animal model of colorectal carcinoma. *J Natl Cancer Inst* 1996;88:430–436.

494. Cheradame S, Etienne MC, Chazal M, et al. Relevance of tumoral folylpolyglutamate synthetase and reduced folates for optimal 5-fluorouracil efficacy. Experimental data. *Eur J Cancer* 1997;33:950–959.

495. Drake JC, Voeller DM, Allegra CJ, et al. The effect of dose and interval between 5-fluorouracil and leucovorin on the formation of thymidylate synthase ternary complex in human cancer cells. *Br J Cancer* 1995;71:1145–1150.

496. Keyomarsi K, Moran R. Folinic acid augmentation of the effects of fluoropyrimidines on murine and human leukemic cells. *Cancer Res* 1986;46:5229–5235.

497. Mini E, Moroson BA, Bertino JR. Cytotoxicity of floxuridine and 5-fluorouracil in human T-lymphoblast leukemia cells. Enhancement by leucovorin. *Cancer Treat Rep* 1987; 71:381–389.

498. Park JG, Collins JM, Gazdar AF, et al. Enhancement of fluorinated pyrimidine induced cytotoxicity by leucovorin in human colorectal carcinoma cell lines. *J Natl Cancer Inst* 1988;80:1560–1564.

499. Matherly LH, Czajkowski CA, Muench SP, et al. Role for cytosolic folate binding proteins in compartmentation of endogenous tetrahydrofolates and the formyltetrahydrofolate-mediated enhancement of 5-fluoro-2'-deoxyuridine antitumor activity in vitro. *Cancer Res* 1990;50:3262–3269.

500. Nadal JC, van Groeningen CJ, Pinedo HM, et al. In vivo potentiation of 5-fluorouracil by leucovorin in murine colon carcinoma. *Biomed Pharmacother* 1988;42:387–393.

501. Radparvar S, Houghton PJ, Houghton JA. Effect of polyglutamylation of 5,10-methylenetetrahydrofolate on the binding of 5-fluoro-2-deoxyuridylate to thymidylate synthase purified from a human colon adenocarcinoma xenograft. *Biochem Pharmacol* 1989;38:335–342.

502. Houghton PJ, Houghton JA, Hazelton BJ, et al. Biochemical mechanisms in colon xenografts. Thymidylate synthase as a target for therapy. *Invest New Drugs* 1989;7:59–69.

503. Nadal JC, van Groeningen CJ, Pinedo HM, et al. Schedule-dependency of in vivo modulation of 5-fluorouracil by leucovorin and uridine in murine colon carcinoma. *Invest New Drugs* 1989;7:163–172.

504. Wright JE, Dreyfuss A, El-Magharbel I, et al. Selective expansion of 5,10-methylenetetrahydrofolate pools and modulation of 5-fluorouracil antitumor activity by leucovorin in vivo. *Cancer Res* 1989;49:2592–2596.

505. Carlsson G, Gustavsson BG, Spears CP, et al. 5-Fluorouracil plus leucovorin as adjuvant treatment of an experimental liver tumor in rats. *Anticancer Res* 1990;10:813–816.

506. Houghton JA, Williams LG, Cheshire PJ, et al. Influence of dose of [6RS]-leucovorin on reduced folate pools and 5-fluorouracil-mediated thymidylate synthase inhibition in human colon adenocarcinoma xenografts. *Cancer Res* 1990; 50:3940–3946.

507. Houghton JA, Williams WG, deGraaf SS, et al. Comparison of the conversion of 5-formyltetrahydrofolate and 5-methyltetrahydrofolate to 5,10-methylenetetrahydrofolates and tetrahydrofolates in human colon tumors. *Cancer Commun* 1989;1:167–174.

508. Martin DS, Stolf RL, Colofiore JR. Failure of high dose leucovorin to improve therapy with a maximally tolerated dose of 5-fluorouracil. A murine study with clinical relevance. *J Natl Cancer Inst* 1988;80:496–501.

509. Bertrand R, Jolivet J. Lack of interference by the unnatural isomer of 5-formyltetrahydrofolate with the effects of the natural isomer in leucovorin preparations. *J Natl Cancer Inst* 1989;81:1175–1178.

510. Straw JA, Szapary D, Wynn WT. Pharmacokinetics of the diastereoisomers of leucovorin after intravenous and oral administration to normal subjects. *Cancer Res* 1984;44:3114–3119.

511. Machover D, Goldschmidt E, Chollet P, et al. Treatment of advanced colorectal and gastric adenocarcinomas with 5-fluorouracil and high-dose folinic acid. *J Clin Oncol* 1986; 4:685–696.

512. Trave F, Rustum YM, Petrelli NJ, et al. Plasma and tumor tissue pharmacology of high dose intravenous leucovorin calcium in combination with fluorouracil in patients with advanced colorectal carcinoma. *J Clin Oncol* 1988;6:1181–1188.

513. Newman EA, Straw JA, Doroshow JH. Pharmacokinetics of diastereoisomers of (6R,S)-folinic acid (leucovorin) in humans during constant high-dose intravenous infusion. *Cancer Res* 1989;49:5755–5760.

514. Priest DG, Schmitz JC, Bunni MA, et al. Pharmacokinetics of leucovorin metabolites in human plasma as a function of dose administered orally and intravenously. *J Natl Cancer Inst* 1991;83:1806–1812.

515. Haller DG, Catalano PJ, Macdonald JS, et al. Fluorouracil, leucovorin and levamisole adjuvant therapy for colon cancer. Five-year final report of INT-0089. *Proc Am Soc Clin Oncol* 1998;17:265a.

516. Elias L, Crissman HA. Interferon effects upon the adenocarcinoma MCA 38 and HL-60 cell lines. Antiproliferative responses and synergistic interactions with halogenated pyrimidine antimetabolites. *Cancer Res* 1988;48:4868–4873.

517. Elias L, Sandoval JM. Interferon effects upon fluorouracil metabolism by HL-60 cells. *Biochem Biophys Res Commun* 1989;163:867–874.

518. Wadler S, Wersto R, Weinberg V, et al. Interaction of fluorouracil and interferon in human colon cancer cell lines. Cytotoxic and cytokinetic effects. *Cancer Res* 1990;50:5735–5739.

519. Schwartz EL, Hoffman M, O'Connor CJ, et al. Stimulation of 5-fluorouracil metabolic activation by interferon-α in human colon carcinoma cells. *Biochem Biophys Res Commun* 1992;182:1232–1239.

520. Schwartz EL, Baptiste N, O'Connor CJ, et al. Potentiation of the antitumor activity of 5-fluorouracil in colon carcinoma cells by the combination of interferon and deoxyribonucleosides results from complementary effects on thymidine phosphorylase. *Cancer Res* 1994;54:1472–1478.

521. Horowitz RW, Heerdt BG, Hu X, et al. Combination therapy with 5-fluorouracil and IFN-alpha2a induces a nonrandom increase in DNA fragments of less than 3 megabases in HT29 colon carcinoma cells. *Clin Cancer Res* 1997;3:1317–1322.

522. Morita T, Tokue A. Biomodulation of 5-fluorouracil by

interferon-alpha in human renal carcinoma cells. Relationship to the expression of thymidine phosphorylase. *Cancer Chemother Pharmacol* 1999;44:91–96.

523. Houghton JA, Adkins DA, Rahman A, et al. Interaction between 5-fluorouracil, [6R,S]leucovorin, and recombinant human interferon-α2a in cultured colon adenocarcinoma cells. *Cancer Commun* 1991;3:225–231.

524. Houghton JA, Morton CL, Adkins DA, et al. Locus of the interaction among 5-fluorouracil, leucovorin and interferon-α2a in colon carcinoma cells. *Cancer Res* 1993;53:4243–4250.

525. Houghton JA, Cheshire PJ, Morton CL, et al. Potentiation of 5-fluorouracil-leucovorin activity by alpha2a-interferon in colon adenocarcinoma xenografts. *Clin Cancer Res* 1995;1:33–40.

526. Neefe JR, Glass J. Abrogation of interferon-induced resistance to interferon-activated major histocompatibility complex-unrestricted killers by treatment of a melanoma cell line with 5-fluorouracil. *Cancer Res* 1991;51:3159–3163.

527. Reiter Z, Ozes ON, Blatt LM, et al. A dual antitumor effect of a combination of interferon-α or interleukin-2 and 5-fluorouracil on natural killer (NK) cell-mediated cytotoxicity. *Clin Immunol Immunopathol* 1992;62:103–111.

528. Guglielmi A, Aschele C, Mori A, et al. In vitro synergism between 5-fluorouracil and natural beta interferon in human colon carcinoma cells. *Clin Cancer Res* 1995;1: 1337–1344.

529. Marumo K, Oya M, Murai M. Biochemical modulation of 5-fluorouracil with murine interferon-alpha/beta against murine renal cell carcinoma. *Int J Urol* 1997;4:163–168.

530. Koshiji M, Adachi Y, Taketani S, et al. Mechanisms underlying apoptosis induced by combination of 5-fluorouracil and interferon-gamma. *Biochem Biophys Res Commun* 1997; 240:376–381.

531. van der Wilt CL, Smid K, Aherne GW, et al. Biochemical mechanisms of interferon modulation of 5-fluorouracil activity in colon cancer cells. *Eur J Cancer* 1997;33:471–478.

532. Ismail A, Van Groeningen CJ, Hardcastle A, et al. Modulation of fluorouracil cytotoxicity by interferon-alpha and -gamma. *Mol Pharmacol* 1998;53:252–261.

533. Aquino A, Prete SP, Greiner JW, et al. Effect of the combined treatment with 5-fluorouracil, gamma-interferon or folinic acid on carcinoembryonic antigen expression in colon cancer cells. *Clin Cancer Res* 1998;4:2473–2481.

534. Wadler S, Lembersky B, Atkins M, et al. Phase II trial of fluorouracil and recombinant interferon alfa-2a in patients with advanced colorectal carcinoma. An Eastern Cooperative Oncology Group study. *J Clin Oncol* 1991;9:1806–1810.

535. Makower D, Wadler S, Haynes H, et al. Interferon induces thymidine phosphorylase/platelet-derived endothelial cell growth factor expression in vivo. *Clin Cancer Res* 1997; 3:923–929.

536. Grem JL, Jordan E, Robson ME, et al. Phase II study of fluorouracil, leucovorin, and interferon alfa-2a in metastatic colorectal carcinoma. *J Clin Oncol* 1993;9:1737–1745.

537. Hill M, Norman A, Cunningham D, et al. Royal Marsden Phase III trial of fluorouracil with or without interferon α-2b in advanced colorectal cancer. *J Clin Oncol* 1995;13: 1297–1302.

538. Hill M, Norman A, Cunningham D, et al. Impact of protracted venous infusion 5-fluorouracil with or without interferon α-2b on tumor response, survival, and quality of life in advanced colorectal cancer. *J Clin Oncol* 1995;13:2317–2323.

539. Phase III randomized study of two fluorouracil combinations with either interferon α-2a or leucovorin for advanced colorectal cancer. Corfu-A study group. *J Clin Oncol* 1995;13:921–928.

540. Seymour MT, Slevin ML, Kerr ML, et al. Randomized trial assessing the addition of interferon α-2a to fluorouracil and leucovorin in advanced colorectal cancer. Colorectal Cancer Working Party of the United Kingdom Medical Research Council. *J Clin Oncol* 1996;14:2280–2288.

541. Dufour P, Husseini F, Dreyfus B, et al. 5-Fluorouracil versus 5-fluorouracil plus alpha-interferon as treatment of metastatic colorectal carcinoma. A randomized study. *Ann Oncol* 1996;7:575–579.

542. Kosmidis PA, Tsavaris N, Skarlos D, et al. Fluorouracil and leucovorin with or without interferon alfa-2b in advanced colorectal cancer. Analysis of a prospective randomized phase III trial. Hellenic Cooperative Oncology Group. *J Clin Oncol* 1996;14:2682–2687.

543. Hausmaninger H, Moser R, Samonigg H, et al. Biochemical modulation of 5-fluorouracil by leucovorin with or without interferon-alpha-2c in patients with advanced colorectal cancer. Final results of a randomised phase III study. *Eur J Cancer* 1999;35:380–385.

544. Wolmark N, Bryant J, Smith R, et al. Adjuvant 5-fluorouracil and leucovorin with or without interferon alfa-2a in colon carcinoma. National Surgical Adjuvant Breast and Bowel Project protocol C-05. *J Natl Cancer Inst* 1998;90:1810–1816.

545. Danhauser LL, Freimann JH Jr, Gilchrist TL, et al. Phase I and plasma pharmacokinetic study of infusional 5-fluorouracil combined with recombinant interferon alfa-2a in patients with advanced cancer. *J Clin Oncol* 1993;11:751–761.

546. Meadows LM, Walther P, Ozer H. Interferon and 5-fluorouracil, possible mechanisms of antitumor action. *Semin Oncol* 1991;18:71–76.

547. Schuller J, Czejka M. Pharmacokinetic interaction of 5-fluorouracil and interferon alpha-2b with or without folinic acid. *Med Oncol* 1995;12:47–53.

548. Yee LK, Allegra CJ, Steinberg SM, et al. Decreased catabolism of 5-fluorouracil in peripheral blood mononuclear cells during therapy with 5-fluorouracil, leucovorin, and interferon α-2a. *J Natl Cancer Inst* 1992;84:1820–1825.

549. O'Dwyer PJ, King SA, Hoth DF, et al. Role of thymidine in biochemical modulation. A review. *Cancer Res* 1987;47: 3911–3919.

550. Vogel SJ, Presant CA, Ratkin FA, et al. Phase I study of thymidine plus 5-fluorouracil infusions in advanced colorectal carcinoma. *Cancer Treat Rep* 1979;63:1–5.

551. Chen J-J, Jones ME. Effect of 6-azauridine on de novo pyrimidine biosynthesis in cultured Ehrlich ascites cells. *J Biol Chem* 1979;254:4908–4914.

552. Ahluwalia GS, Grem JL, Ho Z, et al. Metabolism and action of amino acid analog anti-cancer agents. *Pharmacol Ther* 1990;46:243–271.

553. O'Dwyer PJ, Alonso MT, Leyland-Jones B. Acivicin. A new glutamine antagonist in clinical trials. *J Clin Oncol* 1984; 2:1064–1071.

554. Moyer JD, Handschumacher RE. Selective inhibition of pyrimidine synthesis and depletion of nucleotide pools by n-(phosphonacetyl)-L-aspartate. *Cancer Res* 1979;39:3089–3094.

555. Moyer JD, Smith PA, Levy EJ, et al. Kinetics of n-(phosphonacetyl)-L-aspartate and pyrazofurin depletion of pyrimidine ribonucleotide and deoxyribonucleotide pools and their relationship to nucleic acid synthesis in intact and permeabilized cells. *Cancer Res* 1982;42:4525–4531.

556. Ardalan B, Glazer RI, Kensler TW, et al. Synergistic effect of 5-fluorouracil and n-(phosphonacetyl)-L-aspartate on cell growth and ribonucleic acid synthesis in human mammary carcinoma. *Biochem Pharmacol* 1981;30:2045–2049.

557. Anukarahanonta T, Holstege A, Keppler DOR. Selective enhancement of 5-fluorouridine uptake and action in rat hepatomas in vivo following pretreatment with D-galactosamine and 6-azauridine or n-(phosphonacetyl)-L-aspartate. *Eur J Cancer* 1980;16:1171–1180.

558. Major PP, Egan EM, Sargent L, et al. Modulation of 5-FU metabolism in human MCF-7 breast carcinoma cells. *Cancer Chemother Pharmacol* 1982;8:87–91.

559. Liang C-M, Donehower RC, Chabner BA. Biochemical interactions between n-(phosphonacetyl)-L-aspartate and 5-fluorouracil. *Mol Pharmacol* 1982;21:224–230.

560. Erichsen C, Christensson PI, Jakobsson B, et al. Effect of n-phosphonacetyl-L-aspartate and D-glucosamine on the incorporation of 5-fluorouridine into normal tissues and an adenocarcinoma in the rat. *Anticancer Res* 1987;7:77–80.

561. Martin DS, Stolfi RL, Sawyer RC, et al. Therapeutic utility of utilizing low doses of n-(phosphonacetyl)-L-aspartic acid in combination with 5-fluorouracil. A murine study with clinical relevance. *Cancer Res* 1983;43:2317–2321.

562. Grem JL, King SA, O'Dwyer PJ, et al. Biochemistry and clinical activity of n-(phosphonacetyl)-L-aspartate. A review. *Cancer Res* 1988;48:4441–4454.

563. Johnson RK, Swyrd EA, Stark GR. Effects of n-(phosphonacetyl)-L-aspartate on murine tumors and normal tissues in vivo and in vitro and the relationship of sensitivity to rate of proliferation and level of aspartate transcarbamylase. *Cancer Res* 1978;38:371–378.

564. Jayaram HN, Cooney DA, Vistica DT, et al. Mechanisms of sensitivity or resistance of murine tumors to n-(phosphonacetyl)-L-aspartate. *Cancer Treat Rep* 1979;63:1291–1302.

565. Weber G. Biochemical strategy of cancer cells and the design of chemotherapy. GHA Clowes Memorial Lecture. *Cancer Res* 1983;43:3466–3492.

566. Buroker TR, Moertel CG, Fleming TR, et al. A controlled evaluation of recent approaches to biochemical modulation or enhancement of 5-fluorouracil therapy in colorectal carcinoma. *J Clin Oncol* 1985;3:1624–1631.

567. Karle JM, Anderson LW, Erlichman C, et al. Serum uridine levels in patients receiving n-(phosphonacetyl)-L-aspartate. *Cancer Res* 1980;40:2938–2940.

568. Chan TCK, Markman M, Cleary S, et al. Plasma uridine changes in cancer patients treated with the combination of dipyridamole and n-phosphonacetyl-L-aspartate. *Cancer Res* 1986;46:3168–3172.

569. Monks A, Cysyk RL. Uridine regulation by the isolated rat liver. Perfusion with an artificial oxygen carrier. *Am J Physiol* 1982;242:R465–R470.

570. Gasser T, Moyer JD, Handschumacher RE. Novel single-pass exchange of circulating uridine in rat liver. *Science* 1981;213:777–778.

571. Casper ES, Vale K, Williams LJ, et al. Phase I and clinical pharmacological evaluation of biochemical modulation of 5-fluorouracil with n-(phosphonacetyl)-L-aspartic acid. *Cancer Res* 1983;43:2324–2329.

572. Jayaram HN, Cooney DA. Analogs of L-aspartic acid in chemotherapy for cancer. *Cancer Treat Rep* 1979;63:1095–1108.

573. Miller AA, Moore EC, Hurlbert RB, et al. Pharmacological and biochemical interactions of n-(phosphonacetyl)-L-aspartate and 5-fluorouracil in beagles. *Cancer Res* 1986;43:2565–2570.

574. Kemeny N, Seiter K, Martin D, et al. A new syndrome. Ascites, hyperbilirubinemia, and hypoalbuminemia after biochemical modulation of fluorouracil with n-phosphonacetyl-L-aspartate (PALA). *Ann Intern Med* 1991;115:946–951.

575. Fleming RA, Capizzi RL, Muss HB, et al. Phase I study of N-(phosphonacetyl)-L-aspartate with fluorouracil and with or without dipyridamole in patients with advanced cancer. *Clin Cancer Res* 1996;2:1107–1114.

576. Moore EC, Friedman J, Valdivieso M, et al. Aspartate carbamoyltransferase activity, drug concentrations, and pyrimidine nucleotides in tissues from patients treated with n-(phosphonacetyl)-L-aspartate. *Biochem Pharmacol* 1982;31:3317–3321.

577. O'Dwyer PJ, Paul AR, Walczak J, et al. Phase II study of biochemical modulation of fluorouracil by low-dose PALA in patients with colorectal cancer. *J Clin Oncol* 1990;8:1497–1503.

578. O'Dwyer PJ, Ryan LM, Valone FH, et al. Phase III trial of biochemical modulation of 5-fluorouracil by IV or oral leucovorin or by interferon in advanced colorectal cancer. An ECOG/CALGB phase III trial. *Proc Am Soc Clin Oncol* 1996;15:207.

579. Martin DS, Stolfi RL, Sawyer RC, et al. Improved therapeutic index with sequential n-phosphonacetyl-L-aspartate plus high-dose methotrexate plus high-dose 5-fluorouracil and appropriate rescue. *Cancer Res* 1983;43:4653–4661.

580. Kemeny N, Schneider A, Martin DS, et al. Phase I trial of n-(phosphonacetyl)-L-aspartate, methotrexate and 5-fluorouracil with leucovorin rescue in patients with advanced cancer. *Cancer Res* 1989;49:4636–4639.

581. O'Dwyer PJ, Hudes GR, Colofiore J, et al. Phase I trial of fluorouracil modulation by n-phosphonacetyl-L-aspartate and 6-methylmercaptopurine riboside. Optimization of 6-methylmercaptopurine riboside dose and schedule through biochemical analysis of sequential tumor biopsy specimens. *J Natl Cancer Inst* 1991;83:1235–1240.

582. Pizzorno G, Wiegand RA, Lentz SK, et al. Brequinar potentiates 5-fluorouracil antitumor activity in a murine model colon 38 tumor by tissue-specific modulation of uridine nucleotide pools. *Cancer Res* 1992;52:1660–1665.

583. Peters GM, Kraal I, Pinedo HM. In vitro and in vivo studies on the combination of brequinar sodium (DUP 785, NSC 268390) with 5-fluorouracil. Effects of uridine. *Br J Cancer* 1992;65:229–233.

584. Chen T-L, Erlichman C. Biochemical modulation of 5-fluorouracil with or without leucovorin by a low dose of brequinar in MGH-U1 cells. *Cancer Chemother Pharmacol* 1992;30:370–376.

585. Peters GJ, Schwartsmann G, Nadal JC, et al. In vivo inhibition of the pyrimidine de novo enzyme dihydroorotic acid dehydrogenase by brequinar sodium (DUP 785, NSC 268390) in mice and patients. *Cancer Res* 1990;50:4644–4649.

586. Buzaid AC, Pizzorno G, Marsh JC, et al. Biochemical modulation of 5-fluorouracil with brequinar. Results of a phase I study. *Cancer Chemother Pharmacol* 1995;36:373–378.

587. Moran RG, Danenberg PV, Heidelberger C. Therapeutic response of leukemic mice treated with fluorinated pyrimidines and inhibitors of deoxyuridylate synthesis. *Biochem Pharmacol* 1982;31:2929–2935.

588. Engstrom PF, MacIntyre JM, Mittelman A, et al. Chemotherapy of advanced colorectal carcinoma. Fluorouracil alone vs two drug combinations using fluorouracil, hydroxyurea, semustine, dacarbazine, razoxane, and mitomycin. A phase III trial by the Eastern Cooperative Oncology Group. *Am J Clin Oncol* 1984;7:313–318.

589. Engstrom PF, MacIntyre JM, Schutt AJ, et al. Chemotherapy of large bowel carcinoma—fluorouracil plus hydroxyurea vs methyl-CCNU, oncovin, fluorouracil and streptozotocin. An Eastern Cooperative Oncology Group Study. *Am J Clin Oncol* 1985;8:358–361.

590. Di Costanzo F, Gasperoni S, Malacarne P, et al. High-dose folinic acid and 5-fluorouracil alone or combined with hydroxyurea in advanced colorectal cancer. A randomized trial of the Italian Oncology Group For Clinical Research. *Am J Clin Oncol* 1998;21:369–375.

591. Santelli J, Valeriote F. In vivo potentiation of 5-fluorouracil cytotoxicity against AKR leukemia by purines, pyrimidines and their nucleosides and deoxynucleosides. *J Natl Cancer Inst* 1980;64:69–72.

592. Iigo M, Kuretani K, Hoshi A. Relationship between antitumor effect and metabolites of 5-fluorouracil in combination treatment with 5-fluorouracil and guanosine in ascites sarcoma 180 tumor system. *Cancer Res* 1983;43:5687–5694.

593. Iigo M, Yamaizumi Z, Nishimura S, et al. Mechanism of potentiation of antitumor activity of 5-fluorouracil by guanine ribonucleotides against adenocarcinoma 755. *Eur J Cancer Clin Oncol* 1987;23:1059–1065.

594. Parker WB, Klubes P. Enhancement by uridine of the anabolism of 5-fluorouracil in mouse T-lymphoma (S-49) cells. *Cancer Res* 1985;45:4249–4256.

595. Tuchman M, Ramnaraine ML, O'Dea RF. Effects of uridine and thymidine on the degradation of 5-fluorouracil, uracil and thymine by rat liver dihydropyrimidine dehydrogenase. *Cancer Res* 1985;45:5553–5556.

596. Nabeya Y, Isono K, Moriyama Y, et al. Ribose-transfer activity from uridine to 5-fluorouracil in Ehrlich ascites tumor cells. *Jpn J Cancer Res* 1990;81:692–700.

597. Chu MYW, Naguib FNM, Iltzsch MH, et al. Potentiation of FdUrd antineoplastic activity by the uridine phosphorylase inhibitors benzylacyclouridine and benzyloxybenzylacyclouridine. *Cancer Res* 1984;44:1852–1856.

598. Darnowski JW, Handschumacher RE. Tissue-specific enhancement of uridine utilization and 5-fluorouracil therapy in mice by benzylacyclouridine. *Cancer Res* 1985;45:5364–5368.

599. Ashour OM, Naguib FNM, Khalifa MMA, et al. Enhancement of 5-fluoro-2'-deoxyuridine antitumor efficacy by the uridine phosphorylase inhibitor-5-(benzyloxybenzyl)barbituric acid acyclonucleoside. *Cancer Res* 1995;55:1092–1098.

600. Pu T, Robertson JM, Lawrence TS. Current status of radiation sensitization by fluorinated pyrimidines. *Oncology* 1995;9:707–735.

601. Garrett C, Wataya Y, Santi D. Thymidylate synthetase. Catalysis of dehalogenation of 5-bromo- and 5-iodo-2'-deoxyuridylate. *Biochemistry* 1979;18:2798.

602. Heidelberger C, Griesback I, Ghobar A. The potentiation of 5-iodo-2'-deoxyuridine of the tumor-inhibitory activity of 5-fluoro-2'-deoxyuridine. *Cancer Chemother Rep* 1960;6:37.

603. Burchenal JH, Oettgen HF, Reppert JA, et al. Studies on the synergism of fluorinated pyrimidines and certain pyrimidine and purine derivatives against transplanted mouse leukemia. *Cancer Chemother Rep* 1960;6:1.

604. Benson AB, Trump DL, Cummings KB, et al. Modulation of 5-iodo-2'-deoxyuridine metabolism and cytotoxicity in human bladder cancer cells by fluoropyrimidines. *Biochem Pharmacol* 1985;34:3925.

605. Bagshawe KD, Boden GM, Britton DW, et al. A cytotoxic DNA precursor is taken up selectively by human cancer xenografts. *Br J Cancer* 1987;55:299.

606. Mancini WR, Stetson PL, Lawrence TS, et al. Variability of 5-bromo-2'-deoxyuridine incorporation into DNA of human glioma cell lines and modulation with fluoropyrimidines. *Cancer Res* 1991;51:870.

607. Lawrence TS, Davis MA, Maybaum J, et al. Modulation of iododeoxyuridine-mediated radiosensitization by 5-fluorouracil in human colon cancer cells. *Int J Radiat Oncol Biol Phys* 1992;22:49.

608. Vazquez-Padua MA, Risueno C, Fischer PH. Regulation of the activation of fluorodeoxyuridine by substrate competition and feedback inhibition in 647V cells. *Cancer Res* 1989;49:618.

609. Calabresi P, Creasey WA, Prusoff WH, et al. Clinical and pharmacological studies with 5-iodo-2'-deoxyuridine. *Cancer Res* 1963;23:583.

610. Papac R, Jacobs E, Wong F, et al. Clinical evaluation of the pyrimidine nucleosides 5-fluoro-2'-deoxyuridine and 5-iodo-2'-deoxyuridine. *Cancer Chemother Rep* 1960;6:143.

611. Young CW, Ellison RR, Sullivan RD, et al. The clinical evaluation of 5-fluorouracil and 5-fluoro-2'-deoxyuridine in solid tumors in adults. *Cancer Chemother Rep* 1960;6:17.

612. Kinsella TJ, Russo A, Mitchell JB, et al. A phase I study of intravenous iododeoxyuridine as a clinical radiosensitizer. *Int J Radiat Oncol Biol Phys* 1985;111:1941.

613. Kinsella TJ, Collins J, Rowland J, et al. Pharmacology and phase I/II study of continuous intravenous infusions of iododeoxyuridine and hyperfractionated radiotherapy in patients with glioblastoma multiforme. *J Clin Oncol* 1988;6:871.

614. Belanger K, Klecker RW Jr, Rowland J, et al. Incorporation of iododeoxyuridine into DNA of granulocytes in patients. *Cancer Res* 1986;46:6509.

615. Speth PAJ, Kinsella TJ, Chang AE, et al. Selective incorporation of iododeoxyuridine into DNA of hepatic metastases versus normal human liver. *Clin Pharmacol Ther* 1988;44:369.

616. Speth PAJ, Kinsella TJ, Belanger K, et al. Fluorodeoxyuridine modulation of the incorporation of iododeoxyuridine into DNA of granulocytes. A phase I and clinical pharmacology study. *Cancer Res* 1988;48:2933.

617. McGinn CJ, Kunugi KA, Tutsch KD, et al. Leucovorin modulation of 5-iododeoxyuridine radiosensitization. A phase I study. *Clin Cancer Res* 1986;2:1299–1305.

618. Remick SC, Benson AB, Weese JL, et al. Phase I trial of hepatic artery infusion of 5-iodo-2'-deoxyuridine and 5-fluorouracil in patients with advanced hepatic malignancy. Biochemically based combination therapy. *Cancer Res* 1989;49:6437.

619. Weber G. Biochemical strategy of cancer cells and the design of chemotherapy. *Cancer Res* 1983;43:3466.

620. Paterson ARP, Jakobs ES, Ng CYC, et al. Nucleoside transport inhibition in vitro and in vivo. In: Gerlach E, Becker BF, eds. *Topics and perspectives in adenosine research.* Berlin: Springer-Verlag, 1987:89–101.

621. Griffith DA, Jarvis SM. Nucleoside and nucleobase transport systems of mammalian cells. *Biochim Biophys Acta* 1996;1286:153–181.

622. Grem JL, Fischer PH. Augmentation of 5-fluorouracil cytotoxicity in human colon cancer cells by dipyridamole. *Cancer Res* 1985;45:2967–2972.

623. Fisher PH, Pamukcu R, Bittner G, et al. Enhancement of the sensitivity of human colon cancer cells to growth inhibition by acivicin achieved through inhibition of nucleic acid precursor salvage of dipyridamole. *Cancer Res* 1984;44: 3355–3359.

624. Chan TC, Howell SB. Mechanism of synergy between n-phosphonacetyl-L-aspartate and dipyridamole in a human ovarian carcinoma cell line. *Cancer Res* 1985;45:3598–3604.

625. van Mouwerik TJ, Pangallo CA, Willson JKV, et al. Augmentation of methotrexate cytotoxicity in human colon cancer cells achieved through inhibition of thymidine salvage by dipyridamole. *Biochem Pharmacol* 1987;36:809–814.

626. Grem JL, Fischer PH. Modulation of fluorouracil metabolism and cytotoxicity by nitrobenzylthioinosine. *Biochem Pharmacol* 1986;35:2651–2654.

627. Grem JL, Fischer PH. Alteration of fluorouracil metabolism in human colon cancer cells by dipyridamole with a selective increase in fluorodeoxyuridine monophosphate levels. *Cancer Res* 1986;46:6191–6199.

628. Lonn U, Lonn S, Nylen U, et al. 5-Fluoropyrimidine-induced DNA damage in human colon adenocarcinoma and its augmentation by the nucleoside transport inhibitor dipyridamole. *Cancer Res* 1989;49:1085–1089.

629. Budd GT, Jayaraj A, Grabowski D, et al. Phase I trial of dipyridamole with 5-fluorouracil and folinic acid. *Cancer Res* 1990;50:7206–7211.

630. Bailey H, Wilding G, Tutsch KD, et al. A phase I trial of 5-fluorouracil, leucovorin, and dipyridamole given by concurrent 120-h continuous infusions. *Cancer Chemother Pharmacol* 1992;30:297–302.

631. Fischer PH, Willson JKV, Risueno C, et al. Biochemical assessment of the effects of acivicin and dipyridamole given as a continuous 72-hour intravenous infusion. *Cancer Res* 1988;48:5591–5596.

632. Willson JKV, Fischer PH, Remick SC, et al. Methotrexate and dipyridamole combination chemotherapy based upon inhibition of nucleoside salvage in humans. *Cancer Res* 1989;49:1866–1889.

633. Köhne C-H, Hiddemann W, Schüller J, et al. Failure of orally administered dipyridamole to enhance the antineoplastic activity of fluorouracil in combination with leucovorin in patients with advanced colorectal cancer. A prospective randomized trial. *J Clin Oncol* 1995;13:1201–1208.

634. Schabel FM, Trader MW, Laster WR Jr, et al. *cis*-Dichlorodiammineplatinum(II) combination chemotherapy and cross-resistance studies with tumors of mice. *Cancer Treat Rep* 1979;63:1459–1473.

635. Dionet C, Verrelle P. Curability of mouse L1210 leukemia by combination of 5-fluorouracil, cis-diamminedichloroplatinum(II), and low doses of gamma-rays. *Cancer Res* 1984;44:652–656.

636. Beaupain R, Dionet C. Effects of combined treatments of cis-diamminedichloroplatinum(II), 5-fluorouracil, and x-rays on growth of human cancer nodules maintained in continuous organotypic culture. *Cancer Res* 1985;45:3150–3154.

637. Scanlon KJ, Newman EM, Lu Y, et al. Biochemical basis for cisplatin and 5-fluorouracil synergism in human ovarian carcinoma cells. *Proc Natl Acad Sci U S A* 1986;83:8923–8925.

638. Pratesi G, Gianni L, Manzotti C, et al. Sequence dependence of the antitumor and toxic effects of 5-fluorouracil and cis-diamminedichloroplatinum combination on primary colon tumors in mice. *Cancer Chemother Pharmacol* 1988;20:237–241.

639. Palmeri S, Trave F, Russello O, et al. The role of drug sequence in therapeutic selectivity of the combination of 5-fluorouracil and cisplatin. *Sel Cancer Ther* 1989;5:169–177.

640. Esaki T, Nakano S, Tatsumoto T, et al. Inhibition by 5-fluorouracil of cis-diamminedichloroplatinum(II)-induced DNA interstrand cross-link removal in a HST-1 human squamous carcinoma cell line. *Cancer Res* 1992;52:6501–6506.

641. Kuroki M, Nakano S, Mitsugi K, et al. In vivo comparative therapeutic study of optimal administration of 5-fluorouracil and cisplatin using a newly established HST-1 human squamous-carcinoma cell line. *Cancer Chemother Pharmacol* 1992;29:273–276.

642. Tsai C-M, Hsiao S-H, Frey CM, et al. Combination cytotoxic effects of cis-diamminedichloroplatinum(II) and 5-fluorouracil with and without leucovorin against human non-small cell lung cancer cell lines. *Cancer Res* 1993; 53:1079–1084.

643. Johnston PG, Geoffroy F, Drake J, et al. The cellular interaction of 5-fluorouracil and cisplatin in a human colon carcinoma cell line. *Eur J Cancer* 1996;32A:2148–2154.

644. Loehrer PJS, Turner S, Kubilis P, et al. A prospective randomized trial of fluorouracil versus fluorouracil plus cisplatin in the treatment of metastatic colorectal cancer. A Hoosier Oncology Group Trial. *J Clin Oncol* 1988;6:642–648.

645. Lokich JJ, Ahlgren HD, Cantrell J, et al. A prospective randomized comparison of protracted infusional 5-fluorouracil with or without weekly bolus cisplatin in metastatic colorectal carcinoma. *Cancer* 1991;67:14–19.

646. Kemeny N, Israel K, Niedzwiecki D, et al. Randomized study of continuous infusion fluorouracil versus fluorouracil plus cisplatin in patients with metastatic colorectal cancer. *J Clin Oncol* 1990;8:313–318.

647. Diaz-Rubio E, Jimeno J, Anton A, et al. A prospective randomized trial of continuous infusion 5-fluorouracil (5-FU) versus 5-FU plus cisplatin in patients with advanced colorectal cancer. A trial of the Spanish Cooperative Group for Digestive Tract Tumor Therapy (T.T.D.). *Am J Clin Oncol* 1992;15:56–60.

648. Hansen RM, Ryan L, Anderson T, et al. Phase III study of bolus versus infusion fluorouracil with or without cisplatin

in advanced colorectal cancer. *J Natl Cancer Inst* 1996;88:668–674.

649. Raymond E, Buquet-Fagot F, Djelloul C, et al. Antitumor activity of oxaliplatin in combination with 5-fluorouracil and the thymidylate synthase inhibitor AG337 in human colon, breast and ovarian cancers. *Anticancer Drugs* 1997;8:876–885.

650. Fischel JL, Etienne MC, Formento P, et al. Search for the optimal schedule for the oxaliplatin/5-fluorouracil association modulated or not by folinic acid. Preclinical data. *Clin Cancer Res* 1998;4:2529–2535.

651. de Gramont A, Vignoud J, Tournigand C, et al. Oxaliplatin with high-dose leucovorin and 5-fluorouracil 48-hour continuous infusion in pretreated metastatic colorectal cancer. *Eur J Cancer* 1997;33:214–219.

652. deBraud F, Munzone E, Nole F, et al. Synergistic activity of oxaliplatin and 5-fluorouracil in patients with metastatic colorectal cancer with progressive disease while on or after 5-fluorouracil. *Am J Clin Oncol* 1998;21:279–283.

653. Andre T, Louvet C, Raymond E, et al. Bimonthly high-dose leucovorin, 5-fluorouracil infusion and oxaliplatin (FOLFOX3) for metastatic colorectal cancer resistant to the same leucovorin and 5-fluorouracil regimen. *Ann Oncol* 1998;9:1251–1253.

654. de Gramont A, Figer A, Seymour M, et al. Leucovorin and fluorouracil with or without oxaliplatin as first-line treatment in advanced colorectal cancer. *J Clin Oncol* 2000; 18:2938–2947.

655. Laurie JA, Moertel CG, Fleming TR, et al. Surgical adjuvant therapy of large-bowel carcinoma. An evaluation of levamisole and fluorouracil. *J Clin Oncol* 1989;7:1447–1456.

656. Moertel CG, Fleming TR, Macdonald JS, et al. Fluorouracil plus levamisole as effective adjuvant therapy after resection of stage III colon carcinoma. A final report. *Ann Intern Med* 1995;122:321–326.

657. Zoetmulder FAN, Taal BG, Van Tinteren H, et al. Adjuvant 5FU plus levamisole improves survival in stage II and III colonic cancer, but not in rectal cancer. Interim analysis of the Netherlands Adjuvant Colorectal Cancer Project (NACCP). *Proc Am Soc Clin Oncol* 1999;18:266a.

658. Grem JL. Levamisole as a therapeutic agent for colorectal carcinoma. *Cancer Cells* 1990;2:131–137.

659. Bandealy MT, Gonin R, Loehrer PJ, et al. Prospective randomized trial of 5-fluorouracil versus 5-fluorouracil plus levamisole in the treatment of metastatic colorectal cancer. A Hoosier Oncology Group Trial. *Clin Cancer Res* 1998;4:935–939.

660. De Brabander M, Vandebroek J, Wassenaar H, et al. Immunological alterations induced by adjuvant treatment of postoperative colon carcinoma Duke's B or C with levamisole in combination with 5-FU. *Anticancer Res* 1995;15:2271–2277.

661. Grem JL, Allegra CJ. Toxicity of levamisole and 5-fluorouracil in human colon carcinoma cells. *J Natl Cancer Inst* 1989;81:1413–1417.

662. Kovach JS, Svingen PA, Schaid DJ. Levamisole potentiation of fluorouracil antiproliferative activity mimicked by orthovanadate, an inhibitor of tyrosine phosphatase. *J Natl Cancer Inst* 1992;84:515–519.

663. Kimmel DW, Wijdicks EF, Rodriguez M. Multifocal inflammatory leukoencephalopathy associated with levamisole therapy. *Neurology* 1995;45:374–376.

664. Savarese DM, Gordon J, Smith TW, et al. Cerebral demyelination syndrome in a patient treated with 5-fluorouracil and levamisole. The use of thallium SPECT imaging to assist in noninvasive diagnosis—a case report. *Cancer* 1996;77:387–394.

665. Luppi G, Zoboli A, Barbieri F, et al. Multifocal leukoencephalopathy associated with 5-fluorouracil and levamisole adjuvant therapy for colon cancer. A report of two cases and review of the literature. The INTACC Intergruppo Nazionale Terpia Adiuvante Colon Carcinoma. *Ann Oncol* 1996;7:412–415.

666. Yeo W, Tong MM, Chan YL. Multifocal cerebral demyelination secondary to fluorouracil and levamisole therapy. *J Clin Oncol* 1999;17:431–433.

667. Moertel CG, Fleming TR, Macdonald JS, et al. Hepatic toxicity associated with fluorouracil plus levamisole adjuvant therapy. *J Clin Oncol* 1993;11:2386–2390.

668. Norum J. 5-Fluorouracil/levamisole induced intrahepatic fat infiltration imitating liver metastasis. *Acta Oncol* 1995;34:971–972.

669. Cascinu S, Catalano V, Latini L, et al. A randomized trial of adjuvant therapy of stage III colon cancer. Levamisole and 5-fluorouracil versus 5-fluorouracil alone. *Proc Am Soc Clin Oncol* 1999;18:240a.

670. Brunetti I, Falcone A, Calabresi P, et al. 5-Fluorouracil enhances azidothymidine cytotoxicity. In vitro, in vivo and biochemical studies. *Cancer Res* 1990;50:4026–4031.

671. Weber G, Ichikawa S, Nagai M, et al. Azidothymidine inhibition of thymidine kinase and synergistic cytotoxicity with methotrexate and 5-fluorouracil in a rat hepatoma and human colon cancer cells. *Cancer Commun* 1990;2:129–133.

672. Weber G, Nagai M, Prajfa N, et al. AZT: a biochemical response modifier of methotrexate and 5-fluorouracil cytotoxicity in human ovarian and pancreatic carcinoma cells. *Cancer Commun* 1991;3:127–132.

673. Tosi P, Calabresi P, Goulette FA, et al. Azidothymidine-induced cytotoxicity and incorporation into DNA in the human colon tumor cell line HCT-8 is enhanced by methotrexate in vitro and in vivo. *Cancer Res* 1992;52:4069–4073.

674. Andreuccetti M, Allegrini G, Antonuzzo A, et al. Azidothymidine in combination with 5-fluorouracil in human colorectal cell lines. In vitro synergistic cytotoxicity and DNA-induced strand-breaks. *Eur J Cancer* 1996;32A:1219–1226.

675. Yasuda C, Kato M, Kuroda D, et al. Experimental studies on potentiation of the antitumor activity of 5-fluorouracil with 3'-azido-3'-deoxythymidine for the gastric cancer cell line MKN28 in vivo. *Jpn J Cancer Res* 1997;88:97–102.

676. Posner MR, Darnowski JW, Calabresi P, et al. Oral azidothymidine, continuous infusion 5-fluorouracil and oral leucovorin. A phase I study. *J Natl Cancer Inst* 1990;82:1710–1714.

677. Beitz JG, Darnowski JW, Cummings FJ, et al. Phase I trial of high-dose infused zidovudine combined with leucovorin plus fluorouracil. *Cancer Invest* 1995;13:464–469.

678. Clark J, Sikov W, Cummings F, et al. Phase II study of 5-fluorouracil, leucovorin and azidothymidine in patients with metastatic colorectal cancer. *J Cancer Res Clin Oncol* 1996;122:554–558.

679. Falcone A, Lencioni M, Brunetti I, et al. Maximum tolerable doses of intravenous zidovudine in combination with 5-fluorouracil and leucovorin in metastatic colorectal cancer

patients. Clinical evidence of significant antitumor activity and enhancement of zidovudine-induced DNA single strand breaks in peripheral nuclear blood cells. *Ann Oncol* 1997;8:539–545.

680. Kano Y, Akutsu M, Tsunoda S, et al. Schedule-dependent interaction between paclitaxel and 5-fluorouracil in human carcinoma cell lines in vitro. *Br J Cancer* 1996;74:704–710.

681. Johnson KR, Wang L, Miller MC III, et al. 5-Fluorouracil interferes with paclitaxel cytotoxicity against human solid tumor cells. *Clin Cancer Res* 1997;3:1739–1745.

682. Grem JL, Nguyen D, Monahan BP, et al. Sequence-dependent antagonism between fluorouracil and paclitaxel in human breast cancer cells. *Biochem Pharmacol* 1999;58:477–486.

683. Heidelberger C, Griesvach L, Montag BJ, et al. Studies on fluorinated pyrimidines. II. Effects on transplanted tumors. *Cancer Res* 1958;18:305–317.

684. Vietti T, Eggerding F, Valeriote F. Combined effect of x-radiation and 5-fluorouracil on survival of transplanted leukemic cells. *J Natl Cancer Inst* 1971;47:865–870.

685. Byfield JE, Calabro-Jones P, Klisak I, et al. Pharmacologic requirements for obtaining sensitization of human tumor cells in vitro to combined 5-fluorouracil or ftorafur and x-rays. *Int J Radiat Oncol Biol Phys* 1982;8:1923–1933.

686. Weinberg MJ, Rauth AM. 5-Fluorouracil infusions and fractionated doses of radiation. Studies with a murine squamous cell carcinoma. *Int J Radiat Oncol Biol Phys* 1987;13:1691–1699.

687. Ishikawa T, Tanaka Y, Ishitsuka H, et al. Comparative antitumor activity of 5-fluorouracil and 5'-deoxyfluorouridine in combination with radiation therapy in mice bearing colon 26 adenocarcinoma. *Cancer Res* 1989;80:583–591.

688. Smalley SR, Kimler BF, Evans RG. 5-Fluorouracil modulation of radiosensitivity in cultured human carcinoma cells. *Int J Radiat Oncol Biol Phys* 1991;20:207–211.

689. Bruso CE, Shewach DS, Lawrence TS. Fluorodeoxyuridine-induced radiosensitization and inhibition of DNA double-strand break repair in human colon cancer cells. *Int J Radiat Oncol Biol Phys* 1990;19:1411–1417.

690. Lawrence T, Heimburger D, Shewach DL. The effects of leucovorin and dipyridamole on fluoropyrimidine-induced radiosensitization. *Int J Radiat Oncol Biol Phys* 1991;20:377–381.

691. Miller EM, Kinsella TJ. Radiosensitization by fluorodeoxyuridine. Effects of thymidylate synthase inhibition and cell synchronization. *Cancer Res* 1992;52:1687–1694.

692. Davis MA, Tang HY, Maybaum J, et al. Dependence of fluorodeoxyuridine-mediated radiosensitization on S phase progression. *Int J Radiat Biol* 1995;67:509–517.

693. Lawrence TS, Davis MA, Loney TL. Fluoropyrimidine-mediated radiosensitization depends on cyclin E-dependent kinase activation. *Cancer Res* 1996;56:3203–3206.

694. Lawrence TS, Tepper JE, Blackstock AW. Fluoropyrimidine-radiation interactions in cells and tumors. *Semin Radiat Oncol* 1997;7:260–266.

695. Rich TA. Irradiation plus 5-fluorouracil. Cellular mechanisms of action and treatment schedules. *Semin Radiat Oncol* 1997;7:267–273.

696. Epidermoid anal cancer. Results from the UKCCCR randomized trial of radiotherapy alone versus radiotherapy, 5-fluorouracil and mitomycin C. UKCCCR Anal Cancer Trial Working Party. *Lancet* 1996;348:1049–1054.

697. Bartelink H, Roelofsen F, Eschwege F, et al. Concomitant radiotherapy and chemotherapy is superior to radiotherapy alone in the treatment of locally advanced anal cancer. Results of a phase III randomized trial of the European Organization for Research and Treatment of Cancer Radiotherapy and Gastrointestinal Cooperative Groups. *J Clin Oncol* 1997;15:2040–2049.

698. Morris M, Eifel PJ, Lu J, et al. Pelvic radiation with concurrent chemotherapy compared with pelvic and para-aortic radiation for high-risk cervical cancer. *N Engl J Med* 1999;340:1137–1143.

699. Herskovic A, Martz K, al-Sarraf M, et al. Combined chemotherapy and radiotherapy compared with radiotherapy alone in patients with cancer of the esophagus. *N Engl J Med* 1992;326:1593–1598.

700. Cooper JS, Guo MD, Herskovic A, et al. Chemoradiotherapy of locally advanced esophageal cancer. Long-term follow-up of a prospective randomized trial (RTOG 85-01). Radiation Therapy Oncology Group. *JAMA* 1999;281:1623–1627.

701. O'Connell MJ, Martenson JA, Wieand HS, et al. Improving adjuvant therapy for rectal cancer by combining protracted infusion fluorouracil with radiation therapy after curative surgery. *N Engl J Med* 1994;33:502–507.

702. Au JL, Sadee W. The pharmacology of ftorafur. *Recent Results Cancer Res* 1981;76:100–114.

703. Benvenuto JA, Liehr JG, Winkler T, et al. Human urinary metabolites of 1-(tetrahydro-2-furanyl)-5-fluorouracil (ftorafur). *Cancer Res* 1980;40:2814–3870.

704. Au JL, Sadee W. Stereoselective metabolism of ftorafur. *Cancer Chemother Pharmacol* 1981;7:55–59.

705. El Sayed YM, Sadee W. Metabolic activation of ftorafur. The microsomal oxidative pathway. *Biochem Pharmacol* 1982;31:3006–3008.

706. El Sayed YM, Sadee W. Metabolic activation of R,S-1-(tetrahydro-2-furanyl)-5-fluorouracil (ftorafur) to 5-fluorouracil by soluble enzymes. *Cancer Res* 1983;43:4039–4044.

707. Hornbeck CL, Griffiths JC, Floyd RA, et al. Serum concentrations of 5-FU, ftorafur, and a major serum metabolite following ftorafur chemotherapy. *Cancer Treat Rep* 1981;65:69–72.

708. Benvenuto J, Lu K, Hall SW, et al. Metabolism of 1-(tetrahydro-2-furanyl)-5-fluorouracil (ftorafur). *Cancer Res* 1978;38:3867–3870.

709. Hall SW, Valdivieso M, Benjamin RS. Intermittent high single dose ftorafur. A phase I clinical trial with pharmacologic-toxicity correlations. *Cancer Treat Rep* 1977;61:1495–1498.

710. Antilla MI, Sotaniemi EA, Kaiaralcoma MI, et al. Pharmacokinetics of ftorafur after intravenous and oral administration. *Cancer Chemother Pharmacol* 1983;10:150–153.

711. Belitsky GA, Bukhman VM, Konopleva IA. Changes in toxic and antitumor properties of ftorafur by induction or inhibition of the microsomal enzyme activity. *Cancer Chemother Pharmacol* 1981;6:183–187.

712. Fujimoto S, Kashizulia T, Amenmuja K, et al. Intensive chemotherapy for patients with digestive tract cancer using hepatic drug-metabolizing enzyme induction. *Gann* 1979;25:971–979.

713. Blokhina NG, Vozny EK, Garin AM. Results of treatment of malignant tumors with ftorafur. *Cancer* 1972;30:390–392.

714. Karev NI. Experience with ftorafur treatment in breast cancer. *Neoplasm* 1972;19:347–350.

715. Valdivieso M, Bodey GP, Gottleib JA, et al. Clinical evaluation of ftorafur. *Cancer Res* 1976;36:1821–1824.

716. Buroker T, Padilla F, Groppe C, et al. Phase II evaluation of ftorafur in previously untreated colorectal cancer. A Southwest Oncology Group study. *Cancer* 1979;44:48–51.

717. Friedman MA, Ignoffo RJ. A review of the United States clinical experience of the fluoropyrimidine, ftorafur (NSC 148958). *Cancer Treat Rev* 1980;7:205–213.

718. Wada T, Koyama H, Teresarwa T. Recent advances in chemotherapy for advanced breast cancer. *Recent Results Cancer Res* 1981;76:316–324.

719. Ansfield FJ, Kallas GJ, Singson JP. Phase I–II studies of oral tegafur (ftorafur). *J Clin Oncol* 1983;1:107–110.

720. Kajanti MJ, Pyrhönen SO, Maiche AG. Oral tegafur in the treatment of metastatic breast cancer. A phase II study. *Eur J Cancer* 1993;29A:863–866.

721. Palmeri S, Gebbia V, Russo A, et al. Oral tegafur in the treatment of gastrointestinal tract cancers. A phase II study. *Br J Cancer* 1990;61:475–478.

722. Bjerkeset T, Fjosne HE. Comparison of oral ftorafur and intravenous 5-fluorouracil in patients with advanced cancer of the stomach, colon or rectum. *Oncology* 1986;43:212–215.

723. Wooley PV, Macdonald JS, Smythe T, et al. A phase II trial of ftorafur, adriamycin and mitomycin C (FAM II) in advanced gastric adenocarcinoma. *Cancer* 1979;44:1211–1214.

724. Hortobagyi GN, Blumenschein GR, Tashima CK, et al. Ftorafur, Adriamycin, cyclophosphamide and BCG in the treatment of metastatic breast cancer. *Cancer* 1979;44:398–405.

725. Queisser W, Schnitzler G, Schaefer J, et al. Comparison of ftorafur with 5-fluorouracil in combination chemotherapy of advanced gastrointestinal carcinoma. *Recent Results Cancer Res* 1981;79:82–92.

726. Nakajima T, Takahashi T, Takagi K, et al. Comparison of 5-fluorouracil with ftorafur in adjuvant chemotherapies with combined inductive and maintenance therapies for gastric cancer. *J Clin Oncol* 1984;2:1366–1371.

727. Marenich AF, Perevodchikova NI, Grigorova TM, et al. Comparative evaluation of two regimens of combination chemotherapy in patients with stage III–IV ovarian cancer. *Vestn Akad Med Nauk USSR* 1984;5:28–32.

728. Manzuik LV, Perevodchikova NI, Gorbunova VA, et al. Initial clinical experience with oral ftorafur and oral 6R,S-leucovorin in advanced colorectal carcinoma. *Eur J Cancer* 1993;29A:1793–1794.

729. Fuji S, Ikenaka K, Fukushima M, et al. Effect of uracil and its derivatives on antitumor activity of 5-fluorouracil and 1-(2-tetrahydrofuryl)-5-fluorouracil. *Jpn J Cancer Res* 1979;69:763–772.

730. Tang SG, Hornbeck CL, Byfield JE. Enhanced accumulation of 5-fluorouracil in human tumors in athymic mice by co-administration of ftorafur and uracil. *Int J Radiat Oncol Biol Phys* 1984;10:1687–1689.

731. Ho DH, Cobington WP, Pazdur R, et al. Clinical pharmacology of combined oral uracil and ftorafur. *Drug Metab Dispos* 1992;20:936–940.

732. Fujita K, Munakata A. Concentration of 5-fluorouracil in renal cells from cancer patients administered a mixture of 1-(2-tetrahydrofuryl)-5-fluorouracil and uracil. *Int J Clin Pharmacol Res* 1991;11:171–174.

733. Takayama H, Konami T, Konishi T, et al. Studies on 5-FU concentration in serum and bladder tumor tissue after oral administration of UFT. *Acta Urol Jpn* 1986;32:1449–1453.

734. Ota K, Taguchi T, Kimura K. Report on nationwide pooled data and cohort investigation in UFT phase II study. *Cancer Chemother Pharmacol* 1988;22:333–338.

735. Taguchi T. Experience with UFT in Japan. *Oncology (Huntingt)* 1997;11:30–34.

736. Kubota Y, Hosaka M, Fukushima S, et al. Prophylactic oral UFT therapy for superficial bladder cancer. *Cancer* 1993;71:1842–1845.

737. Ho DH, Pazdur R, Covington W, et al. Comparison of 5-fluorouracil pharmacokinetics in patients receiving continuous 5-fluorouracil infusion and oral uracil plus N1-(2'-tetrahydrofuryl)-5-fluorouracil. *Clin Cancer Res* 1998;4:2085–2088.

738. Muggia FM, Wu X, Spicer D, et al. Phase I and pharmacokinetic study of oral UFT, a combination of the 5-fluorouracil prodrug tegafur and uracil. *Clin Cancer Res* 1996;2:1461–1467.

739. Pazdur R, Lassere Y, Rhodes V, et al. Phase II trial of uracil and tegafur plus oral leucovorin. An effective oral regimen in the treatment of metastatic colorectal carcinoma. *J Clin Oncol* 1994;12:2296–2300.

740. Gonzalez Baron M, Feliu J, Garcia Giron C, et al. UFT modulated with leucovorin in advanced colorectal cancer. Oncopaz experience. *Oncology* 1997;54:24–29.

741. Ichikura T, Tomimatsu S, Okusa Y, et al. Thymidylate synthase inhibition by an oral regimen consisting of tegafur-uracil (UFT) and low-dose leucovorin for patients with gastric cancer. *Cancer Chemother Pharmacol* 1996;38:401–405.

742. Meropol NJ, Sonnichsen DS, Birkhofer MJ, et al. Bioavailability and phase II study of oral UFT plus leucovorin in patients with relapsed or refractory colorectal cancer. *Cancer Chemother Pharmacol* 1999;43:221–226.

743. Sulkes A, Benner SE, Canetta RM. Uracil-ftorafur. An oral fluoropyrimidine active in colorectal cancer. *J Clin Oncol* 1998;16:3461–3475.

744. Pazdur R, Douillard J-Y, Skillings JR, et al. Multicenter phase III study of 5-fluorouracil or UFT™ in combination with leucovorin in patients with metastatic colorectal cancer. *Proc Am Soc Clin Oncol* 1999;18:263a.

745. Carmichael J, Popiela T, Radstone D, et al. Randomized comparative study of Orzel®, (oral uracil/tegafur (UFT™) plus leucovorin (LV)) versus parenteral 5-fluorouracil plus LV in patients with metastatic colorectal cancer. *Proc Am Soc Clin Oncol* 1999;18:264a.

746. Smith R, Wickerham DL, Wieand HS, et al. UFT plus calcium folinate vs 5-FU plus calcium folinate in colon cancer. *Oncology (Huntingt)* 1999;13(suppl 3):44–47.

747. Eda H, Fujimoto K, Watanabe S-I, et al. Cytokines induce uridine phosphorylase in mouse colon 26 carcinoma cells and make the cells more susceptible to 5'-deoxy-5-fluorouridine. *Jpn J Cancer Res* 1993;84:341–347.

748. Eda H, Fujimoto K, Watanabe S-I, et al. Cytokines induce thymidine phosphorylase in tumor cells and make the cells more susceptible to 5'-deoxy-5-fluorouridine. *Cancer Chemother Pharmacol* 1993;32:333–339.

749. Cook AF, Holman MJ, Kramer MJ, et al. Fluorinated pyrimidine nucleosides. 3. Synthesis and antitumor activity of a series of 5'-deoxy-5-fluoropyrimidine nucleosides. *J Med Chem* 1979;22:1330–1335.

750. Bollag W, Hartman HR. Tumor inhibitory effects of a new fluorouracil derivative. 5'-Deoxy-5-fluorouridine. *Eur J Cancer* 1980;16:427–432.

751. Armstrong RD, Diasio RB. Metabolism and biological activity of 5'-deoxy-5-fluorouridine, a novel fluoropyrimidine. *Cancer Res* 1980;40:3333–3338.

752. Ishitsuka H, Miwa M, Takemoto F, et al. Role of uridine phosphorylase for antitumor activity of 5'-deoxy-5-fluorouridine. *Jpn J Cancer Res (Gann)* 1980;71:112–123.

753. Kono A, Hara Y, Sugata S, et al. Activation of 5'-deoxyfluorouridine by thymidine phosphorylase in human tumors. *Chem Pharm Bull (Tokyo)* 1983;31:175–178.

754. Armstrong RD, Cadman E. 5'-Deoxyfluorouridine selective toxicity for human tumor cells compared to human bone marrow. *Cancer Res* 1983;43:2525–2528.

755. Connolly KM, Diasio RB, Armstrong RD, et al. Decreased immunosuppression associated with anticancer activity of 5'-deoxy-5-fluorouridine compared to 5-fluorouracil and 5-fluorouridine. *Cancer Res* 1983;43:2529–2535.

756. Miwa M, Nishimura J, Kayamiyama T, et al. Conversion of 5'-deoxyuridine to 5-FU by pyrimidine nucleoside phosphorylase in normal and tumor tissues from rodents bearing tumors and cancer patients. *Jpn J Cancer Chemother* 1987;14:2924–2929.

757. Peters GJ, Braakhuis BJM, de Bruijn EA, et al. Enhanced therapeutic efficacy of 5'-deoxy-5-fluorouridine in 5-fluorouracil resistant head and neck tumours in relation to 5-fluorouracil metabolising enzymes. *Br J Cancer* 1989;59:327–334.

758. Geng YM, Gheuens E, de Bruijn EA. Activation and cytotoxicity of 5'-deoxy-5-fluorouridine in c-Ha-ras transfected NIH 3T3 cells. *Biochem Pharmacol* 1991;41:301–303.

759. Tevaearai HT, Laurent PL, Suardet L, et al. Interactions of interferon-α-2a with 5'-deoxy-5-fluorouridine in colorectal cancer cells in vitro. *Eur J Cancer* 1992;28:368–372.

760. Nio Y, Kimura H, Tsubone M, et al. Antitumor activity of 5'-deoxy-5-fluorouridine in human digestive organ cancer xenografts and pyrimidine nucleoside phosphorylase activity in normal and neoplastic tissues from human digestive organs. *Anticancer Res* 1992;12:1141–1146.

761. el Khouni MH, el Kouni MM, Naguib NM. Differences in activities and substrate specificity of human and murine pyrimidine nucleoside phosphorylases. Implications for chemotherapy with 5 fluoropyrimidines. *Cancer Res* 1993;53:3687–3693.

762. el Khouni MH, Naguib FNM, Chu SH, et al. Effect of the n-glycosidic bond conformation and modifications in the pentose moiety on the binding of nucleoside ligands to uridine phosphorylase. *Mol Pharmacol* 1988;34:104–110.

763. Zimmerman M, Seidenberg JI. Thymidine phosphorylase and nucleoside deoxyribosyltransferase in normal and malignant tissues. *J Biol Chem* 1960;239:2618–2621.

764. Veres Z, Szabolcs A, Szinai I, et al. Enzymatic cleavage of 5-substituted-2'-deoxyuridines by pyrimidine nucleoside phosphorylases. *Biochem Pharmacol* 1986;35:1057–1059.

765. Vertongen F, Fondu P, Van den Heule B, et al. Thymidine kinase and thymidine phosphorylase activities in various types of leukemia and lymphoma. *Tumour Biol* 1984;5:303–311.

766. Sommadossi J-P, Aubert C, Cano J-P, et al. Kinetics and metabolism of a new fluoropyrimidine, 5'-deoxy-5-fluorouridine, in humans. *Cancer Res* 1983;43:930–933.

767. de Bruijn EA, van Oosterom AT, Tjaden UR, et al. Pharmacology of 5'-deoxy-5-fluorouridine in patients with resistant ovarian cancer. *Cancer Res* 1985;45:5931–5935.

768. Schaaf LJ, Dobbs BR, Edwards IR, et al. The pharmacokinetics of doxifluridine and 5-fluorouracil after single intravenous infusions of doxifluridine to patients with colorectal cancer. *Eur J Clin Pharmacol* 1988;34:439–443.

769. Fossa SD, Flokkmann A, Heier M, et al. Phase I/II tolerability/pharmacokinetic study with one-hour intravenous infusion of doxifluridine (5'-dFUrd) 3 g/m² vs 5 g/m² q × 5 per month. *Cancer Chemother Pharmacol* 1986;18:252–256.

770. Malet-Martino MC, Servin P, Bernadou J, et al. Human urinary excretion of doxifluridine and metabolites during a 5-day chemotherapeutic schedule using fluorine-19 nuclear magnetic resonance spectrometry. *Invest New Drugs* 1987;5:273–279.

771. Martino R, Bernadou J, Malet-Martino MC, et al. Excretion of doxifluridine catabolites in human bile assessed by 19F NMR spectrometry. *Biomed Pharmacother* 1987;41:104–106.

772. Reece PA, Olver IN, Morris RG, et al. Pharmacokinetic study of doxifluridine given by 5-day stepped-dose infusion. *Cancer Chemother Pharmacol* 1990;25:274–278.

773. Abele R, Alberto P, Seematter RJ, et al. Phase I clinical study with 5'-deoxy-5'-fluorouridine, a new fluoropyrimidine derivative. *Cancer Treat Rep* 1982;1307–1313.

774. Hurteloup P, Armand JP, Cappelaere P, et al. Phase II clinical evaluation of doxifluridine. *Cancer Treat Rep* 1986;70:1339–1340.

775. Fossa SD, Dahl O, Hoel R, et al. Doxifluridine (5'dFUR) in patients with advanced colorectal carcinoma. *Cancer Chemother Pharmacol* 1985;15:161–163.

776. Alberto P, Mermillod B, Germano G, et al. A randomized comparison of doxifluridine and fluorouracil in colorectal cancer. *Eur J Cancer Clin Oncol* 1998;24:559–563.

777. Alberto P, Jungi WF, Siegenthaler P, et al. A phase II study of doxifluridine in patients with advanced breast cancer. *Eur J Cancer Clin Oncol* 1988;24:565–566.

778. Heier MS, Fossa SD. Wernicke-Korsakoff-like syndrome in patients with colorectal carcinoma treated with high-dose doxifluridine. *Acta Neurol Scand* 1986;73:449–457.

779. Schuster D, Heim ME, Dombernowski P, et al. Prospective randomized phase III trial of doxifluridine versus 5-fluorouracil in patients with advanced colorectal cancer. *Onkologie* 1991;14:333–337.

780. Bajetta E, Colleoni M, Rosso R, et al. Prospective randomised trial comparing fluorouracil versus doxifluridine for the treatment of advanced colorectal cancer. *Eur J Cancer* 1993;29A:1658–2663.

781. Alberto P, Winkelmann JJ, Paschoud N, et al. Phase I study of oral doxifluridine using two schedules. *Eur J Cancer Clin Oncol* 1989;25:905–908.

782. Bajetta E, Colleoni M, Di Bartolomeo M, et al. Doxifluridine and leucovorin. An oral treatment combination in advanced colorectal cancer. *J Clin Oncol* 1995;13:2613–2619.

783. Blum JL, Jones SE, Buzdar AU, et al. Multicenter Phase II study of capecitabine in paclitaxel-refractory metastatic breast cancer. *J Clin Oncol* 1999;17:485–493.

784. Budman DR, Meropol NJ, Reigner B, et al. Preliminary studies of a novel oral fluoropyrimidine carbamate. Capecitabine. *J Clin Oncol* 1998;16:1795–1802.

785. Mackean M, Planting A, Twelves C, et al. Phase I and pharmacologic study of intermittent twice-daily oral therapy with capecitabine in patients with advanced and/or metastatic cancer. *J Clin Oncol* 1998;16:2977–2985.

786. Ishikawa T, Utoh M, Sawada N, et al. Tumor selective delivery of 5-fluorouracil by capecitabine, a new oral fluoropyrimidine carbamate, in human cancer xenografts. *Biochem Pharmacol* 1998;55:1091–1097.

787. Ishikawa T, Sekiguchi F, Fukase Y, et al. Positive correlation between the efficacy of capecitabine and doxifluridine and the ratio of thymidine phosphorylase to dihydropyrimidine dehydrogenase activities in tumors in human cancer xenografts. *Cancer Res* 1998;58:685–690.

788. Miwa M, Ura M, Nishida M, et al. Design of a novel oral fluoropyrimidine carbamate, capecitabine, which generates 5-fluorouracil selectively in tumours by enzymes concentrated in human liver and cancer tissue. *Eur J Cancer* 1998;34:1274–1281.

789. Cassidy J, Dirix L, Bissett D, et al. A Phase I study of capecitabine in combination with oral leucovorin in patients with intractable solid tumors. *Clin Cancer Res* 1998;4:2755–2761.

790. Reigner B, Verweij J, Dirix L, et al. Effect of food on the pharmacokinetics of capecitabine and its metabolites following oral administration in cancer patients. *Clin Cancer Res* 1998;4:941–948.

791. Twelves C, Glynne-Jones R, Cassidy J, et al. Effect of hepatic dysfunction due to liver metastases on the pharmacokinetics of capecitabine and its metabolites. *Clin Cancer Res* 1999;5:1696–1702.

792. Cox JV, Pazdur R, Thibault A, et al. A Phase III Trial of XELODA™ (Capecitabine) in previously untreated advanced/metastatic colorectal cancer. *Proc Am Soc Clin Oncol* 1999;18:265a.

793. Twelves C, Harper P, Van Cutsem E, et al. A Phase III Trial (S014796) of Xeloda™ (Capecitabine) in previously untreated advanced/metastatic colorectal cancer. *Proc Am Soc Clin Oncol* 1999;18:263a.

794. Porter DJ, Chestnut WG, Merrill BM, et al. Mechanism-based inactivation of dihydropyrimidine dehydrogenase by 5-ethynyluracil. *J Biol Chem* 1992;267:5236–5242.

795. Spector T, Harrington JA, Porter DJ. 5-Ethynyluracil (776C85). Inactivation of dihydropyrimidine dehydrogenase in vivo. *Biochem Pharmacol* 1993;46:2243–2248.

796. Baccanari DP, Davis ST, Knick VC, et al. 5-Ethynyluracil (776C85). A potent modulator of the pharmacokinetics and antitumor efficacy of 5-fluorouracil. *Proc Natl Acad Sci U S A* 1993;90:11064–11068.

797. Cao S, Rustum YM, Spector T. 5-Ethynyluracil (776C85). Modulation of 5-fluorouracil efficacy and therapeutic index in rats bearing advanced colorectal carcinoma. *Cancer Res* 1994;54:1507–1510.

798. Cao S, Baccanari DP, Joyner SS, et al. 5-Ethynyluracil (776C85). Effects on the antitumor activity and pharmacokinetics of tegafur, a prodrug of 5-fluorouracil. *Cancer Res* 1995;55:6227–6230.

799. Spector T, Cao S, Rustum YM, et al. Attenuation of the antitumor activity of 5-fluorouracil by (R)-5-fluoro-5,6-dihydrouracil. *Cancer Res* 1995;55:1239–1241.

800. Arellano M, Malet-Martino M, Martino R, et al. 5-Ethynyl-uracil (GW776). Effects on the formation of the toxic catabolites of 5-fluorouracil, fluoroacetate and fluorohydroxypropionic acid in the isolated perfused rat liver model. *Br J Cancer* 1997;76:1170–1180.

801. Adams ER, Leffert JJ, Craig DJ, et al. In vivo effect of 5-ethynyluracil on 5-fluorouracil metabolism determined by 19F nuclear magnetic resonance spectroscopy. *Cancer Res* 1999;59:122–127.

802. Khor SP, Amyx H, Davis ST, et al. Dihydropyrimidine dehydrogenase inactivation and 5-fluorouracil pharmacokinetics: allometric scaling of animal data, pharmacokinetics and toxicodynamics of 5-fluorouracil in humans. *Cancer Chemother Pharmacol* 1997;39:233–238.

803. Schilsky RL, Hohneker J, Ratain MJ, et al. Phase I clinical and pharmacologic study of eniluracil plus fluorouracil in patients with advanced cancer. *J Clin Oncol* 1998;16:1450–1457.

804. Baker SD, Khor SP, Adjei AA, et al. Pharmacokinetic, oral bioavailability, and safety study of fluorouracil in patients treated with 776C85, an inactivator of dihydropyrimidine dehydrogenase. *J Clin Oncol* 1996;14:3085–3096.

805. Smith I, Johnston S, O'Brien M, et al. High activity with eniluracil (776C85) and continuous low dose oral 5-fluorouracil (1 mg/m^2 × 2 daily) as first-line chemotherapy in patients with advanced breast cancer. A phase II study. *Proc Am Soc Clin Oncol* 1999;18:106a.

806. Mani S, Beck T, Chevlen E, et al. A phase II open-label study to evaluate a 28-day regimen of oral 5-fluorouracil plus 776C85 for the treatment of patients with previously untreated metastatic colorectal cancer. *Proc Am Soc Clin Oncol* 1998;17:281a.

807. Grem J, Harold N, Bi D, et al. A Phase I and pharmacologic study of weekly oral fluorouracil given with eniluracil (GW776C85) and leucovorin in patients with solid tumors. *Proc Am Soc Clin Oncol* 1999;18:173a.

808. Shirasaka T, Shimamato Y, Ohshimo H, et al. Development of a novel form of an oral 5-fluorouracil derivative (S-1) directed to the potentiation of the tumor selective cytotoxicity of 5-fluorouracil by two biochemical modulators. *Anticancer Drugs* 1996;7:548–557.

809. Shirasaka T, Shimamoto Y, Fukushima M. Inhibition by oxonic acid of gastrointestinal toxicity of 5-fluorouracil without loss of its antitumor activity in rats. *Cancer Res* 1993;53:4004–4009.

810. Shirasaka T, Nakano K, Takechi T, et al. Antitumor activity of 1 M tegafur-0.4 M 5-chloro-2,4-dihydroxypyridine- 1 M potassium oxonate (S-1) against human colon carcinoma orthotopically implanted into nude rats. *Cancer Res* 1996;56:2602–2606.

811. Suzuki M, Sekiguchi I, Sato I, et al. Combined effects of S-1, a new form of oral tegafur, plus modulators on ovarian cancer in nude rats. *Chemotherapy* 1996;42:452–458.

812. Takechi T, Nakano K, Uchida J, et al. Antitumor activity and low intestinal toxicity of S-1, a new formulation of oral tegafur, in experimental tumor models in rats. *Cancer Chemother Pharmacol* 1997;39:205–211.

813. Fukushima M, Satake H, Uchida J, et al. Preclinical antitumor efficacy of S-1. A new oral formulation of 5-fluorouracil on human tumor xenografts. *Int J Oncol* 1998;13:693–698.

814. Konno H, Tanaka T, Baba M, et al. Therapeutic effect of 1 M tegafur-0.4 M 5-chloro-2,4-dihydroxypyridine-1 M

potassium oxonate (S-1) on liver metastasis of xenotransplanted human colon carcinoma. *Jpn J Cancer Res* 1999; 90:448–453.

815. Cao S, Lu K, Toth K, et al. Persistent induction of apoptosis and suppression of mitosis as the basis for curative therapy with S-1, an oral 5-fluorouracil prodrug in a colorectal tumor model. *Clin Cancer Res* 1999;5:267–274.

816. Fukushima M, Shimamoto Y, Kato T, et al. Anticancer activity and toxicity of S-1, an oral combination of tegafur and two biochemical modulators, compared with continuous i.v. infusion of 5-fluorouracil. *Anticancer Drugs* 1998;9:817–823.

817. Sakata Y, Ohtsu A, Horikoshi N, et al. Late phase II study of novel oral fluoropyrimidine anticancer drug S-1 (1 M Tegafur-0.4 M Gimestat-1 M Otastat Potassium) in advanced gastric cancer patients. *Eur J Cancer* 1998;34:1715–1720.

818. Kurihara M, Koizumi W, Hasegawa K, et al. Late phase II study of S-1, a novel oral fluoropyrimidine derivative, in patients with advanced gastric cancer. *Proc Am Soc Clin Oncol* 1998;17:262a.

819. Baba H, Ohtsu A, Sakata Y, et al. Late phase II study of S-1 in patients with advanced colorectal cancer in Japan. *Proc Am Soc Clin Oncol* 1998;17:277a.

820. Endo S, Niwa H, Kida A, et al. Late phase II study of S-1 in patients with head and neck cancer. *Proc Am Soc Clin Oncol* 1999;18:395a.

821. Taguchi T, Morimoto K, Horikoshi N, et al. An early phase II clinical study of S-1 in patients with breast cancer. S-1 cooperative study group (breast cancer working group). *Gann* 1998;25:1035–1043.

822. Matsushima E, Yoshida K, Kitamura R. Determination of S-1 (combined drug of tegafur, 5-chloro-2,4-dihydroxypyridine and potassium oxonate) and 5-fluorouracil in human plasma and urine using high-performance liquid chromatography and gas chromatography-negative ion chemical ionization mass spectrometry. *J Chromatogr B Biomed Sci Appl* 1997;691:95–104.

823. Horikoshi N, Aiba K, Nakano Y. Pharmacokinetic study of S-1, a new oral fluoropyrimidine consisting of DPD inhibitor and G.I. protector. *Proc Am Soc Clin Oncol* 1998;17:234a.

824. Noordhuis P, Van Groeningen CJ, Voorn DA, et al. Toxicity of S-1 (Ftorafur:CDHP:Oxonic acid = 1:0.4:1) during

treatment is associated with prolonged exposure to 5-fluorouracil. *Proc Am Assoc Cancer Res* 1999;40:158a.

825. Hoff PM, Wenske CA, Medgyesy DC, et al. Phase I and pharmacokinetic study of the novel oral fluoropyrimidine, S-1. *Proc Am Soc Clin Oncol* 1999;18:173a.

826. Fujii S, Fukushima M, Shimamoto Y, et al. Antitumor activity of BOF-A2, a new 5-fluorouracil derivative. *Jpn J Cancer Res* 1989;80:173–181.

827. Tatsumi K, Yamauchi T, Kiyono K, et al. 3-Cyano-2,6-dihydroxypyridine (CNDP), a new potent inhibitor of dihydrouracil dehydrogenase. *J Biochem* 1993;114:912–918.

828. Hirohashi M, Kido M, Yamamoto Y, et al. Synthesis of 5-fluorouracil derivatives containing an inhibitor of 5-fluorouracil degradation. *Chem Pharm Bull* 1993;41:1498–1506.

829. Miyauchi S, Imaoka T, Utsunomiya T, et al. Oral administration of BOF-A2 to rats with lung transplanted tumors results in increased 5-fluorouracil levels. *Jpn J Cancer Res* 1994;85:665–668.

830. Okayasu T, Sugiyama K, Miyauchi S. Inhibition of catabolic pathway of 5-fluorouracil by 3-cyano-2,6-dihydroxypyridine in human lung cancer tissues. *Jpn J Cancer Res* 1994;85:101–105.

831. Murata R, Shibamoto Y, Miyauchi S, et al. The combined antitumour effect of a new 5-fluorouracil derivative, BOF-A2, and radiation in vivo. *Br J Cancer Suppl* 1996; 27:S114–S116.

832. Shibamoto Y, Murata R, Miyauchi S, et al. Combined effect of clinically relevant doses of emitefur, a new 5-fluorouracil derivative, and radiation in murine tumours. *Br J Cancer* 1996;74:1709–1713.

833. Yoneda K, Yamamoto T, Ueta E, et al. The inhibitory action of BOF-A2, a 5-fluorouracil derivative, on squamous cell carcinoma. *Cancer Lett* 1999;137:17–25.

834. Nakai Y, Furuse K, Ohta M, et al. Efficacy of a new 5-fluorouracil derivative, BOF-A2, in advanced non-small cell lung cancer. A multi-center phase II study. *Acta Oncol* 1994;33:523–526.

835. Matei C, Hoff PM, Brito R, et al. Phase I trial of oral BOF-A2 plus leucovorin in advanced colorectal cancer. Antitumor activity in fluorouracil-resistant patients. *Proc Am Soc Clin Oncol* 1998;17:230a.

9

CYTIDINE ANALOGS

ROCIO GARCIA-CARBONERO
DAVID P. RYAN
BRUCE A. CHABNER

Nucleoside analogs compete with their physiologic counterparts for incorporation into nucleic acids and have earned an important place in the treatment of acute leukemia. The most important of these are the arabinose nucleosides, a unique class of antimetabolites originally isolated from the sponge *Cryptothethya crypta*[1] but now produced synthetically.[2] They differ from the physiologic deoxyribonucleosides by the presence of a β-OH group in the 2' position of the sugar (Fig. 9-1). Several arabinose nucleosides have useful antitumor and antiviral effects. The most active cytotoxic agent of this class is cytosine arabinoside (ara-C, cytarabine). A related nucleoside, adenine arabinoside, has antitumor and antiviral action,[3] and its analog, 2-fluoro-ara-adenosine monophosphate, has strong activity in lymphomas and in chronic lymphocytic leukemia.[4] Another member of the group is arabinosyl-5-azacytidine, a synthetic analog that failed in the clinic.[5]

CYTOSINE ARABINOSIDE

Ara-C is one of the most effective agents in the treatment of acute myelogenous leukemia[6] and is incorporated into virtually all standard induction regimens for this disease, generally in combination with an anthracycline (daunorubicin hydrochloride or idarubicin hydrochloride). Ara-C is also a component of consolidation and maintenance regimens after remission is attained. Clear clinical evidence now exists that a dose-response effect is present for ara-C both as induction[7] and consolidation[8] therapy in acute myelogenous leukemia. High-dose ara-C confers particular benefit in patients with certain cytogenetic abnormalities related to the core binding factor that regulates hematopoiesis (t8:21, inv 16, del 16, t 16:16)[9] (Table 9-1). Ara-C is also active against other hematologic malignancies, including non-Hodgkin's lymphoma,[10] acute lymphoblastic leukemia,[11] and chronic myelogenous leukemia,[12] but has little activity as a single agent against solid tumors. This limited spectrum of activity has been attributed to the lack of metabolic activation of this agent in solid tumors and its selective action against rapidly dividing cells. The essential features of ara-C pharmacology are described in Table 9-2.

Mechanism of Action

In human cells, ara-C acts as an analog of deoxycytidine and has multiple effects on DNA synthesis. Ara-C undergoes phosphorylation to form arabinosylcytosine triphosphate (ara-CTP), which competitively inhibits DNA polymerase α in opposition to the normal substrate deoxycytidine 5'-triphosphate (dCTP).[13] This competitive inhibition has been demonstrated with crude DNA polymerase from calf thymus[13] and with purified enzyme from human leukemic cells,[14] as well as with enzyme from a variety of murine tumors.[15,16] Ara-CTP has an affinity for human leukemia cell DNA polymerase α in the range of 1×10^{-6} mol per L, and the inhibition is reversible in cell-free systems by the addition of dCTP or in intact cells by the addition of deoxycytidine, the precursor of dCTP.[17] When present at high intracellular concentrations, ara-CTP also inhibits DNA polymerase β.[18] The effects of ara-C on DNA polymerase activity extend not only to semiconservative DNA replication but also to DNA repair. Repair of ultraviolet light damage to DNA, a function that depends on polymerase α, is blocked more potently than the repair of photon- or γ radiation–induced strand breaks,[19,20] the repair of which is accomplished by a different polymerase. In addition to having an effect on eukaryotic DNA polymerases, ara-CTP is a potent inhibitor of viral RNA-directed DNA polymerase [K_i (inhibition constant) = 0.1 μmol per L].

More important than the effects of ara-C on DNA synthesis, however, is its incorporation into DNA, a feature that correlates closely with cytotoxicity[21,22] (Fig. 9-2). In fact, a preponderance of evidence suggests that this is the major cytotoxic lesion in ara-C–treated cells. Drugs that

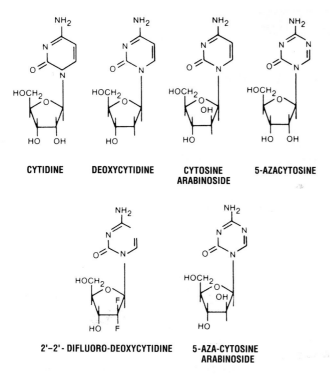

FIGURE 9-1. Structure of cytidine analogs.

prevent ara-C incorporation into DNA, such as aphidicolin, also block its cytotoxicity.[23] A given level of ara-C incorporation can be achieved by various combinations of concentrations (C) and times (T) of exposure that yield a specific C × T product. A linear relationship exists between picomoles of ara-C incorporated and the log of cell survival for a wide range of drug concentrations and durations of exposure. Thus drug toxicity is a direct function of incorporation into DNA, and the latter varies directly with the C × T product.[24] Once the nucleotide is incorporated into DNA, tumor cells do not seem to be able to excise it,[25] and the incorporated ara-C inhibits template function and

chain elongation.[23,26,27] In experiments with purified enzyme and calf thymus DNA, the consecutive incorporation of two ara-C or two arabinosyl-5-azacytidine (ara-5–aza-C) residues effectively stopped chain elongation by DNA polymerase α.[14] At high concentrations of ara-C one finds a greater than expected proportion of ara-C residues at the 3'-terminus, which confirms a direct effect on chain termination.[25] These observations support the hypothesis that ara-C incorporation into DNA is a prerequisite for drug action and is responsible for cytotoxicity.

Ara-C also causes an unusual reiteration of DNA segments.[28] Human lymphocytes exposed to ara-C in culture synthesize small reduplicated segments of DNA, which results in multiple copies of limited portions of DNA. These reduplicated segments increase the possibility of recombination, crossover, and gene amplification; gaps and breaks are observed in karyotype preparations after ara-C treatment. The same mechanism, reiteration of DNA synthesis after its inhibition by an antimetabolite, may explain the high frequency of gene reduplication induced by methotrexate sodium, 5-fluorouracil, and hydroxyurea (see Chapters 7, 8, and 11). In summary, although ara-C has multiple effects on DNA synthesis, the most important seems to be its incorporation into DNA.

Other biochemical actions of ara-C have been described, including inhibition of ribonucleotide reductase[29] and formation of ara-CDP-choline, an analog of cytidine 5'-diphosphocholine (CDP-choline) that inhibits synthesis of membrane glycoproteins and glycolipids.[30] Ara-C also has the interesting property of promoting differentiation of leukemic cells in tissue culture, an effect that is accompanied by decreased c-*myc* oncogene expression.[31,32] These changes in morphology and oncogene expression occur at concentrations above the threshold for cytotoxicity and may simply represent terminal injury of cells. Molecular analysis of clinical bone marrow samples from patients in remission has revealed persistence of leukemic markers,[33] which sug-

TABLE 9-1. COMPLETE REMISSION (CR) DURATION BY CYTOGENETIC GROUP ACCORDING TO CYTOSINE ARABINOSIDE (ARA-C) DOSE RANDOMIZATION

Cytogenetic Group	Ara-C Dose	No. of Patients	Median Time of CR (mo)	% 5-yr CR Estimate (95% CI)	% Cure Estimate
Group CBF[a]	3 g/m²	18	NR	78 (59–97)	66
	400 mg/m²	20	NR	57 (34–80)	52
	100 mg/m²	19	14.3	16 (0–32)	23
Group NL[b]	3 g/m²	45	18.2	40 (25–54)	47
	400 mg/m²	48	21.4	37 (13–51)	32
	100 mg/m²	47	12.5	20 (8–32)	12
Group other[c]	3 g/m²	27	13.3	21 (5–37)	17
	400 mg/m²	31	10.6	13 (1–25)	10
	100 mg/m²	30	9.6	13 (0–26)	3

CI, confidence interval; NR, not reached.
[a]Core binding factor type [t(8;21), t(16;16), inv(16), and del(16)].
[b]Normal karyotype.
[c]Other karyotype abnormalities.

TABLE 9-2. KEY FEATURES OF CYTOSINE ARABINOSIDE (ARA-C) PHARMACOLOGY

Mechanism of action:	Inhibits DNA polymerase α, is incorporated into DNA, and terminates DNA chain elongation.
Metabolism:	Activated to triphosphate in tumor cells.
	Degraded to inactive ara-U by deamination.
	Converted to ara-CDP choline derivative.
Pharmacokinetics:	Plasma: $t_{1/2\alpha}$ 7–20 min, $t_{1/2\beta}$ 2 h; CSF: $t_{1/2}$ 2 h
Elimination:	Deamination in liver, plasma, and peripheral tissues—100%
Drug interactions:	Methotrexate sodium increases ara-CTP formation.
	Tetrahydrouridine, 3-deazauridine inhibit deamination.
	Ara-C blocks DNA repair, enhances activity of alkylating agents.
	Fludarabine phosphate increases ara-CTP formation.
Toxicity:	Myelosuppression
	Gastrointestinal epithelial ulceration
	Intrahepatic cholestasis, pancreatitis
	Cerebellar and cerebral dysfunction (high dose)
	Conjunctivitis (high dose)
	Hidradenitis
	Noncardiogenic pulmonary edema
Precautions:	High incidence of cerebral-cerebellar toxicity with high-dose ara-C in the elderly, especially in those with compromised renal function.

ara-U, uracil arabinoside; ara-CDP, arabinosylcytosine diphosphate; ara-CTP, arabinosylcytosine triphosphate; CSF, cerebrospinal fluid; $t_{1/2}$, half-life.

gests that differentiation may have occurred in response to ara-C in clinical use.

The molecular mechanism of cell death after ara-C exposure is unclear. Both normal and malignant cells undergo apoptosis in experimental models.[34,35] A complex system of interacting transduction signals ultimately determines whether a cell exposed to a cytotoxic agent is destined to die. Exposure of leukemic cells to ara-C stimulates the formation of ceramide, a potent inducer of apoptosis.[36] On the other hand, an increase in protein kinase C (PKC) activity is observed in leukemic cells in response to ara-C *in*

vitro.[37] This is thought to be due to ara-C induction of diacylglycerol, which in turn induces PKC activity. Because PKC activation is known to oppose apoptosis in hematopoietic cells, the lethal actions of ara-C may depend, at least partially, on its relative effects on the PKC and sphingomyelin pathways. Transcriptional regulation of gene expression is another key mechanism through which the growth and differentiation of mammalian cells are controlled. The induction of some transcription factors, such as AP-1 (a dimer of jun-fos or jun-jun proteins) and NF-kB, has been temporally associated with ara-C–induced apoptosis.[38,39]

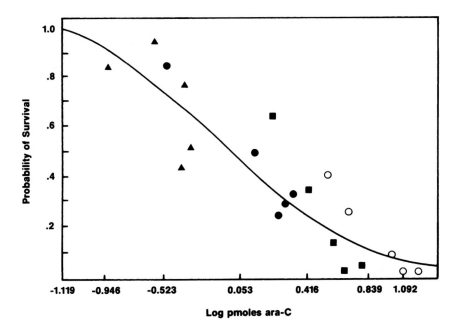

FIGURE 9-2. Relationship between acute myelogenous leukemia blast clonogenic survival and incorporation of tritium-labeled cytosine arabinoside (ara-C) in DNA at ara-C concentrations of 10^{-7} mol per L (▲), 10^{-6} mol per L (●), 10^{-5} mol per L (■), and 10^{-4} mol per L (○) during periods of 1, 3, 6, 12, and 24 hours. (From Kufe DW, Spriggs DR. Biochemical and cellular pharmacology of cytosine arabinoside. *Semin Oncol* 1985;12:34.)

Whether increased expression of these transcription factors plays a direct role in the molecular signaling that leads to anticancer drug–induced programmed cell death is not clear, however. The ability of PKC inhibitors to promote ara-C–induced apoptosis despite antagonizing *c-jun* up-regulation illustrates the fact that apoptosis can occur by a mechanism that does not involve the induction of *c-jun* expression.[40] Some have also reported that induction of pRb phosphatase activity by DNA-damaging drugs, including ara-C, is at least one of the mechanisms responsible for p53-independent, Rb-mediated G_1 arrest and apoptosis.[41] The resulting hypophosphorylated pRb binds to and inactivates the E2F transcription factor, which inhibits the transcription of numerous genes involved in cell-cycle progression.[42]

Cellular Pharmacology and Metabolism

Ara-C penetrates cells by a carrier-mediated process shared by physiologic nucleosides.[43,44] Several different classes of transporters for nucleosides have been identified in mammalian cells[45]; the most extensively characterized in human tumors is identified by its binding to nitrobenzylthioi-

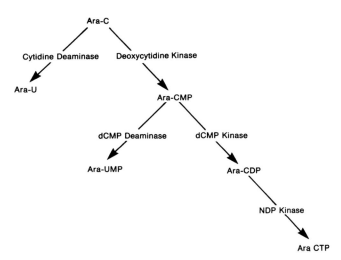

FIGURE 9-4. Metabolism of cytosine arabinoside (ara-C) by tumor cells. The conversion of arabinosyluracil monophosphate (ara-UMP) to a triphosphate has not been demonstrated in mammalian cells. (ara-CDP, arabinosylcytosine diphosphate; ara-CMP, arabinosylcytosine monophosphate; ara-CTP, arabinosylcytosine triphosphate; ara-U, uracil arabinoside; dCMP, deoxycytidine monophosphate; NDP, nucleoside diphosphate.)

nosine (NBMPR). The number of transport sites on the cell membrane is greater in acute myelocytic leukemia than in acute lymphocytic leukemia cells and can be enumerated by incubation of cells with NBMPR. A steady-state level of intracellular drug is achieved within 90 seconds at 37°C. Studies of Wiley et al.[44,46] and others[45,47,48] suggest that the NBMPR transporter plays a limiting role in the action of this agent, in that the formation of the ultimate toxic metabolite ara-CTP is strongly correlated with the number of transporter sites on leukemic cells[46] (Fig. 9-3). At drug concentrations above 10 μmol per L, the transport process becomes saturated, and further entry takes place by passive diffusion.[49]

As shown in Figure 9-4, ara-C must be converted to its active form, ara-CTP, through the sequential action of three enzymes: (a) deoxycytidine (CdR) kinase, (b) deoxycytidine monophosphate (dCMP) kinase, and (c) nucleoside diphosphate (NDP) kinase. Ara-C is subject to degradation by cytidine deaminase, forming the inactive product uracil arabinoside (ara-U); arabinosylcytosine monophosphate (ara-CMP) is likewise degraded by a second enzyme, dCMP deaminase, to the inactive arabinosyluracil monophosphate (ara-UMP). Each of these enzymes, with the exception of NDP kinase, has been examined in detail because of its possible relevance to ara-C resistance.

The first activating enzyme, CdR kinase, is found in lowest concentration (Table 9-3) and is believed to be rate limiting in the process of ara-CTP formation. The enzyme is a 30.5-kd protein that phosphorylates deoxycytidine, deoxyguanosine, deoxyadenosine, ara-C, dideoxycytidine, fludarabine, gemcitabine, and other cytidine and purine analogs. The complementary DNA (cDNA) coding for CdR kinase has been cloned as well as cDNAs with specific

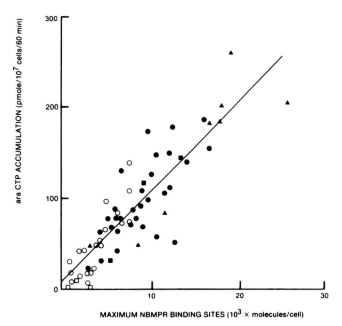

FIGURE 9-3. Correlation between accumulation of arabinosylcytosine triphosphate (ara-CTP) and nucleoside transport capacity measured by the maximal number of nitrobenzylthioinosine (NBMPR) binding sites on leukemic cells ($r = 0.87$; $p < .0001$). Ara-CTP accumulation was measured after incubation of cells with 1 μmol per L of tritium-labeled cytosine arabinoside for 60 minutes. (●, acute myelogenous leukemia; ○, non-T-cell acute lymphoblastic leukemia; ▲, T-cell leukemia/lymphoma, lymphoblastic leukemia; ■, acute undifferentiated leukemia; ▫, chronic lymphocytic leukemia.) (From Wiley JS, Taupin J, Jamieson GP, et al. Cytosine arabinoside transport and metabolism in acute leukemias and T-cell lymphoblastic lymphoma. *J Clin Invest* 1985;75:632.)

TABLE 9-3. KINETIC PARAMETERS OF CYTOSINE ARABINOSIDE (ARA-C)–METABOLIZING ENZYMES

Enzyme	Substrate	K_m (mol/L)	Activity in AML Cells (nmol/h/mg Protein at 37°C)
CdR kinase	Ara-C	2.6×10^{-5} }	15.4 ± 16
	CdR	7.8×10^{-6} }	
dCMP kinase	Ara-CMP	6.8×10^{-4} }	1,990 ± 1,500
	dCMP	1.9×10^{-3} }	
dCDP kinase	Ara-CDP	? }	Not known
	Other NDPs	? }	
CR deaminase	Ara-C	8.8×10^{-5} }	372 ± 614
	CdR	1.1×10^{-5} }	
dCMP deaminase	Ara-CMP	Ara-CMP has higher K_m than dCMP;	1,250 (5 patients)
	dCMP	exact K_m not determined	

AML, acute myelogenous leukemia; Ara-C, ara-CDP, arabinosylcytosine diphosphate; ara-CMP, arabinosylcytosine monophosphate; CdR, deoxycytidine; CR, cytidine; dCDP, deoxycytidine diphosphate; dCMP, deoxycytosine monophosphate; NDPs, nucleoside diphosphates.

mutations that lead to ara-C resistance in experimental cells.[50,51] The rate-limiting role of CdR kinase in ara-C activation is illustrated by the fact that transfection of malignant cell lines with retroviral vectors containing CdR kinase cDNA substantially increases their susceptibility to ara-C, 2-chloro-2'-deoxyadenosine, 2-fluoro-9-β-D-arabinofuranosyladenine, and less potently to gemcitabine.[52] Moreover, some investigators have demonstrated higher ara-C cytotoxicity in intradermal and intracerebral gliomas transduced with CdR kinase in rat models than in the same tumor models with no CdR kinase transduction.[53] This transduction of genes that sensitize tumor cells to prodrugs *in vivo* represents a potential strategy for cancer gene therapy.

CdR kinase activity is highest during the S phase of the cell cycle.[54] The K_m, or affinity constant, for ara-C is 20 μmol per L, compared with the higher affinity or 7.8 μmol per L for the physiologic substrate CdR.[55] This enzyme is strongly inhibited by dCTP but weakly inhibited by ara-CTP. This lack of "feedback" inhibition allows accumulation of the ara-C nucleotide to higher concentrations. Protein kinase C-α, the activity of which is increased after ara-C exposure, has been implicated in phosphorylation of deoxycytidine kinase, increasing its overall activity at concentrations of substrate greater than the K_m. This observation raises the possibility that ara-C at high doses may potentiate its own metabolism by induction of the PKC activator diacylglycerol.[56]

The second activating enzyme, dCMP kinase,[57] is found in several hundred–fold higher concentration than CdR kinase. Its affinity for ara-CMP is low (K_m = 680 μmol per L) but greater than the affinity for the competitive physiologic substrate dCMP. Because of its relatively poor affinity for ara-CMP, this enzyme could become rate limiting at low ara-C concentrations. The third activating enzyme, the diphosphate kinase, appears not to be rate limiting because the intracellular pool of arabinosylcytosine diphosphate (ara-CDP) is only a fraction of the ara-CTP pool.[58]

Opposing the activation pathway are two deaminases found in high concentration in some tumor cells as well as normal tissues. Cytidine deaminase is widely distributed in mammalian tissues, including intestinal mucosa, liver, and granulocytes.[59–62] It is found in granulocyte precursors and in leukemic myeloblasts in lower concentrations than in mature granulocytes, but even in these immature cells the deaminase level exceeds the activity of CdR kinase, the initial activating enzyme.[55,61] The second degradative enzyme, dCMP deaminase (Fig. 9-4), regulates the flow of physiologic nucleotides from the dCMP pool into the deoxyuridine monophosphate pool that is ultimately converted to deoxyribothymidine 5'-phosphate (dTMP) by thymidylate synthase.[63] The enzyme dCMP deaminase is strongly activated by intracellular dCTP (K_m = 0.2 μmol per L) and strongly inhibited by deoxythymidine triphosphate in concentrations of 0.2 μmol per L or greater. Ara-CTP weakly activates this enzyme (K_m = 40 μmol per L)[64] and thus would not promote degradation of its own precursor nucleotide, ara-CMP. The affinity of dCMP deaminase for ara-CMP is somewhat higher than that of dCMP kinase for the same substrate, but the activity of these competitive enzymes depends greatly on their degree of activation or inhibition by regulatory triphosphates (dCTP), and dCMP deaminase concentration in leukemic myeloblasts is slightly less than that of dCMP kinase (Table 9-3).

The balance between activating and degrading enzymes thus is crucial in determining the quantity of drug converted to the active intermediate, ara-CTP. This enzymatic balance varies greatly among cell types.[55] Kinase activity is higher and deaminase lower in lymphoid leukemia than in acute myeloblastic leukemia. Enzyme activities vary also with cell maturity; deaminase increases dramatically with maturation of granulocyte precursors, whereas kinase activity decreases correspondingly.[61] Thus admixture of normal granulocyte precursors with leukemic cells in human bone marrow samples complicates the interpretation of enzyme measurements unless normal and leukemic cells are separated. In general, cytidine deaminase (D) activity greatly exceeds kinase (K) (the kinase/deaminase ratio averages 0.03) in human acute myeloblastic leukemia, whereas the enzyme activities are approximately equal in acute lymphoblastic leukemia and Burkitt's lymphoma. Thus the biochemical setting seems to favor drug activation by lymphoblastic leukemia cells if these initial enzymes play a rate-limiting role.

In fact, this may not be the case. Chou et al.[58] found that human acute myeloblastic leukemia cells formed 12.8 ng of ara-CTP per 10^6 cells after 45 minutes of incubation with 1×10^{-5} mol per L ara-C. Acute lymphoblastic leukemia cells formed less ara-CTP, 6.3 ng per 10^6 cells, and as expected, the more mature chronic myelocytic and chronic lymphocytic leukemia cells formed lesser amounts of ara-CTP (4.7 to 5.2 ng per 10^6 cells). From this study and others,[46,48] the likelihood is that other factors, such as transport across the cell membrane, may limit ara-CTP formation.

In addition to its activation to ara-CTP, ara-C is converted intracellularly to ara-CDP-choline,[65] an analog of the physiologic CDP-choline lipid precursor. However, ara-C does not inhibit incorporation of choline into phospholipids of normal or transformed hamster embryo fibroblasts.[30] Ara-CMP does inhibit the transfer of galactose, N-acetylglucosamine, and sialic acid to cell surface glycoproteins. Further, ara-CTP inhibits the synthesis of cytidine monophosphate–acetylneuraminic acid, an essential substrate in sialylation of glycoproteins, although high ara-CTP concentrations (0.1 to 1 mmol per L) are needed to produce this effect.[66] Thus ara-C treatment could alter membrane structure, antigenicity, and function.

Biochemical Determinants of Cytosine Arabinoside Resistance

The foregoing consideration of ara-C metabolism and transport makes it clear that a number of factors could affect ara-C response. Not surprisingly, many of these factors have been implicated in various preclinical models of ara-C resistance. The most frequent abnormality found in resistant leukemic cells recovered from mice treated with ara-C has been decreased activity of CdR kinase.[67,68] In cultured cells exposed to a mutagen and then to low concentrations of ara-C, some single-step mutants developed high-level resistance to ara-C through loss of activity of CdR kinase, whereas other resistant clones exhibited markedly expanded dCTP pools, presumably through increased cytidine-5'-triphosphate (CTP) synthetase activity or through deficiency of dCMP deaminase.[69–72] As mentioned earlier, specific mutations and deletions in the CdR kinase coding cDNAs derived from resistant cells have been described by Owens et al.[51]

The role of cytidine deaminase in experimental models of resistance is less clear. Retrovirus-mediated transfer of the cytidine deaminase cDNA into 3T3 murine fibroblast cells significantly increases drug resistance to ara-C and other nucleoside analogs such as 5-aza-2'-deoxycytidine, and gemcitabine. This phenotype of increased cytidine deami-

nase activity and drug resistance is reversed by the cytidine deaminase inhibitor tetrahydrouridine.[73] Other genes, including proto-oncogenes, may affect ara-C response. Transfection of rodent fibroblasts and human mammary HBL 100 cells with *c-H-ras* conferred resistance to ara-C, an event attributed to decreased activity of CdR kinase.[74] On the other hand, *N-ras* or *K-ras* mutations strongly correlated with increased ara-C sensitivity in the screening of human tumor cell lines from the National Cancer Institute's *in vitro* Antineoplastic Drug Screen.[75]

Although various metabolic lesions have been implicated as causing ara-C resistance in animals, their relevance to resistance in human leukemia is less certain. Studies have described specific biochemical changes in drug-resistant patients with leukemia, including deletion of CdR kinase,[76] increased cytidine deaminase,[77] a decreased number of nucleoside transport sites,[46] and increased dCTP pools.[78] Other clinical investigators have not been able to correlate resistance with either CdR kinase or cytidine deaminase,[79,80] but with the exception of Wiley et al.,[46] who correlated clinical response with *in vitro* transport, few have examined transport. All studies have shown extreme variability in enzyme levels among patients with acute myelocytic or lymphocytic leukemia (Fig. 9-5). Thus no

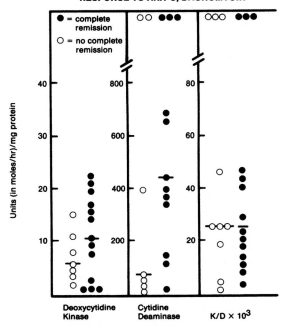

FIGURE 9-5. Response as a function of deoxycytidine kinase and cytidine deaminase activities and their ratio in patients with acute myelogenous leukemia. (ara-C, cytosine arabinoside; K/D, kinase/deaminase ratio.) (From Chang P, Wiernik PH, Reich SD, et al. Prediction of response to cytosine arabinoside and daunorubicin in acute nonlymphocytic leukemia. In: Mandelli F, ed. *Therapy of acute leukemias: proceedings of the second international symposium, Rome, 1977.* Rome: Lombardo Editore, 1979:148.)

TABLE 9-4. CORRELATION OF *IN VITRO* ARA-CTP POOLS AND RETENTION OF ARA-CTP 4 HOURS AFTER DRUG REMOVAL WITH DURATION OF COMPLETE RESPONSE OF PREVIOUSLY UNTREATED PATIENTS WITH ACUTE NONLYMPHOCYTIC LEUKEMIA[a]

	No. of Patients	Ara-CTP Retention at 4 Hours after Removal of ara-C (% of Peak ara-CTP)	Median Duration of CR (mo)
All patients	80	18.4	21.4
≥20% retention	36	42.0	44.8
<20% retention	44	13.9	12.2

ara-C, cytosine arabinoside; ara-CTP, arabinosylcytosine triphosphate; CR, complete response.
[a]Patients were treated with protocol using ara-C (100 mg/m²/day × 10).
Data from Preisler HD, Rustum Y, Priore RL. Relationship between leukemic cell retention of cytosine arabinoside triphosphate and the duration of remission in patients with acute non-lymphocytic leukemia. *Eur J Cancer Clin Oncol* 1985;21:23.

agreement exists as to the specific changes responsible for resistance in human leukemia.

Although *specific biochemical lesions* associated with resistance in humans are unclear, the current understanding of ara-C action suggests that the ultimate formation of ara-CTP and the duration of its persistence in leukemic cells determine response.[58,81] Chou et al.[58] found greater ara-CTP formation in leukemic cells of responders when these cells were incubated *in vitro* with ara-C, but in other series of patients no correlation was seen between remission induction or duration of complete remission and ara-CTP formation.[82–84]

Priesler et al.[85] found a strong correlation between duration of remission and the ability of cells to *retain* ara-CTP *in vitro* after removal of ara-C from the medium (Table 9-4). Attempts to monitor ara-CTP formation in leukemic cells taken from patients during therapy have yielded useful information on rates of nucleotide formation and disappearance (the intracellular ara-CTP half-life is approximately 3 hours) but have not disclosed useful correlations of ara-CTP levels with response.[84,86] Again, considerable variability has been observed in the rates of formation of ara-CTP, and this rate does not correlate well with plasma ara-C concentrations in individual patients (Fig. 9-6).

Although specific steps in ara-C activation and degradation exert a strong influence on its ultimate action, the cellular response to ara-C–mediated DNA damage also governs whether the genotoxic insult results in cell death. In this sense, overexpression of Bcl-2 and Bcl-X$_L$ in leukemic blasts have been associated with *in vitro* resistance to ara-C–mediated apoptosis.[87] The intracellular metabolism of ara-C and its initial effects on DNA are not modified by Bcl-2 expression, which suggests that Bcl-2 primarily regulates the more distal steps in the ara-C–induced cell death pathway. Although the precise mechanism by which these proteins prevent ara-C–induced cytotoxicity remains to be elucidated, Bcl-2 and Bcl-X$_L$ have been shown to antagonize ara-C–mediated cell death by a mechanism that prevents the activation of *Caenorhabditis elegans* death–like proteases, such as Yama/CPP32 protease, which are involved in the execution of apoptosis.[87] The fact that antisense oligo-

nucleotides directed against Bcl-2 increase the susceptibility of leukemic blasts to ara-C–induced apoptosis *in vitro*,[88] and that patients whose blasts express high levels of Bcl-2 respond poorly to ara-C–containing regimens,[89] further illustrates the potential role of Bcl-2 in ara-C resistance.

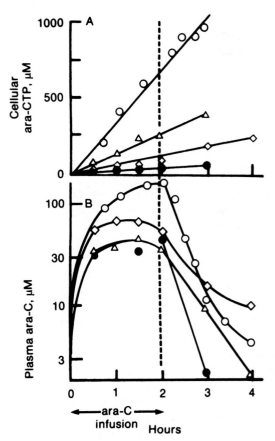

FIGURE 9-6. Pharmacokinetics of arabinosylcytosine triphosphate (ara-CTP) in leukemia cells and of cytosine arabinoside (ara-C) in plasma. Blood samples were drawn at the indicated times during and after infusion of ara-C, 3 g per m², to patients with acute leukemia in relapse. Symbols for each analysis are the same for individual patients. [From Plunkett W, Liliemark JO, Estey E, et al. Saturation of ara-CTP accumulation during high-dose ara-C therapy: pharmacologic rationale for intermediate-dose ara-C. *Semin Oncol* 1987;14(2[Suppl 1]):159.]

Exceptions are seen, however, in which even high levels of Bcl-2 expression apparently fail to prevent cell death.

Phosphorylation of apoptotic or DNA damage response factors may also determine the outcome of ara-C exposure. Studies have shown that phosphorylation of Bcl-2 is required for its antiapoptotic function, and a functional role for PKC-α in Bcl-2 phosphorylation and suppression of apoptosis has been postulated,[90] although this observation has not been confirmed by others.[91] Altered phosphorylation of transcription factors also influences the cellular response to ara-C toxic insult. Ara-C–induced activation of PKC and mitogen-activated protein kinase (MAPK) has been reported to increase c-*jun* expression and phosphorylation,[37,92] and hyperphosphorylation of the AP-1 transcription factor has been associated with ara-C resistance in human myeloid leukemic cell lines *in vitro*.[93]

Clinical studies of determinants of ara-C response are complicated by the fact that ara-C is almost always given in combination with an anthracycline or an anthraquinone. Thus a complete response or long remission duration does not necessarily imply sensitivity to ara-C. A lack of response does imply resistance to both agents in the combination, except for the not-infrequent cases in which failure can be attributed to infection or inability to administer full dosages of drug. With these limitations, the duration of complete response is probably the most appropriate and important single yardstick of drug sensitivity, because it reflects the fractional cell kill during induction therapy.

Cell Kinetics and Cytosine Arabinoside Cytotoxicity

In addition to biochemical factors that determine response, cell kinetic properties exert an important influence on the results of ara-C treatment. As an inhibitor of DNA synthesis, ara-C has its greatest cytotoxic effects during the S phase of the cell cycle,[94] perhaps due to the requirement for its incorporation into DNA and the greater activity of anabolic enzymes during S phase. The duration of exposure of cells to ara-C is directly correlated with cell kill, because the longer exposure period allows ara-C to be incorporated into the DNA of a greater percentage of cells as they pass through S phase (Fig. 9-7). The cytotoxic action of ara-C is not only cell-cycle phase–dependent but is also dependent on the rate of DNA synthesis. That is, cell kill in tissue culture is greatest if cells are exposed during periods of maximal rates of DNA synthesis, as in the recovery period after exposure to a cytotoxic agent. In experimental situations it has been possible to schedule sequential doses of ara-C to coincide with the peak in recovery of DNA synthesis and thus to improve the therapeutic results.[95–97]

Burke and colleagues[96,98] have attempted to exploit kinetic patterns of leukemic cell recovery after ara-C by optimizing sequential doses of drug. Thus retreatment 8 to 10 days after an initial dose of ara-C has yielded a promis-

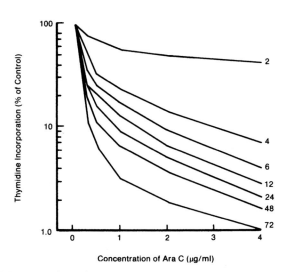

FIGURE 9-7. Thymidine incorporation into DNA of M19 human melanoma cells as a function of drug concentration and duration of exposure to cytosine arabinoside (ara-C). The exposure duration in hours is indicated by the numbers adjacent to the individual curves. The data indicate a near linear relationship between inhibition of thymidine incorporation and drug concentration but a lesser dependence on time for intervals longer than 12 hours, perhaps because of the cell-cycle dependence of the drug. Thus, most replicating cells are exposed to ara-C during their period of DNA synthesis if the exposure time is 12 hours or longer.

ing improvement in the duration of unmaintained remission in adult patients with leukemia in uncontrolled studies.[98]

In humans, the influence of tumor cell kinetics on response is unclear. Although earlier studies showed that the complete remission rate seems to be *higher* in patients who have a high percentage of cells in S phase,[99] remissions are *longer* in patients with leukemias that have long cell-cycle time.[100]

Clinical Pharmacology—Assay Methods

A number of assay methods have been used to measure ara-C concentration in plasma.[101–105] The preferred method for assay of ara-C and its primary metabolite ara-U is high-pressure liquid chromatography, which has the requisite specificity and adequate (0.1 μmol per L) sensitivity.[106,107] An alternative method using gas chromatography–mass spectrometry combines high specificity with greater sensitivity (4 nmol per L) but requires derivatization of samples and thus prolonged performance time.[108] Because of the presence of cytidine deaminase in plasma, the deaminase inhibitor tetrahydrouridine must be added to plasma samples immediately after blood samples are obtained.

Pharmacokinetics

The important factors that determine ara-C pharmacokinetics are its high aqueous solubility and its susceptibility to deamination in liver, plasma, granulocytes, and gastrointestinal tract. Ara-C is amenable to use by multiple schedules and routes of administration and has shown clinical activity in dosages ranging from 3 mg per m^2 twice weekly to 3 g per m^2 every 12 hours for 6 days. Remarkably, over this wide dosage range, its pharmacokinetics remains quite constant and predictable.

Distribution

As a nucleoside, ara-C is transported across cell membranes by active transport and distributes quickly into total-body water.[109,110] It crosses into the central nervous system (CNS) with surprising facility for a water-soluble compound and reaches steady-state levels at 20% to 40% of those found simultaneously in plasma during constant intravenous infusion.[102] At conventional doses of ara-C (100 mg per m^2 by 24-hour infusion), spinal fluid levels reach 0.2 µmol per L, which is probably above the cytotoxic threshold for leukemic cells. High doses of ara-C yield proportionately higher ara-C levels in the spinal fluid.[111–113]

Plasma Pharmacokinetics

The pharmacokinetics of ara-C is characterized by rapid disappearance from plasma owing to deamination, with some variability seen among individual patients.[102,104,108,110] Peak plasma concentrations reach 10 µmol per L after bolus doses of 100 mg per m^2 and are proportionately higher (up to 150 µmol per L) for doses up to 3 g per m^2 given over a 1- or 2-hour infusion[111,114] (Fig. 9-8). Thereafter, the

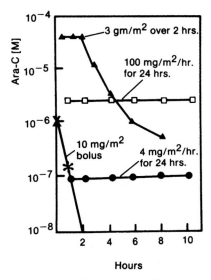

FIGURE 9-8. Cytosine arabinoside (ara-C) pharmacokinetics in plasma after doses of 3 g per m^2 given over 2 hours, 100 mg per m^2 per hour by continuous infusion for 24 hours, 4 mg per m^2 per hour (a conventional antileukemic dose) by continuous intravenous infusion, and 10 mg per m^2 subcutaneously or intravenously as a bolus.

plasma concentration of ara-C declines, with a half-life of 7 to 20 minutes. A second phase of drug disappearance has been detected after high-dose ara-C infusion, with a terminal half-life of 30 to 150 minutes, but the drug concentration during this second phase has cytotoxic potential only in patients treated with high-dose ara-C.[113,115] Seventy percent to 80% of a given dose is excreted as ara-U,[102] which, within minutes of drug injection, becomes the predominant compound found in plasma. Ara-U has a longer half-life in plasma (3.2 to 5.8 hours) than does ara-C and may enhance the activation of ara-C through feedback inhibition of ara-C deamination in leukemic cells.[115]

The steady-state level of ara-C in plasma achieved by constant intravenous infusion remains proportional to dose for dose rates up to 2 g per m^2 per day. At this dosage, steady-state plasma levels approximate 5 µmol per L. Above this rate of infusion, the deamination reaction is saturated and ara-C plasma levels rise unpredictably, which leads to severe toxicity in some patients.[116] To accelerate the achievement of a steady-state concentration, one may give a loading dose of three times the hourly infusion rate before infusion.[110] Equivalent drug exposure (area under the curve) is achieved by subcutaneous or intravenous infusion of ara-C,[117] although one study has reported higher ara-CTP concentrations in leukemia cells after subcutaneous administration.[118]

Owing to the presence of high concentrations of cytidine deaminase in the gastrointestinal mucosa and liver, orally administered ara-C provides much lower plasma levels than does direct intravenous administration. Three- to tenfold higher doses must be given in animals to achieve an equal biologic effect. The oral route, therefore, is not routinely used in humans.

Ara-C may also be administered by intraperitoneal infusion for treatment of ovarian cancer.[119] After instillation of 100 µmol per L of drug, ara-C levels fall in the peritoneal cavity with a half-life of approximately 2 hours. Simultaneous plasma levels are 100- to 1,000-fold lower, presumably due to deamination of ara-C in liver before it reaches the systemic circulation. In 21-day continuous infusion, patients tolerated up to 100 µmol per L intraperitoneal concentrations but developed peritonitis at higher concentrations.[120]

Cerebrospinal Fluid Pharmacokinetics

After intravenous administration of 100 mg per m^2 of ara-C, parent drug levels reach 0.1 to 0.3 µmol per L in the cerebrospinal fluid (CSF), with a decline in levels thereafter characterized by a half-life of 2 hours. Proportionately higher CSF levels are reached by intravenous high-dose ara-C regimens; for example, a 3-g-per-m^2 infusion intravenously over 1 hour yields peak CSF concentrations of 4 µmol per L,[114] whereas the same dose over 24 hours yields peak CSF ara-C concentrations of 1 µmol per L.[116]

Ara-C is effective when administered intrathecally for the treatment of metastatic neoplasms. A number of dosing schedules for giving intrathecal ara-C have been recommended, but twice weekly or weekly schedules of administration are the most widely used. The dose of ara-C ranges from 30 to 50 mg per m². The dose is generally adjusted in pediatric patients according to age (15 mg for children below 1 year of age, 20 mg for children between 1 and 2 years, 30 mg for children between 2 and 3 years, and 40 mg for children older than 3 years). The clinical pharmacology of ara-C in the CSF following intrathecal administration differs considerably from that seen in the plasma following a parenteral dose. Systematically administered ara-C is rapidly eliminated by biotransformation to the inactive metabolite ara-U. In contrast, little conversion of ara-C to ara-U takes place in the CSF following an intrathecal injection. The ratio of ara-U to ara-C is only 0.08, a finding that is consistent with the very low levels of cytidine deaminase present in the brain and cerebrospinal fluid. Following an intraventricular administration of 30 mg of ara-C, peak levels exceed 2 mmol per L, and levels decline slowly, with the terminal half-life being approximately 3.4 hours.[102] Concentrations above the threshold for cytotoxicity (0.1 μg per mL, or 0.4 μmol per L) are maintained in the CSF for 24 hours. The CSF clearance is 0.42 mL per minute, which is similar to the CSF bulk flow rate. This finding suggests that drug elimination occurs primarily by this route. Plasma levels following intrathecal administration of 30 mg per m² of ara-C are less than 1 μmol per L, which illustrates again the advantage of intracavitary therapy with a drug that is rapidly cleared in the systemic circulation.

Depocytarabine (DTC 101) is a depot formulation in which ara-C is encapsulated in microscopic Gelfoam particles (DepoFoam) for sustained release into the cerebrospinal fluid, so that the need for repeated lumbar punctures is avoided. The encapsulation of ara-C in DepoFoam results in a 55-fold increase in CSF half-life after intraventricular administration in rats, from 2.7 hours to 148 hours. Cytotoxic concentrations of free ara-C (more than 0.4 μmol per L) in CSF were maintained for more than 1 month following a single intrathecal dose administration of 2 mg of DTC 101 in rhesus monkeys. A phase I trial of DTC 101 given intraventricularly has been performed in patients with leptomeningeal metastasis. Free ara-C CSF concentration decreased biexponentially. Ara-C concentration was maintained above the threshold for cytotoxicity for an average of 12 ± 3 days. The maximum tolerated dosage was 75 mg administered every 3 weeks and the dose-limiting toxicity was headache and arachnoiditis.[121] Preliminary results of a randomized study involving patients with lymphomatous meningitis demonstrate a possible prolongation of time to neurologic progression in patients treated with 50 mg of depocytarabine every 2 weeks compared with patients treated with standard intrathecal ara-C.[122]

Alternate Schedules of Administration

Although ara-C is used most commonly in regimens of 100 to 200 mg per m² per day for 7 days, other high- and low-

dose schedules have been used in treating leukemia. The more effective of these newer regimens have been high-dose schemes, usually 2 to 3 g per m² every 12 hours for 6 doses.[123] High-dose ara-C is used primarily in the consolidation phase for acute myelocytic leukemia.[8] The rationale for the higher-dose regimen initially rested on the assumption that ara-C phosphorylation is the rate-limiting intracellular step in the drug's activation and could be promoted by raising intracellular concentrations to the K_m of deoxycytidine kinase for ara-C, or approximately 20 μmol per L. Above this level, further increases in ara-C do not lead to increased ara-CTP, because the phosphorylation pathways become saturated.[48,124]

Others have examined the clinical activity of low-dose ara-C, particularly in elderly patients with myelodysplastic syndromes.[125] These regimens have used dosages in the range of 3 to 20 mg per m² per day for up to 3 weeks. The rationale for low-dose regimens has been based primarily on the expectation that they would produce less toxicity; low concentrations of ara-C were also thought to promote leukemic cell differentiation (or apoptosis) in tissue culture. In isolated cases, the persistence of chromosomal markers for the leukemic cell line in remission granulocytes has been documented,[126,127] findings that support differentiation. In general, although the low-dose regimens produce less toxicity, particularly at the lower end of the dose spectrum, the therapeutic results have been disappointing, in that less than 20% of patients achieve a clinical remission.[128] The problem is that continuous exposure of normal myeloid precursor cells to drug concentrations as low as 10 nmol per L inhibits proliferation.[129] After intravenous doses as low as 3 mg per m², peak plasma levels reach 100 nmol per L and remain above the inhibitory concentration (10 nmol per L) for 30 to 60 minutes. Thus low-dose ara-C regimens have not avoided the myelosuppressive effects of standard schedules.

Toxicity

The primary determinants of ara-C toxicity are drug concentration and duration of exposure. Because ara-C is cell-cycle-phase–specific, the duration of cell exposure to the drug is critical in determining the fraction of cells killed.[130] In humans, single-bolus doses of ara-C as large as 4.2 g per m² are well tolerated because of the rapid inactivation of the parent compound and the brief period of exposure, whereas constant infusion of drug for 48 hours using total doses of 1 g per m² produces severe myelosuppression.[131]

Myelosuppression and gastrointestinal epithelial injury are the primary toxic side effects of ara-C. With the conventional 5- to 7-day courses of treatment, the period of maximal toxicity begins during the first week of treatment and lasts 14 to 21 days. The primary targets of ara-C are platelet production and granulopoiesis, although anemia also occurs. Little acute effect is seen on the lymphocyte count, although a depression of cell-mediated immunity is found in patients receiving ara-C.[132] Megaloblastic changes consistent with suppression of DNA synthesis are observed in both the white and red cell precursors.[133]

Gastrointestinal symptoms, including nausea, vomiting, and diarrhea, are frequent during the period of drug administration but subside quickly after treatment. Severe gastrointestinal lesions occur in patients treated with ara-C as part of complex chemotherapy regimens, and the specific contribution of ara-C is difficult to ascertain in these cases. All parts of the gastrointestinal tract are affected. Oral mucositis also occurs and may be severe and prolonged in patients receiving more than 5 days of continuous treatment. Clinical symptoms of diarrhea, ileus, and abdominal pain may be accompanied by gastrointestinal bleeding, electrolyte abnormalities, and protein-losing enteropathy. Radiologic evidence of dilatation of the terminal ileum, termed typhlitis, may be associated with progressive abdominal pain and bowel perforation. Pathologic findings include denudation of the epithelial surface and loss of crypt cell mitotic activity. Reversible intrahepatic cholestasis occurs frequently in patients receiving ara-C for induction therapy but requires cessation of therapy in fewer than 25% of patients.[134,135] It is manifested primarily as an increase in hepatic enzymes in the serum, together with mild jaundice, and rapidly reverses with discontinuation of treatment. Ara-C has been implicated as the cause of pancreatitis in a small number of patients.[136]

Toxicity of High-Dose Cytosine Arabinoside

High-dose ara-C significantly increases the incidence and severity of bone marrow and gastrointestinal toxic effects.[7] Hospitalization for fever and neutropenia is required in 71% of the treatment courses in patients receiving 3 g per m[2] per 12 hours given on alternative days for six doses, and platelet transfusions are required in 86%.[8] Treatment-related deaths, primarily due to infection, occurred in 5% of the patients treated with this schedule.[8] In addition, high-dose ara-C produces pulmonary toxicity, including noncardiogenic pulmonary edema, in approximately 10% of patients, and a surprisingly high incidence of *Streptococcus viridans* pneumonia is seen, especially in pediatric populations.[137–139] The pulmonary edema syndrome is frequently irreversible.

Cholestatic jaundice and elevation of serum glutamic-oxaloacetic transaminase, serum glutamic-pyruvic transaminase, and alkaline phosphatase, with underlying cholestasis and passive congestion on liver biopsy, are also frequently observed with the high-dose regimen.[140] These changes, however, are generally clinically unimportant and reversible. A more dangerous toxicity involving cerebral and cerebellar dysfunction occurs in 10% of patients receiving 3 g per m[2] for 6 doses[8] and in two-thirds of patients receiving 4.5 g per m[2] for 12 doses.[141] Age over 40 years, abnormal alkaline

phosphatase activity in serum, and compromised renal function[142] are risk factors associated with an increased susceptibility to CNS toxicity, which is manifested as slurred speech, unsteady gait, dementia, and coma.[141] Patients with two or more of these risk factors treated with high-dose ara-C develop CNS toxicity in 37% of the cases, whereas the incidence is less than 1% when fewer than two of these criteria are present.[142] Symptoms of neurologic toxicity resolve within several days in approximately 20% of patients and gradually recede in approximately 40%; however, a permanent disability is present in the remaining 40%, and occasional patients have died of CNS toxicity.[8] Progressive brainstem dysfunction[143] and an ascending peripheral neuropathy[144] also have been reported after high-dose ara-C. Conjunctivitis, responsive to topical steroids, also has been a frequent side effect of high-dose ara-C.[145] Rarely, skin rash[146] and even anaphylaxis have been noted.[147] Neutrophilic eccrine hydradenitis, an unusual febrile cutaneous reaction manifested as plaques or nodules during the second week after chemotherapy, is being reported with increasing frequency[148] after high-dose ara-C. Finally, reports have appeared sporadically in the literature of cardiac toxicity associated with ara-C, generally at high dosages. Findings have included arrhythmias, pericarditis, and congestive heart failure. None of these reports provide conclusive evidence for a cause-effect relationship.[149]

Toxicity of Intrathecal Cytosine Arabinoside

Ara-C given intrathecally is infrequently associated with fever and seizures occurring within 24 hours of administration and arachnoiditis occurring within 4 to 7 days.[150] Rarely, it causes a progressive brainstem toxicity that may be fatal.[151] Intrathecal ara-C should be used with caution in patients who have previously experienced methotrexate neurotoxicity.

Although ara-C causes chromosomal breaks in cultured cells and in the bone marrow of patients receiving therapy,[152] it is not an established carcinogen in humans. The drug is teratogenic in animals.[153]

Drug Interactions

Ara-C has synergistic antitumor activity with a number of other antitumor agents in animal tumor models. These other agents include alkylating agents [cyclophosphamide[154] and carmustine (BCNU)[155]], cisplatin,[156] purine analogs,[157,158] methotrexate,[159,160] and etoposide.[161] In the past, ara-C and 6-thioguanine (6-TG) were frequently combined in the treatment of acute leukemia. This interaction seems to be highly schedule dependent. Ara-C, as an inhibitor of DNA synthesis, blocks the incorporation of 6-TG into DNA; however, if ara-C is given 12 hours before 6-TG, enhanced incorporation of the purine analog is observed.[162] On the other hand, evidence exists that 6-TG,

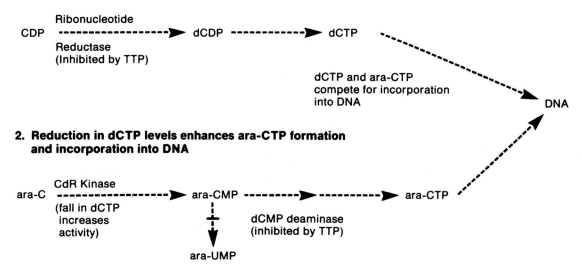

FIGURE 9-9. Interactions of thymidine and cytosine arabinoside (ara-C). (ara-CMP, arabinosylcytosine monophosphate; ara-CTP, arabinosylcytosine triphosphate; ara-UMP, arabinosyluracil monophosphate; CDP, cytidine diphosphate; CdR, deoxycytidine; dCDP, deoxycytidine diphosphate; dCMP, deoxycytidine monophosphate; dCTP, deoxycytidine triphosphate; TTP, thymidine triphosphate.)

given before or with ara-C, enhances ara-C incorporation into DNA by blocking the exonuclease activity inherent in DNA polymerase.[163]

The basis for ara-C potentiation of alkylating agents and cisplatin is thought to be inhibition of repair of DNA-alkylator adducts, although this hypothesis has not been proven. The hypothesis is consistent with the finding that ara-C exposure preceding cisplatin is synergistic—perhaps allowing for inhibition of repair[164]—whereas ara-C after cisplatin is not.[156]

Tetrahydrouridine, a potent inhibitor of cytidine deaminase ($K_i = 3 \times 10^{-8}$ mol per L),[62] also enhances ara-CTP formation in acute myelocytic leukemia cells *in vitro* but not in chronic lymphocytic leukemia cells, which lack the target enzyme.[165] Tetrahydrouridine enhances the growth-inhibitory effects of sublethal concentrations of ara-C in experiments with the sarcoma 180 cell line, which contains high amounts of cytidine deaminase.[166] Initial clinical evaluation of the combination indicates that tetrahydrouridine in intravenous doses of 50 mg per m² markedly prolongs the plasma half-life of ara-C from 10 to 120 minutes and causes a corresponding enhancement of toxicity to bone marrow.[167,168] In combination with tetrahydrouridine, the tolerable dosage of ara-C is reduced 30-fold to 0.1 mg per kg per day for 5 days. Whether the combination has greater therapeutic effects and a better therapeutic ratio than ara-C alone is unclear.

Inhibitors of ribonucleotide reductase—such as hydroxyurea,[169] 2,3-dihydro-1 *H*-imidazolo(1,2-*b*)pyrazole,[170] and thymidine triphosphate[171]—all enhance ara-C toxicity by decreasing dCTP pools (Fig. 9-9). A decrease in dCTP

should have several beneficial effects on ara-C activity. CdR kinase, the enzyme that converts ara-C to ara-CMP (Fig. 9-4), is inhibited by dCTP, whereas dCMP deaminase, which would convert ara-CMP to the inactive ara-UMP, is inhibited by the fall in dCTP; a decrease in dCTP pools should thus increase ara-CTP formation. Second, because ara-CTP and dCTP compete for the same active site on DNA polymerase, a decrease in dCTP pools should lead to a relative increase in the amount of ara-C incorporated into DNA.

Experimental studies have confirmed that synergy between ara-C and thymidine occurs in some but not all tumor cell lines[171,172] and experimental chemotherapy settings.[173,174] The combination of ara-C and thymidine has received limited clinical evaluation in patients with refractory leukemia and lymphoma, and the initial results have not been favorable, as only 7 of 26 patients in the largest study achieved remission.[174-176] Thymidine (75 g per m² per day) is extremely cumbersome to administer because of the massive fluid load required.[174,175] Tumor cells may develop resistance to both agents by a single-step mutation related to expansion of the dCTP pool as a result of increased *de novo* synthesis of pyrimidines.[69]

The conversion of ara-C to its active form, ara-CTP, is also augmented by pretreatment with methotrexate, according to studies of the murine lymphoma cell lines L1210 and L5178Y.[159,160] Simultaneous administration of ara-C and methotrexate is associated with greater retention of ara-CTP in tumor cells and better therapeutic results than achieved with schedules using ara-C alone or ara-C and methotrexate administered 24 hours apart.[177] In a study involving pediatric patients with acute lymphoblastic leukemia, however, the administration of methotrexate and ara-C resulted in red blood cell methotrexate levels that were markedly lower than levels in patients treated with methotrexate alone. Moreover, patients with red blood cell methotrexate levels below the median had a significantly worse event-free survival and overall survival than those with levels above the median. These data suggest that ara-C given in combination with methotrexate may have antagonistic effects.[178] The biochemical basis for this interaction is unclear.

Ara-C is commonly used in combination with daunorubicin or etoposide for the treatment of acute myelocytic leukemia. In experimental systems, minute (0.01 μmol per L) concentrations of ara-C cause an increase in levels of topoisomerase II, enhance the rate of protein-associated DNA strand breaks induced by etoposide,[161] and increase their cytotoxicity. Ara-C has no apparent direct effect on topoisomerase II activity.[179]

Ara-CTP formation, a requisite step for cytotoxicity, is markedly augmented by prior exposure of leukemic cells to fludarabine (fluoro-ara-adenine) phosphate, but this combination decreases the intracellular levels of fluoro-arabynosyl-adenine-triphosphate (F-ara-ATP).[157,180] The former effect is thought to be the consequence of the inhibition of ribonucleotide reductase by fludarabine triphosphate. Approximately a 50% increase in leukemic cell ara-CTP is associated with pretreatment of chronic lymphocytic leukemia patients with fludarabine. Ara-C also may shorten the plasma half-life of fludarabine.[158] Clinical studies performed during treatment of patients with acute myelogenous leukemia demonstrated that the accumulation of ara-CTP in circulating leukemia blasts was increased by a median of twofold when fludarabine was infused 4 hours before ara-C. The augmentation was dependent on the cellular concentration of fludarabine triphosphate. Fludarabine at 15 mg per m^2 infused over 30 minutes consistently produced cellular fludarabine triphosphate levels that maximized ara-CTP accumulation in acute myelocytic leukemia blasts.[181]

Considerable interest has focused on the use of ara-C in combination with hematopoietic growth factors (HGFs). The theoretical gain of this combination would be that administration of HGFs before the administration of a cell-cycle–specific drug, such as ara-C, would recruit leukemia cells into the susceptible S phase of the cell cycle, which would thereby enhance cytotoxicity. In fact, several *in vitro* studies have shown that cytokines, particularly interleukin 3 and granulocyte-macrophage colony-stimulating factor, stimulate myeloid leukemia proliferation[182] and increase leukemic blast susceptibility to ara-C–induced apoptosis.[183] Growth regulatory molecules might also affect the therapeutic index by increasing the ara-CTP to dCTP ratio[184] and the ara-C incorporation into DNA.[185] Conflicting results have been observed in *in vivo* studies, however, and several randomized clinical trials have shown no advantage in response rate or survival in patients with acute myelo-

cytic leukemia treated with HGFs in combination with ara-C compared with patients treated with ara-C alone.[186]

As resistance to a broad range of chemotherapeutic agents, including ara-C, may arise from defects in damage recognition and apoptosis pathways, a major field of investigations has been the modulation of signal transduction–apoptotic pathways. Staurosporine, a highly potent but nonspecific inhibitor of PKC (20 to 50 nmol per L), significantly potentiated ara-C–mediated apoptosis in human myeloid leukemia cell lines HL-60 and U937 but was ineffective when given alone at these concentrations.[187] In contrast, coadministration of another nonspecific PKC inhibitor, H7, and two highly selective PKC inhibitors, calphostin C and chelerythrine, also increased the extent of DNA fragmentation observed in ara-C treated cells but only at concentrations that were themselves sufficient to induce DNA damage.[187] Sustained exposure to bryostatin 1, a macrocyclic lactone PKC activator, also enhanced ara-C–mediated apoptosis. These apparently conflicting observations may be explained by the phenomenon of down-regulation of PKC expression after sustained activation.[188] Moreover, agents that down-regulate or inhibit PKC circumvent resistance of Bcl-2–overexpressing leukemia cells to ara-C–induced apoptosis and activation of the protease cascade. This finding suggests the possibility that modulation of the phosphorylation status of Bcl-2 contributes to this effect.[91]

OTHER CYTIDINE ANALOGS

One objective of analog development in the general area of cytidine antimetabolites has been to find compounds that preserve the inhibitory activity of ara-C but are resistant to deamination. This goal is based primarily on the assumptions that the rapid metabolism of ara-C and its short half-life in plasma constitute an inconvenience because they require continuous infusion of drug rather than intermittent bolus administration—and that deamination may play a role in tumor cell resistance. As reviewed earlier in this chapter, the evidence that nucleoside deamination is responsible for resistance is limited to the study of Steuart and Burke[77] and has not been confirmed by subsequent work. Nonetheless, a number of deaminase-resistant analogs have been developed, and several, including cyclocytidine (O^2,2'-cyclocytidine)[189] and N^4-behenoyl ara-C,[190] have shown antileukemic activity in limited clinical trials. Representative compounds are listed in Table 9-5. Cyclocytidine proved to have undesirable side effects, including hypotension and parotid pain, and did not show activity superior to that of ara-C in its initial trials. The lipid-soluble conjugates, such as the behenoyl derivative, may have the additional advantage of ready diffusion into the cell in view of evidence that ara-C transport by an active transporter may be a limiting factor in leukemia cells.

TABLE 9-5. ALTERNATIVE FORMS OF CYTIDINE ANTIMETABOLITE CHEMOTHERAPY

	Rationale	Effect	Reference
Entrapment of ara-C in liposomes	Prevents deamination; preferential uptake by tumor cells	Acts as depot form of ara-C with slow release	194, 312
N^4-Palmitoyl-ara-C	Resistant to deaminase, highly lipid soluble, active orally	Greater ara-C nucleotide formation *in vitro*, longer $t_{1/2}$	313
2'-Azido-2'-deoxy-ara-C	Resistant to deaminase	Has antitumor activity	314
5'-(Cortisone-21-phosphoryl) ester of ara-C	Resistant to deaminase, combines two active drugs, targets to steroid receptor + cells	Less active than ara-C *in vivo*	315
5'-Acyl esters of ara-C (e.g., 5'-palmitate ester)	Lipid-soluble, depot form, resistant to deamination	Prolonged $t_{1/2}$, has antitumor activity, but clinical formulation difficult owing to poor aqueous solubility	316
N^4-Behenoyl-ara-C	Resistant to deamination	Active in human acute leukemia	190
Ara-C conjugate with poly-H^5-(2-hydroxyethyl)-L-glutamine	Slow release of ara-C *in vivo*	Increased *in vivo* activity in mice	317
Dihydro-5-azacytidine	Resistant to chemical degradation	—	318
5-Aza-arabinosylcytosine	Resistant to deamination	Broad solid tumor spectrum in mice	319
5-Aza-2'-deoxycytidine	Activated by deoxycytidine kinase	Antileukemic activity in humans	320
2'-2'-Difluorodeoxycytidine	Longer intracellular half-life, different mechanism of action	Broad solid tumor spectrum in experimental tumors	321

ara-C, cytosine arabinoside; $t_{1/2}$, half-life.

The N^4-acyl compounds are extensively incorporated into membrane lipids and may have novel effects as analogs of the physiologic lipid conjugate ribo-cytidine diphosphate-L-palmitin, a precursor of membrane lipids. An orally active ester, 1-β-D-arabinofuranosylcytosine-5'-stearylphosphate, which is cleaved to ara-C by plasma or tissue esterases (or both), yields prolonged elevation of plasma ara-C levels after single oral doses of the parent compound.[191]

The unique cytidine nucleoside 5-(β-D-ribofuranosyl) isocytosine, or isocytidine, competes with cytidine for incorporation into RNA and DNA. It is activated by cytidine kinase, but because of its poor affinity for this enzyme, high doses are required to express antitumor activity.[192] This agent is highly active against some ara-C–resistant tumors, probably due to increased utilization of ribonucleotide pathways for activation of cytidine to dCTP pools in these cells. An initial phase I trial of this agent failed to disclose antitumor activity. The dose-limiting toxicity was hepatic necrosis at dosages above 120 mg per m² daily for 5 days.[193]

A hybrid of ara-C and 5-azacytidine, 5-aza-cytosine arabinoside[194] (Fig. 9-1), is activated by the same pathway as ara-C and is incorporated into DNA, where it inhibits DNA synthesis. It is not deaminated and has broad activity against human xenografts in nude mice and against murine solid tumors, but it failed to demonstrate clinical activity. A related analog, 5-aza-2'-deoxycytidine (Decitabine), is incorporated into DNA and, like 5-azacytidine, inhibits DNA methylation and promotes differentiation.[195] In human K562 cells, Decitabine was a more effective inducer of erythroid differentiation than its related analog 5-azacytidine, with less acute cell toxicity.[196] In addition, Decitabine showed a greater antileukemic activity than ara-C when the two drugs were compared *in vitro* on a panel of human leu-

kemia cell lines of different phenotypes,[197] and also in some animal tumor models.[198] Decitabine has entered human clinical trials. Encouraging antileukemic activity has been observed in patients with untreated and heavily pretreated acute myelocytic leukemia and acute lymphoblastic leukemia, and the drug has been shown to induce trilineage responses in patients with advanced myelodysplastic syndromes.[199,200] Its most frequent side effects are myelosuppression and moderate emesis, with no other major extrahematologic toxicities.[199,200]

5-Azacytidine

The success of ara-C as an antileukemic agent has encouraged the search for other cytidine analogs, particularly those that would not require activation by deoxycytidine kinase (the enzyme deleted in many ara-C–resistant tumors). Considering ribonucleosides with structural changes in the basic pyrimidine ring was logical, because these would be activated in all likelihood by uridine-cytidine kinase, an entirely separate enzyme. Considerable enthusiasm greeted the introduction of 5-azacytidine, an analog of cytidine synthesized by Sorm and colleagues in 1963[201] and later isolated as a product of fungal cultures.[202] The compound was found to be toxic to both bacterial and mammalian cells. In clinical trials, however, its only important cytostatic action was exerted against acute myelocytic leukemia,[203–205] and this is the only malignant disease for which it is now occasionally used. Although responses to 5-azacytidine have been reported in patients with various solid tumors, including carcinoma of the breast and colon and malignant melanoma, the clinical activity has been too meager and the toxicity too significant to warrant further clinical trials as a cytotoxic agent for these tumors.[206] Other

TABLE 9-6. KEY FEATURES OF 5-AZACYTIDINE PHARMACOLOGY

Mechanism of action:	Incorporated into DNA and RNA; prevents DNA methylation.
Metabolism:	Activated to a triphosphate. Degraded to inactive, unstable 5-aza-uridine by cytidine deaminase.
Pharmacokinetics and elimination:	Plasma half-lives not known, but the drug is chemically unstable and is rapidly deaminated.
Drug interactions:	Tetrahydrouridine inhibits deamination, increases toxicity.
Toxicity:	Myelosuppression Nausea, vomiting after bolus dose Hepatocellular dysfunction Muscle tenderness, weakness Lethargy, confusion, coma
Precautions:	Hepatic failure may occur in patients with underlying liver dysfunction. Use with caution in patients with altered mental status.

actions of 5-azacytidine have awakened interest among biologists and clinicians, however, particularly its ability to inhibit DNA cytosine methylation and, as a consequence, to promote expression of "suppressed" genes. For example, the drug is able to promote the synthesis of fetal hemoglobin, an effect believed to be mediated by hypomethylation of the γ-globin gene in erythroid precursor cells.[207,208] The use of 5-azacytidine for gene demethylation in inherited diseases—a subject of considerable interest in molecular genetics—has been limited by its bone marrow toxicity and by concerns about carcinogenesis. The important features of the pharmacokinetics and clinical effects of 5-azacytidine are summarized in Table 9-6.

Structure and Mechanism of Action

The biochemistry and pharmacology of 5-azacytidine have been reviewed in depth by Glover and Leyland-Jones.[209] The analog 5-azacytidine differs from cytidine in the presence of a nitrogen at the 5 position of the heterocyclic ring (Fig. 9-10). This substitution renders the ring chemically unstable and leads to spontaneous decomposition of the compound in neutral or alkaline solution, with a half-life of approximately 4 hours. The product of this ring opening, *N*-formylamidinoribofuranosylguanylurea, may recyclyze to form the parent compound but is also susceptible to further spontaneous decomposition to ribofuranosylurea.[210] This spontaneous chemical instability is important in the drug's use in two ways: (a) the ultimate antitumor activity of the drug has been attributed to its incorporation into nucleic acids and subsequent spontaneous decomposition, and (b) the preparation formulated for clinical application

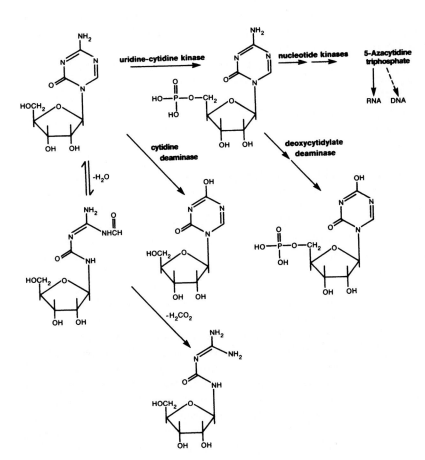

FIGURE 9-10. Metabolic activation and degradation of 5-azacytidine.

must be administered within several hours of its dissolution in dextrose and water or saline.[211] In buffered solutions such as Ringer's lactate and at acidic pH, the agent is considerably more stable, with a half-life of 65 hours at 25°C and 94 hours at 20°C.[212]

The mechanism of 5-azacytidine action has not been firmly established, although the balance of evidence suggests that, as a triphosphate, it competes with CTP for incorporation into RNA,[213] the primary event that leads to a number of different effects on RNA processing and function.[214] These effects include an inhibition of the formation of ribosomal 28 S and 18 S RNA from higher-molecular-weight species,[215] defective methylation[216] and acceptor function of transfer RNA,[217] disassembly of polyribosomes,[218] and a marked inhibition of protein synthesis.[219]

Other effects of 5-azacytidine, however, may be relevant to its antitumor activity. This analog is also incorporated into DNA,[220,221] although to a lesser extent than into RNA. The consequences of 5-azacytidine incorporation into DNA are not fully understood, but one important effect is the inhibition of DNA methylation. The methylation of cytosine residues in DNA inactivates specific genes, whereas treatment of cells with 5-azacytidine leads to a reduction in cytosine methylation and enhanced expression of a broad variety of genes, depending on the cell type studied.[222,223]

Cellular Pharmacology

The analog 5-azacytidine readily enters mammalian cells by a facilitated nucleoside transport mechanism shared with the physiologic nucleosides uridine and cytidine.[221] The initial step in its activation consists of conversion to a monophosphate by uridine-cytidine kinase (Fig. 9-10), which is found in low concentration in human acute myelocytic leukemia cells,[210] has low affinity for 5-azacytidine (K_m = 0.2 to 11 mmol per L),[224,225] and probably represents the rate-limiting step in 5-azacytidine activation. Either uridine[226] or cytidine is capable of preventing 5-azacytidine toxicity in the whole animal and in tissue culture[227] by competitively inhibiting its phosphorylation. Deletion of uridine-cytidine kinase has been observed in mutant Novikoff hepatoma cells resistant to 5-azacytidine,[221] as well as in other resistant cell types.[228] Cytidine deaminase, found in 10- to 30-fold higher concentration than uridine-cytidine kinase in leukemic cells, degrades 5-azacytidine to 5-azauridine. The role of this enzyme in resistance to 5-azacytidine has not been defined.

Further activation of 5-azacytidine monophosphate (5-aza-CMP) to a triphosphate probably occurs by the enzyme dCMP kinase and nucleoside diphosphate kinase. One hour after exposure of cells to the drug, 60% to 70% of acid-soluble radioactivity was identified as 5-azacytidine triphosphate.[221]

Both drug concentration and duration of exposure are important determinants of 5-azacytidine cytotoxicity in tissue culture, a finding consistent with a preferential action on rapidly dividing cells. In tissue culture experiments it has greatest lethality for cells in the S phase of the cell cycle and relatively little effect against nondividing cells.[229,230] Dose-survival curves *in vivo* for L1210 and normal hematopoietic cells are both biphasic, however, which indicates perhaps the presence of more than a single site or mechanism of cytotoxic action.[231]

In addition to its cytotoxic effects, 5-azacytidine has other biologic actions of possible importance in its clinical use. Through its inhibition of DNA methylation, it has been found to induce the synthesis of various proteins, including hepatic enzymes (tyrosine aminotransferase),[232] metallothionein,[233] β- and γ-globin,[207] histocompatibility proteins,[234,235] and T-cell surface markers.[236] It can reactivate repressed genes coding for thymidine kinase,[237] hypoxanthine-guanine phosphoribosyl transferase,[238] or DNA repair[239] and in doing so may convert drug-resistant cells to drug-sensitive, or vice versa. Probably through its effects on DNA methylation, 5-azacytidine is able to increase the immunogenicity of tumor cells,[234] induce senescence in cell lines,[240] and increase the phenotypic diversity of tumor cell lines in mice.[237] The drug has mutagenic and teratogenic effects,[229,241,242] but it is not known to be carcinogenic in humans.

Assay Methods

At present, no assay method specific for 5-azacytidine has been developed for clinical use. Future attempts to develop such methods will undoubtedly be complicated by the chemical instability of the drug, its very limited lipid solubility (which will complicate attempts at extraction and concentration from plasma), and the presence in serum of cytidine deaminase, an enzyme that hydrolyzes 5-azacytidine.

Clinical Pharmacology and Pharmacokinetics

The limited information available on 5-azacytidine pharmacokinetics in animals and humans is based on studies using drug labeled with radioactive carbon (^{14}C)[211,243–245] and provides an incomplete understanding of drug disposition because of the drug's extensive metabolism and chemical decomposition. After subcutaneous injection [^{14}C]5-azacytidine is well absorbed, as judged by radioactivity levels in plasma.[236] Radioactivity distributes into a volume approximately equal to or greater than total-body water (0.58 to 1.15 L per kg) with little plasma protein binding. Peak plasma levels of 0.1 to 1.0 mmol per L are reached by drug infusion at a rate of 2 to 6 mg per hour in adult patients. The primary half-life of radioactivity in plasma is approximately 3.5 hours after bolus intravenous injection, but after 30 minutes less than 2% of radioactivity is associated with intact drug.[211] Isolated measurements of radioactivity in the CSF indicate poor penetration of drug, with a CSF to plasma ratio of less than 0.1.

TABLE 9-7. 5-AZACYTIDINE IN THE TREATMENT OF ACUTE MYELOGENOUS LEUKEMIA

Reference	Dosage (mg/m²/day)	Bolus (B) or Infusion (I)	Toxicity	CR Rate
203	150–200 × 5 days	B	N, V, D, M	5/14 (36%)
204	300–400 × 5 days	B	N, V, D, M	3/18 (17%)
205	150–200 × 5 days	I	M	11/45 (24%)
206	200–250 × 5 days	B	N, V, M, Neuro	5/18 (28%)

CR, complete remission; D, diarrhea; M, myelosuppression; N, nausea; Neuro, neuromuscular symptoms (see text); V, vomiting.

The identity of metabolites is unclear in humans. 5-Azacytidine is known to be susceptible to deamination by cytidine deaminase,[246,247] an enzyme found in high concentrations in liver, granulocytes, and intestinal epithelium and in lower concentration in plasma. A number of metabolic products have been identified in the urine of beagle dogs, including 5-azacytosine, 5-azauracil, and ring cleavage products.[243] The last-named may result from decomposition of the parent compound or of its deamination product, 5-azauridine.

Toxicity

A number of schedules of administration have been used for 5-azacytidine,[203–206] including single weekly intravenous doses of up to 750 mg per m², daily doses of 150 to 200 mg per m² for 5 to 10 consecutive days, and continuous infusion of similar daily doses for up to 5 days (Table 9-7). With each of these schedules, the primary toxicity has been leukopenia, although nausea and vomiting have been extremely bothersome for patients receiving the drug in bolus doses, which has led some investigators to favor continuous intravenous infusion.[205] The latter schedule is also supported by cell kinetic considerations, in view of the drug's greater activity in the S phase of the cell cycle and its very rapid metabolism in humans. The continuous infusion of 5-azacytidine requires fresh preparation of drug at frequent intervals, usually every 3 to 4 hours, because of the chemical instability of the agent. The response rate to 5-azacytidine in previously treated patients with acute myelocytic leukemia has varied from 17% to 36% and seems to be approximately equivalent for the bolus and continuous-infusion schedules.

Maximal dosages, as shown in Table 9-7, produce profound leukopenia and somewhat lesser thrombocytopenia. Hepatotoxicity also has been observed, particularly in patients with preexisting hepatic dysfunction.[248]

A syndrome of neuromuscular toxicity was observed by Levi and Wiernik[249] in patients receiving 200 mg per m² per day by intravenous bolus injection. Whether this peculiar reaction was related to the somewhat higher dosage of drug is unclear, but neurotoxicity has been reported only sporadically by other investigators using this agent.[205] Several less worrisome acute toxic reactions have been associated with 5-azacytidine, including transient fever, a pruritic skin rash, and rarely hypotension during or immediately after bolus intravenous administration.[204]

Low-dose 5-azacytidine has been used in experimental trials to raise fetal hemoglobin levels in patients with sickle cell anemia and thalassemia, but concerns regarding possible carcinogenicity have discouraged routine use to treat these diseases and it has been largely replaced by hydroxyurea for this indication. When given as a continuous infusion of 2 mg per kg per day for 5 days, one cycle per month, the drug regularly produces a reticulocytosis of fetal hemoglobin–containing cells and an increase in hemoglobin content in blood of 2 to 3 g per 100 mL.[250] On this schedule, little myelosuppression, nausea, or vomiting occur.

Gemcitabine

Gemcitabine (2,2-difluorodeoxycytidine, dFdC) is the most important cytidine analog to enter clinical trials since ara-C (Fig. 9-11). It has become the standard first-line therapy for patients with advanced pancreatic cancer,[251] and it is rapidly becoming incorporated into first-line regimens in non–small cell lung cancer and transitional cell carcinoma of the bladder.[252–256] The drug was selected for development on the basis of its impressive activity against murine solid tumors and human xenografts in nude mice.[257] In tissue culture it is generally more potent than ara-C; the 50% inhibition concentration values for human leukemic cells range from 3 to 10 nmol per L for 48-hour exposure compared with 26 to 52 nmol per L for ara-C.[258] Although its metabolism to triphosphate status and its effects on DNA in general mimic those of ara-C, differences are found in kinetics of inhibition and additional sites of action of the newer compound, and clearly the spectrum of activity is different.

Cellular Pharmacology, Metabolism, and Mechanism of Action

Gemcitabine retains many of the characteristics of ara-C. Its key features are shown in Table 9-2. Influx of gemcitabine through the cell membrane occurs via active nucleoside

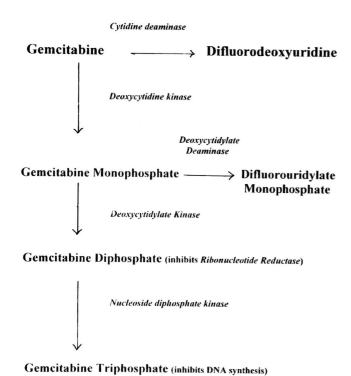

FIGURE 9-11. Key steps in gemcitabine metabolism.

transporters,[259] and deoxycytidine kinase phosphorylates gemcitabine intracellularly to produce difluorodeoxycytidine monophosphate (dFdCMP), from which point it is converted to its diphosphate and triphosphate difluorodeoxycytidine (dFdCDP, dFdCTP) (Fig. 9-1).[260] Its affinity for deoxycytidine kinase is threefold lower than that of deoxycytidine itself, whereas it has a 50% lower affinity for cytidine deaminase than does deoxycytidine.[261] Cytidine deaminase conversion of gemcitabine to difluorodeoxyuri-

dine (dFdU) represents the main catabolic pathway.[262] To a lesser extent, pyrimidine nucleoside phosphorylase clears gemcitabine by cleaving the pyrimidine base from the furanose ring.

As with ara-C, *in vitro* studies of gemcitabine suggest potent inhibition of DNA synthesis as its mechanism of action,[257,260,263] but kinetic studies indicate that the killing effects of gemcitabine are not confined to the S phase of the cell cycle, and the drug is as effective against confluent cells as it is against cells in log-phase growth.[264] The cytotoxic activity may be a result of several actions on DNA synthesis: dFdCTP competes with dCTP as a weak inhibitor of DNA polymerase[263]; dFdCDP is a potent inhibitor of ribonucleotide reductase, which results in depletion of deoxyribonucleotide pools necessary for DNA synthesis[265]; and dFdCTP is incorporated into DNA and, after the incorporation of one more nucleotide, leads to DNA strand termination.[266] This "extra" nucleotide may be important in hiding the dFdCTP from DNA repair enzymes, because incorporation of gemcitabine into DNA appears to be resistant to the normal mechanisms of DNA repair.[267] These effects on DNA synthesis represent the main action of gemcitabine, and emerging evidence demonstrates that incorporation of dFdCTP into DNA is critical for gemcitabine-induced apoptosis.[268,269]

Several important differences exist between ara-C and gemcitabine (Fig. 9-12). First, dFdCTP has a biphasic elimination from leukemic cells with α half-life ($t_{1/2\alpha}$) = 3.9 hours and β half-life ($t_{1/2\beta}$) = 16 hours, whereas ara-CTP has a monophasic elimination with $t_{1/2}$ = 0.7 hours.[260] Also, dFdCDP is a stronger inhibitor of ribonucleotide reductase (50% inhibition concentration of 4 µmol per L), and exposure to the drug blocks incorporation of labeled cytidine into the cellular pool of dCTP.[265] Further, dFdC causes a

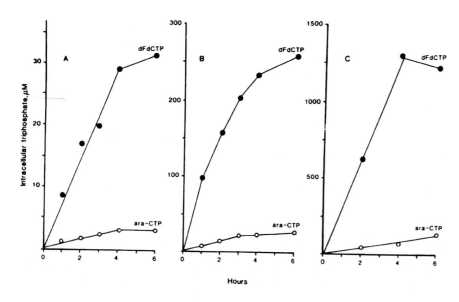

FIGURE 9-12. Accumulation of difluorodeoxycytidine triphosphate (dFdCTP) and arabinosylcytosine triphosphate (ara-CTP) as a function of time after incubation of cells with either dFdCTP or ara-C at drug concentrations of 1 µmol per L **(A)**, 10 µmol per L **(B)**, and 100 µmol per L **(C)**. (Adapted from Heinemann V, Hertel LW, Grindey GB, et al. Comparison of the cellular pharmacokinetics and toxicity of 2',2'-difluorodeoxycytidine and 1-beta-D-arabinofuranosylcytosine. *Cancer Res* 1988;48:4024–4031.)

decrease in all intracellular deoxynucleotide triphosphates, consistent with inhibition of ribonucleotide reductase. The significance of ribonucleotide reductase inhibition is uncertain. Some cell lines selected for resistance to other inhibitors of this enzyme, such as hydroxyurea and deoxyadenosine, do not show cross-resistance to dFdC.[270] On the other hand, resistance to gemcitabine has been demonstrated through overexpression of ribonucleotide reductase.[271] Nevertheless, the significance of ribonucleotide reductase inhibition may be in its self-potentiating effects.[272] Deamination of dFdCMP by dCMP deaminase requires activation by dCTP. As dCTP pools become depleted by the effect of gemcitabine on ribonucleotide reductase, less deamination of gemcitabine diphosphate occurs and intracellular accumulation of gemcitabine metabolites increases. Furthermore, high intracellular concentration of dFdCTP appears to inhibit dCMP deaminase directly.[262]

The activity of dFdCTP on DNA repair mechanisms may allow for increased cytotoxicity of other chemotherapeutic agents, particularly platinum compounds. Cisplatin works by creating interstrand and intrastrand cross-links. A mechanism of resistance may be removal of these cross-links by nucleotide excision repair (NER). Preclinical studies of tumor cell lines show that cisplatin-DNA adducts are enhanced in the presence of gemcitabine.[273] In cisplatin-resistant tumor cell lines, which have increased expression of NER, the addition of gemcitabine to cisplatin decreased tumor survival over that seen with cisplatin alone. This effect was proportional to dFdCTP concentration, which suggests that gemcitabine suppresses the repair of cisplatin adducts by its inhibitory effect on NER.[274] Alternatively, cisplatin may be augmenting the incorporation of dFdCTP into DNA, which results in synergistic antitumor activity.[275] Phase II studies of the use of gemcitabine and cisplatin in lung cancer and transitional cell cancer have found promising clinical activity and have led to ongoing phase III studies.

Mechanisms of Resistance

Resistance to gemcitabine is not fully understood. *In vitro* studies have suggested several possible mechanisms. Gemcitabine resistance has been induced in ovarian cancer cell lines by making the cells deficient in deoxycytidine kinase.[276] Interestingly, gemcitabine resistance in deoxycytidine kinase–deficient cells can be overcome by up-regulation of thymidine kinase 2, which can also phosphorylate gemcitabine.[277] Induction of cytidine deaminase and large quantities of heat-shock protein have also conferred gemcitabine resistance to cells.[278,279] Lastly, inhibition of nucleoside transporters can prevent the influx of gemcitabine through the cell membrane.[259] Resistance to gemcitabine has not been associated with increased P-glycoprotein expression.[280] No important studies of clinical resistance to gemcitabine have been carried out as of this writing.

Pharmacokinetic Data

In animals, gemcitabine pharmacokinetics is largely determined by deamination, which proceeds more rapidly in mice than in rats or dogs.[281] Gemcitabine half-life in mice is 0.28 hours compared with 1.38 hours in dogs. In both species the predominant elimination product is dFdU. Grunewald and colleagues have found that in both *in vitro* cell lines and cells taken from patients during treatment maximal accumulation of dFdCTP occurs when plasma (or tissue culture) drug concentrations are in the range of 15 to 20 µmol per L, a level achieved during 3-hour infusions of 300 mg per m^2.[282]

Abbruzzese et al. performed a phase I study of gemcitabine given weekly as a 30-minute infusion on days 1, 8, and 15 followed by a 1 week rest in patients with refractory solid tumors.[283] The maximum tolerated dose (MTD) was 1,000 mg per m^2 per week. The dose-limiting toxicity was myelosuppression characterized by thrombocytopenia with relative sparing of granulocytes. Pharmacokinetic analysis showed a $t_{1/2}$ of 8 minutes for the parent compound and a biphasic elimination of dFdU, with $t_{1/2\alpha} = 27$ minutes and $t_{1/2\beta} = 14$ hours. No relationship was found between degree of myelosuppression and any of the pharmacokinetic parameters. The area under the curve of plasma dFdC was proportional to the dose over a range of 10 to 1,000 mg per m^2 per week. Clearance was dose independent but varied widely among individuals (39 to 1,239 L per hour per m^2 at a dose of 1,000 mg per m^2).

Although a higher gemcitabine dose of 2,200 mg per m^2 administered over 30 minutes on days 1, 8, and 15 can be safely given to less heavily treated or chemonaïve patients, no improvement in efficacy has been demonstrated.[284] This lack of dose responsiveness may be due to the ability of cells to generate the active metabolite. In the case of ara-C, the ability of peripheral blood mononuclear cells to accumulate ara-CTP saturates at ara-C concentrations of greater than 10 µmol per L.[285] A similar series of studies with gemcitabine have demonstrated that activation of gemcitabine by deoxycytidine kinase to dFdCTP is saturated at infusion rates of approximately 10 mg per m^2 per minute.[282,286] This "dose-rate infusion" produced steady-state dFdC levels of 15 to 20 µmol per L in plasma. In leukemic patients, the MTD for "dose-rate infusion" is 4,800 mg per m^2 infused over 480 minutes.[287,288] Biphasic elimination of gemcitabine was seen in the leukemic cells at this infusion rate, and inhibition of DNA synthesis was proportional to the intracellular level of dFdCTP. Based on these results, a phase I study using constant dose-rate infusion of gemcitabine on days 1, 8, and 15 every 28 days was carried out in patients with metastatic solid tumors.[289] Although the MTD was estimated to be 2,250 mg per m^2 over 225 minutes, the recommended

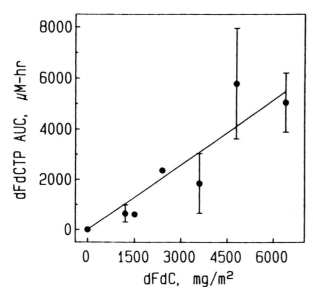

FIGURE 9-13. Relationship between dose of gemcitabine (diflu-orodeoxycytidine, dFdC) and area under the curve (AUC) of difluorodeoxycytidine triphosphate (dFdCTP) in circulating leukemia cells during gemcitabine infusion. Shown is the mean ± standard error of the mean of the AUC observed for patients at each dose during this phase I study of dose-rate infusion of gemcitabine in patients with leukemia. (Adapted from Grunewald R, Kantarjian H, Du M, et al. Gemcitabine in leukemia: a phase I clinical, plasma, and cellular pharmacology study. *J Clin Oncol* 1992;10:406–413.)

phase II dose of gemcitabine administered as a dose-rate infusion is 1,500 mg per m^2 over 150 minutes due to the occurrence of cumulative neutropenia and thrombocytopenia at higher doses. The dose-rate infusion resulted in higher levels of dFdCTP in circulating leukemic cells than a fixed infusion duration of 30 minutes (Fig. 9-13).

In a proof-of-concept study, Tempero and colleagues performed a randomized phase II study of constant dose-rate infusion at 10 mg per m^2 per minute versus dose-intense infusion over 30 minutes in patients with advanced pancreatic cancer.[290] Patients were randomized to receive gemcitabine 1,500 mg per m^2 over 150 minutes or 2,200 mg per m^2 over 30 minutes. Constant dose-rate infusion resulted in a statistically significant increase in the level of gemcitabine triphosphate within peripheral blood mononuclear cells (336 mmol per L versus 114 mmol per L). Furthermore, activity appeared to be enhanced with the constant dose-rate infusion, as 1-year survival increased from 0% to 23%.

Toxicity

The dose-limiting toxicity of gemcitabine is invariably hematologic, and the toxicity profile differs according to schedule. In general, the longer-duration infusions lead to greater myelosuppression. The MTD for a daily × 5 schedule every 21 days is 12 mg per m^2 per day or 60 mg per m^2

per cycle.[291] The MTD for twice-weekly doses of gemcitabine administered for 3 weeks with a 1-week rest period depends on the time of infusion. When the drug is administered over 5 minutes, the MTD is 150 mg per m^2, and when it is administered as a 30-minute infusion, the MTD is 75 mg per m^2.[292] For a 24-hour infusion given weekly in 3 out of 4 weeks, the MTD is 180 mg per m^2 per dose.[293] The weekly dose schedule has gained popularity and is implemented as a 30-minute infusion in 3 out of 4 weeks. The MTD for chemonaïve patients is 2,200 mg per m^2 per week, and the MTD for pretreated patients is 800 to 1,000 mg per m^2 per week.[283,284] A dose of 1,000 mg per m^2 is recommended for treatment of a variety of solid tumors.

The safety of gemcitabine has been evaluated in a database including 22 studies using the once-weekly treatment regimen.[294] Nine hundred and seventy-nine patients received at least one dose of gemcitabine and were evaluable for toxicity. World Health Organization (WHO) grade 3 and 4 neutropenia occurred in 19.3% and 6% of patients, respectively. WHO grade 3 and 4 thrombocytopenia occurred in 4.1% and 1.1% of patients, respectively. Clinically significant consequences of hematologic toxicity were uncommon, as only 1.1% of patients experienced WHO grade 3 infection and 0.7% of patients required platelet transfusions. Among nonhematologic toxicities, flulike symptoms including fever, headache, back pain, and myalgias occur in approximately 45% of patients. The duration of these symptoms was short and less than 1% of patients discontinued therapy due to flulike symptoms. Asthenia is also common, occurring in 42% of patients. A transient, mild elevation in liver function test results (WHO grade 1 or 2 elevations in alanine aminotransferase) was detected in 41% of cycles.

Although severe nonhematologic reactions are rare, several specific syndromes complicating gemcitabine therapy are emerging. Hemolytic-uremic syndrome has been reported as a complication of gemcitabine therapy,[295–297] and a review of the manufacturer's database estimated an overall incidence rate of 0.015%.[298] Patients who are treated for prolonged periods (i.e., longer than 1 year) may be at higher risk for developing hemolytic-uremic syndrome. Acute respiratory distress syndrome has been reported in patients treated with gemcitabine.[299] One reported case of "capillary leak" pulmonary toxicity responded to treatment with corticosteroids.[300]

Radiation Sensitization

Due to its inhibition of ribonucleotide reductase and DNA polymerase, gemcitabine may have strong radiosensitization effects. Preclinical studies of gemcitabine have shown potent radiosensitization effects in human colon, pancreatic, head and neck, and cervical cancer cell lines.[301–304] These effects parallel the intracellular depletion of deoxyadenosine triphosphate and are most prominent when gemcitabine is administered before radiation therapy. Interestingly, the radio-sensitization effect had no correlation with dFdCMP incorporation into DNA, which suggests that the inhibition of ribonucleotide reductase is the key mechanism of action.[305] Furthermore, the radiation-sensitizing effect occurred at gemcitabine levels 1,000 times lower than the peak level achieved with intravenous administration.[56] *In vitro* studies suggest that maximal enhancement of radiation sensitization occurs when gemcitabine is administered before radiation, and *in vivo* studies suggest that this effect is most pronounced when the time interval is 24 to 60 hours.[301,306,307]

Preliminary clinical data have confirmed the marked synergistic toxicity of gemcitabine and radiation, and have also yielded promising early results. Administration of gemcitabine 300 mg per m^2 every week during radiotherapy to patients with head and neck cancer caused grade 3 to 4 skin toxicity in seven of eight patients and mucositis in all patients. Nevertheless, seven of eight patients had clinical and pathologic complete responses.[308] The combination of gemcitabine 800 mg per m^2 on days 5, 12, and 19 every 28 days; cisplatin 20 mg per m^2 on days 1 to 5 every 28 days; and radiation on weeks 2, 3, 4 and 6, 7, 8 caused grade 3 or 4 mucositis in all four patients treated and grade 4 hematologic toxicity in three of eight courses.[309]

In a phase I trial of twice-weekly gemcitabine and concurrent radiation in patients with advanced pancreatic cancer, the MTD was 40 mg per m^2 administered over 30 minutes on Monday and Thursday of each week.[310] The dose-limiting toxicities were grade 3 neutropenia, thrombocytopenia, nausea, and vomiting. Antitumor activity was seen in three patients, who achieved a partial response. When the drug was administered as a weekly 24-hour infusion with concurrent radiation to patients with gastrointestinal cancers, dose-limiting toxicities included grade 3 diarrhea, grade 3 nausea, and grade 3 hematologic toxicity at a dose of 150 mg per m^2.[311]

REFERENCES

1. Bergmann W, Feeney R. Contributions to the study of marine products: XXXII. The nucleosides of sponges. *J Org Chem* 1951;16:981.
2. Roberts WK, Dekker CA. A convenient synthesis of arabinosylcytosine (cytosine arabinoside). *J Org Chem* 1967; 32:84.
3. Lee WW, Benitez A, Goodman L, et al. Potential anticancer agents: XL. Synthesis of the beta-anomer of 9-(D-arabinofuranosyl) adenine. *J Am Chem Soc* 1960;82:2648.
4. Warrell RP, Berman E. Phase I and II study of fludarabine phosphate in leukemia: therapeutic efficacy with delayed central nervous system toxicity. *J Clin Oncol* 1986;4:74.
5. Dalal M, Plowman J, Breitman TR, et al. Arabinofuranosyl-5-azacytosine: antitumor and cytotoxic properties. *Cancer Res* 1986;46:831.
6. Ellison RR, Holland JF, Weil M, et al. Arabinosyl cytosine: a useful agent in the treatment of acute leukemia in adults. *Blood* 1968;32:507.
7. Bishop JF, Matthews JP, Young GA, et al. A randomized study of high-dose cytarabine in induction in acute myeloid leukemia. *Blood* 1996;87:1710.
8. Mayer RJ, Davis RB, Schiffer CA, et al. Intensive chemotherapy in adults with acute myeloid leukemia. *N Engl J Med* 1994;331:896.
9. Bloomfield CD, Lawrence D, Byrd JC, et al. Frequency of prolonged remission duration after high-dose cytarabine by cytogenetic subtype. *Cancer Res* 1998;58:4173.
10. Cadman E, Farber L, Berd D, et al. Combination therapy for diffuse leukocytic lymphoma that includes antimetabolites. *Cancer Treat Rep* 1977;61:1109.
11. Bryan JH, Henderson ES, Leventhal BG. Cytosine arabinoside and 6-thioguanine in refractory acute lymphocytic leukemia. *Cancer* 1974;33:539.
12. Guilhot F, Chastang C, Michallet M, et al. Interferon alfa-2b combined with cytarabine versus interferon alone in chronic myelogenous leukemia. *N Engl J Med* 1997;337:223.
13. Furth JJ, Cohen SS. Inhibition of mammalian DNA polymerase by the 5'-triphosphate of 9-β-D-arabinofuranosylcytosine and the triphosphate of 9-β-D-arabinofuranosyladenine. *Cancer Res* 1968;28:2061.
14. Townsend AJ, Cheng YC. Sequence-specific effects of ara-5-aza-CTP and ara-CTP on DNA synthesis by purified human DNA polymerases in vitro: visualization of chain elongation on a defined template. *Mol Pharmacol* 1987;32:330.
15. Kimball AP, Wilson MJ. Inhibition of DNA polymerase by β-D-arabinosylcytosine and reversal of inhibition by deoxycytidine-5'-triphosphate. *Proc Soc Exp Biol* 1968;127:429.
16. Graham FL, Whitmore GF. Studies in mouse L-cells on the incorporation of 1-β-D-arabinofuranosylcytosine into DNA and on inhibition of DNA polymerase by 1-β-D-arabinofuranosylcytosine-5'-triphosphate. *Cancer Res* 1970;30:2636.
17. Chu MY, Fischer GA. A proposed mechanism of action of 1-β-D-arabinofuranosylcytosine as an inhibitor of the growth of leukemic cells. *Biochem Pharmacol* 1962;11:423.
18. Yoshida S, Yamada M, Masaki S. Inhibition of DNA polymerase-α and -β of calf thymus by 1-β-D-arabinofuranosylcytosine-5'-triphosphate. *Biochim Biophys Acta* 1977;477:144.
19. Fram RJ, Kufe DW. Effect of 1-β-D-arabinofuranosyl cytosine and hydroxyurea on the repair of x-ray-induced DNA single-strand breaks in human leukemic blasts. *Biochem Pharmacol* 1985;34:2557.
20. Fram RJ, Kufe DW. Inhibition of DNA excision repair and the repair of x-ray-induced DNA damage by cytosine arabinoside and hydroxyurea. *Pharmacol Ther* 1985;31:165.
21. Kufe WE, Major PP, Egan EM, et al. Correlation of cytotoxicity with incorporation of araC into DNA. *J Biol Chem* 1980;255:8997.
22. Fram RJ, Egan EM, Kufe DW. Accumulation of leukemic cell DNA strand breaks with adriamycin and cytosine arabinoside. *Leuk Res* 1983;7:243.
23. Kufe DW, Munroe D, Herrick D, et al. Effects of 1-β-D-arabinofuranosylcytosine incorporation on eukaryotic DNA template function. *Mol Pharmacol* 1984;26:128.
24. Kufe DW, Spriggs DR. Biochemical and cellular pharmacology of cytosine arabinoside. *Semin Oncol* 1985;12:34.

25. Major P, Egan E, Herrick D, et al. The effect of araC incorporation on DNA synthesis. *Biochem Pharmacol* 1982;31:2937.

26. Mikita T, Beardsley GP. Functional consequences of the arabinosylcytosine structural lesion in DNA. *Biochemistry* 1988;27:4698.

27. Ross DD, Cuddy DP, Cohen N, et al. Mechanistic implications of alterations in HL-60 cell nascent DNA after exposure to 1-β-D-arabinofuranosylcytosine. *Cancer Chemother Pharmacol* 1992;31:61.

28. Woodcock DM, Fox RM, Cooper IA. Evidence for a new mechanism of cytotoxicity of 1-β-D-arabinofuranosylcytosine. *Cancer Res* 1979;39:418.

29. Moore EC, Cohen SS. Effects of arabinonucleotides on ribonucleotide reduction by an enzyme system from rat tumor. *J Biol Chem* 1967;242:2116.

30. Hawtrey AO, Scott-Burden T, Robertson G. Inhibition of glycoprotein and glycolipid synthesis in hamster embryo cells by cytosine arabinoside and hydroxyurea. *Nature* 1974;252:58.

31. Mitchell T, Sarabin E, Kufe D. Effects of 1-β-D-arabinofuranosylcytosine on proto-oncogene expression in human U-937 cells. *Mol Pharmacol* 1986;30:398.

32. Bianchi Scarra GL, Romani M, Civiello DA, et al. Terminal erythroid differentiation in the K-562 cell line by 1-β-D-arabinofuranosylcytosine: accompaniment by c-myc messenger RNA decrease. *Cancer Res* 1986;46:6327.

33. Vogelstein ER, Burke PJ, Schiffer CA, et al. Differentiation of leukemia cells to polymorphonuclear leukocytes in patients with acute nonlymphocytic leukemia. *N Engl J Med* 1986;315:15.

34. Anilkumar TV, Sarraf CE, Hunt T, et al. The nature of cytotoxic drug-induced cell death in murine intestinal crypts. *Br J Cancer* 1992;65:552.

35. Gunji H, Kharbanda S, Kufe D. Induction of internucleosomal DNA fragmentation in human myeloid leukemia cells by 1-β-D-arabinofuranosylcytosine. *Cancer Res* 1991; 51:741.

36. Strum JC, Small GW, Pauig SB, et al. 1-β-D-arabinofuranosylcytosine stimulates ceramide and diglyceride formation in HL-60 cells. *J Biol Chem* 1994;269:15493.

37. Kharbanda S, Datta R, Kufe D. Regulation of c-jun gene expression in HL-60 leukemia cells by 1-β-D-arabinofuranosylcytosine. Potential involvement of a protein kinase C dependent mechanism. *Biochemistry* 1991;30:7947.

38. Brach MA, Kharbanda SM, Herrmann F, et al. Activation of the transcription factor kB in human KG-1 myeloid leukemia cells treated with 1-β-D-arabinofuranosylcytosine. *Mol Pharmacol* 1992;41:60.

39. Kharbanda SM, Sherman ML, Kufe DW. Transcriptional regulation of c-jun gene expression by arabinofuranosylcytosine in human myeloid leukemia cells. *J Clin Invest* 1990;86:1517.

40. Bullock G, Ray S, Reed J, et al. Evidence against a direct role for the induction of c-jun expression in the mediation of drug-induced apoptosis in human acute leukemia cells. *Clin Cancer Res* 1995;1:559.

41. Dou QP, An B, Will P. Induction of a retinoblastoma phosphatase activity by anticancer drugs accompanies p53-independent G_1 arrest and apoptosis. *Proc Natl Acad Sci U S A* 1995;92:9019.

42. Ikeda M, Jakoi L, Nevins J. A unique role for the Rb protein in controlling E2F accumulation during cell growth and differentiation. *Proc Natl Acad Sci U S A* 1996;93:3215.

43. Plagemann PGW, Marz R, Wolhueter RM. Transport and metabolism of deoxycytidine and 1-β-D-arabinofuranosylcytosine into cultured Novikoff rat hepatoma cells, relationship to phosphorylation and regulation of triphosphate synthesis. *Cancer Res* 1978;38:978.

44. Wiley JS, Jones SP, Sawyer WH, et al. Cytosine arabinoside influx and nucleoside transport sites in acute leukemia. *J Clin Invest* 1982;69:479.

45. Belt JA, Noel DL. Isolation and characterization of a mutant of L1210 murine leukemia deficient in nitrobenzylthioinosine-insensitive nucleoside transport. *J Biol Chem* 1988;263:13819.

46. Wiley JS, Taupin J, Jamieson GP, et al. Cytosine arabinoside transport and metabolism in acute leukemias and T-cell lymphoblastic lymphoma. *J Clin Invest* 1985;75:632.

47. Tanaka M, Yoshida S. Formation of cytosine arabinoside-5'-triphosphate in cultured human leukemic cell lines correlates with nucleoside transport capacity. *Jpn J Cancer Res* 1987;78:851.

48. White JC, Rathmell JP, Capizzi RL. Membrane transport influences the rate of accumulation of cytosine arabinoside in human leukemia cells. *J Clin Invest* 1987;79:380.

49. Jamieson GP, Snook MB, Wiley JS. Saturation of intracellular cytosine arabinoside triphosphate accumulation in human leukemic blast cells. *Leuk Res* 1990;14:475.

50. Chottiner EG, Shewach SDS, Datta NS, et al. Cloning and expression of human deoxycytidine kinase cDNA. *Proc Natl Acad Sci U S A* 1991;88:1531.

51. Owens JK, Shewach DS, Ullman B, et al. Resistance to 1-β-D-arabinofuranosylcytosine in human T lymphoblasts mediated by mutations within the deoxycytidine kinase gene. *Cancer Res* 1992;52:2389.

52. Hapke DM, Stegmann APA, Mitchell BS. Retroviral transfer of deoxycytidine kinase into tumor cell lines enhances nucleoside toxicity. *Cancer Res* 1996;56:2343.

53. Manome Y, Wen PY, Dong Y, et al. Viral vector transduction of the human deoxycytidine kinase cDNA sensitizes glioma cells to the cytotoxic effects of cytosine arabinoside in vitro and in vivo. *Nat Med* 1996;2:567.

54. Gandhi V, Plunkett W. Cell cycle-specific metabolism of arabinosyl nucleosides in K562 human leukemia cells. *Cancer Chemother Pharmacol* 1992;31:11.

55. Coleman CN, Stoller RG, Drake JC, et al. Deoxycytidine kinase: properties of the enzyme from human leukemic granulocytes. *Blood* 1975;46:791.

56. Wang L, Kucera GL. Deoxycytidine kinase is phosphorylated in vitro by protein kinase Cα. *Biochim Biophys Acta* 1994;1224:161.

57. Hande KR, Chabner BA. Pyrimidine nucleoside monophosphate kinase from human leukemic blast cells. *Cancer Res* 1978;38:579.

58. Chou T-C, Arlin Z, Clarkson BD, et al. Metabolism of 1-β-D-arabinofuranosylcytosine in human leukemic cells. *Cancer Res* 1977;37:3561.

59. Chou T-C, Hutchison DJ, Schmid FA, et al. Metabolism and selective effects of 1-β-D-arabinofuranosylcytosine in L1210 and host tissues in vivo. *Cancer Res* 1975;35:225.

60. Camiener GW, Smith CG. Studies of the enzymatic deamination of cytosine arabinoside: I. Enzyme distribution and specific specificity. *Biochem Pharmacol* 1965;14:1405.

61. Chabner B, Johns D, Coleman C, et al. Purification and properties of cytidine deaminase from normal and leukemic granulocytes. *J Clin Invest* 1974;53:922.

62. Stoller RG, Myers CE, Chabner BA. Analysis of cytidine deaminase and tetrahydrouridine interaction by use of ligand techniques. *Biochem Pharmacol* 1978;27:53.

63. Jackson RC. The regulation of thymidylate biosynthesis in Novikoff hepatoma cells and the effects of Amethopterin, 5-fluorodeoxyuridine, and 3-deazauridine. *J Biol Chem* 1978;253:7440.

64. Ellims P, Kao AH, Chabner BA. Deoxycytidylate deaminase: purification and kinetic properties of the enzyme isolated from human spleen. *J Biol Chem* 1981;256:6335.

65. Lauzon GJ, Paran JH, Paterson ARP. Formation of 1-β-D-arabinofuranosylcytosine diphosphate choline in cultured human leukemic RPMI 6410 cells. *Cancer Res* 1978; 38:1723.

66. Myers-Robfogel MW, Spatato AC. 1-β-D-Arabinofuranosylcytosine nucleotide inhibition of sialic acid metabolism in WI-38 cells. *Cancer Res* 1980;40:1940.

67. Chu MY, Fischer GA. Comparative studies of leukemic cells sensitive and resistant to cytosine arabinoside. *Biochem Pharmacol* 1965;14:333.

68. Drahovsky D, Kreis W. Studies on drug resistance: II. Kinase patterns in P815 neoplasms sensitive and resistant to 1-β-D-arabinofuranosylcytosine. *Biochem Pharmacol* 1970;19:940.

69. De Saint Vincent BR, Dechamps M, Buttin G. The modulation of the thymidine triphosphate pool of Chinese hamster cells by dCMP deaminase and UDP reductase. *J Biol Chem* 1980;255:162.

70. De Saint Vincent BR, Buttin G. Studies on 1-β-D-arabinofuranosyl cytosine–resistant mutants of Chinese hamster fibroblasts: III. Joint resistance to arabinofuranosyl cytosine and to excess thymidine—a semidominant manifestation of deoxycytidine triphosphate pool expansion. *Somatic Cell Genet* 1979;5:67.

71. De Saint Vincent BR, Buttin G. Studies on 1-β-D-arabinofuranosyl cytosine–resistant mutants of Chinese hamster fibroblasts: IV. Altered regulation of CTP synthetase generates arabinosylcytosine and thymidine resistance. *Biochim Biophys Acta* 1980;610:352.

72. Cohen A, Ullman B. Analysis of the drug synergism between thymidine and arabinosyl cytosine using mouse S-49 T lymphoma mutants. *Cancer Chemother Pharmacol* 1985;14:70.

73. Eliopoulos N, Cournoyer D, Momparler RL. Drug resistance to 5-aza-2'-deoxycytidine, 2',2'-difluorodeoxycytidine, and cytosine arabinoside conferred by retroviral-mediated transfer of human cytidine deaminase cDNA into murine cells. *Cancer Chemother Pharmacol* 1998;42:373.

74. Riva C, Khyari SE, Rustum Y, et al. Resistance to cytosine arabinoside in cells transfected with activated Ha-ras oncogene. *Anticancer Res* 1995;15:1297.

75. Koo H, Monks A, Mikheev A, et al. Enhanced sensitivity to 1-β-D-arabinofuranosylcytosine and topoisomerase II inhibitors in tumor cell lines harboring activated ras oncogenes. *Cancer Res* 1996;56:5211.

76. Tattersall MNH, Ganeshaguru K, Hoffbrand AV. Mechanisms of resistance of human acute leukaemia cells to cytosine arabinoside. *Br J Haematol* 1974;27:39.

77. Steuart CD, Burke PJ. Cytidine deaminase and the development of resistance to arabinosylcytosine. *Nature New Biol* 1971;233:109.

78. Chiba P, Tihan T, Szekeres T, et al. Concordant changes of pyrimidine metabolism in blasts of two cases of acute myeloid leukemia after repeated treatment with araC in vivo. *Leukemia* 1990;4:761.

79. Chang P, Wiernik PH, Reich SD, et al. Prediction of response to cytosine arabinoside and daunorubicin in acute nonlymphocytic leukemia. In: Mandelli F, ed. *Therapy of acute leukemias: proceedings of the second international symposium, Rome, 1977.* Rome: Lombardo Editore, 1979:148.

80. Smyth JF, Robins AB, Leese CL. The metabolism of cytosine arabinoside as a predictive test for clinical response to the drug in acute myeloid leukaemia. *Eur J Cancer* 1976;12:567.

81. Estey E, Plunkett W, Dixon D, et al. Variables predicting response to high dose cytosine arabinoside therapy in patients with refractory acute leukemia. *Leukemia* 1987; 1:580.

82. Ross DD, Thompson BW, Joneckis CC, et al. Metabolism of araC by blast cells from patients with ANLL. *Blood* 1986;68:76.

83. Rustum YM, Riva C, Preisler HD. Pharmacokinetic parameters of 1-β-D-arabinofuranosylcytosine and their relationship to intracellular metabolism of araC, toxicity, and response of patients with acute nonlymphocytic leukemia treated with conventional and high-dose araC. *Semin Oncol* 1987;14:141.

84. Estey EH, Keating MJ, McCredie KB, et al. Cellular ara-CTP pharmacokinetics, response, and karyotype in newly diagnosed acute myelogenous leukemia. *Leukemia* 1990;4:95.

85. Preisler HD, Rustum Y, Priore RL. Relationship between leukemic cell retention of cytosine arabinoside triphosphate and the duration of remission in patients with acute nonlymphocytic leukemia. *Eur J Cancer Clin Oncol* 1985;21:23.

86. Plunkett W, Iacoboni S, Keating MJ. Cellular pharmacology and optimal therapeutic concentrations of 1-β-D-arabinofuranosylcytosine 5'-triphosphate in leukemic blasts during treatment of refractory leukemia with high-dose 1-β-D-arabinofuranosylcytosine. *Scand J Haematol* 1986;34:51.

87. Ibrado AM, Uang Y, Fang G, et al. Overexpression of Bcl-2 or Bcl-xL inhibits araC-induced CPP32/Yama protease activity and apoptosis of human acute myelogenous leukemia HL-60 cells. *Cancer Res* 1996;56:4743.

88. Keith FJ, Bradbury DA, Zhu Y, et al. Inhibition of bcl-2 with antisense oligonucleotides induces apoptosis and increases the sensitivity of AML blasts to araC. *Leukemia* 1995;9:131.

89. Campos L, Rouault J, Sabido O, et al. High expression of bcl-2 protein in acute myeloid leukemia cells is associated with poor response to chemotherapy. *Blood* 1993;81:3091.

90. Ruvolo PR, Deng X, Carr BK, et al. A functional role for mitochondrial protein kinase Cα Bcl2 phosphorylation and suppression of apoptosis. *J Biol Chem* 1998;273:25436.

91. Wang S, Vrana JA, Bartimole TM, et al. Agents that downregulate or inhibit protein kinase C circumvent resistance to

1-β-D-arabinofuranosylcytosine–induced apoptosis in human leukemia cells that overexpress Bcl-2. *Mol Pharmacol* 1997;52:1000.

92. Kharbanda S, Emoto Y, Kisaki H, et al. 1-β-D-arabinofuranosylcytosine activates serine/threonine protein kinases and c-jun gene expression in phorbol ester-resistant myeloid leukemia cells. *Mol Pharmacol* 1994;46:67.

93. Kolla SS, Studzinski GP. Constitutive DNA binding of the low mobility forms of the AP-1 and SP-1 transcription factors in HL60 cells resistant to 1-β-D-arabinofuranosylcytosine. *Cancer Res* 1994;54:1418.

94. Karon M, Chirakawa S. The locus of action of 1-β-D-arabinofuranosylcytosine in the cell cycle. *Cancer Res* 1970;29:687.

95. Young RC, Schein PS. Enhanced antitumor effect of cytosine arabinoside given in a schedule dictated by kinetic studies in vivo. *Biochem Pharmacol* 1973;22:277.

96. Burke PJ, Karp JE, Vaughan WP, et al. Recruitment of quiescent tumor by humoral stimulatory activity: requirements for successful chemotherapy. *Blood Cells* 1982;8:519.

97. Aglietta M, Colly L. Relevance of recruitment-synchronization in the scheduling of 1-β-D-arabinofuranosylcytosine in a slow-growing acute myeloid leukemia of the rat. *Cancer Res* 1979;39:2727.

98. Vaughan WP, Karp JE, Burke PJ. Two-cycle-timed sequential chemotherapy for adult acute nonlymphocytic leukemia. *Blood* 1984;64:975.

99. Preisler HD, Azarnia N, Raza A, et al. Relationship between percent of marrow cells in S phase and the outcome of remission induction therapy for acute nonlymphocytic leukemia. *Br J Haematol* 1984;56:399.

100. Raza A, Preisler HD, Day R, et al. Direct relationship between remission duration in acute myeloid leukemia and cell cycle kinetics: a leukemia intergroup study. *Blood* 1990;76:2191.

101. Boutagy J, Harvey DJ. Determination of cytosine arabinoside in human plasma by gas chromatography with a nitrogen-sensitive detector and by gas chromatography-mass spectrometry. *J Chromatogr* 1978;146:283.

102. Ho DHW, Frei E III. Clinical pharmacology of 1-β-D-arabinofuranosylcytosine. *Clin Pharmacol Ther* 1971;12:944.

103. Mehta BM, Meyers MB, Hutchison DJ. Microbiologic assay for cytosine arabinoside (NSC-63878): the use of a mutant of *Streptococcus faecium* var. *durans* resistant to methotrexate (NSC-740) and 6-mercaptopurine (NSC-755). *Cancer Chemother Rep* 1975;59:515.

104. Van Prooijen HC, Vierwinden G, van Egmond J, et al. A sensitive bioassay for pharmacokinetic studies of cytosine arabinoside in man. *Eur J Cancer* 1976;12:899.

105. Piall EM, Aherne GW, Marks VM. A radioimmunoassay for cytosine arabinoside. *Br J Cancer* 1979;40:548.

106. Sinkule JA, Evans WE. High-performance liquid chromatographic assay for cytosine arabinoside, uracil arabinoside, and some related nucleosides. *J Chromatogr* 1983;274:87.

107. Liversidge GG, Nishihata T, Higuchi T, et al. Simultaneous analysis of 1-β-D-arabinofuranosyluracil and sodium salicylate in biologic samples by high-performance liquid chromatography. *J Chromatogr* 1983;276:375.

108. Harris AL, Potter C, Bunch C, et al. Pharmacokinetics of cytosine arabinoside in patients with acute myeloid leukaemia. *Br J Clin Pharmacol* 1979;8:219.

109. Van Prooijen R, van der Kleijn E, Haanen C. Pharmacokinetics of cytosine arabinoside in acute leukemia. *Clin Pharmacol Ther* 1977;21:744.

110. Wau SH, Huffman DH, Azarnoff DL, et al. Pharmacokinetics of 1-β-D-arabinofuranosylcytosine in humans. *Cancer Res* 1974;34:392.

111. Lopez JA, Nassif E, Vannicola P, et al. Central nervous system pharmacokinetics of high-dose cytosine arabinoside. *J Neurooncol* 1985;3:119.

112. Slevin ML, Piall EM, Aherne GW, et al. Effect of dose and schedule on pharmacokinetics of high-dose cytosine arabinoside in plasma and cerebrospinal fluid. *J Clin Oncol* 1983;1:546.

113. Beithaupt H, Pralle H, Eckhardt T, et al. Clinical results and pharmacokinetics of high-dose cytosine arabinoside (HD ARA-C). *Cancer* 1982;50:1248.

114. Early AP, Preisler HD, Slocum H, et al. A pilot study of high-dose of 1-β-D-arabinofuranosylcytosine for acute leukemia and refractory-lymphoma: clinical response and pharmacology. *Cancer Res* 1982;42:1587.

115. Capizzi RL, Yang JL, Ching E, et al. Alterations of the pharmacokinetics of high-dose araC by its metabolite, high araU in patients with acute leukemia. *J Clin Oncol* 1983;1:763.

116. Donehower RC, Karp JE, Burke PJ. Pharmacology and toxicity of high-dose cytarabine by 72-hour continuous infusion. *Cancer Treat Rep* 1986;70:1059.

117. Slevin ML, Piall EM, Aherne GW, et al. Subcutaneous infusion of cytosine arabinoside: a practical alternative to intravenous infusion. *Cancer Chemother Pharmacol* 10:112, 1983.

118. Liliemark JO, Paul CY, Gahrton CG, et al. Pharmacokinetics of 1-β-D-arabinofuranosylcytosine 5'-triphosphate in leukemic cells after intravenous and subcutaneous administration of 1-β-D-arabinofuranosylcytosine. *Cancer Res* 1985;45:2373.

119. Markman M. The intracavitary administration of cytarabine to patients with nonhematopoietic malignancies: pharmacologic rationale and results of clinical trials. *Semin Oncol* 1985;12[Suppl 3]:177.

120. Kirmani S, Zimm S, Cleary SM, et al. Extremely prolonged continuous intraperitoneal infusion of cytosine arabinoside. *Cancer Chemother Pharmacol* 1990;25:454.

121. Chamberlain MC, Khatibi S, Kim JC, et al. Treatment of leptomeningeal metastasis with intraventricular administration of Depot cytarabine (DTC 101). *Arch Neurol* 1993;50:261.

122. Howell SB, Glantz MJ, LaFollette S, et al. A controlled trial of Depocyt™ for the treatment of lymphomatous meningitis. *Proc Am Soc Clin Oncol* 1999;18:11a(abst 34).

123. Capizzi RL, Powell BL, Cooper MR, et al. Dose-related pharmacologic effects of high-dose araC and its use in combination with asparaginase for the treatment of patients with acute nonlymphocytic leukemia. *Scand J Haematol* 1986;34[Suppl 44]:17.

124. Plunkett W, Iacoboni S, Estey E, et al. Pharmacologically directed araC therapy for refractory leukemia. *Semin Oncol* 1985;12[Suppl 3]:20.

125. Wisch JS, Griffin JD, Kufe DN. Response of preleukemic syndromes to continuous infusion of low-dose cytarabine. *N Engl J Med* 1983;309:1599.

126. Tilly H, Bastard C, Bizet M, et al. Low-dose cytarabine: persistence of a clonal abnormality during complete remission of acute nonlymphocytic leukemia. *N Engl J Med* 1986;314:246.

127. Beran M, Hittelman WN, Andersson BS, et al. Induction of differentiation in human myeloid leukemia cells with cytosine arabinoside. *Leuk Res* 1986;10:1033.

128. Cheson BD, Jasperse DM, Simon R, et al. A critical appraisal of low-dose cytosine arabinoside in patients with acute nonlymphocytic leukemia and myelodysplastic syndromes. *J Clin Oncol* 1986;4:1857.

129. Raijmakers R, DeWitte T, Linssen P, et al. The relation of exposure time and drug concentration in their effect on cloning efficiency after incubation of human bone marrow with cytosine arabinoside. *Br J Haematol* 1986;62:447.

130. Skipper HE, Schabel FM Jr, Wilcox WS. Experimental evaluation of potential anticancer agents: XXI. Scheduling of arabinosyl cytosine to take advantage of its S-phase specificity against leukemia cells. *Cancer Chemother Rep* 1967;51:125.

131. Frei E III, Bickers JN, Hewlett JS, et al. Dose schedule and antitumor studies of arabinosyl cytosine (NSC 63878). *Cancer Res* 1969;29:1325.

132. Mitchell MS, Wade ME, DeConti RC, et al. Immunosuppressive effects of cytosine arabinoside and methotrexate in man. *Ann Intern Med* 1969;70:535.

133. Talley RW, Vaitkevicius VK. Megaloblastosis produced by a cytosine antagonist, 1-β-D-arabinofuranosyl cytosine. *Blood* 1963;21:352.

134. Slavin RE, Dias MA, Saral R. Cytosine arabinoside-induced gastrointestinal toxic alterations in sequential chemotherapeutic protocols. *Cancer* 1978;42:1747.

135. Goode UB, Leventhal B, Henderson E. Cytosine arabinoside in acute granulocytic leukemia. *Clin Pharmacol Ther* 1971;12:599.

136. Altman A, Dinndorf P, Quinn JJ. Acute pancreatitis in association with cytosine arabinoside therapy. *Cancer* 1982;49:1384.

137. Anderson BS, Luna MA, Yee C, et al. Fatal pulmonary failure complicating high-dose cytosine arabinoside therapy in acute leukemia. *Cancer* 1990;65:1079.

138. Weisman SJ, Scoopo FJ, Johnson GM, et al. Septicemia in pediatric oncology patients: the significance of viridans streptococcal infections. *J Clin Oncol* 1990;8:453.

139. Rudnick SA, Cadman EC, Capizzi RL, et al. High-dose cytosine arabinoside (HD ARA-C) in refractory acute leukemia. *Cancer* 1979;44:1189.

140. George CB, Mansour RP, Redmond J, et al. Hepatic dysfunction and jaundice following high-dose cytosine arabinoside. *Cancer* 1984;54:2360.

141. Herzig RH, Hines JD, Herzig GP, et al. Cerebellar toxicity with high-dose cytosine arabinoside. *J Clin Oncol* 1987;5:927.

142. Rubin EH, Anderson JW, Berg DT, et al. Risk factors for high-dose cytarabine neurotoxicity: an analysis of a cancer and leukemia group B trial in patients with acute myeloid leukemia. *J Clin Oncol* 1992;10:948.

143. Shaw PJ, Procopis PG, Menser MA, et al. Bulbar and pseudobulbar palsy complicating therapy with high-dose cytosine arabinoside in children with leukemia. *Med Pediatr Oncol* 1991;19:122.

144. Paul M, Joshua D, Rahme N, et al. Fatal peripheral neuropathy associated with axonal degeneration after high-dose cytosine arabinoside in acute leukemia. *Br J Haematol* 1991;79:521.

145. Castleberry RP, Crist WM, Holbrook T, et al. The cytosine arabinoside syndrome. *Pediatr Oncol* 1981;9:257.

146. Hopen G, Mondino BJ, Johnson BL, et al. Corneal toxicity with systemic cytarabine. *Am J Ophthalmol* 1981;91:500.

147. Rassiga AL, Schwartz HJ, Forman WB, et al. Cytarabine-induced anaphylaxis: demonstration of antibody and successful desensitization. *Arch Intern Med* 1980;140:425.

148. Flynn TC, Harris TJ, Murphy GF, et al. Neutrophilic eccrine hidradenitis: a distinctive rash associated with cytarabine therapy and acute leukemia. *J Am Acad Dermatol* 1984;11:584.

149. Reykdal S, Sham R, Kouides P. Cytarabine-induced pericarditis: a case report and review of the literature of the cardio-pulmonary complications of cytarabine. *Leuk Res* 1995;19:141.

150. Eden OB, Goldie W, Wood T, et al. Seizures following intrathecal cytosine arabinoside in young children with acute lymphoblastic leukemia. *Cancer* 1978;42:53.

151. Kleinschmidt-DeMasters BK, Yeh M. "Locked-in syndrome" after intrathecal cytosine arabinoside therapy for malignant immunoblastic lymphoma. *Cancer* 1992;70:2504.

152. Bell WR, Whang JJ, Carbone PP, et al. Cytogenetic and morphologic abnormalities in human bone marrow cells during cytosine arabinoside therapy. *Blood* 1966;27:771.

153. Dixon RL, Adamson RH. Antitumor activity and pharmacologic disposition of cytosine arabinoside (NSC 63878). *Cancer Chemother Rep* 1965;48:11.

154. Schabel FM Jr. In vivo leukemic cell kill kinetics and curability in experimental systems. In: *The proliferation and spread of neoplastic cells.* Baltimore: Williams & Wilkins, 1968:379.

155. Tyrer DD, Kline I, Vendetti JM, et al. Separate and sequential chemotherapy of mouse leukemia L1210 with 1-β-D-arabinofuranosylcytosine hydrochloride and 1,3-bis-(2-chloroethyl)-1-nitrosourea. *Cancer Res* 1968;27:873.

156. Kern DH, Morgan CR, Hildebrand-Zanki SU. In vitro pharmacodynamics of 1-β-D-arabinofuranosylcytosine: synergy of antitumor activity with cis-diamminedichloroplatinum(II). *Cancer Res* 1988;48:117.

157. Burchenal JH, Dollinger MR. Cytosine arabinoside in combination with 6-mercaptopurine, methotrexate, or fluorouracil in L1210 mouse leukemia. *Cancer Chemother Rep* 1967;51:435.

158. Gandhi V, Kemena A, Keating MJ, et al. Fludarabine infusion potentiates arabinosylcytosine metabolism in lymphocytes of patients with chronic lymphocytic leukemia. *Cancer Res* 1992;52:897.

159. Cadman E, Eiferman F. Mechanism of synergistic cell killing when methotrexate precedes cytosine arabinoside. *J Clin Invest* 1979;64:788.

160. Hoovis ML, Chu MY. Enhancement of the antiproliferative action of 1-β-D-arabinofuranosylcytosine by methotrexate in murine leukemic cells (L5178Y). *Cancer Res* 1973;33:521.

161. Chresta CM, Hicks R, Hartley JA, et al. Potentiation of etoposide-induced cytotoxicity and DNA damage in CCRF-

CEM cells by pretreatment with non-cytotoxic concentrations of arabinosyl cytosine. *Cancer Chemother Pharmacol* 1992;31:139.

162. LePage GA, White SC. Scheduling of arabinosylcytosine (araC) and 6-thioguanine (TG). *Proc Am Assoc Cancer Res* 1972;13:11.

163. Lee MYW, Byrnes JJ, Downey KM, et al. Mechanism of inhibition of deoxyribonucleic acid synthesis by 1-β-D-arabinofuranosyladenosine triphosphate and its potentiation by 6-mercaptopurine ribonucleoside 5'-monophosphate. *Biochemistry* 1980;19:213.

164. Swinnen LJ, Barnes DM, Fisher SG, et al. 1-β-D-arabinofuranosylcytosine and hydroxyurea: production of cytotoxic synergy with cis-diamminedichloroplatinum(II) and modifications in platinum-induced DNA interstrand crosslinking. *Cancer Res* 1989;49:1383.

165. Ho DHW, Carter CJ, Brown NS, et al. Effects of tetrahydrouridine on the uptake and metabolism of 1-β-D-arabinofuranosylcytosine in human normal and leukemic cells. *Cancer Res* 1980;40:2441.

166. Chabner BA, Hande KR, Drake JC. AraC metabolism: implications for drug resistance and drug interactions. *Bull Cancer* 1979;66:89.

167. Kreis W, Woodcock TM, Gordon CS. Tetrahydrouridine: physiologic disposition and effect upon deamination of cytosine arabinoside in man. *Cancer Treat Rep* 1977; 61:1347.

168. Wong PP, Currie VE, Mackey RW, et al. Phase I evaluation of tetrahydrouridine combined with cytosine arabinoside. *Cancer Treat Rep* 1979;63:1245.

169. Rauscher F III, Cadman E. Biochemical and cytokinetic modulation of L1210 and HL-60 cells by hydroxyurea and effect on 1-β-D-arabinofuranosylcytosine metabolism and cytotoxicity. *Cancer Res* 1983;43:2688.

170. Grant S, Bhalla K, Rauscher F III, et al. Potentiation of 1-β-D-arabinofuranosylcytosine metabolism and cytotoxicity by 2,3-dihydro-1H-imidazolo[1,2-b]pyrazole in the human promyelocytic leukemia cell, HL-60. *Cancer Res* 1983; 43:5093.

171. Harris AW, Reynolds EC, Finch LR. Effects of thymidine on the sensitivity of cultured mouse tumor cells to 1-β-D-arabinofuranosylcytosine. *Cancer Res* 1979;39:538.

172. Grant S, Lehman C, Cadman E. Enhancement of 1-β-D-arabinofuranosylcytosine accumulation with L1210 cells and increased cytotoxicity following thymidine exposure. *Cancer Res* 1980;40:1525.

173. Danhauser LL, Rustum YM. Effect of thymidine on the toxicity, antitumor activity and metabolism of 1-β-D-arabinofuranosylcytosine in rats bearing a chemically induced colon carcinoma. *Cancer Res* 1980;40:1274.

174. Fram R, Major P, Egan E, et al. A phase I-II study of combination therapy with thymidine and cytosine arabinoside. *Cancer Chemother Pharmacol* 1983;11:43.

175. Blumenreich MS, Chou TC, Andreeff M, et al. Thymidine as a kinetic and biochemical modulator of 1-β-D-arabinofuranosylcytosine in human acute nonlymphocytic leukemia. *Cancer Res* 1984;44:825.

176. Zittoun R, Zittoun J, Marquet J, et al. Modulation of 1-β-D-arabinofuranosylcytosine metabolism by thymidine in human acute leukemia. *Cancer Res* 1985;45:5186.

177. Roberts D, Peck C, Hillard S, et al. Methotrexate-induced changes in the level of 1-β-D-arabinofuranosylcytosine triphosphate in L1210 cells. *Cancer Res* 1979;39:4048.

178. Graham ML, Shuster JJ, Kamen BA, et al. Changes in red blood cell methotrexate pharmacology and their impact on outcome when cytarabine is infused with methotrexate in the treatment of acute lymphocytic leukemia in children: a Pediatric Oncology Group Study. *Clin Cancer Res* 1996;2:331.

179. Bakic M, Chan D, Andersson BS, et al. Effect of 1-β-D-arabinofuranosylcytosine on nuclear topoisomerase II activity and on the DNA cleavage and cytotoxicity produced by 4'-(9-acridinylamino)methanesulfon-m-anisidide and etoposide in m-AMSA-sensitive and -resistant human leukemia cells. *Biochem Pharmacol* 1987;36:4067.

180. Kemena A, Gandhi V, Shewach DS, et al. Inhibition of fludarabine metabolism by arabinosylcytosine during therapy. *Cancer Chemother Pharmacol* 1992;31:193.

181. Gandhi V, Estey E, Du M, et al. Minimum dose of fludarabine for the maximal modulation of 1-β-D-arabinofuranosylcytosine triphosphate in human leukemia blasts during therapy. *Clin Cancer Res* 1997;3:1539.

182. Karp JE, Burke PJ, Donehower RC. Effects of rhGM-CSF on intracellular araC pharmacology in vitro in acute myelocytic leukemia: comparability with drug-induced humoral stimulatory activity. *Leukemia* 1990;4:553.

183. Bhalla K, Tang C, Ibrado AM, et al. Granulocyte-macrophage colony-stimulating factor/interleukin-3 fusion protein (pIXY 321) enhances high-dose ara-C-induced programmed cell death or apoptosis in human myeloid leukemia cells. *Blood* 1992;80:2883.

184. Bhalla K, Holladay C, Arlin Z, et al. Treatment with interleukin-3 plus granulocyte-macrophage colony-stimulating factors improves the selectivity of araC in vitro against acute myeloid leukemia blasts. *Blood* 1991;78:2674.

185. Hiddemann W, Kiehl M, Zuhlsdorf M, et al. Granulocyte-macrophage colony-stimulating factor and interleukin-3 enhance the incorporation of cytosine arabinoside into the DNA of leukemic blasts and the cytotoxic effect on clonogenic cells from patients with acute myeloid leukemia. *Semin Oncol* 1992;19:31.

186. Stone RM, Berg DT, George SL, et al. Granulocyte-macrophage colony-stimulating factor after initial chemotherapy for elderly patients with primary acute myelogenous leukemia. *N Engl J Med* 1995;332:1671.

187. Grant S, Turner AJ, Bartimole TM, et al. Modulation of 1-β-D-arabinofuranosyl cytosine-induced apoptosis in human myeloid leukemia cells by staurosporine and other pharmacologic inhibitors of protein kinase C. *Oncol Res* 1994;6:87.

188. Jarvis WD, Povirk LF, Turner AJ, et al. Effects of bryostatin 1 and other pharmacological activators of protein kinase C on 1-β-D-arabinofuranosyl cytosine-induced apoptosis in HL-60 human promyelocytic leukemia cells. *Biochem Pharmacol* 1994;47:839.

189. Ho DHW. Biochemical studies of a new antitumor agent, O^2, 2'-cyclocytidine. *Biochem Pharmacol* 1974;23:1235.

190. Ueda T, Nakamura T, Ando S, et al. Pharmacokinetics of N^4-behenoyl-of 1-β-D-arabinofuranosylcytosine in patients with acute leukemia. *Cancer Res* 1983;43:3412.

191. Kodama K, Morozumi M, Saitoh K, et al. Antitumor activity and pharmacology of 1-β-D-arabinofuranosylcytose-5'-

stearyl-phosphate: an orally active derivative of 1-β-D-arabinofuranosylcytosine. *Jpn J Cancer Res* 1989;80:679.

192. Chow TC, Burchenal JH, Fox JJ, et al. Metabolism and effects of 5-(β-D-ribofuranosyl)isocytosine in P815 cells. *Cancer Res* 1979;39:721.

193. Woodcock TM, Chou TC, Tan CTC, et al. Biochemical, pharmacological, and phase I clinical evaluation of pseudoisocytidine. *Cancer Res* 1980;40:4243.

194. Allen TM, Mehra T, Hansen C, et al. Stealth liposomes: an improved sustained release system for 1-β-D-arabinofuranosylcytosine. *Cancer Res* 1992;52:2431.

195. Covey JM, Zaharko DS. Comparison of the in vitro cytotoxicity (L1210) of 5-aza-2'-deoxycytidine with its therapeutic and toxic effects in mice. *Eur J Cancer Clin Oncol* 1985;21:109.

196. Attadia V, Saglio G, Fusco A, et al. Effects of 5-aza-2'-deoxycytidine on erythroid differentiation and globin synthesis of the human leukemic cell line K562. In: Momparler RL, de Vos D, eds. *5-aza-2'-deoxycytidine: preclinical and clinical studies.* Haarlem, The Netherlands: PHC, 1990:89.

197. Momparler RL, Onetto-Pothier N, Momparler LF. Comparison of the anti-leukemic activity of cytosine arabinoside and 5-aza-2'-deoxycytidine against human leukemic cells of different phenotype. *Leukemia Res* 1990;14:755.

198. Richel DJ, Colly LP, Lurvink E, et al. Comparison of the anti-leukemic activity of 5-aza-2'-deoxycytidine and arabinofuranosyl-cytosine arabinoside in rats with myelocytic leukemia. *Br J Cancer* 1988;58:730.

199. Pinto A, Zagonel V. 5-aza-2'-deoxycytidine (Decitabine) and 5-azacytidine in the treatment of acute myeloid leukemias and myelodysplastic syndromes: past, present and future trends. *Leukemia* 1993;7:51.

200. Kantarjian HM, O'Brien SM, Estey E, et al. Decitabine studies in chronic and acute myelogenous leukemia. *Leukemia* 1997;11:S35.

201. Sorm F, Piskala A, Cihak A, et al. 5-Azacytidine, a new highly effective cancerostatic. *Experientia* 1964;20:202.

202. Hanka LJ, Evans JS, Mason DJ, et al. Microbiological production of 5-azacytidine: 1. Production and biological activity. *Antimicrob Agents Chemother* 1966;6:619.

203. Karon M, Sieger L, Leimbrock S, et al. 5-Azacytidine: a new active agent for the treatment of acute leukemia. *Blood* 1973;42:359.

204. McCredie KB, Bodey GP, Burgess MA, et al. Treatment of acute leukemia with 5-azacytidine (NSC-102816). *Cancer Chemother Rep* 1973;57:319.

205. Vogler WR, Miller DS, Keller JW. 5-Azacytidine (NSC-102816): a new drug for the treatment of myeloblastic leukemia. *Blood* 1976;48:331.

206. Von Hoff DD, Slavik M, Muggia FM. A new anticancer drug with effectiveness in acute myelogenous leukemia. *Ann Intern Med* 1976;85:237.

207. Humphries RK, Dover G, Young NS, et al. 5-Azacytidine acts directly on both erythroid precursors and progenitors to increase production of fetal hemoglobin. *Tsitologiia* 1985;27:805.

208. Galanello R, Stamatoyannopoulos G, Papayannopoulou T. Mechanism of Hb F stimulation by S-stage compounds: in vitro studies with bone marrow cells exposed to 5-azacytidine, araC, or hydroxyurea. *J Clin Invest* 1988;81:1209.

209. Glover AB, Leyland-Jones B. Biochemistry of azacytidine: a review. *Cancer Treat Rep* 1987;71:959.

210. Beisler J. Isolation, characterization, and properties of a labile hydrolysis product of the antitumor nucleoside, 5-azacytidine. *J Med Chem* 1978;21:204.

211. Israili ZH, Vogler WR, Mingioli ES, et al. The disposition and pharmacokinetics in humans of 5-azacytidine administered intravenously as a bolus or by continuous infusion. *Cancer Res* 1976;36:1453.

212. Notari RE, De Young JL. Kinetics and mechanisms of degradation of the antileukemic agent 5-azacytidine in aqueous solutions. *J Pharm Sci* 1975;64:1148.

213. Vesely J, Cihak A. 5-Azacytidine: mechanism of action and biological effects in mammalian cells. *Pharmacol Ther* 1978;2:813.

214. Glazer RI, Peale AL, Beisler JA, et al. The effects of 5-azacytidine and dihydro-5-azacytidine on nucleic ribosomal RNA and poly(A) RNA synthesis in L1210 cells in vitro. *Mol Pharmacol* 1980;17:111.

215. Weiss JW, Pitot HC. Inhibition of ribosomal precursor RNA maturation by 5-azacytidine and 8-azaguanine in Novikoff hepatoma cells. *Arch Biochem Biophys* 1974;165:588.

216. Lee T, Karon MR. Inhibition of protein synthesis in 5-azacytidine-treated HeLa cells. *Biochem Pharmacol* 1976;25:1737.

217. Kalousek F, Raska K, Jurovik M, et al. Effect of 5-azacytidine on the acceptor activity of sRNA. *Colln Czech Chem Commun* 1966;31:1421.

218. Cihak A, Vesela H, Sorm F. Thymidine kinase and polyribosomal distribution in regenerating rat liver following 5-azacytidine. *Biochim Biophys Acta* 1968;166:277.

219. Cihak A, Vesely J. Prolongation of the lag period preceding the enhancement of thymidine and thymidylate kinase activity in regenerating rat liver by 5-azacytidine. *Biochem Pharmacol* 1972;21:3257.

220. Li LH, Olin EJ, Buskirk HH, et al. Cytotoxicity and mode of action of 5-azacytidine on L1210 leukemia. *Cancer Res* 1970;30:2760.

221. Plagemann PGW, Behrens M, Abraham D. Metabolism and cytotoxicity of 5-azacytidine in cultured Novikoff rat hepatoma and P388 mouse leukemia cells and their enhancement by preincubation with pyrazofurin. *Cancer Res* 1978;38:2458.

222. Adams RL, Burdon RH. DNA methylation in eukaryotes. *CRC Crit Rev Biochem* 1982;13:349.

223. Jones PA, Taylor SM, Wilson V. DNA modification, differentiation, and transformation. *J Exp Zool* 1983;228:287.

224. Drake JC, Stoller RG, Chabner BA. Characteristics of the enzyme uridine-cytidine kinase isolated from a cultured human cell line. *Biochem Pharmacol* 1977;26:64.

225. Lee T, Karon M, Momparler RL. Kinetic studies on phosphorylation of 5-azacytidine with the purified uridine-cytidine kinase from calf thymus. *Cancer Res* 1974;34:2481.

226. Vadlamudi S, Padarathsingh M, Bonmassar E, et al. Reduction of antileukemic and immunosuppressive activities of 5-azacytidine in mice by concurrent treatment with uridine. *Proc Soc Exp Biol Med* 1970;133:1232.

227. Vadlamudi S, Choudry JN, Waravdekar VS, et al. Effect of combination treatment with 5-azacytidine and cytidine on the life span and spleen and bone marrow cells of leukemic (L1210) and nonleukemic mice. *Cancer Res* 1970;30:362.

228. Vesely J, Cihak A, Sorm F. Biochemical mechanisms of drug resistance: IV. Development of resistance to 5-azacytidine and simultaneous depression of pyrimidine metabolism in leukemic mice. *Int J Cancer* 1967;2:639.

229. Li LH, Olin EJ, Fraser TJ, et al. Phase specificity of 5-azacytidine against mammalian cells in tissue culture. *Cancer Res* 1970;30:2770.

230. Lloyd HH, Dalmadge EA, Wikoff LJ. Kinetics of the reduction in viability of cultured L1210 leukemic cells exposed to 5-azacytidine (NSC-102816). *Cancer Chemother Rep* 1972; 56:585.

231. Presant CA, Vietti TJ, Valeriote F. Kinetics of both leukemic and normal cell population reduction following 5-azacytidine. *Cancer Res* 1975;35:1926.

232. Cihak A, Lamar C, Pitot HC. Studies on the mechanism of the stimulation of tyrosine aminotransferase activity in vivo by pyrimidine analogs: the role of enzyme synthesis and degradation. *Arch Biochem Biophys* 1973;156:176.

233. Stallings RL, Crawford BD, Tobey RA, et al. 5-Azacytidine-induced conversion to cadmium resistance correlated with early S phase replication of inactive metallothionein genes in synchronized CHO cells. *Somat Cell Mol Genet* 1986; 12:423.

234. Carlow DA, Kerbel RS, Feltis JT, et al. Enhanced expression of class I major histocompatibility complex gene (Dk) products on immunogenic variants of a spontaneous murine carcinoma. *J Natl Cancer Inst* 1985;75:291.

235. Bonal FJ, Pareja E, Martin J, et al. Repression of class I H-2K, H-2D antigens or GR9 methylcholanthrene-induced tumour cell clones is related to the level of DNA methylation. *J Immunogenet* 1986;13:179.

236. Richardson B, Kahl L, Lovett EJ, et al. Effect of an inhibitor of DNA methylation on T cells: I. 5-Azacytidine induces T4 expression on T8+ T cells. *J Immunol* 1986;137:35.

237. Liteplo RG, Alvarez E, Frost P, et al. Induction of thymidine kinase activity in a spontaneously enzyme-deficient murine tumor cell line by exposure in vivo to the DNA-hypomethylating agent 5-aza-2'-deoxycytidine: implications for mechanisms of tumor progression. *Cancer Res* 1985;45:5294.

238. Jones PA, Taylor SM, Mohandas T, et al. Cell cycle-specific reactivation of an inactive X-chromosome locus by 5-azadeoxycytidine. *Proc Natl Acad Sci U S A* 1982;79:1215.

239. Jeggo PA, Holliday R. Azacytidine-induced reactivation of a DNA repair gene in Chinese hamster ovary cells. *Mol Cell Biol* 1986;6:2944.

240. Holliday R. Strong effects of 5-azacytidine on the in vitro lifespan of human diploid fibroblasts. *Exp Cell Res* 1986;166:543.

241. Karon M, Benedict W. Chromatid breakage: differential effect of inhibitors of DNA synthesis during G_2 phase. *Science* 1972;178:62.

242. Seifertova M, Vesely J, Cihak A. Enhanced mortality in offspring of male mice treated with 5-azacytidine prior to mating: morphological changes in testes. *Neoplasma* 1976; 23:53.

243. Coles E, Thayer PS, Reinhold V, et al. Pharmacokinetics and excretion of 5-azacytidine (NSC-102816) and its metabolites. *Proc Am Assoc Cancer Res* 1974;16:91.

244. Chan KK, Staroscik JA, Sadee W. Synthesis of 5-azacytidine-6-³C and -6-¹⁴C. *J Med Chem* 1977;20:598.

245. Troetel WM, Weiss AJ, Stambaugh JE, et al. Absorption, distribution, and excretion of 5-azacytidine (NSC-102816) in man. *Cancer Chemother Rep* 1972;56:405.

246. Chabner BA, Drake JC, Johns DC. Deamination of 5-azacytidine by a human leukemia cell cytidine deaminase. *Biochem Pharmacol* 1973;22:2763.

247. Neil GL, Moxley TE, Kuentzel SL, et al. Enhancement by tetrahydrouridine (NSC-112907) of the oral activity of 5-azacytidine (NSC-102816) in L1210 leukemic mice. *Cancer Chemother Rep* 1975;59:459.

248. Bellet RE, Mastrangelo MJ, Engstrom PF, et al. Hepatotoxicity of 5-azacytidine (NSC-102816): a clinical and pathologic study. *Neoplasma* 1973;20:303.

249. Levi J, Wiernik P. A comparative clinical trial of 5-azacytidine and guanazole in previously treated adults with acute nonlymphocytic leukemia. *Cancer* 1976;38:36.

250. Ley TJ, DeSimone J, Keller GH, et al. 5-Azacytidine selectively increases gamma-globin synthesis in a patient with beta + thalassemia. *N Engl J Med* 1982;307:1469.

251. Burris HA 3rd, Moore MJ, Andersen J, et al. Improvements in survival and clinical benefit with gemcitabine as first-line therapy for patients with advanced pancreas cancer: a randomized trial. *J Clin Oncol* 1997;15:2403.

252. Stadler WM, Murphy B, Kaufman D, et al. Phase II trial of gemcitabine (GEM) plus cisplatin (CDDP) in metastatic urothelial cancer (UC). *Proc Annu Meet Am Soc Clin Oncol* 1997;16:A1152(abst).

253. Rosell R, Tonato M, Sandler A. The activity of gemcitabine plus cisplatin in randomized trials in untreated patients with advanced non-small cell lung cancer. *Semin Oncol* 1998; 25:27.

254. Castellano D, Lianes P, Paz-Ares L, et al. A phase II study of a novel gemcitabine plus cisplatin regimen administered every three weeks for advanced non-small-cell lung cancer. *Ann Oncol* 1998;9:457.

255. Anton A, Diaz-Fernandez N, Gonzalez Larriba JL, et al. Phase II trial assessing the combination of gemcitabine and cisplatin in advanced non-small cell lung cancer (NSCLC). *Lung Cancer* 1998;22:139.

256. Lippe P, Tummarello D, Monterubbianesi MC, et al. Weekly gemcitabine and cisplatin in advanced non-small-cell lung cancer: a phase II study. *Ann Oncol* 1999;10:217.

257. Hertel LW, Boder GB, Kroin JS, et al. Evaluation of the antitumor activity of gemcitabine (2',2'-difluoro-2'-deoxycytidine). *Cancer Res* 1990;50:4417.

258. Bouffard DY, Laliberte J, Momparler RL. Comparison of antineoplastic activity of 2-2-difluoro-2-deoxycytidine and cytosine arabinoside against human myeloid and lymphoid leukemic cells. *Anticancer Drugs* 1991;2:49.

259. Mackey JR, Mani RS, Selner M, et al. Functional nucleoside transporters are required for gemcitabine influx and manifestation of toxicity in cancer cell lines. *Cancer Res* 1998;58:4349.

260. Heinemann V, Hertel LW, Grindey GB, et al. Comparison of the cellular pharmacokinetics and toxicity of 2',2'-difluorodeoxycytidine and 1-beta-D-arabinofuranosylcytosine. *Cancer Res* 1988;48:4024.

261. Bouffard DY, Laliberte J, Momparler RL. Kinetic studies on 2',2'-difluorodeoxycytidine (gemcitabine) with purified

human deoxycytidine kinase and cytidine deaminase. *Biochem Pharmacol* 1993;45:1857.

262. Heinemann V, Xu YZ, Chubb S, et al. Cellular elimination of 2',2'-difluorodeoxycytidine 5'-triphosphate: a mechanism of self-potentiation. *Cancer Res* 1992;52:533.

263. Gandhi V, Plunkett W. Modulatory activity of 2',2'-difluorodeoxycytidine on the phosphorylation and cytotoxicity of arabinosyl nucleosides. *Cancer Res* 1990;50:3675.

264. Rockwell S, Grindey GB. Effect of 2',2'-difluorodeoxycytidine on the viability and radiosensitivity of EMT6 cells in vitro. *Oncol Res* 1992;4:151.

265. Heinemann V, Xu YZ, Chubb S, et al. Inhibition of ribonucleotide reduction in CCRF-CEM cells by 2',2'-difluorodeoxycytidine. *Mol Pharmacol* 1990;38:567.

266. Huang P, Chubb S, Hertel LW, et al. Action of 2',2'-difluorodeoxycytidine on DNA synthesis. *Cancer Res* 1991; 51:6110.

267. Gandhi V, Legha J, Chen F, et al. Excision of 2',2'-difluorodeoxycytidine (gemcitabine) monophosphate residues from DNA. *Cancer Res* 1996;56:4453.

268. Huang P, Plunkett W. Fludarabine- and gemcitabine-induced apoptosis: incorporation of analogs into DNA is a critical event. *Cancer Chemother Pharmacol* 1995;36:181.

269. Huang P, Plunkett W. Induction of apoptosis by gemcitabine. *Semin Oncol* 1995;22:19.

270. Cory AH, Hertel LW, Kroin JS, et al. Effects of 2',2'-difluorodeoxycytidine (gemcitabine) on wild type and variant mouse leukemia L1210 cells. *Oncol Res* 1993;5:59.

271. Goan YG, Zhou B, Hu E, et al. Overexpression of ribonucleotide reductase as a mechanism of resistance to 2',2'-difluorodeoxycytidine in human KB cancer cell line. *Proc Annu Meet Am Assoc Cancer Res* 1999;40:A4473.

272. Iwasaki H, Huang P, Keating MJ, et al. Differential incorporation of ara-C, gemcitabine, and fludarabine into replicating and repairing DNA in proliferating human leukemia cells. *Blood* 1997;90:270.

273. Van Moorsel CJ, Veerman G, Kuiper CM, et al. Mechanism of synergism between gemcitabine and cisplatin in ovarian and non-small cell lung cancer cell lines. *Proc Annu Meet Am Assoc Cancer Res* 1996;37:A2537(abst).

274. Yang LY, Li L, Liu XM, et al. Gemcitabine suppresses the repair of cisplatin adducts in plasmid DNA by extracts of cisplatin-resistant human colon carcinoma cells. *Proc Annu Meet Am Assoc Cancer Res* 1995;36:A2124(abst).

275. Van Moorsel CJA, Lakerveld B, Smid K, et al. Effects of gemcitabine on formation and repair of platinum-DNA adducts in ovarian cancer cell lines. *Proc Annu Meet Am Assoc Cancer Res* 1999;40:A3889.

276. Ruiz van Haperen VW, Veerman G, van Moorsel CJ, et al. Induction of in vivo resistance against gemcitabine (dFdC, 2',2'-difluoro-deoxycytidine). *Adv Exp Med Biol* 1998; 431:637.

277. Van der Wilt CL, Loves W, Padron JM, et al. Upregulation of not only deoxycytidine kinase, but also thymidine kinase 2 decreases resistance against gemcitabine. *Proc Annu Meet Am Assoc Cancer Res* 1999;40:A4475.

278. Sliutz G, Karlseder J, Tempfer C, et al. Drug resistance against gemcitabine and topotecan mediated by constitutive hsp70 overexpression in vitro: implication of quercetin as sensitiser in chemotherapy. *Br J Cancer* 1996;74:172.

279. Neff T, Blau CA. Forced expression of cytidine deaminase confers resistance to cytosine arabinoside and gemcitabine. *Exp Hematol* 1996;24:1340.

280. Waud WR, Gilbert KS, Grindey GB, et al. Lack of in vivo crossresistance with gemcitabine against drug-resistant murine P388 leukemias. *Cancer Chemother Pharmacol* 1996;38:178.

281. Shipley LA, Brown TJ, Cornpropst JD, et al. Metabolism and disposition of gemcitabine, and oncolytic deoxycytidine analog, in mice, rats, and dogs. *Drug Metab Dispos* 1992;20:849.

282. Grunewald R, Abbruzzese JL, Tarassoff P, et al. Saturation of 2',2'-difluorodeoxycytidine 5'-triphosphate accumulation by mononuclear cells during a phase I trial of gemcitabine. *Cancer Chemother Pharmacol* 1991;27:258.

283. Abbruzzese JL, Grunewald R, Weeks EA, et al. A phase I clinical, plasma, and cellular pharmacology study of gemcitabine. *J Clin Oncol* 1991;9:491.

284. Fossella FV, Lippman SM, Shin DM, et al. Maximum-tolerated dose defined for single-agent gemcitabine: a phase I dose-escalation study in chemotherapy-naive patients with advanced non-small-cell lung cancer. *J Clin Oncol* 1997; 15:310.

285. Plunkett W, Liliemark JO, Adams TM, et al. Saturation of 1-beta-D-arabinofuranosylcytosine 5'-triphosphate accumulation in leukemia cells during high-dose 1-beta-D-arabinofuranosylcytosine therapy. *Cancer Res* 1987;47:3005.

286. Grunewald R, Kantarjian H, Keating MJ, et al. Pharmacologically directed design of the dose rate and schedule of 2',2'-difluorodeoxycytidine (gemcitabine) administration in leukemia. *Cancer Res* 1990;50:6823.

287. Grunewald R, Kantarjian H, Du M, et al. Gemcitabine in leukemia: a phase I clinical, plasma, and cellular pharmacology study. *J Clin Oncol* 1992;10:406.

288. Abbruzzese JL, Gravel D, Tarassoff P, et al. Pharmacologically directed strategy for dose intensification of gemcitabine: a Phase I trial. *Proc Annu Meet Am Assoc Cancer Res* 1993;34:A2233(abst).

289. Touroutoglou N, Gravel D, Raber MN, et al. Clinical results of a pharmacodynamically-based strategy for higher dosing of gemcitabine in patients with solid tumors. *Ann Oncol* 1998;9:1003.

290. Tempero M, Plunkett W, Ruiz van Haperen V, et al. Randomized phase II trial of dose intense gemcitabine by standard infusion vs. fixed dose rate in metastatic pancreatic carcinoma. *Proc Annu Meet Am Soc Clin Oncol* 1999;18:A1048.

291. O'Rourke TJ, Brown TD, Havlin K, et al. Phase I clinical trial of gemcitabine given as an intravenous bolus on 5 consecutive days [Letter]. *Eur J Cancer* 1994;30A:417.

292. Poplin EA, Corbett T, Flaherty L, et al. Difluorodeoxycytidine (dFdC), gemcitabine: a Phase I study. *Invest New Drugs* 1992;10:165.

293. Anderson H, Thatcher N, Walling J, et al. A phase I study of a 24 hour infusion of gemcitabine in previously untreated patients with inoperable non-small-cell lung cancer. *Br J Cancer* 1996;74:460.

294. Aapro MS, Martin C, Hatty S. Gemcitabine—a safety review. *Anticancer Drugs* 1998;9:191.

295. Casper ES, Green MR, Kelsen DP, et al. Phase II trial of gemcitabine (2,2'-difluorodeoxycytidine) in patients with adenocarcinoma of the pancreas. *Invest New Drugs* 1994; 12:29.

296. Brodowicz T, Breiteneder S, Wiltschke C, et al. Gemcitabine-induced hemolytic uremic syndrome: a case report [Letter]. *J Natl Cancer Inst* 1997;89:1895.

297. Flombaum CD, Mouradian JA, Casper ES, et al. Thrombotic microangiopathy as a complication of long-term therapy with gemcitabine. *Am J Kidney Dis* 1999;33:555.

298. Fung MC, Storniolo AM, Nguyen B, et al. A review of hemolytic uremic syndrome in patients treated with gemcitabine therapy. *Cancer* 1999;85:2023.

299. Pavlakis N, Bell DR, Millward MJ, et al. Fatal pulmonary toxicity resulting from treatment with gemcitabine. *Cancer* 1997;80:286.

300. Vander Els NJ, Miller V. Successful treatment of gemcitabine toxicity with a brief course of oral corticosteroid therapy. *Chest* 1998;114:1779.

301. Shewach DS, Hahn TM, Chang E, et al. Metabolism of 2'-2'-difluoro-2'-deoxycytidine and radiation sensitization of human colon carcinoma cells. *Cancer Res* 1994;54:3218.

302. Lawrence TS, Chang EY, Hahn TM, et al. Radiosensitization of pancreatic cancer cells by 2',2'-difluoro-2'-deoxycytidine. *Int J Radiat Oncol Biol Phys* 1996;34:867.

303. Mohideen MN, McCall A, Kamradt M, et al. Activity of gemcitabine and its radiosensitization of human cervical cancer cells. *Proc Annu Meet Am Soc Clin Oncol* 1997; 16:A865(abst).

304. Rosier JF, Beauduin M, Bruniaux M, et al. The effect of 2'-2' difluorodeoxycytidine (dFdC, gemcitabine) on radiation-induced cell lethality in two human head and neck squamous carcinoma cell lines differing in intrinsic radiosensitivity. *Int J Radiat Biol* 1999;75:245.

305. Shewach DS, Keena D, Rubsam LZ, et al. Mechanism of radiosensitization by 2',2'-difluorodeoxycytidine. *Proc Annu Meet Am Assoc Cancer Res* 1996;37:A4196(abst).

306. Shewach DS, Lawrence TS. Gemcitabine and radiosensitization in human tumor cells. *Invest New Drugs* 1996;14:257.

307. Milas L, Fujii T, Hunter N, et al. Enhancement of tumor radioresponse in vivo by gemcitabine. *Cancer Res* 1999;59:107.

308. Eisbruch A, Shewach DS, Urba S, et al. Phase I trial of radiation (RT) concurrent with low-dose gemcitabine (GEM) for head and neck cancer: high mucosal and pharyngeal toxicity. *Proc Annu Meet Am Soc Clin Oncol* 1997;17:A1377.

309. Merlano M, Benasso M, Corvo R, et al. Gemcitabine (GEM), cisplatin (PT) and radiotherapy (RT) in squamous cell carcinoma of the head and neck. *Proc Annu Meet Am Soc Clin Oncol* 1997;17:A1445.

310. Blackstock AW, Bernard SA, Richards F, et al. Phase I trial of twice-weekly gemcitabine and concurrent radiation in patients with advanced pancreatic cancer. *J Clin Oncol* 1999;17:2208.

311. Kudrimoti M, Regine W, John W, et al. Concurrent infusional gemcitabine and radiation in the treatment of advanced unresectable GI malignancy: a phase I/II study. *Proc Am Soc Clin Oncol* 1999;18:A928.

312. Schwendener RA, Schott H. Treatment of L1210 murine leukemia with liposome-incorporated N4-hexadecyl-1-beta-D-arabinofuranosyl cytosine. *Int J Cancer* 1992;51(3):466.

313. Tsuruo T, Iida H, Tsukagoshi S, et al. Comparison of cytotoxic effect and cellular uptake of 1-beta-D-arabinofuranosylcytosine and its N^4-acyl derivatives, using cultured KB cells. *Cancer Res* 1979;39(3):1063.

314. Bobek M, Cheng YC, Bloch A. Novel arabinofuranosyl derivatives of cytosine resistant to enzymatic deamination and possessing potent antitumor activity. *J Med Chem* 1978;21(7):597.

315. Hong CI, Nechaev A, West CR. Synthesis and antitumor activity of 1-beta-D-arabinofuranosylcytosine conjugates of cortisol and cortisone. *Biochem Biophys Res Commun* 1979;88(4):1223.

316. Ho DH, Neil GL. Pharmacology of 5'-esters of 1-beta-D-arabinofuranosylcytosine. *Cancer Res* 1977;37(6):1640.

317. Kato Y, Saito M, Fukushima H, et al. Antitumor activity of 1-beta-D-arabinofuranosylcytosine conjugated with polyglutamic acid and its derivative. *Cancer Res* 1984;44(1):25.

318. Holoye PY, Dhingra HM, Umsawasdi T, et al. Phase II study of 5,6-dihydro-5-azacytidine in extensive, untreated non-small cell lung cancer. *Cancer Treat Rep* 1987; 71(9):859.

319. Ahluwalia GS, Cohen MB, Kang GJ, et al. Arabinosyl-5-azacytosine: mechanisms of native and acquired resistance. *Cancer Res* 1986;46(9):4479.

320. Rivard GE, Momparler RL, Demers J, et al. Phase I study on 5-aza-2'-deoxycytidine in children with acute leukemia. *Leuk Res* 1981;5(6):453.

321. Lund B, Kristjansen PE, Hansen HH. Clinical and preclinical activity of 2',2'-difluorodeoxycytidine (gemcitabine). *Cancer Treat Rev* 1993;19(1):45.

10

PURINE ANTIMETABOLITES

KENNETH R. HANDE

GUANINE ANALOGS

The guanine analog 6-mercaptopurine (6-MP) was one of the first antineoplastic agents developed.[1] Over 50 years later, it is still used as primary therapy for children with acute lymphoblastic leukemia. The antimetabolite 6-thioguanine (6-TG) is given for remission induction and maintenance treatment of acute myelogenous leukemia. It is currently being evaluated as a primary treatment for acute lymphoblastic leukemia.[2] Azathioprine, a prodrug of 6-MP with better immunosuppressive activity than 6-MP,[3] is widely given as an immunosuppressant in clinical transplantation. These three drugs are closely related in structure (Fig. 10-1), metabolism, mechanism of action, and toxicity. Due to their similarities, they are discussed together in this section. The key pharmacologic features of these drugs are summarized in Tables 10-1 through 10-3.

Mechanism of Action

The compound 6-MP is a structural analog of hypoxanthine with a substitution of a thiol for the naturally occurring 6-hydroxyl group (Fig. 10-1). 6-MP undergoes extensive hepatic and cellular metabolism after dosing.[4] Three major competing transformation routes are present: one anabolic and two catabolic. 6-MP is activated intracellularly by the enzyme hypoxanthine-guanine phosphoribosyl transferase (HGPRT) to form 6-thioinosine monophosphate (TIMP). TIMP inhibits *de novo* purine synthesis[5] (Fig. 10-2). TIMP is sequentially metabolized to thioguanosine monophosphate and then to 6-thioguanosine triphosphate. 6-TG triphosphate (6-TGTP) is incorporated into DNA and RNA. Present evidence suggests that the cytotoxic effect of 6-MP occurs through incorporation of 6-TGTP into DNA. Cells incorporating 6-TGTP survive, but the abnormal DNA templates compromise subsequent replication.[6] The quantity of 6-MP metabolite present in DNA correlates with cytotoxicity.[7] Incorporation of 6-TGTP into DNA triggers programmed cell death by a process involving the mismatch repair pathway.[8,9] The cytotoxicity of 6-TG depends on (a) incorporation of 6-TG into DNA, (b) miscoding during DNA replication, and (c) recognition of the abnormal base pairs by proteins of the postreplicative mismatch repair system.

6-TG is activated in a manner similar to that outlined for 6-MP.[10] Thioguanine is converted to 6-thioguanylic acid (TGMP) by HGPRT. TGMP is subsequently incorporated into RNA and DNA in its deoxytriphosphate form. Incorporation of fraudulent nucleotides into DNA is believed to be the primary mechanism of cytotoxicity,[11] triggering apoptosis by a process involving the mismatch repair pathway, as with 6-MP.[8] Thioguanine is more directly converted into cytotoxic thioguanine nucleotides than is 6-MP.[2] Significantly higher cellular concentrations of thioguanine nucleotides are seen after 6-TG administration than after 6-MP.[12] Methylated thioinosine monophosphate formation is greater with 6-MP.

Azathioprine (Fig. 10-1) is rapidly cleaved by nonenzymatic mechanisms to 6-MP and methyl-4-nitro-5-imidazole derivatives (Fig. 10-2). The thioimidazole metabolites may contribute to the immunosuppressive effects of azathioprine.[13] Although incorporation of false nucleotides into DNA and inhibition of purine synthesis by 6-MP ribonucleotides are the probable mechanism for cytotoxicity, the mechanism by which azathioprine and 6-MP modify the immune response is less well understood. Azathioprine inhibits T-lymphocyte activity to a greater extent than B-lymphocyte activity. It interferes with the synthesis of some cytokines, such as interleukin 2. When azathioprine yields 6-MP *in vivo*, the imidazole ring reacts with glutathione and cysteine residues. The alkylation of lymphocyte thiol groups may be important in azathioprine immunosuppression.

Clinical Pharmacology

6-Mercaptopurine

6-MP is commercially available in 50-mg tablets, which also contain the inactive ingredients corn and potato starch, lactose, magnesium stearate, and stearic acid. An

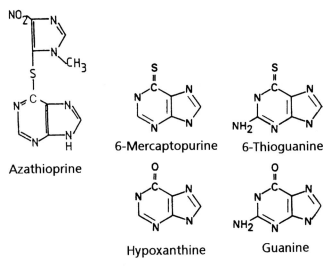

FIGURE 10-1. Structure of the naturally occurring purine guanine and related antineoplastic agents 6-mercaptopurine, 6-thioguanine, and azathioprine.

intravenous preparation of 6-MP has been formulated for research purposes but is not yet available for general clinical use. 6-MP is relatively insoluble and unstable in alkaline solutions.

Advances in high-performance liquid chromatography (HPLC) in the 1980s have allowed specific, sensitive assays for measurement of clinically relevant thiopurine concentrations. Plasma 6-MP, 6-TG, and metabolite concentrations as low as 0.1 μmol per L can be measured using HPLC techniques.[14,15] Using these assays, accurate kinetics of oral and intravenous preparations have been determined. After oral administration of commonly used doses of 6-MP (75 mg per m²), peak plasma concentrations of 0.3 to 1.8 μmol per L are seen within a mean of 2.2 hours.[16] The vol-

TABLE 10-1. KEY FEATURES OF 6-MERCAPTOPURINE

Mechanism of action:	Incorporation of metabolites into DNA correlates with cytotoxicity
Metabolism:	Activation: conversion to thiopurine nucleotides
	Catabolism: conversion to 6-thiouric acid by xanthine oxidase
	Catabolism: conversion to 6-methylthiopurine by thiopurine methyltransferase (TPMT)
Pharmacokinetics:	Half-life: 50 min
	Poor and variable oral bioavailability
Elimination:	Metabolism at conventional doses by xanthine oxidase and TPMT
Drug interactions:	Allopurinol decreases 6-mercaptopurine elimination and concomitant use requires dosage reduction (by 75%)
Toxicity:	Myelosuppression
	Mild gastrointestinal effects (nausea, vomiting)
	Rare hepatotoxicity
Precautions:	Dosage reductions with allopurinol
	Increased toxicity in individuals with genetic deficiency of TPMT (genetic screening possible)

TABLE 10-2. KEY FEATURES OF 6-THIOGUANINE

Mechanism of action:	Incorporation of fraudulent nucleotides into DNA
Metabolism:	Activation: conversion to thiopurine nucleotides
	Catabolism: conversion to 6-thioxanthine by guanase
	Catabolism: conversion to 2-amino-6-methyl thiopurine by thiopurine methyltransferase (TPMT)
Pharmacokinetics:	Half-life: 90 min
	Poor and variable bioavailability
Elimination:	Hepatic metabolism
Drug interactions:	None well defined
Toxicity:	Myelosuppression
	Mild gastrointestinal effects (nausea, vomiting)
	Rare hepatotoxicity
Precautions:	Increased toxicity in individuals with genetic deficiency of TPMT

ume of distribution exceeds that of total-body water (0.9 L per kg). Little penetration into the cerebrospinal fluid (CSF) occurs. With high-dose oral 6-MP (500 mg per m²), plasma 6-MP concentrations of 5 to 12 μmol per L are achieved.[17] In human leukemic cell culture models, concentrations of 1 to 10 μmol per L are cytotoxic. After intravenous dosing, the half-life of 6-MP is 50 to 100 minutes.[18,19] After intravenous dosing at 1 g per m² over 8 hours, plasma concentrations of 6-MP reach 25 μmol per L and CSF concentrations 3.8 μmol per L.[19] Only weak protein binding is noted with 6-MP (20% bound).

Oral absorption of 6-MP is incomplete and highly variable.[20] At a dose of 75 mg per m², the mean 6-MP bioavailability is only 16% (range, 5% to 37%).[11] Clearance of 6-MP occurs primarily through two routes of metabolism. 6-MP is oxidized to the inactive metabolite 6-thiouric acid by xanthine oxidase (Fig. 10-2). 6-MP also undergoes S-methylation by the enzyme thiopurine methyltransferase

TABLE 10-3. KEY FEATURES OF AZATHIOPRINE

Mechanism of action:	Similar to that of 6-mercaptopurine; immunosuppressive activity may be due to alkylation of lymphocyte thiol groups; interferes with synthesis of various cytokines
Metabolism:	Rapidly converted to 6-mercaptopurine (6-MP) by nonenzymatic mechanisms
Pharmacokinetics:	See 6-mercaptopurine (see Table 10-1)
Elimination:	Rapid metabolism to 6-mercaptopurine, and subsequent elimination similar to that of 6-MP
Drug interactions:	Allopurinol decreases elimination. Concomitant use with allopurinol requires azathioprine dosage reductions (by 75% or more)
Toxicity:	Myelosuppression
	Mild gastrointestinal effects (nausea, vomiting)
	Rare hepatotoxicity
Precautions:	Dosage reduction with allopurinol
	Increased toxicity in individuals with genetic deficiency of thiopurine methyltransferase

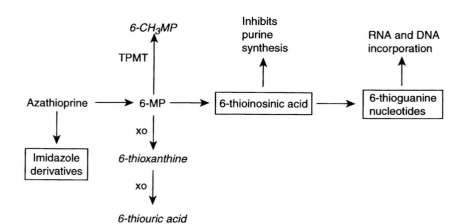

FIGURE 10-2. Mechanism of activation and catabolism of azathioprine and 6-mercaptopurine (6-MP). Active metabolites are indicated by surrounding boxes. Inactive (or less active) metabolites are indicated by italic print. (6-CH₃MP, 6-methyl mercaptopurine; TPMT, thiopurine methyltransferase; XO, xanthine oxidase.)

(TPMT) to yield 6-methyl mercaptopurine. The intestinal mucosa and liver contain high concentrations of the enzyme xanthine oxidase. The low bioavailability of 6-MP is due to a large first-pass effect as drug is absorbed through the intestinal wall into the portal circulation and metabolized by xanthine oxidase. The concomitant administration of allopurinol (an inhibitor of xanthine oxidase) increases 6-MP bioavailability fivefold.[21] Interestingly, allopurinol does not alter the plasma kinetics of intravenously administered 6-MP, although more 6-MP and less thiouric acid are excreted in the urine after allopurinol therapy.[22] Methotrexate sodium, often used with 6-MP in maintenance treatment of acute lymphoblastic leukemia, is a weak inhibitor of xanthine oxidase. Concomitant use of methotrexate results in a small increase in the bioavailability of 6-MP. The modest increase in bioavailability, however, is thought not to be clinically significant.[23] The plasma concentration × time profile of 6-MP differs in the same patient when studied on repeated occasions.[24] Food intake decreases oral drug absorption. 6-MP clearance rates of 600 to 900 mL per minute per m² have been measured after intravenous 6-MP administration.[16,19,22] Due to poor bioavailability, apparent clearance rates after oral administration are fivefold greater.[16,17,20]

High-dose oral 6-MP (500 mg per m²) has been used in an attempt to saturate the first-pass metabolism of 6-MP and thereby increase bioavailability.[17] Even at a dose of 500 mg per m² of 6-MP, xanthine oxidase is not saturated and no improvement in bioavailability is seen. In contrast to the results mentioned earlier, however, Kato et al.[25] found that the variability in oral 6-MP absorption decreased and bioavailability improved as the dose of 6-MP was increased from 50 mg to 175 mg per m². This same group has suggested that rectal administration of 6-MP, by eliminating the first-pass metabolism of orally absorbed drug, can increase the bioavailability of 6-MP more than fourfold.[26] Food intake and oral antibiotic use can reduce the oral absorption of 6-MP.[27,28]

As previously mentioned, two catabolic pathways for 6-MP metabolism exist that significantly affect drug activity:

one via xanthine oxidase (just discussed) and a second via TPMT. Patient-to-patient variation in TPMT activity can result in significant changes in 6-MP metabolism and in drug toxicity. As seen in Figure 10-2, TPMT catalyzes the S-methylation of 6-MP to a relatively inactive metabolite, 6-methyl mercaptopurine (6-CH₃MP). TPMT activity across individuals is controlled by a common genetic polymorphism.[29] The frequency distribution of TPMT activity in large population studies is trimodal. One in 300 subjects has very low enzyme activity; 11% of the population have intermediate activity; and the rest have high enzyme activity. A single genetic locus with two alleles (one for low and one for high activity) is responsible for the trimodal distribution.[30] TPMT activity in erythrocytes correlates with activity in other tissues, such as lymphocytes, kidney, and liver.[31] Lymphoblasts from individuals heterozygous for the normal TMTP gene have lower TMPT activity than lymphoblasts from homozygous patients.[32] Patients with low TPMT activity are more susceptible to 6-MP– and 6-TG–induced myelosuppression.[33] Marked myelosuppression in patients receiving 6-MP, 6-TG, or azathioprine therapy may be a result of genetic deficiency in TPMT activity in that patient.[34] In patients with no TMPT activity, the dosage of 6-MP, but not the dosage of other chemotherapeutic agents given for their leukemia, should be reduced. Some data suggest that blacks may have less TPMT activity than whites,[35] which could increase toxicity in that population. A reciprocal relationship between TPMT activity and the formation of 6-thiopurine nucleotides has been demonstrated. Lennard et al.[36] have suggested that children with high TPMT activity are at greater risk of disease relapse due to decreased drug activation.

The TPMT gene has now been cloned.[37] Eight TPMT polymorphisms associated with reduced enzyme activity have been identified.[38] In describing gene mutations, the convention has been adopted that the nonmutated gene is designated TPMT*1* and mutated genes are designated TPMT*2* through TPMT*8* based on the order in which they were first described. In white populations, the most common mutation genotype associated with low enzyme activity is TPMT*3*, which is found in more than 80% of heterozygotes.[39] Genetic testing using polymerase chain reaction methods can now identify TPMT-deficient and heterozygous patients.[40] This test, as opposed to direct measurement of TPMT activity in red blood cells, is not affected by prior blood transfusions to the patient.

Several studies have suggested that variability in oral absorption of 6-MP may affect the risk of relapse in children with acute lymphoblastic leukemia.[41–43] In a study by Koren et al.,[41] patients with low- or standard-risk acute lymphoblastic leukemia who achieved an area under the curve (AUC) of less than 21 mg per mL × minutes after daily exposure to 6-MP had a poorer survival than patients achieving a higher 6-MP AUC. These authors suggested that plasma 6-MP concentrations be monitored to ensure adequate drug exposure to improve cure rates in acute lymphoblastic leukemia. However, reservations about this study are warranted. First, 6-MP is not the active metabolite, and plasma levels of 6-MP may not necessarily reflect active intracellular metabolite concentrations. Measurement of intracellular thiopurine nucleotide levels may be a better predictor for response. Second, Koren et al. used a "standard" AUC in their calculations (the AUC measured divided by the administered dose). Such normalization may be invalid when correlation between oral dose and AUC is poor, as is found with 6-MP. Other studies have failed to correlate 6-MP plasma concentrations with leukemic response rate.[20]

The compound 6-MP was originally formulated as an oral preparation due to its limited solubility. Because of the previously mentioned difficulties with poor oral bioavailability and the availability of a suitable preparation, intravenous 6-MP was reevaluated in the 1980s.[44,45] The use of intravenous 6-MP may be advantageous for several reasons: (a) the poor and variable bioavailability of oral 6-MP, (b) achievement of higher blood and CSF concentrations, and (c) elimination of the potential for patient noncompliance.

6-Thioguanine

6-TG is available as 40-mg tablets for oral use. An intravenous preparation is investigational. As with 6-MP, the absorption of 6-TG in humans is variable and incomplete (mean bioavailability is 30% with a range of 14% to 46%).[46] Peak plasma levels of 0.03 to 5 μmol per L occur 2 to 4 hours after ingestion[34]; the median drug half-life is 90 minutes, but wide variability is reported.[47] Intravenously administered 6-TG has been evaluated. Clearance of drug (600 to 1,000 mL per minute per m^2) appears to be dose dependent, which suggests saturation of clearance at doses over 10 mg per m^2 per hour.[48,49] Plasma concentrations of 4 to 10 mmol per L can be achieved.

The catabolism of 6-TG differs from that of 6-MP. 6-TG is not a substrate for xanthine oxidase. 6-TG is converted to 6-thiohypoxanthine (an inactive metabolite) by the action of the enzyme guanase. Because 6-TG inactivation is not dependent on the action of xanthine oxidase, an inhibitor of xanthine oxidase such as allopurinol does not block the detoxification of 6-TG. In humans, methylation of 6-TG via TPMT is more extensive than is that of 6-MP. The product of methylation, 2-amino-6-methylthiopurine, is substantially less active and less toxic than 6-TG.

Azathioprine

Azathioprine is rapidly degraded by nonenzymatic mechanisms to 6-MP. The metabolic pathways thereafter are identical to those of 6-MP.[50] In transplant patients taking 2 mg per kg per day azathioprine, peak 6-MP plasma concentrations are low (75 ng per mL) and plasma drug half-life is short (1.9 hours).[51] The time to peak drug concentration is less than 2 hours after oral administration. Plasma concentrations of 6-MP exceed those of azathioprine within an hour of drug administration.[50] Renal function impairment does not alter the plasma kinetics of either azathioprine or 6-MP.

Toxicity

6-Mercaptopurine

The dose-limiting toxicity of 6-MP is myelosuppression, which occurs 1 to 4 weeks after the onset of therapy and is reversible when the drug is discontinued. Platelets, granulocytes, and erythrocytes are all affected. Weekly monitoring of blood counts during the first 2 months of therapy is recommended. 6-MP is also an immunosuppressant and inhibits allograft rejection. Immunity to infectious agents or vaccines is subnormal in patients receiving 6-MP. Gastrointestinal mucositis and stomatitis are modest. Approximately one-fourth of treated patients experience nausea, vomiting, and anorexia. Gastrointestinal side effects appear to be more common in adults than in children.[52] Hepatotoxicity is seen in a small number of patients receiving 6-MP.[53] Hepatotoxicity is usually mild and reversible, and has a clinical picture consisting primarily of cholestatic jaundice, although elevations of alkaline phosphatase and transaminase may be seen. Increased transaminase levels are noted in roughly 15% of patients.[54] Frank hepatic necrosis can occur after high doses of 6-MP.[55] Jaundice usually appears 1 or 2 months into therapy but can occur as early as 1 week after drug initiation. At very high doses (more than 1,000 mg per m^2), the limited solubility of 6-MP can cause precipitation of drug in the renal tubules with hematuria and crystalluria.[56] 6-MP has teratogenic properties. Women receiving 6-MP in the first trimester of pregnancy may have an increased incidence of abortion; the risk of malformation in offspring surviving exposure during the first trimester is not known.[57] In a series of 28 women receiving 6-MP after the first trimester of pregnancy, three mothers died before giving birth, one abortion occurred, and one child was stillborn. No abnormal fetuses were found.

6-Thioguanine

As with 6-MP, the primary toxicity of 6-TG is myelosuppression. Blood counts should be taken frequently, as a delayed effect may occur during oral drug administration. In a phase I trial of 6-TG administered intravenously daily for 5 days, leukopenia and thrombocytopenia were the dose-limiting toxicities seen at 55 to 65 mg per m² per day.[58] Higher doses result in mucositis. 6-TG produces gastrointestinal toxicities similar to those of 6-MP but less frequently. Jaundice and hepatic venoocclusive disease have been reported with 6-TG therapy.[59]

Azathioprine

Adverse effects from azathioprine are similar to those seen with 6-MP. These include leukopenia, diarrhea, nausea, abnormal liver function tests, and skin rashes. Frequent measurement of blood count is warranted throughout therapy (weekly during the first 8 weeks of therapy). A hypersensitivity reaction generally characterized by fever, severe nausea, diarrhea, and vomiting has been reported.[60] Patients develop toxicity within 4 weeks of starting azathioprine.[61] Long-term immunosuppressive therapy, including use of azathioprine, results in an increased frequency of secondary infections and an increased risk of malignant tumors.[62] Acute myeloid leukemia associated with karyotypic changes of 7q-/-7 has been reported.[63] Risk of cancer development increases with longer duration of azathioprine use [for less than 5 years' use, the relative risk (RR) = 1.3; for 5 to 10 years' use, RR = 2.0; for more than 10 years' use, RR = 4.4].[64]

Toxicity from azathioprine, primarily myelosuppression and gastrointestinal intolerance, requires dosage adjustment or discontinuation of treatment in up to 40% of patients.[54,65] Several studies[65–67] indicate that patients heterozygous for mutant TPMT are at high risk for toxicity and dose modification. In a study by Black et al.,[65] all patients heterozygous for the TMPT3 allele required discontinuation of therapy within 1 month. The authors suggested that molecular testing for TMPT would be a cost-effective way of identifying the 10% of the population at high risk for toxicity.

Clinical Use and Drug Interactions

The guanine analog 6-mercaptopurine was originally used as remission induction therapy for acute lymphoblastic leukemia in children. Currently, it is a regular component of maintenance therapy for this disease. It is occasionally used in adult lymphocytic leukemia. It has little role in treatment of solid tumors or myeloid leukemias. 6-MP is usually given orally at a dosage of 60 to 100 mg per m² daily by

mouth for several weeks. Although dosage reductions have been suggested for patients with hepatic and renal function impairment, no good data exist justifying such dosage adjustments. Dosage adjustment for patients with mutant TPMT are appropriate. 6-TG is used as a second-line agent for acute myelogenous leukemia. It is given orally at a dose of roughly 75 mg per m² (2 mg per kg). If no toxicity occurs, the dose may be increased to 90 mg per m². Although theoretical advantages exist for intravenous administration of 6-TG, further investigation of such therapy is required. Studies have explored the use of 6-TG as a substitute for 6-MP in treatment of acute lymphoblastic leukemia.[12,49]

Azathioprine is used as an immunosuppressant to prevent rejection of organ transplants and in the treatment of illnesses believed to be autoimmune in character (lupus erythematosus, rheumatoid arthritis, ulcerative colitis, etc.). Azathioprine is available in 50-mg tablets and 100-mg vials for intravenous administration. Dosages of 3 to 5 mg per kg daily are commonly used. Dosages should be adjusted, however, to the minimal needed to prevent organ rejection and control disease. Intravenous drug should be used only in patients unable to tolerate oral therapy. Again, identifying patients heterozygous for TMPT3 mutations may be appropriate. In patients with TMPT3 mutations, treatment with lower dosages of 6-MP or azathioprine should be considered.

As previously mentioned,[21] allopurinol inhibits the catabolism of 6-MP and increases its bioavailability. Oral doses of 6-MP and azathioprine should be reduced by at least 75% in patients who are also receiving allopurinol. Combined use of standard-dose azathioprine (or 6-MP) and allopurinol results in life-threatening toxicity.[68] Methotrexate causes a modest increase in 6-MP bioavailability but not to an extent significant enough to warrant dosage reduction.[23] The biochemical interactions of 6-MP and methotrexate, including reasons for their synergy in maintenance treatment of childhood acute lymphoblastic leukemia, are discussed more fully in Chapter 7 on antifolates.

ADENOSINE ANALOGS

The adenosine analogs are examples of agents developed through rational drug design. Their availability has improved the treatment options for several types of chronic leukemias and lymphomas. Adenosine analogs were initially evaluated in follow-up of observations of patients with a rare congenital illness who are unable to synthesize the enzyme adenosine deaminase (ADA).

ADA catalyzes the deamination of adenosine to inosine and of deoxyadenosine to deoxyinosine. Lack of ADA results in accumulation of deoxyadenosine, which is cytotoxic to lymphocytes. Clinically, congenital deficiency of ADA leads to lymphocyte dysfunction and severely impaired cellular immunity. The effect of deoxyadenosine

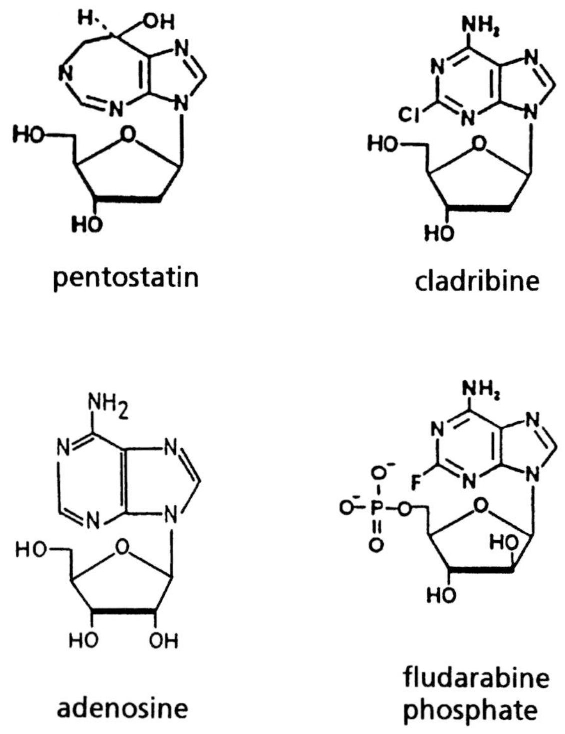

FIGURE 10-3. Structure of adenosine and the adenosine analogs fludarabine (9-β-D-arabinofuranosyl-2-fluoroadenosine monophosphate), pentostatin (2-deoxycoformycin), and cladribine (2-chlorodeoxyadenosine).

on lymphocytes prompted investigators to evaluate adenosine analogs in the treatment of lymphocytic malignancies. Three adenosine analogs with documented clinical utility are fludarabine phosphate, pentostatin, and 2'-chlorodeoxyadenosine (cladribine) (Fig. 10-3). Key pharmacologic features of the adenosine analogs are listed in Tables 10-4 through 10-6.

TABLE 10-4. KEY FEATURES OF FLUDARABINE

Mechanism of action:	Incorporation into DNA as a false nucleotide
	Inhibition of DNA polymerase, DNA primase, and DNA ligase
	DNA chain termination
Metabolism:	Rapid dephosphorylation of fludarabine phosphate in plasma to F-ara-A
	Activation of F-ara-A to F-ara-ATP within cells
Pharmacokinetics:	Rapid dephosphorylation to F-ara-A
	Half-life of F-ara-A: 6–30 h
Elimination:	Primarily renal excretion of F-ara-A
Drug interactions:	Increases cytotoxicity of cytarabine and cisplatin
Toxicity:	Myelosuppression
	Immunosuppression
	Neurotoxicity at high doses
	Rare: interstitial pneumonitis and hemolytic anemia
Precautions:	Dosage reduction for patients with renal failure

F-ara-A, 9-β-D-arabinofuranosyl-2-fluoroadenine; F-ara-ATP, 9-β-D-arabinofuranosyl-2-fluoroadenine triphosphate.

TABLE 10-5. KEY FEATURES OF PENTOSTATIN (DEOXYCOFORMYCIN)

Mechanism of action:	Inhibition of adenosine deaminase with subsequent accumulation of dATP pools
	Inhibition of DNA replication and repair by dATP
Metabolism:	Minimal
Pharmacokinetics:	Clearance rate of 8 mL/min/m², which decreases with decreasing creatinine clearance
Elimination:	Majority of drug is excreted unchanged in the urine
Drug interactions:	None recognized
Toxicity:	Well tolerated at low doses
	At high doses: nausea, immunosuppression, nephrotoxicity, central nervous system disturbances
Precautions:	Dosage reductions for patients with renal failure

dATP, deoxyadenosine triphosphate.

Fludarabine

Over the past decade, fludarabine has become an effective agent for the treatment of chronic lymphocytic leukemia (CLL), prolymphocytic leukemia, indolent non-Hodgkin's lymphoma, cutaneous T-cell lymphoma, Waldenström's macroglobulinemia, and, in combination with cytosine arabinoside, acute myelogenous leukemia.[69–74] Fludarabine was developed through chemical modifications of adenosine arabinoside (ara-A) designed to avoid the rapid deamination of ara-A by adenosine deaminase. The 2-fluoroderivative of ara-A is relatively resistant to deamination and retains cytotoxic activity, but is poorly soluble in water. The monophosphate analog, 9-β-D-arabinofuranosyl-2-fluoroadenine monophosphate (F-ara-AMP), is resistant to adenosine deaminase and has improved aqueous solubility (Fig. 10-3). Key features of fludarabine are summarized in Table 10-4.

TABLE 10-6. KEY FEATURES OF CLADRIBINE (2-CHLORODEOXADENOSINE)

Mechanism of action:	Activated to 2-CdATP that is incorporated into DNA, producing DNA strand breaks
	2-CdATP inhibits ribonucleotide reductase
	Triggers apoptosis by activating caspaces
Metabolism:	Activation to 2-CdATP within cells
Pharmacokinetics:	Significant variability in cladribine plasma AUC
	40–50% oral bioavailability
	50% urinary excretion
Drug interactions:	Increases toxicity or cytosine arabinoside
Toxicity:	Myelosuppression
	Fever
	Immunosuppression
	Renal failure at high doses

AUC, area under the (concentration × time) curve; 2-CdATP, 2-chloro-2'-deoxyadenosine 5'triphosphate.

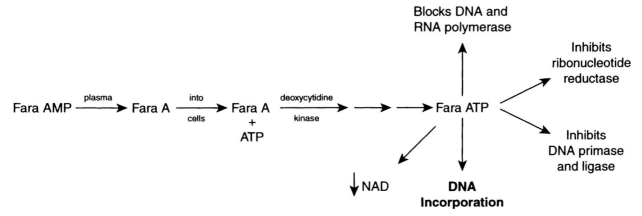

FIGURE 10-4. Activation of fludarabine. (ATP, adenosine triphosphate; F-ara-A, 9-β-D-arabinofuranosyl-2-fluoroadenine; F-ara-AMP, 9-β-D-arabinofuranosyl-2-fluoroadenine monophosphate; F-ara-ATP, 9-β-D-arabinofuranosyl-2-fluoroadenine triphosphate; NAD, nicotinamide adenine dinucleotide.)

Mechanism of Action

After intravenous administration, fludarabine phosphate is rapidly dephosphorylated in plasma to the nucleoside 2-fluoro-ara-A (Fig. 10-4).[75] This compound enters cells via carrier-mediated transport[76] and is phosphorylated to its active form, 9-β-D-arabinofuranosyl-2-fluoroadenine triphosphate (F-ara-ATP). Phosphorylation, initiated by deoxycytidine kinase, is necessary for the cytotoxic and therapeutic activity of fludarabine.[77] Mutant cell lines that lack deoxycytidine kinase are resistant to the cytotoxicity and therapeutic activity of fludarabine. Once activated, F-ara-ATP inhibits several intracellular enzymes important in DNA replication, including DNA polymerase,[78] ribonucleotide reductase,[79] DNA primase,[80] and DNA ligase I.[81] In addition, fludarabine is incorporated into DNA. Once incorporated, fludarabine is an effective DNA chain terminator,[78] primarily at the 3' end of DNA. Incorporation of fludarabine into DNA is required for drug-induced DNA fragmentation.[82] The amount of fludarabine incorporated is linearly correlated with loss of clonagenicity.[78] Excision of the 3'-terminal fludarabine does not easily occur,[83] and the presence of this false nucleotide leads to apoptosis.

Although the effects of fludarabine on DNA synthesis account for its activity in dividing cells, fludarabine is also cytotoxic in diseases with very low growth fractions, such as CLL or indolent lymphomas. This raises the question of how an "S-phase" agent is active in nondividing cells. Although the specific mechanism(s) by which fludarabine induces cell death among quiescent cells is under investigation, proposed mechanisms of action include fludarabine's ability to inhibit RNA polymerases by incorporation into RNA, depletion of nicotinamide adenine dinucleotide with resultant decrease in cellular energy stores, and interference with normal DNA repair processes.[84,85] The most suggestive evidence indicates that fludarabine triggers apoptosis after incorporation into DNA during the DNA repair process.[86,87]

Clinical Pharmacology

Plasma concentrations of parent F-ara-AMP and F-ara-A have been determined using HPLC.[88,89] After rapid intravenous administration or a 30-minute drug infusion, parent drug (F-ara-AMP) undergoes rapid conversion (2 to 4 minutes) to F-ara-A. Peak plasma F-ara-A concentrations of 0.3 to 1.0 mg per L are achieved after doses of 80 to 250 mg fludarabine.[75,88–92] Wide variations in terminal drug half-life (7 to 33 hours) and AUC are found. Drug clearance is linear with no change with repeated doses. Children may have a lower volume of distribution and clearance than adults.[88] F-ara-A is excreted primarily in the urine (30% to 60%) with no metabolites. Total-body clearance of F-ara-A is significantly lower in patients with renal impairment than in patients with normal kidney function (total-body clearance = 51.82 ± 6.70 mL per minute per m² versus 73.53 ± 3.79 mL per minute per m²).[88] Therefore, a dosage reduction is recommended for patients with renal dysfunction. Oral bioavailability is roughly 75%, and oral formulations for commercial use are being developed.[93]

Toxicity

The dose-limiting toxicities of fludarabine are myelosuppression and infectious complications from immunosuppression.[72,73,94] Reversible leukopenia and thrombocytopenia have been reported after fludarabine administration with a median time to nadir of 13 days (range, 3 to 25 days) and 16 days (range, 2 to 32 days), respectively. Twenty percent to 50% of treated patients have a neutrophil count nadir of less than 1,000 per mm³ at standard dosages of 25 mg per m² per day for 5 days. Platelet nadirs of less than 50 to 100,00 per mm³ are seen in 20% of patients.[69,70,95,96] Up to 25% of patients treated with fludarabine have a febrile episode. Many are fevers of unknown origin but one-third of patients have a serious documented infection.

Fludarabine is immunosuppressive. Therapy is associated with an increased risk of opportunistic infections. CD4 and CD8 T-lymphocytic subpopulations decrease to levels of 150 to 200 per mm^3 after three courses of therapy.[97] The most frequent infectious complications are respiratory. Infections with *Cryptococcus, Listeria monocytogenes, Pneumocystis carinii,* cytomegalovirus, herpes simplex virus, varicella zoster, and *Mycobacterium,* organisms associated with T-cell dysfunction, are seen.[98,99] Previous therapy, advanced disease, and neutropenia are risk factors. The use of prednisone with fludarabine has been reported to increase infectious complications.[73] The development of autoimmune hemolytic anemia has been seen with fludarabine use.[100,101] Hemolysis has been noted after any treatment cycle but is most common during cycles 1 to 3 (71% of cases). Death from hemolysis has been reported. Corticosteroids are used for treatment. Acute tumor lysis is a rare complication in patients with CLL and indolent lymphomas treated with fludarabine.[102]

Other reported fludarabine toxicities include mild nausea and vomiting, infection, peripheral sensorimotor neuropathy, and hepatocellular toxicity with elevations in serum transaminases. An irreversible neurotoxicity syndrome with cortical blindness, optic neuritis, encephalopathy, generalized seizures, and coma has been described.[103] This occurs in patients receiving high drug doses (more than 40 mg per m^2 per day for 5 days). Mild, reversible neurotoxicity, however, is seen at lower dosages with increased frequency in elderly patients.[104] Neurotoxicity is reported in 16% of patients.[103] Pulmonary toxicity characterized by fever, cough, and hypoxia, and diffuse interstitial pneumonitis has also been reported.[105]

Clinical Use

Fludarabine has demonstrated clinical activity in a variety of low-grade lymphoproliferative malignancies, including CLL, hairy cell leukemia, Waldenström's macroglobulinemia, and non-Hodgkin's lymphoma.[69,71,72] Response rates from 32% to 57% have been reported among patients with refractory CLL treated with fludarabine at doses of 15 to 30 mg per m^2 per day for 5 days every 28 days. The median duration of disease control is 65 to 91 weeks. Among patients with previously untreated CLL, fludarabine has produced responses in more than 70% of patients, including complete responses in one-third. A median survival of 63 months has been reported.[80] The exact role of fludarabine in management of CLL in previously untreated patients has not yet been completely defined.[106] The National Cancer Institute has initiated a phase III comparison of chlorambucil versus fludarabine versus fludarabine plus chlorambucil in treatment of CLL. Preliminary results[107] indicate that the combination regimen is associated with excess hematologic toxicity. Patients treated with fludarabine have a higher complete response rate than those receiving chlorambucil but a similar partial response rate.

No survival difference has been noted to date. In a multicenter, randomized trial, fludarabine produced a higher response rate and longer disease-free survival in patients with CLL than did CAP [cyclophosphamide, doxorubicin hydrochloride (Adriamycin), and prednisone] chemotherapy. Among previously untreated patients, median survival was slightly longer with fludarabine, although the difference did not reach statistical significance.[70]

Approximately half of patients with indolent non-Hodgkin's lymphoma respond to fludarabine.[72,73,96,108] Response rates of patients with intermediate- and high-grade non-Hodgkin's lymphoma are significantly lower (0% to 10%). A 33% response rate has been reported in patients with mantle cell lymphomas.[109] Activity has also been reported in Waldenström's macroglobulinemia (30% response rate),[69] cutaneous T-cell lymphomas,[110] and, in combination with cytosine arabinoside, in acute myelogenous leukemia,[111] in which complete response rates of 35% to 60% have been reported.

Drug Interactions

Fludarabine is synergistic with at least two other antineoplastic agents, cytosine arabinoside and cisplatin. Fludarabine increases intracellular accumulation of cytosine arabinoside.[112] Increased incorporation of arabinosylcytidine triphosphate into DNA occurs through modulation of deoxynucleotide triphosphate pools by fludarabine.[113] Fludarabine also acts with cytosine arabinoside to inhibit DNA polymerase α.[114] Fludarabine increases the cytotoxicity of cisplatin *in vivo* by inhibiting repair of cisplatin-induced DNA strand breaks.[87]

Pentostatin (Deoxycoformycin)

Pentostatin, or 2'-deoxycoformycin, is a purine analog originally prepared from a streptomycin antibiotic culture but now chemically synthesized.[115] It was originally developed after the recognition that children with inherited deficiency of the enzyme ADA have severe lymphopenia. Pentostatin was identified as a potent ADA inhibitor[115] and was subsequently tried as therapy for lymphocytic leukemias.[116] No activity was noted in patients with acute leukemias. The drug was found useful, however, in therapy of hairy cell leukemia and some indolent lymphomas.[72] The key pharmacologic features of pentostatin are listed in Table 10-5.

Mechanism of Action

The specific mechanism for pentostatin cytotoxicity is unknown but is believed to involve the accumulation of deoxyadenosine and deoxyadenosine triphosphate after ADA inhibition. Pentostatin binds tightly to ADA with a slow dissociation rate of 60 hours.[117] Abnormally high levels of deoxyadenosine triphosphate, which build up with

ADA inhibition, exert a negative feedback on ribonucleotide reductase, which results in an imbalance in deoxynucleotide pools. This imbalance inhibits DNA synthesis and alters DNA replication and repair. S-adenosylhomocysteine hydrolase is also inhibited, which blocks normal cellular methylation reactions.[118] These mechanisms are relevant to proliferating cells. The mechanism of action of pentostatin on nonproliferating cells is unclear.

Pentostatin enters cells via the nucleoside transport system[119] with a rate of cellular uptake that parallels that of other nucleosides.[120] Pentostatin exerts tight-binding inhibition of ADA.[121] When administered at dosages intended to produce total-body ADA inhibition in acute lymphocytic leukemia, serious renal, pulmonary, and central nervous system toxicity is encountered.[122] Thus, toxicity has limited the usefulness of this drug in conditions associated with high ADA activity, such as acute leukemias.[123] However, pentostatin has been found to be very active in hairy cell leukemia, in which cellular ADA levels are lower.[124] Clinical responses are seen in patients with hairy cell leukemia at dosages much lower than those necessary to treat T-cell leukemias.[125]

Clinical Pharmacology

Pentostatin is reasonably stable after reconstitution at neutral pH. Care must be taken if the drug is extensively diluted with 5% dextrose in water, however, as pentostatin's stability is compromised at pH values less than 5.[126] Pentostatin has a large volume of distribution but little protein binding.[127] Pentostatin has a terminal elimination half-life of 2.6 to 15 hours.[128,129] Plasma levels of pentostatin 1 hour after administration exceed the ADA-inhibitory concentration by approximately 10^6, a finding that supports the recommendation for an intermittent infusion schedule.[130] Only a relatively small amount of pentostatin is metabolized, and 40% to 80% of the drug is excreted in urine unchanged within 24 hours.[128] Plasma clearance averages 68 mL per minute per m^2 and correlates with creatinine clearance. For patients with impaired renal function (creatinine clearance of less than 60 mL per minute), drug half-life is prolonged (approximately 18 hours). Dose reductions are probably necessary for patients with impairment in renal function,[130] although this has not been carefully studied. Pentostatin is not bioavailable by the oral route.[126] Pentostatin crosses the blood–brain barrier, and CSF concentrations are 10% to 13% of serum drug concentrations.[131]

Toxicity

Toxic effects seen at high doses (10 mg or more per m^2 per day) include nausea and vomiting, immunosuppression, conjunctivitis, renal impairment, hepatic enzyme elevation, and central nervous system disturbances, among which are somnolence, confusion, and coma.[122] At dosages used to treat hairy cell leukemia (4 mg per m^2 biweekly), the incidence of these side effects is low and therapy is usually well toler-

ated.[132] Reported toxicities included worsening of neutropenia with initiation of therapy. Up to 70% of patients treated at the current recommended dosage develop neutropenia,[131] whether as part of their disease or from therapy. Mild to moderate lethargy, rash, and reactivation of herpes zoster late in therapy have been reported.[133] Renal toxicity, seen in early trials, is minimized with the use of lower drug dosages and adequate hydration. Cardiac complications in elderly patients after pentostatin therapy have been described but appear to be uncommon.[134] Patients with poor performance status or impaired renal function have a higher incidence of life-threatening toxicity. The most common nonmyelosuppressive drug toxicities are nausea and vomiting (40% to 70% of patients). Nausea and vomiting may be delayed (12 to 72 hours) after administration. Elevation in transaminase concentrations occurs after drug administration but levels usually return to normal.[116] Keratoconjunctivitis has been reported.

Clinical Use

In clinical trials, pentostatin delivered in low doses produces responses, including pathologic complete responses, in more than 90% of patients with hairy cell leukemia, even those refractory to splenectomy and interferon-α therapy.[135] It is currently approved by the Food and Drug Administration for treatment of hairy cell leukemia. Because of its activity in hairy cell leukemia, pentostatin has also been evaluated for treatment of a number of other closely related disorders, including CLL,[136] adult T-cell leukemia/lymphoma,[137] cutaneous T-cell lymphoma,[138] Waldenström's macroglobulinemia,[139] and refractory multiple myeloma.[140,141] Although activity has been reported, further trials are needed to determine the usefulness of pentostatin in treating these disorders.[127]

Cladribine

Mechanism of Action

Cladribine, or 2-chlorodeoxyadenosine (2-CdA; Leustatin), is a purine nucleoside analog with demonstrated activity in low-grade lymphoproliferative diseases, childhood leukemias, and multiple sclerosis. Its important pharmacologic features are noted in Table 10-6. Substitution of chlorine at the 2 position of deoxyadenosine produces 2-CdA or cladribine (Fig. 10-3), which is relatively resistant to enzymatic deamination by adenosine deaminase. Intracellular transport of cladribine occurs via nucleoside delivery mechanisms.[142] Cladribine is a prodrug and needs intracellular phosphorylation to active nucleotides. The 5'-triphosphate metabolite (2-chloro-2'-deoxyadenosine 5'triphosphate, 2-CdATP) accumulates in cells rich in deoxycytidine kinase[143] (Fig. 10-5). This compound is incorporated into DNA, producing DNA strand breaks and inhibition of DNA synthesis.[144] High intracellular concentrations

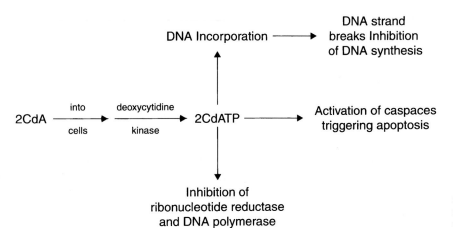

FIGURE 10-5. Activation of cladribine (2-chlorodeoxyadenosine or 2-CdA). (2-CdATP, 2-chloro-2'-deoxyadenosine 5'triphosphate.)

of 2-CdATP also inhibit DNA polymerases[145] and ribonucleotide reductase,[78] which causes an imbalance in deoxyribonucleotide triphosphate pools with subsequent impairment of DNA synthesis and repair. The cytotoxic activity of cladribine, however, appears independent of cell division.[144] The mechanism by which CdATP triggers apoptosis in nondividing cells has not been clear. Cysteine proteases, referred to as caspaces, are active in apoptosis. The caspaces activate endonucleases, which causes cleavage of genomic DNA.[146,147] Leoni et al.[148] have suggested that 2-CdATP cooperates with cytochrome C and protease activating factor 1 to initiate the caspace cascade, which leads to DNA degradation, even in the absence of cell division. Cladribine is cytotoxic to a variety of cell lines in culture.[149]

Clinical Pharmacology

Concentrations of cladribine in plasma have been assayed by radioimmunoassay techniques[150] or HPLC.[151] Liquid chromatography can identify a major cladribine metabolite, 2-chlorodeoxyinosine, in addition to the parent compound, but the radioimmunoassay is more sensitive. Cladribine is a prodrug. It is activated within the cell to cladribine nucleotides. Intracellular drug concentrations are several hundred–fold higher than plasma concentrations.[152] Cladribine nucleotides are retained in leukemic cells with an intracellular half-life of 9 to 30 hours. The long intracellular half-life supports the use of intermittent drug administration.[153] Unfortunately, no correlations have been found between the plasma AUC of cladribine or intracellular cladribine concentrations and the response to treatment.[154]

After a 2-hour infusion of 0.12 mg per kg cladribine, peak serum concentrations of nearly 50 mg per mL are achieved.[155] A linear dose-concentration relationship is present up to dosages of 2.5 mg per m² per hour.[153] Cladribine clearance rates of 664 to 978 mL per hour per kg have been reported, with significant interpatient variability (±50%). The drug is weakly bound to plasma protein (20%). Renal clearance accounts for 50% of total drug clearance, with 20% to 30% of drug excreted as unchanged cladribine

within the first 24 hours.[156,157] Little information is available regarding dosage adjustments for renal or hepatic insufficiency. Given the high renal drug clearance, however, caution should be used in giving cladribine to patients with renal failure. Chlorodeoxyinosine is the major metabolite formed. It accounts for only 1% to 3% of administered drug.[153]

Bioavailability of subcutaneously administered cladribine is excellent (100%).[158] Oral administration has been evaluated, and bioavailability averages 50%. Significant patient-to-patient variability (±28%) exists in the AUC achieved after administration of drug by any method.[156,159] A drug-drug interaction between cladribine and cytosine arabinoside has been reported. Pretreatment of patients with cladribine increases the intracellular accumulation of cytosine arabinoside triphosphate, the active metabolite of cytosine arabinoside, by 40%.[160] Other pyrimidine analogs, such as gemcitabine, may be similarly affected.

Toxicity

Myelosuppression is usually the dose-limiting toxicity of cladribine. The standard dosage has been 0.7 mg per kg per cycle (usually as a continuous 7-day infusion at 0.1 mg per m² per day).[161] Nausea, alopecia, and hepatic and renal toxicity rarely occur at this dosage. Fever (temperature higher than 100°F) has been seen in two-thirds of patients treated with cladribine, mostly during the period of neutropenia. Myelosuppression and immunosuppression with development of opportunistic infections are the major adverse events. Severe (grade 3 or 4) neutropenia and lymphopenia occur in half of treated patients. Neutrophil counts decrease 1 to 2 weeks after the start of therapy and persist for 3 to 4 weeks.[162] Twenty percent of patients develop grade 3 or 4 thrombocytopenia. Infections, often opportunistic infections such as with *Candida* or *Aspergillus*, occur in 15% to 40% of patients.[162–164] Betticher et al.[165] have shown that reducing the dose of cladribine from 0.7 to 0.5 mg per kg per cycle decreased the rate of grade 3 myelosuppression (33% to 8%) and the infection rate (30% to 7%). No change in lymphoma response rate was noted with this dose reduction.

Toxicities other than myelosuppression and infections are rare but have been reported. After high-dose cladribine treatment (five to ten times the recommended therapeutic dose), renal failure has developed 1 to 2 weeks after therapy. Autoimmune hemolytic anemia has been reported in CLL patients receiving cladribine.[166] Eosinophilia,[167] nausea, and fatigue have been noted. Progressive irreversible motor weakness with paraparesis was noted 1 to 5 months after high-dose cladribine therapy in some patients.

Clinical Use

Cladribine entered clinical testing in the mid-1980s. Its spectrum of activity appears similar to that of other adenosine analogs (e.g., fludarabine). Initial studies demonstrated activity in CLL[168,169] and in hairy cell leukemia.[161,170] Cladribine is also effective for low-grade non-Hodgkin's lymphomas,[171] cutaneous T-cell lymphoma,[172] Waldenström's macroglobulinemia,[173] and blast-phase chronic myelogenous leukemia.[174] The optimal dosage and route of drug administration is currently under study. As previously mentioned, doses of 0.5 mg per kg per cycle may be as effective as higher doses but with reduced toxicity.[165] Subcutaneous[175] and oral routes[176] of drug administration have demonstrated activity. Cladribine has been tested in treatment of nonhematologic disorders, such as multiple sclerosis[177] and rheumatoid arthritis.[178]

ALLOPURINOL

Allopurinol has no antineoplastic activity. It is frequently used in treating patients with malignant disease, however, to prevent hyperuricemia and uric acid nephropathy. The clinical use of allopurinol in cancer chemotherapy and its potential interactions with various antitumor agents are

TABLE 10-7. KEY FEATURES OF ALLOPURINOL

Mechanism of action:	Limits conversion of xanthine and hypoxanthine to uric acid by inhibiting xanthine oxidase
	Causes feedback inhibition of *de novo* purine synthesis
Metabolism:	Rapid metabolic conversion to oxipurinol, which is the active metabolite
Pharmacokinetics:	Allopurinol half-life: 0.7–1.6 h
	Oxipurinol half-life: 14–28 h
Elimination:	Allopurinol: metabolism to oxipurinol
	Oxipurinol: renal excretion
Drug interactions:	Prolongs half-life of 6-mercaptopurine (6-MP) and azathioprine by decreasing rate of metabolic elimination
	Prevents formation of toxic 5-fluorouracil metabolites
	May impair hepatic microsomal enzyme function
Toxicity:	Rash
	Hypersensitivity syndrome (toxic epidermal neurolysis, renal failure, hepatic failure)
	Rare: xanthine nephropathy
Precautions:	Reduce doses of 6-MP or azathioprine
	Reduce allopurinol doses for renal insufficiency
	Stop drug for rash
	Do not use to treat asymptotic hyperuricemia

summarized in this section. The key features of allopurinol are summarized in Table 10-7.

Mechanism of Action

Allopurinol (4-hydroxpyrazolo [3,4-D] pyrimidine) and its major metabolic product oxipurinol (4,6-dihydroxypyrazolo [3,4-D] pyrimidine) are analogs of hypoxanthine and xanthine, respectively. Both inhibit the enzyme xanthine oxidase and block the conversion of hypoxanthine and xanthine to uric acid (Fig. 10-6). Allopurinol binds to xanthine oxidase and undergoes internal conversion to oxipurinol, simulta-

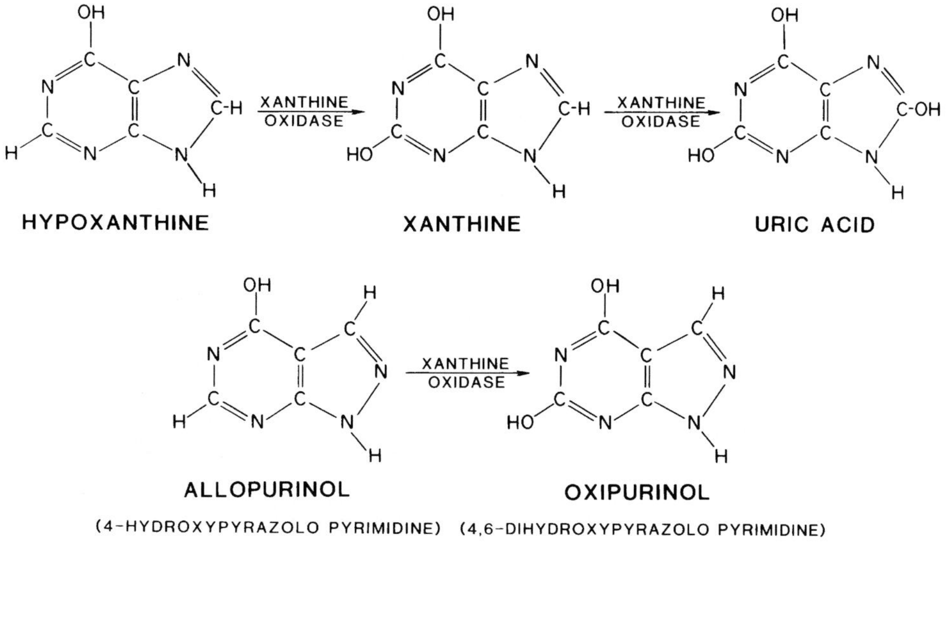

FIGURE 10-6. Metabolic pathway for the conversion of hypoxanthine and xanthine to uric acid and of allopurinol to oxipurinol.

PURINE METABOLISM

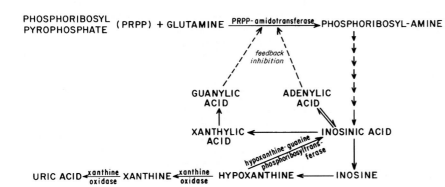

FIGURE 10-7. Feedback inhibition of *de novo* purine biosynthesis. Inhibition of xanthine oxidase by allopurinol causes an increase in serum hypoxanthine concentrations, which in turn causes increased concentrations of inosinic, xanthylic, adenylic, and guanylic acids. Guanylic and adenylic acids are inhibitors of phosphoribosylpyrophosphate (PRPP) aminotransferase.

neously reducing xanthine oxidase.[179] Oxipurinol inhibits xanthine oxidase by attaching at the active site of the enzyme in a stoichiometric fashion, one molecule of oxipurinol for each functionally active site of xanthine oxidase [K_i (inhibition constant) = 5.4×10^{-10} mol per L].

Allopurinol reduces serum uric acid concentrations not only by inhibiting xanthine oxidase but also by decreasing the rate of *de novo* purine biosynthesis. Administration of allopurinol to patients with primary gout lowers serum uric acid concentrations and results in a concomitant rise in serum xanthine and hypoxanthine concentrations.[180,181] Conversion of hypoxanthine to inosinic acid and subsequently to adenylic and guanylic acid is increased (Fig. 10-7). Adenylic and guanylic acid are allosteric inhibitors of 5-phospho-α-D-ribosyl aminotransferase,[182,183] the critical enzyme involved in *de novo* purine synthesis. Total purine excretion (xanthine plus hypoxanthine plus uric acid) decreases by 30% to 40% after initiation of allopurinol therapy. Allopurinol and oxipurinol are also converted to their respective ribonucleotides. This leads to decreased intercellular concentrations of 5-phospho-α-D-ribosyl, which also contributes to decreased purine synthesis.[184] The effect of allopurinol on *de novo* purine synthesis is negligible in treatment of the tumor lysis syndrome in which release of purines from DNA occurs.

Clinical Pharmacology

Oral allopurinol tablets are commercially available in 100-mg and 300-mg doses (Zyloprim). An intravenous preparation is now available. Allopurinol is well absorbed orally (70% to 80% of the administered dose).[185,186] The oral bioavailability of oxipurinol has been thought to be less (40%).[187] A rapid-release oxipurinol preparation has been developed, however, that has bioavailability nearly comparable to that of allopurinol.[188] After oral administration of 300 mg of allopurinol, plasma oxipurinol concentrations of 10 to 40 μmol per L (1.5 to 6.5 mg per L) are achieved within 1 to 3 hours.[189] Linear absorption is noted with doses of up to 900 mg.[190] Administration of allopurinol by rectal supposi-

tory has been tested. Absorption by this route of administration is poor and clinically unsuitable.[185]

The plasma half-life of allopurinol is short (30 to 100 minutes)[189] with rapid conversion of allopurinol to oxipurinol. The volume of distribution of both allopurinol and oxipurinol is roughly that of total-body water with little binding of either drug to plasma proteins.[186] A small amount of allopurinol is excreted directly in the urine (clearance rate of 13 to 19 mL per minute),[189] but most of an administered dose of allopurinol is metabolized to oxipurinol. In patients with normal renal function, steady-state oxipurinol plasma concentrations are 15 mg per L (100 mmol per L) at an allopurinol dosage of 300 mg per day. This is in excess of the concentration needed to inhibit xanthine oxidase (25 mmol per L).[188] Impaired renal clearance of oxipurinol leads to a prolonged oxipurinol plasma half-life (14 to 28 hours). Oxipurinol clearance and drug half-life are closely tied to creatinine clearance.[191] Patients with renal failure have delayed oxipurinol excretion and require a dosage reduction to prevent drug accumulation. Maintenance doses of allopurinol should be reduced to maintain serum oxipurinol levels comparable to those in patients with normal renal function (Table 10-8).[191,192]

TABLE 10-8. ADULT MAINTENANCE DOSES OF ALLOPURINOL

Creatinine Clearance (mL/min)	Maintenance Dose of Allopurinol (mg)
0	100 every 3 d
10	100 every 2 d
20	100 daily
40	150 daily
60	200 daily
80	250 daily
100	300 daily
120	350 daily
140	400 daily

From Hande KR, Noone RM, Stone WJ. Severe allopurinol toxicity. Description and guidelines for prevention in patients with renal insufficiency. *Am J Med* 1984;76:47–56.

Hemodialysis removes oxipurinol from the body with a clearance rate of roughly 78 mL per minute.[193] A routine 4-hour dialysis lowers serum oxipurinol concentrations by 40%.[193] A 200-mg dose of allopurinol is recommended to replace drug lost by hemodialysis.

Oxipurinol clearance rates vary with the dietary protein intake of patients. A low-protein diet (19 g per day) can decrease oxipurinol clearance (64%) and increase the oxipurinol plasma half-life nearly threefold compared with a high-protein diet (268 g per day).[194,195] These changes are believed to be due to the adaptive response of the kidney to protein restriction. This study suggests that malnourished patients given routine allopurinol doses have increased plasma concentrations of oxipurinol.

Toxicity

Allopurinol therapy is well tolerated in most patients and produces few side effects. Skin rash is seen in 2% of patients on allopurinol.[196] In patients allergic to allopurinol, oxipurinol may be tried as an alternative therapy for xanthine oxidase inhibition. Cross-sensitivity between allopurinol and oxipurinol has been noted, however.[197] In patients allergic to allopurinol, the drug should be avoided if possible. Nevertheless, desensitization to allopurinol has been successfully accomplished in allergic patients for whom no substitute is available.[198] Gastrointestinal intolerance, fever, and alopecia are rare complications of allopurinol therapy.[199] A severe, potentially life-threatening hypersensitivity syndrome resulting from allopurinol use has been reported.[191] Patients usually have fever (87% of reported cases), eosinophilia (73%), skin rash (92%) including toxic epidermal neurolysis, renal dysfunction, and hepatic failure (68%). Death has been reported in 21% of published cases. This hypersensitivity syndrome usually appears 2 to 4 weeks after the initiation of treatment with 300 to 400 mg per day of allopurinol. Over 80% of patients developing this syndrome have underlying renal failure when allopurinol therapy is initiated. Steady-state concentrations of oxipurinol are elevated in this situation and may play a role in the development of the toxicity syndrome. The hope is that adjustments of allopurinol dosages for renal insufficiency (Table 10-8) will lower the risk for drug toxicity.[192]

Xanthine nephropathy is a rare complication of allopurinol therapy in cancer patients. The normal urinary excretion of either xanthine or hypoxanthine is less than 30 mg per day.[200] In patients with primary gout who are taking allopurinol, the renal excretion of total oxypurines (xanthine plus hypoxanthine) increases to 40 mg to 500 mg per day with 55% to 70% of the total excretion being xanthine.[181] Development of xanthine nephropathy has occurred in patients receiving allopurinol who have had rapid tumor lysis[201,202] and in occasional patients with Lesch-Nyhan syndrome. *De novo* purine biosynthesis does not contribute in a significant manner to the acute purine load seen after rapid tumor lysis. Therefore, the fall in uric acid excretion in this situation can be accompanied by a nearly equal rise in the excretion of xanthine and hypoxanthine. In two reported cases of xanthine nephropathy, serum xanthine concentrations have reached levels of 6 mg to 14 mg per dL after chemotherapy[203,204]; such levels are over 200-fold higher than normal plasma xanthine concentrations. These high xanthine concentrations may lead to concomitantly high urinary xanthine concentrations, which results in xanthine precipitation in the renal tubule in a manner similar to uric acid deposition.

Even though xanthine precipitation is a potential complication of allopurinol therapy in patients who have massive tumor lysis, allopurinol treatment is beneficial to such patients. It enables them to excrete a larger total purine load. Because the solubility of a single purine, such as xanthine, hypoxanthine, or uric acid, is independent of the others, dividing the purine load among these three purines by the use of allopurinol increases the total amount of purine that can be excreted in the urine. Xanthine concentrations in excess of 5 mg per dL may cause a falsely low uric acid measurement as determined by the uricase method.[204] Elevated xanthine concentrations do not affect uric acid measurements determined by the phosphotungstate calorimetric assay.

Clinical Uses

Gout

In the treatment of primary gout, allopurinol produces a fall in serum uric acid concentration and a decrease in urinary uric acid excretion 1 or 2 days after initiation of therapy and produces a maximal reduction in serum urate levels within 4 to 14 days.[180,181] In addition to lowering serum and urinary uric acid concentrations, therapy with allopurinol also produces a decrease in the frequency of urate stone formation and shrinkage in size of gouty tophi. Although allopurinol administration generally improves the clinical symptoms in patients with primary gout, an acute arthritic flare may occasionally occur after initiation of allopurinol therapy and may require temporary treatment with colchicine. A dosage of 300 mg allopurinol per day is effective in a majority of patients with primary gout but occasional patients require higher drug dosages. A once-daily dose of 300 mg of allopurinol is clinically as effective as three equally divided doses of 100 mg.[205] In patients who do not respond to 300 mg of allopurinol per day, dosages of 600 to 1,000 mg per day are usually effective in lowering serum uric acid concentrations.

Hyperuricemia Secondary to Tumor Lysis

With rapid tumor lysis after cancer treatment, a sudden, temporary rise in uric acid production occurs that is not due to increased *de novo* synthesis but is due to cell destruction with release of preformed purines. Uric acid is sparingly soluble in both water and urine. The rapid release of uric acid after tumor cell death may lead to a marked increase in urinary excretion of uric acid with subsequent renal failure due to the precipitation of urate crystals in the distal renal tubules, where concentration and acidification are maximal. The incidence of urate stones as a complication of untreated chronic myeloproliferative disease has been established at 40%.[206] The incidence of uric acid nephropathy and complications of tumor lysis in various other neoplastic diseases and situations, however, has not been extensively investigated.[207] The development of hyperuricemia after treatment of leukemias and lymphomas is so common that hydration and allopurinol therapy are recommended before chemotherapy for these diseases is begun.

The use of allopurinol in preventing secondary hyperuricemia due to tumor lysis has been empiric. DeConti and Calabresi[208] and Krakoff and Meyer[209] used doses of 200 mg to 800 mg of allopurinol daily before the initiation of chemotherapy and demonstrated that these doses are effective in preventing elevations of serum uric acid in most cases. If marked tumor lysis and hyperuricemia are expected after chemotherapy, optimal management consists of lowering serum uric acid levels before initiating treatment. If rapid antineoplastic treatment is required, however, significant oxipurinol blood levels can be achieved within 30 minutes of an intravenous allopurinol infusion and within 2 to 4 hours of oral allopurinol administration.[189] Allopurinol is usually given before cytoreductive treatment of all leukemias and lymphomas. Dosages of 300 mg to 400 mg per m² per day should be given for 2 to 3 days, with dosage subsequently reduced to 300 mg to 400 mg per day. These dosages prevent marked increases in uric acid excretion after chemotherapy,[210,211] although clinically significant tumor lysis is still seen in 5% of patients with high-grade lymphomas and laboratory evidence of lysis is found in 40%.[212]

Drug Interactions

Xanthine oxidase catalyzes the conversion of both azathioprine and 6-MP to the inactive metabolite, 6-thiouric acid. Concomitant administration of allopurinol with either of these two agents results in increased 6-MP plasma concentrations and increased toxicity. This drug interaction is primarily seen when azathioprine or 6-MP is given orally and is less apparent when 6-MP is administered intravenously.[20] Oral doses of 6-MP or azathioprine should be reduced by at least 65% to 75% when allopurinol is used concomitantly. White blood cell counts should be taken frequently. Even with azathioprine dosage reductions of 67%, myelosuppression is seen in over one-third of patients also treated with allopurinol.[213] Inactivation of 6-TG occurs through

the enzyme guanase and not via xanthine oxidase, so that no dosage reduction is needed when allopurinol and 6-TG are used in combination.

Both allopurinol and oxipurinol are reabsorbed in the renal tubules. The concomitant use of the uricosuric agent probenecid with allopurinol results in a shorter oxipurinol plasma half-life due to more rapid renal excretion of the drug.[214] When thiazides are used with allopurinol, an increase in the rate of orotic acid excretion is noted, and the risk of allopurinol hypersensitivity reactions also seems to increase. However, no prolongation of oxipurinol half-life has been noted in volunteers with normal renal function who are also receiving thiazides.[215]

Allopurinol can antagonize the antitumor effect of 5-fluorouracil (5-FU) both *in vitro* and *in vivo*.[216] Allopurinol causes an increase in plasma concentrations of orotic acid. The 5-fluorouracil is converted to its active metabolite, 5-fluorouridine monophosphate, through the action of the enzyme orotate phosphoribosyltransferase. Orotic acid is an inhibitor of orotate phosphoribosyltransferase, and the elevated levels of orotic acid found after allopurinol administration decrease the activation of 5-FU. Certain tumor cell lines, however, seem to activate 5-FU through a different series of enzyme reactions.

REFERENCES

1. Burchenal JH, Murphy ML, Ellison RR, et al. Clinical evaluation of a new antimetabolite, 6-mercaptopurine, in the treatment of leukemia and allied diseases. *Blood* 1953; 8:965–999.
2. Lancaster DL, Lennard L, Rowland K, et al. Thioguanine versus mercaptopurine for therapy of childhood lymphoblastic leukaemia: a comparison of haematological toxicity and drug metabolite concentrations. *Br J Haematol* 1998;102:439–443.
3. Murray JE, Merrill JP, Harrison JH, et al. Prolonged survival of human kidney homografts by immunosuppressive drug therapy. *N Engl J Med* 1963;268:1315–1323.
4. Lennard L. The clinical pharmacology of 6-mercaptopurine. *Eur J Clin Pharmacol* 1992;43:329–339.
5. Fernandes JF, LePage GA, Linder A. The influence of azaserine and 6-mercaptopurine on the in vivo metabolism of ascites tumor cells. *Cancer Res* 1956;16:154–161.
6. Ling Y-H, Chan JY, Beattie KL, et al. Consequences of 6-thioguanine incorporation into DNA on polymerase, ligase, and endonuclease reaction. *Mol Pharmacol* 1992;42:802–807.
7. Tidd DM, Patterson ARP. Distinction between inhibition of purine nucleotide synthesis and the delayed cytotoxic reaction of 6-mercaptopurine. *Cancer Res* 1974;34:733–737.
8. Waters TR, Swann PF. Cytotoxic mechanism of 6-thioguanine: L Mut S, the human mismatch binding heterodimer binds to DNA containing S⁶-methythioguanine. *Biochemistry* 1997;36:2501–2506.
9. Swann PF, Waters TR, Moulton DC, et al. Role of postreplicative DNA mismatch repair in the cytotoxic action of thioguanine. *Science* 1996;273:1109–1111.

10. Fairchild CR, Maybaum J, Kennedy KA. Concurrent unilateral chromatic damage and DNA strand breakage in response to 6-thioguanine treatment. *Biochem Pharmacol* 1986;35:3533–3541.

11. Pan BF, Nelson JA. Characterization of the DNA damage in 6-thioguanine treated cells. *Biochem Pharmacol* 1990;40:1063–1069.

12. Erb N, Harms DO, Janka-Schaab G. Pharmacokinetics and metabolism of thiopurines in children with acute lymphoblastic leukemia receiving 6-thioguanine versus 6-mercaptopurine. *Cancer Chemother Pharmacol* 1998;42:266–272.

13. Elion GB. Significance of azathioprine metabolites. *Proc R Soc Med* 1972;65:257–260.

14. Ding TL, Benet LZ. Determination of 6-mercaptopurine and azathioprine in plasma by high-performance liquid chromatography. *J Chromatogr* 1979;163:281–288.

15. Lavi L, Holcenberg JS. A rapid sensitive high performance liquid chromatography assay for 6-mercaptopurine metabolites in red blood cells. *Anal Biochem* 1985;144:514–521.

16. Zimm S, Collins JM, Riccardi R, et al. Variable bioavailability of oral mercaptopurine. Is maintenance chemotherapy in acute lymphoblastic leukemia being optimally delivered? *N Engl J Med* 1983;308:1005–1009.

17. Arndt CAS, Balis FM, McCully CL, et al. Bioavailability of low-dose vs high-dose 6-mercaptopurine. *Clin Pharmacol Ther* 1988;43:588–591.

18. Loo TL, Luce JK, Sullivan MP, et al. Clinical pharmacologic observations on 6-mercaptopurine and 6-mercaptopurine ribonucleotide. *Clin Pharmacol Ther* 1968;9:180–194.

19. Jacqz-Aigrain E, Nafa S, Medard Y, et al. Pharmacokinetics and distribution of 6-mercaptopurine administered intravenously in children with lymphoblastic leukaemia. *Eur J Clin Pharmacol* 1997;53:71–74.

20. Balis FM, Holcenberg JS, Poplack DG, et al. Pharmacokinetics and pharmacodynamics of oral methotrexate and mercaptopurine in children with lower risk acute lymphoblastic leukemia; a joint Children's Cancer Group and Pediatric Oncology Branch study. *Blood* 1998;92:3569–3577.

21. Zimm S, Collins JM, O'Neill D, et al. Chemotherapy: inhibition of first-pass metabolism in cancer interaction of 6-mercaptopurine and allopurinol. *Clin Pharmacol Ther* 1983;34:810–817.

22. Zimm S, Ettinger LJ, Holcenberg JS, et al. Phase I and clinical pharmacological study of mercaptopurine administered as a prolonged intravenous infusion. *Cancer Res* 1985;45:1869–1873.

23. Balis FM, Holcenberg JS, Zimm S, et al. The effect of methotrexate on the bioavailability of oral 6-mercaptopurine. *Clin Pharmacol Ther* 1987;41:384–387.

24. Lafolie P, Hayder S, Bjork O, et al. Intraindividual variation in 6-mercaptopurine pharmacokinetics during oral maintenance therapy of children with acute lymphoblastic leukemia. *Eur J Clin Pharmacol* 1991;40:599–601.

25. Kato Y, Matsushita T, Chiba K, et al. Dose-dependent kinetics of orally administered 6-mercaptopurine in children with leukemia. *J Pediatr* 1991;119:311–316.

26. Kato Y, Matsushita T, Uchida H, et al. Rectal bioavailability of 6-mercaptopurine in children with acute lymphoblastic leukemia: partial avoidance of "first-pass" metabolism. *Eur J Clin Pharmacol* 1992;42:619–622.

27. Burton NK, Barnett MJ, Aherne GW, et al. The effect of food on the oral administration of 6-mercaptopurine. *Cancer Chemother Pharmacol* 1986;18:90–91.

28. Burton NK, Aherne GW. The effect of cotrimoxazole on the absorption of orally administered 6-mercaptopurine in the rat. *Cancer Chemother Pharmacol* 1986;16:81–84.

29. Weinshilboum RM. Methyltransferase pharmacogenetics. *Pharmacol Ther* 1989;43:77–90.

30. Weinshilboum RM, Sladek SK. Mercaptopurine pharmacogenetics: monogenic inheritance of erythrocyte thiopurine methyltransferase activity. *Am J Hum Genet* 1980;32:651–662.

31. Szumlanski CL, Honchel R, Scott MC, et al. Human liver thiopurine methyltransferase pharmacogenetics: biochemical properties, liver-erythrocyte correlation and presence of isoenzymes. *Pharmacogenetics* 1992;2:148–159.

32. Coulthard SA, Howell C, Robson J, et al. The relationship between thiopurine methyltransferase activity and genotype in blasts from patients with acute leukemia. *Blood* 1998;92:2856–2862.

33. Lennard L, Rees CA, Lilleyman JS, et al. Childhood leukemia: a relationship between intracellular 6-mercaptopurine metabolites and neutropenia. *Br J Clin Pharmacol* 1983;16:359–363.

34. Lennard L, VanLoon JA, Weinshilboum RM. Pharmacogenetics of acute azathioprine toxicity: relationship to thiopurine methyltransferase genetic polymorphism. *Clin Pharmacol Ther* 1989;46:149–154.

35. Jones CD, Smart C, Titus A, et al. Thiopurine methyltransferase activity in a sample population of black subjects in Florida. *Clin Pharmacol Ther* 1993;53:348–353.

36. Lennard L, Lilleyman JS, Van Loon JA, et al. Genetic variation in response to 6-mercaptopurine for childhood acute lymphoblastic leukemia. *Lancet* 1991;336:225–229.

37. Szumlanski C, Otterness D, Her C, et al. Thiopurine methyltransferase pharmacogenetics: human gene cloning and characterization of a common polymorphism. *DNA Cell Biol* 1996;15:17–30.

38. Otterness D, Szumlanski C, Lennard L, et al. Human thiopurine methyltransferase pharmacogenetics: gene sequences polymorphisms. *Clin Pharmacol Ther* 1997;62:60–73.

39. Tai HL, Krynetski EY, Yates CR, et al. Thiopurine 5-methyltransferase deficiency: two nucleotide transitions define the most prevalent mutant allele associated with loss of catalytic activity in Caucasians. *Am J Hum Genet* 1996;58:694–702.

40. Yates CR, Krynetski EY, Loennechen T, et al. Molecular diagnosis of thiopurine 5-methyltransferase deficiency: genetic basis for azathioprine and mercaptopurine intolerance. *Ann Intern Med* 1997;126:608–614.

41. Koren G, Ferrazini G, Sulh H, et al. Systemic exposures to mercaptopurine as a prognostic factor in acute lymphocytic leukemia. *N Engl J Med* 1990;323:17–21.

42. Hayder S, Lafolie P, Bjork O, et al. 6-Mercaptopurine plasma levels in children with acute lymphoblastic leukemia: relationship to relapse risk and myelotoxicity. *Ther Drug Monit* 1989;11:617–622.

43. Lennard L, Lilleyman JS. Variable 6-mercaptopurine metabolism and treatment outcome in childhood lymphoblastic leukemia. *J Clin Oncol* 1989;7:1816–1823.

44. Pinkel D. Intravenous mercaptopurine; life begins at 40. *J Clin Oncol* 1993;11:1826–1831.

45. Lokick J, Moore C, Anderson N, et al. Phase I–II trial of 14 day infusional 6-mercaptopurine in advanced colorectal cancer. *Eur J Cancer* 1998;34:584–585.

46. LePage GA, Whitecar JP. Pharmacology of 6-thioguanine in man. *Cancer Res* 1971;31:1627–1631.

47. Brox LW, Birkett L, Belch A. Clinical pharmacology of oral thioguanine in acute myelogenous leukemia. *Cancer Chemother Pharmacol* 1981;6:35–38.

48. Konits PH, Egorin MJ, Van Echo DA, et al. Phase II evaluation and plasma pharmacokinetics of high dose intravenous 6-thioguanine in patients with colorectal carcinoma. *Cancer Chemother Pharmacol* 1982;8:199–203.

49. Kitchen BJ, Balis FM, Poplack DG, et al. A pediatric phase I trial and pharmacokinetic study of thioguanine administered by continuous i.v. infusion. *Clin Cancer Res* 1997;3:713–717.

50. Liliemark J, Petterson B, Lafolie P, et al. Determination of plasma azathioprine and 6-mercaptopurine in patients with rheumatoid arthritis treated with oral azathioprine. *Ther Drug Monit* 1990;12:339–343.

51. Chan CLC, Erdmen GR, Gruber SA, et al. Azathioprine metabolism: pharmacokinetics of 6-mercaptopurine, 6-thiouric acid and 6-thioguanine nucleotides in renal transplant patients. *J Clin Pharm* 1990;30:358–363.

52. Burchenal JH, Ellison RR. Pyrimidine and purine antagonists. *Clin Pharmacol Ther* 1961;2:523–541.

53. Einhorn M, Davidson I. Hepatotoxicity of 6-mercaptopurine. *JAMA* 1964;188:802–806.

54. Kirsschner BS. Safety of azathioprine and 6-mercaptopurine in pediatric patients with inflammatory bowel disease. *Gastroenterology* 1998;115:813–821.

55. Clark PN, Hsia YE, Huntsman RG. Toxic complications of treatment with 6-mercaptopurine. *BMJ* 1960;1:393–395.

56. Duttera MJ, Caralla RL, Gallelli JF. Hematuria and crystalluria after high-dose 6-mercaptopurine administration. *N Engl J Med* 1972;287:292–294.

57. Blatt J, Muluhill JJ, Ziegler JL, et al. Pregnancy outcome following cancer chemotherapy. *Am J Med* 1980;69:828–832.

58. Kovach JS, Rubin J, Creagan ET, et al. Phase I trial of parenteral 6-thioguanine given on 5 consecutive days. *Cancer Res* 1986;46:5959–5962.

59. Gill RA, Onstad GR, Cardmore JM, et al. Hepatic veno-occlusive disease caused by 6-thioguanine. *Ann Intern Med* 1982;96:58–60.

60. Cochrane D, Adamson AR, Halsey JP. Adverse reactions to azathioprine mimicking gastroenteritis. *J Rheumatol* 1987;14:1075–1077.

61. Fields CK, Robinson JW, Roy TM, et al. Hypersensitivity reaction to azathioprine. *South Med J* 1998;91:471–474.

62. Silman AJ, Petrie J, Hazelman B, et al. Lymphoproliferative cancer and other malignancy in patients with rheumatoid arthritis treated with azathioprine: a 20 year follow-up study. *Ann Rheum Dis* 1988;47:988–992.

63. Kwong AL, Au WY, Liang RH. Acute myeloid leukemia after azathioprine treatment for autoimmune disease association with -7/7q-. *Cancer Genet Cytogenet* 1998;104:94–97.

64. Confavreux C, Saddier P, Grimaud J, et al. Risk of cancer from azathioprine therapy in multiple sclerosis: a case-control study. *Neurology* 1996;46:1607–1612.

65. Black AJ, McLeod HL, Capell HA, et al. Thiopurine methyltransferase genotype predicts therapy-limiting severe toxicity from azathioprine. *Ann Intern Med* 1998;129:716–718.

66. Stolk JN, Boerbooms AM, deAbreu RA, et al. Reduced thiopurine methyltransferase activity and development of side effects of azathioprine treatment in patients with rheumatoid arthritis. *Arthritis Rheum* 1998;41:1858–1866.

67. Lennard L, Welch JC, Lilleyman JS. Thiopurine drugs in the treatment of childhood leukaemia: the influence of inherited thiopurine methyltransferase activity on drug metabolism and cytotoxicity. *Br J Clin Pharmacol* 1997;44:455–461.

68. Kennedy DT, Hayney MS, Lake KD. Azathioprine and allopurinol: the price of an avoidable drug interaction. *Ann Pharmacother* 1996;30:951–954.

69. Sorensen JM, Vena DA, Fallavollita A, et al. Treatment of refractory chronic lymphocytic leukemia with fludarabine phosphate via the group C protocol mechanism of the National Cancer Institute: five-year follow-up report. *J Clin Oncol* 1997;15:458–465.

70. Johnson S, Smith AG, Loffler H, et al. Multicentre prospective randomized trial of fludarabine versus cyclophosphamide, doxorubicin, and prednisone (CAP) for treatment of advanced-stage chronic lymphocytic leukaemia. The French Cooperative Group on CLL. *Lancet* 1996;347:1432–1438.

71. Leblond V, Ben-Othman T, Deconinck E, et al. Activity of fludarabine in previously treated Waldenström's macroglobulinemia: a report of 71 cases. *J Clin Oncol* 1998;16:2060–2064.

72. Fidias P, Chabner BA, Grossbard ML. Purine analogs for the treatment of low-grade lymphoproliferative disorders. *Oncologist* 1996;1:125–139.

73. Adkins JC, Peters DH, Markham A. Fludarabine. An update of its pharmacology and use in the treatment of haematological malignancies. *Drugs* 1997;53:1005–1037.

74. Gandhi V, Nowak B, Keating MJ, et al. Fludarabine potentiates metabolism of cytarabine in patients with acute myelogenous leukemia during therapy. *J Clin Oncol* 1993;11:116–124.

75. Danhauser L, Plunkett W, Keating M, et al. 9-β-D-arabinofuranosyl-2-fluoroadenine 5'-monophosphate pharmacokinetics in plasma and tumor cells of patients with relapsed leukemia and lymphoma. *Cancer Chemother Pharmacol* 1986;18:145–152.

76. Sirotnak FM, Chello PL, Dorick DM, et al. Specificity of systems mediating transport of adenosine, 9-β-D-arabinofuranosyl-2-fluoroadenine, and other purine nucleoside analogues in L1210 cells. *Cancer Res* 1983;43:104–109.

77. Dow LW, Bell DE, Poulakos L, et al. Differences in metabolism and cytotoxicity between 9-β-D-arabinofuranosyladenine and 9-β-D-arabinofuranosyl-2-fluoroadenine in human leukemic lymphoblasts. *Cancer Res* 1980;40:1405–1410.

78. Huang P, Chubb S, Plunkett W. Termination of DNA synthesis by 9-beta-D-arabinofuranosyl-2-fluoroadenine. A mechanism for cytotoxicity. *J Biol Chem* 1990;265:16617–16625.

79. Parker WB, Ashok RB, Shen SX, et al. Interaction of the 2-halogenated dATP analogs (F, Cl, and Br) with human DNA polymerase, DNA primase and ribonucleotide reductase. *Mol Pharmacol* 1988;34:485–491.

80. Catapan CV, Chandler KB, Fernandes DJ. Inhibition of primer RNA formation in CCRF-CEM leukemia cells by fludarabine triphosphate. *Cancer Res* 1991;51:1829–1835.

81. Yang SW, Huang P, Plunkett W, et al. Dual mode of inhibition of purified DNA ligase I from human cells by 9-beta-D-arabinofuranosyl-2-fluoroadenine triphosphate. *J Biol Chem* 1992;267:2345–2349.

82. Huang P, Robertson LE, Wright S, et al. High molecular weight DNA fragmentation: a critical event in nucleoside analog-induced apoptosis in leukemic cells. *Clin Cancer Res* 1995;1:1005–1013.

83. Kamiya K, Huang P, Plunkett W. Inhibition of the 3'→5' exonucleases of human DNA polymerase epsilon by fludarabine-terminated DNA. *J Biol Chem* 1996;271:19428–19435.

84. Plunkett W, Gandhi V. Cellular metabolism of nucleoside analogs in CLL: implications for drug development. In: Cheson BE, ed. *Chronic lymphocytic leukemia: scientific advances and clinical developments.* New York: Marcel Dekker, 1993:197–219.

85. Plunkett W, Begleiter A, Liliemark O, et al. Why do drugs work in CLL? *Leuk Lymphoma* 1996;22[Suppl 2]:1–11.

86. Sandoval A, Consoli U, Plunkett W. Fludarabine-mediated inhibition of nucleotide excision repair induces apoptosis in quiescent human lymphocytes. *Clin Cancer Res* 1996;2: 1731–1741.

87. Li L, Keating MJ, Plunkett W, et al. Fludarabine mediated repair inhibition of cisplatin-induced DNA lesions in human chronic myelogenous leukemia-blast crisis K567 cells: induction of synergistic cytotoxicity independent of reversal of apoptosis resistance. *Mol Pharmacol* 1997;52: 798–806.

88. Malspeis L, Grever MR, Staubus AE, et al. Pharmacokinetics of 2-F-ara-A (9-β-D-arabinofuranosyl-2-fluoroadenine) in cancer patients during the phase I clinical investigation of fludarabine phosphate. *Semin Oncol* 1990;17[Suppl 8]:18–32.

89. Kemena A, Fernandez M, Bauman J, et al. A sensitive fluorescence assay for quantitation of fludarabine and metabolites in biological fluids. *Clin Chim Acta* 1991;200:95–106.

90. Danhauser L, Plunkett W, Liliemark J, et al. Comparison between the plasma and intracellular pharmacology of 1-β-D-arabinofuranosyl-2-fluoroadenine 5'-monophosphate in patients with relapsed leukemia. *Leukemia* 1987;1:638–643.

91. Hersh MR, Kuhn JG, Phillips JL, et al. Pharmacokinetic study of fludarabine phosphate (NSC 312887). *Cancer Chemother Pharmacol* 1986;17:277–280.

92. Avramis VI, Champagne J, Sato J, et al. Pharmacology of fludarabine phosphate after a phase I/II trial by a loading bolus and continuous infusion in pediatric patients. *Cancer Res* 1990;50:7226–7231.

93. Kemena A, Keating M, Plunkett W. Oral bioavailability of plasma fludarabine and fludarabine triphosphate (F-ara-ATP) in peripheral CLL cells. *Onkologie* 1991;14:83.

94. Von Hoff DD. Phase I clinical trials with fludarabine phosphate. *Semin Oncol* 1990;17[Suppl 8]:33–38.

95. Juliusson G. Complications in the treatment of CLL with purine analogues. *Hematol Cell Ther* 1997;39[Suppl I]:41–44.

96. Hochster HS, Kim KM, Green MD, et al. Activity of fludarabine in previously treated non-Hodgkin's low-grade lymphoma: results of an Eastern Cooperative Oncology Group study. *J Clin Oncol* 1992;10:28–32.

97. Keating MJ, O'Brien S, Lerner S, et al. Long-term follow-up of patients with chronic lymphocytic leukemia (CLL)

98. Anaissie EJ, Kontoyiannis DP, O'Brien S, et al. Infections in patients with chronic lymphocytic leukemia treated with fludarabine. *Ann Intern Med* 1998;129:559–566.

99. Byrd JC, Hargis JB, Kester KE, et al. Opportunistic pulmonary infections with fludarabine in previously treated patients with low-grade lymphoid malignancies: a role for *Pneumocystis carinii* pneumonia prophylaxis. *Am J Hematol* 1995;49:135–142.

100. Weiss RB, Freiman J, Kweder SL, et al. Hemolytic anemia after fludarabine therapy for chronic lymphocytic leukemia. *J Clin Oncol* 1998;16:1885–1889.

101. Gonzalez H, Leblond V, Azar N, et al. Severe autoimmune hemolytic anemia in eight patients treated with fludarabine. *Hematol Cell Ther* 1998;40:113–118.

102. Cheson BD, Frame JN, Vena D, et al. Tumor lysis syndrome: an uncommon complication of fludarabine therapy of chronic lymphocytic leukemia. *J Clin Oncol* 1998;16: 2313–2320.

103. Cheson BD, Vena DA, Foss FM, et al. Neurotoxicity of purine analogs: a review. *J Clin Oncol* 1994;12:2216–2228.

104. Cohen RB, Abdallah JM, Gray JR, et al. Reversible neurologic toxicity in patients treated with standard-dose fludarabine phosphate for mycosis fungicides and chronic lymphocytic leukemia. *Ann Intern Med* 1993;118:114–116.

105. Hurst PG, Habib MP, Garewal H, et al. Pulmonary toxicity associated with fludarabine monophosphate. *Invest New Drugs* 1987;5:207–210.

106. Cheson BD. The purine analogs—a therapeutic beauty contest. *J Clin Oncol* 1992;3:352–355.

107. Rai K, Peterson B, Kolitz J, et al. Fludarabine induces a high complete remission rate in previously untreated patients with active chronic lymphocytic leukemia. A randomized inter-group study. *Blood* 1995;86:607a(abst).

108. Redman JR, Cabanillas F, Velasquez WS, et al. Phase II trial of fludarabine phosphate in lymphoma: an effective new agent in low-grade lymphoma. *J Clin Oncol* 1992;10:790–794.

109. Decaudin D, Bossq J, Tertian G, et al. Phase II trial of fludarabine monophosphate in patients with mantle-cell lymphomas. *J Clin Oncol* 1998;16:579–583.

110. Foss FM, Ihde DC, Linnoila IR, et al. Phase II trial of fludarabine phosphate and interferon alfa-2a in advanced mycosis fungoides/Sezary syndrome. *J Clin Oncol* 1994;12: 2051–2059.

111. Estey E, Plunkett W, Gandhi V, et al. Fludarabine and arabinosylcytosine therapy of refractory and relapsed acute myelogenous leukemia. *Leuk Lymphoma* 1993;9:343–350.

112. Seymour JF, Huang P, Plunkett W, et al. Influence of fludarabine on pharmacokinetics and pharmacodynamics of cytarabine: implications for a continuous infusion schedule. *Clin Cancer Res* 1996;2:653–658.

113. Gandhi V, Estey E, Du M, et al. Minimum dose of fludarabine for the maximal modulation of 1-beta-D-arabinofuranosylcytosine triphosphate in human leukemia blasts during therapy. *Clin Cancer Res* 1997;3:1539–1545.

114. Gandhi V, Huang P, Chapman AJ, et al. Incorporation of fludarabine and 1-beta-D-arabinofuranosylcytosine 5'-triphosphates by DNA polymerase alpha: affinity, interaction and consequences. *Clin Cancer Res* 1997;3:1347–1355.

receiving fludarabine regimens as initial therapy. *Blood* 1998;92:1165–1171.

115. Agarwal RP. Inhibitors of adenosine deaminase. *Pharmacol Ther* 1982;17:399–429.

116. Grever MR, Siaw MFE, Jacob WF, et al. The biochemical and clinical consequences of 2-deoxycoformycin in refractory lymphoproliferative malignancy. *Blood* 1981;57:406–417.

117. Jackson RC, Leopold WR, Ross DA. The biochemical pharmacology of (2'R)-chloropentostatin, a novel inhibitor of adenosine deaminase. *Adv Enzyme Regul* 1986;25:125–139.

118. O'Dwyer PJ, Wagner B, Leyland-Jones B, et al. 2'-Deoxycoformycin (pentostatin) for lymphoid malignancies. *Ann Intern Med* 1988;108:733–743.

119. Chello PL, Sirotnak FM, Yang CH, et al. Initial rate kinetics and evidence for durability of mediated transport of adenosine, related purine nucleosides and nucleoside analogues in L1210 cells. *Cancer Res* 1983;43:97–103.

120. Wiley JS, Smith CL, Jamieson GP. Transport of 2'deoxycoformycin in human leukemic and lymphoma cells. *Biochem Pharmacol* 1991;42:708–710.

121. Agarwal RP, Spector T, Parks RE. Tight-binding inhibitors—IV. Inhibition of adenosine deaminase by various inhibitors. *Biochem Pharmacol* 1977;26:359–367.

122. Smyth JF, Prentice HG, Proctor S, et al. Deoxycoformycin in the treatment of leukemias and lymphomas. *Ann N Y Acad Sci* 1985;451:123–128.

123. Huang AT, Logue GL, Engelbrecht HL. Two biochemical markers in lymphocyte subpopulations. *Br J Haematol* 1976;34:631–638.

124. Johnston JB, Glazer RI, Pugh L, et al. The treatment of hairy-cell leukaemia with 2'-deoxycoformycin. *Br J Haematol* 1986;63:525–534.

125. Spiers AS, Parekh SJ, Bishop MB. Hairy-cell leukemia: induction of complete remission with pentostatin (2'deoxycoformycin). *J Clin Oncol* 1984;2:1336–1342.

126. Al-Razzak KA, Benedetti AE, Waugh WN, et al. Chemical stability of pentostatin (NSC-218321), a cytotoxic and immunosuppressant agent. *Pharm Res* 1990;7:452–460.

127. Kane BJ, Kuhn JG, Roush MK. Pentostatin: an adenosine deaminase inhibitor for the treatment of hairy cell leukemia. *Ann Pharmacother* 1992;26:939–946.

128. Smyth JF, Paine RM, Jackman AL, et al. The clinical pharmacology of the adenosine deaminase inhibitor 2'deoxycoformycin. *Cancer Chemother Pharmacol* 1980;5:93–101.

129. Schneider R, Korngold G, Vale K, et al. Clinical and pharmacologic investigation of deoxycoformycin. *Proc Am Assoc Cancer Res* 1980;21:185(abst).

130. Malspeis L, Weinrib AB, Staubus AE, et al. Clinical pharmacokinetics of 2'-deoxycoformycin. *Cancer Treat Symp* 1984;2:7–15.

131. Major PP, Agarwal RP, Kufe DW. Deoxycoformycin: neurological toxicity. *Cancer Chemother Pharmacol* 1981;5: 193–196.

132. Cassileth PA, Cheuvart B, Spiers ASD, et al. Pentostatin induces durable remissions in hairy cell leukemia. *J Clin Oncol* 1991;9:243–246.

133. Gribbin TE. New purine analogues for the treatment of chronic B-cell malignancies. *Henry Ford Hosp Med J* 1991;39:98–102.

134. Grem JL, King SA, Chun HG, et al. Cardiac complications observed in elderly patients following 2'deoxycoformycin therapy. *Am J Hematol* 1991;38:245–247.

135. Ho AD, Thaler J, Mandelli F, et al. Response to pentostatin in hairy cell leukemia refractory to interferon alpha. *J Clin Oncol* 1989;7:1533–1538.

136. Cheson BD. Current approaches to the chemotherapy of B-cell chronic lymphocytic leukemia: a review. *Am J Hematol* 1989;32:72–77.

137. Lofters W, Campbell M, Gibbs WN, et al. 2'-Deoxycoformycin therapy in adult T-cell leukemia/lymphoma. *Cancer* 1987;60:2605–2608.

138. Cummings FJ, Kim K, Neiman RS, et al. Phase II trial of pentostatin in refractory lymphomas and cutaneous T-cell disease. *J Clin Oncol* 1991;9:565–571.

139. Riddell S, Johnston JB, Rayner HL, et al. Response of Waldenström's macroglobulinemia to pentostatin (2'-deoxycoformycin). *Cancer Treat Rep* 1985;70:546–548.

140. Belch RA, Henderson JF, Brox LW. Treatment of multiple myeloma with deoxycoformycin. *Cancer Chemother Pharmacol* 1985;14:49–52.

141. Grever MR, Crowley J, Salmon S, et al. Phase II investigation of pentostatin in multiple myeloma: a Southwest Oncology Group study. *J Natl Cancer Inst* 1990;82:1778–1779.

142. Avery TL, Rehg JE, Lumm WC, et al. Biochemical pharmacology of 2-chlorodeoxyadenosine in malignant human hematopoietic cell lines and therapeutic effects of 2-bromodeoxyadenosine in drug combinations in mice. *Cancer Res* 1989;49:4972–4978.

143. Kawasaki H, Carrera CJ, Piro LO, et al. Relationship of deoxycytidine kinase and cytoplasmic 5' nucleotidase to the chemotherapeutic efficacy of 2-chlorodeoxyadenosine. *Blood* 1993;81:597–601.

144. Seto S, Carrera CJ, Kubota M, et al. Mechanism of deoxyadenosine and 2-chlorodeoxyadenosine toxicity to nondividing human lymphocytes. *J Clin Invest* 1985;75:377–383.

145. Hentosh P, Kools R, Blakley RL. Incorporation of 2-halogen-2'-deoxyadenosine 5-triphosphates into DNA during replication by human polymerases alpha and beta. *J Bio Chem* 1990;265:4033–4040.

146. Cohen GM. Caspace: the executioners of apoptosis. *Biochem J* 1997;326:1–16.

147. Liu X, Zou H, Slaughter C, et al. DFF, a heterodimeric protein that functions down stream of caspace-3 to trigger DNA fragmentation during apoptosis. *Cell* 1997;89:175–184.

148. Leoni LM, Chao Q, Cottam HB, et al. Induction of an apoptotic program in cell free extracts by 2-chloro-2'deoxyadenosine 5' triphosphate and cytochrome C. *Proc Natl Acad Sci U S A* 1998;95:9567–9571.

149. Beutler E, Piro LD, Saven A, et al. 2-Chlorodeoxyadenosine (2-CdA): a potent chemotherapeutic and immunosuppressive nucleoside. *Leuk Lymphoma* 1991;5:1–8.

150. Carson DA, Wasson DB, Beutler E. Antileukemic and immunosuppressive activity of 2-chloro-2'-deoxyadenosine. *Proc Natl Acad Sci U S A* 1984;81:2232–2236.

151. Liliemark J, Pettersson B, Juliusson G. Determination of 2-chloro-2'-deoxyadenosine in human plasma. *Biomed Chromatogr* 1991;5:262–264.

152. Liliemark J, Juliusson G. Cellular pharmacokinetics of 2-chloro-2'-deoxyadenosine nucleotides: comparison of intermittent and continuous intravenous infusion and subcutaneous and oral administration in leukemia patients. *Clin Cancer Res* 1995;1:385–390.

153. Liliemark J. The clinical pharmacokinetics of cladribine. *Clin Pharmacokinet* 1997;32:120–131.

154. Albertioni F, Lindemalm S, Reichelova V, et al. Pharmacokinetics of cladribine and its 5′ monophosphate and 5′ triphosphate in leukemic cells of patients with chronic lymphocytic leukemia. *Clin Cancer Res* 1998;4:653–658.

155. Liliemark J, Juliusson G. On the pharmacokinetics of 2-chloro-2′-deoxyadenosine in humans. *Cancer Res* 1991; 51:5570–5572.

156. Kearns CM, Blakley RL, Santana VM, et al. Pharmacokinetics of cladribine (2-chlorodeoxyadenosine) in children with acute leukemia. *Cancer Res* 1994;54:1235–1239.

157. Albertioni F, Pettersson B, Reichelovà V, et al. Analysis of 2-chloro-2′-deoxyadenosine in human blood samples and urine by high-performance liquid chromatography using solid phase extraction. *Ther Drug Monit* 1995;16:413–418.

158. Lilliemark J, Albertioni F, Hansen M, et al. On the bioavailability of oral and subcutaneous 2-chloro2′-deoxyadenosine in humans: alternative routes of administration. *J Clin Oncol* 1992;10:1514–1518.

159. Saven A, Kawasaki H, Carrera CJ, et al. 2-Chlorodeoxyadenosine dose escalation in nonhematological malignancies. *J Clin Oncol* 1993;11:671–678.

160. Gandhi V, Estey E, Keating MJ, et al. Chlorodeoxyadenosine and arabinosylcytosine in patients with acute myelogenous leukemia: pharmacokinetic, pharmacodynamic, and molecular interactions. *Blood* 1996;87:256–264.

161. Piro LD, Carrera CJ, Carson DA, et al. Lasting remission in hairy-cell leukemia induced by a single infusion of 2-chlorodeoxyadenosine. *N Engl J Med* 1990;322:1117–1121.

162. Cheson BD. Infectious and immunosuppressive complications of purine analog therapy. *J Clin Oncol* 1995;13:2431–2448.

163. Van den Neste E, Delannoy A, Vandercam B, et al. Infectious complications after 2-chlorodeoxyadenosine therapy. *Eur J Haematol* 1996;56:235–240.

164. Hoffman M, Tallman MS, Hakimian D, et al. 2-Chlorodeoxyadenosine is an active salvage therapy in advanced indolent non-Hodgkin's lymphoma. *J Clin Oncol* 1994;12:788–792.

165. Betticher DC, von Rohr A, Ratschiller D, et al. Fewer infections, but maintained antitumor activity with lower-dose vs standard-dose cladribine in pretreated low-grade non-Hodgkin's lymphoma. *J Clin Oncol* 1998;16:850–858.

166. Chasty RC, Myint H, Oscier DG, et al. Autoimmune haemolysis in patients with B-CLL treated with chlorodeoxyadenosine (CDA). *Leuk Lymphoma* 1998;29:391–398.

167. Larfars G, Uden-Blohme AM, Samuelsson J. Fludarabine, as well as 2-chlorodeoxyadenosine, can induce eosinophilia during treatment of lymphoid malignancies. *Br J Haematol* 1996;94:709–712.

168. Piro LD, Carrera CJ, Beutler E, et al. 2-Chlorodeoxyadenosine: an effective new agent for the treatment of chronic lymphocytic leukemia. *Blood* 1988;72:1069–1073.

169. Saven A, Lemon RH, Kosty M, et al. 2-Chlorodeoxyadenosine activity in patients with untreated chronic lymphocytic leukemia. *J Clin Oncol* 1995;13:570–574.

170. Saven A, Piro LD. Complete remissions in hairy-cell leukemia with 2-chlorodeoxyadenosine after failure with 2-deoxycoformycin. *Ann Intern Med* 1983;119:278–283.

171. Kay AC, Saven A, Carrera CJ, et al. 2-Chlorodeoxyadenosine treatment of low-grade lymphomas. *J Clin Oncol* 1992;10:371–377.

172. Kuzel TM, Hurria A, Samuelson E, et al. Phase II trial of 2-chlorodeoxyadenosine for the treatment of cutaneous T-cell lymphoma. *Blood* 1996;87:906–911.

173. Dimopoulos MA, Kantarjian H, Weber D, et al. Primary therapy of Waldenström's macroglobulinemia with 2-chlorodeoxyadenosine. *J Clin Oncol* 1994;12:2694–2698.

174. Dann EJ, Anastasi J, Larson RA. High-dose cladribine therapy for chronic myelogenous leukemia in the accelerated or blast phase. *J Clin Oncol* 1998;16:1498–1504.

175. Betticher DC, Ratschiller D, Hsu Schmitz SF, et al. Reduced dose of subcutaneous cladribine induces identical response rates but decreased toxicity in pretreated chronic lymphocytic leukaemia. Swiss Group of Clinical Cancer Research (SAKK). *Ann Oncol* 1998;9:721–726.

176. Juliusson G, Christiansen I, Hansen MM, et al. Oral cladribine as primary therapy for patients with B-cell chronic lymphocytic leukemia. *J Clin Oncol* 1996;14:2160–2166.

177. Romine JS, Sipe JC, Koziol JA, et al. A double-blind, placebo-controlled, randomized trial of cladribine in relapsing-remitting multiple sclerosis. *Proc Assoc Am Physicians* 1999;111:35–44.

178. Schirmer M, Mur E, Pfeiffer KP, et al. The safety profile of low-dose cladribine in refractory rheumatoid arthritis. A pilot trial. *Scand J Rheumatol* 1997;26:376–379.

179. Spector T. Inhibition of urate production by allopurinol. *Biochem Pharmacol* 1977;26:355–358.

180. Yu TF, Gutman AB. Effect of allopurinol on serum and urinary uric acid in primary and secondary gout. *Am J Med* 1964;37:885–898.

181. Klinenberg JG, Goldfinger SE, Seegmiller JE. The effectiveness of the xanthine oxidase inhibitor allopurinol in the treatment of gout. *Ann Intern Med* 1965;62:639–647.

182. Caskey CT, Ashton DM, Wyngaarden JB. Enzymology of feedback inhibition of glutamine phosphoribosylpyrophosphate aminotransferase by purine ribonucleotide. *J Biol Chem* 1964;239:2570–2579.

183. Kelley WN, Rosenbloom FM, Miller J, et al. An enzymatic basis for variation in response to allopurinol. *N Engl J Med* 1968;278:287–293.

184. Fox IH, Wyngaarden JB, Kelley WN. Depletion of erythrocyte phosphoribosylpyrophosphate in man; a newly observed effect of allopurinol. *N Engl J Med* 1970;283:1177–1182.

185. Applebaum SJ, Mayersohn M, Dorr RT, et al. Allopurinol kinetics and bioavailability; intravenous, oral and rectal administration. *Cancer Chemother Pharmacol* 1982;8:93–98.

186. Elion GB, Kovensky A, Hitching GH, et al. Metabolic studies of allopurinol, an inhibitor of xanthine oxidase. *Biochem Pharmacol* 1966;15:863–880.

187. Elion GB, Yu FT, Gutman AB, et al. Renal clearance of oxipurinol, the chief metabolite of allopurinol. *Am J Med* 1968;45:69–77.

188. Walter-Sack I, deUries JX, Frei M, et al. Uric acid lowering effect of oxipurinol sodium in hyperuricemic patients—therapeutic equivalence to allopurinol. *J Rheumatol* 1996;23:498–501.

189. Hande KR, Reed E, Chabner BA. Allopurinol kinetics. *Clin Pharmacol Ther* 1978;23:598–605.

190. Graham S, Day RO, Wong H, et al. Pharmacodynamics of oxipurinol after administration of allopurinol to healthy subjects. *Br J Clin Pharmacol* 1996;41:299–304.

191. Hande KR, Noone RM, Stone WJ. Severe allopurinol toxicity; description and guidelines for prevention in patients with renal insufficiency. *Am J Med* 1984;76:47–56.

192. Kumar A, Edward N, White MI, et al. Allopurinol, erythema multiforme and renal insufficiency. *BMJ* 1996; 312:173–174.

193. Hayes CP, Metz EN, Robinson RR, et al. The use of allopurinol to control hyperuricemia in patients on chronic intermittent hemodialysis. *Trans Am Soc Artif Intern Organs* 1965;11:247–251.

194. Berlinger WG, Park G, Spector R. The effect of dietary protein on the clearance of allopurinol and oxipurinol. *N Engl J Med* 1985;313:771–776.

195. Park GD, Berlinger WG, Spector R, et al. Sustained reductions in oxipurinol renal clearance during a restricted diet. *Clin Pharmacol Ther* 1987;41:616–621.

196. Boston Collaborative Drug Surveillance Program. Excess of ampicillin rash associated with allopurinol or hyperuricemia. *N Engl J Med* 1972;286:505–507.

197. Lockard O, Harmon C, Nolph K, et al. Allergic reaction to allopurinol with cross-reactivity to oxipurinol. *Ann Intern Med* 1976;85:333–335.

198. Fam AG, Lewtas J, Stein J, et al. Desensitization to allopurinol in patients with gout and cutaneous reactions. *Am J Med* 1992;93:299–302.

199. McInnes GT, Lawson DH, Jick HJ. Acute adverse reactions attributed to allopurinol in hospitalized patients. *Ann Rheum Dis* 1981;40:245–249.

200. Goldfinger S, Klinenberg JF, Seegmiller JE. The renal excretion of oxipurines. *J Clin Invest* 1965;44:623–628.

201. Band PR, Silverberg DS, Henderson JF, et al. Xanthine nephropathy in a patient with lymphosarcoma treated with allopurinol. *N Engl J Med* 1970;283:354–357.

202. Ablin A, Stephens B, Hirata T, et al. Nephropathy, xanthinuria and orotic aciduria complicating Burkitt's lymphoma treated with chemotherapy and allopurinol. *Metabolism* 1972;21:771–778.

203. Green ML, Fujimoto WY, Seegmiller JE. Urinary xanthine stones—a rare complication of allopurinol therapy. *N Engl J Med* 1969;280:426–427.

204. Hande KR, Perini R, Putterman G, et al. Hyperxanthinemia interferes with serum uric acid determinations by the uricase method. *Clin Chem* 1979;25:1492–1494.

205. Rodnan GP, Robin JA, Tolchin SF, et al. Allopurinol and gouty hyperuricemia. *JAMA* 1975;231:1143–1147.

206. Rieselbach RE, Bentzel CJ, Cotlove E, et al. Uric acid excretion and renal function in the acute hyperuricemia of leukemia. *Am J Med* 1964;37:872–884.

207. Hande KR. Hyperuricemia, uric acid nephropathy and the tumor lysis syndrome. In: McKinney TD, ed. *Renal complications of neoplasia.* New York: Praeger, 1986:134–156.

208. DeConti RC, Calabresi P. Use of allopurinol for prevention and control of hyperuricemia in patients with neoplastic disease. *N Engl J Med* 1966;274:481–486.

209. Krakoff IH, Meyer RL. Prevention of hyperuricemia in leukemia and lymphoma: use of allopurinol, a xanthine oxidase inhibitor. *JAMA* 1965;193:1–6.

210. Hande KR, Hixon C, Chabner B. Postchemotherapy purine excretion in lymphoma patients receiving allopurinol. *Cancer Res* 1981;41:2273–2279.

211. Andreoli S, Clark J, McGuire W, et al. Purine excretion during tumor lysis in children with acute lymphocytic leukemia receiving allopurinol; relationship to acute renal failure. *J Pediatr* 1986;109:292–298.

212. Hande KR, Garrow GC. Acute tumor lysis syndrome in patients with high-grade non-Hodgkin's lymphoma. *Am J Med* 1993;94:133–139.

213. Cummins D, Sekar M, Halil O, et al. Myelosuppression associated with azathioprine-allopurinol interaction after heart and lung transplantation. *Transplantation* 1996;61:1661–1662.

214. Tjandramaga TB, Cucinell SA, Israili ZH. Observations on the disposition of probenecid in patients receiving allopurinol. *Pharmacology* 1972;8:259–272.

215. Hande KR. Evaluation of a thiazide-allopurinol drug interaction. *Am J Med Sci* 1986;29:213–216.

216. Woolley PV, Ayoob MJ, Smith FP, et al. A controlled trial of the effect of 4-hydroxypyrozolopyrimidine (allopurinol) on the toxicity of a single bolus dose of 5-fluorouracil. *J Clin Oncol* 1985;3:103–109.

11

HYDROXYUREA

LUIS PAZ-ARES
ROSS C. DONEHOWER

In the more than 30 years since \hydroxyurea (HU) was first evaluated clinically, this drug has remained of interest for both clinical and laboratory investigators. A number of unique and surprisingly diverse biologic effects have been identified for HU, which have led to exploration of its clinical utility in treating a wide range of malignant and nonmalignant diseases. Its use has been encouraged by the fact that the drug can be administered orally and that the toxicity in most patients is very modest. HU has been an invaluable probe for the laboratory study of its intracellular target, ribonucleotide reductase (RR), the enzyme catalyzing the rate-limiting step in the *de novo* synthesis of deoxyribonucleotide triphosphates (dNTPs) in DNA synthesis and an important enzyme in DNA repair processes. The key features of this drug are shown in Table 11-1.

HU (Fig. 11-1) was originally synthesized in Germany in 1869,[1] but its potential biologic significance was not recognized until 1928 when leukopenia and megaloblastic anemia were observed in experimental animals treated with this compound.[2] In the 1950s the drug was evaluated in a large number of experimental murine tumor models and was found to have broad antitumor activity against both leukemia and solid tumors.[3,4] Clinical trials with HU began in the 1960s. Based on studies of the structure-activity relationships,[5] a number of other aliphatic and aromatic compounds containing both the carbonyl group and the —NOH group were synthesized and tested in experimental tumor systems.[6-11] Other structural classes have been studied as well,[12,13] and although several of these compounds are more potent inhibitors of RR *in vitro* than HU, no significant therapeutic advantage could be demonstrated in experimental systems. Several of these other inhibitors of RR have reached clinical trial, including guanazole and various thiosemicarbazones, but none has demonstrated clear advantages over HU.[14-17]

The principal use of HU has been as a myelosuppressive agent in the myeloproliferative syndromes, particularly chronic myelogenous leukemia (CML) and polycythemia vera. The efficacy of HU as initial therapy for CML has

been known for a number of years,[18-21] although its use had been traditionally reserved for patients whose disease was no longer responsive to busulfan. Currently, HU is preferred over busulfan as initial chemotherapy treatment in CML for several reasons. As suggested by the initial uncontrolled studies, HU prolongs the chronic phase of CML, delaying blastic transformation, and improves survival. A prospective, randomized multicenter study performed by the German CML Study Group involving patients with early chronic-phase disease has shown the advantage of HU over busulfan in duration of the chronic phase (47 versus 37 months) and survival (58.2 versus 45.4 months).[22] A subsequent trial performed by the same group confirmed these results.[23] Data from the International Bone Marrow Transplant Registry also showed that busulfan therapy, but not HU therapy, given before allogeneic stem cell transplantation adversely affects posttransplantation survival.[24] In addition, because HU has less effect on hematopoietic stem cells, the prolonged cytopenias occasionally observed with busulfan are rarely encountered with HU.[20,21] Finally, the leukemogenic potential of HU may be less than that of busulfan.

The role of conventional chemotherapy agents in the treatment of CML has dramatically changed since the introduction of interferon-α. Four randomized trials from Japan, the United Kingdom, Italy, and Germany compared interferon-α therapy with chemotherapy (HU or busulfan).[23,25-27] In all trials, rates of major and complete cytogenetic responses and rates of survival were significantly higher among patients receiving interferon-α than among those receiving conventional chemotherapy. A recent meta-analysis of seven randomized trials comparing interferon-α treatment with chemotherapy confirmed better survival with interferon-α treatment than with either HU ($p = .001$) or busulfan ($p < .001$).[28] Five-year survival rates were 57% with interferon-α and 42% with chemotherapy. A detailed analysis of these studies reveals that the evidence for superiority of interferon-α over HU comes from trials in which the cytokine was given in combination with che-

TABLE 11-1. KEY FEATURES OF HYDROXYUREA

Mechanism of action:	Inhibitor of ribonucleotide reductase by inactivation of the tyrosyl free radical on the M-2 subunit.
	Allosteric inhibition of other enzymes in the replitase complex by cross-inhibition.
	Regulation of gene expression.
Pharmacokinetics:	Nonlinear at high doses.
	Bioavailability of essentially 100%.
	Elimination half-life of 3.5–4.5 h.
	Rapid distribution to tissues and extracellular fluid compartments.
Elimination/ metabolism:	Renal excretion predominates, although interpatient variability is significant.
	Several enzyme systems capable of metabolism of hydroxyurea exist, but the extent of metabolism in humans is not known.
Drug interactions:	Increases metabolism of cytosine arabinoside (ara-C) to active metabolite and the incorporation of arabinosylcytosine triphosphate into DNA.
	Enhances the effects of other antimetabolites.
	Increases the phosphorylation of antiviral nucleosides and favors their incorporation into viral DNA.
	Enhances effects of ionizing radiation.
Toxicity:	Myelosuppression, with white blood cells affected to a greater extent than platelets or red blood cells.
	Gastrointestinal effects (nausea, vomiting, changes in bowel habits, ulceration).
	Dermatologic effects (pigmentation, leg ulcers, erythema, rash, atrophy).
	Renal effects, rare.
	Hepatic effects, occasionally severe.
	Neurologic effects, rare.
	Acute interstitial lung disease, rare.
Precautions:	Decrease dosage in renal failure until patient tolerance demonstrated.
	When given with concomitant radiotherapy, anticipate increased tissue reaction.
	Use with caution when combined with ara-C or other antimetabolites.
	Use with caution in pregnant or lactating women.

motherapy [HU or, less frequently, busulfan or cytosine arabinoside (cytarabine, or ara-C)].[29] In fact, the only trial that compared monotherapy treatment with interferon-α and treatment with HU did not show significant differences in outcome.[23] Taken collectively, these data suggest that in patients for whom bone marrow transplantation is not an option, the combination of interferon-α and HU (or ara-C or both) is a reasonable choice for initial treatment of CML.[29,30] For patients who are not candidates for interferon-α therapy, who opt for a less toxic treatment alternative, or whose disease has unfavorable prognostic features, single-agent HU treatment is a reasonable option.

Since the introduction of HU by the Polycythemia Vera Study Group in the 1970s, data have accumulated on the efficacy and safety of this drug in the treatment of essential thrombocythemia and polycythemia vera.[31–33] With careful management, HU has been found to be effective in controlling thrombocytosis and elevated hematocrit of polycythemia vera patients, as well as diminishing the risk of thrombosis relative to a control group.[34,35] The trend for improved survival in patients given HU may suggest a decrease in events related to thrombosis, which further supports the view that in patients with essential thrombocythemia, as well as polycythemia vera, HU can effectively lessen the risk of thrombosis.[32,35] Other purported advantages for HU included a lower risk of leukemogenesis than with treatment using ^{32}P or the bifunctional alkylating agent chlorambucil.[31] Increasing concern has been expressed, however, about the risk of secondary leukemia with HU treatment in these diseases. Some authors have not found an increased risk of leukemic conversion with HU treatment,[33,36,38] but a significant risk has been noted in other studies, particularly in patients also exposed to other drugs.[32,37,39,40] Adequately designed controlled prospective studies are required to resolve this issue, but existing data suggest that long-term risk of leukemia may be increased. All these controversies make the choice of optimal therapy for these two diseases an area of active debate. Therapy for individual patients must be chosen on the basis of age, concurrent medical problems, and degree of risk from the disease to minimize treatment-related complications and maximize potential benefit. HU (with phlebotomy) is possibly the treatment of choice for high-risk polycythemia vera patients, whereas nonleukemogenic alternatives (interferon and anagrelide hydrochloride) may be considered for

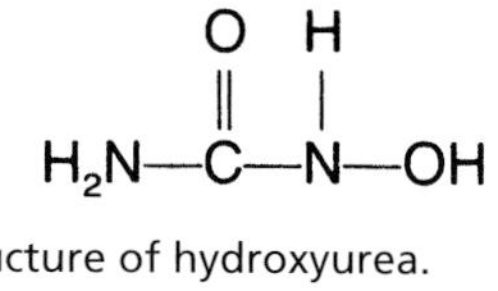

$$
\underset{\text{H}_2\text{N}}{}-\overset{\overset{\text{O}}{\|}}{\text{C}}-\overset{\overset{\text{H}}{|}}{\text{N}}-\text{OH}
$$

FIGURE 11-1. Structure of hydroxyurea.

younger patients and those at low risk of thrombotic complications. Likewise, the risk-benefit analysis of HU treatment in patients with high-risk essential thrombocythemia may favor the use of HU for elderly patients and anagrelide for younger ones.

HU has been evaluated as therapy for a number of advanced solid tumors, and although responses were seen in early studies of several diseases, including malignant melanoma, squamous cell cancer of the head and neck, renal cell carcinoma, transitional cell carcinoma of the urothelium, and prostate cancer, the level of activity was modest. HU cannot be considered to be standard therapy either as a single agent or as part of the standard chemotherapy regimen for any solid tumor.[41] A number of studies of solid tumor disease have focused on the potential role of HU as a biochemical modulator of the effects of other antimetabolites such as ara-C, gemcitabine hydrochloride, fludarabine phosphate, and 5-fluorouracil (5-FU), or DNA-damaging agents such as etoposide or cisplatin.[42] Perhaps the most widely studied interaction has been that with 5-FU, in which the synergistic effect of HU is attributed to decreases in deoxyuridine nucleotides (deoxyuridine monophosphate, deoxyuridine triphosphate). This may result in enhanced 5-fluorodeoxyuridylate thymidylate synthase inhibition by decreasing competitive substrate, as well as in decreased repair of DNA strand breaks after excision of uracil residues. A number of pilot clinical trials have been performed, but a specific role for this combination remains to be defined.

HU has been studied extensively as a potential radiosensitizing agent. The rationale for this was based initially on studies demonstrating that HU was able to synchronize cells in a radiation-sensitive phase of the cell cycle.[43] This effect also may occur as a result of HU inhibition of the repair of radiation-induced DNA damage.[44,45] This interaction has been studied clinically since the 1970s in several diseases, including cervical carcinoma, primary brain tumors, head and neck cancer, and non–small cell lung cancer. The most convincing evidence for a benefit from the addition of HU was seen in early studies of locally advanced cancer of the uterine cervix, in which a consistent advantage has been found in progression-free survival for women with stage III to IVA disease.[46–48] More recent trials, however, have shown the superiority of cisplatin-based chemotherapy over HU as concomitant treatment to radiotherapy in this specific setting.[49–51] Promising results have also been reported with the use of HU-containing schedules and concurrent radiotherapy in treatment of locally advanced head and neck cancer.[52,53]

Several groups of investigators have been evaluating the use of HU and other S-phase–specific chemotherapeutic agents to treat sickle cell anemia for a number of years. Initially, uncontrolled studies demonstrated an increase in the production of fetal hemoglobin, accompanied by an amelioration of symptoms, in patients treated with HU.[54,55]

This effect is also demonstrable *in vitro* by the incubation of HU with erythroid progenitors.[56] Whether the induction of fetal hemoglobin represents a response to inhibition of DNA synthesis in red cell progenitors or a specific alteration of hemoglobin F transcription is uncertain.[57,58] Convincing evidence now exists that induction of hemoglobin F is not the only, and perhaps not the major, contributor to the drug's efficacy.[59,60] The benefit from HU may be due in part to its ability to suppress both erythropoiesis and myelopoiesis. A marked decrease in the endothelial adhesion of patients' red blood cells is observed after 2 weeks of HU therapy, coincident with a decrease in absolute reticulocyte levels, and occurs before hemoglobin F levels start to raise.[59] A strong inverse correlation between neutrophil count and crisis rate have been noticed.[61] In terms of clinical efficacy, a randomized, double-blind study has demonstrated that long-term treatment with HU decreases the incidence of painful crisis by 44% in adult patients with sickle cell disease.[61,62] HU treatment also reduced the frequency of acute chest syndrome and hospitalization, and the need for blood transfusion. This establishes HU as the first clinically acceptable drug shown to decrease crises in sickle cell disease. HU appears to be as effective in children with sickle cell disease and in patients with sickle cell–β-thalassemia and sickle cell–hemoglobin C disease, although only a small number of individuals have been treated and the studies were uncontrolled.[63–66]

HU may serve as an important model for agents that contribute to inhibition of the replication of human immunodeficiency virus (HIV) by a mechanism other than targeting of a viral enzyme or a structural protein. The ability of HU to decrease intracellular levels of dNTPs first led Lori et al. to propose using the compound to inhibit HIV replication.[67] Subsequent studies have confirmed this effect and have focused on the anti-HIV mechanism of action of HU and its synergistic interactions with other antiretroviral compounds, particularly the nucleoside reverse transcriptase inhibitors such as didanosine.[68–72] Currently available clinical data, including those from several uncontrolled studies and four randomized trials, reveal that HU has little activity as a single agent but produces a pronounced inhibition of HIV replication when combined with didanosine or with didanosine plus stavudine in patients who have not been heavily pretreated.[72–76] Importantly, HU appears to maintain the activity of the nucleoside reverse transcriptase inhibitors even in the presence of genotypic mutations of the HIV characteristically associated with resistance.[70,72,73] The anti-HIV effect of HU is not consistently accompanied by an increase in the CD4+ lymphocyte count. The lack of such an increase has been attributed to the cytostatic activity of the drug and has uncertain clinical relevance. The antiviral activity of HU is induced at low doses, typically 1,000 mg orally daily, that cause minimal toxicity. Questions about the role of the compound in the treatment of HIV infection that remain to be answered include its effectiveness in boosting immune function, the most appropriate dosage regimen, the timing of individual doses, its role in salvage therapy, and the risk associated with long-term use in this context.

Finally, the revisited interest in HU as salvage treatment for chronic plaque psoriasis is probably worth mentioning.[77] One-half to two-thirds of the patients obtain a clinically valuable response, usually evident within 2 to 3 weeks of starting treatment. Disease refractoriness to other forms of therapy does not appear to preclude response to HU.

MECHANISM OF ACTION AND CELLULAR PHARMACOLOGY

The primary site of cytotoxic action for HU is inhibition of the RR enzyme system. This highly regulated enzyme system is responsible for the conversion of ribonucleotide diphosphates to the deoxyribonucleotide form, which can subsequently be used in either *de novo* DNA synthesis or DNA repair.[78] HU can be shown to inhibit RR *in vitro*,[79–81] and the extent of inhibition of DNA synthesis observed in HU-treated cells correlates closely with the size of the decreased deoxyribonucleotide pools.[82–84] This enzyme has an important role as a rate-limiting reaction in the regulation of DNA synthesis. In human and other mammalian cells this unique enzyme consists of two different subunits, usually referred to as M-1 and M-2.[85–88] Protein M-1 is a dimer with a molecular weight of 170 kd and contains the binding site for the substrates as well as the allosteric effector sites.[88] This subunit is responsible for the complex regulation of the enzyme by cellular nucleotide pools. Although considerable variability exists among enzymes from various tissue sources, the general regulatory effects are summarized in Table 11-2.[89–91] The reduction of all substrates is inhibited and the enzyme complex dissociates in the presence of deoxyadenosine triphosphate.[86] Protein M-1 is present at a relatively constant level throughout the cell cycle, except in cells in G_0 or those that have undergone terminal differentiation, in which it is markedly decreased.[92] The gene coding for this protein can be mapped to chromosome 11.[93,94]

TABLE 11-2. REGULATORY EFFECTS OF NUCLEOTIDE TRIPHOSPHATE ON RIBONUCLEOTIDE REDUCTASE

Substrate	Activators	Inhibitors
CDP	ATP	dATP, dGTP
UDP		dUTP, dTTP, dATP
ADP	dGTP, GTP	dATP, dTTP
GDP	dTTP	dATP, dGTP

ADP, adenosine diphosphate; ATP, adenosine triphosphate; CDP, cytidine diphosphate; dATP, deoxyadenosine triphosphate; dGTP, deoxyguanosine triphosphate; dTTP, deoxythymidine triphosphate; dUTP, deoxyuridine triphosphate; GDP, guanosine diphosphate; GTP, guanosine triphosphate; UDP, uridine diphosphate.

Protein M-2 is the catalytic subunit of the enzyme and exists as a dimer with a molecular weight of 88 kd. This unique protein contains stoichiometric amounts of iron and a stable organic free radical localized to a tyrosine residue. The fully conserved tyrosyl radical is essential to enzyme activity and is localized in proximity to and stabilized by the binuclear nonheme iron complex.[79,95,96] The cellular concentration of M-2 protein is variable throughout the cell cycle; it peaks in S phase, which suggests that functional enzyme activity is dependent on the concentration of M-2 protein.[97,98] The M-2 subunit sequences have been mapped to chromosome 2 in human cells and seem to be in the same amplification unit as the gene for ornithine decarboxylase.[99,100] Studies have identified two genes encoding for the equivalent of the M-1 subunit in *Saccharomyces cerevisiae*, RR1 and RR3.[101] The expression of RR1 is largely cell-cycle regulated, but RR3 is induced by DNA damage and is under the control of a different promoter system than RR1. Two genes are also found that encode for the equivalent of the mammalian M-2 subunit in the same organism: RR2 and RR4.[102] RR4 can also be induced by DNA damage. It has nonoverlapping functions with RR2, and one cannot substitute for the other, even when overexpressed. In fact, RR4 has been proposed to play a key role in the assembly of the diiron-tyrosyl radical cofactor in RR2.[103]

HU seems to enter cells by passive diffusion.[104,105] The inhibition of RR occurs as a result of inactivation of the tyrosyl free radical on the M-2 subunit, with disruption of the enzyme's iron-binding center.[79,106–108] The fact that this inhibition can be partially reversed *in vitro* by ferrous iron[109] and that cytotoxicity can be enhanced by iron-chelating agents[110,111] emphasizes the importance of the nonheme iron cofactor in this process. In *Escherichia coli*, the susceptibility of the tyrosyl radical to inactivation by HU is dependent on the regulatory state of the enzyme.[112] The magnitude of the decreases in cellular deoxyribonucleotide pools seen after HU exposure correlates closely with the degree of inhibition of DNA synthesis.[82,113] HU selectively kills cells in S phase, and within an S-phase population of cells, those that are most rapidly synthesizing DNA are most sensitive.[114–117] The cytotoxic effects of HU correlate with dose or concentration achieved,[82–84] as well as with duration of drug exposure.[115,118] The cell kinetic effects that follow HU exposure involve partial synchronization in G_1 or S phase. Cells progress normally through the cell cycle until they reach the G_1-S interface. Rather than being prevented from entering S phase, as was once thought, cells enter S phase at a normal rate but are accumulated there as a result of the inhibition of DNA synthesis.[119–121] In a Burkitt's lymphoma cell line, cell death has been attributed to apoptosis.[122]

HU induces the expression of proinflammatory cytokine genes, including those for tumor necrosis factor and, to a lesser extent, interleukin 1 and interleukin 6, in *ex vivo* experiments in the rat.[123] This effect was specific to certain genes, because the expression of other cytokines (interleukin 2, interleukin 4, interleukin 10, interferons) was not affected. Further evidence that HU can regulate gene expression comes from a study of Huang et al. These authors showed that the drug modulates the expression of the β-globin gene in patients with β-thalassemia.[124] The mechanism through which HU affects gene expression, in particular whether such action is secondary to RR inhibition, remains to be clarified.

Jiang et al. have demonstrated that HU may be transformed *in vivo* to nitric oxide (NO), which is a known RR inhibitor itself.[125] The possibility therefore exists that the RR inhibition observed after HU exposure may be both direct and mediated through the NO metabolite. Indeed, HU-borne NO may be the intermediate effector in other actions of the drug.[126] Against this hypothesis is the fact that the pharmacologic profile of HU is quite different from that of classical NO donors.

Several of the enzymes involved in DNA polymerization and DNA precursor synthesis are assembled in a replitase complex during S phase of the cell cycle to channel metabolites to enzymes sequentially during the synthetic process.[127–129] Replitase contains DNA polymerases, thymidine kinase, dihydrofolate reductase, nucleoside-5'-phosphate kinase, thymidylate synthase, and RR. Cross-inhibition is a phenomenon observed with enzymes of the replitase complex, in which inhibition of one enzyme in the complex leads to inhibition of a second, unrelated enzyme. This occurs only in intact cells and only in S phase. Evidence suggests that this is the result of a direct allosteric, structural interaction from a remote site within the complex, because disruptions of deoxyribonucleotide pools do not explain the findings.[130] HU appears to be able to inhibit DNA polymerases, thymidylate synthase, and thymidine kinase by this mechanism under certain conditions.

A potentially important consequence of HU action is the acceleration of the loss of extrachromosomally amplified genes present in double-minute chromosomes.[131] Evidence indicates that such acentric extrachromosomal elements are common in the gene amplification process. Exposure to HU at clinically achievable concentrations leads to enhanced loss of both amplified oncogenes[132] and drug-resistance genes.[133] Strategies for use of this phenomenon clinically are under consideration.

MECHANISMS OF CELLULAR RESISTANCE

The principal mechanism by which cells achieve resistance to HU is elevation in cellular RR activity. As noted above, the cellular levels of the M-1 subunit do not change during the cell cycle, whereas levels of the M-2 subunit increase during DNA synthesis, which suggests that functional enzyme activity depends on the M-2 protein. The site of action of HU specifically involves the M-2 subunit, and the increased RR activity seen in resistant cells is due principally to overexpression of this protein.[134–139] Transfection of the human M-2 gene into drug-sensitive KB cells confers resistance by increasing the enzyme activity, and subsequently the dNTP intracellular pools.[140,141] Transfection of the M-1 gene does not result in a decreased sensitivity to HU, although transfected cells resist dNTP inhibition of RR activity, probably due to an alteration of the function of effector binding sites or the affinity of activator-inhibitor provisions.[139–141] Several different molecular mechanisms can contribute to the increased RR activity in HU-resistant cells. A number of cell lines have amplifications of the gene coding for M-2 protein accompanied by an elevation in M-2 messenger RNA (mRNA) and M-2 protein levels.[134,142] As is the case with other examples of drug resistance, the mRNA levels and protein expression are often elevated much above the extent to which the gene has been amplified.[134,136] It also seems that posttranscriptional modifications can occur during drug selection, which results in an increased translational efficiency. An increase in M-2 protein biosynthetic rate can then occur with no further increase in mRNA levels.[134,136] Indeed, an overexpression of eukaryotic initiation factor 4E causes a specific translational enhancement of M-2 in Chinese hamster ovary cells.[143] The resulting cells display an altered cell-cycle phenotype similar to that of cells selected for M-2 overexpression with HU. Only when high levels of resistance to HU are reached does amplification of the M1 gene and overexpression of the protein become manifest.[134,138] This dissociation of M-1 and M-2 expression results from the fact that they are regulated by different mechanisms[98,135] and are coded for by genes on different chromosomes. Cells selected for resistance to HU with increased M-2 expression often have coamplification or expression of ornithine decarboxylase, presumably as a result of the proximity of these genes on chromosome 2.[99,142]

The suggestion has been made that some examples of HU resistance may be the result of the production of an RR with decreased sensitivity to HU inhibition.[144,145] Subsequent studies, however, have not supported this possibility.[146] In bacteria, mechanisms other than those affecting RR have been associated with HU resistance and include increased expression of a phosphotransferase that inactivates the drug[147] and amplification of a gene coding for a phosphoinositide-specific phospholipase.[148] The relationship of this enzyme to drug resistance in humans is not clear.

In most studies, HU resistance has been associated with parallel decreased sensitivity to other RR inhibitors and often to other antimetabolites.[149–151] Interestingly, some inhibitors of the M-2 subunit, including the new compound triapine (3-aminopyridine-2-carboxaldehyde thiosemicarbazone, or 3-AP), retain their antitumor effect in HU-resistant cell lines.[17,149] In addition, some of these cell lines with increased RR activity display an increased sensitivity to nucleotide analogs such as 6-thioguanine (via increased conversion to the deoxynucleotide and enhancement of its incorporation into DNA)[152] or gemcitabine (via increased drug uptake by the cells).[151]

DRUG INTERACTIONS

HU has been studied both in the laboratory and in the clinic as a modulator of ara-C metabolism and cytotoxicity.[42,153,154] Studies have shown a significant increase in formation of arabinosylcytosine triphosphate[153] and its incorporation into DNA[154] in HU-treated cells. The assumption was that this was the result of the decreased cellular levels of deoxycytidine triphosphate expected after HU exposure and the resultant effect that this might have on ara-C metabolism. Certain studies, however, have shown that in some cell lines modulation at the level of deoxycytidine kinase is the result of decreased deoxycytidine, the competitive substrate, rather than decreased feedback inhibition by deoxycytidine triphosphate.[154] Other nucleotide analogs such as gemcitabine, fludarabine, and cladribine appear to interact significantly with HU as evidenced by increased levels of RR activity and of dNTP pools in several cells resistant to the mentioned compounds.[155,156] Some of these drugs, such as gemcitabine and fludarabine, are also RR inhibitors but act at a different site of the M-2 subunit. Iwakasi et al. have shown that nucleotide analogs that inhibit RR (fludarabine, gemcitabine) are preferentially incorporated within replicating DNA in CCRF-CEM cells.[157] By contrast, 60% of DNA ara-C, which does not inhibit RR, was incorporated by repair synthesis. A large proportion of ara-C was incorporated into replicating DNA when cells were pretreated with HU. Therefore, pretreatment with HU affords a better opportunity for analog triphosphates generated by the salvage pathway to compete with dNTPs for incorporation into DNA, and a therapeutic benefit is suggested for combinations of ara-C and RR inhibitors in malignancies with relatively large growth fractions. Clinically, the doses of ara-C must be modified downward when given in combination with HU. No randomized clinical trial has purely assessed the contribution of HU to combination therapy with ara-C. A controlled phase III trial, however, has shown the superiority of interferon-α and HU plus ara-C over interferon-α and HU in patients with newly diagnosed CML.[30] HU also has been shown to increase the toxicity of fludarabine in a small clinical pilot study.[42]

As noted earlier, the major clinical interest in HU in treatment of solid tumors has been in combination with 5-FU. Synergy has been demonstrated in experimental tumor models, presumably based on the ability of HU to lower cellular pools of deoxyuridine monophosphate, the competitive substrate for inhibition of thymidylate synthase by 5-fluorodeoxyuridylate.[18] A number of clinical trials of this combination have been performed, but its role remains uncertain. These two G_1-S arresting agents, 5-FU and HU, have been show *in vitro* to interfere with the cytotoxic effects of antimitotic agents (vinblastine sulfate, colchicine, nocodazole) that produce mitotic arrest and apoptosis.[158] The antimetabolites perturb the ability of the antimitotic drugs to induce bcl-2 phosphorylation and c-raf-1 activation, and to increase the p21[WAF1/CIP1] protein levels, which prevents the majority of cells from progressing to the G_2-M phase.

HU has been evaluated in both clinical and laboratory studies in combination with chemotherapy agents that produce DNA damage, such as alkylating agents, cisplatin, and inhibitors of topoisomerase II.[42] Although synergy has been observed in preclinical testing, the clinical role for such combinations remains speculative. Synchronization in the G_1-S phase drives cells to a condition of increased sensitivity to radiation. Besides, HU exerts a radiosensitizing action through other mechanisms, because it selectively kills cells in the S phase of the cell cycle and significantly affects DNA repair mechanisms after radiation damage.

HU exerts its anti-HIV activity through several mechanisms.[67–73] HU decreases the activation of CD4 T lymphocytes, which limits HIV integration and production.[72] The cytostatic effects of HU also reduce CD8 activation and ultimately prevent CD8 exhaustion and CD4 killing. The antiviral effects of HU related to its ability to block human immunodeficiency virus 1 DNA synthesis and replication in human lymphocytes by decreasing intracellular deoxynucleotides.[67] Synergy has consistently been observed between HU and the 2'-3' dideoxynucleotides, particularly didanosine, in inhibiting viral replication *in vitro* and in clinical trials.[68–76] The depletion of cellular dNTPs by HU favors incorporation into viral DNA of an increased proportion of the nucleoside reverse transcriptase inhibitor. In addition, HU enhances the intracellular phosphorylation of antiviral nucleosides, which increases their activity *in vitro*.[68,70]

CLINICAL PHARMACOLOGY

As the clinical usage of the drug has expanded, a more complete understanding of the clinical pharmacology of HU has become available (Table 11-3). Prior studies had been limited by the use of relatively insensitive colorimetric methods,[159,160] although appropriately sensitive methods, including an HPLC assay with electromechanical detection, have now been developed.[161–168] HU is generally administered orally, and doses are titrated in response to changes in peripheral white blood cell counts. Although significant interpatient variability is observed, peak concentrations of 0.1 to 2.0 mmol per L are achieved 1.0 to 1.5 hours after doses of 15 to 80 mg per kg.[163–168] Oral bioavailability is excellent (80% to 100%), and comparable

TABLE 11-3. SUMMARY OF PHARMACOKINETIC PARAMETERS OF HYDROXYUREA

Study	Dose	Route	N	PK Model	F (%)	$t_{1/2}$ (h)	V_d (L/kg)	C_{max}, C_{min} (mmol/L)	Clearance
Tracewell et al.[167]	1,520 mg/m² q6h 84–315 mg/m² (48–72 h infants)	p.o. i.v.	8 46	Nonlinear[a]	79.2	1.6–4.2[b]	0.186 × body weight (kg) + 25.4		CL_R = 90.8 mL/min CL_{NR} v_{max} = 97 μmol/L/h K_m = 0.32 mmol/L
Veale et al.[169]	1,000 mg/h q6h 1,000 mg/h (48 h infants)	p.o. i.v.	9 9					$C_{ss,av}$ = 1.730 $C_{max,ss}$ = 2 $C_{min,ss}$ = 1	CL = 126.8 mL/min
Villani et al.[163]	500 mg q12h	p.o.	9	Linear One-compartment		2.5		$C_{ss,av}$ = 0.045 $C_{max,ss}$ = 0.135 $C_{min,ss}$ = 0.0085	CL/F = 0.18 L/kg/h
Rodriguez et al.[162]	2,000 mg	p.o. and i.v.	29	Linear Two-compartment	108	3.32 3.39	V_{ss} = 19.71 mg/m²		CL/F = 124 mL/min CL = 106 mL/min

C_{max}, maximum plasma concentration; $C_{max,ss}$, maximum plasma concentration at steady state; C_{min}, minimum plasma concentration; $C_{min,ss}$, minimum plasma concentration at steady state; $C_{ss,av}$, average steady-state plasma concentration; CL, clearance; CL_R, renal clearance; CL_{NR}, nonrenal clearance; F, bioavailability; K_m, binding affinity; N, number of patients; PK, pharmacokinetic; $t_{1/2}$, half-life; V_d, volume of distribution; v_{max}, maximum volume; V_{ss}, steady-state volume.

[a]One-compartment pharmacokinetic model with parallel Michaelis-Menten metabolism and first-order renal excretion.

[b]$t_{1/2}$ was concentration dependent (nonlinear pharmacokinetics).

plasma concentrations are seen after oral and intravenous dosing.[162,167] After attainment of peak plasma concentrations, HU disappears rapidly from plasma. The elimination half-life ranges from 3.5 to 4.5 hours.[167,168] Data available from a comprehensive population pharmacokinetic study of multiple oral and intravenous dosing are best described by a one-compartment model with parallel Michaelis-Menten metabolism and first-order renal excretion.[167] Renal clearance at standard doses is 60 to 90 mL per minute in an average patient, and pharmacokinetics are nonlinear with dose. The volume of distribution is described by the formula 0.186 × (body weight) + 25.4 L. Other studies using a unique dose level (1,000 or 2,000 mg daily) described a correct fit by a one- or two-compartment linear model.[162,163]

Several high-dose 24- to 120-hour continuous-infusion regimens for HU administration, with or without initial loading, have been evaluated.[169–171] Continuous infusion of 1 g per hour for 24 hours is capable of sustaining plasma concentrations in excess of 1 mmol per L. Other investigators have evaluated patient tolerance of long-term infusions and have found that 0.5 g per m² per day was tolerated for 12 weeks, 1 g per m² per day was tolerated for 5 weeks, 1.66 g per m² per day was tolerated for 3 weeks, and 2.5 g per m² per day was tolerated for 1 week.[172] Based on the available data, from the standpoint of pharmacokinetics and bioavailability, administering HU parenterally has no clear advantages, except in those patients with impaired gastrointestinal function.[162]

Although precise guidelines are not available, the prudent course is to modify dosages for patients with abnormal renal function until individual tolerance can be assessed. Unfortunately, pharmacokinetic studies of patients with altered renal function have not been performed to provide guidelines. The full extent and significance of HU metabolism in humans has not been established. Data from several experimental animal systems suggest that the metabolism of HU does occur, but none of these conversions has been demonstrated conclusively in humans. HU is degraded by urease, an enzyme found in intestinal bacteria.[173] Hydroxylamine (NH_2OH), a product of this reaction, has not been identified in humans. Acetohydroxamic acid is found in the plasma of patients receiving HU therapy,[173] however, and may represent the product of a reaction between hydroxylamine and acetylcoenzyme A, a major thioester in mammalian tissues. The conversion of HU to urea in mice has also been reported.[174] An enzyme system capable of this conversion is found in mouse liver, with the greatest activity localized in the mitochondrial subcellular fraction.[175] Similar activity has not been demonstrated in human liver.

HU distributes rapidly to tissues. Studies in rats and mice using radiolabeled HU demonstrate that the drug is found in body tissues in quantities proportional to weight 30 to 60 minutes after injection.[174] The drug readily enters cerebrospinal fluid and third-space collections of fluid such as ascites or pleural effusions. Ratios for simultaneous plasma and cerebrospinal fluid concentrations of 4:1 to 9:1 and for plasma and ascites concentrations of 2:1 to 7.5:1 have been observed.[164] The significance of these ratios is uncertain because they were single points taken at arbitrary times after drug administration, and the time course of disappearance from these extravascular sites was not evaluated. HU is excreted in significant quantities in human breast milk and should be used only with caution, if at all, in women who are breast-feeding infants.[176]

TOXICITY

Regardless of which schedule of administration is used, the dose-limiting toxicity of HU is myelosuppression. This is the direct result of inhibition of DNA synthesis in bone marrow, and megaloblastic changes can be detected in granulocyte and erythroid precursors within 48 hours of the first dose.[19,177] In patients with nonhematologic malignancies, the peripheral white blood cell count begins to fall in 2 to 5 days. Patients with leukemia or myeloproliferative syndromes experience a more rapid fall in white blood cell counts. The rapidity of the effect on the circulating leukemia cell population and the brief duration of its action have been the basis for the use of HU in patients with acute nonlymphocytic leukemia who present with markedly elevated peripheral blood blast counts or in patients with dangerously elevated platelet counts, as in essential thrombocythemia. Whether this provides an advantage over the prompt institution of standard ara-C–containing leukemia therapy has not been demonstrated conclusively.

All patients on dosages of 80 mg per kg per day become leukopenic within 14 days, whereas the incidence is 70% for patients receiving half that amount.[178,179] Intermittent dosing with the higher doses decreases the hematologic toxicity, but the impact on therapeutic effect has not been fully evaluated. Reversal of the HU effect on peripheral white blood cell counts occurs rapidly, but the nadir in platelet count may occur 7 to 10 days later. Treatment of the myeloproliferative syndromes usually begins with much lower dosages of 0.5 to 2.0 g per day, which are titrated to the clinical response. At the low dosages commonly used to treat HIV infection (1.0 to 1.2 g per day), clinically relevant marrow toxicity requiring dose adjustment or discontinuation are rare.

The gastrointestinal side effects of nausea, vomiting, anorexia, and either diarrhea or constipation rarely require discontinuation of therapy at the dosages usually used clinically. Oral mucositis and ulceration of the gastrointestinal tract are less common but may be higher in patients receiving concomitant radiation and HU than in those receiving either therapy alone.

Patients who have taken HU for an extended period may develop one of several dermatologic changes. These include hyperpigmentation, erythema of the face and hands, a more diffuse maculopapular rash, or dry skin with atrophy.[180] Changes in the nails may include atrophy or the formation of multiple pigmented nail bands.[180,181] More severe skin reactions include an ulcerative dermatitis resembling lichen planus.[182] Skin ulcerations, usually in the legs, may occur in patients undergoing long-term treatment for myeloproliferative diseases.[183] Healing or improvement of these ulcers requires cessation of treatment, and anecdotal evidence indicates that topical treatment with granulocyte-macrophage colony-stimulating factor may be beneficial.[184] When concomitant radiation therapy is given, patients receiving HU seem to have an increased tissue reaction and may have a recurrence or "recall" of erythema or hyperpigmentation in previously irradiated areas.[185] Alopecia has been seen rarely.

A number of other, less frequent drug-related effects have been either reported anecdotally or mentioned briefly in the clinical studies already discussed. Transient abnormalities of renal function have been noted in a number of studies and include elevations of serum urea nitrogen and creatinine, proteinuria, and an active urine sediment.[186] Renal failure or severe, prolonged periods of kidney dysfunction have not been reported. Liver function test abnormalities, on the other hand, have been more significant, and occasionally the patient has progressed to clinical jaundice. A more typical pattern has been transient elevation of hepatocellular enzymes.[187] Headache, drowsiness, confusion, and dizziness also have been reported but are of uncertain significance. The frequency of sensorial neuropathy, rarely seen with single-agent HU therapy, is significant in regimens combining HU with didanosine, stavudine, or both.[188] Several cases of acute interstitial lung disease and alveolitis have been reported.[189,190] Drug-induced fever has also been noted.[191]

Due to the mechanism of action of HU, of particular concern are the effects on growth and development and its mutagenic potential (teratogenic and carcinogenic), especially in patients with nonmalignant diseases, who frequently need long-term drug administration. Although the number of studies is limited and the median follow-up is shorter than 3 years, no growth failures or chronic organ damage has been observed in children with sickle cell disease treated with HU. A single study has demonstrated an increased incidence of chromosomal abnormalities in patients treated with HU.[192] HU treatment, especially when HU is combined with other agents, is associated with an incidence of leukemia of 3% to 12% in patients with myeloproliferative syndromes.[30–40] This risk is possibly higher than in patients not treated with cytotoxic drugs and appears to be proportional to the intrinsic leukemogenic risk of the underlying condition (higher in polycythemia vera than in essential thrombocythemia). To date, no secondary leukemia or cancer has occurred in patients with sickle cell disease who have been treated with HU, but fewer than 300 patients have been treated for 5 years.[64] HU has been given for more than 5 years to 64 children with cyanotic heart disease without any reports of tumors.[193] In any case, due to the limited available data, HU should be considered to have uncertain carcinogen potential and should be used with caution to treat nonmalignant diseases. HU is a potent teratogen in all animal species tested so far and qualifies as a universal teratogen; it should not be used in women of childbearing age unless the possibility of pregnancy can be excluded. However, a number of patients who conceived while receiving HU for a variety of hematologic conditions completed normal pregnancies after discontinuation of the drug.[194]

REFERENCES

1. Dresler WFC, Stein R. Uber den Hydroxylharnstoff. *Justus Liebigs Ann Chem* 1869;150:242.
2. Rosenthal F, Wislicki L, Koller L. Uber die Beziehungen von schwersten Blutgiften zu Abbauprodukten des Eiweisses: ein Beitrag zum Entstehungmechanismus der pernizosen Anemie. *Klin Wochenschr* 1928;7:972.
3. Tarnowski GS, Stock CC. Chemotherapy studies on the RC and S790 mouse mammary carcinomas. *Cancer Res* 1958;18:1.
4. Stearns B, Losee KA, Bernstein J. Hydroxyurea: a new type of potential antitumor agent. *J Med Chem* 1963;6:201.
5. Young CW, Schochetman G, Hodas S, et al. Inhibition of DNA synthesis by hydroxyurea: structure-activity relationships. *Cancer Res* 1967;27:535.
6. Gale GR, Hynes JB. Effects of certain arylhydroxamic acids on deoxyribonucleic acid synthesis by Ehrlich ascites tumor cells in vitro. *J Med Chem* 1968;11:191.
7. Gale GR, Hynes JB, Smith AB. Synthesis of additional arylhydroxamic acids which inhibit nucleic acid biosynthesis in vitro. *J Med Chem* 1970;13:571.
8. Van't Riet B, Wampler GL, Elford HL. Synthesis of hydroxy- and amino-substituted benzohydroxamic acids: inhibition of ribonucleotide reductase and antitumor activity. *J Med Chem* 1979;22:589.
9. Elford HL, Wampler GL, van't Riet B. New ribonucleotide reductase inhibitors with antineoplastic activity. *Cancer Res* 1979;39:844.
10. Flora KP, van't Riet B, Wampler GL. Antitumor activity of amidoximes (hydroxyurea analogs) in murine tumor systems. *Cancer Res* 1978;38:1291.
11. Chou JT, Beck WT, Khwaja T, et al. Synthesis and anticancer activity of novel cyclic *N*-hydroxyureas. *J Pharm Sci* 1977;66:1556.
12. Brockman RW, Shaddix S, Laster WR Jr, et al. Inhibition of ribonucleotide reductase, DNA synthesis, and L1210 leukemia by guanazole. *Cancer Res* 1970;30:2358.
13. Agrawal KC, Sartorelli AC. α-[*N*]-Heterocyclic carboxaldehyde thiosemicarbazones. In: Sartorelli AC, Johns DG, eds. *Handbook of experimental pharmacology*, vol 38. New York: Springer-Verlag, 1975:793.
14. DeConti RC, Toftness BR, Agrawal KC, et al. Clinical and pharmacologic studies with 5-hydroxy-2-formylpiridine thiosemicarbazone. *Cancer Res* 1972;32:1455.
15. Yakar D, Holland JF, Ellison RR, et al. Clinical pharmacological trial of guanazole. *Cancer Res* 1973;33:972.
16. Veale D, Carmichael J, Cantwell BM, et al. A phase I and pharmacokinetic study of didox: a ribonucleotide reductase inhibitor. *Br J Cancer* 1988;58:70.
17. Finch RA, Liu MC, Cory AH, et al. Triapine (3-aminopyridine-2-carboxaldehyde thiosemicarbazone; 3-AP): an inhibitor of ribonucleotide reductase with antineoplastic activity. *Adv Enzyme Regul* 1999;39:3.
18. Fishbein WN, Carbone PP, Freireich EJ, et al. Clinical trials of hydroxyurea in patients with cancer and leukemia. *Clin Pharmacol Ther* 1964;5:574.
19. Kennedy BJ, Yarbro JW. Metabolic and therapeutic effects of hydroxyurea in chronic myelogenous leukemia. *JAMA* 1966;195:1038.
20. Kennedy BJ. Hydroxyurea therapy in chronic myelogenous leukemia. *Cancer* 1972;29:1052.
21. Bolin RW, Robinson WA, Sutherland J, et al. Busulfan versus hydroxyurea in long term therapy of chronic myelogenous leukemia. *Cancer* 1982;50:1683.
22. Hehlmann R, Heimpel H, Hasford J, et al. Randomized comparison of busulfan and hydroxyurea in chronic myelogenous leukemia: prolongation of survival by hydroxyurea. The German CML Study Group. *Blood* 1993;82:398.
23. Hehlmann R, Heimpel H, Hasford J, et al. Randomized comparison of interferon-alpha with busulfan and hydroxyurea in chronic myelogenous leukemia. The German CML Study Group. *Blood* 1994;84:4064.
24. Goldman JM, Szydlo R, Horowitz MM, et al. Choice of pretransplant treatment and timing of transplants for chronic myelogenous leukemia in chronic phase. *Blood* 1993;82:2235.
25. Ohnishi K, Ohno R, Tomonaga M, et al. A randomized trial comparing interferon-α with busulfan for newly diagnosed chronic myelogenous leukemia in chronic phase. *Blood* 1995;86:906.
26. Allan NC, Richards SM, Shepherd PC. UK Medical Council randomized multicentre trial of interferon-α for chronic myeloid leukaemia: improved survival irrespective of cytogenetic response. The UK Medical Research Council's Working Parties for Therapeutic Trials in Adult Leukaemia. *Lancet* 1995;345:1392.
27. Interferon alfa-2a as compared with conventional chemotherapy for the treatment of chronic myeloid leukemia. The Italian Cooperative Study Group on Chronic Myeloid Leukemia. *N Engl J Med* 1994;330:820.
28. Interferon alfa versus chemotherapy for chronic myeloid leukemia: a meta-analysis of seven randomized trials: Chronic Myeloid Leukemia Triallists' Collaborative group. *J Natl Cancer Inst* 1997;89:1616.
29. Silver RT, Woolf SH, Hehlmann R, et al. An evidence-based analysis of the effect of busulfan, hydroxyurea, interferon and allogenic bone marrow transplantation in treating the chronic phase of chronic myeloid leukemia: developed for the American Society of Hematology. *Blood* 1999;94:1517.
30. Guilhot F, Chastang C, Michallet M, et al. Interferon alfa-2b combined with cytarabine versus interferon alone in chronic myelogenous leukemia. *N Engl J Med* 1997;337:223.
31. Wasserman LR. The management of polycythemia vera. *Br J Haematol* 1971;21:371.
32. Steckers Y, Preudhomme C, Lai JL, et al. Acute myeloid leukemia and myelodysplastic syndromes following essential thrombocythemia treated with hydroxyurea: high proportion of cases with 17p depletion. *Blood* 1998;91:616.
33. Frutchman SM, Mack K, Kaplan ME, et al. From efficacy to safety: a Polycythemia Vera Study Group Report on Hydroxyurea in patients with polycythemia vera. *Semin Hematol* 1997;34:17.
34. Barbui T, Finazzi G. Risk factors and prevention of vascular complications in polycythemia vera. *Semin Thromb Hemost* 1997;23:455.
35. Cortelazzo S, Finazzi G, Ruggieri M, et al. Hydroxyurea for patients with essential thrombocythemia and a high risk of thrombosis. *N Engl J Med* 1995;332:1132.

36. Lofvenberg E, Nordenson I, Wahlin A. Cytogenetic abnormalities and leukemia transformation in hydroxyurea-treated patients with Philadelphia chromosome negative myeloproliferative disease. *Cancer Genet Cytogenet* 1990; 49:57.

37. Weinfeld A, Swolin B, Westin J. Acute leukemia after hydroxyurea in polycythemia vera and allied disorders. *Eur J Hematol* 1994;52:134.

38. Murphy S, Peterson P, Iland H, et al. Experience of the Polycythemia Vera Study Group with essential thrombocythemia: a final report on diagnostic criteria, survival, and leukemic transition to treatment. *Semin Hematol* 1997; 34:29.

39. Najean Y, Rain JD, for the French Polycythemia Study Group. Treatment of polycythemia vera: the use of hydroxyurea and pipobroman in 292 patients under the age of 65 years. *Blood* 1997;90:3370.

40. Najean Y, Rain JD. Treatment of the polycythemia vera. A short survey. *Haematologica* 1998;83[Suppl 10]:295.

41. Donehower RC. An overview of the clinical experience with hydroxyurea. *Semin Oncol* 1992;19:11.

42. Schilsky RL, Ratain MJ, Vokes EE, et al. Laboratory and clinical studies of biochemical modulation by hydroxyurea. *Semin Oncol* 1992;19:84.

43. Sinclair WK. The combined effect of hydroxyurea and x-rays on Chinese hamster cells in vitro. *Cancer Res* 1968; 28:198.

44. Fram RJ, Kufe DW. Effect of 1-beta-D-arabinofuranosyl cytosine and hydroxyurea on the repair of x-ray-induced DNA single-strand breaks in human leukemia blasts. *Biochem Pharmacol* 1985;34:2557.

45. Fram RJ, Kufe DW. Inhibition of DNA excision repair and the repair of x-ray-induced DNA damage by cytosine arabinoside and hydroxyurea. *Pharmacol Ther* 1985;31:165.

46. Hreshchyshyn MM, Aron BS, Boronow RC, et al. Hydroxyurea or placebo combined with radiation to treat stages IIIB and IV cervical cancer confined to the pelvis. *Int J Radiat Oncol Biol Phys* 1979;5:317.

47. Piver MS, Vongtama V, Emrich LJ. Hydroxyurea plus pelvic radiation versus placebo plus pelvic radiation in surgically staged stage IIIB cervical cancer. *J Surg Oncol* 1987;35:129.

48. Stehman FB, Bundy BN, Thomas G, et al. Hydroxyurea versus misonidazole with radiation in cervical carcinoma: long-term follow-up of a Gynecologic Oncology Group Trial. *J Clin Oncol* 1993;11:1523.

49. Rose PG, Bundy BN, Watkins EB, et al. Concurrent cisplatin-based radiotherapy and chemotherapy for locally advanced cervical cancer. *N Engl J Med* 1999;340:1144.

50. Whitney RC, Sause W, Bundy BN, et al. Randomized comparison of fluorouracil plus cisplatin versus hydroxyurea as an adjunct to radiation therapy in stage IIB-IVA carcinoma of the cervix with negative para-aortic lymph nodes: a Gynecologic Oncology Group and Southwest Oncology Group study. *J Clin Oncol* 1999;17:1339.

51. Monaghan J. Time to add chemotherapy to radiotherapy for cervical cancer. *Lancet* 1999;353:1288.

52. Haraf DJ, Vokes EE, Panje WR, et al. Survival and analysis of failure following hydroxyurea, 5-fluorouracil and concomitant radiation therapy in poor prognosis head and neck cancer. *Am J Clin Oncol* 1991;14:419.

53. Haraf DJ, Kies M, Rademaker AW, et al. Radiation therapy with concomitant hydroxyurea and fluorouracil in stage II and III head and neck cancer. *J Clin Oncol* 1999;17:638.

54. Charache S, Dover GJ, Moyer MA, et al. Hydroxyurea-induced augmentation of fetal hemoglobin production in patients with sickle cell anemia. *Blood* 1987;69:109.

55. Charache S, Dover GJ, Moore RD, et al. Hydroxyurea: effect on hemoglobin F production in patients with sickle cell anemia. *Blood* 1992;79:2555.

56. Fibache E, Burke KP, Schechter AN, et al. Hydroxyurea increases fetal hemoglobin in cultured erythroid cells derived from normal individuals and patients with sickle cell anemia or beta-thalassemia. *Blood* 1993;81:1630.

57. Miller BA, Platt O, Hope S, et al. Influence of hydroxyurea on fetal hemoglobin production in vitro. *Blood* 1987; 70:1824.

58. Galanello R, Stamatoyannopoulos G, Papayannopoulou T. Mechanism of Hb F stimulation by S-stage compounds: in vitro studies with bone marrow cells exposed to 5-azacytidine, ARA-C, or hydroxyurea. *J Clin Invest* 1988;81:1209.

59. Bridges KR, Barabino GD, Brugnara C, et al. A multiparameter analysis of sickle erythrocytes in patients undergoing hydroxyurea therapy. *Blood* 1996;88:4701.

60. Adragna NC, Fonseca P, Lauf PK. Hydroxyurea affects cell morphology, cation transport, and red blood cell adhesion in cultured vascular endothelial cells. *Blood* 1994;83:533.

61. Charache S, Barton FB, Moore RD, et al. Hydroxyurea and sickle cell anemia: clinical utility of a myelosuppressive "switching agent." *Medicine* 1996;75:320.

62. Charache S, Terrin ML, Moore RD, et al. Effect of hydroxyurea on the frequency of painful crises in sickle cell anemia. *N Engl J Med* 1995;332:1372.

63. Kinney TR, Helms RW, O'Branski EE, et al. Safety of hydroxyurea in children with sickle cell anemia: results of the HUG-KIDS study, a phase I/II trial. *Blood* 1999; 94:1550.

64. Steinberg MH. Management of sickle cell disease. *N Engl J Med* 1999;340:1021.

65. Voskaridou E, Kalotychou V, Loukopoulos D. Clinical and laboratory effects of long-term administration of hydroxyurea to patients with sickle cell/β-thalassemia. *Br J Hematol* 1995;89:479.

66. Steinberg MH, Nagel RL, Brugnara C. Cellular effects of hydroxyurea in Hb SC disease. *Br J Hematol* 1997;98:1078.

67. Lori F, Malykh A, Cara A, et al. Hydroxyurea as an inhibitor of human immunodeficiency virus-type 1 replication. *Science* 1994;266:801.

68. Gao WY, Johns DG, Mitsuya H. Anti-human immunodeficiency virus type 1 activity of hydroxyurea in combination with 2'-3' dideoxynucleotides. *Mol Pharmacol* 1994;46:767.

69. Malley SD, Grange JM, Hamedi-Sangsari F, et al. Synergistic anti-human immunodeficiency virus type 1 effect of hydroxamate compounds with 2'-3' dideoxyinosine in infected resting human lymphocytes. *Proc Natl Acad Sci U S A* 1994;91:11017.

70. Palmer S, Cox S. Increased activation of the combination of 3'-azido-3'-deoxythymidine. *Antimicrob Agents Chemother* 1997;41:460.

71. Gao WY, Johns DG, Chokekuchai S, et al. Disparate actions of hydroxyurea in potentiation of purine and pyrim-

idine 2'-3'-dideoxynucleoside activities against replication of HIV. *Proc Natl Acad Sci U S A* 1995;92:8333.

72. Lori F. Hydroxyurea and HIV: 5 years later—from antiviral to immune-modulation effects. *AIDS* 1999;13:1433.

73. Lori F, Malykh AG, Foli A. Combination of a drug targeting the cell with a drug targeting the virus controls human immunodeficiency virus type I resistance. *AIDS Res Hum Retroviruses* 1997;13:1403.

74. Rutschmann OT, Opravil M, Iten A, et al. A placebo controlled trial of didanosine plus stavudine, with and without hydroxyurea, for HIV infection. The Swiss HIV Cohort Study. *AIDS* 1998;12:F71.

75. Federici ME, Lup S, Cahn P, et al. Hydroxyurea in combination regimens for the treatment of antiretroviral-naïve, HIV-infected adults. Paper presented at: 12th International AIDS Conference, June 28–July 3, 1998; Geneva, Switzerland. Abst 287.

76. Frank I, Boucher H, Fiscus S, et al. Phase I/II dosing study of once daily hydroxyurea alone vs didanosine alone vs ddI + hydroxyurea. Paper presented at: 6th Conference of Retroviruses and Opportunistic Infections; January 31–February 4, 1999; Chicago, IL. Abstr 402.

77. Smith CH. Use of hydroxyurea in psoriasis. *Clin Exp Dermatol* 1999;24:2.

78. Thelander L, Reichard P. Reduction of ribonucleotides. *Annu Rev Biochem* 1979;48:133.

79. Graslund A, Ehrenberg A, Thelander L. Characterization of the free radical of mammalian ribonucleotide reductase. *J Biol Chem* 1982;257:5711.

80. Elford HL. Effect of hydroxyurea on ribonucleotide reductase. *Biochem Biophys Res Commun* 1968;33:129.

81. Turner MK, Abrams R, Lieberman I. Meso-α,β diphenylsuccinate and hydroxyurea as inhibitors of deoxycytidylate synthesis in extracts of Ehrlich ascites and L cells. *J Biol Chem* 1966;241:5777.

82. Nicander B, Reichard P. Relations between synthesis of deoxyribonucleotides and DNA replication in 3T6 fibroblasts. *J Biol Chem* 1986;260:5376.

83. Skoog L, Nordenskjold B. Effects of hydroxyurea and 1-β-D-arabinofuranosyl cytosine on deoxynucleoside triphosphate pools in mouse embryo cells. *Eur J Biochem* 1971;19:81.

84. Plagemann PGW, Erbe J. Intracellular conversions of deoxyribonucleotides by Novikoff rat hepatoma cells and effects of hydroxyurea. *J Cell Physiol* 1974;83:321.

85. Hopper S. Ribonucleotide reductase of rabbit bone marrow: I. Purification, properties, and separation into two protein fractions. *J Biol Chem* 1972;247:3336.

86. Cory JG, Fleischer AE, Munro JB III. Reconstitution of the ribonucleotide reductase in mammalian cells. *J Biol Chem* 1978;253:2898.

87. Change C-H, Cheng Y-C. Demonstration of two components and association of adenosine diphosphate-cytidine diphosphate reductase from cultured human lymphoblast cells (Molt-4F). *Cancer Res* 1979;39:436.

88. Thelander L, Eriksson S, Akerman M. Ribonucleotide reductase from calf thymus. *J Biol Chem* 1980;255:7426.

89. Moore EC, Hurlbert RB. Regulation of mammalian deoxyribonucleotide biosynthesis by nucleotides as activators and inhibitors. *J Biol Chem* 1966;241:4802.

90. Eriksson S, Thelander L, Akerman M. Allosteric regulation of calf thymus ribonucleotide diphosphate reductase. *Biochemistry* 1979;18:2948.

91. Chang C-H, Cheng Y-C. Effects of nucleoside triphosphates on human ribonucleotide reductase from Molt-4F cells. *Cancer Res* 1979;39:5087.

92. Mann GJ, Musgrove EA, Fox RM, et al. Ribonucleotide reductase M1 subunit in cellular proliferation, quiescence, and differentiation. *Cancer Res* 1988;48:5151.

93. Brissenden JR, Caras I, Thelander L, et al. The structural gene for the M1 subunit of ribonucleotide reductase maps to chromosome 11, band 15 in human and to chromosome 7 in mouse. *Exp Cell Res* 1988;174:302.

94. Engstrom Y, Francke U. Assignment of the structural gene for subunit M1 of human ribonucleotide reductase to the short arm of chromosome 11. *Exp Cell Res* 1985;158:477.

95. Sjoberg B-M, Graslund A. Ribonucleotide reductase. *Adv Inorg Biochem* 1983;5:87.

96. Thelander M, Graslund A, Thelander L. Subunit M2 of mammalian ribonucleotide reductase. *J Biol Chem* 1985;260:2737.

97. Eriksson S, Graslund A, Skog S, et al. Cell cycle dependent regulation of mammalian ribonucleotide reductase. *J Biol Chem* 1984;259:11695.

98. Engstrom Y, Eriksson S, Jildevik I, et al. Cell cycle-dependent expression of mammalian ribonucleotide reductase. *J Biol Chem* 1985;260:9114.

99. Yang-Feng TL, Barton DE, Thelander L, et al. Ribonucleotide reductase M2 subunit sequences mapped to four different chromosomal sites in humans and mice: functional locus identified by its amplification in hydroxyurea-resistant cell lines. *Genomics* 1987;1:77.

100. Ask A, Persson L, Rehnholm A, et al. Development of resistance to hydroxyurea during treatment of human myelogenous leukemia K562 cells with α-difluoromethylornithine as a result of coamplification of genes for ornithine decarboxylase and ribonucleotide reductase R2 subunit. *Cancer Res* 1993;53:5263.

101. Elledge SJ, Davis RWD. Two genes differentially regulated in the cell cycle and by DNA damaging agents encode alternative regulatory subunits of ribonucleotide reductase. *Genes Dev* 1990;4:740.

102. Huang M, Elledge SJ. Identification of RNR4, encoding a second essential small subunit of RR in *Saccharomyces cerevisiae*. *Mol Cell Biol* 1997;17:6105.

103. Nguyen H-H, Ge J, Perlstein DL, et al. Purification of ribonucleotide reductase subunits Y1, Y2, Y3, and Y4 from yeast: Y4 plays a key role in diiron cluster assembly. *Proc Natl Acad Sci U S A* 1999;96:1239.

104. Morgan JS, Creasey DC, Wright JA. Evidence that the antitumor agent hydroxyurea enters mammalian cells by a diffusion mechanism. *Biochem Biophys Res Commun* 1986;134:1254.

105. Tagger AY, Boux J, Wright JA. Hydroxy [^{14}C] urea up-take by normal and transformed human cells: evidence for a mechanism of passive diffusion. *Biochem Cell Biol* 1987;65:925.

106. Akerblom L, Ehrenberg A, Graslund A, et al. Overproduction of the free radical of ribonucleotide reductase in hydroxyurea-resistant mouse fibroblast 3T6 cells. *Proc Natl Acad Sci U S A* 1981;78:2159.

107. Nyholm S, Thelander L, Graslund A. Reduction and loss of the iron center in the reaction of the small subunit of mouse ribonucleotide reductase with hydroxyurea. *Biochemistry* 1993;32:11569.

108. McClarty GA, Chan AK, Choy BK, et al. Increased ferritin gene expression is associated with increased ribonucleotide reductase gene expression and the establishment of hydroxyurea resistance in mammalian cells. *J Biol Chem* 1990; 265:7539.

109. Moore EC. The effects of ferrous iron and dithioerythritol on inhibition by hydroxyurea of ribonucleotide reductase. *Cancer Res* 1969;29:291.

110. Satyamoorthy K, Chitnis M, Basrur V. Sensitization of P388 murine leukemia cells to hydroxyurea cytotoxicity by hydrophobic iron-chelating agents. *Anticancer Res* 1986; 6:329.

111. Satyamoorthy K, Chitnis MP, Basrur VS, et al. Potentiation of hydroxyurea cytotoxicity in human chronic myeloid leukemia cells by iron-chelating agent. *Leuk Res* 1986;10:1327.

112. Karlsson M, Sahlin M, Sjoberg BM. *Escherichia coli* ribonucleotide reductase: radical susceptibility to hydroxyurea is dependent on the regulatory state of the enzyme. *J Biol Chem* 1992;267:12622.

113. Bianchi V, Pontis E, Reichard P. Changes of deoxyribonucleoside triphosphate pools induced by hydroxyurea and their relation to DNA synthesis. *J Biol Chem* 1986; 261:16037.

114. Farber E, Baserga R. Differential effects of hydroxyurea on survival of proliferating cells in vivo. *Cancer Res* 1969; 29:136.

115. Sinclair WK. Hydroxyurea: differential lethal effects on cultured mammalian cells during the cell cycle. *Science* 1965;150:1729.

116. Ford SS, Shackney SE. Lethal and sublethal effects of hydroxyurea in relation to drug concentration duration of drug exposure in sarcoma 180 in vitro. *Cancer Res* 1977;37:2628.

117. Kim JH, Gelbard AS, Perez AG. Action of hydroxyurea on the nucleic acid metabolism and viability of HeLa cells. *Cancer Res* 1967;27:1301.

118. Moran RE, Straus MJ. Cytokinetic analysis of L1210 leukemia after continuous infusion of hydroxyurea in vivo. *Cancer Res* 1979;39:1616.

119. Maurer-Schultze B, Siebert M, Bassukas ID. An in vivo study on the synchronizing effect of hydroxyurea. *Exp Cell Res* 1988;174:230.

120. Walters RA, Tobey RA, Hildebrand CE. Hydroxyurea does not prevent synchronized G1 Chinese hamster cells from entering DNA synthetic period. *Biochem Biophys Res Commun* 1976;69:212.

121. Cress AR, Gerner EW. Hydroxyurea inhibits ODC induction, but not the G_1 to S-phase transition. *Biochem Biophys Res Commun* 1979;87:773.

122. Johnson CA, Forster TH, Winterford CM, et al. Hydroxyurea induces apoptosis and regular DNA fragmentation in a Burkitt's lymphoma cell line. *Biochim Biophys Acta* 1992;1136:1.

123. Navarra P, Grohmann U, Nocentini G, et al. Hydroxyurea induces the gene expression and synthesis of proinflammatory cytokines in vivo. *J Pharmacol Exp Ther* 1997;280:477.

124. Huang SZ, Ren ZR, Chen MJ, et al. Treatment of beta-thalassemia with hydroxyurea (HU)-effects of HU on globin gene expression. *Sci China B* 1994;37:1350.

125. Jiang J, Jordan SJ, Barr DP, et al. In vivo production of nitric oxide in rats after administration of hydroxyurea. *Mol Pharmacol* 1997;52:1081.

126. Guittet O, Roy B, Lepoivre M. Nitric oxide: a radical molecule in quest of free radicals in proteins. *Cell Mol Life Sci* 1999;55:1054.

127. Reddy GP, Pardee AB. Multienzyme complex for metabolic channeling in mammalian DNA replication. *Proc Natl Acad Sci U S A* 1980;77:3312.

128. Reddy GP, Pardee AB. Inhibitor evidence for allosteric interaction in the replitase multienzyme complex. *Nature* 1983;304:86.

129. Allen JR, Reddy GP, Lasser GW, et al. T4 ribonucleotide reductase. Physical and kinetic linkage to other enzymes of deoxyribonucleotide biosynthesis. *J Biol Chem* 1980;255:7583.

130. Plucinski TM, Fager RS, Reddy GP. Allosteric interaction of components of the replitase complex is responsible for enzyme cross-inhibition. *Mol Pharmacol* 1990;38:114.

131. Von Hoff DD, Waddelow T, Forseth B, et al. Hydroxyurea accelerates loss of extrachromosomally amplified genes from tumor cells. *Cancer Res* 1991;51:6273.

132. Eckhardt SG, Dai A, Davidson KK, et al. Induction of differentiation in HL60 cells by the reduction of extrachromosomally amplified c-myc. *Proc Natl Acad Sci U S A* 1994; 91:6674.

133. Nevaldine BH, Rizwana R, Hahn PJ. Differential sensitivity of double minute chromosomes to hydroxyurea treatment in cultured methotrexate-resistant mouse cells. *Mutation Res* 1999;406:55.

134. Choy BK, McClarty GA, Chan AK, et al. Molecular mechanisms of drug resistance involving ribonucleotide reductase: hydroxyurea resistance in a series of clonally related mouse cell lines selected in the presence of increasing drug concentrations. *Cancer Res* 1988;48:2029.

135. Wright JA, Alam TG, McClarty GA, et al. Altered expression of ribonucleotide reductase and role of M2 gene amplification in hydroxyurea-resistant hamster, mouse, rat, and human cell line. *Somat Cell Mol Genet* 1987;13:155.

136. McClarty GA, Chan AK, Engstrom Y, et al. Elevated expression of M1 and M2 components and drug-induced posttranscriptional modulation of ribonucleotide reductase in a hydroxyurea-resistant mouse cell line. *Biochemistry* 1987;26:8004.

137. McClarty GA, Tonin PN, Srinivasan PR, et al. Relationships between reversion of hydroxyurea resistance in hamster cells and the coamplification of ribonucleotide reductase M2 component, ornithine decarboxylase and P5-8 genes. *Biochem Biophys Res Commun* 1988;154:975.

138. Cocking JM, Tonin PN, Stokoe NM, et al. Gene for M1 subunit of ribonucleotide reductase is amplified in hydroxyurea-resistant hamster cells. *Somat Cell Mol Genet* 1987; 13:221.

139. Wadler S, Zhang H, Cammer M, et al. Quantification of ribonucleotide reductase expression in wild-type and hydroxyurea-resistant cell lines employing in situ reverse transcriptase polymerase chain reaction and a computerized image system. *Anal Biochem* 1999;267:24.

12

ANTIMICROTUBULE AGENTS

ERIC K. ROWINSKY
ROSS C. DONEHOWER

Microtubules are one of the most strategic subcellular targets of anticancer therapy. Although they are principally recognized as being important for their role in separating the duplicate set of chromosomes during mitosis, microtubules also play critical roles in many interphase functions such as maintenance of cell shape and scaffolding, intracellular transport, secretion, neurotransmission, and possibly the relay of signals between cell surface receptors and the nucleus.[1-6] For the most part, antimicrotubule agents are structurally complex, naturally occurring alkaloids or semisynthetic compounds. Despite their early promise, only two antimicrotubule agents, the vinca alkaloids vincristine sulfate and vinblastine sulfate, were widely used until the late 1980s. The identification of other classes of antimicrotubule agents, however, that possess novel mechanisms of cytotoxic action and unique spectra of antitumor activity, such as the taxanes, epothilones, semisynthetic vinca analogs like vinorelbine tartrate, and estramustine phosphate sodium, has resulted in a resurgence of interest in the microtubule as an important target in cancer chemotherapy.

MICROTUBULE STRUCTURE

Microtubules are composed of molecules of tubulin, each of which is a heterodimer consisting of two tightly linked globular subunits.[1-3] These subunits are related proteins (each consisting of approximately 450 amino acids with a molecular weight of 50,000) called α-tubulin and β-tubulin.[7,8] When tubulin molecules assemble into microtubules, they form linear "protofilaments" with the β-tubulin subunit of one tubulin molecule in contact with the α-tubulin subunit of the next[1,2,9-12] (Fig. 12-1). Microtubules consist of 13 protofilaments aligned side by side around an apparently empty central core. All protofilaments are aligned in parallel with the same "polarity," that is, one end at which assembly is rapid (plus end) and one end at which growth is slow or net disassembly occurs (minus end).

Although at least six forms of both α- and β-tubulins are found in humans, each encoded by a different gene, they are similar proteins and copolymerize *in vitro*.[12-14] They can have distinct locations in the cell, however, and may perform different functions. Both α- and β-tubulin proteins may undergo posttranslational modifications, including acetylation and detyrosylation.[13-16] These modifications, which occur only on microtubule polymers and not on free tubulin proteins, may account for the distinct functional differences of microtubules in various tissues. Modified regions of polymerized tubulin provide sites for the binding of microtubule-associated proteins (MAPs), which stabilize microtubules against disassembly and mediate interactions with other cellular components.[17,18] Two major classes of MAPs can be isolated in association with microtubules from brain tissue, which is rich in tubulin: high-molecular-weight proteins that have molecular weights of 200,000 to 300,000 and τ proteins that have molecular weights of 40,000 to 60,000. Both classes of MAPs have two binding domains, one of which binds to microtubules. Because this domain also binds to free tubulin molecules simultaneously, MAPs facilitate the initial nucleation step of tubulin polymerization. The other domain appears to be involved in linking the microtubule to other cellular components.

Microtubule assembly and disassembly are in dynamic equilibrium, the direction of which is determined by several factors, including the concentration of free tubulin and various chemical mediators such as Mg^{2+}, guanosine triphosphate (GTP) (promotion of assembly), and Ca^{2+} (inhibition of assembly).[1,2,16-25] If the polymerization reaction is followed *in vitro*, an initial lag phase is noted, after which microtubules form rapidly until a plateau phase is reached. The lag phase is observed because the rate of elongation exceeds the rate of nucleation of new microtubules during the early phase of polymerization. In the intact cell, microtubules usually grow from a specific nucleating site or microtubule-organizing center, which, in most cases, is the centrosome. During rapid polymerization, the high con-

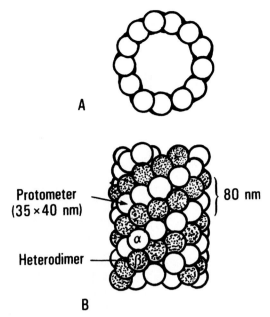

FIGURE 12-1. Model of a microtubule in cross-sectional (A) and longitudinal (B) views. Thirteen protofilaments are in each microtubule. The protofilaments are made up of heterodimers consisting of α- and β-tubulin subunits.

centration of free tubulin results in net assembly until the plateau phase is reached, at which time a critical concentration of tubulin is attained and the rates of both polymerization and depolymerization are balanced.

Each tubulin molecule is associated with two molecules of GTP. One is tightly bound to the α-tubulin subunit, and the second is on the β-tubulin subunit and is readily exchangeable with free guanosine diphosphate (GDP).[19] The assembly of tubulin into microtubules at the plus end occurs spontaneously *in vitro* and is accompanied by the delayed hydrolysis of one molecule of bound GTP to GDP.[20–25] The energy provided by the hydrolysis of GTP is not required for polymerization. Instead, this reaction lowers the critical concentration of the free subunit required for net polymerization at the plus end, which results in the tighter binding of free tubulin at the plus end. On the other hand, the minus end is bound tightly to the microtubule-organizing center, which prevents both assembly and disassembly of subunits at that end.

The plus end of individual microtubules *in vitro* switches spontaneously from a slowly growing to a rapidly shrinking state.[26–29] This behavior, known as *dynamic instability*, occurs because GTP is hydrolyzed only after each tubulin subunit is polymerized. GTP subunits tend to be found only at the growing end of the microtubule, and the rate of growth depends on the availability of GTP subunits. Once the GTP "cap" is lost from the end of a microtubule, the end loses subunits more rapidly. Depolymerization occurs approximately 100-fold faster at a GDP cap than at a GTP cap, and therefore, once rapid depolymerization occurs, the GTP cap is difficult to regain.

Cells modify the rate of dynamic instability of microtubules to perform specific functions.[30,31] In mitosis, for example, the rates of both microtubule assembly and disassembly are increased ("treadmilling") so that chromosomes can readily attach to growing microtubules at their plus ends, thereby forming mitotic spindles. In contrast, MAPs suppress dynamic instability during differentiation by binding to the microtubules and stabilizing them against depolymerization. This stability allows the cell to organize its cytoplasm.

VINCA ALKALOIDS

The vinca alkaloids are naturally occurring or semisynthetic nitrogenous bases that are present in minute quantities in the pink periwinkle plant *Catharanthus roseus* G. Don (formerly *Vinca rosea* Linn). The early medicinal uses of *C. roseus* for controlling hemorrhage, scurvy, toothaches, and diabetes and for the healing of chronic wounds led to the screening of these compounds for their hypoglycemic activity, which turned out to be of little importance compared with their cytotoxic properties.[32,33] The vinca alkaloids were demonstrated to induce cytotoxicity by disrupting microtubules. Until 1994, only two vinca alkaloids, vincristine (VCR) and vinblastine (VBL), were approved for the treatment of malignant diseases in the United States. A third vinca alkaloid, vindesine (VDS, desacetyl VBL carboxyamide), a semisynthetic derivative and human metabolite of VBL, was introduced in the 1970s. Although VDS is active against several tumor types, most notably non–small cell lung cancer, it has been available only for investigational purposes in the United States and has not demonstrated a unique role in cancer therapeutics. Other vinca alkaloids with antitumor activity include vinleurosine and vinrosidine; however, further clinical development of these compounds has been abandoned due to their unpredictable toxicities. Two semisynthetic derivatives of VBL, vinorelbine (VRL, 5'-nor-hydro VBL) and vinzolidine, have undergone clinical evaluation.[34] These compounds, especially VRL, which was approved for the treatment of non–small cell lung cancer in 1994, are of interest for several reasons. First, VRL has broad antitumor activity as a single agent and may not be completely cross-resistant with VCR and VBL. In addition, both VRL and vinzolidine may be administered orally in contrast to other available vinca alkaloids, which are administered parenterally. The key features of the vinca alkaloids are given in Tables 12-1 and 12-2.

Structures

The vinca alkaloids have a large dimeric asymmetrical structure composed of a dihydroindole nucleus (vindoline), which is the major alkaloid in the periwinkle, linked by a

TABLE 12-1. KEY FEATURES OF VINCA ALKALOIDS

	Vincristine Sulfate	Vinblastine Sulfate	Vindesine Sulfate	Vinorelbine Tartrate
Mechanism of action:	Inhibit polymerization of tubulin			
Standard dosage (mg/m²):	1–1.4 q3wk	6–8/wk	3–4 q1–2wk	15–30 q1–2wk
Pharmacokinetics and elimination:	See Table 12-2			
Principal toxicity:	Peripheral neuropathy Constipation SIADH	Neutropenia Thrombocytopenia Alopecia Peripheral neuropathy (mild) SIADH	Neutropenia Peripheral neuropathy (moderate) Alopecia	Neutropenia Peripheral neuropathy (moderate) Constipation
Precautions:	Patients with abnormal liver function should be treated with caution. See section on dosage and schedule for specific dosing guidelines.			

SIADH, syndrome of inappropriate antidiuretic hormone secretion.

carbon-carbon bond to an indole nucleus (catharanthine), which is found in much lower quantities in the plant (Fig. 12-2). VCR and VBL are structurally identical, with the exception of the substituent (R_1) attached to the nitrogen of the vindoline nucleus, where VCR possesses a formyl group and VBL has a methyl group. VCR and VBL vary dramatically, however, in their spectra of antitumor activity and toxicities. VBL and VDS differ in two substituents (R_2 and R_3) attached to the vindoline nucleus, whereas in VRL it is the catharanthine ring that is modified.

Mechanism of Action

The vinca alkaloids induce cytotoxicity by interacting with tubulin.[35] However, they are also capable of many other biochemical and biologic activities that may or may not be related to their effects on microtubules, including competition for transport of amino acids into cells; inhibition of purine biosynthesis; inhibition of RNA, DNA, and protein synthesis; disruption of lipid metabolism; elevation of oxidized glutathione; inhibition of glycolysis; alterations in the release of antidiuretic hormone; inhibition of release of histamine by mast cells and enhanced release of epinephrine;

inhibition of calcium-calmodulin–regulated cyclic adenosine monophosphate phosphodiesterase; and disruption in the integrity of the cell membrane and membrane function.[3,4,36–47]

Despite their diverse biochemical and biologic properties, the cytotoxic activity of the vinca alkaloids is primarily due to their ability to disrupt microtubules, especially microtubules comprising the mitotic spindle apparatus, which thereby induces metaphase arrest in dividing cells. In support of this mechanism of action, strong correlations have been observed between cytotoxicity and the dissolution of the mitotic spindles. The accumulation of mitotic figures correlates with both drug concentration and duration of treatment.[48–51] Although the vinca alkaloids are generally classified as mitotic inhibitors, this mechanism may not be the only important mechanism of cytotoxicity *in vivo*. The vinca alkaloids also affect microtubules involved in chemotaxis and directional migration; intracellular transport and movement of organelles such as mitochondria and secretory granules, especially in neural cells; secretory processes; membrane trafficking; and transmission of receptor signals. They also disrupt the structural integrity of some cells, particularly platelets that are rich in

TABLE 12-2. VINCA ALKALOIDS: PHARMACOKINETIC PARAMETERS

	Vincristine Sulfate	Vinblastine Sulfate	Vindesine Sulfate	Vinorelbine Tartrate
Standard adult dosage range (mg/m²/wk)	1.0–1.4	6–8	3–4	15–30
Optimal pharmacokinetic model	Triexponential	Triexponential	Triexponential	Triexponential
Elimination half-lives				
α (min)	<5	<5	<5	<5
β (min)	50–155	53–99	55–99	49–168
γ (h)	23–85	20–64	20–24	18–49
Clearance (L/h/kg)	0.16	0.74	0.25	0.4–1.29
Primary mechanism of drug disposition	Hepatic metabolism and biliary excretion	Hepatic metabolism and biliary excretion	Hepatic metabolism and biliary excretion	Hepatic metabolism and biliary excretion
References	146, 151	146, 151	146, 151	168, 191–195

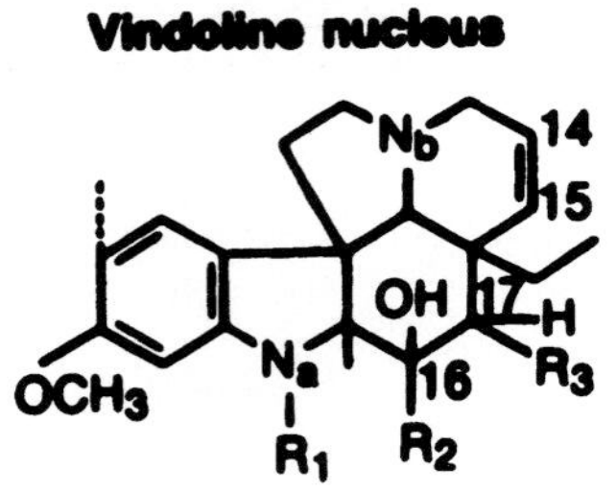

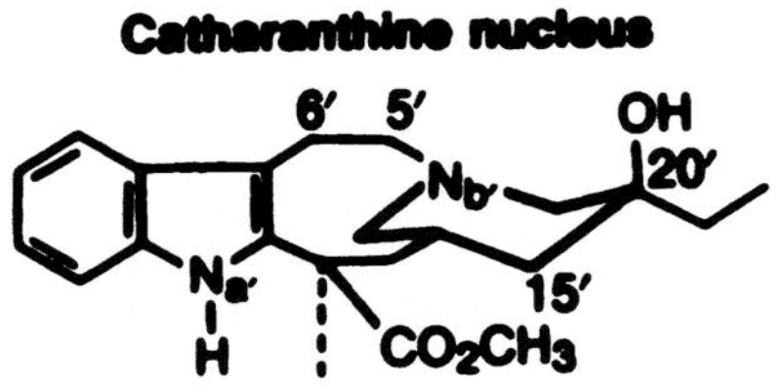

	R_1	R_2	R_3
Vindesine	$-CH_3$	$-CONH_2$	$-OH$
Vincristine	$-CHO$	$-CO_2CH_3$	$-OCOCH_3$
Vinblastine	$-CH_3$	$-CO_2CH_3$	$-OCOCH_3$

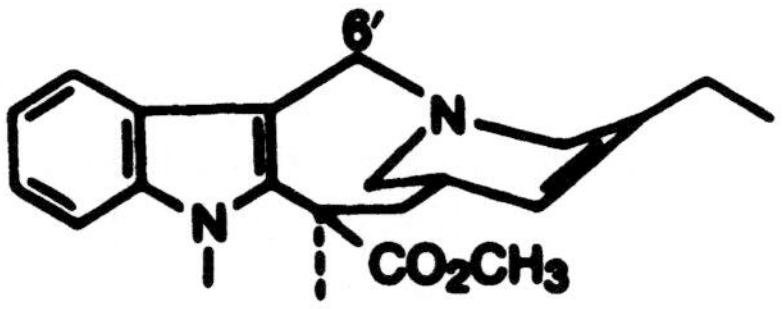

Vinorelbine	$-CH_3$	$-CO_2CH_3$	$-OCOCH_3$

FIGURE 12-2. Structural modifications of the vindoline nucleus and catharanthine nucleus in various vinca alkaloids. (From Rahmani R, Zhou XJ. Pharmacokinetics and metabolism of vinca alkaloids. In: Workman P, Graham MA, eds. *Cancer surveys, pharmacokinetics and cancer chemotherapy*, vol 17. Plainview, NY: Cold Spring Harbor Laboratory Press, 1993:269, with permission.)

tubulin and depend on microtubules for structure.[52–57] Therefore, the fact that the vinca alkaloids induce morphologic changes and cytotoxicity in both normal and neoplastic cells in the G_1 and S phase of the cell cycle, as well as in the mitotic phases, is not surprising.[48,58–64]

The vinca alkaloids bind to sites on tubulin that are similar to the binding sites for maytansine, another complex plant alkaloid.[35,65] The binding sites of the vinca alkaloids, however, appear to be distinct from the binding sites of other compounds such as the taxanes,[66,67] GTP and GDP,[35] derivatives of 5,6-diphenylpyridazine-3-one,[68] and the site on the tubulin heterodimer shared by colchicine, podophyllotoxin, steganacin, combretastatin, and many synthetic compounds.[35,69–72] This was well established in early studies which demonstrated that the vinca alkaloids and colchicine may be bound simultaneously and that the vinca alkaloids may stabilize the colchicine-binding properties of tubulin without affecting the tubulin-colchicine reaction itself.[73–77]

At least two different classes of vinca alkaloid binding sites in tubulin have been identified.[73] High-affinity sites [K_a (dissociation constant) = 5.3×10^5 mol per L^{-1}], which are found in very low density at the ends of microtubules (16.8 ± 4.3 per microtubule out of a potential number of 17,000 tubulin dimers per average 10-μm microtubule), are responsible for the substoichiometric disruption of the microtubule assembly process and most likely represent the intrinsic binding sites on tubulin.[73,78,79] The binding of the vinca alkaloids to these sites results in the inhibition of microtubule assembly. The binding of one molecule of VBL per microtubule may inhibit the rate of microtubule assembly by as much as 50%.[79] Kinetic studies of this type of inhibition have shown that the major effect of low concentrations of the vinca alkaloids on microtubules at steady state is to decrease the rate constants for both dissociation and association of tubulin dimers at the plus (assembly) end of the microtubule, which thereby produces a "kinetic cap."[80] The vinca alkaloids also appear to decrease the association rate constant at the minus end without affecting the dissociation rate constant at that end, the net affect being a depolymerization at the minus end.[81] The other binding site is a low-affinity, high-capacity site (K_a = 3 to 4×10^3 mol per L^{-1}) that has a density of 1.4 to 1.7 sites per heterodimer and is situated along the wall of the microtubule.[73,79,82] The difference in the affinities of the vinca alkaloids for the two classes of binding site may be due to partial concealment of the intrinsic site in the microtubule wall or to a conformational difference in the core of the microtubule compared with its end.

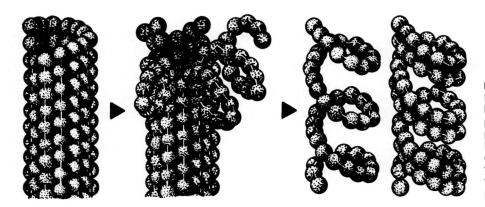

FIGURE 12-3. Model of the vinca alkaloid–induced disassembly of microtubules containing microtubule-associated protein into spiraled protofilaments comprised of one or two spirals. (From Donoso JA, Haskins KM, Himes RH. Effect of microtubule proteins on the interaction of vincristine with microtubules and tubulin. *Cancer Res* 1979;39:1604, with permission.)

The low-affinity binding site may be responsible for the splaying of microtubules into spiral aggregates or spiral protofilaments, which leads to the disintegration of microtubules.[80] This splaying occurs at high (stoichiometric) drug concentrations by a propagated mechanism. Initial drug binding to a limited number of sites weakens the lateral interactions between the protofilaments and exposes new sites.[79–83] Spiral protofilaments may then associate to form paracrystalline structures. The proposal has been made that MAPs stabilize the longitudinal interactions between dimers in the protofilaments as they splay apart after binding the vinca alkaloid, as illustrated in Figure 12-3.[84]

The relationships between the inhibitory effects of vinca alkaloids on cell proliferation, mitotic arrest, mitotic spindle disruption, and depolymerization of microtubules have been characterized in a series of elegant studies.[85–89] Although the antiproliferative effects of the vinca alkaloids are noted over a wide range of concentrations, the drug concentration that inhibits cell proliferation is directly related to the concentration that induces metaphase arrest in 50% of the cells. The inhibition of proliferation and blockage of cells in metaphase at the lowest effective drug concentrations occur with little or no microtubule depolymerization or disorganization of the mitotic spindle apparatus. With increasing drug concentrations, the organization of microtubules and chromosomes in arrested mitotic spindles deteriorates in a manner that is common to all derivatives. These results indicate that the antiproliferative effects of the vinca alkaloids at their lowest effective concentrations are due to the inhibition of mitotic spindle function. This results from drug-induced alterations in the dynamics of tubulin addition and loss at the ends of mitotic spindle microtubules rather than by simple depolymerization of the microtubules. Similar effects have been demonstrated with nocodazole, podophyllotoxin, and the taxanes.[88,89]

The explanation for the differential effects of the various vinca alkaloids in both normal tissues and tumors is not clear. VCR, the most potent of the analogs in humans and the most neurotoxic, has the greatest affinity for tubulin.[90] Although the vinca alkaloids may demonstrate similar potencies against preparations of tubulin derived from any given tissue, these agents have different biologic activities *in vivo*, possibly due to their differential effects on various tubulin isoforms, differences in cofactors that influence interactions with tubulin (e.g., MAPs, cytoplasmic cofactors), and differences in tissue permeation and cellular retention.[84,91–101] For example, the higher cellular retention of VCR compared with VBL in cultured leukemia cells may explain why VCR is more potent than VBL during short treatment periods, whereas the drugs are equitoxic with more prolonged exposures.[92,96–101] The magnitude of intracellular GTP also may be an important factor in influencing the interactions between vinca alkaloids and tubulin,[91] and the proposal has been made that variations in VCR retention among tumors and normal tissues may be related to differences in GTP hydrolysis.[100,101] Pharmacokinetic differences among the vinca alkaloids, which are discussed later in this chapter, also may account for differences in biologic effects *in vivo*.

Cellular Pharmacology

The vinca alkaloids are rapidly taken up into cells. In murine leukemia cells, the intracellular concentrations of VCR are 5- to 20-fold higher than the extracellular concentration, and the ratio of intracellular to extracellular concentrations for several vinca alkaloids ranges from 150- to 500-fold in various murine and human hematopoietic tumor cell lines.[91,102,103] Marked differences exist in cellular retention among the vinca alkaloids; VCR is accumulated to a much greater degree than either VBL or VDS.[92,104,105] In addition, the degree of cellular accumulation of the vinca alkaloids has been demonstrated to be directly related to drug lipophilicity, although a number of factors undoubtedly play a role.[106]

The vinca alkaloids originally were felt to enter cells by both energy- and temperature-dependent active transport processes; K_m (Michaelis-Menten constant) values of 6.45 and 9.2 µmol per L were reported for VCR in human leukemia (CCRF-CEM) and murine leukemia (L1210, P388) cell lines, respectively.[103,106] In subsequent studies, a temperature-independent, nonsaturable mechanism, analogous

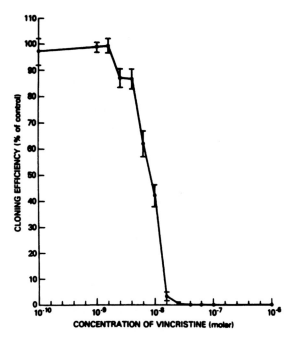

FIGURE 12-4. Cytotoxicity of vincristine (VCR) for L1210 murine leukemia cells as measured by cloning efficiency. Cells were placed in soft agar containing VCR at the specified concentration; the number of colonies was counted 14 days later and expressed as a percentage of the number of colonies that developed from unexposed (control) cells. (From Jackson DV, Bender RA. Cytotoxic thresholds of vincristine in a murine and human leukemia cell line in vitro. *Cancer Res* 1979;39:4346, with permission.)

to a simple diffusion process, has been determined to be primarily responsible for intracellular transport.[106–108] The temperature-dependent, saturable process appears to be less important.[108] The intracellular accumulation of the vinca alkaloids is both a requirement for cytotoxicity and a determinant of resistance. Cytotoxicity is directly related to the extracellular concentration of drug when the duration of treatment is kept constant; for prolonged exposure to VCR, the concentration yielding 50% inhibition lies in the range of 1 to 5 nmol per L (Fig. 12-4).[109–111] The duration of drug exposure above a critical threshold concentration, however, may be the most important determinant of cytotoxicity for the vinca alkaloids.

In addition to their direct cytotoxic effects on tumor cells, the vinca alkaloids, taxanes, and other experimental antimitotics also inhibit angiogenesis with surprising potency. *In vitro*, 0.1 to 1.0 pmol per L VBL blocked endothelial proliferation, chemotaxis, and spreading on fibronectin, all essential steps in angiogenesis,[112] but other normal cells such as fibroblasts and lymphoid tumors were unaffected at these minute concentrations. In combination with anti–vascular endothelial growth factor receptor antibodies, low doses of VBL significantly augmented antitumor response, even in tumors resistant to direct cytotoxic effects of the drug.[113] In these experiments, the combination of drug and antibody produced early and marked

endothelial necrosis, followed by tumor regression. Whether these antiangiogenic effects play a role in clinical responses to the vinca class of drugs remains unanswered.

Mechanisms of Resistance

Resistance to the vinca alkaloids develops rapidly *in vitro* in the presence of the drugs and arises by at least two different mechanisms. The clinical relevance of these mechanisms, however, is not known. In most experimental models, drug resistance is associated with decreased drug accumulation and retention.[114] This is the result of the phenomenon of pleiotropic or multidrug resistance (MDR), a phenotype characterized by cross-resistance to other structurally bulky natural products such as the anthracyclines, epipodophyllotoxins, taxanes, dactinomycin (actinomycin D), and colchicine. Initial studies attributed the MDR phenotype to overexpression of the *mdr-1* gene.[114,115] These cells may have homogeneously staining chromosomal regions or double-minute chromosomes, which indicates the presence of an amplified gene that codes for a membrane P-glycoprotein (Pgp or P-170).[116,116a] Cells that are resistant to the vinca alkaloids on the basis of MDR have an increased capacity to expel natural products as a result of Pgp's functioning as an energy-dependent plasma membrane transport efflux pump.[114,117,118] Pgp forms a channel in the membrane through which drugs are transported, and drug resistance is proportional to the amount of Pgp.[117–120] Pgp is constitutively overexpressed by various normal tissues, including renal tubular epithelium, colonic mucosa, adrenal medulla, and other epithelial tissues.[121] In addition, Pgp has been detected in human cancers, particularly in tumors derived from tissues in which the protein is constitutively expressed, such as kidney and large bowel cancers. It is also found in posttreatment lymphomas, leukemias, and multiple myeloma, which suggests a role in drug resistance.

The specific Pgp associated with resistance to the vinca alkaloids shows slight antigenic and amino acid sequence differences and a different peptide map after digestion than does Pgp from cells selected for resistance to colchicine or paclitaxel.[122–124c] In fact, two forms of the protein are produced by a single clone of VCR-resistant cells, and these forms undergo posttranslational *N*-glycosylation and phosphorylation, which leads to further structural diversity.[124] This diversity may explain the greater degree of resistance for the specific agent used compared with the resistance to other drugs conferred by MDR, and it also may explain the variable patterns of resistance among cells of the MDR type. Another important feature of MDR is that it is functionally reversible after treatment with various agents that have distinctly different structural and functional characteristics, such as the calcium-channel blockers, calmodulin inhibitors, detergents, progestational and antiestrogenic agents, antibiotics, antihypertensives, antiarrhythmics, antimalarials, and immunosuppressives.[115] These agents bind directly to Pgp, thereby blocking the efflux of the cytotoxic drugs and increasing intracellular drug concentrations. Resistance to the vinca alkaloids is also conferred by the multidrug resistance protein (MRP)[124d,124e] and the breast cancer resistance protein.[124f,124g]

The cytotoxic effect of the vinca alkaloids is manifested as apoptosis, or programmed cell death. Vinca-induced apoptosis, however, does not depend on the presence of an intact p53 checkpoint; sensitivity of isogenic cell lines differing only in p53 status are the same.[125] The loss of p21, a protein that controls entry into M phase at the G_2-M checkpoint, enhances sensitivity of tumor cells to vincas and taxanes,[126] possibly by hastening entry of drug-damaged cells into mitosis. Low doses of DNA-damaging agents, such as doxorubicin hydrochloride, actually decrease sensitivity to the antimitotic drugs in p21-competent cells by induction of the checkpoint protein, and sensitivity can be restored by transfection of functional p21, even in the absence of p53.[127] These correlates of vinca and taxane response have not been extended to clinical chemotherapy.

Another mechanism of resistance to antimicrotubule agents *in vitro* results from alterations in α- and β-tubulin proteins.[128–132] Whether these changes are due to mutations or posttranslational modifications such as phosphorylation or acetylation is not known. These alterations result in either decreased drug binding or increased resistance to microtubule disassembly.[128–132] Resistance may also be related to the overexpression of the β-III isotype of β-tubulin.[133] Some have also speculated that changes in the GTP-binding domain of tubulin may be the structural basis for this type of resistance.[132] Another important feature of this type of resistance to the vinca alkaloids is that collateral sensitivity is conferred to the taxanes, which inhibit microtubule disassembly.

Clinical Pharmacology

Analytical Assays

Information about the pharmacology of the vinca alkaloids in humans has been limited in the past by lack of sensitive, specific, and reliable analytic assays capable of measuring the minute plasma concentrations that result from the administration of milligram-quantity doses of these agents. Pharmacologic studies were performed initially with radio-labeled drugs; however, interpretation of the results has been compromised by the chemical instability of these agents. Several vinca alkaloids, particularly VCR and VBL, may undergo spontaneous degradation under mild conditions, forming degradative products that can be separated using high-pressure liquid chromatography (HPLC).[134,135] Therefore, investigators have used radiolabeled compounds coupled to HPLC for further separation to define the plasma disappearance of the vinca alkaloids.[136–143] The

extent to which the formation of degradative products occurs *in vivo*, however, is not known.

Radioimmunoassay and enzyme-linked immunosorbent assay (ELISA) methods using antiserum raised against the vinca alkaloids are capable of detecting picomolar drug concentrations.[144–156] Because polyclonal antisera raised against the vinca alkaloids cannot distinguish between the parent compounds and related derivatives, these assays may not provide sufficient quantitative information about degradation products and metabolites. However, more refined radioimmunoassay and ELISA methods using monoclonal antibodies have considerably greater sensitivity and specificity.[152,157–160]

Advances in HPLC methods for extraction (solid-phase and liquid-liquid) and detection (electrochemical and fluorescence) have made this the most feasible method for separating vinca alkaloids from their metabolites.[161–166]

Pharmacokinetics

General

The vinca alkaloids are usually administered intravenously as a bolus injection or as a brief infusion, and their pharmacokinetic behavior in plasma optimally fits open three-compartment models.[167] Pharmacokinetic characteristics include large volumes of distribution, high clearance rates, and long terminal half-lives ($t_{1/2}$). Pertinent pharmacokinetic parameters of the vinca alkaloids are summarized in Table 12-2. In comparative studies of VCR, VBL, and VDS, VCR has had the longest terminal $t_{1/2}$ and the lowest clearance rate, VBL has had the shortest terminal $t_{1/2}$ and the highest clearance rate, and VDS has had intermediate values.[146,151] The proposal has been made that the longer terminal $t_{1/2}$ and lower clearance rate of VCR account for its greater propensity to induce neurotoxicity.[146,151] At conventional adult dosages, peak plasma concentrations (C_{peak}), which persist for only a few minutes, range from 100 to 500 nmol per L, and plasma levels remain above 1 to 2 nmol per L for relatively long durations.[146,168]

Vincristine

After standard doses of VCR administered intravenously as a bolus injection, plasma disposition is triphasic, with α half-life ($t_{1/2α}$) values of less than 5 minutes due to extensive and rapid tissue binding. Consequently, the apparent volumes of distribution (V_d) are high (central V_d of 0.328 ±0.1061 L per kg and $V_{dγ}$ (V_d for the terminal γ phase) of 8.42 ± 3.17 L per kg), which indicates extensive tissue binding.[146,151] The β half-life ($t_{1/2β}$) values range from 50 to 155 minutes, and γ half-life ($t_{1/2γ}$) values are even more variable, ranging from 23 to 85 hours.[141,146,151,167,169]

Considerable interest has arisen in using protracted VCR administration schedules, because prolonged infusions may closely simulate the optimal *in vitro* conditions required for cytotoxicity.[110,111,169,170] For example, VCR concentrations of 100 to 400 nmol per L are achieved only briefly after intravenous bolus injection, and levels generally decline to less than 10 nmol per L in 2 to 4 hours. Exposure to 100 nmol per L VCR for 3 hours is required to kill 50% of L1210 murine or CEM human lymphoblastic leukemia cells, whereas treatment durations of 6 to 12 hours are required to achieve this degree of cytotoxicity at 10 nmol per L, and no lethal effects occur at VCR concentrations below 2 nmol per L.[111] A 0.5-mg intravenous bolus injection of VCR followed by a continuous infusion at dosages of 0.5 to 1.0 mg per m² per day for 5 days results in steady-state VCR concentrations ranging from 1 to 10 nmol per L, and terminal $t_{1/2}$ after discontinuation of the infusions ranging from 10.5 hours (1.0 mg per m²) to 21.7 hours (0.5 mg per m²).[169,170] Although peak VCR plasma concentrations achieved with prolonged infusions are lower than levels achieved with bolus injections, more prolonged schedules are associated with a greater duration of drug exposure above a critical threshold concentration.[169,170]

VCR pharmacokinetics in children is similar to that in adults, although significant interindividual and intraindividual variability has been observed,[171] perhaps related to steroid induction of P-450 metabolism in leukemic patients.

Other drugs known to interaction with vincristine, and presumably the other vincas, include phenytoin (Dilantin) and carbamazepine,[172] which induce P-450 3A4 and increase VCR clearance, and itraconzole,[173] which inhibits the same P-450 isoenzyme group and enhances VCR toxicity.

The tissue distribution of VCR has been studied in animals. In dogs and rodents, the spleen accumulates VCR to a greater extent than any other tissue.[136,150,174] In the monkey, the tissue with the highest VCR concentration is the pancreas.[139] Although tritium-labeled VCR was shown to enter the central nervous system of primates rapidly after intravenous injection in one study,[139] poor drug penetration across the blood–brain barrier has been documented in most clinical studies. Inhibition of Pgp, however, may allow entry of VCR into the brain.[136,140,147,148,174] In humans, VCR concentrations in cerebrospinal fluid are 20- to 30-fold lower than concurrent plasma concentrations and usually do not exceed 1.1 nmol per L.[148]

Approximately 48% of VCR is bound to plasma proteins.[137] VCR also undergoes extensive binding to formed blood elements, especially platelets and red blood cells, which led in the past to the use of VCR-loaded platelets for treating disorders of platelet consumption such as idiopathic thrombocytopenia purpura and thrombotic thrombocytopenia purpura.[175,176]

VCR is metabolized primarily in the liver and is excreted in the feces.[104,105,136,137] Within 72 hours after the administration of radiolabeled VCR, 12% of the labeled material is excreted in the urine, 50% of which consists of metabolites; approximately 70% is excreted in the feces, 40% of which consists of metabolites. VCR is rapidly excreted into bile with an initial bile to plasma concentration ratio of 100:1

that declines to 20:1 at 72 hours posttreatment.[136] Metabolites accumulate rapidly in the bile, so that only 46.5% of the total biliary product is the parent compound.[136] As many as 6 to 11 metabolites have been detected in both humans[136,142,149,177] and animals.[136,177,178] Most, however, have not been structurally identified. The metabolites 4-deacetylvincristine and N-deformylvincristine have been isolated from human bile,[177,178] whereas 4-deacetylvincristine, and both 4'-deoxy-3'-hydroxyvincristine and 3',4'-epoxyvincristine N-oxide have been tentatively identified after incubation of VCR with bile.[134,135]

The specific contribution of P-450–mediated metabolism of vincristine is uncertain, although its importance is suggested by observations of enhanced clearance with phenytoin and increased toxicity with the 3A inducer, itraconazole. Transfection of tumor cells with 3A4 increases resistance to VBL, whereas lines selected for VBL resistance may show increased 3A4 activity.[179] Specific 3A4 metabolites have not been identified in humans, however.

Vinblastine

The pharmacologic behavior of VBL also reflects its extensive tissue binding and resembles that of VCR. Although plasma protein binding has been reported to range from 43% to 99.7%, it most likely approaches the high end of this range.[141,143,180] VBL binds extensively to formed blood elements, with 50% of radiolabeled drug bound to platelets, red blood cells, and white blood cells within 20 minutes after an intravenous injection.[181,182] Extensive platelet binding is most likely due to the high concentrations of tubulin in platelets.

Plasma disappearance fits a triexponential model with a rapid distribution phase ($t_{1/2\alpha}$ less than 5 minutes) due to rapid tissue binding.[143] VBL is more avidly sequestered in tissues than VCR, as demonstrated by retention of 73% of radioactivity in the body 6 days after an injection of the radiolabeled agent.[143] Values for $t_{1/2\alpha}$ and $t_{1/2\beta}$ have been reported to range from 53 to 99 minutes and 20 to 24 hours, respectively.[143,151,167] High steady-state levels and long terminal $t_{1/2}$ values have been reported after prolonged (5-day) infusions of VBL: 1.1 nmol per L at 1 mg per m² per day ($t_{1/2}$ = 28 days); 3.3 nmol per L at 1.7 mg per m² per day ($t_{1/2}$ = 3 days); and 6.6 nmol per L at 2 mg per m² per day ($t_{1/2}$ = 6 days).[167,170,183,184]

VBL mainly undergoes hepatic metabolism and biliary excretion. Over a 9-day period after the administration of radiolabeled VBL to dogs, 30% to 36% of total radioactivity is recovered in bile and 12% to 17% is found in urine.[185] Fecal excretion of the parent compound is relatively low, which indicates that metabolism is significant. *In vitro* studies indicate that the cytochrome P-450 CYP3A isoform is primarily responsible for biotransformation of VBL.[186] At least one metabolite, desacetylvinblastine (VDS), which may be as active as the parent compound, has been identified in both dogs and humans.[141,185] Small quantities of VDS also have been detected in both urine and feces.

Vindesine

After intravenous administration of VDS by bolus injection, plasma disposition is characterized by a triexponential process.[140,143,144,146,151,187,188] As with the other vinca alkaloids, VDS is rapidly distributed to body tissues, and the $t_{1/2\alpha}$ is less than 5 minutes. Values for $t_{1/2\beta}$ and $t_{1/2\gamma}$ range from 55 to 99 minutes and 20 to 24 hours, respectively. Clearance is low, which indicates that drug accumulation may occur with short-interval, repetitive dosing schedules. The large V_d, low renal clearance rate, and long terminal $t_{1/2}$ of VDS also suggest that it undergoes extensive tissue binding and delayed elimination. Although peak plasma VDS concentrations that range from 0.1 to 1.0 μmol per L are achieved with bolus injections, levels typically decline to less than 0.1 μmol per L in 1 to 2 hours after treatment. Plasma levels achieved with bolus injection are approximately 16-fold higher than levels achieved with prolonged infusions[188]; however, optimal steady-state VDS concentrations for cytotoxicity (0.01 to 0.1 μmol per L) are readily achieved with prolonged infusion schedules (1.2 to 2.0 mg per m^2 per day for 2 to 5 days).[145,153,170,187–189]

The liver is the main organ involved in VDS metabolism and disposition, and the cytochrome P-450 mixed function oxidase CYP3A may be the principal isoform involved in biotransformation.[104,138,145,190] VDS concentrations in bile are much higher than simultaneously measured plasma levels, and biliary and renal clearance rates have been reported to be 29 and 12 mL per minute, respectively.[145] Renal excretion accounts for only 1% to 13% of drug disposition.[140,153,187]

Vinorelbine

VRL disposition in plasma has been described by both biexponential and triexponential pharmacokinetic models.[106,168,191–196] A rapid decay of VRL concentrations occurs in the first hour posttreatment, followed by slower elimination phases ($t_{1/2\gamma}$ = 18 to 49 hours). Consequently, the plasma clearance rate is high, approaching hepatic blood flow. The V_d at steady state is large (20 to 75.6 L per kg).[168,191–195]

VRL is extensively bound to platelets, lymphocytes, and plasma proteins, including α$_1$-acid glycoprotein, albumin, and lipoprotein.[197] The magnitude of protein binding ranges from 80% to 91%, and the unbound fraction averages 14%. Because of substantial binding to platelets, the percentage of drug bound in blood is approximately 98%. Initially, VRL concentrations are higher in red blood cells than in plasma, but levels decay faster in red blood cells, so the plasma to red blood cell VRL ratio is approximately 2 after 2 hours.[189]

Tissue-distribution studies in several animal species have shown that VRL is widely distributed, and high levels are found in all tissues (tissue to plasma ratios of 20 to 80) except in brain. In addition, VLR's distribution in tissues, except for fatty tissues, is greater than that of other vinca alkaloids. VRL concentrations achieved in human lung are approximately 300-fold greater than plasma levels and 3.4- and 13.8-fold higher than lung tissue concentrations achieved with VDS and VCR, respectively.[191,198] High tissue concentrations are also sustained for relatively long durations (more than 5 days in monkeys).[191]

As with the other vinca alkaloids, the principal route of excretion for tritium-labeled VRL in animals and humans is the feces (33% to 80%), whereas urinary excretion represents only 16% to 30% of drug elimination.[191,192] Approximately 95% of the radioactivity excreted in the urine is in the form of unchanged VRL.[194] Fecal excretion occurs slowly (more than 3 to 4 weeks in monkeys and humans), whereas complete urinary excretion occurs rapidly (more than 50% within 24 hours). The recovery of VRL is incomplete (approximately 80% of total dose) even after prolonged collections,[191,192] which is similar to the recoveries reported with other vinca alkaloids.[140,141,146,199] This suggests that tissue binding and metabolism are substantial. Indeed, the results of *in vitro* metabolic studies using animals and human hepatocyte suspensions have demonstrated that the liver plays a major role in drug metabolism and excretion.[191,192,200–202] Although the structures of all VRL metabolites have not been identified, comparison of radiochromatograms of extracellular supernatants with standards suggest the presence of deacetylvinorelbine and N-oxide derivatives.[192,201] Although VRL N-oxide does not appear to be an active cytotoxic agent, deacetylvinorelbine may be as active as VRL.[202] This finding is probably of minor clinical significance, however, because metabolites have not been detected in blood and only small quantities have been found in urine.[193,194]

VRL total body clearance (1.2 L per hour per kg) and terminal $t_{1/2}$ (26 hours) are the same in elderly patients (over 65) and younger patients, provided that patients have normal hepatic function.[196] Clearance is adversely affected in patients who have liver metastases that replace more than 75% of the organ[203]; clearance can be predicted in such patients by the monoethylglycinexylidide clearance test, which assess P-450 3A4 metabolic function. Although VRL clearance is not accurately predicted by bilirubin concentrations in serum, markedly elevated levels were associated with significant reductions in clearance in the few patients studied. A 50% reduction in dosage is recommended for patients with bilirubin levels above 1.5 mg per deciliter and a 75% reduction for levels higher than 3 mg per dL.

VRL is active when given orally. Animal studies have shown that 100% of total radioactivity is absorbed after the ingestion of tritium-labeled VRL, whereas human studies using powder-filled capsules and liquid-filled gelatin capsules have shown that the bioavailability of the parent compound is 43% and 27%, respectively.[195,204] In humans, peak plasma levels are achieved within 1 to 2 hours after an oral dose, and erratic pharmacokinetic behavior is not noted, which indicates that oral administration may be feasible. Concurrent food consumption reduces bioavailability by 20%.[205] The maximum tolerated dosage orally is 80 mg per m^2 in a single dose per week. Divided doses decrease bioavailability. Drug concentrations in blood increase disproportionately at doses of 120 mg per m^2.[205]

Doses and Schedules

The vinca alkaloids are most commonly administered by direct intravenous injection or through the side-arm tubing of a running intravenous infusion. These agents should be administered by trained oncology personnel, because drug extravasation may cause severe soft tissue injury.

Vincristine

VCR is routinely administered to children (more than 10 kg) as a bolus intravenous injection at a dosage of 2.0 mg per m^2 weekly. For smaller children, a dosage of 0.05 mg per kg weekly is used. For adults, the conventional weekly dose is 1.4 mg per m^2. A restriction of the absolute single dose of VCR to 2.0 mg per m^2, which is commonly referred to as *capping*, has been adopted based on early reports of substantial neurotoxicity at higher doses. This restriction is largely based on empiricism, however, and available evidence suggests that the practice of capping should be reconsidered.[206] The fact that the cumulative dose may be a more critical factor than single dose has readily been appreciated; however, significant interpatient variability exists, and some patients are able to tolerate much higher VCR doses with little or no toxicity.[207,208] This may be due to large interindividual differences in drug exposure, which may vary as much as 11-fold.[209,210] This explanation, however, does not justify capping VCR doses at 2.0 mg in all patients.

The common feeling is that VCR dosing should be adjusted based on toxicity; however, dosages should not be reduced for mild peripheral neurotoxicity, particularly if VCR is being used in potentially curative situations. Instead, VCR dosing may have to be modified for signs and symptoms indicative of more serious neurotoxicity, including severe symptomatic sensory changes, motor and cranial nerve deficits, and ileus, until toxicity resolves. In clearly palliative settings, reducing dosage, lengthening dosing intervals, or selecting an alternative drug may be justified in the event of moderate neurotoxicity. A routine prophylactic regimen to prevent gastrointestinal toxicity is also recommended.

Based on *in vitro* data indicating that the duration of VCR exposure above a critical threshold concentration is an important determinant for cytotoxicity, prolonged infusion schedules have been evaluated.[111,170,211] After a 0.5-mg-per-m^2 intravenous injection of VCR, total daily VCR doses of 0.25 to 0.50 mg per m^2 as a 5-day infusion are generally well tolerated.[170] In children, the administration of VCR as a 5-day infusion has permitted a twofold increase in the dose that can be safely administered without major toxicity compared with bolus schedules.[211]

VCR is a potent vesicant and should not be administered intramuscularly, subcutaneously, or intraperitoneally. Direct intrathecal injection of VCR or other vinca alkaloids, which has occurred as an inadvertent clinical mishap, induces a severe myeloencephalopathy characterized by ascending motor and sensory neuropathies, encephalopathy, and rapid death[212,213] (see Toxicity). Administration of VCR 0.4 mg per day as a 5-day infusion by the hepatic intraarterial route also has been associated with profound toxicity, including disorientation and diarrhea.[214]

Although the issue has not been evaluated carefully, the major role of the liver in the disposition and metabolism of VCR implies that dose modifications should be considered for patients with hepatic dysfunction.[210] Firm guidelines for dose modifications have not been established, however. A 50% dosage reduction is recommended for patients with plasma total bilirubin levels between 1.5 and 3.0 mg per dL and at least a 75% dosage reduction for serum total bilirubin levels above 3.0 mg per dL. Dosage reductions for renal dysfunction are not indicated.[215]

Vinblastine

VBL has been administered intravenously on various schedules. The most commonly used schedule administers a bolus injection at a dose of 6 mg per m^2 per day in cyclic combination-chemotherapy regimens. Approved initial dose recommendations for weekly dosing are 2.5 and 3.7 mg per m^2 for children and adults, respectively, followed by gradual dose escalation in increments of 1.8 and 1.25 mg per m^2, respectively, each week. Dosage escalations should be based on hematologic tolerance. The recommendation is also that maximal weekly doses of 18.5 mg per m^2 in adults and 12.5 mg per m^2 in children not be exceeded; however, these doses are substantially higher than most patients can tolerate due to myelosuppression, even on less frequent schedules of administration. Because the severity of the leukopenia that may occur with identical VBL doses varies widely, VBL probably should not be given more frequently than once each week. Oral administration may result in unpredictable toxicity.[216]

Five-day continuous infusions of VBL have been used at dosages ranging from 1.5 to 2.0 mg per m^2 per day, which achieve plasma concentrations of approximately 2 nmol per L.[170] In one study of VBL on this administration schedule, patients who were more likely to respond to treatment had longer terminal-phase $t_{1/2}$ values.[217] Little, if any, evidence exists, however, to support the notion that prolonged infusion schedules are more effective than bolus schedules.

Although specific guidelines have not been established, VBL dosages should be modified for patients with hepatic dysfunction, especially biliary obstruction, due to the importance of the liver in drug disposition (see Vincristine under Doses and Schedules). Dosage reductions in patients with renal dysfunction are not indicated.[215]

Vindesine

VDS has been administered intravenously on many schedules, including weekly and biweekly bolus and prolonged infusion schedules. The agent also has been given in fractionated doses as either an intermittent or a continuous infusion over 1 to 5 days. VDS is most commonly administered as a single intravenous dose of 2 to 4 mg per m[2] every 7 to 14 days, which is associated with both antitumor activity and tolerable toxicity.[218,219] Intermittent or continuous-infusion schedules usually administer VDS dosages of 1 to 2 mg per m[2] per day for 1 to 2 days or 1.2 mg per m[2] per day for 5 days every 3 to 4 weeks.[167,170] More prolonged schedules (up to 21 days) also have been evaluated.

Although specific dosing guidelines have not been established for patients with hepatic or renal dysfunction, the pharmacologic similarities of VDS and other vinca alkaloids and the increased toxicity of VDS noted in patients with abnormal liver function mandate that dosage reductions be strongly considered for patients with severe hepatic dysfunction, especially biliary obstruction (see Vincristine under Doses and Schedules for guidelines). Dosage reductions in patients with renal dysfunction are not indicated.[215]

Vinorelbine

VRL is most commonly administered intravenously at a dose of 30 mg per m[2] on a weekly or biweekly schedule as a slow injection through a side-arm port into a running infusion or as a short infusion over 20 minutes.[220] Oral doses of 80 to 100 mg per m[2] given weekly are generally well tolerated.[195] An acceptable oral formulation, however, is not yet available. Other dosing schedules that have been evaluated include long-term oral administration of low doses and intermittent high-dose and prolonged intravenous infusion schedules.[220–222] Like the other vinca alkaloids, the clearance of VRL is impaired in patients with hepatic dysfunction, and dosage reductions should be considered in this setting.[203,223] Recommendations include a 50% dosage reduction for serum total bilirubin concentrations between 1.5 and 3 mg per dL and a 75% dosage reduction for patients with plasma total bilirubin concentrations above 3.0 mg per dL. Dosage reductions are not recommended for patients with renal insufficiency.

Toxicity

The principal toxicities of the vinca alkaloids differ dramatically despite their structural and pharmacologic similari-

ties. Several potential explanations for their selective effects in various normal and neoplastic tissues are discussed in the section entitled Mechanism of Action in this chapter.

Vincristine

Neurologic

Peripheral neurotoxicity is the principal toxicity of VCR.[224–226] Neurotoxicity is typically cumulative, and its severity is related to both total dose and duration of treatment. Initially, only symmetrical sensory impairment and paresthesias in the distal extremities may be encountered. However, neuritic pain and motor dysfunction, loss of deep tendon reflexes, foot and wrist drop, ataxia, and paralysis may occur with continued use. These effects are almost always symmetrical and may persist for months after treatment is stopped. The manifestations of advanced motor neurotoxicity are usually irreversible or minimally reversible. Patients also may complain of bone, back, and limb pain. In adults, neuropathic effects may begin after cumulative doses of as little as 5 to 6 mg and may be profound after cumulative doses of 15 to 20 mg. Children may be less susceptible than adults, but the elderly are particularly susceptible. Severe neurotoxicity has been observed after the administration of VCR to patients with antecedent neurologic disorders such as hereditary motor and sensory neuropathy type I, Charcot-Marie-Tooth disease, and childhood poliomyelitis.[226–229]

Despite the pathologic findings of axonal degeneration and demyelination, peripheral nerve conduction velocities are generally normal except in patients with severe motor dysfunction. Electrophysiologic testing often reveals diminished amplitudes in sensory and motor nerve action potentials and normal or slightly abnormal latencies in either motor or sensory fibers even with marked clinical symptoms.[224–226,230] Muscle sampling may show increased insertional activity, spontaneous fibrillation potentials, and an impaired interference pattern, particularly in distal muscles, which reflects denervation.[225,230] Unmyelinated fibers may be the most sensitive to the toxic effects of VCR, which explains the early loss of deep tendon reflexes.[231,232]

VCR also may affect cranial nerves, which results in hoarseness due to vocal cord paralysis,[233] diplopia, facial palsy, and jaw, pharyngeal, and parotid pains. Although the uptake of the vinca alkaloids into the brain is low due to low cerebrovascular permeability and extensive drug binding to plasma constituents,[136,147,234] VCR may cause central nervous system toxicity, manifested by depression, confusion, agitation, hallucinations, seizures, and coma.[224–226,235] VCR also has been implicated as a cause of inappropriate antidiuretic hormone secretion (SIADH), possibly due to direct affects on the hypothalamus, neurohypophyseal tract, or posterior pituitary gland (see later section on endocrine toxicity).[236] In addition, visual effects, including transient cortical blindness, retinal changes, and optic atrophy with cortical blindness, have been described.[237,238] VCR also has been implicated in causing a partially reversible hearing loss,[239] as well as neurologic syndromes characterized by ataxia and athetosis.[240]

Acute severe autonomic effects are uncommon but may result as a consequence of high single doses (more than 2 mg per m²) or in patients with hepatic dysfunction. Autonomic effects include paralytic ileus (see Gastrointestinal), urinary retention (see Genitourinary), cardiac autonomic dysfunction, orthostatic hypotension, and arterial hypotension and hypertension (see Cardiovascular).[241–243] An acute necrotizing myopathy also has been observed.[244]

Many attempts have been made to decrease or prevent neurotoxicity with various types of agents such as thiamine, vitamin B$_{12}$, pyridoxine, and folinic acid with no convincing success.[213,245–248] Folinic acid (not folic acid) has been shown to protect mice against an otherwise lethal dose of VCR and has been used successfully in several cases of VCR overdosage in humans; however, it has not been studied prospectively.[245,247] Concurrent administration of a mixture of gangliosides with VCR also has been reported to reduce the peripheral neurotoxicity produced with standard dosages of VCR.[249] Another agent used to prevent neurotoxicity for which results are encouraging is glutamic acid, based on its ability to enhance microtubule formation *in vitro*, as well as its possible competition with VCR for carrier-mediated membrane transport.[248] In a randomized clinical trial, coadministration of glutamic acid and VCR reduced the incidence of paresthesias and loss of the Achilles tendon reflex. However, glutamic acid has not been shown to be helpful in ameliorating VCR-related gastrointestinal and hematologic toxicities.

The inadvertent administration of VCR intrathecally, often a mistake made in patients who are intended to receive intrathecal methotrexate, causes an ascending myeloencephalopathy and is usually fatal. Reports of the results of immediate cerebrospinal fluid withdrawal and lavage with Ringer's lactate supplemented with fresh frozen plasma (15 mL per L) at a rate of 55 mL per hour for 24 hours provide encouragement for this treatment, in that two patients thus treated survived with significant paraplegia but intact cerebral function.[250,251] To prevent this catastrophic mistake, pharmacy, nursing, and physicians should all be trained not to administer intrathecal methotrexate and intravenous vincristine in a single setting,[252] and the drugs should not be delivered together to patient care staff.

Gastrointestinal

Constipation, abdominal cramps, nausea, vomiting, mucositis, diarrhea, paralytic ileus, intestinal necrosis, and perforation occur infrequently.[240–243,253] Constipation due to autonomic dysfunction may result in the impaction of stool in the upper colon. An empty rectum may be noted on digital examination, and an abdominal radiograph may be useful in diagnosing this condition. This condition may be respon-

sive to high enemas and laxatives. A routine prophylactic regimen to prevent constipation is therefore recommended for all patients receiving VCR. Paralytic ileus also may occur, particularly in pediatric patients. The ileus, which may mimic a "surgical abdomen," usually resolves with conservative therapy alone after termination of treatment. Patients who receive high dosages of VCR or have hepatic dysfunction may be especially prone to develop severe gastrointestinal complications due to autonomic neurotoxicity. Although success with drugs used prophylactically to minimize toxicity, including lactulose,[254] caerulein,[255] metaclopramide,[256] and the cholecystokinin analog sincalide,[257] has been reported anecdotally, these agents also may alter the pharmacokinetic behavior of the vinca alkaloids by affecting biliary excretion and/or enterohepatic recirculation, which may ultimately result in increased drug clearance.[258]

Genitourinary

VCR-induced autonomic neurotoxicity may produce bladder atony, thereby causing polyuria, dysuria, incontinence, and urinary retention.[242] Therefore, the suggestion has been made that other drugs that are known to cause urinary retention, particularly in the elderly, should be discontinued if possible for several days after treatment with VCR.

Endocrine

VCR has been implicated as a cause of SIADH by directly affecting the hypothalamus, neurohypophyseal tract, or posterior pituitary.[236] Patients who are receiving intensive hydration are particularly prone to severe hyponatremia due to SIADH, which may result in generalized seizures. This entity has been associated with elevated plasma antidiuretic hormone levels and usually remits within 2 to 3 days. Hyponatremia generally responds to fluid restriction, as with hyponatremia associated with SIADH due to other causes.

Cardiovascular

Hypertension and hypotension, presumably due to autonomic neurotoxicity, have been observed.[241,243] VCR has been implicated rarely in causing acute cardiac ischemia and massive myocardial infarctions.[259] The mechanism for these effects is not known.

Hematologic

Severe myelosuppression is rare but may be a major manifestation of inadvertent VCR overdosage.[260] Mild to modest anemia, leukopenia, and thrombocytopenia, however, may occur with conventional VCR doses and schedules.[261] VCR also may increase circulating platelets due to the endoreduplication of megakaryocytes.[262]

Dermatologic

VCR may cause alopecia and rashes in as many as 20% of patients. Because VCR is considerably irritating to dermal tissues, extreme care should be taken to prevent drug extravasation into soft tissues. If extravasation is suspected, the injection should be discontinued immediately, and aspiration of any residual drug remaining in the tissues should be attempted. Application of local heat and injection of hyaluronidase 150 mg subcutaneously in a circumferential manner around the needle site may reduce the discomfort.[263] Corticosteroids also have been used successfully in treating drug extravasation.[264]

Miscellaneous

Fever without any obvious cause and pain in tumor sites have been observed after treatment with VCR.[265] Severe hepatic toxicity has been reported with VCR used in combination with dactinomycin.[266]

Vinblastine

Hematologic

Myelosuppression, particularly neutropenia, is the principal toxicity of VBL. Thrombocytopenia and anemia are less common. Nadir blood counts usually occur in 4 to 10 days, with recovery in 7 to 21 days posttreatment.

Gastrointestinal

Stomatitis and pharyngitis are more common with VBL than with VCR. VBL infrequently causes nausea, vomiting, anorexia, pain, diarrhea, and hemorrhagic enterocolitis. Other gastrointestinal effects that are probably due to autonomic neurotoxicity include constipation, ileus, and abdominal pain. These effects are more common with high VBL doses (more than 20 mg) and with combination-chemotherapy regimens consisting of VBL and cisplatin.[267,268]

Neurologic

Neurotoxicity is much less common with VBL than VCR and is usually noted in patients receiving protracted therapy. It is similar to the neurotoxicity induced by VCR, with sensory dysfunction and loss of deep tendon reflexes as the most common manifestations (see Toxicity: Vincristine: Neurologic). Both neurosensory and autonomic effects are more common when patients are heavily pretreated and when VBL is administered as a prolonged infusion alone or in combination with cisplatin.[267-269]

Cardiovascular

Hypertension is the most common cardiovascular effect of VBL. Myocardial infarctions and cerebrovascular events also have been noted with VBL alone or in combination-chemotherapy regimens, particularly those that also include cisplatin and bleomycin sulfate.[259,270] Raynaud's phenomenon may be a lingering effect, especially in patients treated with the combination of VBL, cisplatin, and bleomycin (PVB).[271-274] In one long-term follow-up study, symptomatic Raynaud's phenomenon developed in 44% of patients with germ cell malignancies who were treated with PVB, and an even higher percentage developed abnormal vasoconstrictive responses to cold stimuli.[273] This toxicity occurs less frequently when etoposide is substituted for VBL.[274] Calcium-channel–blocking agents such as nifedipine have been reported to ameliorate the symptoms of Raynaud's phenomenon induced by VBL.[272]

Pulmonary

Acute pulmonary edema has been observed.[275] Acute respiratory distress, acute bronchospasm, interstitial pulmonary infiltrates, and dyspnea also have been noted, particularly when VBL is combined with mitomycin C.[276]

Dermatologic

Mild alopecia is common. Like VCR, VBL is a vesicant, and drug extravasation should be managed similarly (see Toxicity: Vincristine: Dermatologic). Several antidotes have been recommended for VBL extravasation, including corticosteroids,[264] diethylstilbestrol,[277] and hyaluronidase,[263] and a generally conservative approach is advised. VBL also may cause photosensitivity reactions, possibly as a result of corneal irritation.

Endocrine

Although SIADH is more commonly associated with VCR, it also has been reported after treatment with VBL.[167,278]

Miscellaneous

Pain in sites of tumor may occur.

Vindesine

VDS exhibits varying degrees of the toxicities shared by VCR and VBL. The principal dose-limiting toxicities are hematologic and neurologic. These adverse effects are more profound in patients with hepatic dysfunction.[188]

Hematologic

Neutropenia is the most common toxicity of VDS, with nadir neutrophil counts occurring in approximately 7 days and complete recovery in approximately 14 days after treatment. Thrombocytopenia is less common. Myelosuppression has been demonstrated to correlate best with the clearance of VDS and not with peak drug levels.[188] Ineffective erythropoiesis and thrombocytosis also have been described.[279]

Neurologic

Neurotoxicity, characterized by a peripheral neuropathy similar to that described for VCR, is generally noted after three to four courses of treatment.[167,280] Neurosensory manifestations predominate, but motor dysfunction also may occur. Constipation, paralytic ileus, urinary retention, postural hypotension, myalgias, vertigo, and jaw pain are observed less frequently.[280] The most common finding on neurologic examination and electrophysiologic testing after treatment with VDS doses of 0.5 to 3.0 mg per m² is the diminution of proprioceptive reflexes in the lower extremities with attendant diminution of the ankle jerk reflex.[280] Central nervous system effects, including cortical blindness, hemiplegia, and disorientation, also have been reported.[280,281]

Gastrointestinal
Stomatitis, nausea, and vomiting are commonly noted after treatment with high doses of VDS; diarrhea is rare. Autonomic dysfunction may result in constipation and paralytic ileus.[167]

Dermatologic
Alopecia is usually observed after multiple treatments. Various types of skin rashes also have been noted infrequently.[167,278] As with the other vinca alkaloids, VDS is a potent vesicant, and care must be taken to avoid drug extravasation into subcutaneous tissues (see Toxicity: Vincristine: Dermatologic). A relatively high incidence (27%) of local reactions at the injection site without apparent infiltration of the drug also has been noted.[278] These reactions may be prevented by liberally flushing the infusion catheter with 5% dextrose solution before and after drug administration.[282]

Miscellaneous
As with VDS and VBL, SIADH has been described with VDS treatment (see Toxicity: Vincristine: Endocrine).[167,282] Dyspnea associated with a normal lung scan and electrocardiogram has been noted 1 to 5 hours after the administration of VDS used in combination with mitomycin C.[283]

Vinorelbine

Similar to VDS, VRL shares many of the principal toxicities of VCR and VBL, particularly hematologic toxicity and neurotoxicity.

Hematologic
The dose-limiting toxicity of VRL on all schedules is neutropenia.[220] Neutrophil count nadirs occur 7 to 10 days after treatment, and recovery is usually complete in 7 to 14 days. As with other vinca alkaloids, myelosuppression is not cumulative and is readily reversible soon after treatment is discontinued. Mild to moderate anemia is common, and clinically significant thrombocytopenia is rare. Thrombocytosis that is not associated with a coagulopathy also may occur.

Neurologic
VRL has been demonstrated to have a lower affinity for axonal microtubules than for mitotic spindle microtubules compared with both VCR or VBL.[284] Clinical results also indicate that neurotoxicity is less prominent with VRL than with VCR. A mild to moderate peripheral neuropathy, characterized by paresthesias and hyperesthesia, occurs in

7% to 31% of patients.[167,285] Constipation occurs in as many as 30% of patients, with severe toxicity (e.g., paralytic ileus) in 2% to 3%. As with the other vinca alkaloids, the incidence of neurotoxicity increases with the duration of treatment. In a study of patients with non–small cell lung cancer randomized to treatment with either VRL alone, VRL and cisplatin, or VDS and cisplatin, the incidence of severe neurotoxicity was significantly lower in both the single-agent VRL and VRL-cisplatin arms than in the VDS-cisplatin arm.[286] Furthermore, the addition of cisplatin did not significantly increase the incidence of severe toxicity above that observed with VRL alone. Muscle weakness is noted occasionally after 3 to 6 months of treatment; however, these effects usually resolve after VRL is discontinued. Tumor pain and jaw pain also have been noted.

Gastrointestinal
The most common gastrointestinal toxicity of VRL is constipation. Although as many as 38% of patients experience nausea and vomiting, the incidence of severe toxicity is low (2% to 8%).[167,285] Mild to moderate stomatitis and diarrhea occur in less than 20% of patients. Rarely, patients may develop clinical signs and laboratory evidence of mild pancreatitis after VRL.[287] Gastrointestinal effects are more common with oral administration.[195]

Local Toxicity
Like the other vinca alkaloids, VRL is a vesicant. Injection-site reactions, including erythema, pain, and venous discoloration, occur in approximately 33% of patients[167,285]; however, severe local toxicity is uncommon (less than 2%). The risk of phlebitis may increase if veins are not adequately flushed after treatment.

Miscellaneous
In addition to injection-site pain, pain of unspecified etiology occurs in approximately 13% of patients.[285] Chest pain with or without electrocardiographic changes suggestive of ischemia has been observed in 6% of patients. Many of the patients who experience chest pain, however, have either a history of cardiovascular disease or thoracic neoplasms, and it has not been possible to determine whether the chest pain is due to drug-related phenomena, cancer, or exacerbation of underlying atherosclerotic cardiovascular disease. Respiratory reactions, characterized by dyspnea, have been reported in approximately 5% of patients.[285] These respiratory reactions may be classified into two types. One type is an acute reaction with bronchospasm, resembling an allergic reaction. The second type is a subacute reversible reaction associated with cough and dyspnea and occasionally with interstitial infiltrates. This reaction typically occurs within 1 hour after treatment. The use of steroids has been felt to be beneficial in severe cases, and several patients have been retreated without sequelae. No evidence exists that VRL causes chronic pulmonary toxicity. Asymptomatic

and transient elevations in liver function test results, particularly alkaline phosphatase levels, have been noted. Alopecia occurs in approximately 10% of patients. Hand-foot syndrome[288] and SIADH[289] are other rare toxicities associated with VRL administration.

Drug Interactions

Pharmacokinetic interactions of the vinca alkaloids and other drugs have not been studied in detail. The enhancement of methotrexate sodium (MTX) accumulation by tumor cells in the presence of VCR and VBL has been well described.[290,291] The effect is mediated by the blockage of MTX efflux from the cell by the vinca alkaloid. MTX reaches higher steady-state intracellular levels in both acute myeloblastic and lymphoblastic leukemia cells in the presence of VCR,[291,292] but the minimal VCR concentration required to achieve this effect in myeloblasts (0.1 μmol per L) is realized only momentarily during clinical treatment, and even higher concentrations are needed to enhance MTX uptake in lymphoblasts. The schedule of VCR followed by MTX has not demonstrated therapeutic synergism in the L1210 murine leukemia model.[293] Therapeutic synergism is noted with the sequence of MTX followed by VCR, however, but this interaction is not likely to be due to the enhancement of MTX uptake. Thus very little justification exists for routine use of VCR pretreatment in high-dose MTX protocols. The vinca alkaloids and other antimicrotubule agents (e.g., taxanes) also have been demonstrated to inhibit the influx of the epipodophyllotoxins into cells, which results in less cytotoxicity *in vitro*[294]; however, the clinical implications of this preclinical observation have not been evaluated.

Seizures associated with a reduction in plasma phenytoin concentrations by 50% have been observed during treatment with the vinca alkaloids.[295,296] Reduced phenytoin levels have been noted within 24 hours after treatment with VCR, and low phenytoin levels have persisted for up to 10 days, perhaps through substrate competition for CYP3A4 metabolism. Other drug interactions related to CYP3A4 are discussed earlier. The concurrent use of erythromycin and the vinca alkaloids, particularly VBL, has been associated with unusually severe toxicity, possibly due to the inhibitory effects of erythromycin on the cytochrome P-450–mediated metabolism of the vinca alkaloids.[297]

If VCR is used in combination with L-asparaginase, it should be given 12 to 24 hours before the enzyme; administration of L-asparaginase with or before VCR may reduce VCR clearance, thereby increasing toxicity.

TAXANES

The taxanes are an important new class of anticancer agents that exert their cytotoxic effects on microtubules by a unique mechanism of action. Both paclitaxel, the prototypical taxane, which has been approved worldwide for the treatment of several malignancies, and docetaxel, a potent semisynthetic analog, have significant activity in a broad range of tumor types that are generally refractory to conventional therapies, including chemotherapy-resistant epithelial ovarian cancer, advanced breast cancer, small and non–small cell lung cancer, bladder cancer, germ cell malignancies, and head and neck cancer.[298]

Paclitaxel was discovered as part of a National Cancer Institute program in which extracts of thousands of plants were screened for anticancer activity. In 1963, a crude extract with antitumor activity was isolated from the bark of the Pacific yew, *Taxus brevifolia*, a slowly growing evergreen found in the old-growth forests of the Pacific Northwest, and paclitaxel was identified as the active constituent of the extract in 1971.[299] Paclitaxel is also isolated from other members of the *Taxus* genus and produced by *Taxomyces andreanae*, a fungal endophyte isolated from the inner bark of the Pacific yew.[300] Although the supply of paclitaxel originally came from the bark of the tree only, alternate sources, including nonbark biomass, ornamental *Taxus* species, and especially partial synthesis from a readily available precursor, 10-deacetylbaccatin III, derived from the needles of more abundant yew species such as the European yew, *Taxus baccata*, are producing sufficient quantities of the drug to meet commercial demands.[301] Docetaxel, which is also derived semisynthetically from 10-deacetylbaccatin III, is slightly more water soluble than paclitaxel and is a more potent antimicrotubule agent *in vitro*.[301,302] The key features of paclitaxel are given in Table 12-3, and its pharmacokinetics is given in Table 12-4.

Structures

The structures of paclitaxel and docetaxel are shown in Figure 12-5. The taxanes are complex alkaloid esters consisting of a taxane system linked to a four-member oxetane ring at positions C-4 and C-5.[303] The taxane rings of both paclitaxel and docetaxel, but not 10-deacetylbaccatin III, are linked to an ester at the C-13 position. Structure-function studies suggest that analogs without this linkage have little interaction with mammalian tubulin, although they still stabilize microtubules of the amoeba *Physarum polycephalum*.[304] Furthermore, the moieties at the C-2' and C-3' positions are critical with respect to the antimicrotubule effects of the taxanes.[305] Acetyl substitution at C-2' results in a significant loss of activity. Neither the acetyl group at C-10 nor the phenyl group at C-5' are required for in vitro activity,[303,305] and the structures of paclitaxel and docetaxel differ in linkages at these positions.

Mechanism of Action

The binding site for taxanes on microtubules is different from the binding sites for exchangeable GTP, colchicine,

TABLE 12-3. KEY FEATURES OF PACLITAXEL

Mechanism of action:	High-affinity binding to microtubules, with enhanced microtubule formation at high drug concentrations. Inhibition of mitosis.
Dosage:	135–175 mg/m^2 over 24 hours, 175 mg/m^2 over 3 h, 250 mg/m^2 over 24 h with G-CSF, or 140 mg/m^2 over 96 h
Pharmacokinetics:	See Table 12.4. Saturable elimination and distribution, particularly evident with short (3-h) schedule.
Elimination:	Predominantly by hepatic hydroxylation (P-450 enzymes) and biliary excretion of metabolites. Less than 10% of dose eliminated intact in the urine.
Toxicities:	Acute hypersensitivity reactions
	Neutropenia
	Mucositis, especially with prolonged (96-h) infusion
	Thrombocytopenia
	Alopecia
	Sensory neuropathy
	Cardiac conduction disturbances
Precautions:	Patients given 3- or 24-h infusion should receive premedication with corticosteroids and antihistamines. Dosage should be modified in patients with abnormal hepatic function (see section on doses and schedules later in this chapter).

G-CSF, granulocyte colony-stimulating factor.

podophyllotoxin, and vinblastine.[67,306–310] Paclitaxel binds to the *N*-terminal 31 amino acids of the β-tubulin subunit in tubulin oligomers or polymers.[66,67,299–310] Photoaffinity labeling of microtubules with taxane analogs has identified Arg 282 as the photolinking site.[311] Crystal models of the β-tubulin *N*-terminus indicate that His 227 and Asp 224 are critical to binding the C-2 benzoyl side chain of paclitaxel.[312–315] Alternative molecules, such as the epothilones[315] and eleutherobins[316] occupy the same binding sites, albeit with a somewhat altered core and side chain structure. The effects of taxanes on microtubules differ from those of the vincas. Unlike colchicine and the vinca alkaloids, which prevent microtubule assembly, submicromolar concentrations of the taxanes decrease the lag time and shift the dynamic equilibrium between tubulin dimers and microtubules toward microtubule assembly and stabilize microtubules against depolymerization,[89,306–322] thereby inhibiting the dynamic reorganization of the

TABLE 12-4. PACLITAXEL PHARMACOKINETIC PARAMETERS[a]

Schedule (Reference)	Model	$t_{1/2\alpha}$ (h)	$t_{1/2\beta}$ (h)	$t_{1/2\gamma}$ (h)	CL (mL/min/m^2)	$V_{d,ss}$ (L/m^2)	C_{peak} (µmol/L) (dose)
3-h (419)	Triphasic	0.22	1.6	11.1	169	74	6.0–14.2 (210–300 mg/m^2)
3-h (405)	Triphasic, saturable	0.20	1.4	14.4	294	98	2.5 (135 mg/m^2)
		0.27	2.3	18.8	212	99	4.3 (175 mg/m^2)
24-h		0.09	2.2	49.8	363	657	0.2 (135 mg/m^2)
		0.14	2.0	23.6	393	269	0.4 (175 mg/m^2)
3-h (420)	Saturable elimination and distribution			9.2[b]	246[b]		3.3 (135 mg/m^2)
				6.5[b]	190[b]		5.9 (175 mg/m^2)
				7.4[b]	193[b]		7.6 (225 mg/m^2)
24-h				16.2[b]	232[b]		0.3 (135 mg/m^2)
				14.6[b]	232[b]		0.5 (175 mg/m^2)
6-h (400, 402, 404)	Biphasic	0.36	6.4	—	195	59	2.2–13.0 (170–275 mg/m^2)
24-h (403)	Biphasic	0.27	3.9	—	359	55	0.6–0.9 (200–275 mg/m^2)
24-h (407)	Biphasic with saturable elimination and distribution				161[c]		(<400 mg/m^2)
					123[c]		(>400 mg/m^2)
24-h (418)							0.2–3.4 (110–390 mg/m^2)
96-h (395)					437		0.05–0.08 (120–160 mg/m^2)

C_{peak}, peak plasma concentration; CL, systemic clearance; $t_{1/2}$, half-life; $V_{d,ss}$, volume of distribution at steady state.
[a]Parameter values represent mean data from referenced reports.
[b]Apparent values calculated by noncompartmental analysis.
[c]Pediatric study demonstrating saturable pharmacokinetics. Clearance values listed are for doses <400 mg/m^2 (161 mL/min/m^2) and doses >400 mg/m^2 (123 mL/min/m^2).

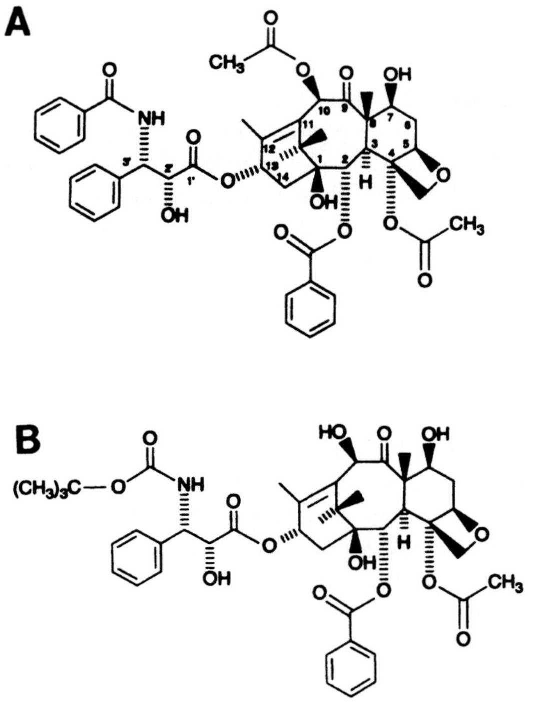

FIGURE 12-5. Structures of the taxanes: **(A)** paclitaxel; **(B)** docetaxel.

microtubule network. At low concentrations (10 to 100 nmol per L), paclitaxel suppresses the dynamic instability of microtubules at the plus end, with only a minimal increase in polymer mass[323] that leads to a block in progression through mitosis. At higher concentrations above 100 nmol per L, the taxanes induce polymerization of tubulin in the presence or absence of factors that are usually essential for this function, such as exogenous GTP or MAPs.[308,319] These microtubules are stable even after treatment with calcium or at low temperatures, factors that usually promote disassembly.[306,307,317,318] The effects of paclitaxel on increase in microtubule mass are maximal when drug concentrations are equimolar with tubulin or when the stoichiometry approaches 1 mole paclitaxel per mole of polymerized tubulin dimer.[89,309,318,321] The binding of paclitaxel to polymerized tubulin is reversible with a binding constant of approximately 0.9 μmol per L.[324] Docetaxel, which most likely shares the same tubulin-binding site as paclitaxel, has a 1.9-fold higher effective affinity for the site.[321] The assembly of GDP- or GTP-tubulin induced by docetaxel also proceeds with a critical protein concentration that is 2.1-fold lower than that of paclitaxel.[321]

At submicromolar concentrations, the taxanes induce microtubule bundling in cells and in cell-free tubulin preparations.[66,67,306,310,321,325–329] The taxanes also induce the formation of numerous abnormal mitotic asters, which, unlike mitotic asters formed under physiologic conditions, do not require centrioles for nucleation.[67,324,327–331] At identical drug concentrations, the initial slope of the assem-

bly reaction and the amount of polymer formed is greater for docetaxel.[332] The cytotoxic effects of docetaxel are also severalfold greater than paclitaxel *in vitro* and in tumor xenografts.[320,332] These characteristics may not translate into a greater therapeutic index for docetaxel, however, because greater potency also may result in more severe toxicity at identical drug concentrations *in vivo*. In addition, the taxanes may not be completely cross-resistant.[333]

The taxanes inhibit proliferation of cells by inducing a sustained mitotic block at the metaphase-anaphase boundary at much lower concentrations than those required to increase microtubule polymer mass and microtubule bundle formation.[322,323] Half-maximal inhibition of HeLa cell proliferation and a 50% blockage in mitotic metaphase occur at 8 nmol per L paclitaxel, whereas the mass of microtubules increases half-maximally at 80 nmol per L paclitaxel and attains maximal levels at 300 nmol per L.[322] These inhibitory effects at low drug concentrations are associated with the formation of an incomplete metaphase plate of chromosomes and an arrangement of spindle microtubules resembling the abnormal organization that occurs at low concentrations of the vinca alkaloids.[85,322] Aberrant mitotic spindle morphology and mitotic block resulting from the stabilization of microtubule dynamics may be due to the inhibitory effects of the taxanes on intrinsic microtubule processes such as dynamic instability (see Microtubule Structure) and treadmilling, which is the balanced net addition of tubulin at one end of the microtubule and the net loss of tubulin at the other end. Treadmilling, which is used by the assembly end of the mitotic spindle to probe the cytoplasm during prometaphase until linkage with a chromosomal kinetochore is established, may be especially sensitive to the stabilization of microtubule dynamics by the taxanes. Although the taxanes bind stoichiometrically to tubulin at high drug concentrations, the inhibition of microtubule dynamics and mitosis at low drug concentrations results from the binding of low numbers of taxane molecules per microtubule. Under conditions associated with the most sensitive mitotic block (3 to 10 nmol per L paclitaxel), intracellular paclitaxel concentrations are 40% to 70% less than the concentrations of tubulin in the microtubule.[89,322]

The taxanes also may induce many other effects *in vitro* and *in vivo* that may or may not be related to their disruptive effects on microtubules. Although the taxanes primarily block cell-cycle traverse in the mitotic phases, paclitaxel prevents the transition from G_0 to S phase in fibroblasts during stimulation of DNA synthesis by growth factors and appears to delay traverse of sensitive leukemia cells through the nonmitotic phases of the cell cycle.[327,329] This indicates that the integrity of microtubules may be critical for the transmission of proliferative signals.[4–6] Explanations that have been proposed to account, in part, for the inhibitory effects of paclitaxel in the nonmitotic cell-cycle phases include the disruption of tubulin in the cell membrane and direct inhibitory effects on the disassembly of the interphase cytoskeleton.[334,335] These effects may result in the disruption of many vital cell functions such as locomotion, intracellular transport, and transmission of proliferative transmembrane signals. Indeed, in Walker 256 carcinosarcoma cells, paclitaxel inhibits shape changes and locomotion, factors that may be related to the invasiveness and metastatic potential of tumors.[336] The agent also has been shown to inhibit steroidogenesis in human Y-1 adrenocortical and MLTC-1 Leydig tumors by decreasing the intracellular transport of cholesterol to cholesterol side-chain cleavage enzymes.[337] The effects on locomotion, shape changes, and intracellular transport appear to be related to perturbations in microtubule dynamics.

The taxanes also inhibit specific functions in nonmalignant tissues, which may be mediated through their effects on microtubule dynamics. For example, paclitaxel inhibits relevant morphologic and biochemical processes in human neutrophils, including chemotaxis, migration, spreading, polarization, hydrogen peroxide generation, and killing of phagocytized microorganisms.[338,339] In addition, the agent antagonizes the effects of microtubule-disrupting drugs on lymphocyte function and cyclic adenosine monophosphate (cAMP) metabolism and inhibits the proliferation of stimulated human lymphocytes.[340–342] Paclitaxel mimics the effects of endotoxic bacterial lipopolysaccharide on macrophages, which results in a rapid decrement in tumor necrosis factor α (TNF-α) receptors and TNF-α release.[343] Paclitaxel also induces the expression of the gene for TNF-α, but these activities are not related to the effects of paclitaxel on microtubule assembly, which raises the issue of what role these cytokines play in the antitumor activity of the taxanes.[344] In addition, paclitaxel inhibits chorioretinal fibroblast proliferation and contractility in an *in vitro* model of proliferative vitreoretinopathy and neointimal smooth muscle cell proliferation after angioplasty in a rat model.[345,346] These activities may be relevant to the treatment of traction retinal detachment and proliferative vitreoretinopathy, and prevention of the restenosis of blood vessels after angioplasty. Finally, paclitaxel inhibits secretory functions in many specialized cells, such as insulin secretion in isolated rat islets of Langerhans, protein secretion in rat hepatocytes, and the nicotinic receptor–stimulated release of catecholamines from chromaffin cells of the adrenal medulla.[347–351]

After the disruption of microtubules and other cellular processes by the taxanes, the precise means by which cell death occurs is not clear. Morphologic features and a DNA fragmentation pattern that are characteristic of programmed cell death, or apoptosis, in paclitaxel-treated cells indicate that the taxanes trigger apoptosis as do many other chemotherapeutic agents.[352] Some investigators have proposed that taxanes produce apoptosis by at least two different mechanisms. At low concentrations (less than 10 nmol per L) apoptosis may occur in the absence of mitotic arrest

and without induction of raf-1 kinase, both of which characterize the action of paclitaxel at higher concentrations.[353,354] Glucocorticoids antagonize the apoptotic effect of the drug at all concentrations.[353]

The pathways responsible for initiating apoptosis are incompletely understood and seem to depend on a variety of factors, including drug concentration, duration of cell exposure, and the cell line studied.[355] At high concentrations paclitaxel induces expression of the c-jun terminal kinase; mutations of this kinase reduce cytotoxicity.[356]

Whether taxane-induced apoptosis requires a functional p53 pathway is unclear and probably depends on the cell line under study. The consensus seems to be that in most cell lines, disruption of p53 has little effect on drug sensitivity.[355] Inhibition of p53 function by transfection of the viral E6 gene,[125] expression of dominant mutant p53,[357] and attempts to correlate p53 status of glioma and lymphoma cell lines with drug sensitivity have all failed to demonstrate a role for p53. Others, however, have found evidence for a role of p53 in ovarian cancer[358] and colorectal cancer cell lines.[359] Finally, overexpression of p21, a downstream effector of p53, appears to block cells in G_2 and prevent progression into the more drug-vulnerable mitotic phase of the cell cycle, decreasing taxane sensitivity.[360,361]

Overexpression of elements of the apoptotic cascade also influence susceptibility to taxane-induced cell death. Increased expression of the antiapoptotic protein Bcl-2 protects against taxane injury in myeloma cells.[362] On the other hand, paclitaxel itself induces phosphorylation, and thereby inactivation, of Bcl-2, an effect that may be secondary to mitotic arrest.[363] Overexpression of other proteins, BAD and BAX, enhances sensitivity of ovarian cancer cells[364,365]; BAD and BAX bind to and inactivate the proapoptotic proteins Bcl-2 and Bcl-X_L. Whether these proteins have any role in determining clinical response is unclear.

Other modulators of these apoptotic pathway proteins include growth factor signaling pathways. For example, a number of tumor growth factors activate the phosphotidylinositol-3 (PI-3) kinase pathway. One component of the PI-3 kinase pathway, Akt kinase, may further influence sensitivity of cells to taxanes by phosphorylating BAD and preventing it from binding to Bcl-X_L.[366]

Growth factor signaling may contribute to taxane resistance by raising the cell threshold for apoptosis. Insulin-like growth factor I protects responsive breast cancer cell lines from anthracyclines or taxanes, possibly by activating the PI-3 kinase pathway and inducing phosphorylation (and inactivation) of antiapoptotic factors.[367] Transfection of cells with Her-2, an epidermal growth factor–like growth factor, increases taxane resistance,[368] and high expression of Her-2 in random cell lines correlates with resistance.[369] Consistent with this relationship, Herceptin, an anti–Her-2 antibody, partially restores sensitivity of these cell lines.[369]

Both paclitaxel and docetaxel have been shown to enhance the cytotoxic effects of ionizing radiation *in vitro* at clinically achievable concentrations (less than 50 nmol per L), which may be due to the inhibition of cell-cycle progression in the G_2 and M phases, the most radiosensitive period of the cell cycle.[370–373] A number of clinical trials are under way to explore this interaction.[374]

Mechanisms of Resistance

Two general mechanisms of acquired taxane resistance have been described in cells made resistant by prolonged treatment at low drug concentrations. As for the vinca alkaloids, several drug-resistant Chinese hamster ovary cell lines with structurally altered α- and β-tubulins and an impaired ability to polymerize tubulin dimers into microtubules have been described (see Vinca Alkaloids: Mechanisms of Resistance).[128–133,375–377] These cells lack normal microtubules in their interpolar mitotic spindles and have an inherently slow rate of microtubule assembly when grown in the absence of drug. These mutants are also collaterally sensitive to the vinca alkaloids.

Selection of paclitaxel-resistant cells *in vitro* is also associated with changes in β-tubulin isotype expression.[133,378–380] Six different isotypes of β-tubulin are expressed in nonmalignant tissues, with the class I isotype comprising 80% to 99% of cellular β-tubulin. The β-III isotype, a minor component of cellular β-tubulin, increases the dynamic instability of microtubules, impairs rates of microtubule assembly, and increases resistance to taxanes.[133] Human ovarian cancer specimens from patients resistant to paclitaxel contained increased β-III,[381] as did leukemia,[378] prostate,[133,379] and ovarian cancer[380,381] cell lines selected for resistance. Further proof that β-III tubulin can cause taxane resistance is provided by experiments which show that antisense oligonucleotides to class III RNA decreased expression of this protein and increased drug sensitivity by 40% in a resistant cell line.[382]

Others have found that mutations affecting the β-tubulin class I genes can lead to resistance. Research groups led by Fojo[383] and Cabral[384] have described paclitaxel-resistant Chinese hamster ovary cells that contained mutated β-tubulin alleles, with mutations involving the putative taxane binding sites; specifically, leucines at positions 215, 217, and 228[384] were mutated to histidine, arginine, or phenylalanine. Low-level expression led to resistance, whereas high-level expression of any of these mutations caused impairment of assembly, cell-cycle arrest, and failure to proliferate, a condition reversed by incubation with paclitaxel.[384]

A second mechanism of acquired taxane resistance fits the general pattern of MDR.[115–124,385–390] The particular species of Pgp found in paclitaxel-resistant murine macrophage cells is similar, but not identical, to that found in vinblastine- and colchicine-resistant cells derived from the same parental line.[122,385–388] These cells are cross-resistant with many other natural products, and resistance to both paclitaxel and docetaxel conferred by *mdr*-1 can be reversed by many classes of drugs, including the calcium-channel blockers, tamoxifen citrate, cyclosporine A, antiarrhythmic agents, and even the principal component of the vehicle used to formulate paclitaxel, Cremophor EL (polyoxyethylated castor oil).[385–392] In fact, plasma concentrations of Cremophor EL achieved with 3-hour infusions of paclitaxel at 135 to 175 mg per m^2 in most patients are capable of reversing MDR *in vitro*.[391–393] The precise role of MDR in conferring resistance to the taxanes in breast cancer and other tumor types in the clinic is being addressed in studies in which Pgp immunoreactivity and MDR expression in tumor biopsy specimens are being correlated with resistance to previously administered anthracyclines and paclitaxel. Preliminary results suggest a lack of complete cross-resistance between the taxanes and anthracyclines in women with breast cancer,[394,395] which may have been anticipated if MDR is a clinically significant mechanism of taxane resistance, and raises the possibility that Cremophor EL may be a built-in modulator of MDR. The feasibility of administering paclitaxel with known MDR modulators such as verapamil hydrochloride, cyclosporine A, and the nonimmunomodulatory cyclosporine analog PSC833 is being evaluated.[396–398]

Other changes in tumor cells selected for drug resistance have included up-regulation of caveolin-1, a principal component of membrane-derived vesicles involved in transmembrane transport of small molecules and in intracellular signaling. Caveolae act as a scaffold for intracellular kinases. One cell line, ninefold resistant to paclitaxel, had a 3.4-fold increase in caveolin-1 but no change in MDR-1 expression. Increased caveolin-1 was also found in cells selected for resistance to epothilone B, a related microtubule inhibitor.

As described previously, taxanes are exported by the MRP-1 transporter, previously described in this chapter, but not the BCRP.

Clinical Pharmacology

Analytical Assays

At the time paclitaxel entered clinical development, the only preclinical pharmacologic data available were obtained with a biochemical assay that exploited the ability of paclitaxel to induce tubulin to form cold-resistant polymers that hydrolyze GTP at 0°C.[399] This assay had a suboptimal lower limit of sensitivity of 0.1 μmol per L and was too complex for monitoring large clinical trials. Several HPLC methods were developed subsequently that permitted the characterization of the pharmacokinetic behavior of paclitaxel on many administration schedules during early clinical trials.[400–404] The variable extraction efficiencies, suboptimal lower limits of sensitivity (50 nmol per L or more), and other assay performance characteristics, however, generally rendered them inadequate for monitoring plasma levels in patients receiving low drug doses and prolonged infusions. More sensitive HPLC assays with lower limits of detection ranging from 7 to 30 nmol per L in plasma have become available, and several of these assays are capable of simultaneously measuring metabolites.[405–407] Similarly, sensitive HPLC methods enabling the quantification of docetaxel in biologic fluids are available.[408–413] One rapid, selective, and reproducible HPLC assay that uses solid-phase extraction (C2 ethyl microcolumns) and ultraviolet detection has a lower limit of sensitivity of 12 nmol per L in plasma and a coefficient of variation of 11% or less.[408,409]

More rapid and sensitive immunologic assays, including indirect competitive inhibition enzyme immunoassays (CIEIAs) and ELISAs, were originally developed for detecting taxanes in plant extracts.[414,415] The CIEIA, which is more sensitive (0.3 nmol per L) than available HPLC assays, may be used to monitor plasma concentrations in clinical trials that use prolonged infusion schedules yielding low taxane concentrations. CIEIAs that use monoclonal antibodies to the taxane ring are also available.[415] Nevertheless, the degree of cross-reactivity of these antibodies to the taxanes and their metabolites is not known.

Pharmacokinetics

General

The taxanes are generally administered by intravenous infusion at dosages of 90 mg per m^2 over 1 hour every week, or 135 to 250 mg per m^2 over 3 or 24 hours once every 3 weeks (paclitaxel), or 40 mg per m^2 over 1 hour every week, or 75 to 100 mg per m^2 over 1 hour (docetaxel) every 3 weeks. Pharmacokinetic features of both agents include large V_d values, rapid uptake in almost all tissues except for the central nervous system, high clearance rates, long terminal $t_{1/2}$ values, and significant hepatic metabolism and biliary excretion. Models of paclitaxel pharmacokinetics have incorporated both saturable metabolism and either saturable tissue uptake or saturable intracellular binding as key elements that explain the nonlinear pharmacokinetics.[416]

Paclitaxel

Early studies focused on the development of prolonged infusion (6- to 24-hour) schedules due to a high incidence of acute hypersensitivity reactions (HSRs) noted with shorter infusions.[298,417] Pertinent pharmacokinetic parameters are summarized in Table 12-4.[395,400–402,407,418–420] In early studies of prolonged (6- and 24-hour) infusions, substantial interpatient variability was noted, but neither nonlinear nor dose-dependent behavior was observed over broad dose ranges. Plasma drug disappearance was characterized by a biphasic process. Values for $t_{1/2\alpha}$ and $t_{1/2\beta}$ averaged 0.34 and 5.8 hours, respectively. Peak plasma concentrations with 1- to 96-hour infusion schedules are in the range of levels

(more than 0.05 to 0.1 µmol per L) capable of inducing significant biologic effects, including toxicity, *in vitro*.

The results of a prospective randomized trial demonstrating that the incidence of major HSRs is equivalent in patients receiving paclitaxel over 3 hours and over 24 hours with premedication[421] resulted in a reevaluation of shorter schedules, especially 1- and 3-hour infusions, which were largely abandoned during early development. From a pharmacologic prospective, the results of this study and more recent trials involving both adults and children indicate that the pharmacokinetic behavior of paclitaxel is nonlinear.[405,407,420] The pharmacokinetics of drugs such as paclitaxel that truly exhibit a nonlinear pharmacokinetic behavior at higher plasma concentrations is more likely to appear linear with prolonged infusion schedules that yield low plasma concentrations. When plasma levels are much lower than K_m, the Michaelis-Menten constant, elimination or distribution processes are not saturated, and pharmacokinetics appears linear (first order). Nonlinear (zero-order) pharmacokinetics, however, becomes more apparent with shorter infusion schedules, which results in higher plasma concentrations that approach or exceed the K_m values of saturable elimination or distribution processes. A combination of saturable distribution and saturable elimination processes appear to be responsible for paclitaxel's nonlinear pharmacokinetic behavior, with tissue distribution becoming effectively saturated at relatively lower drug concentrations (less than 175 mg per m^2 over 3 hours) compared with elimination processes (175 mg per m^2 or higher). This nonlinear pharmacokinetic profile may have important clinical implications. For example, dosage escalations, especially on shorter administration schedules, may result in disproportionate increases in both area under the curve (AUC) and C_{peak}, as well as disproportionate increases in toxicity, whereas dosage reductions may result in disproportionate decreases in AUC or C_{peak}, thereby possibly decreasing antitumor activity. Cremophor EL, the emulsifier used to formulate clinical dosage of paclitaxel, may contribute to the nonlinearity of pharmacokinetics by binding paclitaxel in plasma at high Cremophor concentrations and further by inhibiting secretion of drug and metabolites into bile.[422,423]

V_d values for paclitaxel are much larger than the volume of total-body water, which suggests extensive binding of drug to plasma proteins or other tissue constituents, possibly tubulin. Plasma protein binding is extensive (more than 95%).[400,402,404] At clinically relevant concentrations (0.1 to 0.6 µmol per L), protein binding is concentration independent, which indicates nonspecific hydrophobic binding. Albumin and α_1-acid glycoprotein contribute equally to the binding, with a minor contribution from lipoproteins.[424] None of the drugs that are commonly administered with paclitaxel, such as ranitidine, dexamethasone, diphenhydramine, doxorubicin, 5-fluorouracil, and cisplatin, alters protein binding.[424] Despite extensive binding to plasma proteins, paclitaxel is readily eliminated from the plasma compartment, a finding which suggests lower-affinity, reversible binding. Drug binding to platelets is extensive and saturable, whereas binding to red blood cells is insignificant.[425]

The tissue distribution of paclitaxel has not been studied extensively in humans. Limited data from early clinical trials indicate that biologically relevant drug concentrations (more than 0.1 μmol per L) are achieved in third-space fluid collections such as ascites.[402] The penetration of paclitaxel into the central nervous system, as manifested by detection in the cerebrospinal fluid, is negligible, which may explain paclitaxel's virtual lack of central nervous system toxicity.[418] Paclitaxel has been measured in resected human brain tumors shortly after treatment, however, which may be due to disruptions in the blood–brain barrier due to malignant disease.[426] Tissue-distribution studies in animals using radiolabeled drug have revealed high tissue to plasma paclitaxel ratios in virtually all tissues except brain and testes, which are generally considered "tumor sanctuary" sites.[427–429] Although peripheral neurotoxicity is a principal nonhematologic effect, radioactivity has not been detected in the peripheral nervous system of rats after treatment with tritium-labeled paclitaxel.[427]

The principal mechanisms of systemic clearance were not determined during early clinical trials, but renal clearance was demonstrated to contribute minimally to systemic clearance (5% to 10%).[400,402–404,420,430] Although metabolites have been found in the plasma of patients receiving 3-hour infusions,[420] extrahepatic excretion of metabolites contributes minimally to clearance. In contrast, high concentrations of paclitaxel and metabolites are excreted in the bile of both rodents and humans.[431–433] In humans, 30% of an administered dose of paclitaxel is recovered as either paclitaxel or metabolites from bile collected for 24 hours after treatment.[432–434] Because paclitaxel is widely distributed to peripheral compartments and biliary collections were not carried out for long periods after treatment in humans, conceivably hepatic metabolism and biliary excretion account for a much greater share of total clearance. This is the case in rats, in which 98% of total radioactivity can be recovered from feces collected for 6 days after treatment with paclitaxel labeled with radioactive carbon (^{14}C).[435]

All human paclitaxel metabolites that have been identified have intact side chains at taxane ring positions C-2 and C-13, whereas low concentrations of baccatin III, which lacks the side chain at position C-13, are found in rat bile.[431,432] Most metabolites are hydroxylated derivatives. The major metabolites in human plasma and bile are 6α-hydroxypaclitaxel, a product of CYP2C8, one of the P-450 microsomal isoenzymes; p-hydroxyphenyl-C3'-paclitaxel, a product of CYP3A4; and the dihydroxymetabolite (6α- and C3'-dihydroxypaclitaxel). Considerable variation in the relative amounts of each metabolite is found among

patients, perhaps due to individual differences in isoenzyme activity and its induction or inhibition as a result of drug interactions (see subsequent discussions of this topic).[433,436–440] For example, prolonged treatment with corticosteroids induces CYP3A4 and leads to increased dihydroxypaclitaxel,[433] whereas biricodar, an inhibitor of MDR-1 and multidrug resistance protein, inhibits the same enzyme, delays clearance, and significantly lowers the maximum tolerated dosage.[441] The metabolites are much less active against L1210 leukemia than paclitaxel, but some are as active as paclitaxel in stabilizing microtubules against disassembly in a cell-free system. One possible explanation for this discrepancy is that these hydroxylated metabolites, which are more polar than paclitaxel, are not taken up by the cell as readily as the parent compound.

Drug tolerance is clearly affected by hepatic dysfunction. For patients with a serum bilirubin of 3 mg per dL or higher, the maximum tolerated dose of paclitaxel given as a 24-hour infusion is 50 mg per m^2,[434] approximately one-third of the usual dose (135 to 175 mg per m^2). Neutropenia, the primary dose-limiting toxicity, correlates with the duration of exposure to plasma concentrations above 0.05 μmol per L. For patients with hepatic dysfunction and serum bilirubin above 3 mg per dL, these doses (50 mg per m^2) produced suprathreshold concentrations of drug for greater than 20 hours, a duration equal to that produced by the higher doses in patients with normal liver function. More detailed studies are needed to clarify changes in pharmacokinetics and drug metabolism in patients with hepatic dysfunction. Very little paclitaxel is excreted in the urine, and anephric patients clear paclitaxel at undiminished rates.[442]

Docetaxel

Although the pharmacokinetic behavior of docetaxel has been studied on several administration schedules, dosing schedules of single 1-hour infusions every 3 weeks have received the most attention.[409–413,443–445] Docetaxel was formulated initially as a 15-mg per mL solution in a mixture of ethanol and polysorbate 80 (50/50 volume/volume). This formulation, however, has been replaced by a second formulation containing docetaxel (40 mg per mL) in polysorbate 80 alone. The pharmacologic behavior of both formulations is similar.[412,443] The pharmacokinetic behavior of docetaxel on 1- or 2-hour schedules is linear at doses of 115 mg per m^2 or less and optimally fits a three-compartment model. Values for $t_{1/2\gamma}$ range from 11.4 to 13.6 hours.[409,411–413] In an analysis of pooled pharmacokinetic data using a population approach, an optimal three-compartment model generated the following pharmacokinetic estimates: $t_{1/2\gamma}$, 10.4 hours; clearance, 35 L per hour per m^2; and V_d at steady state, 67.3 L per m^2.[444,445] As with paclitaxel, both V_d and clearance rate are high, which indicates extensive protein binding or drug distribution. Docetaxel binds rapidly and avidly to plasma proteins (more than 90%), especially to albumin, α$_1$-acid glycoprotein, and lipoproteins.[446,447] In addition, peak plasma concentrations generally exceed levels required to induce relevant biologic effects *in vitro*.

Limited information is available about the distribution of docetaxel in humans. In rats and dogs, tissue-distribution studies using [^{14}C]docetaxel have demonstrated a rapid initial distribution phase of plasma radioactivity with an apparent $t_{1/2}$ of 10 minutes.[448] In mice, autoradiographic studies indicate that docetaxel rapidly accumulates in almost all tissues except for the central nervous system.[448] Immediately after treatment, tissue uptake of radioactivity is highest in the liver, bile, and intestines, a finding that is consistent with substantial hepatobiliary extraction and excretion. High levels of radioactivity are also found in the stomach, which indicates the possibility of gastric excretion, as well as in the spleen, bone marrow, myocardium, skeletal muscles, and pancreas.

The metabolism and elimination of docetaxel are similar to those of paclitaxel. In humans, urinary excretion accounts for a small percentage of drug disposition, averaging 2% in one study.[443] Both hepatic metabolism and biliary excretion are also important. In both dogs and mice treated with [^{14}C]docetaxel, fecal excretion of radioactivity accounts for 70% to 80% of the administered dose, whereas urinary excretion accounts for 10% or less.[412,449] Fecal excretion occurs primarily in the first 48 hours posttreatment and is nearly complete by 96 hours (mouse) or 168 hours (dog). In mice, less than 3% of the dose is excreted in the feces as the parent compound in the first 24 hours, and the excretion of three metabolites accounts for 75% of the administered dose. Similar profiles have been noted in humans treated with [^{14}C]docetaxel.[445,446,450] Approximately 80% of the administered dose of total radioactivity is excreted in the feces within 7 days after treatment, with the majority of excretion occurring in the first 48 hours, whereas 5% of total radioactivity is recovered from urine. Radioactivity in salivary secretions is low, and no radioactivity is detected in respiratory secretions. Several metabolites have been detected in the bile and feces of both humans and rats, as well as in microsomal and liver perfusion studies.[449–453] As with paclitaxel, the hepatic cytochrome P-450 mixed-function oxidases are responsible for the bulk of drug metabolism, and CYP3A, CYP2B, and CYP1A isoforms may play major roles in biotransformation.[451–453] The main metabolic pathway consists of oxidation of the tertiary butyl group on the side chain at the C-13 position of the taxane ring as well as cyclization of the side chain[450]; all metabolites appear to maintain their 10-deacetylbaccatin III or 7-epi isomer structural backbones.[454] These metabolites seem to be much less active than docetaxel.[451,454]

Pharmacodynamics

Both linear and nonlinear (sigmoidal maximal effect E_{max}) models have adequately described the relationships between the principal toxicity of both docetaxel and paclitaxel, neutropenia, and relevant pharmacokinetic parameters such as AUC and concentration at steady state (C_{ss}).[400,404,455,456] Analyses of pharmacologic and toxicity data from patients receiving paclitaxel on 3- and 24-hour schedules, however, indicate that the severity of neutropenia correlates best with the duration that plasma concentrations exceed critical threshold levels ranging from 0.05 to 0.1 µmol per L.[405,420] The severity of neuromuscular toxicity also has been directly related to both AUC and C_{ss} in patients receiving paclitaxel on 24-hour schedules.[455,457] Mucositis, the principal toxicity of paclitaxel on a more prolonged 96-hour schedule, has been found to be directly related to paclitaxel C_{ss} and clearance rate.[395]

Doses and Schedules

Paclitaxel

The most critical issues regarding the clinical use of paclitaxel concern optimal dosing and scheduling. Although clear evidence of schedule dependency was not observed in preclinical screening studies, optimal results were noted in a murine leukemia model when mice were treated every 3 hours, which functionally approximates a continuous-administration schedule.[298] The duration of treatment also has been one of the most important parameters influencing cytotoxicity *in vitro*.[458] Because evaluations were limited initially to 24-hour schedules due to the high incidence of HSRs in patients receiving shorter schedules without premedication and the 24-hour schedule was the first schedule to be approved for patients with recurrent or refractory ovarian cancer, most available information regarding paclitaxel's clinical activity pertains to the 24-hour schedule. However, prominent antitumor activity also has been observed with the 1-hour and 3-hour schedules in patients with recurrent or refractory breast and ovarian cancers. In fact, the incidence of HSRs and response rates are equivalent in women with recurrent or refractory ovarian cancer treated with 3- and 24-hour schedules of paclitaxel with premedication, and the 3-hour schedule has been approved for patients with recurrent and refractory breast and ovarian cancers.[421] Regardless, the equivalency of both schedules in the setting of recurrent or refractory ovarian cancer does not signify that both schedules are equivalent in patients with other tumor types and in other settings. Intriguing results also have been obtained for patients with advanced breast cancer who received paclitaxel on more prolonged schedules, particularly 96-hour infusion schedules.[395]

Paclitaxel is usually administered at a dose of 175 mg per m^2 over 3 hours or 135 to 175 mg per m^2 over 24 hours every 3 weeks. A schedule of 1-hour infusion of 80 to 100 mg per m^2 weekly has gained increasing acceptance for breast, lung, and ovarian cancer because of its minimal acute myelosuppression, neurotoxicity, alopecia, and acute side effects.[459,460] Discontinuance of corticosteroid pretreatment may be possible with this schedule. Due to paclitaxel's aqueous insolubility, it is formulated in Cremophor EL (polyoxyethylated castor oil) 50% and dehydrated alcohol 50%. Only glass or polyolefin containers and nitroglycerin tubing (polyethylene lined) are recommended for administration, because significant amounts of the plasticizer diethylhexylphthalate may be leached from polyvinyl chloride–containing tubing and plastic solution bags after contact with Cremophor EL. The following premedication is recommended (see Toxicity: Paclitaxel: Hypersensitivity Reactions): dexamethasone 20 mg orally or intravenously 12 and 6 hours before treatment; diphenhydramine 50 mg intravenously 30 minutes before treatment; and a histamine H_2 antagonist such as cimetidine 300 mg, famotidine 20 mg, or ranitidine 150 mg intravenously 30 minutes before treatment. Although higher paclitaxel doses have not been determined to be superior to lower doses, early phase II studies were performed using higher paclitaxel doses, 250 mg per m² over 24 hours, which usually caused severe neutropenia and often required administration of hematopoietic growth factors (see Toxicity: Paclitaxel: Hematologic).

The high molecular weight, bulky chemical structure, and principal hepatic metabolism of the taxanes render them ideal candidates for intracavitary administration. The feasibility of administering paclitaxel intraperitoneally as a single dose every 3 weeks and weekly has been studied.[461] Dose escalation above 125 mg per m² on a single dosing schedule results in severe abdominal pain, but systemic toxicity is mild at doses less than 175 mg per m². From a pharmacologic perspective, intraperitoneal drug concentrations are several orders of magnitude higher than levels required to induce pertinent microtubule effects *in vitro*. Paclitaxel concentrations of this magnitude are also maintained for several days, which indicates that intraperitoneal clearance of drug is very slow. Of considerable importance, biologically relevant paclitaxel concentrations are also readily achieved and sustained in the plasma for several days after treatment, which is encouraging, because the achievement of relevant systemic concentrations appears to be important in order for a drug to be advantageous when given by the intraperitoneal route.

Because patients with abnormal renal and hepatic functions were not eligible to participate in early trials of paclitaxel, only limited information is available pertaining to the pharmacologic behavior and toxicity of paclitaxel in patients with excretory organ dysfunction. Renal clearance accounts for a small proportion (less than 10%) of total clearance, and therefore dose modifications have not been necessary in patients with severe renal dysfunction.[462,463] In contrast, the magnitude of excretion of both paclitaxel and metabolites into bile is similar to that of other anticancer agents, such as the vinca alkaloids, in which dose modifications are required for hepatic excretory dysfunction. Data from a prospective evaluation of patients with hepatic dysfunction indicate that those with moderate elevations in total bilirubin are more likely to develop severe myelosuppression than are patients without hepatic dysfunction.[434,464] Reducing paclitaxel dosages by at least 50% to 75% in patients with moderate or severe hepatic excretory dysfunction (hyperbilirubinemia) seems prudent.

The severity of hematologic and nonhematologic toxicities does not seem to be affected by age[465,466]; however, the pharmacologic behavior of paclitaxel in elderly patients has not been evaluated prospectively.

Docetaxel

Although several administration schedules have been evaluated, docetaxel is most commonly administered intravenously at a dose of 100 mg per m² as a 1-hour infusion every 3 weeks. Lower doses of docetaxel (60 to 75 mg per m²) given as a 1-hour infusion may be associated with a lower incidence of both hematologic and nonhematologic toxicities; however, the relative therapeutic advantage of high versus low doses is not clear. Docetaxel may be given in dosages of 35 to 45 mg per m² per week, which result in modest neutropenia and less fluid retention than with higher dose regimens.[467] Despite the use of a polysorbate 80 formulation instead of Cremophor EL, occurrence of a relatively high rate of HSRs, as well as a fluid retention syndrome, has led to the use of several premedication regimens. The most frequent is dexamethasone 8 mg orally twice daily for 5 days starting one day before docetaxel administration, with or without both H_1 and H_2 histamine antagonists given intravenously 30 minutes before docetaxel. Use of corticosteroids greatly prevents fluid retention, including the pleural and peritoneal effusions commonly seen after multiple cycles of docetaxel (see later).

Although docetaxel treatment has not been evaluated rigorously in patients with excretory organ dysfunction, the principal role of the liver in drug metabolism and excretion indicates that dosage should be modified in such patients (see Doses and Schedules: Paclitaxel for guidelines). The results of a study involving patients with liver metastases with and without elevations in plasma levels of hepatocellular enzymes or alkaline phosphatase indicate that docetaxel clearance is reduced, which predisposes these patients to more severe neutropenia, mucositis, and rashes than experienced by patients with or without liver metastases and no liver function test abnormalities.[468]

Toxicity

Despite having similar structural features, paclitaxel and docetaxel differ in their toxicity spectra. Myelosuppression, primarily neutropenia, is the principal toxicity of both agents, but the types and frequencies of several nonhematologic side effects are different.

Paclitaxel

Hypersensitivity Reactions
The incidence of major HSRs in early phase I trials approached 25% to 30%.[417,469] Most affected patients have

manifestations of type I HSRs, including dyspnea with bronchospasm, urticaria, and hypotension. Major HSRs usually occur within 2 to 3 minutes after treatment and almost always occur within the first 10 minutes; the majority occur after the first or second dose. One fatality has been reported, but all other patients have recovered completely after cessation of treatment and occasionally after treatment with antihistamines, fluids, and vasopressors. Although minor reactions, such as flushing and rashes, also have been noted in as many as 40% of patients, minor HSRs do not portend the development of major reactions.[417,469]

Initial observations suggested that HSRs were mediated by the release of histamine or other vasoactive substances, as with the HSRs caused by radiographic contrast agents. Although HSRs may be caused by either paclitaxel itself or its Cremophor EL vehicle, the latter has been felt to be responsible, because it induces histamine release and similar manifestations in dogs, and other drugs formulated in it, such as cyclosporine A and vitamin K, induce similar reactions. The phase I trials were completed using 24-hour infusions and premedication with corticosteroids and histamine H_1 and H_2 antagonists (see Doses and Schedules: Paclitaxel), because similar regimens have proven effective in preventing repeated reactions to radiographic contrast agents. Although these measures are not fully protective, the incidence of major HSRs ranges from 1% to 3%.[469] In an assessment of the relative safety and efficacy of two different paclitaxel doses (135 versus 175 mg per m²) and two schedules (24 versus 3 hours) with standard premedication in women with recurrent or refractory ovarian cancer, the incidence of major HSRs was low and similar (2.1% versus 1.0%) in women receiving paclitaxel for 3 hours or 24 hours, respectively.[421] Patients who experience major HSRs may be rechallenged with paclitaxel without recurrence after receiving multiple high doses of corticosteroids, although this approach has not been always successful.[470]

Hematologic

Neutropenia is the principal toxicity of paclitaxel.[469] The onset is usually on days 8 to 10, and recovery is typically complete by days 15 to 21. Neutropenia is not cumulative, which suggests that paclitaxel does not irreversibly damage immature hematopoietic cells. At doses of 200 to 250 mg per m² given over 24 hours, neutropenia is usually severe even in patients who have received minimal prior myelosuppressive therapy or were previously untreated, with neutrophil counts below 500 per μL in most courses. This dose range was initially recommended for phase II studies because the duration of severe neutropenia (less than 500 per μL) was usually short (less than 5 days) and treatment delays for unresolved toxicity were rare. Although the rate of febrile or infectious sequelae was originally reported to be low at

these doses (less than 10% of courses) relative to the rate of severe neutropenia,[469,471,472] these complications occurred more frequently in later studies. Therefore, hematopoietic colony-stimulating factors are used commonly to prevent complications of neutropenia in trials of doses in this range. For most patients, particularly those who have received large doses of other chemotherapy agents previously, the maximum tolerated dose without hematopoietic colony-stimulating factors is 175 to 200 mg per m². A critical pharmacologic determinant of the severity of neutropenia is the duration that plasma drug concentrations are maintained above biologically relevant levels (0.05 to 0.1 μmol per L), which may explain why neutropenia is more severe with longer infusions.[405,420] This does not imply that shorter infusions should always be used, because the optimal dose and schedule have not been determined for most tumors. Notwithstanding these differences, the main clinical determinant of the severity of neutropenia is the extent of prior myelotoxic therapy. Severe thrombocytopenia and anemia are rare.

Neurologic

Paclitaxel induces a peripheral neuropathy that is characterized by sensory symptoms such as numbness and paresthesia in a glove-and-stocking distribution.[469,473] Symmetric distal loss of sensation carried by both large (proprioception, vibration) and small (temperature, pin prick) fibers is often present. Symptoms may begin as soon as 24 to 72 hours after treatment with higher doses (more than 250 mg per m²) but usually occur only after multiple courses at 135 to 250 mg per m². Severe neurotoxicity precludes repetitive treatment with paclitaxel doses above 250 mg per m² over 3 or 24 hours,[473] but severe neurotoxicity is rare at conventional doses (less than 200 mg per m²), even in patients who previously received other neurotoxic agents such as cisplatin.

The distal symmetric length-dependent neurologic deficits suggest that paclitaxel causes a sensory and motor axonal loss similar to the "dying-back" neuropathies that may have its origin in the cell body or in axonal transport, but a few patients have the simultaneous onset of symptoms in the arms and legs, involvement of the face (perioral numbness), the predominance of large fiber loss, and diffuse areflexia suggestive of a neuronopathy. Both types of neuropathy depend on the dose of paclitaxel or its combination with cisplatin.[473,474] Motor and autonomic dysfunction also may occur, especially at high doses and in patients with preexisting neuropathies caused by diabetes mellitus and alcoholism. In addition, optic nerve disturbances, characterized by scintillating scotomata, may occur.[475] Transient myalgia, usually noted 2 to 5 days after therapy, is common at doses above 170 mg per m², and myopathy has been noted with high doses of paclitaxel (more than 250 mg per m^2) in combination with cisplatin.[473,474]

Cardiac

Paclitaxel causes cardiac rhythm disturbances, but the importance of these effects is not known.[476,477] The most common effect, a transient asymptomatic bradycardia, was noted in 29% of patients in one trial.[471] Isolated asymptomatic bradycardia without hemodynamic effects does not appear to be an indication for discontinuing paclitaxel. More important bradyarrhythmias, including Mobitz type I (Wenckebach syndrome), Mobitz type II, and third-degree heart block, also have been noted, but the incidence in a large National Cancer Institute database was only 0.1%.[477] All events occurred in patients enrolled in trials that required continuous cardiac monitoring, which indicates that second- and third-degree heart block is likely underreported, because continuous cardiac monitoring is not usually performed. Most documented episodes have been asymptomatic and reversible. These bradyarrhythmias are probably caused by paclitaxel, because related taxanes affect cardiac automaticity and conduction, and similar disturbances have occurred in humans and animals who have ingested various species of yew plants.[477]

Myocardial infarction, cardiac ischemia, atrial arrhythmias, and ventricular tachycardia also have been noted.[476,477] Whether a direct causal relationship exists between paclitaxel and ventricular and atrial tachycardias and ischemic events is uncertain. Also, no evidence exists that paclitaxel induces cumulative toxicity, nor that it augments the acute cardiac effects of the anthracyclines[477]; however, the frequency of congestive cardiotoxicity in patients treated with paclitaxel and doxorubicin in one trial has been higher than expected from the anthracycline alone.[478] In patients treated with paclitaxel and an anthracycline, potential drug effects on ventricular function should be evaluated at lower cumulative anthracycline doses than might otherwise be done with anthracyclines alone.

Once cardiac effects were documented, eligibility in most early trials was restricted to patients with no history of cardiac disease. This broadly described population, however, undoubtedly excludes many patients who might otherwise be good candidates for paclitaxel, and the precise risks for cardiotoxicity in this population are not known. Routine cardiac monitoring during paclitaxel therapy is not necessary but is advisable for patients who may not be able to tolerate the drug's potential bradyarrhythmic effects, such as those with atrioventricular conduction defects or ventricular dysfunction.

Miscellaneous

Drug-related gastrointestinal effects such as vomiting and diarrhea are infrequent.[469] Higher doses may cause mucosi-

tis, especially in patients with leukemia, who may be more prone to mucosal barrier breakdown,[418] or in patients receiving 96-hour infusions.[395] Rare cases of neutropenic enterocolitis also have been noted, particularly in patients given high doses of paclitaxel in combination with doxorubicin and cyclophosphamide.[479,480] Like other chemotherapeutic agents, paclitaxel induces alopecia of the scalp, but all body hair is often lost with cumulative therapy. Inflammation at the injection site, along the course of an injected vein, and in areas of previous drug extravasation, as well as inflammatory skin reactions over previously radiated sites (radiation recall), may occur.[469,481,482]

Docetaxel

Hematologic

Neutropenia is the principal toxicity of docetaxel. At 100 mg per m^2 of docetaxel (1-hour schedule), neutrophil count nadirs are less than 500 per microliter in 50% to 80% of courses in previously untreated patients and in 83% of courses in heavily pretreated patients.[483–487] The onset of neutropenia is early, with nadirs usually on day 9 and complete recovery generally by days 15 to 21. Treatment delays are rarely required. Febrile neutropenia necessitating hospitalization and parenteral antibiotics has been reported in 11% to 14% of courses.[484,485] Neutropenia is not cumulative. Unlike with paclitaxel, the severity of neutropenia correlates with the AUC of parent compound in plasma but does not seem to be related to the infusion duration; however, experience with longer infusion schedules has been limited. Significant effects on platelets and red blood cells are uncommon.

Hypersensitivity Reactions

Because docetaxel is not formulated in Cremophor EL, HSRs were not originally anticipated to be a major problem. However, both major and minor HSRs occur in approximately 25% of patients receiving docetaxel without premedication.[486] Whether docetaxel's polysorbate 80 formulation, the taxane moiety itself, or both are responsible for HSRs is not known. These reactions are similar to HSRs induced by paclitaxel. Major HSRs, characterized by dyspnea, bronchospasm, and hypotension, usually occur during the first two courses and within minutes after the start of treatment.[488–490] Symptoms generally resolve within 15 minutes after cessation of treatment; however, treatment is usually able to be resumed without further consequence, occasionally after administration of diphenhydramine. The manifestations of minor HSRs include flushing, chest tightness, and low-back pain. Preliminary results indicate that the incidence and severity of HSRs are reduced somewhat by several premedication regimens, including (a) dexamethasone 10 mg given orally 12 and 6 hours before treatment; and (b) dexamethasone 8 mg given orally twice daily for 5 days beginning 1 day before treatment, with or without both H_1 and H_2 histamine antagonists administered 30 minutes before treatment.[488–490]

Fluid Retention

Docetaxel induces a cumulative fluid-retention syndrome characterized by edema, weight gain, pleural effusions, and ascites.[483–488] Neither hypoalbuminemia nor cardiac, renal, or hepatic dysfunction is found, and capillary filtration studies with technetium 99m–labeled albumin and capillaroscopy suggest that docetaxel causes a capillary permeability abnormality.[491] Plasma renin concentrations also have been elevated in some patients.[484] Fluid retention is not usually significant at cumulative doses of less than 400 mg per m^2, but the incidence and severity increase sharply at cumulative doses of 400 mg per m^2 or higher, which often results in the delay or termination of treatment. Both peripheral edema and third-space fluid collections usually resolve slowly after treatment is stopped. The aggressive use of diuretics may be helpful in managing fluid retention; however, preliminary studies suggest that the incidence of fluid retention may be reduced by using lower single-treatment doses of docetaxel (less than 60 to 75 mg per m^2) or an alternate administration schedule (e.g., divided doses on days 1 and 8 every 3 weeks). Premedication with dexamethasone 8 mg orally twice daily for 5 days beginning 1 day before docetaxel reduces the incidence of fluid retention and increases the median number of courses before the onset of this toxicity.[488–490]

Dermatologic

Between 50% and 75% of patients receiving docetaxel develop skin toxicity, typically characterized by an erythematous pruritic maculopapular rash that affects the forearms and hands.[409–413,483–489,492] Other cutaneous effects include superficial desquamation of the hands and feet and onychodystrophy characterized by brown discoloration, ridging, onycholysis, soreness, and brittleness of the fingernails. Docetaxel also induces palmar-plantar erythrodysesthesia that may be responsive to pyridoxine or cooling.[493,494] The use of premedication may decrease the incidence of skin toxicity.[488] Alopecia occurs in most patients. Drug extravasation may produce localized pain and discoloration without necrosis.[410] Phlebitis also has been reported.

Neurologic

Although the incidence of neurotoxicity was reported to be low in early clinical trials, mild to moderate peripheral neurotoxicity has been reported in approximately 40% of previously untreated patients in phase II studies.[483,484] The incidence of peripheral neuropathy may be higher in patients who were previously treated with

platinum compounds and approached 74% in one trial.[485] Nonetheless, severe toxicity is rare after repetitive treatment with single doses of 100 mg per m^2 or less, except in patients with antecedent disorders such as alcohol abuse.[484] The peripheral neuropathy is similar to that induced by paclitaxel, predominately affecting large fiber sensory function.[495,496] Patients typically complain of paresthesias and numbness. Peripheral motor dysfunction resulting in extremity weakness also may occur. Transient myalgias are often noted in the peritreatment period.[485]

Miscellaneous

Asthenia has been observed in as many as 58% to 67% of patients.[483,497] Although malaise is usually mild to moderate in severity, it is occasionally severe enough to warrant dosage reduction or discontinuation of treatment. Cardiac conduction disturbances and ischemia have been noted in the peritreatment period, but no convincing evidence exists that directly links docetaxel to these episodes.[411,483,485] The incidence of stomatitis appears to be higher with docetaxel than with paclitaxel, particularly with prolonged infusions. Nausea, vomiting, and diarrhea occur, but severe gastrointestinal effects are rare.

Drug Interactions

Interactions of taxanes and noncytotoxic inducers or inhibitors of P-450 cytochrome isoenzymes have been discussed in a previous section (see Pharmacokinetics). The taxanes also display significant interactions with other antineoplastic drugs, as the result of effects on cell cycle. Sequence-dependent interactions have been described between the taxanes and other chemotherapy agents. The sequence of cisplatin followed by paclitaxel (24-hour schedule) induced more profound neutropenia than the reverse drug sequence in phase I studies.[498] This could be explained by a 33% reduction in the clearance rate of paclitaxel after cisplatin. The cisplatin-paclitaxel sequence also was suboptimal *in vitro* with respect to cytotoxicity.[499,500] The mechanisms for these sequence-dependent effects *in vitro* are not entirely clear; however, paclitaxel has been shown to inhibit the repair of cisplatin-DNA adducts. Another possibility is that treatment with cisplatin before paclitaxel is antagonistic, because cisplatin inhibits cell-cycle progression in the G_2 phase, thereby preventing further progression into the mitotic phases, which may be the optimal period of cell sensitivity to the taxanes. Regardless of the precise mechanism, these observations formed the rationale for the selection of the sequence of paclitaxel followed by cisplatin for subsequent clinical trials of the paclitaxel-cisplatin chemotherapy combination.

Another potential mechanism for this interaction is the modulation of cytochrome P-450–dependent paclitaxel-metabolizing enzymes by cisplatin. Platinum compounds may depress the activities of cytochrome P-450 mixed-function oxidases.[501] The ability to modulate cytochrome P-450 mixed-function oxidases is not shared by all the platinum compounds. For example, carboplatin does not appear to be capable of modulating P-450 systems and does not modify the pharmacokinetics of paclitaxel.[501,502]

The potential for sequence-dependent interactions also has been examined during developmental studies of paclitaxel-doxorubicin and paclitaxel-cyclophosphamide combinations for breast cancer.[480,503–505] Mucositis is more prominent when paclitaxel (24-hour infusion) is administered before doxorubicin than with the reverse sequence.[503–505] Paclitaxel decreases the clearance of doxorubicin when infused before the anthracycline, and the sequence of paclitaxel then doxorubicin is associated with greater myelosuppression than the reverse sequence.[505] Paclitaxel has similar inhibitor effects on epirubicin hydrochloride clearance.[506,507] Paclitaxel 175 mg per m^2 over 3 hours, immediately preceding bolus epirubicin 90 mg per m^2, decreased total-body clearance of epirubicin by 25%, increased the AUC by one-third, and delayed neutrophil recovery, as compared with the opposite sequence.[507] Similarly, both neutropenia and thrombocytopenia have been more profound with the sequence of cyclophosphamide before paclitaxel (24-hour schedule) than with the reverse sequence.[480] The mechanism for these differential effects is not clear, however, because both pharmacologic and cytotoxicity studies have failed to demonstrate differences between the sequences. Although these studies may potentially be used as paradigms to assess other taxane-based chemotherapy combinations, one should emphasize that sequence-dependent interactions have been noted only with prolonged paclitaxel infusions and not with short (e.g., 3-hour infusion) schedules. Sequence-dependent effects also have not been observed with docetaxel-based drug combinations in which docetaxel is administered as a 1-hour infusion.[508]

Drug interactions may also result from effects on cell cycle. As noted previously, the cytotoxicity of taxanes is prevented by blocking progression of cells into mitosis. Pretreatment of cells with 5-fluorouracil blocks their progression through S phase and prevents mitotic block, reducing cell kill by paclitaxel.[509] A farnesyltransferase inhibitor increases the entry of cells into mitosis, possibly through its effects on signaling proteins, and enhances the growth-inhibitory effects of taxanes and epothilones.[510] Surprisingly, paclitaxel, which promotes tubulin polymerization, and vinblastine, which inhibits the same process, are synergistic against cells in culture when drugs are added simultaneously, but antagonistic when added sequentially.[511] Finally, β-lapachone, a novel topoisomerase I inhibitor in preclinical development, and paclitaxel are synergistic *in vitro* and in xenograft experiments when the two drugs are used together, or when paclitaxel follows β-lapachone, but not in the reverse sequence (first paclitaxel, then β-lapachone).[512] The mechanism is uncertain, but it is believed to be related to enhanced cell entry into mitosis after β-lapachone.

Another possible source of drug interactions is the effects of other classes of concurrently administered drugs on the metabolism of the taxanes. Various pharmacologic inducers of cytochrome P-450 mixed-function oxidases such as phenytoin and phenobarbital accelerate the metabolism of both paclitaxel and docetaxel in human microsomal studies.[436–438,449–454] Preliminary clinical observations also have indicated the possibility of interactions between paclitaxel and inducers of cytochrome P-450 enzymes. For example, rapid drug clearance in some patients has been associated with the use of anticonvulsant agents.[457] Similarly, plasma paclitaxel concentrations and toxicity were much lower than predicted in patients with malignant brain tumors treated with 96-hour infusions of paclitaxel, possibly due to the induction of taxane metabolism by the anticonvulsant agents.[513] Conversely, many types of pharmacologic agents that are capable of inhibiting cytochrome P-450 mixed-function oxidases interfere with the microsomal metabolism of both paclitaxel and docetaxel *in vitro*.[436,438,449–453] For example, diazepam, an inhibitor of CYP3A isoforms, inhibits paclitaxel's major metabolic pathway, whereas several inhibitors of CYP2C isoforms such as orphenadrine citrate, erythromycin, testosterone, and troleandomycin may be potent inhibitors of a minor metabolic pathway. Both ketoconazole and fluconazole also have been shown to inhibit the metabolism of paclitaxel *in vitro*.[429] (See also Pharmacokinetics.)

Concern has also arisen that H$_2$ histamine antagonist premedications may be an important source of drug interactions. Use of these agents with the taxanes may produce variable pharmacologic and toxicologic effects, because these agents differentially inhibit cytochrome P-450 metabolism, with cimetidine being the most potent inhibitor. However, H$_2$ histamine antagonists do not appear to alter the metabolism and pharmacologic disposition of the taxanes in animal and *in vitro* studies.[429,514] In addition, the results of a clinical trial in which patients were randomized to receive either cimetidine or famotidine premedication before their first course of paclitaxel and then crossed over to the alternate premedication during their second course have failed to show significant toxicologic and pharmacologic differences between these H$_2$ histamine antagonists.[515]

NOVEL ANTIMICROTUBULE AGENTS IN EARLY CLINICAL DEVELOPMENT

Dolastatins

The dolastatins constitute a series of oligopeptides isolated from the sea hare, *Dolabella auricularia*. These agents interact with tubulin in the vinca alkaloid–binding domain. The most potent of these compounds is dolastatin 10, which inhibits tubulin polymerization, tubulin-dependent GTP hydrolysis, and the binding of radiolabeled vinca alkaloids to tubulin and stabilizes the colchicine-binding activity of tubulin.[516] It also inhibits the binding of radiolabeled VCR to tubulin in a noncompetitive manner, in contrast with the competitive inhibition observed with VBL, rhizoxin,[516a–516f] and maytansine.[516] Rhizoxin has demonstrated good antitumor activity *in vitro* and against several human tumor xenografts, particularly when given intravenously as a bolus injection. *In vitro* studies indicate that drug resistance may be conferred by the MDR phenotype.[517] Pharmacologic studies using tritium-labeled dolastatin 10 have revealed an elimination $t_{1/2}$ of 3.7 hours and a low urinary excretion (less than 2%) in mice.[518] Dolastatin 10 is also highly protein bound (more than 81%) in human, dog, and mouse plasma. After incubation with whole-liver homogenates, dolastatin 10 is rapidly converted to more polar products, including a dihydroxy derivative. Clinical development of dolastatin 10 also has begun.

Others

Various other natural products that are currently being evaluated for antineoplastic activity include compounds that interact with tubulin in the vinca alkaloid–binding domain, such as dolastatin 15, phomopsin A, halichondrin B, homohalichondrin B, and spongistatin 1, and agents that interact with tubulin at the colchine-binding domain, such as the natural products combretastatin and steganacin and synthetic pyridine and pyridazine derivatives.[68,69,72,519,520]

ESTRAMUSTINE

Estramustine, which is essentially an estradiol molecule linked to a nor-nitrogen mustard through a carbamate ester group (Fig. 12-6), was synthesized in the mid-1960s as an alkylating agent specifically for the treatment of advanced prostate carcinoma.[521] The estradiol portion of the molecule was designed to facilitate uptake by steroid receptors in malignant cells, which was followed by the intracellular release of the nitrogen mustard alkylating moiety. In its proprietary form, the approved agent, estramustine phosphate, has a phosphate at the 17β-position of the steroid D ring, which renders it more water soluble and therefore more feasible for clinical administration.

Mechanism of Action

Although estrogens are released after the administration of estramustine, the drug inhibits growth of a number of cell lines and tumors that lack estrogen receptors and fail to respond to estrogen.[522–525] Not only is estramustine capable of inducing cytotoxicity in estrogen receptor–negative tumor cells, but drug binding is not inhibited by 1,000-fold excess concentrations of estradiol.[522] Other observations are also not congruent with alkylating activity as the principal mechanism of estramustine, including the drug's lack of alkylating activity *in vitro* at concentrations that induce cytotoxicity and the absence of direct DNA damage after treatment at lethal concentrations, noncovalent binding of the drug, the reversibility of various effects, the sensitivity of alkylating agent–resistant cells to estramustine, and the principal clinical toxicities of estramustine, which are atypical for an alkylating agent.[522,523,526]

After treatment with estramustine was demonstrated to produce metaphase arrest,[527,528] it became apparent that the antineoplastic effects of estramustine are mediated through inhibitory and dissociative effects on microtubule structure and function rather than through covalent interactions with proteins and nucleic acids. Estramustine binds to MAPs, including high-molecular-weight and τ proteins, and induces the dissociation of

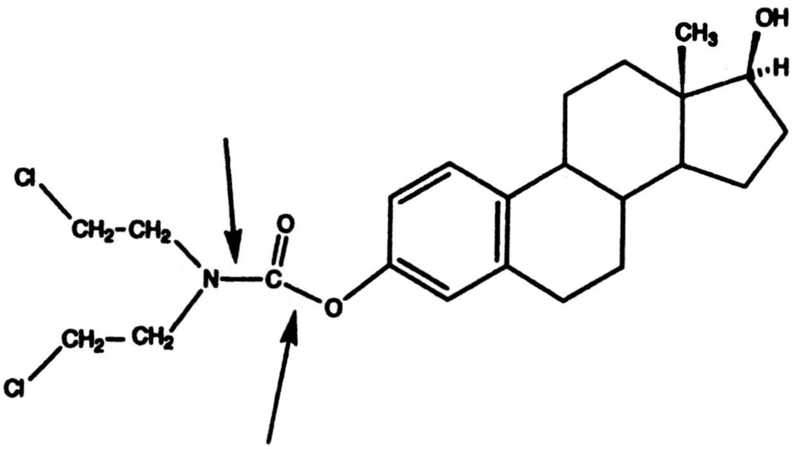

FIGURE 12-6. Structure of estramustine. Arrows show the bonds that separate the estrogenic portion of the molecule from the nitrogen mustard. (From Tew KD, Glusker JP, Hartley-Asp B, et al. Preclinical and clinical perspectives on the use of estramustine as an antimitotic drug. *Pharmacol Ther* 1992;56:323, with permission.)

MAPs from microtubules. These actions result in the inhibition of microtubule assembly and the subsequent disassembly of microtubules.[529–531] Overall, estramustine binds with different avidity to MAPs isolated from various tumor cells and tissues. The binding constants for some of these MAPs have been estimated to range from 10 to 15 µmol per L,[530,532] which are not inconsistent with the concentrations of estramustine that induce antimicrotubule effects and cytotoxicity. In addition to affecting MAPs, estramustine has been shown to interact directly with tubulin.[533]

Estramustine binds to specific proteins in tissues, commonly referred to as *estramustine binding proteins* (EMBPs). An EMBP with a heterodimeric structure and a molecular weight of 46,000 was originally isolated from prostate tissue. Higher-molecular-weight EMBP-like proteins have been found in other tissues and tumors, however, such as prostate adenocarcinoma and astrocytoma.[534] Evidence also exists that EMBP levels in prostate cancer are related to neither the androgen concentrations nor the androgen dependency of the tumors.[535] Instead, EMBP levels correlated with the degree of tumor cell differentiation.

Estramustine also has been demonstrated to enhance the effects of radiation *in vitro*.[536–538] These radiation-enhancing effects are most prominent after prolonged treatment of cells with estramustine before irradiation and may be related to the degree of accumulation of cells in the G_2-M phase of the cell cycle as a result of estramustine.[527]

Mechanisms of Resistance

The mechanisms for cellular resistance to estramustine differ from mechanisms of acquired resistance characterized for other antimicrotubule agents. Estramustine-resistant cells do not possess the MDR phenotype.[523,539–541] First, although the degree of resistance for cells with acquired drug resistance on the basis of MDR is usually several hundred–fold to many thousand–fold, resistance to estramustine does not usually exceed fourfold to fivefold. Second, estramustine-resistant cells exhibit no cross-resistance with other antimicrotubule agents and natural products, to which resistance is conferred by the MDR phenotype. Finally, estramustine-resistant cells do not express increased Pgp messenger RNA or protein levels. In fact, estramustine has been demonstrated to be a modulator of MDR, albeit a less effective one than verapamil.[539–541] In addition, neither modified expression of glutathione *S*-transferase nor increased intracellular levels of glutathione appear to account for estramustine resistance *in vitro*.[523]

The results of drug efflux studies indicate that some estramustine-resistant clones have altered patterns of estramustine extrusion.[523] Although the precise mechanism for

the enhanced efflux of estramustine from resistant cells is not known, Pgp is not increased in these cells.

Clinical Pharmacology

The pharmacokinetic and biologic $t_{1/2}$ values of estramustine are long. In humans treated with radiolabeled estramustine phosphate by intravenous injection, the terminal $t_{1/2}$ values range from 20 to 24 hours.[542] Immediately after injection, estramustine phosphate predominates in plasma; however, it is dephosphorylated to estramustine so that the dephosphorylated compound is the predominate species at 4 hours after treatment. The phosphate moiety appears to be lost in the gastrointestinal tract, liver, and other phosphatase-rich tissues such as the prostate. Peak plasma concentrations in multiple-dose studies in which 600 mg per m^2 was given three times daily have been 326 ng per mL for estramustine (the dephosphorylated estrone derivative), 82 ng per mL for estramustine phosphate, 36 ng per mL for estramustine, 162 ng per mL for estrone, and 17 ng per mL for estradiol.[543]

At least 75% of an oral dose of estramustine phosphate is bioavailable.[542,544] The compound is excreted into the bile, feces, and urine as metabolites of both the alkylating and estrogenic moieties. Within 48 hours after the administration of radiolabeled estramustine phosphate, urinary excretion accounts for 23% of total drug disposition.[545] In addition, only small quantities of unmetabolized drug are found, which indicates that drug disposition is principally due to nonrenal mechanisms. In the liver, the steroidal component of the molecule is conjugated primarily as the glucuronide and excreted into the bile, feces, and urine.

Doses and Schedules

Estramustine phosphate is approved for the treatment of metastatic prostate cancer, particularly for hormonally unresponsive disease. It is available for oral use as a 140-mg capsule. The recommended daily dose of estramustine phosphate is 14 mg per kg given in three or four divided oral doses, although most patients are usually treated in the dosing range of 10 to 16 mg per kg. Patients should be instructed to take estramustine phosphate with water at least 1 hour before or 2 hours after meals. Milk and calcium-rich foods or drugs should be avoided due to the possibility of calcium phosphate salt formation. A parenteral formulation is also available for investigational purposes.

Toxicity

Gastrointestinal toxicities are the most common adverse effects of estramustine phosphate. At conventional dosages, nausea and vomiting are usually transient and responsive to antiemetic treatment. Nausea and vomiting are the dose-limiting toxicities of the oral formulation, however, and intractable vomiting, which may require the termination of therapy, is noted occasionally after 6 to 8 weeks of treatment. Diarrhea may occur in as many as 15% to 30% of patients.

Cardiovascular effects are potentially the most hazardous toxicities of estramustine phosphate, and such problems may occur in 10% of patients who have not been treated with estrogens.[526,546,547] Patients with depressed cardiac function may develop worsening symptoms of congestive heart failure during treatment, presumably due to the salt-retaining effects of the estrogenic portion of the drug. Other rare cardiovascular complications include thromboembolism, cardiac ischemia, and cerebrovascular events. Thus, patients with preexisting cardiac and cerebrovascular disease, as well as hypertension, should be monitored closely.

Gynecomastia and nipple tenderness are experienced by most patients, but these effects can be prevented by prophylactic breast irradiation.

Myelosuppression is uncommon. Other rare effects include abnormalities of liver function test results, fever, urticaria, and other skin rashes.

Drug Interactions

Drugs that reduce glutathione may enhance the activity of estramustine.[545] In addition, the combination of estramustine and other antimicrotubule agents, including VBL and paclitaxel, may produce synergistic cytotoxicity *in vitro*.[548–550]

REFERENCES

1. Dustin P. *Microtubules*, 2nd ed. New York: Springer-Verlag, 1984.
2. Hyams JF, Lloyd CW. *Microtubules*. New York: Wiley-Liss, 1993.
3. Wilson L. Microtubules as drug receptors: pharmacological properties of microtubule protein. *Ann N Y Acad Sci* 1975;253:213.
4. Crossin KL, Carney DH. Microtubule stabilization by Taxol inhibits initiation of DNA synthesis by thrombin and epidermal growth factor. *Cell* 1981;27:341.
5. De Asua LJ, Otto AM. Microtubule-disrupting agents can independently affect the prereplicative period and entry into S phase stimulated by prostaglandin F and fibroblastic growth factor. *J Cell Physiol* 1983;115:15.
6. Teng M, Bartholomew JC, Bissell MJ. Synergism between antimicrotubule agents and growth stimulants in enhancement of cell cycle traverse. *Nature* 1977;268:739.
7. Ponstingl H, Krauhs E, Little M, et al. Complete amino acid sequence of alpha-tubulin from porcine brain. *Proc Natl Acad Sci U S A* 1981;78:2757.
8. Krauhs E, Little M, Kempf T, et al. Complete amino acid sequence of beta-tubulin from porcine brain. *Proc Natl Acad Sci U S A* 1981;78:4156.
9. Amos LA, King A. Arrangement of subunits in flagellar microtubules. *J Cell Sci* 1974;14:523.
10. Amos LA, Baker TS. The three dimension structure of tubulin protofilaments. *Nature* 1979;279:607.
11. Mandelkow E-M, Schulthesiss R, Rapp R, et al. On the surface lattice of microtubule: halt starts, protofilament number, seam and handedness. *J Cell Biol* 1986;102:1067.
12. Raff EC. Genetics of microtubule systems. *J Cell Biol* 1984;99:1.
13. Sullivan KF. Structure and utilization of tubulin isotypes. *Annu Rev Cell Biol* 1988;4:687.
14. Ludena RF. Are tubulin isotypes functionally significant? *Mol Biol Cell* 1983;4:445.
15. Gundersen GG, Khawja S, Bulinski JC. Postpolymerization detyrosination of alpha-tubulin: a mechanism for subcellular differentiation of microtubules. *J Cell Biol* 1987;105:251.
16. Schulze E, Asai DJ, Bulinski JC, et al. Post-translational modification and microtubule stability. *J Cell Biol* 1987;105:2167.
17. Olmsted JB. Microtubule-associated proteins. *Annu Rev Cell Biol* 1986;2:421.
18. Vallee RB, Bloom GS, Theurkauf WE. Microtubule associated proteins: subunits of the cytomatrix. *J Cell Biol* 1984;99:38s.
19. Penningroth SM, Kirschner MW. Nucleotide binding and phosphorylation in microtubule assembly in vitro. *J Mol Biol* 1977;115:643.
20. Weisenberg RC, Deery WJ, Dickinson PJ. Tubulin-nucleotide interactions during the polymerization and depolymerization of microtubules. *Biochemistry* 1976;15:4248.
21. Farrell KW, Jordan MA, Miller HP, et al. Phase dynamics at microtubule ends: the coexistence of microtubule length changes and treadmilling. *J Cell Biol* 1987;104:1035.
22. Mitchison TJ. Localization of exchangeable GTP binding site at the plus end of microtubules. *Science* 1993;261:1044.
23. McIntosh JR, Euteneuer U. Tubulin hooks as probes for microtubule polarity: an analysis of the method and evaluation of data on microtubule polarity in the mitotic spindle. *J Cell Biol* 1984;98:525.
24. Carlier M-F. Role of nucleotide hydrolysis in the polymerization of actin and tubulin. *Cell Biophys* 1988;12:105.
25. Mandelkow E-M, Mandelkow E. Microtubule oscillations. *Cell Motil Cytoskeleton* 1992;22:235.
26. Sammak PJ, Borisy GG. Direct observation of microtubule dynamics in living cells. *Nature* 1988;332:724.
27. Erickson HP, O'Brien ET. Microtubule dynamic instability and GTP hydrolysis. *Annu Rev Biophys Biomol Struct* 1992;21:145.
28. Mandelkow E-M, Mandelkow E, Milligan RA. Microtubule dynamics and microtubule caps—a time resolved cryo-electron microscopy study. *J Cell Biol* 1991;114:977.
29. Mitchison T, Kirschner M. Dynamic instability of microtubule growth. *Nature* 1984;312:237.
30. MacRae TH. Towards an understanding of microtubule function and cell organization: an overview. *Biochem Cell Biol* 1992;70:835.
31. Greer K, Rosenbaum JL. Post-translational modifications of tubulin. In: Warner FD, McIntosh JR, eds. *Cell movement: kinesin, dynein, and microtubule dynamics*, vol. 2. New York: Wiley-Liss, 1989:46.
32. Johnson IS, Armstrong JG, Gorman M, et al. The *Vinca* alkaloids: a new class of oncolytic agents. *Cancer Res* 1967;23:1390.

33. Johnson IS. Historical background of *Vinca* alkaloid research and areas of future interest. *Cancer Chemother Rep* 1968;52:455.

34. Budman DR. New vinca alkaloids and related compounds. *Semin Oncol* 1992;19:639.

35. Correia JJ. Effects of antimitotic agents on tubulin-nucleotide interactions. *Pharmacol Ther* 1991;52:127.

36. Beck WT. Alkaloids. In: Fox BW, Fox M, eds. Antitumor drug resistance. Berlin: Springer-Verlag, 1984:589.

37. Beck WT. Increase by vinblastine of oxidized glutathione in cultured mammalian cells. *Biochem Pharmacol* 1983;29:2333.

38. Cline MJ. Effect of vincristine on synthesis of ribonucleic acid and protein in leukaemic leucocytes. *Br J Haematol* 1968;14:21.

39. Creasey WA, Markiw ME. Biochemical effects of the *Vinca* alkaloids: II. A comparison of the effects of colchicine, vinblastine and vincristine on the synthesis of ribonucleic acids in Ehrlich ascites carcinoma cells. *Biochim Biophys Acta* 1964;87:601.

40. Creasey WA, Markiw ME. Biochemical effects of the *Vinca* alkaloids: III. The synthesis of ribonucleic acid and the incorporation of amino acids in Ehrlich ascites cells in vitro. *Biochim Biophys Acta* 1965;103:635.

41. Kennedy MS, Insel PA. Inhibitors of microtubule assembly enhance beta adrenergic and prostaglandin E1-stimulated cyclic AMP accumulation in S49 lymphoma cells. *Mol Pharmacol* 1979;16:215.

42. Kotani M, Koizumi Y, Yamada T, et al. Increase of cyclic adenosine 3',5'-monophosphate concentration in transplantable lymphoma cells by *Vinca* alkaloids. *Cancer Res* 1978;38:3094.

43. Malawista SE, Bensch KG, Sato H. Vinblastine and griseofulvin reversibly disrupt the living mitotic spindle. *Science* 1968;160:770.

44. Pike MC, Kredich NM, Snyderman R. Influence of cytoskeletal assembly on phosphatidylcholine synthesis in intact phagocytic cells. *Cell* 1980;20:373.

45. Schellenberg RR, Gillespie E. Effect of colchicine, vinblastine, griseofulvin, and deuterium oxide upon phospholipid metabolism in concanavalin A-stimulated lymphocytes. *Biochim Biophys Acta* 1980;619:522.

46. Schroeder F, Fontaine RN, Feller DJ, et al. Drug-induced surface membrane phospholipid composition in murine fibroblasts. *Biochim Biophys Acta* 1981;643:76.

47. Watanabe K, Williams EF, Law JS, et al. Effect of the *Vinca* alkaloids on calcium-calmodulin regulated cyclic adenosine 3',5'-monophosphate phospho-diesterase activity from brain. *Biochem Pharmacol* 1981;30:335.

48. Bruchovsky N, Owen AA, Becker AJ, et al. Effects of vinblastine on the proliferative capacity of L cells and their progress through the division cycle. *Cancer Res* 1965;25:1232.

49. Howard SMH, Theologides A, Sheppard JR. Comparative effects of vindesine, vinblastine, and vincristine on mitotic arrest and hormone response of L1210 leukemia cells. *Cancer Res* 1980;40:2695.

50. Lengsfeld AM, Schultze B, Maurer W. Time-lapse studies of the effects of vincristine on HeLa cells. *Eur J Cancer* 1980;17:307.

51. Tucker RW, Owellen RJ, Harris SB. Correlation of cytotoxicity and mitotic spindle dissolution by vinblastine in mammalian cells. *Cancer Res* 1977;37:4346.

52. Mareel MM, Storme GA, De Bruyne GK, et al. Vinblastine, vincristine, and vindesine: anti-invasive effect on MO4 mouse fibrosarcoma cells in vitro. *Eur J Cancer Clin Oncol* 1982;18:199.

53. Zakhireh B, Malech HL. The effect of colchicine and vinblastine on the chemotactic response of human monocytes. *J Immunol* 1980;125:2143.

54. Samson FE Jr. Mechanisms of axoplasmic transport. *J Neurobiol* 1971;2:347.

55. Sterle M, Pipan N. Influence of antimicrotubular drugs on the Golgi apparatus of stomach secretory mucoid cells and small intestine absorptive cells. *Virchows Arch* [B] 1990;58:317.

56. Behnke O. An electron microscope study of the rat megakaryocyte: II. Some aspects of platelet release and microtubules. *J Ultrastruct Res* 1969;26:111.

57. White JG. Effect of colchicine and *Vinca* alkaloids on human platelets: I. Influence on platelet microtubules and contractile function. *Am J Pathol* 1968;53:281.

58. Palmer CG, Livengood D, Warren AK, et al. The action of vincaleukoblastine on mitosis in vitro. *Exp Cell Res* 1960; 20:198.

59. Krishan A, Frei E III. Morphological basis for the cytolytic effect of vinblastine and vincristine on cultured human leukemic lymphoblasts. *Cancer Res* 1975;35:497.

60. Madoc-Jones H, Mauro F. Interphase action of vinblastine and vincristine: differences in their lethal action through the mitotic cycle of cultured mammalian cells. *J Cell Physiol* 1968;72:185.

61. Schrek R. Cytotoxicity of vincristine to normal and leukemic cells. *Am J Clin Pathol* 1974;62:1.

62. Schrek R, Stefani SS. Toxicity of microtubular drugs to leukemic lymphocytes. *Exp Mol Pathol* 1981;34:369.

63. Strychmans PA, Lurie PM, Manaster J, et al. Mode of action of chemotherapy in vivo on human acute leukemia: II. Vincristine. *Eur J Cancer* 1973;9:613.

64. Rosner F, Hirshaut Y, Grunwald HW, et al. In vitro combination chemotherapy demonstrating potentiation of vincristine cytotoxicity by prednisone. *Cancer Res* 1975;35:700.

65. Huang AB, Lin CM, Hamel E. Maytansine inhibits nucleotide binding at the exchangeable site of tubulin. *Biochem Biophys Res Commun* 1985;128:1239.

66. Rao S, Horwitz SB, Ringel I. Direct photoaffinity labeling of tubulin with taxol. *J Natl Cancer Inst* 1992;84:785.

67. Rao S, Krauss NE, Heerding JM, et al. 3'-(*p*-Azidobenzamido) Taxol photolabels the *N*-terminal 31 amino acids of beta-tubulin. *J Biol Chem* 1994;269:3132.

68. Batra JK, Powers LJ, Hess FD, et al. Derivatives of 5,6-dephenyl-pyridazine-3-one: synthetic antimitotic agents which interact with plant mammalian tubulin at a new drug binding site. *Cancer Res* 1986;46:1889.

69. Temple C Jr, Rener GA, Waud W, et al. Antimitotic agents: structure-activity studies with some pyridine derivatives. *J Med Chem* 1992;35:3686.

70. Hoebeke J, Nijen GV, DeBrabander M. Interaction of nocodazole (R 17934), a new antitumoral drug, with rat brain tubulin. *Biochem Biophys Res Commun* 1976;69:319.

71. Batra JK, Jurd L, Hamel E. Structure-function studies with derivatives of 6-benzyl-1,3-benzodioxole, a new class of synthetic compounds which inhibit tubulin polymerization and mitosis. *Mol Pharmacol* 1986;27:94.

72. Sackett DL. Podophyllotoxin, steganacin, and combretastatin: natural products that bind at the colchicine site of tubulin. *Pharmacol Ther* 1993;59:163.

73. Himes RH. Interactions of the *Catharanthus (Vinca)* alkaloids with tubulin and microtubules. *Pharmacol Ther* 1991;51:256.

74. Bryan J. Definition of three classes of binding sites in isolated microtubule crystals. *Biochemistry* 1972;11:2611.

75. Wilson L, Creshwell KM, Chin D. The mechanism of action of vinblastine: binding of ³H-vinblastine to embryonic chick brain tubulin and tubulin from sea urchin sperm tail outer doublet microtubules. *Biochemistry* 1975;14:5586.

76. Bhattacharyya B, Wolff J. Tubulin aggregation and disaggregation: mediation by two distinct vinblastine-binding sites. *Proc Natl Acad Sci U S A* 1976;73:2375.

77. Wilson L. Properties of cochicine binding protein from chick embryo brain: interactions with vinca alkaloids and podophyllotoxin. *Biochemistry* 1970;9:4999.

78. Jordan MA, Wilson L. Kinetic analysis of tubulin exchange at microtubule ends at low vinblastine concentrations. *Biochemistry* 1990;29:2730.

79. Wilson L, Jordan MA, Morse A, et al. Interaction of vinblastine with steady-state microtubules in vitro. *J Mol Biol* 1982;159:125.

80. Jordan MA, Margolis RL, Himes RH, et al. Identification of a distinct class of vinblastine binding sites on microtubules. *J Mol Biol* 1986;187:61.

81. Panda D, Jordan MA, Chin Chu K, et al. Differential effects of vinblastine on polymerization and dynamics at opposite microtubule ends. *J Biol Chem* 1996;271(47):29807.

82. Singer WD, Jordan MA, Wilson L. Binding of vinblastine to stabilized microtubules. *Mol Pharmacol* 1989;36:366.

83. Rai SS, Wolf J. Localization of critical histidyl residues required for vinblastine-induced tubulin polymerization and for microtubule assembly. *J Biol Chem* 1998;273(47):31131.

84. Donoso JA, Haskins KM, Himes RH. Effect of microtubule proteins on the interaction of vincristine with microtubules and tubulin. *Cancer Res* 1979;39:1604.

85. Jordan MA, Thrower D, Wilson L. Mechanism of inhibition of cell proliferation by *Vinca* alkaloids. *Cancer Res* 1991;51:2212.

86. Toso RJ, Jordan MA, Farrell KW, et al. Kinetic stabilization of the microtubule dynamic instability in vitro by vinblastine. *Biochemistry* 1993;32:1285.

87. Wendell KL, Wilson L, Jordan MA. Mitotic block in HeLa cells by vinblastine: ultrastructural changes in the kinetocore-microtubule attachment and in centrosomes. *J Cell Sci* 1993;104:261.

88. Jordan MA, Thrower D, Wilson L. Effects of vinblastine, podophylotoxin and nocodazole on mitotic spindles: implications for the role of microtubule dynamics in mitosis. *J Cell Sci* 1992;102:401.

89. Wilson L, Miller HP, Farrell KW, et al. Taxol stabilization of microtubules in vitro: dynamics of tubulin addition and loss at opposite microtubule ends. *Biochemistry* 1985;24:5254.

90. Lobert S, Vulevic B, Correia JJ. Interaction of vinca alkaloids with tubulin: a comparison of vinblastine, vincristine, and vinorelbine. *Biochemistry* 1996;35(21):6806.

91. Bowman LC, Houghton JA, Houghton PJ. GTP influences the binding of vincristine in human tumor cytosols. *Biochem Biophys Res Commun* 1986;135:695.

92. Ferguson PJ, Cass CE. Differential cellular retention of vincristine and vinblastine by cultured human promyelocytic leukemia HL-60/C-1 cells: the basis of differential toxicity. *Cancer Res* 1985;45:5480.

93. Himes RH, Kersey RN, Heller-Bettinger I, et al. Action of the *Vinca* alkaloids vincristine and vinblastine, and desacetyl vinblastine amide on microtubules in vitro. *Cancer Res* 1976;36:3798.

94. Houghton JA, Meyer WH, Houghton BJ. Scheduling of vincristine: drug accumulation and response of xenografts of childhood rhabdomyosarcoma determined by frequency of administration. *Cancer Treat Rep* 1987;71:717.

95. Jordan MA, Himes RH, Wilson L. Comparison of the effects of vinblastine, vincristine, vindesine, and vinepidine on microtubule dynamics and cell proliferation in vitro. *Cancer Res* 1985;45:2741.

96. Ferguson PJ, Philips JR, Seiner M, et al. Biochemical effects of Navelbine on tubulin and associated proteins. *Cancer Res* 1984;44:3307.

97. Gout PW, Wijcik LL, Beer CT. Differences between vinblastine and vincristine in distribution in the blood of rats and binding by platelets and malignant cells. *Eur J Cancer* 1978;14:1167.

98. Lengsfeld AM, Dietrich J, Schultze-Maurer B. Accumulation and release of vinblastine and vincristine in HeLa cells: light microscopic, cinematographic, and biochemical study. *Cancer Res* 1982;42:3798.

99. Gout PW, Noble RL, Bruchovsky N, et al. Vinblastine and vincristine-growth-inhibitory effects correlate with their retention by cultured Nb2 node lymphoma cells. *Int J Cancer* 1984;34:245.

100. Bowman LC, Houghton JA, Houghton PJ. Formation and stability of vincristine-tubulin complex in kidney cytosols. Role of GTP and GTP hydrolysis. *Biochem Pharmacol* 1988;37:1251.

101. Houghton JA, Williams LG, Houghton PJ. Stability of vincristine complexes in cytosols derived from xenografts of human rhabdomyosarcoma and normal tissues of the mouse. *Cancer Res* 1985;45:3761.

102. Ferguson PJ, Phillips JR, Steiner M, et al. Differential activity of vincristine and vinblastine against cultured cells. *Cancer Res* 1984;45:5480.

103. Bleyer WA, Frisby SA, Oliverio VT. Uptake and binding of vincristine by murine leukemia cells. *Biochem Pharmacol* 1975;24:633.

104. Rahamani R, Zhou XJ, Placidi M, et al. In vivo and in vitro pharmacokinetics and metabolism of vinca alkaloids in rat: I. Vindesine (4-desacetyl-vinblastine 3-carboxyamide). *Eur J Drug Metab Pharmacol* 1990;15:49.

105. Zhou XJ, Martin M, Placidi M, et al. In vivo and in vitro pharmacokinetics and metabolism of vinca alkaloids: II. Vinblastine and vincristine. *Eur J Drug Metab Pharmacol* 1990;15:323.

106. Rahmani R, Zhou XJ. Pharmacokinetics and metabolism of vinca alkaloids. In: Workman P, Graham MA, eds. *Cancer surveys, pharmacokinetics and cancer chemotherapy*, vol 17. Plainview, NY: Cold Spring Harbor Laboratory Press, 1993:269.

107. Zhou XJ, Rahamani R. Preclinical and clinical pharmacology of *Vinca* alkaloids. *Drugs* 1992;44[Suppl 4]:1.

108. Bender RA, Kornreich WD. Cellular entry of vincristine in

murine leukemia cells. *Proc Am Assoc Cancer Res* 1981; 22:227(abst).

109. Beck WT, Cirtain MC, Lefko JL. Energy-dependent reduced drug binding as a mechanism of *Vinca* alkaloid resistance in human leukemia lymphoblasts. *Mol Pharmacol* 1983;24:485.

110. Bender RA, Kornreich WD, Wodinsky I. Correlates of vincristine resistance in four murine tumor cell lines. *Cancer Lett* 1982;15:335.

111. Jackson DV, Bender RA. Cytotoxic thresholds of vincristine in a murine and human leukemia cell line in vitro. *Cancer Res* 1979;39:4346.

112. Vacca A, Iurlaro M, Ribatti D, et al. Antiangiogenesis is produced by nontoxic doses of vinblastine. *Blood* 1999; 94(12):4143.

113. Klement G, Baruchel S, Rak J, et al. Continuous low-dose therapy with vinblastine and VEGF receptor-2 antibody induces sustained tumor regression without overt toxicity. *J Clin Invest* 2000;105(8):R15.

114. Beck WT. Cellular pharmacology of *Vinca* alkaloid resistance and its circumvention. *Adv Enzyme Regul* 1984;22:207.

115. Moscow JA, Cowan KH. Multidrug resistance. *J Natl Cancer Inst* 1988;80:14.

116. Beck WT, Mueller TJ, Tanzer LR. Altered cell surface membrane glycoproteins in *Vinca*-alkaloid-resistant human leukemic lymphoblasts. *Cancer Res* 1979;39:2070.

116a. Cornwell MM, Tsuruo T, Gottesman MM, et al. ATP-binding properties of P-glycoprotein from multidrug-resistant KB cells. *FASEB J* 1987;1:51.

117. Cornwell MM, Safa AR, Felsted RL, et al. Membrane vesicles from multidrug-resistant human cancer cells contain a specific 150- to 170-kDa protein detected by photoaffinity labeling. *Proc Natl Acad Sci U S A* 1986;83:3847.

118. Safa AR, Glover CJ, Meyers MB, et al. Vinblastine photoaffinity labeling of a high molecular weight surface membrane glycoprotein specific for multidrug-resistant cells. *J Biol Chem* 1986;261:6137.

119. Qian X-D, Beck WT. Progesterone photoaffinity labels P-glycoprotein in multidrug resistant human leukemic lymphoblasts. *J Biol Chem* 1990;265:18753.

120. Yusa K, Tsuruo T. Reversal mechanism of multidrug resistance by verapamil: direct binding of verapamil to P-glycoprotein on specific sites and transport of verapamil outward across the plasma membrane of K562/ADM cells. *Cancer Res* 1989;49:5002.

121. Fojo AT, Ueda K, Slamon DJ, et al. Expression of a multidrug-resistance gene in human tumors and tissues. *Proc Natl Acad Sci U S A* 1987;84:265.

122. Greenberger LM, Williams SS, Horwitz SB. Biosynthesis of heterogeneous forms of multidrug resistance associated glycoproteins. *J Biol Chem* 1987;262:13685.

123. Choi K, Chen C, Kriegler M, et al. An altered pattern of cross-resistance in multidrug-resistant human cells results from spontaneous mutations in the *mdr*1 (P-glycoprotein) gene. *Cell* 1988;53:519.

124. Hamada H, Hagiwara KI, Nakajima T, et al. Phosphorylation of the M_r 170,000 to 180,000 glycoprotein specific to multidrug-resistant tumor cells: effects of verapamil, trifluoroperazine, and phorbol esters. *Cancer Res* 1987;47:2860.

124a. Samuels BL, Hollis DR, Rosner GL, et al. Modulation of vinblastine resistance in metastatic renal cell carcinoma with cyclosporine A or tamoxifen: a cancer and leukemia group B study. *Clin Cancer Res* 1997;3(11):1977.

124b. Van Asperen J, Schinkel AH, Beijnen JH, et al. Altered pharmacokinetics of vinblastine in Mdr1a P-glycoprotein-deficient mice. *J Natl Cancer Inst* 1996;88(14):994.

124c. Drion N, Lemaire M, Lefauconnier J-M, et al. Role of P-glycoprotein in the blood-brain transport of colchicine and vinblastine. *J Neurochem* 1996;67(4):1688.

124d. Loe DW, Almquist KC, Deeley RG, et al. Multidrug resistance protein (MRP)-mediated transport of leukotriene C4 and chemotherapeutic agents in membrane vesicles. *J Biol Chem* 1996;271(16):9675.

124e. Evers R, de Haas M, Sparidans R, et al. Vinblastine and sulfinpyrazone export by the multidrug resistance protein MRP2 is associated with glutathione export. *Br J Cancer* 2000;83(3):375.

124f. Ross DD, Yang W, Abruzzo LV, et al. Atypical multidrug resistance: breast cancer resistance protein messenger RNA expression in mitoxantrone-selected cell lines. *J Natl Cancer Inst* 1999;91(5):429.

124g. Robey RW, Medina-Perez WY, Nishiyama K, et al. Overexpression of the ATP-binding cassette half-transporter, ABCG2 (MXR/BCRP/ABCP1), in flavopiridol-resistant human breast cancer cells. *Clin Cancer Res* (in press).

125. Fan S, Cherney B, Reinhold W, et al. Disruption of p53 function in immortalized human cells does not affect survival or apoptosis after taxol or vincristine treatment. *Clin Cancer Res* 1998;4(4):1047.

126. Blagosklonny MV, Robey R, Bates S, et al. Pretreatment with DNA-damaging agents permits selective killing of checkpoint-deficient cells by microtubule-active drugs. *J Clin Invest* 2000;105(4):533.

127. Stewart ZA, Mays D, Pietenpol JA. Defective G1-S cell cycle checkpoint function sensitizes cells to microtubule inhibitor-induced apoptosis. *Cancer Res* 1999;59(15):3831.

128. Houghton JA, Houghton PJ, Hazelton BJ, et al. In situ selection of a human rhabdomyosarcoma resistant to vincristine with altered alpha-tubulins. *Cancer Res* 1985;45:2706.

129. Minotti AM, Barlow SB, Cabral F. Resistance to antimitotic drugs in Chinese hamster ovary cells correlates with changes in the level of polymerized tubulin. *J Biol Chem* 1991;266:3987.

130. Cabral FR, Brady RC, Schiber MJ. A mechanism of cellular resistance to drugs that interfere with microtubule assembly. *Ann N Y Acad Sci* 1986;466:748.

131. Cabral FR, Barlow SB. Mechanisms by which mammalian cells acquire resistance to drugs that affect microtubule assembly. *FASEB J* 1989;3:1593.

132. Cabral FR, Barlow SB. Resistance to the antimitotic agents as genetic probes of microtubule structure and function. *Pharmacol Ther* 1991;52:159.

133. Ranganathan S, Dexter DW, Benetatos CA, et al. Cloning and sequencing of human βIII-tubulin cDNA: induction of betaIII isotype in human prostate carcinoma cells by acute exposure to antimicrotubule agents. *Biochim Biophys Acta* 1998;1395(2):237.

134. Sethi VS, Thimmaiah KN. Structural studies of the degradation products of vincristine dihydrogen sulfate. *Cancer Res* 1985;45:5386.

135. Thimmaiah KN, Sethi VS. Chemical characterization of the

degradation products of vinblastine dihydrogen sulfate. *Cancer Res* 1985;45:5382.

136. Castle MC, Margileth DA, Oliverio VT. Distribution and excretion of [³H]vincristine in the rat and the dog. *Cancer Res* 1976;36:3684.

137. Bender RA, Castle MC, Margileth DA, et al. The pharmacokinetics of [³H]vincristine in man. *Clin Pharmacol Ther* 1977;22:430.

138. Culp HW, Daniels WD, McMahon RE. Disposition and tissue levels of [³H]vindesine in rats. *Cancer Res* 1977;37:3053.

139. El Dareer SM, White VM, Chen FP, et al. Distribution and metabolism of vincristine in mice, rats, dogs and monkeys. *Cancer Treat Rep* 1977;61:1269.

140. Owellen RJ, Root MA, Hains FO. Pharmacokinetics of vindesine and vincristine in humans. *Cancer Res* 1977;37:2603.

141. Owellen RJ, Hartke CA, Hains FO. Pharmacokinetics and metabolism of vinblastine in humans. *Cancer Res* 1977; 37:2597.

142. Jackson DV, Castle MC, Bender RA. Biliary excretion of vincristine. *Clin Pharmacol Ther* 1978;24:101.

143. Owellen RJ, Hartke CA. The pharmacokinetics of 4-acetyl tritium vinblastine in two patients. *Cancer Res* 1975;35:975.

144. Nelson RL, Dyke RW, Root MA. Clinical pharmacokinetics of vindesine. *Cancer Chemother Pharmacol* 1979;2:243.

145. Hande K, Gay J, Gober J, et al. Toxicity and pharmacology of bolus vindesine injection and prolonged vindesine infusion. *Cancer Treat Rev* 1980;7:25.

146. Nelson RL, Dyke RW, Root MA. Comparative pharmacokinetics of vindesine, vincristine, and vinblastine in patients with cancer. *Cancer Treat Rev* 1980;7[Suppl]:17.

147. Jackson DV, Castle MC, Poplack DG, et al. Pharmacokinetics of vincristine in the cerebrospinal fluid of subhuman primates. *Cancer Res* 1980;40:722.

148. Jackson DV, Sethi VS, Spurr CL, et al. Pharmacokinetics of vincristine in the cerebrospinal fluid of humans. *Cancer Res* 1981;41:1466.

149. Sethi VS, Jackson DV, White DR, et al. Pharmacokinetics of vincristine sulfate in adult cancer patients. *Cancer Res* 1981;41:3551.

150. Sethi VS, Kimball JC. Pharmacokinetics of vincristine sulfate in children. *Cancer Chemother Pharmacol* 1981;6:111.

151. Nelson RL. The comparative clinical pharmacology and pharmacokinetics of vindesine, vincristine, and vinblastine in human patients with cancer. *Med Pediatr Oncol* 1982;10:115.

152. Hacker MP, Dank JR, Ershler WB. Vinblastine pharmacokinetics measured by a sensitive enzyme-linked immunosorbent assay. *Cancer Res* 1984;44:478.

153. Rahmani R, Kleisbauer JP, Cano JP, et al. Clinical pharmacokinetics of vindesine infusion. *Cancer Treat Rep* 1985;69:839.

154. Labinjoki SP, Verajankorva HM, Huthikangas AE, et al. An enzyme-linked immunosorbent assay for the antineoplastic agent vincristine. *J Immunoassay* 1986;7:113.

155. Ratain MJ, Vogelzang NJ. Phase I and pharmacological study of vinblastine by prolonged continuous infusion. *Cancer Res* 1986;46:4827.

156. Ratain MJ, Vogelzang NJ. Limited sampling for vinblastine pharmacokinetics. *Cancer Treat Rep* 1987;71:935.

157. Pontarotti PA, Rahmani R, Martin M, et al. Monoclonal antibodies to antitumor vinca alkaloids: thermodynamics and kinetics. *Mol Immunol* 1985;22:277.

158. Rahmani R, Barbet J, Cano JP. An ¹²⁵I-radiolabeled probe for vinblastine and vinblastine radioimmunoassays. *Clin Chim Acta* 1983;129:57.

159. Rahmani R, Martin M, Barbet J, et al. Radioimmunoassay and preliminary pharmacokinetic studies of rats of 5'-noranhydrovinblastine. *Cancer Res* 1984;44:5609.

160. Huhtikangas A, Lehtola T, Lapinjoki S, et al. Specific radioimmunoassay for vincristine. *Planta Med* 1987;53:85.

161. Bloemhof H, Van Jijk KN, De Graff SSN, et al. Sensitive method for the determination of vincristine in human serum by high-performance liquid chromatography. *J Cancer* 1990;46:262.

162. Vendrig DEMM, Teeuwsen J, Hothuis JJM. Analysis of *Vinca* alkaloids in plasma and urine using high-performance liquid chromatography with electrochemical detection. *J Chromatogr Biomed Appl* 1988;424:83.

163. De Smet M, Van Belle SJP, Storme GA, et al. High-performance liquid chromatographic determination of the *Vinca* alkaloids in plasma and urine. *J Chromatogr Biomed Appl* 1985;345:309.

164. Jehl F, Debs J, Herlin C, et al. Determination of navelbine and desacetylnavelbine in biological fluids by high-performance liquid chromatography. *J Chromatogr Biomed Appl* 1990;525:225.

165. Van Tellinger O, Beijnen JH, Nooijen WJ, et al. Plasma pharmacokinetics of vinblastine and the investigational *Vinca* alkaloid N-(deacetyl-O-4-vinblastoyl-23-ethyl isoleucinate) in mice as determined by high-performance liquid chromatography. *Cancer Res* 1993;53:2061.

166. Robieux I, Vitali V, Aita P, et al. Sensitive high-performance liquid chromatographic method with fluorescence detection for measurement of vinorelbine plasma concentrations. *J Chromatogr* 1996;675:183.

167. Rowinsky EK, Donehower RC. The clinical pharmacology and use of antimicrotubule agents in cancer chemotherapeutics. *Pharmacol Ther* 1991;52:35.

168. Rahmani R, Bruno R, Iliadis A, et al. Clinical pharmacokinetics of the antitumor drug Navelbine (5'-noranhydrovinblastine). *Cancer Res* 1987;47:5796.

169. Jackson DV Jr. The periwinkle alkaloids. In: Lokich JJ, ed. *Cancer chemotherapy by infusion.* Chicago: Precept Press, 1990:155.

170. Jackson DV, Sethi VS, Spurr CL, et al. Pharmacokinetics of vincristine infusion. *Cancer Treat Rep* 1981;65:1043.

171. Gidding CEM, Meeuwen-de Boer GJ, Koopmans P, et al. Vincristine pharmacokinetics after repetitive dosing in children. *Cancer Chemother Pharmacol* 1999;44:203.

172. Villikka K, Kivistö KT, Mäenpää H, et al. Cytochrome P450-inducing antiepileptics increase the clearance of vincristine in patients with brain tumors. *Clin Pharmacol Ther* 1999;66(6):589.

173. Gillies J, Hung KA, Fitzsimons E, et al. Severe vincristine toxicity in combination with itraconazole. *Clin Lab Haematol* 1998;20(2):123.

174. Owellen RJ, Donigian DW. ³H-Vincristine: preparation and preliminary pharmacology. *J Med Chem* 1972;15:894.

175. Linares M, Cervero A, Sanchez M, et al. Slow infusion of vincristine in the treatment of refractory thrombocytopenia purpura. *Acta Haematol* 1988;80:173.

176. Ahn YS, Harrington WJ, Mylvaganam R, et al. Slow infu-

sion of vinca alkaloids in the treatment of idiopathic thrombocytopenia purpura. *Ann Intern Med* 1984;100:192.

177. Sethi VS, Castle MC, Surratt P, et al. Isolation and partial characterization of human urinary metabolites of vincristine sulfate. *Proc Am Assoc Cancer Res* 1981;22:173(abst).

178. Houghton JA, Williams LG, Torrance PM, et al. Determinants of intrinsic sensitivity to *Vinca* alkaloids in xenografts of pediatric rhabdomyosarcomas. *Cancer Res* 1984;44:582.

179. Yao D, Ding S, Burchell B, et al. Detoxication of vinca alkaloids by human P450 CYP3A4-mediated metabolism: implications for the development of drug resistance. *J Pharmacol Exp Ther* 2000;294(1):387.

180. Steele WH, Barber HE, Dawson AA, et al. Protein binding of prednisone and vinblastine in the serum of normal subjects. *Br J Clin Pharmacol* 1982;13:595.

181. Greenius HF, McIntyre RW, Beer CT. The preparation of vinblastine-4-acetyl-*t* and its distribution in the blood of rats. *J Med Chem* 1968;11:254.

182. Hebden HF, Hadfield JR, Beer CT. The binding of vinblastine by platelets in the rat. *Cancer Res* 1970;30:1417.

183. Young JA, Howell S, Green MR. Pharmacokinetics and toxicity of 5-day continuous infusion of vinblastine. *Cancer Chemother Pharmacol* 1984;12:43.

184. Lu K, Yap HY, Watts S, et al. Comparative clinical pharmacology of vinblastine (VBL) in patients with advanced breast cancer: single versus continuous infusion. *Proc Am Assoc Cancer Res* 1979;20:371(abst).

185. Creasey WA, Marsh JC. Metabolism of vinblastine (VBL) in the dog. *Proc Am Assoc Cancer Res* 1973;14:57(abst).

186. Zhou-Pan XR, Seree E, Zhou XJ, et al. Involvement of human liver cytochrome P450 3A in vinblastine metabolism: drug interactions. *Cancer Res* 1993;53:5121.

187. Jackson DV Jr, Sethi VS, Long TR, et al. Pharmacokinetics of vindesine bolus and infusion. *Cancer Chemother Pharmacol* 1994;13:114.

188. Ohnuma T, Norton L, Andrejczuk A, et al. Pharmacokinetics of vindesine given as an intravenous bolus and 24-hour infusion in humans. *Cancer Res* 1985;45:464.

189. Rahmani R, Martin M, Favre R, et al. Clinical pharmacokinetics of vindesine: repeated treatments by intravenous bolus injections. *Eur J Cancer Clin Oncol* 1984;20:1409.

190. Zhou XJ, Zhou-Pan XR, Gauthier T, et al. Human liver microsomal cytochrome P450 3A isoenzymes mediated vindesine biotransformation: metabolic drug interactions. *Biomed Pharmacol* 1993;4:853.

191. Krikorian A, Rahmani R, Bromet M, et al. Pharmacokinetics and metabolism of Navelbine. *Semin Oncol* 1989;16[Suppl 4]:21.

192. Bore P, Rahmani R, van Cantfort J, et al. Pharmacokinetics of a new anticancer drug, Navelbine, in patients. *Cancer Chemother Pharmacol* 1987;23:247.

193. Jehl F, Quoix E, Monteil H, et al. Human pharmacokinetics of Navelbine (NAV), a new *Vinca* alkaloid, as determined by high performance liquid chromatography (HPLC). *Proc Am Soc Clin Oncol* 1990;9:252(abst).

194. Jehl F, Quoix E, Leveque D, et al. Pharmacokinetic and preliminary metabolic fate of Navelbine in humans as determined by high performance liquid chromatography. *Cancer Res* 1991;51:2073.

195. Rowinsky EK, Noe DA, Lucas VS, et al. A phase I, pharmacokinetic and absolute bioavailability study of oral vinorelbine (Navelbine) in solid tumor patients. *J Clin Oncol* 1994;12:1754.

196. Sorio R, Robieux I, Galligioni E, et al. Pharmacokinetics and tolerance of vinorelbine in elderly patients with metastatic breast cancer. *Eur J Cancer* 1997;33(2):301.

197. Urien S, Bree F, Breillout F, et al. Vinorelbine high-affinity binding to human platelets and lymphocytes: distribution in human blood. *Cancer Chemother Pharmacol* 1988;23:247.

198. Leveque D, Quoiz E, Dumont P, et al. Pulmonary distribution of vinorelbine in patients with non-small-cell lung cancer. *Cancer Chemother Pharmacol* 1993;33:176.

199. Rahmani R, Gueritte F, Martin M, et al. Comparative pharmacokinetics of antitumor *Vinca* alkaloids: intravenous bolus injections of navelbine and related alkaloids to cancer patients and rats. *Cancer Chemother Pharmacol* 1986;16:223.

200. Leveque D, Merle-Melet M, Bresler L, et al. Biliary elimination and pharmacokinetics of vinorelbine in micropigs. *Cancer Chemother Pharmacol* 1993;32:487.

201. Zhou XJ, Lacarelle B, de Souza G, et al. In vitro biotransformation of navelbine by animal and hepatic subcellular fractions. *Bull Cancer* 1990;77:586(abst).

202. Sahnoun Z, Durand A, Placid M, et al. Research of navelbine metabolites in the patient using high performance liquid chromatography. *Bull Cancer* 1990;77:598.

203. Robieux I, Sorio R, Borsatti E, et al. Pharmacokinetics of vinorelbine in patients with liver metastases. *Clin Pharmacol Ther* 1996;59(1):32.

204. Favre R, Delgado J, Besenval M, et al. Phase I trial of escalating doses of orally administered Navelbine (NVB): II. Clinical results. *Proc Am Soc Clin Oncol* 1989;8:246(abst).

205. Rowinsky EK, Lucas VS, Hsieh AY, et al. The effects of food and divided dosing on the bioavailability of oral vinorelbine. *Cancer Chemother Pharmacol* 1996;39:9.

206. Sulkes A, Collins JM. Reappraisal of some dosage adjustment guidelines. *Cancer Treat Rep* 1987;71:229.

207. Costa G, Hreshchyshyn MM, Holland JF. Initial clinical studies with vincristine. *Cancer Chemother Rep* 1962;24:39.

208. Holland JF, Scharlan C, Gailani S, et al. Vincristine treatment of advanced cancer: a cooperative study of 392 cases. *Cancer Res* 1973;33:1258.

209. Desai ZR, Van den Berg HW, Bridges JM, et al. Can severe vincristine neuropathy be prevented? *Cancer Chemother Pharmacol* 1982;8:211.

210. Van den Berg HW, Desai ZR, Wilson R, et al. The pharmacokinetics of vincristine in man: reduced drug clearance associated with raised serum alkaline phosphatase and dose-limiting elimination. *Cancer Chemother Pharmacol* 1982;8:215.

211. Pinkerton CR, McDermott B, Philip T, et al. Continuous vincristine infusion as part of a high dose chemoradiotherapy regimen: drug kinetics and toxicity. *Cancer Chemother Pharmacol* 1988;22:271.

212. Slyter H, Liwnicz B, Herrick MK, et al. Fatal myeloencephalopathy caused by intrathecal vincristine. *Neurology* 1980;30:867.

213. Dyke RW. Treatment of inadvertent intrathecal administration of vincristine. *N Engl J Med* 1989;321:1270.

214. Jackson DV Jr, Richards F, Spurr CL, et al. Hepatic intra-arterial infusions of vincristine. *Cancer Chemother Pharmacol* 1984;13:120.

215. Kinzel PE, Dorr RT. Anticancer drug renal toxicity and

elimination: dosing guidelines for altered renal function. *Cancer Treat Rev* 1995;21:33.

216. Falkson G, Van Dyk JJ, Falkson FC. Oral vinblastine sulfate (NSC 49842) in malignant disease. *S Afr Cancer Bull* 1968; 2:78.

217. Zeffrin J, Yagoda A, Kelsen D, et al. Phase I-II trial of 5-day continuous infusion of vinblastine sulfate. *Anticancer Res* 1984;4:411.

218. Gralla RJ, Tan CTC, Young CW. Vindesine: a review of phase II trials. *Cancer Chemother Pharmacol* 1979;2:247.

219. Ohnuma T, Greenspan EM, Holland JF. Initial clinical study with vindesine: tolerance to weekly IV bolus and 24-hour infusion. *Cancer Treat Rep* 1980;64:25.

220. Cvitkovic E, Izzo J. The current and future place of vinorelbine in cancer therapy. *Drugs* 1982;44[Suppl 2]:34.

221. Fields S, Burris H, Shaffer D, et al. Phase I clinical trial of chronic oral Navelbine administration. *Ann Oncol* 1992;3[Suppl 1]:125(abst).

222. Khayat D, Covelli A, Variol P, et al. Phase I and pharmacologic study of intravenous (i.v.) vinorelbine in patients with solid tumors. *Proc Am Soc Clin Oncol* 1995;14:469(abst).

223. Robieux I, Sorio R, Vitali V, et al. Pharmacokinetics of vinorelbine in breast cancer patients with liver metastases. *Proc Am Soc Clin Oncol* 1995;14:458(abst).

224. Legha SS. Vincristine neurotoxicity: pathophysiology and management. *Med Toxicol* 1986;1:421.

225. Tuxen MK, Hansen SW. Neurotoxicity secondary to antineoplastic drugs. *Cancer Treat Rev* 1994;20:191.

226. Miller BR. Neurotoxicity and vincristine. *JAMA* 1985; 253:2045.

227. Griffiths JD, Stark RJ, Ding JC, et al. Vincristine neurotoxicity in Charcot-Marie-Tooth Syndrome. *Med J Aust* 1985;143:305.

228. McGuire SA, Gospe SM Jr, Dahl G. Acute vincristine neurotoxicity in the presence of hereditary motor and sensory neuropathy type I. *Med Pediatr Oncol* 1989;17:520.

229. Olek MJ, Bordeaux B, Leshner RT. Charcot-Marie-Tooth disease type I diagnosed in a 5-year old boy after vincristine neurotoxicity, resulting in maternal diagnosis. *J Am Osteopath Assoc* 1999;99(3):165.

230. Casey EB, Jellife AM, Le Quesne PM, et al. Vincristine neuropathy, clinical and electrophysiological observations. *Brain* 1973;96:69.

231. Donoso JA, Green LS, Heller-Bettinger E, et al. Action of the *Vinca* alkaloids vincristine, vinblastine, and desacetyl vinblastine amide on axonal fibrillar organelles in vitro. *Cancer Res* 1977;37:1401.

232. Goldstein BD, Lowndes HE. Motor nerve function in vincristine neuropathy: lack of evidence of a dying-back neuropathy. *Pharmacologist* 1978;20:162.

233. Ryan SP, DelPrete SA, Weinstein PW, et al. Low-dose vincristine-associated bilateral vocal cord paralysis. *Conn Med* 1999;63(10):583.

234. Greig NH, Soncrant TT, Shetty HU, et al. Brain uptake and anticancer activities of vincristine and vinblastine are restricted by their low cerebrovascular permeability and binding to plasma constituents in rat. *Cancer Chemother Pharmacol* 1990;26:263.

235. Hurwitz RL, Mahoney DH Jr, Armstrong DL, et al. Reversible encephalopathy and seizures as a result of conventional vincristine administration. *Med Pediatr Oncol* 1988;16:216.

236. Stuart MJ, Cuaso C, Miller M, et al. Syndrome of recurrent increased secretion of antidiuretic hormone following multiple doses of vincristine. *Blood* 1975;45:315.

237. Bird RL, Rohrbaugh TM, Raney B Jr, et al. Transient cortical blindness secondary to vincristine therapy in children. *Cancer* 1983;47:37.

238. Ripps H, Mehaffey L III, Siegel IM, et al. Vincristine-induced changes in the retina of the isolated arterially perfused cat eye. *Exp Eye Res* 1989;48:771.

239. Yousif H, Richardson SG, Saunders WA. Partially reversible nerve deafness due to vincristine. *Postgrad Med J* 1990;66:688.

240. Carpentieri R, Lockhart LH. Ataxia and athetosis as side effects of chemotherapy with vincristine in non-Hodgkin's lymphomas. *Cancer Treat Rep* 1978;62:561.

241. Hironen HE, Saknu TT, Heinonen E, et al. Vincristine treatment of acute lymphoblastic leukemia induces transient autonomic cardioneuropathy. *Cancer* 1988;64:801.

242. Gottlieb RJ, Cuttner J. Vincristine-induced bladder atony. *Cancer* 1971;28:674.

243. Carmichael SM, Eagleton L, Ayers CR, et al. Orthostatic hypotension during vincristine therapy. *Arch Intern Med* 1970;126:290.

244. Blain PG. Adverse effects of drugs on skeletal muscle. *Adverse Drug React Bull* 1984;104:384.

245. Grush OC, Morgan SK. Folinic acid rescue for vincristine toxicity. *Clin Toxicol* 1979;14:71.

246. Jackson DV Jr, Pope EK, McMahan RA, et al. Clinical trial of pyridoxine to reduce vincristine neurotoxicity. *J Neurooncol* 1986;4:37.

247. Jackson DV Jr, McMahan RA, Pope EK, et al. Clinical trial of folinic acid to reduce vincristine neurotoxicity. *Cancer Chemother Pharmacol* 1986;17:281.

248. Jackson DV, Wells HB, Atkins JN, et al. Amelioration of vincristine neurotoxicity by glutamic acid. *Am J Med* 1988;84:1016.

249. Helmann K, Hutchinson GE, Henry K. Reduction of vincristine toxicity by Cronassial. *Cancer Chemother Pharmacol* 1987;20:21.

250. Ferayan AA, Russell NA, Wohaibi MA, et al. Cerebrospinal fluid lavage in the treatment of inadvertent intrathecal vincristine injection. *Childs Nerv Syst* 1999;15:87.

251. Michelagnoli MP, Bailey CC, Wilson I, et al. Potential salvage therapy for inadvertent intrathecal administration of vincristine. *Br J Haematol* 1997;99(2):364.

252. Fernandez CV, Esau R, Hamilton D, et al. Intrathecal vincristine: an analysis of reasons for recurrent fatal chemotherapeutic error with recommendations for prevention. *J Pediatr Hematol Oncol* 1998;20(6):587.

253. Sharma RK. Vincristine and gastrointestinal transit. *Gastroenterology* 1988;95:1435.

254. Harris AC, Jackson JM. Lactulose in vincristine-induced constipation. *Med J Aust* 1972;2P:573.

255. Agosti A, Bertaccini G, Paulucci R, et al. Caerulein treatment for paralytic ileus. *Lancet* 1971;1:395.

256. Garewal HS, Dalton WS. Metoclopramide in vincristine-induced ileus. *Cancer Treat Rep* 1985;69:1309.

257. Jackson DV, Wu WC, Spurr CL. Treatment of vincristine-induced ileus with sincalide, a cholecystokinin analogue. *Cancer Chemother Pharmacol* 1982;8:83.

258. Castle MC. Plant alkaloids: the *Vinca* alkaloids. In: Woolley

PV, ed. *Cancer management in man: biological response modifiers, chemotherapy, antibiotics, hyperthermia, supporting measures.* Dordrecht, The Netherlands: Kluwer Academic Publishers, 1987:147.

259. Kantor AF, Greene MH, Boice JD, et al. Are *Vinca* alkaloids associated with myocardial infarction? *Lancet* 1981;1:1111.

260. Kaufman IA, Khung FH, Koenig HM, et al. Overdosage with vincristine. *J Pediatr* 1976;89:671.

261. Steurer G, Kuzmitis R, Pavelka M, et al. Early onset thrombocytopenia during combination chemotherapy in testicular cancer is induced by vincristine. *Cancer* 1989;63:51.

262. Bunn PA, Ford SS, Shackney SE. The effects of colcemide on hematopoiesis in the mouse. *J Clin Invest* 1975;58:1280.

263. Dorr RT, Alberts DS. *Vinca* alkaloid skin toxicity: antidote and drug disposition studies in the mouse. *J Natl Cancer Inst* 1985;74:113.

264. Bellone JD. Treatment of vincristine extravasation. *JAMA* 1981;245:343.

265. Ishii E, Hara T, Mizumo Y, et al. Vincristine-induced fever in children with leukemia and lymphoma. *Cancer* 1988;61:660.

266. Green DM, Norkool P, Breslow NE, et al. Severe hepatic toxicity after treatment with vincristine and dactinomycin using single-dose or divided schedules: a report from the National Wilms' Tumor Study. *J Clin Oncol* 1990;9:1525.

267. Bostrom B. Severe ileus from cisplatin and vinblastine infusion in neuroblastoma. *J Clin Oncol* 1988;6:1356.

268. Hansen SW. Autonomic neuropathy after treatment with cisplatin, vinblastine, and bleomycin for germ cell tumors. *BMJ* 1990;300:511.

269. Hansen SW, Helweg-Larsen S, Trajoborg W. Long-term neurotoxicity in patients treated with cisplatin, vinblastine, and bleomycin for metastatic germ cell cancer. *J Clin Oncol* 1989;7:1457.

270. Subar M, Muggia FM. Apparent myocardial ischemia associated with vinblastine administration. *Cancer Treat Rep* 1986;70:690.

271. Teutsch C, Lipton A, Harvey HA. Raynaud's phenomenon as a side effect of chemotherapy with vinblastine and bleomycin for testicular carcinoma. *Cancer Treat Rep* 1977;61:925.

272. Hantel A, Rowinsky EK, Donehower RC. Nifedipine and oncologic Raynaud's phenomenon. *Ann Intern Med* 1988;108:767.

273. Hansen SW, Disen N. Raynaud's phenomenon in patients treated with cisplatin, vinblastine, and bleomycin for germ cell cancer: measurement of vasoconstrictor response to cold. *J Clin Oncol* 1985;7:940.

274. Williams SD, Birch R, Einhorn LH, et al. Disseminated germ cell tumors: chemotherapy with cisplatin plus bleomycin plus either vinblastine or etoposide. A trial of the Southeastern Cancer Study Group. *N Engl J Med* 1987;316:1435.

275. Israel RH, Olson JP. Pulmonary edema associated with intravenous vinblastine. *JAMA* 1978;240:1585.

276. Ballen KK, Weiss ST. Fatal acute respiratory failure following vinblastine and mitomycin administration for breast cancer. *Am J Med Sci* 1988;295:558.

277. Cutts JH. Protective action of diethylstilbestrol on toxicity of vinblastine in rats. *J Natl Cancer Inst* 1968;41:919.

278. Miller TP, Jones SE, Chester A. Phase II trial of vindesine in the treatment of lymphomas, breast cancer, and other solid tumors. *Cancer Treat Rep* 1980;64:1001.

279. Jumean HG, Camitta B, Holcenberg J, et al. Deacetyl vinblastine amide sulfate induced ineffective erythropoiesis. *Cancer* 1979;44:64.

280. Obrist R, Paravicini U, Hartmann D, et al. Vindesine: a clinical trial with special reference to neurological side effects. *Cancer Chemother Pharmacol* 1979;2:233.

281. Heran F, Defer G, Brugieres P, et al. Cortical blindness during chemotherapy: clinical, CT, and MR correlations. *J Comput Assist Tomogr* 1990;14:262.

282. Antony A, Robinson WA, Roy C, et al. Inappropriate antidiuretic hormone secretion after high dose vinblastine. *J Urol* 1980;123:783.

283. Kris MG, Pablo D, Gralla RJ, et al. Dyspnea following vinblastine or vindesine administration in patients receiving mitomycin plus vinca alkaloid combination therapy. *Cancer Treat Rep* 1984;68:1029.

284. Binet S, Fellous A, Lataste H, et al. In situ analysis of the action of Navelbine on various types of microtubules using immunofluorescence. *Semin Oncol* 1989;16[Suppl 4]:5.

285. Hohneker JA. A summary of vinorelbine (Navelbine) safety data from North American clinical trials. *Semin Oncol* 1994;21[Suppl 10]:42.

286. Le Chevalier T, Brisgand D, Douillard J-Y, et al. Randomized study of vinorelbine and cisplatin versus vindesine and cisplatin versus vinorelbine alone in non–small cell lung cancer: results of a European multicenter trial including 612 patients. *J Clin Oncol* 1994;12:360.

287. Raderer M, Kornek G, Scheithauer W. Correspondence re: Vinorelbine-induced pancreatitis: a case report. *J Natl Cancer Inst* 1998;90(4):329.

288. Hoff PM, Valero V, Ibrahim N, et al. Hand-foot syndrome following prolonged infusion of high doses of vinorelbine. *Cancer* 1998;82:965.

289. Garrett CA, Simpson TA Jr. Syndrome of inappropriate antidiuretic hormone associated with vinorelbine therapy. *Ann Pharmacother* 1998;32(12):1309.

290. Bender RA, Bleyer WA, Frisby SA. Alteration of methotrexate uptake in human leukemia cells by other agents. *Cancer Res* 1975;35:1305.

291. Zager RF, Frisby SA, Oliverio VT. The effects of antibiotics and cancer chemotherapeutic agents on the cellular transport and antitumor activity of methotrexate in L1210 murine leukemia. *Cancer Res* 1973;33:1670.

292. Warren RD, Nichols AP, Bender RA. The effect of vincristine on methotrexate uptake and inhibition of DNA synthesis by human lymphoblastoid cells. *Cancer Res* 1977;37:2993.

293. Bender RA, Nichols AP, Norton L, et al. Lack of therapeutic synergism of vincristine and methotrexate in L1210 murine leukemia in vivo. *Cancer Treat Rep* 1978;62:997.

294. Yalowich JC. Effect of microtubule inhibition on etoposide accumulation and DNA damage in human K562 cells in vitro. *Cancer Res* 1987;47:1010.

295. Bolin R, Riva R, Albani R, et al. Decreased phenytoin level during antineoplastic therapy: a case report. *Epilepsia* 1983;24:75.

296. Jarosinski PF, Moscow JA, Alexander MS, et al. Altered phenytoin clearance during intensive chemotherapy for acute lymphoblastic leukemia. *J Pediatr* 1988;112:996.

297. Tobe SW, Siu LL, Jamal SA, et al. Vinblastine and erythromycin: an unrecognized serious drug interaction. *Cancer Chemother Pharmacol* 1995;35:188.

298. Rowinsky EK, Onetto N, Canetta RM, et al. Taxol: the prototypic taxane, an important new class of antitumor agents. *Semin Oncol* 1992;119:646.

299. Wani MC, Taylor HL, Wall ME, et al. Plant antitumor agents: VI. The isolation and structure of Taxol, a novel antileukemic and antitumor agent from *Taxus brevifolia*. *J Am Chem Soc* 1971;93:2325.

300. Stierle A, Strobel G, Stierle D. Taxol and taxane production by *Taxomyces andreanae*, an endophytic fungus of Pacific yew. *Science* 1993;260:214.

301. Denis J-N, Greene AE. A highly efficient approach to natural Taxol. *J Am Chem Soc* 1988;110:5917.

302. Mangatal L, Adeline MT, Guenard D, et al. Application of the vicinal oxyamination reaction with asymmetric induction to the hemisynthesis of Taxol and analogues. *Tetrahedron* 1989;45:4177.

303. Kingston DGI, Samaranayake G, Ivey CA. The chemistry of Taxol, a clinically useful anticancer agent. *J Nat Prod* 1990;53:1.

304. Lataste H, Senilh V, Wright M, et al. Relationships between the structures of Taxol and baccatine III derivatives and their in vitro action of the disassembly of mammalian brain and *Pysarum* amoebal microtubules. *Proc Natl Acad Sci U S A* 1984;81:4090.

305. Gueritte-Voegelein F, Guenard D, Lavelle F, et al. Relationships between the structures of Taxol analogues and their antimitotic activity. *J Med Chem* 1991;34:992.

306. Schiff PB, Fant J, Horwitz SB. Promotion of microtubule assembly in vitro by Taxol. *Nature* 1979;22:665.

307. Schiff PB, Horwitz SB. Taxol stabilizes microtubules in mouse fibroblast cells. *Proc Natl Acad Sci U S A* 1980;77:1561.

308. Schiff PB, Horwitz SB. Taxol assembles tubulin in the absence of exogenous guanosine 5'-triphosphate or microtubule-associated protein. *Biochemistry* 1981;20:3247.

309. Parness J, Horwitz SB. Taxol binds to polymerized microtubules in vitro. *J Cell Biol* 1981;91:479.

310. Rao S, Orr GA, Chaudhary AG, et al. Characterization of the taxol binding site on the microtubule. 2-(m-Azidobenzoyl)taxol photolabels a peptide (amino acids 217-231) of beta-tubulin. *J Biol Chem* 1995;270(35):20235.

311. Rao S, He L, Chakravarty S, et al. Characterization of the Taxol binding site on the microtubule. Identification of Arg(282) in beta-tubulin as the site of photoincorporation of a 7-benzophenone analogue of Taxol. *J Biol Chem* 1999;274(53):37990.

312. Nogales E, Wolf SG, Downing KH. Structure of the alpha beta tubulin dimer by electron crystallography. *Nature* 1998;391:199.

313. Nogales E, Whittaker M, Milligan RA, et al. High-resolution model of the microtubule. *Cell* 1999;96:79.

314. Amos LA, Löwe J. How Taxol stabilises microtubule structure. *Chem Biol* 1999;6:R65.

315. He L, Jagtap PG, Kingston DGI, et al. A common pharmacophore for Taxol and the epothilones based on the biological activity of a taxane molecule lacking a C-13 side chain. *Biochemistry* 2000;39:3972.

316. McDaid HM, Bhattacharya SK, Chen X-T, et al. Structure-activity profiles of eleutherobin analogs and their cross-resistance in Taxol-resistant cell lines. *Cancer Chemother Pharmacol* 1999;44:131.

317. Thompson WC, Wilson L, Purich DL. Taxol induces microtubule assembly at low temperatures. *Cell Motil* 1981;1:445.

318. Collins CA, Vallee RB. Temperature-dependent reversible assembly of taxol-treated microtubules. *J Cell Biol* 1987;105:2847.

319. Hamel E, del Campo AA, Lowe MC, et al. Interactions of Taxol, microtubule-associated proteins and guanine nucleotides in tubulin polymerization. *J Biol Chem* 1981;256:11887.

320. Ringel I, Horwitz SB. Studies with RP56976 (Taxotere): a semisynthetic analogue of taxol. *J Natl Cancer Inst* 1991;83:288.

321. Diaz JF, Andreu JM. Assembly of purified GDP-tubulin into microtubules induced by Taxol and Taxotere: reversibility, ligand stoichiometry and competition. *Biochemistry* 1993;32:2747.

322. Jordan MA, Toso RJ, Thrower D, et al. Mechanism of mitotic block and inhibition of cell proliferation by Taxol at low concentrations. *Proc Natl Acad Sci U S A* 1993;90:9552.

323. Yvon AMC, Wadsworth P, Jordan MA. Taxol suppresses dynamics of individual microtubules in living human tumor cells. *Mol Biol Cell* 1999;10:947.

324. De Brabander M, Geuens G, Nuydens R, et al. Taxol induces the assembly of free microtubules in living cells and blocks the organizing capacity of the centrosomes and kinetochores. *Proc Natl Acad Sci U S A* 1981;78:5608.

325. Manfredi JJ, Fant J, Horwitz SB. Taxol induces the formation of unusual arrays of cellular microtubules in colchicine-pretreated J774.2 cells. *Eur J Cell Biol* 1986;42:126.

326. Albertini DF. In vivo and in vitro studies of the role of HMW-MAPs in Taxol-induced microtubule bundling. *Eur J Cell Biol* 1984;33:134.

327. Rowinsky EK, Donehower RC, Jones RJ, et al. Microtubule changes and cytotoxicity in leukemic cell lines treated with Taxol. *Cancer Res* 1988;48:4093.

328. Roberts JR, Rowinsky EK, Donehower RC, et al. Demonstration of the cell cycle positions for Taxol-induced asters and "bundles" by sequential measurement of fluorescence, DNA content, and autoradiographic labeling of Taxol-sensitive and -resistant cells. *J Histochem Cytochem* 1989;37:1659.

329. Roberts JR, Allison DC, Dooley WC, et al. Effects of Taxol on cell cycle traverse: taxol-induced polyploidization as a marker for drug resistance. *Cancer Res* 1990;50:710.

330. Mole-Bajer J, Bajer AS. Action of Taxol on mitosis: modification of microtubule arrangements and function of the mitotic spindle in the *Haemanthus* endosperm. *J Cell Biol* 1983;95:527.

331. Schatten G, Schatten H, Bestor TH, et al. Taxol inhibits the nuclear movements during fertilization and induces asters in unfertilized sea urchin eggs. *J Cell Biol* 1982;94:455.

332. Bissery M-C, Guenard D, Gueritte-Voegelein F, et al. Experimental antitumor activity of Taxotere (RP 56976, NSC 628503), a Taxol analogue. *Cancer Res* 1991;51:4845.

333. Garcia P, Braguer D, Carles G, et al. Comparative effects of Taxol and Taxotere on different human carcinoma cell lines. *Cancer Chemother Pharmacol* 1994;34:335.

334. Rubin RW, Quillen M, Corconan JJ, et al. Tubulin as a major cell surface protein in human lymphoid cells of leukemic origin. *Cancer Res* 1982;42:1384.

335. Quillen M, Castello C, Krishan A, et al. Cell surface tubulin in leukemic cells: molecular structure surface binding, turnover, cell cycle expression, and origin. *J Cell Biol* 1985;101:2345.

336. Keller HU, Zimmerman A. Shape changes and chemokinesis of Walker 256 carcinosarcoma cells in response to colchicine, vinblastine, nocodazole, and Taxol. *Invasive Metastasis* 1986;6:33.

337. Rainey WE, Kramer RE, Mason JI, et al. The effect of

Taxol, a microtubule-stabilizing drug, on steroidogenic cells. *J Cell Physiol* 1985;123:17.

338. Roberts RL, Nath J, Friedman MM, et al. Effects of Taxol on human neutrophils. *J Immunol* 1982;129:1295.

339. Iannone A, Wolberg G, Reynolds-Vaughn R, et al. Taxol inhibits *N*-formyl-methionyl-leucyl-phenylalanine (FMLP)-induced neutrophil polarization and H_2O_2 production while decreasing [^{3}H]FMLP binding. *Agents Actions* 1987;21:278.

340. Wolberg G, Stopford CR, Zimmerman TP. Antagonism by Taxol of effects of microtubule-disrupting agents on lymphocyte cAMP metabolism and cell function. *Proc Natl Acad Sci U S A* 1984;81:3496.

341. Cuthbert JA, Shay JW. Microtubule and lymphocyte responses: effect of colchicine and Taxol on mitogen-induced human lymphocyte activation and proliferation. *J Cell Physiol* 1983;116:127.

342. Chuang LT, Lotzova E, Heath J, et al. Alteration of lymphocyte microtubule assembly, cytotoxicity and activation by the anticancer drug Taxol. *Cancer Res* 1994;54:1286.

343. Ding AH, Porteu F, Sanchez E, et al. Shared actions of endotoxin and Taxol on TNF receptors and TNF release. *Science* 1990;248:370.

344. Burkhart CA, Berman JW, Swindell CS, et al. Relationship between Taxol and other taxanes on induction of tumor necrosis factor-alpha gene expression and cytotoxicity. *Cancer Res* 1994;22:5779.

345. Van Bockxmeer FM, Martin CE, Thompson DE, et al. Taxol for the treatment of proliferative vitreoretinopathy. *Invest Ophthalmol Vis Sci* 1985;26:1140.

346. Sollott SJ, Cheng L, Pauly RR, et al. Taxol inhibits neointimal smooth muscle cell accumulation after angioplasty in the rat. *J Clin Invest* 1995;95:1869.

347. Howell SL, Hii CS, Shaikh S, et al. Effects of Taxol and nocodazole on insulin secretion from isolated rat islands of Langerhans. *Bioscience Rep* 1982;2:795.

348. Oda K, Kehara Y. Taxol, a potent promotor of microtubule assembly, inhibits secretion of plasma proteins in cultured rat hepatocytes. *Biochem Biophys Res Commun* 1982;107:561.

349. Kaufman SS, Tuma DJ, Vanderhoof JA. Reduced effect of Taxol on plasma protein secretion by developing rat liver. *Toxicol Appl Pharmacol* 1986;82:233.

350. Thuret-Carnahan J, Bossu J-L, Feltz A, et al. Effect of Taxol on secretory cells: functional, morphological, and electrophysiological correlates. *J Cell Biol* 1985;100:1863.

351. McKay DB. Structure-activity study on the actions of Taxol and related taxanes on primary cultures of adrenal medullary cells. *J Pharmacol Exp Ther* 1989;248:1302.

352. Donaldson KL, Gollsby G, Kiener PA, et al. Activation of p34^{cdc2} coincident with Taxol-induced apoptosis. *Cell Growth Diff* 1994;5:1041.

353. Fan W. Possible mechanisms of paclitaxel-induced apoptosis. *Biochem Pharmacol* 1999;57:1215.

354. Torres K, Horwitz SB. Mechanisms of Taxol-induced cell death are concentration dependent. *Cancer Res* 1998;58(16):3620.

355. Blagosklonny MV, Fojo T. Molecular effects of paclitaxel: myths and reality (a critical review). *Int J Cancer* 1999;83:151.

356. Lee L-F, Li G, Templeton DJ, et al. Paclitaxel (Taxol)-induced gene expression and cell death are both mediated by the activation of c-Jun NH_2-terminal kinase (JNK/SAPK). *J Biol Chem* 1998;273(43): 28253.

357. Borbé R, Rieger J, Weller M. Failure of Taxol-based combination chemotherapy for malignant glioma cannot be overcome by G2/M checkpoint abrogators or altering the p53 status. *Cancer Chemother Pharmacol* 1999;44:217.

358. Giannakakou P, Poy G, Zhan Z, et al. Paclitaxel selects for mutant or pseudo-null p53 in drug resistance associated with tubulin mutations in human cancer. *Oncogene* 2000;19:3078.

359. Rakovitch E, Mellado W, Hall EJ, et al. Paclitaxel sensitivity correlates with p53 status and DNA fragmentation, but not G2/M accumulation. *Int J Radiat Oncol Biol Phys* 1999;44(5):1119.

360. Li W, Fan J, Banerjee D, et al. Overexpression of p21^{waf1} decreases g2-M arrest and apoptosis induced by paclitaxel in human sarcoma cells lacking both p53 and functional rb protein. *Mol Pharmacol* 1999;55:1088.

361. Schmidt M, Lu Y, Liu B, et al. Differential modulation of paclitaxel-mediated apoptosis by p21^{Waf1} and p27^{Kip1}. *Oncogene* 2000;19:2423.

362. Gazitt Y, Rothenberg ML, Hilsenbeck SG, et al. Bcl-2 overexpression is associated with resistance to paclitaxel, but not gemcitabine, in multiple myeloma cells. *Int J Oncol* 1998;13(4):839.

363. Scatena CD, Stewart ZA, Mays D, et al. Mitotic phosphorylation of Bcl-2 during normal cell cycle progression and taxol-induced growth arrest. *J Biol Chem* 1998;273(46):30777.

364. Strobel T, Tai Y-T, Korsmeyer S, et al. BAD partly reverses paclitaxel resistance in human ovarian cancer cells. *Oncogene* 1998;17:2419.

365. Strobel T, Kraeft SK, Chen LB, et al. BAX expression is associated with enhanced intracellular accumulation of paclitaxel: a novel role for BAX during chemotherapy-induced cell death. *Cancer Res* 1998;58(21):4776.

366. Page C, Lin HJ, Jin Y, et al. Overexpression of Akt/AKT can modulate chemotherapy-induced apoptosis. *Anticancer Res* 2000;20(1A):407.

367. Gooch JL, Van Den Berg CL, Yee D. Insulin-like growth factor (IGF)-I rescues breast cancer cells from chemotherapy-induced cell death—proliferative and anti-apoptotic effects. *Breast Cancer Res Treat* 1999;56(1):1.

368. Yu D, Liu B, Tan M, et al. Overexpression of c-erbB-2/neu in breast cancer cells confers increased resistance to Taxol via mdr-1-independent mechanisms. *Oncogene* 1996;13:1359.

369. Yu D, Liu B, Jing T, et al. Overexpression of both p185^{c-erB2} and p170^{mdr-1} renders breast cancer cells highly resistant to Taxol. *Oncogene* 1998;16:2087.

370. Tishler RB, Schiff PB, Geard CR, et al. Taxol: a novel radiation sensitizer. *Int J Radiat Oncol Biol Phys* 1992;22:613.

371. Tishler RB, Geard CR, Hall EJ, et al. Taxol sensitizes human astrocytoma cells to radiation. *Cancer Res* 1992;52:3495.

372. Steren A, Sevin BU, Perras J, et al. Taxol sensitizes human ovarian cancer cells to radiation. *Gynecol Oncol* 1993;48:252.

373. Choy H, Rodrieguez F, Wilcox B, et al. Radiation sensitizing effects of Taxotere (RP 56976). *Proc Am Assoc Cancer Res* 1992;33:500(abst).

374. Herscher LL, Hahn SM, Kroog G, et al. A phase I study of paclitaxel as a radiation sensitizer in the treatment of non–small cell lung cancer and mesothelioma. *J Clin Oncol* 1998;16:635.

375. Brewster F, Warr JR. Verapamil reversal of vincristine resistance and cross-resistance patterns of vincristine-resistant Chinese hamster ovary cells. *Cancer Treat Rep* 1987;71:353.

376. Cabral F, Wible L, Brenner S, et al. Taxol-requiring mutants

of Chinese hamster ovary cells with impaired mitotic spindle activity. *J Cell Biol* 1983;97:30.

377. Cabral FR. Isolation of Chinese hamster ovary cell mutants requiring the continuous presence of Taxol for cell division. *J Biol* 1983;97:22.

378. Jaffrezou J-P, Dumontet C, Derry WB, et al. Novel mechanisms of resistance of paclitaxel (Taxol®) in human K562 leukemia cells by combined selection with PSC833. *Oncol Res* 1995;7:517.

379. Ranganathan S, Benetatos CA, Colarusso PJ, et al. Altered beta-tubulin isotype expression in paclitaxel-resistant human prostate carcinoma cells. *Br J Cancer* 1998;77(4):562.

380. Nicoletti MI, Valoti G, Giannakakou P, et al. Expression of β-tubulin isotypes in human ovarian carcinoma xenografts and in a sub-panel of human cancer cell lines from the NCI-Anticancer Drug Screen. Correlation with sensitivity to microtubule active agents. *Clin Cancer Res* (*in press*).

381. Kavallaris M, Kuo DYS, Burkhart CA, et al. Taxol-resistant epithelial ovarian tumors are associated with altered expression of specific beta-tubulin isotypes. *J Clin Invest* 1997;100(5):1282.

382. Kavallaris M, Burkhart CA, Horwitz SB. Antisense oligonucleotides to class III beta-tubulin sensitize drug-resistant cells to taxol. *Br J Cancer* 1999;80(7):1020.

383. Giannakakou P, Sackett DL, Kang Y-K, et al. Paclitaxel-resistant human ovarian cancer cells have mutant beta-tubulins that exhibit impaired paclitaxel-driven polymerization. *J Biol Chem* 1997;272:17118.

384. Gonzalez-Garay ML, Chang L, Blade K, et al. A β-tubulin leucine cluster involved in microtubule assembly and paclitaxel resistance. *J Biol Chem* 1999;274(34):23875.

385. Horwitz SB, Cohen D, Rao S, et al. Taxol: mechanisms of action and resistance. *J Natl Cancer Inst Monogr* 1993;15:55.

386. Horwitz SB, Lothstein L, Mellado W, et al. Taxol: mechanisms of action and resistance. *Ann N Y Acad Sci* 1986;466:733.

387. Roy SN, Horwitz SB. A phosphoglycoprotein with Taxol resistance in J774.2 cells. *Cancer Res* 1985;45:3856.

388. Greenberger LM, Lothstein L, Williams SS, et al. Distinct P-glycoprotein precursors are overproduced in independently isolated drug-resistant cell lines. *Proc Natl Acad Sci U S A* 1988;85:3762.

389. Lehnert M, Emerson S, Dalton W, et al. In vitro evaluation of chemosensitizers for clinical reversal of P-glycoprotein-associated Taxol resistance. *J Natl Cancer Inst Monogr* 1993;15:63.

390. Racker E, Wu L-T, Westcott D. Use of slow Ca^{2+} blockers to enhance inhibition by Taxol of growth of drug-sensitive and -resistant Chinese hamster ovary cells. *Cancer Treat Rep* 1986;70:275.

391. Woodcock DM, Jefferson S, Linsenmeyer ME. Reversal of the multidrug resistance phenotype with Cremophor EL, a common vehicle for water-insoluble vitamins and drugs. *Cancer Res* 1990;50:4199.

392. Chervinsky DS, Brecher ML, Hoelcle MJ. Cremophor-EL enhances Taxol efficacy in a multi-drug resistant c1300 neuroblastoma cell line. *Anticancer Res* 1993;13:93.

393. Webster L, Linenmyer M, Millward M, et al. Measurement of Cremophor EL following taxol: plasma levels sufficient to reverse drug exclusion mediated by the multidrug-resistant phenotype. *J Natl Cancer Inst* 1993;85:1685.

394. Seidman A, Crown J, Reichman B, et al. Paclitaxel as a second and subsequent chemotherapy for metastatic breast cancer: activity independent of prior anthracycline response. *J Clin Oncol* 1995;13:1152.

395. Wilson WH, Berg S, Bryant G, et al. Paclitaxel in doxorubicin-refractory or mitoxantrone-refractory breast cancer: a phase I/II trial of 96-hour infusion. *J Clin Oncol* 1994;12:1621.

396. Tolcher A, Cowan KH, Solomon D, et al. Phase I crossover study of paclitaxel with r-verapamil in patients with metastatic breast cancer. *J Clin Oncol* 1996;14:1173.

397. Chico I, Kang MH, Bergan R, et al. Phase I study of infusional paclitaxel with the P-glycoprotein antagonist PSC 833. *J Clin Oncol* 2001;19:832.

398. Fisher GA, Bartlett NL, Lum BL, et al. Phase I trial of Taxol with high-dose cyclosporine as a modulator of multidrug resistance. *Proc Am Soc Clin Oncol* 1994;13:144(abst).

399. Hamel E, Lin CM, Johns DG. Tubulin-dependent biochemical assay for the antineoplastic agent Taxol and applications to measurements of the drug in the serum. *Cancer Treat Rep* 1982;66:1381.

400. Longnecker SM, Donehower RC, Cates AE, et al. High performance liquid chromatographic assay for Taxol (NSC 125973) in human plasma and urine pharmacokinetics in a phase I trial. *Cancer Treat Rep* 1986;71:53.

401. Grem JL, Tutsch KD, Simon KJ, et al. Phase I study of Taxol administered as a short IV infusion daily for 5 days. *Cancer Treat Rep* 1987;71:1179.

402. Wiernik PH, Schwartz EL, Strauman JJ, et al. Phase I clinical and pharmacokinetic study of taxol. *Cancer Res* 1987;47:2486.

403. Wiernik PH, Schwartz EL, Einzig A, et al. Phase I trial of Taxol given as a 24-hour infusion every 21 days: responses observed in metastatic melanoma. *J Clin Oncol* 1987;5:1232.

404. Brown T, Havlin K, Weiss G, et al. A phase I trial of taxol given by 6-hour intravenous infusion. *J Clin Oncol* 1991;9:1261.

405. Huizing MT, Keung ACF, Rosing H, et al. Pharmacokinetics of paclitaxel and metabolites in a randomized comparative study in platinum-pretreated ovarian cancer patients. *J Clin Oncol* 1993;11:2127.

406. Willey TA, Bekos EJ, Gaver RC, et al. High-performance liquid chromatographic procedure for the quantitative determination of paclitaxel (Taxol) in human plasma. *J Chromatogr* 1993;621:231.

407. Sonnichsen D, Hurwitz C, Pratt C, et al. Saturable pharmacokinetics and paclitaxel pharmacodynamics in children with solid tumors. *J Clin Oncol* 1994;12:532.

408. Vergniol JC, Bruno R, Montay G, et al. Determination of Taxotere in human plasma by a semi-automated high performance liquid chromatographic method. *J Chromatogr* 1992;582:273.

409. Extra J-M, Rousseau F, Bruno R, et al. Phase I and pharmacokinetic study of Taxotere (RP 56976; NSC 628503) given as a short intravenous infusion. *Cancer Res* 1993;53:1037.

410. Pazdur R, Newman RA, Newman BM, et al. Phase I trial of Taxotere: five-day schedule. *J Natl Cancer Inst* 1992; 84:1781.

411. Bissett D, Setanoians A, Cassidy J, et al. Phase I and pharmacokinetic study of Taxotere (RP 56976) administered as a 24-hour infusion. *Cancer Res* 1993;53:523.

412. Bruno R, Sanderink GJ. Pharmacokinetics and metabolism of Taxotere (docetaxel). In: Workman P, Graham MA, eds. *Cancer*

surveys: pharmacokinetics and cancer chemotherapy, vol 17. Plainview, NY: Cold Spring Harbor Laboratory Press, 1993:305.

413. Burris H, Kuhn J, Kalter S, et al. Phase I clinical trial of Taxotere administered as either a 2-hour or 6-hour intravenous infusion. *J Clin Oncol* 1993;11:950.

414. Grothaus PG, Raybould TJG, Bignami GS, et al. An enzyme immunoassay for the determination of Taxol and taxanes in *Taxus* sp. tissues and human plasma. *J Immunol Methods* 1993;158:5.

415. Leu J-G, Chen B-X, Schiff PB, et al. Characterization of polyclonal and monoclonal anti-Taxol antibodies and measurement of Taxol in serum. *Cancer Res* 1993;53:1388.

416. Karlsson MO, Molnar V, Freijs A, et al. Pharmacokinetic models for the saturable distribution of paclitaxel. *Drug Metab Dispos* 1999;27(10):1220.

417. Weiss R, Donehower RC, Wiernik PH, et al. Hypersensitivity reactions from Taxol. *J Clin Oncol* 1990;8:1263.

418. Yang CPH, Galbiati F, Volonté D, et al. Upregulation of caveolin-1 and caveolae organelles in taxol-resistant A549 cells. *FEBS Lett* 1998;439:368.

419. Schiller JH, Storer B, Tutsch K, et al. Phase I trial of 3-hour infusion of paclitaxel with or without granulocyte colony-stimulating factor. *J Clin Oncol* 1994;12:241.

420. Gianni L, Kearns C, Gianni A, et al. Nonlinear pharmacokinetics and metabolism of paclitaxel and its pharmacokinetic/pharmacodynamic relationships in humans. *J Clin Oncol* 1995;13:180.

421. Eisenhauer E, ten Bokkel Huinink W, Swenerton KD, et al. European-Canadian randomized trial of Taxol in relapsed ovarian cancer: high vs low dose and long vs short infusion. *J Clin Oncol* 1994;12:2654.

422. Van Tellingen O, Huizing MT, Panday VR, et al. Cremophor EL causes (pseudo-) non-linear pharmacokinetics of paclitaxel in patients. *Br J Cancer* 1999;81(2):330.

423. Sparreboom A, Van Tellingen O, Nooijen WJ, et al. Nonlinear pharmacokinetics of paclitaxel in mice results from the pharmaceutical vehicle Cremophor EL. *Cancer Res* 1996;56:2112.

424. Kumar GN, Walle UK, Bhalla KN, et al. Binding of taxol to human plasma, albumin, and alpha 1-acid glycoprotein. *Res Commun Chem Pathol Pharmacol* 1993;80:337.

425. Wild MD, Walle K, Walle T. Extensive and saturable accumulation of paclitaxel (Taxol) by the human platelet. *Cancer Chemother Pharmacol* 1995;36:41.

426. Helmans JJ, Beijnen JH, Eeltink CM, et al. Paclitaxel (Taxol) concentrations in glioma. *Ann Oncol* 1994;5[Suppl 5]:199(abst).

427. Lesser G, Grossman SA, Eller S, et al. The neural and extra-neural distribution of systemically administered [^{3}H]paclitaxel in rats: a quantitative autoradiographic study. *Cancer Chemother Pharmacol* 1995;37:173.

428. Eiseman JL, Eddington ND, Leslie J, et al. Plasma pharmacokinetics and tissue distribution of paclitaxel in CD2F1 mice. *Cancer Chemother Pharmacol* 1994;34:465.

429. Klecker RW, Jamis-Dow CA, Egorin MJ, et al. Effect of cimetidine, probenecid, and ketoconazole on the distribution, biliary secretion, and metabolism of ^{3}H-Taxol in the Sprague-Dawley rat. *Drug Metab Dispos Biol Fate* 1994;22:254.

430. Walle T, Walle UK, Kumar GN, et al. Taxol metabolism and disposition in cancer patients. *Drug Metab Dispos* 1995;23:506.

431. Monsarrat B, Mariel E, Crois S, et al. Taxol metabolism: isolation and identification of three major metabolites in rat bile. *Drug Metab Dispos* 1990;18:895.

432. Monsarrat B, Alvinerie P, Dubois J, et al. Hepatic metabolism and biliary clearance of Taxol in rats and humans. *J Natl Cancer Inst Monogr* 1993;15:39.

433. Monsarrat B, Chatelut E, Royer I, et al. Modification of paclitaxel metabolism in a cancer patient by induction of cytochrome P450 3A4. *Drug Metab Dispos* 1998;26(3):229.

434. Venook AP, Egorin MJ, Rosner GL, et al. Phase I and pharmacokinetic trial of paclitaxel in patients with hepatic dysfunction: Cancer and Leukemia Group B 9264. *J Clin Oncol* 1998;16(5):1811.

435. Gaver RC, Deeb G, Willey T, et al. The disposition of paclitaxel (Taxol) in the rat. *Proc Am Assoc Cancer Res* 1993;34:390(abst).

436. Cresteil T, Monsarrat B, Alvinerie P, et al. Taxol metabolism by human liver microsomes: identification of cytochrome p450 isoenzymes involved in its biotransformation. *Cancer Res* 1994;54:386.

437. Harris JW, Rahman A, Kim B-R, et al. Metabolism of Taxol by human hepatic microsomes and liver slices: participation of cytochrome P450 3A4 and an unknown P450 enzyme. *Cancer Res* 1994;15:4026.

438. Harris JW, Katki A, Anderson LW, et al. Isolation, structural determination, and biological activity of 6 α hydroxytaxol, the principal human metabolite of Taxol. *J Med Chem* 1994;37:706.

439. Desai PB, Duan JZ, Zhu YW, et al. Human liver microsomal metabolism of paclitaxel and drug interactions. *Eur J Drug Metab Pharmacokinet* 1998;23(3):417.

440. Connichsen DS, Liu Q, Schuetz EG, et al. Variability in human cytochrome P450 paclitaxel metabolism. *J Pharmacol Exp Ther* 1995;275:566.

441. Rowinsky EK, Smith L, Wang YM, et al. Phase I and pharmacokinetic study of paclitaxel in combination with biricodar, a novel agent that reverses multidrug resistance conferred by overexpression of both MDR1 and MRP. *J Clin Oncol* 1998;16:2964.

442. Woo MH, Gregornik D, Shearer PD, et al. Pharmacokinetics of paclitaxel in an anephric patient. *Cancer Chemother Pharmacol* 1999;43:92.

443. Aapro MS, Zulian G, Alberto P, et al. Phase I and pharmacokinetic study of RP 56976 in a new ethanol-free formulation of Taxotere. *Ann Oncol* 1992;3[Suppl 3]:53(abst).

444. Bruno R, Dorr MB, Montay G, et al. Design and implementation of population pharmacokinetic studies during the development of docetaxel (RP 56976), a new anticancer drug. *Clin Pharmacol Ther* 1994;55:161(abst).

445. Rosing H, Lustig V, van Warmerdam LJC, et al. Pharmacokinetics and metabolism of docetaxel administered as a 1-h intravenous infusion. *Cancer Chemother Pharmacol* 2000;45:213.

446. De Valeriola D, Brassinne C, Cpillard C. Study of excretion balance, metabolism, and protein binding of C^{14} radiolabeled Taxotere (RP 56976, NSC 628503) in cancer patients. *Proc Am Assoc Cancer Res* 1993;34:373(abst).

447. Schellens JHM, Ma J, Bruno R, et al. Pharmacokinetics of cisplatin and Taxotere (docetaxel) and WBC DNA-adduct formation of cisplatin in the sequence Taxotere/cisplatin and cisplatin/Taxotere in a phase I/II study in solid tumor patients. *Proc Am Soc Clin Oncol* 1994;13:132(abst).

448. Marland M, Gaillard C, Sanderink G, et al. Kinetics distribution, metabolism and excretion of radiolabelled Taxotere (^{14}C-RP 56976) in mice and dogs. *Proc Am Assoc Cancer Res* 1993;34:393(abst).

449. Gaillard C, Monsarrat B, Vuilhorgne M, et al. Docetaxel (Taxotere) metabolism in the rat in vivo and in vitro. *Proc Am Assoc Cancer Res* 1994;35:428(abst).

450. Sparreboom A, Van Tellingen O, Scherrenburg EJ, et al. Isolation, purification and biological activity of major docetaxel metabolites from human feces. *Drug Metab Dispos* 1996;24(6):655.

451. Gires P, Gaillard C, Martin S, et al. [^{14}C]docetaxel (Taxotere) disposition in the isolated perfused rat liver and effect of enzyme induction. *Eur J Drug Metab Pharmacokinet* 1994;19[Suppl 2]:29(abst).

452. Marre F, De Sousa G, Placidi M, et al. Elucidation of hepatic biotransformation of Taxotere using human "in vitro" models. *Bull Cancer* 1993;80:527(abst).

453. Zhou-Pan XR, Marre F, Zhou XJ, et al. Preliminary characterization of Taxotere metabolism using human liver microsomal fractions. *Maimonide* 1992;1:S23(abst).

454. Commercon A, Bourzat JD, Bezard D, et al. Partial synthesis of major human metabolites of docetaxel. *Tetrahedron* 1994;50:10289.

455. Rowinsky EK, Chaudhry V, Forastiere AA, et al. A phase I and pharmacologic study of Taxol and cisplatin with granulocyte colony-stimulating factor: neuromuscular toxicity is dose-limiting. *J Clin Oncol* 1993;11:2010.

456. Rowinsky EK. The pharmacology of Taxol. *J Natl Cancer Inst Monogr* 1993;15:25.

457. Hurwitz CA, Relling MV, Weitman SD, et al. Phase I trial of paclitaxel in children with refractory solid tumors: a Pediatric Oncology Group study. *J Clin Oncol* 1993;11:2324.

458. Arbuck SA, Canetta R, Onetto N, et al. Current dosage and schedule issues in the development of paclitaxel (Taxol). *Semin Oncol* 1993;20[Suppl 3]:31.

459. Fennelly D, Aghajanian C, Shapiro F, et al. Phase I and pharmacologic study of paclitaxel administered weekly in patients with relapsed ovarian cancer. *J Clin Oncol* 1997;15(1):187.

460. Seidman AD, Hudis CA, Albanel J, et al. Dose-dense therapy with weekly 1-hour paclitaxel infusions in the treatment of metastatic breast cancer. *J Clin Oncol* 1998;16(10):3353.

461. Markman M, Rowinsky E, Hakes T, et al. Phase I trial of Taxol administered by the intraperitoneal route: a Gynecologic Oncology Group study. *J Clin Oncol* 1992;10:1485.

462. Schilder LE, Egorin ME, Zuhowski EG, et al. The pharmacokinetics of Taxol in a dialysis patient. *Proc Am Soc Clin Oncol* 1994;13:136(abst).

463. Fazeny B, Olsen SJ, Willey T, et al. Pharmacokinetic assessment of paclitaxel in an ovarian cancer patient on hemodialysis. *Proc Am Soc Clin Oncol* 1994;13:136(abst).

464. Venock AP, Egorin M, Braun TD, et al. Paclitaxel (Taxol) in patients with liver dysfunction (CALGB 9264). *Proc Am Soc Clin Oncol* 1994;13:139(abst).

465. Zaheer W, Lichtman SM, DeMarco L, et al. The use of Taxol in elderly patients. *Proc Am Soc Clin Oncol* 1994;13:441(abst).

466. Bicher A, Sarosy G, Kohn E, et al. Age does not influence Taxol dose intensity in recurrent carcinoma of the ovary. *Cancer* 1993;71[Suppl 2]:594.

467. Hainsworth JD, Burris HA 3rd, Erland JB, et al. Phase I trial of docetaxel administered by weekly infusion in patients with advanced refractory cancer. *J Clin Oncol* 1998;16:2164.

468. Francis P, Bruno R, Seidman A, et al. Pharmacodynamics of docetaxel (Taxotere) in patients with liver metastases. *Proc Am Soc Clin Oncol* 1994;13:138(abst).

469. Rowinsky EK, Eisenhauer EA, Chaudhry V, et al. Clinical toxicities encountered with Taxol. *Semin Oncol* 1993;20[Suppl 3]:1.

470. Peereboom D, Donehower RC, Eisenhauer EA, et al. Successful retreatment with Taxol after major hypersensitivity reactions. *J Clin Oncol* 1993;11:885.

471. McGuire WP, Rowinsky EK, Rosenshein NB, et al. Taxol: a unique antineoplastic agent with significant activity in advanced ovarian epithelial neoplasms. *Ann Intern Med* 1989;111:273.

472. Holmes FA, Walters RS, Theriault RL, et al. Phase II trial of Taxol, an active drug in metastatic breast cancer. *J Natl Cancer Inst* 1991;83:1797.

473. Rowinsky EK, Chaudhry V, Cornblath DR, et al. The neurotoxicity of taxol. *J Natl Cancer Inst Monogr* 1993;15:107.

474. Chaudhry V, Rowinsky EK, Sartorius SE, et al. Peripheral neuropathy from Taxol and cisplatin combination chemotherapy: clinical and electrophysiological studies. *Ann Neurol* 1994;35:490.

475. Capri G, Munzone E, Tarenzi E, et al. Optic nerve disturbances: a new form of paclitaxel neurotoxicity. *J Natl Cancer Inst* 1994;86:1099.

476. Rowinsky EK, McGuire WP, Guarnieri T, et al. Cardiac disturbances during the administration of Taxol. *J Clin Oncol* 1991;9:1704.

477. Arbuck SG, Strauss H, Rowinsky EK, et al. A reassessment of the cardiac toxicity associated with Taxol. *J Natl Cancer Inst Monogr* 1993;15:117.

478. Gianni L, Straneo G, Capri F, et al. Optimal dose and sequence finding study of paclitaxel (P) by 3 h infusion with bolus doxorubicin (D) in untreated metastatic breast cancer patients (Pts). *Proc Am Soc Clin Oncol* 1994;13:74(abst).

479. Pestalozzi BC, Sotos GA, Choyke PL, et al. Typhlitis resulting from treatment with Taxol and doxorubicin in patients with metastatic breast cancer. *Cancer* 1993;71:1797.

480. Kennedy MJ, Zahurak ML, Donehower RC, et al. Phase I and pharmacologic study of sequences of paclitaxel and cyclophosphamide supported by granulocyte colony-stimulating factor in women with previously treated metastatic breast cancer. *J Clin Oncol* 1996;14:783.

481. Ajani JA, Dodd LG, Daugherty K, et al. Taxol-induced soft-tissue injury secondary to extravasation: characterization by histopathology and clinical course. *J Natl Cancer Inst* 1994;86:51.

482. Shenkier T, Gelmon K. Paclitaxel and radiation recall dermatitis [Letter]. *J Clin Oncol* 1994;12:439.

483. Fosella FV, Lee JS, Murphy WK, et al. Phase II study of docetaxel for recurrent or metastatic non–small cell lung cancer. *J Clin Oncol* 1994;12:1238.

484. Francis PA, Rigas JR, Kris MG, et al. Phase II trial of docetaxel in patients with stage III and IV non–small cell lung cancer. *J Clin Oncol* 1994;12:1232.

485. Frances P, Schneider J, Hann L, et al. Phase II trial of docetaxel in patients with platinum-refractory advanced ovarian cancer. *J Clin Oncol* 1994;12:2201.

486. Verweij J, Clavel M, Chevalier B. Paclitaxel (Taxol) and docetaxel (Taxotere): not simply two of a kind. *Ann Oncol* 1994;5:495.

487. Chevallier B, Fumoleau P, Kerbrat P, et al. Docetaxel is a major cytotoxic drug for the treatment of advanced breast cancer: a phase II trial of the Clinical Screening Cooperative Group of the European Organization for Research and Treatment of Cancer. *J Clin Oncol* 1995;13:314.

488. Eisenhauer EA, Lu F, Muldal A, et al. Predictors and treatment of docetaxel toxic effects. *Ann Oncol* 1994;5[Suppl 5]:202(abst).

489. Galindo E, Kavanagh J, Fossella F, et al. Docetaxel (Taxotere) toxicities: analysis of a single institution experience of 168 patients (623 courses). *Proc Am Soc Clin Oncol* 1994;13:164(abst).

490. Wanders J, Schrijvers D, Bruntsh U, et al. The EORTC-ECTG experience with acute hypersensitivity reactions (HSR) in Taxotere studies. *Proc Am Soc Clin Oncol* 1993;12:73(abst).

491. Oulid-Aissa D, Behar A, Spielmann M, et al. Management of fluid retention syndrome in patients treated with Taxotere (docetaxel): effect of premedication. *Proc Am Soc Clin Oncol* 1994;13:465(abst).

492. Tomiak E, Piccart MJ, Kerger J, et al. Phase I study of docetaxel administered as a 1-hour intravenous infusion on a weekly basis. *J Clin Oncol* 1994;12:1458.

493. Vukeljia SJ, Baker WJ, Burris III HA, et al. Pyridoxine therapy for palmar-plantar erythrodysthesia associated with Taxotere. *J Natl Cancer Inst* 1993;85:1432.

494. Zimmerman GC, Keeling JH, Lowry M, et al. Prevention of docetaxel-induced erythrodysthesia with local hypothermia. *J Natl Cancer Inst* 1994;86:557.

495. Balmaceda C, Forsyth P, Seidman AD, et al. Peripheral neuropathy in patients receiving Taxotere chemotherapy. *Ann Neurol* 1993;34:313(abst).

496. Frelich RJ, Balmaceda C, Rubin M, et al. Motor neuropathy due to Taxotere and Taxol. *Neurology* 1994;44[Suppl 2]:A217(abst).

497. Catimel G, Verweij J, Mattijssen V, et al. Docetaxel (Taxotere): an active drug for the treatment of patients with advanced squamous cell carcinoma of the head and neck. *Ann Oncol* 1994;5:533.

498. Rowinsky EK, Gilbert M, McGuire WP, et al. Sequences of Taxol and cisplatin: a phase I and pharmacologic study. *J Clin Oncol* 1991;9:1692.

499. Rowinsky EK, Citardi M, Noe DA, et al. Sequence-dependent cytotoxicity between cisplatin and the antimicrotubule agents Taxol and vincristine. *J Cancer Res Clin Oncol* 1993; 119:737.

500. Parker RJ, Dabholkar MD, Lee K-B, et al. Taxol effect on cisplatin sensitivity and cisplatin cellular accumulation in human ovarian cancer cells. *J Natl Cancer Inst Monogr* 1993;15:83.

501. LeBlanc GA, Sundseth SS, Weber GF, et al. Platinum anticancer drugs modulate P-450 mRNA levels and differentially alter hepatic drug and steroid hormone metabolism in male and female rats. *Cancer Res* 1992;52:540.

502. Huizing MT, Giaccone G, van Warmerdam LJ, et al. Pharmacokinetics of paclitaxel and carboplatin in a dose-escalating and dose-sequencing study in patients with non–small-cell lung cancer. The European Cancer Centre. *J Clin Oncol* 1997;15:317.

503. Sledge GW, Robert N, Goldstein LJ, et al. Phase I trial of Adriamycin and Taxol in metastatic breast cancer. *Eur J Cancer* 1993;29A[Suppl 6]:S81(abst).

504. Holmes FA, Newman RA, Madden V, et al. Schedule dependent pharmacokinetics (PK) in a phase I trial of Taxol (T) and doxorubicin (D) as initial chemotherapy for metastatic breast cancer. In: *Proceedings of the 8th NCI-EORTC Symposium on New Drugs in Cancer Therapy, Amsterdam, March 15–18, 1994.* Dordrecht, The Netherlands: Kluwer, 1994:197(abst).

505. Holmes FA, Madden T, Newman RA, et al. Sequence-dependent alteration of doxorubicin pharmacokinetics by paclitaxel in a phase I study of paclitaxel and doxorubicin in patients with metastatic breast cancer. *J Clin Oncol* 1996;14:2713.

506. Venturini M, Lunardi G, Del Mastro L, et al. Sequence effect of epirubicin and paclitaxel treatment on pharmacokinetics and toxicity. *J Clin Oncol* 2000;18(10):2116.

507. Esposito M, Venturini M, Vannozzi MO, et al. Comparative effects of paclitaxel and docetaxel on the metabolism and pharmacokinetics of epirubicin in breast cancer patients. *J Clin Oncol* 1999;17(4):1132.

508. Verweij J, Planting AST, Van der Berg MEL, et al. A phase I study of docetaxel (Taxotere) and cisplatin in patients with solid tumors. *Proc Am Soc Clin Oncol* 1994;13:148(abst).

509. Grem JL, Nguyen D, Monahan BP, et al. Sequence-dependent antagonism between fluorouracil and paclitaxel in human breast cancer cells. *Biochem Pharmacol* 1999;58:477.

510. Moasser MM, Sepp-Lorenzino L, Kohn NE, et al. Farnesyl transferase inhibitors cause enhanced mitotic sensitivity to taxol and epothilones. *Proc Natl Acad Sci U S A* 1998;95:1369.

511. Giannakakou P, Villalba L, Li H, et al. Combinations of paclitaxel and vinblastine and their effects on tubulin polymerization and cellular cytotoxicity: characterization of a synergistic schedule. *Int J Cancer* 1998;75:57.

512. Li CJ, Li Y-Z, Ventura Pinto A, et al. Potent inhibition of tumor survival in vivo by β-lapachone plus taxol: combining drugs imposes different artificial checkpoints. *Proc Natl Acad Sci U S A* 1999;96(23):13369.

513. Fettel MR, Grossman SA, Balmaceda C, et al. Clinical and pharmacological study of preirradiation taxol administered as a 96-hour infusion in adults with newly diagnosed glioblastoma multiforme. *Proc Am Soc Clin Oncol* 1994;13:179.

514. James-Dow CA, Klecker RW, Katki AG, et al. Metabolism of Taxol by human and rat liver in vitro. A screen for drug interactions and interspecies differences. *Cancer Chemother Pharmacol* 1995;36:107.

515. Slichenmyer W, McGuire W, Donehower R, et al. Pretreatment H$_2$ receptor antagonists that differ in P450 modulation activity: comparative effects on paclitaxel clearance rates. *Cancer Chemother Pharmacol* 1995;36:227.

516. Bai R, Roach MC, Jararam SK, et al. Differential effects of active isomers, segments, and analogues of dolastatin-10 on ligand interactions with tubulin: correlations with cytotoxicity. *Biochem Pharmacol* 1993;45:1503.

516a. Takahashi M, Iwasaki S, Kobayashi H, et al. Studies on macrocyclic lactone antibiotics: XI. Antimitotic and antitubulin activity of new antitumor antibiotics, rhizoxin and its homologues. *J Antibiot* 1987;40:66.

516b. Sawada T, Kobayashi H, Hashimoto Y, et al. Identification of the fragment photoaffinity-labeled with azidodansylrhizoxin as Met-363-Lys-379 on beta-tubulin. *Biochem Pharmacol* 1993;45:1387.

516c. Hamel E. Natural products which interact with tubulin in the vinca domain: maytansine, rhizoxin, phomopsin A, dolastatin 10 and 15 and halichondrin B. *Pharmacol Ther* 1992;55:31.

516d. Tsuro T, Oh-hara T, Iida H, et al. Rhizoxin, a macrocyclic lactone antibiotic, as a new antitumor agent against human and murine tumor cells and their vincristine-resistant sublines. *Cancer Res* 1986;46:381.

516e. Graham MA, Bissett D, Setanoians A, et al. Preclinical and phase I studies with rhizoxin to apply a pharmacokinetically guided-dose escalation scheme. *J Natl Cancer Inst* 1992;84:494.

516f. Bissett D, Graham MA, Setanoians A, et al. Phase I and pharmacokinetic study of rhizoxin. *Cancer Res* 1992;52:2894.

517. Toppmeyer DL, Slapak CA, Croop J, et al. Role of P-glycoprotein in dolastatin-10 resistance. *Biochem Pharmacol* 1994;48:609.

518. Newman RA, Fuentes A, Covey JM, et al. Preclinical pharmacology of the natural marine product dolastatin 10 (NSC 376128). *Drug Metab Dispos Biol Fate* 1994;22:428.

519. Hendriks HR, Plowman J, Berger DP, et al. Preclinical antitumor activity and animal toxicology studies of rhizoxin, a novel tubulin-interacting agent. *Ann Oncol* 1992;3:755.

520. Bai R, Cichacz ZA, Herald CL, et al. Spongistatin 1, a highly cytotoxic, sponge-derived, marine natural product that inhibits mitosis, microtubule assembly, and the binding of vinblastine to tubulin. *Mol Pharmacol* 1993;44:757.

521. Jonsson G, Hogberg B. Treatment of advanced prostatic carcinoma with estracyt: a preliminary report. *Scand J Urol Nephrol* 1971;5:103.

522. Tew KD. The mechanism of action of estramustine. *Semin Oncol* 1983;10:21.

523. Tew KD, Glusker JP, Hartley-Asp B, et al. Preclinical and clinical perspectives on the use of estramustine as an antimitotic drug. *Pharmacol Ther* 1992;56:323.

524. Muntzing J, Jensen G, Hogberg B. Pilot study on the growth inhibition by estramustine phosphate (Estracyt) of rat mammary tumors sensitive and insensitive to oestrogens. *Acta Pharmacol Toxicol* 1979;44:1.

525. Petrow V, Padilla GM. Design of cytotoxic steroids for prostate cancer. *Prostate* 1986;9:169.

526. Benson R, Hartley-Asp B. Mechanisms of action and clinical uses of estramustine. *Cancer Invest* 1990;8:375.

527. Hartley-Asp B. Estramustine-induced mitotic arrest in two human prostatic carcinoma cell lines, DU 145 and PC-3. *Prostate* 1984;5:93.

528. Tew KD, Hartley-Asp B. Cytotoxic properties of estramustine unrelated to alkylating and steroid constituents. *Urology* 1984;23:28.

529. Friden B, Wallin M, Deinum J, et al. Effect of estramustine phosphate on the assembly of trypsin-treated microtubules and microtubules reconstituted from purified tubulin with either tau, MAP-2 or the tubulin-binding fragment of MAP-2. *Arch Biochem Biophys* 1987;257:123.

530. Sterns ME, Tew KD. Estramustine binds MAP-2 to inhibit microtubule assembly in vitro. *J Cell Sci* 1988;89:331.

531. Wallin M, Deinum J, Friden B. Interaction of estramustine phosphate with microtubule-associated proteins. *Fed Eur Biochem Soc Lett* 1985;179:289.

532. Sterns W, Wang M, Tew KD, et al. Estramustine binds a MAP-1-like protein to inhibit microtubule assembly in vitro and disrupts microtubule organization in DU 145 cells. *J Cell Biol* 1988;107:2647.

533. Dahllof B, Billstrom A, Cabral F, et al. Estramustine depolymerizes microtubules by binding to tubulin. *Cancer Res* 1993;53:4573.

534. Bergenheim AT, Bjork P, Bergh J, et al. Estramustine-binding protein and specific binding of the anti-mitotic compound estramustine in astrocytoma. *Cancer Res* 1994;54:4974.

535. Shiina H, Sumi H, Ishibe T, et al. Study of estramustine binding protein: its relationship to androgen dependency and histological differentiation in human prostatic carcinoma tissue. *Urol Int* 1994;52:213.

536. Kim JH, Khil MS, Kim SH, et al. Clinical and biological studies of estramustine phosphate as a novel radiation sensitizer. *Int J Radiat Oncol Biol Phys* 1994;29:555.

537. Yoshida D, Piepmeir J, Weinstein M. Estramustine sensitizes human glioblastoma cells to irradiation. *Cancer Res* 1994;54:1415.

538. Eklov S, Essand M, Carlsson J, et al. Radiation sensitization by estramustine studies on cultured human prostatic cancer cells. *Prostate* 1992;21:287.

539. Speicher LA, Sheridan VR, Godwin AK, et al. Resistance to the antimitotic drug estramustine is distinct from the multidrug resistant phenotype. *Br J Cancer* 1991;64:267.

540. Speicher LA, Barone LR, Chapman AE, et al. P-glycoprotein binding and modulation of the multidrug-resistant phenotype by estramustine. *J Natl Cancer Inst* 1994;86:688.

541. Yang CP, Shen HJ, Horwitz SB. Modulation of the function of P-glycoprotein by estramustine. *J Natl Cancer Inst* 1994;86:723.

542. Forshell GP, Muntzing J, Ek A, et al. The absorption, metabolism and excretion of Estracyt (NSC-89199) in patients with prostatic cancer. *Invest Urol* 1976;14:128.

543. Kirdini RY, Karr JP, Murphy GP, et al. Prostate cancer: plasma concentrations of estramustine and its metabolites. *N Y State J Med* 1980;80:1390.

544. Nilsson T, Jonsoon G. Clinical results with estramustine phosphate (NSC-89199): a comparison of the intravenous and oral preparations. *Cancer Chemother Rep* 1975;59:229.

545. Kirdini RY, Muntzing J, Varkarakis MJ, et al. Studies on the antiprostatic action of Estracyt, a nitrogen mustard of estradiol. *Cancer Res* 1974;34:1025.

546. Lundgren R, Sundin T, Leinstedt E, et al. Cardiovascular complications of estrogen therapy for nondisseminated prostatic carcinoma. *Scand J Urol Nephrol* 1986;20:101.

547. Murphy GP, Slack NH, Mittelman A, et al. Experiences with estramustine phosphate (Estracyt, Emcyt) in prostatic cancer. *Semin Oncol* 1983;10:34.

548. Tew KD, Woodworth A, Stearns ME. Relationship of glutathione depletion and inhibition of glutathione-S-transferase activity to the antimitotic properties of estramustine. *Cancer Treat Rep* 1986;70:715.

549. VanBell SJP, Schalleier D, deWasch G, et al. Broad phase II study of the combination of two microtubular inhibitors: estramustine and vinblastine. *Proc Am Soc Clin Oncol* 1988;7:207(abst).

550. Speicher LA, Barone L, Tew KD. Combined activity of estramustine and Taxol in human prostatic carcinoma cell lines. *Cancer Res* 1992;52:4433.

13

ALKYLATING AGENTS

KENNETH D. TEW
O. MICHAEL COLVIN
BRUCE A. CHABNER

The alkylating agents are antitumor drugs that act through the covalent bonding of alkyl groups (one or more saturated carbon atoms) to cellular molecules. Historically, the alkylating agents have played an important role in the development of cancer chemotherapy. The nitrogen mustards mechlorethamine (HN_2, "nitrogen mustard") and tris(β-chloroethyl)amine (HN_3) were the first nonhormonal agents to show significant antitumor activity in humans.[1–3] The clinical trials of nitrogen mustards in patients with lymphomas evolved from clinical observations of the effects of sulfur mustard gas used in World War I. This compound was found to produce lymphoid aplasia in addition to the expected irritation of the lungs and mucous membranes and was evaluated as an antitumor agent.[4] The related, but less reactive nitrogen mustards, the bischloroethyl-amines (Fig. 13-1), were found to be less toxic and to cause regressions of lymphoid tumors in mice. The first clinical studies produced some dramatic tumor regressions in lymphoma patients, and the antitumor effects were confirmed by an organized multiinstitution study.[1–3] The demonstration of the clinical utility of the nitrogen mustards encouraged further efforts to find chemical agents with antitumor activity, which led to the wide variety of antitumor agents in use today. At present, alkylating agents occupy a central position in cancer chemotherapy, both in conventional combination regimens and in high-dose protocols with bone marrow transplantation. Because of their linear dose-response curve in cell culture experiments, these drugs [particularly the combination of cyclophosphamide, melphalan, and carmustine (bischloroethylnitrosourea, BCNU)] have become the primary tools used in allogeneic transplantation protocols for acute leukemia and in autologous transplantation for lymphomas and breast cancer.

CHEMISTRY

Mechanisms of Alkylating Reactions

Traditionally, alkylating reactions have been classified as S_N1 (nucleophilic substitution, first order, Fig. 13-2) or S_N2 (nucleophilic substitution, second order, Fig. 13-2). In the S_N1 reaction a highly reactive intermediate is initially formed, and then this intermediate reacts rapidly with a nucleophile to produce the alkylated product. In this reaction, the rate-limiting step is the initial formation of the reactive intermediate. Thus the reaction exhibits first-order kinetics with regard to the concentration of the original alkylating agent, and the rate is essentially independent of the concentration of the substrate; hence, the designation S_N1.

The S_N2 alkylation reaction represents a bimolecular nucleophilic displacement. The rate of this reaction is dependent on the concentration of both the alkylating agent and the target nucleophile. Therefore, the reaction follows second-order kinetics. The terms S_N1 and S_N2 are defined kinetically but normally are used in reference to the mechanism of action.

Those compounds that alkylate via a highly reactive intermediate, such as the aliphatic nitrogen mustard mechlorethamine, would be expected to be less selective in their alkylation targets than the less reactive S_N2 reagents, such as the alkyl alkane sulfonate busulfan. No simple relationship exists, however, between the therapeutic or toxic effects of an alkylating agent and its chemical reactivity. The clinically useful agents include drugs that alkylate through an S_N1 mechanism, agents that alkylate through an S_N2 mechanism, and some compounds that alkylate through reactions with characteristics of both an S_N1 and an S_N2 mechanism.[5–7] As a class, the alkylating agents share a common target (DNA) and are cytotoxic, mutagenic, and carcinogenic. The activity of most alkylating agents is enhanced by hyperthermia, by nitroimidazoles, and by glutathione depletion. They differ greatly, however, in their toxicity profiles and antitumor activity. These differences are undoubtedly the result of differences in pharmacokinetic features, lipid solubility, ability to penetrate the central nervous system (CNS), membrane transport properties, detoxification reactions, and specific enzymatic reactions capable of repairing alkylation sites on DNA.[8,8a] For example, the nitrosoureas produce a specific

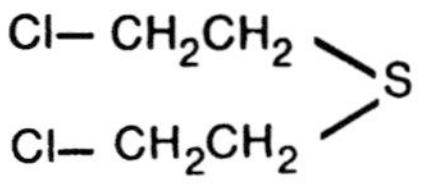

A

Bischloroethylsulfide (sulfur mustard).

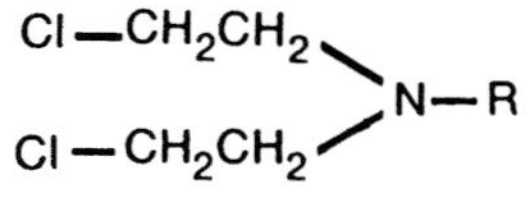

B

Bischloroethylamine (nitrogen mustard general structure). —R = —CH_3 in mechlorethamine. —R = —CH_2CH_2Cl in tris(β-chloroethyl)amine.

FIGURE 13-1. Structures of bischloroethylsulfide and bischloroethylamine. **A:** Bischloroethylsulfide (sulfur mustard). **B:** Bischloroethylamine (nitrogen mustard general structure).

site of alkylation on the O-6 position of guanine; resistance to this group of agents is correlated with the presence of a guanine-O^6-alkyl transferase.[9] Clinically, the nitrosoureas do not share cross-resistance with nitrogen mustard in the treatment of lymphomas. The selectivity of a given alkylating agent obviously depends on a number of other chemical and pharmacologic factors. If the agent is an S_N1 type reacting through an alkylating intermediate with a brief existence, the biologic half-life and membrane-penetrating properties of this intermediate may determine the selectivity. In the complex environment of the cell, especially the nucleus, chemical half-lives of nanoseconds and nanometer distances may be important in determining sites of alkylation. Application of techniques such as magnetic resonance imaging and mass spectrometry to the study of the alkylation mechanism and the chemical nature of the intermediates involved are making possible a detailed understanding of these alkylation reactions.[6,7] Such approaches, coupled with improved techniques of localizing and studying cellular damage[10,11] and determining sites and mechanisms of detoxification,[12–14] should eventually make it possible to predict the sites of alkylation of an agent and to understand and modify the biologic consequences of such alkylations.

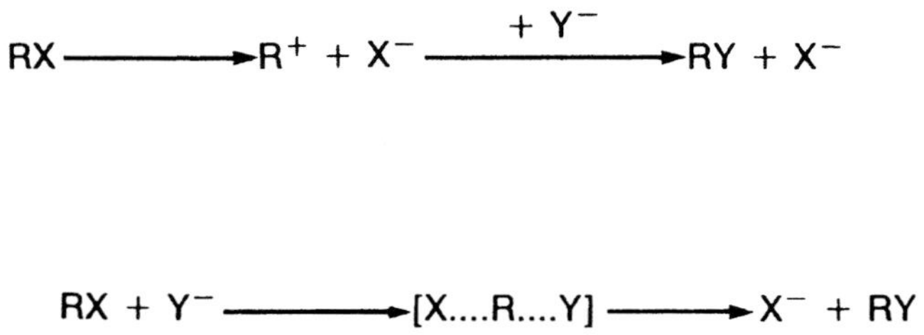

FIGURE 13-2. S_N1 and S_N2 reactions.

Types of Alkylating Agents Used Clinically

The important pharmacologic properties of the clinically useful alkylating agents are summarized in Table 13-1.

Nitrogen Mustards

The most commonly used alkylating agents have been the bischloroethylamines or nitrogen mustards. The first nitrogen mustard to be used extensively in the clinic was mechlorethamine (Fig. 13-1), sometimes referred to by its original code name HN_2 or by the term *nitrogen mustard.* The mechanism of alkylation by the nitrogen mustards is shown in Figure 13-3. In the initial step, chlorine is lost and the β-carbon reacts with the nucleophilic nitrogen atom to form the cyclic, positively charged, and very reactive aziridinium moiety. Reaction of the aziridinium ring with a nucleophile (electron-rich atom) yields the initial alkylated product. Formation of a second aziridinium by the remaining chloroethyl group allows for a second alkylation, which produces a cross-link between the two alkylated nucleophiles.

After introduction of mechlorethamine, a great many analogs were synthesized in which the methyl group was replaced by a variety of chemical groups. Most of these compounds proved to have less antitumor activity than mechlorethamine, but four derivatives seem to have a higher therapeutic index and a broader range of clinical activity and can be administered both orally and intravenously. These drugs, which for the most part have replaced mechlorethamine in clinical use, are melphalan (L-phenylalanine mustard), chlorambucil, cyclophosphamide, and ifosfamide (Fig. 13-4). The latter two agents are unique in requiring metabolic activation and undergo a complex series of activation and degradation reactions (to be described in detail later in this chapter).

As can be seen from the structures, these derivatives have electron-withdrawing groups substituted on the nitrogen atom. This alteration reduces the nucleophilicity of the nitrogen and renders the molecules less reactive. Melphalan and chlorambucil retain alkylating activity and seem to be more tumor selective than nitrogen mustard. Cyclophosphamide and ifosfamide, on the other hand, possess no alkylating activity and must be metabolized to produce alkylating compounds. Cyclophosphamide has been the most widely used alkylating agent and has activity against a variety of tumors.[15] In 1972, ifosfamide,[16] an isomeric analog of cyclophosphamide, was introduced into clinical use. It has greater activity against testicular cancer and soft tissue sarcomas.[17,18] Melphalan has been widely used in the treatment of ovarian cancer,[19] multiple myeloma,[20] and carcinoma of the breast.[21] Chlorambucil has been most

TABLE 13-1. KEY FEATURES OF SELECTED ALKYLATING AGENTS

	Cyclophosphamide	Chlorambucil	Melphalan	BCNU	Busulfan
Mechanism of action:	All agents produce alkylation of DNA through the formation of reactive intermediates that attack nucleophilic sites.				
Mechanisms of resistance:	Increased capacity to repair alkylated lesions, e.g., guanine O^6-alkyl transferase (nitrosoureas, busulfan)				
	Increased expression of glutathione-associated enzymes, including γ-glutamyl cysteine synthetase, γ-glutamyl transpeptidase, and glutathione-S-transferases				
	Increased aldehyde dehydrogenase (cyclosphamide)				
	Decreased expression or mutation of p53				
Dose/schedule (mg/m²):	400–2,000 i.v. 100 p.o. qd	1–3 p.o. qd	8 p.o. qd × 5 d	200 i.v.	2–4 mg daily
Oral bioavailability:	100%	50%	30% (variable)	Not known	50% or greater
Pharmacokinetics: primary elimination $t_{1/2}$ (h)	3–10 (parent) 1.6 (aldophosphamide) 8.7 (phosphoramide mustard)	1.5 (parent) 2.5 (phenylacetic acid)	1.5 (parent)	0.25 to 0.75[a] (nonlinear increase with dose from 170 to 720 mg/m²)	
Metabolism:	Microsomal hydroxylation Hydrolysis to phosphoramide mustard (active) and acrolein Excretion as inactive oxidation products	Chemical decomposition to active phenyl acetic acid mustard and to inert dechlorination products	Chemical decomposition to inert dechlorination products 20–35% excreted unchanged in urine	Chemical decomposition to active and inert products	Enzymatic conjugation with glutathione
Toxicity:					
Myelosuppression	Acute, platelets spared	Acute	Delayed, nadir at 4 wk	Delayed, nadir 4–6 wk	Acute and delayed
Alopecia Pulmonary fibrosis Venoocclusive disease Leukemogenesis Infertility Teratogenesis	Seen with all alkylating agents ⟶				
Other	Cystitis; cardiac toxicity; IADH	—	—	Renal injury	Addisonian syndrome, seizures
Precautions:	Use MESNA with high-dose therapy	—	$t_{1/2}$ prolonged in patients with renal dysfunction	—	Monitor AUC with high-dose therapy
Drug interactions:	Expect increased cytotoxicity with radiation sensitizers, and glutathione depletion		Cimetidine decreases bioavailability by 30%	—	Induces phenytoin (Dilantin) metabolism

AUC, area under the concentration × time curve; BCNU, bischloroethylnitrosourea; IADH, inappropriate antidiuretic hormone syndrome; MESNA, 2-mercaptoethane sulfonate; $t_{1/2}$, half-life.
[a]See reference 276a.

widely used in the treatment of chronic lymphocytic leukemia,[22,23] lymphomas,[22,24] and ovarian carcinoma.[25]

Aziridines

The aziridines are analogs of the putative ring-closed intermediates of the nitrogen mustards but are less reactive chemically. Compounds bearing two or more aziridine groups, such as those shown in Figure 13-5 [thiotepa (triethylenethiophosphoramide),[26,27] triethylenemelamine,[28,29] and trenimon[30]], have shown clinical activity against human tumors. The antitumor activity of these compounds seems to be comparable to that of the nitrogen mustards.

Thiotepa in particular has been used in the treatment of carcinoma of the breast[31] and the ovary[32] and for the intrathecal treatment of meningeal carcinomatosis.[33] At standard dosages, the aziridines have no therapeutic advantage over the nitrogen mustards. Thiotepa is used with increasing frequency as a component of high-dose chemotherapy regimens.

These aziridine compounds were originally tested for antitumor activity because the nitrogen mustards alkylate through an aziridine intermediate. Both thiotepa and its primary desulfurated metabolite TEPA (triethylenephosphoramide) have cytotoxic activity *in vitro*. Although the mechanism of action of these compounds has not been

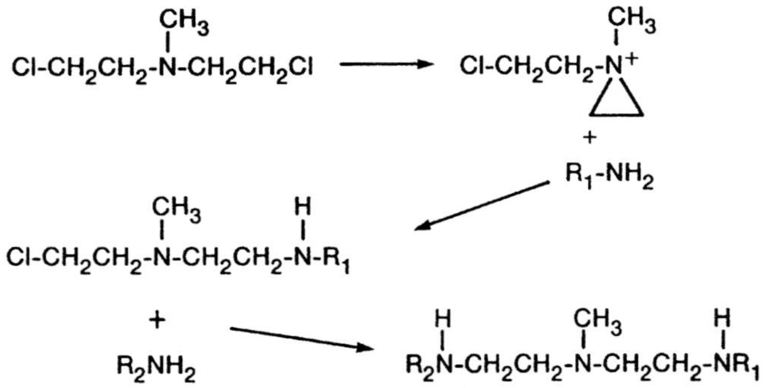

FIGURE 13-3. Alkylation mechanism of nitrogen mustards. (From Colvin M. Molecular pharmacology of alkylating agents. In: Cooke ST, Prestayko AW. *Cancer and chemotherapy*, vol 3. New York: Academic Press, 1981:291.)

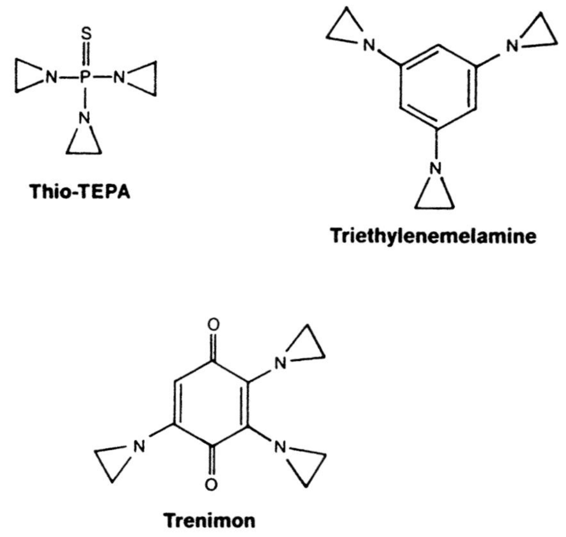

FIGURE 13-5. Aziridine antitumor agents.

explored thoroughly, they presumably alkylate through opening of the aziridine rings, as shown for the nitrogen mustards. The reactivity of the aziridine groups is increased by protonation and thus is enhanced at low pH.

Epoxides

Epoxides, such as dianhydrogalactitol (Fig. 13-6), have antitumor activity against a variety of animal tumors. Dianhydrogalactitol has undergone phase I trials,[34,35] and in phase II trials has shown activity in patients with brain tumors,[36,37] but it is ineffective against other solid tumors.[38–41] A related compound, dibromodulcitol, has modest activity against breast cancer.[42]

The epoxides are chemically similar to the aziridines and presumably alkylate in a similar fashion. Like the aziridines and busulfan, the epoxides exhibit S_N2 alkylation kinetics. In the physiologic pH range the reactivity of the epoxides is less pH dependent than that of the aziridines because the epoxides protonate less readily.

Dihalogenated polyhydroxyl compounds such as dibromodulcitol (Fig. 13-6) spontaneously produce the corresponding diepoxides in aqueous solution, and diepoxides are probably responsible for their antitumor activity.[43–45]

Alkyl Alkane Sulfonates

The major clinical representative of the alkyl alkane sulfonates is busulfan (Fig. 13-7), which is widely used for the treatment of chronic myelogenous leukemia.[46] Its alkylation mechanism is shown in Figure 13-8. Compounds with one to eight methylene units between the sulfonate groups have antitumor activity, but maximal activity is shown by the compound with four methylene units.[47,48]

Busulfan exhibits S_N2 alkylation kinetics. The compound reacts more extensively with thiol groups of amino acids and proteins[49] than do the nitrogen mustards, and these findings have prompted the suggestion that the alkyl alkane sulfonates may exert their cytotoxic activities through such thiol reactions rather than through interactions with DNA.[49,50] Brookes and Lawley[51] were able to demonstrate the reaction of busulfan with the N-7 position of guanosine, but the ability to cross-link DNA is uncertain.[52]

In contrast to the nitrogen mustards and nitrosoureas, busulfan displays a more marked effect on myeloid cells

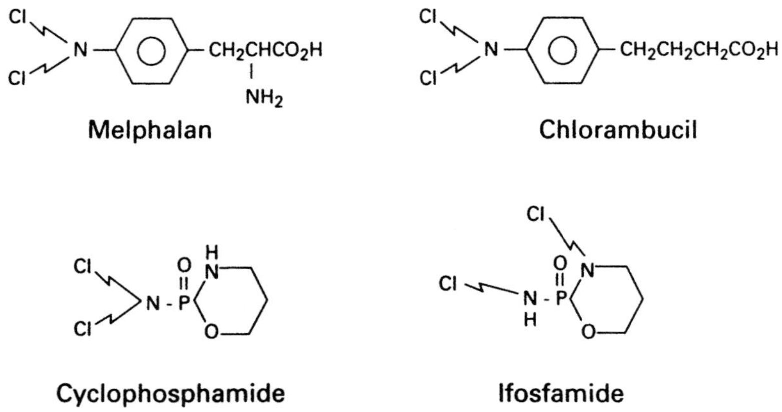

Melphalan

Chlorambucil

Cyclophosphamide

Ifosfamide

FIGURE 13-4. Structures of four analogs of mechlorethamine.

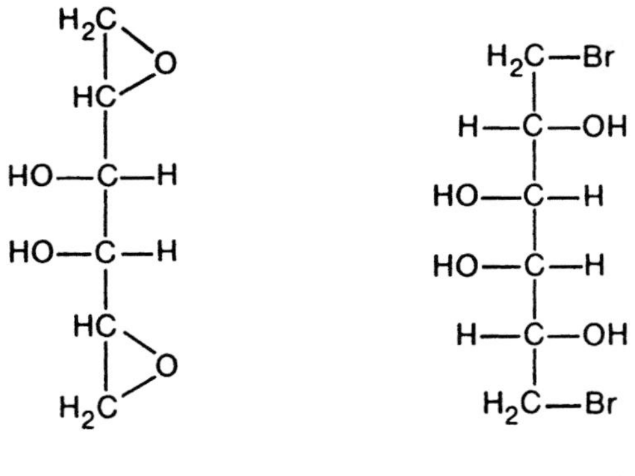

Dianhydrogalactitol   **Dibromodulcitol**

FIGURE 13-6. Structures of epoxides.

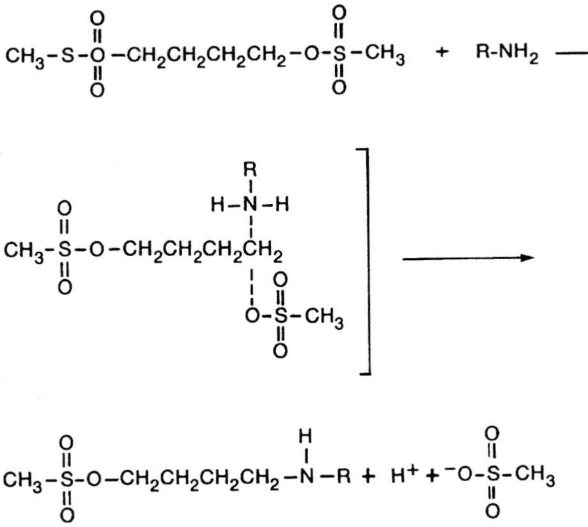

FIGURE 13-8. Alkylation mechanism of alkane sulfonates. (From Colvin M. Molecular pharmacology of alkylating agents. In: Cooke ST, Prestayko AW. *Cancer and chemotherapy*, vol 3. New York: Academic Press, 1981:291.)

than on lymphoid cells.[53] This specificity is manifest clinically in the activity of busulfan against chronic myelogenous leukemia. Busulfan also is markedly cytotoxic to hematopoietic stem cells. This effect is seen clinically in the prolonged aplasia that may follow busulfan administration and can be shown experimentally in stem cell cloning systems.[54] The pharmacologic bases for these properties of busulfan are not understood. Busulfan is used in experimental high-dose protocols, with bone marrow transplantation.[55]

Nitrosoureas

The nitrosourea antitumor agents in current use were developed on the basis of the observations that methylnitrosoguanidine and methylnitrosourea exhibited modest antitumor activity in experimental animal tumor models.[56] Careful structure-function studies have demonstrated that chloroethyl derivatives such as chloroethylnitrosourea and BCNU (Fig. 13-9) possess greater antitumor activity than methylnitrosourea and other alkyl derivatives and that the nitrosourea derivatives are more active than the nitrosoguanidines.[56–58]

These chloroethylnitrosoureas eradicated intracranially inoculated tumors[58] because of their lipophilic character and ability to cross the blood–brain barrier. In its initial trials, BCNU showed significant activity against brain tumors, colon cancer, and the lymphomas.[59,60] Subsequently, cyclohexylchloroethylnitrosourea (CCNU, lomustine) and methylcyclohexylchloroethylnitrosourea (methyl-CCNU, semustine) (Fig. 13-9) had greater activity against solid tumors in experimental animals.[61] Methyl-CCNU has been

used in adjuvant treatment of colon cancer but has no obvious role at present in clinical chemotherapy.[62] Several new nitrosoureas have been tested in patients in Europe and Japan, but none has an established place in standard cancer treatment regimens.[63]

The nitrosoureas show partial cross-resistance with other alkylating agents.[58] A number of studies have confirmed that these drugs are indeed alkylating agents, and the mechanism of the alkylation reaction has been established (Fig. 13-10).

At physiologic pH, proton abstraction by a hydroxyl ion initiates spontaneous decomposition of the molecule to yield an isocyanate compound[64] and a diazonium hydroxide molecule.[65] The chloroethyl diazonium ion or the chloroethyl carbonium ion generated may then alkylate biologic

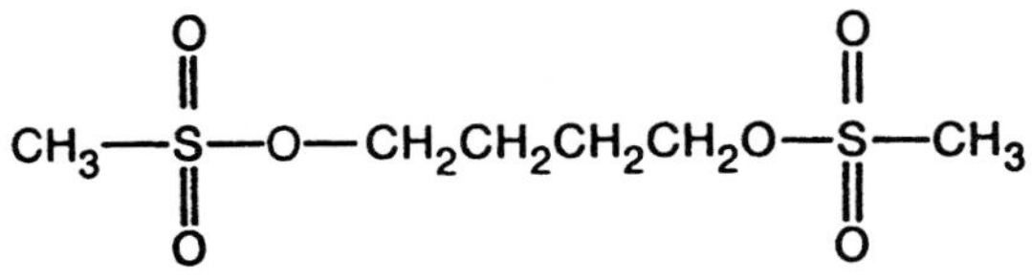

Chloroethylnitrosourea

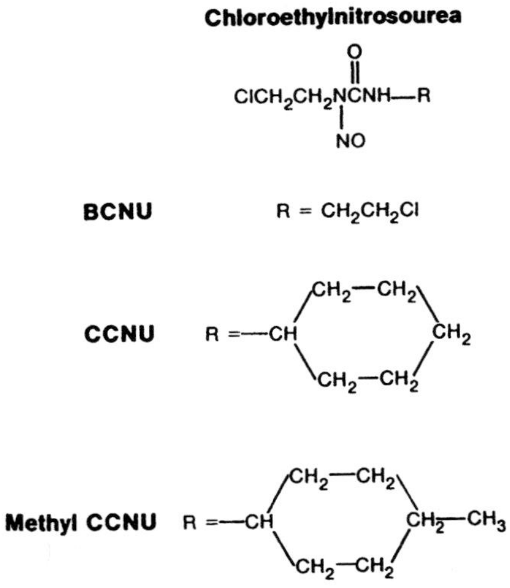

FIGURE 13-9. Structures of nitrosoureas. (BCNU, bischloroethylnitrosourea; CCNU, cyclohexylchloroethylnitrosourea.)

FIGURE 13-7. Structure of busulfan.

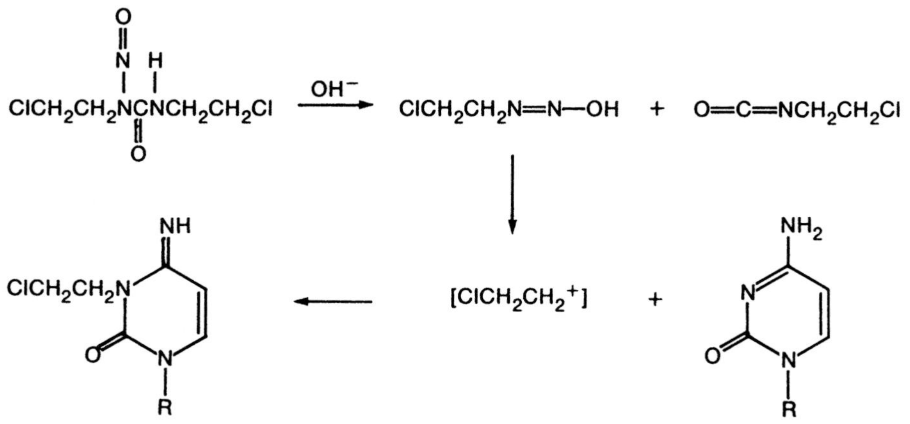

FIGURE 13-10. Alkylation of nucleoside by bischloroethylnitrosourea (BCNU).

molecules. The alkylation of nitrogens in cytidylate and guanylate units in DNA yields chloroethylamino groups on the nucleotide, and these are capable, through a dehalogenation step, of a second alkylation to produce DNA-DNA and DNA-protein cross-links.[66,67]

Isocyanates result from the spontaneous breakdown of many of the methyl- and chloroethylnitrosoureas. These electrophilic species show specificity for the nucleophilic sulfhydryl and amino groups of proteins and can inhibit enzymes such as DNA polymerase,[68] DNA ligase,[69] RNA synthetic and processing enzymes,[70] and glutathione reductase.[71] Both chlorozotocin and streptozotocin (Fig. 13-11) undergo internal carbamoylation[72] at the 1- or 3-OH group of the glucose ring, with the net result that little release of carbamoylating species occurs. Nevertheless, these two agents possess significant antitumor activity, and because of this, carbamoylation is believed to be of only marginal importance to the therapeutic efficacy of clinically used nitrosoureas. A nitrosourea with no alkylating activity, N,N^1 bis(*trans*-4-hydroxycyclohexyl)-N^1-nitrosourea, possesses significant carbamoylating potential and causes cellular damage consistent with an imbalance of cellular thiol-disulfide status.[73] These biochemical effects, together with other preclinical data, suggest that carbamoylation may be responsible for many of the toxicities associated with nitrosourea therapy.[65,74,75]

Streptozotocin (Fig. 13-11), a methylnitrosourea isolated from *Streptomyces,* is remarkable for its potent antileu-

kemic activity in mice,[76] its lack of bone marrow toxicity,[77] and its strong diabetogenic effect in animals.[78] Because of this specific toxicity to pancreatic beta cells, streptozotocin was tested against islet cell carcinoma of the pancreas in humans and showed clinically significant activity.[79,80] The dose-limiting toxicities in humans have been gastrointestinal and renal, and the drug has considerably less hematopoietic toxicity than the other nitrosoureas.

In an effort to increase the antitumor effects of streptozotocin while preserving the bone marrow–sparing effect, chlorozotocin (in which the 1-methyl group has been replaced by a chloroethyl group; see Fig. 13-11) was synthesized and tested.[81,82] This compound and similar nitrosoureas bearing a glucose moiety have reduced bone marrow toxicity in mice[83] but do cause hematopoietic suppression in humans.[84]

Currently, BCNU is only occasionally used in the treatment of lymphomas,[85] lung cancer,[86] colon cancer,[87] and drug-resistant multiple myeloma.[88] As predicted from the animal studies, the nitrosoureas have shown significant activity against brain tumors.[89] When used as an adjuvant to radiation therapy, they enhance survival in patients with grade III and IV astrocytomas.[90] The severe hematopoietic depression (especially thrombocytopenia) produced by these agents is a significant limiting factor in their use. BCNU has been used in high-dose protocols for bone marrow transplantation regimens.[91]

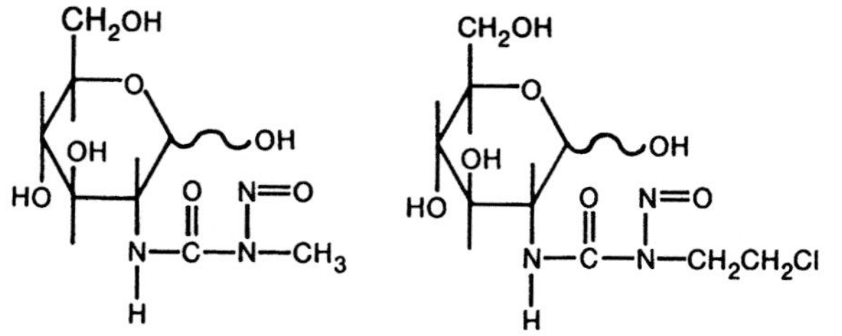

Alkylating Agent–Steroid Conjugates

Under the rationale that steroid receptors may serve to localize and concentrate appended drug species in hormone-responsive cancers, a number of synthetic conjugates of mustards and steroids have been developed. Of these drugs, two have made the transition into clinical application. Prednimustine is an ester–linked conjugate of chlorambucil and prednisolone. Estramustine is a carbamate ester–linked conjugate of nornitrogen mustard and estradiol. The difference in this linkage group is critical to the behavior of the drug, both mechanistically and clinically.

FIGURE 13-11. Structures of streptozotocin and chlorozotocin.

Serum esterases are prevalent and readily cleave the ester link of prednimustine with the ultimate release of the hormone and the active alkylating drug. Therapeutic advantage has been seen to accrue with prednimustine, primarily because of the altered human pharmacokinetics; half-life is prolonged as a consequence of slow hydrolysis of the ester bond.[92] In addition, the elimination phase of chlorambucil in patient plasma was significantly longer after administration of prednimustine than after chlorambucil.[93] Thus prednimustine acts as a prodrug, delivering alkylating components over a prolonged period.

The pharmacology of estramustine is governed by the presence of the carbamate in the steroid-mustard linkage. The presence of this group adds great stability to the parent molecule, with the result that no proton abstraction can occur and no alkylating functionality ensues.[94,95] Both the preclinical and clinical data (dose-limiting toxicities do not include myelosuppression) are consistent with the lack of alkylating activity. Indeed, detailed studies of the mechanism of action have indicated that the drug has antimitotic properties[96] and as such falls outside the scope of this chapter. Pharmacokinetic studies indicate that the parent compound (estramustine phosphate) is hydrolyzed to estramustine and further converted to estradiol and estrone, which raises the possibility of hormonal actions.[96a] The antimicrotubule properties of estramustine have led to its use in combination with other existing antimitotic drugs such as vinblastine sulfate and paclitaxel. The former has produced encouraging results in hormone-refractory prostate cancer either alone or in combination with vinblastine or mitoxantrone hydrochloride.[97-98a] Estramustine binds to the P-glycoprotein that mediates multidrug resistance and in so doing blocks efflux of the natural-product drugs that serve as substrates of the pump.[99] Because of its radiosensitizing properties, it is being tested with radiotherapy for treatment of locally advanced prostate cancer.

Prodrugs of Alkylating Agents

Therapy with alkylating agents is compromised by their high level of toxicity to normal tissues and their lack of tumor selectivity. Efforts to improve selectivity have led to the synthesis of antibody-enzyme conjugates that bind to tumor surface antigens. At the cell surface, the enzymes, which include peptidases or nitro-reductases, cleave circulating alkylating prodrugs, which releases active cytotoxins.[99a] The concept of antibody-directed enzyme prodrug therapy (ADEPT) is illustrated by the use of an antibody linked to the peptidase carboxypeptidase G-2, which liberates an active alkylator from an inactive γ-glutamyl conjugate. The peptidase can be linked to any antibody that localizes selectively to a tumor cell membrane. An alternative is to deliver the carboxypeptidase G-2 gene to tumor cells via a viral vector. Expression of the peptidase on the cell surface then leads to prodrug activation and cell kill.[99b] A third alternative exploits the high level of glutathione-*S*-transferase (GST) *pi*-1 in tumor cells. In this case, the prodrug consists of the alkylating agent conjugated to a glutathione molecule; it is then cleaved by the enzyme, which creates a cytotoxic intracellular species,[99c] as shown in Figure 13-12. In still other experiments, the gene for a cytochrome P-450 isoenzyme is delivered to tumors by a viral vector and enhances tumor cell activation of cyclophosphamide.[99d] An effective *in vivo* strategy for gene delivery to tumors is critical to the success of this approach and has yet to be demonstrated in humans. Many of these new agents have begun testing in humans.

CELLULAR PHARMACOLOGY

Sites of Alkylation

A radioactive alkylating agent, mechlorethamine, administered to an animal covalently binds to a wide variety of biologic molecules,[100] including nucleic acids, proteins, amino acids, and nucleotides. The rates of alkylation of cellular nucleophiles are most dependent on their potential energy states, which can be defined as "hard" or "soft" based on the polarization of their reactive centers.[101] The aziridinium ion is highly polarized and is a hard electrophile (highly positively charged at the electrophilic center). Such ions react most readily with hard nucleophiles, in which the high-energy transition state of the reaction (a potential energy barrier to the reaction) is most favorable. In specific terms, an active alkylating species from a nitrogen mustard demonstrates selectivity for nucleophiles in the following order: (a) oxygens of phosphates, (b) oxygens of bases, (c) amino groups of purines, (d) amino groups of proteins, (e) sulfur atoms of methionine, and (f) thiol groups of cysteinyl residues of glutathione.[102] The least-favored reactions still occur but at slower rates unless they are catalyzed by enzymes such as the GSTs.[12-14] Which of these alkylated molecules represents the critical target responsible for the cytotoxic actions of the agent is difficult to ascertain. The action of these compounds could be due to inactivation of enzymes, depletion of critical amino acids or nucleic acid precursors, damage to nucleic acids, alteration of cell membranes, or a combination of these actions. Because the alkylating agents generally are active at very low doses, the antitumor effect appears unlikely to be due to depletion of low-molecular-weight compounds such as amino acids, unless a particular target is present in very small quantities or specifically localized in tumors. Although these possibilities cannot be definitely eliminated, the cytotoxicity is most likely due to alkylation of DNA. Because one of the consistently observed biochemical effects of alkylating agents at cytotoxic levels is the inhibition of DNA synthesis,[103,104] a

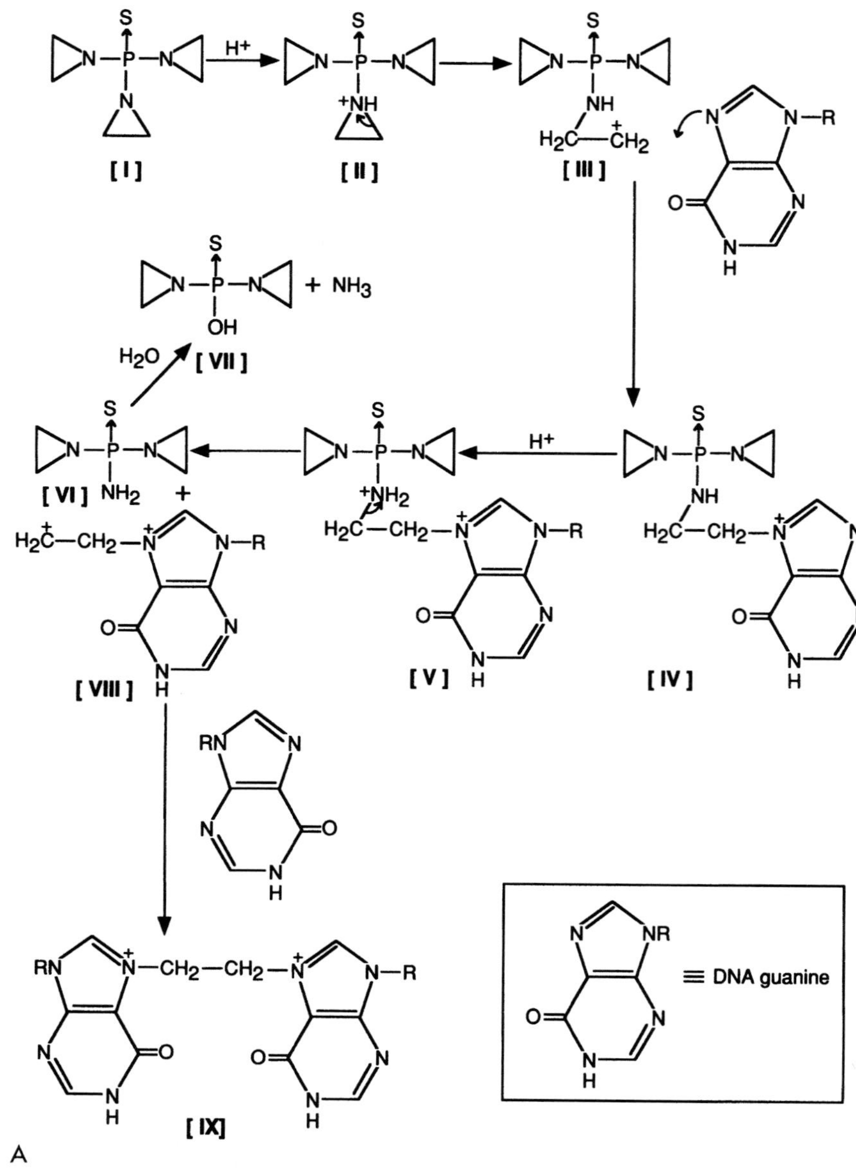

FIGURE 13-12. Alternative mechanisms of cross-linking by thiotepa. **A:** Alkylation and cross-linking by sequential reactions of a single aziridine group. (*continued*)

number of studies have focused on the mechanism of this inhibition. Conflicting reports have appeared, but the evidence favors the hypothesis that the inhibition is due to damage to the nucleic acid template rather than to inactivation of DNA polymerase or other enzymes responsible for DNA synthesis.[105–109]

In the DNA molecule the phosphoryl oxygens of the sugar phosphate backbone are obvious electron-rich targets for alkylation. A number of studies have shown that alkylation of the phosphate groups does occur[110–112] and can result in strand breakages from hydrolysis of the resulting phosphotriesters. Although the biologic significance of the strand breakage due to phosphate alkylation remains uncertain, the process is so slow that it seems unlikely that it is a major determinant of cytotoxicity, even for monofunctional agents.[113]

Extensive studies with carcinogenic alkylating agents such as methyl methane sulfonate have shown that virtually all the oxygen and nitrogen atoms of the purine and pyrimidine bases of DNA can be alkylated to varying degrees. The relative significance to carcinogenesis or cytotoxicity of alkylation of each of these sites remains uncertain. Various reports[114–116] have indicated that alkylation of the O-6 atom and of the extracyclic nitrogen of guanosine may be of particular importance for carcinogenesis.

Studies of the base specificity of alkylation by the chemotherapeutic alkylating agents have been much less extensive. Busulfan and mechlorethamine alkylate the N-7 position of guanosine and guanylic acid. Di(guanin-7-yl) derivatives (two guanine molecules abridged at the N-7 position by an alkylating agent) have been isolated from acid hydrolysates of the reaction mixtures.[51,117]

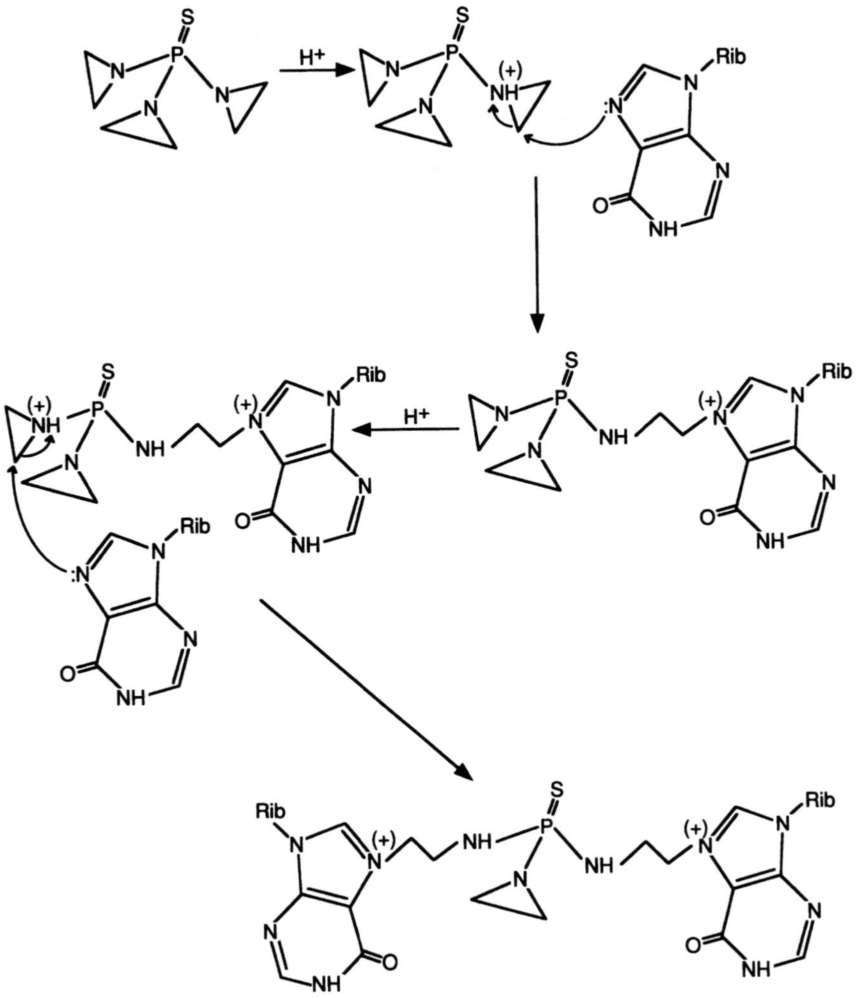

FIGURE 13-12. (*continued*) **B:** Cross-linking produced by sequential alkylating reactions of two aziridine groups from the same parent drug molecule.

B

N,N-Diethyl-2-chloroethylamine hydrochloride, a monofunctional nitrogen mustard, reacts in solution with (in decreasing order of reactivity) the N-7 of guanosine, the N-1 of adenosine, the N-3 of deoxycytidine, and the N-3 of thymidine.[118] Reaction of the nitrogen mustard with native DNA, however, initially produces only N-7–alkylated guanine. After extensive alkylation and denaturation of the DNA has taken place, alkylation of the N-1 of adenosine occurs. The reason for the enhanced alkylation of the N-7 position of deoxyguanosine is uncertain, but it may be due to base stacking and charge transfer that enhance the nucleophilic character of the N-7 position.[119]

Base sequence influences the alkylating reaction. The N-7 position of deoxyguanosine is most electronegative and, therefore, most vulnerable to attack by the aziridinium cation intermediate of the nitrogen mustards when the base is flanked by deoxyguanosines on its 3' and 5' sides. The preferred sites of alkylation may differ among the various alkylating agents. The key site of DNA attack for the nitrosoureas as well as nonclassic methylating agents such as procarbazine and dacarbazine seems to be the O-6

methyl group of guanine[9]; enhanced repair of this site is associated with drug resistance.[120]

DNA Cross-Linking

On the basis of their isolation of the di(guanin-7-yl) products, Brookes and Lawley[119,121] postulated that the bifunctional alkylating agents such as the nitrogen mustards produced interstrand and intrastrand DNA-DNA cross-links and that these cross-links were responsible for the inactivation of the DNA and for the cytotoxicity of the bifunctional alkylating agents. On the basis of the Watson-Crick DNA model, these authors suggested that the appropriate spatial relationship for cross-linking by nitrogen mustards or sulfur mustard between the N-7 positions of deoxyguanylic acid residues in complementary DNA strands occurred in the base sequences shown in Figure 13-13.

The importance of cross-linking is supported by the fact that the bifunctional alkylating agents, with few exceptions, are much more effective antitumor agents than the analogous monofunctional agents, as originally described by

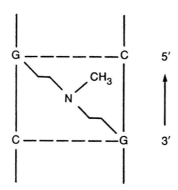

FIGURE 13-13. Cross-linking of DNA by nitrogen mustard. (Modified and reproduced from Brookes P, Lawley PD. The reaction of mono- and di-functional alkylating agents with nucleic acids. *Biochem J* 1961;80:486, with permission.)

Loveless and Ross.[122] Furthermore, increasing the number of alkylating units on the molecule beyond two does not usually increase the antitumor activity of the compound.

Direct evidence that DNA cross-linking occurs as the result of treatment of DNA or cells with bifunctional alkylating agents was provided initially by relatively insensitive physical techniques, including sedimentation velocity studies and denaturation-renaturation studies.[122–127] These techniques, however, could not detect DNA interstrand cross-linking in mammalian cells exposed to therapeutic levels of alkylating agents *in vitro* or in tissues after *in vivo* drug administration. In 1976, a more sensitive assay for DNA interstrand cross-linking in cells, the alkaline elution method,[128] was reported that has the necessary sensitivity to detect DNA cross-linking in cells and tumor-bearing animals exposed to minimal cytotoxic levels of alkylating agents.[10,129,130] These studies, and others using ethidium bromide fluorescence to detect cross-links, have shown that DNA cross-linking by bifunctional alkylating agents correlates with cytotoxicity and that DNA in drug-resistant cells has lower levels of cross-linkage.[131,132] Thus, evidence increasingly supports the hypothesis that DNA interstrand cross-linking is the major mechanism of alkylating agent cytotoxicity.

Work by Ludlum et al.[66] and Kohn[67] suggests that the chloroethylnitrosoureas cross-link via a unique mechanism. The spontaneous decomposition of the chloroethylnitrosoureas generates a chloroethyldiazonium hydroxide entity[65] that can alkylate either the N-3 position of the deoxycytidylic acid residue or the N-7 position of a deoxyguanylic acid residue to produce an alkylating chloroethylamine group on the nucleotide in the DNA strand. This group could then alkylate an adjacent nucleotide (presumably deoxycytidylate or deoxyguanylate) on the complementary DNA strand, producing an interstrand cross-link. Based on considerations of resistance, that is, the role of guanine-O^6-alkyl transferase, alkylation at this site is also probably involved in the DNA cross-links.

The alkaline elution technique also has detected DNA-protein as well as DNA-DNA cross-links,[133] which supports data from previous investigators.[134–136] Ewig and Kohn's work[133] indicates that DNA-protein cross-links do not play a major role in cytotoxicity.

Although DNA-DNA cross-links likely mediate the cytotoxic effects of alkylating agents, the monofunctional DNA alkylations greatly exceed cross-links in number and are potentially cytotoxic. This hypothesis is supported by the fact that certain clinically effective agents, such as procarbazine and dacarbazine, are monofunctional alkylating compounds and do not produce cross-links in experimental systems. The basis of the cytotoxic effects of monofunctional alkylation is probably single-strand DNA breaks. Although apurinic sites in the DNA lead to spontaneous hydrolysis of an adjacent phosphodiester bond, this process is probably too slow to be of biologic significance.[113] Endonucleases produce single-strand breaks at apurinic sites,[137,138] however, and may be responsible for the toxic and therapeutic effects of the monofunctional agents. The presence of apurinic sites may produce cross-links, but the low frequency of these cross-links makes it unlikely that they are responsible for the antitumor activity of the monofunctional agents.[139]

The assumption has usually been that the alkylation of nucleic acids is randomly distributed along the DNA molecule. However, specific regions of the DNA may be selectively susceptible to alkylation. One determinant of regional specificity of DNA alkylations may be chromatin structure[11,140]; areas of active transcription seem to be most vulnerable.

Intranuclear DNA exists in a tight complex with highly basic proteins (histones), other nonhistone proteins, and RNA. This complex, called *chromatin,* has a beaded appearance in electron micrographs and is composed of tightly packed spheres of nucleic acid and protein, called *nucleosomes,* that contain highly active regions for transcription of RNA and more linear intervening regions, called *linker segments.* Characteristic histones and nonhistone proteins are associated with the nucleosome and linker regions and are believed to modify the accessibility of DNA to alkylation and to enzymatic repair of alkylation. The nucleosome, containing the more active region of DNA, is more highly susceptible to alkylation by nitrosoureas and other alkylating agents and is less easily repaired than the linker region. Agents that preferentially alkylate transcriptionally active regions of nucleosomal DNA are thus believed to have greater toxicity for cells.

The glycosylated nitrosourea chlorozotocin, which has somewhat reduced myelotoxicity, has the interesting property of producing greater alkylation of nucleosomal DNA than of linker regions in tumor cells, and the opposite pattern in bone marrow cells.[141] This differential effect on tumor versus normal tissue may account for the improved therapeutic ratio of this new agent in preclinical studies. Lesser myelosuppression also has been observed in phase I and II trials in humans.[84]

Although the significance of this regional specificity is not known, such localization of alkylation might play an important role in the cellular effect of the alkylating agents.

The mechanism of alkylation by thiophosphates such as thiotepa likely begins with protonation of the aziridine N, which leads to ring opening (Fig. 13-12). Cross-linking can proceed by one of several mechanisms, either activation of the free chloroethyl carbon or activation of a second aziridine ring on the original molecule.

In summary, the preponderance of evidence supports the hypothesis that the major factor in the cytotoxicity of most of the clinically effective alkylating agents is interstrand DNA cross-linking, which results in inactivation of the DNA template, cessation of DNA synthesis, and, ultimately cell death. Cell checkpoint proteins, including most prominently p53, are responsible for the recognition of DNA alkylation and strand breaks. Recognition of DNA damage leads to a halt in cell-cycle progression and initiation of programmed cell death. Cells containing mutated p53 are resistant to alkylating agents.[142] The details of alkylating agent interaction with DNA are still being elucidated and may depend on the specific alkylating agent and on the target cell under consideration. As discussed, monofunctional alkylations undoubtedly play a role in cytotoxicity, and the relative roles of cross-links and monofunctional alkylations in the antitumor and toxic effects of the alkylating agents remain to be elucidated. An increased knowledge of alkylation mechanisms and targets may make it possible to improve the therapeutic index of these agents. For example, cross-linking activity seems in many instances to be associated with antitumor effect, whereas monofunctional alkylations are usually associated with general cytotoxicity and carcinogenicity. Thus, if the ratio of cross-links to monofunctional alkylations produced by a drug can be increased, the carcinogenicity of the agent likely will be reduced relative to the antitumor activity.

Cellular Uptake

The uptake of alkylating agents into cells is a potential critical determinant of cellular specificity. The cellular uptake of only a few alkylating agents has been examined, however. Wolpert and Ruddon[143] and Goldenberg and Vanstone[144] demonstrated that the uptake of mechlorethamine by Ehrlich ascites tumor cells and by L5178Y lymphoblasts is by active transport systems. These systems are temperature dependent, accumulate drug against a concentration gradient, and are sensitive to metabolic inhibitors. The natural substrate for the lymphoblast transport system seems to be choline,[145] whose structural resemblance to protonated mechlorethamine (the drug would be protonated at physiologic pH) is shown in Figure 13-14.

Melphalan is transported into several cell types by at least two active transport systems, which also carry leucine and other neutral amino acids across the cell mem-

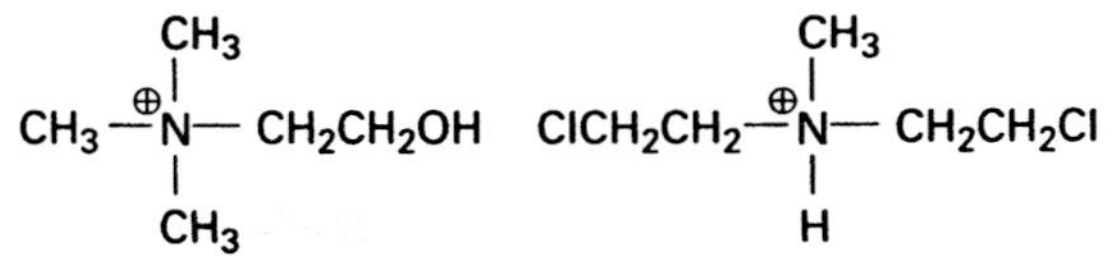

FIGURE 13-14. Structures of choline and mechlorethamine.

brane.[146–148] High levels of leucine in the medium protect cells from the cytotoxic effects of melphalan by competing with melphalan for transport into the target cells.[149] Because appreciable levels of leucine are present in plasma and extracellular fluid, this competition may have pharmacologic significance. Although murine leukemia cells contain at least two transport systems for melphalan and L-leucine, one of these systems is lacking in murine granulocyte precursors (CFU-Cs).[150] This system, missing in CFU-Cs but present in leukemia cells, is identified by its capacity to transport the amino acid analog 2-amino-bicyclo[2,2,]heptane-2-carboxylic acid (BCH). These unexpected findings have prompted a search for cytotoxic analogs of BCH that might be taken up by tumor cells but not by normal granulocyte precursors. In contrast to mechlorethamine and melphalan, which are carried by active transport systems, the highly lipid-soluble nitrosoureas BCNU and CCNU enter cells by passive diffusion.[151]

Tumor Resistance

The emergence of alkylating agent–resistant tumor cells is a major problem that limits the clinical effectiveness of these drugs. One mechanism for drug resistance is that of decreased drug entry into the cell. Numerous studies have shown that L5178Y lymphoblast cells resistant to mechlorethamine may have decreased uptake of the drug.[136,143,152–154] Murine L1210 leukemia cells that are resistant to melphalan have a specific mutation in the lower-affinity, higher-velocity L-transport system, which results in a decreased affinity of the carrier protein for leucine and melphalan.

Among other mechanisms of resistance to alkylating agents, changes in sulfhydryl content have been implicated in experimental tumors. For example, the increased non-protein sulfhydryl content of Yoshida sarcoma cells appears to be responsible for resistance to mechlorethamine.[155] Calcutt and Connors[156] found that tumor cells resistant to alkylating agents possessed a higher ratio of protein-free to protein-bound thiol compounds and suggested that the increased thiol content might function with and inactivate the alkylating agent intracellularly. Increased thiol content of melphalan-resistant ovarian carcinoma cells has been reported,[157] which has led to the experimental use of buthionine sulfoximine, an inhibitor of glutathione synthesis, to reverse resistance to cyclophosphamide, melphalan, and the nitrosoureas in experimental tumors.[158] This reversing agent has entered clinical trials. Although increased intracellular glutathione content may be found in resistant cells, enzymatic detoxification mechanisms that conjugate alkylating intermediates or metabolize them to inactive derivatives have been identified in drug-resistant mutants. Examples of such mechanisms include elevated glutathione transferase levels in mechlorethamine-resistant cells[159] and increased aldehyde dehydrogenase activity, which converts aldophosphamide to its inactive carboxyphosphamide, in cells resistant to cyclophosphamide.[160–162]

Another potential mechanism to explain resistance of cells to alkylating agents is the enhanced repair of the lesions generated by alkylation. Because DNA appears to be the most critical target for the alkylating agents, the repair of DNA has been a major focus of study.[10] Enhanced excision of alkylated nucleotides from DNA appears responsible for the resistance of bacteria to alkylating agents.[124,126] Mammalian cells are capable of such excision repair of sulfur mustard–alkylated nucleotides.[163]

With the exception of guanine-O^6-alkyl transferase in nitrosourea-resistant cells, the specific enzymes responsible for repair of alkylating agent DNA lesions have not yet been identified. Considerable speculation exists, based on analogies to the mammalian heat-shock proteins and the recA DNA repair system in bacteria, that exposure to alkylating agents leads to induction of a series of defensive responses, including decrease in drug-activating enzymes (the P-450 system), increase in glutathione transferase, and increase in DNA repair capacity. This pattern of changes has been most clearly demonstrated in preneoplastic liver nodules after exposure to alkylating carcinogens.[164]

As mentioned previously, cell death after DNA damage is dependent on recognition of that damage by p53, which blocks cell-cycle progression, initiates attempts to repair damage, and ultimately activates apoptotic pathways. Defects in damage recognition or apoptosis may lead to relative resistance.[164a] Probably multiple mechanisms of cellular resistance occur in a given tumor cell population and are responsible for the drug resistance seen clinically. Goldenberg[165] found that L5178Y lymphoma cells resistant to mechlorethamine are 18.5-fold more resistant to mechlorethamine than the wild-type sensitive cells but are uniformly two- to threefold more resistant to a variety of other alkylating agents. On this basis, Goldenberg suggested that specific resistance to mechlorethamine occurred because of decreased transport into the cell, whereas the general cross-resistance was due to other mechanisms, such as enhanced repair capacity. This hypothesis is consistent with the observation of Schabel et al.[166] in experimental animal tumors and with clinical experience. In both situations, varying degrees of cross-resistance between alkylating agents are seen, but a tumor that is resistant to one alkylating agent may remain significantly responsive to another. This finding forms the rational basis for the use of combinations of alkylating agents in high-dose chemotherapy regimens before bone marrow transplantation.[167]

Reversal of Resistance

Drug Modulation

In recent times, much attention has been focused on the discovery and development of drugs that might serve to reverse the resistant phenotype expressed by malignant cells. Because of the plurality of factors that can contribute to the acquired resistant phenotype, a number of distinct (but sometimes overlapping) approaches have been adopted. Because alterations in reduced glutathione (GSH) metabolism have been implicated in resistance to a number of alkylating agents, drugs that modulate GSH-associated enzymes have attracted interest and have met with some degree of preclinical success.

For most alkylating agents, essentially four separate approaches have been adopted: (a) precursors of GSH have been given to replete GSH in normal tissues, thus reducing the host toxicity; (b) specific inhibitors of GSH biosynthetic enzymes have been administered to decrease intracellular GSH; (c) inhibitors of detoxifying enzymes such as GSTs have been given to decrease the tumor cell's ability to protect itself against alkylating metabolites; and (d) other precursor thiols have been administered to protect normal tissues.

Because GSH cannot readily cross cell membranes, early efforts to increase intracellular GSH relied on administration of the constituent amino acids, especially cysteine. More recently, a number of monoesters of GSH have been synthesized that are able to traverse the cell membrane and enhance intracellular GSH.[168] In animal studies, the GSH-monoethyl ester successfully modulated anticancer drugs such as BCNU, cyclophosphamide, and mitomycin C.[169] Primarily, the ester protected liver, lungs, and spleen. At least in the murine system, it afforded no protection to marrow progenitor cells, a major dose-limiting concern to the therapeutic application of GSH repletion.

The obverse approach to repletion is depletion of GSH, in an attempt to gain a therapeutic advantage through specific effects in tumor cells. A number of oxidizing agents, including diethylmaleate, phorone, and dimethylfumarate, have been used and, although successful in achieving tumor cell GSH depletion, have proved to be too toxic to use clinically. The toxicities and complications associated with the use of nonspecific depletors of GSH were circumvented by the design and synthesis of agents that acted as inhibitors of certain enzymes involved in the synthesis of GSH. The direct interference with GSH synthetase results in the buildup of 5-oxoproline, and this has the consequence of marked acidosis in patients.[170] By far the most effective approach to reducing the GSH biosynthetic capacity of a cell has been achieved by administering amino acid sulfoximines,[171,172] which inhibit γ-glutamylcysteine synthetase. The lead compound to emerge from these studies was L-buthionine (*SR*)-sulfoximine (BSO), the *R*-stereoisomer of which is the active inhibitor of γ-glutamylcysteine synthetase.[173] A large number of reports now detail low levels of GSH in tumor cells, which perhaps reflects an increased requirement for the thiol in these malignant tissues. That a drug such as BSO would have an impact on the cytotoxic efficacy of existing anticancer drugs seems reasonable. Therefore, even though treatment of tumor-bearing animals with BSO would be expected to affect the GSH status of both tumor and normal tissues, the possibility of therapeutic advantage remains feasible. This concept gained credibility by the observation that in certain animal models BSO caused differential sensitization of tumor. Bone marrow cells appeared to be less affected by combinations of melphalan and BSO than was a syngeneic tumor.[174] In a phase I trial of BSO (maximum tolerated dose, 1,500 mg per m^2 every 12 hours for six doses), first alone and then in subsequent cycles with melphalan,[175] the only side effect of note was a single instance of hepatotoxicity, which was probably related to the concomitant use of the antibiotic norfloxacin. This indicates the need for caution in the use of BSO with medications that produce hepatotoxic electrophiles, such as acetaminophen. In patients who had biochemical evidence of glutathione depletion in peripheral blood mononuclear cells, melphalan cycles produced severe neutropenia. Five of eight patients had greater than 80% depletion of white blood cell GSH 72 to 96 hours after initiation of BSO therapy, with full recovery of GSH by 48 hours after drug administration. In two of four patients tested, tumor cells in ascitic fluid had greater than 80% GSH depletion. Thus BSO, at the dosages tested, produced GSH depletion in both normal and malignant tissues in about half of patients without serious side effects other than myelosuppression. In future studies, determining if GSH depletion correlates with pharmacologic effect in normal and malignant tissues will be critical. In addition, the precise scheduling of BSO doses, as well as alkylating agent treatment, will depend on documenting the degree and time course of GSH depletion. By relating the pharmacokinetics of BSO to its effects on tissue stores of GSH, one may be able to individualize treatment schedules based on BSO pharmacokinetics. Experiences with phase I and II evaluation of BSO efficacy have been summarized in a review by Bailey.

An alternative approach to depleting GSH is to inhibit the enzymes that use GSH as a cofactor. Because GST overexpression was determined to be at least one contributing mechanism to the alkylating agent–resistant phenotype, a rationale was established for the use of GST inhibitors as modulating agents. The plant phenolic acid ethacrynic acid (EA) is the first such inhibitor to be developed to the stage of clinical trial. One of the pragmatic reasons that focused the early efforts on EA was that the drug had already been studied extensively as a diuretic and had already gained U.S. Food and Drug Administration approval.

EA conjugates to GSH through a nucleophilic attack at the drug's α,β-unsaturated ketone by a mechanism similar to that described for acrolein. The Michael addition chemistry that governs the thioether formation is just one of the possible mechanisms by which EA inhibits GST; however, it is the most important. Although this reaction can occur spontaneously, it also can be catalyzed by all three major classes of GSTs,[176] particularly the π isozyme.

Preclinical studies initially demonstrated that EA was effective at sensitizing a Walker 256 rat breast carcinoma and HT29 human colon cancer cell line to chlorambucil[177] and improved the efficacy of alkylating agent treatment of the HT29 xenograft in nude mice.[178] An overall assessment of the preclinical data positively influenced the decision to take EA into clinical trial.

To determine the dose-limiting toxicities in humans, a phase I trial was carried out using EA in combination with thiotepa. Twenty-seven patients with a variety of advanced neoplasms were treated with 52 courses.[179] The major toxicity of EA was diuresis (which was observed at every dose level). Severe metabolic abnormalities occurred at 75 mg per m^2. At 50 mg per m^2, the diuretic effects were manageable. Myelosuppression was the most important effect of the combination. Two of seven courses of EA, 50 mg per m^2, and thiotepa, 55 mg per m^2, were associated with grade 3 or 4 neutropenia or thrombocytopenia or both. Glutathione transferase activity in the white blood cells decreased to a mean nadir of 37% of control after EA administration, with recovery by 6 hours. Chronic lymphocytic leukemia was chosen for phase II studies of this combination on the basis of the observation that, in chronic lymphocytic leukemia lymphocytes, GST activity was twofold higher in cells from chlorambucil-resistant patients than in chronic lymphocytic leukemia cells from untreated patients and in lymphocytes from normal individuals.[180]

Quite a different approach to modulation of alkylator toxicity was suggested in studies by the United States Army, which examined over 4,000 synthetic thiol derivatives as radioprotectors.[181] From these, researchers selected WR2721, 5-2-(3-aminopropylamino)-ethylphosphorothioic acid, the dephosphorylation of which yields the active thiol WR1065, a molecule with structural homology similar to GSH. The major advantage of the phosphorothioate is its apparent selective uptake in normal tissues and a lack of protection for malignant tissues. The WR compounds only weakly reverse DNA-platinum adducts and weakly bind to cisplatin in solution.[182] Although the reason for the high therapeutic index is not clear, one hypothesis is that normal tissues, because of their greater alkaline phosphatase activity, preferentially activate the prodrug by dephosphorylation, which produces higher localized concentrations of WR1065.[183] By forming conjugates with alkylating electrophiles and protecting normal tissues, WR2721 enhances the dose-modifying factor of cisplatin, melphalan, cyclophosphamide, nitrogen mustard, BCNU, and 5-fluorouracil.[184] Clinical trials of WR2721 have focused on regimens containing cyclophosphamide and cisplatin.

These trials, as well as the clinical pharmacology and use of WR2721 for radioprotection, are reviewed in detail in Chapter 25. The results to date indicate that WR2721, given as a single dose at 740 mg per m^2 before 1,500 mg per m^2 of cyclophosphamide, does afford protection from granulocytopenia, decreasing the duration and increasing the nadir granulocyte count.[185] More recent studies suggest that WR2721 decreases myelosuppression, neurotoxicity, and nephrotoxicity of the cisplatin-cyclophosphamide combination without compromising the antitumor effect. Hospers et al. have reviewed the ongoing clinical trials with WR2721 and alkylating agents.[186]

Nitrosourea Modulation

A modulatory approach specific for nitrosoureas has resulted from studies of DNA repair. In the 1960s, evidence suggested that nitrosoureas had curative potential in many murine tumors.[187] The lack of success of these same agents in managing human neoplasms led to the uncovering of a mammalian alkyltransferase (AGT) specific for the "repair" of alkylated guanines. AGT binds irreversibly to O^6-guanine alkyl adducts and removes them from DNA, inactivating itself in the process. This enzyme was expressed (Mer+) at high levels (more than 200 molecules per cell) in most human tumors but was relatively deficient (Mer-) in murine tumors.[188] The human enzyme has 208 amino acids, with a cysteine-containing conserved sequence responsible for the thiol exchange reaction with the drug-induced alkyl group.[189] Because the DNA repair reactions generally involve multiple steps including excision and synthesis, AGT catalysis does not directly qualify as a complete repair function in itself but may be rate limiting in the process. Relatively nontoxic agents thus could deplete AGT and enhance the therapeutic utility of nitrosoureas.

Initially, streptozotocin as a methylating nitrosourea was combined with BCNU. Methylating nitrosoureas, because of their inability to cross-link DNA, are generally at least one log unit less cytotoxic than chloroethylnitrosoureas. The methylation of guanine at the O-6 position by streptozotocin, however, served to irreversibly consume and inactivate AGT, and a maximal increase in antitumor effect was observed when streptozotocin was given 1 hour before BCNU.[190]

Methylated oligonucleotides that interact directly with AGT were then tested for their potential to enhance chloroethylnitrosoureas. O^6-methylguanine is itself an effective inhibitor.[191,192] Although a high degree of variability was seen in the extent of enzyme inhibition, the base analog did not become incorporated into DNA,[191–193] a factor of some significance with regard to potential mutagenicity and car-

cinogenicity of these alkylated bases. The interaction of AGT with O^6-methylguanine is stoichiometric, time dependent, and irreversible. The first-order rate constant for the reaction is so slow as to make accurate calculation difficult, but it has been estimated to be 10^7 to 10^8 times slower than the reaction with O^6-methyl adduct in double-stranded DNA.[194] Presumably, this reflects certain steric substrate requirements for maximal enzyme activity.

In cultured human leukemic cells, O^6-methylguanine at a concentration of 0.5 mmol per L induced a threefold increase in sensitivity to both methyl- and chloroethylnitrosoureas.[195] Addition of the base analog either before or after treatment with the nitrosourea enhanced sensitivity, which suggests that inhibiting the regeneration of the AGT after the initial depletion was valuable.

The relative success of O^6-methylguanine in modulating AGT activity led to the screening of a number of modified bases as potential inhibitors of the enzyme. The specific utility of O^6-methylguanine is hampered by its low solubility in water and its corresponding low potency in animals.[196] A comparison of the chemical reactions of methyl and benzyl groups indicated that the latter were more readily displaced in bimolecular displacement reactions.[197] This would seem to be in conflict with the inverse correlation between the rate of repair of alkylated bases and the size of the alkyl side chain. For example, branched-chain derivatives such as O^6-isobutylguanine are known to react very slowly with AGT.[198] The bulkiness of the side chain interferes sterically with the reactive center of the incoming nucleophile, which for AGT is the activated thiol of the electron-donating cysteine. In the case of the benzyl derivative, however, the steric hindrance of the benzene ring is considerably offset by the propensity of the benzene ring to delocalize the charge in the transition state for a displacement reaction. For these reasons, the usual order of reactivity for the alkylation displacement reactions is benzyl > methyl > *n*-propyl > isobutyl,[197] and this corresponds to the reactivity of these alkyl species with AGT. At 50 μmol per L, O^6-benzylguanine produced more than 90% inhibition of AGT within 20 minutes of incubation with human colon carcinoma cells. This compared with 80% inhibition by 200 μmol per L O^6-methylguanine.[199] Nitrogen mustards and platinum agents that produce only limited damage at the O-6 position of guanine were unaffected by the concomitant administration of O^6-benzylguanine. Of some clinical significance, a number of Mer+ brain tumor cell lines were sensitized to nitrosoureas used in the therapeutic management of the disease. The enhancement ratios reported for O^6-benzylguanine were equivalent or superior to those found for other modulating agents. Thus the *in vitro* observations supported the continued development of O^6-benzylguanine, as did clinical evidence that response to nitrosoureas and methylating agents is inversely related to the tumor level of AGT.[199a] Phase I trials of O^6-benzylguanine have been completed[199b,199c] and reveal the following: (a) the optimal dose of O^6-benzylguanine, as determined by AGT depletion in human tumors *in vivo*, is 120 mg per m²; (b) the well-tolerated dose of BCNU in combination with the modifier is 40 mg per m², much below the standard dose of BCNU of 120 to 200 mg per m²; (c) surrogate measurements of AGT depletion in peripheral white blood cells do not reflect the depletion in tumors, which are more resistant than normal tissues to AGT depletion; and (d) O^6-benzylguanine is rapidly metabolized to O^6-benzyl 8-oxo-guanine, an equipotent inhibitor with a longer half-life than the parent.[199d] Further trials in Japan have revealed a benzylguanine-resistant polymorphism of AGT in 10% to 15% of the Japanese population but not in whites.[199e] In an interesting segue from these studies, Gerson et al. have proposed that benzylguanine-resistant variants of AGT could be transfected into normal hematopoietic stem cells to protect the host and allow dose escalation of O^6-benzylguanine–alkylating agent combinations.[199f]

CLINICAL PHARMACOLOGY

The primary characteristics of the clinical pharmacokinetics of standard alkylating agents are given in Table 13-1. Although some agents are too reactive chemically to provide more than momentary exposure of tumor cells to parent drug, the best examples being mechlorethamine and BCNU, others are stable in their parent form and require metabolic activation, as in the case of cyclophosphamide and ifosfamide. The clinician must possess a working knowledge of the chemical and metabolic fate of individual alkylating agents to adjust doses for organ dysfunction and to plan rational regimens for organ perfusion or intracavitary instillation.

Activation, Decomposition, and Metabolism

Decomposition versus Metabolism

A principal route of degradation of most of the reactive alkylating agents is spontaneous hydrolysis of the alkylating entity (i.e., alkylation by water).[200–210] For example, mechlorethamine rapidly undergoes reaction to produce 2-hydroxyethyl-2-chloroethylmethylamine (Fig. 13-15A) and bis-2-hydroxyethylmethylamine (Fig. 13-15B).[200] Likewise, both melphalan and chlorambucil undergo similar hydrolysis to form the monohydroxyethyl and bishydroxyethyl products, although less rapidly than the aliphatic nitrogen mustards.[201,202]

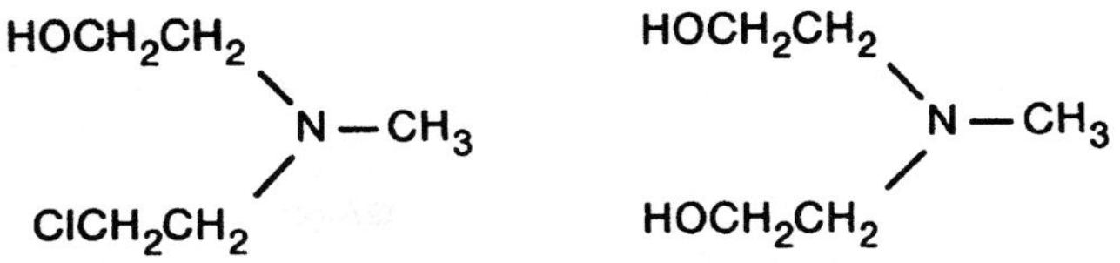

FIGURE 13-15. Hydrolysis products of mechlorethamine.

Most alkylating agents also undergo some degree of enzymatic metabolism. For example, if mechlorethamine radiolabeled in the methyl group is administered to mice, approximately 15% of the radioactivity can be recovered as exhaled carbon dioxide, which indicates that enzymatic demethylation is occurring. A major route of metabolism of chlorambucil is oxidation of the butyric acid side chain to produce phenylacetic acid mustard (Fig. 13-16).[203–205] Phenylacetic acid mustard undergoes hydrolysis to produce the mono- and bishydroxyethyl products. Melphalan is similarly converted to mono- and dihydroxy metabolites. Its monohydroxy metabolite has one-twentieth the activity of the parent compound.

Cyclophosphamide and Ifosfamide

The widely used drugs cyclophosphamide and ifosfamide are activated to alkylating and cytotoxic metabolites by the mixed-function oxidases in hepatic microsomes.[206–209] The complex metabolic transformations that cyclophosphamide undergoes are illustrated in Figure 13-17.[210,211] The initial metabolic step is the oxidation of the ring carbon adjacent to the ring nitrogen to produce 4-hydroxycyclophosphamide. The latter is a hemiaminal, which spontaneously ring-opens and establishes an equilibrium with the amino aldehyde aldophosphamide.

The 4-hydroxycyclophosphamide and aldophosphamide may be oxidized by soluble enzymes to produce 4-ketocyclophosphamide and carboxyphosphamide, respectively. These compounds have little cytotoxic activity and represent inactivated urinary excretion products. They account between them for approximately 80% of a dose of administered cyclophosphamide.[212,213]

The aldophosphamide that has escaped enzymatic oxidation by aldehyde dehydrogenase can enter tumor cells and eliminate acrolein to produce phosphoramide mustard,[214] an active alkylating agent that appears to be responsible for the biologic effects of cyclophosphamide.[215,216]

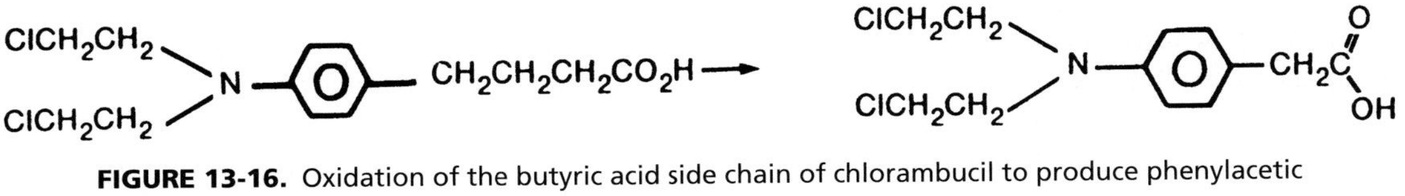

FIGURE 13-16. Oxidation of the butyric acid side chain of chlorambucil to produce phenylacetic acid mustard.

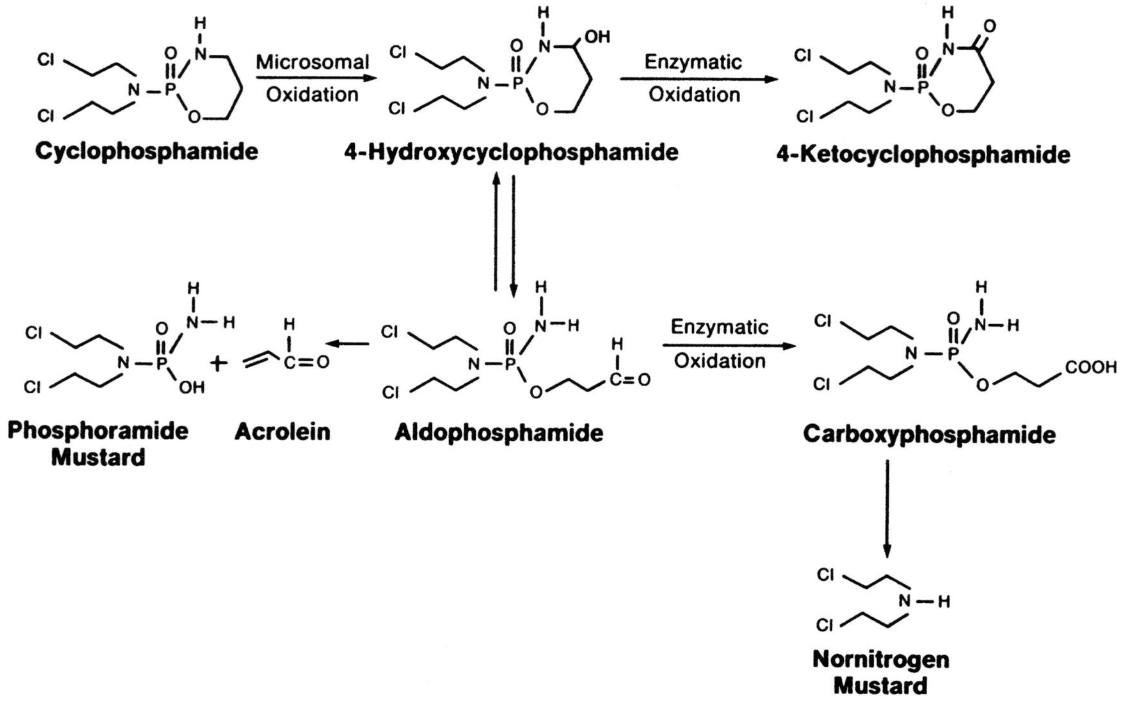

FIGURE 13-17. Metabolism of cyclophosphamide.

The 4-hydroxycyclophosphamide/aldophosphamide is cytotoxic both *in vitro* and *in vivo* but is not an alkylating agent. This compound seems to serve as a transport form to deliver the highly polar phosphoramide mustard efficiently into cells, because 4-hydroxycyclophosphamide is one-fourth to one-tenth as potent as phosphoramide mustard.[216] Furthermore, the amount of DNA cross-linking produced by the two compounds corresponds to their relative cytotoxic potency, and cytotoxicity from the two compounds correlates with similar degrees and types of DNA cross-linking.[217] The high therapeutic index, selectivity of action, and other unique properties of cyclophosphamide are most likely attributable to the properties of 4-hydroxy-cyclophosphamide/aldophosphamide, but circulating phosphoramide mustard may play a significant role in the effects of the drug.[210] 4-Hydroperoxycyclophosphamide, a chemically stable form of 4-hydroxycyclophosphamide, has been used for selective purging of tumor cells from bone marrow and has a cytotoxicity for these cells that is 3 to 4 log units greater than that for myeloid precursor cells.[218]

A related oxazaphosphorine, ifosfamide (Fig. 13-4), requires hepatic P-450 mixed-function oxidase for activation to its active intermediates, which are found in plasma and urine.[219] Like cyclophosphamide, it undergoes hepatic activation to an aldehyde form that decomposes in plasma and peripheral tissues to yield acrolein and its alkylating metabolite.[220] Hydroxylation proceeds at a slower rate for ifosfamide than for cyclophosphamide, which results in a longer plasma half-life for the parent compound. Dechloro-

ethylation of ifosfamide produces inactive metabolites and competes with the activation step as a major pathway of elimination.[221] Both cyclophosphamide (above doses of 4 g per m^2) and ifosfamide (above doses of 5 g per m^2) exhibit dose-dependent nonlinear pharmacokinetics, with significant delays in elimination at higher doses.[222]

Nitrosoureas

The base-catalyzed decomposition of nitrosoureas to generate the alkylating chloroethyldiazonium hydroxide entity[65] has been mentioned, and the products generated by this decomposition in aqueous solution are illustrated in Figure 13-18. The nitrosoureas also undergo metabolic transformation. Hill et al.[223] demonstrated that BCNU is enzymatically denitrosated by hepatic microsomes, a finding of possible clinical significance.[224] Enhancement of microsomal activity in vivo by phenobarbital abolished the therapeutic effect of BCNU against the 9L intracerebral rat tumor and decreased the therapeutic activity of CCNU and BCNU against this tumor. The phenobarbital-treated rats had increased plasma clearance of BCNU, with lower plasma levels and lower area under the concentration × time curve (AUC) plasma values of BCNU. CCNU and methyl-CCNU undergo hydroxylation of their cyclohexyl ring to produce a series of metabolites that represent the major circulating species after treatment with these drugs.[225,226] These metabolites have increased alkylating activity but diminished carbamoylating effects.[227,228] The

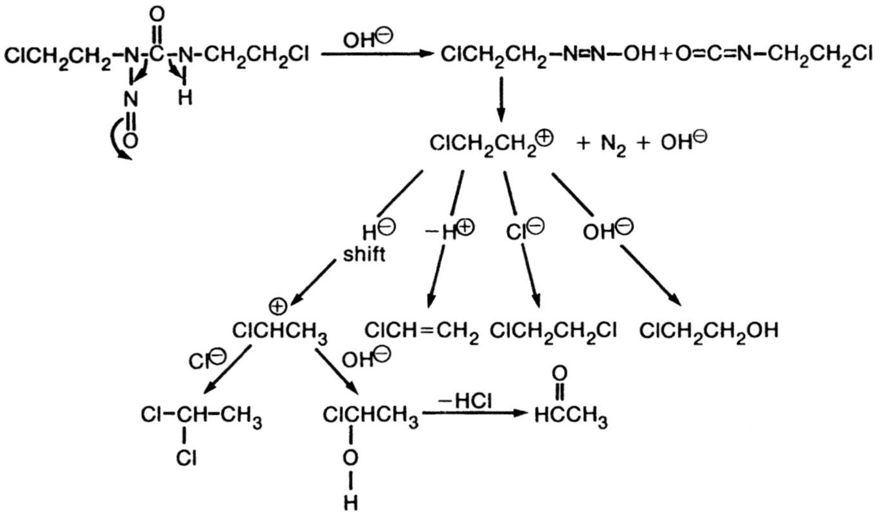

FIGURE 13-18. Decomposition of bischloroethylnitrosourea (BCNU) in buffered aqueous solution.

plasma clearance of parent BCNU decreases and the plasma half-life increases as doses escalate from standard-dose (225 mg per m²) to high-dose regimens (720 mg per m²) (Table 13-1).

Clinical Pharmacokinetics

Because of the lack of definitive techniques for measuring specific drug and metabolite molecules, the data on the clinical pharmacology of the alkylating agents have been relatively limited. Recently, however, gas chromatography–mass spectrometry and high-pressure liquid chromatography (HPLC) have generated more definitive pharmacokinetic information (Table 13-1).

Melphalan

The clinical pharmacology of melphalan has been examined by several groups. Alberts and colleagues[229] studied the pharmacokinetics of melphalan in patients who received 0.6 mg of the drug per kg intravenously. The peak levels of melphalan, as measured by HPLC, were 4.5 to 13 µmol per L (1.4 to 4.1 µg per mL), and the mean terminal-phase half-life ($t_{1/2\beta}$) of the drug in the plasma was 1.8 hours. The 24-hour urinary excretion of the parent drug averaged 13% of the administered dose. Inactive mono- and dihydroxy metabolites appear in plasma within minutes of drug administration.

Other studies have demonstrated low and variable systemic availability of the drug after oral dosing.[202,230] Food slows its absorption. After oral administration of melphalan, 0.6 mg per kg, much lower peak levels of drug of approximately 1 µmol per L (0.3 µg per mL) were seen. The time to achieve peak plasma levels varied considerably and occurred as late as 6 hours after dosing. The low bioavailability was due to incomplete absorption of the drug from the gastrointestinal tract, because 20% to 50% of an

oral dose could be recovered in the feces.[230] No drug or drug products were found in the feces after intravenous administration. Not only does oral melphalan show unpredictable bioavailability, but its AUC is reduced one-third by concomitant administration of cimetidine.[231]

After conventional oral doses of 0.15 to 0.25 mg per kg,[232] peak plasma levels of 0.16 to 0.625 µmol per L (50 to 190 ng per mL) occurred 0.7 to 2.3 hours after drug administration. The same plasma levels were found after the initial dose of drug and after the second dose in a 5-day schedule, which indicates that no accumulation of the drug in plasma occurs with daily administration. In this study the magnitude and time of peak plasma levels appear to be more consistent than was seen using higher doses as reported by Alberts et al.[229] Cornwell and colleagues[233] pointed out that, among patients receiving intravenous melphalan, the incidence of severe myelosuppression is increased in those with a blood urea nitrogen level greater than 30 mg per dL, which suggests that these patients have altered drug excretion. The half-life of melphalan in plasma is significantly prolonged in anephric dogs.[234] Thus, as an approximation, intravenous doses of this agent should be reduced by 50% in patients with an elevated blood urea nitrogen level.

The drug has been administered experimentally by intraperitoneal instillation, and this route yields a gradient of 100:1 between peritoneal fluid and plasma.[235] This form of therapy is potentially useful for the treatment of ovarian cancer. The drug also has proven effective for treatment of in-transit limb metastases of malignant melanoma; in these studies it was administered with hyperthermia and tumor necrosis factor via isolated limb perfusion.[235a]

Chlorambucil

After the oral administration of 0.6 mg per kg of chlorambucil,[202,203] peak levels of 2.0 to 6.3 µmol per L (0.6 to 1.9

µg per mL) occurred within 1 hour. Peak plasma levels of phenylacetic acid mustard, an alkylating metabolite of uncertain but potential importance, ranged from 1.8 to 4.3 µmol per L (0.5 to 1.18 µg per mL), and the peak levels of this metabolite were achieved 2 to 4 hours after dosing. The terminal-phase half-lives for chlorambucil and phenylacetic acid mustard were 92 and 145 minutes, respectively. Less than 1% of the administered dose of chlorambucil was excreted in the urine as either chlorambucil (0.54%) or as phenylacetic acid mustard (0.25%). Approximately 50% of the radioactivity from carbon 14–labeled chlorambucil administered orally was excreted in the urine in 24 hours. Of this material, over 90% appeared to be the monohydroxy and dihydroxy hydrolysis products of chlorambucil and phenylacetic acid mustard. Thus, orally administered chlorambucil is absorbed more completely and more rapidly than melphalan and has a similar terminal-phase half-life.

Cyclophosphamide

The study of the clinical pharmacology of cyclophosphamide has been complicated by the inactivity of the parent compound and by the complex array of metabolites. These metabolites have proved difficult to isolate and measure, and their properties are not yet completely established. The pharmacokinetics and bioavailability of the parent compound have been well established by a number of studies[236–243] (Table 13-2).

Cyclophosphamide seems to be reasonably well absorbed after oral administration to humans. D'Incalci et al.[236] found the systemic availability of the unchanged drug after oral administration of 100-mg doses (1 to 2 mg per kg) to be 97% of that after intravenous injection of the same dose. Juma and colleagues[237] found the systemic availability of the drug to be somewhat less and more variable (mean 74%, range 34% to 90%) after oral administration of larger doses of 300 mg (3 to 6 mg per kg). A more recent comparison of oral versus intravenous cyclophosphamide

in the same patient revealed no difference in the AUC for the primary cytotoxic metabolites, hydroxycyclophosphamide and phosphoramide mustard, after drug administration by the two different routes.[243] After intravenous administration, the peak plasma levels of the parent compound are dose dependent, with peak levels of 4, 50, and 500 nmol per mL reported after the administration of 1 to 2,[236] 6 to 15,[237] and 60 mg per kg,[238] respectively. The terminal-phase half-life of cyclophosphamide varies considerably among patients, with a range of 3 to 10 hours reported by a number of authors. In patients less than 19 years of age, the primary half-life for cyclophosphamide is 1.5 hours.[242] No significant change is seen in cyclophosphamide clearance rates in successive cycles of therapy,[239] although Moore et al.[240] observed a doubling of clearance rates on the second day of a 2-day course of high-dose cyclophosphamide. Less than 15% of the parent drug is eliminated in the urine; the major site of clearance is the liver. A strategy for estimation of the AUC of cyclophosphamide, based on plasma sampling at 1, 4, and 24 hours, should prove useful in examining the relationships between pharmacokinetics, organ function, and toxicity, which are poorly understood.[241]

The pharmacokinetics of the metabolites has been clarified in recent years. Initial measurements of total plasma alkylating activity showed considerable variation across patients, but similar ranges of alkylating activity of the equivalent of 10 to 80 nmol of nitrogen mustard per mL after doses of 40 to 60 mg of cyclophosphamide per kg have been found by several investigators.[237,244,245] Peak alkylating levels are achieved 2 to 3 hours after drug administration, and Juma et al.[237] found the terminal half-life of plasma alkylating activity to be 7.7 hours. All investigators have noted a plateau-like level of plasma alkylating activity maintained for at least 6 hours.

The predominant metabolites found in plasma are nornitrogen mustard and phosphoramide mustard, with lesser concentrations of the putative transport forms aldophosphamide and 4-hydroxycyclophosphamide (Table 13-2).

TABLE 13-2. CLINICAL PHARMACOKINETICS OF CYCLOPHOSPHAMIDE AND METABOLITES

Subject of Study	Cyclophosphamide Dose (mg/kg)	Peak Plasma Concentration, (µmol/L)	Plasma $t_{1/2}$ (h)	References
Cyclophosphamide	1–2	4	—	236
	6–15	50	3–10	237
	60	500	—	238
Total alkylating activity	40–60	10–80	7.7	237, 244, 245
Phosphoramide mustard	60–75	50–100	—	238
	4–12	3–18	8.7	247
Nornitrogen mustard	60–75	200–500	—	238, 247
	4–9	4–15	3.31	—
Aldophosphamide/4-hydroxycyclo-phosphamide	10	1.4	1–5	242, 243, 248,
	20	2.6	—	250, 251

$t_{1/2}$, half-life.

Of some significance is the fact that reports[246] have questioned the reliability and applicability of earlier gas chromatography methods[238,247] for measuring levels of phosphoramide mustard and nornitrogen mustard in patient plasma. Because of these concerns, the actual quantitation of these metabolites and their half-lives (Table 13-2) remain approximate.

Fenselau et al.[248] identified aldophosphamide as the cyanohydrin derivative in the plasma of patients receiving cyclophosphamide, and Wagner et al.[249] identified a mercaptan derivative of 4-hydroxycyclophosphamide in the plasma of cyclophosphamide-treated patients. Because the two primary metabolites are in equilibrium, the formation of either derivative should allow the measurement of the total of the two metabolites. Wagner et al.[250] used the mercaptan derivatization technique to estimate that peak plasma levels of 1.4 and 2.6 nmol of total 4-hydroxycyclophosphamide/ aldophosphamide per mL are achieved in humans after injection of doses of 10 and 20 mg of radiolabeled cyclophosphamide per kg, respectively. Subsequent studies have determined that 4-hydroxycyclophosphamide/aldophosphamide has a half-life of approximately 1.5 hours in children[242] and 1 to 5 hours in adults receiving conventional[243] or high-dose[251] cyclophosphamide. The AUC for 4-hydroxycyclophosphamide and aldophosphamide at conventional doses of drug ranged from 3 to 19 nmol per mL × hours and seems to be independent of either peak plasma levels or the plasma half-life of the parent drug or hydroxycyclophosphamide; this indicates that ultimately most parent compound is eliminated by this route.[242]

The relative roles of each of the known active metabolites, 4-hydroxycyclophosphamide/aldophosphamide, phosphoramide mustard, and nornitrogen mustard, in the therapeutic and toxic effects of the parent compound remain unclear. Usually greater than 100 nmol per mL for 30 minutes or greater than 50 nmol per mL × hours of exposure of phosphoramide mustard and nornitrogen mustard is required *in vitro* to achieve a significant cytotoxic effect on murine L1210 leukemia cells. 4-Hydroxycyclophosphamide demonstrates significant cytotoxicity at levels of 10 to 30 nmol per mL for 30 minutes (5 to 15 nmol per mL × hours of exposure).[252] Also, phosphoramide mustard is considerably less immunosuppressive than cyclophosphamide, both on a molar basis and relative to the degree of hematopoietic suppression produced.[253] Furthermore, *in vivo*, phosphoramide mustard and nornitrogen mustard do not exhibit the characteristically high therapeutic index of cyclophosphamide, whereas 4-hydrocyclophosphamide does.[254] This presumably reflects the polar nature of these metabolites and their relatively poor cellular uptake. Thus, the available clinical pharmacologic data suggest that the major antitumor and immunosuppressive effects of cyclophosphamide are mediated by 4-hydroxycyclophosphamide.

Because the initial metabolism of cyclophosphamide is by the hepatic microsomal enzymes, modulation of the activity of these enzymes *in vivo* might be expected to alter the pharmacokinetics of the drug. Pretreatment with phenobarbital reduces the plasma half-life of the parent compound in both humans and experimental animals.[255,256] Also, with repeated doses of cyclophosphamide, the plasma half-life can be shown to become progressively shorter,[236,239] which indicates that cyclophosphamide can induce the microsomal enzymes responsible for its metabolism. The wide variation in the plasma half-life of cyclophosphamide seen in patients is likely due to differing previous drug exposure and the consequent differences in hepatic microsomal activity. For example, Egorin et al.[257] found consistently short plasma half-lives of cyclophosphamide (less than 2 hours) in a group of patients with brain tumors who had had long-term phenobarbital exposure.

In the mouse, phenobarbital pretreatment decreases the AUC plasma concentration for alkylating metabolites[258] and decreases the toxicity of cyclophosphamide. Sladek,[259] however, was unable to find any effect of phenobarbital on the toxicity or therapeutic effect of cyclophosphamide in tumor-bearing rats. Because the rate of cyclophosphamide metabolism in humans is closer to the rate in the rat than to that in the mouse, the toxicity and therapeutic index of cyclophosphamide in humans probably are not significantly altered by modulations of the rate of metabolism.

Two authors have reported increased and prolonged plasma levels of cyclophosphamide metabolites in patients with renal failure,[245,260] and on this basis a reduction in dosage has been recommended for such patients. That these elevated metabolite levels are associated with increased toxicity has not been established, however. Administration of full doses of cyclophosphamide to patients with severe renal impairment does not result in an increase in hematologic or other toxicity.[261]

Ifosfamide

The clinical pharmacology of ifosfamide has been studied by Creaven and Allen and colleagues[262–264] and has been summarized by Brade et al.[265] After single doses of 3.8 to 5.0 g per m², the terminal half-life of ifosfamide was 15 hours, considerably longer than the previously cited values of 3 to 10 hours for cyclophosphamide. At ifosfamide doses of 1.6 to 2.4 g per m², however, the half-life of the drug was similar to that of cyclophosphamide. Creaven et al.[262] found similar values for alkylating activity in plasma after the administration of 3.8 g ifosfamide and 1.1 g cyclophosphamide per m². Also, the alkylating activity excreted in the urine was similar for these doses of the two analogs and ranged from 6% to 15% for ifosfamide, although urinary excretion may approach 50% at high single doses.[265] These findings are consistent with the previous results of Allen and Creaven,[219] which indicate that microsomal activation of ifosfamide to alkylating metabolites proceeds more slowly than the activation of cyclophosphamide and that high doses of ifosfamide seem to saturate the activation mechanism. As with cyclophosphamide, ifosfamide clearance increases during continuous infusion or with multiple daily doses. Pharmacokinetics reaches a steady state 2 to 3 days after drug administration is begun.[266]

Norpoth[267] reported that cleavage of the chloroethyl group from the side chain and ring nitrogen is a quantitatively more significant pathway for ifosfamide metabolism than for cyclophosphamide metabolism in humans. Whereas less than 10% of an administered dose of cyclophosphamide is dechlorethylated,[213] as much as 50% of a dose of ifosfamide may be excreted in the urine as dechlorethylated products. These findings suggest that the less rapid oxidative activation at C-4 of ifosfamide allows the chloroethyl group cleavage to become a significantly competing pathway in the *in vivo* metabolism of the drug. Although oxidation at C-4 of both cyclophosphamide and ifosfamide leads to ring opening and creation of compounds with alkylating activity, the products of side-chain cleavage have little alkylating activity. Thus, at doses below 3.8 g per m², the rates of metabolism of cyclophosphamide and ifosfamide are similar, but a lower proportion of the ifosfamide is converted into alkylating and biologically active metabolites.

Thiotepa

Studies using gas chromatographic analysis specific for thiotepa have revealed that after parenteral administration of the agent at 30 to 300 mg per m² in adults and children, it is rapidly desulfurated to TEPA and other alkylating species.[268–273] The conversion of thiotepa to TEPA is mediated by mixed-function P-450 oxygenases as confirmed *in vitro* by incubation of thiotepa with hepatic microsomes. This biotransformation pathway is shared with many compounds containing the P-S moiety and results in the replacement of the sulfur with oxygen. Aside from individual variability, the plasma terminal half-life of intact thiotepa is a relatively consistent 1.2 to 2 hours. TEPA appears in plasma within 5 minutes of thiotepa administration. In 120 minutes its plasma concentration reaches that of thiotepa, but it persists longer, with a half-life of 3 to 21 hours, so that after 24 hours, TEPA concentration × time exceeds that of the parent drug. In 24 hours, only 1.5% of the administered thiotepa is excreted in the urine unchanged, together with 4.2% as TEPA and 23.5% as other alkylating species.[268] Although both thiotepa and TEPA have cytotoxic activity, the nadirs of leukopenia, which occurs at approximately 2 weeks, and of thrombocytopenia, which occurs at 3 weeks, correlate best with the AUC of the parent drug. Thiotepa clearance is enhanced by administration of clofibrate or phenobarbital, which induces P-450, although data are insufficient to provide guidelines for dosage adjustment in the presence of these drugs.

The pharmacokinetics in children resembles that in adults.[269,272] Although some suggestion is seen of saturability of hepatic metabolism as conventional doses increase in the range of 60 to 80 mg per m², the primary elimination half-life in children receiving transplant dosages of 300 mg per m² per day for 3 days was 1.3 hours, a value consistent with that observed at conventional dosages. In these children, the total plasma clearance averaged 11.25 L per hour per m², and the volume of distribution was 19.4 L per m². Similar pharmacokinetic studies of high-dose thiotepa have not been performed in adults.

Nitrosoureas

In initial studies of the clinical pharmacology of BCNU, the unchanged compound could not be detected in plasma, even as early as 5 minutes after drug administration.[274] Levin et al.,[275] however, studied the pharmacokinetics of BCNU in humans and found that after short-term infusion (15 to 75 minutes) of 60 to 170 mg per m², initial peak levels of up to 5 μmol per L of BCNU were achieved. The plasma concentration decay curves were biexponential, with a distribution-phase half-life of 6 minutes and a second-phase half-life of 68 minutes. Because the half-life for degradation of BCNU in plasma *in vitro* is approximately 15 minutes, the relatively long plasma half-life *in vivo* probably reflects return of BCNU to the plasma from a peripheral compartment. With high-dose BCNU, longer elimination half-lives of 22 to 45 minutes have been reported.[276,276a]

A new analog of BCNU, fotemustine (diethyl-1-[3-(2-chloroethyl)-3-nitrosoureido]-ethylphosphonate), has a longer plasma half-life in rats, greater ability to penetrate tumor cells, and evidence of clinical activity against malignant gliomas.[63]

Busulfan

The pharmacokinetics of busulfan have been studied using a variety of sensitive methods.[277–277d] The parent compound is measured by gas chromatography after extraction and derivatization with TFTP (2,3,5,6-tetrafluorothiophenol).[277b] A similar derivatization was used by Grochow et al. to measure busulfan by liquid chromatography, using a C8 Radial Pak column.[277c] The liquid chromatographic methods are in general less sensitive than gas chromatography or gas chromatography–mass spectrometry, with lower limits of detection of 20 to 100 μg per L compared with 0.5 to 1.0 μg per L. Busulfan is eliminated primarily by enzymatic conjugation with glutathione.[277] A number of downstream metabolic products, including 3-hydroxysulfolane, tetrahydrothiophene-1-oxide, and sulfolane, have been identified in rat and human urine.[277a] None of these metabolites has antitumor activity. The drug is well absorbed, with bioavailability approaching 100% for standard doses of 2 to 6 mg per day.[277d] At the high doses used in bone marrow transplant regimens, oral absorption is less consistent. An intravenous preparation of busulfan is under clinical development.

The drug exhibits circadian rhythmicity in its pharmacokinetics, particularly in children, with higher drug levels and slower elimination in the evening. The primary elimination half-life is approximately 2.5 hours in both children and adults, although interpatient variability is considerable at both low and high doses.

The relationship between dose and AUC appears to be a linear over a broad dose range and within specific age groups. Clearance declines with age, however, which leads to underdosing of children in high-dose regimens.[278] Busulfan clearance for patients older than 18 years averages 2.64 to 2.9 mL per minute per kg, whereas for children aged 2 to 14 clearance averages 4.4 to 4.5 mL per minute per kg, and for children age 3 or younger it is 6.8 to 8.4 mL per minute per kg.[277d] Thus, larger doses must be used in the younger age groups to achieve the desired cytotoxic exposure. Vassal et al.[277d] advise a dosage of 1 mg per kg every 6 hours for 4 days in adults to achieve an AUC of 6,500 ng per hour per mL, whereas children should be treated with dosages based on body surface area and age. Children aged 2 to 14 should receive 37.5 mg per m² every 6 hours for 16 doses; and infants (less than 2 years), 2.34 mg per kg or 47 mg per m² every 6 hours for 16 doses.

Other important pharmacokinetic parameters for high-dose busulfan include a volume of distribution of 0.6 L per kg in adults, 1 L per kg in children aged 2 to 14, and 1.4 to 1.6 L per kg in infants. Although data are incomplete, young children with hepatic disease (e.g., lysosomal storage disease) have a more prolonged half-life (4.9 hours) than their counterparts with normal liver function (2.3 hours).[277d] Because of its high lipid solubility and low level of protein binding, busulfan penetrates readily into the brain and cerebrospinal fluid. The ratio of drug concentration in cerebrospinal fluid to plasma approximates 1.[279] Positron-labeled busulfan has been used to track uptake into the brain, revealing that approximately 20% of a standard dose rapidly enters the CNS.[280] This access to the brain may enhance the activity of this drug against leukemia and lymphoma cells in the CNS, but it also may explain its propensity to cause seizures in up to 15% of patients receiving high doses. Prophylaxis with anticonvulsants is advised in patients receiving high-dose busulfan. Busulfan enhances the clearance of phenytoin [Dilantin] and, in some patients, lowers the drug's plasma concentration below the therapeutic range, which increases the risk of seizures[281]; thus, phenytoin levels should be monitored in the setting of busulfan therapy or an alternative, non–P-450 metabolized anticonvulsant should be used (see Chapter 22).

Pharmacokinetic studies have provided insight into a second important toxicity associated with high-dose busulfan, namely, hepatic venoocclusive disease (VOD). This potentially fatal complication results from injury to vascular endothelium, with intravascular coagulation and hepatic failure. At the recommended total dose of 600 mg per m² for pediatric patients and 16 mg per kg for adults over 4 days, approximately 20% of patients develop VOD. Grochow et al.[277c] found that five of six patients with VOD had a drug exposure (AUC) greater than the mean of 2,012 μmol × minutes per L, which indicates the need to monitor drug concentrations in plasma and to adjust dosage accordingly. Considerations in routine monitoring have not been thoroughly evaluated in prospective studies as of this writing and include the methods of measurement, sampling strategy, variability of intraindividual measurements, and changes in pharmacokinetics during the 4-day period of drug administration. The reader is referred to the excellent discussion in Grochow and Ames.[276a]

TOXICITY

Hematopoietic Suppression

The usual dose-limiting toxicity of the alkylating agents is suppression of hematopoiesis. Characteristically, this suppression involves all formed elements of the blood—leukocytes, platelets, and red cells. However, the degree, time course, and cellular pattern of the hematopoietic suppression produced by the various alkylating agents differ. Figure 13-19A shows the pattern and time course of the decrease in circulating leukocytes and platelets after the administration of 0.1 mg mechlorethamine per kg per day for 4 days.[282] In contrast to this pattern is that which occurs after administration of 60 mg of cyclophosphamide per kg per day, also given for 4 days (Fig. 13-19B).[283] Although the depth of the leukocyte nadir produced by cyclophosphamide is similar to that produced by nitrogen mustard, the return of the leukocyte count to normal is more rapid, and the platelet count is not depressed to clinically hazardous levels. Clinically significant depression of the platelets may be seen when the dose of the drug exceeds 30 mg per kg, but a relative platelet sparing is very characteristic of cyclophosphamide.

Even at the very high doses (200 mg per kg or greater) of cyclophosphamide used in preparation for bone marrow transplantation, some recovery of endogenous hematopoietic elements occurs within 21 to 28 days. This stem cell–sparing property of cyclophosphamide is further reflected by the fact that cumulative damage to the bone marrow is rarely (if ever) seen when cyclophosphamide is given as a single agent, and repeated high doses of the drug can be given without progressive lowering of leukocyte and platelet counts. In contrast to cyclophosphamide, busulfan (Myleran) seems to be especially damaging to bone marrow stem cells,[53,54] and prolonged hypoplasia of the bone marrow may be seen after busulfan administration. Phenylalanine mustard seems to be more damaging to hematopoietic stem cells than cyclophosphamide,

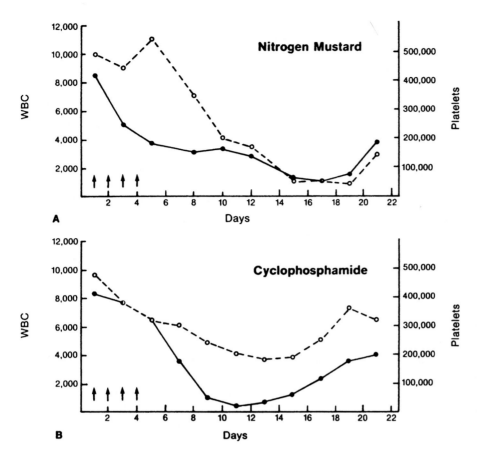

FIGURE 13-19. Leukopenia and thrombocytopenia after administration of mechlorethamine, 0.1 mg per kg per day for 4 days **(A)**, or cyclophosphamide, 60 mg per kg per day for 4 days **(B)**. [●, white blood count (WBC); ○, platelets.] (Modified and reproduced from Nissen-Meyer R, Host H. A comparison between the hematologic side effects of cyclophosphamide and nitrogen mustard. *Cancer Chemother Rep* 1960;9:51, with permission.)

in that a longer recovery period for hematopoietic cells is seen both in animals[284] and in humans, and a cumulative bone marrow depression may occur with repeated doses of melphalan.

The hematopoietic depression produced by the nitrosoureas is characteristically delayed. The onset of leukocyte and platelet depression occurs 3 to 4 weeks after drug administration and may last an additional 2 to 3 weeks.[59] Thrombocytopenia appears earlier and usually is more severe than leukopenia. Even if the nitrosourea is given at 6-week intervals, hematopoietic recovery may not occur between courses, and the drug dose often must be decreased when repeated courses are used.

The differences in the time course and patterns of hematopoietic depression produced by the various alkylating agents are remarkable and indicate that these agents have selectivities for different hematopoietic precursors. Thus, cyclophosphamide seems to spare hematopoietic stem cells, busulfan is especially damaging to these stem cells, and the nitrosoureas seem to damage a hematopoietic precursor whose differentiation or maturation period is 3 to 4 weeks. The biochemical basis for the stem cell–sparing effect of cyclophosphamide is now known to be the presence of a high level of the enzyme aldehyde dehydrogenase in the early bone marrow progenitor cells. The mechanistic and biochemical bases for the profound effect

of busulfan and the nitrosoureas on marrow stem cells remain unknown.

Nausea and Vomiting

Although nausea and vomiting are not usually life-threatening toxic reactions, they are a frequent side effect of alkylating agent therapy and are poorly controlled by conventional antiemetics. These side effects are a major source of patient discomfort and a significant cause of lack of drug compliance and even discontinuation of therapy.[285] Some evidence has been presented that the nausea and vomiting produced by alkylating agents are centrally mediated and are not due to direct gastrointestinal toxicity.[286] The frequency and degree of this reaction are highly variable among patients. Some tolerate high doses of alkylating agents without nausea and vomiting, whereas others are severely incapacitated by low doses of these drugs. The overall frequency of nausea and vomiting increases, however, as the dose of alkylating agent is increased. The time of onset of these side effects is also variable. Some patients may experience nausea within a few minutes of the administration of the drug, but in others the onset of this symptom is often delayed for several hours. In particular, the nausea and vomiting seen after cyclophosphamide administration is usually delayed and may occur as late as 8 hours after drug administration. For this reason, ensuring that the patient receives sustained antiemetic coverage is important (see Chapter 23).

Interstitial Pneumonitis and Pulmonary Fibrosis

Pulmonary fibrosis as a complication of long-term busulfan therapy was described initially by Ohner et al.[287] The characteristic clinical presentation of this syndrome is the gradual onset of fever, a nonproductive cough, and dyspnea, followed by tachypnea and cyanosis, progressing to severe pulmonary insufficiency and death.[288,289] The chest radiograph shows a diffuse intraalveolar or interstitial process or a combination of these changes. The histologic changes include atypia of the alveolar and bronchiolar epithelia, hyperplasia of type II pneumocytes, and interstitial and intraalveolar edema and fibrosis.[290] The pulmonary diffusion capacity may be depressed before the onset of clinical symptoms.[291] If busulfan is stopped before the onset of clinical symptoms, the pulmonary function may stabilize, but if clinical symptoms are manifest, the condition may be rapidly fatal.[289]

A similar type of pulmonary damage has been described occasionally in patients after treatment with a number of other antineoplastic drugs,[292] especially after cyclophosphamide[293–295] and after BCNU and methyl-CCNU in cumulative doses exceeding 1,000 mg per m².[296–300] In addition, BCNU given in high single doses of 900 to 1,500 mg per m², in association with autologous bone marrow transplantation, was reported to cause the onset of pulmonary infiltrates, hyaline membrane formation, and fibrosis within 3 weeks of treatment in 3 of 14 patients.[301] Gallium 67 scans may detect drug-induced pulmonary lesions before they are apparent on chest radiographs.[302] Reports also have appeared of development of pulmonary fibrosis after therapy with melphalan,[303] chlorambucil,[304,305] and mitomycin C, an alkylating antibiotic.[306] Although the precise mechanism of the pulmonary toxicity is not known, this effect presumably is due to direct cytotoxicity of the alkylating agents to pulmonary epithelium, which results in alveolitis and fibrosis.[289] The finding of a similar pulmonary toxicity as a major limitation of bleomycin sulfate therapy[289] and reports of interstitial pulmonary damage after 6-mercaptopurine[307,308] and azathioprine[309] therapy have demonstrated that such effects are not limited to the alkylating agents.

Renal and Bladder Toxicity

A toxicity that seems to be unique to the oxazaphosphorines (cyclophosphamide and ifosfamide) is hemorrhagic cystitis, which may range from a mild cystitis to severe bladder damage with massive hemorrhage.[310–312] This toxicity is due to the excretion of toxic metabolites in the urine, with subsequent direct irritation of the bladder mucosa.[310,313] Acrolein may be responsible for cyclophosphamide-induced cystitis, because in rats this complication is also produced by the cyclophospha-

mide analog diethyl cyclophosphamide, which yields acrolein as its only alkylating metabolite.[314] The incidence and severity of the complication can be lessened by adequate hydration and frequent bladder emptying. In dogs, the bladder damage from high doses of cyclophosphamide can be prevented by continuous irrigation of the bladder with a solution containing *N*-acetylcysteine,[315] and this technique has been used successfully in patients receiving high doses of cyclophosphamide and ifosfamide.[316] Parenteral administration of *N*-acetylcysteine and other sulfhydryl-containing compounds has been shown to prevent or diminish bladder damage in rodents,[317,318] and this approach is now being used in humans.[319] The most effective agent for preventing oxazaphosphorine-induced cystitis is 2-mercaptoethane sulfonate (MESNA), which dimerizes to an inactive metabolite in plasma but hydrolyzes in urine to yield the active parent that conjugates with alkylating species and prevents cystitis. MESNA should be administered routinely to all patients receiving ifosfamide and to any patient who is receiving high-dose cyclophosphamide or has a history of drug-induced cystitis.[320] MESNA is given in divided doses every 4 hours in dosages of 60% of those of the alkylating agent. Experiments in animals and clinical evaluation indicate that the systemic administration of sulfhydryl compounds does not impair the antitumor or immunosuppressive effect of cyclophosphamide.[317,318]

The danger of hemorrhagic cystitis increases with the magnitude of an acute dose of cyclophosphamide, and it may occur in some patients receiving more than 50 mg per kg despite adequate hydration. In the authors' experience, however, some of the most severe cases of hemorrhagic cystitis have occurred suddenly in patients receiving daily oral cyclophosphamide for many months or years who fail to maintain adequate hydration. Therefore, such patients must be monitored carefully. We also have seen patients who did not show evidence of bladder damage at the time of cyclophosphamide administration but who developed bladder hemorrhage several months later on receiving a subsequent course of therapy with other antitumor agents such as cytosine arabinoside or methotrexate sodium. Such patients presumably sustain subclinical bladder damage at the time of cyclophosphamide administration and have persistent abnormalities of the bladder mucosa, as described by Forni et al.[311] The bladder hemorrhage is precipitated by the mucosal irritation of the second drug. Various techniques of cauterization of the bladder have been used for severe hemorrhagic cystitis produced by cyclophosphamide, but continuous irrigation of the bladder to prevent intravesicular clots and transfusion to replace blood loss have usually been effective. In cases of severe refractory bleeding, instillation of dilute alum (1% solution) or dilute formalin may reduce hemorrhage but carries the risk of augmenting fibrosis and destruction of the urinary epithelium.[321–323] If all local measures fail, cystectomy may be necessary to prevent fatal hemorrhage. Although the major urologic damage produced by cyclophosphamide is in the bladder, the damage in severe cases may extend up the ureters to the renal pelvises, and urinary epithelial casts may be seen after cyclophosphamide therapy.[324] The analog ifosfamide produces a similar type of bladder damage but is more likely than cyclophosphamide to produce renal damage. At high doses of ifosfamide, severe renal tubular damage with elevation of serum urea and creatinine has been seen, and a Fanconi-like syndrome has been described after ifosfamide therapy.[325,326] Chronic cystitis due to cyclophosphamide has been associated with the later development of malignant transitional cell tumors of the bladder.[327]

A toxic effect of cyclophosphamide that is probably related to a renal tubular effect is water retention.[328] This syndrome is usually seen in patients receiving cyclophosphamide doses of 50 mg per kg or greater and is characterized by a marked fall in urinary output 6 to 8 hours after drug administration, significant weight gain, a marked increase in urine osmolality, and a decrease in serum osmolality. In extreme cases, the patient may develop pleural and pericardial effusions. The onset of water retention coincides with the peak excretion of alkylating metabolites in the urine, an observation consistent with the hypothesis that the effect is due to a direct action of the metabolites on the renal tubules. The syndrome is self-limited, and by 12 to 16 hours fluid retention is reversed and excess fluid is excreted. For preservation of high urinary output and avoidance of the possible induction of symptomatic hyponatremia, continuous infusion of furosemide is effective in maintaining a diuresis and promoting free water clearance, although K^+ supplementation is required to prevent hypokalemia.[329] The complication of water retention has been seen most frequently in young children treated with high doses of cyclophosphamide,[330] especially those who have been hydrated with salt-free glucose solutions before treatment.

Preclinical toxicologic testing of the nitrosoureas disclosed nephrotoxicity in mice, dogs, and monkeys,[331] but initial clinical trials failed to confirm this complication in humans. The use of more prolonged courses of treatment, however, has now made it clear that all three commonly used nitrosoureas can produce a dose-related renal toxicity that can result in renal failure and death.[332–334] Total doses of more than 1,200 mg of BCNU or methyl-CCNU per m^2 caused renal toxicity in 14 of 17 patients reported by Schacht and Baldwin,[333] and Harmon et al.[334] found that all 6 children who received more than 1,500 mg of methyl-CCNU per m^2 either developed overt renal failure or had macroscopic evidence of renal damage (shrunken kidneys) at death. In patients developing clinical evidence of toxicity, increases in serum creatinine usually appear after the completion of therapy and may be first detected up to 2 years after treatment.

Renal biopsy findings in affected patients resemble those in radiation nephritis[334] and include prominent glomerulosclerosis, basement membrane thickening, and severe tubular loss, with varying amounts of interstitial fibrosis. Proteinuria and urinary sediment abnormalities are not consistently associated with nitrosourea-induced renal damage.

Alopecia

Alopecia has been associated predominantly with cyclophosphamide (E. Frei III, *personal communication*, 1975).[335–337] It occurs infrequently with busulfan.

The degree of alopecia after cyclophosphamide administration may be quite severe, especially when this drug is used in combination with vincristine sulfate or doxorubicin hydrochloride. Regrowth of the hair inevitably occurs after cessation of therapy but may be associated with a change in the color and greater curl.[338] The use of a tourniquet[339] or ice pack applied to the scalp[340] during and for a short period after cyclophosphamide administration may reduce the subsequent alopecia.

Allergic Reactions

Because of the ability of the alkylating agents to bind readily to biologic molecules, these compounds would be expected to act as haptens and produce allergic reactions. An increasing number of reports of skin eruption, angioneurotic edema, urticaria, and anaphylactic reactions after systemic administration of alkylating agents have appeared.[341–345] Topical application of nitrogen mustard, as for treatment of mycosis fungoides, causes sensitization to subsequent applications of the same drug in many patients and also can sensitize patients to other chloroethyl-containing agents administered systemically.[346] Although these complications occur infrequently, the clinician must observe patients carefully for evidence of sensitization and be aware of the possibility of an anaphylactic reaction when administering these drugs. Data are as yet insufficient to determine patterns of cross-reactivity between alkylating agents or to suggest strategies for desensitization to the alkylating agents.

Gonadal Atrophy

Alkylating agents have profound toxic effects on reproductive tissue; these are discussed in greater detail in Chapter 4. A depletion of testicular germ cells but preservation of Sertoli's cells was described by Spitz[347] in the first extensive review of the histologic effects of mechlorethamine in patients. This toxic effect and its functional counterpart of aspermia have subsequently been well documented in both animals[348] and humans.[349,350] Miller[350] found aspermia in nine of nine men under treatment for lymphoma with chlorambucil and two of two patients being treated with cyclophosphamide. Testicular biopsies in these patients demonstrated the germinal aplasia with preservation of Sertoli's cells described by Spitz.[347] Fairley et al.[351] and Kumar et al.[352] made similar observations in men treated with cyclophosphamide. Sherins and DeVita[353] studied reproductive capacity in men after treatment for lymphoma with drug combinations that included either mechlorethamine or cyclophosphamide. A very high incidence of aspermia (10 of 16 cases) or oligospermia (2 of 16 cases) was found in these patients up to 3 years after cessation of therapy. In the patients with total absence of germ cells, an increase in plasma levels of follicle-stimulating hormone was found. However, four men who were in remission and off therapy for 2 to 7 years showed complete spermatogenesis, which indicates that the testicular damage by alkylating agents is reversible. One of Sherins and DeVita's patients and at least two men in other studies[354,355] have fathered children after cyclophosphamide therapy.

Amenorrhea as a complication of busulfan therapy was reported by Galton et al.[356] Several reports subsequently documented the high incidence of amenorrhea and ovarian atrophy associated with cyclophosphamide therapy.[352,353,357,358] The most extensive study, reported by Kyoma et al.,[359] was of 18 premenopausal women treated with prolonged daily cyclophosphamide after radical breast surgery. Seventeen of the patients (94%) developed amenorrhea, and menstruation returned in only two of these. In this study and others,[353] amenorrhea developed after lower doses in older patients than in younger patients and was less likely to be reversible in the older patients. A high incidence of amenorrhea after melphalan therapy also has been established.[21,360] Pathologic examination of the ovaries after alkylating agent–induced amenorrhea reveals the absence of mature or primordial follicles. Endocrinologic studies demonstrate the decreased estrogen and progesterone levels and elevated serum follicle-stimulating hormone and luteinizing hormone levels typical of menopause.

Teratogenesis

Virtually all alkylating agents are teratogenic.[361–363] Studies have been carried out in a number of systems, both *in vivo* and in embryo culture *in vitro*.[364–367] The teratogenic action seems to be due to direct cytotoxicity to the developing embryo by the same mechanisms operative in tumor cells,[368,369] and the antimetabolites exhibit similar teratogenic effects.

Because of the demonstrated teratogenicity of the alkylating agents in animals, appropriate concern has existed about the potential effects of their administration to patients during pregnancy. In 1968, Nicholson[370] reviewed literature reports of women treated with cytotoxic agents during pregnancy. In the 25 instances in which the alkylating agents were given during the first trimester of pregnancy and the status of the fetus was recorded, 4 cases of fetal malformation occurred. No instances of malformed fetuses were reported when alkylating agents or other cytotoxic drugs were administered during the second or third trimester. Thus, administration of alkylating agents during the first trimester presents a definite risk of a malformed viable infant, but the administration of such drugs during the second and third trimesters does not increase the risk of fetal malformation above normal. Other reports confirm the risk of malformation in children born to mothers who had received chlorambucil,[371] cyclophosphamide,[372] or nitrogen mustard and procarbazine[373] during the first trimester and the birth of normal infants to mothers receiving alkylating agents during the second or third trimester.[374,375]

Carcinogenesis

Carcinogenesis as a complication of cancer chemotherapy is covered in detail in Chapter 5. Case reports began appearing during the early 1970s of development of a fulminant acute myeloid leukemia in patients treated with alkylating agents. These leukemias are characterized by a preceding phase of myelodysplasia, loss of part or all of chromosome 5 or 7, and a poor response to treatment. The initial reports described this association in patients with multiple myeloma[376,377] and lymphomas,[378] and the possibility that the development of acute leukemia might be part of the natural history of these diseases had to be considered. A number of cases of acute leukemia after alkylating agent therapy have now been reported in patients with other malignancies, however, as well as in patients treated for nonmalignant diseases. Most of the cases described have been in patients treated with melphalan,[377,379] cyclophosphamide (which is much less leukemogenic than melphalan),[378,380,381] chlorambucil,[382,383] and the nitrosoureas.[384] This circumstance probably reflects the fact that these have been the most widely used of the alkylating agents. Also, the preponderance of patients with multiple myeloma, Hodgkin's disease, and carcinoma of the ovary in the reports of leukemogenesis is probably due to the fact that patients with these diseases may have good responses and are often treated with alkylating agents for a number of years. Reimer et al.[385] predicted that the rate of occurrence of acute leukemia in patients with ovarian cancer who survive for 10 years after treatment with alkylating agents might be as high as 5% to 10%, and in patients receiving high-dose therapy, the rate seems to be substantially higher. Similar rates of second malignancy occur in patients with Hodgkin's disease treated with MOPP chemotherapy, which contains mechlorethamine and the highly carcinogenic procarbazine (as well as vincristine and prednisone).[386] Melphalan seems to be more carcinogenic than cyclophosphamide in women with ovarian cancer. In one series the incidence of acute leukemia in patients treated with melphalan was 93-fold higher than in an age-matched untreated population and was two- to threefold greater than for women receiving cyclophosphamide.[387] Acute leukemia has been the most frequently described second malignancy and usually develops 1 to 4 years after drug exposure. Other malignancies, including solid tumors, also have been reported to develop in patients treated with alkylating agents.[386,388]

Organ Toxicity in High-Dose Chemotherapy

At conventional dosages, alkylating agents produce myelosuppression as their dose-limiting toxicity. Gastrointestinal epithelial damage and other toxicities (cystitis, pulmonary fibrosis, leukemogenesis) may become significant problems with long-term treatment but rarely limit initial therapy. For this reason, and because of their steep dose-response to tumor-killing curves, the alkylating agents have become a logical tool, either alone or in combination, for high-dose chemotherapy regimens in which bone marrow toxicity is expected and is accommodated by bone marrow transplantation, stem cell reconstitution from peripheral blood monocytes, and growth factor rescue.[389–392] In this high-dose setting, toxicities that affect the gut, lung, liver, and CNS become dose limiting and life-threatening. A list of the dose-limiting extramedullary tox-

icities of the alkylating agents is given in Table 13-3. Melphalan produces severe gastrointestinal toxicity.[393] A number of alkylating agents, including the nitrosoureas, busulfan, thiotepa, cyclophosphamide, and mitomycin C, produce venoocclusive disease of the liver in which endothelial damage to small venules leads to thrombosis, hepatic congestion, hepatocellular necrosis, and liver failure.[394] Venoocclusive disease due to busulfan may be avoided by dosage adjustment based on pharmacokinetic monitoring, which detects patients with slow busulfan clearance.[395]

The highly lipid-soluble alkylators, especially ifosfamide, busulfan, the nitrosoureas, and thiotepa, cause CNS dysfunction, including seizures, altered mental status, cerebellar dysfunction, cranial nerve palsies, and coma.[396–398] High-dose ifosfamide is most frequently the cause of neurotoxicity. In addition to affecting the CNS, ifosfamide may produce painful and acute exacerbation of peripheral sensory neuropathies and motor dysfunction of the distal extremities.[399] At the nonmyeloablative clinical doses, con-

TABLE 13-3. ALKYLATING AGENTS IN HIGH-DOSE CHEMOTHERAPY

Dose-Limiting Extramedullary Toxicities of Single Agents

Drug	MTD[a] (mg/m²)	Fold Increase Over Standard Dose	Major Organ Toxicities
Cyclophosphamide	7,000	7.0	Cardiac
Ifosfamide	16,000	2.7	Renal, CNS
Thiotepa	1,000	18.0	GI, CNS
Melphalan	180	5.6	GI
Busulfan	640	9.0	GI, hepatic
BCNU	1,050	5.3	Lung, hepatic
Cisplatin	200	2.0	PN, renal
Carboplatin	2,000	5.0	Renal, PN, hepatic
Etoposide	3,000	6.0	GI

Combination High-Dose Chemotherapy Regimens

Regimen	Dose	Major Toxicities	Regimen MTD[b]	References
Cyclophosphamide	6,000			
BCNU	300	Lung, GI	0.47	445
Etoposide	750			
Busulfan	640	Lung, GI, hepatic	1.0	446
Cyclophosphamide	8,000			
Ifosfamide	16,000			
Carboplatin	1,800	Renal, hepatic, GI	0.8	447
Etoposide	1,500			
Cyclophosphamide	5,250			
Etoposide	1,200	GI, renal	0.68	448
Cisplatin	180			
Cyclophosphamide	6,000			
Thiotepa	500	GI, cardiac	0.59	449
Carboplatin	800			
Cyclophosphamide	5,625			
BCNU	600	Lung, hepatic, renal	0.57	450
Cisplatin	165			

BCNU, bischloroethylnitrosourea; CNS, central nervous system; GI, gastrointestinal; MTD, maximum tolerated dose; PN, peripheral neuropathy.
[a]See references 91, 438–444.
[b]See Eder et al.[449] for calculation of regimen MTD.

two types of clinical application. The first use has been for the suppression of the recipient immune response before organ transplantation. Since the demonstration by Santos and colleagues[429] that matched sibling bone marrow can be successfully transplanted into recipients who have been pretreated with large doses of cyclophosphamide, this drug has been one of several agents used for bone marrow transplantation, the others being methotrexate and cyclosporin A. Cyclophosphamide also has been shown to be effective in controlling kidney graft rejection[430] but has been less widely used for this application than the antimetabolite immunosuppressive agents.

The other use of alkylating agents in patients with nonmalignant disease has been in the treatment of immunologic disorders. Osborne et al.,[431] in 1947, reported the successful treatment of a patient with systemic lupus erythematosus using nitrogen mustard. Subsequently, the alkylating agents have been tried in a wide variety of diseases thought to be autoimmune in nature, with variable results. Cyclophosphamide has been shown to be an effective agent in the treatment of Wegener's granulomatosis,[432] rheumatoid arthritis,[433,434] idiopathic thrombocytopenic purpura,[435] and membranous glomerulonephritis.[436,437] Because of the severe side effects, however, including carcinogenesis, the role of alkylating agents in the treatment of nonmalignant disease must be considered carefully.

REFERENCES

1. Rhoads CP. Nitrogen mustards in treatment of neoplastic disease. *JAMA* 1946;131:656.
2. Jacobson LP, Spurr CL, Barron ESQ, et al. Studies on the effect of methyl-bis(beta-chloroethyl)amine hydrochloride on neoplastic diseases and allied disorders of the hemapoietic system. *JAMA* 1946;132:263.
3. Goodman LS, Wintrobe MM, Dameshek W, et al. Use of methyl-bis(beta-chloroethyl)amine hydrochloride for Hodgkin's disease, lymphosarcoma, leukemia. *JAMA* 1946; 132:126.
4. Adair CPJ, Bagg HJ. Experimental and clinical studies on the treatment of cancer by dichloroethylsulphide (mustard gas). *Ann Surg* 1931;93:190.
5. Ross WLJ. Alkylating agents. In: *Biological alkylating agents.* London: Butterworths, 1962:3.
6. Colvin M, Brundrett RB, Kan MN, et al. Alkylating properties of phosphoramide mustard. *Cancer Res* 1976; 36:1121.
7. Brundrett RB, Cowens JW, Colvin M. Chemistry of nitrosoureas: decomposition of deuterated 1,3-bis(2-chloroethyl)-1-nitrosoureas. *J Med Chem* 1976;19:958.
8. Harris AL. DNA repair and resistance to chemotherapy. *Cancer Surv* 1985;4:601.
8a. Russo JE, Hilton J, Colvin OM. The role of aldehydehydrogenase iso-enzymes in cellular resistance to the alkylating agent cyclophosphamide. In: Weiner H, Flynn TG, eds. *Enzymology and molecular biology of carbonyl metabolism*, vol 2. New York: Alan R Liss, 1989:65.
9. Brent TP, Houghton PJ, Houghton JA. O^6-Alkylguanine-DNA alkyltransferase activity correlates with the therapeutic response of human rhabdomyosarcoma xenografts to 1-(2-chloroethyl)-3-(*trans*-4-methylcyclohexyl)-1-nitrosourea. *Proc Natl Acad Sci U S A* 1985;82:2987.
10. Ewig RAG, Kohn KW. DNA damage and repair in mouse leukemia L1210 cells treated with nitrogen mustard, 1,3-bis(2-chloroethyl)-1-nitrosourea, and other nitrosoureas. *Cancer Res* 1977;37:2114.
11. Sudhaker S, Tew KD, Schein PS, et al. Nitrosourea interaction with chromatin and effect on poly (adenosine diphosphate ribose) polymerase activity. *Cancer Res* 1979; 39:1411.
12. Ciaccio PJ, Tew KD, LaCreta FP. The spontaneous and glutathione-*S*-transferase-mediated reaction of chlorambucil with glutathione. *Cancer Commun* 1990;2:279.
13. Ciaccio PJ, Tew KD, LaCreta FP. The enzymatic conjugation of chlorambucil with glutathione is catalyzed by human glutathione-*S*-transferase enzymes and inhibition by ethacrynic acid. *Biochem Pharmacol* 1991;42:2410.
14. Bolton MG, Colvin OM, Hilton J. Specificity of isozymes of murine glutathione-*S*-transferase for the conjugation of glutathione with L-phenylalanine mustard. *Cancer Res* 1991;51:2410.
15. Friedman OM, Myles A, Colvin M. Cyclophosphamide and certain structurally related phosphoramide mustards. In: Rosowsky A, ed. *Advances in cancer chemotherapy*, vol 1. New York: Marcel Dekker, 1979:179.
16. Drings P, Fritsch H. Erfahrungen mit Iphosphamide in hoher Einzeldosis bei metastasierten soliden Tumoren. *Verh Dtsch Ges Inn Med* 1972;78:166.
17. Brade W, Seeber S, Herdrich K. Comparative activity of ifosfamide and cyclophosphamide. *Cancer Chemother Pharmacol* 1986;18[Suppl 2]:1.
18. Wiltshaw E, Westbury G, Harmer C, et al. Ifosfamide plus MESNA with and without Adriamycin in soft tissue sarcoma. *Cancer Chemother Pharmacol* 1986;18[Suppl 2]:10.
19. Frick JC, Tretter P, Tretter W, et al. Disseminated carcinoma of the ovary treated by L-phenylalanine mustard. *Cancer* 1968;21:508.
20. Costa G, Engle RL Jr, Schilling A, et al. Melphalan and prednisone: an effective combination for the treatment of multiple myeloma. *Am J Med* 1973;54:589.
21. Fisher B, Sherman B, Rockette H, et al. L-Phenylalanine mustard (L-PAM) in the management of premenopausal patients with primary breast cancer. *Cancer* 1979;44:847.
22. Goldin D, Israels L, Nabarro J, et al. Clinical trials of p-(di-2-chloroethylamino)-phenylbutyric acid (CB 1348) in malignant lymphoma. *BMJ* 1955;2:172.
23. Rundles RW, Striggle J, Bell W, et al. Comparison of chlorambucil and Myleran in chronic lymphocytic and granulocytic leukemia. *Am J Med* 1959;27:424.
24. Zdink E, Stutzman L. Chlorambucil therapy for lymphomas and chronic lymphocytic leukemia. *JAMA* 1965; 191:444.
25. Wiltshaw E. Chlorambucil in the treatment of primary adenocarcinoma of the ovary. *J Obstet Gynaecol Br Commonw* 1964;72:586.

26. Baterman JC. Chemotherapy of solid tumors with triethylene thiophosphoramide. *N Engl J Med* 1955;252:879.

27. Ultmann JE, Hyman GA, Crandall C, et al. Methylene thiophosphoramide thio-TEPA in the treatment of neoplastic disease. *Cancer* 1957;10:902.

28. Rundles RW, Barton WB. Triethylene melamine in the treatment of neoplastic disease. *Blood* 1952;7:483.

29. Sykes MP, Rundles RW, Pierce VK, et al. Triethylene melamine in the management of far advanced ovarian cancer. *Surg Gynecol Obstet* 1955;101:133.

30. Morack G, Nissen E, Pockrandt H, et al. Ergebnisse einer gezielten zytostatischen Behandlung des Ovarialkarzinoms. *Zentralbl Gynaekol* 1978;100:367.

31. Perloff M, Hart RD, Holland JF. Vinblastine, Adriamycin, thio-TEPA, and Halotestin (VATH). *Cancer* 1978; 42:2534.

32. Greenspan EM. Thio-TEPA and methotrexate chemotherapy of advanced ovarian carcinoma. *J Mount Sinai Hosp N Y* 1968;35:52.

33. Gutin PH, Levi JA, Wiernik PH, et al. Treatment of malignant meningeal disease with intrathecal thioTEPA: a phase II study. *Cancer Treat Rep* 1977;61:885.

34. Haas CD, Stephens RC, Hollister M, et al. Phase I evaluation of dianhydrogalactitol (NSC-132313). *Cancer Treat Rep* 1976;60:611.

35. Vogel CL, Winton EF, Moore MR, et al. Phase I trial of dianhydrogalactitol administered IV in a weekly schedule. *Cancer Treat Rep* 1976;60:895.

36. Espana P, Wiernik PH, Walker M. Phase II study of dianhydrogalactitol in malignant glioma. *Cancer Treat Rep* 1978;62:1199.

37. Chiuten DF, Rosencweig M, Von Hoff DD, et al. Clinical trials with hexitol derivatives in the U.S. *Cancer* 1981; 47:442.

38. Thigpen JT, Lamson MK. Phase II trial of dianhydrogalactitol in advanced soft tissue and bony sarcomas: a Southwest Oncology Group Study. *Cancer Treat Rep* 1979; 63:553.

39. Thigpen JT, Al-Serraf M, Hewlett JS. Phase II trial of dianhydrogalactitol in metastatic malignant melanoma: a Southwest Oncology Group Study. *Cancer Treat Rep* 1979; 63:525.

40. Edmonson JH, Frytak S, Letendre L, et al. Phase II evaluation of dianhydrogalactitol in advanced head and neck carcinomas. *Cancer Treat Rep* 1979;63:2081.

41. Hoogstraten R, O'Bryan R, Jones S. 1,2:5,6-Dianhydrogalactitol in advanced breast cancer. *Cancer Treat Rep* 1978;62:841.

42. Tormey DC, Falkson G, Simon RM. A randomized comparison of two sequentially administered regimens to a single regimen in metastatic breast cancer. *Cancer Clin Trials* 1979;2:247.

43. Elson LA, Jarman M, Ross WCJ. Toxicity, haematological effects and antitumor activity of epoxides derived from disubstituted hexitols: mode of action of mannitol, Myleran and dibromomannitol. *Eur J Cancer* 1968; 4:617.

44. Seller C, Ecklardt IP, Kralovanszky J, et al. Clinical and pharmacologic experience with dibromodulcitol (NSC-104800), a new antitumor agent. *Cancer Chemother Rep* 1969;53:377.

45. Andrews NL, Weiss AJ, Wilson W, et al. Phase II study of dibromodulcitol (NSC-104800). *Cancer Chemother Rep* 1974;58:653.

46. Galton D. Myleran in chronic myeloid leukaemia. *Lancet* 1953;264:208.

47. Haddow A, Timmis GM. Myleran in chronic myeloid leukaemia—chemical constitution and biological action. *Lancet* 1953;1:207.

48. Timmis GM, Hudson RF. Part I: chemistry of alkylating agents: discussion. *Ann N Y Acad Sci* 1958;68:727.

49. Roberts JJ, Warwick GP. Mode of action of alkylating agents: formation of *S*-ethylcysteine from ethyl methanesulphonate in vivo. *Nature* 1957;179:1181.

50. Roberts JJ, Warwick GP. Metabolic and chemical studies of "Myleran": formation of 3-hydroxytetrahydrothiophene-1,1-dioxide in vivo, and reactions with thiols in vitro. *Nature* 1959;184:1288.

51. Brookes P, Lawley PD. The alkylation of guanosine and guanylic acid. *J Chem Soc* 1961;1961:3923.

52. Mitchell MP, Walker IG. Studies on the cytotoxicity of Myleran and dimethyl Myleran. *Can J Biochem* 1972;50:1074.

53. Elson LA. Hematological effects of the alkylating agents. *Ann N Y Acad Sci* 1958;68:826.

54. Fried W, Kede A, Barone J. Effects of cyclophosphamide and busulfan on spleen-colony-forming units and on hematopoietic stroma. *Cancer Res* 1977;37:1205.

55. Tutschka PJ, Copelan EA, Klein JP. Bone marrow transplantation for leukemia following a new busulfan and cyclophosphamide regimen. *Blood* 1987;70:1382.

56. Skinner WA, Gram HF, Greene MO, et al. Potential anticancer agents—XXXI. The relationship of chemical structure to antileukemic activity with analogues. *J Med Pharmaceut Chem* 1960;2:299.

57. Hyde KA, Acton E, Skinner WA, et al. Potential anticancer agents—LXII. The relationship of chemical structure to antileukemia activity with analogues of 1-methyl-3-nitro-1-nitrosoguanidine (NSC-9369), part II. *J Med Pharmaceut Chem* 1962;5:1.

58. Schabel FM Jr, Johnston TP, McCaleb GS, et al. Experimental evaluation of potential anticancer agents: VIII. Effects of certain nitrosoureas on intracerebral L1210 leukemia. *Cancer Res* 1963;23:226.

59. DeVita VT, Carbone PP, Owens AH Jr, et al. Clinical trials with 1,3-bis(2-chloroethyl)-1-nitrosourea, NSC-409962. *Cancer Res* 1965;25:1876.

60. Nissen NI, Pajak TF, Glidewell O, et al. A comparative study of a BCNU containing 4-drug program versus MOPP versus 3-drug combination in advanced Hodgkin's disease. *Cancer* 1979;43:31.

61. Schabel FM Jr. Nitrosoureas: a review of experimental antitumor activity. *Cancer Treat Rep* 1976;60:665.

62. Wolmark N, Fisher B, Rockette H, et al. Postoperative adjuvant chemotherapy of BCG for colon cancer: results from NSABP Protocol C-01. *J Natl Cancer Inst* 1988; 80:30.

63. Frenay M, Giroux B, Khoury S, et al. Phase II study of fote-

mustine in recurrent supratentorial malignant gliomas. *Eur J Cancer* 1991;27:852.

64. Montgomery J, Ruby J, McCaleb GS, et al. The modes of decomposition of 1,3-bis(2-chloroethyl)-1-nitrosourea and related compounds. *J Med Chem* 1967;10:668.

65. Colvin M, Brundrett RB, Cowens JW, et al. A chemical basis for the antitumor activity of chloroethylnitrosoureas. *Biochem Pharmacol* 1976;25:695.

66. Ludlum DB, Kramer BS, Wang J, et al. Reaction of 1,3-bis(2-chloroethyl)-1-nitrosourea with synthetic polynucleotides. *Biochemistry* 1975;14:5480.

67. Kohn KW. Interstrand cross-linking of DNA by 1,3-bis(2-chloroethyl)-1-nitrosourea and other 1-(2-haloethyl)-1-nitrosoureas. *Cancer Res* 1977;37:1450.

68. Baril BB, Baril EF, Lazlo J, et al. Inhibition of rat liver DNA polymerase by nitrosourea and isocyanates. *Cancer Res* 1975;35:1.

69. Kann HE Jr, Kohn KW, Lyles JM. Inhibition of DNA repair by the 1,3-bis(2-chloroethyl)-1-nitrosoureas breakdown product, 2-chloroethyl isocyanate. *Cancer Res* 1974;34:398.

70. Kann HE Jr, Kohn KW, Widerlite L, et al. Effects of 1,3-bis(2-chloroethyl)-1-nitrosourea and related compounds on nuclear RNA metabolism. *Cancer Res* 1974;34:1982.

71. Babson JR, Reed DJ. Inactivation of glutathione reductase by 2-chloroethyl nitrosourea derived isocyanates. *Biochem Biophys Res Commun* 1978;83:754.

72. Hammer CF, Loranger RA, Schein PS. The structures and decomposition products of chlorozotocin: new intramolecular carbamates of 2-amino-2-deoxyhexoses. *J Organ Chem* 1981;46:1521.

73. Tew KD, Kyle G, Johnson A, et al. Carbamoylation of glutathione reductase and changes in cellular and chromosome morphology in a rat cell line resistant to nitrogen mustards but collaterally sensitive to nitrosoureas. *Cancer Res* 1985;45:2326.

74. Bowdon BJ, Grimsley J, Lloyd HH. Interrelationships of some chemical, physicochemical, and biological activities of several 1-(2-haloethyl)-1-nitrosoureas. *Cancer Res* 1974;34:194.

75. Panasci LC, Green D, Nagourney R, et al. A structure-activity analysis of chemical and biological parameters of chloroethylnitrosoureas in mice. *Cancer Res* 1977;37:2615.

76. Schein PS, Cooney DA, Vernon ML. The use of nicotinamide to modify the toxicity of streptozotocin diabetes without loss of antitumor activity. *Cancer Res* 1967;27:2324.

77. Schein PS. 1-Methyl-1-nitrosourea and dialkylnitrosamine depression of nicotinamide adenine dinucleotide. *Cancer Res* 1969;29:226.

78. Rakietan N, Rakietan M, Nadkarni M. Studies on the diabetogenic action of streptozotocin (NSC-37917). *Cancer Chemother Rep* 1963;29:91.

79. Broder LE, Carter SK. Pancreatic islet cell carcinoma. *Ann Intern Med* 1973;79:108.

80. Moertel CG, Hanley JA, Johnson LA. Streptozocin alone compared with streptozocin plus fluorouracil in the treatment of advanced islet-cell carcinoma. *N Engl J Med* 1980;303:1189.

81. Schein PS, O'Connell MJ, Blom J, et al. Clinical antitumor activity and toxicity of streptozotocin (NSC-85998). *Cancer* 1974;34:993.

82. Anderson T, McMenamim M, Schein P. Chlorozotocin, 2-[3-(2-chloroethyl)-3-nitrosoureido]-D-glucopyranose, an antitumor agent with modified bone marrow toxicity. *Cancer Res* 1975;35:761.

83. Fox PA, Panasci LC, Schein PS. Biological and biochemical properties of 1-(2-chloroethyl)-3-(beta-l-glucopyranosyl)-1-nitrosourea (NSC-D-254157), a nitrosourea with reduced bone marrow toxicity. *Cancer Res* 1977;37:783.

84. Gralla RJ, Tan CTC, Young CW. Phase I trial of chlorozotocin. *Cancer Treat Rep* 1979;63:17.

85. Hansen HH, Selawry OS, Pajak TF, et al. The superiority of CCNU in the treatment of advanced Hodgkin's disease. *Cancer* 1981;47:14.

86. Cohen MH, Ihde DC, Bunn PA, et al. Cyclic alternating combination chemotherapy of small cell bronchogenic carcinoma. *Cancer Treat Rep* 1979;63:163.

87. Moertel CG. Therapy of advanced gastrointestinal cancer with the nitrosoureas. *Cancer Chemother Rep 3* 1973;4(3):27

88. Cornwell CG III, Pajak TF, Kochwa S, et al. Comparison of oral melphalan, CCNU and BCNU with and without vincristine and prednisone in the treatment of multiple myeloma. *Cancer* 1982;50:1669.

89. Levin VA, Wilson CB. Nitrosourea pharmacodynamics in relation to the central nervous system. *Cancer Treat Rep* 1976;60:725.

90. Eyre HJ, Eltingham JR, Gehan EA, et al. Randomized comparisons of radiotherapy and carmustine versus procarbazine versus decarbazine for the treatment of malignant gliomas following surgery: a Southwest Oncology Group Study. *Cancer Treat Rep* 1986;70:1085.

91. Phillips GL, Wolff SN, Fay JW, et al. Intensive 1,3-bis(2-chloroethyl)-1-nitrosourea (BCNU) monochemotherapy and autologous bone marrow transplantation for malignant gliomas. *J Clin Oncol* 1986;4:639.

92. Hartley-Asp B, Gunnarsson PO, Liljekvist J. Cytotoxicity and metabolism of prednimustine, chlorambucil and prednisolone in a Chinese hamster cell line. *Cancer Chemother Pharmacol* 1986;16:85.

93. Bastholt L, Johansson C-J, Pfeiffer P, et al. A pharmacokinetic study of prednimustine as compared with prednisolone plus chlorambucil in cancer patients. *Cancer Chemother Pharmacol* 1991;28:205.

94. Tew KD. The mechanism of action of estramustine. *Semin Oncol* 1983;10:21.

95. Punzi JS, Duax WL, Strong P, et al. Molecular conformation of estramustine and two analogues. *Mol Pharmacol* 1992;41:569.

96. Tew KD, Glusker JP, Hartley-Asp B, et al. Preclinical and clinical perspectives on the use of estramustine as an antimitotic drug. *Pharmacol Ther* 1993;56:323.

96a. Edman K, Svensson L, Eriksson B, et al. Determination of estramustine phosphate and its metabolites estromustine, estramustine, estrone and estradiol in human plasma by liquid chromatography with florescence detection and gas chromatography with nitrogen-phosphorus and mass spectrometric detection. *J Chromatogr B Biomed Sci Appl* 2000; 738(2):267.

97. Hudes GR, Greenberg R, Kriegel RL, et al. Phase II study of estramustine and vinblastine, two microtubule inhibitors, in hormone-refractory prostate cancer. *J Clin Oncol* 1992;10:1754.

98. Seidman A, Scher HI, Petrylak D, et al. Estramustine and vinblastine: use of prostate-specific antigen as a clinical trial end point for hormone-refractory prostate cancer. *J Urol* 1992;147:931.

98a. Hudes G, Einhorn L, Ross E, et al. Vinblastine versus vinblastine plus oral estramustine phosphate for patients with hormone-refractory prostate cancer: a Hoosier Oncology Group and Fox Chase Network phase III trial. *J Clin Oncol* 1999;17(10):3160.

99. Speicher LA, Barone LR, Chapman AE, et al. P-glycoprotein binding and modulation of the multidrug-resistant phenotype by estramustine. *J Natl Cancer Inst* 1994; 86:688.

99a. Deonarain MP, Epenetos AA. Targeting enzymes for cancer therapy: old enzymes in new roles. *Br J Cancer* 1994; 70:786.

99b. Niculescu-Duvaz D, Niculescu-Duvaz I, Friedlow F, et al. Self-immolative nitrogen mustard prodrugs for suicide gene therapy. *J Med Chem* 1998;41:5297.

99c. Morgan AS, Sanderson PE, Borch RF, et al. Tumor efficacy and bone marrow-sparing properties of TER286, a cytotoxin activated by glutathione S-transferase. *Cancer Res* 1998;58:2568.

99d. Chase M, Chung RY, Chiocca EA. An oncolytic viral mutant that delivers the CYP2B1 transgene and augments cyclophosphamide chemotherapy. *Nat Biotechnol* 1998; 16:444.

100. Skipper HE, Bennett LL, Langham WH. Overall tracer studies with C^{14}-labeled nitrogen mustard in normal and leukemic mice. *Cancer* 1951;4:1025.

101. Pearson RG, Songstad J. Application of the principle of hard and soft acids and bases to organic chemistry. *J Am Chem Soc* 1967;89:1827.

102. Coles B. Effects of modifying structure on electrophilic reactions with biological nucleophiles. *Drug Metab Rev* 1985;15:1307.

103. Drysdale RB, Hopkins A, Thompson RY, et al. Some effects of nitrogen and sulphur mustards on the metabolism of nucleic acids in mammalian cells. *Br J Cancer* 1958; 12:137.

104. Wheeler GP. Studies related to the mechanism of action of cytotoxic alkylating agents: a review. *Cancer Res* 1962; 22:651.

105. Goldstein NO, Rutman RJ. The effect of alkylation on the in vitro thymidine-incorporating system of Lettré-Ehrlich cells. *Cancer Res* 1964;24:1363.

106. Tomisek AJ, Simpson BT. Effect of in vivo cyclophosphamide treatment on the DNA-primary ability of DNA from Fortner plasmacytoma. *Proc Am Assoc Cancer Res* 1966; 7:71.

107. Ruddon RW, Johnson JM. The effect of nitrogen mustard on DNA template activity in purified DNA and RNA polymerase systems. *Mol Pharmacol* 1968;4:258.

108. Wheeler GP, Alexander JA. Effects of nitrogen mustard and

cyclophosphamide upon the synthesis of DNA in vivo and in cell-free preparation. *Cancer Res* 1969;29:98.

109. Roberts JJ, Brent TP, Crathorn AR. Evidence for the inactivation and repair of the mammalian DNA template after alkylation by mustard gas and half mustard gas. *Eur J Cancer* 1971;7:515.

110. Bannon P, Verly W. Alkylation of phosphates and stability of phosphate triesters in DNA. *Eur J Biochem* 1972;31:103.

111. Lawley PD. Reaction of N-methyl-N-nitrosourea (MNUA) with P-labelled DNA: evidence for formation of phosphotriesters. *Chem Biol Interact* 1973;7:127.

112. Singer B, Fraenkel-Courat H. Human pancreatic enzymes: purification and characterization of a nonelastolytic enzyme, protease E, resembling elastase. *Biochemistry* 1975;14:722.

113. Verly WG. Monofunctional alkylating agents and apurinic sites in DNA. *Biochem Pharmacol* 1974;23:3.

114. Loveless A. Possible relevance of O-6 alkylating of deoxyguanosine to the mutagenicity and carcinogenicity of nitrosamines and nitrosamides. *Nature* 1969;233:206.

115. Gerchman LL, Ludlum DB. The properties of O^6-methylguanine in templates for RNA polymerase. *Biochim Biophys Acta* 1973;308:310.

116. Weinstein IB, Jeffrey AM, Jennette KW, et al. Benzo[a]pyrene diol epoxides as intermediates in nucleic acid binding in vitro and in vivo. *Science* 1976;195:592.

117. Tong WP, Ludlum DB. Crosslinking of DNA by busulfan formation of diguanyl derivatives. *Biochim Biophys Acta* 1980;608:174.

118. Price CC, Gaucher GM, Koneru P, et al. Relative reactivities for monofunctional nitrogen mustard alkylation of nucleic acid components. *Biochim Biophys Acta* 1968; 166:327.

119. Brookes P, Lawley PD. The reaction of mono- and difunctional alkylating agents with nucleic acids. *Biochem J* 1961;80:486.

120. Silber JR, Blank A, Bobola MS, et al. O-6-methylguanine-DNA methyltransferase-deficient phenotype in human gliomas: frequency and time to tumor progression after alkylating agent-based chemotherapy. *Clin Cancer Res* 1999;5:807.

121. Brookes P, Lawley PD. The action of alkylating agents on deoxyribonucleic acid in relation to biological effects of the alkylating agents. *Exp Cell Res* 1963;9[Suppl]:512.

122. Loveless A, Ross WCJ. Chromosome alteration and tumour inhibition by nitrogen mustards: the hypothesis of cross-linking alkylation. *Nature* 1950;166:113.

123. Geiduschek EP. "Reversible" DNA. *Proc Natl Acad Sci U S A* 1961;47:950.

124. Kohn KW, Steigbiel NH, Spears CL. Cross-linking and repair of DNA in sensitive and resistant strains of *E. coli* treated with nitrogen mustard. *Proc Natl Acad Sci U S A* 1965;53:1154.

125. Kohn KW, Spears CL, Doty P. Intra-strand crosslinking of DNA by nitrogen mustard. *J Mol Biol* 1966;19:266.

126. Lawley PD, Brookes P. Cytotoxicity of alkylating agents towards sensitive and resistant strains of *Escherichia coli* in relation to extent and mode of alkylation of cellular macromolecules and repair of alkylation lesions in deoxyribonucleic acid. *Biochem J* 1968;109:433.

127. Venitt S. Interstrand cross-links in the DNA of *Escherichia coli* B/r and Bs-1 and their removal by the resistant strain. *Biochem Biophys Res Commun* 1968;31:355.

128. Kohn KW, Erickson LC, Ewig RAG, et al. Fractionation of DNA from mammalian cells by alkaline elution. *Biochemistry* 1976;15:4629.

129. Ross WE, Ewig RAG, Kohn KW. Differences between melphalan and nitrogen mustard in the formation and removal of DNA cross-links. *Cancer Res* 1978;38:1502.

130. Thomas CB, Osieka R, Kohn KW. DNA cross-linking by in vivo treatment with 1-(2-chloroethyl)-3-(4-methylcyclohexyl)-1-nitrosourea of sensitive and resistant human colon carcinoma xenografts in nude mice. *Cancer Res* 1978;38:2448.

131. Erickson LC, Bradley MO, Ducore JM, et al. DNA cross-linking and cytotoxicity in normal and transformed human cells treated with antitumor nitrosourea. *Proc Natl Acad Sci U S A* 1980;77:467.

132. Garcia ST, McQuillan A, Panasci I. Correlation between the cytotoxicity of melphalan and DNA crosslinks as detected by the ethidium bromide fluorescence assay in the F_1 variant of B_{16} melanoma cells. *Biochem Pharmacol* 1988;37:3189.

133. Ewig RAG, Kohn KW. DNA-protein crosslinking and DNA interstrand crosslinking by haloethylnitrosourea in L1210 cells. *Cancer Res* 1978;38:3197.

134. Rutman RJ, Steele WJ, Price CC. Experimental chemotherapy studies: I. Chemical and metabolic investigations of chloroquine mustard. *Cancer Res* 1961;21:1124.

135. Berenbaum MC. Histochemical evidence for crosslinking of DNA by alkylating agents in vivo. *Biochem Pharmacol* 1962;11:1035.

136. Klatt P, Stehlin JS Jr, McBride C, et al. The effect of nitrogen mustard treatment on the DNA of sensitive and resistant Ehrlich tumor cells. *Cancer Res* 1969;29:286.

137. Verly WG, Paquette Y. An endonuclease for depurinated DNA in *Escherichia coli* B. *Cancer J Biochem* 1972;50:217.

138. Hadi SM, Goldthwait DA. Endonuclease II of *Escherichia coli*: degradation of partially depurinated DNA. *Biochemistry* 1971;10:4986.

139. Burnotte J, Verly WG. Crosslinking of methylated DNA by moderate heating at neutral pH. *Biochim Biophys Acta* 1972;262:449.

140. Tew KD, Sudhakar S, Schein PS, et al. Binding of chlorozotocin and 1-(2-chloroethyl)-3-cyclohexyl-1-nitrosourea to chromatin and nucleosomal fractions of HeLa cells. *Cancer Res* 1978;38:3371.

141. Tew KD, Smulson ME, Schein PS. Molecular pharmacology of nitrosoureas. *Recent Results Cancer Res* 1981;76:130.

142. Lowe SW, Ruley HE, Jacks T, et al. P53-dependent apoptosis modulates the cytotoxicity of anticancer agents. *Cell* 1993;74:957.

143. Wolpert MK, Ruddon RW. A study on the mechanisms of resistance to nitrogen mustard (HN2) in Ehrlich ascites tumor cells: comparison of uptake of HN_2-^{14}C into sensitive and resistant cells. *Cancer Res* 1969;29:873.

144. Goldenberg GJ, Vanstone CL. Transport carrier for nitrogen mustard in HN2-sensitive and -resistant L5178Y lymphoblasts. *Clin Res* 1969;17:665.

145. Goldenberg GJ, Vanstone CL, Bihler I. Transport of nitrogen mustard on the transport-carrier for choline in L5178Y lymphoblasts. *Science* 1971;172:1148.

146. Goldenberg GJ, Lee M, Lam H-YP, et al. Evidence for carrier-mediated transport of melphalan by L5178Y lymphoblasts in vitro. *Cancer Res* 1977;37:755.

147. Vistica DT, Rabon A, Rabinowitz M. Effect of L-alpha-amino-gamma-guanidinobutyric acid on melphalan therapy of the L1210 murine leukemia. *Cancer Lett* 1979;6(6):345.

148. Begleiter A, Lam H-YP, Grover J, et al. Evidence for active transport of melphalan by two amino acid carriers in L5178Y lymphoblasts in vitro. *Cancer Res* 1979;39:353.

149. Vistica DT, Toal JN, Rabinowitz M. Amino acid conferred protection against melphalan: characterization of melphalan transport and correlation of uptake with cytotoxicity in cultured L1210 murine leukemia cells. *Biochem Pharmacol* 1978;27:2865.

150. Vistica DT. Cytotoxicity as an indicator for transport mechanism: evidence that murine bone marrow progenitor cells lack a high affinity leucine carrier that transports melphalan in murine L1210 leukemia cells. *Blood* 1980;56:427.

151. Begleiter A, Lam H-YP, Goldenberg GJ. Mechanism of uptake of nitrosourea by L5178Y lymphoblasts in vitro. *Cancer Res* 1977;37:1022.

152. Goldenberg GJ, Vanstone CL, Israels LG, et al. Evidence for a transport carrier of nitrogen mustard in nitrogen mustard-sensitive and -resistant L5178Y lymphoblasts. *Cancer Res* 1970;30:2285.

153. Rutman RJ, Chun EHL, Lewis FA. Permeability differences as a source of resistance to alkylating agents in Ehrlich tumor cells. *Biochem Biophys Res Commun* 1968;32:650.

154. Redwood WR, Colvin M. Transport of melphalan by sensitive and resistant L1210 cells. *Cancer Res* 1980;40:1144.

155. Hirono I. Non-protein sulphydryl group in the original strain and subline of the ascites tumour resistant to alkylating reagents. *Nature* 1960;186:1059.

156. Calcutt G, Connors TA. Tumour sulphydryl levels and sensitivity to the nitrogen mustard Merophan. *Biochem Pharmacol* 1963;12:839.

157. Hamilton TC, Winker MA, Lovie KG, et al. Augmentation of Adriamycin, melphalan and cisplatin cytotoxicity in drug-resistant and -sensitive human ovarian carcinoma cell lines by buthionine sulfoximine mediated glutathione depletion. *Biochem Pharmacol* 1985;34:2583.

158. Somfai-Relle S, Suzukake K, Vistica BP, et al. Reduction in cellular glutathione by buthionine sulfoximine and sensitization of murine tumor cells resistant to L-phenylalanine mustard. *Biochem Pharmacol* 1984;33:485.

159. Robson CN, Lewis AD, Wolf CR, et al. Reduced levels of drug-induced DNA crosslinking in nitrogen mustard-resistant Chinese hamster ovary cells expressing elevated glutathione *S*-transferase activity. *Cancer Res* 1987;47:6022.

160. Sladek NE. Bioassay and relative cytotoxic potency of cyclophosphamide metabolites generated in vitro and in vivo. *Cancer Res* 1973;33:1150.

161. Connors TA, Cox PJ, Farmer PB, et al. Some studies of the active intermediate formed in the microsomal metabolism of cyclophosphamide and isophosphamide. *Biochem Pharmacol* 1974;23:115.

162. Hilton J. Role of aldehyde dehydrogenase in cyclophosphamide-resistant L1210 leukemia. *Cancer Res* 1984;44:5156.

163. Crathorne AR, Roberts JJ. Mechanism of the cytotoxic action of alkylating agents in mammalian cells and evidence for the removal of alkylated groups from deoxyribonucleic acid. *Nature* 1966;211:150.

164. Cowan K, Batist G, Tulpule A, et al. Similar biochemical changes associated with multidrug resistance in human breast cancer cells and carcinogen-induced resistance in xenobiotics in rats. *Proc Natl Acad Sci U S A* 1986;83:9328.

164a. Kirsch D, Kastan M. Tumor-suppressor p53: implications for tumor development and prognosis. *J Clin Oncol* 1998;16:3158.

165. Goldenberg GJ. The role of drug transport in resistance to nitrogen mustard and other alkylating agents in L5178Y lymphoblasts. *Cancer Res* 1975;35:687.

166. Schabel FM Jr, Trader MW, Laster WR Jr, et al. Patterns of resistance and therapeutic synergism among alkylating agents. *Antibiot Chemother* 1978;23:200.

167. Antman K, Eder JP, Elias A, et al. High-dose combination alkylating agent preparative regimen with autologous bone marrow support: the Dana-Farber Cancer Institute/Beth Israel Hospital experience. *Cancer Treat Rep* 1987;71:19.

168. Puri RN, Meister A. Transport of glutathione as γ-glutamylcysteinylglycyl ester, into liver and kidney. *Proc Natl Acad Sci U S A* 1983;80:5258.

169. Teicher BA, Crawford JM, Holden SA, et al. Glutathione monoethylester can selectively protect liver from high-dose BCNU or cyclophosphamide. *Cancer* 1988;62:1275.

170. Meister A. Glutathione deficiency produced by inhibition of its synthesis, and its reversal: applications in research and therapy. *Pharmacol Ther* 1991;51:155.

171. Sekura R, Meister A. Covalent interaction of L-2-amino-4-oxo-5-chlorpentanoate at the glutamate binding site of γ-glutamylcystein synthetase. *J Biol Chem* 1977;252:2600.

172. Griffith WO, Meister A. Differential inhibition of glutamine and γ-glutamylcysteine synthetase by alpha alkyl analogues of methionine sulfoximine that induce convulsions. *J Biol Chem* 1978;253:2333.

173. Campbell EB, Hayward ML, Griffith OW. Analytical and preparative separation of the diastereomers of L-buthionine (*SR*)-sulfoximine, a potent inhibitor of glutathione biosynthesis. *Anal Biochem* 1991;194:268.

174. Kramer RA, Greene K, Ahmed S, et al. Chemosensitization of L-phenylalanine mustard by the thiol-modulating agent buthionine sulfoximine. *Cancer Res* 1987;47:1583.

175. O'Dwyer PJ, Hamilton TC, Young RC, et al. Depletion of glutathione in normal and malignant human cells in vivo by buthionine sulfoximine: clinical and biochemical results. *J Natl Cancer Inst* 1992;84:264.

176. Habig WH, Pabst MJ, Jakoby WB. Glutathione-S-transferases: the first enzymatic step in mercapturic acid formation. *J Biol Chem* 1974;249:7130.

177. Tew KD, Bomber AM, Hoffman SJ. Ethacrynic acid and piriprost as enhancers of cytotoxicity in drug-resistant and -sensitive cell lines. *Cancer Res* 1988;48:3622.

178. Clapper ML, Hoffman SJ, Tew KD. Sensitization of human colon tumor xenografts to L-phenylalanine mustard using ethacrynic acid. *J Cell Pharmacol* 1990;1:71.

179. O'Dwyer PJ, LaCreta F, Nash S, et al. Phase I study of thiotepa in combination with the glutathione transferase inhibitor ethacrynic acid. *Cancer Res* 1991;51:6059.

180. Schisselbauer J, Silber R, Papadopoulous E, et al. Characterization of lymphocyte glutathione-S-transferase isozymes in chronic lymphocytic leukemia (CLL). *Cancer Res* 1990;50:3569.

181. Davidson DE, Grenan MM, Sweeney TR. Biological characteristics of some improved radioprotectors. In: Brady L, ed. *Cancer management*, vol 5. New York: Masson Publishers, 1980:309.

182. Treskes M, Nijtmans LG, Fischinger-Schepman AM, et al. Effects of the modulating agent WR2721 and its main metabolites on the formation and stability of cisplatin-DNA adducts in vitro in comparison to the effects of thiosulfate and diethyldithiocarbamate. *Biochem Pharmacol* 1992;43:1013.

183. Yuhas JM, Spellman JM, Culo F. The role of WR-2721 in radiotherapy and/or chemotherapy. *Cancer Clin Trials* 1980;3:211.

184. Tew KD, Houghton PJ, Houghton JA, eds. *Preclinical and clinical modulation of anticancer drugs*. Boca Raton, FL: CRC Press, 1993:chap 3.

185. Glover D, Glick JH, Weiler C. WR2821 protects against the hematologic toxicity of cyclophosphamide: a controlled phase II trial. *J Clin Oncol* 1986;4:584.

186. Hospers GA, Eisenhauer EA, de Vries EG. The sulfhydryl containing compounds WR-2721 and glutathione as radio- and chemoprotective agents. A review, indications for use and prospects. *Br J Cancer* 1999;80:629.

187. Skipper HE, Schabel FM Jr, Trader MW, et al. Experimental evaluation of potential anticancer agents: VI. Anatomical distribution of leukemic cells and failure of chemotherapy. *Cancer Res* 1961;21:1154.

188. Day RS III, Ziolkowski CHJ, Scudiero DA, et al. Defective repair of alkylated DNA by human tumor and SV-40-transformed human cell strains. *Nature* 1980;288:724.

189. Tano K, Shiota S, Collier J, et al. Isolation and structural characterization of a cDNA clone encoding the human DNA repair protein for O^6-alkylguanine. *Proc Natl Acad Sci U S A* 1990;87:686.

190. Futscher BW, Micetich KC, Barnes DM, et al. Inhibition of a specific DNA repair system and nitrosourea cytotoxicity in resistant human cancer cells. *Cancer Commun* 1989;1:65.

191. Dolan ME, Corsico CD, Pegg AE. Exposure of HeLa cells to O^6-alkylguanines increases sensitivity to the cytotoxic effects of alkylating agents. *Biochem Biophys Res Commun* 1985;132:178.

192. Dolan ME, Morimoto K, Pegg AE. Reduction of O^6-alkylguanine-DNA-alkyltransferase activity in HeLa cells treated with O^6-alkylguanines. *Cancer Res* 1985;45:6413.

193. Karran P. Possible depletion of a DNA repair enzyme in human lymphoma cells by subversive repair. *Proc Natl Acad Sci U S A* 1985;82:5285.

194. Yarosh DB, Hurst-Calderone S, Babich MA, et al. Inactivation of O^6-methylguanine-DNA methyltransferase and

sensitization of human tumor cells to killing by chloroethyl-nitrosourea by O^6-methylguanine as a free base. *Cancer Res* 1986;46:1663.

195. Gerson SL, Trey JE. Modulation of nitrosourea resistance in myeloid leukemias. *Blood* 1988;71:1487.

196. Dolan ME, Larkin GL, English HF, et al. Depletion of O^6-alkylguanine-DNA alkyltransferase activity in mammalian tissues and human tumor xenografts in nude mice by treatment with O^6-methylguanine. *Cancer Chemother Pharmacol* 1989;25:103.

197. Gould ES. *Mechanism and structure in organic chemistry.* New York: Rinehart and Winston, 1959.

198. Yarosh DB. The role of O^6-methylguanine-DNA methyltransferase in cell survival, mutagenesis and carcinogenesis. *Mutat Res* 1985;145:1.

199. Dolan ME, Moschel RC, Pegg AE. Depletion of mammalian O^6-alkylguanine-DNA alkyltransferase activity by O^6-benzylguanine provides a means to evaluate the role of this protein in protection against carcinogenic and therapeutic alkylating agents. *Proc Natl Acad Sci U S A* 1990; 87:5368.

199a. Dolan ME, Pegg AE. O^6-Benzylguanine and its role in chemotherapy. *Clin Cancer Res* 1997;8:837.

199b. Schilsky RS, Dolan ME, Bertucci D, et al. Phase I clinical and pharmacological study of O^6-benzylguanine followed by carmustine in patients with advanced cancer. *Clin Cancer Res* 2000;6(8):3025.

199c. Friedman HS, Kokkinakis DM, Pluda J, et al. Phase I trial of O^6-benzylguanine for patients undergoing surgery for malignant glioma. *J Clin Oncol* 1998;16:3570.

199d. Dolan ME, Roy SK, Fasanmade AA, et al. O^6-Benzylguanine in humans: metabolic, pharmacokinetic and pharmacodynamic findings. *Clin Oncol* 1998;16:1803.

199e. Gerson SL, Schupp J, Liu L, et al. Leukocyte O^6-alkylguanine-DNA alkyltransferase from human donors is uniformly sensitive to O^6-benzylguanine. *Clin Cancer Res* 1999;5:521.

199f. Reese JS, Davis BM, Liu L, et al. Simultaneous protection of G156A methylguanine DNA methyltransferase gene-transduced hematopoietic progenitors and sensitization of tumor cells using O^6-benzylguanine and temozolomide. *Clin Cancer Res* 1999;5:163.

200. Bartlett PD, Ross SD, Swain CG. Kinetics and mechanisms of the reactions of tertiary β-chloroethylamines in solution: III. β-Chloroethyldiethylamine and tris-β-chloroethylamine. *J Am Chem Soc* 1949;71:1415.

201. Chang SY, Alberts DS, Farquhar D, et al. Hydrolysis and protein binding of melphalan. *J Pharm Sci* 1978;67:682.

202. Alberts DS, Chang SY, Chen H-SG, et al. Comparative pharmacokinetics of chlorambucil and melphalan in man. *Recent Results Cancer Res* 1980;74:124.

203. Alberts DS, Chang SY, Chen H-SG, et al. Pharmacokinetics and metabolism of chlorambucil in man: a preliminary report. *Cancer Treat Rev* 1979;6[Suppl]:9.

204. McLean A, Woods RC, Catovsky D, et al. Pharmacokinetics and metabolism of chlorambucil in patients with malignant disease. *Cancer Treat Rev* 1979;6[Suppl]:33.

205. Everett JL, Roberts JJ, Ross WCJ. Aryl-2-halogenoalkylamines: XII. Some carboxylic derivatives of *N, N*-di-2-chloroethylaniline. *J Chem Soc* 1953:2386.

206. Arnold H, Bourseaux F, Brock N. Neuartige Krebs-Chemotherapeutika aus der Gruppe der zyklischen *N*-Lost-Phosphamidester. *Naturwissenschaften* 1958;45:64.

207. Foley GE, Friedman OM, Drolet BP. Studies on the mechanism of action of Cytoxan: I. Evidence of activation in vivo. *Proc Am Assoc Cancer Res* 1960;3:111.

208. Brock N, Hohorst H-J. Uber die Aktivierung von Cyclophosphamid in vivo und in vitro. *Arzneimittelforschung* 1963;13:1021.

209. Cohen JL, Jao JY. Enzymatic basis of cyclophosphamide activation by hepatic microsomes of the rat. *J Pharmacol Exp Ther* 1970;174:206.

210. Friedman OM, Myles A, Colvin M. Cyclophosphamide and related phosphoramide mustards: current status and future prospects. In: Rosowsky A, ed. *Advances in cancer chemotherapy.* New York: Marcel Dekker, 1979:159.

211. Colvin M. A review of the pharmacology and clinical use of cyclophosphamide. In: Pinedo HM, ed. *Clinical pharmacology of antineoplastic drugs.* Amsterdam: Elsevier, 1978:245.

212. Struck RF, Kirk MC, Mellett LB, et al. Urinary metabolites of the antitumor agent cyclophosphamide. *Mol Pharmacol* 1971;7:519.

213. Bakke JE, Feil WJ, Fjelstul CE, et al. Metabolism of cyclophosphamide by sheep. *J Agric Food Chem* 1972;20:384.

214. Colvin M, Padgett CA, Fenselau C. A biologically active metabolite of cyclophosphamide. *Cancer Res* 1973;33:915.

215. Maddock CL, Handler AH, Friedman OM, et al. Primary evaluation of alkylating agent cyclohexylamine salt of *N,N*-bis(2-chloroethyl)phosphorodiamidic acid (NSC-69945; OMF-59) in experimental antitumor assay systems. *Cancer Chemother Rep* 1966;50:629.

216. Hohorst H-J, Draeger A, Peter G, et al. The problem of oncostatic specificity of cyclophosphamide (NSC-27271): studies on reactions that control the alkylating and cytotoxic activity. *Cancer Treat Rep* 1976;60:309.

217. Colvin M, Hilton J. Pharmacology of cyclophosphamide and metabolites. *Cancer Treat Rep* 1982;65[Suppl 3]:89.

218. DeJong JP, Nikkels PGJ, Brockbank KGM, et al. Comparative in vitro effects of cyclophosphamide derivatives on murine bone marrow-derived stromal and hemopoietic progenitor cell classes. *Cancer Res* 1985;45:4001.

219. Allen LM, Creaven PJ. In vitro activation of isophosphamide (NSC 109724), a new oxazaphosphorine, by rat-liver microsomes. *Cancer Chemother Rep* 1972;56:603.

220. Low JE, Borch RF, Sladek NE. Further studies on the conversion of 4-hydroxyoxaphosphorines to reactive mustards and acrolein in inorganic buffers. *Cancer Res* 1983;43:5815.

221. Colvin M. The comparative pharmacology of cyclophosphamide and ifosfamide. *Semin Oncol* 1982;9[Suppl 1]:2.

222. Chen TL, Kennedy MG, Karaly SB, et al. Nonlinear pharmacokinetics of cyclophosphamide and 4-hydroxycyclophosphamide aldophosphamide in patients with metastatic breast cancer receiving high dose chemotherapy followed by autologous bone marrow transplantation. *Drug Metab Dispos* 1997;25:544.

223. Hill DL, Kirk MC, Struck RF. Microsomal metabolism of nitrosoureas. *Cancer Res* 1975;35:296.

224. Levin VA, Stearns J, Byrd A, et al. The effect of phenobarbital pretreatment on the antitumor activity of 1,3-bis(2-

chloroethyl)-1-nitrosourea (BCNU), 1-(2-chloroethyl)-3-cyclohexyl-1-nitrosourea (CCNU) and 1-(2-chloroethyl)-3-(2,6-dioxo)-3-piperidyl-1-nitrosourea (PCNU), and on the plasma pharmacokinetics and biotransformation of BCNU. *J Pharmacol Exp Ther* 1979;208:1.

225. May HE, Boose R, Reed DJ. Hydroxylation of the carcinostatic 1-(2-chloroethyl)-3-cyclohexyl-1-nitrosourea (CCNU) by rat liver microsomes. *Biochem Biophys Res Commun* 1974;57:426.

226. Hilton J, Walker MD. Hydroxylation of 1-(2-chloroethyl)-3-cyclohexyl-1-nitrosourea. *Biochem Pharmacol* 1975;24:2153.

227. Wheeler GP, Johnston TP, Bowdon BJ, et al. Comparison of the properties of metabolites of CCNU. *Biochem Pharmacol* 1977;26:2331.

228. Reed DJ, May HE. Cytochrome P-450 interactions with the 2-chloroethylnitrosoureas and procarbazine. *Biochimie* 1978;60:989.

229. Alberts DS, Chang SY, Chen H-SG, et al. Kinetics of intravenous melphalan. *Clin Pharmacol Ther* 1979;26:73.

230. Tattersall MHN, Weinberg A. Pharmacokinetics of melphalan following oral or intravenous administration in patients with malignant disease. *Eur J Cancer* 1978;14:507.

231. Sviland L, Robinson A, Proctor SJ, et al. Interaction of cimetidine with oral melphalan. A pharmacokinetic study. *Cancer Chemother Pharmacol* 1987;20:173.

232. Pallante SL, Fenselau C, Mennel RG, et al. Quantitation by gas chromatography-chemical ionization-mass spectrometry of phenylalanine mustard in plasma of patients. *Cancer Res* 1980;40:2268.

233. Cornwell GG III, Pajak TF, McIntyre OR, et al. Influence of renal failure on myelosuppressive effects of melphalan: cancer and leukemia group B experience. *Cancer Treat Rep* 1982;66:475.

234. Alberts DS, Chen HSG, Benz D, et al. Effect of renal dysfunction in dogs on the disposition and marrow toxicity of melphalan. *Br J Cancer* 1981;43:330.

235. Howell SB, Pfeifle CE, Olshen RA. Intraperitoneal chemotherapy with melphalan. *Ann Intern Med* 1984;101:14.

235a. Alexander HR Jr, Bartlett DL, Libutti SK, et al. Isolated hepatic perfusion with tumor necrosis factor and melphalan for unresectable cancers confined to the liver. *J Clin Oncol* 1998;16(4):1479.

236. D'Incalci M, Bolis G, Facchinetti T, et al. Decreased half-life of cyclophosphamide in patients under continual treatment. *Eur J Cancer* 1979;19:7.

237. Juma FD, Rogers HJ, Trounce JR. Pharmacokinetics of cyclophosphamide and alkylating activity in man after intravenous and oral administration. *Br J Clin Pharmacol* 1979;8:209.

238. Jardine I, Fenselau C, Appler M, et al. Quantitation by gas chromatography–chemical ionization mass spectrometry of cyclophosphamide, phosphoramide mustard, and nornitrogen mustard in the plasma and urine of patients receiving cyclophosphamide therapy. *Cancer Res* 1978;38:408.

239. Erlichman C, Soldin SJ, Hardy RW, et al. Disposition of cyclophosphamide on two consecutive cycles of treatment in patients with ovarian carcinoma. *Arzneimittelforschung* 1988;38:839.

240. Moore MJ, Hardy RW, Thiessen JJ, et al. Rapid development of enhanced clearance after high-dose cyclophosphamide. *Clin Pharmacol Ther* 1988;44:622.

241. Egorin MJ, Forrest A, Belani CP, et al. A limited sampling strategy for cyclophosphamide pharmacokinetics. *Cancer Res* 1989;49:3129.

242. Sladak NE, Doeden D, Powers JF, et al. Plasma concentrations of 4-hydroxycyclophosphamide and phosphoramide mustard in patients repeatedly given high doses of cyclophosphamide in preparation for bone marrow transplantation. *Cancer Treat Rep* 1984;68:1247.

243. Struck RF, Alberts DS, Horne K, et al. Plasma pharmacokinetics of cyclophosphamide and its cytotoxic metabolites after intravenous versus oral administration in a randomized, crossover trial. *Cancer Res* 1987;47:2723.

244. Brock N, Gross R, Hohorst H-J, et al. Activation of cyclophosphamide in man and animals. *Cancer* 1971;27:1512.

245. Bagley CM Jr, Bostick FW, DeVita VT Jr. Clinical pharmacology of cyclophosphamide. *Cancer Res* 1973;33:226.

246. Phillipou G, Seaborn CJ, Raniolo E. Reproducibility of methods relating to cyclophosphamide metabolic structures. *J Natl Cancer Inst* 1993;85:1249.

247. Juma FD, Rogers HJ, Trounce JR. The pharmacokinetics of cyclophosphamide, phosphoramide mustard and nor-nitrogen mustard studied by gas chromatography in patients receiving cyclophosphamide therapy. *Br J Clin Pharmacol* 1980;10:327.

248. Fenselau C, Kan M-NN, Subba Rao S, et al. Identification of aldophosphamide as a metabolite of cyclophosphamide in vitro and in vivo in humans. *Cancer Res* 1977;37:2538.

249. Wagner T, Peter G, Voelcker G, et al. Characterization and quantitative estimation of activated cyclophosphamide in blood and urine. *Cancer Res* 1977;37:2592.

250. Wagner T, Heydrich D, Voelcker G, et al. Characterization and quantitative estimation of activated cyclophosphamide in blood and urine. *Cancer Res Clin Oncol* 1980;96:79.

251. Graham MI, Shaw IC, Souhami RL, et al. Decreased plasma half-life of cyclophosphamide during repeated high-dose administration. *Cancer Chemother Pharmacol* 1983;10:192.

252. Crook R, Souhami RL, McLean AEM. Cytotoxicity, DNA crosslinking, and single strand breaks induced by activated cyclophosphamide and acrolein in human leukemia cells. *Cancer Res* 1980;46:5029.

253. Sensenbrenner LL, Marini JJ, Colvin M. Comparative effects of cyclophosphamide, isophosphamide, 4-methylcyclophosphamide and phosphoramide mustard on murine hematopoietic and immunocompetent cells. *J Natl Cancer Inst* 1979;62:975.

254. Brock N. Comparative pharmacologic study in vitro and in vivo with cyclophosphamide (NSC-26271), cyclophosphamide metabolites, and plain nitrogen mustard compounds. *Cancer Treat Rep* 1976;60:301.

255. Field RB, Gang M, Kline I, et al. The effect of phenobarbital or 2-diethylaminoethyl-2,2-diphenylvalerate on the activation of cyclophosphamide in vivo. *J Pharmacol Exp Ther* 1972;180:475.

256. Jao JY, Jusko WJ, Cohen JL. Phenobarbital effects on cyclophosphamide pharmacokinetics in man. *Cancer Res* 1972; 32:2761.

257. Egorin M, Kaplan R, Salcman M, et al. Plasma and cerebrospinal fluid (CSF) pharmacokinetics of cyclophosphamide (CYC) in patients treated with and without dimethyl sulfoxide (DMSO). *Proc Am Assoc Cancer Res* 1981;22:210.

258. Alberts DS, van Daalen Wetters T. The effects of phenobarbital on cyclophosphamide antitumor activity. *Cancer Res* 1976;36:2785.

259. Sladek N. Therapeutic efficacy of cyclophosphamide as a function of its metabolism. *Cancer Res* 1972;32:535.

260. Mouridsen HT, Jacobson E. Pharmacokinetics of cyclophosphamide in renal failure. *Acta Pharmacol Toxicol* 1975;36:409.

261. Humphrey RL, Kvols LK. The influence of renal insufficiency on cyclophosphamide-induced hematopoietic depression and recovery. *Proc Am Assoc Cancer Res* 1974;15:84.

262. Creaven PJ, Allen LM, Alford DA, et al. Clinical pharmacology of isophosphamide. *Clin Pharmacol Ther* 1974; 16:77.

263. Allen LM, Creaven PJ. Pharmacokinetics of ifosfamide. *Clin Pharmacol Ther* 1975;17:492.

264. Nelson RL, Allen LM, Creaven PJ. Pharmacokinetics of divided-dose ifosfamide. *Clin Pharmacol Ther* 1976; 19:365.

265. Brade WP, Herdrich K, Varini M. Ifosfamide—pharmacology, safety and therapeutic potential. *Cancer Treat Rev* 1985;12:1.

266. Boddy AV, Cole M, Pearson ADJ, et al. The kinetics of the auto-induction of ifosfamide metabolism during continuous infusion. *Cancer Chemother Pharmacol* 1995;36:53.

267. Norpoth K. Studies on the metabolism of isophosphamide (NSC-109724) in man. *Cancer Treat Rep* 1976;60:437.

268. Cohen BE, Egorin ME, Kohlhepp EA, et al. Human plasma pharmacokinetics and urinary excretion of thiotepa and its metabolites. *Cancer Treat Rep* 1986;70:859.

269. Heideman RL, Cole DE, Balis F, et al. Phase I and pharmacokinetic evaluation of thiotepa in the cerebrospinal fluid and plasma of pediatric patients: evidence for dose-dependent plasma clearance of thiotepa. *Cancer Res* 1989;49:736.

270. Hogan B. Pharmacokinetics of thiotepa and tepa in the conventional dose-range and its correlation to myelosuppressive effects. *Cancer Chemother Pharmacol* 1991; 27:373.

271. O'Dwyer PJ, LaCreta F, Engstrom PF, et al. Phase I/pharmacokinetic reevaluation of thiotepa. *Cancer Res* 1991; 51:3171.

272. Kletzel M, Kearns GL, Thompson HC Jr. Pharmacokinetics of high-dose thiotepa in children undergoing autologous bone marrow transplantation. *Bone Marrow Transplant* 1992;10:171.

273. O'Dwyer PJ, LaCreta F, Schilder R, et al. Phase I trial of thiotepa in combination with recombinant human granulocyte-macrophage colony-stimulating factor. *J Clin Oncol* 1992;10:1352.

274. DeVita VT, Denham C, Davidson JD, et al. The physiological disposition of the carcinostatic 1,3-bis(2-chloroethyl)-1-nitrosourea (BCNU) in man and animals. *Clin Pharmacol Ther* 1965;8:566.

275. Levin VA, Hoffman W, Weinkam RJ. Pharmacokinetics of BCNU in man: a preliminary study of 20 patients. *Cancer Treat Rep* 1978;62:1305.

276. Henner WD, Peters WP, Eder JP, et al. Pharmacokinetics and immediate effects of high-dose carmustine in man. *Cancer Treat Rep* 1986;70:877.

276a. Jones RB et al. Nitrosoureas. In: Grochow LB, Ames MM, eds. *A clinician's guide to chemotherapy pharmacokinetics and pharmacodynamics*. Baltimore: Williams & Wilkins, 1998:331.

277. Hassan M, Ehrsson H. Urinary metabolites of busulfan in the rat. *Drug Metab Dispos* 1987;15:399.

277a. Hassan M, Öberg G, Ehrsson H, et al. Pharmacokinetic and metabolic studies of high-dose busulphan in adults. *Eur J Clin Pharmacol* 1989;36:525.

277b. Chen T-L, Grochow LB, Hurowitz LA, et al. Determination of busulfan in human plasma by gas chromatography with electron-capture detection. *J Chromatogr* 1988; 425:303.

277c. Grochow LB, Jones RJ, Brundrett RB, et al. Pharmacokinetics of busulfan: correlation with veno-occlusive disease in patients undergoing bone marrow transplantation. *Cancer Chemother Pharmacol* 1989;25:55.

277d. Vassal G, Fischer A, Challine D, et al. Busulfan disposition below the age of three: alteration in children with lysosomal storage disease. *Blood* 1993;82:1030.

278. Grochow LB, Krivit W, Whitley CB, et al. Busulfan disposition in children. *Blood* 1990;75:1723.

279. Hassan M, Ehrsson H, Smedmyr B, et al. Cerebrospinal fluid and plasma concentrations of busulfan during high-dose therapy. *Bone Marrow Transplant* 1989;4:113.

280. Hassan M, Thorell J-O, Warne N, et al. ^{11}C-labeling of busulphan. *Appl Radiat Isot* 1991;42:1055.

281. Grigg AP, Shepherd JD, Phillips GL. Busulphan and phenytoin. *Ann Intern Med* 1989;111:1049.

282. Nissen-Meyer R, Host H. A comparison between the hematological side effects of cyclophosphamide and nitrogen mustard. *Cancer Chemother Rep* 1960;9:51.

283. Mullins GM, Colvin M. Intensive cyclophosphamide therapy in solid tumors. *Cancer Chemother Rep* 1975; 59:411.

284. Botnick LE, Hannon EC, Hellman S. Multisystem stem cell failure after apparent recovery from alkylating agents. *Cancer Res* 1978;38:1942.

285. Penta JS, Poster DS, Bruno S, et al. Clinical trials with antiemetic agents in cancer patients receiving chemotherapy. *J Clin Pharmacol* 1981;21:11S.

286. Borison HL, Brand ED, Orkand RK. Emetic action of nitrogen mustard (mechlorethamine hydrochloride) in dogs and cats. *Am J Physiol* 1968;192:410.

287. Ohner H, Schwartz R, Rubio F, et al. Interstitial pulmonary fibrosis following busulfan therapy. *Am J Med* 1961; 31:134.

288. Burn WA, McFarland W, Matthews MJ. Busulfan-induced pulmonary disease. *Am Rev Respir Dis* 1970;101:408.

289. Willson JKV. Pulmonary toxicity of antineoplastic drugs. *Cancer Treat Rep* 1978;62:2003.

290. Koss LG, Melamed MR, Mayer K. The effect of busulfan on human epithelia. *Am J Clin Pathol* 1965;44:385.

291. Littler WA, Ogilvie C. Lung function in patients receiving busulfan. *BMJ* 1970;4:530.

292. Kreisman H, Wolkove N. Pulmonary toxicity of antineoplastic therapy. *Semin Oncol* 1992;19:508.

293. Mark GJ, Lehimgar-Zadeh A, Ragsdale BD. Cyclophosphamide pneumonitis. *Thorax* 1978;33:89.

294. Patel AR, Shah PC, Rhee HC, et al. Cyclophosphamide therapy and interstitial pulmonary fibrosis. *Cancer* 1976;38:1542.

295. Radin AE, Haggard ME, Travis LB. Lung changes and chemotherapeutic agents in childhood. *Am J Dis Child* 1970;120:337.

296. Bailey CC, Marsden HB, Jones PH. Fatal pulmonary fibrosis following 1,3-bis(2-chloroethyl-1-nitrosourea (BCNU) therapy. *Cancer* 1978;42:74.

297. Crittenden D, Tranum BL, Hunt A. Pulmonary fibrosis after prolonged therapy with 1,3-bis(2-chloroethyl)-1-nitrosourea. *Chest* 1977;72:372.

298. Holoye PY, Jenkins DE, Greenberg SD. Pulmonary toxicity in long-term administration of BCNU. *Cancer Treat Rep* 1976;60:1691.

299. Lee W, Moore RP, Wampler GL. Interstitial pulmonary fibrosis as a complication of prolonged methyl-CCNU therapy. *Cancer Treat Rep* 1978;62:1355.

300. Hundley RF, Lukens JN. Nitrosourea-associated pulmonary fibrosis. *Cancer Treat Rep* 1979;63:2128.

301. Litam JP, Dail DH, Spitzer G, et al. Early pulmonary toxicity after administration of high-dose BCNU. *Cancer Treat Rep* 1981;65:39.

302. Moinuddin M. Radionuclide scanning in the detection of drug-induced lung disorders. *J Thorac Imag* 1991;6:62.

303. Codling BW, Chakera TM. Pulmonary fibrosis following therapy with melphalan for multiple myeloma. *J Clin Pathol* 1972;25:668.

304. Jacobs S. The Hamman-Rich syndrome following treatment of lymphoma with chlorambucil. *J La State Med Soc* 1975;127:311.

305. Cole RC, Myers TJ, Klatsky AU. Pulmonary disease with chlorambucil therapy. *Cancer* 1978;41:455.

306. Orwoll ES, Kiessling PJ, Patterson JR. Interstitial pneumonia from mitomycin. *Ann Intern Med* 1978;89:352.

307. Lampert F. Lungenveranderungen bei der akuten lymphoblastischen Leukamie. *Radiologe* 1968;8:308.

308. Okita H, Ito L, Taketomi T, et al. Four patients with leukemia who showed especially atypical type of interstitial pneumonia, probably caused following the administration of antileukemic drugs [author's translation]. *Jpn J Clin Hematol* 1974;15:764.

309. Rubin G, Baume P, Vandenberg R. Azathioprine and acute restrictive lung disease. *Aust N Z J Med* 1972;2:272.

310. Philips FS, Sternberg SS, Cronin AP, et al. Cyclophosphamide and urinary bladder toxicity. *Cancer Res* 1961;21:1577.

311. Forni AM, Koss LG, Geller W. Cytological study of the effect of cyclophosphamide on the epithelium of the urinary bladder in man. *Cancer* 1964;17:1348.

312. Rubin JS, Rubin RT. Cyclophosphamide hemorrhagic cystitis. *J Urol* 1966;96:313.

313. Bellin HJ, Cherry JM, Koss LG. Effects of a single dose of cyclophosphamide: V. Protection effect of diversion of the urinary stream on dog bladder. *Lab Invest* 1974;30:43.

314. Cox PJ. Cyclophosphamide cystitis—identification of acrolein as the causative agent. *Biochem Pharmacol* 1979;28:2045.

315. Primack A. Amelioration of cyclophosphamide-induced cystitis. *J Natl Cancer Inst* 1971;47:223.

316. Van Dyk JJ, Falkson HC, van Der Merwe AM, et al. Unexpected toxicity in patients treated with iphosphamide. *Cancer Res* 1972;32:921.

317. Botta JA Jr, Nelson LW, Weikel JN Jr. Acetylcysteine in the prevention of cyclophosphamide-induced cystitis in rats. *J Natl Cancer Inst* 1973;51:1051.

318. Kline I, Gang M, Venditti JM. Protection with *N*-acetylcysteine (NAC) against isophosphamide (ISOPH, NSC-10924) host toxicity and enhancement of therapy in early murine leukemia L1210. *Proc Am Assoc Cancer Res* 1972;13:29.

319. Scheef W, Klein HO, Brock N, et al. Controlled clinical studies with an antidote against the urotoxicity of oxazaphosphorines: preliminary results. *Cancer Treat Rep* 1979;63:501.

320. Andriole GL, Sandlund JT, Miser JS, et al. The efficacy of Mesna (2-mercaptoethane sodium sulfonate) as a uroprotectant in patients with hemorrhagic cystitis receiving further oxazaphosphorine chemotherapy. *J Clin Oncol* 1987;5:799.

321. Godec CJ, Gleich P. Intractable hematuria and formalin. *J Urol* 1983;130:688.

322. Ostroff EB, Chenault OW Jr. Alum irrigation for the control of massive bladder hemorrhage. *J Urol* 1982;128:929.

323. Goel AK, Rao MS, Bhagwat S, et al. Intravesical irrigation with alum for the control of massive bladder hemorrhage. *J Urol* 1985;133:956.

324. Fernbach DJ. Chemotherapy for acute leukemia in children: comparison of cyclophosphamide (NSC-26271) and 6-mercaptopurine (NSC-755). *Cancer Chemother Rep* 1967;51:381.

325. DeFronzo RA, Abeloff M, Braine H, et al. Renal dysfunction after treatment with isophosphamide (NSC-109724). *Cancer Chemother Rep* 1974;58(3):375.

326. Moncrieff M, Foot A. Fanconi syndrome after ifosfamide. *Cancer Chemother Pharmacol* 1989;23:121.

327. Manohoran A. Carcinoma of the urinary bladder in patients receiving cyclophosphamide. *Aust N Z J Med* 1984;14:507.

328. DeFronzo RA, Braine HG, Colvin M, et al. Water intoxication in man after cyclophosphamide therapy. *Ann Intern Med* 1973;78:861.

329. Green TP, Mirkin BL. Prevention of cyclophosphamide-induced antidiuresis by furosemide infusion. *Clin Pharmacol Ther* 1981;29:634.

330. Harlow PJ, DeClerck YA, Shore NA, et al. A fatal case of inappropriate ADH secretion induced by cyclophosphamide therapy. *Cancer* 1979;44:896.

331. Carter SK, Newman JW. Nitrosoureas: 1,3-bis(2-chloro-

ethyl)-1-nitrosourea (NSC-409962; BCNU) and 1-(2-chloroethyl)-3-cyclohexyl-1-nitrosourea (NSC-70937; CCNU)—clinical brochure. *Cancer Chemother Rep 3* 1968;1:115.

332. Silver HKB, Morton DL. CCNU nephrotoxicity following sustained remission in oat cell carcinoma. *Cancer Treat Rep* 1979;63:226.

333. Schacht RG, Baldwin DS. Chronic interstitial nephritis and renal failure due to nitrosourea (NU) therapy. *Kidney Int* 1978;14:661.

334. Harmon WE, Cohen HJ, Schneeberger EE, et al. Chronic renal failure in children treated with methyl CCNU. *N Engl J Med* 1979;300:1200.

335. Bierman HR, Kelly KH, Knudson AG Jr, et al. The influence of 1,4-dimethylsulfonoxy-1,4-dimethylbutane (CB 2348, dimethyl Myleran) in neoplastic disease. *Ann N Y Acad Sci* 1958;68:1211.

336. Feil VS, Lamoureaux CJH. Alopecia activity of cyclophosphamide metabolites and related compounds in sheep. *Cancer Res* 1974;34:2596.

337. Nathanson L, Hall TC, Rutenberg A, et al. Clinical toxicologic study of cyclohexylamine salt of *N*, *N*-bis(2-chloroethyl)-phosphorodiamidic acid (NSC-69945; OMF-59). *Cancer Chemother Rep* 1967;51:35.

338. Ganci L, Serrou B. Changes in hair pigmentation associated with cancer chemotherapy. *Cancer Treat Rep* 1980; 64:193.

339. Hennessy JD. Alopecia and cytotoxic drugs. *BMJ* 1966; 2:1138.

340. Dean JC, Salmon SE, Griffith KS. Prevention of doxorubicin-induced hair loss with scalp hypothermia. *N Engl J Med* 1980;301:1427.

341. Lakin JD, Cahill RA. Generalized urticaria to cyclophosphamide: type I hypersensitivity to an immunosuppressive agent. *J Allergy Clin Immunol* 1976;58:160.

342. Ross WE, Chabner BA. Allergic reaction to cyclophosphamide in a mechlorethamine-sensitive patient. *Cancer Treat Rep* 1977;61:495.

343. Karchmer RK, Hansen BL. Possible anaphylactic reaction to intravenous cyclophosphamide. *JAMA* 1977; 237:475.

344. Legha SS, Hall S. Acute cyclophosphamide hypersensitivity reaction: possible lack of cross-sensitivity to mechlorethamine and isophosphamide. *Cancer Treat Rep* 1978; 62:180.

345. Cornwell GG III, Pajak TF, McIntyre OR. Hypersensitivity reactions to IV melphalan during treatment of multiple myeloma: cancer and leukemia group B experience. *Cancer Treat Rep* 1979;63:399.

346. Weiss RB, Bruno S. Hypersensitivity reactions to cancer chemotherapeutic agents. *Ann Intern Med* 1981;94:66.

347. Spitz S. The histological effects of nitrogen mustards on human tumors and tissues. *Cancer* 1948;1:383.

348. DeRooij DG, Kramer MR. The effects of three alkylating agents on the seminiferous epithelium of rodents. *Virchows Arch (Zellpathol)* 1969;4:267.

349. Richter P, Calamera JC, Morgenfeld MC, et al. Effect of chlorambucil on spermatogenesis in the human with malignant lymphoma. *Cancer* 1970;25:1026.

350. Miller DG. Alkylating agents and human spermatogenesis. *JAMA* 1971;217:1662.

351. Fairley KF, Barrie JU, Johnson W. Sterility and testicular atrophy related to cyclophosphamide therapy. *Lancet* 1972;1:568.

352. Kumar R, Biggart JD, McEvoy J, et al. Cyclophosphamide and reproductive function. *Lancet* 1972;1:1212.

353. Sherins RJ, DeVita VT. Effect of drug treatment for lymphoma on male reproductive capacity. *Ann Intern Med* 1973;79:216.

354. Hinkes E, Plotkin D. Reversible drug-induced sterility in a patient with acute leukemia. *JAMA* 1973;223:1490.

355. Blake DA, Heller RH, Hsu SH, et al. Return of fertility in a patient with cyclophosphamide-induced azoospermia. *Johns Hopkins Med J* 1976;139:20.

356. Galton DAG, Till M, Wiltshaw E. Busulfan (1,4-dimethylsulfonoxy-butane, Myleran): summary of clinical results. *Ann N Y Acad Sci* 1958;68:967.

357. Miller JJ, Williams GF, Leissring JC. Multiple late complications of therapy with cyclophosphamide, including ovarian destruction. *Am J Med* 1971;50:530.

358. Fosdick WM, Parson JL, Hill DF. Long-term cyclophosphamide therapy in rheumatoid arthritis. *Arthritis Rheum* 1968;11:151.

359. Kyoma H, Wada T, Nishizawa T, et al. Cyclophosphamide-induced ovarian failure and its therapeutic significance in patients with breast cancer. *Cancer* 1977;39:1403.

360. Rose DP, Davis TE. Ovarian function in patients receiving adjuvant chemotherapy for breast cancer. *Lancet* 1977; 1:1174.

361. Haskin D. Some effects of nitrogen mustard on the development of external body form in the fetal rat. *Anat Rec* 1948;102:493.

362. Bodenstein D. The effects of nitrogen mustard on embryonic amphibian development. *J Exp Zool* 1948;108:93.

363. Bodenstein D, Goldin A. A comparison of the effects of various nitrogen mustard compounds on embryonic cells. *J Exp Zool* 1948;108:75.

364. Murphy ML, Karnofsky DA. Effect of azaserine and other growth-inhibiting agents on fetal development of the rat. *Cancer* 1956;9:955.

365. Murphy ML, Del Moro A, Lacon C. The comparative effects of five poly-functional alkylating agents on the rat fetus, with additional notes. *Ann N Y Acad Sci* 1958; 68:762.

366. Klein NW, Vogler MA, Chatot CL, et al. The use of cultured rat embryos to evaluate the teratogenic activity of serum: cadmium and cyclophosphamide. *Teratology* 1958;21:199.

367. Gibson JE, Becker BA. Teratogenicity of structural truncates of cyclophosphamide in mice. *Teratology* 1971; 4:141.

368. Sadler TW, Kochhar DM. Chlorambucil-induced cell death in embryonic mouse limb buds. *Toxicol Appl Pharmacol* 1976;37:237.

369. Brummett ES, Johnson EM. Morphological alterations in the developing fetal rat limb due to maternal injection of chlorambucil. *Teratology* 1979;20:279.

370. Nicholson HO. Cytotoxic drugs in pregnancy. *J Obstet Gynaecol Br Commonw* 1968;75:307.

371. Steege JF, Caldwell DS. Renal agenesis after first trimester exposure to chlorambucil. *South Med J* 1980;73:1414.

372. Toledo TM, Harper RC, Moser RH. Fetal effects during cyclophosphamide and irradiation therapy. *Ann Intern Med* 1971;74:87.

373. Garrett MJ. Teratogenic effects of combination chemotherapy. *Ann Intern Med* 1974;80:667.

374. Ortega J. Multiple agent chemotherapy including bleomycin of non-Hodgkin's lymphoma during pregnancy. *Cancer* 1977;40:2829.

375. Lergier JE, Jiminez E, Maldonado N, et al. Normal pregnancy in multiple myeloma treated with cyclophosphamide. *Cancer* 1974;34:1018.

376. Kyle RA, Pierce RV, Bayrd ED. Multiple myeloma and acute myelomonocytic leukemia. *N Engl J Med* 1970;283:1121.

377. Rosner F, Grunwald H. Multiple myeloma terminating in acute leukemia. *Am J Med* 1974;57:927.

378. Rosner F, Grunwald H. Hodgkin's disease and acute leukemia. *Am J Med* 1975;58:339.

379. Einhorn N. Acute leukemia after chemotherapy (melphalan). *Cancer* 1978;41:444.

380. Seiidenfeld AM, Smythe HA, Ogryzlo MA, et al. Acute leukemia in rheumatoid arthritis treated with cytotoxic agents. *J Rheumatol* 1976;3:295.

381. Hochberg MC, Shulman LE. Acute leukemia following cyclophosphamide therapy for Sjögren's syndrome. *Johns Hopkins Med J* 1978;142:211.

382. Steigbigel RT, Kim H, Potolsky A, et al. Acute myeloproliferative disorder following long-term chlorambucil therapy. *Arch Intern Med* 1974;134:728.

383. Cardamone JM, Kimmerle RI, Marshall EY. Development of acute erythroleukemia in B-cell immunoproliferative disorders after prolonged therapy with alkylating drugs. *Am J Med* 1974;57:837.

384. Cohen RJ, Wiernik PH, Walker MD. Acute nonlymphocytic leukemia associated with nitrosourea chemotherapy: report of two cases. *Cancer Treat Rep* 1976;60:1257.

385. Reimer RR, Hoover R, Fraumeni JF Jr, et al. Acute leukemia after alkylating-agent therapy of ovarian cancer. *N Engl J Med* 1977;297:177.

386. Tucker MA, Coleman CN, Cox RS, et al. Risk of second cancers after treatment for Hodgkin's disease. *N Engl J Med* 1988;318:76.

387. Green MH, Harris EL, Gershenson DM, et al. Melphalan may be a more potent leukemogen than cyclophosphamide. *Ann Intern Med* 1986;105:360.

388. Penn I. Second malignant neoplasms associated with immunosuppressive medications. *Cancer* 1976;37:1024.

389. Lazarus HM, Herzig RH, Graham-Pole J, et al. Intensive melphalan chemotherapy and cryopreserved autologous bone marrow transplantation for the treatment of refractory cancer. *J Clin Oncol* 1983;1:359.

390. Leff RS, Thompson JM, Mosley KR, et al. Phase II trial of high-dose melphalan and autologous bone marrow transplantation for metastatic colon carcinoma. *J Clin Oncol* 1986;4:1586.

391. Takvorian T, Canellos GP, Ritz J, et al. Prolonged disease-free survival after autologous bone marrow transplantation in patients with non-Hodgkin's lymphoma with a poor prognosis. *N Engl J Med* 1987;316:1499.

392. Morgan M, Dodds A, Atkinson K, et al. The toxicity of busulfan and cyclophosphamide as the preparative regimen for bone marrow transplantation. *Br J Haematol* 1990;77:529.

393. McElwain TJ, Hedley DW, Gordon MY, et al. High dose melphalan and non-cryopressed autologous bone marrow treatment of malignant melanoma and neuroblastoma. *Exp Hematol* 1979;7[Suppl 5]:360.

394. Rollins BJ. Hepatic venoocclusive disease. *Am J Med* 1988;81:297.

395. Grochow LB, Piantadosi S, Santos G, et al. Busulfan dose adjustment decreases the risk of venoocclusive disease in patients undergoing bone marrow transplantation. *Proc Am Assoc Cancer Res* 1992;33:200.

396. Phillips GL, Fay JW, Wolff SN, et al. 1,3-Bis (2-chloroethyl)-1-nitrosourea (BCNU) and autologous bone marrow transplantation (BMTX) for refractory malignancy. *Proc Am Assoc Cancer Res* 1980;21:180.

397. Takvorian T, Parker LM, Hochberg FH, et al. Single high dose of BCNU with autologous bone marrow (ABM). *Proc Am Soc Clin Oncol* 1980;21:341.

398. Steinberg SS, Philips FS, Scholler J. Pharmacological and pathological effects of alkylating agents. *Ann N Y Acad Sci* 1958;68:811.

399. Patel SR, Forman AD, Benjamin RS. High-dose ifosfamide-induced exacerbation of peripheral neuropathy. *J Natl Cancer Inst* 1994;86:305.

400. Bethlenfalvay NC, Bergin JJ. Severe cerebral toxicity after intravenous nitrogen mustard therapy. *Cancer* 1972;29:366.

401. Pratt CB, Green AA, Horowitz ME, et al. Central nervous system toxicity following the treatment of pediatric patients with ifosfamide/mesna. *J Clin Oncol* 1986;4:1253.

402. Curtin JP, Koonings PP, Gutierrez M, et al. Ifosfamide-induced neurotoxicity. *Gynecol Oncol* 1991;42:193.

403. Goren MP, Right RK, Pratt CB, et al. Dechlorethylation of ifosfamide and neurotoxicity. *Lancet* 1986;2:1219.

404. Antman KH, Montella D, Rosenbaum C, et al. Phase II trial of ifosfamide with mesna in previously treated metastatic sarcoma. *Cancer Treat Rep* 1985;69:499.

405. Pratt CB, Goren MP, Meyer WH, et al. Ifosfamide neurotoxicity is related to previous treatment for pediatric solid tumors. *J Clin Oncol* 1990;8:1399.

406. Thigpen T. Ifosfamide-induced central nervous system toxicity [Editorial]. *Gynecol Oncol* 1991;42:191.

407. Colvin M, Santos GW. High dose cyclophosphamide administration in man. *Proc Am Assoc Cancer Res* 1970;11:17.

408. Buckner CD, Rudolph RJ, Fefer A, et al. High dose cyclophosphamide therapy for malignant disease. *Cancer* 1972;29:357.

409. Steinherz LJ, Steinherz PG. Cyclophosphamide cardiotoxicity. *Cancer Bull* 1985;37:231.

410. Slavin RE, Millan JC, Mullins GM. Pathology of high dose intermittent cyclophosphamide therapy. *Hum Pathol* 1975;6:693.

411. Hektoen L, Corper HJ. The effect of mustard gas (dichloroethyl-sulphide) on antibody formation. *J Infect Dis* 1921;28:279.

412. Philips FS, Hopkins FH, Freeman MLH. Effects of tris(beta-chloroethyl)amine on antibody-production in goats. *J Immunol* 1947;55:289.

413. Spurr CL. Influence of nitrogen mustards on the antibody response. *Proc Soc Exp Biol Med* 1947;64:259.

414. Makinodan T, Santos GW, Quinn RP. Immunosuppressive drugs. *Pharmacol Rev* 1970;22:189.

415. Sensenbrenner LL, Owens AH Jr, Heiby JR, et al. Comparative effects of cytotoxic agents on transplanted hematopoietic and antibody-producing cells. *J Natl Cancer Inst* 1973;50:1027.

416. Berenbaum CC, Brown IN. Dose-response relationships for agents inhibiting the immune response. *Immunology* 1964;7:65.

417. Santos GW, Owens AH Jr. 19S and 7S antibody production in the cyclophosphamide- or methotrexate-treated rat. *Nature* 1966;209:622.

418. Owens AH Jr, Santos GW. The effect of cytotoxic drugs on graft-versus-host disease in mice. *Transplantation* 1971; 11:378.

419. Many A, Schwartz RS. On the mechanisms of immunological tolerance in cyclophosphamide-treated mice. *Clin Exp Immunol* 1970;6:87.

420. Larman SP, Weidanz WO. The effect of cyclophosphamide on the ontogeny of the humoral immune response in chickens. *J Immunol* 1970;105:614.

421. Turk JL, Paulter LW. Selective depletion of lymphoid tissue by cyclophosphamide. *Clin Exp Immunol* 1972; 10:285.

422. Turk JL. Studies on the mechanism of action of methotrexate and cyclophosphamide on contact sensitivity in the guinea pig. *Int Arch Allergy* 1964;24:191.

423. Maguire HC, Ettore VL. Enhancement of dinitrochlorobenzene (DNCB) contact sensitization by cyclophosphamide in the guinea pig. *J Invest Dermatol* 1967; 48:39.

424. Stevenson HC, Fauci AS. XII. Differential effects of in vitro cyclophosphamide on human lymphocyte subpopulations involved in B-cell activation. *Immunology* 1980; 39:391.

425. Shand FL, Howard JG. Cyclophosphamide inhibited B-cell receptor regeneration as a basis for drug-induced tolerance. *Nature* 1978;271:255.

426. Ozer H, Cowens JW, Nussbaum A, et al. Human immunoregulatory T subset function defined in vitro by cyclophosphamide metabolites. *Fed Proc* 1981;40:1075.

427. Mullins GM, Anderson PN, Santos GW. High dose cyclophosphamide therapy in solid tumors. *Cancer* 1975; 36:1950.

428. Santos GW. Immunological toxicity of cancer chemotherapy. *Recent Results Cancer Res* 1974;49:20.

429. Santos GW, Sensenbrenner LL, Anderson PN, et al. HL-A-identical marrow transplants in aplastic anemia, acute leukemia, and lymphosarcoma employing cyclophosphamide. *Transplant Proc* 1976;8:607.

430. Starzl TE, Groth CG, Putman CW, et al. Cyclophosphamide for clinical renal and hepatic transplantation. *Transplant Proc* 1973;5:511.

431. Osborne EO, Jordon JW, Hoak FC, et al. Nitrogen mustard therapy in cutaneous blastomatous disease. *JAMA* 1947;135:1123.

432. Reza MJ, Dornfield L, Goldberg LS, et al. Long-term follow-up of patients treated with cyclophosphamide. *Arthritis Rheum* 1975;18:501.

433. Cooperating Clinics Committee of the American Rheumatism Association. A controlled trial of cyclophosphamide in rheumatoid arthritis. *N Engl J Med* 1970;283:883.

434. Townes AS, Sowa JM, Schulman LE. Controlled trial of cyclophosphamide in rheumatoid arthritis (RA): an 11-month double-blind crossover study. *Arthritis Rheum* 1972;15:129.

435. Laros RK Jr, Penner JA. "Refractory" thrombocytopenic purpura treated successfully with cyclophosphamide. *JAMA* 1971;215:445.

436. Weinerman B, Maxwell I, Hryniuk W. Intermittent cyclophosphamide treatment of autoimmune thrombocytopenia. *Can Med Assoc J* 1974;111:1100.

437. Barratt TM, Soothill JF. Controlled trial of cyclophosphamide in steroid-sensitive relapsing nephrotic syndrome of childhood. *Lancet* 1970;2:279.

438. Gianni AM, Bregni M, Siena S, et al. Recombinant human granulocyte-macrophage colony-stimulating factor reduces hematologic toxicity and widens clinical applicability of high-dose cyclophosphamide treatment in breast cancer and non-Hodgkin's lymphoma. *J Clin Oncol* 1990;8:768.

439. Elias AN, Eder JP, Shea T, et al. High-dose ifosfamide with mesna uroprotection: a phase I study. *J Clin Oncol* 1990;8:170.

440. Lazarus HM, Reed MD, Spitzer TR, et al. High-dose IV thiotepa and cryopreserved autologous bone marrow transplantation for therapy of refractory cancer. *Cancer Treat Rep* 1987;71:689.

441. Peters WP, Henner WD, Grochow LB, et al. Clinical and pharmacologic effects of high-dose single-agent busulfan with autologous bone marrow support in the treatment of solid tumors. *Cancer Res* 1987;47:6402.

442. Ozols RF, Corden BJ, Jacob J, et al. High-dose cisplatin in hypertonic saline. *Ann Intern Med* 1984;100:19.

443. Shea TC, Flaherty M, Elias A, et al. A phase I clinical and pharmacokinetic study of carboplatin and autologous bone marrow support. *J Clin Oncol* 1989;7:651.

444. Reid JM, Pendergrass TW, Krailo MD, et al. Plasma pharmacokinetics and cerebrospinal fluid concentrations of idarubicin and idarubicinol in pediatric leukemia patients: a Children's Cancer Study Group report. *Cancer Res* 1990; 50:6525.

445. Kessinger A, Armitage JO, Smith DM, et al. High-dose therapy and autologous peripheral blood stem cell transplantation for patients with lymphoma. *Blood* 1989; 74:1260.

446. Jones RJ, Piantadosi S, Mann RB, et al. High-dose cytotoxic therapy and bone marrow transplantation for relapsed Hodgkin's disease. *J Clin Oncol* 1990;8:527.

447. Wilson WH, Jain V, Bryant G, et al. Phase I and II study of high-dose ifosfamide, carboplatin and etoposide with autologous bone marrow rescue in lymphomas and solid tumors. *J Clin Oncol* 1992;10:1712.

448. Dunphy FR, Spitzer G, Buzdar AU, et al. Treatment of estrogen receptor-negative or hormonally refractory breast cancer with double high-dose chemotherapy intensification and bone marrow support. *J Clin Oncol* 1990;8:1207.

449. Eder JP, Elias A, Shea TC, et al. A phase I–II study of cyclophosphamide, thiotepa, and carboplatin with autologous bone marrow transplantation in solid tumor patients. *J Clin Oncol* 1990;8:1239.

450. Peters WP, Shpall EJ, Jones RB, et al. High-dose combination alkylating agents with bone marrow support as initial treatment for metastatic breast cancer. *J Clin Oncol* 1988;6:1368.

14

NONCLASSIC ALKYLATING AGENTS

HENRY S. FRIEDMAN
STEVEN D. AVERBUCH
JOANNE KURTZBERG

Classic alkylating agents, such as the prototype nitrogen-mustard compounds, typically contain a chloroethyl group, and their biologic activity results from polyfunctional alkylation of biologic macromolecules. Compounds with diverse chemical structures are also capable of covalent binding to biologic macromolecules, and they also have important clinical activity. These compounds, referred to as the *nonclassic alkylating agents*, include procarbazine (PCB), dacarbazine (DTIC), hexamethylmelamine (HMM), pentamethylmelamine (PMM), and temozolomide (TMZ).

Although these agents lack bifunctionality, as Newell and co-workers[1] point out, they share a common structural feature, an *N*-methyl group, which is important for activity. These agents are essentially prodrugs and must undergo complex metabolic transformation to active intermediates; their precise cellular mechanisms of action and clinical pharmacology are not completely understood, but they are clinically useful, and indeed, PCB and DTIC are part of curative regimens for lymphomas. Additionally, TMZ was recently approved for treatment of patients with recurrent anaplastic astrocytoma, the first new agent approved for malignant gliomas in more than 30 years.

PROCARBAZINE

PCB was synthesized as part of an effort to develop new monoamine-oxidase inhibitors at the Hoffman-LaRoche Laboratories,[2] and it was found to have antitumor activity in rodent preclinical testing.[3,4] Early clinical trials demonstrated significant efficacy for PCB in the treatment of Hodgkin's disease and lymphomas, with little activity against solid tumors.[5–9] PCB has been used widely in combination with other agents in the treatment of Hodgkin's and non-Hodgkin's lymphomas,[10–13] and to a lesser extent, in small cell lung carcinoma[14–16] and melanoma.[17,18] Building on earlier experience with the treatment of brain tumors,[19–21] recent trials have demonstrated considerable

activity against high-grade glioma.[22–24] Nevertheless, there is still little known about PCB's cellular mechanism of action, and information regarding its clinical pharmacology is incomplete.

Mechanism of Action and Cellular Pharmacology

PCB, a prodrug, must undergo metabolism to active species. It enters cells by passive diffusion and thereafter is rapidly converted to cytotoxic metabolites by several possible routes.[25–39] Although selected tumor cells may contain cytosolic enzymes capable of activating PCB,[29] the parent drug is weakly cytotoxic for most tumor cell lines in culture, and its activity is markedly enhanced by allowing chemical decomposition of the drug[25] or cocultivation of tumor cells with rat hepatocytes.[31] However, it is not clear that the cytotoxic species generated by *in vitro* incubation with hepatic microsomes or intact hepatocytes is the same as that produced in humans.

As indicated in Figure 14-1, potential pathways of activation include chemical decomposition (I) as well as microsomal oxidation (II–V). The active end products have not been identified with certainty; they may be diazonium ions (R—$N^+\equiv N$), methyl or *N*-isopropylbenzamide free radicals, or other species capable of covalently binding to DNA.[40–43] Although most evidence favors a cytotoxic pathway involving the production of methyl or benzylazoxy intermediates by liver cytochrome P-450, with release of these metabolites into plasma and their subsequent uptake and further decomposition to diazonium ions *in situ*, free-radical species (either a methyl radical or an isopropylbenzylamide radical) can be generated by pathways II and V in the presence of rat liver cytochrome P-450.[44] Thus, it is not clear which of the several putative and positively identified metabolites are responsible for cytotoxicity. The metabolic pathways will be considered again with respect to PCB pharmacokinetics in humans in the section Clinical Pharmacology.

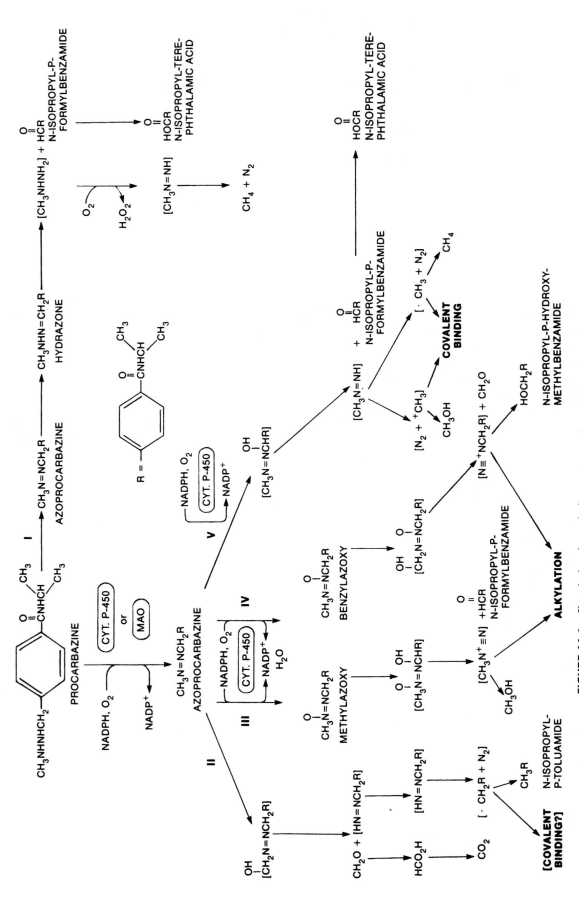

FIGURE 14-1. Chemical and metabolic reactions of procarbazine, leading to the generation of reactive intermediates. I, Chemical breakdown of procarbazine in aqueous solution; II, III, IV, and V, proposed metabolic activation pathways *in vivo*. Intermediates not identified *in vitro* or *in vivo* are indicated by brackets. See text for detailed description. (CYT, cytochrome; MAO, monoamine oxidase; NADP, nicotinamide adenine dinucleotide phosphate; NADPH, nicotinamide adenine dinucleotide phosphate.)

Several additional cellular effects of PCB and its metabolites have been demonstrated, although it is unclear whether these contribute directly to cytotoxicity. Hydrogen peroxide and formaldehyde are two potentially toxic products generated from PCB and are thought to cause cytotoxicity by interaction with DNA.[45] However, the data demonstrating azoPCB activity in the absence of hydrogen peroxide generation strongly argue against a role for this toxic byproduct in the cytotoxic activity of PCB.[25,46] Earlier reports and more recent studies using alkaline elution techniques have demonstrated that PCB and its metabolites are capable of causing chromatid and single-strand DNA breaks in murine tumor cells *in vitro*.[29,47–49] The number of breaks depends on the dosage and time elapsed after treatment, and it has been suggested that the breaks occur during, or soon after, DNA synthesis.[50] Because the percentage of cells undergoing mitosis is also diminished as a function of dosage and time after PCB,[48] it is likely that the most susceptible phase in the cell cycle may be the premitotic G_2 phase. However, this has not been confirmed using current technology, such as cell sorting by flow cytometry. In addition, a G_2 block may simply indicate the physiologic response of cells to DNA injury. Chromatid translocations (sister chromatid exchange) are also observed in murine tumor cells *in vivo* after PCB treatment, although this effect is not observed *in vitro* after PCB.[47,48] Again, this result suggests that differences exist in the toxic metabolites generated *in vitro* versus *in vivo*.

In addition to these effects on nuclear DNA, PCB can inhibit DNA, RNA, and protein synthesis *in vitro* and *in vivo*.[26,47,51] Single doses of PCB administered to mice bearing transplanted tumors inhibited DNA incorporation of thymidine by 35% to 70%.[26,47] Maximal inhibition occurred within several hours, and complete recovery was achieved by 8 to 24 hours. *De novo* purine synthesis and pyrimidine-nucleotide synthesis are inhibited, but there is no effect on nucleoside or nucleotide kinases. PCB produces a similar time course and degree of inhibition for the RNA (uracil) incorporation of orotic acid and for nuclear RNA synthesis. Protein synthesis inhibition due to PCB is relatively delayed, reaching a maximum at 12 to 16 hours, and this effect is believed to be a result of the inhibition of nucleic acid synthesis.[26,47,51,52] PCB seems to inhibit normal transfer RNA (tRNA) methylation, and the resulting altered tRNA synthesis and function may well account for some of the effects on nucleic acid and protein synthesis.[43,53]

The most compelling evidence to date suggests that the cytotoxicity of PCB is mediated by its role as a methylating agent. Adult Fisher rats treated with radiolabeled PCB developed large amounts of O^6-[^{14}C]methylguanine compared with 7-[^{14}C]methylguanine.[54] O^6-methylguanine is a known mutagenic and carcinogenic adduct[55–57] also thought to contribute to cytotoxicity.[58] Accordingly, the observation that administration of PCB to athymic nude mice bearing xenografts derived from human malignant gliomas and medulloblastoma resulted in greater growth delays in those tumors lacking O^6-alkylguanine-DNA alkyl transferase (AGT),[59] the enzyme mediating repair of O^6-methylguanine,[60] is particularly convincing. Four of five tumor lines with AGT levels had growth delays of less than 20 days after PCB, whereas all five lines with undetectable AGT levels had growth delays of more than 30 days. Furthermore, O^6-methylguanine was found in significantly higher levels in two sensitive lines with low-AGT levels as compared with O^6-methylguanine levels in a resistant line with a high-AGT level.

Mechanisms of Resistance

Recent studies have shed light on the cellular mechanism(s) of resistance to PCB. Resistance develops rapidly in tumor cells[3] after exposure to PCB, and one study suggested a direct correlation between the rate of DNA synthesis and the rapidity of resistance development.[26] Resistant cells also were found to contain additional chromosomes.[61] The previously mentioned inverse correlation between central nervous system (CNS) xenograft response to PCB and AGT activity suggests that resistance to this methylating agent is secondary to AGT-mediated repair of O^6-methylguanine, similar to nitrosourea resistance mediated by this enzyme.[60] However, an alternative method of resistance has recently been defined. Friedman et al.[61a] established a methylator-resistant human glioblastoma multiforme xenograft, D-245 MG (PR), in athymic nude mice by serially treating the parent xenograft, D-245 MG, with PCB. D-245 MG xenografts were sensitive to PCB, TMZ, *N*-methyl-*N*-nitrosourea, 1,3-bis(2-chloroethyl)-1-nitrosourea, 9-aminocamptothecin, topotecan, CPT-11, cyclophosphamide, and busulfan. D-245 MG (PR) xenografts were resistant to PCB, TMZ, *N*-methyl-*N*-nitrosourea, and busulfan, but they were sensitive to the other agents. D-245 MG and D-245 MG (PR) xenografts displayed no AGT alkyl transferase activity, and their levels of glutathione and glutathione-*S*-transferase were similar. D-245 MG xenografts expressed the human mismatch-repair proteins hMSH2 and hMLH1, whereas D-245 MG (PR) expressed hMLH1 but not hMSH2.

These results indicate conclusively that this resistance to PCB and other methylators was secondary to an *in vivo*–acquired mismatch repair deficiency. This observation is consistent with other reports demonstrating methylator resistance in human tumor cells resulting from mismatch repair deficiency.[61b,61c]

Drug Interactions

Because PCB undergoes extensive hepatic microsomal metabolism and because it inhibits monoamine oxidase, which is widespread in tissues and plasma, there are many potential drug-drug and drug-food interactions. The activ-

**TABLE 14-1. KEY FEATURES OF PROCARBAZINE (PCB)
[*N*-ISOPROPYL-α-(2-METHYLHYDRAZINO)-*p*-TOLUAMIDE, IBENZMETHYZIN,
NATULAN, MATULANE, NSC-77213]**

Mechanism of action:	Metabolic activation required: methylation of nucleic acids; inhibition of DNA, RNA, and protein synthesis.
Metabolism:	Converted to azoPCB by erythrocyte and liver microsomes.
	Subsequent metabolism to *N*-isopropyl-*p*-formylbenzamide, *N*-isopropyl-*p*-hydroxymethyl benzamide, *N*-isopropyl-*p*-toluamide, *N*-isopropyl-*N*-isopropylterephthalamic acid (inactive), methane, and carbon dioxide.
	Possible formation of methyldiazene free radical "active intermediate."
Pharmacokinetics:	Half-life = 7 min.
	Approximately 100% bioavailability from oral route, peak plasma concentration reached within 60 min.
	Equilibration between plasma and cerebrospinal fluid in 15–30 min.
Elimination:	Renal elimination of ≥75% in 24 h.
Drug and food interactions:	PCB may inhibit hepatic microsomal drug metabolism and therefore potentiate activity of barbiturates, antihistamines, narcotics, and phenothiazines.
	Alcohol use may cause "disulfiram-like" reaction.
	Sympathomimetics, tricyclic antidepressants, or tyramine-rich foods may cause severe hypertension due to PCB inhibition of monoamine oxidase.
Toxicity:	Myelosuppression.
	Gastrointestinal (nausea and vomiting); rare hepatic dysfunction.
	Neurotoxicity (drowsiness, depression, agitation, paresthesias).
	Cutaneous or pulmonary hypersensitivity (rare).
	Azoospermia; anovulation.
	Carcinogenesis (associated with secondary malignancy in treated patients).
	Teratogenesis.
Precautions:	Dose modification may be necessary in hepatic and/or renal dysfunction.
	Avoid alcohol.
	Avoid tyramine-rich foods, sympathomimetics, tricyclic antidepressants, hypnotics, antihistamines, narcotics, phenothiazines.

ity of other drugs that are inactivated by microsomal metabolism may be enhanced in the presence of PCB, as shown by a prolonged pentobarbital-induced sleep time in animals.[62–65] Therefore, patients taking barbiturates, phenothiazines, narcotics, and other hypnotics or sedatives may experience potentiated effects of these agents. Conversely, these drugs and others, such as cimetidine, that affect hepatic metabolism may increase or decrease PCB metabolism and thereby alter PCB activity and toxicity.[45,66,67] Pretreatment of rats with phenobarbital before PCB administration resulted in increased PCB clearance and a slight decrease in concentrations of the azo metabolite. Inasmuch as phenobarbital or phenytoin pretreatment increased the survival of tumor-bearing mice treated with PCB (Table 14-1), it may be presumed that microsomal enzyme induction resulted in increased production of active PCB metabolites.[46] It is not known whether this drug interaction may be useful clinically to achieve therapeutic advantage through biochemical modulation of PCB activity.

Monoamine oxidase inhibition[68] and pyridoxal phosphate depletion[69] by PCB cause CNS depression. This also may potentiate the sedative effects of other CNS depressants. This inhibition of monoamine oxidase also predisposes patients to acute hypertensive reactions after concomitant therapy with tricyclic antidepressants and sympathomimetic drugs, as well as after ingestion of tyramine-rich foods, such as red wine, bananas, ripe cheese, and yogurt. Finally, a disulfiram-like reaction manifest by sweating, facial flushing, and headache may occur in patients who ingest alcohol while taking PCB.

Clinical Pharmacology

PCB hydrochloride is supplied in capsules containing the equivalent of 50 mg of the base for oral administration. As a single agent, the usual dose is 100 to 200 mg per m² of body surface area, given daily until myelosuppression occurs. As part of the mechlorethamine, vincristine, PCB, and prednisone (MOPP) combination regimen for Hodgkin's disease, the daily dose of PCB is 100 mg per m² of body surface area daily for 14 days.[10]

The pharmacokinetics and metabolism of PCB have been studied mostly in laboratory animals, and information regarding pharmacokinetics in humans is incomplete.[62,70–73] After oral administration, the drug is rapidly and completely absorbed from the gastrointestinal tract. The biodistribution of PCB is not well known; however, earlier studies using drug that was isotopically labeled at different sites on the molecule showed high levels of radioactivity in the liver, kidney, intestine, and skin at 30 and 60 minutes after drug administration.[72] There is also rapid equilibration of [^{14}C]PCB (labeled in the benzyl ring) between

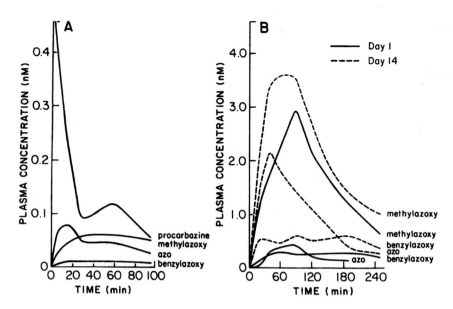

FIGURE 14-2. A: Procarbazine (PCB) disappearance and azo and azoxy metabolite kinetics in rat plasma after administration of PCB, 150 mg per kg, intraperitoneal. **B:** Plasma concentrations of azo and azoxyprocarbasine metabolites in a patient after the administration of PCB, 250 mg per kg per day, orally, on days 1 and 14 of a 14-day treatment schedule. (From Shiba DA, Weinkam RJ. Quantitative analysis of PCB, PCB metabolites and chemical degradation products with application to pharmacokinetic studies. *J Chromatogr* 1982; 229:397.)

plasma and cerebrospinal fluid (CSF) in dogs and humans.[62] After the intravenous (i.v.) administration of 150 mg [14C]PCB, the plasma half-life ($t_{1/2}$) of parent drug was approximately 7 minutes in humans, whereas studies in dogs and rats demonstrated $t_{1/2}$ of 12 and 24 minutes, respectively.[70] Because single-bolus i.v. dosages of PCB produce a spectrum of toxicity, primarily neurotoxicity,[74] distinct from the myelosuppression seen after oral administration, it is likely that a first-pass effect of orally administered drug through the portal circulation significantly influences drug metabolism and pharmacokinetics. This is supported by the observation of almost complete conversion of PCB to the azo metabolite in isolated liver perfusion studies.[35,71] After the intraperitoneal (i.p.) injection of 150 mg PCB in rats, the azo metabolite appears in plasma within minutes, peaking at 10 to 20 minutes and then decreasing slowly over several hours concomitant with the appearance of the methyl and benzylazoxy isomers[28] (Fig. 14-2A). Preliminary data in humans show that the methylazoxy isomer is the major plasma metabolite after a single 250 mg per kg oral dose of PCB. This compound peaks at approximately 90 minutes and seems to have an initial plasma half-life of approximately 60 minutes. AzoPCB and the benzylazoxy isomer are present in relatively equal but lesser concentrations compared to the methylazoxy isomer. Interestingly, PCB treatment seems to alter its own metabolism, a change that may, in turn, influence its activity.[28,46,63] The total and relative plasma concentrations of PCB metabolites are markedly changed after the administration of a fourteenth daily oral dose of PCB[28] (Fig. 14-2B). Of note was the significant increase in azoPCB concentration, suggesting that prior PCB exposure induces this metabolite's production or delays its clearance. Shiba and Weinkam[46] also observed that prior treatment with PCB enhances PCB antitumor activity in rats.

In all species examined, the major urinary metabolite of PCB is the biologically inactive *N*-isopropylterephthalamic acid.[62,66,70–72] Approximately 70% of radioactivity administered in the form of [14C]PCB was recovered, primarily as the acid, in the urine during the first 24 hours. There is minimal fecal excretion (4% to 12% over 96 hours), and approximately 30% of radioactivity labeled in the *N*-methyl group appears as respiratory $^{14}CO_2$.[72,75]

The complex pharmacokinetic and excretion characteristics of PCB reflect the rapid and extensive enzymatic metabolism of this compound, which is necessary for antitumor activity and presumably is responsible for host organ toxic reactions. The proposed metabolic routes for PCB were discussed in detail in the previous edition of this text[76] and were reviewed in detail by Prough and Tweedie[29] (Fig. 14-1). The understanding of PCB metabolism is improving as a result of improved experimental techniques and analytical methods, including high-pressure liquid chromatography (HPLC) and mass spectroscopy.[27,28,33–37,77,78] Again, most of the information in this area is derived from studies in animals *in vivo* and *in vitro*. However, there do not seem to be any major discrepancies in these results in animals as compared with the literature describing human metabolism.[46,62,70,72,79] Nonetheless, the information is not sufficient to allow assignment of quantitative importance to the several possible alternate routes of metabolism (Fig. 14-1).

PCB is not stable in aqueous solution, decomposing by rapid metal-catalyzed oxidation to azoPCB with the production of hydrogen peroxide.[29,33,45,62,77] In the presence of light, isomerization to the biologically inactive hydrazone (*N*-isopropyl-*p*-formylbenzamide methylhydrazine) occurs slowly. This is followed by hydrolysis to yield the aldehyde, *N*-isopropyl-*p*-formylbenzamide, and methylhydrazine. The former compound is further oxidized to *N*-isopropyl-terephthalamic acid. Earlier studies suggested that this route of chemical decomposition was responsible for the biologic activity of PCB,[45,62,70] but subsequent investigations have shown that the chemical decomposition products are relatively stable under physiologic conditions and that they account for a small proportion of the compounds formed *in vitro* and *in vivo* as compared to cytochrome P-450–mediated metabolism.[25,26,29,33–38] Because of PCB's chemical degradation to potentially toxic compounds under common conditions, such as aqueous solvent, trace metal contamination, and air and light exposure, extreme care must be taken in the formulation and storage of PCB solutions intended for parenteral administration. These considerations also apply when evaluating the results of PCB studies *in vitro* and *in vivo*.

In biologic systems, the oxidation of PCB to azoPCB occurs by microsomal cytochrome P-450 oxidoreductase or by mitochondrial monoamine oxidase enzymatic conversion[32,34,71,80,81] (Fig. 14-1). Isolated rat liver perfusion studies, as well as incubation of drug with rat liver microsomes, disclose extensive metabolism of the drug and suggest that the liver is the predominant site of the initial metabolism of PCB.[29,34–38] The subsequent metabolism of azoPCB may occur by several different routes. Isozymic cytochrome P-450–mediated *N*-oxidation results in the formation of methyl and benzylazoxy isomers[27,34,82,83] (Fig. 14-1, pathways III and IV). The former is produced in higher quantitative yield during *in vitro* reactions and is the predominant metabolite of azoPCB in rat and human plasma.[28,29] It has been proposed that hydroxylation of either carbon atom adjacent to the azoxy function results in unstable compounds that react to produce the reactive alkylating alkyldiazonium ion [R—N$^+$≡N]. Further microsomal metabolism of the azoxy compounds results in formation of *N*-isopropyl-*p*-formylbenzamide or *N*-isopropyl-*p*-hydroxymethylbenzamide. These compounds are then oxidized to the major urinary metabolite, *N*-isopropylterephthalamic acid.[27–29,62,70] Alternatively, Moloney and associates[40] recently demonstrated a pathway of metabolic activation of the terminal *N*-methyl group of azoPCB that does not involve azoxy formation (Fig. 14-1, pathway V). This pathway involves a P-450–mediated oxidation of the benzyl carbon atom adjacent to the azo function with subsequent formation of *N*-isopropyl-*p*-formylbenzamide and a putative unstable methyldiazene intermediate. The proposed intermediate could form either a methyl radical or a carbonium ion, both of which are covalent binding species. If, instead, hydrogen abstraction occurs, as in the presence of reduced glutathione, then methane is formed as a final metabolic product.[38,73] Another pathway that would produce a free-radical intermediate and not involve azoxy formation is the oxidation of the methyl carbon adjacent to the azo function (Fig. 14-1, pathway II). This metabolic route would ultimately lead to formation of CO_2 and *N*-isopropyl-*p*-toluamide, a metabolite identified in rat plasma and brain after the administration of PCB.[33,71–73,75,76] Because

the azoxy metabolites are the predominant products found in plasma, however, it is likely that pathways III and IV predominate in humans.

Toxicity

After oral administration, PCB causes anorexia and mild nausea and vomiting, which is probably of central origin and often abates with continued use.[84] In some patients, it is often helpful to escalate the dosage in a stepwise fashion over the first several days of drug administration to minimize these gastrointestinal side effects. Mild to moderate myelosuppression in the form of reversible leukopenia and thrombocytopenia is the most common dose-limiting toxicity of PCB given orally. Depression of peripheral leukocyte and platelet counts becomes apparent after 1 week of therapy and may persist for 2 weeks or longer after discontinuation of the drug.[85] PCB also may cause hemolysis in individuals with glucose-6-phosphate dehydrogenase deficiency.[86] PCB generally does not cause mucosal injury to the rapidly proliferating gastrointestinal epithelium.

Patients receiving PCB orally may occasionally experience neurotoxicity manifest by drowsiness, depression, agitation, paresthesias of the extremities,[87] and reversible orthostatic hypotension.[8] These effects are probably a result of central monoamine oxidase inhibition and may be related to drug-induced depletion of pyridoxal phosphate.[68,69,88] When PCB is administered intravenously, neurotoxic effects become more pronounced and are dose limiting. After a single high-dose i.v. bolus (2 g per m^2) or a 5-day continuous infusion of PCB, patients experienced severe nausea and vomiting, confusion, and even coma lasting several days.[74,88] Myelosuppression does not occur when PCB is administered in this way. However, there is also a parallel lack of clinical antitumor effect, which emphasizes the importance of first-pass hepatic metabolism for activation of PCB to antiproliferative intermediates. The pattern of toxicity after small, intermittent i.v. doses is more like that seen after oral administration,[1,6] although it is unlikely that this schedule offers any clinical benefit over that of conventional oral dosing.

PCB also may cause hypersensitivity reactions, including maculopapular skin rash, eosinophilia, pulmonary infiltrates, or, rarely, transient hepatic dysfunction.[5,7,89–93] The skin rash usually responds to concomitant glucocorticosteroid treatment, and the PCB may be continued without exacerbation of rash or further sequelae. In contrast, PCB-induced interstitial pneumonitis usually necessitates discontinuation of the drug.

PCB has potent immunosuppressive properties[94] that may contribute to the infectious complications. These immunosuppressive properties have been used to therapeutic advantage for the treatment of lupus erythematosus and in the suppression of graft-versus-host disease after bone marrow transplantation.[95] With the use of newer agents developed for these indications and with the increasing

TABLE 14-2. EXPERIMENTAL BIOCHEMICAL MODULATION OF PROCARBAZINE (PCB) EFFICACY AND TOXICITY IN MICE BEARING L1210 LEUKEMIA, i.p.

Treatment	Modulation	Life-span increase (%)[a]	Sperm count (%)[b]	Reference
PCB 200 mg/kg, i.p., daily × 3	None	122		43
PCB 200 mg/kg, i.p., daily × 3	Phenytoin 60 mg/kg, p.o., for 7 d	146[c]		43
PCB 200 mg/kg, i.p., daily × 3	Phenobarbital 48 mg/kg, p.o., for 7 d	140[c]		43
PCB 400 mg/kg, i.p.	None	125	45	108
PCB 400 mg/kg, i.p.	N-Acetylcysteine 189.9 mg/kg, i.p.	128	85	108
PCB 400 mg/kg, i.p.	Sodium ascorbate 307.4 mg/kg, i.p.	125	90	108

[a]% mean treated/control.
[b]Mean expressed as a percentage of control mice given 0.9% NaCl.
[c]Significant at the 95% confidence limit compared to mice treated with PCB alone.

concern over serious late toxic reactions to PCB, this drug should probably not be used for nonneoplastic diseases.

The successful use of PCB-containing chemotherapy combinations resulting in curative and long-term disease-free survival has directed increasing attention and concern to the chronic and late toxicities of this agent. PCB has profound azoospermic,[96,97] teratogenic,[98] mutagenic,[99,100] and carcinogenic[101,102] properties in experimental animals, and most of these effects have been associated with PCB use in humans.

PCB is highly toxic to reproductive organs, causing azoospermia and anovulation.[103–107] More than 90% of men receiving PCB in combination with classic alkylating agents, such as in MOPP combination chemotherapy for Hodgkin's disease, have irreversible azoospermia. Approximately 50% of women thus treated have permanent drug-induced ovarian failure. In pregnant animals, administration of PCB causes congenital skeletal and CNS abnormalities.[98,108] Although evidence for direct causation of lethal and nonlethal mutations in human fetuses is lacking, women of childbearing potential should be advised against pregnancy during chemotherapy. In women treated with MOPP chemotherapy who regain normal ovarian function, there seems to be no impairment of fertility nor any increased birth defects in offspring.[106,107,109,110]

Mutagenesis and carcinogenesis resulting from PCB have been demonstrated experimentally *in vitro* and *in vivo*.[99–102] Nonlymphocytic leukemias and adenocarcinomas developed in rodents and nonhuman primates after PCB administration, and, accordingly, the finite increased incidence of secondary leukemias and solid malignancies in patients after treatment with MOPP combination chemotherapy pointed to PCB as the responsible carcinogen.[111–113] Because this regimen also contains an alkylating agent with carcinogenic properties, it is difficult to assign a direct cause of secondary malignancies to PCB alone.[113] Indeed, studies in experimental systems suggest that additive or interactive effects of classic alkylating agents with PCB may account for the observed mutagenesis.[114]

The mechanisms of PCB gonadal toxicity and somatic genotoxicity are mostly thought to be the same as for its antitumor activity. As for the latter, metabolic conversion of PCB is necessary for its toxic and carcinogenic effects on normal tissue, although it is not clear which metabolic pathways are mechanistically important, nor is it known whether there may be separate mechanisms for anticancer activity and for normal organ toxicity. Yost and associates[115,116] recently proposed separate mechanisms for PCB spermatotoxicity and anticancer activity based on different activating metabolic pathways. Furthermore, these authors exploited this difference by using antioxidants that protected against PCB spermatotoxicity but did not compromise its antileukemic activity in mice (Table 14-2). These studies, as well as those of Prough and Tweedie[29] and Shiba and Weinkam,[46] which show improved therapeutic benefit from phenobarbital induction of PCB metabolism, suggest that anticancer and toxic effects of PCB may be separable and, therefore, susceptible to modulation for therapeutic advantage. Further investigations of PCB's metabolism and molecular mechanisms of action are necessary to develop clinically useful approaches to lessen toxicity successfully and improve efficacy.

DACARBAZINE

History

DTIC was chemically synthesized as a result of a rational attempt to develop agents capable of interfering with the synthesis of purines. As reviewed by Montgomery,[117] a series of compounds designed as analogs of aminoimidazole carboxamide (AIC), an intermediate in purine ring synthesis, was synthesized in the late 1950s and had significant antitumor activity in experimental testing. The addition of nitrous acid to form a 5-diazoimidazole derivative seemed to confer this antitumor activity, and the further addition of a third nitrogen group to form the 5-triazene resulted in a light-sensitive compound that spontaneously converted back to the diazo analog. Dimethyl substitution of the triazine resulted in a more stable but still light-sensitive derivative, DTIC, which was highly active and was developed for clinical use.[118]

TABLE 14-3. KEY FEATURES OF DACARBAZINE [5-(3,3-DIMETHYL-1-TRIAZENO) IMIDAZOLE-4-CARBOXAMIDE, DTIC, DIC, NSC-45388]

Mechanism of action:	Metabolic activation probably required; methylation of nucleic acids; direct DNA damage; inhibition of purine synthesis.
Metabolism:	Oxidative *N*-methylation to 5-aminoimidazole-4-carboxamide via formation of 5(3-hydroxymethyl-3-methyltriazen-1-yl)imidazole-4-carboxamide and 5-(3-methyltriazen-2-yl)imidazole-4-carboxamide.
	$t_{1/2\alpha}$ = 3 min; $t_{1/2\beta}$ = 41 min.
	V_d = 0.6 L/kg; Cl = 15 mL/kg/min.
	20% protein bound.
	Variable oral absorption.
	Poor CSF penetration (plasma/CSF ratio = 7:1 at equilibrium).
Elimination:	Renal excretion: 50% as unchanged dacarbazine and 9–18% as 5-aminoimidazole-4-carboxamide.
	Minor hepatobiliary and pulmonary excretion.
Drug and food interactions:	*Corynebacterium parvum* may prolong $t_{1/2}$.
Toxicity:	Myelosuppression.
	Gastrointestinal (nausea and vomiting).
	Influenza-like syndrome (fever, myalgia, and malaise).
	Infrequent alopecia, cutaneous hypersensitivity, or photosensitivity.
	Rare hepatic vein thrombosis and hepatic necrosis.
	Possible carcinogenesis and teratogenesis.
Precautions:	Dose modification may be necessary in hepatic and/or renal dysfunction.

Cl, clearance; CSF, cerebrospinal fluid; $t_{1/2}$, half-life; V_d, apparent volume of distribution.

DTIC is an active single agent in the treatment of metastatic malignant melanoma, producing remissions in 16% to 31% of patients with this disease,[119] and it is also active as a single agent in Hodgkin's disease.[120] Thus, in the United States, DTIC is approved for use in these two diseases. It is frequently used alone or in combination with agents such as nitrosoureas, bleomycin, and vinca alkaloids in melanoma,[121–124] and it is most commonly used as part of the doxorubicin, bleomycin, vinblastine, and DTIC (ABVD) and actinomycin D, bleomycin, and vincristine regimens for Hodgkin's disease.[125,126] In addition, DTIC has demonstrated activity in the treatment of sarcomas,[127–129] childhood neuroblastoma,[130,131] and primary brain tumors.[132] It may be the most active agent alone or in combination for the treatment of malignant amine precursor uptake and decarboxylation and other neuroendocrine tumors.[133–135] The key features of DTIC are summarized in Table 14-3.

General Mechanism of Action and Cellular Pharmacology

The exact mechanism underlying DTIC's antitumor activity remains an enigma. Although DTIC was developed as a purine antimetabolite, there is abundant evidence that its antitumor activity does not result from interference with purine synthesis. The drug is active against several cell lines resistant to the purine analogs 6-thioguanine and 6-mercaptopurine, and it does not demonstrate cell-cycle schedule dependence observed with other antimetabolites.[117] Second, the AIC portion of the molecule is not necessary for antitumor activity.[136,137] In fact, most of the mechanistic studies and structure-activity relationship determinations in biologic systems have been performed using 1-phenylamine analogs of DTIC.[138–143] Most studies in tissue culture show that the parent DTIC compound has little activity,[137,144,145] and it is well established that host metabolic activation to methylating species is necessary for antitumor activity.[138–143,146,147] As discussed in detail below, DTIC undergoes demethylation[1] to form 5(3-methyltriazeno)imidazole-4-carboxamide (MTIC), which subsequently tautomerizes and eliminates the reactive methyldiazonium ion $CH_3N^+\equiv N$ as the active methylating intermediate (Fig. 14-3). Alkylation of nucleic acids and the production of alkali-labile DNA lesions have been demonstrated *in vitro*,[145,148–150] and 7-methylguanine has been recovered from the urine of rats and humans after DTIC administration.[151] Recently, dose-dependent formation of 7-[^{14}C]methylguanine was found in several organs after a single i.p. injection of [^{14}C-methyl]DTIC in rats.[152] There are several questions remaining as to whether nucleophilic alkylation by MTIC accounts for the antitumor specificity of DTIC therapy.[140,142,153,154] MTIC also has been shown to inhibit purine-nucleoside incorporation into DNA,[155] but this may be a result of DNA alkylation and cell damage.

Several *in vitro* studies showed direct cytotoxicity with DTIC, but these effects were probably due to light activation of the parent compound to toxic species.[144,145,147,156–159] When incubated with tumor cells in culture, DTIC inhibits DNA, RNA, and protein synthesis.[160] Because this effect is enhanced in the presence of light,[148] it is likely that photodecomposition of the DTIC to toxic species is involved in inhibition of macromolecular synthesis. This explana-

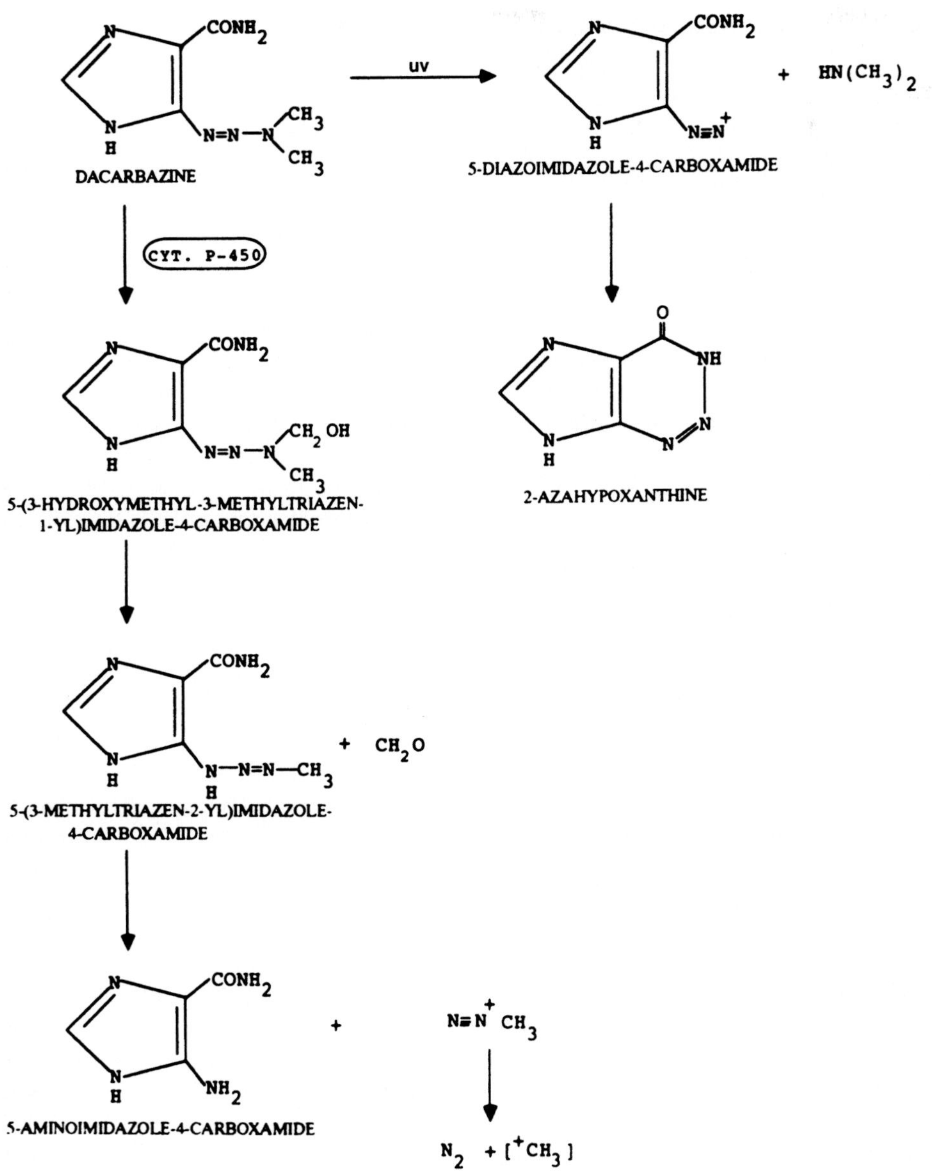

FIGURE 14-3. Light-activated and metabolic reactions of dacarbazine leading to the generation of reactive intermediates. (CYT, cytochrome; uv, ultraviolet.)

tion has recently been contested by the results of Lonn and Lonn.[161–163] In experiments on human cell lines performed in the dark, these workers showed that DTIC directly damages DNA in the presence of functioning DNA polymerase α.[161] Furthermore, they showed that cytotoxicity was enhanced if DNA repair processes were inhibited by the addition of 3-aminobenzamide or a specific calmodulin inhibitor, W7.[162,163]

The mechanism for cellular uptake of DTIC or its activated metabolic intermediates has not been studied. Similarly, the effect of DTIC on the cell cycle is unclear. The drug seems to be active in all phases[158–160] and may cause progression delay through the G_2 phase of the cell cycle.[164]

There is mounting evidence to suggest that, similar to PCB, the production of O^6-methylguanine is the primary cytotoxic event after administration of DTIC. Xenografts, or cell lines with negligible levels of AGT, are more sensitive to DTIC than are xenografts or cell lines with high levels of AGT.[165–171] Furthermore, DTIC depletes AGT levels in human colon cancer HT 29 xenografts in athymic mice[172] and in human peripheral blood cells in patients treated for metastatic melanoma.[173]

In addition to the cytotoxic activity, DTIC and other dimethyltriazene analogs[143,174–179] can inhibit metastatic spread of tumors and increase survival time *in vivo*. The analog with the best activity against the primary tumor may not necessarily be the agent with the best antimetastatic effect, suggesting that the underlying mechanisms are different. Although the mechanism of this apparent antimetastatic property is unknown, it may be associated with the ability of DTIC to enhance tumor immunogenicity.[180–185] DTIC analogs induce tumor cells to differentiate *in vitro*,[186] but again, the significance of this property is unknown.

Mechanisms of Resistance

Questions regarding the nature and mechanisms of inherent or acquired cellular resistance to DTIC have not been adequately addressed. In human melanoma cells *in vitro*, Hayward and Parson[155] showed an enhanced toxicity of MTIC in the presence of 3-aminobenzamide, an inhibitor of DNA repair. Taken together with the results of Lonn and Lonn,[161–163] a corollary explanation for tumor cell resistance to triazenes may be an increase in activity of calmodulin-mediated DNA excision-repair enzymes or a decrease in DNA polymerase α. Tumor cells that are selected for DTIC resistance *in vivo* also display increased immunogenicity, although there seem to be different mechanisms accounting for these two characteristics.[137,183,187]

The previously mentioned work[165–171] supporting O^6-methylguanine as the major cytotoxic lesion produced by DTIC strongly suggests that elevated levels of AGT may be responsible for resistance to this agent. The inverse relationship between AGT levels and response to DTIC in human xenografts also may be operational in clinical tumor resistance to DTIC.[165–171]

Drug Interactions

At present, there are no known drug or food interactions with DTIC that are of clinical importance. Because DTIC has been used in conjunction with immune adjuvants in the treatment of malignant melanoma, there has been some interest in the influence of these agents on DTIC pharmacology. Farquhar and co-workers[188] described an inhibition of DTIC *N*-demethylase in rats pretreated with bacillus Calmette-Guérin (BCG), suggesting that patients receiving both agents may be less able to activate DTIC. In four patients with melanoma, BCG did not seem to influence DTIC pharmacokinetics, although altered metabolism per se was not examined.[189] In contrast, patients receiving *Corynebacterium parvum* adjuvant immunotherapy did show a prolongation of DTIC serum half-life[190] consistent with *C. parvum*'s ability to depress hepatic microsomal *N*-demethylation of a variety of drugs.[191] Although the initial step for metabolic activation of DTIC is catalyzed by microsomal cytochrome P-450, the interaction of phenobarbital, or other commonly used cytochrome P-450 inducing agents, with DTIC has not been reported.

DTIC activity against L1210 murine leukemia is potentiated by alkylating agents, such as melphalan, and by doxorubicin.[117] Activity is also enhanced when DTIC is combined with the nitrosoureas bischloromethyl-nitrosourea (BCNU) and chloroethylcyclo-hexylnitrosourea (CCNU). The mechanism(s) for the potentiation observed using these combinations may be related to the ability of nitrosoureas to deplete AGT and thereby sensitize cells to methylating agents.

Clinical Pharmacology

DTIC is supplied in sterile vials containing 100 or 200 mg DTIC for i.v. administration. As a single agent, a dose of up to 1,500 mg per m² of body surface area may be given as a single bolus as opposed to the more frequently used schedule of 250 mg per m² daily for 5 days every 3 to 4 weeks.[121,123,129,192] The latter schedule was developed in an attempt to minimize the gastrointestinal toxicity from DTIC, which tends to lessen with repeated administration. Most studies, however, fail to show any significant schedule dependency with respect to antitumor efficacy or toxicity.[121,123] DTIC also has been used by intraarterial infusion for the regional treatment of malignant melanoma involving liver, pelvis, the maxillofacial region, and extremities with high response rates in uncontrolled series.[193–196] It is not known whether *in situ* melanoma cells in humans are capable of metabolizing DTIC[148,197]; otherwise, these results are difficult to interpret because DTIC requires metabolic activation for its antitumor activity.

Initial studies of DTIC pharmacokinetics and metabolism in rodents, dogs, and humans used radiochemical[146,151,152,198,199] and colorimetric methods.[200–202] More recently, improved experimental methods, such as HPLC[142,189,190,203] and mass spectroscopy,[204] have been used to study triazine pharmacology. Because of the scarcity of clinical studies using adequately sensitive and specific techniques, knowledge of DTIC pharmacology in humans remains incomplete. After oral administration, the drug is absorbed slowly and variably[201,202]; therefore, i.v. administration is the preferred route. Intravenous boluses of 2.65 to 6.85 mg per kg (approximately 120 to 300 mg per m²) produced peak plasma concentrations of nearly 10 to over 30 µg per mL, respectively.[189] After i.v. administration of DTIC, Breithaupt and co-workers[189] found a biphasic plasma disappearance of the parent drug consistent with a two-compartment model with an initial half-life of 3 minutes and a terminal half-life of 41 minutes (Fig. 14-4). This is in contrast to a terminal half-life of 3.2 hours found in an earlier study using HPLC[190] analysis and 5 hours found in a study using colorimetric analysis.[148] Approximately 20% of DTIC is loosely bound to plasma protein.[201] In humans, the mean volume of distribution for DTIC was 0.6 L per kg, and the total-body clearance was 15.4 mL per kg per minute.[189] In one study, approximately 50% of an i.v. dose of DTIC was recovered in the urine as parent drug, and the renal clearance was calculated to be between 5 and 10 mL per kg per minute,[189] confirming earlier reports[201,202] that tubular secretion may be involved in the renal excretion of DTIC. Hepatobiliary excretion of DTIC is probably of some importance,[148] but this has not been adequately studied. Altered schedules of i.v. drug administration did not change the area under the curve (concentration × time), confirming a lack of schedule dependence for DTIC pharmacokinetics.[189]

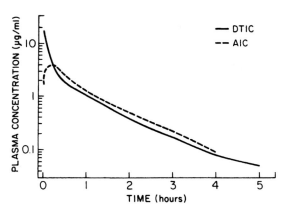

FIGURE 14-4. Plasma concentrations of dacarbazine (DTIC) and 5-aminoimidazole-4-carboxamide (AIC) in a patient after administration of dacarbazine, 6.34 mg per kg, intravenous. [From Breithaupt H, Dammann A, Aigner K. Pharmacokinetics of dacarbazine (DTIC) and its metabolite 5-aminoimidazole-4-carboxamide (AIC) following different dose schedules. *Cancer Chemother Pharmacol* 1982;9:103.]

Loo and co-workers[148] reported increased plasma half-lives in a single patient with hepatic and renal dysfunctions. There are no specific guidelines for DTIC dosing in hepatic or renal dysfunction; however, dosage modifications may be necessary in some patients with moderately severe liver or renal, or both, abnormalities.

In rats,[152] dogs,[201] and humans,[121] DTIC penetrates poorly into the CSF. At equilibrium, the ratio between plasma and spinal fluid was 7 to 1. This finding may explain the lack of DTIC activity against intracranial L1210 leukemia.[117] It fails to explain, however, the observations that DTIC inhibits tumor cell dissemination to the CNS in mice[176,179] and that the drug has activity against transplantable murine ependymoblastoma[205] and against primary and metastatic brain tumors in humans.[119,122,132]

The major metabolite of DTIC found in plasma and urine is AIC (Fig. 14-4),[146,189,198,199,201] with cumulative excretion in the urine accounting for 9% to 20% of parent compound in several patients studied.[189,199] AIC is also formed from DTIC in the presence of liver microsomes[148,157,206] and by some tumor cells.[148,207] After the i.p. administration of [^{14}CO-methyl]DTIC to rats or mice, 4% of the dose is recovered as respiratory $^{14}CO_2$ in 6 hours, and 9% of the dose is recovered as $^{14}CO_2$ in 24 hours.[152,208,209] Presumably, the expired radiolabeled $^{14}CO_2$ is derived from the formaldehyde produced after *N*-demethylation of DTIC. These findings, as well as the identification of 5-(3-hydroxymethyl-3-methyltriazen-1-yl) imidazole-4-carboxamide (HMTIC) as a urinary metabolite of DTIC in rats,[152,210–212] are consistent with a metabolic pathway for DTIC, as shown in Figure 14-3.

As discussed previously, DTIC activation requires an initial oxidation of an *N*-methyl group by microsomal nicotinamide adenine dinucleotide phosphate (reduced form) (NADPH) cytochrome P-450 mixed-function oxidase to form HMTIC. Loss of formaldehyde results in the formation of MTIC, which then spontaneously tautomerizes to AIC and the methyldiazonium ion, $CH_3N^+{\equiv}N$, as the active methylating agent (Fig. 14-3).[138–143,146,147] The methyldiazonium ion is also a postulated end product in the activation of PCB (Fig. 14-1). Alternatively, an *N*-hydroxy metabolite of a monomethyltriazene analog preliminarily has been identified as a candidate for a cytotoxic intermediate.[142] It is not clear which of the DTIC metabolic intermediates, HMTIC, MTIC, or the putative (*N*-hydroxymonomethyltriazeno)imidazole-4-carboxamide, is the predominant active form of the drug *in vivo*.

Further analogs of DTIC and phenyltriazenes have been developed and tested.[117,207–213] Shealy[213] examined the activity of several synthesized analogs with *N*-substitution of the triazeno group. He and his co-workers found that in addition to DTIC, 5-bis(2-chloroethyl)triazenoimidazole-4-carboxamide had significant activity against L1210 murine leukemia.[214] Other investigators showed that increasing the alkyl side-chain length beyond pentyl weakened the antitumor activity against Ehrlich carcinoma.[215,216] Studies of structure-activity relationships have shown that lipophilic and steric properties of an analog may determine its oxidative metabolism and antitumor activity.[209–211] Para derivatives of (3,3-dimethyl-1-triazeno)benzoic acid had significantly greater activity than did ortho or meta derivatives,[176,178,208] and it is quite possible that some of the structurally related differences noted may be a result of altered antimetastatic rather than selective antitumor effects of the compounds.[178,179] At present, DTIC remains the only dimethyltriazene available for clinical use.

DTIC is susceptible to photodecomposition to 5-diazoimidazole-4-carboxamide, which then spontaneously cyclizes to form the purine analog azahypoxanthine[117,217] (Fig. 14-3). Both of these photodecomposition products may be cytotoxic to cells in tissue culture,[144,145,147,156–159] although another report[218] has questioned the results of these earlier studies. Nonetheless, DTIC probably should be protected from light during *in vitro* studies. The importance of light protection for DTIC solutions before clinical use is also controversial. Again, earlier reports suggested an enhanced DTIC toxicity when solutions were exposed to light,[217,219] whereas more recent studies show that DTIC solutions are stable for more than 24 hours when not protected from light[220] and that light exposure before drug administration did not alter *in vivo* activity or toxicity.[218]

Toxicity

The most frequent toxic reaction to DTIC treatment is moderately severe nausea and vomiting, which occurs in 90% of patients.[129,221] These symptoms appear soon after infusion and may persist for up to 12 hours. The severity of gastrointestinal toxicity decreases with successive doses when the drug is given on a 5-day schedule and if the initial dose is decreased.[221] Above 1,200 mg per m² as a rapid intravenous bolus, DTIC frequently causes severe, but short-lived, watery diarrhea.[121,192] After rapid infusion of a high dose (greater than 1,380 mg per m²) of DTIC, hypotension may occur.[192]

Myelosuppression is a common dose-related toxicity of DTIC, although the degree of leukopenia and thrombocytopenia is variably mild to moderate. Significant myelosuppression occurs when more than 1,380 mg per m² is given as a single i.v. bolus,[192] whereas studies using a 5-day administration schedule reported increasing frequency of myelosuppression above a total of 1,000 mg per m².[121,129] In the latter, nadir leukopenia and thrombocytopenia occurred on day 25, with complete recovery by day 40. This delayed bone marrow recovery is not common, however, and usually there is sufficient recovery so that DTIC may be administered every 21 to 28 days.

Less frequent toxic reactions include a flulike syndrome of fever up to 39°C, myalgias, and malaise lasting several days after DTIC treatment. Headache, facial flushing, facial paresthesias, pain along the injection vein, alopecia, and abnormal hepatic and renal function tests rarely occur. Photosensitivity to DTIC has been reported in several patients, especially after high-dose therapy.[192,222] This toxicity was reproduced in an animal model[218] and is probably due to the fact that DTIC is photodecomposed to toxic intermediates. Therefore, patients should be advised to avoid sunlight exposure for several days after DTIC therapy. Cases of hepatic vein occlusion associated with fever, eosinophilia, and hepatic necrosis and resulting in death have been attributed to DTIC as a distinct clinical pathologic syndrome.[223–227] The mechanism for this toxicity is unknown, but an allergic etiology has been suggested.[226,227]

DTIC causes a number of immunologic effects *in vitro* and *in vivo*. The drug markedly depresses antibody responses and allograft rejection in mice for up to 60 days after a single injection.[180,228] This is probably a specific effect of DTIC, because structure activity studies showed different patterns of immunodepression depending on which phenyltriazene analog was tested.[229] DTIC apparently does not directly suppress natural killer cell activity in mice.[230] As discussed previously in the context of a possible mechanism for DTIC's antimetastatic properties, the drug can significantly alter the immunogenicity of tumor cells in mice.[180–182] After DTIC treatment, L1210 or L5178 lymphomas were found to be highly immunogenic, such that large inocula of the DTIC-resistant tumors were rejected by immunocompetent animals. DTIC-treated cells were actually less susceptible to natural killer cell cytolysis *in vitro*[231]; however, tumor rejection may be a result of the development of cytotoxic lymphocytes *in vivo*.[181,185] Antigenic alteration of DTIC-exposed cells also may explain the induction of tumor cell immunogenicity.[182–184,232] Drug-induced somatic mutation has been suggested as the underlying mechanism,[187] although significant chromosomal alterations as a result of triazine exposure were not observed *in vitro*.[233]

DTIC has mutagenic, carcinogenic, and teratogenic properties in experimental systems.[234,235] In rodents, DTIC causes lymphoma and tumors of the thymus, lung, uterus, or mammary glands when given orally or by single or multiple injections.[137,236–238] MTIC treatment also caused similar tumors but in a lower frequency compared with DTIC.[237] It is not firmly established whether DTIC is carcinogenic for humans. In a retrospective analysis of patients receiving either MOPP or ABVD (plus or minus radiation therapy) for Hodgkin's disease, Valagussa et al.[239] reported no treatment-associated secondary malignancies in patients receiving ABVD. Subsequently, isolated cases of acute leukemia occurring after DTIC therapy have been reported,[240,241] but these remain quite rare. Finally, DTIC causes dose-dependent fetal malformations and fetal resorptions when administered to pregnant rats and rabbits.[242,243] Teratogenic effects were observed in the urogenital system, skeleton, eye, and cardiovascular system.

TEMOZOLOMIDE

History

Several series of 1,2,4-triazines and -triazinones were synthesized in England in the 1960s and 1970s, and selected compounds proved to have activity against murine tumors.[244–248] The most promising was mitozolomide, which was active against a broad spectrum of murine tumors,[247] but it produced severe and unpredictable thrombocytopenia in clinical trials and was abandoned as a clinical candidate.[248]

Selection of the next generation of imidazotetrazinones focused on TMZ, the 3-methyl derivative of mitozolomide (Fig. 14-5). This compound, with a different spectrum of activity against murine tumors,[249] was less active and con-

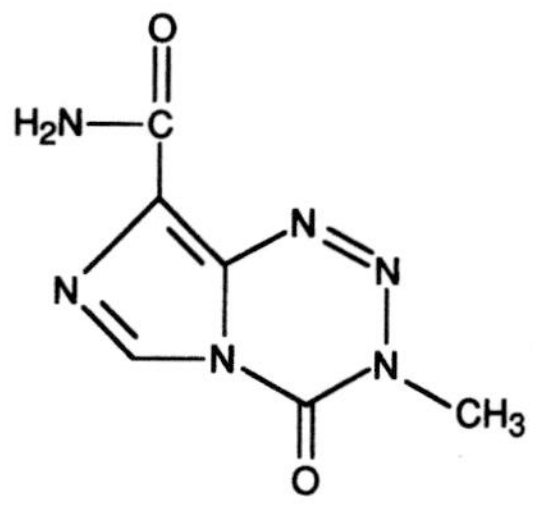

FIGURE 14-5. Structure of temozolomide.

TABLE 14-4. KEY FEATURES OF TEMOZOLOMIDE {8-CARBAMOYL-3-METHYLIMIDAZO [5,1-D]-1,2,3,5-TETRAZIN-4(3H)-ONE}

Mechanism of action:	Methylation of nucleic acids
Metabolism:	Chemical conversion of 5(3-methyltria-zeno)imidazole-4-carboxamide
Pharmacokinetics (i.v. or p.o.):	Volume of distribution: 28.3 L
	Elimination half-life: 1.8 h
	Distribution half-life: 0.26 h
	Clearance: 11.76 L/h[253]
Drug and food inter-actions:	Unknown
Toxicity:	Myelosuppression
	Nausea and vomiting
	Elevated hepatic transaminases

siderably less toxic than mitozolomide and displayed superb delivery to all body tissues, including the brain.[250,251] TMZ was rationally advanced to clinical trial, in part based on the realization that under physiologic conditions the ring opens with resulting generation of the monomethyl triazine MTIC, the same metabolite formed by metabolic dealkylation of DTIC.[252] The inefficient demethylation of DTIC in humans (despite rapid demethylation in mice) coupled with the conversion of TMZ to MTIC without need for this metabolic step suggested a potential benefit for the use of TMZ. See Table 14-4 for key features of TMZ.

Phase I trials of intravenous and subsequently oral TMZ began in 1987 with a single-dose schedule and demonstrated the dose-limiting toxicity to be myelosuppression with trivial clinical benefits observed.[253] However, based on preclinical data supporting a multiple-dose regimen, another phase I trial using a 5-day schedule was conducted, with myelosuppression again the dose-limiting toxicity. Greater clinical activity was noted with four responses (two partial and two complete) in 23 patients with metastatic melanoma and two partial responses in four patients with high-grade glioma.[253]

Further evaluation in 28 patients with primary brain tumors revealed five radiographic responses in ten patients with recurrent astrocytoma (the majority of which were high-grade). Similarly, four radiographic responses were seen in seven patients with newly diagnosed high-grade glioma.[254] It should be noted that radiographic criteria for response were not the conventionally accepted partial or complete response criteria. Nevertheless, these results are provocative and justified further studies in patients with CNS tumors, particularly gliomas.

This O'Reilly study was extended to 75 patients (48 with recurrent disease and 27 with new diagnoses).[255] Improvements on computed tomography (CT) were seen in 12 (25%) of the patients with recurrent disease and in eight (30%) of the patients with new diagnoses. Twenty-two percent of patients with recurrences and 43% of those with newly diagnosed tumors survived to 1 year.

The Cancer Research Campaign (CRC) conducted a multicenter phase II study in which TMZ demonstrated activity in patients with recurrent and progressive high-grade glioma.[256] Objective responses, measured by improvement in neurologic status, were seen in 11 (11%) of 103 patients who received TMZ; five of these patients had improvement on CT or magnetic resonance imaging (MRI) scans.[256] Objective responses were observed in patients diagnosed with anaplastic astrocytoma, glioblastoma multiforme (grade IV), and unclassified high-grade astrocytoma (grades III–IV).

The Schering-Plough Research Institute conducted a randomized, multicenter, open-label phase II study of TMZ and PCB in 225 patients with glioblastoma multiforme (GBM) at first relapse.[257] The primary objectives were to compare the progression-free survival at 6 months and safety of TMZ and PCB in adult patients with GBM who had failed conventional treatment. The 6-month progression-free survival rate was significantly higher for patients who received TMZ (21%) than for those who received PCB (8%) ($p = .008$). Median progression-free survival for TMZ patients (12.4 weeks) was significantly longer than for PCB patients (8.32 weeks; $p = .0063$). The 6-month overall survival rate for TMZ patients was 60% versus 44% for PCB patients ($p = .019$).

The Schering-Plough Research Institute also conducted an open-label, multicenter phase II trial comprised of 162 patients with malignant astrocytoma at first relapse.[258] The primary protocol end point, progression-free survival at 6 months, was 46% [95% confidence limit (CL), 38% to 54%]. The median progression-free survival was 5.4 months, and 24% of patients remained progression-free at 12 months based on Kaplan-Meier estimates.

Duke participated in a Schering-Plough Research Institute multicenter phase II trial evaluating the activity of TMZ *before* radiation therapy in the treatment of newly diagnosed high-grade glioma.[259] Eligibility criteria included residual enhancing disease on postoperative MRI and a Karnofsky performance score (KPS) greater than or equal to 70%. Thirty-three patients with GBM evaluated for tumor response revealed three with complete response, 14 with partial response, four with stable disease, and 12 with progressive disease. Five patients with anaplastic astrocytoma evaluated for response revealed one with partial response, two with stable disease, and two with progressive disease.

The efficacy of TMZ has also been evaluated in a study of patients with advanced metastatic melanoma, including patients with brain metastases.[260] Among 56 patients (49 with evaluable lesions), complete responses occurred in three, all with lung metastases only, and partial responses occurred in nine, yielding a response rate of 21%. Stable disease was observed in an additional eight patients.

General Mechanism of Action and Cellular Pharmacology

The spontaneous conversion of TMZ is initiated by the effect of water at the highly electropositive C^4 position of

TMZ. This activity opens the ring, releases CO_2, and generates the reactive methylating agent MTIC. The initial proposal was that this effect of water was catalyzed in the close environment of the major groove of DNA,[261,262] but confirming this mechanism has been difficult, and it is known that TMZ converts readily to MTIC in free solution in the absence of DNA.[263] MTIC degrades to the methyldiazonium cation, which transfers the methyl group to DNA and to the final degradation product AIC, which is excreted via the kidneys.[264,265] The methylation of DNA appears to be the principal mechanism responsible for the cytotoxicity of TMZ to malignant cells (see below). The methyldiazonium cation can also react with RNA and with soluble and cellular protein.[266] However, the methylation of RNA and the methylation or carbamoylation of protein do not appear to have any known significant role in the antitumor activity of TMZ.[266] Further studies are required to clarify the role of these targets in the biochemical mechanism of action of TMZ.

The spontaneous conversion of TMZ and MTIC is dependent on pH. Under acidic conditions, TMZ is stable; however, its chemical stability decreases at a pH of greater than 7.0 and is converted rapidly to MTIC in that environment.[265] In contrast, MTIC is more stable under basic conditions and rapidly degrades to the methyldiazonium cation and AIC at a pH of less than 7.0.[265] A comparison of the half-life of TMZ in phosphate buffer (pH, 7.4; $t_{1/2}$ = 1.83 hours)[253,265] indicates that the conversion of TMZ to MTIC is a chemically controlled reaction with little or no enzymatic component. The spontaneous conversion of TMZ may contribute to its highly reproducible pharmacokinetics in comparison with other alkylating agents such as DTIC and PCB, which must undergo metabolic conversion in the liver and are thus subject to interpatient variation in metabolic rates of conversion.[262,265]

Among the lesions produced in DNA after treatment of cells with TMZ, the most common is methylation at the N^7 position of guanine, followed by methylation at the O^3 position of adenine and the O^6 position of guanine.[265] Although the N^7-methylguanine and O^3-methyladenine adducts probably contribute to the antitumor activity of TMZ in some, if not all, sensitive cells, their role is controversial.[267] The critical role of the O^6-methylguanine adduct, which accounts for 5% of the total adducts formed by TMZ,[265] in the agent's antitumor activity is supported by the correlation between the sensitivity of tumor cell lines to TMZ and the activity of the DNA repair protein AGT, which specifically removes alkyl groups at the O^6 position of guanine. Cell lines that have low levels of AGT are sensitive to the cytotoxicity of temozolomide, whereas cell lines that have high levels of this repair protein are much more resistant to it.[268–271] This correlation also has been observed in human glioblastoma xenograft models.[272–274] The preferential alkylation of guanine and adenine and the correlation of sensitivity to the drug with the ability to repair the O^6-

alkylguanine lesion also have been seen with triazine, DTIC, and the nitrosourea alkylating agents BCNU and CCNU.[271,275,276]

The cytotoxic mechanism of temozolomide appears to be related to the failure of the DNA mismatch repair system to find a complementary base for methylated guanine. This system involves the formation of a complex of proteins that recognize, bind to, and remove methylated guanine.[277–279] The proposed hypothesis is that when this repair process is targeted to the DNA strand opposite the O^6-methylguanine, it cannot find a correct partner, thus resulting in long-lived nicks in the DNA.[280] These nicks accumulate and persist into the subsequent cell cycle, where they ultimately inhibit initiation of replication in the daughter cells, blocking the cell cycle at the G_2M boundary.[280–284] In murine[281] and human[285] leukemia cells, sensitivity to temozolomide correlates with increased fragmentation of DNA and apoptotic cell death.

DNA adducts formed by temozolomide and the subsequent DNA damage or alteration of specific genes may cause cell death or reduce the metastatic potential of tumor cells. For example, mutations caused by adduct formation may result in altered surface antigens on tumor cells that contribute enhanced immunogenicity in the host.[180,286,287] The effects of enhanced immunologic response range from complete tumor rejection to reduced growth rates and reduced metastatic potential.[288] Additional evidence suggests that temozolomide can reduce the metastatic potential of Lewis lung carcinoma cells[289] and induce differentiation in the K562 erythroleukemia cell line.[186,290] It has been postulated that temozolomide-induced DNA damage and subsequent cell-cycle arrest may reduce the metastatic properties of some tumor cells.[290–292]

Mechanism of Resistance

AGT DNA Repair Protein

Several studies have shown that AGT is the primary mechanism of resistance to temozolomide and other alkylating agents.[169,293] AGT functions as the first line of defense against temozolomide by removing the alkyl groups from the O^6 position of guanine, in effect reversing the cytotoxic lesion of temozolomide.[294] AGT levels can be correlated with the sensitivity of tumor cell lines to temozolomide and the alkylating agents BCNU and DTIC.[276,285,295–298] The role of AGT in resistance to temozolomide is also evidenced by the ability of the virally transfected human AGT gene to confer a high level of resistance to temozolomide and other methylating and chloroethylating agents on cells that are devoid of endogenous AGT activity.[299]

AGT levels in human tumor tissues and normal tissue specimens derived from brain, lung, and ovary vary widely over a 100-fold range, with some human tumors having no detectable activity.[300–303] Some specimens from all tumor types examined in these studies have demonstrated a complete absence of AGT activity: As many as 22% of primary brain tumor specimens have no detectable AGT activity.[300] Similar findings with respect to AGT levels in brain tumor cells have been observed in *in vitro* models.[304] AGT activity has been localized to both the cytoplasm and the nucleus of the cell, although the function of cytoplasmic AGT and its mechanism of transport to the nucleus are unknown.[301] AGT transfers the methyl group to an internal cysteine residue, acting as methyltransferase and methyl acceptor protein. In the process, AGT becomes irreversibly inactivated, and new AGT must be synthesized to restore AGT activity.[60] Therefore, the number of O^6-methylguanine adducts that can be repaired is limited by the number of AGT molecules of the protein available.[60]

Deficiency in Mismatch Repair Pathway

Although AGT is clearly important in the resistance of cells to temozolomide, some cell lines that express low levels of AGT are nevertheless resistant, indicating that other resistance mechanisms may be involved.[305,306] A deficiency in the mismatch repair pathway as a result of mutations in any one of the four proteins that recognize and repair DNA (i.e., GTBP, hMSH2, hPMS2, and hMLH1) can render cells tolerant to methylation and to the cytotoxic effects of temozolomide. This deficiency in the mismatch repair pathway results in a failure to recognize and repair the O^6-methylguanine adducts produced by temozolomide and other methylating agents.[61a,269,307] The DNA damage that results from failure to repair the O^6-methylguanine adducts produces a particular type of genomic instability, microsatellite instability, that is associated with some familial and sporadic cancers, such as hereditary nonpolyposis colorectal cancer.[308,309] The high level of resistance in tumor cells that are deficient in mismatch repair is unrelated to the level of AGT and is, therefore, unaffected by AGT inhibitors.

Nucleotide Excision Repair

Another possible mechanism of resistance to temozolomide is nucleotide excision repair. Unlike the case with the O^6-methylguanine adduct, the N^7-methylguanine and O^3-methyladenine adducts introduced into DNA by temozolomide will block DNA synthesis and lead directly to cell death unless repaired by the system of adduct-specific enzymes involved in DNA nucleotide excision repair.[310] Studies have shown that treatment of human tumor cells with temozolomide induced an increase in the activity of an enzyme, PARP, believed to be involved in nucleotide excision repair,[311,312] and inhibition of PARP has been reported to enhance the cytotoxicity of methylating agents.[313,314] Several studies with inhibitors of PARP and with cell lines deficient in either mismatch repair or exci-

sion repair have indicated a role of the repair of N^7-methylguanine and O^3-methyladenine adducts in the resistance to the antitumor activity of temozolomide and other alkylating agents.[267,269,313,314] However, the importance of these adducts in the antitumor activity of the drug may be secondary to that of the O^6-MG adduct, except in cells that are deficient in base excision repair.[168,315,316]

Drug Interactions

There are no known adverse reactions with other drugs. It is expected that compounds that deplete AGT will increase temozolomide toxicity.

Clinical Pharmacology and Toxicity

Temozolomide is supplied in capsules containing 5, 25, 100, or 250 mg for oral use. In the initial phase I trial in the United Kingdom, temozolomide was administered as a single i.v. dose at doses of 50 to 200 mg per m² and subsequently was given orally to fasted patients as a single dose, up to a total dose of 200 to 1,200 mg per m². Additionally, oral doses of 750 to 1,200 mg per m² were divided into 5 equal doses and administered daily for 5 days at 4-week intervals.

The pharmacokinetics of temozolomide were evaluated in the United Kingdom phase I trials.[253] After intravenous administration, plasma temozolomide concentrations declined biexponentially consistent with a two-compartment open model and a terminal elimination half-life of 1.8 hours. After oral administration, plasma temozolomide concentrations were consistent with a one-compartment oral model, with rapid absorption and maximum plasma concentrations occurring 0.7 hour after treatment. The clearance of temozolomide was 11.8 L per hour, and the pharmacokinetics were independent of the dosage (with a linear relationship between dose and area under the time × concentration curve). Oral bioavailability was considered to be complete.

In 1993, Schering-Plough began the worldwide development of temozolomide using machine-filled capsules that were prepared according to good manufacturing practices, which differed from the hand-filled capsules used in the initial study. Several phase I studies have evaluated the safety and tolerability of that new temozolomide formulation (Temodal). Data from these studies have confirmed the safety, tolerability, and pharmacokinetics of temozolomide reported in the CRC phase I study (Table 14-3).[317–325]

Phase I studies of temozolomide also were expanded to include pediatric cancer patients. A phase I study was conducted to define the multiple-dose pharmacokinetics of temozolomide in this population. In this study, 19 patients between 3 and 17 years old were given temozolomide over a dosage range of 100 to 240 mg per m² per day. Temozolomide was absorbed rapidly, had an AUC that increased in a

TABLE 14-5. KEY FEATURES OF HEXAMETHYLMELAMINE (HMM, NSC-13875)

Mechanism of action:	Possible alkylation of nucleic acids; inhibition of DNA and RNA synthesis.
Metabolism:	Microsomal hydroxylation to hydroxymethylmelamine and microsomal demethylation to methylmelamine derivatives and formaldehyde.
Pharmacokinetics:	$t_{1/2\alpha}$ = 0.5 h; $t_{1/2\beta}$ = 4.7–10.2 h.
	Variable oral absorption, peak plasma concentration at 0.5–3.0 h.
	94% protein bound.
	Poor CSF penetration, whereas demethylated metabolites have higher CSF penetration.
Elimination:	Hepatic (extensive first-pass effect) and renal.
	Minor respiratory and fecal.
Drug and food interactions:	Barbiturates may enhance metabolism.
	Cimetidine may inhibit metabolism.
Toxicity:	Gastrointestinal (nausea and vomiting).
	Neurotoxicity (mood alterations, hallucinations, peripheral neuropathy).
	Mild myelosuppression (leukopenia and thrombocytopenia).
Precautions:	None.

CSF, cerebrospinal fluid; $t_{1/2}$, half-life.

dosage-related manner, and showed no evidence of accumulation. The plasma half-life, whole-body clearance, and volume of distribution were independent of dosage (Table 14-4).[317] Compared with adult patients treated with 200 mg per m² per day, children appeared to have a higher AUC (48.7 vs. 34.5 mg per hour per mL), most likely because children have a larger ratio of body surface area to volume. Despite higher concentrations at dosages equivalent to those used in adult patients, the bone marrow function in pediatric patients appears to allow greater exposure to the drug before dose-limiting bone marrow toxicity develops.[317]

The effects of food and gastric pH on the pharmacokinetics and bioavailability of orally administered temozolomide also have been evaluated. Administration of temozolomide after ingestion of food resulted in a small decrease in its oral bioavailability.[322] When temozolomide was taken after a meal, a slight (9%), but statistically significant, reduction occurred in the rate and extent of its absorption (Table 14-5). Because AUC confidence levels were within the bioequivalence guidelines of 80% to 125%, it is unlikely that the slight reduction observed in the oral bioavailability of temozolomide in the presence of a meal has any clinical effect on the antitumor activity of temozolomide.

The oral bioavailability, maximum plasma concentration, and half-life of temozolomide were not affected by an increase in gastric pH of 1 to 2 units, resulting from the administration of ranitidine every 12 hours on either the first 2 or the last 2 days of the 5-day temozolomide dosing schedule.[324]

Subsequent phase I trials sponsored by Schering-Plough in adult[319–324] and pediatric patients[317,326] with advanced cancer also have confirmed that hematologic toxicity, specifically thrombocytopenia and neutropenia, is dose-limiting. Neutropenia or thrombocytopenia appeared 21 to 28 days after the first dose of each cycle and recovered to grade 1 myelosuppression within 7 to 14 days. Grade 4 toxicity occurred at cumulative oral dosages of more than 1,000 mg per m² over 5 days, but little other toxicity was seen.[320] Grade 3 or 4 myelosuppression occurred in less than 10% of patients studied.

The effect of prior treatment with chemotherapy, radiation, or both, on the maximum tolerated dose (MTD) of temozolomide has been evaluated.[319,323] In one of these studies,[323] 24 patients stratified according to prior exposure to chemotherapy and radiation were given a dosage of 100 mg per m² per day of temozolomide for 5 days, which was escalated to 150 and 200 mg per m² per day in the absence of myelosuppression. The MTD for temozolomide was established as 150 mg per m² per day.[323] The other similar phase I study, reported by the National Cancer Institute, evaluated the safety of temozolomide in patients who were stratified on the basis of prior exposure to nitrosourea.[319] The MTD for patients with prior exposure to nitrosourea was 150 mg per m² per day, and the MTD for patients without such prior exposure was 250 mg per m² per day. An evaluation of the pharmacokinetics of temozolomide showed that its clearance from the plasma was significantly less in patients with prior exposure to nitrosourea than it was in patients without such prior exposure.[319] This may have contributed to the lower dose of temozolomide that was tolerated by these patients and had a notable effect on the dosing recommendation for these patients.[319]

The results of these studies indicated that a dosage of 200 mg per m² of temozolomide given on a 5-day schedule and repeated every 28 days is appropriate for patients who are not pretreated with radiation, chemotherapy, or both.

Patients who are pretreated with chemotherapy receive a lower starting dose of temozolomide (i.e., 150 mg per m²), which can be escalated to 200 mg per m² in subsequent courses in the absence of grade 3 or 4 myelosuppression.[323]

HEXAMETHYLMELAMINE

History

The *N*-methyl–substituted *s*-triazine derivatives HMM and PMM are the third clinically important group of nonclassic alkylating agents that require biochemical activation for their antitumor activity.[1] HMM, a structural analog of the alkylating agent triethylenemelamine (TEM), was synthesized in the early 1950s.[327] It was initially shown to have activity against experimental rodent sarcomas.[328,329] PMM, a urinary metabolite of HMM (Fig. 14-6), also has *in vivo* antitumor activity against L1210 leukemia, sarcoma 180, or Lewis lung carcinoma with a therapeutic index equal to

HMM.[330] PMM was developed for clinical trials because its greater aqueous solubility allowed for i.v. formulation.[331] For both of these compounds, the presence of the *N*-methyl groups is necessary for antitumor activity, although their precise metabolism and mechanism of action remain uncertain.[1,332]

HMM has been approved for treatment of patients with ovarian cancer who have failed first-line regimens. The results of trials were reviewed by Blum and co-workers[333] and more recently by Foster and co-workers.[334] As a single agent, HMM has unquestioned activity against advanced ovarian cancer, with an overall objective response rate of 21%.[334] In previously untreated patients, the response rate exceeds 30%, and some patients have pathologically proven complete remissions of modest duration.[335,336] The precise role for HMM in combination chemotherapy regimens for advanced ovarian cancer remains controversial,[337] although these regimens clearly have high activity.[334,337–339] As a second-line therapy in ovarian carcinoma, HMM has activity against alkylating agent–resistant tumors.[340–344] HMM also

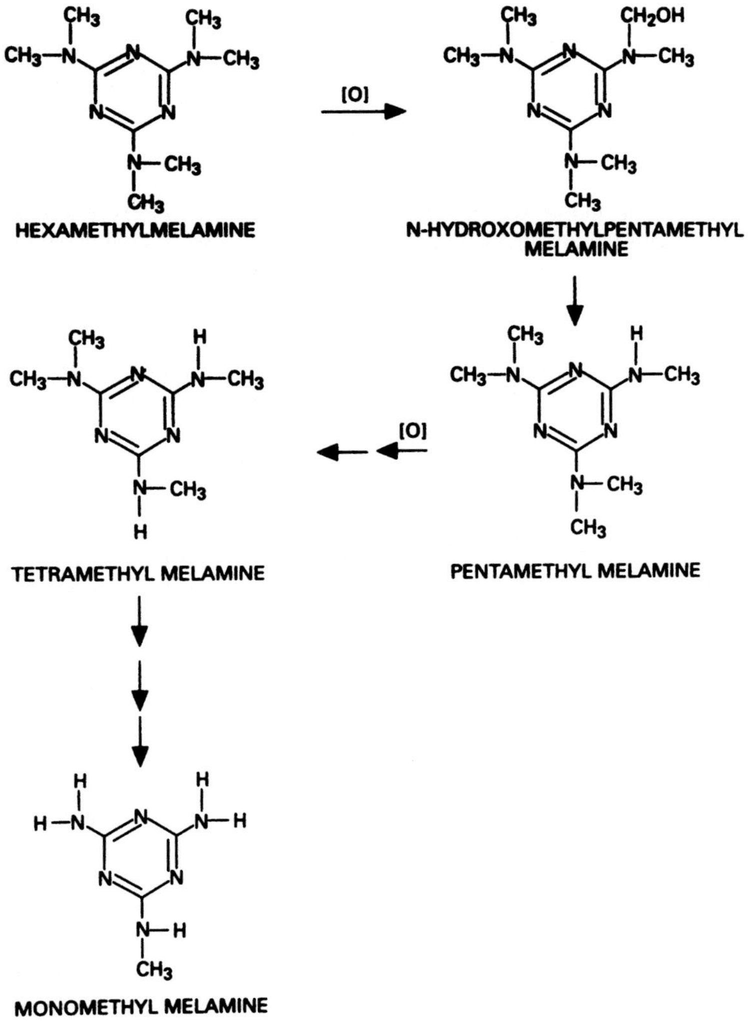

FIGURE 14-6. Metabolic reactions of hexamethylmelamine, leading to the generation of hydroxylated and demethylated intermediates.

has activity against non–small cell and small cell lung carcinoma, breast cancer, endometrial cancer, refractory lymphomas,[334] bilharzial bladder carcinoma,[345] and, when combined with prednisone, possibly against multiple myeloma.[346] Because of significant neurotoxicity and only scattered responses observed during initial clinical trials,[347] PMM has not undergone further clinical investigation. However, because of the clinical activity of HMM and PMM and because of the lack of cross-resistance with classic alkylating agents, there remains an interest in achieving a greater understanding of HMM pharmacology and structure-activity relationships so that analogs with higher therapeutic ratios may be developed. The key features of HMM are summarized in Table 14-5.

General Mechanism of Action and Cellular Pharmacology

The cellular mechanism of HMM antitumor activity is unknown. Because of the structural similarity to TEM and the *N*-methyl structural requirement for activity, most attention has been directed to the HMM methyl groups as reactive sites of the molecule. However, neither HMM or its metabolites showed reactivity with 4-(*p*-nitrobenzyl)pyridine, an acceptor for alkylating species, in a chemical assay.[348] After i.v. administration to mice, ring and methyl ^{14}C–labeled drug resulted in recovery of covalently bound acid-precipitable material, presumably nucleic acids, proteins, or both.[349–352] HMM undergoes extensive demethylation with the formation of formaldehyde *in vivo* (Fig. 14-6).[332,348,349,353] The latter may be reused in the one-carbon pool for *de novo* purine or pyrimidine biosynthesis; this may explain why methyl-labeled HMM showed greater covalent binding than did ring-labeled HMM.[349,351] It is unlikely that the formaldehyde formed from HMM metabolism is responsible for cytotoxicity, because the HMM analog trimethylomelamine, which produces equal plasma concentrations of formaldehyde, has no antitumor activity,[349,354] and *in vitro* studies in L1210 leukemia and PC 6 plasmacytoma failed to show a correlation between formaldehyde production or formaldehyde-induced DNA-protein cross-links and cytotoxicity.[354,355] Alternatively, the *N*-hydroxy metabolite *N*-hydroxymethylpentamethylmelamine (HMPMM) has been suggested as an active intermediate that has cytotoxic activity *in vitro*[332,351,354,356–358] and antitumor activity *in vivo*.[332] HMPMM has been identified as a metabolite of HMM *in vitro*[359] and *in vivo*.[360] HMM, PMM, and HMPMM have been shown to inhibit DNA and RNA synthesis,[356,357,361] whereas DNA-protein and DNA-DNA cross-linking probably does not account for the cytotoxicity of these compounds.[352,358]

There are few studies that specifically examine HMM cellular pharmacology. As mentioned above, HMM and PMM may be cytotoxic *in vitro*[356,357,362]; however, this is clearly the case when a metabolic activating system is present that converts parent drug to active intermediates.[332,351,354,355,358] One study has suggested that HMM and PMM enter cells by simple diffusion, and some *in vitro* tumor cell systems have been shown to metabolize HMM and PMM,[363] whereas others have not.[357,358]

Mechanisms of Resistance

Virtually nothing is known about cellular mechanisms of HMM resistance except for the facts that, clinically, many alkylator-resistant tumors do not exhibit cross-resistance to HMM[340–344] and Chinese hamster ovary cells with a multi-drug-resistant phenotype do not exhibit cross-resistance to HMM.[364] There are no studies investigating altered transport or altered DNA repair as a possible mechanism of resistance. Because studies have shown that oxidative HMM metabolism may be regulated by cellular glutathione[365,366] and because elevated glutathione levels have been associated with alkylating agent resistance, it would be of interest to determine the role of glutathione in the cellular pharmacology of HMM.

Drug Interactions

HMM and PMM are extensively metabolized *in vivo*, and there are many potential drug-drug interactions that may occur and may have clinical significance. In rodents, pretreatment with phenobarbital enhances HMM microsomal metabolism[367,368] and antagonizes HMM antitumor activity. It may be expected that barbiturates or other known inducers of liver microsomal enzymes would alter the metabolism, and perhaps activity, of HMM in humans, although there is no information available to support this. Hande and co-workers[369] have shown that cimetidine, through inhibition of microsomal metabolism, caused a dose-dependent prolongation of HMM half-life that was associated with increased toxicity. HMM pharmacokinetics were not altered by concomitant doxorubicin or cyclophosphamide.[370]

Clinical Pharmacology

Because of its poor aqueous solubility, HMM is supplied in capsules of 50 and 100 mg for oral administration. Usual dosages are 4 to 12 mg per kg daily for 14 to 21 days each month, although longer periods of continuous administration have been used.[335,340,347] HMM has been solubilized in a lipid emulsion[371–373] for i.v. administration, and this formulation is being evaluated clinically.[374,375] PMM was formulated for parenteral administration, and a single i.v. dose of up to 1,500 mg per m^2 every 3 weeks and 1,000 mg per m^2 three times a week every 3 weeks were the MTDs in several phase I clinical studies.[347,376–380]

HMM and PMM metabolism and pharmacokinetics have been studied extensively in experimental animals and humans. The analytical methods most frequently used to detect the parent compounds and their demethylated metabolites involved separation procedures, such as cation exchange, followed by gas chromatography with a nitrogen detector[381,382] or with mass spectroscopy.[383] These methods provide high sensitivity and specificity in contrast to earlier, less-specific methods that used ultraviolet spectral detection for HMM concentration determinations.[384] HPLC analysis for HMM, PMM, and their metabolites also has been described.[350,361,385–387] Dubois and co-workers[360] have used a sensitive, reverse-phase HPLC method to measure HMM and HMPMM in plasma obtained from mice.

HMM and PMM display dose-dependent and species-dependent pharmacokinetics.[388,389] After oral administration, HMM has extremely variable bioavailability with a 100-fold variation in peak blood levels.[390] Several studies have suggested that extensive first-pass hepatic metabolism or intestinal wall metabolism, rather than poor absorption, may account for the variable bioavailability.[391–393] In patients, the peak plasma levels are achieved 0.5 to 3.0 hours after the oral dose, with concentrations ranging between 0.2 and 20.8 μg per mL. The initial half-life of parent drug plasma disappearance in one study was 0.5 hour.[370] In several studies, the terminal half-life varied between 4.7 and 13.0 hours, and the AUC ranged from 70.2 to 3,607.0 μg per mL/minute.[347,390] The plasma half-life of ring-labeled [14C]HMM is 13 hours, significantly longer than the intact parent molecule.[353] In one study, HMM pharmacokinetics was not influenced by the presence of ascites.[370]

PMM pharmacokinetics after i.v. administration have been studied in animals[361,388,389,391,394,395] and during several phase I clinical trials.[347,376,379,380,383,386,387,391,396] The plasma levels were dose-dependent,[376,380,388] and clearance was reduced at higher dosages and in the presence of hepatic dysfunction. Plasma decay of the parent drug was biphasic according to a two-compartment model (Fig. 14-7A). In humans, the initial and terminal half-lives for PMM were approximately 30 and 100 to 143 minutes,[376,380,383,386,387,389,391,396] respectively, with much more rapid elimination found in mice, rats, and rabbits.[361,388,389,391,394] After a 24-hour infusion of ring-labeled [14C]PMM, the 14C plasma half-life was 12 hours.[379] In this study, the mean apparent volume of distribution was 2.04 L per kg, and the mean total clearance was 14 mL per kg per minute. Benvenuto and co-workers[396] have shown variable pharmacokinetic parameters for each of the demethylated PMM metabolites (Fig. 14-7A).

In a small series of patients given an oral dosage, the highest concentrations of HMM were found in tissues containing significant fat, whereas lower concentrations (equal to plasma) were found in primary tumor.[397] Small metastatic deposits contained significantly higher HMM concentrations compared to larger metastases or primary tumor. After i.p. administration to mice bearing ovarian carcinoma, HMM and PMM were widely distributed among all organs examined.[352,394] HMM measured in CSF in one patient[398] was found to be 6% of the plasma concentration. Lesser methylated melamine metabolites were found in the CSF in higher concentrations with CSF and plasma ratios approaching 1. After a single i.p. dose in mice, the concentration of HMM or PMM in brain was approximately four times that measured in plasma,[394] although in another study, brain PMM concentrations were constantly higher than the concentrations of HMM.[361] HMM and PMM showed moderate protein binding of 94% and 70%, respectively.[395,399]

The major elimination route for HMM and PMM is hepatic metabolism, with less than 1% of parent compound found in the urine,[353,367,382,383] although the majority (approximately 70% to 90%) of administered drug is excreted in the urine when radiolabel recovery or total drug

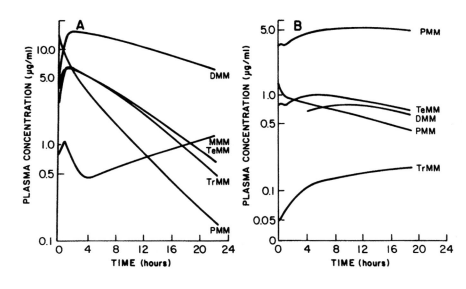

FIGURE 14-7. A: Plasma concentration of pentamethylmelamine (PMM) and demethylated metabolites in a patient with normal liver function after the administration of PMM, 1 g per m², intravenous. **B:** Plasma concentration of PMM and demethylated metabolites in a patient with abnormal liver function (bilirubin = 2) after the administration of PMM, 640 mg per m², intravenous. (DMM, dimethylmelamine; MMM, monomethylmelamine; TeMM, tetramethylmelamine; TrMM, trimethylmelamine.) (From Benvenuto JA, Stewart DJ, Benjamin RS, et al. Pharmacology of pentamethylmelamine in humans. *Cancer Res* 1981;41:566.)

and metabolites are measured.[379,384,391] Benvenuto and co-workers[396] found that reduced clearance of PMM correlated with the severity of liver dysfunction, which was associated with a higher incidence of neurologic toxicity (Fig. 14-7B). Ring-labeled [^{14}C]HMM produced no detectable respiratory 14 CO_2,[353] although up to 30% of the administered dosage was recovered as respiratory $^{14}CO_2$ if the *N*-methyl group contained the radiolabel.[367] Fecal elimination was minimal.

Many *in vitro* and *in vivo* studies in several species have demonstrated rapid and extensive metabolism of HMM and PMM.[356,358–360,363,367–369,382,384,386,389,392,395,396] The metabolic route based on these studies is shown in Figure 14-6. It is now recognized that microsomal *N*-demethylation takes place after hydroxylation of the methyl group,[359] and this latter compound (HMPMM) has been identified *in vivo*.[360] This microsomal oxidation is catalyzed by inducible, NADPH-dependent cytochrome P-450, which seems to be regulated by cellular glutathione.[365,366,395] Presumably, analogous hydroxylation and demethylation account for the subsequent metabolism of PMM and lesser methylated melamines. Additionally, mitochondrial metabolism of HMM has been demonstrated in hepatic and intestinal preparations.[378] In contrast to 5-azacytidine,[400] the *s*-triazine ring is not metabolically cleaved.

Examination of the structure-activity relationships for these compounds shows that the *in vivo* antitumor activity declines as the number of methyl groups decreases.[330–332] Thus, tetramethylmelamine retains some activity, but trimethylmelamine is inactive. Substitution of the methyl group with ethyl or other constituents also renders the compound inactive.[332] Because the hydroxymethyl metabolite is more cytotoxic *in vitro* and this may represent the pharmacologically active intermediate of HMM or PMM,[351,352,356–358] a trihydroxy-trimethyl analog that does not require metabolic activation has been synthesized. This analog has equivalent, or superior, activity to HMM and PMM in preclinical studies,[331,385,401,402] but comparative clinical trials have yet to be performed.

Toxicity

The major toxicity of HMM and PMM is dose-limiting gastrointestinal toxicity consisting of nausea and vomiting, anorexia, and diarrhea,[334,347,376,377,379,380,403,404] which worsens with cumulative dosing,[335,336,340] precluding continuous administration. The mechanism for this toxicity is most likely central, because high concentrations of PMM and other demethylated metabolites are readily detected in the CNS, and i.v. administration of PMM causes just as severe gastrointestinal toxicity.[347] Another consequence of high-CNS drug and metabolite concentrations is a 25% or greater incidence of neurotoxicity[334,336,347,376–378,403,404] consisting of mood changes, such as lethargy, depression, agitation, hallucinations, or even coma, in addition to

peripheral neuropathy. The trihydroxy-trimethyl analog of PMM has much lower CNS concentrations (brain to plasma ratio of 0.08, compared with 1.04 for PMM), and this compound has demonstrated less gastrointestinal and neurotoxicity in initial phase I clinical studies.[399]

Prolonged administration of HMM also results in myelosuppression, with leukopenia observed more frequently than thrombocytopenia.[335,336] This is rarely a dose-limiting toxicity, and it may be avoided with shorter courses of treatment. There have been reports of cutaneous hypersensitivity, and possible hepatic toxicity in patients with liver metastases has been reported.[376] The immunologic, mutagenic, and carcinogenic activities of HMM or PMM have not been well studied. HMM, in combination with other agents, did not alter lymphocyte populations in ovarian cancer patients.[405] HMM was weakly mutagenic in an *in vitro* assay.[405] Although TEM had significant tumor-initiating activity, HMM and PMM had none.[406] Acute nonlymphocytic leukemia has been described after HMM treatment in combination[407] and as a single agent.[408] Chronic oral HMM administration decreased fertility in male rats and affected embryos in female rats at high dosages.[409] In this study, several minor and occasional major teratogenic effects were observed.

REFERENCES

1. Newell D, Gescher A, Harland S, et al. *N*-Methyl antitumor agents: a distinct class of anticancer drugs? *Cancer Chemother Pharmacol* 1987;19:91.
2. Zeller P, Gutmann H, Hegedus B, et al. Methylhydrazine derivatives, a new class of cytotoxic agents. *Experientia* 1963;19:129.
3. Bollag W, Grunberg E. Tumour inhibitory effects of a new class of cytotoxic agents: methylhydrazine derivatives. *Experientia* 1963;19:130.
4. Bollag W. The tumor-inhibitory effects of the methylhydrazine derivative Ro 4-6467/1 (NSC-77213). *Cancer Chemother Rep* 1963;33:1.
5. Martz G, D'Allessandri A, Keel HJ, et al. Preliminary clinical results with a new anti-tumor agent Ro 4-6467 (NSC-77213). *Cancer Chemother Rep* 1963;33:5.
6. Mathe G, Schweisguth O, Schneider M, et al. Methyl hydrazine in the treatment of Hodgkin's disease. *Lancet* 1963;2:1077.
7. Brunner KW, Young CW. A methylhydrazine derivative in Hodgkin's disease and other malignant neoplasms: therapeutic and toxic effects studies in 51 patients. *Ann Intern Med* 1965;63:69.
8. Samuels ML, Leary WV, Alexanian R, et al. Clinical trials with *N*-isopropyl-(2-methylhydrazino)-*p*-toluamide hydrochloride in malignant lymphoma and other disseminated neoplasia. *Cancer* 1967;20:1187.
9. Spivack SD. PCB. *Ann Intern Med* 1974;81:795.
10. DeVita VT, Serpick AA, Carbone PP. Combination chemotherapy in the treatment of advanced Hodgkin's disease. *Ann Intern Med* 1970;73:881.

11. Stolinsky DC, Solomon J, Pugh R, et al. Clinical experience with PCB in Hodgkin's disease, reticulum cell sarcoma, and lymphosarcoma. *Cancer* 1970;26:984.

12. DeVita VT, Canellos GP, Chabner B, et al. Advanced diffuse histiocytic lymphoma, a potentially curable disease. *Lancet* 1975;1:248.

13. DeVita VT, Hubbard SM, Longo DL. The chemotherapy of lymphomas: looking back, moving forward—the Richard and Hinda Rosenthal Foundation award lecture. *Cancer Res* 1987;47:5810.

14. Samuels ML, Leary WV, Howe CD. PCB (NSC-77213) in treatment of advanced bronchogenic carcinoma. *Cancer Chemother Rep* 1969;53:135.

15. Gersel Pedersen A, Sorenson S, Aabo K, et al. Phase II study of PCB in small cell carcinoma of the lung. *Cancer Treat Rep* 1982;66:273.

16. Daniels JR, Chak LY, Sikic BI, et al. Chemotherapy of small cell carcinoma of lung: a randomized comparison of alternating and sequential combination chemotherapy programs. *J Clin Oncol* 1984;2:1192.

17. Luce JK. Chemotherapy of malignant melanoma. *Cancer* 1972;30:1604.

18. Carmo-Pereira J, Costa FO, Henriques E. Combination cytotoxic chemotherapy with PCB, vincristine, and lomustine in disseminated malignant melanoma: 8 years follow-up. *Cancer Treat Rep* 1984;68:1211.

19. Kumar AR, Renaudin J, Wilson CB, et al. PCB hydrochloride in the treatment of brain tumors. *J Neurosurg* 1974;40:365.

20. Gutin PH, Wilson CB, Kumar AR, et al. Phase II study of PCB, CCNU, and vincristine combination chemotherapy in the treatment of brain tumors. *Cancer* 1975;35:1398.

21. Levin VA, Rodriguez LA, Edwards MSB, et al. Treatment of medulloblastoma with PCB, hydroxyurea, and reduced radiation dose to whole brain and spine. *J Neurosurg* 1988;68:383.

22. Rodriguez LA, Prados M, Silver P, et al. Reevaluation of PCB for the treatment of recurrent malignant central nervous system tumors. *Cancer* 1989;64:2420.

23. Newton HB, Junck L, Bromberg J, et al. PCB chemotherapy in the treatment of recurrent malignant astrocytomas after radiation and nitrosourea. *Neurology* 1990;40:1743.

24. Newton HB, Bromberg J, Junck L, et al. Comparison between BCNU and PCB chemotherapy for treatment of gliomas. *J Neurooncol* 1993;15:157.

25. Gale GR, Simpson JG, Smith AB. Studies of the mode of action of *N*-isopropyl-alpha-(2-methylhydrazino)-*p*-toluamide. *Cancer Res* 1967;27:1186.

26. Gutterman J, Huang AT, Hochstein P. Studies on the mode of action of *N*-isopropyl-alpha-(2-methylhydrazine)-*p*-toluamide. *Proc Soc Exp Biol Med* 1969;130:797.

27. Cummings SW, Guengerich FP, Prough RA. The characterisation of *N*-isopropyl-*p*-hydroxymethylbenzamide formed during the oxidative metabolism of azoPCB. *Drug Metab Dispos* 1982;10:459.

28. Shiba DA, Weinkam RJ. Quantitative analysis of PCB, PCB metabolites and chemical degradation products with application to pharmacokinetic studies. *J Chromatogr* 1982;229:397.

29. Prough RA, Tweedie DJ. PCB. In: Powis G, Prough RA, eds. *Metabolism and action of anti-cancer drugs*. London: Taylor & Francis, 1987:29.

30. Lee IP, Dixon RL. Effects of PCB on spermatogenesis determined by velocity sedimentation cell separation. *J Pharmacol Exp Ther* 1972;181:219.

31. Alley MC, Powis G, Appel PL, et al. Activation and inactivation of cancer chemotherapeutic agents by rat hepatocytes cocultured with human tumor cell lines. *Cancer Res* 1984;44:549.

32. Prough RA, Coomes ML, Dunn DL. The microsomal metabolism of carcinogenic and/or therapeutic hydrazines. In: Ullrich V, Roots I, Hildebrandt A, et al, eds. *Microsomes and drug oxidations*. Oxford: Pergamon Press, 1977:500.

33. Weinkam RJ, Shiba DA. Metabolic activation of PCB. *Life Sci* 1978;22:937.

34. Dunn DL, Lubet RA, Prough RA. Oxidative metabolism of *N*-isopropyl-alpha-(2-methylhydrazino)-*p*-toluamide hydrochloride (PCB) by rat liver microsomes. *Cancer Res* 1979;39:4555.

35. Prough RA, Wittkop JA, Reed DJ. Evidence for the hepatic metabolism of some monoalkylhydrazines. *Arch Biochem Biophys* 1969;131:369.

36. Baggiolini M, Dewald B, Aebi H. Oxidation of *p*-N1-methylhydrazinomethyl)-*N*-isopropylbenzamide to the methylazo derivative and oxidative cleavage of the N^2-C bond in the isolated perfused rat liver. *Biochem Pharmacol* 1969;18:2187.

37. Kuttab SH, Tanglerpaibul S, Vouros P. Studies on the metabolism of PCB by mass spectroscopy. *Biomed Mass Spectrom* 1982;9:78.

38. Molony SJ, Prough RA. Studies on the pathway of methane formation from PCB, a 2-methylbenzyl hydrazine derivative, by rat liver microsomes. *Arch Biochem Biophys* 1983;221:577.

39. Lam H, Begleiter A, Stein W, et al. On the mechanism of uptake of PCB by L5178Y lymphoblasts in vivo. *Biochem Pharmacol* 1978;27:1883.

40. Moloney SJ, Wiebkin P, Cummings SW, et al. Metabolic activation of the terminal *N*-methyl group of *N*-isopropyl-alpha-(2-methylhydrazino)-*p*-toluamide hydrochloride (PCB). *Carcinogenesis* 1985;6:397.

41. Kreis W, Yen Y. An antineoplastic C^{14}-labeled methylhydrazine derivative in P815 mouse leukemia: a metabolic study. *Experientia* 1965;21:284.

42. Matsumoto H, Higa HH. Studies on methylazoxymethanol, the aglycone of cycasin: methylation of nucleic acids in vitro. *Biochem J* 1966;98:20C.

43. Kreis W. Metabolism of an antineoplastic methylhydrazine derivative in a P815 mouse neoplasm. *Cancer Res* 1970;30:82.

44. Sinha BK. Metabolic activation of PCB: evidence for carbon-centered free radical intermediates. *Biochem Pharmacol* 1984;33:2777.

45. Berneis K, Kofler M, Bollag W, et al. The degradation of deoxyribonucleic acid by new tumor inhibiting compounds: the intermediate formation of hydrogen peroxide. *Experientia* 1963;19:132.

46. Shiba DA, Weinkam RJ. The in vivo cytotoxic activity of PCB and PCB metabolites against L1210 ascites leukemia cells in CDF_1 mice and the effects of pretreatment with PCB, phenobarbital, diphenylhydantoin, and methylprednisolone upon in vivo PCB activity. *Cancer Chemother Pharmacol* 1983;11:124.

47. Therman E. Chromosome breakage by 1-methyl-2-benzyl-hydrazine in mouse cancer cells. *Cancer Res* 1972;32:1133.

48. Rutishauser A, Bollag W. Cytological investigations with a new class of cytotoxic agent: methylhydrazine derivatives. *Experientia* 1963;19:131.

49. Erikson JM, Ducore JM, Prough RA. Genotoxic and cytotoxic effect of PCB (*N*-isopropyl-alpha-(2-methylhydrazino)-*p*-toluamide) and its metabolites in L1210 cells. *Proc Am Assoc Cancer Res* 1987;28:3.

50. Blijleven WG, Vogel E. The mutational spectrum of PCB on *Drosophila melanogaster*. *Mutat Res* 1977;45:47.

51. Sartorelli AC, Tsunamura S. Studies on the biochemical mode of action of a cytotoxic methylhydrazine derivative, *N*-isopropyl-alpha-(2-methylhydrazino)-*p*-toluamide. *Mol Pharmacol* 1966;2:275.

52. Koblet H, Diggelmann H. The action of ibenzmethyzin on protein synthesis in the rat liver. *Eur J Cancer* 1968;4:45.

53. Revel M, Littauer U. The coding properties of methyldeficient phenylalanine transfer RNA from *Escherichia coli*. *J Mol Biol* 1966;15:389.

54. Meer L, Schold SC, Kleihues P. Inhibition of the hepatic O^6-alkylguanine-DNA alkyltransferase in vivo by pretreatment with antineoplastic agents. *Biochem Pharmacol* 1989;38:929.

55. Rossi SC, Conrad M, Voigt JM, et al. Excision repair of O^6-methylguanine synthesised at the rat H-rasN-methyl-*N*-nitrosourea activation site and introduced in *Escherichia coli*. *Carcinogenesis (Lond)* 1989;10:373.

56. Swenberg JA, Bedell MA, Billings KC, et al. Cell-specific differences in O^6-alkylguanine DNA repair activity during continuous exposure to carcinogen. *Proc Natl Acad Sci U S A* 1982;79:5499.

57. Bedell MA, Lewis JG, Billings KC, et al. Cell specificity in hepatocarcinogenesis: O^6-methylguanine preferentially accumulates in target cell DNA during continuous exposure of rats to 1,2-dimethylhydrazine. *Cancer Res* 1982;42:3079.

58. Hall J, Kataoka H, Stephenson C, et al. O^6-Methylguanine and methylphosphotriesters to the cytotoxicity of alkylating agents in mammalian cells. *Carcinogenesis (Lond)* 1988;9:1587.

59. Schold SC Jr, Brent TP, von Hofe E, et al. O^6-Alkylguanine-DNA alkyltransferase and sensitivity to PCB in human brain tumor xenografts. *J Neurosurg* 1989;70:573.

60. Pegg AE. Mammalian O^6-alkylguanine-DNA alkyltransferase: regulation and importance in response to alkylating carcinogenic and therapeutic agents. *Cancer Res* 1990;50:6119.

61. Huang A, Gutterman J, Hochstein P. Cytogenetic changes induced by PCB in Ehrlich ascites tumor cells. *Experientia* 1969;25:203.

61a. Friedman HS, Johnson SP, Dong Q, et al. Methylator resistance mediated by mismatch repair deficiency in a glioblastoma multiforme xenograft. *Cancer Res* 1997;57:2933.

61b. Kat A, Thilly WG, Fang WH, et al. An alkylation-tolerant mutator human cell line is deficient in strand specific mismatch repair. *Proc Natl Acad Sci U S A* 1993;90:6424.

61c. Koi M, Umar A, Chauhan DP, et al. Human chromosome 3 corrects mismatch repair deficiency and microsatellite instability and reduces *N*-methyl-*N'*-nitro-*N*-nitrosoguanidine tolerance in colon tumor cells with homozygous hMLH1 mutation. *Cancer Res* 1994;54:4308.

62. Oliverio VT, Denham C, DeVita VT, et al. Some pharmacologic properties of a new antitumor agent, *N*-isopropylalpha-(2-methylhydrazino)-*p*-toluamide hydrochloride (NSC-77213). *Cancer Chemother Rep* 1964;42:1.

63. Eade N, MacLeod S, Renton K. Inhibition of hepatic microsomal drug metabolism by the hydrazines Ro4-4602, MK486, and PCB hydrochloride. *Can J Physiol Pharmacol* 1972;50:721.

64. Lee IP, Lucier GW. The potentiation of barbiturate-induced narcosis by PCB. *J Pharmacol Exp Ther* 1976;196:586.

65. Reed D. Effects in vivo of lymphoma ascites tumors and PCB, alone and in combination, upon hepatic drug-metabolizing enzymes of mice. *Biochem Pharmacol* 1976;25:153.

66. Schwartz DE. Comparative metabolic studies with natulan, methylhydrazine, and methylamine in rats. *Experientia* 1966;22:212.

67. Hande KR, Noone RM. Cimetidine prolongs the half-life of PCB and hexamethylmelamine. *Proc Am Assoc Cancer Res* 1983;24:287.

68. DeVita V, Hahn M, Oliverio V. Monoamine oxidase inhibition by a new carcinostatic agent, PCB. *Proc Soc Exp Biol Med* 1965;120:561.

69. Chabner BA, DeVita VT, Considine N, et al. Plasma pyridoxal phosphate depletion by the carcinostatic PCB. *Proc Soc Exp Biol Med* 1969;132:1119.

70. Raaflaub J, Schwartz DE. Uber den Metabolismus eines cytostatisch wirksamen methylhydrazin-derivates (Natulan). *Experientia* 1965;21:44.

71. Baggliolini M, Bickel HM, Messiha FS. Demethylation in vivo of Natulan, a tumor-inhibiting methylhydrazine derivative. *Experientia* 1965;21:334.

72. Schwartz DE, Bollag W, Obrecht P. Distribution and excretion studies of PCB in animals and man. *Arzneimittel-Forsch* 1967;17:1389.

73. Dost FN, Reed DJ. Methane formation in vivo from *N*-isopropyl-alpha-(2-methylhydrazino)-*p*-toluamide hydrochloride, a tumor-inhibiting methylhydrazine derivative. *Biochem Pharmacol* 1967;16:1741.

74. Chabner BA, Sponzo R, Hubbard S, et al. High dose intermittent intravenous infusion of PCB (NSC-77213). *Cancer Chemother Rep* 1973;57:361.

75. Gescher A, Raymont C. Studies of the metabolism of *N*-methyl containing antitumor agents: $^{14}CO_2$ breath analysis after administration of ^{14}C-labelled *N*-methyl drugs, formaldehyde and formate in mice. *Biochem Pharmacol* 1981;30:1245.

76. Weinkam RJ, Shiba DA. Nonclassical alkylating agents: PCB. In: Chabner BA, ed. *Pharmacologic principles of cancer treatment*. Philadelphia: Saunders, 1982:340.

77. Gorsen RM, Weiss AJ, Manthei RW. Analysis of PCB and metabolites by gas chromatography-mass spectrometry. *J Chromatogr* 1980;221:309.

78. Rucki RJ, Ross A, Moros SA. Application of an electrochemical detector to the determination of PCB hydrochloride by high-performance liquid chromatography. *J Chromatogr* 1980;190:359.

79. Wolff T, Dislerath LM, Worthington MT, et al. Substrate specificity of human liver cytochrome P-450 debrisoquine hydroxylase probed using immunochemical inhibition and chemical modeling. *Cancer Res* 1985;45:2116.

80. Wittkop JA, Prough RA, Reed DJ. Oxidative demethylation of *N*-methylhydrazines by rat liver microsomes. *Arch Biochem Biophys* 1969;134:308.

81. Coomes MW, Prough RA. The mitochondrial metabolism of 1,2-disubstituted hydrazines, PCB and 1,2-dimethylhydrazine. *Drug Metab Dispos* 1983;11:550.

82. Wiebkin P, Prough RA. Oxidative metabolism of *N*-isopropyl-alpha-(2-methylazo)-*p*-toluamide (azoPCB) by rodent liver microsomes. *Cancer Res* 1980;40:3524.

83. Prough RA, Brown MI, Dannan GA, et al. Major isozymes of rat liver microsomal cytochrome P-450 involved in the *N*-oxidation of *N*-isopropyl-alpha-(2-methylazo)-*p*-toluamide, the azo derivative of PCB. *Cancer Res* 1984;44:543.

84. DeVita V, Serpick A, Carbone P. Preliminary clinical studies with ibenz-methyzin. *Clin Pharmacol Ther* 1966;7:542.

85. Hoagland HC. Hematologic complications of cancer chemotherapy. *Semin Oncol* 1982;9:95.

86. Sponzo RW, Arseneau J, Canellos GP. PCB-induced oxidative haemolysis: relationship to in vivo red cell survival. *Br J Haematol* 1974;27:587.

87. Weiss HD, Walker MD, Wiernik PH. Neurotoxicity of commonly used antineoplastic agents. *N Engl J Med* 1974;291:75.

88. Casimir A, Kavanagh J, Liu F, et al. Phase I trial of intravenous PCB administered as a 5 day continuous infusion: correlation with plasma levels of pyridoxal phosphate. *Proc Am Assoc Cancer Res* 1983;24:144.

89. Lokich JJ, Moloney WC. Allergic reaction to PCB. *Clin Pharmacol Ther* 1972;13:573.

90. Jones SE, Moore M, Blank N, et al. Hypersensitivity of PCB (Matulane) manifested by fever and pleuro pulmonary reaction. *Cancer* 1972;29:498.

91. Weiss RB. Hypersensitivity reactions to cancer chemotherapy. *Semin Oncol* 1982;9:5.

92. Dunagin WG. Clinical toxicity of chemotherapeutic agents: dermatologic toxicity. *Semin Oncol* 1982;9:14.

93. Garbes ID, Henderson ES, Gomez GA, et al. PCB-induced interstitial pneumonitis with a normal chest x-ray: a case report. *Med Pediatr Oncol* 1986;14:238.

94. Liske R. A comparative study of the action of cyclophosphamide and PCB on the antibody production in mice. *Clin Exp Immunol* 1973;15:271.

95. Sullivan KM, Shulman HM, Storb R, et al. Chronic graft-versus-host disease in 52 patients: adverse natural course and successful treatment with combination immunosuppression. *Blood* 1981;57:26.

96. Parvinen L. Early effects of PCB (*N*-isopropyl-L-(2-methylhydrazino)-*p*-toluamide hydrochloride) on rat spermatogenesis. *Exp Mol Pathol* 1979;30:1.

97. Chryssanthou CP, Wallach RC, Atchison M. Meiotic chromosomal changes and sterility produced by nitrogen mustard and PCB in mice. *Fertil Steril* 1983;39:97.

98. Chaube S, Murphy M. Fetal malformations produced in rats by PCB. *Teratology* 1969;2:23.

99. Pueyo C. Natulan induces forward mutations to L-arabinose–resistance in *Salmonella typhimurium*. *Mutat Res* 1979;67:189.

100. Gatehouse DG, Paes DJ. A demonstration of the in vitro bacterial mutagenicity of PCB, using the microtitre fluctuation test and large concentrations of S9 fraction. *Carcinogenesis* 1983;4:347.

101. Kelly MG, O'Gara RW, Yancey ST, et al. Comparative carcinogenicity of *N*-isopropyl-alpha-(2-methylhydrazino)-*p*-toluamide HCl (PCB hydrochloride), its degradation products, other hydrazines, and isonicotinic acid hydrazide. *J Natl Cancer Inst* 1969;42:337.

102. Sieber SM, Correa P, Dalgard DW, et al. Carcinogenic and other adverse effects of PCB in nonhuman primates. *Cancer Res* 1978;38:2125.

103. Schilsky RL, Lewis BJ, Sherins RJ, et al. Gonadal dysfunction in patients receiving chemotherapy for cancer. *Ann Intern Med* 1980;93:109.

104. Chapman RM. Effect of cytotoxic therapy on sexuality and gonadal function. *Semin Oncol* 1982;9:84.

105. Waxman JH, Terry YA, Wrigley PF, et al. Gonadal function in Hodgkin's disease: long-term follow up of chemotherapy. *Br Med J* 1982;285:1612.

106. Schilsky RL, Sherins RJ, Hubbard SM, et al. Long-term follow up of ovarian function in women treated with MOPP chemotherapy for Hodgkin's disease. *Am J Med* 1981;71:552.

107. Horning SJ, Hoppe RT, Kaplan HS, et al. Female reproductive potential after treatment for Hodgkin's disease. *N Engl J Med* 1981;304:1377.

108. Johnson JM, Thompson DJ, Haggerty GC, et al. The effect of prenatal PCB treatment on brain development in the rat. *Teratology* 1985;32:203.

109. Andrieu JM, Ochoa-Molina ME. Menstrual cycle, pregnancies and offspring before and after MOPP therapy for Hodgkin's disease. *Cancer* 1983;52:435.

110. Lacher MJ, Toner K. Pregnancies and menstrual function before and after combined radiation and chemotherapy for Hodgkin's disease. *Cancer Invest* 1986;4:93.

111. Glicksman AS, Pajak TF, Gottlieb A, et al. Second malignant neoplasms in patients successfully treated for Hodgkin's disease: a Cancer and Leukemia Group B study. *Cancer Treat Rep* 1982;66:1035.

112. Grunwald HW, Rosner F. Acute myeloid leukemia following treatment of Hodgkin's disease. *Cancer* 1982;50:676.

113. Henry-Amar M. Quantitative risk of second cancer in patients in first complete remission from early stages of Hodgkin's disease. *Natl Cancer Inst Monogr* 1988;6:65.

114. Goldstein LS. Dominant lethal mutations induced in mouse spermatogonia by mechlorethamine, PCB, and vincristine administered in 2-drug and 3-drug combinations. *Mutat Res* 1987;191:171.

115. Yost GS, Horstman MG, El Walily AF, et al. PCB spermatogenesis toxicity: Deuterium isotope effects point to regioselective metabolism in mice. *Toxicol Appl Pharmacol* 1985;80:316.

116. Horstman MG, Meadows GG, Yost GS. Separate mechanisms for PCB spermatotoxicity and anticancer activity. *Cancer Res* 1987;47:1547.

117. Montgomery JA. Experimental studies at Southern Research Institute with DTIC (NSC-45388). *Cancer Treat Rep* 1976;60:125.

118. Shealy YF, Montgomery JA, Laster WR Jr. Antitumor activity of triazenoimidazoles. *Biochem Pharmacol* 1962;11:674.

119. Comis RL. DTIC (NSC 45388) in malignant melanoma: a perspective. *Cancer Treat Rep* 1976;60:165.

120. Frei E, Luce JK, Talley RW, et al. 5-(3,3-Dimethyl-1-tria-

zeno)imidazole-4-carboxamide (NSC-45388) in the treatment of lymphoma. *Cancer Chemother Rep* 1972;56:667.

121. Cowan DH, Bergsagel DE. Intermittent treatment of metastatic malignant melanoma with high dose 5-(3,3-dimethyl-1-triazeno)-imidazole-4-carboxamide (NSC-45388). *Cancer Chemother Rep* 1971;55:175.

122. Einhorn LH, Furnas B. Combination chemotherapy for disseminated melanoma with DTIC, vincristine, and methyl-CCNU. *Cancer Treat Rep* 1977;61:881.

123. Pritchard KI, Quirt IC, Cowan DH, et al. DTIC therapy in metastatic melanoma: a simplified dose schedule. *Cancer Treat Rep* 1980;64:1123.

124. Carey RW, Anderson JR, Green M, et al. Treatment of metastatic malignant melanoma with vinblastine, dacarbazine, and cisplatin: a report from the cancer and leukemia group B. *Cancer Treat Rep* 1986;70:329.

125. Bonadonna G, Zucali R, Monfardini S, et al. Combination chemotherapy of Hodgkin's disease with adriamycin, bleomycin, vinblastine and imidazole carboxamide versus MOPP. *Cancer* 36:252, 1975.

126. Bonadonna G, Valagussa P, Santoro A. Alternating non-cross-resistant combination chemotherapy or MOPP in stage IV Hodgkin's disease: a report of 8-year results. *Ann Intern Med* 1986;104:739.

127. Gottlieb JA, Benjamin RS, Baker LH, et al. Role of DTIC (NSC-45388) in the chemotherapy of sarcoma. *Cancer Treat Rep* 1976;60:199.

128. Vogel CL, Primack A, Owor R, et al. Effective treatment of Kaposi's sarcoma with 5-(3,3-dimethyl-1-triazeno) imidazole-4-carboxamide (NSC 45388). *Cancer Chemother Rep* 1973;57:65.

129. Luce JK, Thurman WG, Isascs BL, et al. Clinical trials with the anti-tumor agent 5-(3,3-dimethyl-1-triazeno)imidazole-4-carboxamide (NSC-45388). *Cancer Chemother Rep* 1970;54:119.

130. Finklestein JZ, Albo V, Ertel I, et al. 5-(3,3-Dimethyl-1-triazeno)imidazole-4-carboxamide (NSC-45388) in the treatment of solid tumors in children. *Cancer Chemother Rep* 1975;59:351.

131. Finklestein JZ, Klemperer MR, Evans A, et al. Multiagent chemotherapy for children with metastatic neuroblastoma: a report from Children's Cancer Study Group. *Med Pediatr Oncol* 1979;6:179.

132. Eyre HJ, Eltringham JR, Gehan EA, et al. Randomized comparisons of radiotherapy and carmustine versus PCB versus dacarbazine for the treatment of malignant gliomas following surgery: a Southwest Oncology Group Study. *Cancer Treat Rep* 1986;70:1085.

133. Kessinger A, Foley JF, Lemon HM. Therapy of malignant APUD cell tumors: effectiveness of DTIC. *Cancer* 1983;51:790.

134. Averbuch SD, Steakley CS, Young RC, et al. Malignant pheochromocytoma: effective treatment with a combination of cyclophosphamide, vincristine, and dacarbazine. *Ann Intern Med* 1988;109:267.

135. Altimari AF, Badrinath K, Reisel HJ, et al. DTIC therapy in patients with malignant intra-abdominal neuroendocrine tumors. *Surgery* 1987;102:1009.

136. Clarke DA, Barcley RK, Stock CC, et al. Triazenes as inhibitors of mouse sarcoma 180. *Proc Soc Exp Biol Med* 1955;90:484.

137. Schmid FA, Hutchison DJ. Chemotherapeutic, carcinogenic, and cell-regulatory effects of triazenes. *Cancer Res* 1974;34:1671.

138. Audette RCS, Connors TA, Mandel HG, et al. Studies on the mechanism of action of the tumour inhibitory triazenes. *Biochem Pharmacol* 1973;22:1855.

139. Connors TA, Goddard PM, Merai K, et al. Tumour inhibitory triazenes: structural requirements for an active metabolite. *Biochem Pharmacol* 1976;25:241.

140. Gescher A, Hickman JA, Simmonds RJ, et al. Studies of the mode of action of antitumour triazenes and triazines: II. Investigation of the selective toxicity of 1-aryl-3,3-dimethyltriazenes. *Biochem Pharmacol* 1981;30:89.

141. Lown JW, Singh R. Mechanism of action of antitumor 3(2-haloethyl) aryltriazenes on deoxyribonucleic acid. *Biochem Pharmacol* 1982;31:1257.

142. Farina P, Gescher A, Hickman JA, et al. Studies of the mode of action of the antitumour triazenes and triazines-IV: the metabolism of 1-(4-acetylphenyl)-3,3-dimethyltriazene. *Biochem Pharmacol* 1982;31:1887.

143. Sava G, Giraldi T, Lassiani L, et al. Mechanism of the anti-leukemic effects of 1-*p*-carboxamidophenyl-3,3-dimethyltriazene and its in vitro metabolites. *Biochem Pharmacol* 1982;31:3629.

144. Beal DD, Skibba JL, Whitnable KK, et al. Effects of 5-(3,3-dimethyl-1-triazeno)imidazole-4-carboxamide and its metabolites on Novikoff hepatoma cells. *Cancer Res* 1976;36:2827.

145. Saunders PP, Chao LY. Fate of the ring moiety of 5-(3,3-dimethyl-1-triazeno)imidazole-4-carboxamide in mammalian cells. *Cancer Res* 1974;34:2464.

146. Skibba JL, Beal DD, Ramirez G, et al. *N*-Demethylation of the antineoplastic agent 4(5)-(3,3-dimethyl-1-triazeno)imidazole-5(4)-carboxamide by rats and man. *Cancer Res* 1970;30:147.

147. Metelmann HR, Von Hoff DD. Application of a microsomal drug activation system in a human tumor cloning assay. *Invest New Drugs* 1983;1:27.

148. Loo TL, Householder GE, Gerulath AH, et al. Mechanism of action and pharmacology studies with DTIC (NSC-45388). *Cancer Treat Rep* 1976;60:149.

149. Nagasawa HT, Shirota FN, Mizuno NS. The mechanism of alkylation of DNA by 5-(3-methyl-1-triazeno)imidazole-4-carboxamide (MIC), a metabolite of DIC (NSC-45388). *Chem Biol Interact* 1974;8:403.

150. Mizuno NS, Decker RW. Alteration of DNA by 5-(3-methyl-1-triazeno)imidazole-4-carboxamide (NSC-407347). *Biochem Pharmacol* 1976;25:2643.

151. Skibba JL, Bryan GT. Methylation of nucleic acids and urinary excretion of ^{14}C-labelled 7-methylguanine by rats and man after administration of 4(5)-(3,3-dimethyl-1-triazeno)imidazole-5(4)-carboxamide. *Toxicol Appl Pharmacol* 1971;18:707.

152. Meer L, Janzer RC, Kleihues P, et al. In vivo metabolism and reaction with DNA of the cytostatic agent, 5-(3,3-dimethyl-1-triazeno)-imidazole-4-carboxamide (DTIC). *Biochem Pharmacol* 1986;35:3243.

153. Hansch C, Hatheway GJ, Quinn FR, et al. Antitumour 1-(*x*-aryl)3,3-dialkyltriazenes: 2. On the role of correlation analysis in decision making in drug modification: toxicity

quantitative structure activity relationships of 1-(*x*-phenyl) 3,3-dialkyltriazenes in mice. *J Med Chem* 1978;21:574.

154. Hickman JA. Investigation of the mechanism of action of antitumour dimethyltriazenes. *Biochimie* 1978;60:997.

155. Hayward IP, Parson PG. Epigenetic effects of the methylating agent 5-(3-methyl-1-triazeno)-imidazole carboxamide in human melanoma cells. *Aust J Exp Biol Med Sci* 1984;62:597.

156. Saunders PP, Schultz GA. Studies of the mechanism of action of the antitumor agent 5(4)-(3,3-dimethyl-1-triazeno)imidazole-4(5)-carboxamide in *Bacillus subtilis. Biochem Pharmacol* 1970;19:911.

157. Gerulath AH, Loo TL. Mechanism of action of 5-(3,3-dimethyl-1-triazeno)imidazole-4-carboxamide (NSC-45388) in mammalian cells in culture. *Biochem Pharmacol* 1972; 21:2335.

158. Gerulath H, Barranco SC, Humphrey RM. The effects of treatments with (3,3-dimethyl-1-triazeno)imidazole-4-carboxamide in darkness and in light on survival and progression of Chinese hamster ovary cells in vitro. *Cancer Res* 1974;34:1921.

159. Saunders PP, DeChang W, Chao LY. Mechanisms of 5-(3,3-dimethyl-1-triazeno)imidazole-4-carboxamide (dacarbazine) cytotoxicity toward Chinese hamster ovary cells in vitro are dictated by incubation conditions. *Chem Biol Interact* 1986;58:319.

160. Shirakawa S, Frei E III. Comparative effects of the antitumor agents 5-(dimethyltriazeno)imidazole-4-carboxamide and 1,3-bis(2-chloroethyl)-1-nitrosourea on cell cycle of L1210 leukemia cells in vivo. *Cancer Res* 1970;30:2173.

161. Lonn U, Lonn S. Prevention of dacarbazine damage of human neoplastic cell DNA by aphidi colin. *Cancer Res* 1987;47:26.

162. Lonn U, Lonn S. Inhibition of poly (ADP-ribose) synthetase potentiates cell dacarbazine cytotoxicity. *Biochem Biophys Res Commun* 1987;142:1089.

163. Lonn U, Lonn S. W-7, a calmodulin inhibitor, potentiates dacarbazine cytotoxicity in human neoplastic cells. *Int J Cancer* 1987;39:638.

164. Wodinsky I, Swiniarski J, Kensler CJ. Spleen colony studies of leukemia L1210: IV. Sensitivities of L1210 and L1210/6-MP to triazenoimidazole carboxamides—a preliminary report. *Cancer Chemother Rep* 1968;52:393.

165. Hayward IP, Parsons PG. Comparison of virus reactivation, DNA base damage, and cell cycle effects in autologous melanoma cells resistant to methylating agents. *Cancer Res* 1984;44:55.

166. Gibson NW, Hartley JA, LaFrance RJ, et al. Differential cytotoxicity and DNA-damaging effects produced in human cells of the Mer+ and Mer– phenotypes by a series of alkyltriazenylimidazoles. *Carcinogenesis (Lond)* 1986;7:259.

167. Lunn JM, Harris AL, Brown PM, et al. Potential of the cytotoxic action of DTIC: involvement of O^6-methylguanine–DNA-methyltransferase. *Br J Cancer* 1986;54:186.

168. Catapano CV, Broggini M, Erba E, et al. In vitro and in vivo methazolostone-induced DNA damage and repair in L1210 leukemia sensitive and resistant to chlorethylnitrosoureas. *Cancer Res* 1987;47:4884.

169. D'Incalci M, Citti L, Taverna P, et al. Importance of DNA repair enzyme O^6-alkyltransferase (AT) in cancer chemotherapy. *Cancer Treat Rev* 1988;15:279.

170. Lunn JM, Harris AL. Cytotoxicity of 5-(3-methyl-1-triazeno)imidazole-4-carboxamide) (MTIC) on Mer+, Mer+, Rem– and Mer– cells: differential potentiation by 3-acetamidobenzamide. *Br J Cancer* 1988;57:54.

171. Foster BJ, Newell DR, Lunn JM, et al. Correlation of dacarbazine and CB10-277 activity against human melanoma xenografts with O^6-alkyltransferase. *Proc Am Assoc Cancer Res* 1990;31:401.

172. Mitchell RB, Dolan ME. Effect of temozolomide and dacarbazine on O^6-alkylguanine–DNA alkyltransferase activity and sensitivity of human tumor cells and xenografts to 1,3-bis(2-chloroethyl)-1-nitrosourea. *Cancer Chemother Pharmacol* 1993;32:59.

173. Lee SM, Thatcher N, Dougal M, et al. Dosage and cycle effects of dacarbazine (DTIC) and fotemustine on O^6-alkylguanine–DNA alkyltransferase in human peripheral blood mononuclear cells. *Br J Cancer* 1993;67:216.

174. Colombo T, D'Incalci M. Comparison of the antitumour activity of DTIC and 1-*p*-(3,3-dimethyl-1-triazeno)benzoic acid potassium salt on murine transplantable tumours and their hematological toxicity. *Cancer Chemother Pharmacol* 1984;13:139.

175. Giraldi T, Houghton PJ, Taylor DM, et al. Antimetastatic action of some triazine derivatives against the Lewis lung carcinoma in mice. *Cancer Treat Rep* 1978;62:721.

176. Sava G, Giraldi T, Lassiani L, et al. Mechanism of the antimetastatic action of dimethyl triazenes. *Cancer Treat Rep* 1979;63:93.

177. Giraldi T, Sava G, Cuman R, et al. Selectivity of the antimetastatic and cytotoxic effects of 1-*p*-(3,3-dimethyl-1-triazeno)benzoic acid potassium salt, (±)1,2-di(3,5-dioxopiperazin-1-yl)propane, and cyclophosphamide in mice bearing Lewis lung carcinoma. *Cancer Res* 1981;41:2524.

178. Sava G, Giraldi T, Lassiani L, et al. Metabolism and mechanism of the antileukemic action of isomeric aryldimethyltriazenes. *Cancer Treat Rep* 1982;66:1751.

179. Sava G, Giraldi T, Perissin L, et al. Infiltration of liver and brain by tumor cells in leukemic mice: prevention by dimethyltriazenes and cyclophosphamide. *Tumori* 1984;70:477.

180. Bonmassar E, Bonmassar A, Vadlamudi S, et al. Immunological alteration of leukemic cells in vitro after treatment with an antitumor drug. *Proc Natl Acad Sci U S A* 1970;66:1089.

181. Nicolin A, Bini A, Coronetti E, et al. Cellular immune responses to a drug treated L51784 lymphoma subline. *Nature* 1974;251:654.

182. Pucetti P, Romani L, Taramelli D, et al. Drug mediated changes of tumour cell immunogenicity and antigenicity. *Int J Tissue React* 1982;4:189.

183. Fioretti MC, Nardelli B, Bianchi R, et al. Antigenic changes of a murine lymphoma by in vivo treatment with triazine derivatives. *Cancer Immunol Immunother* 1981;11:283.

184. Contessa AR, Bonmassar A, Giampietri A, et al. In vitro generation of a highly immunogenic subline of L1210 leukemia following exposure to 5-(3,3'-dimethyl-1-triazeno)imidazole-4-carboxamide. *Cancer Res* 1981;41:2476.

185. Franco P, Veronese F, Levi F, et al. Antibody-dependent cellular cytotoxicity against drug-induced antigens in L5178Y mouse lymphoma. *Br J Cancer* 1982;46:173.

186. Tisdale MJ. Induction of haemoglobin synthesis in the

human leukemia cell line K562 by monomethyl-triazenes and imidazotetrazinones. *Biochem Pharmacol* 1985;34:2077.

187. Fioretti MC, Bianchi R, Romani L, et al. Drug-induced immunogenic changes of murine leukemia cells: dissociation of onset of resistance and emergence of novel immunogenicity. *J Natl Cancer Inst* 1983;71:1247.

188. Farquhar D, Loo TL, Gutterman JU, et al. Inhibition of drug metabolizing enzymes in the rat after bacillus Calmette-Guérin treatment. *Biochem Pharmacol* 1976;25:1529.

189. Breithaupt H, Dammann A, Aigner K. Pharmacokinetics of dacarbazine (DTIC) and its metabolite 5-aminoimidazole-4-carboxamide (AIC) following different dose schedules. *Cancer Chemother Pharmacol* 1982;9:103.

190. Benvenuto JA, Hall SW, Farquhar D, et al. High-pressure liquid chromatography in pharmacological studies of anticancer drugs. *Chromatogr Sci* 1979;10:377.

191. Lipton A, Hepner GW, White DS, et al. Decreased hepatic drug demethylation in patients receiving chemo-immunotherapy. *Cancer* 1978;41:1680.

192. Buesa JM, Gracia M, Valle M, et al. Phase I trial of intermittent high-dose dacarbazine. *Cancer Treat Rep* 1984;68:499.

193. Savlov ED, Hall TC, Oberfield RA. Intra-arterial therapy of melanoma with dimethyl triazeno imidazole carboxamide (NSC-45388). *Cancer* 1971;28:1161.

194. Einhorn LH, McBride CM, Luke JK, et al. Intra-arterial infusion therapy with 5-(3,3-dimethyl-1-triazeno)imidazole-4-carboxamide (NSC-45388) for malignant melanoma. *Cancer* 1973;32:749.

195. Jortay AM, Lejeune FJ, Kenis Y. Regional chemotherapy of maxillofacial malignant melanoma with intracarotid artery infusion of DTIC. *Tumori* 1977;63:299.

196. Aigner K, Hild P, Henneking K, et al. Regional perfusion with cisplatinum and dacarbazine. *Rec Res Cancer Res* 1983;86:239.

197. Mizuno NS, Humphrey EW. Metabolism of 5-(3,3-dimethyl-1-triazeno)imidazole-4-carboxamide (NSC45388) in human and animal tumor tissue. *Cancer Chemother Rep* 1972; 56:465.

198. Householder GE, Loo TL. Disposition of 5-(3,3-dimethyl-1-triazeno)imidazole-4-carboxamide, a new antitumor agent. *J Pharmacol Exp Ther* 1971;179:386.

199. Skibba JL, Ramirez G, Beal DD, et al. Metabolism of 4(5)-(3,3-dimethyl-1-triazeno)imidazole-5(4)-carboxamide to 4(5)amino-imidazole-5(4)-carboxamide in man. *Biochem Pharmacol* 1970;19:2043.

200. Loo TL, Stasswender EA. Colorimetric determination of dialkyltriazenoimidazoles. *J Pharm Sci* 1967;56:1016.

201. Loo TL, Luce JK, Jardine H, et al. Pharmacologic studies of the antitumor agent 5-(dimethyl-triazeno)imidazole-4-carboxamide. *Cancer Res* 1968;28:2448.

202. Skibba JL, Ramirez G, Beal DD, et al. Preliminary clinical trial and the physiologic disposition of 4(5)-(3,3-dimethyl-1-triazeno)imidazole-5(4)-carboxamide in man. *Cancer Res* 1969;29:1944.

203. Fiore D, Jackson AJ, Didolkar MS, et al. Simultaneous determination of dacarbazine, its photolytic degradation product, 2-azahypoxanthine, and the metabolite 5-aminoimidazole-4-carboxamide in plasma and urine by high-pressure liquid chromatography. *Antimicrob Agents Chemother* 1985;27:977.

204. Farina P, Benfenati BR, Torti L, et al. Metabolism of the anticancer agent 1-(4-acetylphenyl)-3,3-dimethyltriazene. *Biomed Mass Spectrom* 1983;10:485.

205. Venditti JM. Antitumor activity of DTIC (NSC 45388) in animals. *Cancer Treat Rep* 1976;60:135.

206. Hill DL. Microsomal metabolism of triazenylimidazoles. *Cancer Res* 1975;35:3106.

207. Shealy YF, Krauth CA, Holum B, et al. Synthesis and properties of the antileukemic agent 5(or 4)-3,3-bis(2-chloroethyl)1-triazenoimidazole-4(or 5)carboxamide. *J Pharm Sci* 1969;57:83.

208. Sava G, Giraldi T, Lassiani L, et al. Metabolism and mechanism of the antileukemic action of isomeric aryldimethyltriazenes. *Cancer Treat Rep* 1982;66:1751.

209. Ray SK, Basak SC, Raychaudhury C, et al. The utility of information content, hydrophobicity, and van der Waals volume in the design of barbiturates and tumor inhibitory triazenes: a comparative study. *Arzheim Forsch* 1983;33:352.

210. Steven MFG. DTIC: a springboard to new antitumour agents. In: Reinhoudt DW, Connors TA, Pinedo HM, et al., eds. *Structure-activity relationships of antitumour agents.* The Hague: Martinus Nijhoff, 1983:183.

211. Wilman DEV, Cox PJ, Goddard PM, et al. Tumor inhibitory triazenes: 3. Dealkylation within an homologous series and its relation to antitumor activity. *J Med Chem* 1984;27:870.

212. Vaughan K, Tang Y, Llanos G, et al. Studies of the mode of action of antitumor triazenes and triazines: 6. 1-Aryl-3-(hydroxymethyl)-3-methyltriazenes: synthesis, chemistry and antitumor properties. *J Med Chem* 1984;27:357.

213. Shealy YF. Synthesis and biological activity of 5-amino imidazoles and 5-triazenoimidazoles. *J Pharm Sci* 1970; 59:1533.

214. Shealy YF, Krauth CA. Complete inhibition of mouse leukemia L1210 by 5(or 4)-(3,3bis(2-chloroethyl)-triazeno)imidazole-4(or 5)-carboxamide. *Nature* 1966;210:208.

215. Hano K, Akashi A, Yamamoto I, et al. Antitumor activity of 4(or 5) aminoimidazole-5(or 4)-carboxamide derivatives. *Gann* 1965;56:417.

216. Wilman DEV, Goddard PM. Tumor inhibitory triazenes: 2. Variation of antitumor activity within an homologous series. *J Med Chem* 1980;23:1052.

217. Baird GM, Willoughby MLN. Photodegradation of dacarbazine. *Lancet* 1978;2:681.

218. Dorr RT, Soble M, Alberts DS, et al. Experimental dacarbazine (DTIC) antitumor activity and skin toxicity in relation to light exposure and pharmacologic antidotes. *Cancer Treat Rep* 1987;71:267.

219. Koriech O, Shukla V. Reduced toxicity of DTIC with administration in the dark. *Proc Am Assoc Cancer Res* 1980;21:168.

220. Bosanquet AG. Stability of solutions of antineoplastic agents during preparation and storage for in vitro assays: general considerations, the nitrosoureas and alkylating agents. *Cancer Chemother Pharmacol* 1985;14:83.

221. Moore GE, Meiselbaugh D. DTIC (NSC 45388) toxicity. *Cancer Treat Rep* 1976;60:219.

222. Beck TM, Hart NE, Smith CE. Photosensitivity reaction following DTIC administration: report of two cases. *Cancer Treat Rep* 1980;64:725.

223. Fosch PJ, Cazarnetzki BM, Macher E, et al. Hepatic failure in a patient treated with DTIC for malignant melanoma. *J Cancer Res Clin Oncol* 1979;95:281.

224. Greenstone MA, Dowd PM, Mikhailidis DP, et al. Hepatic vascular lesions associated with dacarbazine treatment. *Br Med J* 1981;282:1744.

225. Feaux de Lacroix W, Runne U, Hauk H, et al. Acute liver dystrophy with thrombosis of hepatic veins: a fatal complication of dacarbazine treatment. *Cancer Treat Rep* 1983; 67:779.

226. McClay E, Lusch CJ, Mastrangelo MJ. Allergy-induced hepatic toxicity associated with dacarbazine. *Cancer Treat Rep* 1987;71:219.

227. Ceci G, Bella M, Melissari M, et al. Fatal hepatic vascular toxicity of DTIC: is it really a rare event? *Cancer* 1988;61:1988.

228. Puccetti P, Giampietri A, Fioretti MC. Long-term depression of two primary immune responses induced by a single dose of 5-(3,3-dimethyl-1-triazeno)-imidazole-4-carboxamide (DTIC). *Experientia* 34:799, 1978.

229. Nardelli B, Puccetti P, Romani L, et al. Chemical xenogenication of murine lymphoma cells with triazine derivatives: immunotoxicological studies. *Cancer Immunol Immunother* 17:213, 1984.

230. Mantovani A, Luini W, Peri G, et al. Effect of chemotherapeutic agents on natural cell-mediated cytotoxicity in mice. *J Natl Cancer Inst* 61:1255, 1978.

231. Romani L, Migliorati G, Bonmassar E, et al. Susceptibility of murine lymphoma cells treated with 5-(3,3-dimethyl-1-triazenyl)-1*H* imidazole-4-carboxamide to NK-mediated cytotoxicity in vitro. *Int J Immunopharmacol* 1985;5:299.

232. Marelli O, Canti G, Franco P, et al. L1210/DTIC antigenic subline: studies at the clone level. *Eur J Cancer Clin Oncol* 1986;22:1401.

233. Vernole P, Caporossi D, Tedeschi B, et al. Sister-chromatid exchanges in human lymphocytes exposed to 1-*p*-(3-methyltriazeno)benzoic acid potassium salt. *Mutat Res* 1988; 208:233.

234. Tamaro M, Dolzani L, Monti-Bragadin C, et al. Mutagenic activity of the dacarbazine analogue *p*-(3,3-dimethyl-1-triazeno)benzoic acid potassium salt in bacterial cells. *Pharmacol Res Commun* 1986;18:491.

235. Singh B, Gupta RS. Mutagenic responses of thirteen anticancer drugs on mutation induction at multiple genetic loci and on sister chromatid exchanges in Chinese hamster ovary cells. *Cancer Res* 1983;43:577.

236. Skibba JL, Erturk E, Bryan GT. Induction of thymic lymphosarcomas and mammary adenocarcinomas in rats by oral administration of the antitumor agent 4(5)-(3,3-dimethyl-1-triazeno)-imidazole-5(4)-carboxamide. *Cancer* 1970;26:1000.

237. Beal DD, Skibba JL, Croft WA, et al. Carcinogenicity of the antineoplastic agent, 5-(3,3-dimethyl-1-triazeno)-imidazole-4-carboxamide, and its metabolites in rats. *J Natl Cancer Inst* 1975;54:951.

238. Weisburger JH, Griswold DP, Prejean JD, et al. I: Tumor induction by cytostatics? The carcinogenic properties of some of the principal drugs used in clinical cancer chemotherapy. *Rec Res Cancer Res* 1975;52:1.

239. Valagussa P, Santoro A, Fossati Bellani F, et al. Absence of treatment-induced second neoplasms after ABVD in Hodgkin's disease. *Blood* 1982;59:488.

240. Brusamolino E, Papa G, Valagussa P, et al. Treatment-related leukemia in Hodgkin's disease: a multi-institution study on 75 cases. *Hematol Oncol* 1987;5:83.

241. Carey RW, Kunz VS. Acute nonlymphocytic leukemia (ANLL) following treatment with dacarbazine for malignant melanoma. *Am J Hematol* 1987;25:119.

242. Chaube S, Swinyard CA. Urogenital anomalies in fetal rats produced by the anticancer agent 4(5)-(3,3-dimethyl-1-triazeno)-imidazole-4-carboxamide. *Anat Rec* 1976;186:461.

243. Thompson DJ, Molello JA, Sterbing RJ, et al. Reproduction and teratology studies with oncolytic agents in the rat and rabbits: II. 5-(3,3-Dimethyl-1-triazeno)-imidazole-4-carboxamide (DTIC). *Toxicol Appl Pharmacol* 1975;33:281.

244. Baldwin RW, Partridge MW, Stevens MFG. Pyrazolotriazines: a new class of tumour-inhibitory agents. *J Pharm Pharmacol* 1966;18S:1S.

245. Stevens MFG. Second-generation azolotetrazinones. In: *New avenues in developmental cancer chemotherapy.* London: Academic Press, 1987:335.

246. Stevens MFG, Hickman JA, Stone R, et al. Antitumor imidazotetrazines: 1. Synthesis and chemistry of 8-carbamoyl-3(2-chloroethyl)imidazo[5,2-D]-1,2,3,5-tetrazin-4(3*H*)-one, a novel broad-spectrum antitumor agent. *J Med Chem* 1984;27:196.

247. Hickman JA, Stevens MFG, Gibson NW, et al. Experimental antitumor activity against murine tumor model systems of 8-carbamoyl-3(2-chloroethyl)imidazo[5,1-D]-1,2,3,5-tetrazin-4(3*H*)-one (mitozolomide), a novel broad-spectrum agent. *Cancer Res* 1985;45:3008.

248. Newlands ES, Backledge G, Slack JA, et al. Phase I clinical trial of mitozolomide. *Cancer Treat Rep* 1985;69:801.

249. Horspool KR, Stevens MFG, Newton CG, et al. Antitumor imidazotetrazines: 20. Preparation of the 8-acid derivative of mitozolomide and its utility in the preparation of active antitumor agents. *J Med Chem* 1990;30:1393.

250. Stevens MFG, Hickman JA, Langdon SP, et al. Antitumor activity and pharmacokinetics in mice of 8-carbamoyl-3(2-chloroethyl)imidazo[5,1-D]-1,2,3,5-tetrazin-4(3*H*)-one (CCRG81045; MB39831), a novel drug with potential as an alternative to dacarbazine. *Cancer Res* 1987;47:5846.

251. Stevens MFG, Newlands ES. From triazines and triazenes to temozolomide. *Eur J Cancer* 1993;29A:1045.

252. Tsang LL, Quarterman CP, Gescher A, Slack JA. Comparison of the cytotoxicity in vitro of temozolomide and dacarbazine, prodrugs of 3-methyl-(trizen-1-yl) imidazole-4 carboxamide. *Cancer Chemother Pharmacol* 1991;27:342.

253. Newlands ES, Blackledge GP, Slack JA, et al. Phase I trial of temozolomide (CCRG81045: MB39831: NSC-362856). *Br J Cancer* 1992;65:287.

254. O'Reilly SM, Newlands ES, Glaser MG, et al. Temozolomide: a new oral cytoxic chemotherapeutic agent with promising activity against primary brain tumours. *Eur J Cancer* 1993;29A:940.

255. Newlands ES, O'Reilly SM, Glaser MG, et al. The Charing Cross Hospital experience with temozolomide in patients with gliomas. *Eur J Cancer* 1996;32A:2236.

256. Bower M, Newlands ES, Bleehen NM, et al. Multicentre CRC phase II trial of temozolomide in recurrent or progres-

sive high-grade glioma. *Cancer Chemother Pharmacol* 1997;40:484.

257. Yung A, Levin VA, Brada M, et al. Randomized, multicenter, open-label, Phase II, comparative study of temozolomide and procarbazine in the treatment of patients with glioblastoma multiforme at first relapse. *Br J Cancer* 2000;83:588–593.

258. Yung A, Prados M, Poisson M, for the Temodal Brain Tumor Group. Multicenter Phase II trial of temozolomide in patients with malignant astrocytoma at first relapse. *J Clin Oncol* 1999;17:2762–2769.

259. Friedman HS, McLendon RE, Kerby T, et al. DNA mismatch repair and *O*6-alkylguanine-DNA alkytransferase analysis and response to Temodal in newly diagnosed malignant glioma. *J Clin Oncol* 1998;6:3851.

260. Blehen NM, Newlands ES, Lee SM, et al. Cancer Research Campaign phase II trial of temozolomide in metastatic melanoma. *J Clin Oncol* 1995;13:910.

261. Clark AS, Stevens MFG, Sansom CE, et al. Anti-tumor imidazotetrazines. Part XXI. Mitozolomide and temozolomide: probes for the major groove of DNA. *Anti-Cancer Drug Design* 1990;5:63.

262. Lowe PR, Sansom CE, Schwalbe CH, et al. Antitumor imidazotetrazines. 25. Crystal structure of 8-carbamoyl-3-methylimidazo[5,1-*d*]-1,2,3,4-tetrazin-4(3*H*)-one (temozolomide) and structural comparisons with the related drugs mitozolomide and DTIC. *J Med Chem* 1992;35:3377.

263. Clark AS, Deans B, Stevens MGF, et al. Antitumor imidazotetrazines. 32. Synthesis of novel imidazotetrazinones and related bicyclic heterocycles to probe the mode of action of the antitumor drug temozolomide. *J Med Chem* 1995; 38:1493.

264. Spassova MK, Golovinsky EV. Pharmacobiochemistry of arylalkyltriazenes and their application in cancer chemotherapy. *Pharmacol Ther* 1985;27:333.

265. Denny BJ, Wheelhouse RT, Stevens MFG, et al. NMR and molecular modeling investigation of the mechanism of activation of the antitumor drug temozolomide and its interaction with DNA. *Biochem* 1994;33:9045.

266. Bull VL, Tisdale MJ. Antitumor imidazotetrazines—XVI. Macromolecular alkylation by 3-substituted imidazotetrazinones. *Biochem Pharmacol* 1987;36:3215.

267. Liu L, Chatterjee S, Gerson S. Blockade of base excision repair appears to mediate cytotoxicity to temozolomide in mismatch repair deficient tumor cells. *Proc Am Assoc Cancer Res* 1997;38:288(abst 1536).

268. D'Atri S, Bonmassar E, Franchi A, et al. Repair of DNA methyl adducts and sensitivity to temozolomide of acute myelogenous leukemia (AML) cells. *Exp Hematol* 1991; 19:530 (abst 276).

269. Wedge SR, Porteous JK, Newlands ES. 3-Aminobenzamide and/or *O*6-benzylguanine evaluated as an adjunct to temozolomide or BCNU treatment in cells of variable mismatch repair status and *O*6-alkylguanine-DNA alkyltransferase activity. *Br J Cancer* 1996;1030.

270. Wedge SR, Porteous JK, May BL, et al. Potentiation of temozolomide and BCNU cytotoxicity by *O*6-benzylguanine: a comparative study *in vitro*. *Br J Cancer* 1996;73:482.

271. Dolan ME, Mitchell RB, Mummert C, et al. Effect of *O*6-benzylguanine analogues on sensitivity of human tumor cells to the cytotoxic effects of alkylating agents. *Cancer Res* 1991;51:3367.

272. Friedman HS, Dolan ME, Pegg AE, et al. Activity of temozolomide in the treatment of central nervous system tumor xenografts. *Cancer Res* 1995;55:2853.

273. Plowman J, Waud WR, Koutsoukos AD, et al. Preclinical antitumor activity of temozolomide in mice: efficacy against human brain tumor xenografts and synergism with 1,3-bis (2-chloroethyl)-1-nitrosourea. *Cancer Res* 1994;54:3793.

274. Wedge SR, Porteous JK, Newlands ES. Effect of single and multiple administration of an *O*6-benzylguanine/temozolomide combination: an evaluation in a human melanoma xenograft model. *Cancer Chemother Pharmacol* 1997;40:266.

275. Dolan ME, Moschel RC, Pegg AE. Depletion of mammalian *O*6-alkylguanine-DNA alkyltransferase activity by *O*6-benzylguanine provides a means to evaluate the role of this protein in protection against carcinogenic and therapeutic alkylating agents. *Proc Natl Acad Sci U S A* 1990;87:5368.

276. D'Atri S, Piccioni D, Castellano A, et al. Chemosensitivity to triazine compounds and *O*6-alkylguanine-DNA alkyltransferase levels: studies with blasts of leukaemic patients. *Ann Oncol* 1995;6:389.

277. Drummond JT, Li G-M, Longley MJ, et al. Isolation of an hMSH2-p160 heterodimer that restores DNA mismatch repair to tumor cells. *Science* 1995;268:1909.

278. Palombo F, Gallinari P, Iaccarino I, et al. GTBP, a 160-kilodalton protein essential for mismatch-binding activity in human cells. *Science* 1995;268:1912.

279. Li G-M, Modrich P. Restoration of mismatch repair to nuclear extracts of H6 colorectal tumor cells by a heterodimer of human MutL homologs. *Proc Natl Acad Sci U S A* 1995;92:1950.

280. Karran P, Macpherson P, Ceccotti S, et al. *O*6-methylguanine residues elicit DNA repair synthesis by human cell extracts. *J Biol Chem* 1993;268:15878.

281. Taverna P, Catapano CV, Citti L, et al. Influence of *O*6-methylguanine on DNA damage and cytotoxicity of temozolomide in L1210 mouse leukemia sensitive and resistant to chloroethylnitrosoureas. *Anticancer Drugs* 1992;3:401.

282. Karran P, Hampson R. Genomic instability and tolerance to alkylating agents. *Cancer Surv* 1996;28:69.

283. Karran P, Bignami M. Self-destruction and tolerance in resistance of mammalian cells to alkylation damage. *Nucleic Acids Res* 1992;20:2933.

284. Ceccotti S, Dogliottie E, Gannon J, et al. *O*6-methylguanine in DNA inhibits replication in vitro by human cell extracts. *Biochem* 1993;32:13664.

285. Tentori L, Graziani G, Gilberti S, et al. Triazine compounds induce apoptosis in *O*6-alkylguanine-DNA alkyltransferase deficient leukemia cell lines. *Leukemia* 1995;9:1888.

286. Puccetti P, Romani L, Fioretti MC. Chemical xenogenization of experimental tumors. *Cancer Metastasis Rev* 1987; 6:93.

287. Bianchi R, Citti L, Beghetti R, et al. *O*6-methylguanine-DNA methyltransferase activity and induction of novel immunogenicity in murine tumor cells treated with methylating agents. *Cancer Chemother Pharmacol* 1992;29:277.

288. Allegrucci M, Fuschiotti P, Puccetti P, et al. Changes in the tumorigenic and metastatic properties of murine melanoma cells treated with a triazine derivative. *Clin Exp Metastasis* 1989;7:329.

289. Tentori L, Leonetti C, Aquino A. Temozolomide reduces the metastatic potential of Lewis lung carcinoma (3LL) in mice: role of α-6 integrin phosphorylation. *Eur J Cancer* 1995;31A:746.

290. Tisdale MJ. Antitumor imidazotetrazines-X. Effect of 8-carbamoyl-3-methylimidazo[5,1-*d*]-1,2,3,5-tetrazine-4-(3H)-one (CCRG 81045; M&B 39831; NSC 362856) on DNA methylation during induction of haemoglobin synthesis in human leukaemia cell line K562. *Biochem Pharmacol* 1986;35:311.

291. Tisdale MJ. Antitumor imidazotetrazines and gene expression. *Acta Oncol* 1988;27:511.

292. Tisdale MJ. Antitumor imidazotetrazines-XVIII. Modification of the level of 5-methylcytosine in DNA by 3-substituted imidazotetrazinones. *Biochem Pharmacol* 1989;38:1097.

293. Pegg AE, Dolan ME, Moschel RC. Structure, function, and inhibition of O⁶-alkylguanine-DNA alkyltransferase. *Prog Nucleic Acid Res Mol Biol* 1995;51:167.

294. Pegg AE. Alkylation and subsequent repair of DNA after exposure of dimethylnitrosamine and related carcinogens. *Rev Biochem Toxicol* 1983;5:83.

295. Tisdale MJ. Antitumor imidazotetrazines-XV. Role of guanine O⁶ alkylation in the mechanism of cytotoxicity of imidazotetrazinones. *Biochem Pharmacol* 1987;36:457.

296. Baer JC, Freeman AA, Newlands ES, et al. Depletion of O⁶-alkylguanine-DNA alkyltransferase correlates with potentiation of temozolomide and CCNU toxicity in human tumor cells. *Br J Cancer* 1993;67:1299.

297. Redmond SMS, Joncourt F, Buser K, et al. Assessment of P-glycoprotein, glutathione-based detoxifying enzymes and O⁶-alkylguanine-DNA alkyltransferase as potential indicators of constitutive drug resistance in human colorectal tumors. *Cancer Res* 1991;51:2092.

298. Franchi A, Papa G, D'Atri S, et al. Cytotoxic effects of dacarbazine in patients with acute myelogenous leukemia: a pilot study. *Haematologica* 1992;77:146.

299. Wang G, Weiss, Sheng P, et al. Retrovirus-mediated transfer of the human O⁶-methylguanine-DNA-methyltransferase gene into a murine hematopoietic stem cell line and resistance to the toxic effects of certain alkylating agents. *Biochem Pharmacol* 1996;51:1221.

300. Citron M, Decker R, Chen S, et al. O⁶-methylguanine-DNA methyltransferase in human normal and tumor tissue from brain, lung and ovary. *Cancer Res* 1991;51:4131.

301. Belanich M, Randall T, Pastor MA, et al. Intracellular localization and intracellular heterogeneity of the human DNA repair protein O⁶-methylguanine-DNA methyltransferase. *Cancer Chemother Pharmacol* 1996;37:547.

302. Wiestler O, Kleihues P, Pegg A. O⁶-alkylguanine-DNA alkyltransferase activity in human brain and brain tumors. *Carcinogenesis* 1984;5:121.

303. Frosina G, Rossi O, Arena G, et al. O⁶-alkylguanine-DNA alkyltransferase activity in human brain tumors. *Cancer Lett* 1990;55:153.

304. Yarosh D. The role of O⁶-methylguanine-DNA methyltransferase in cell survival, mutagenesis and carcinogenesis. *Mutat Res* 1985;145:1.

305. Walker MC, Masters JRW, Margison GP. O⁶-alkylguanine-DNA alkyltransferase activity in nitrosourea sensitivity in human cancer cell lines. *Br J Cancer* 1990;66:840.

306. Bobola MS, Tseng SH, Blank A, et al. Role of O⁶-meth-ylguanine-DNA methyltransferase in resistance of human brain tumor cell lines to the clinically relevant methylating agents temozolomide and streptozotocin. *Clin Cancer Res* 1996;2:735.

307. Liu L, Markowitz S, Willson JKV, et al. Mismatch repair mutator phenotype confers resistance to temozolomide in human cancer cell lines. *Proc Am Assoc Cancer Res* 1996;37:365(abst 2491).

308. Ionov Y, Peinado MA, Malkhosyan S, et al. Ubiquitous somatic mutations in simple repeated sequences reveal a new mechanism for colonic carcinogenesis. *Nature* 1993;363:558.

309. Aaltonen LA, Peltomaki P, Leach FS, et al. Clues to the pathogenesis of familial colorectal cancer. *Science* 1993; 260:812.

310. Margison GP, O'Connor PJ. Biological consequences of reactions with DNA: role of specific lesions. *Handbook Exp Pharmacol* 1989;94:547.

311. Tisdale MJ. Antitumor imidazotetrazines-XI. Effect of 8-carbamoyl-3-methylimidazo [5,1-*d*]-1,2,3,5-tetrazine-4(3H)-one (CCRG 81045; M&B 39831; NSC 362856) on poly (ADP-ribose) metabolism. *Br J Cancer* 1985;52:789.

312. Durkacz BW, Omidiji O, Gray DA, et al. (ADP-ribose)n participates in DNA excision repair. *Nature* 1980;283:593.

313. Wu Z, Chan C-L, Eastman A, et al. Expression of O⁶-methylguanine-DNA methyltransferase in a DNA excision repair-deficient Chinese hamster ovary cell line and its response to certain alkylating agents. *Cancer Res* 1992; 52:32.

314. Boulton S, Pemberton LC, Porteous JK, et al. Potentiation of temozolomide-induced cytotoxicity: a comparative study of the biological effects of poly(ADP-ribose) polymerase inhibitors. *Br J Cancer* 1995;72:849.

315. Deans B, Tisdale MJ. Antitumor imidazotetrazines. XXVIII 3-methyladenine DNA glycosylane activity in cell lines sensitive and resistant to temozolomide. *Cancer Lett* 1992;63:151.

316. Imperatore L, Damia G, Taverna P, et al. 3T3 NIH murine fibroblasts and B78 murine melanoma cells expressing the *Escherichia coli* N3-methyladenine-DNA glycosylase I do not become resistant to alkylating agents. *Carcinogenesis* 1994;15:533.

317. Estlin EJ, Lashford L, Ablett S, et al. Phase I study of temozolomide in paediatric patients with advanced cancer. *Br J Cancer* 1988;78:652.

318. Baker SD, Wirth P, Statkevich P, et al. Absorption, metabolism and exretion of ¹⁴C-temozolomide in patients with advanced cancer. *Proc Am Soc Clin Oncol* 1997;16:214a (abst 749).

319. Dhodapkar JR, Rubin J, Reid JM, et al. Phase I trial of temozolomide (NSC 362856) in patients with advanced cancer. *Clin Cancer Res* 1997;3:1093.

320. Eckardt JR, Weiss GR, Burris HA, et al. Phase I and pharmacokinetic trial of SCH52365 (temozolomide) given orally daily × 5 days. *Proc Am Soc Clin Oncol* 1995;14:484 (abst 1579).

321. Brada M, Moore S, Judson I, et al. A phase I study of SCH 52365 (temozolomide) in adult patients with advanced cancer. *Proc Am Soc Clin Oncol* 1995;14:470 (abst 1521).

322. Reidenberg P, Willalona M, Eckhardt G, et al. Phase I clinical and pharmacokinetic study of temozolomide in

advanced cancer patients stratified by extent of prior therapy. *Ann Oncol* 1996;7:99(abst 344).

323. Reidenberg P, Statkevich P, Judson I, et al. Effect of food on the oral bioavailability of temozolomide, a new chemotherapeutic agent. *Clin Pharmacol Ther* 1996;59:70(abst PIII-44).

324. Statkevich P, Judson I, Batra V, et al. Effect of ranitidine (R) on the pharmacokinetics (PK) of temozolomide (T). *Clin Pharmacol Ther* 1997;61:72(abst PI-39).

325. Baker SD, Statkevich P, Rowinsky E, et al. Pharmacokinetics (PK) and pharmacodynamics (PD) of temozolomide (TEM) administered as a single oral dose. *Pharm Res* 1996;13S:487(abst PPDM 8378).

326. Nicholson HS, Krailo M, Ames MM, et al. Phase I study of temozolomide in children and adolescents with recurrent solid tumors: a report from the Children's Cancer Group (CCG). *J Clin Oncol* 1998;16:3037.

327. Kaiser DW, Thurston JT, Dudley JR, et al. Cyanuric chloride derivatives: II. Substituted melamines. *J Am Chem Soc* 1951;73:2984.

328. Hendry JA, Homer RF, Rose FL, et al. Cytotoxic agents: III. Derivatives of ethylenimines. *Br J Pharmacol* 1951;6:357.

329. Buckley SM, Srock CC, Crossley ML, et al. Inhibition of the Crocker mouse sarcoma 180 by certain ethylenimine derivatives and related compounds. *Cancer* 1952;5:144.

330. Lake LM, Grunden EE, Johnson BM. Toxicity and antitumor activity of hexamethylmelamine and its *N*-demethylated metabolites in mice with transplantable tumor. *Cancer Res* 1975;35:2858.

331. Cumber AJ, Ross WCJ. Analogues of hexamethylmelamine: the antineoplastic activity of derivatives with enhanced water solubility. *Chem Biol Interact* 1977;17:349.

332. Rutty CJ, Connors TA. In vitro studies with hexamethylmelamine. *Biochem Pharmacol* 1977;26:2385.

333. Blum RH, Livingston RB, Carter SK. Hexamethylmelamine—a new drug with activity in solid tumors. *Eur J Cancer* 1973;9:195.

334. Foster BJ, Harding BJ, Leyland-Jones B, et al. Hexamethylmelamine: a critical review of an active drug. *Cancer Treat Rev* 1986;13:197.

335. Wilson WL, Bisel HF, Cole D, et al. Prolonged low-dosage administration of hexamethylmelamine (NSC-13875). *Cancer* 1970;25:568.

336. Wharton JT, Rutledge F, Smith JP, et al. Hexamethylmelamine: an evaluation of its role in the treatment of ovarian cancer. *Am J Obstet Gynecol* 1979;133:833.

337. Foster BJ, Clagett-Carr K, Marsoni S, et al. Role of hexamethylmelamine in the treatment of ovarian cancer: where is the needle in the haystack? *Cancer Treat Rep* 1986;70:1003.

338. Neijt JP, ten Bokkel Huinink WW, van der Burg MEL, et al. Randomized trial comparing two combination chemotherapy regimens (CHAP-5 vs CP) in advanced ovarian carcinoma. *J Clin Oncol* 1987;5:1157.

339. Hainsworth JD, Grosh WW, Burnett LS, et al. Advanced ovarian cancer: long-term results of treatment with intensive cisplatin-based chemotherapy of brief duration. *Ann Intern Med* 1988;108:165.

340. Johnson BL, Fisher RI, Bender RA, et al. Hexamethylmelamine in alkylating agent-resistant ovarian carcinoma. *Cancer* 1978;42:2157.

341. Bonomi PD, Mladineo J, Morrin B, et al. Phase II trial of hexamethylmelamine in ovarian carcinoma resistant to alkylating agents. *Cancer Treat Rep* 1979;63:137.

342. Bolis G, D'Incalci M, Belloni C, et al. Hexamethylmelamine in ovarian cancer resistant to cyclophosphamide and adriamycin. *Cancer Treat Rep* 1979;63:1375.

343. Omura GA, Greco FA, Birch R. Hexamethylmelamine in mustard-resistant ovarian adenocarcinoma. *Cancer Treat Rep* 1980;64:530.

344. Vogl SE, Pagano M, Davis TE, et al. Hexamethylmelamine and cisplatin in advanced ovarian cancer after failure of alkylating-agent therapy. *Cancer Treat Rep* 1982;66:1285.

345. Gad-el-Mawla N, Ziegler JL, Hamza R, et al. Randomized phase II trial of hexamethylmelamine versus pentamethylmelamine in carcinoma of the Bilharzial bladder. *Cancer Treat Rep* 1984;68:793.

346. Oken MM, Lenhard RE, Tsiatsis AA, et al. Contribution of prednisone to the effectiveness of hexamethylmelamine in multiple myeloma. *Cancer Treat Rep* 1987;71:807.

347. Foster BJ, Clagett-Carr K, Hoth D, et al. Pentamethylmelamine: review of an aqueous analogue of hexamethylmelamine. *Cancer Treat Rep* 1986;70:383.

348. Worzalla JF, Johnson BM, Ramirez G, et al. *N*-Demethylation of the antineoplastic agent hexamethylmelamine by rats and man. *Cancer Res* 1973;33:2810.

349. Rutty CJ, Connors TA, Hoang-Nam N, et al. In vivo studies with hexamethylmelamine. *Eur J Cancer* 1978;14:713.

350. Garattini E, Broggini M, Coccia P, et al. Biochemical studies on the ability of pentamethylmelamine to interact in vivo with DNA and proteins in a sensitive murine ovarian reticular cell sarcoma. *Biochem Pharmacol* 1984;33:2715.

351. Ames MM, Sanders ME, Tiede WS. Role of *N*-methylolpentamethylmelamine in the metabolic activation of hexamethylmelamine. *Cancer Res* 1983;43:500.

352. Garattini E, Colombo T, Donelli MG, et al. Distribution, metabolism, and irreversible binding of hexamethylmelamine in mice bearing ovarian carcinoma. *Cancer Chemother Pharmacol* 1983;11:51.

353. Worzalla JF, Kaiman BD, Johnson BM, et al. Metabolism of hexamethylmelamine-ring-C14 in rats and man. *Cancer Res* 1974;34:2669.

354. Ross D, Langdon SP, Gescher A, et al. Studies of the mode of action of antitumor triazenes and triazines-V. The correlation of the in vitro cytotoxicity and in vivo antitumor activity of hexamethylmelamine analogues with their metabolism. *Biochem Pharmacol* 1984;33:1131.

355. Ross WE, McMillan DR, Ross CF. Comparison of DNA damage by methylmelamines and formaldehyde. *J Natl Cancer Inst* 1981;67:217.

356. Rutty CJ, Abel G, Harrap KR. In vitro cytotoxicity of hexamethylmelamine and its analogues. *Br J Cancer* 1979;40:317.

357. D'Incalci M, Erba E, Balconi G, et al. Time dependence of the in vitro cytotoxicity of hexamethylmelamine and its metabolites. *Br J Cancer* 1980;41:630.

358. Miller KJ, McGovern RM, Ames MM. Effect of a hepatic activation system on the antiproliferative activity of hexamethylmelamine against human tumor cell lines. *Cancer Chemother Pharmacol* 1985;15:49.

359. Gescher A, D'Incalci M, Fanelli R, et al. *N*-Hydroxymethyl-

pentamethylmelamine, a major in vitro metabolite of hexamethylmelamine. *Life Sci* 1980;26:147.

360. Dubois J, Atassi G, Hanocq M, et al. Pharmacokinetics and metabolism of hexamethylmelamine in mice after i.p. administration. *Cancer Chemother Pharmacol* 1986;18:226.

361. Morimoto M, Green D, Rahman A, et al. Comparative pharmacology of pentamethylmelamine and hexamethylmelamine in mice. *Cancer Res* 1980;40:2762.

362. Rutty CJ, Abel G. In vitro cytotoxicity of the methylmelamines. *Chem Biol Interact* 1980;29:235.

363. Begleiter A, Grover J, Goldenberg GJ. Uptake and metabolism of hexamethylmelamine and pentamethylmelamine L5178Y lymphoblasts in vitro. *Cancer Res* 1980;40:4489.

364. Gupta RS. Genetic, biochemical, and cross-resistance studies with mutants of Chinese hamster ovary cells resistant to the anticancer drugs VM-26 and VP16-213. *Cancer Res* 1983;43:1568.

365. Borm PJA, Mingels MJJ, Frankhuijzen-Sierevogel AC, et al. Cellular and subcellular studies of the biotransformation of hexamethylmelamine in rat and isolated hepatocytes and intestinal epithelial cells. *Cancer Res* 1984;44:2820.

366. Brindley C, Gescher A, Langdon SP, et al. Studies of the mode of action of antitumor triazenes and triazines-III. Metabolism studies on hexamethylmelamine. *Biochem Pharmacol* 1982;31:625.

367. Worzalla JF, Lee DM, Johnson RO, et al. Effect of microsomal enzyme-inducing chemicals on the metabolism of hexamethylmelamine (HMM NSC-13875) in rats and hamsters. *Proc Am Assoc Cancer Res* 1973;33:2810.

368. Paoline A, D'Incalci M. Effect of phenobarbital pretreatment on the metabolism and antitumor activity of hexamethylmelamine. *Cancer Treat Rep* 1986;70:513.

369. Hande K, Combs G, Swingle R, et al. Effect of cimetidine and ranitidine on the metabolism and toxicity of hexamethylmelamine. *Cancer Treat Rep* 1986;70:1443.

370. D'Incalci M, Beggiolin G, Sessa C, et al. Influence of ascites on the pharmacokinetics of hexamethylmelamine and *N*-demethylated metabolites in ovarian cancer patients. *Eur J Clin Oncol* 1981;17:1331.

371. Ames MM, Kovach JS. Parenteral formulation of hexamethylmelamine potentially suitable for use in man. *Cancer Treat Rep* 1982;66:1579.

372. Wickes AD, Howell SB. Pharmacokinetics of hexamethylmelamine administered via the ip route in an oil emulsion vehicle. *Cancer Treat Rep* 1985;69:657.

373. Gordon IL, Kar R, Opfell RW, et al. Pharmacokinetics of hexamethylmelamine in intralipid following hepatic regional administration in rabbits. *Cancer Res* 1987;47:5070.

374. Ames MM, Kovach JS, Moertel CG. Clinical evaluation of a new formulation of hexamethylmelamine (H) suitable for intravenous administration. *Proc Am Assoc Cancer Res* 1986;27:167.

375. van Harskamp G, Hulshoff A, de Bruyn DPM, et al. A phase I clinical and pharmacological study of intravenous hexamethylmelaminechloride. *Proc Am Soc Clin Oncol* 1986;5:51.

376. Ihde DC, Dutcher JS, Young RC, et al. Phase I trial of pentamethylmelamine: a clinical and pharmacologic study. *Cancer Treat Rep* 1981;65:755.

377. Van Echo DA, Chiuten DF, Whitacre M, et al. Phase I trial of pentamethylmelamine in patients with previously treated malignancies. *Cancer Treat Rep* 1980;64:1335.

378. Goldberg RS, Griffin JP, McSherry JW, et al. Phase I study of pentamethylmelamine. *Cancer Treat Rep* 1980;64:1319.

379. Casper ES, Gralla RJ, Lynch GR, et al. Phase I and pharmacological studies of pentamethylmelamine administered by 24-hour intravenous infusion. *Cancer Res* 1981;41:1402.

380. Muindi JRF, Newell DR, Smith IE, et al. Pentamethylmelamine (PMM): phase I clinical and pharmacokinetic studies. *Br J Cancer* 1983;47:27.

381. D'Incalci M, Morazzoni P, Pantarotto C. Gas chromatographic determination of hexamethylmelamine in mouse plasma. *Anal Biochem* 1979;99:441.

382. Ames MM, Powis G. Determination of pentamethylmelamine and hexamethylmelamine in plasma and urine by nitrogen-phosphorous gas-liquid chromatography. *J Chromatogr* 1979;174:245.

383. Dutcher JS, Jones RB, Boyd MR. A sensitive and specific assay for pentamethylmelamine in plasma: applicability to clinical studies. *Cancer Treat Rep* 1980;64:99.

384. Bryan GT, Gorske AL. Use of ion-exchange chromatography in the spectrophotometric assay for the antineoplastic agent, hexamethylmelamine, in biological fluids. *J Chromatogr* 1968;34:67.

385. Rutty IR, Abel G, et al. Preclinical toxicology, pharmacokinetics and formulation of N^2,N^4,N^6-trihydroxymethyl-N^2,N^4,N^6-trimethylamine (Trimelamol), a water-soluble cytotoxic *s*-triazine which does not require metabolic activation. *Cancer Chemother Pharmacol* 1986;17:251.

386. Jones B, Deesen P, Lacher M, et al. Pharmacokinetics of pentamethylmelamine (PMM) and its demethylated metabolites. *Proc AACR ASCO* 1980;21:186.

387. Benvenuto JA, Stewart DJ, Benjamin RS, et al. High performance liquid chromatographic analysis of pentamethylmelamine and its metabolites in biological fluids. *J Chromatogr* 1981;222:518.

388. Colombo T, Torti L, D'Incalci M. Dose-dependent pharmacokinetics of PMM in the rat. *Cancer Chemother Pharmacol* 1981;5:201.

389. Rutty CJ, Newell DR, Muindi JRF, et al. The comparative pharmacokinetics of pentamethylmelamine in man, rat, and mouse. *Cancer Chemother Pharmacol* 1982;8:105.

390. D'Incalci M, Bolis G, Mangioni C, et al. Variable oral absorption of hexamethylmelamine in man. *Cancer Treat Rep* 1978;62:2117.

391. Ames MM, Powis G, Kovach JS, et al. Disposition and metabolism of pentamethylmelamine and hexamethylmelamine in rabbits and humans. *Cancer Res* 1979;39:5016.

392. Klippert PJ, Hulshoff A, Mingels MJJ, et al. Low oral bioavailability of hexamethylmelamine in the rat due to simultaneous hepatic and intestinal metabolism. *Cancer Res* 1983;43:3160.

393. Bryan GT, Worzalla JF, Gorske AL, et al. Plasma levels and urinary excretion of hexamethylmelamine following oral administration to human subjects with cancer. *Clin Pharmacol Ther* 1968;9:777.

394. Broggini M, Rossi C, Colombo T, et al. Hexamethylmelamine and pentamethylmelamine tissue distribution in M5076/73A ovarian cancer-bearing mice. *Cancer Treat Rep* 1982;66:127.

395. Broggini M, Colombo T, D'Incalci M, et al. Pharmacoki-

netics of hexamethylmelamine and pentamethylmelamine in mice. *Cancer Treat Rep* 1981;65:669.

396. Benvenuto JA, Stewart DJ, Benjamin RS, et al. Pharmacology of pentamethylmelamine in humans. *Cancer Res* 1981;41:566.

397. D'Incalci M, Farina P, Sessa C, et al. Hexamethylmelamine distribution in patients with ovarian and other pelvic cancers. *Cancer Treat Rep* 1982;66:231.

398. D'Incalci M, Sessa C, Begglilin G, et al. Cerebrospinal fluid levels of hexamethylmelamine and *N*-demethylated metabolites. *Cancer Treat Rep* 1981;65:350.

399. Judson IR, Rutty CJ, Abel G, et al. Low central nervous system penetration of N^2,N^4,N^6-trihydroxymethyl-N^2,N^4,N^6-trimethylmelamine (Trimelamol): a cytotoxic *s*-triazine with reduced neurotoxicity. *Br J Cancer* 1986;53:601.

400. Beisler JA. Isolation, characterization, and properties of a labile hydrolysis product of the antitumor nucleoside, 5-azacytidine. *J Med Chem* 1978;21:204.

401. Connors TA, Cumber AJ, Ross WCJ, et al. Regression of human lung tumor xenografts induced by water-soluble analogues of hexamethylmelamine. *Cancer Treat Rep* 1977;61:927.

402. Boven E, Nauta MM, Schluper HMM, et al. Superior effi-cacy of trimelmol to hexamethylmelamine in human ovarian cancer xenografts. *Cancer Chemother Pharmacol* 1986;18:124.

403. Louis J, Louis NB, Linman JW, et al. The clinical pharmacology of hexamethylmelamine: phase I study. *Clin Pharmacol Ther* 1967;8:55.

404. Ajani JA, Cabanillas FF, Bodey GP. Phase I trial of pentamethylmelamine. *Cancer Treat Rep* 1982;66:1227.

405. Kohorn EI, Klein-Angerer S. The effect of chemotherapy on lymphocyte subpopulations and cell-mediated cytotoxicity in patients with ovarian cancer. *Gynecol Oncol* 1984;19:60.

406. Ashby J, Callander RD, Rose FL. Weak mutagenicity to *Salmonella* of the formaldehyde-releasing anti-tumor agent hexamethylmelamine. *Mutat Res* 1985;142:121.

407. Johnson DH, Porter LL, List AF, et al. Acute nonlymphocytic leukemia after treatment of small cell lung cancer. *Am J Med* 1986;81:962.

408. Grubb BP, Thant M. Case report: acute myelocytic leukemia in a patient treated with hexamethylmelamine. *Am J Med Sci* 1986;292:393.

409. Thompson DJ, Dyke II, Molello JA. Reproduction studies on hexamethylmelamine in the rat and rabbit. *Toxicol Appl Pharmacol* 1984;72:245.

15

CISPLATIN AND ANALOGS

EDDIE REED

Cisplatin, *cis*-diamminedichloroplatinum(II), is the primary molecule in a family of cytotoxic compounds that are based on elemental platinum. These compounds are among the most widely used and most effective anticancer drugs. They are responsible for the high rate of cure of germ cell tumors of the testes, for high remission rates in ovarian cancer, and, when used in combination with other drugs or irradiation, for improved local control of a wide variety of tumors of the upper airway, esophagus, cervix, and anus. They are potent cytotoxins as well as radiation sensitizers. The physical chemistry of cisplatin and its interactions with cellular macromolecules have been reviewed extensively in previous editions of this book.[1,2] A summary of the main points includes the following. The antitumor activity of this class of compounds was discovered by Rosenberg and colleagues, during the study of the effects of electric current on bacterial growth.[3,4] Platinum is in the third row of transition metals in the periodic table and has eight electrons in the outer *d* shell. Due to the nature of the orbitals around the platinum atom, the atom has bond angles and a spatial configuration that are relatively fixed. The spatial configuration depends on whether the oxidation state of platinum is +2 or +4. These states are usually designated Pt(II) and Pt(IV).

Although the development of Pt(IV) analogs has generated a great deal of interest, clinical activity has been seen primarily with cisplatin analogs that are in the Pt(II) state, namely cisplatin and carboplatin (Fig. 15-1). The reason for this is not clear. Pt(II) complexes can have distinct *cis* and *trans* isomers, and generally *trans* isomers are much less cytotoxic than *cis* isomers. For example, *trans*-diamminedichloroplatinum(II) is much less potent in cell culture systems than cisplatin and has not been developed clinically.

The biologic actions of Pt(II) complexes are due to displacement reactions, which cause the platinum to become stably bound to DNA, RNA, proteins, and other biomolecules. All of the active antitumor complexes are bifunctional in that they can form, by successive displacement reactions, two stable bonds under physiologic conditions so as to produce a covalent cross-link between two nucleophilic atoms of a macromolecule. In this respect, the Pt(II) complexes are similar to bifunctional alkylating agents such as nitrogen mustards. Ligand displacement reactions in platinum complexes occur with retention of the spatial configuration of the fixed bond angles, unlike with alkylating agents, in which configuration typically becomes inverted. The stability of the binding of different ligands to Pt(II) varies greatly. Although the binding to sulfur or nitrogen sites is essentially irreversible under physiologic conditions, the stability of binding to halogens is much lower, in the order $I^- > Br^- > Cl^-$, and the stability of binding to water is weaker still.

Cisplatin's transit across cellular membranes can be explained by the chemistry of its reactions in water and biologic fluids. Aquation and hydrolysis equilibria of cisplatin in an aqueous milieu at physiologic pH yield products that have a neutral charge (Fig. 15-2). Neutral molecules have one chloro-leaving group and one hydroxy-leaving group. Such molecules could theoretically cross cell membranes based on chemistry alone. Once inside cells, pH and pKa values suggest that these neutral species would be readily converted to charged aquo-hydroxy species, which would result in intracellular trapping of drug. Therefore, chemically, no need exists for an active transport mechanism for cisplatin, unlike with some alkylating agents. As discussed below, however, evidence exists that membrane proteins may play a role in cellular drug accumulation or cellular efflux of drug or both. The detailed aquation chemistry of cisplatin has not been replicated for any of the cisplatin analogs.

Cisplatin binds to RNA more extensively than to DNA and to DNA more extensively than to protein, when binding is assessed as moles of drug per gram of macromolecule. In most systems, the binding to DNA correlates well with cisplatin-induced cell kill. Reports from the early development of cisplatin, however, observed that some cell lines (Burkitt's lymphoma cells and others) showed cisplatin-induced cell lysis before significant DNA damage could develop.

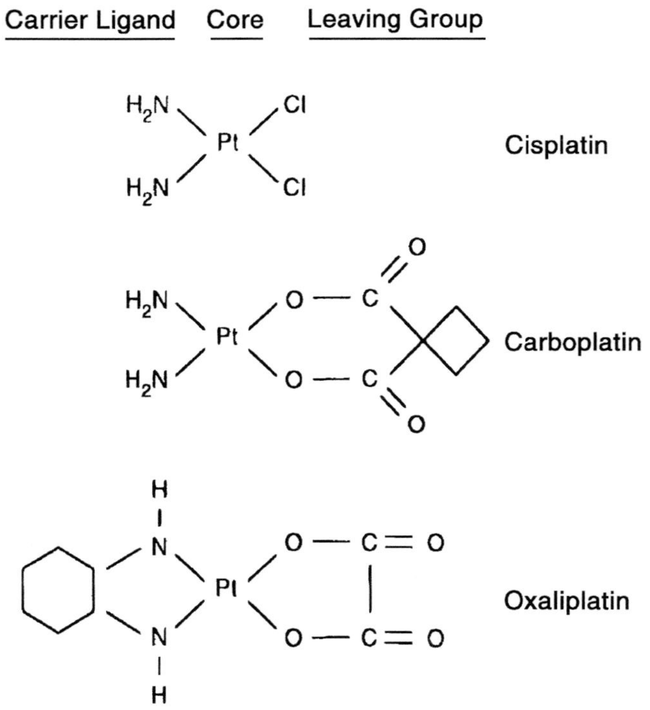

FIGURE 15-1. Two-dimensional structures are shown for cisplatin, carboplatin, and oxaliplatin. The core structures are the same, based on the *cis* configuration of Pt(II). The leaving groups are different for the three compounds. The carrier ligand is different for oxaliplatin.

In the reaction of cisplatin with DNA, the two chloride ligands can react with two different sites to produce cross-links or adducts. Generally, if the two sites are on the same DNA strand, the lesion is referred to as a *DNA adduct*. If the sites are on different DNA strands, the lesion is referred to as a *DNA cross-link*. Cisplatin has been noted to bind to all DNA bases but has preference for the N-7 positions of adenine and guanine. This is due to the high nucleophilicity of the N-7 sites of these purine bases. The bond distance between the chloride-leaving groups of cisplatin is fixed at approximately 3 Å, whereas the corresponding bond distance for alkylating agents can range between 7 and 10 Å. This results in a situation in which bifunctional binding of cisplatin to DNA distorts DNA to conform to the fixed stereochemistry of the cisplatin molecule. DNA-platinum-protein cross-links may occur as well but appear to have a minor role in platinum biology.

When cisplatin is exposed to isolated DNA *in vitro*, to cultured cells, or to human patients, the pattern of cisplatin-DNA binding shows a consistent distribution of types of lesions. Approximately 60% of lesions are d(GpG)-diammineplatinum(II) intrastrand adducts, approximately 30% are d(ApG) adducts, approximately 10% are d(GpXpG) adducts, and less than 2% are in the form of interstrand cross-links (Table 15-1). A d(GpA) lesion is never seen, presumably due to steric hindrance by the methyl group on the adenine ring. The intrastrand adduct results in specific three-dimensional changes in the DNA double helix, with bending of the double strand toward the major groove at an angle that has been variably reported as between 55 and 70 degrees.[5] Limited local denaturation occurs as well. This kinking in the DNA is thought to provide the basis for recognition by a range of nuclear proteins, including DNA repair proteins, high mobility group (HMG) proteins, and others.

The chemistry of protein interactions with the platinum-DNA adduct has been studied by a number of groups. In

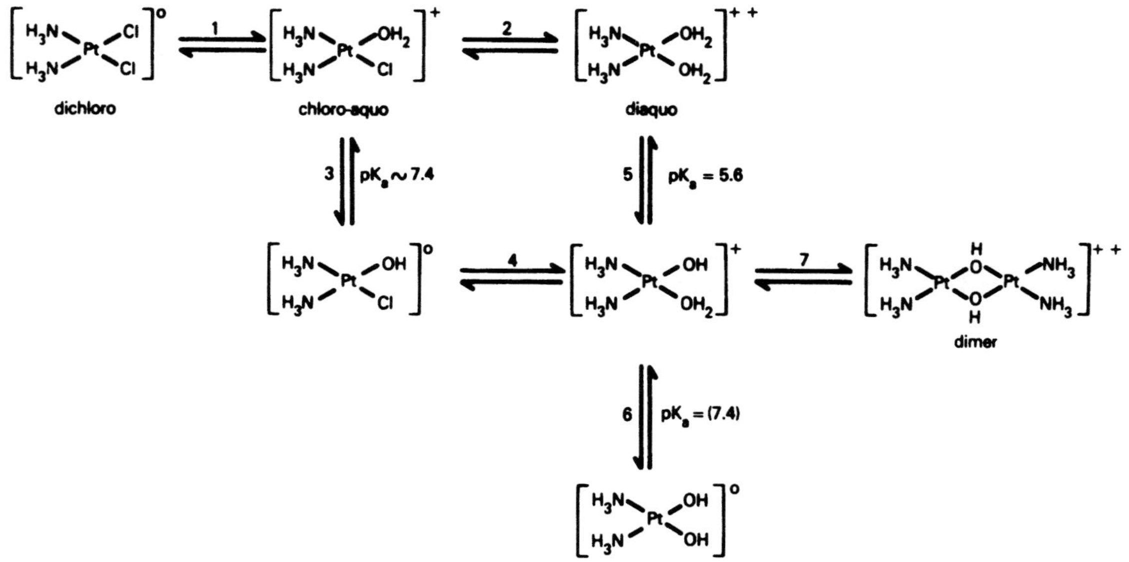

FIGURE 15-2. Aquation and hydrolysis equilibria of cisplatin (pKa values are from ref. 187). Note that reactions 3 and 6 are favored at physiologic pH and yield products that have a neutral charge and that theoretically could readily cross cell membranes.

TABLE 15-1. TYPES OF DNA LESIONS CAUSED BY CISPLATIN AND CARBOPLATIN (OXALIPLATIN NOT FULLY CHARACTERIZED)

DNA lesion	% of total DNA damage	Comment
N7-d(GpG)-intrastrand adduct	~60%	Possibly lethal to cells
N7-d(ApG)-intrastrand adduct	~30%	Possibly lethal to cells
N7-d(GpXpG)-intrastrand adduct	~10%	Potential lethality unclear
N7-d(X)-d(X)-interstrand cross-link	<2%	Biologic importance unclear
		Levels correlate with cellular toxicity

nucleotide excision repair, a group of proteins are associated with DNA damage recognition and excision for a range of DNA lesions that include cisplatin.[6–8] The two lead proteins in this activity are XPC and hHR23B. This heterodimer is sometimes referred to as the DNA damage sensor and repair-recruitment factor.[6] In mismatch repair, the hMSH2 homodimer generates a ringed structure that appears to wrap around the platinum-DNA lesion at the site of the damage. Here, too, DNA damage recognition is based on a class of lesions that may kink DNA—and platinum-DNA damage belongs to that class—rather than being specific for platinum-DNA damage. Once bound to the site of damage, the hMSH2 homodimer may recruit other proteins and thereby send the signal for cellular apoptosis to be initiated.[9] Lippard's group has examined the potential for HMG proteins to interfere with the normal functioning of DNA damage-recognition proteins.[10,11] They have focused on three-dimensional changes caused by cisplatin that may attract HMG proteins. In their studies of adducted DNA constructs, recognition of the three-dimensional alterations by HMG1 is highly dependent on the presence of phenylalanine at position 37 of the protein.[11] Mutant variants of HMG1 with alanine at the same position show dramatically reduced binding to the site of DNA damage. Although HMGs have a number of very important intracellular functions, the biologic significance of HMGs with respect to platinum-DNA damage is not yet clear.

Differences in replicative bypass of lesions may be related to the three-dimensional structure of the DNA adduct. Scheeff et al. showed through molecular modeling that cisplatin and oxaliplatin (discussed further later) had very similar types of distortion of the DNA double helix, with one major exception. The 1,2-diaminocyclohexane ring of oxaliplatin tended to protrude directly into the narrowed major groove of the damaged DNA, forming a less polar major groove in the area of the adduct.[12] This has been suggested to cause reduced recognition and reduced repair of oxaliplatin-DNA adducts. This "carrier ligand" effect has been studied extensively by Chaney and colleagues, as discussed later. Other work suggests that cisplatin may enhance recombination within cellular DNA, through a unique interaction between a cisplatin-DNA-histone complex and topoisomerase I.[13]

The debate as to the nature of the true cytotoxic lesion formed by platinum binding to DNA has yet to be com-

pletely resolved. Various reports have suggested that the d(GpG) lesion may be more cytotoxic and that the d(ApG) lesion may be more mutagenic—and vice versa.[2] Several reports generated data from cisplatin and from carboplatin using isolated DNA and cultured Chinese hamster ovary cells.[14–16] These studies have provided indirect evidence that the d(ApG) adduct may be the primary lesion-causing cytotoxicity in their system, although other lesions could not be ruled out (Fig. 15-3). Cisplatin, carboplatin, and oxaliplatin form the same DNA lesions in approximately the same percentages, although the time frames are different for the three drugs, with carboplatin and oxaliplatin taking more time than cisplatin.[17,18]

That carrier ligand influences platinum analog pharmacology is a concept pioneered by Chaney and colleagues.[19–22] Carrier ligand may influence platinum whole-animal and intracellular pharmacology, as well as DNA repair and replicative bypass of DNA lesions. These matters are discussed independently later. From the work of Chaney and others,

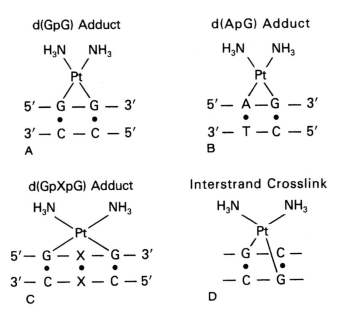

FIGURE 15-3. Bifunctional adducts of cisplatin with DNA. Lesions indicated in panels **A, B,** and **C** represent different intrastrand adducts, which together account for more than 90% of total platinum binding to DNA. The lesion indicated in panel **D** is the interstrand cross-link measured by alkaline elution and accounts for less than 5% of total platinum binding to DNA. See text for discussion.

TABLE 15-2. KEY FEATURES OF CISPLATIN AND ANALOG CHEMISTRY

Rigid stereochemistry is in a planar conformation, with leaving groups in the *cis* positions.

Bond angles and bond lengths are rigid, with ~3 Å between the two leaving groups.

DNA bends to accommodate the stereochemistry of the drug, forming a kink in the double helix.

The kinking of the platinum-DNA complex causes recognition by appropriate proteins.

Some nuclear proteins (high mobility group proteins and select transcription factors) may bind to the kinked DNA and block access to the site of damage. This block to appropriate proteins (repair proteins, for example) may facilitate the development of cellular resistance.

Clinical activity (and differences in clinical profiles) are related to four properties:

Cis versus *trans* configuration

Pt(II) versus Pt(IV) oxidation state

Nature of leaving groups (cisplatin vs. carboplatin)

Nature of carrier ligand (cisplatin vs. oxaliplatin)

oxaliplatin has emerged as the third platinum analog with clear clinical efficacy. When cisplatin is compared with carboplatin, the primary difference is the leaving group. When cisplatin is compared with oxaliplatin, the primary difference is the carrier ligand moiety; the leaving group of oxaliplatin bears some similarity to that of carboplatin (Fig. 15-1).

Four major chemistry principles appear to influence the clinical activity of platinum compounds. *Cis* isomers are active, whereas *trans* isomers are not. Analogs in the Pt(II) oxidation state have been clinically successful, whereas Pt(IV) analogs have not. The leaving group appears to influence the reactivity and thus the clearance and toxicity of the analog (cisplatin vs. carboplatin). The carrier ligand also appears to have substantial impact on stability, recognition by repair processes, clinical distribution, patterns of toxicity, and efficacy. Table 15-2 summarizes several important points regarding the chemistry of platinum-based anticancer agents.

PLATINUM-DNA DAMAGE IN CELLS AND IN TISSUES

Study of platinum-DNA adduct in clinical and preclinical systems was made possible by a series of technical innovations that allowed measurement of platinum-DNA damage after therapeutic levels of drug exposure, without the use of radioisotopes. These methods included the enzyme-linked immunosorbent assay of Poirier,[23,24] the high-pressure liquid chromatography assays of Eastman and Fichtinger-Schepman,[25,26] and atomic absorption spectrophotometry (AAS) with Zeeman background correction.[27]

In recent years, further elucidation of the relationships between DNA damage and biologic effect have been pursued by a number of groups. In tissue culture conditions, the direct relationship between platinum-DNA damage level and cell kill is unquestioned in most cell lines.[21,28,29] Consistent with this principle, reduction in a cell's ability to remove platinum damage from cellular DNA is associated with markedly increased cell kill in a wide range of systems.[7,29–31] Conversely, enhanced DNA repair is associated with enhanced cellular resistance to platinum compounds.[28,32–34]

Reductions in a cell's ability to remove platinum-DNA adduct from cellular DNA can be effected by direct inhibitors of DNA repair,[35] by biologic agents,[36–38] by agents that influence cellular signaling pathways,[39–41] by glucose-related stress,[29] and possibly by other mechanisms.[1,2] Whether a final common pathway exists for all of these approaches toward reducing a cell's ability to remove platinum-DNA adduct is not clear. A number of studies, however, point to the impact that each of these approaches may have on cellular signaling pathways, even though that effect may be indirect. In turn, an increased recognition that cellular signaling pathways impact DNA adduct repair has been apparent in reports by several groups.[39,42,43]

In previous editions of this book, the early work on platinum-DNA adduct and its relationship(s) to defined clinical and biologic end points has been detailed. Poirier's group was the first to show a relationship between platinum-DNA damage levels in tissues obtained from patients and clinical outcomes.[24,44,45] Adduct levels in peripheral blood cell DNA were shown to correlate with disease response in ovarian cancer, testicular cancer, and breast and colon cancers. Fichtinger-Schepman and colleagues performed several studies to suggest that one could measure adduct levels in blood cells *ex vivo* and that a linear relationship existed between *ex vivo* levels and adduct levels formed in clinical blood specimens.[46,47] The studies of Poirier and colleagues, and those of Fichtinger-Schepman and colleagues, were all performed in the setting of a relatively simple treatment regimen.

Perera and colleagues analyzed adduct levels along with several other molecular end points in a cohort of testicular cancer patients that underwent a complex multiagent treatment regimen.[48–50] Perera found no statistically significant relationship between adduct level and disease response in this cohort, but a statistically significant relationship was seen between sister chromatid exchange levels and disease response,[50] which suggests that total DNA damage was the relevant end point in her studies.

The original observations by Poirier were confirmed in independent blinded studies by Reed and colleagues.[51,52] AAS was used to measure peripheral blood adduct levels in a cohort of 49 patients with 24 different tumor types. When adduct levels were assessed 24 hours after the first dose of therapy, the relationship to disease response was direct, with a two-sided p value of .007. Schellens et al. studied a group of 45 patients with a variety of tumor types and assessed adduct levels through an analysis of area under the concentration × time curve (AUC).[53] Platinum-DNA adduct AUC was directly related to a favorable clinical response, regardless of tumor type, with a two-sided *p* value of less than .0001. All of the above studies were conducted in adult patients.

More recent platinum-DNA adduct studies in the clinic have focused on the relationships that may occur in children[54,55] as well as in adults,[56] and how adduct levels may be related to traditional pharmacokinetic/pharmacodynamic assessments of cisplatin, carboplatin, or one of the platinum analogs. Peng and colleagues studied platinum-DNA adduct levels in peripheral blood leucocytes in 24 children with solid tumors after cisplatin- or carboplatin-based therapy.[54] Adduct was measured by enzyme-linked immunosorbent assay. The authors found considerable interindividual variation in adduct level that was not correlated with the AUC for cisplatin. This suggests that the variation in DNA adduct levels among individuals was not a pharmacokinetic effect and was probably dependent on cellular/tissue factors. This is consistent with the previous observations of Reed and Poirier in adult patients.[24,57] Tonda et al. studied 27 children treated with carboplatin in a range of doses and assessed platinum-DNA adduct by AAS.[55] They found that, at lower doses of carboplatin, DNA adduct could not be measured in peripheral blood cells using this technique. In each of these studies, the perception was that cohort sample size was too small to assess any possible relationship between adduct level and disease response.

Fichtinger-Schepman and colleagues studied the relationship between DNA adduct levels formed *ex vivo*, those formed in xenografts, and those formed in a clinical setting.[58] Tumor fragments from human patients were treated with cisplatin *ex vivo*, and cisplatin-DNA adduct levels were measured by ^{32}P postlabeling. Fragments were also xenografted into mice, the mice were treated with cisplatin, and adduct levels were measured in tumor tissues. Positive correlations were found between the DNA adduct levels measured *ex vivo* and the clinical response to treatment (*p* <.05), and between *ex vivo* DNA adduct levels and adduct levels measured in xenografted tumors (*p* <.02).

Poirier's group has investigated the development of platinum-DNA adduct in the mitochondria of cultured cells,[59,60] maternal and fetal rodent tissues,[61,62] maternal and fetal patas monkeys,[63,64] and maternal human tissues.[65] In cultured Chinese hamster ovary cells, cisplatin-DNA adduct levels were sixfold higher in mitochondrial DNA than in nuclear DNA.[59] Further, no evidence was found of removal of mitochondrial DNA adduct at 54 hours after the cisplatin exposure.[60] In rats, cisplatin was given to pregnant females at 18 days of gestation, and animals were sacrificed 24 hours later.[61] In maternal and fetal brain, DNA adduct levels were 7- to 50-fold higher in mitochondrial DNA than in nuclear DNA. In fetal liver, mitochondrial DNA adduct levels were 2- to 16-fold higher. Fetal kidney,

liver, and lung contained fewer cisplatin-DNA adducts than the corresponding maternal tissues, but fetal brain contained higher adduct levels.[62]

In patas monkeys, cisplatin was administered in the third trimester of pregnancy.[63,64] Adduct could be measured in a wide range of fetal tissues, including adrenal gland, brain, heart, kidney, liver, skin, spleen, and thymus. In monkeys, however, maternal tissues showed approximately twice as much DNA damage as fetal tissues. Platinum-DNA adduct has been measured in peripheral blood and placenta of a pregnant human patient,[64] as well as in cord blood of another individual.[65] In both human cases, the patient had ovarian cancer that was diagnosed during pregnancy.

Although DNA adduct once held promise as a potentially useful tool to assist in the clinical development of drugs in this class, current data do not support its clinical use, primarily due to potential drug interactions. The use of DNA adduct in the preclinical setting is probably worthwhile, however, and should be further explored to answer critical questions regarding the potential efficacy of new compounds and new approaches of combining platinum drugs with modulatory or synergizing agents.

GADD (growth arrest and DNA damage) genes are said to be induced by an array of DNA-damaging agents and other agents that generate cellular stress. In squamous carcinoma cells xenografted into nude mice, GADD153 protein levels at baseline were 4.5 times higher in tumor cells than in stromal cells.[66] After treatment with cisplatin, however, GADD153 levels increased in stromal cells by 72%, compared with a 50% increase in tumor cells. In this setting, levels of cisplatin-DNA adduct were sixfold higher in stromal cells than in tumor cells. The authors calculated that tumor cells were 25-fold more effective in inducing GADD153 at the same level of DNA adduct.

PLATINUM-DNA DAMAGE AND DNA REPAIR

Platinum-DNA damage is repaired by the nucleotide excision DNA repair pathway, designated NER. The specific sequence of steps has been worked out and is elegantly summarized in several reviews.[6–8] Generally, platinum-DNA damage is recognized by the XPA-hHR23B heterodimer, which is considered as a DNA damage sensor and repair-recruitment factor. Basal transcription factor IIH (TFIIH) is recruited to the site of the damage. TFIIH is a complex of nine different proteins. Among the proteins within TFIIH are XPB and XPD, which are helicases that induce strand separation at the site of the lesion. XPA appears to be important in recruiting other DNA repair proteins to this platinum-DNA-protein complex, which is now in the "open" DNA conformation. Replication protein A (RPA) stabilizes the "open" DNA complex. "Open" means that the DNA strands have been separated at and around the site of the platinum-DNA lesion and are held in place by the protein machinery that includes TFIIH.

XPG makes the 3' cut in the DNA strand that has the covalent damage. ERCC1-XPF is a heterodimer that makes the 5' cut in the DNA strand that has the covalent damage. The ERCC1-XPF heterodimer executes the last "substep" in this process. Typically, the damage-containing oligomer ranges from 24 to 32 bases in length. After excision of the damage, a number of general replication factors fill the DNA gap, and the ends of the new DNA are ligated to close the gap. Although this damage recognition/excision process is rate limiting to NER, what is rate limiting to cisplatin damage recognition/excision is not clear.

NER has two subpathways: global genomic repair and transcription-coupled repair. For cisplatin, global genomic repair tends to be higher in cisplatin-resistant cells than in cisplatin-sensitive cells.[67–69] Further, transcription-coupled repair tends to be increased in cisplatin-resistant cells, to an even greater extent than global genomic repair. Whereas differences in global genomic repair between sensitive and resistant human ovarian cancer cells may be approximately two- to threefold, differences in transcription-coupled repair may be more than eightfold between the same cell lines.[68,69] One should note that, in transcription-coupled repair, DNA damage is recognized by the RNA polymerase II protein complex, which then recruits the normal NER protein machinery.[6]

In most reports, cells that have substantial differences in NER for cisplatin-DNA damage have a more than tenfold difference in their relative sensitivities to cisplatin, platinum analogs, and other heavy metals.[28,70,71] Such metals include cadmium, gallium, vanadium, and others. In contrast, cells that show differences in mismatch repair without changes in NER tend to have differences in cisplatin sensitivity of two- to threefold.[72,73] In the original observation linking mismatch repair (MMR) to cisplatin resistance, cell lines were used that had been previously shown to have greater than eightfold differences in NER activity as well.[68,74]

MMR is the DNA repair pathway responsible for the repair of slipped intermediates and of base mismatches in cellular DNA.[75–77] The primary function of MMR is to maintain integrity of the genome for purposes of DNA replication. MMR proteins are probably also responsible for sending cellular signals that initiate apoptosis in response to unrepaired bulky covalent DNA damage such as cisplatin-DNA adduct.

One group has presented a scheme of how signaling by MMR proteins may lead to apoptosis and demonstrated that this may occur through a p53-dependent or p53-independent pathway.[9,78] These pathways are illustrated in Figure 15-4. In their model, cisplatin could induce p53-dependent apoptosis through a mechanism that does not include MMR. Alternatively, unrepaired cisplatin-DNA damage could cause MLH1 to signal through ATM, to initiate a p53-dependent cascade or a p53-independent cas-

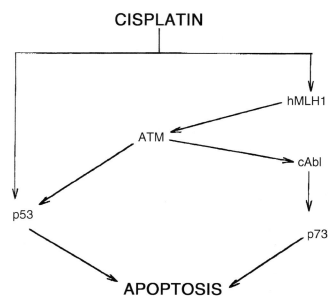

FIGURE 15-4. Flow diagram showing several critical genes involved in cisplatin-induced apoptosis, based on the work of Wang and his group.[9,78] Mismatch repair may initiate apoptosis through recognition of unrepaired platinum-DNA adduct and go through a p53-dependent or p53-independent pathway.

cade. ATM is the gene associated with ataxia telangiectasia. Other important genes in the p53-independent cascade include cAbl and p73. Hence, MMR proteins have a sensing function to detect cisplatin-DNA damage; this sensing allows the initiation of a signaling cascade that results in apoptosis. Cells that have lost MMR function (particularly hMLH1 and hMSH3) appear to have enhanced resistance to cisplatin, although only approximately two- to threefold over baseline.[72,73] Whereas MMR proteins appear to be very effective in the recognition of cisplatin-DNA damage, this is not the case for oxaliplatin-DNA damage.[79]

Replicative bypass of bulky DNA lesions is an important mechanism for cell survival but also a mechanism for the induction of mutagenesis. Chaney's group has performed a series of elegant studies to assess this biologic occurrence and the way it may relate to MMR.[19,79,80] In one study, the carrier ligand for the platinum analog was shown to be an important variable in the interaction between DNA damage recognition proteins, DNA polymerases, and the DNA adduct for that specific platinum analog.[19,81] Translesion DNA synthesis past these adducts was greatest for diene analogs of cisplatin, followed by oxaliplatin, followed by cisplatin, followed by JM216, which demonstrated the least amount of translesional DNA synthesis in an *in vitro* system.[19]

Chaney's group studied the roles of hMLH1, hMSH3, and hMSH6 in the replicative bypass of DNA lesions caused by cisplatin and by oxaliplatin.[79,80] Defects in hMLH1 or hMSH3 resulted in a 1.5- to 4.8-fold increase in cisplatin resistance and a 2.5- to 6-fold increase in replicative bypass of cisplatin-DNA adducts. No differences in replicative bypass were seen for oxaliplatin-DNA adducts under any conditions studied. Defects in hMSH6 did not result in increased replicative bypass for either agent. Chaney and colleagues also have studied nucleotide excision repair of platinum compounds in human cells. For cisplatin, oxaliplatin, and JM216, the kinetics of repair of platinum-DNA damage were the same when an *in vitro* repair system was used.[21]

In human gallbladder carcinoma cells, transfection of v-src induced resistance to cisplatin and induced an increased ability to repair cisplatin-DNA interstrand cross-links as measured by alkaline elution.[82] Increased expression of BRCA1 has been observed in a cisplatin-resistant human breast cancer cell line as well as several ovarian cancer cell lines.[82] In this latter study, antisense to BRCA1 partially reversed the cisplatin resistance phenotype. BRCA1 is essential for gene-specific repair of oxidative DNA damage.[83]

Within NER, one of the critical genes is ERCC1. A defect in ERCC1 results in the most severe DNA repair deficiency phenotype known.[6,7] Studies have been performed to assess the potential use of ERCC1 as a marker for the NER process in human cells and tissues. Two early reports showed statistically significant correlations between tumor tissue messenger RNA (mRNA) levels of ERCC1 and of XPA, and clinical resistance to platinum compounds in advanced-stage ovarian cancer.[81,84] Another report showed that mRNA levels of ERCC1 were directly related to cisplatin resistance in human gastric cancer.[85] Additional reports showed similar relationships in ovarian cancer for other genes involved in the rate-limiting step of NER—the DNA damage–recognition and excision step. In ovarian cancer tissues, these NER genes appear to be highly expressed, or expressed to low levels, in concert,[86,87] a finding that suggests some degree of coordinate regulation of these genes. Coordinate regulation of ERCC1, XPB, XPD, and CSB was most clearly shown in malignant and nonmalignant human brain tissue specimens.[88,89]

In vitro, the absence of a functional ERCC1 is associated with the total loss of repair of cisplatin-DNA adduct.[30] Also, the intracellular levels of expression of ERCC1 correlate with cisplatin-DNA adduct repair in human ovarian cancer cells.[90] Molecular and pharmacologic factors that influence mRNA expression of ERCC1 influence cellular sensitivity to cisplatin and cisplatin-DNA adduct repair.[35,36,39–41] Intrinsic aspects of ERCC1 that influence its level of mRNA expression and impact the DNA repair phenotype include a polymorphism at codon 118,[91,92] and the degree to which alternative splicing occurs within the cells, involving exon VIII.[93,94] Allelic loss or allelic gain of ERCC1 appears to have no influence on the cisplatin resistance phenotype in ovarian cancer patients.[95] Likewise, gene copy number of XPA appears to have no impact.[96] UCN-01 is a novel anticancer agent that inhibits DNA repair. It mediates its effect through inhibition of the NER complex and specifically ERCC1-XPA interaction,[97] and enhances cisplatin activity.

Clinical evidence is growing that DNA repair is important in clinical specimens, including MMR as well as NER. Howell's group assessed tumor samples from 38 human ovarian cancer patients before and after treatment with cisplatin chemotherapy for the percentage of cells that expressed detectable hMLH1 protein.[98] After therapy, hMLH1 staining was reduced in 66% of the cases ($p = .0005$). This supports the concept that platinum-based therapy may have selected for preexisting mismatch repair–deficient cells, which resulted in enrichment of this genotype. Observations of this type, along with the clinical observations regarding NER discussed earlier, suggest that NER abnormalities and MMR abnormalities may occur in the same clinical tissues at the same time, and both could affect clinical response.

PLATINUM AND APOPTOSIS

Cisplatin induces apoptosis in a wide range of cell types, and the apoptotic effect may be modulated by cytokines. That effect may vary depending on the cell type and the specific cytokine. In the T98G malignant glioma cell line, interleukin 6 (IL-6) inhibits cisplatin-induced apoptosis, whereas interleukin 1α and interleukin 1β enhanced sensitivity to cisplatin.[99] Dedoussis et al. showed that IL-6 expression was related to intracellular glutathione levels and that anti–IL-6 antibodies reduced those levels and reversed the cisplatin resistance phenotype in a human leukemia cell line.[99] In ovarian cancer cells, IL-6 inhibits cisplatin-induced apoptosis but does not influence intracellular levels of Bcl-2 protein in these cells.[100] In gastric cancer cell lines, cisplatin and tumor necrosis factor were synergistic in a fashion which suggest that tumor necrosis factor sensitized to cisplatin, but not the reverse.[101] Tumor necrosis factor β is associated with increased apoptosis in a number of cell systems. Cross-resistance to cisplatin and to tumor necrosis factor β was observed in an L1210 murine leukemia cell line that had been selected for resistance to cisplatin.[102]

Fas and Fas ligand have been implicated in apoptotic pathways in a number of cell types. Anti-Fas antibody, which activates the Fas receptor, was found to synergize with cisplatin in the induction of apoptosis in the T24 human bladder cancer cell line.[103] Activation of the APO-1/Fas system was also found to be important in cisplatin-induced apoptosis in human brain tumor cells.[104] Activation of the Fas ligand system was shown to be associated with an increase in cisplatin-related apoptosis in human proximal tubular epithelial cells,[105] which contributes to an understanding of cisplatin-related renal toxicity.

In a separate study of cisplatin-induced apoptosis in renal tubular cells, cell death was preceded by a loss of cytoskeletal F-actin stress fibers and a reduction of mRNA encoding for fibronectin, collagen a2 type IV, and laminin B2.[106] Whereas blocking the cytoskeletal changes was associated with a reduction in DNA fragmentation, blocking apoptosis with bcl-2 did not prevent cisplatin-induced breakdown in the cytoskeleton. Hence, cisplatin-related kidney toxicity is more complex than simply the induction of apoptosis in renal tubule cells and may involve functional changes secondary to cytoskeletal loss.

Bax is an apoptosis-promoting member of the bcl-2 gene family. When bax was transfected into the IMC-3 human head and neck squamous cell carcinoma cell line, these cells became more sensitive to cisplatin-induced apoptosis.[107] Although bcl-2 antagonizes the induction of apoptosis in some cell lines, its transfection into human testicular germ cell lines sensitized these cells to cisplatin-induced apoptosis and resulted in reciprocal down-regulation of Bcl-X(L).[108]

Apoptosis may be caspase dependent or caspase independent, depending on the system studied. Henkels and Turchi assessed whether this switch may occur as a function of the level of resistance of cells from the same genomic background.[109] They studied the A2780 human ovarian cancer cell line and the two derived sublines CP70 and C30. The apoptosis-related factors bcl-2, bcl-x, bcl-xL, bcl-xS, and bax showed different patterns of expression over time within the same cells after cisplatin exposure. Measurement of isoforms of bax showed a different pattern in sensitive A2780 cells than in the cisplatin-resistant CP70 or C30 cells. Analysis of the data suggested that, whereas A2780 cells followed a caspase-3–independent pathway of apoptosis, CP70 and C30 cells probably followed a caspase-3–dependent pathway. In rats, caspase inhibitors protect more than 80% of auditory hair cells from cisplatin-induced apoptosis and protect rat spinal ganglia cells in culture,[110] which suggests a possible therapeutic use for such a compound.

Apoptosis may also diverge based on p53. It may be p53 dependent or p53 independent. EAT/mcl-1 has sequence similarity to Bcl-2 and shows increased expression during the differentiation of the multipotent human embryonic carcinoma cell line NCR-G3. When transfected into cells, EAT/mcl-1 appeared to inhibit p53-independent apoptosis in response to cisplatin treatment.[111] Evidence to support the existence of a p53-independent apoptotic pathway was reported in studies of murine L1210 cell lines, in which extreme cisplatin resistance was shown to be unrelated to cell-cycle perturbations and was independent of p53 deficiency.[112] Although these two examples are noteworthy, several studies reinforce earlier observations that the induction of apoptosis is p53 dependent in many normal and malignant cell types.[113–118] In cells in which apoptosis is p53 dependent, activation of the cellular cyclic adenosine monophosphate response may be associated with protection from cisplatin-induced apoptosis.[119] Generally, mutant p53 is associated with resistance to apoptosis and decreased sensitivity to cisplatin.

Protein kinase C (PKC) may play a role in the regulation of the caspase-dependent apoptotic pathway. Cisplatin was found to cause a time- and dose-dependent increase in the catalytic fragments of several isoforms of PKC, including PKC delta, PKC epsilon, and PKC zeta.[120] In response to cisplatin, PKC activators activated caspase-3, whereas PKC inhibitors blocked caspase 3 activation. Another gene whose functions have been implicated in cisplatin-induced apoptosis is WAF1/cip1, a DNA damage–response gene, down-regulation of which resulted in increased sensitivity to cisplatin in human glioma cells.[121]

Several pharmacologic maneuvers may modify a cell's ability to enter the cell cycle and thus increase that cell's sensitivity to cisplatin-induced apoptosis.[122–128] Inhibition of telomerase activity,[122,123] hypoxia,[126] caffeine use,[127] and mitochondrial depletion[128] all enhance cytotoxicity, whereas inhibition of protein synthesis decreases drug-induced apoptosis.[124]

One group of investigators posed the question of whether cisplatin-induced apoptosis results in strand cleavage at preferred sites in cellular DNA. The authors studied circular DNA structures in human epidermoid KB-VI cells and quantitated double minutes and episomes using scanning electron microscopy.[129] The profile observed was most consistent with preferential cleavage at matrix attachment regions in cellular DNA, which suggests an ordered DNA cleavage process during apoptosis.

Interference of one cancer drug with another is one possible explanation for treatment failure. Judson and colleagues studied the effect of cisplatin on paclitaxel-induced apoptosis in cisplatin-resistant human ovarian cancer cells.[130] The authors assessed apoptotic effect by DNA fragmentation assays, fluorescence microscopy, and flow cytometry. They found that cisplatin blocked paclitaxel-induced apoptosis in these cells at a point downstream of Bcl-2 degradation and in a manner independent of paclitaxel's effect on microtubule stabilization.

Apoptosis is only one of several cellular properties that may impact greatly on the cisplatin sensitivity/resistance phenotype. Other important factors that have been studied extensively include cytosolic inactivation of drug, alterations in transmembrane cellular accumulation of drug, and altered DNA damage repair and/or damage tolerance. All of these factors have been reviewed in previous chapters of this book and can be investigated in detail therein. These four areas of interest are summarized in Table 15-3.

CLINICAL PHARMACOLOGY

The clinical pharmacology of cisplatin and carboplatin have been studied extensively, and major clinically important points are summarized in Tables 15-4 and 15-5. This is the collective work of a large number of investigators over many

TABLE 15-3. MECHANISMS OF CELLULAR RESISTANCE TO PLATINUM COMPOUNDS

Alterations in transmembrane cellular accumulation of drug

No specific transmembrane carrier for cisplatin has ever been identified.

Altered cellular accumulation has been associated with inhibition of a variety of membrane proteins, including Na,K–adenosine triphosphatase.

Transmembrane transit of drug can be explained by the chemistry of cisplatin in water.

Cytosolic inactivation of drug

Glutathione conjugation of activated platinum occurs, with possible active transport out of the cell for drug conjugated to reduced glutathione by the multidrug resistance protein class of adenosine triphosphate–dependent transporters.

Metallothioneins find and inactivate platinum.

Other sulfhydryl-containing groups, such as proteins, inactivate drug.

DNA repair

Nucleotide excision repair increases (NER; this pathway is responsible for the repair of cisplatin-DNA damage).

Clinical data show enhanced messenger RNA expression in platinum-resistant tumors.

Increased NER is associated with high levels of resistance (more than tenfold over baseline) in cultured cells.

Defective mismatch repair (MMR) may be responsible for recognition of platinum-DNA adducts and for the linkage of unrepaired DNA damage, to apoptotic pathways.

Clinical data show enrichment of MMR-defective cells in tumors after platinum therapy.

Defective MMR associated with low levels of resistance (two- to threefold over baseline) in cultured cells.

Translesional DNA synthesis is observed to occur preferentially in cisplatin-resistant cells.

In many cell lines, increased NER and defective MMR occur in tandem.

Resistance to apoptosis

Resistance may be mediated through loss of MMR protein(s), specifically MLH1.

Apoptotic response may be p53 dependent and caspase dependent, although not in all cases.

TABLE 15-4. KEY FEATURES OF CISPLATIN

Dosage:	50–75 mg/m² i.v., every 3–4 wk.
	Other dosing regimens may be used in selected situations.
	Usually administered in normal saline, with vigorous i.v. prehydration (at least 0.5 L of saline with 125 mg mannitol).
Mechanism of action:	Covalently binds to DNA bases and disrupts DNA function.
	Toxicity may be related to DNA damage and/or protein damage.
Metabolism:	Inactivated intracellularly and in the bloodstream by sulfhydryl groups.
	Drug covalently binds to glutathione, metallothionein, and sulfhydryls on proteins.
Pharmacokinetics:	After i.v. bolus, $t_{1/2\alpha}$ = 20–30 min; $t_{1/2\beta}$ = approximately 60 min; $t_{1/2\gamma}$ = approximately 24 h.
Elimination:	Approximately 25% of an i.v. dose is excreted from the body during the first 24 h.
	Of that portion eliminated, excretion is renal >90%, and bile <10%.
	Extensive long-term protein binding has been observed in many tissues.
Drug interactions:	Thiosulfates administered i.v. may inactivate drug systemically.
	Amifostine (WR2721) may also act to inactivate drug, but preferentially in normal tissues.
	May show enhanced efficacy—and worsened toxicity—with a range of other cytotoxic agents.
Toxicity:	Renal insufficiency with cation wasting
	Nausea and vomiting
	Peripheral neuropathy
	Auditory impairment
	Myelosuppression (thrombocytopenia > WBC > RBC)
	Visual impairment (rare)
	Hypersensitivity (rare)
	Seizures (rare)
Precautions:	Use with caution in the presence of other nephrotoxic drugs (aminoglycosides, etc.).
	Monitor blood electrolytes and cations.
	Maintain high urine flow during cisplatin administration.
	Aggressive premedication with antiemetics is recommended.
	Caution should be used if the 24-h creatinine clearance is <60 mL/min. Consideration should be given to using alternative agents in this setting, although cisplatin can be safely administered if extensive precautions are used.

RBC, red blood cell count; $t_{1/2}$, half-life; WBC, white blood cell count.

years, and specific citations of their work are included in previous reviews.[1,2,130–133a] Oxaliplatin is the third platinum analog with accepted clinical utility, and its clinical pharmacology is summarized in Table 15-6. It has not been studied as extensively as its two predecessors. Whereas the cellular pharmacology of compounds of carrier ligand specificity was pioneered by Chaney and colleagues,[19–22] the clinical development of oxaliplatin has been championed primarily by Cvitkovic and his group.[134–136]

Oxaliplatin appears to have activity in ovarian cancer[135] and is particularly active in colorectal cancer when used in combination with 5-fluorouracil and leucovorin.[134,136–143] Limited studies have examined oxaliplatin's clinical pharmacology,[136,144,145] and reports have begun to appear that suggest unusual toxicities for this agent, which may be rare in occurrence.[146,147]

In treatment of ovarian cancer, oxaliplatin was combined with cisplatin in a program of 2-hour infusions for both drugs at doses of 130 mg per m² and 100 mg per m², respectively, on day 1.[135] This regimen was repeated every 3 weeks. In this phase II study of heavily pretreated patients, responses were seen in cisplatin-sensitive and cisplatin-resistant patients, and the response rate was 23% in the cisplatin-resistant group.

In colon cancer, oxaliplatin is usually given in combination with 5-fluorouracil and leucovorin, with the oxaliplatin given as a 6-hour infusion. In a study involving 151 colorectal cancer patients whose tumors were consid-

TABLE 15-5. KEY FEATURES OF CARBOPLATIN

Dosage:	Generally dosed by AUC, in mg/m² × min. Usual dosing range is 4–6 mg/m² × min.
	Calvert formula is generally used for calculating the AUC. A measured creatinine clearance is recommended. Calvert formula is: AUC (carboplatin) = dose/(creatinine clearance + 25).
	The older dosing method is: 1 mg cisplatin = 4 mg carboplatin. This approach is not recommended. AUC dosing is associated with greater patient safety, particularly with respect to myelosuppression.
Mechanism of action:	Covalent binding to DNA.
Metabolism:	Conversion to a DNA-reactive species occurs more quickly in cells than in i.v. solutions, which suggests the activity of esterases in cleavage of the dicarboxylate side group.
Pharmacokinetics:	After i.v. bolus, $t_{1/2\alpha}$ = 12–24 min; $t_{1/2\beta}$ = 1.3–1.7 h; $t_{1/2\gamma}$ = 22–40 h.
Elimination:	Approximately 90% is excreted in the urine in 24 h.
Drug interactions:	See cisplatin.
Toxicity:	Myelosuppression is more prominent than with cisplatin.
	Nausea and vomiting may occur but are much less prominent than with cisplatin.
	Nephrotoxicity can occur, particularly at higher dosages and in patients with prior renal dysfunction.
Precautions:	AUC dosing very important in the setting of preexistent renal dysfunction.

AUC, area under the concentration × time curve; $t_{1/2}$, half-life.

ered initially to be unresectable because of large liver metastases, this three-drug regimen was administered, followed by attempted surgical resection in patients showing response to chemotherapy.[137] In the 77 patients who went to surgery, median survival was 48 months. In separate phase III studies of the use of the oxaliplatin, 5-fluorouracil, and leucovorin combination as first-line therapy in metastatic colorectal carcinoma, objective response rates were statistically significantly higher for the three-drug combination, than for 5-fluorouracil and leucovorin only.[138] In one study the difference was a 59% objective response rate versus 23%, and in the other the

TABLE 15-6. KEY FEATURES OF OXALIPLATIN

Dosage:	80–100 mg/m² q2wk; or 100–135 mg/m² q3wk.
	Given as a 2-, 4-, or 6-h infusion; 6-h infusions are used most commonly.
	Administer in a 5% dextrose i.v. solution.
Mechanism of action:	DNA damage. May have unique properties based on unique carrier ligand.
	1,2-diaminocyclohexane carrier ligand is the nonleaving group.
	The leaving group ester linkages are similar to those of carboplatin.
Metabolism:	Not fully characterized. Drug accumulates in red blood cells of humans and rats but does not accumulate in plasma (cisplatin accumulates in plasma with repeated dosing).
Pharmacokinetics:	With a 4-h infusion:
	Free platinum levels decrease in a triphasic fashion
	Terminal $t_{1/2}$ = 27.3 h
	Volume of distribution = 349 L
	Total clearance = 222 mL/min; renal clearance = 121 mL/min
Elimination:	Renal elimination is important. Characterization in humans is not complete.
Drug interactions:	Most effective in gastrointestinal malignancies, given in combination with fluorouracil analogs.
	Synergizes with antimetabolites; additional studies warranted.
Toxicity:	When given with 5-fluorouracil, major toxicities include:
	Myelosuppression (neutropenia primarily)
	Diarrhea ± stomatitis
	Peripheral neuropathy (sensory much greater than motor)
	Nausea and vomiting—mild to moderate
	Rare toxicities: anaphylaxis, hemolytic anemia
Precautions:	Similar to those for cisplatin and carboplatin.

$t_{1/2}$, half-life.

difference was a 50.7% response rate versus 22.3%.[138] Infusion of 5-fluorouracil has usually been chronomodulated in these studies.

The major points of comparison for cisplatin, carboplatin, and oxaliplatin are listed in Tables 15-4, 15-5, and 15-6. Similarities and differences are seen in the respective clinical profiles of these three agents in terms of toxicity and efficacy. Because much more is known about cisplatin and carboplatin, the clinical summary below is based on the large literature regarding the clinical pharmacology of these two agents. How much of this pertains to oxaliplatin is not yet clear.

The stabilities of cisplatin and carboplatin in intravenous solutions have been studied by a number of groups. Solutions examined have included 0.9% NaCl, 5% dextrose, 5% dextrose and 0.9% NaCl, 5% dextrose and 0.45% NaCl, and 5% dextrose and 0.225% NaCl. In solutions that contain 0.9% NaCl, cisplatin is stable for up to 6 hours (more than 90% of original drug can be recovered). Lower NaCl concentrations are associated with greater rates of drug loss. A solution of 0.9% NaCl should be used for intravenous administration as well as intraperitoneal administration of cisplatin. Bicarbonate-containing solutions should be avoided because they are very reactive with cisplatin. Use of glass containers and plastic bags is acceptable. In contrast, carboplatin stability may be decreased in the presence of NaCl. Intravenous solutions that do not contain NaCl may be more appropriate for carboplatin administration.

No consensus exists on how long the intravenous infusion of cisplatin or carboplatin must be. In the Medicine Branch of the National Cancer Institute, each drug may be infused over an approximately 60-minute period. Other institutions commonly use longer (up to 4 hours) or shorter (15 to 30 minutes) infusion times, and no apparent differences in drug effect have been observed. Of note, continuous intravenous infusion of cisplatin (over a period of 24 hours or longer) has been studied and is associated with lessened toxicity and lessened efficacy.

Cisplatin and carboplatin dosing have been reasonably standardized over the past few years. For cisplatin, older dosing regimens ranged from daily times 5 (usually 20 mg per m^2 per dose) to a single intravenous infusion, with multiple variations in between. In most malignancies in which it is useful, the current standard dosing regimen for cisplatin is 50 to 75 mg per m^2 per dose, repeated every 3 to 4 weeks, alone or in combination with other agents. For cisplatin used alone, reports have been published of cisplatin regimens of 100 mg per m^2 per dose, but these reports show a high rate of drug-related toxicity.[148] For carboplatin, the standard dosing is based on AUC and generally ranges from 4 to 6 min × mg per m^2 with occasional use of an AUC of 7.5. For bone marrow transplantation regimens, carboplatin doses up to 18 min × mg per m^2 have been used.

Cisplatin and carboplatin have substantial differences in toxicity profile but similarities are also present. Cisplatin is much more emetogenic and more neurotoxic. However, carboplatin is not devoid of these properties. Vigorous premedication with antiemetics (usually H_3-receptor antagonists) is a must for cisplatin use, and premedication is advised for carboplatin. Neurotoxicity is a major side effect of cisplatin and can be ameliorated somewhat by the use of amifostine. Neurotoxicity is not common with carboplatin at standard doses, but does occur. Manifestations of cisplatin neurotoxicity may include peripheral neuropathy, auditory impairment, visual disturbances, and, less commonly, cortical blindness, seizures, papilledema, and retrobulbar neuritis. Auditory impairment may be subtle. For example, some patients complain of the loss of the ability to focus on one single conversation in a restaurant—one may lose the ability to filter out extraneous auditory input. Both agents tend to cause preferentially more thrombocytopenia in their respective myelosuppression profiles, but cisplatin shows this effect much less than carboplatin.

Kidney damage is more common with cisplatin but can occur with carboplatin as well.[149] Therefore, vigorous intravenous hydration is particularly important when cisplatin is given but is also important when carboplatin is used. Intravenous hydration and mannitol administration are useful for the preemptive management of platinum-related renal toxicity, but the routine use of furosemide is not recommended. Furosemide may increase urine flow, but it reduces total-body water, which may increase systemic drug levels and have a detrimental effect on cisplatin handling within the kidney.

Milligram dose reductions for carboplatin can be readily performed by delivering the total dose based on AUC. If this is done, AUC should be based on a calculated creatinine clearance. Patients who have received cisplatin or carboplatin in the past may have a "disconnect" between the serum creatinine value and true renal function.[150] Patients with a normal serum creatinine may have a markedly reduced measured creatinine clearance, particularly if they have received large cumulative doses of platinum agents in the past.

Cation loss in the urine is a common component of cisplatin-related renal toxicity and may include Mg^{2+}, Ca^{2+}, and other heavy metals. The treating physician should consider regular replacement of these cations, along with administration of over-the-counter supplements that include zinc, selenium, etc. The use of B vitamins to lessen cisplatin-related neurotoxicity has been advocated within the lay ovarian cancer community. One study has addressed this in a prospective randomized trial. Ovarian cancer patients were randomized to receive or not to receive 100 mg per day of vitamin B_6 while receiving multiagent platinum-based chemotherapy.[151] The group that received B_6 experienced less neurotoxicity and tolerated the treatment regimen quite well. However, the median disease-free survival rate and percentage of complete responders in the group given B$_6$ were statistically significantly lower than in the group that did not receive B$_6$.[151]

Reported clinical phase III and pharmacologic studies comparing cisplatin with carboplatin were given a detailed critical assessment to determine the relative roles of cisplatin and carboplatin in the treatment of malignant disease.[133a] This review assessed all reported data between 1966 and 1997. The authors concluded that carboplatin and cisplatin were of clinically equivalent efficacy in treating suboptimally debulked ovarian cancer, non–small cell lung cancer, and extensive-stage small cell lung cancer. Cisplatin was determined to be clinically superior in treating germ cell, head and neck, and esophageal cancers. Further studies were felt to be needed with regard to optimally debulked ovarian cancer, limited-stage small cell lung cancer, and bladder, cervical, and endometrial cancers. Oxaliplatin is particularly active in colorectal cancer.[137,138]

Regional administration of cisplatin and of carboplatin was once a popular approach, but it may be of less utility than was initially anticipated. Regional routes of administration include intraperitoneal, intraarterial, intravesicular, and intrapleural. Although some continue to be strong proponents of these types of treatment, these routes should be used only in very selected cases. Although pharmacologic advantage can be easily demonstrated with any of these regional approaches, clear advantages in clinical efficacy have been demonstrated in very few studies. A consensus has developed that intraperitoneal therapy may have a clinical advantage for ovarian cancer patients with small-volume disease (less than 0.3 cm), confined to the abdomen and pelvis.[152] Whether the clinical advantage of intraperitoneal administration is sufficiently great, however, that intraperitoneal therapy can be routinely recommended over other nonintraperitoneal treatment approaches in this patient subset is not clear. Intraperitoneal therapy may often be complicated by peritonitis, adhesions, catheter clotting, and other problems.

Selected clinical circumstances may be found in which installation of cisplatin or carboplatin into a third-space cavity may be a reasonable palliative treatment approach. Sixty-eight patients with malignant pleural effusions from non–small cell lung cancer were studied to determine the pharmacokinetics of cisplatin and etoposide in the pleural space.[153] All pleural fluid was drained from the space, then cisplatin (80 mg per m^2) and etoposide (80 mg per m^2) were instilled. The β half-life of free platinum in the intrapleural space was 10.51 hours, which suggests intense local exposure to drug. The authors felt this approach to be associated with definite clinical benefit in this patient subset. A similar approach was taken by Ratto et al., but involved only 10 patients.[154] In this study, cisplatin (100 mg per m^2) was infused into the pleural space with or without hyperthermia, in patients with malignant mesothelioma. Ratto and colleagues confirmed an apparent pharmacologic advantage for intracavitary over systemic treatment in this setting as well.

Continuous hyperthermic peritoneal perfusion was developed by Alexander's group to assess the efficacy of a number of cytotoxic agents, as well as biologic agents, in the setting of uniform delivery of heat to the peritoneal surface.[155–157] The authors have reported a pharmacologic advantage for this approach for a number of agents, including cisplatin, carboplatin, tumor necrosis factor, and other agents. One study in rats suggested that, when cisplatin is administered by local injection, the coadministration of epinephrine results in four- to tenfold higher intratumoral levels of platinum, as measured by atomic absorption spectrometry.[158] A possible effect of epinephrine on intratumoral blood flow parameters was not assessed.

Amifostine (WR2721) is a sulfhydryl prodrug in clinical use as a protector against platinum-induced neural and renal toxicity.[159–163] Two studies have investigated the effect of amifostine on cisplatin pharmacology and DNA damage in tumor-bearing nude mice.[164,165] Cisplatin-DNA adduct levels were measured in normal and in tumor tissues. When cisplatin was given in combination with amifostine, cisplatin exposure resulted in lower cisplatin-DNA adduct levels in normal tissues than when cisplatin was used alone.[164] The DNA adduct levels measured in tumor tissues were not significantly different in mice treated with cisplatin alone and in those given the combination. Ueda and colleagues performed a similar study, also in mice, using sodium malate as the quenching agent.[166] They observed preferential distribution of radioactive carbon–labeled sodium malate into normal tissues, which was associated with a 55% decrease in measurable tissue platinum levels in those tissues. Platinum levels in tumor tissues were no different in groups of mice treated with cisplatin alone and with cisplatin plus sodium malate.

When pharmacokinetic studies are conducted, the handling of the blood sample can be of critical importance. This factor was studied by Johnsson et al.[167] They observed that whole blood can be stored for up to 2 hours at 4°C or 20°C without change in the free fraction of platinum. After that time, gradual reduction in free fraction is seen. If blood is stored at –70°C before ethanol deproteinization or ultrafiltration, the free fraction of platinum remains unchanged for approximately 3 months. If stored at –20°C, the free fraction may decrease substantially by 14 days.

The cellular and tissue handling of platinum compounds may be similar to that of other heavy metals, and uptake appears to be via adenosine triphosphate–dependent ion pumps. Tokuchi et al. studied 21 patients with small cell lung cancer to determine whether thallium-201 uptake may be predictive of disease response in this cancer.[168] They observed a direct relationship between the retention index of thallium-201 and response to platinum-based chemotherapy. Further, ouabain, an inhibitor of the Na,K–adenosine triphosphatase pump, reduced cellular sensitivity to cisplatin in their *in vitro* system and inhibited intracellular uptake of thallium. Consistent with the above, Potdevin and colleagues showed that cisplatin and carboplatin induced a dose-dependent inhibition of Na$^+$-coupled glucose uptake in renal brush border membrane vesicles,[169] which again demonstrated the biologic association between platinum actions at the cell membrane and Na$^+$ transport.

Kroning et al. studied cells from different parts of the nephron and showed differences in cellular transport characteristics for cisplatin, different sensitivities to cisplatin, and different levels of expression of the antiapoptotic protein Bcl-X(L) in proximal and distal renal tubule cell lines.[170] The greater sensitivity to cisplatin in distal tubule cells was independent of the differences in cellular uptake of drug.

The chinchilla appears to be a good model for cisplatin-related hearing loss in humans.[1,2] Studies in chinchilla show that carboplatin may also have defined patterns of damage to both inner hair cells and outer hair cells in the cochlea. Carboplatin produces a selective loss of inner hair cells and causes a one-third reduction in the amplitude of conduction within the eight nerve fiber at moderately large doses.[171] At these doses (50 mg per kg intraperitoneally in the chinchilla), no changes were seen in conduction threshold nor in latency of conduction.[171] The dose of carboplatin needed to destroy outer hair cells is approximately four to five times greater than that needed to damage inner hair cells.[172]

The list of agents that may enhance cisplatin or carboplatin cytotoxicity in certain cell systems is increasing and includes 1-α,25-dihydroxyvitamin D$_3$,[173] hyperthermia,[174] interleukin 1α,[175] amphotericin B,[176] digitonin,[177] amifostine,[178] aphidicolin,[179] tamoxifen,[180,181] interferon-β,[182] and x-irradiation,[183] as well as a long list of cytotoxic anticancer agents.[1,2]

Like other DNA-reactive drugs, platinum compounds are known to be carcinogenic and teratogenic in animals[184] and are associated with secondary leukemias in humans.[185,186] This topic is considered in greater detail in Chapter 5 and effects on fertility are discussed in Chapter 4. The platinum compounds are also potent radiosensitizers, an important property in their clinical use; this topic is covered in Chapter 25 (Radiation Modifiers).

SUMMARY

Platinum compounds continue to be the mainstay of curative and palliative therapy for a wide range of adult malignancies. The recent success of oxaliplatin therapy strongly suggests that carrier ligand effects can contribute in a major way to the successful clinical development of agents in this class. Toxicities continue to be an important barrier to clinical success, and methods to ameliorate those toxicities should be actively investigated.

REFERENCES

1. Reed E, Kohn KW. Cisplatin and platinum analogs. In: Chabner BA, Collins J, eds. *Cancer chemotherapy—principles and practice*. Philadelphia: JB Lippincott, 1990:465–490.
2. Reed E, Dabholkar M, Chabner BA. Platinum analogues. In: Chabner BA, Longo DL, eds. *Cancer chemotherapy*, 2nd ed. Philadelphia: Lippincott–Raven Publishers, 1996:357–378.
3. Rosenberg B, Van Camp L, Krigas T. Inhibition of cell division in Escherichia coli by electrolysis products from a platinum electrode. *Nature* 1965;205:698.
4. Rosenberg B, Van Camp L, Trosko JE, et al. Platinum compounds: a new class of potent antitumor agents. *Nature* 1969;222:385–386.
5. Gelasco A, Lippard SJ. NMR solution structure of a DNA dodecamer duplex containing a cis-diammineplatinum(II) d(GpG) intrastrand cross-link, the major adduct of the anticancer drug cisplatin. *Biochemistry* 1998;37:9230–9239.
6. De Laat WL, Jaspers NG, Hoeijmakers JH. Molecular mechanism of nucleotide excision repair. *Genes Dev* 1999;13:768–785.
7. Reed E. Platinum-DNA adduct, nucleotide excision repair, and platinum based anti-cancer chemotherapy. *Cancer Treat Rev* 1998;24:331–344.
8. Sancar A. Mechanisms of DNA excision repair. *Science* 1994;266:1954–1956.
9. Gong JG, Costanzo A, Yang HQ, et al. The tyrosine kinase c-Abl regulates p73 in apoptotic response to cisplatin-induced DNA damage. *Nature* 1999;399:806–809.
10. Jamieson ER, Jacobson MP, Barnes CM, et al. Structural and kinetic studies of a cisplatin-modified DNA icosamer binding to HMG1 domain B. *J Biol Chem* 1999;274:12346–12354.
11. Ohndorf U-M, Rould MA, He Q, et al. Basis for recognition of cisplatin-modified DNA by high-mobility-group proteins. *Nature* 1999;399:708–712.
12. Scheeff ED, Briggs JM, Howell SB. Molecular modeling of the intrastrand guanine-guanine DNA adducts produced by cisplatin and oxaliplatin. *Mol Pharmacol* 1999;56:633–643.
13. Kobayashi S, Furukawa M, Dohi C, et al. Topology effect for DNA structure of cisplatin: topological transformation of cisplatin-closed circular DNA adducts by DNA topoisomerase I. *Chem Pharm Bull (Tokyo)* 1999;47:783–790.
14. Fichtinger-Schepman AM, van Dijk-Knijnenburg HC, van der Velde-Visser SD, et al. Cisplatin and carboplatin DNA adducts: is PT-AG the cytotoxic lesion? *Carcinogenesis* 1995;16:2447–2453.
15. Blommaert FA, van Dijk-Knijnenburg HC, Dijt FJ, et al. Formation of DNA adducts by the anticancer drug carboplatin: different nucleotide sequence preferences in vitro and in cells. *Biochemistry* 1995;34:8474–8480.
16. Blommaert FA, Floot BG, van Dijk-Knijnenburg HC, et al. The formation and repair of cisplatin-DNA adducts in wild-type and cisplatin resistant L1210 cells: comparison of immunocytochemical determination with detection in isolated DNA. *Chem Biol Interact* 1998;108:209–225.
17. Saris CP, van de Vaart PJ, Rietbrock RC, et al. In vitro formation of DNA adducts by cisplatin, lobaplatin and oxaliplatin in calf thymus DNA in solution and in cultured human cells. *Carcinogenesis* 1996;17:2763–2769.

18. Micetich KC, Barnes D, Erickson LC. A comparative study of the cytotoxicity and DNA-damaging effects of *cis*-diammino(1,1cyclobutanedicarboxylato)-platinum(II) and *cis*-diamminedichloroplatinum(II) on L1210 cells. *Cancer Res* 1985;45:4043–4047.

19. Vaisman A, Lim SE, Patrick SM, et al. Effect of DNA polymerases and high mobility group protein 1 on the carrier ligand specificity for translesion synthesis past platinum-DNA adducts. *Biochemistry* 1999;38:11026–11039.

20. Luo FR, Wyrick SD, Chaney SG. Cytotoxicity, cellular uptake, and cellular biotransformations of oxaliplatin in human colon carcinoma cells. *Oncol Res* 1998;10:595–603.

21. Reardon JT, Vaisman A, Chaney SG, et al. Efficient nucleotide excision repair of cisplatin, oxaliplatin, and bis-aceto-ammine-dichloro-cyclohexylamine-platinum(IV) (JM216) platinum intrastrand DNA diadducts. *Cancer Res* 1999;59:3968–3971.

22. Luo FR, Wyrick SD, Chaney SG. Comparative neurotoxicity of oxaliplatin, ormaplatin and their biotransformation products using a rat dorsal root ganglia in vitro explant culture model. *Cancer Chemother Pharmacol* 1999;44:29–38.

23. Poirier MC, Lippard SJ, Zwelling LA, et al. Antibodies elicited against cis-diamminedichloroplatinum(II)-DNA adducts formed in vivo and in vitro. *Proc Natl Acad Sci U S A* 1982; 79:6443–6447.

24. Reed E, Ozols RF, Tarone R, et al. Platinum-DNA adducts in leukocyte DNA correlate with disease response in ovarian cancer patients receiving platinum-based chemotherapy. *Proc Natl Acad Sci U S A* 1987;84:5024–5028.

25. Eastman A. Reevaluation of interaction of cis-dichloro(ethylene-diammine)platinum(II) with DNA. *Biochemistry* 1986;25:3912–3915.

26. Fichtinger-Schepman AM, van der Veer JL, den Hartog JH, et al. Adducts of the antitumor drug *cis*-diamminedichloroplatinum(II), with DNA: formation, identification and quantitation. *Biochemistry* 1985;24:707–713.

27. Reed E, Sauerhoff S, Poirier MC. Quantitation of platinum-DNA binding in human tissues following therapeutic levels of drug exposure—a novel use of graphite furnace spectrometry. *Atomic Spectrosc* 1988;9:93–95.

28. Parker RJ, Eastman A, Bostick-Bruton F, et al. Acquired cisplatin resistance in human ovarian cancer cells is associated with enhanced repair of cisplatin-DNA lesions and reduced drug accumulation. *J Clin Invest* 1991;87:772–777.

29. Yamada M, Tomida A, Yun J, et al. Cellular sensitization to cisplatin and carboplatin with decreased removal of platinum-DNA adduct by glucose-regulated stress. *Cancer Chemother Pharmacol* 1999;44:59–64.

30. Lee KB, Parker RJ, Bohr VA, et al. Cisplatin sensitivity/resistance in UV-repair deficient Chinese hamster ovary cells of complementation groups 1 and 3. *Carcinogenesis* 1993;14:2177–2180.

31. Benchekroun MN, Parker R, Dabholkar M, et al. Effects of interleukin-1-alpha on DNA repair on human ovarian carcinoma (NIH:OVARCAR-3) cells: implications in the mechanism of sensitization of *cis*-diamminedichloroplatinum (II). *Mol Pharmacol* 1995;47:1255–1260.

32. Masumoto N, Nakano S, Fujishima H, et al. V-src induces cisplatin resistance by increasing the repair of cisplatin-DNA interstrand cross-links in human gallbladder adenocarcinoma cells. *Int J Cancer* 1999;80:731–737.

33. Eastman A, Schulte N, Sheibani N, et al. Mechanisms of resistance to platinum drugs. In: Nicolini M, ed. *Platinum and other metal coordination compounds in cancer chemotherapy*. Boston: Martinus Nijhoff, 1988:178–196.

34. Dabholkar M, Parker R, Reed E. Determinants of cisplatin sensitivity in non-malignant, non-drug-selected human T cell lines. *Mutation Res* 1992;274(1):45–56.

35. Li Q, Bostick-Bruton F, Reed E. Modulation of ERCC-1 mRNA expression by pharmacological agents in human ovarian cancer cells. *Biochem Pharmacol* 1999;57:347–353.

36. Li Q, Bostick-Bruton F, Reed E. Effect of interleukin-1 and tumor necrosis factor on cisplatin-induced ERCC1 mRNA expression in a human ovarian carcinoma cell line. *Anticancer Res* 1998;18:2283–2287.

37. Benchekroun MN, Parker R, Reed E, et al. Inhibition of DNA repair and sensitization of cisplatin in human ovarian cancer cells by interleukin-1-alpha. *Biochem Biophys Res Commun* 1993;195:294–300.

38. Buell JR, Reed E, Lee KB, et al. Synergistic effect and molecular basis of tumor necrosis factor and cisplatin cytotoxicity and hyperthermia against gastric cancer cells. *Ann Surg Oncol* 1997;4:141–148.

39. Li Q, Gardner K, Zhang L, et al. Cisplatin induction of ERCC1 mRNA expression in A2780/CP70 human ovarian cancer cells. *J Biol Chem* 1998;273:23419–23425.

40. Li Q, Tsang B, Gardner K, et al. Phorbol ester exposure activates an AP-1 associated increase in ERCC1 mRNA expression in human ovarian cancer cells. *Cell Mol Life Sci* 1999;55:456–466.

41. Li Q, Ding L, Yu JJ, et al. Cisplatin and phorbol ester independently induce ERCC1 protein in human ovarian tumor cells. *Int J Oncol* 1998;13:987–992.

42. Burger H, Nooter K, Boersma AW, et al. Distinct p53-independent apoptotic cell death signalling pathways in testicular germ cell tumor cell lines. *Int J Cancer* 1999;81:620–628.

43. Singh RA, Sodhi A. Expression and activation of RAS and mitogen-activated protein kinases in macrophages treated in vitro with cisplatin: regulation by kinases, phosphatases, and Ca^{2+}/calmodulin. *Immunol Cell Biol* 1999;77:356–363.

44. Reed E, Yuspa SH, Zwelling LA, et al. Quantitation of cisplatin-DNA intrastrand adducts in testicular and ovarian cancer patients receiving cisplatin chemotherapy. *J Clin Invest* 1986;77:545–550.

45. Reed E, Ostchega Y, Steinberg S, et al. An evaluation of platinum-DNA adduct levels relative to known prognostic variables in a cohort of ovarian cancer patients. *Cancer Res* 1990;50:2256–2260.

46. Fichtinger-Schepman AMJ, van Oosterom AT, Lohman PHM, et al. *Cis*-diamminedichloroplatinum(II)-induced adducts in peripheral leukocytes from seven cancer patients: quantitative immunochemical detection of the adduct induction and removal after a single dose of *cis*-diamminedichloroplatinum(II). *Cancer Res* 1987;47:3000–3004.

47. Fichtinger-Schepman AMJ, van Oosterom AT, Lohman PHM, et al. Interindividual human variation in cisplatinum sensitivity, predictable in an in vitro assay? *Mutat Res* 1987;190:59–62.

48. Perera FB, Tang D, Reed E, et al. Multiple biologic markers in testicular cancer patients treated with platinum-based chemotherapy. *Cancer Res* 1992;52:3558–3565.

49. Motzer RJ, Reed E, Tang D, et al. Platinum-DNA adducts assayed in leukocytes of germ cell tumor patients measured by atomic absorbance spectroscopy and enzyme linked immunosorbent assay. *Cancer* 1994;73:2843–2852.

50. Tang DL, Motzer RJ, Warburton D, et al. A study of five biological markers and clinical response in 36 testicular cancer patients treated with platinum-based chemotherapy. *Proc Am Assoc Cancer Res* 1992;33:263(abst 1577).

51. Parker RJ, Gill I, Tarone R, et al. Platinum-DNA damage in leukocyte DNA of patients receiving carboplatin and cisplatin chemotherapy, measured by atomic absorption spectrometry. *Carcinogenesis* 1991;12:1253–1258.

52. Reed E, Parker RJ, Gill I, et al. Platinum-DNA adduct in leukocyte DNA of a cohort of 49 patients with 24 different types of malignancy. *Cancer Res* 1993;53:3694–3699.

53. Schellens JH, Ma J, Planting AS, et al. Relationship between the exposure to cisplatin, DNA-adduct formation in leucocytes and tumor response in patients with solid tumors. *Br J Cancer* 1996;73:1569–1575.

54. Peng B, Tilby MJ, English MW, et al. Platinum-DNA adduct formation in leucocytes of children in relation to pharmacokinetics after cisplatin and carboplatin therapy. *Br J Cancer* 1997;76:1466–1473.

55. Tonda ME, Murry DJ, Rodman JH. Formation of platinum-DNA adducts in pediatric patients receiving carboplatin. *Pharmacotherapy* 1996;16:631–637.

56. Bonetti A, Apostoli P, Zaninelli M, et al. Inductively coupled plasma mass spectroscopy quantitation of platinum-DNA adducts in peripheral blood leukocytes of patients receiving cisplatin or carboplatin based chemotherapy. *Clinical Cancer Res* 1996;2:1829–1835.

57. Reed E. Alkylating agents and platinum—is clinical resistance simply a "tumor cell" phenomenon? *Curr Opin Oncol* 1991;3(6):1055–1059.

58. Welters MJP, Braakhuis BJM, Jacobs-Bergmans AJ, et al. The potential of platinum-DNA adduct determination in ex vivo treated tumor fragments for the prediction of sensitivity to cisplatin chemotherapy. *Ann Oncol* 1999;10:97–103.

59. Olivero OA, Semino C, Kassim A, et al. Preferential binding of cisplatin to mitochondrial DNA of Chinese hamster ovary cells. *Mutat Res* 1995;346:221–230.

60. Olivero OA, Chang PK, Lopez-Larraza DM, et al. Preferential formation and decreased removal of cisplatin-DNA adducts in Chinese hamster ovary cell mitochondrial DNA as compared to nuclear DNA. *Mutat Res* 1997;391:79–86.

61. Giurgiovich AJ, Diwan BA, Olivero OA, et al. Elevated mitochondrial cisplatin-DNA adduct levels in rat tissues after transplacental cisplatin exposure. *Carcinogenesis* 1997;18:93–96.

62. Giurgiovich AJ, Diwan BA, Lee KB, et al. Cisplatin-DNA adduct formation in maternal and fetal rat tissues after transplacental cisplatin exposure. *Carcinogenesis* 1996;17:1665–1669.

63. Giurgiovich AJ, Anderson LM, Dones AB, et al. Transplacental cisplatin exposure induces persistent fetal mitochondrial and genomic DNA damage in patas monkeys. *Reprod Toxicol* 1997;11:95–100.

64. Shamkhani H, Anderson LM, Henderson CE, et al. DNA adducts in human and patas monkey maternal and fetal tissues induced by platinum drug chemotherapy. *Reprod Toxicol* 1994;8:207–216.

65. Koc O, McFee M, Reed E, et al. Detection of platinum-DNA adducts in cord blood lymphocytes following *in utero* platinum exposure. *Eur J Cancer* 1994;30A:716–717.

66. Johnsson A, Strand C, Los G. Expression of GADD153 in tumor cells and stromal cells from xenografted tumors in nude mice treated with cisplatin: correlation with cisplatin-DNA adducts. *Cancer Chemother Pharmacol* 1999;43:348–352.

67. Bohr VA, Reed E, Zhen W. Gene specific damage and repair of platinum adducts and crosslinks. In: Howell SB, ed. *Platinum and other metal coordination compounds in cancer chemotherapy*. New York: Plenum Press, 1992:231–240.

68. Zhen W, Link CJ Jr, O'Connor PM, et al. Increased gene-specific repair of cisplatin interstrand crosslinks in cisplatin resistant human ovarian cancer cells. *Mol Cell Biol* 1992;12:3689–3698.

69. Jones JC, Zhen W, Reed E, et al. Preferential DNA repair of cisplatinum lesions in active genes in CHO cells. *J Biol Chem* 1991;266:7101–7107.

70. Parker RJ, Vionnet JA, Bostick-Bruton F, et al. Ormaplatin sensitivity/resistance in human ovarian cancer cells made resistant to cisplatin. *Cancer Res* 1993;53:242–247.

71. Lee KB, Parker RJ, Reed E. Effect of cadmium on human ovarian cancer cells with acquired cisplatin resistance. *Cancer Lett* 1995;88:57–66.

72. Fink D, Aebi S, Howell SB. The role of DNA mismatch repair in drug resistance. *Clinical Cancer Res* 1998;4:1–6.

73. Aebi S, Fink D, Gordon R, et al. Resistance to cytotoxic drugs in DNA mismatch repair-deficient cells. *Clinical Cancer Res* 1997;3:1763–1767.

74. Drummond JT, Anthoney A, Brown R, et al. Cisplatin and Adriamycin resistance are associated with MutL-alpha and mismatch repair deficiency in an ovarian tumor cell line. *J Biol Chem* 1996;271:19645–19648.

75. Modrich P. Mismatch repair, genetic stability and cancer. *Science* 1994;266:1959–1960.

76. Drummond JT, Li G-M, Longley MJ, et al. Isolation of an hMSH2-p160 heterodimer that restores DNA mismatch repair to tumor cells. *Science* 1995;268:1909–1912.

77. Karran P. Appropriate partners make good matches. *Science* 1995;268:1857–1858.

78. Nehma A, Baskaran R, Nebel S, et al. Induction of JNK and c-Abl signalling by cisplatin and oxaliplatin in mismatch repair-proficient and -deficient cells. *Br J Cancer* 1999;79:1104–1110.

79. Vaisman A, Varchenko M, Umar A, et al. The role of hMLH1, hMSH3, and hMSH6 defects in cisplatin and oxaliplatin resistance: correlation with replicative bypass of platinum-DNA adducts. *Cancer Res* 1998;58:3579–3585.

80. Raymond E, Faivre S, Woynarowski JM, et al. Oxaliplatin: mechanism of action and antineoplastic activity. *Semin Oncol* 1998;25:4–12.

81. Dabholkar M, Bostick-Bruton F, Weber C, et al. ERCC1 and ERCC2 expression in malignant tissues from ovarian cancer patients. *J Natl Cancer Inst* 1992;84:1512–1517.

82. Masumoto N, Nakano S, Fujishima H, et al. V Induces cisplatin resistance by increasing the repair of cisplatin-DNA interstrand cross-links in human gallbladder adenocarcinoma cells. *Int J Cancer* 1999;80:731–737.

83. Husain A, He G, Venkatraman ES, et al. BRCA1 up-regulation is associated with repair mediated resistance to cis-diamminedichloroplatinum(II). *Cancer Res* 1998;58:1120–1123.

84. Dabholkar M, Vionnet JA, Bostick-Bruton F, et al. mRNA Levels of XPAC and ERCC1 in ovarian tumor tissue correlates with response to platinum containing chemotherapy. *J Clin Invest* 1994;94:703–708.

85. Metzger R, Leichman CG, Danenberg KD, et al. ERCC1 mRNA levels complement thymidylate synthase mRNA levels in predicting response and survival for gastric cancer patients receiving combination cisplatin and fluorouracil chemotherapy. *J Clin Oncol* 1998;16:309–316.

86. Reed E. The chemotherapy of ovarian cancer. *PPO Updates* 1996;10(7):1–12.

87. Reed E. Ovarian cancer: molecular abnormalities. In: Bertino JR, ed. *The encyclopedia of cancer.* San Diego: Academic Press, 1996:1192–1200.

88. Dabholkar MD, Berger MS, Vionnet JA, et al. Malignant and non-malignant brain tissues differ in their mRNA expression patterns for ERCC1 and ERCC2. *Cancer Res* 1995;55:1261–1266.

89. Dabholkar MD, Berger MS, Vionnet JA, et al. Comparative analyses of relative ERCC3 and ERCC6 mRNA levels in gliomas and adjacent non-neoplastic brain. *Mol Carcinog* 1996;17:1–7.

90. Li Q, Yu JJ, Mu C, et al. Association between the level of ERCC1 expression and the repair of cisplatin-induced DNA damage in human ovarian cancer cells. *Anticancer Res* 2000;20(2A):645–652.

91. Yu JJ, Mu C, Lee KB, et al. A nucleotide polymorphism in ERCC1 gene in human ovarian cancer cell lines and tumor tissues. *Mutat Res Genomics* 1997;382:13–20.

92. Yu JJ, Lee KB, Mu C, et al. Comparison of two human ovarian carcinoma cell lines (A2780/CP70 and MCAS) that are equally resistant to platinum, but differ at codon 118 of the ERCC1 gene. *Int J Oncol* 2000;6(3):555–560.

93. Yu JJ, Mu C, Dabholkar M, et al. Alternative splicing of ERCC1 and cisplatin-DNA adduct repair in human tumor cell lines. *Int J Mol Med* 1998;1:617–620.

94. Dabholkar M, Vionnet J, Parker RJ, et al. Expression of an alternatively spliced ERCC1 mRNA species is related to reduced DNA repair efficiency in human T lymphocytes. *Oncol Rep* 1995;2:209–214.

95. Yu JJ, Bicher A, Bostick-Bruton F, et al. Absence of evidence for allelic loss or allelic gain for ERCC1 and for XPD in human ovarian cancer cells and tissues. *Cancer Lett* 2000;151(2):127–132.

96. States JC, Reed E. Enhanced XPA mRNA levels in cisplatin-resistant human ovarian cancer are not associated with XPA mutations or gene amplification. *Cancer Lett* 1996; 108:233–237.

97. Jiang H, Yang LY. Cell cycle checkpoint abrogator UCN-01 inhibits DNA repair: association with attenuation of the interaction of XPA and ERCC1 nucleotide excision repair proteins. *Cancer Res* 1999;59:4529–4534.

98. Fink D, Nebel S, Norris PS, et al. Enrichment for DNA mismatch repair-deficient cells during treatment with cisplatin. *Int J Cancer* 1998;321:741–746.

99. Dedoussis GV, Mouzaki A, Theodoropoulou M, et al. Endogenous interleukin 6 conveys resistance to *cis*-diamminedichloroplatinum-mediated apoptosis of the K562 human leukemic cell line. *Exp Cell Res* 1999;249:269–278.

100. Ishioka S, van Haaften-Day C, Sagae S, et al. Interleukin-6

101. (IL-6) does not change the expression of Bcl-2 protein in the prevention of cisplatin induced apoptosis in ovarian cancer cell lines. *J Obstet Gynaecol Res* 1999;25:23–27.

101. Buell JF, Reed E, Lee KB, et al. Synergistic effect and possible mechanisms of tumor necrosis factor and cisplatin cytotoxicity under moderate hyperthermia against gastric cancer cells. *Ann Surg Oncol* 1997;4:141–148.

102. Stoika RS, Yakymovych MY, Yakymovych IA, et al. Cisplatin-resistant derivatives of murine L1210 leukemia cells are not susceptible to growth inhibiting and apoptosis inducing actions of transforming growth factor beta. *Anticancer Drugs* 1999;10:457–463.

103. Mizutani Y, We XX, Yoshida O, et al. Chemoimmunosensitization of the T24 human bladder cancer line to Fas-mediated cytotoxicity and apoptosis by cisplatin and 5-fluorouracil. *Oncol Rep* 1999;6:979–982.

104. Fulda S, Scaffidi C, Pietsch T, et al. Activation of the CD95 (APO-1/Fas) pathway in drug- and gamma-irradiation-induced apoptosis of brain tumor cells. *Cell Death Differ* 1998;5:884–893.

105. Razzaque MS, Koji T, Kumatori A, et al. Cisplatin-induced apoptosis in human proximal tubular epithelial cells is associated with the activation of the Fas/Fas ligand system. *Histochem Cell Biol* 1999;111:359–365.

106. Kruidering M, van de Water B, Zhan Y, et al. Cisplatin effects on F-actin and matrix proteins precede renal tubular cell detachment and apoptosis in vitro. *Cell Death Differ* 1998;5:601–614.

107. Sugimoto C, Fujieda S, Ski M, et al. Apoptosis-promoting gene (bax) transfer potentiates sensitivity of squamous cell carcinoma to cisplatin in vitro and in vivo. *Int J Cancer* 1999;82:860–867.

108. Arriola EL, Rodriguez-Lopez AM, Hickman JA, et al. Bcl-2 overexpression results in reciprocal downregulation of Bcl-X(L) and sensitizes human testicular germ cell tumors to chemotherapy-induced apoptosis. *Oncogene* 1999;18(7):1457–1464.

109. Henkels KM, Turchi JJ. Cisplatin-induced apoptosis proceeds by caspase-3-dependent and -independent pathways in cisplatin-resistant and -sensitive human ovarian cancer cell lines. *Cancer Res* 1999;59:3077–3083.

110. Liu W, Staecker H, Stupak H, et al. Caspase inhibitors prevent cisplatin-induced apoptosis of auditory sensory cells. *Neuroreport* 1998;9:2609–2614.

111. Ando T, Umezawa A, Suzuki A, et al. EAT/mcl-1, a member of the bcl-2 related genes, confers resistance to apoptosis induced by cis-diammine dichloroplatinum (II) via a p53 independent pathway. *Jpn J Cancer Res* 1998;89:1326–1333.

112. Stoika RS, Yakymovych M, Yakymovych I, et al. Cisplatin-resistant derivatives of murine L1210 leukemia cells are not susceptible to growth-inhibiting and apoptosis-inducing actions of transforming growth factor beta1. *Anticancer Drugs* 1999;10:457–463.

113. Siemer S, Ornskov D, Guerra B, et al. Determination of mRNA and protein levels of p53, MDM2, and protein kinase CK2 subunits in F9 cells after treatment with the apoptosis-inducing drugs cisplatin and carboplatin. *Int J Biochem Cell Biol* 1999;31:661–670.

114. Piovesan B, Pennell N, Berinstein NL. Human lymphoblastoid cell lines expressing mutant p53 exhibit decreased sen-

sitivity to cisplatin induced cytotoxicity. *Oncogene* 1998; 17:2339–2350.

115. Han JY, Chung YJ, Park SW, et al. The relationship between cisplatin-induced apoptosis and p53, bcl-2 and bax expression in human lung cancer cells. *Korean J Intern Med* 1999;14:42–52.

116. Jones NA, Turner J, McIlwrath AJ, et al. Cisplatin- and paclitaxel-induced apoptosis of ovarian carcinoma cells and the relationship between bax and bak up-regulation and the functional status of p53. *Mol Pharmacol* 1998;53:819–826.

117. Raaphorst GP, Mao J, Yang H, et al. Evaluation of apoptosis in four human tumour cell lines with differing sensitivities to cisplatin. *Anticancer Res* 1998;18:2945–2951.

118. Segal-Bendirdjian E, Mannone L, Jacquemin-Sablon A. Alteration in p53 pathway and defect in apoptosis contribute independently to cisplatin-resistance. *Cell Death Differ* 1998;5:390–400.

119. Von Knethen A, Lotero A, Brune B. Etoposide and cisplatin induced apoptosis in activated RAW 264.7 macrophages is attenuated by cAMP-induced gene expression. *Oncogene* 1998;17:387–394.

120. Basu A, Akkaraju GR. Regulation of caspase activation and cis-diamminedichloroplatinum(II) induced cell death by protein kinase C. *Biochemistry* 1999;38:4245–4251.

121. Ruan S, Okcu MF, Pong RC, et al. Attenuation of WAF1/ Cip1 expression by an antisense adenovirus expression vector sensitizes glioblastoma cells to apoptosis induced by chemotherapeutic agents 1,3-bis(2-chloroethyl)-1-nitrosourea and cisplatin. *Clin Cancer Res* 1999;5:197–202.

122. Ishibashi T, Lippard SJ. Telomere loss in cells treated with cisplatin. *Proc Natl Acad Sci U S A* 1998;95:4219–4223.

123. Kondo Y, Kondo S, Tanaka Y, et al. Inhibition of telomerase increases the susceptibility of human malignant glioblastoma cells to cisplatin-induced apoptosis. *Oncogene* 1998; 16:2243–2248.

124. Takeda M, Kobayashi M, Shirato I, et al. Involvement of macromolecule synthesis, endonuclease activation and c-fos expression in cisplatin-induced apoptosis of mouse proximal tubule cells. *Toxicol Lett* 1998;94:83–92.

125. Timmer-Bosscha H, de Vries EG, Meijer C, et al. Differential effects of all-trans-retinoic acid, docosahexaenoic acid, and hexadecylphosphocholine on cisplatin-induced cytotoxicity and apoptosis in a cisplatin-sensitive and resistant human embryonal carcinoma cell line. *Cancer Chemother Pharmacol* 1998;41:469–476.

126. Suzuki H, Tomida A, Tsuruo T. A novel mutant from apoptosis-resistant colon cancer HT-29 cells showing hyperapoptotic response to hypoxia, low glucose and cisplatin. *Jpn J Cancer Res* 1998;89:1169–1178.

127. Takahashi M, Yamamoto Y, Hatori S, et al. Enhancement of CDDP cytotoxicity by caffeine is characterized by apoptotic cell death. *Oncol Rep* 1998;5:53–56.

128. Liang BC, Ullyatt E. Increased sensitivity to *cis*-diamminedichloroplatinum induced apoptosis with mitochondrial DNA depletion. *Cell Death Differ* 1998;5:694–701.

129. Schoenlein PV, Barrett JT, Welter D. The degradation profile of extrachromosomal circular DNA during cisplatin-induced apoptosis is consistent with preferential cleavage at matrix attachment regions. *Chromosoma* 1999;108:121–131.

130. Judson PL, Watson JM, Gehrig PA, et al. Cisplatin inhibits

131. Reed E. Anticancer drugs. Sect 7, Platinum analogs. In: DeVita VT, Hellman S, Rosenberg SA, eds. *Cancer principles and practice of oncology.* Philadelphia: JB Lippincott, 1993:390–400.

132. Reed E. Cisplatin. *Cancer Chemother Biol Response Modif* 1999;18:145–152.

133. Dabholkar M, Reed E. Cisplatin. In: Pinedo HM, Chabner BA, Longo DL, eds. *Cancer chemotherapy and biological response modifiers annual,* vol 16. Amsterdam: Elsevier Science, 1996:88–110.

133a. Go RS, Adjei AA. Review of the comparative pharmacokinetics and clinical activity of cisplatin and carboplatin. *J Clin Oncol* 1999;17:409–422.

134. Cvitkovic E, Bekradda M. Oxaliplatin: a new therapeutic option in colorectal cancer. *Semin Oncol* 1999;26:647–662.

135. Soulie P, Bensmaine A, Garrino C, et al. Oxaliplatin/cisplatin (LOHP/CDDP) combination in heavily pretreated ovarian cancer. *Eur J Cancer* 1997;33:1400–1406.

136. Gamelin E, Bouil AL, Boisdron-Celle M, et al. Cumulative pharmacokinetic study of oxaliplatin, administered every three weeks, combined with 5-fluorouracil in colorectal cancer patients. *Clin Cancer Res* 1997;3:891–899.

137. Giacchetti S, Itzhaki M, Gruia G, et al. Long term survival of patients with unresectable colorectal cancer liver metastases following infusional chemotherapy with 5-fluorouracil, leucovorin, oxaliplatin and surgery. *Ann Oncol* 1999;10:663–669.

138. Wiseman LR, Adkins JC, Plosker GL, et al. Oxaliplatin: a review of its use in the management of metastatic colorectal cancer. *Drugs Aging* 1999;14:459–475.

139. Levi F, Zidani R, Brienza S, et al. A multicenter evaluation of intensified, ambulatory, chronomodulated chemotherapy with oxaliplatin, 5-fluorouracil, and leucovorin as initial treatment of patients with metastatic colorectal carcinoma. International Organization for Cancer Chronotherapy. *Cancer* 1999;85:2532–2540.

140. Andre T, Bensmaine MA, Louvet C, et al. Multicenter phase II study of bimonthly high dose leucovorin, fluorouracil infusion, and oxaliplatin for metastatic colorectal cancer resistant to the same leucovorin and fluorouracil regimen. *J Clin Oncol* 1999;17:3560–3568.

141. Giacchetti S, Perpoint B, Zidani R, et al. Phase III multicenter randomized trial of oxaliplatin added to chronomodulated fluorouracil-leucovorin as first line treatment of metastatic colorectal cancer. *J Clin Oncol* 2000;18:136–147.

142. Brienza S, Bensmaine MA, Soulie P, et al. Oxaliplatin added to 5-fluorouracil-based therapy (5-FU +/- FA) in the treatment of 5-FU-pretreated patients with advanced colorectal carcinoma (ACRC): results from the European compassionate-use program. *Ann Oncol* 1999;10:1311–1316.

143. Becouarn Y, Ychou M, Ducreux M, et al. Phase II trial of oxaliplatin as first line chemotherapy in metastatic colorectal cancer patients. Digestive Group of French Federation of Cancer Centers. *J Clin Oncol* 1998;16:2739–2744.

144. Extra JM, Marty M, Brienza S, et al. Pharmacokinetics and safety profile of oxaliplatin. *Semin Oncol* 1998;25(2[Suppl 5]):13–22.

145. Kern W, Braess J, Bottger B, et al. Oxaliplatin pharmacokinetics during a four-hour infusion. *Clin Cancer Res* 1999;5:761–765.

146. Larzilliere I, Brandissou S, Breton P, et al. Anaphylactic reaction to oxaliplatin: a case report. *Am J Gastroenterol* 1999;94:3387–3388.

147. Desrame J, Broustet H, Darodes de Tailly P, et al. Oxaliplatin induced hemolytic anemia. *Lancet* 1999;354:1179–1180.

148. Muggia FM, Braly PS, Brady MF, et al. Phase III randomized study of cisplatin versus paclitaxel versus cisplatin and paclitaxel in patients with suboptimal stage III or IV ovarian cancer: a Gynecologic Oncology Group study. *J Clin Oncol* 2000;18:106–115.

149. Reed E, Jacob J. Carboplatin and renal dysfunction. *Ann Intern Med* 1989;110:409.

150. Reed E, Jacob J, Brawley O. Measures of renal function in cisplatin-related chronic renal disease. *J Natl Med Assoc* 1991;83:522–526.

151. Wiernik PH, Yeap B, Vogl SE, et al. Hexamethylmelamine and low or moderate dose cisplatin with or without pyridoxine for treatment of advanced ovarian carcinoma; a study of the Eastern Cooperative Oncology Group. *Cancer Invest* 1992;10:1–9.

152. Markman M. Intraperitoneal therapy of ovarian cancer. *Semin Oncol* 1998;25:356–360.

153. Tohda Y, Iwanaga T, Takada M, et al. Intrapleural administration of cisplatin and etoposide to treat malignant pleural effusions in patients with non-small cell lung cancer. *Chemotherapy* 1999;45:197–204.

154. Ratto GB, Civalleri D, Esposito M, et al. Pleural space perfusion with cisplatin in the multimodality treatment of malignant mesothelioma: a feasibility and pharmacokinetic study. *J Thorac Cardiovasc Surg* 1999;117:759–765.

155. Ma GY, Bartlett DL, Reed E, et al. Continuous hyperthermic peritoneal perfusion with cisplatin for the treatment of peritoneal mesothelioma. *Cancer J Sci Am* 1997;3:174–179.

156. Bartlett DL, Buell JF, Fraker DL, et al. Phase I trial of continuous hyperthermic peritoneal perfusion with TNF and cisplatin in the treatment of peritoneal carcinomatosis. *Cancer* 1998;83:1251–1261.

157. Cho H-K, Lush RM, Bartlett DL, et al. Pharmacokinetics of cisplatin administered by continuous hyperthermic peritoneal perfusion (CHPP) to patients with peritoneal carcinomatosis. *J Clin Pharmacol* 1999;39:394–401.

158. Dvillard C, Benoit L, Moretto P, et al. Epinephrine enhances penetration and anti-cancer activity of local cisplatin or rat sub-cutaneous and peritoneal tumors. *Int J Cancer* 1999;81:779–784.

159. Capizzi RL. Amifostine reduces the incidence of cumulative nephrotoxicity from cisplatin: laboratory and clinical aspects. *Semin Oncol* 1999;26(2[Suppl 7]):72–81.

160. Mabro M, Faivre S, Raymond E. A risk-benefit assessment of amifostine in cytoprotection. *Drug Safety* 1999;21:367–387.

161. Hensley ML, Schuchter LM, Lindley C, et al. American Society of Clinical Oncology clinical practice guidelines for the use of chemotherapy and radiotherapy protectants. *J Clin Oncol* 1999;17:3333–3355.

162. Van der Jijgh WJ, Korst AE. Amifostine (Ethyol): pharmacokinetic and pharmacodynamic effects in vivo. *Eur J Cancer* 1996;32A[Suppl 4]:S26–S30.

163. Hartmann JT, Kollmannsberger C, Kanz L, et al. Platinum organ toxicity and possible prevention in patients with testicular cancer. *Int J Cancer* 1999;83:866–869.

164. Korst AEC, Boven E, Van Der Sterre MLT, et al. Pharmacokinetics of cisplatin with and without amifostine in tumour-bearing nude mice. *Eur J Cancer* 1998;34:412–416.

165. Fichtner I, Lemm M, Becker M, et al. Effects of amifostine (WR-2721, ethyol) on tumor growth and pharmacology of cytotoxic drugs in human xeno transplanted neuroblastomas. *Anticancer Drugs* 1997;8:174–181.

166. Ueda H, Sugiyama K, Tashiro S, et al. Mechanism of the protective effect of sodium malate on cisplatin-induced toxicity in mice. *Biol Pharm Bull* 1998;21:121–128.

167. Johnsson A, Bjork H, Schuetz A, et al. Sample handling for determination of free platinum in blood after cisplatin exposure. *Cancer Chemother Pharmacol* 1998;41:248–251.

168. Tokuchi Y, Isobe H, Takekawa H, et al. Predicting chemotherapeutic response to small-cell lung cancer of platinum compounds by thallium-201 single-photon emission computerized tomography. *Br J Cancer* 1998;77:1363–1368.

169. Potdevin S, Courjault-Gautier F, Ripoche P, et al. Similar effects of *cis*-diamminedichloroplatinum(II) and *cis*-diammine-1,1-cyclobutanedicarboxylatoplatinum(II) on sodium-coupled glucose uptake in renal brush-border membrane vesicles. *Arch Toxicol* 1998;72(10):663–670.

170. Kroning R, Katz D, Lichtenstein AK, et al. Differential effects of cisplatin in proximal and distal renal tubule epithelial cell line. *Br J Cancer* 1999;79(2):293–299.

171. Burkard R, Trautwein P, Salvi R. The effects of click level, click rate, and level of background masking noise on the inferior caliculus potential (ICP) in the normal and carboplatin-treated chinchilla. *J Acoust Soc Am* 1997;102(6):3620–3627.

172. Hofstetter P, Ding D, Salvi R. Magnitude and pattern of inner and outer hair cell loss in chinchilla as a function of carboplatin dose. *Audiology* 1997;36(6):301–311.

173. Moffatt KA, Johannes WU, Miller GJ. 1Alpha,25dihydroxy-vitamin D3 and platinum drugs act synergistically to inhibit the growth of prostate cancer cell lines. *Clin Cancer Res* 1999;5(3):695–703.

174. Murray TG, Cicciarelli N, McCabe CM, et al. In vitro efficacy of carboplatin and hyperthermia in a murine retinoblastoma cell line. *Invest Ophthalmol Vis Sci* 1997;38(12):2516–2522.

175. Yu WD, Chang MJ, Trump DL, et al. Interleukin-1alpha synergistic in vivo enhancement of cyclophosphamide- and carboplatin-mediated antitumor activity. *Cancer Immunol Immunother* 1997;44(6):316–322.

176. Poulain L, Sichel F, Crouet H, et al. Potentiation of cisplatin and carboplatin cytotoxicity by amphotericin B in different human ovarian carcinoma and malignant peritoneal mesothelioma cells. *Cancer Chemother Pharmacol* 1997;40(5):385–390.

177. Lindner PG, Heath D, Howell SB, et al. Digitonin enhances the efficacy of carboplatin in liver tumor after intra-arterial administration. *Cancer Chemother Pharmacol* 1997;40(5):444–448.

178. Korst AE, Boven E, van der Sterre ML, et al. Influence of single and multiple doses of amifostine on the efficacy and the pharmacokinetics of carboplatin in mice. *Br J Cancer* 1997;75(10):1439–1446.

179. Sargent JM, Elgie AW, Williamson CJ, et al. Aphidicolin

markedly increases the platinum sensitivity of cells from primary ovarian tumors. *Br J Cancer* 1996;74(11):1730–1733.

180. Mastronardi L, Farah JO, Puzzilli F, et al. Tamoxifen modulation of carboplatin cytotoxicity in a human U-138 glioma cell line. *Clin Neurol Neurosurg* 1998;100(2):89–93.

181. Mohammed MQ, Photiou A, Shah P, et al. Activity of platinum drugs against melanoma cell lines: is it modulated in vitro in the presence of tamoxifen? *Anticancer Res* 1995;15(4):1319–1326.

182. Hubner B, Eckert K, Garbe C, et al. Synergistic interactions between interferon beta and carboplatin on SK-MEL 28 human melanoma cell growth inhibition in vitro. *J Cancer Res Clin Oncol* 1995;121(2):84–88.

183. Yang LX, Douple EB, O'Hara JA, et al. Production of DNA double-strand breaks by interactions between carboplatin and radiation: a potential mechanism for radiopotentiation. *Radiat Res* 1995;143(3):309–315.

184. Hennings H, Shores RA, Poirier MC, et al. Enhanced malignant conversion of benign mouse skin tumors by cisplatin. *J Natl Cancer Inst* 1990;82:836–840.

185. Reed E, Evans MK. Acute leukemia following cisplatin-based chemotherapy in a patient with ovarian cancer. *J Natl Cancer Inst* 1990;82:431–432.

186. Reed E. Leukemia following cisplatin therapy—response [Letter]. *J Natl Cancer Inst* 1990;82:795.

187. Lim MC, Martin RB. The nature of *cis* amine Pd(II) and antitumor *cis* amine Pt(II) complexes in aqueous solutions. *Inorg Nucl Chem* 1976;38:1911–1914.

16

BLEOMYCIN

JOHN S. LAZO
BRUCE A. CHABNER

In a search for new antimicrobial and antineoplastic agents, Umezawa and colleagues[1] isolated a number of small glycopeptides from culture broths of the fungus *Streptomyces verticillus*. The most active antitumor agent found in these broths was, in fact, a mixture of peptides now known in clinical usage as *bleomycin*, a drug that has important activity against Hodgkin's disease, non-Hodgkin's lymphoma, testicular cancer, malignant pleural effusions, cancers of the cervix and penis, and head and neck cancer. Bleomycin used in combination with vinblastine sulfate and *cis*-diamminedichloroplatinum has produced a high rate of cure in patients with germinal neoplasms of the testis, and in fact, deletion of bleomycin from this regimen compromises therapeutic efficacy.[2] The drug has attracted great interest because of its unique biochemical action and its virtual lack of toxicity for normal hematopoietic tissue. Its primary pharmacologic and pharmacokinetic features are shown in Table 16-1.

STRUCTURE AND MECHANISM OF ACTION

The bleomycins are a family of peptides with a molecular weight of approximately 1,500 (Fig. 16-1). All contain a unique structural component, bleomycinic acid, and differ only in their terminal alkylamine group. Because of their unusual structure, catalytic properties, and important antitumor activity, the bleomycin antibiotics have been the subject of intensive basic and clinical investigation. Bleomycin A_2, the predominant peptide, has been prepared by total chemical synthesis, as has a series of analogs.[3–5] More than 100 additional bleomycin-like antitumor antibiotics have been isolated or synthesized, but none has yet emerged as superior in clinical activity.

The clinical mixture of bleomycin peptides is formulated as a sulfate salt, and its potency is measured in units (U) of antimicrobial activity. Each unit contains between 1.2 and 1.7 mg of polypeptide protein. The powdered clinical mixture is stable for at least 1 year at room temperature and for 4 weeks after reconstitution in aqueous solution if stored at 4°C.

The multiple glycopeptides found in the clinical preparation of bleomycin have been separated and purified by paper, conventional column, and high-performance liquid chromatography (HPLC).[6,7] The predominant active component, comprising approximately 70% of the commercial preparation, is the A_2 peptide shown in Figure 16-1. The remaining bleomycins differ in the nature of the terminal amine. The native compound isolated from *S. verticillus* is a blue-colored Cu(II) coordinated complex. Bleomycin complexes *in vitro* 1:1 with several endogenous and exogenous metals, including Cu(I), C(II), Fe(II), Fe(III), Co(II), Co(III), Zn(II), Mn(II), and Mn(III). The Co(III) complexes are essentially inert with respect to biologic activity and the exchangeability of their bound metal and thus have been candidates for tumor localization, especially with cobalt 57 (^{57}Co). Unfortunately, the half-life of ^{57}Co is 270 days rather than the desired several hours or days common for clinically useful diagnostic agents. Among endogenous metals, bleomycin has the highest affinity for Cu(II); bleomycin has a fourfold greater affinity for reduced Cu(I) than for Fe(II).[8] In initial clinical trials with Cu(II)·bleomycin, patients experienced profound phlebitis, and the white apobleomycin was soon adopted for clinical use. Nevertheless, after systemic administration, bleomycin appears to speciate rapidly with Cu(II) removed from plasma proteins.[9] The Cu(II)·bleomycin complex is internalized through a poorly described endocytotic system that may include discrete plasma membrane proteins of 250 kd.[10,11] Most investigators believe that the Cu·bleomycin is a prodrug and that cleavage-competent bleomycin is Fe(II)-speciated. Considerable chemical evidence regarding DNA damage produced by Fe(II)·bleomycin exists to support this hypothesis.[8] The primary model was first outlined by Umezawa's group[9] and is schematically represented in Figure 16-2. Cu(II) associated with intracellular Cu(II)·bleomycin is reduced, possibly by intracellular cysteine-rich proteins, to Cu(I), which is released, and the apobleomycin quickly complexes with Fe(II).[12] Nuclear translocation of the

TABLE 16-1. KEY FEATURES OF BLEOMYCIN PHARMACOLOGY

Mechanism of action:	Oxidative cleavage of DNA initiated by hydrogen abstraction
Metabolism:	Activated by microsomal reduction
	Degraded by hydrolase found in multiple tissues
Pharmacokinetics:	$t_{1/2\alpha}$: 24 min; $t_{1/2\beta}$: 2–4 h
Elimination:	Renal: 45–70% in first 24 h
Drug interactions:	None clearly established at a biochemical level.
	Oxygen enhances pulmonary toxicity.
	cis-Platinum induces renal failure and increases risk of pulmonary toxicity.
Toxicity:	Pulmonary interstitial infiltrates and fibrosis
	Desquamation, especially of fingers, elbows
	Raynaud's phenomenon
	Hypersensitivity reactions (fever, anaphylaxis, eosinophilic pulmonary infiltrates)
Precautions:	Pulmonary toxicity increased in patients with:
	Underlying pulmonary disease
	Age greater than 70 yr
	Renal insufficiency
	Prior chest irradiation
	O_2 during surgery
	Reduce dose if creatinine clearance <60 mL/min

$t_{1/2}$, half-life.

Fe(II)·bleomycin complex proceeds with subsequent chromatin damage. The metal coordination chemistry of bleomycin has been the subject of considerable attention, and primarily on the basis of studies using electron paramagnetic resonance (EPR),[13] crystallography,[14] and Fe(II) surrogate metals such as Cu(II), a square-pyramidal complex, as indicated in Figure 16-1, is most favored.[8,9] Six distinct moieties are required for this metal coordination complex, and the N-1 of the pyrimidine, the N of the imidazole, and the secondary amine are undisputed participants.[8] Debate still exists about the arrangement of the remaining ligands, and this presumably will be resolved with further structural analyses. Although many aspects of the cellular scheme found in Figure 16-2 are biologically and chemically appealing, several questions remain unanswered, including the identity of the sulfhydril-rich reductant for Cu(II), the recipient and fate of the Cu(I), the intracellular source of Fe(II), the mode by which the metal-bound bleomycin translocates the plasma membrane, and the nucleus. Therefore, others[15,16] have developed a rival hypothesis to explain the antitumor activity and fate of bleomycin. Even though Cu(II)·bleomycin is not highly cytotoxic,[17,18] persuasive arguments for a potential functional role of Cu(I)·bleomycin in the biologic actions of this antineoplastic agent have been presented.[8,16] Thus the widely embraced concept that Fe(II)-complexed bleomycin

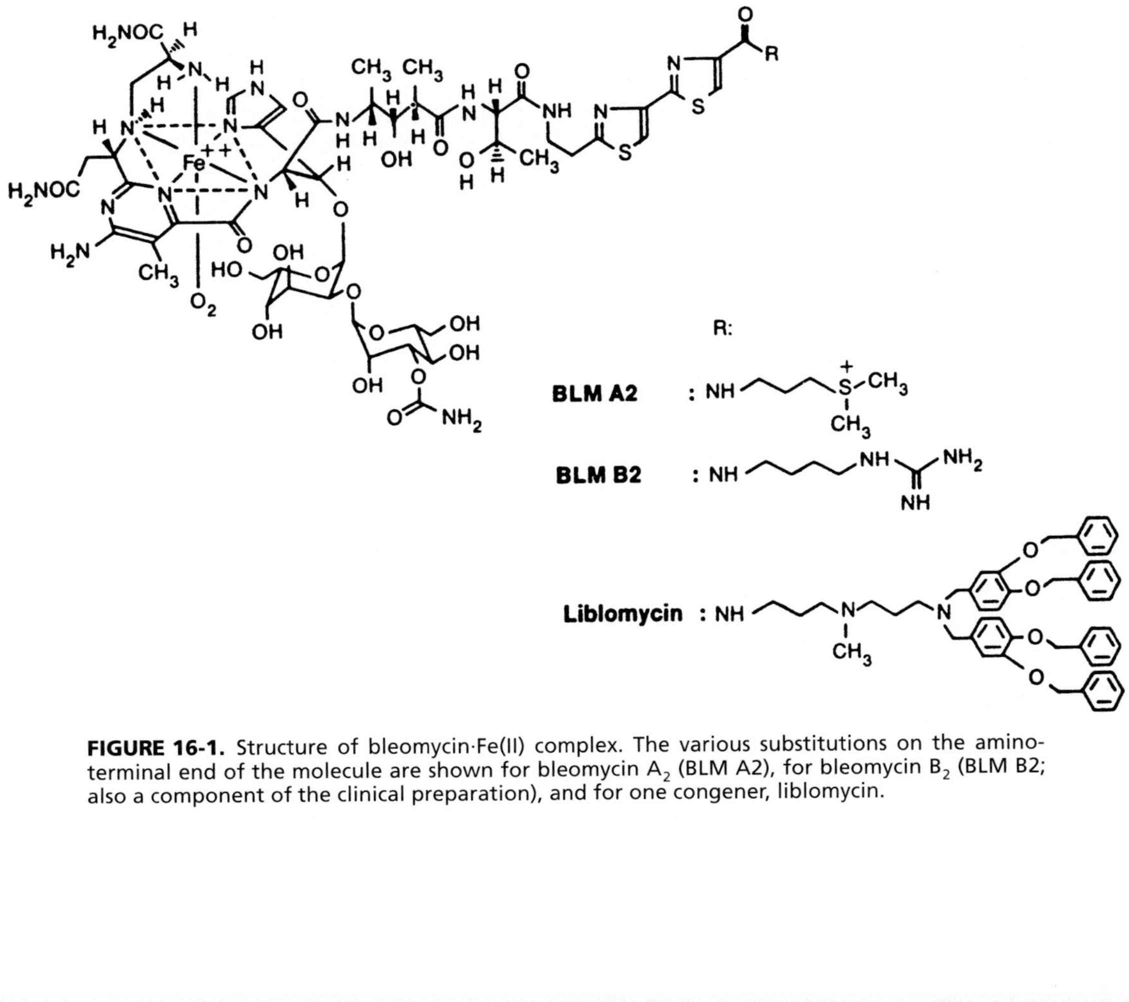

FIGURE 16-1. Structure of bleomycin·Fe(II) complex. The various substitutions on the amino-terminal end of the molecule are shown for bleomycin A_2 (BLM A2), for bleomycin B_2 (BLM B2; also a component of the clinical preparation), and for one congener, liblomycin.

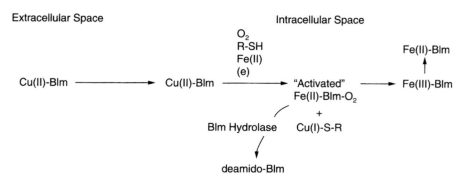

FIGURE 16-2. Schematic representation of bleomycin (Blm) transformation as it moves from the extracellular to the intracellular space. The Cu(II)·Blm complex in the extracellular space is converted to a cytotoxic Fe(II)·Blm·O$_2$ complex in the cell. Inactivation of Blm by Blm hydrolase is also shown.

is the only biologically relevant species may require revision in the future.

MECHANISM OF ACTION

Early mechanistic studies identified a concentration-dependent loss in DNA integrity with loss of cell viability in the absence of marked decreases in either RNA or protein composition. After considering several potential therapeutic targets, including RNA and DNA polymerases and nucleases and DNA ligases, most investigators accepted direct DNA damage as the most attractive candidate for the cytotoxicity and, consequently, the antitumor activity of bleomycin.[8,9] Single- and double-strand DNA damage is readily observed in cultured cells and isolated DNA incubated with bleomycin in solution. This breakage is reflected in the chromosomal gaps, deletions, and fragments seen in cytogenetic studies of whole cells. Nevertheless, as with many antineoplastic agents, reports exist dissociating DNA damage from cell death.[19] Although this may simply reflect rapid DNA repair, other biochemical targets continue to be examined. For example, bleomycin mediates lipid peroxidation, which certainly has been associated with the lethality of other small redox-active molecules. The fact that bleomycin can participate in the oxidative degradation of the three major classes of RNA—transfer RNA, messenger RNA, and ribosomal RNA—in a substrate-specific and ternary-structure–dependent manner is also interesting.[20] The cleavage of RNA

occurs by H abstraction from the oligoribonucleotides[21] in the presence of DNA, and at pharmacologically relevant bleomycin concentrations.[22] This has rekindled interest in the possibility that RNA damage may have therapeutic relevance. Nevertheless, the primacy of DNA damage as the major mechanism of bleomycin cytotoxicity remains.[23]

CHEMISTRY OF BLEOMYCIN-MEDIATED DNA CLEAVAGE

The mechanism by which Fe(II)·bleomycin cleaves DNA has been examined using viral, bacterial, mammalian, and synthetic DNAs. Bleomycin is unlike most DNA-damaging agents because it attacks neither the nucleic bases nor the phosphate linkage. In this multistep process, initially an "activated" Fe(II)·bleomycin·O$_2$ complex is formed that is kinetically competent to cleave DNA. The binding of dioxygen to Fe(II)·bleomycin proceeds most rapidly in the presence of DNA, which stabilizes the complex.[24] The proposed sequence of events responsible for the production of an activated bleomycin has been deduced from *in vitro* studies and is briefly outlined in Figure 16-3. Fe(II) combines with apobleomycin, producing an EPR-silent, high-spin Fe(II)·bleomycin complex. With dioxygen, this is rapidly converted to a ternary Fe(II)·bleomycin·O$_2$ species, which can be trapped with isocyanide, CO, or NO or can be activated by a $1e^-$ reduction. The e^- can be supplied by a second Fe(II)·bleomycin·O$_2$ molecule,[10,18] by H$_2$O$_2$,[10] by

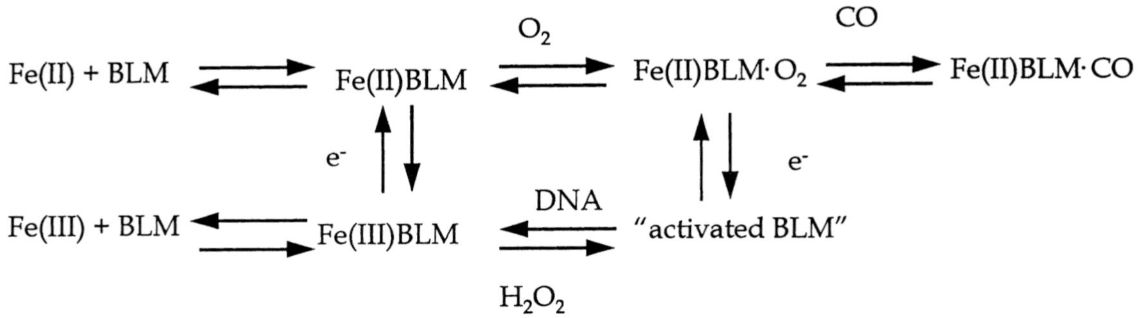

$$Fe(II) + BLM \rightleftharpoons Fe(II)BLM \xrightarrow{O_2} Fe(II)BLM \cdot O_2 \xleftarrow{CO} Fe(II)BLM \cdot CO$$

$$Fe(III) + BLM \leftarrow Fe(III)BLM \xleftarrow{DNA} \text{"activated BLM"}$$

$$H_2O_2$$

FIGURE 16-3. Model for the activation of cleavage-competent bleomycin (BLM).

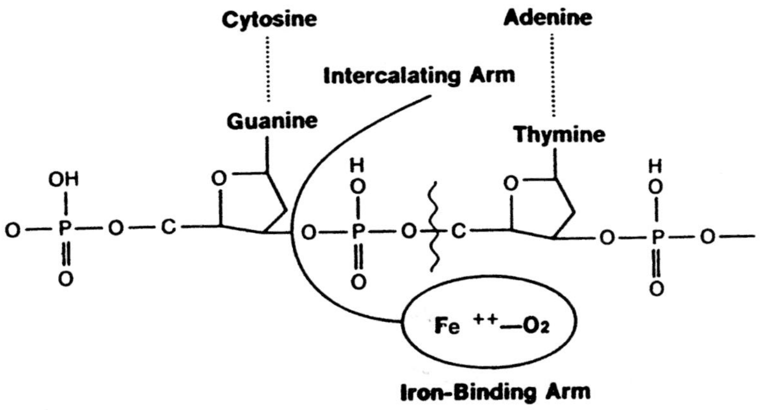

FIGURE 16-4. Intercalation of the bithiazole groups between DNA base pairs, at least one of which contains the GpT of GpC sequence. Also shown is the apposition of the Fe(II)-binding portion of bleomycin to the deoxyribose group, which is cleaved via hydrogen abstraction at the C-4' of the deoxyribose.

microsomal enzymes and nicotinamide-adenine dinucleotide phosphate (reduced form) (NADPH) organic reductant,[25] or by nuclei and nicotinamide-adenine dinucleotide (reduced form) (NADH).[26] Mossbauer studies[25] suggest that the activated bleomycin has a half-life of a few minutes at 0°C, so it is likely to be reasonably long-lived even at 37°C. In the absence of DNA, the activated species will self-destruct. The association constant of Fe(II)·bleomycin for duplex DNA, however, is approximately 10^5 per M.[27] Thus the second step in the DNA cleavage process readily occurs. The interaction of bleomycin with DNA shows nucleotide sequence selectivity[28] and most likely occurs at the minor groove where the primary DNA target, H4', is located.[23] At saturating concentrations of bleomycin, one molecule of drug associates with four or five base pairs of DNA. The binding between bleomycin and DNA appears to be through electrostatic interactions and partial intercalation (insertion between base pairs) of the amino-terminal tripeptide of bleomycin (called the *S tripeptide*)[29,30] (Fig. 16-4). The bithiazole of the S tripeptide bonds to guanine groups in the favored sequence of GpC and GpT.[28,29] The terminal dimethylsulfonium of bleomycin A_2 also participates in DNA binding, as indicated by broadening of the proton magnetic resonance of the sulfonium moiety in the presence of DNA.[28] Almost certainly this also occurs with the highly positively charged terminal amines of the other bleomycins. Evidence for intercalation comes from observations using gel electrophoresis, centrifugal sedimentation, linear dichroism methods, viscometric techniques, and nuclear magnetic resonance spectroscopy. Generally in these studies either bleomycin or its S tripeptide is mixed with DNA, and linear DNA is lengthened or supercoiled circular DNA is relaxed. Both these effects are indicative of unwinding of the double-helical structure as the result of intercalation[30] and can be produced by bithiazole alone or by bleomycin and bleomycin analogs. Fe(II)·bleomycin exhibits a strong preference for the B-form of DNA rather than for the Z-form,[31] consistent with interactions with the minor groove of DNA.

The third step in the action of bleomycin is the generation of single- and double-strand DNA breaks. During the DNA cleavage process, Fe(II)·bleomycin functions catalytically as a ferrous oxidase[32] with the oxidation of Fe(II) to Fe(III); regeneration of the active Fe(II) requires endogenous reductants, including cytochrome P-450 reductase and NADPH,[33] an enzyme found in the nucleus and nuclear membrane. Under very controlled *in vitro* conditions, the short-lived oxygenated iron-bleomycin species[34] participates in almost four cleavage events per bleomycin molecule. Others have estimated the reduction of dioxygen by bleomycin, as monitored by measurement of oxygen consumption, with a maximum velocity of 27 mol oxygen consumed per minute per mole of bleomycin.[32] The K_m (binding affinity) of this reaction for Fe(II) is 1.8 mmol per L.[32]

The mechanism of DNA cleavage has been defined by the DNA fragments produced after incubation of the substrate with activated bleomycin.[23,35–38] Incubation of DNA with bleomycin in an aerobic environment results in the scission of the C-3'—C-4' ribose bond via a Criegee-type rearrangement, which produces three types of product, including a 5'-oligonucleotide terminating at its 3' end with a phosphoroglycolic acid moiety, a 3'-oligonucleotide containing a 5'-phosphate, and a 3'-(thymin-9'-yl)propenal.[10,18] Exposure to Fe(II)·bleomycin produces the release of all four bases (thymine, cytosine, adenine, and guanine)[36] (Fig. 16-5, pathway A). Under anaerobic conditions, the free-base release is accompanied by production of an oxidatively damaged sugar in the intact DNA strand, which yields DNA cleavage only in basic conditions, namely, pH 12 (Fig. 16-5, pathway B). No base propenal is released. Which of these pathways predominates in intact cells is not known, although both free bases and base propenal adducts are detected in most cells. The base propenal compounds have intrinsic cytotoxicity and may contribute to the damage to cells.[39]

Bleomycin produces both single- and double-strand DNA breaks in a ratio of approximately 10:1. The unexpectedly high frequency of double-strand breaks has been addressed in elegant studies of the effect of bleomycin on hairpin-shaped oligonucleotides that have single-strand gaps corresponding to those produced by bleomycin.[40] The highly electronegative 3'-phosphoglycolate and 5'-phosphate groups remaining at

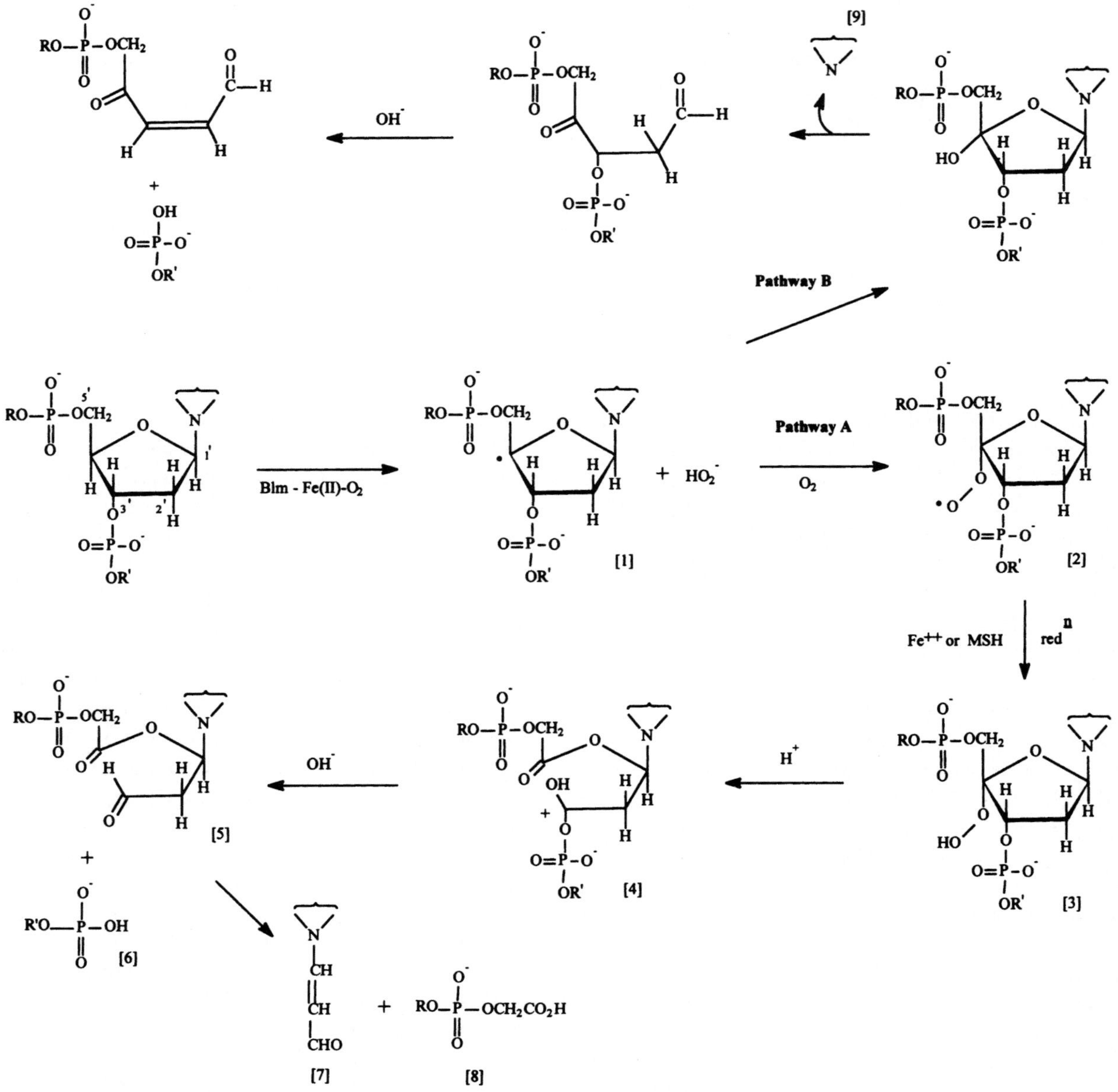

FIGURE 16-5. Scheme for the cleavage of the 3'—4' deoxyribose bond by the activated bleomycin·Fe(II)·O$_2$ complex. The activated drug complex initially abstracts a hydrogen radical from the 4' position to produce the unstable intermediate [1] that decomposes in the presence of oxygen (pathway A) to produce the free base propenal [7], leaving a 3'-phosphoglycolate ester [8] and a 5'-phosphate [6] at the free ends of the broken DNA strand. Under conditions of limited oxygen, a free base [9] is released, and DNA strand scission occurs only in the presence of alkali (pH 12).

the site of DNA single-strand cleavage may promote access of a second bleomycin molecule to the opposing strand and strongly promote the formation of a double-strand break.

Analysis of the products of DNA cleavage, using either viral or mammalian DNA, has consistently shown a preferential release of thymine or thymine-propenal, with lesser amounts of the other three bases or their propenal adducts.[23,41] The propensity for attack at thymine bases probably results from the previously mentioned preference for partial intercalation of bleomycin between base pairs in which at least one strand contains the sequence 5'-GpT-3'. The speci-

ficity for cleavage of DNA at a residue located at the 3' side of G seems to be absolute.[42] A schematic representation of the intercalation and cleavage processes as conceived by Grollman and Takeshita[43] is given in Figure 16-4 and summarizes the structural and sequence specificities discussed in this chapter.

CELLULAR PHARMACOLOGY

The cellular uptake of bleomycin is slow, and large concentration gradients are maintained between extracellular and intracellular spaces.[44] Autoradiographic studies with radioactive carbon–labeled bleomycin have demonstrated early accumulation of labeled material at the cell membrane of murine tumor cells, with gradual appearance of labeling at the nuclear membrane only after 4 hours of exposure.[45] The importance of the plasma membrane as a barrier for the highly cationic bleomycins, which also have a significant size, has been clearly documented by studies using electrical permeabilization techniques.[46] The cytotoxicity of bleomycin was greatly enhanced when an electric pulse was used to increase the total intracellular drug. Moreover, the mode of cell death seems related to the drug content; cells with only a few thousand bleomycin molecules arrest in the G_2-M phase of the cell cycle and become enlarged and polynucleated before dying.[46] In contrast, when cells are electroporated and several million bleomycin molecules are internalized, the morphologic appearance is apoptotic. A bleomycin-binding membrane protein has been identified with a molecular mass of 250 kd that has half-maximal saturation with a bleomycin concentration of 5 µmol per L.[13] This protein may be responsible for the internalization of bleomycin, but additional characterization is necessary to affirm its role in the cytotoxic action of bleomycin. Using a fluorescent mimic of bleomycin or agents that disrupt vacuoles, Mistry et al.[47] and Lazo et al.[10] concluded that the internalized bleomycin is sequestered in cytoplasmic organelles. The process by which the entrapped bleomycin is released from the vesicles is not known.

Once bleomycin is internalized, it either translocates to the nucleus to effect DNA damage or it can be degraded by bleomycin hydrolase, which has been characterized and cloned from several species.[48–51] This homomultimeric enzyme metabolizes and inactivates a broad spectrum of bleomycin analogs. The enzyme cleaves the carboxamide amine from the β-aminoalaninamide, yielding a weakly cytotoxic (less than 1/100) deaminobleomycin.[48] Both the primary amino acid sequence and higher-order structure determined by x-ray crystallography reveal that bleomycin hydrolase is a founding member of what is a growing class of self-compartmentalizing or sequestered intracellular proteases.[52,53] Both yeast and human enzymes are homohexamers with a ring or barrel-like structure that have the papain-like active sites situated within a central channel in a manner resembling the organization of the active sites in the 20S proteosome.[52,53] The central channel, which has a strong positive electrostatic potential in the yeast protein, is slightly negative in human bleomycin hydrolase.[53] The yeast enzyme binds to DNA and RNA but human bleomycin hydrolase lacks this attribute.[50,53,54] The C-terminus requires autoprocessing of the terminal amino acid, and the processed enzyme has both aminopeptidase and peptide ligase activity.[54,55] The kinetic properties of bleomycin hydrolase, such as its pH optimum and salt requirements, are distinct from those of other cysteine proteinases, although the substrate specificity of bleomycin hydrolase is similar to that of cathepsin H.[49] Human bleomycin hydrolase is located on chromosome band 17q11.2 and has one polymorphic site encoding either a valine or isoleucine.[56,57] Bleomycin hydrolase is found in both normal and malignant cells.[50,58] That this is the only enzyme responsible for metabolizing bleomycin was documented with bleomycin-hydrolase-null or "knockout" mice.[59] This inactivating enzyme is present in relatively low concentrations in lung and skin, the two normal tissues most susceptible to bleomycin damage.[48,58] Interestingly, pulmonary bleomycin hydrolase levels are highest in animal species or strains resistant to the pulmonary toxicity of bleomycin.[48] Mice that lack the functional gene are more sensitive to the toxic effects of bleomycin.[59] The enzyme is cytoplasmic but also may be localized to distinct subcellular organelles,[60,61] although the functional significance of this regionalization requires more investigation.

Cells exposed to bleomycin in culture seem to be most susceptible in mitosis or in the G_2, or intermitotic, phase of the cell cycle[62]; in addition, progression of cells through G_2 into mitosis is blocked by the drug.[63] In mouse L cells, S phase is also lengthened before G_2 blockade.[64] Barlogie et al.[65] observed that cell death also occurred in cells exposed during G_1, although cell killing was maximal in G_2.

DNA is more sensitive to DNA cleavage at the G_2-M and G_1 phases of the cell cycle than at S phase, which may reflect differences in chromatin structure.[66] The degree of chromatin compactness dramatically influences bleomycin-induced DNA damage.[67]

Despite the apparent increased toxicity for cells in G_2, no agreement exists regarding preferential kill of logarithmically growing cells as compared with plateau-phase cells; indeed, some workers have observed greater fractional cell kill for plateau-phase cells.[68] The possibility of enhancing cell kill by exposure during G_2 has led to the clinical use of bleomycin by continuous infusion to maximize the chances of tumor cell exposure during the most sensitive phase of the cell cycle. The results of these trials have not been convincing with respect to increasing activity.

The intracellular lesions caused by bleomycin include chromosomal breaks and deletions and both single-strand and (less frequently) double-strand breaks. In nonmitotic cells, DNA is organized into nucleosomes, or small beads, which are joined by long strands, or linker regions. The primary point of attack seems to be in the linker regions of DNA, between nucleosomes.[69] Interestingly, the resulting 180– to 200–base-pair fragments are similar in size to those formed by endonucleases activated during apoptosis.[46] The technique of alkaline elution has been used by Iqbal and co-workers,[70] who observed a biphasic survival curve for cell survival or for DNA single-strand breaks versus dose. The reason for the biphasic characteristics of these curves is unclear, but it may be related to the differing susceptibility of DNA to cleavage by bleomycin during different phases of the cell cycle or the production of small internucleosomal DNA breaks from either direct DNA damage or an apoptotic endonuclease. Clearly, however, cell kill and DNA strand breakage increase in proportion to the duration of drug exposure for at least 6 hours; this finding again implies a greater effectiveness for bleomycin given by prolonged infusion than by intravenous bolus.

Cells are able to repair bleomycin-induced DNA breaks via a complex array of enzymes, including DNA polymerase β. A delay in plating cells after bleomycin exposure increases plating efficiency, presumably by allowing time for repair of potentially lethal damage.[71] Inhibitors of DNA repair, such as caffeine and 3'-aminobenzamide,[72] accentuate DNA strand breakage and cell kill by bleomycin. Indirect evidence suggests that repair processes similar to those required for repair of lesions induced by *ionizing radiation* play a role in limiting damage due to bleomycin,[73,74] whereas cells deficient in repair mechanisms for *ultraviolet radiation* damage have no increased sensitivity to bleomycin. Cells from patients with ataxia-telangiectasia, which arises from an inherited defect in DNA repair, have increased sensitivity to bleomycin.[75] Bleomycin activity is enhanced by heat, by misonidazole,[76] and by calmodulin antagonists such as trifluoperazine.[77]

RESISTANCE

Several intracellular factors have been identified as contributors to bleomycin tumor resistance: increased drug inactivation, decreased drug accumulation, and increased repair of DNA damage. Early studies[78] demonstrated increased rates of bleomycin inactivation in two bleomycin-resistant rat hepatoma cell lines. Morris et al.[79] raised a neutralizing polyclonal antibody to bleomycin hydrolase and demonstrated an increased level of this enzyme in cultured human head and neck carcinoma cells with acquired resistance to bleomycin. Metabolic inactivation of bleomycin also can contribute to intrinsic bleomycin resistance in human colon carcinoma cells.[80] Treatment of tumor-bearing mice with E-64 before treatment with bleomycin inhibited bleomycin metabolism and increased the antitumor activity of bleomycin without increasing pulmonary toxicity.[80] This provides a potentially novel approach to increase the therapeutic activity of bleomycin.

Increased bleomycin hydrolase activity is not the only mechanism of bleomycin resistance.[81] Some cells selected in culture for bleomycin resistance display enhanced DNA repair capacity.[82] A decrease in drug content is also seen in human tumor cells with acquired resistance to bleomycin.[19] Because Fe(III)·bleomycin requires reduction to Fe(II)·bleomycin, sulfhydryl groups on proteins and peptides are potential factors in drug resistance. Tumor lines with elevated levels of glutathione, selected for resistance to doxorubicin, are collaterally sensitive to bleomycin.[83] The evidence for glutathione enhancement of bleomycin activity is not entirely clear; others have found that buthionine sulfoxamine, a glutathione-depleting agent, enhances tumor sensitivity to bleomycin.[84] Increasing the major protein thiol metallothionein produces a small increase in bleomycin sensitivity, consistent with the proposal that this cysteine-rich protein may assist in the removal of Cu(I) from bleomycin.[12] Bleomycin is not affected by P-glycoprotein, the product of the multidrug resistance gene, in contrast to many other natural products.

CLINICAL PHARMACOKINETICS

A number of techniques have been developed for assay of bleomycin in biologic fluids, including microbiologic methods,[85] HPLC,[86] biochemical techniques (degradation of DNA),[87] and radioimmunoassay methods.[88] The most rapid and simplest for clinical studies is the radioimmunoassay, which, using bleomycin labeled with iodine-125 or ^{57}Co, has provided insight into the disposition of bleomycin in humans and has superseded the less sensitive and less specific microbiologic assay techniques. The antibodies described by Broughton and Strong[88] react quantitatively with the component peptides of the clinically used bleomycin formulation. The primary component peptides A_2 and B_2 give 75% to 100% reactivity compared with the mixture in standard curve determinations. HPLC, using the ion-pairing technique, allows resolution of the component peptides but is more time-consuming.

The hallmark of bleomycin pharmacokinetics in patients with normal serum creatinine is a rapid, two-phase drug disappearance from plasma; 45%[89] to 70%[90] of the dose is excreted in the urine within 24 hours. For intravenous bolus doses, the half-lives for plasma disappearance have varied somewhat among the published studies. Alberts et al.[91] reported α and β half-lives of 24 minutes and 4 hours, respectively, whereas Crooke et al.[92] estimated β half-life to be approximately 2 hours. Peak plasma concentrations reach 1 to 10 mU per mL for intravenous bolus doses of 15 U per m².

For patients receiving bleomycin by continuous intravenous infusion, the postinfusion half-life is approximately 3 hours. Intramuscular injection of bleomycin (2 to 10 U per m²) gave peak plasma levels of 0.13 to 0.6 mU per mL, or approximately one-tenth the peak level achieved by the intravenous bolus doses.[93] The mean half-life after intramuscular injection was 2.5 hours, or approximately the same as that after intravenous injection. Peak serum concentrations were reached approximately 1 hour after injection (Fig. 16-6). Bleomycin pharmacokinetics also have been studied in patients receiving intrapleural or intraperitoneal injections. These routes have proved effective in controlling malignant effusions due to breast, lung, and ovarian cancer.[94] Intracavitary bleomycin, in doses of 60 U per m², gives peak plasma levels of 0.4 to 5.0 mU per mL,

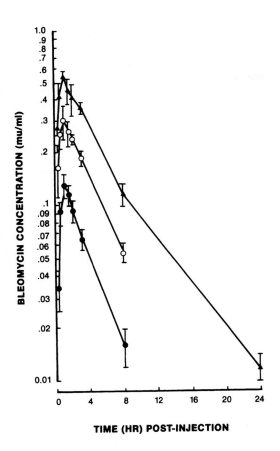

FIGURE 16-6. Pharmacokinetics of bleomycin after intramuscular administration of 2 (●), 5 (○), and 10 (▲) mg of bleomycin per m². (From Oken MM, Crooke ST, Elson MK, et al. Pharmacokinetics of bleomycin after IM administration in man. *Cancer Treat Rep* 1981;65:485.)

with a plasma half-life of 3.4 hours after intrapleural doses and 5.3 hours after intraperitoneal injection.[95] Corresponding intracavitary levels are 10- to 22-fold higher than simultaneous plasma concentrations.[96] Approximately 45% of an intracavitary dose is absorbed into the systemic circulation, and 30% is excreted in the urine as immunoreactive material.

As might be expected, bleomycin pharmacokinetics is markedly altered in patients with abnormal renal function, particularly those with creatinine clearance of less than 35 mL per minute. Alberts et al.[91] noted a terminal half-life of approximately 10 hours in a patient with a slightly elevated creatinine clearance of 1.5 mg per dL, and Crooke et al.[89] reported a patient who showed a creatinine clearance of 10.7 mL per minute and a β half-life of 21 hours. Others have reported a high frequency of pulmonary toxicity in patients with renal dysfunction secondary to cisplatin treatment.[90,97] One report described fatal pulmonary fibrosis that occurred after three doses of 20 U each given to a patient with chronic renal insufficiency (blood urea nitrogen, 48 mg per dL; creatinine, 4.8 mg per dL).[98] The available data are too limited to provide accurate guidelines for dosage adjustment in patients with renal failure. The prudent course is to decrease dosages by 50% for patients with clearances below 25 mL per minute.

CLINICAL TOXICITY AND SIDE EFFECTS

The most important toxic actions of bleomycin affect the lungs and skin; usually little evidence of myelosuppression is apparent except in patients with severely compromised bone marrow function due to extensive previous chemotherapy.[99] In such patients, myelosuppression is usually mild and is seen primarily with high-dose therapy. Fever occurs during the 48 hours after drug administration in one-quarter of patients.[100] Some investigators advocate using a 1-U test dose of bleomycin in patients receiving their initial dose of drug,[101] because rare instances of fatal acute allergic reactions have been reported.

Pulmonary Toxicity

Pulmonary toxicity is manifest as a subacute or chronic interstitial pneumonitis complicated in its later stages by progressive interstitial fibrosis, hypoxia, and death.[102] Pulmonary toxicity, usually manifested with cough, dyspnea, and bibasilar pulmonary infiltrates on chest radiographs, occurs in 3% to 5% of patients receiving a total dose of less than 450 U bleomycin; it increases significantly to a 10% incidence in those treated with greater cumulative doses.[100] Toxicity is also more frequent in patients older than age 70, in those with underlying emphysema, and in patients receiving single doses greater than 25 U per m².[103] The use of bleomycin in single doses of more than 30 U is to be discouraged, because instances of rapid onset of fatal pulmonary fibrosis 7 to 8 weeks after high-dose bleomycin have been reported.[104] Evidence also exists that previous radiotherapy to the chest predisposes to bleomycin-induced pulmonary toxicity.[105] Although the risk of lung toxicity increases with cumulative doses greater than 450 U, severe pulmonary sequelae have been observed at total doses below 100 U. In the standard regimen for treating testicular cancer, bleomycin is given in doses of 30 U per week for 12 doses, and the incidence of fatal pulmonary toxicity in this low-risk population of young male patients is approximately 2%.[2,106]

Pathogenesis of Pulmonary Toxicity

The potential for bleomycin A_2, A_5, A_6, or B_2 to cause pulmonary toxicity is easily demonstrated by intravenous infusion or by direct instillation of the parent molecule into the trachea of a rodent, where it induces an acute inflammatory response, epithelial apoptosis, an alveolar fibrinoid exudate, and, over a period of 1 to 2 weeks, progressive deposition of collagen.[106a,106b] The terminal amines of these bleomycins are sufficient, by themselves, to cause the toxicity in rodents, and the toxic potency of the bleomycins is directly correlated with the potency of their individual terminal amines, with the A_2 aminopropyl-dimethylsulfonium and the A_5 spermidine having greater effect than the B_2 agmatine.[107] These findings raise the possibility that modification of the terminal amine might allow selection of a less toxic analog for clinical use. Several such analogs have been tested, but clinical superiority has not been demonstrated.

The pathogenesis of bleomycin pulmonary toxicity in rodents serves as a model for understanding pulmonary fibrosis, an end result of a broad range of human diseases induced by drugs, autoimmunity, and infection.[106a] The primary model has been the intratracheal instillation of bleomycin in mice or hamsters,[108] although one should note that in clinical drug use the agent is administered intravenously. The drug has direct toxicity to alveolar epithelial cells, causing induction of epithelial apoptosis, intraalveolar inflammation, cytokine release by alveolar macrophages, fibroblast proliferation, and collagen deposition,[108–110] as well as endothelial cell damage in small pulmonary vessels.[111] As changes progress from acute inflammation to interstitial fibrosis, pulmonary function deteriorates, as indicated by a decrease in lung compliance, a decrease in carbon monoxide diffusion capacity, and terminal hypoxia.[112,113] Hydroxyproline deposition parallels the increase in collagen and serves as a quantitative measure of the progression of fibrosis in animal models.[112]

A broad array of cytokines, produced by alveolar macrophages and by endothelial cells in response to bleomycin, have been implicated in the molecular pathogenesis of pulmonary fibrosis. These include transforming growth factor β (TGF-β),[113–115] tumor necrosis factor α (TNF-α),[116–118] interleukin 1β,[118] interleukins 2, 3, 4, 5, and 6,[119,120] and various chemokines. Bleomycin and TGF-β both stimulate the promoter that controls transcription of a collagen precursor.[115] Interleukin 1 augments TGF-β secretion stimulated by bleomycin, whereas TNF-α enhances prostaglandin secretion and fibroblast proliferation.[118]

Genetic experiments have provided further insight into factors that influence susceptibility to fibrosis,[119–122] as well as the central role of cytokines in bleomycin lung toxicity. They illustrate the importance of drug inactivation, fibrin deposition, and cytokine action in mediating lung injury. Travis and colleagues have shown that strains of mice with greatly increased susceptibility to bleomycin toxicity (and simultaneously to radiation toxicity) can be inbred, although the specific genetic defect is still unclear.[121,122] Other experiments have shown that specific genetic lesions do predispose to pulmonary fibrosis. Bleomycin hydrolase knockout mice have significantly greater lung and epidermal toxicity than normal controls.[123] Mice lacking plasminogen activator inhibitor 1, a protein that blocks the activation of the major fibrinolytic protease in plasma and in the alveolar space, have decreased susceptibility to bleomycin pulmonary fibrosis.[124]

Perhaps the most compelling genetic experiments implicate the central role of TGF-β, which is secreted by alveolar macrophages in response to bleomycin.[125] TGF-β is secreted in a complex with a latency-associated peptide and is activated by binding of the complex to αvβ6 integrin found on alveolar epithelial cells and keratinocytes. This binding of the TGF-β complex to its integrin exposes cytokine-binding domains that allow interaction of TGF-β with its receptor(s) and stimulates the production of procollagen by fibroblasts.[126] Mice in which αvβ6 integrin has been knocked out develop an inflammatory alveolar response to bleomycin but do not develop progressive fibrosis.

The stimulus for cytokine and chemokine release is uncertain, although apoptosis of epithelial cells, alveolar macrophages, or lymphocytes may play an important role.[127,128] In mice, genetic deletion of either Fas, which is expressed on pulmonary epithelial cells, or Fas ligand, as expressed on T lymphocytes, does not prevent inflammation but does protect against pulmonary fibrosis.[128] Soluble Fas antigen or anti-Fas ligand antibody also provides protection against fibrosis, presumably by preventing Fas-mediated epithelial apoptosis.

In addition to providing remarkable insights regarding the pathogenesis of pulmonary fibrosis, these experiments suggest a number of new approaches to prevention of bleomycin toxicity. Thus, in various animal models, protection is provided by Fas antigen and anti-Fas ligand antibodies[128]; TNF-α–soluble receptor[129]; TGF-β antibodies[130]; granulocyte-macrophage colony-stimulating factor antibodies[131]; pirfenidone, an inhibitor of platelet-derived growth factor function and procollagen transcription[132,133]; the antioxidant amifostine[134]; relaxin, a collagen matrix–degrading protein that increases collagenase secretion and decreases procollagen synthesis[135]; transgenic expression of *Sh ble*, a yeast protein that binds the iron-bleomycin complex and protects against its toxicity[136]; dehydroproline, an inhibitor of procollagen synthesis[137,138]; and indomethacin.[139] These findings may be applicable to the general problem of preventing drug-induced or idiopathic pulmonary fibrosis in humans,[140] although none of these agents has been shown to be efficacious in a clinical trial.

In general, in animal toxicology experiments, single high doses of bleomycin produce greater pulmonary inflammation and fibrosis than do smaller daily doses or continuous drug infusion,[141,142] but these findings have never been confirmed in humans.

Clinical Syndrome of Pulmonary Toxicity

Clinical symptoms of bleomycin pulmonary injury include a nonproductive cough, dyspnea, and occasionally fever and pleuritic pain. Physical examination usually reveals little auscultatory evidence of pulmonary alveolar infiltrates, and initial chest films are often negative or may reveal an increase in interstitial markings, especially in the lower lobes, with a

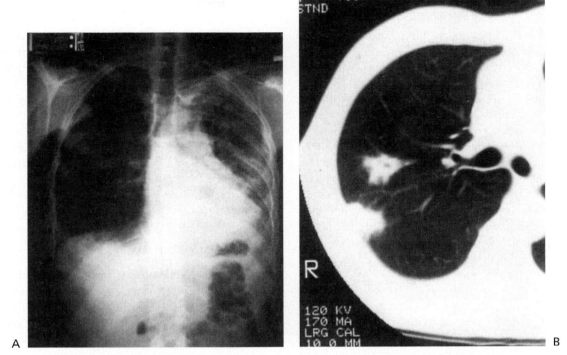

FIGURE 16-7. A: Typical interstitial pulmonary infiltrates, most obvious in left lung, observed during treatment of a patient with testicular carcinoma. **B:** Nodular variant of bleomycin pulmonary toxicity in a patient undergoing treatment for testicular cancer. Computed tomographic scan of chest showing a nodular density with central cavitation. On biopsy, the lesion was found to be composed of granulomas with associated interstitial pneumonitis. Appropriate stains and cultures did not reveal infectious agents. (From Talcott JA, Garnick MB, Stomper PC, et al. Cavitary lung nodules associated with combination chemotherapy containing bleomycin. *J Urol* 1987;138:619.)

predilection for subpleural areas. Chest radiographs, when positive, reveal patchy reticulonodular infiltrates, which in later stages may coalesce to form areas of apparent consolidation. In occasional patients, the initial radiographic changes may be discrete nodules indistinguishable from metastatic tumor; central cavitation of nodules may be present[143,144] (Fig. 16-7). Gallium-67 lung scans or computed tomographic scans (Fig. 16-8) may show the presence

of a diffuse lung lesion at a time of minimal abnormality on plain films of the chest; computed tomographic scans are much more sensitive than posteroanterior chest films in revealing the extent of pulmonary fibrosis. Radiologic findings do not differentiate bleomycin lung toxicity from other forms of interstitial lung disease,[145] however, particularly *Pneumocystis carinii* pneumonia. Arterial oxygen desaturation and an abnormal carbon monoxide diffusion capacity

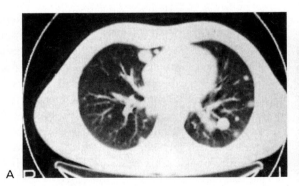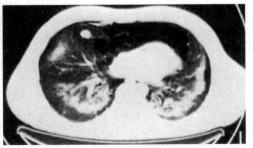

FIGURE 16-8. Computed tomographic scans of the chest before **(A)** and after **(B)** treatment for testicular cancer. The multiple metastatic pulmonary nodules partially regressed with therapy, but the posttreatment film shows dense bilateral pulmonary fibrosis, as well as a large left pneumothorax and pneumomediastinum. The patient died of bleomycin pulmonary toxicity shortly afterward.

are present in symptomatic patients with bleomycin toxicity, as is also the case in patients with other forms of interstitial pulmonary disease. Thus, open lung biopsy is usually required to distinguish between the primary differential diagnostic alternatives, specifically a drug-induced pulmonary lesion, an infectious interstitial pneumonitis, and neoplastic pulmonary infiltration. The findings on histologic examination of human lung after bleomycin treatment closely resemble those previously described in the experimental animal and include an acute inflammatory infiltrate in the alveoli, interstitial and intraalveolar edema, pulmonary hyaline membrane formation, and intraalveolar and, later in the course, interstitial fibrosis. In addition, squamous metaplasia of the alveolar lining cells has been described as a characteristic finding.[146] In rare cases, a true hypersensitivity pneumonitis may develop, characterized by underlying eosinophilic pulmonary infiltrates and a prompt clinical response to corticosteroids.[147]

Pulmonary function tests, particularly a rapid fall in the carbon monoxide diffusing capacity, are of possible value in predicting a high risk of pulmonary toxicity. Most patients treated with bleomycin, however, show a progressive (10% to 15%) fall in diffusion capacity with increasing total dose and a more marked increase in changes above a 240-mg total dose. Whether or not the diffusion capacity test can be used to predict which patients will subsequently develop clinically significant pulmonary toxicity is not clear.[148] As mentioned earlier, at advanced stages in the evolution of bleomycin pulmonary toxicity, the diffusion capacity as well as arterial oxygen saturation and total lung capacity become markedly abnormal. Long-term assessment of pulmonary function in patients treated with bleomycin for testicular cancer has revealed a return to baseline normal values at a median of 4 years after treatment.[149]

Patients who have received bleomycin seem to be at greater risk of respiratory failure during the postoperative recovery period after surgery.[150] In one study, five of five patients treated with 200 U per m² bleomycin (cumulative dose) for testicular cancer died of postoperative respiratory failure; a reduction in inspired oxygen to an fraction of inspired oxygen of 0.24 and a decrease in the volume of fluids administered during surgery prevented mortality in subsequent patients.[150] The sensitivity of bleomycin-treated patients to high concentrations of inspired oxygen is intriguing in view of the molecular action of bleomycin, which is dependent on and mediated by the formation of oxygen-derived free radicals. Current safeguards for anesthesia of bleomycin-treated patients include the use of the minimum tolerated concentration of inspired oxygen and modest fluid replacement to prevent pulmonary edema.

No specific therapy is available for patients with bleomycin-induced lung toxicity. Discontinuation of the drug may be followed by a period of continued progression of the pulmonary findings, with partial reversal of the abnormalities in pulmonary function only after several months. The inflammatory component of the pathologic process does resolve in experimental models,[113] and interstitial infiltrates regress clinically, but the reversibility of pulmonary fibrosis has not been documented. The value of corticosteroids in promoting recovery from bleomycin-induced lung toxicity remains controversial, although beneficial effects have been described in isolated case studies.[151,152] Long-term follow-up of patients with clinical and radiographic evidence of bleomycin-induced pneumonitis suggests a complete resolution of radiographic, clinical, and pulmonary function abnormalities in a small series of eight patients 2 years after completion of treatment for testicular cancer,[153] although in more severe cases pulmonary fibrosis may be only partially reversible.

Cutaneous Toxicity

A more common but less serious toxicity of bleomycin is its effect on skin, which may relate to bleomycin hydrolase levels.[58] Approximately 50% of patients treated with conventional once- or twice-daily doses of this agent develop erythema, induration, and hyperkeratosis and peeling of skin that may progress to frank ulceration.[100] These changes predominantly affect digits, hands, joints, and areas of previous irradiation. Hyperpigmentation, alopecia, and nail changes also occur during bleomycin therapy. These cutaneous side effects do not necessitate discontinuation of therapy, particularly if clear benefit is being derived from the drug. Rarely, patients may develop Raynaud's phenomenon while receiving bleomycin.[154] Other toxic reactions to bleomycin include hypersensitivity reactions, characterized by urticaria, periorbital edema, and bronchospasm.[100]

SCHEDULES OF ADMINISTRATION

Bleomycin has been used in a number of different schedules and routes of administration. The most common route and schedule is bolus intravenous injection. Because of the greater effect of bleomycin on cells in the mitotic and G_2 phases of the cell cycle, the drug has been given by continuous infusion to produce prolonged exposure to toxic concentrations, but a high incidence of pulmonary toxicity has sometimes resulted. For example, continuous infusion of 25 U per day for 5 days produced the expected rapid onset of pulmonary toxicity, particularly in patients with previous chest irradiation,[105,155] but in addition caused hypertensive episodes in 17% of patients and hyperbilirubinemia in 30%.[105] These latter toxicities are rarely seen with conventional bolus doses.

Continuous intraarterial infusion also has been used for patients with carcinoma of the cervix[156] and of the head and neck.[157] One study[156] noted a disappointing 12% response rate to infusion of 20 U per m² per week for courses of up to 3 weeks. Pulmonary toxicity was observed in 20% of patients.

Bleomycin also has been applied topically as a 3.5% ointment in a xipamide (Aquaphor) base. Two-week courses of treatment produced complete regression of Paget's disease of the vulva in four of seven patients,[158] with no serious local toxicity.

As described previously in the discussion of pharmacokinetics, bleomycin can be used to sclerose the pleural space in patients with malignant effusions. After thorough evacuation of fluid from the pleural space, 40 U per m² is dissolved in 100 mL normal saline and instilled through a thoracostomy tube, which is clamped for 8 hours and then returned to suction. In approximately one-third of patients thus treated, the effusion clears completely; this is about the same response rate as obtained with tetracycline instillation.[159,160] The only toxic reactions are fever and pleuritis, both of which resolve in 24 to 48 hours. The intraperitoneal instillation of bleomycin has been used in patients with ovarian cancer, mesothelioma, and other malignancy confined to the peritoneum[95] but with rare responses. Sixty mg of bleomycin per m² was dissolved in 2 L of saline, and the solution was placed in the peritoneal cavity for a 4- to 8-hour dwell time. Side effects included abdominal pain, fever, rash, and mucositis. A limited pharmacokinetic advantage was observed (peritoneal area under the concentration × time curve was sevenfold greater than plasma area under the curve), which provides little justification for this route of administration.

Bleomycin has been instilled into the urinary bladder in doses of 60 U in 30 mL of sterile water.[161] Seven of 26 patients with superficial transitional cell carcinomas had complete disappearance of disease after 7 to 8 weekly treatments, but all had relatively small lesions. The primary toxic reaction was cystitis. Plasma drug level monitoring revealed little evidence of systemic absorption.

RADIATION AND DRUG INTERACTION

Bleomycin is used frequently in combination therapy regimens for treatment of lymphomas and squamous carcinomas of the esophagus and head and neck, primarily because of its lack of myelosuppressive toxicity. The pharmacologic basis of synergism between bleomycin and various agents has received considerable attention[162,163] but is only poorly understood. Administration of bleomycin within 3 hours of irradiation, either before or after, produces greater than additive effects,[164] possibly owing to the production of free-radical damage to DNA by both agents. This interaction has been tested in a randomized clinical trial of radiation therapy plus or minus bleomycin, 5 mg twice weekly, in patients with head and neck cancer.[165] In this study, the group receiving bleomycin had a significantly higher complete response rate and a better 3-year disease-free survival rate. As mentioned earlier, synergistic pulmonary toxicity has been reported in patients receiving bleomycin after previous chest irradiation.

REFERENCES

1. Umezawa H, Maeda K, Takeuchi T, et al. New antibiotics, bleomycin A and B. *J Antibiot (Tokyo)* 1966;19:200.
2. Levi JA, Raghavan D, Harvey V, et al. The importance of bleomycin in combination chemotherapy for good-prognosis germ cell carcinoma. *J Clin Oncol* 1993;11:1300.
3. Saito S, Umezawa Y, Yoshioka T, et al. An improved total synthesis of bleomycin. *J Antibiot (Tokyo)* 1983;36:92.
4. Takita T, Umezawa Y, Saito S, et al. Total synthesis of bleomycin. In: Rich DH, Gross E, eds. *Peptides: synthesis-structure-function*. Rockford, IL: Pierce Chemical Co, 1981:29.
5. Takita T, Umezawa Y, Saito S, et al. Total synthesis of bleomycin A₂. *Tetrahedron Lett* 1982;23:521.
6. Umezawa H, Suhara Y, Takita T, et al. Purification of bleomycin. *J Antibiot (Tokyo)* 1966;19:210.
7. Mistry JS, Sebti SM, Lazo JS. Separation of bleomycins and their deamido metabolites by high-performance cation-exchange chromatography. *J Chromatogr* 1990;514:86.
8. Stubbe J, Kozarich JW. Mechanisms of bleomycin-induced DNA degradation. *Chem Rev* 1987;87:1107.
9. Umezawa H. Advances in bleomycin studies. In: Hecht SM, ed. *Bleomycin: chemical, biochemical, and biological aspects*. New York: Springer-Verlag, 1979:24.
10. Lazo JS, Schisselbauer JC, Herring GM, et al. Involvement of the cellular vacuolar system with the cytotoxicity of bleomycin-like agents. *Cancer Commun* 1990;2:81.
11. Pron G, Belehradek J Jr, Mir LM. Identification of a plasma membrane protein that specifically binds bleomycin. *Biochem Biophys Res Commun* 1993;194:333.
12. Takahashi K, Takita T, Umezawa H. The nature of thiol compounds which trap cuprous ion reductively liberated from bleomycin-Cu(II) in cells. *J Antibiot (Tokyo)* 1987;40:348.
13. Dabrowiak JC, Greenaway FT, Santillo FS, et al. The iron complexes of bleomycin and tallysomycin. *Biochem Biophys Res Commun* 1979;91:721.
14. Takita T, Muraoka Y, Nakatani T, et al. Chemistry of bleomycin: XXI. Metal-complex and its implication for the mechanism of bleomycin action. *J Antibiot (Tokyo)* 1978; 31:1073.
15. Ehrenberg GM, Shipley JB, Heimbrook DC, et al. Copper dependent cleavage of bleomycin. *Biochemistry* 1987; 26:931.
16. Hecht SM. The chemistry of activated bleomycin. *Acc Chem Res* 1986;19:383.
17. Sausville EA, Peisach J, Horwitz SB. Effects of chelating agents and metal ions on the degradation of DNA by bleomycin. *Biochemistry* 1978;17:2740.
18. Sausville EA, Peisach J, Horwitz SB. A role for ferrous ion and oxygen in the degradation of DNA by bleomycin. *Biochem Biophys Res Commun* 1976;73:814.
19. Lazo JS, Schisselbauer JC, Meandzija B, et al. Initial single strand DNA damage and cellular pharmacokinetics of bleomycin A₂. *Biochem Pharmacol* 1989;38:2207.
20. Holes CE, Carter BJ, Hecht SM. Characterization of iron (II)·bleomycin–mediated RNA strand scission. *Biochemistry* 1993;32:4293.
21. Holmes CE, Duff RJ, von der Marvel GA, et al. On the chemistry of DNA degradation by Fe·bleomycin. *Bioorganic Med Chem* 1997;5:1235.

22. Morgan MA, Hecht SM. Iron (II)·bleomycin–mediated degradation of a DNA-RNA heteroduplex. *Biochemistry* 1994;33:10286.

23. Burger RM. Cleavage of nucleic acids by bleomycin. *Chem Rev* 1998;98:1153.

24. Fulmer P, Pettering DH. Reaction of DNA-bound ferrous bleomycin with dioxygen: activation versus stabilization of dioxygen. *Biochemistry* 1994;33:5319.

25. Ciriolo MR, Magliozzo RS, Peisach J. Microsome-stimulated activation of ferrous bleomycin in the presence of DNA. *J Biol Chem* 1987;262:6290.

26. Mahmutoglu I, Kappus H. Redox cycling of bleomycin-Fe(III) by an NADH-dependent enzyme, and DNA damage in isolated rat liver nuclei. *Biochem Pharmacol* 1987; 36:3677.

27. Burger RM, Kent TA, Horwitz SB, et al. Mossbauer study of iron bleomycin and its activation intermediates. *J Biol Chem* 1983;258:1559.

28. Kasai H, Naganawa H, Takita T, et al. Chemistry of bleomycin: XXII. Interaction of bleomycin with nucleic acids, preferential binding to guanine base and electrostatic effect of the terminal amine. *J Antibiot (Tokyo)* 1978;31:1316.

29. Umezawa H, Takita T, Sugiura Y, et al. DNA-bleomycin interaction: nucleotide sequence-specific binding and cleavage of DNA by bleomycin. *Tetrahedron* 1984;40:501.

30. Povirk LF, Hogan M, Dattagupta N. Binding of bleomycin to DNA: intercalation of the bithiazole rings. *Biochemistry* 1979;18:96.

31. Hertzberg RP, Caranfa MJ, Hecht SM. Degradation of structurally modified DNAs by bleomycin group antibiotics. *Biochemistry* 1988;27:3164.

32. Caspary WJ, Niziak C, Lanzo DA, et al. Bleomycin A₂: a ferrous oxidase. *Mol Pharmacol* 1979;16:256.

33. Kilkuskie RE, Macdonald TL, Hecht SM. Bleomycin may be activated for DNA cleavage by NADPH–cytochrome P450 reductase. *Biochemistry* 1984;23:6165.

34. Burger RM, Horwitz SB, Peisach J, et al. Oxygenated iron bleomycin: a short-lived intermediate in the reaction of ferrous bleomycin with O₂. *J Biol Chem* 1979;254:12299.

35. Sugiura Y, Kikuchi TK. Formation of superoxide and hydroxy radicals by bleomycin and iron (II). *J Antibiot (Tokyo)* 1978;31:1310.

36. Sausville E, Stein R, Peisach J, et al. Properties and products of the degradation of DNA by bleomycin. *Biochemistry* 1978;17:2746.

37. Burger RM, Projan SJ, Horwitz SB, et al. The DNA cleavage mechanism of iron-bleomycin. *J Biol Chem* 1986; 261:15955.

38. Rabow L, Stubbe J, Kozarich JW, et al. Identification of the alkali-labile product accompanying cytosine release during bleomycin-mediated degradation of d(CGCGCG). *J Am Chem Soc* 1986;108:7130.

39. Grollman AP, Takeshita M, Pillai KM, et al. Origin and cytotoxic properties of base propenals derived from DNA. *Cancer Res* 1985;45:1127.

40. Keller TJ, Oppenheimer NJ. Enhanced bleomycin-mediated damage of DNA opposite charged nicks: a model for bleomycin-directed double strand scission of DNA. *J Biol Chem* 1987;262:15144.

41. Burger RM, Berkowitz AR, Peisach J, et al. Origin of mal-ondialdehyde from DNA degraded by Fe(II)-bleomycin. *J Biol Chem* 1980;255:11832.

42. Takeshita M, Grollman AP, Ohtsubo E, et al. Interaction of bleomycin with DNA. *Proc Natl Acad Sci U S A* 1978;75:5983.

43. Grollman AP, Takeshita M. Interactions of bleomycin with DNA. In: Weber G, ed. *Advances in enzyme regulation*, vol 18. Oxford: Pergamon Press, 1980:67.

44. Roy SN, Horwitz SB. Characterization of the association of radiolabeled bleomycin A₂ with HeLa cells. *Cancer Res* 1984;44:1541.

45. Fugimito J, Higashi H, Kosaki G. Intracellular distribution of [¹⁴C]bleomycin and the cytokinetic effects of bleomycin in the mouse tumor. *Cancer Res* 1976;36:2248.

46. Touchekti O, Pron G, Belehradek J Jr, et al. Bleomycin, an apoptosis mimetic drug that induces two types of cell death depending on the number of molecules internalized. *Cancer Res* 1993;53:5462.

47. Mistry JS, Jani JP, Morris G, et al. Synthesis and evaluation of fluoromycin: a novel fluorescence-labeled derivative of talisomycin S₁₀ᵦ. *Cancer Res* 1992;52:709.

48. Lazo JS, Humphreys CJ. Lack of metabolism as the biochemical basis of bleomycin-induced pulmonary toxicity. *Proc Natl Acad Sci U S A* 1983;80:3064.

49. Sebti SM, Mignano JE, Jani JP, et al. Bleomycin hydrolase: molecular cloning, sequencing and biochemical studies reveals membership in the cysteine proteinase family. *Biochemistry* 1989;28:6544.

50. Brömme D, Rossi AB, Smeekens SP, et al. Human bleomycin hydrolase: molecular cloning, sequencing, functional expression, and enzymatic characterization. *Biochemistry* 1996;35:6706.

51. Enekel C, Wolf DH. BLH1 codes for a yeast thiol aminopeptidase, the equivalent of mammalian bleomycin hydrolase. *J Biol Chem* 1993;268:7036.

52. Joshua-Tor L, Xu HE, Johnston SA, et al. Crystal structure of a conserved protease that binds DNA: the bleomycin hydrolase, Gal6. *Science* 1995;269:945.

53. Farrell PA, Gonzalez F, Zheng W, et al. Crystal structure of human bleomycin hydrolase, a self-compartmentalizing cysteine protease. *Structure* 1999;7:619.

54. Koldamova RP, Lefterov IM, Gadjeva VG, et al. Essential binding and functional domains of human bleomycin hydrolase. *Biochemistry* 1998;37:2282.

55. Zheng W, Johnston SA, Joshua-Tor L. The unusual active site of Gal6/bleomycin hydrolase can act as a carboxypeptidase, aminopeptidase, and peptide ligase. *Cell* 1998;93:103.

56. Montoya SE, Ferrell RE, Lazo JS. Genomic structure and genetic mapping of the human neutral cysteine protease bleomycin hydrolase. *Cancer Res* 1997;57:4191.

57. Ferrando A, Pendas A, Elena L, et al. Gene characterization, promoter analysis, and chromosomal localization of human bleomycin hydrolase. *J Biol Chem* 1997;272:33298.

58. Takeda A, Nonaka M, Ishikawa A, et al. Immunohistochemical localization of the neutral cysteine protease bleomycin hydrolase in human skin. *Arch Dermatol Res* 1999; 291:238.

59. Schwartz DR, Homanics GE, Hoyt DG. The neutral cysteine protease bleomycin hydrolase is essential for epidermal integrity and bleomycin resistance. *Proc Natl Acad Sci U S A* 1999;96:4680.

60. Koldamova RP, Lefterov LM, DiSabella MT, et al. An evolutionarily conserved cysteine protease, human bleomycin hydrolase, binds to the human homologue of ubiquitin-conjugating enzyme 9. *Mol Pharmacol* 1998;54:954.

61. Nishimura C, Suzuki H, Tanaka N, et al. Intracellular degradation of bleomycin hydrolase in two Chinese hamster cell lines in relation to their peplomycin susceptibility. *Biochim Biophys Acta* 1989;1012:29.

62. Barranco SC, Humphrey RM. The effects of bleomycin on survival and cell progression in Chinese hamster cells in vitro. *Cancer Res* 1971;31:1218.

63. Tobey RA. Arrest of Chinese hamster cells in G_2 following treatment with the antitumor drug bleomycin. *J Cell Physiol* 1972;79:259.

64. Wanatabe M, Takabe Y, Katsumata T, et al. Effects of bleomycin on progression through the cell cycle of mouse L cells. *Cancer Res* 1974;34:2726.

65. Barlogie B, Drewinko B, Schumann J, et al. Pulse cytophotometric analysis of cell cycle perturbation with bleomycin in vitro. *Cancer Res* 1976;36:1182.

66. Olive PL, Banath JP. Detection of DNA double-strand breaks through the cell cycle after exposure to x-rays, bleomycin, etoposide and [125]IdUrd. *Int J Radiat Biol* 1993;64:349.

67. Lopez-Larraza DM, Bianchi NO. DNA response to bleomycin in mammalian cells with variable degrees of chromatin condensation. *Environ Mol Mutagen* 1993;21:258.

68. Twentyman PR. Bleomycin—mode of action with particular reference to the cell cycle. *Pharmacol Ther* 1983;23:417.

69. Kuo MT, Hsu TC. Bleomycin causes release of nucleosomes from chromatin and chromosomes. *Nature* 1978;271:83.

70. Iqbal ZM, Kohn KW, Ewig RAG, et al. Single-strand scission and repair of DNA in mammalian cells by bleomycin. *Cancer Res* 1976;36:3834.

71. Barranco SC, Novak JK, Humphrey RM. Studies on recovery from chemically induced damage in mammalian cells. *Cancer Res* 1975;35:1194.

72. Nakatsugawa S, Dewey WC. The role in cancer therapy of inhibiting recovery from PLD induced by radiation or bleomycin. *Int J Radiat Oncol Biol Phys* 1984;10:1425.

73. Onishi T, Shimada K, Takagi Y. Effects of bleomycin on *Escherichia coli* strains with various sensitivities to radiation. *Biochem Biophys Acta* 1973;312:248.

74. Cramer P, Painter RB. Bleomycin-resistant DNA synthesis in ataxia telangiectasia cells. *Nature* 1981;291:671.

75. Taylor AMR, Rosney CM, Campbell JB. Unusual sensitivity of ataxia telangiectasia cells to bleomycin. *Cancer Res* 1979;39:1046.

76. Ma F, Hiraoka M, Jo S, et al. Response of mammary tumors of C3H/He mice to hyperthermia and bleomycin in vivo. *Radiat Med* 1985;3:230.

77. Lazo JS, Chen DL, Gallicchio VS, et al. Increased lethality of calmodulin antagonists and bleomycin to human bone marrow and bleomycin-resistant malignant cells. *Cancer Res* 1986;46:2236.

78. Mayaki M, Ono T, Hori S, et al. Binding of bleomycin to DNA in bleomycin-sensitive and resistant rat ascites hepatoma cells. *Cancer Res* 1975;35:2015.

79. Morris G, Mistry JS, Jani JP, et al. Neutralization of bleomycin hydrolase by an epitope-specific antibody. *Mol Pharmacol* 1992;42:57.

80. Jani JP, Mistry JS, Morris G, et al. In vivo circumvention of human colon carcinoma resistance to bleomycin. *Cancer Res* 1992;52:2931.

81. Brabbs S, Warr JR. Isolation and characterization of bleomycin-resistant clones of OHO cells. *Genet Res* 1979;34:269.

82. Zuckerman JE, Raffin TA, Brown JM, et al. In vitro selection and characterization of a bleomycin-resistant subline of B16 melanoma. *Cancer Res* 1986;46:1748.

83. Tsuruo T, Hamilton TC, Louie KG, et al. Collateral susceptibility of Adriamycin-, melphalan- and cisplatin-resistant human ovarian tumor cells to bleomycin. *Jpn J Cancer Res* 1986;77:941.

84. Russo A, Mitchell JB, McPherson S, et al. Alteration of bleomycin cytotoxicity by glutathione depletion or elevation. *Int J Radiat Oncol Biol Phys* 1984;10:1675.

85. Umezawa H, Takeuchi T, Hori S, et al. Studies on the mechanism of antitumor effect of bleomycin on squamous cell carcinoma. *J Antibiot (Tokyo)* 1972;25:409.

86. Shiu GK, Goehl TJ. High-performance liquid chromatographic determination of bleomycin A_2 in urine. *J Chromatogr* 1980;181:127.

87. Galvan L, Strong JE, Crooke ST. Use of PM-2 DNA degradation as a pharmacokinetic assay for bleomycin. *Cancer Res* 1979;39:3948.

88. Broughton A, Strong JE. Radioimmunoassay of bleomycin. *Cancer Res* 1976;36:1418.

89. Crooke ST, Luft F, Broughton A, et al. Bleomycin serum pharmacokinetics as determined by a radioimmunoassay and a microbiologic assay in a patient with compromised renal function. *Cancer* 1977;39:1430.

90. Bennett WM, Pastore L, Houghton DC. Fatal pulmonary bleomycin toxicity in cisplatin-induced acute renal failure. *Cancer Treat Rep* 1980;64:921.

91. Alberts DS, Chen HSG, Liu R, et al. Bleomycin pharmacokinetics in man: I. Intravenous administration. *Cancer Chemother Pharmacol* 1978;1:177.

92. Crooke ST, Comis RL, Einhorn LH, et al. Effects of variations in renal function on the clinical pharmacology of bleomycin administered as an IV bolus. *Cancer Treat Rep* 1977;61:1631.

93. Oken MM, Crooke ST, Elson MK, et al. Pharmacokinetics of bleomycin after IM administration in man. *Cancer Treat Rep* 1981;65:485.

94. Paladine W, Cunningham TJ, Sponzo R, et al. Intracavitary bleomycin in the management of malignant effusions. *Cancer* 1976;38:1903.

95. Alberts DS, Chen HSG, Mayersohn M, et al. Bleomycin pharmacokinetics in man: II. Intracavitary administration. *Cancer Chemother Pharmacol* 1979;2:127.

96. Howell SB, Schiefer M, Andrews PA, et al. The pharmacology of intraperitoneally administered bleomycin. *J Clin Oncol* 1987;5:2009.

97. Dalgleish AG, Woods RL, Levi JA. Bleomycin pulmonary toxicity: its relationship to renal dysfunction. *Med Pediatr Oncol* 1984;12:313.

98. McLeod BF, Lawrence HJ, Smith DW, et al. Fatal bleomycin toxicity from a low cumulative dose in a patient with renal insufficiency. *Cancer* 1987;60:2617.

99. Hubbard SP, Chabner BA, Canellos GP, et al. High-dose intravenous bleomycin in treatment of advanced lymphomas. *Eur J Cancer* 1975;11:623.

100. Blum RH, Carter SK, Agre K. A clinical review of bleomycin—a new antineoplastic agent. *Cancer* 1973;31:903.

101. Levy RL, Chiarillo S. Hyperpyrexia, allergic-type response, and death occurring with bleomycin administration. *Oncology* 1980;37:316.

102. Comis RL. Bleomycin pulmonary toxicity: current status and future directions. *Semin Oncol* 1992;19[Suppl 5]:64.

103. Parvinen LM, Kikku P, Maekinen E, et al. Factors affecting the pulmonary toxicity of bleomycin. *Acta Radiol Oncol* 1983;22:417.

104. Dee GJ, Austin JH, Mutter GL. Bleomycin-associated pulmonary fibrosis: rapidly fatal progression without chest radiotherapy. *J Surg Oncol* 1987;35:135.

105. Samuels ML, Johnson DE, Holoye PH, et al. Large-dose bleomycin therapy and pulmonary toxicity: a possible role of prior radiotherapy. *JAMA* 1976;235:1117.

106. Williams SD, Birch R, Einhorn LA, et al. Treatment of disseminated germ cell tumors with cisplatin, bleomycin, and either vinblastine or etoposide. *N Engl J Med* 1987;316:1435.

106a. Harrison JH Jr, Lazo JS. High dose continuous infusion of bleomycin in mice: a new model for drug-induced pulmonary fibrosis. *J Pharmacol Exp Ther* 1987;243:1185.

106b. Hay J, Shahzeidi S, Laurent G. Mechanisms of bleomycin-induced lung damage. *Arch Toxicol* 1991;65:81.

107. Raisfeld IH. Role of terminal substituents in the pulmonary toxicity of bleomycins. *Toxicol Appl Pharmacol* 1981;57:355.

108. Huff RA, Bevan DR. Application of alkaline unwinding to analysis of breaks induced by bleomycin in hamster lung DNA in vivo. *J Appl Toxicol* 1991;11:359.

109. Phan SH, Varani J, Smith D. Rat lung fibroblast collagen metabolism in bleomycin-induced pulmonary fibrosis. *J Clin Invest* 1985;76:241.

110. Conley NS, Yarbro JW, Ferrari HA, et al. Bleomycin increases superoxide anion generation by pig peripheral alveolar macrophages. *Mol Pharmacol* 1986;30:48.

111. Adamson IY, Bowden DH. The pathogenesis of bleomycin-induced pulmonary fibrosis in mice. *Am J Pathol* 1974;77:185.

112. Sikic BI, Young DM, Mimnaugh EG, et al. Quantification of bleomycin pulmonary toxicity in mice by changes in lung hydroxyproline content and morphometric histopathology. *Cancer Res* 1978;38:787.

113. Phan S, Gharaee-Kermani M, McGarry B, et al. Regulation of rat pulmonary artery endothelial cell transforming growth factor-beta production by Il-1beta and tumor necrosis factor-alpha. *J Immunol* 1992;149:103.

114. Hoyt DG, Lazo JS. Alterations in pulmonary mRNA encoding procollagens, fibronectin and transforming growth factor-β precede bleomycin-induced pulmonary fibrosis in mice. *J Pharmacol Exp Ther* 1988;246:765.

115. King SL, Lichter AC, Rowe SW, et al. Bleomycin stimulates pro-alpha (I) collagen promoter through transforming growth factor beta response element by intracellular and extracellular signaling. *J Biol Chem* 1994;269:13156.

116. Everson MP, Chandler DB. Changes in distribution, morphology, and tumor necrosis factor-alpha secretion of alveolar macrophage subpopulations during the development of bleomycin-induced pulmonary fibrosis. *Am J Pathol* 1992; 140:503.

117. Khalil N, Whitman C, Zuo L, et al. Regulation of alveolar macrophage transforming growth factor-beta secretion by corticosteroids in bleomycin-induced pulmonary inflammation in the rat. *J Clin Invest* 1993;92:1812.

118. Piguet PF, Collart MA, Grau GE, et al. Tumor necrosis factor/cachectin plays a key role in bleomycin induced pneumopathy and fibrosis. *J Exp Med* 1989;170:655.

119. Scheule RK, Perkins RC, Hamilton R, et al. A. Bleomycin stimulation of cytokine secretion by the human alveolar macrophage. *Am J Physiol* 1992;262:L386.

120. Baecher AC, Barth RK. PCR analysis of cytokine induction profiles associated with mouse strain variation in susceptibility to pulmonary fibrosis. *Reg Immunol* 1993;5:207.

121. Haston CK, Amos CI, King TM, et al. Inheritance of susceptibility to bleomycin-induced pulmonary fibrosis in the mouse. *Cancer Res* 1996;56:2596.

122. Haston CK, Travis EL. Murine susceptibility to radiation-induced pulmonary fibrosis is influenced by a genetic factor implicated in susceptibility to bleomycin-induced pulmonary fibrosis. *Cancer Res* 1997;57:5286.

123. Schwartz DR, Homanics GE, Hoyt DG, et al. The neutral cysteine protease bleomycin hydrolase is essential for epidermal integrity and bleomycin resistance. *Proc Natl Acad Sci U S A* 1999;96:4680.

124. Eitzman DT, McCoy RD, Zheng X, et al. Bleomycin-induced pulmonary fibrosis in transgenic mice that either lack or overexpress the murine plasminogen activator inhibitor-1 gene. *J Clin Invest* 1996;97(1):232.

125. Munger JS, Huang X, Kawakatsu H, et al. The integrin αvβ6 binds and activates latent TGFβ1: a mechanism for regulating pulmonary inflammation and fibrosis. *Cell* 1999;96:319.

126. Coker RK, Laurent GJ, Shahzeidi S, et al. Transforming growth factors-β_1, -β_2, and -β_3 stimulate fibroblast procollagen production in vitro but are differentially expressed during bleomycin-induced lung fibrosis. *Am J Pathol* 1997;150(3):981.

127. Hamilton RF Jr, Li L, Felder TB, et al. Bleomycin induces apoptosis in human alveolar macrophages. *Am J Physiol* 1995;269:L318.

128. Kuwano K, Hagimoto N, Kawasaki M, et al. Essential roles of the fas-fas ligand pathway in the development of pulmonary fibrosis. *J Clin Invest* 1999;104(1):13.

129. Piguet PK, Besin C. Treatment by human recombinant soluble TNF receptor of pulmonary fibrosis induced by bleomycin or silica in mice. *Eur Respir J* 1994;7:515.

130. Giri SN, Hyde DM, Hollinger MA. Effect of antibody to transforming growth factor beta on bleomycin-induced accumulation of lung collagen in mice. *Thorax* 1993;48:959.

131. Piguet PF, Grau GE, deKossodo S. Role of granulocyte-macrophage colony stimulating factor in pulmonary fibrosis induced in mice by bleomycin. *Exp Lung Res* 1993;19:579.

132. Gurujeyalakshmi G, Hollinger MA, Giri SN. Pirfenidone inhibits PDGF isoforms in bleomycin hamster model of lung fibrosis at the translational level. *Am J Physiol* 1999;276:L311.

133. Iyer SN, Gurujeyalakshmi G, Giri SN. Effects of pirfenidone on procollagen gene expression at the transcriptional level in bleomycin hamster model of lung fibrosis. *J Pharmacol Exp Ther* 1999;289:211.

134. Nici L, Santos-Moore A, Kuhn C, et al. Modulation of bleomycin-induced pulmonary toxicity in the hamster by the antioxidant amifostine. *Cancer* 1998;83(9):2008.

135. Unemori EN, Pickford LB, Salles AL, et al. Relaxin induces an extracellular matrix-degrading phenotype in human lung fibroblasts in vitro and inhibits lung fibrosis in a murine model in vivo. *J Clin Invest* 1996;98(12):2739.

136. Weinbach J, Camus A, Barra J, et al. Transgenic mice expressing the Sh ble bleomycin resistance gene are protected against bleomycin-induced pulmonary fibrosis. *Cancer Res* 1996;56:5659.

137. Phan SH, Thrall RS, Ward PA. Bleomycin-induced pulmonary fibrosis in rats: biochemical demonstration of increased rates of collagen synthesis. *Am Rev Respir Dis* 1980;121:501.

138. Kelley J, Newman RA, Evans JN. Bleomycin-induced pulmonary fibrosis in the rat: prevention with an inhibitor of collagen synthesis. *J Lab Clin Med* 1980;96:954.

139. Thrau RS, McCormick JR, Jack RM, et al. Bleomycin-induced pulmonary fibrosis in the rat: inhibition by indomethacin. *Am J Pathol* 1979;95:117.

140. Witschi H. Exploitable biochemical approaches for the evaluation of toxic lung damage. *Essays Toxicol* 1975;6:125.

141. Sikic BI, Collins JM, Mimnaugh EG, et al. Improved therapeutic index of bleomycin when administered by continuous infusion in mice. *Cancer Treat Rep* 1978;62:2011.

142. Samuels ML, Johnson DE, Holoye PY. Continuous intravenous bleomycin (NSC-125066) therapy with vinblastine (NSC-49842) in stage III testicular neoplasia. *Cancer Chemother Rep* 1975;59:563.

143. Zucker PK, Khouri NF, Rosenshein NB. Bleomycin-induced pulmonary nodules: a variant of bleomycin pulmonary toxicity. *Gynecol Oncol* 1987;28:284.

144. Talcott JA, Garnick MB, Stomper PC, et al. Cavitary lung nodules associated with combination chemotherapy containing bleomycin. *J Urol* 1987;138:619.

145. Richman SD, Levenson SM, Bunn PA, et al. ^{67}Ga-Accumulation in pulmonary lesions associated with bleomycin toxicity. *Cancer* 1975;36:1966.

146. Burkhardt A, Gebbers JO, Holtje WJ. Die bleomycin-lunge. *Dtsch Med Wochenschr* 1977;102:281.

147. Holoye PY, Luna MA, MacKay B, et al. Bleomycin hypersensitivity pneumonitis. *Ann Intern Med* 1978;88:47.

148. Comis RL, Kuppinger MS, Ginsberg SJ, et al. Role of single-breath carbon monoxide-diffusing capacity in monitoring the pulmonary effects of bleomycin in germ-free tumor patients. *Cancer Res* 1979;39:5076.

149. Osanto S, Bukman A, Van Hoek F, et al. Long-term effects of chemotherapy in patients with testicular cancer. *J Clin Oncol* 1992;10:574.

150. Goldiner PL, Carlon GC, Critkovic E, et al. Factors influencing post-operative morbidity and mortality in patients treated with bleomycin. *Br Med J* 1978;1:1664.

151. Yagoda A, Etwbanas E, Tan CTC. Bleomycin, an antitumor antibiotic: clinical experience in 274 patients. *Ann Intern Med* 1972;77:861.

152. Maher J, Daley PA. Severe bleomycin lung toxicity: reversal with high dose corticosteroids. *Thorax* 1993;48:92.

153. Van Barneveld PW, Sleijfer DT, van der Mark TW, et al. Natural course of bleomycin-induced pneumonitis: a follow-up study. *Am Rev Respir Dis* 1987;135:48.

154. Letters to the editor. *Cancer Treat Rep* 1978;62(4):569.

155. Einhorn L, Krause M, Hornbach N, et al. Enhanced pulmonary toxicity with bleomycin and radiotherapy in oat cell lung cancer. *Cancer* 1976;37:2414.

156. Morrow CP, DiSaia PJ, Mangan CF, et al. Continuous pelvic arterial infusion with bleomycin for squamous carcinoma of the cervix recurrent after irradiation therapy. *Cancer Treat Rep* 1977;61:1403.

157. Bitter K. Pharmacokinetic behaviour of bleomycin–cobalt-57 with special regard to intra-arterial perfusion of the maxillofacial region. *J Maxillofac Surg* 1976;4:226.

158. Watring WG, Roberts JA, Lagasse LD, et al. Treatment of recurrent Paget's disease of the vulva with topical bleomycin. *Cancer* 1978;41:10.

159. Kessinger A, Wigton RS. Intracavitary bleomycin and tetracycline in the management of malignant pleural effusions: a randomized study. *J Surg Oncol* 1987;36:81.

160. Maiche AG, Virkkunen P, Kantkanen T, et al. Bleomycin and mitoxantrone in the treatment of malignant pleural effusions. *Am J Clin Oncol* 1992;16:50.

161. Bracken RB, Johnson DE, Rodriquez L, et al. Treatment of multiple superficial tumors of bladder with intravesical bleomycin. *Urology* 1977;9:161.

162. Crooke ST, Bradner WT. Bleomycin, a review. *J Med* 1976;7:333.

163. Blehan NM, Gillies NE, Twentyman PR. The effect of bleomycin and radiation in combination on bacteria and mammalian cells in culture. *Br J Radiol* 1974;47:346.

164. Takabe Y, Miyamoto T, Watanabe M, et al. Synergism of x-ray and bleomycin on Ehrlich ascites tumour cells. *Br J Cancer* 1977;36:391.

165. Fu K, Phillips TL, Silverberg IJ, et al. Combined radiotherapy and chemotherapy with bleomycin and methotrexate for advanced inoperable head and neck cancer: update of a Northern California Oncology Group randomized trial. *J Clin Oncol* 1987;5:1410.

17

ANTITUMOR ANTIBIOTICS

JAAP VERWEIJ
ALEX SPARREBOOM
KEES NOOTER

Over several decades, microbial fermentation has yielded many valuable compounds, such as the anthracyclines, bleomycins, and various unusual nucleosides, which are discussed in separate chapters. In this chapter we consider three relatively long-standing antibiotics of diverse structure. Dactinomycin (actinomycin D or DACT) is still one of the most valuable drugs in pediatric oncology, whereas mitomycin C, although largely replaced by newer classes of agents, is still occasionally used in treating tumors of the gastrointestinal and respiratory tracts, and for intravesicular treatment of bladder cancer. Mithramycin, although an active agent in testicular cancer, has been supplanted by more active and less toxic drugs, and remains of value only because of its hypocalcemic effect.

DACTINOMYCIN

DACT, a product of the *Streptomyces* yeast species, was discovered in 1940,[1] was introduced into the clinic in 1954,[2] and has since been identified as an active cytotoxic drug for gestational choriocarcinoma,[3,4] Wilms' tumor,[5,6] neuroblastoma,[7] childhood rhabdomyosarcoma,[8] and Ewing's sarcoma.[9] Numerous analogs have been isolated from various sources, but none has demonstrated superiority over DACT. Its key pharmacologic features are given in Table 17-1.

Mechanism of Action and Cellular Pharmacology

The structure of DACT[10] is shown in Figure 17-1. It consists of two symmetric polypeptide chains attached to a central phenoxazone ring. Naturally occurring actinomycins differ in the peptide chains but not in the phenoxazone ring.[11] DACT is known to be a strong DNA-binding drug and a potent inhibitor of RNA and protein synthesis. Actual binding to DNA was shown to occur preferentially with guanine-cytidine base pairs.[12] Based on spectroscopy and hydrodynamic studies, Muller and Crothers proposed a model for the DNA-DACT intercalation.[13] In this model, the drug's chromophore (the phenoxazone ring) lies intercalated between base pairs with the peptide lactone rings lying in the minor groove. Structural information obtained by x-ray crystallographic studies and later by nuclear magnetic resonance led to a further refinement of the intercalating model.[14–16]

The most stable complex of DACT with DNA is formed by interaction of the drug with the sequence dGpdC on one DNA strand and the complementary sequence on the other strand. However, DACT may also bind to other base sequences on DNA.[17,18] The crystal structure of the complex formed between DACT and the sequence dGpdC has been solved[19] and involves a nonclassic pseudointercalation of drug inserted between bases of nonpaired strands of the helix. This finding seems to be unique to the d(GC) dinucleotide pair, because two-dimensional proton–magnetic resonance studies on the complex formed between DACT and the hexanucleoside pentaphosphate d(ATGCAT) have revealed a classic intercalation structure[20] confirmed by studies of this complex in the crystalline state.[21] These findings imply that the preferential binding is probably the simple intercalation of a planar ring between adjacent bases. Besides binding to double-strand DNA, DACT is also known to bind to single-strand DNA (ssDNA).[22]

In addition to the structural studies described above, other research has made progress in elucidating the kinetics of DACT binding to DNA. Although early studies suggested that conformational changes in the drug were responsible for the slow, complicated kinetics of association between DACT and DNA,[13] this has now been ruled out.[23] The association rate does not depend on polynucleotide sequence or length but probably reflects the summation of multiple sites of interaction with DNA.

DACT also binds to the ssDNA in the open complex formed by the polymerase and prevents reannealing of

TABLE 17-1. KEY FEATURES OF DACTINOMYCIN

Mechanism of action:	Inhibition of RNA and protein synthesis
Metabolism:	Unknown
Pharmacokinetics:	$t_{1/2\beta}$: 36 h
Elimination:	Renal: 6–30%, Bile: 5–11%
Drug interactions:	None
Toxicity:	Myelosuppression
	Nausea and vomiting
	Mucositis
	Diarrhea
	Necrosis at extravasation
	Radiation sensitization and recall reactions
Precautions:	Avoid extravasation

$t_{1/2}$, half-life.

ssDNA. Results suggest that stabilization of unusual ssDNA hairpins by DACT may be an important aspect of its potent transcription inhibition activity.[24]

The elongation of RNA chains is more seriously impaired than initiation, termination, or release of RNA.[25] RNA synthesis inhibition by DACT has proved to be a useful tool for measuring degradation rates of prelabeled RNA species, as well as dependence of various cellular functions on synthesis of new molecules of RNA or protein.

DACT has been shown to be taken up in tissues by passive diffusion.[26] The response to DACT depends on the ability of the cell to accumulate and retain the drug.[27] Transport of DACT into cells varies among different tumors and cell types and is markedly enhanced by increased temperature or alterations in the membrane lipid bilayer.[28,29] *In vitro* studies in the murine T-cell hybridoma line A1.1 suggest that DACT induces cell death via apoptosis.[30]

Although high doses of DACT inhibited growth in a human embryonal rhabdomyosarcoma cell line and induced cytotoxicity, at low doses the drug induced morphologic and

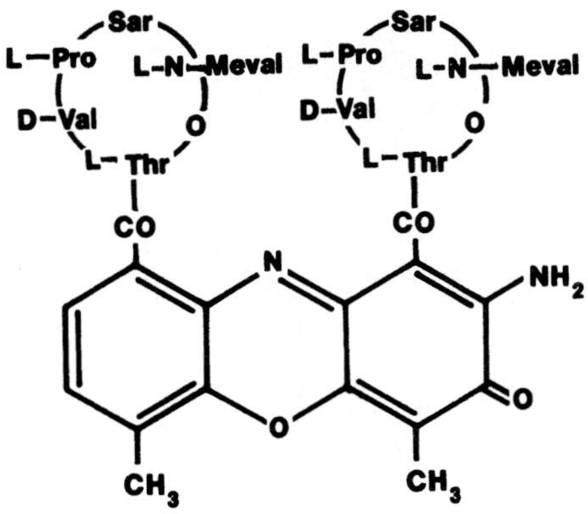

FIGURE 17-1. Structure of dactinomycin. (D-Val, D-valine; L-N-Meval, methylvaline; L-Thr, L-threonine; L-Pro, L-proline; Sar, sarcosine.)

phenotypic differentiation.[31] Apparently, low-dose DACT releases these cells from their differentiation blockade, allowing them to recover normal myogenic development. This suggests a potential role for differentiation therapy in the treatment of rhabdomyosarcomas.

Mechanism of Resistance

Initial studies suggested that resistance to DACT was related to reduced uptake[32] associated with decreased cell membrane permeability.[33] Indeed, detergents such as polysorbate 80[34] and amphotericin B,[35] which increase cell membrane permeability, enhance drug uptake and overcome resistance *in vitro*.

More recent work on resistance, however, has implicated increased efflux.[36] Indeed, Chinese hamster ovary cells were found to be cross-resistant to DACT and to other drugs such as vinca alkaloids,[37] anthracyclines,[37] and epipodophyllotoxins,[38] and a human erythroleukemia cell line was cross-resistant to DACT, vincristine sulfate, and doxorubicin hydrochloride.[39] In several instances, drug resistance could be overcome with verapamil hydrochloride,[39,40] which suggested that DACT resistance is part of the P-glycoprotein multidrug resistance (MDR) phenotype.[41,42] Indeed, human tumor cell lines made resistant to DACT *in vitro* were found to amplify P-glycoprotein–encoding genes.[43,44] Finally, lipophilic agents with low toxicity, recognized and processed by the molecular system involved in MDR and able to reverse MDR by saturating the system at high concentrations, were able to increase accumulation of DACT in MDR WEHI 164 cells.[45] Thus, an increased drug efflux, mediated by overexpression of the P-170 membrane glycoprotein, seems to play an important role in resistance to DACT *in vitro*. This hypothesis requires confirmation in studies of human tumors with *de novo* or acquired resistance to DACT.

Drug Interactions

No pharmacokinetic interactions between DACT and other drugs are known.

Clinical Pharmacology

The pharmacokinetics of DACT have been studied in rat, monkey, and dog[46] using thin-layer chromatography and electrophoresis after administration of tritium-labeled actinomycin D. In these species, serum levels of DACT declined rapidly after administration, with concomitant accumulation of drug in the tissues.

The mean drug half-life in tissues was 47 hours. No metabolites have been identified. Urinary excretion varies from 6% to 31%, and bile excretion varies from 5% to 11%. A very limited study in humans yielded similar results.[47] The half-life of distribution was very short, whereas the plasma elimination half-life was 36 hours. Urinary and fecal excretion were 20% and 14%, respectively. Only 3.3% of the urinary excretion consisted of metabolites. Clearly, more extensive and detailed pharmacokinetic studies are required in humans.

By adsorbing DACT onto polybutylcyanoacrylate nanoparticles, one can achieve a significant increase of drug concentration in muscle, spleen, and liver in Wistar rats, whereas urinary excretion is diminished.[48] Similar results were obtained by liposome entrapment of DACT.[49] Although no slow-release system has yet resulted in a higher efficacy,[49,50] some enhanced activity has been suggested with liposomes when studied in S250 soft tissue sarcoma–bearing rats.[51] Based on pharmacokinetic data and the schedule dependency of DACT activity in tumor-bearing mice,[52] single-dose intermittent schedules have been developed and have been compared with daily administration of DACT for 5 days. The data indicate similar antitumor activity[53] without increased toxicity.[54]

Toxicity

At the usual clinical dosages of 10 to 15 mg per kg per day for 5 days, DACT causes nausea, vomiting, diarrhea, mucositis, and hair loss. The major and dose-limiting side effect is myelosuppression, with a white blood cell and platelet nadir occurring 8 to 14 days after drug administration.[55] Drug extravasation results in soft tissue necrosis.[55] Rare but sometimes severe side effects include a venoocclusive disease–like hepatotoxicity[56–58] that occurs almost exclusively in children treated for Wilms' tumor[59] and immune thrombocytopenia.[60] By inhibiting repair of sublethal radiation-induced damage,[61] DACT acts as a radiosensitizer[62,63] and may also cause radiation recall phenomena, in which patients receiving DACT experience inflammatory reactions in previously irradiated sites. The clinical consequences of such reactions may be serious, especially with the involvement of vital organs.[64] Corticosteroids may ameliorate these reactions.

MITHRAMYCIN (PLICAMYCIN)

Mithramycin (NSC-24559) was isolated from a fermentation broth of *Streptomyces plicatus*.[65] Although the drug had antitumor activity in embryonal cell carcinoma of the testis,[66] its primary use was in the treatment of hypercalcemia of malignancy unresponsive to other therapy,[67] for which recently it has largely been replaced by biphosphonates.[68] Some years ago interest in this agent was rekindled by the observation that in low doses it promoted maturation of myeloblasts,[69] but a study has shown that it is largely ineffective in the blast phase of chronic myeloid leukemia, although it may still be of value in the accelerated phase.[70] The key features of mithramycin are summarized in Table 17-2.

TABLE 17-2. KEY FEATURES OF MITHRAMYCIN

Mechanism of action:	Probably DNA binding inhibiting RNA synthesis
Metabolism:	Unknown
Pharmacokinetics:	$t_{1/2\alpha}$: 1 h
	$t_{1/2\beta}$: 12 h
Elimination:	Renal: 40%
Drug interactions:	None
Toxicity:	Hemorrhagic syndrome
	Nausea and vomiting
	Hepatotoxicity
	Renal toxicity
	Diarrhea
	Stomatitis
Precautions:	None

$t_{1/2}$, half-life.

Mechanism of Action and Cellular Pharmacology

Mithramycin consists of a crystalline aglycone (chromomycinone) with three attached sugar moieties (olivose, oliose, and mycarose) (Fig. 17-2). The drug occurs as a bright yellow crystalline powder, has a molecular weight of 1,085, and is slightly soluble in water. The antineoplastic activity of mithramycin is believed to result from binding to DNA, but the precise mechanism of action is not fully understood. Experimental evidence has shown that the drug forms complexes with DNA in the presence of divalent cations, especially magnesium, thereby inhibiting DNA-

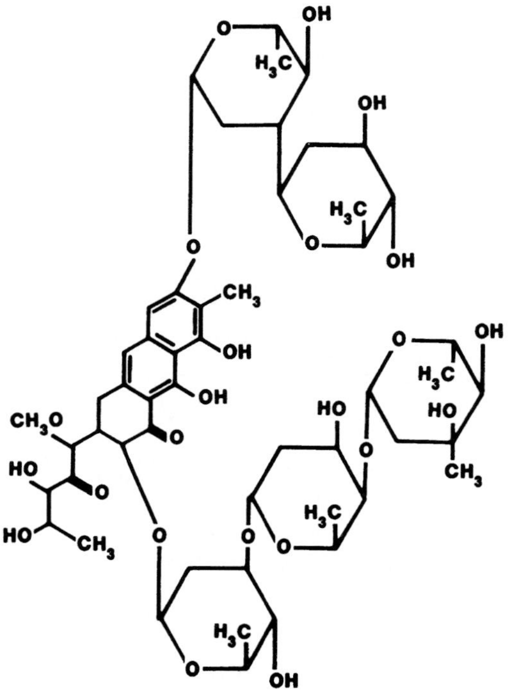

FIGURE 17-2. Structure of mithramycin.

dependent synthesis of RNA.[71,72] Whether or not binding to DNA occurs through intercalation of the DNA structure is not clear.[71,73] Mithramycin binds preferentially to guanine-cytosine base pairs.[74] This is consistent with the observed competition between DACT and mithramycin for binding sites on DNA.[75] The inhibition of DNA-directed RNA synthesis seems to be the principal biochemical effect of mithramycin and occurs within 3 hours of incubation with mithramycin, at a time when DNA synthesis is unaffected. Mithramycin inhibits transcription from the human c-*myc* and promotors *in vitro*[76] as well as *in vivo*.[77] Mithramycin also inhibits binding of transcription-activating proteins or factors to G-C–rich promoter regions of the SV40 virus genome,[78] a finding which suggests that RNA synthesis inhibition may result from anti-promoter actions.

Mechanism of Resistance

Because of its infrequent use, the mechanism of resistance to mithramycin has received very little study. Vinblastine-resistant mutants of Chinese hamster ovary cells showed cross-resistance to mithramycin.[37] In addition, some data obtained in patients with acute leukemias or the blastic phase of chronic myeloid leukemia[79] suggest that mithramycin is involved in the MDR phenotype. Recently, an ATP-binding cassette (ABC) transporter was found to be essential for mithramycin resistance in the producer *Streptomyces argillaceus*. Antibiotic producers must possess a resistance mechanism to ensure the survival of the organism during the biosynthesis of the toxic molecule. Mithramycin is synthesized by *S. argillaceus,* which is highly resistant to mithramycin *in vivo* but sensitive to the related drugs chromomycin and olivomycin. A gene, designated *mtrA,* encoding an adenosine triphosphate–binding protein of the ABC transporter superfamily was found to be responsible for this resistance pattern.[80]

Drug Interactions

No pharmacokinetic interactions between mithramycin and other drugs are known.

Clinical Pharmacology

No sensitive analytical assay is available for mithramycin. Human pharmacokinetic data are limited to the data from a patient with glioblastoma who was given tritium-labeled mithramycin.[81] The initial plasma half-life was approximately 1 hour, followed by a slow decline of plasma radioactivity over the next 12 hours. The urinary excretion was 42% over 15 hours, which indicated that the plasma elimination half-life is approximately 15 hours. The most feasible administration regimen for mithramycin seems to be an alternate-day administration of 50 mg per kg per day for three to eight doses per course, with courses repeated every 4 weeks.[82] For the treatment of hypercalcemia, doses of 15 to 25 mg per kg may be given at 4- to 7-day intervals, as required to control serum calcium.

Toxicity

The most severe side effect of mithramycin is a diffuse hemorrhagic syndrome with thrombocytopenia, capillary endothelial cell swelling, and perivascular leukocyte infiltration.[83] The incidence of this syndrome increases from approximately 5% in patients treated for less than 10 days with doses of 30 mg per kg per day or less to more than 10% if higher doses or longer courses are used.

Decreased platelet aggregation,[84,85] reduced platelet adenosine diphosphate content,[85] reduced levels of coagulation factors II, V, VII, and X with prolonged clotting and prothrombin times,[83] and increased fibrinolytic activity[83] have been reported.

Common side effects include nausea, vomiting, and anorexia; less frequently, diarrhea, stomatitis, and fever are observed.[86] Furthermore, hepatotoxicity[86,87] and renal toxicity[87] are rather common sequelae of high-dose regimens, whereas skin toxicity[88] and neurotoxicity are rare. These side effects are all ameliorated by using an alternate-day regimen.

Because of these side effects, mithramycin has become an unattractive anticancer drug. At lower dosages than required for antitumor activity, however, mithramycin can still be used for the treatment of hypercalcemia. It inhibits bone resorption[89] caused by factors such as parathyroid hormone,[90] prostaglandin E_2,[91] or serum factors in multiple myeloma.[91]

MITOMYCIN C (MUTAMYCIN)

Mitomycin C (MMC) was isolated from *Streptomyces caespitosus* in 1958.[92] The initial clinical studies used daily low-dose schedules, which resulted in unacceptably severe, cumulative myelosuppression. In more recent trials, an intermittent dosing schedule was introduced, using bolus injections every 4 to 8 weeks, which resulted in more manageable hematologic toxicity. With the latter schedule MMC was found to be active against a wide variety of solid tumors, including breast cancer, non–small cell lung cancer, gastric cancer, pancreatic cancer, gallbladder cancer, colorectal cancer, cervical cancer, prostatic cancer, and superficial bladder cancer (Table 17-3). In addition MMC is used as a radiosensitizer in combination with radiotherapy for the treatment of epidermoid anal cancer[111] and head and neck cancer.[112] Several analogs with suggested superior activity to the parent drug have entered clinical trials.[113–115] Key features of MMC are listed in Table 17-4.

TABLE 17-3. SINGLE-AGENT ACTIVITY OF MITOMYCIN C IN SOLID TUMORS

Tumor type	No. of evaluated patients	Response rate (%)	References
Breast	394[a]	18[a]	93
(Non–small cell) lung	356[a]	26[a]	94–97
Stomach	343[a]	29[a]	98, 99
Pancreatic	44	27	100
Gallbladder	30	10	101
Colorectal	272	16	102
Cervical	173[a]	36[a]	103, 104
Prostatic	81	21[a]	105–107
Superficial bladder	276[a,b]	67[a,b]	108–110

[a]Cumulative data.
[b]Intravesical administration.

Mechanism of Action and Cellular Pharmacology

Studies have revealed the absolute stereochemical configuration of MMC[116] (Fig. 17-3). The mitomycins have unique chemical structures in which quinone, aziridine, and carbamate functions are arranged around a pyrrolo[l,2-*a*]indole nucleus. They are the only known naturally occurring compounds containing an aziridine ring. MMC is soluble in both aqueous and organic solvents.

In aqueous solution the drug is unstable; decomposition is strongly pH dependent. Mild acidic conditions result in cleavage of the C-9a-methoxy group, formation of a C-9=C-9a double bond, and opening of the aziridine ring (Fig. 17-4).[117] Protonation of the C-9a-methoxy group is assumed to be the triggering factor in the acid hydrolysis of MMC.[118] The 1,2-disubstituted indoloquinones thus obtained are referred to as *mitosenes*. Extended hydrolysis in dilute acidic solutions also causes replacement of the C-7-amino function by a hydroxyl group.[119] Pronounced acidic conditions lead to cleavage of the C-10-carbamate function in addition to that of the other labile functions already mentioned.[120] Hydrolysis of MMC in alkaline solution leads to replacement of the C-7-aminofunction by a hydroxyl group[121] and to cleavage of the C-10-carbamate function,[120] but has no effect on the C-9a-methoxy or the aziridine groups. Under pronounced alkaline conditions the quinone chromophore is destroyed.[121]

Because of its chemical instability in solution, the clinical formulation of MMC is a lyophilized form containing mannitol (Mutamycin) or sodium chloride (Mitomycin Kyowa) as excipients. After dissolution in water, MMC is administered intravenously. The stability of the reconstituted solutions is limited. Storage of MMC at room temperature in unbuffered solutions (pH 7.0) for 5 days seems justified.[122]

Formation of DNA Adducts

Early studies of the molecular pharmacology of MMC revealed that the drug cross-linked the complementary strands of DNA,[123] and evidence was also obtained for monofunctional alkylation, that is, attachment to a single DNA strand.[124] MMC has been demonstrated to exert its activity primarily as a DNA replication inhibitor, and DNA interstrand cross-linking is regarded as the most highly lethal type of MMC-induced damage,[124] although monofunctional alkylation is by far the most frequently observed interaction.[125] DNA cross-linking and alkylating activity require the chemical or enzymatic reduction of the quinone function, which transforms the drug into a highly reactive alkylator. Although the initial hypothesis regarding the mechanism of this process pointed to a central role of the C-1 aziridine and the C-10 carbamate groups of the molecule,[126] more recent research specified several additional

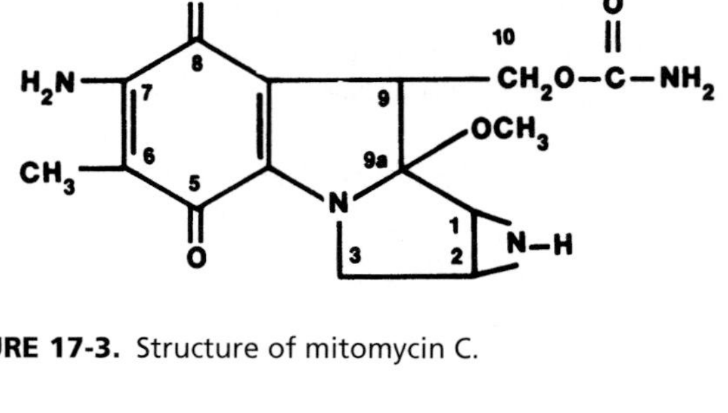

TABLE 17-4. KEY FEATURES OF MITOMYCIN C

Mechanism of action:	Alkylation of DNA
Metabolism:	Hepatic
Pharmacokinetics:	$t_{1/2\alpha}$: 2–10 min
	$t_{1/2\beta}$: 25–90 min
Elimination:	Renal: 1–20%
Drug interaction:	None
Toxicity:	Myelosuppression
	Necrosis at extravasation
	Hemolytic uremic syndrome
	Interstitial pneumonitis
	Cardiomyopathy
Precautions:	Avoid extravasation.

$t_{1/2}$, half-life.

FIGURE 17-3. Structure of mitomycin C.

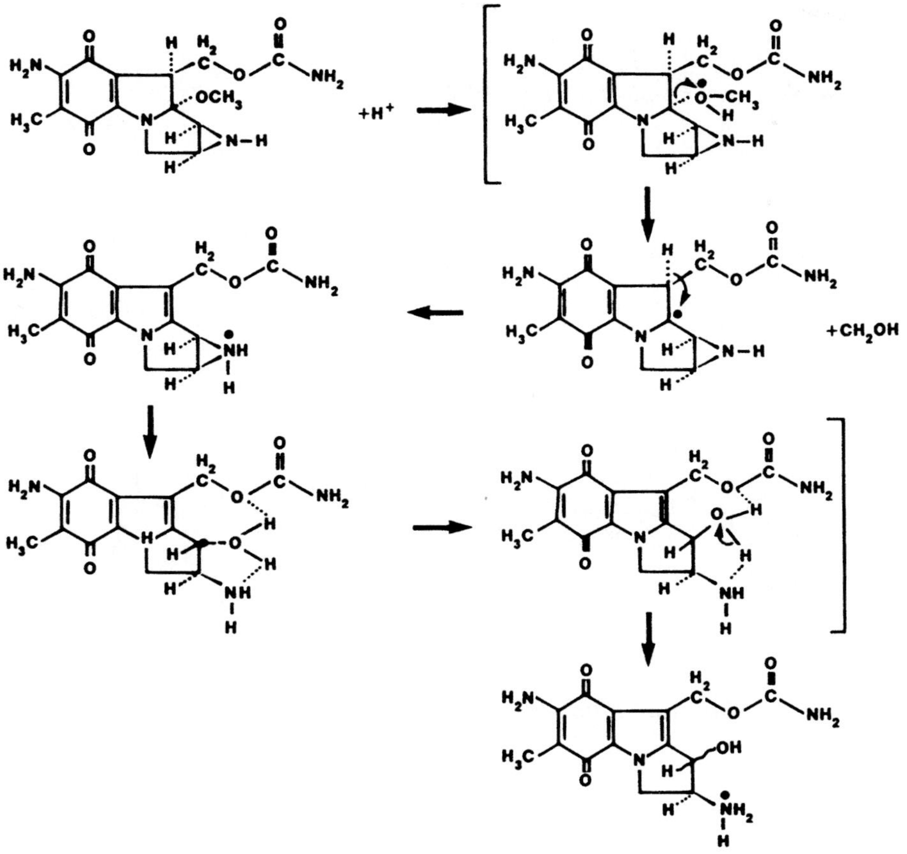

FIGURE 17-4. Mechanism of the acid-catalyzed hydrolysis of mitomycin C (R=H).

reactive electrophiles, featuring a quinone methide[127] (see later) and the oxidized forms aziridinomitosene and leuco-aziridinomitosene.[128] The chemical identity of the DNA cross-links induced by reduced MMC has been determined by isolating cross-linked nucleosides from treated DNA.[129] Monofunctionally alkylated nucleosides (monoadducts) formed alongside the cross-linked adduct were also isolated,[130] in addition to a DNA intrastrand cross-link by a MMC that results from 2,7-diaminomitosene, a major metabolic product of enzymatic activation lacking the aziridine function.[131] This latter adduct was found to be sequence-specific to guanines in the $(G)_n$ tract of DNA, which indicates that selective removal of the aziridine function of MMC results in a switch from minor to major groove alkylation of DNA. Acidic activation of MMC is the second mechanism by which DNA alkylation can be produced.[132]

Reductive Alkylation

The need for reduction of MMC to produce alkylating reactions led in 1972 to the introduction of the term *bioreductive alkylation* to describe a proposed mechanism of drug action.[133] MMC is considered to be a prototype of the bioreductive alkylating agents. Two mechanisms exist through which reductive metabolism mediates the cytotoxic effects of MMC. First, under anaerobic conditions,

one- or two-electron reduction followed by spontaneous loss of methanol leads to the formation of reactive unstable intermediates.

Initially two possible sites of attack on the intermediate by nucleophils (C-1 and C-10) were postulated.[126] This suggested mechanism was later revised.[134] The hypothesis included formation of a hydroquinone and its rearrangement to yield a quinone-methide followed by a nucleophilic addition of DNA leading to a monoalkylated product. Intramolecular displacement of the carbamate group would then result in the cross-linked adduct (Fig. 17-5). The formation of a quinone-methide indeed was confirmed.[135] Although the cross-linking of MMC to DNA in viable cells has been observed and cell extracts dependent on the reduced form of nicotinamide adenine dinucleotide phosphate (NADPH) that are capable of activating MMC have been prepared, reproducing the process in model systems *in vitro* has been difficult. Reduction can be easily accomplished, but covalent binding to DNA has been difficult to reproduce. The addition of a reducing agent increases the binding to DNA[136] by creating conditions favorable for the maintenance of the semiquinone radical, the intermediate that is formed by the first electron uptake of MMC.

For this reason the semiquinone is believed to bind initially to DNA.[136] The existence of the semiquinone radical during the reduction of MMC has been proven in several

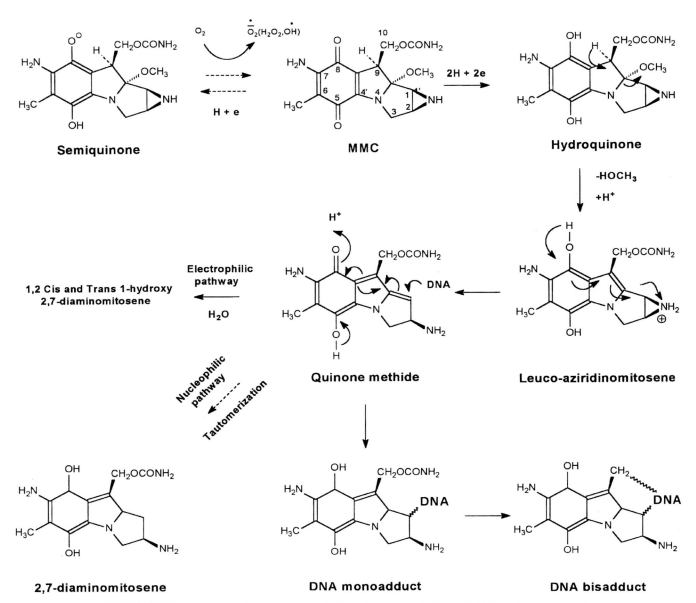

FIGURE 17-5. Proposed pathways of metabolic activation and DNA alkylation of mitomycin C (MMC) after one- or two-electron quinone reduction. (Modified from Reddy MV, Randerath K. ^{32}P-Analysis of DNA adducts in somatic and reproductive tissues of rats treated with the anticancer antibiotic mitomycin C. *Mutat Res* 1987;179:75–88; and Cummings J, Spanswick VJ, Smyth JF. Re-evaluation of the molecular pharmacology of mitomycin C. *Eur J Cancer* 1995;31A:1928–1933.)

studies, and evidence is increasing that one-electron reduction is sufficient to activate both the C-1 and C-10 electrophilic centers.[137–140]

Aerobic Activation

Under aerobic conditions a second mechanism comes into play through which MMC develops its cytotoxic effect. Reductive metabolism again leads to the formation of reduced MMC; however, its aerobic fate is different. Molecular oxygen reacts with either the short-lived semiquinone radical[137,141] or the hydroquinone form to generate the superoxide radical anion,[137,141] hydroxyl radicals,[142,143] or

hydrogen peroxide.[144] Formation of these highly reactive species may lead to cytotoxic effects such as lipid peroxidation or nucleic acid damage and can be prevented by free radical scavengers such as mannitol as well as by protective enzymes such as superoxide dismutase or catalase.

Whether the reactive intermediate of MMC is formed through the radical semiquinone or the dianion (hydroquinone form) depends on the half-life of the radical anion. In an aprotic environment the radical anion may have a considerable lifetime; in protic media, however, it exists only a few milliseconds, with rapid uptake of a second electron. Furthermore, oxygen definitely plays an important role, as it is a specific inhibitor of the two-electron pathway because of interaction with and inactivation of the semiquinone species by oxygen.

Reductive activation of MMC to the semiquinone can be accomplished either by enzyme systems or by chemical reducing agents such as sodium borohydride,[126] molecular hydrogen in combination with platinum dioxide or palladium as a catalyst,[117] or sodium thiosulfate.[126,136] Enzyme systems capable of activating MMC include NADPH–cytochrome P-450 reductase,[145,146] xanthine oxidase,[147] xanthine dehydrogenase,[148] and NADH–cytochrome b_5 reductase[149,150] (for overviews, see Cummings et al.[151] and Ross et al.[152]).

A controversial aspect of the bioreductive activation of mitomycin C concerns the role of an enzyme called DT-diaphorase (DTD). DTD is an obligate two-electron reductase that is characterized by its ability to use both the reduced form of nicotinamide adenine dinucleotide (NADH) and NADPH as electron donors and by its inhibition by dicumarol.[153] A number of studies have implicated DTD in the bioreductive activation of mitomycin C in tumor cell systems, although the initial studies with purified DTD were inconclusive.[154,155] Both MMC-induced cytotoxicity and induction of DNA interstrand cross-links, however, were found to be DTD dependent and could be inhibited by pretreatment of HT-29 colon carcinoma cell lines with dicumarol.[156]

The ability of DTD to metabolize MMC to a reactive cytotoxic species suggests that the level of DTD may be an important determinant of the antitumor activity of MMC. The expression of the NADPH:quinone oxireductase gene (NQO1) encoding for DTD was greatly decreased in resistant colon carcinoma cell lines, and this correlated extremely well with the reduction in DTD activity.[157]

As MMC appears not to be the best substrate for DTD (due to a mechanism-based inhibition of DTD within the pH range of 7.0 to 7.8),[156,158] NQO1 may serve as an important target for the development of novel bioreductive antitumor agents.

In an interesting paper, Nishiyama et al.[159] report that the role of DTD in MMC-induced cytotoxicity *in vitro* may differ from that *in vivo*, where they found an inverse relationship between DTD activity and MMC cytotoxicity with augmentation of the cytotoxicity by the addition of the DTD inhibitor dicumarol.

The NADPH–cytochrome P-450 reductase is a flavoprotein containing 1 mole each of flavin mononucleotide and flavin adenine dinucleotide, and its function is to transfer electrons from NADPH to the various forms of cytochrome P-450. The involvement of this cytochrome P-450 enzyme in MMC activation was first described in 1979.[145] To further define the role of this enzyme, it was transfected into Chinese hamster ovary cells. Results confirmed the significance of the enzyme in MMC activation to toxic species, with greater cytotoxicity occurring under hypoxic conditions.[160,161] This was suggested in earlier studies also, which showed that, under anaerobic conditions, cytotoxicity of MMC was independent of NADPH–cytochrome P-450.[162,163] Also, in EMT-6 cells dicumarol inhibits MMC-induced toxicity in air but paradoxically potentiates toxicity under hypoxic conditions.[164] In addition, the aerobic sensitivity of Chinese hamster ovary cells and human fibroblasts has been associated with elevated NQO1 levels, but sensitive and resistant cells, which had widely different levels of NQO1, demonstrated similar sensitivities to MMC under hypoxic conditions.[165]

These and other data may suggest that the enzymes involved in the reduction of MMC under hypoxic conditions may not be the same as those observed under aerobic conditions, or that the products of reduction, and hence those responsible for alkylation, may differ.

The process of alkylation of DNA nucleotides by MMC has been clarified by work with model nucleophils[166,167] in aqueous solution under reducing conditions that may mimic the *in vivo* process. This approach provided information concerning both the initial reaction site in MMC subject to nucleophilic attack as well as the mechanism of these transformations. Ideal nucleophils were found to be potassium ethyl xanthate[166] and potassium ethyl monothiocarbonate.[167] Both mono- and disubstituted mitosenes with nucleophiles at C-1, C-10, or both of MMC have been identified. This work constituted the first demonstration of chemical reactivity at both C-1 and C-10 of MMC on reductive activation and thus supported the mechanism of action proposed for this drug. Discrimination between the two reaction sites (C-1 and C-10) is possible by decreasing the temperature during the alkylation reaction.[167] Under these milder conditions, substitution at C-1 occurred preferentially. Displacement of the carbamate group at C-10 in the monofunctionally alkylated molecule is readily observed under reductive conditions[167]; this result implies that, after monofunctional alkylation of MMC at C-1, secondary activation of monofunctionally bound MMC at C-10 is probably the main route for the bifunctional binding of MMC to nucleophiles and for cross-linking of DNA.[140,147] The reaction at G-10 leading to alkylation has been examined by means of chemical reduction of MMC in alcoholic solvents, which results in the isolation and identification of C-10-methyl adducts. A mechanism of C-10 alkylation that proceeds through the intermediacy of an iminium ion has been proposed.[168]

Analysis of DNA Adducts

Several studies have been published on covalent interactions between MMC and DNA or DNA fragments.[129,169–172] As with model nucleophils, adducts were characterized as mono- or bifunctional mitosene derivatives. Actual binding sites of MMC in DNA are the N-6 position of adenine residues or either the N-2 or N-7 position of guanine residues.[129,169–171] Reassignment of the previously suggested attachment to the O-6 position of guanine has been reported.[171] Acid-activated MMC was found to alkylate preferentially the guanine N-7 position, in contrast to reductively activated MMC, which preferentially alkylates the guanine N-2 position, possibly because of the different electronic structures of acid- and reduction-activated MMC.

The activation mechanism of MMC can presumably now be evaluated from analysis of the DNA adducts formed *in vivo*.

The question of whether this drug is preferentially activated to a cytotoxic intermediate in hypoxic cells remains unanswered.[173–177] Preferential activation of MMC to cytotoxic metabolites in hypoxic tumor cells has been demonstrated in the murine cell lines EMT-6 and S-180.[143] However, although MMC has the potential to attack selectively the chemotherapy-resistant hypoxic cell components of solid tumors, selective toxicity to hypoxic cells could not be observed *in vivo* using the same EMT-6 cell line[173] or other cell lines and fresh tumors.[174] The proposal was made that this failure might result from the poor penetration of MMC into avascular tumor regions. In the search for agents that are more preferentially toxic to hypoxic cells than MMC, Sartorelli found that the related agent porfiromycin produces a greater differential kill of hypoxic EMT-6 cells in culture than of their oxygenated counterparts[175]; however, porfiromycin was considerably less toxic to aerobic cells than MMC.[176] Because the preferential toxicity for hypoxic cells remains a possibility, a combined regimen of radiation and MMC (or porfiromycin) has been proposed for treating locally advanced solid tumors.[111,112,176,178] Radiation is most effective against aerobic tumor cells, whereas MMC may eradicate the radiation-resistant hypoxic cells.

Induction of Apoptosis

Most anticancer drugs kill cells by a programmed process referred to as apoptosis. The intrinsic threshold of a particular cell for induction of apoptosis may determine its sensitivity to the killing effects of drugs and may constitute an alternative mechanism of drug resistance. A number of (proto)oncogenes and tumor suppressor genes have been shown to be involved in the apoptotic pathway. The p53 tumor suppressor gene is thought to play a central role in drug-induced apoptosis. DNA damage induced by genotoxic drugs such as MMC leads to up-regulation of p53,[179] which is a transcription factor for genes involved in cell-cycle arrest and apoptosis. Cell-cycle arrest allows time for repair, but when the damage is too severe, apoptosis occurs.[180] Although the view is generally accepted that the p53 tumor suppressor gene may play an important role in drug-induced apoptosis, the role of its immediate downstream effector p21/Waf1/Cip1 is less clear. The p53-independent up-regulation of p21 may also have an important role in the induction of apoptosis.[180]

Interestingly, avian and mammalian B and T lymphocytes have a differential sensitivity to a number of anticancer agents. In a chicken embryo model system,[181] differentiating B lymphocytes (bursacytes) appeared more sensitive than T lymphocytes (thymocytes) to the cytotoxic effects of MMC, probably due to early and extensive triggering of apoptosis in the differentiating B lymphocytes.[182] In virally transformed B- and T-lymphoma cell lines, no quantitative differences were found between the B and T cell lines in the induction of cross-links by both MMC and its aminodisulfide analog BMY25067 (or BMS-181174). Analysis of the persistence of the DNA lesions over multiple cell cycles revealed that, in both cell lines, the DNA damage was almost not repaired. At comparable levels of DNA damage, however, the B-lymphoma cells were easily triggered into apoptosis whereas the T-lymphoma cells were not. Apparently, the B-lymphoma cell lines have a lower intrinsic threshold for induction of apoptosis than the T-lymphoma lines.

Mutagenesis

Most anticancer drugs are mutagenic, and the alkylating agents in particular have been subject to research on mutagenicity. Although the majority of DNA damage is repaired by the different cellular DNA repair systems, persisting DNA lesions may lead to enhanced mutagenesis, due to the occurrence of errors on replication of a damaged template. Monofunctionally activated MMC has been shown to cause a substantial increase in the mutation frequency in human Ad293 cells transfected with a shuttle vector plasmid pSP189.[183] The observed bias of mutations of G:C and the formation of guanine monoadducts suggest that monoadducts may be responsible for the mutations. In *Saccharomyces cerevisiae* strains the highest mutagenic activity was found at high P-450 and glutathione content,[184] which confirmed the relevance of metabolizing enzymes and mitochondrial function on MMC's mechanism of action.

Mechanism of Resistance

The mechanisms of resistance to MMC are incompletely understood but probably involve changes in drug accumulation, bioactivation, inactivation of the alkylating species, and DNA excision repair.[185–187] In a series of Chinese hamster ovary cell mutants selected for MMC resistance, a progressive loss of MMC activation capacity and increased capacity for excision repair of DNA was found as cells became more drug resistant.[186] The specific bioactivation enzyme system deficient in the resistant cells was not identified in these studies, although the primary activation mechanism in the sensitive parent was sensitive to dicumarol and therefore probably to DTD. In some resistant cell lines, MMC shares in the MDR phenotype that encompasses doxorubicin, vincristine, and other natural products and that is mediated by overexpression of the drug efflux protein P-170.[187,188] On the other hand, several drugs known to reverse MDR induced by other drugs were not capable of reversing MMC-induced MDR, which suggests yet unexplained differences in MDR.[189] One subline of the HCT 116 human colon carcinoma cell line resistant to MMC had an increased expression of a 148,000-molecular-weight membrane protein, the level of which correlated with the degree of MMC resistance.[185] The investigators observed no *in vitro* cross-resistance to other natural product–type cytotoxic agents. The increased expression of this cell surface protein in drug-resistant phenotypes may be a useful marker for MMC resistance.

Finally, in the MDR leukemia cell line P388/R-84, increased glutathione transferase–dependent drug detoxification was found to represent another mechanism of MMC resistance.[190,191]

Drug Interactions

No pharmacokinetic interactions between MMC and other drugs are known. A suggested interaction with furosemide[192] was excluded in a pharmacokinetic study.[193]

Clinical Pharmacology

Although MMC was isolated in 1958, detailed pharmacokinetic data were not available for many years due to the absence of suitable analytic methodologies with sufficient assay sensitivity. Analytic methods based on bioassays measuring cytotoxicity in repair-deficient mutant Chinese hamster ovary cells,[194] adenosine triphosphate bioluminescence assays,[195] or reversed-phase high-pressure liquid chromatography assays with ultraviolet (365 nm),[192,196–205] polarographic,[206] or mass-spectrometric detection[207] have been developed and are more sensitive than the microbiologic assay used in earlier work.[208,209] Currently, high-pressure liquid chromatography assays with ultraviolet detection are the most widely used and have lower limits of quantitation of around 5 ng per mL with a 25-µL sample volume. All investigators have reported a biexponential decline of the plasma concentration-time curves, which corresponds to a two-compartment model with linear pharmacokinetics up to doses as high as 60 mg per m².[210]

The reader is referred to the excellent review of MMC pharmacokinetics by Dorr[210] for further information. After a rapid distribution half-life (2 to 10 minutes), elimination half-life is 25 to 90 minutes (mean, 54 minutes). A remarkable observation in two studies was an unexplained increase in total-body clearance and decrease in area under the plasma concentration × time curve of MMC after combination chemotherapy that included 5-fluorouracil and doxorubicin.[201,211] No correlations have been found between pharmacokinetic data of MMC and a wide variety of clinical parameters.[192,201,202]

Most important, impaired liver or renal function does not seem to change the pharmacokinetic behavior of MMC, and therefore neither change requires dosage reduction. Urinary recovery after intravenous administration ranged from 1% to 20%, which cannot explain the rapid plasma clearance. Therefore, the suggestion has been made that MMC is rapidly cleared from plasma by biodegradation. The liver is thought to be the major organ of biotransformation,[209] but the spleen, kidney, brain, and heart may also be involved in this process.[208,209] The presence of oxygen markedly reduced the rate of metabolism of MMC in liver homogenates, compared with metabolism in a similar anaerobic system.[208] As biotransformation is required for activity, this supports the theory of a more pronounced metabolic activation under anaerobic conditions.

Intraarterial hepatic infusions,[203] isolated liver perfusion with MMC[212] or intraarterial infusion with Rhizoma Bletillae embolization,[213] and entrapment of MMC into microspheres[214–217] have been reported in an attempt to enhance local drug delivery, but have failed to yield a more favorable balance between tumor exposure and systemic exposure than intravenous infusions.

As mentioned, MMC is more cytotoxic to hypoxic than aerobic cells. The oxygen-transport–modifying drug BW12C increases tumor hypoxia and might thereby increase MMC cytotoxicity. In a phase I and pharmacokinetic study, administration of BW12C did not change MMC pharmacokinetics nor increase side effects.[218] Although MMC is absorbed after oral administration, absorption is rather erratic by this route.[219–221] Intravesical MMC therapy to treat superficial bladder cancer results in extremely low plasma levels, with virtually no systemic side effects and a significant exposure at the target site (bladder).[108,222–224] MMC uptake in bladder tissues is linearly related to drug concentration in urine, and based partly on this finding a phase III trial has been initiated with intravesical MMC in bladder cancer patients.[225] Enhancement of MMC instillation therapy has been achieved in experimental models through electromotive drug delivery[226] or by simultaneous application of microwave-induced hyperthermia.[227] MMC administered intraperitoneally is rapidly absorbed through the serosal surface into plasma, and hence effective control of local lesions through attainment of high drug levels in the peritoneal cavity is infeasible.[227] A variety of drug delivery systems have been devised to achieve sustained intraperitoneal delivery of MMC, including activated carbon particles,[228] poly(L-lactic acid) microcapsules,[229] the Pluronic F127 triblock copolymer,[230] and galactoxyloglucan gels.[231] Studies have also focused on rectal (suppository) MMC administration[232] and hypoxic pelvic perfusion with or without hemofiltration,[233] but no clear pharmacologic benefits could be found.

Toxicity

The most significant and frequent side effect of MMC is a delayed myelosuppression, which seems to be directly related to schedule and total dose.[234] Below a total dose of

50 mg, hematologic toxicity is rare. At higher doses thrombocytopenia is more frequent than leukocytopenia and anemia. Other toxic reactions usually include mild and infrequent anorexia, nausea, vomiting, and diarrhea. Alopecia, stomatitis, and rashes also occur infrequently. Extravasation results in tissue necrosis with very disabling ulcers that may require plastic surgery.[235] High doses of MMC may result in lethal venoocclusive liver disease.[236]

Other more frequent and potentially lethal side effects include hemolytic uremic syndrome, interstitial pneumonitis, and cardiac failure. An MMC-induced hemolytic uremic syndrome has been observed in over 200 reported cases.[237] The exact pathogenesis still remains unclear. The incidence seems to be less than 10%[237,238] and is dose dependent, with rare instances at doses below 30 mg per m^2 and most cases at cumulative doses above 50 mg per m^2.[238] No consistently effective treatment for this syndrome is available. Although recovery after temporary hemodialysis has been reported,[239,240] most other treatments have been unsuccessful.

Because red blood cell transfusion aggravates hemolysis and may precipitate pulmonary edema,[241,242] it should be avoided if possible. Data suggest at least a temporary benefit of staphylococcal protein A immunoperfusion to remove immune complexes, although consistent recovery has not been achieved.[243]

Pulmonary toxicity of MMC consists of an interstitial pneumonitis with dry cough and progressive dyspnea, and chest films show diffuse bilateral interstitial reticular infiltrates.[237] Discontinuation of MMC administration may occasionally lead to recovery from this side effect, but often progressive respiratory failure occurs. Corticosteroid treatment may be helpful in preventing progression of pulmonary dysfunction. The incidence of pulmonary toxicity is approximately 7% of the treated population. Cardiac failure secondary to MMC occurs in a similar percentage of treated patients, and the incidence rises with cumulative doses above 30 mg per m^2.[244,245] *In vitro* studies have suggested that this side effect may be related to an inhibition of endothelial cell proliferation.[246]

Analogs

The MMC analog N7[2-(nitrophenyldithio)-ethyl]MMC or BMS-181174 (BMY25067) (Fig. 17-6) was much more active than MMC *in vitro* (even in cells that were resistant to MMC), as active *in vivo*, and seemed to have fewer side effects in preclinical testing than MMC. Unfortunately, clinical studies could not confirm the greater activity.[247] BMS-181174 was of particular interest because it shows antitumor activity against both aerobic and anaerobic cells. The metabolic activation and mechanism of action of BMS-181174 clearly differed from that of MMC.[248] In contrast to MMC, which is more toxic to cells under hypoxic conditions, BMS-181174 was more cytotoxic

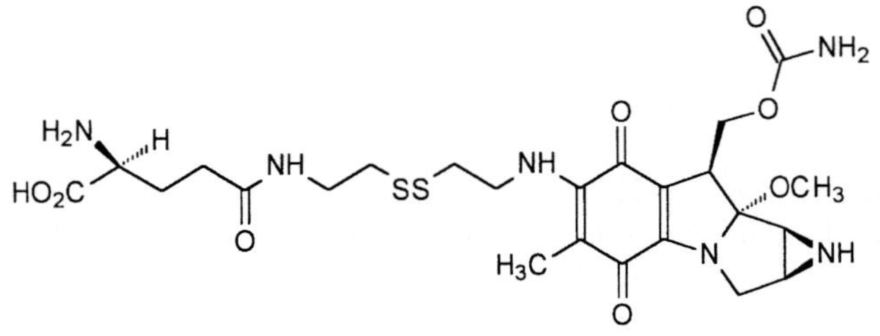

BMS-181174 (BMY-25067)

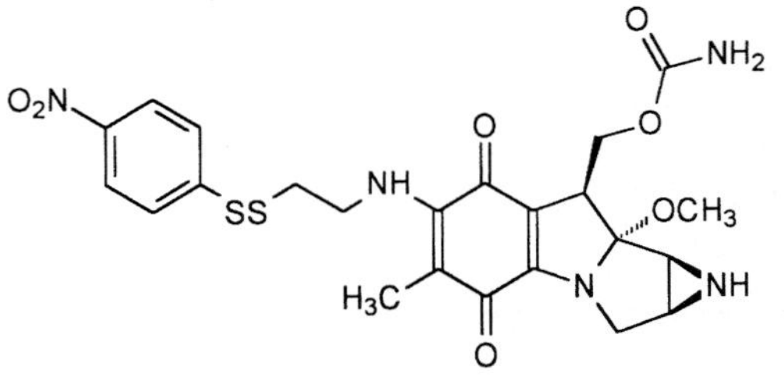

KW-2149

FIGURE 17-6. Structures of the mitomycin C analogs BMS-181174 (BMY25067) and KW-2149.

under aerobic conditions.[248] In anaerobic conditions BMS-181174 was also more toxic than MMC. The cytotoxicity of BMS-181174 was primarily due to DNA cross-linking. Because of its side effects in humans, the development of BMS-181174 was discontinued.

The same holds for the MMC analog KW-2149 (7-*N*-[2-[Y-L-glutamylamino]ethyldithioethyl]mitomycin C), which could be activated to a DNA cross-linking species by an extracellular serum factor.[249] Human serum had high activity, and mouse serum had low activity. KW-2149 activation resulted in a compound with a much higher rate of cellular uptake and a greatly increased DNA binding. This route of activation of KW-2149 is quite different from the one for MMC and may explain the cytotoxicity of the analog to MMC-resistant cells. The remarkable species difference in serum factor activation may also have accounted for the much more pronounced pulmonary toxicity seen in humans, which has led to discontinuation of development despite impressive activity in non–small cell lung cancer.[250]

REFERENCES

1. Waksman SA, Woodruff HB. Bacteriostatic and bactericidal substances produced by a soil *Actinomyces. Proc Soc Exp Biol Med* 1940;45:609–614.
2. Farber S, Tock R, Sears EM, et al. Advances in chemotherapy of cancer in man. *Adv Cancer Res* 1956;4:1–71.
3. Lewis JL. Chemotherapy of gestational choriocarcinoma. *Cancer* 1972;30:1517–1521.
4. Goldstein DP, Berkowitz RS. The management of gestational trophoblastic neoplasma. In: Goldstein DS, ed. *Cur-*

rent problems in obstetrics and gynecology. Chicago: Year Book Medical Publishers, 1980:25–26.

5. D'Angio GJ, Breslow N, Beckewith JB, et al. Treatment of Wilms' tumor. Results of the third National Wilms' Tumor Study. *Cancer* 1989;64:349–360.

6. Wolf JA, D'Angio G, Hartman J, et al. Long-term evaluation of single versus multiple courses of actinomycin D therapy of Wilms' tumor. *N Engl J Med* 1974;290:84–86.

7. Tan CT, Dargeon HW, Burchenal JH. The effect of actinomycin D on cancer in childhood. *Pediatrics* 1959;24:544–561.

8. Heyn R, Holland R, Joo P, et al. Treatment of rhabdomyosarcoma in children with surgery, radiotherapy and chemotherapy. *Med Pediatr Oncol* 1977;3:21–32.

9. Senyszyn JJ, Johnson RE, Curran RE. Treatment of metastatic Ewing's sarcoma with actinomycin D (NSC-3053). *Cancer Chemother Rep* 1970;54:103–107.

10. Brockmann H. Structural differences of the actinomycins and their derivatives. *Ann N Y Acad Sci* 1960;89:323–335.

11. Sengupta SK, Anderson JE, Kelley C. Carbon-7 substituted actinomycin D analogues as improved antitumor agents: synthesis and DNA-binding and biological properties. *J Med Chem* 1982;25:1214–1219.

12. Kamawata J, Imoniski M. Interaction of actinomycin with DNA. *Nature* 1960;187:1112–1113.

13. Muller W, Crothers D. Studies on the binding of actinomycin and related compounds to DNA. *J Mol Biol* 1968; 35:251–290.

14. Sobell HM, Jam SC. Stereochemistry of actinomycin D binding to DNA: II. Detailed molecular model of actinomycin-DNA complex and its implications. *J Mol Biol* 1972;68:21–34.

15. Liu X, Chen H, Patel DJ. Solution structure of actinomycin-DNA complexes: drug intercalation at isolated G-C sites. *J Biomol NMR* 1991;1:323–347.

16. Yu C, Tseng YY. NMR study of the solution confirmation of actinomycin D. *Eur J Biochem* 1992;209:181–187.

17. Wells RD, Larson JE. Studies on the binding of actinomycin D to DNA and DNA model polymers. *J Mol Biol* 1970;49:319–342.

18. Waterloh K, Fox KR. Secondary (non-GpC) binding sites for actinomycin on DNA. *Biochim Biophys Acta* 1992; 1131:300–306.

19. Takusagawa F, Dabrow M, Neidle S, et al. The structure of a pseudo intercalated complex between actinomycin and the DNA binding sequence d(GpC). *Nature* 1982;296:466–469.

20. Brown S, Mullis K, Levenson C, et al. Aqueous solution structure of an intercalated actinomycin D–dATGCAT complex by two-dimensional and one-dimensional proton NMR. *Biochemistry* 1984;23:403–408.

21. Takusagawa F, Goldstein BM, Youngster S, et al. Crystallization and preliminary x-ray study of a complex between dATAGCAT and actinomycin D. *J Biol Chem* 1984;259: 4714–4715.

22. Wadkins RM, Jovin TM. Actinomycin D and 7-aminoactinomycin D binding to single-stranded DNA. *Biochemistry* 1991;30:9469–9478.

23. Brown SC, Shafer RH. Kinetic studies of actinomycin D binding to mono-, oligo- and polynucleotides. *Biochemistry* 1987;26:277–281.

24. Wadkins RM, Vladu B, Tung CS. Actinomycin D binds to metastable hairpins in single-stranded DNA. *Biochemistry* 1998;37:11915–11923.

25. Reich E, Franklin RM, Shatkin AJ, et al. Action of actinomycin D on animal cells and virus. *Proc Natl Acad Sci U S A* 1962;48:1238–1245.

26. Kessel D, Wodinsky I. Uptake in vivo and in vitro of actinomycin D by mouse leukemias as factors in survival. *Biochem Pharmacol* 1968;17:161–164.

27. Inaba M, Johnson RK. Decreased retention of actinomycin D as the basis for cross resistance in anthracycline resistant sublines of P. 388 leukemia. *Cancer Res* 1977;37:4629–4634.

28. Bowen D, Goldmann ID. The relationship among transport, intracellular binding, and inhibition of RNA synthesis by actinomycin D in Ehrlich ascites tumor cells in vitro. *Cancer Res* 1975;35:3054–3060.

29. Polet H. Role of the cell-membrane in the uptake of ^{3}H-actinomycin D by mammalian cells in vitro. *J Pharmacol Exp Ther* 1975;192:270–279.

30. Cotter TG, Glynn JM, Echeverri F, et al. The induction of apoptosis by chemotherapeutic agents occurs in all phases of the cell cycle. *Anticancer Res* 1992;12:773–780.

31. Marchal JA, Prados J, Melguizo C, et al. Actinomycin D treatment leads to differentiation and inhibits proliferation in rhabdomyosarcoma cells. *J Lab Clin Med* 1997; 130:42–50.

32. Peterson RHF, Neil JAO, Bielder L. Some biochemical properties of Chinese hamster cells sensitive and resistant to actinomycin D. *J Cell Biol* 1974;63:773–779.

33. Bosman HH. Mechanism of cellular drug resistance. *Nature* 1971;233:566–569.

34. Riehm H, Biedler JL. Potentiation of drug effect by Tween 80 in Chinese hamster cells resistant to actinomycin D and daunomycin. *Cancer Res* 1972;32:1195–1200.

35. Medoff J, Medoff G, Goldstein MN, et al. Amphotericin B-induced sensitivity to actinomycin D in drug-resistant HeLa cells. *Cancer Res* 1976;35:2548–2552.

36. Goldberg IH, Beerman TA, Poor R. Antibiotics: nucleic acids as targets in chemotherapy. In: Becker FF, ed. *Cancer*, vol 5. New York: Plenum Press, 1978:427–456.

37. Gupta RS. Cross-resistance of vinblastine- and taxol-resistant mutants of Chinese hamster ovary cells to other anticancer drugs. *Cancer Treat Rep* 1985;69:515–521.

38. Gupta RS. Podophyllotoxin-resistant mutants of Chinese hamster ovary cells: cross-resistance studies with various microtubule inhibitions and podophyllotoxin analogues. *Cancer Res* 1983;43:505–512.

39. Okabe-Kado J, Hayashi M, Honma Y, et al. Effects of inducers of erythroid differentiation of human leukemia K562 cells on vincristine-resistant K562/VCR cells. *Leuk Res* 1983;7:481–485.

40. Gupta RS, Murray W, Gupta R. Cross resistance pattern towards anticancer drugs of a human carcinoma multidrug-resistant cell line. *Br J Cancer* 1988;58:441–447.

41. Diddens H, Gekeler V, Neumann M, et al. Characterization of actinomycin-D-resistant CHO cell lines exhibiting a multidrug-resistance phenotype and amplified DNA sequences. *Int J Cancer* 1987;40:635–642.

42. Pastan I, Gottesman M. Multiple-drug resistance in human cancer. *N Engl J Med* 1987;316:1388–1393.

43. LaQuaglia MP, Kopp EB, Spengler BA, et al. Multidrug resistance in human neuroblastoma cells. *J Pediatr Surg* 1991;26:1107–1112.

44. Tishler DM, Raffel C. Development of multidrug resistance in a primitive neuroectodermal tumor cell line. *J Neurosurg* 1992;76:502–506.

45. Hofsli E, Nissen-Meyer J. Reversal of multidrug resistance by lipophilic drugs. *Cancer Res* 1990;50:3997–4002.

46. Galbraith WM, Mellet LB. Tissue disposition of ³H-actinomycin D (NSC-3053) in the rat, monkey and dog. *Cancer Chemother Rep* 1975;59:1061–1069.

47. Tattersall MHM, Sodergren JE, Sengupta SK, et al. Pharmacokinetics of actinomycin D in patients with malignant melanoma. *Clin Pharmacol Ther* 1975;17:701–708.

48. Kante B, Couvreur P, Lenaerts V, et al. Tissue distribution of [3H]actinomycin D adsorbed on polybutylcyanoacrylate nanoparticles. *Int J Pharm* 1980;7:45–53.

49. Kaye SB, Boden JA, Ryman BE. The effect of liposome (phospholipid vesicle) entrapment of actinomycin D and methotrexate on the in vivo treatment of sensitive and resistant solid murine tumors. *Eur J Cancer Clin Oncol* 1981;177:279–289.

50. Kedar A, Mayhew EG, Moore RM, et al. Failure of actinomycin D entrapped in liposomes to prolong survival in renal cell adenocarcinoma-bearing mice. *Oncology* 1981;38:311–314.

51. Brasseur F, Couvreur P, Kante B, et al. Actinomycin D adsorbed on polymethylcyanoacrylate nanoparticles: increased efficiency against an experimental tumor. *Eur J Cancer Clin Oncol* 1980;16:1441–1445.

52. Galbraith WM, Mellet LB. Disposition of ³H-actinomycin D in tumor-bearing mice. *Cancer Res* 1976;36:1242–1245.

53. Benjamin RS, Hall SW, Burgess MA. A pharmacokinetically based phase I–II study of single dose actinomycin D (NSC-8053). *Cancer Treat Rep* 1976;60:289–291.

54. Blatt J, Trigg ME, Pizzo PA, et al. Single dose actinomycin D in childhood solid tumors. *Cancer Treat Rep* 1981;65:145–147.

55. Frei E. The clinical use of actinomycin. *Cancer Chemother Rep* 1974;58:49–54.

56. White L, Tobias V, Hughes DW. Actinomycin D-induced hepatotoxicity. *Pediatr Hematol Oncol* 1989;6:53–57.

57. Zoubek A, Wiesbauer P, Pracher AC, et al. Veno-occlusive disease der Leber als Behandlungskomplikation bei Kindern mit Wilmstumor. *Padiatr Padol* 1992;27:47–50.

58. Hadzar V, Kutluk T, Akyuz C, et al. Veno-occlusive disease-like hepatotoxicity in two children receiving chemotherapy for Wilms' tumor and clear sarcoma of kidney. *Pediatr Hematol Oncol* 1998;15:85–89.

59. Kanwar VS, Albuqurque MLC, Ribeiro RC, et al. Veno-occlusive disease of liver after chemotherapy for rhabdomyosarcoma: case report with review of the literature. *Med Pediatr Oncol* 1995;24:334–340.

60. Yu LC, Warrier RP, Gaumer R, et al. Actinomycin-induced immune thrombocytopenia. *Clin Pediatr* 1990;29:196–197.

61. Elkind MM, Ben Hur E. DNA lesions and mammalian cell killing—cause and effect. *Isr J Chem* 1972;10:1255–1272.

62. D'Angio GJ, Farber S, Maddock CI. Potentiation of x-ray effects by actinomycin D. *Radiology* 1959;73:175–177.

63. Concannon JP, Dalbow MH, Weil V, et al. Radiation and actinomycin D mortality studies: circadian variations in

64. Littman P, Rosenstock JG, Baily C. Radiation myelitis following craniospinal irradiation with concurrent actinomycin D therapy. *Med Pediatr Oncol* 1978;5:145–151.

65. Rao KV, Cullen WP, Sobin BA. Mithramycin: an antibiotic with antitumor properties. *Proc Am Assoc Cancer Res* 1960;3:143.

66. Kennedy BJ, Griffen VO, Lober P. The specific effect of mithramycin on embryonal carcinoma of the testis. *Cancer Res* 1965;18:1631–1636.

67. Slayton RE, Shnider B, Eliase E, et al. New approach to the treatment of hypercalcemia: the effect of short term treatment with mithramycin. *Clin Pharmacol Ther* 1971;12:833–837.

68. Ostenstad B, Andersen OK. Disodium pamidronate versus mithramycin in the management of tumour-associated hypercalcemia. *Acta Oncol* 1992;31:861–864.

69. Koller CA, Miller DM. Preliminary observations on the therapy of the myeloid blast phase of chronic granulocytic leukemia with plicamycin and hydroxy urea. *N Engl J Med* 1986;315:1433–1438.

70. Johnson PR, Yin JA, Narayanan MN, et al. Failure of mithramycin to control the myeloid blast phase of chronic granulocytic leukemia: a report on nine patients and review of the literature. *Hematol Oncol* 1991;9:9–15.

71. Dasgupta D, Shashiprabha BK, Podder SK. Mode of action of antitumor antibiotic: part II—evidence for intercalation of mithramycin between DNA bases in the presence of Mg²⁺. *Indian J Biochem Biophys* 1979;16:18–21.

72. Miller DM, Polansky DA, Thomas SD, et al. Rapid communication: mithramycin selectively inhibits transcription of G-C containing DNA. *Am J Med Sci* 1987;294:388–394.

73. Dalgleish DG, Fey G, Kersten W. Circular dichroism studies of complexes of the antibiotics daunomycin, nogalamycin, chromomycin and mithramycin with DNA. *Biopolymers* 1974;13:1757–1766.

74. Van de Sande JH, Lin CC, Jorgenson KF. Reverse binding on chromosomes produced by a guanine-cytosine specific DNA binding antibiotic: olivomycin. *Science* 1977;195:400–402.

75. Blau L, Bittman R. Equilibrium and kinetic measurements of actinomycin binding to deoxyribonucleic acid in the presence of competing drugs. *Mol Pharmacol* 1975;11:716–721.

76. Hardenbol P, van Dijke MW. In vitro inhibition of c-myc transcription by mithramycin. *Biochem Biophys Res Commun* 1992;185:553–558.

77. Jones DE, Cui DM, Miller DM. Expression of beta-galactosidase under the control of the human c-myc promoter in transgenic mice is inhibited by mithramycin. *Oncogene* 1995;10:2323–2330.

78. Ray R, Snyder RC, Thomas S, et al. Mithramycin blocks protein binding and function of the SV40 early promoter. *J Clin Invest* 1989;83:2003–2007.

79. Carulli G, Petrini M, Marini A, et al. P-glycoprotein and drug resistance in acute leukemias and in the blastic crisis of chronic myeloid leukemia. *Haematologica* 1990;75:516–521.

80. Fernandez E, Lombo F, Mendez C, et al. An ABC transporter is essential for resistance to the antitumor agent mithramycin in the producer *Streptomyces argillaceus*. *Mol Gen Genet* 1996;251:692–698.

81. Ransohoff J, Martin BF, Medrek TJ, et al. Preliminary study of mithramycin (NSC-24559) in primary tumors of the central neoplasms. *Cancer* 1970;26:755–766.

82. Kennedy BJ. Mithramycin therapy in advanced testicular neoplasms. *Cancer* 1970;26:755–766.

83. Monto RW, Talley RW, Caldwell MJ, et al. Observations on the mechanism of hemorrhagic toxicity in mithramycin (NSC-24559) therapy. *Cancer Res* 1969;29:697–704.

84. Ahr DJ, Scialla SJ, Kimball DB. Acquired platelet dysfunction following mithramycin therapy. *Cancer* 1978;41:448–454.

85. Kubisz P, Klener P, Cronberg S. Influence of mithramycin on some platelet functions in vitro. *Acta Haematol* 1980;63:101–106.

86. Zojer N, Keck AV, Pechersdorfer M. Comparative tolerability of drug therapies for hypercalcemia of malignancy. *Drug Saf* 1999;21:389–406.

87. Slavik M, Carter SK. Chromomycin A3, mithramycin and olivomycin: antitumor antibiotics of related structure. *Adv Pharmacol Chemother* 1975;12:1–30.

88. Purpora D, Ahern MJ, Shverman M. Toxic epidermal necrolysis after mithramycin. *N Engl J Med* 1978;299:1412–1413.

89. Kiang DT, Kennedy BJ. Effect of mithramycin on the bone metabolism. *J Clin Endocrinol Metab* 1979;48:341–344.

90. Minkin C. Inhibition of parathyroid hormone stimulated bone resorption in vitro by the antibiotic mithramycin. *Calcif Tissue Res* 1973;13:249–257.

91. Rubenstein M. The use of mithramycin to impair release from bone of ^{45}Ca induced by prostaglandin E_2 and multiple myeloma sera. *Proc Am Soc Clin Oncol* 1980;21:17.

92. Wakaki S, Marumo H, Tomioka K. Isolation of new fractions of antitumor mitomycins. *Antibiot Chemother* 1958;8:228–240.

93. Hortobagyi GN. Mitomycin: its evolving role in the treatment of breast cancer. *Oncology* 1993;50[Suppl 1]:1–8.

94. Israel L, Chahinian P, Depierre A. Response of 65 measurable epidermoid bronchogenic tumors of known spontaneous doubling time to four chemotherapeutic regimens: strategic deductions. *Med Pediatr Oncol* 1975;1:83–93.

95. Cohen MM, Perevodchikova MI. Single agent chemotherapy of lung cancer. In: Muggia FC, Rozencweig M, eds. *Lung cancer: progress in therapeutic research*, vol 11. New York: Raven Press, 1979:343–374.

96. Veeder MH, Jett JR, Su JQ, et al. A phase III trial of mitomycin C alone versus mitomycin C, vinblastine and cisplatin for metastatic squamous cell lung carcinoma. *Cancer* 1992;70:2281–2287.

97. Spain RC. The case for mitomycin in non-small cell lung cancer. *Oncology* 1993;50[Suppl 1]:35–52.

98. Comis RL, Carter SK. A review of chemotherapy in gastric cancer. *Cancer* 1974;34:1576–1586.

99. Baker LM, Izbicki DO, Vaitkevicius VK. Phase II study of porfiromycin versus mitomycin C utilizing acute intermittent schedules. *Med Pediatr Oncol* 1976;2:207–213.

100. Zimmerman SE, Smith FP, Schein PS. Chemotherapy of pancreatic carcinoma. *Cancer* 1981;47:1724–1728.

101. Taal BG, Audisio RA, Bleiberg H, et al. Phase II trial of mitomycin C (MMC) in advanced gallbladder and biliary tree carcinoma. An EORTC Gastro Intestinal Tract Cancer Cooperative Group study. *Ann Oncol* 1993;4:607–609.

102. Rozencweig M, Bleiberg H, Kenis Y. Mitomycin C therapy in advanced colorectal cancer. In: Ogawa M, Rozencweig M, Staquet MJ, eds. *Mitomycin C: current impact on cancer chemotherapy*. Amsterdam: Excerpta Medica, 1982:76–88.

103. Baker L. Study of mitomycin C in cervical cancer in the United States. In: Carter SK, Crooke ST, eds. *Mitomycin C: current status and new developments*. New York: Academic Press, 1979:159–162.

104. Wasserman TH, Carter SK. The integration of chemotherapy into combined modality treatment of solid tumors. VIII Cervical cancer. *Cancer Treat Rep* 1977;4:25–46.

105. Jones WG, Fossa SD, Bona AV, et al. Mitomycin C in the treatment of metastatic prostate cancer: report on an EORTC phase II study. *World J Urol* 1986;4:182–185.

106. Veronesi A, Dal Bo V, Lo Re G, et al. Mitomycin C treatment of advanced hormone-resistant prostatic carcinoma: a phase II study. *Cancer Chemother Pharmacol* 1989;23:115–116.

107. Dik P, Blom JH, Schroder FH. Mitomycin C and aminoglutethimide in the treatment of metastatic prostatic cancer: a phase II study. *Br J Urol* 1992;70:542–545.

108. Mishina T, Watanable H. Mitomycin C bladder installations for bladder tumors. In: Carter SK, Crooke ST, eds. *Mitomycin C: current status and new developments*. New York: Academic Press, 1979:193–285.

109. Harrison GSM, Green DF, Newling DWW, et al. A Phase II study of intravesical mitomycin C in the treatment of superficial bladder cancer. *Br J Urol* 1983;55:676–679.

110. Issell BF, Pront GR, Soloway MS, et al. Mitomycin C intravesical therapy in noninvasive bladder cancer after failure on thiotepa. *Cancer* 1984;53:1025–1028.

111. Cummings BJ. Anal cancer. *Int J Radiat Oncol Biol Phys* 1990;19:1309–1315.

112. Keane TJ, Cummings BJ, O'Sullivan B, et al. A randomized trial of radiation therapy compared to split course radiation therapy combined with mitomycin C and 5-fluorouracil as initial treatment for advanced laryngeal and hypopharyngeal squamous carcinoma. *Int J Radiat Oncol Biol Phys* 1993;25:613–618.

113. Bradner WT, Rose WC, Schurig JE, et al. Antitumor activity and toxicity in animals of H-7[2-(4-nitrophenyldithio)ethyl] mitomycin C (BMY 25067). *Invest New Drugs* 1990;8:[Suppl 1]:1–7.

114. Xu BH, Singh SV. Effect of buthionine sulfoxime and ethacrynic acid on cytotoxic activity of mitomycin C analogues BMY 25282 and BMY 25067. *Cancer Res* 1992;52:6666–6670.

115. Philips RM, Hulbert PB, Bibby MC, et al. In vitro activity of the novel indoloquinone EO-9 and the influence of pH on cytotoxicity. *Br J Cancer* 1992;65:359–364.

116. Shirahata K, Hirayama N. Revised absolute configuration of MMC: x-ray analysis of 1-*N*-(*p*-bromobenzoyl)MMC. *J Am Chem Soc* 1983;105:7199–7202.

117. Beijnen JH, Underberg WJM. Degradation of mitomycin C in acidic solution. *Int J Pharm* 1985;24:219–229.

118. Underberg WJM, Lingeman H. Aspects of the chemical stability of mitomycin C and porfiromycin in acidic solution. *J Pharm Sci* 1983;72:549–553.

119. Stevens CL, Taylor KG, Munk ME, et al. Chemistry and structure of mitomycin C. *J Med Chem* 1964;8:1–10.

120. Garrett ER. The physical chemical characterization of the products, equilibria and kinetics of the complex transforma-

tions of the antibiotic porfiromycin. *J Med Chem* 1963; 6:488–501.

121. Beijnen JH, den Hartigh J, Underberg WJM. Qualitative aspects of the degradation of mitomycins in alkaline solution. *J Pharm Biomed Anal* 1985;3:71–79.

122. Beijnen JH, Rosing H, Underberg WJM. Stability of mitomycins in infusion fluids. *Acta Pharm Chem Sci Ed* 1985;13:58–66.

123. Iyer VN, Szybalski W. A molecular mechanism of mitomycin action: linking of complementary DNA strands. *Proc Natl Acad Sci U S A* 1963;50:355–362.

124. Tomasz M, Palom Y. The mitomycin bioreductive antitumor agents: cross-linking and alkylation of DNA as the molecular basis of their activity. *Pharmacol Ther* 1997; 76:73–87.

125. Reddy MV, Randerath K. ^{32}P-Analysis of DNA adducts in somatic and reproductive tissues of rats treated with the anticancer antibiotic mitomycin C. *Mutat Res* 1987;179:75–88.

126. Iyer VN, Szybalski W. Mitomycin and porfiromycin: chemical mechanism of activation and cross-linking of DNA. *Science* 1964;145:55–58.

127. Cummings J, Spanswick VJ, Smyth JF. Re-evaluation of the molecular pharmacology of mitomycin C. *Eur J Cancer* 1995;31A:1928–1933.

128. Suresh Kumar G, Lipman R, Cummings J, et al. Mitomycin C-DNA adducts generated by DT-diaphorase: revised mechanism of the enzymatic reductive activation of mitomycin C. *Biochemistry* 1997;36:14128–14136.

129. Tomasz M, Lipman R, Chowdary D, et al. Isolation and structure of a covalent cross-link adduct between mitomycin C and DNA. *Science* 1987;235:1204–1208.

130. Bizanek R, McGuinness BF, Nakanishi K, et al. Isolation and structure of an intrastrand cross-link adduct of mitomycin C and DNA. *Biochemistry* 1992;31:3084–3091.

131. Suresh Kumar G, Musser SM, Cummings J, et al. 2,7-Diaminomitosene, a monofunctional mitomycin derivative, alkylates DNA in the major groove: structure and base-sequence specificity of the DNA adduct and mechanism of the alkylation. *J Am Chem Soc* 1996;118:9209–9217.

132. Tomasz M, Lipman R. Alkylation reaction of mitomycin C at acid pH. *J Am Chem Soc* 1979;101:6063–6067.

133. Lin AJ, Cosby LA, Shansky CW, et al. Potential bioreductive alkylating agents: 1. Benzoquinone derivatives. *J Med Chem* 1972;15:1247–1252.

134. Moore HW, Czerniak R. Naturally occurring quinones as potential bioreductive alkylating agents. *Med Res Rev* 1981;1:249–280.

135. Lin AJ, Sartorelli AC. 2,3-Dimethyl-5,6-bis(methylene)-1,4-benzoquinone: the active intermediate of bioreductive alkylating agents. *J Org Chem* 1973;38:813.

136. Tomasz M, Mercado CM, Olson J, et al. The mode of interaction of mitomycin C with desoxyribonucleic acid and other polynucleotides in vitro. *Biochemistry* 1974;13:4878–4887.

137. Kalyanaraman B, Perez-Reyes E, Mason RP. Spin trapping and direct electron spin resonance investigations of the redox metabolism of quinone anticancer drugs. *Biochim Biophys Acta* 1980;630:119–130.

138. Andrews PA, Pan SS, Bachur NR. Electrochemical reductive activation of mitomycin C. *J Am Chem Soc* 1986; 108:4158–4166.

139. Egbertson M, Danishefsky SJ. Modeling of the electrophilic activation of mitomycins: chemical evidence for the intermediacy of a mitosene semiquinone as the active electrophile. *J Am Chem Soc* 1987;109:2204–2205.

140. Kohn H, Zein N, Lin XQ, et al. Mechanistic studies on the mode of reaction of mitomycin C under catalytic and electrochemical reductive conditions. *J Am Chem Soc* 1987; 109:1833–1840.

141. Bachur NR, Gordon SL, Gee MV. A general mechanism for microsomal activation of quinone anticancer agents to free radicals. *Cancer Res* 1978;38:1745–1750.

142. Lown JW, Chen HH. Evidence for the generation of free hydroxyl radicals from certain quinone antitumor antibiotics upon reductive activation in solution. *Can J Chem* 1981;59:390–395.

143. Kennedy KA, Rockwell S, Sartorelli AC. Preferential activation of mitomycin C to cytotoxic metabolites by hypoxic tumor cells. *Cancer Res* 1980;40:2356–2360.

144. Tomasz MA. H_2O_2 generation during the redox cycle of MMC and DNA-bound MMC. *Chem Biol Interact* 1976;13:89–97.

145. Bachur NR, Gordon SL, Gee MV, et al. NADPH cytochrome P-450 reductase activation of quinone anticancer agents to free radicals. *Proc Natl Acad Sci U S A* 1979; 76:954–957.

146. Keyes SR, Fracasso PM, Heimbrook DC, et al. Role of NADPH cytochrome c reductase and DT-diaphorase in the biotransformation of mitomycin C. *Cancer Res* 1984;44: 5638–5643.

147. Pan SS, Andrews PA, Glover CJ, et al. Reductive activation of MMC and MMC metabolites catalysed by NADPH-cytochrome P-450 reductase and xanthine oxidase. *J Biol Chem* 1984;259:959–966.

148. Gustafson DL, Pritsos CA. Bioactivation of mitomycin C by xanthine dehydrogenase from EMT6 mouse mammary carcinoma tumors. *J Natl Cancer Inst* 1992;84:1180–1185.

149. Fisher JF, Olsen RA. Mechanistic aspects of mitomycin C activation by flavoprotein transhydrogenases. *Dev Biochem* 1982;21:240.

150. Belcourt MF, Hodnick WF, Rockwell S, et al. The intracellular location of NADH: cytochrome b_5 reductase modulates the cytotoxicity of the mitomycins to Chinese hamster ovary cells. *J Biol Chem* 1998;273:8875–8881.

151. Cummings J, Spanswick VJ, Tomasz M, et al. Enzymology of mitomycin C metabolic activation in tumour tissue. Implications for enzyme-directed bioreductive drug development. *Biochem Pharmacol* 1998;56:405–414.

152. Ross D, Beall HD, Siegel D, et al. Enzymology of bioreductive drug activation. *Br J Cancer* 1996;74:S1–S8.

153. Ernster L. DT-diaphorase. *Methods Enzymol* 1967;10: 309–317.

154. Schlager JJ, Powis G. Mitomycin C is not metabolized by but is an inhibitor of human kidney NAD(P)H: (quinone-acceptor)oxidoreductase. *Cancer Chemother Pharmacol* 1988;22:126–130.

155. Workman P, Walton MI, Powis G, et al. DT-diaphorase: questionable role in mitomycin C resistance, but a target for novel bioreductive drugs. *Br J Cancer* 1989;60:800–802.

156. Siegel D, Gibson NW, Preusch PC, et al. Metabolism of mitomycin C by DT-diaphorase: role in mitomycin C-

induced DNA damage and cytotoxicity in human colon carcinoma cells. *Cancer Res* 1990;50:7483–7489.

157. Traver RD, Panenberg KD, Horiksohi T, et al. Level of protein activity and gene expression of DT-diaphorase (DTD) in human colon carcinoma cell lines. *Proc Am Assoc Cancer Res* 1991;32:13.

158. Siegel D, Senekowitsch C, Beall H, et al. Bioreductive activation of mitomycin C by DT-diaphorase. *Biochemistry* 1992;31:7879–7885.

159. Nishiyama M, Saeki S, Aogi K, et al. Relevance of DT-diaphorase activity to mitomycin C (MMC) efficacy on human cancer cells: differences in in vitro and in vivo systems. *Int J Cancer* 1993;53:1013–1016.

160. Sawamura AO, Aoyama T, Tamakoshi K, et al. Transfection of human cytochrome P-450 reductase cDNA and its effects on the sensitivity to toxins. *Oncology* 1996;53:406–411.

161. Belcourt MF, Hodnick WF, Rockwell S, et al. Differential toxicity of mitomycin C and porfiromycin to aerobic and hypoxic Chinese hamster ovary cells overexpressing human NADPH:cytochrome c (P-450) reductase. *Proc Natl Acad Sci U S A* 1996;93:456–460.

162. Hoban PR, Walton MI, Robson CN, et al. Decreased NADPH: cytochrome P-450 reductase activity and impaired drug activation in a mammalian cell line resistant to mitomycin C under aerobic but not hypoxic conditions. *Cancer Res* 1990;50:4692–4697.

163. Bligh HFJ, Bartoszek A, Robson CN, et al. Activation of mitomycin C by NADPH: cytochrome P 450-reductase. *Cancer Res* 1990;50:7789–7792.

164. Keyes SR, Rockwell S, Sartorelli AC. Modification of the metabolism and cytotoxicity of bioreductive alkylating agents by dicoumarol in aerobic and hypoxic tumor cells. *Cancer Res* 1989;49:3310–3313.

165. Dulhanty AM, Whitmore GF. Chinese hamster ovary cell lines resistant to mitomycin C under aerobic but not hypoxic conditions are deficient in DT-diaphorase. *Cancer Res* 1991;51:1860–1865.

166. Hornemann U, Iguchi K, Keller PJ, et al. Reactions of mitomycin C with potassium ethyl xanthate in neutral aqueous solution. *J Org Chem* 1984;48:5026.

167. Bean M, Kohn H. Studies on the reaction of mitomycin C with potassium ethyl monothiocarbonate under reductive conditions. *J Org Chem* 1984;48:5033.

168. Tomasz M, Lipman R. Reductive metabolism and alkylating activity of mitomycin C induced by rat liver microsomes. *Biochemistry* 1981;20:5056–5061.

169. Hashimoto Y, Shudo K, Okamoto T. Modification of deoxyribonucleic acid with reductively activated MMC: structures of modified nucleotides. *Chem Pharm Bull* 1983;31:861–869.

170. Tomasz M, Jung M, Verdine G, et al. Circular dichroism spectroscopy as a probe for the stereochemistry of aziridine cleavage reactions of mitomycin C: application to adducts of mitomycin C with DNA constituents. *J Am Chem Soc* 1984;106:7367–7370.

171. Tomasz M, Lipman R, Verdine G, et al. Reassignment of the guanine-binding mode of reduced mitomycin C. *Biochemistry* 1986;25:4337–4343.

172. Tomasz M, Chowdary D, Lipman R, et al. Reaction of DNA with chemically or enzymatically activated DNA: isolation and structure of the major covalent adduct. *Proc Natl Acad Sci U S A* 1986;83:6702–6706.

173. Rockwell S. Effects of mitomycin C alone and in combination with x-rays on EMT-6 mouse mammary tumors in vivo. *J Natl Cancer Inst* 1983;71:765–771.

174. Ludwig CU, Peng YM, Beaudry JN, et al. Cytotoxicity of mitomycin C on clonogenic human carcinoma cells is not enhanced by hypoxia. *Cancer Chemother Pharmacol* 1984;12:146–150.

175. Sartorelli AC. The role of mitomycin antibiotics in the chemotherapy of solid tumors. *Biochem Pharmacol* 1986;35:67–70.

176. Fracasso PM, Sartorelli AC. Cytotoxicity and DNA lesions produced by mitomycin C and porfiromycin in hypoxic and aerobic EMT-6 and Chinese hamster ovary cells. *Cancer Res* 1986;46:3939–3944.

177. Rockwell S. Effects of some proliferative and environmental factors on the toxicity of mitomycin C to tumor cells in vitro. *Int J Cancer* 1986;38:229–235.

178. Keyes SR, Rockwell S, Sartorelli AC. Enhancement of mitomycin C cytotoxicity to hypoxic tumor cells by dicoumarol in vivo and in vitro. *Cancer Res* 1985;45:213–216.

179. Beard SE, Capaldi SR, Gee P. Stress responses to DNA damaging agents in the human colon carcinoma cell line, RKO. *Mutat Res* 1996;371:1–13.

180. Kawasaki T, Tomita Y, Bilim V, et al. Abrogation of apoptosis induced by DNA-damaging agents in human bladder cancer cell lines with p21/WAF1/CIP1 and/or p53 gene alterations. *Int J Cancer* 1996;68:501–505.

181. Hemendinger RA, Bloom SE. Selective mitomycin C and cyclophosphamide induction of apoptosis in differentiating B lymphocytes compared to T lymphocytes in vivo. *Immunopharmacology* 1996;35:71–82.

182. Muscarella DE, Bloom SE. Involvement of gene-specific DNA damage and apoptosis in the differential toxicity of mitomycin C analogs towards B-lineage versus T-lineage lymphoma cells. *Biochem Pharmacol* 1997;53:811–822.

183. Maccubbin AE, Mudipalli A, Nadadur SS, et al. Mutations in a shuttle vector plasmid exposed to monofunctionally activated mitomycin C. *Environ Mol Mutagen* 1997;29:143–151.

184. Rossi C, Poli P, Candi A, et al. Modulation of mitomycin C mutagenicity on Saccharomyces cerevisiae by glutathione, cytochrome P-450, and mitochondria interactions. *Mutat Res* 1997;390:113–120.

185. Willson IKV, Long BH, Marks ME, et al. Mitomycin C resistance in a human colon carcinoma cell line associated with cell surface protein alternations. *Cancer Res* 1984;44:5880–5885.

186. Dulhanty AM, Li M, Whitmore GF. Isolation of Chinese hamster ovary cell mutants deficient in excision repair and mitomycin C bioactivation. *Cancer Res* 1989;49:117–122.

187. Giavazzi R, Kartner N, Hart IR. Expression of cell surface p-glycoprotein by an Adriamycin-resistant murine fibrosarcoma. *Cancer Res* 1983;43:145–147.

188. Dorr RT, Liddil JD, Trent JM, et al. Mitomycin C resistant L-1210 leukemia cells: association with pleiotropic drug resistance. *Biochem Pharmacol* 1987;36:3115–3120.

189. Dorr RT, Liddil JD. Modulation of mitomycin C-induced multidrug resistance in vitro. *Cancer Chemother Pharmacol* 1991;27:290–294.

190. Singh SV, Xu BH, Maurya AK, et al. Modulation of mitomycin C resistance by glutathione transferase inhibitor ethacrynic acid. *Biochim Biophys Acta* 1992;1137:257–263.

191. Xu BH, Singh SV. Potentiation of mitomycin C cytotoxicity by glutathione depletion in a multi-drug resistant mouse leukemia cell line. *Cancer Lett* 1992;66:49–53.

192. Verweij J, den Hartigh J, Stuurman M, et al. Relationship between clinical parameters and pharmacokinetics of mitomycin C. *J Cancer Res Clin Oncol* 1987;113:91–94.

193. Verweij J, Kerpel-Fronius S, Stuurman M, et al. Absence of interaction between furosemide and mitomycin C. *Cancer Chemother Pharmacol* 1987;19:84–86.

194. Marshall RS, Erlichman C, Rauth AM. A bioassay to measure cytotoxicity of plasma from patients treated with mitomycin C. *Cancer Res* 1985;45:5939–5943.

195. Nguyen HN, Sevin BU, Averette HE, et al. The use of ATP bioluminescence assays in selecting a drug screen panel for chemotherapy testing of uterine cancer cell lines. *Gynecol Oncol* 1992;45:185–191.

196. Eksborg S, Ehrsson H, Lindfors A. Liquid chromatographic determination of mitomycin C in human plasma and urine. *J Chromatogr* 1983;274:263–270.

197. Tjaden UR, De Bruijn EA, Van der Hoeven RA, et al. Automated analysis of mitomycin C in body fluids by high-performance liquid chromatography with on-line sample pre-treatment. *J Chromatogr* 1987;420:53–62.

198. Song D, Au JL. Direct injection isocratic high-performance liquid chromatographic analysis of mitomycin C in plasma. *J Chromatogr B Biomed Sci Appl* 1996;676:165–168.

199. Joseph G, Biederbick W, Woschee U, et al. Sensitive and convenient high-performance liquid chromatographic method for the determination of mitomycin C in human plasma. *J Chromatogr B Biomed Sci Appl* 1997;698:261–267.

200. Paroni R, Arcelloni C, De Vecchi E, et al. Plasma mitomycin C concentrations determined by HPLC coupled to solid-phase extraction. *Clin Chem* 1997;43:615–658.

201. Den Hartigh J, McVie JG, Van Oort WJ, et al. Pharmacokinetics of mitomycin C in humans. *Cancer Res* 1983;43:5017–5021.

202. Van Hazel GA, Scott M, Rubin J. Pharmacokinetics of mitomycin C in patients receiving the drug alone or in combination. *Cancer Treat Rep* 1983;67:805–810.

203. Hu E, Howell SB. Pharmacokinetics of intra-arterial mitomycin C in humans. *Cancer Res* 1983;43:4474–4477.

204. Schilcher RB, Young JD, Ratanatharatorn V, et al. Clinical pharmacokinetics of high dose mitomycin C. *Cancer Chemother Pharmacol* 1984;13:186–198.

205. Buice RG, Niell HB, Sidhu P, et al. Pharmacokinetics of mitomycin C in non-oat cell carcinoma of the lung. *Cancer Chemother Pharmacol* 1984;13:1–4.

206. Tjaden UR, Langenberg JP, Ensing K, et al. Determination of mitomycin C in plasma, serum and urine by high-performance liquid chromatography with ultra-violet and electrochemical detection. *J Chromatogr* 1982;232:355–367.

207. Niessen WM, Bergers PJ, Tjaden UR, et al. Phase-system switching as an on-line sample pretreatment in the bioanalysis of mitomycin C using supercritical fluid chromatography. *J Chromatogr* 1988;454:243–251.

208. Schwarz HS, Philips FS. Pharmacology of mitomycin C: II. Renal excretion and metabolism by tissue homogenates. *J Pharmacol Exp Ther* 1961;133:335–342.

209. Fujita H. Comparative studies on the blood level, tissue distribution excretion and inactivation of anticancer drugs. *Jpn J Clin Oncol* 1971;12:151–162.

210. Dorr RT. New findings in the pharmacokinetics, metabolic, and drug-resistance aspects of mitomycin C. *Semin Oncol* 1988;15[Suppl 4]:32–41.

211. Verweij J, Stuurman M, de Vries J, et al. The difference in pharmacokinetics of mitomycin C, given either as a single agent or as a part of combination chemotherapy. *J Cancer Res Clin Oncol* 1986;112:282–284.

212. Marinelli A, De Brauw LM, Beerman H, et al. Isolated liver perfusion with mitomycin C in the treatment of colorectal cancer metastases confined to the liver. *Jpn J Clin Oncol* 1996;26:341–350.

213. Zhan XX, Thorpe PE, Agrawal DK, et al. Pharmacokinetic, angiographic, and histologic comparison of catheter-directed chemoembolization versus systemic chemotherapy in a canine mode. *Can J Physiol Pharmacol* 1996;74:1117–1125.

214. Pfeifle CE, Howell SB, Ashburn WL, et al. Pharmacologic studies of intra-hepatic artery chemotherapy with degradable starch microspheres. *Cancer Drug Deliv* 1986;3:1–14.

215. Ensminger WE, Gyves JW, Stetson P, et al. Phase I study of hepatic arterial degradable starch microspheres and mitomycin. *Cancer Res* 1985;45:4464–4467.

216. Milano G, Boublil JL, Bruneton JM, et al. Systemic blood levels after intra-arterial administration of micro-encapsulated mitomycin C in cancer patients. *Eur J Drug Metab Pharmacol* 1985;10:197–201.

217. Czejka MJ, Jager W, Schuller J. Pharmacokinetics of mitomycin C in patients after bolus injection and chemobolisation of the hepatic artery with Spherex Starch particles. *Eur J Drug Metab Pharmacokinet* 1992;17:85–87.

218. Dennis IF, Ramsay JRS, Workman P, et al. Pharmacokinetics of BW12C and mitomycin C, given in combination in a phase I study in patients with advanced gastrointestinal cancer. *Cancer Chemother Pharmacol* 1993;32:67–72.

219. Bradner WT. Oral activity of mitomycin C (NSC 26980) on Walker 256 (intramuscular) tumor. *Cancer Chemother Rep* 1968;52:389–391.

220. Crooke ST, Henderson M, Samson M, et al. Phase I study of oral mitomycin C. *Cancer Treat Rep* 1976;60:1633–1636.

221. Van Oosterom AT, de Bruyn EA, Kuin CM, et al. Clinical and pharmacological data of mitomycin C after oral administration. In: *Proceedings of the 5th NCI/EORTC New Drug Symposium*, 1986(abst 8.08).

222. Wajsman Z, Dhafir RA, Pfeffer M, et al. Studies of mitomycin C absorption after intravesical treatment of superficial bladder tumors. *J Urol* 1984;132:30–33.

223. Dalton JT, Wientjes MG, Badalament RA, et al. Pharmacokinetics of intravesical mitomycin C in superficial bladder cancer patients. *Cancer Res* 1991;51:5144–5152.

224. Wientjes MG, Badalament RA, Wang RC, et al. Penetration of mitomycin C in human bladder. *Cancer Res* 1993;53:3314–3320.

225. Gao X, Au JL, Badalament RA, et al. Bladder tissue uptake of mitomycin C during intravesical therapy is linear with drug concentration in urine. *Clin Cancer Res* 1998;4:139–143.

226. Di Stasi SM, Vespasiani G, Giannantoni A, et al. Electromotive delivery of mitomycin C into human bladder wall. *Cancer Res* 1997;57:875–880.

227. Colombo R, Da Pozzo LF, Lev A, et al. Neoadjuvant combined microwave-induced local HT and topical chemotherapy versus chemotherapy alone for superficial bladder cancer. *J Urol* 1996;155:1227–1232.

228. Hagiwara A, Takahashi T, Lee R, et al. Chemotherapy for carcinomatous peritonitis and pleuritis with MMC-CH, mitomycin C adsorbed on activated carbon particles. *Cancer* 1987;59:245–251.

229. Iwa T, Ohira M, Yamada T, et al. Intra-abdominal administration of 5-FU poly(L-lactic acid) microspheres for management of carcinomatous peritonitis. *J Clin Exp Med* 1985;135:1095–1096.

230. Miyazaki S, Ohkawa Y, Takada M, et al. Antitumor effect of Pluronic F-127 gel containing mitomycin C on sarcoma-180 ascites tumour in mice. *Chem Pharm Bull* 1992;40:2224–2226.

231. Suisha F, Kawasaki N, Miyazaki S, et al. Xyloglucan gels as sustained release vehicles for the intraperitoneal administration of mitomycin C. *Int J Pharm* 1998;172:27–32.

232. Pokorny RM, Wrightson WR, Lewis RK, et al. Suppository administration of chemotherapeutic drugs with concomitant radiation for rectal cancer. *Dis Colon Rectum* 1997;40:1414–1420.

233. Guadagni S, Aigner KR, Palumbo G, et al. Pharmacokinetics of mitomycin C in pelvic stopflow infusion and hypoxic pelvic perfusion with and without hemofiltration: a pilot study of patients with recurrent unresectable rectal cancer. *J Clin Pharmacol* 1998;38:936–944.

234. Crooke ST, Bradner WT. Mitomycin C: a review. *Cancer Treat Res* 1976;3:121–139.

235. Argenta LC, Manders EK. Mitomycin C extravasation injuries. *Cancer* 1983;51:1080–1082.

236. Lazarus HM, Gottfried MR, Herzig RH, et al. Veno-occlusive disease of the liver after high-dose mitomycin C therapy and autologous bone marrow transplantation. *Cancer* 1982;49:1789–1795.

237. Verweij J, Van der Burg MEL, Pinedo HM. Mitomycin C-induced hemolytic uremic syndrome: six case reports and review of the literature on renal, pulmonary and cardiac side effects of the drug. *Radiother Oncol* 1987;8:33–41.

238. Verweij J, de Vries J, Pinedo HM. Mitomycin C-induced renal toxicity, a dose-dependent side effect? *Eur J Cancer Clin Oncol* 1987;23:195–199.

239. Hamner RW, Verani R, Weinman EJ. Mitomycin associated renal failure. *Arch Intern Med* 1983;143:803–807.

240. Verweij J, Boven E, van der Meulen J, et al. Recovery from mitomycin C-induced haemolytic uraemic syndrome. *Cancer* 1984;54:2878–2881.

241. Jones BG, Fielding JWL, Newman CE, et al. Intravascular haemolysis and renal impairment after blood transfusion in two patients on long-term 5-fluorouracil and mitomycin C. *Lancet* 1980;1:1275–1277.

242. Gulati SC, Sordillo P, Kempin S, et al. Microangiopathic hemolytic anemia observed after treatment of epidermoid carcinoma with mitomycin C and 5-flourouracil. *Cancer* 1980;45:2252–2257.

243. Korec S, Schein PS, Smith FP, et al. Treatment of cancer-associated hemolytic uremic syndrome with staphylococcal protein A immunoperfusion. *J Clin Oncol* 1986;4:210–215.

244. Verweij J, van Zanten T, Souren T, et al. Prospective study of the dose relationship of mitomycin C-induced interstitial pneumonitis. *Cancer* 1987;60:756–761.

245. Verweij J, Funke-Küpper AJ, Teule GJJ, et al. A prospective study on the dose dependency of cardiotoxicity induced by mitomycin C. *Med Oncol Tumor Pharmacother* 1988;5:159–163.

246. Dirix LY, Libura M, Libura J, et al. In vitro toxicity studies with mitomycins and bleomycin on endothelial cells. *Anticancer Drugs* 1997;8:859–868.

247. Macaulay VM, O'Byrne KJ, Green JA, et al. Phase I study of the mitomycin C analogue BMS-181174. *Br J Cancer* 1998;77:2020–2027.

248. Rockwell S, Kemple B, Kelley M. Cytotoxicity of BMS-181174. Effects of hypoxia, dicoumarol, and repair deficits. *Biochem Pharmacol* 1995;50:1239–1243.

249. Masters JRW, Know RJ, Hartley JA, et al. KW-2149 (7-N-[2-[Y-L-glutamylamino]ethyldithioethyl]mitomycin C). A new mitomycin C analogue activated by serum. *Biochem Pharmacol* 1997;53:279–285.

250. Dirix L, Catimel G, Koier I, et al. Phase I and pharmacologic study of a novel mitomycin C analogue KW-2149. *Anticancer Drugs* 1995;6:53–63.

18

ANTHRACYCLINES AND ANTHRACENEDIONES

JAMES H. DOROSHOW

DAUNORUBICIN (DAUNOMYCIN) AND DOXORUBICIN

The anthracycline antibiotics doxorubicin and daunorubicin, initially discovered over 30 years ago,[1,2] are among the most widely used antineoplastic agents in current clinical practice; their antineoplastic spectrum of action compares favorably with that of the alkylating agents and the taxanes. Doxorubicin hydrochloride and daunorubicin hydrochloride are especially active against the hematopoietic malignancies such as acute lymphocytic leukemia and acute myelogenous leukemia (AML), Hodgkin's and non-Hodgkin's lymphoma, and multiple myeloma, as well as carcinomas of the breast, lung, ovary, stomach, and thyroid, sarcomas of bone and soft tissue origin, and various childhood malignancies. The key features of the two most commonly used anthracyclines, daunorubicin and doxorubicin, are summarized in Table 18-1, and the structures of the anthracyclines now in use are shown in Figure 18-1. Doxorubicin is currently used principally for the treatment of solid tumors, especially breast cancer and lymphoma, whereas daunorubicin is routinely used as part of chemotherapeutic induction programs for AML and acute lymphocytic leukemia. The doxorubicin analog epirubicin is similar to the parent compound with respect to its acute toxicity profile and spectrum of antitumor efficacy but is significantly less potent and only slightly less cardiotoxic. The modestly decreased cardiac toxicity of epirubicin is only a marginal advantage, because other means are currently available to lessen the risk of anthracycline-induced heart damage. Idarubicin, a daunorubicin analog, has significant activity in the treatment of AML but is less active against solid tumors and thus is an appropriate alternate anthracycline only in the setting of acute leukemia.

In the clinic, the anthracyclines doxorubicin and daunorubicin have no known antagonistic interactions with any of the other commonly used anticancer agents. Furthermore, these drugs are active over a wide range of doses and in a variety of administration schedules; essentially equivalent antitumor activity is observed whether the anthracycline is given as a single large bolus dose once a month, as a weekly intravenous bolus, or as a prolonged infusion.[3,4] Changes in drug scheduling, however, do change the pattern of normal tissue injury. The combination of broad antitumor activity, lack of antagonism with other antitumor agents, and flexibility in dose and schedule make doxorubicin and daunorubicin very useful in the design of drug combinations. As a result, anthracycline-containing combination chemotherapy protocols have become standard therapy for cancers of the breast, ovary, thyroid, and stomach; bone and soft tissue sarcomas; essentially all hematologic malignancies; and many childhood solid tumors. Although the acute toxicities associated with anthracycline administration, such as myelosuppression, mucositis, and alopecia, are important in clinical practice, the toxic reaction that causes the greatest concern is the unique, cumulative cardiac injury produced by these drugs. Elucidation of the biochemical mechanisms of this cardiac toxicity has resulted in the identification of an iron-chelating agent with its own modest antineoplastic activity, dexrazoxane (ICRF-187), which can block the cardiac toxicity of the anthracycline antibiotics in a wide range of animal models. Prospective, randomized clinical trials have shown that this agent is highly effective in reducing the cardiac toxicity of doxorubicin. This development, as well as the demonstration of a steep dose-response curve for doxorubicin in the treatment of solid tumors[5] and the feasibility of using colony-stimulating factors with or without peripheral blood progenitor support to ameliorate the bone marrow toxicity of the anthracyclines, has permitted a significant increase in the dose intensity and duration of anthracycline therapy and may further increase the clinical utility of this family of drugs.[6–8]

General Mechanism of Action and Cellular and Molecular Pharmacology

Transmembrane Transport

The initial studies of anthracycline cellular pharmacokinetics reported the existence of a carrier-mediated transport

TABLE 18-1. KEY FEATURES OF DAUNORUBICIN AND DOXORUBICIN

Mechanism of action:	Pleiotropic effects, including (a) activation of signal transduction pathways, (b) generation of reactive oxygen intermediates, (c) stimulation of apoptosis, and (d) inhibition of DNA topoisomerase II catalytic activity.
Metabolism:	Reduction of side-chain carbonyl to alcohol resulting in some loss of cytotoxicity.
	One-electron reduction to semiquinone free-radical intermediate by flavoproteins leading to aerobic production of superoxide anion, hydrogen peroxide, and hydroxyl radical.
	Two-electron reduction resulting in formation of aglycone species that can be conjugated for export in bile.
Pharmaco-kinetics:	*Doxorubicin*: V_d = 25 L; protein binding = 60–70%; CSF/plasma ratio, very low; $t_{1/2\alpha}$ = 10 min; $t_{1/2\beta}$ = 1–3 h; $t_{1/2\gamma}$ = 30 h. Circulates predominantly as parent drug; doxorubicinol is most common metabolite, although a substantial fraction of patients form doxorubicin 7-deoxyaglycone and doxorubicinol 7-deoxyaglycone; substantial interpatient variation in biotransformation; no apparent dose-related change in clearance; clearance higher in men than in women.
	Daunorubicin: V_d, protein binding, and CSF/plasma ratio similar to those of doxorubicin; $t_{1/2\alpha}$ = 40 min; $t_{1/2\beta}$ = 20–50 h. Metabolism to daunorubicin faster than for equivalent doxorubicin metabolism, although interpatient variation remains high.
Elimination:	Only 50–60% of parent drug accounted for by known routes of elimination, which include reduction of the side-chain carbonyl by hepatic aldo-keto reductases, aglycone formation, and excretion of biliary conjugates and metabolites. A substantial fraction of the parent compound is bound to DNA and cardiolipin in tissues and is slowly dissociated, which contributes to prolonged disappearance. Although changes in anthracycline pharmacokinetics may be difficult to demonstrate in patients with mild alterations in liver function, drug clearance is definitely decreased in the presence of significant hyperbilirubinemia or in patients with marked burden of metastatic tumor in liver.
Drug interactions:	Heparin binds to doxorubicin, causing aggregation; coadministration of both drugs leads to increased doxorubicin clearance. In rodents, phenobarbital has been shown to increase, and morphine to decrease, doxorubicin disappearance; drugs that diminish hepatic reduced glutathione pools (acetaminophen and BCNU) sensitize the liver to anthracycline toxicity.
Toxicity:	Myelosuppression.
	Mucositis.
	Alopecia.
	Cardiac toxicity.
	Severe local tissue damage after drug extravasation.
Precautions:	Acute and chronic cardiac decompensation can occur. Most common is cumulative dose-related congestive cardiomyopathy, which is more frequent in patients with underlying hypertensive heart disease and in those previously receiving mediastinal radiation with a cardiac dose of >2,000 cGy.
	Radiation sensitization of normal tissues, including chest wall and esophagus, is common and effects may occur many years after radiation exposure.
	Extravasation damage to extremities has resulted in loss of limb function.

BCNU, bischloroethylnitrosourea (carmustine); CSF, cerebrospinal fluid; $t_{1/2}$, half-life; V_d, apparent volume of distribution.

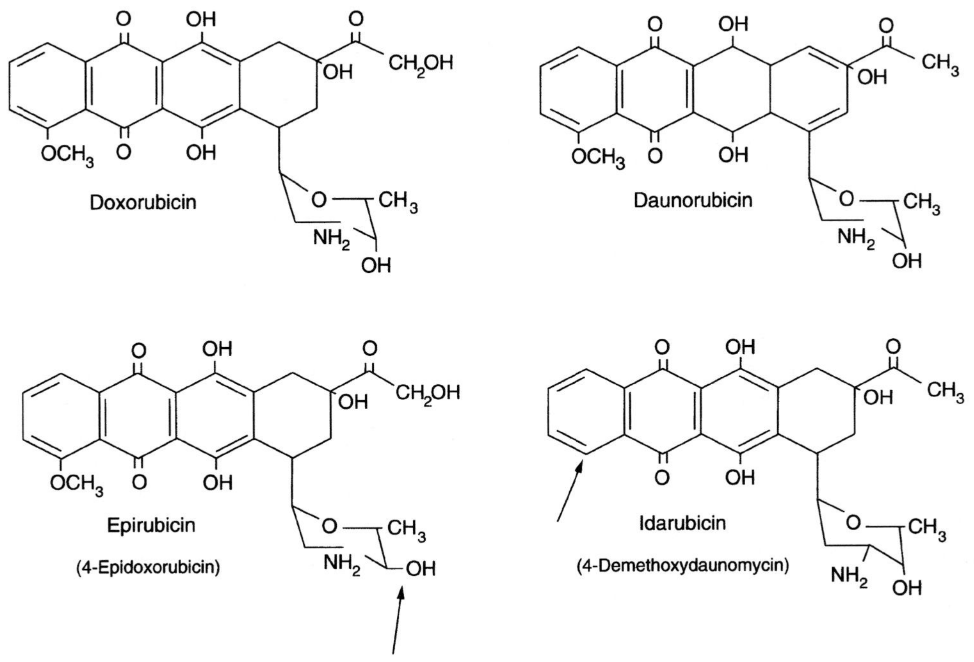

FIGURE 18-1. Structures of the four anthracyclines in current clinical use. For epirubicin and idarubicin, arrows point to the sites where these new drugs differ from doxorubicin and daunomycin, respectively.

system. This was based on the apparent saturation kinetics for uptake, and the K_m (Michaelis-Menten constant) and V_{max} (maximum reaction velocity) for this carrier were calculated. However, the physical properties of doxorubicin vary over the concentration range at which these studies were done; both doxorubicin and daunorubicin, like other planar molecules, self-associate by ring stacking, forming polymers.[9] As a result, progressively less of the added drug is available for uptake into the cell.[10] For doxorubicin and daunorubicin, transmembrane movement is by free diffusion of the un-ionized drug.[11] Furthermore, the uptake of the less polar daunorubicin is substantially faster than that of doxorubicin, which is itself substantially faster than that of its polar alcohol metabolite.[12]

The daunosamine sugar can become protonated within the physiologic pH range with a pKa of 7.6.[13,14] For this reason, both extracellular and intracellular pH can have a significant impact on anthracycline uptake and cytotoxicity.[15–17] For example, intracellular acidosis would result in enhanced drug accumulation because un-ionized drug would enter, would become protonated, and would be unable to diffuse out of the cell. Conversely, relative acidification of the extracellular fluid would result in a shift of drug out of the cell. In this regard, one should point out that tumor masses as small as 1 cm can exhibit extracellular pHs as low as 6.0 to 6.5.[18] More recent *in vivo* measurements using phosphorus-31 magnetic resonance spectroscopy have demonstrated that the intracellular pH of tumor cells in xenograft models is most frequently neutral to alkaline, whereas the extracellular pH is acidic.[14] Thus, the fact that simultaneous alkalinization of intra- and extracellular pH has been demonstrated to enhance the uptake and cytotoxicity of doxorubicin in cell culture and in SCID (severe combined immunodeficiency disease) mice carrying the human MCF-7 breast carcinoma is not surprising.[14,16] Furthermore, the acidification of intracellular organelles, including lysosomes, the Golgi network, and endosomes, in doxorubicin-resistant tumor cells significantly increases drug sequestration in these sites away from targets critical for tumor cell killing; blockade of sodium/proton exchange in acidic organelles produces a redistribution of doxorubicin into the cytoplasm and nucleus that can partially restore doxorubicin sensitivity in cells expressing the multidrug resistance phenotype.[19,20]

The cellular pharmacology of the anthracyclines is also characterized by the ability of essentially all nucleated cells to accumulate these drugs to an extraordinary degree.[21] Ratios between the intracellular and extracellular concentration of daunorubicin and doxorubicin are routinely on the order of 30- to 1,000-fold both at the end of a short-term *in vitro* incubation and in leukemic blasts at the end of an anthracycline infusion.[22] The accumulation of the anthracyclines is due to DNA binding, rapid association with cell membranes, and storage in several different intracellular compartments; furthermore, significant differences

are seen in degree of accumulation based on cell and tissue type.[21] This phenomenon is important for understanding both the pharmacokinetics of these drugs and the therapeutic efficacy of prolonged intravenous infusions.

In addition to the diffusion of the anthracyclines across the cell membrane, active drug efflux occurs in some cells. The initial demonstration of adenosine triphosphate (ATP)–dependent drug efflux resulted from the elucidation of the role of the multidrug resistance transporter in acquired anthracycline resistance.[23–26] Cells expressing the *MDR1* gene product efflux anthracyclines using the P-170 glycoprotein, a membrane protein capable of pumping a wide range of natural products, including the anthracyclines, out of cells. The P-170 glycoprotein has ATP binding sites, and drug efflux is dependent on the presence of adequate intracellular ATP pools. Other ATP-dependent drug efflux mechanisms capable of transporting anthracyclines against a concentration gradient have been discovered and may contribute to tumor cell drug resistance and to transport of the anthracycline antibiotics in normal host tissues, including the liver. These efflux mechanisms transport unmodified and/or glutathione-conjugated drug molecules.[27–35]

As is apparent from the studies reviewed earlier, although the general processes by which anthracyclines cross cell membranes have been examined in outline form, the kinetics of this process has not been established definitively, as is the case for methotrexate. The major barrier to such studies is the tendency for these drugs to bind to many intracellular proteins, DNA, phospholipids, and, perhaps, glycosaminoglycans. Because only free drug is presumably available for transport, efflux should be examined as a function of free, not total or bound, drug. This has rarely been done, however, in studies of drug efflux using anthracycline-resistant cell lines. Furthermore, the elucidation of several different energy-dependent efflux proteins in both tumor cells and normal tissues complicates the interpretation of prior studies, while at the same time providing continuing opportunities for additional evaluations of cellular pharmacokinetic processes.

DNA Intercalation, Topoisomerase II Interactions, and Other Effects on DNA

DNA Intercalation

Considerable controversy remains regarding the mechanism of action of the anthracyclines and thus regarding the importance of various intracellular targets. No disagreement exists, however, with the observation that the bulk of intracellular drug is in the nucleus and that a portion of the anthracycline in the nucleus is intercalated into the DNA double helix (Fig. 18-2). Detailed studies of daunorubicin affinity for DNA have identified a preference for dGdC-rich regions that are flanked by A:T base pairs.[36] In short, defined DNA sequences prepared by polymerase chain reaction, daunorubicin binds preferentially to either

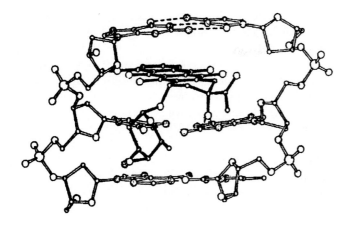

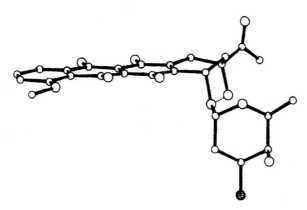

FIGURE 18-2. Three-dimensional view of daunomycin free and intercalated into DNA. This view shows the planar nature of the drug chromophore and how this is critical to DNA intercalation.

5'(A or T)GC or 5'(A or T)CG triplets.[37] The consensus sequence for highest doxorubicin affinity is 5'-TCA.[38] With respect to DNA interactions, the anthracycline molecule (Fig. 18-1) can be separated by function into three domains: the planar ring, which actually intercalates into DNA; the side chain (and its associated D ring), which provides an important hydrogen bonding function; and the daunosamine sugar, which binds to the minor groove and plays a critical role in base recognition and sequence specificity.[37]

The assumption had generally been that all of the drug within the nucleus is intercalated. When tumor cells exposed to doxorubicin or daunorubicin are examined by fluorescence microscopy, an intense nuclear fluorescence is observed, and many investigators have assumed that the intensity of this fluorescence is a measure of the amount of drug intercalated into DNA. Anthracycline fluorescence is quenched significantly on intercalation, however, and in fact, this quenching has been used to measure intercalation.[39] Thus, the nuclear fluorescence of the anthracyclines is likely to be due to binding of the drug to components of the nucleus by a nonintercalative mechanism. In fact, sta-

ble, covalently bound doxorubicin-DNA adducts (containing the daunosamine sugar) have been produced under conditions favored by the iron-dependent redox chemistry in which doxorubicin participates.[40]

Because the anthracyclines concentrate in the nucleus and are good DNA intercalators, DNA intercalation was presumed initially to play an important role in their mechanism of action. Several proposals were advanced to describe how DNA intercalation might lead to tumor cell kill, the best documented of which were studies demonstrating inhibition of RNA and DNA polymerases by the anthracyclines.[41,42] Unfortunately, the drug concentrations required for inhibition of these enzymes are far in excess of that which can be achieved *in vivo*, which probably explains the lack of correlation between inhibition of RNA and DNA synthesis and the cytotoxicity of doxorubicin.[43]

Topoisomerase II Interactions

An important advance in our understanding of anthracycline-DNA interactions occurred with the demonstration that anthracyclines cause protein-associated DNA breaks measured by filter elution, which in some cell lines are correlated with cytotoxicity.[44–46] Subsequent investigations have shown that the formation of protein-associated DNA breaks is caused by the formation of a ternary drug-DNA-enzyme "cleavable complex" involving the anthracycline antibiotic and DNA topoisomerase II, an enzyme associated with the nuclear matrix that plays a critical role in releasing torsional strain in DNA as well as in chromosome condensation.[47] Anthracyclines inhibit topoisomerase II by trapping DNA strand passage intermediates, which can be detected as protein-associated DNA single- and double-strand breaks linked to the enzyme.[48,49] Previously the presumption had been that through intercalation the anthracyclines altered the three-dimensional conformation of DNA, which arrested the cycle of topoisomerase II action at the point of DNA cleavage. Topoisomerase II–associated DNA cleavage, however, can be demonstrated at doxorubicin concentrations (10^{-8} mol per L) well below the dissociation constant for DNA intercalation,[50] as well as with anthracycline analogs that do not intercalate into DNA.[51] Thus, anthracyclines may stimulate topoisomerase II–mediated DNA cleavage by a nonintercalative mechanism. Studies evaluating the interaction of the anthracyclines with topoisomerase II have demonstrated that doxorubicinone actively inhibits the purified enzyme, which suggests that the anthracycline sugar is not required for enzyme inhibition. Because the daunosamine sugar plays an important role in DNA binding, DNA intercalation may possibly be dissociated further as a mechanism of action.[49] Research has demonstrated that the anthracyclines produce topoisomerase-related DNA cleavage in specific regions of the DNA (with an adenine at the 3'-end of one break site); this may provide a clue to gene-specific effects of these drugs.[52] Clearly, as is described subsequently, anthracycline resistance may be associated with alterations in the level or function of topoisomerase II, which indicates a potentially important role for this enzyme in anthracycline action.[53–55]

Molecular studies performed both in human cell lines and in yeast model systems have more clearly defined the role of the α isoform of topoisomerase II in the production of protein-associated DNA cleavage after doxorubicin exposure.[56,57] Overexpression of the antisense construct of topoisomerase IIα in human U937 monocytic leukemia cells down-regulates topoisomerase IIα messenger RNA (mRNA) levels by more than 70% with a concomitant reduction in the cytotoxicity of daunorubicin. Furthermore, a detailed reexamination of doxorubicin-related single-strand cleavage and topoisomerase-DNA complex formation has confirmed this process to be ATP-dependent and specific for topoisomerase II (not I),[58] an observation originally described more than a decade earlier.[59]

Although anthracycline interactions with DNA topoisomerase II clearly occur in many mammalian cell lines, the formation of cleavable complexes alone probably is only potentially lethal and is not in itself sufficient for tumor cell killing. Although the initial correlations of protein-associated single-strand cleavage and cytotoxicity in L1210 cells, which were performed at clinically relevant drug concentrations, suggested a direct relationship between topoisomerase II–mediated DNA damage and cytotoxicity for doxorubicin,[44,60] subsequent investigations have demonstrated a dissociation between tumor cell killing and the kinetics of DNA break formation and disappearance for doxorubicin and its analogs.[61] In some cell lines, only DNA double-strand cleavage can be associated with cytotoxicity,[62] and in others, DNA single-strand cleavage is modest and double-strand cleavage essentially undetectable at even supralethal drug concentrations.[63,64] Furthermore, evidence from several different model systems does not provide uniform support for a causal relationship between the level of topoisomerase II and the sensitivity of human cell lines to doxorubicin *in vitro*.[65,66] Finally, correlations between topoisomerase IIα content or activity in primary tumors and clinical outcome for breast cancer patients treated with anthracyclines have not been demonstrable.[67,68]

In addition to stabilizing the cleavable complex, the anthracyclines and a number of other antineoplastic compounds can inhibit the catalytic activity of the enzyme without trapping the complex, as has been appreciated for some time.[48,69] This observation, important for the development of new anthracyclines as well as combination regimens, underlies the demonstration that certain anthracycline analogs (not doxorubicin) antagonize the cytotoxicity and DNA cleavage of etoposide through inhibition of cleavable complex formation.[70–72] Furthermore, certain anthracycline analogs have been found that inhibit both topoisomerase I and topoisomerase II, which may explain their nonoverlapping resistance profiles and altered spectrum of action.[73–75] Doxorubicin is

also known to exhibit more cytotoxicity than expected per DNA break. This might mean either that doxorubicin-associated breaks are qualitatively different from those produced by other topoisomerase II–active drugs or that other mechanisms of action might be operating in parallel. Thus, questions remain regarding the precise role of cleavable complex formation in the cytotoxicity of the anthracycline antibiotics.

Other Effects on DNA

In addition to the physicochemical effects of the anthracyclines on DNA and their interactions with topoisomerase II, doxorubicin has been demonstrated to produce other, previously undescribed effects on DNA. Among the most important of these findings is the observation that doxorubicin and daunorubicin form DNA-anthracycline complexes that significantly modify the ability of a specific class of nuclear enzymes, the helicases, to dissociate duplex DNA into DNA single strands in an ATP-dependent fashion. The entire process of strand separation is thus hindered, which limits replication.[76] This effect occurs at clinically relevant drug concentrations (less than 1 μmol per L) and parallels, at least in part, the cytotoxic spectrum of several anthracycline analogs.[77] The mechanism of helicase inhibition involves the formation of an irreversible ternary complex between anthracyclines that possess an unblocked daunosamine sugar, DNA, and the helicase.[78] Given the diversity of human DNA helicases, differential effects of the anthracyclines could be related to their interactions with this class of nuclear enzymes. In the absence of significant DNA double-strand cleavage, doxorubicin interferes with DNA unwinding and produces nonoligosomal fragmentation of nascent DNA during continuous exposure to very low drug concentrations.[64,79] This DNA effect is associated with tumor cell differentiation and suppression of c-*myc* oncogene expression by both doxorubicin and certain of its analogs, and suggests yet another potential growth-inhibitory pathway for the anthracyclines.[80,81]

As is reviewed subsequently, research has also demonstrated that doxorubicin can undergo cycles of reduction and oxidation in essentially all intracellular compartments, including the nucleus and the mitochondrion. Doxorubicin redox cycling has been shown to oxidize DNA bases in human chromatin and in intact tumor cells, which may provide a cytotoxic mechanism unrelated to strand cleavage.[82–84] Mitochondrial DNA is also susceptible to oxidative stress *in vitro* and in the rat after doxorubicin administration, in which the production of 8-hydroxyguanosine, a byproduct of hydroxyl-radical attack on DNA, is significantly increased in cardiac and to a lesser extent in liver mitochondria relative to the level observed in nuclear DNA from these two organs.[85–87] Evidence of DNA base oxidation has also been demonstrated in patients treated with anthracycline antibiotics. Urinary hydroxymethyluracil (an oxidative byproduct of thymine) has been observed within 24 hours of drug treatment in patients receiving combination chemotherapy that included an anthracycline.[88,89] After bolus therapy with the anthracycline analog epirubicin hydrochloride, a wide variety of oxidized DNA bases can be found in chromatin isolated from patient lymphocytes using gas chromatography–mass spectroscopy (GC-MS).[90] In patients receiving a 96-hour infusion of doxorubicin, producing steady-state drug levels of 0.1 μmol per L, a two- to fivefold increase in 5-OH-hydantoin, 5-OH-uracil, and 5,6-di-OH-uracil was observed by GC-MS in peripheral blood mononuclear cells beginning 72 hours after the initiation of treatment.[91] These data are important because of the inhibitory effects of oxidized DNA bases on the action of DNA polymerases and other DNA repair mechanisms as well as their mutagenic properties and their potentially adverse consequences for the synthesis of genes comprising the mitochondrial respiratory chain.[92,93]

Finally, studies suggest that treatment with doxorubicin (or epirubicin) when used in combination with cyclophosphamide, is associated with a dramatically increased risk of a second malignancy, specifically acute monocytic or myelomonocytic leukemia.[94–96] Thus, one must remember that both doxorubicin and daunorubicin are both mutagens and carcinogens[97]; only recently have investigators begun to map the base substitutions and deletions produced by doxorubicin, which appear to occur adjacent to preferential doxorubicin DNA binding sequences. The mechanism of specific doxorubicin-induced mutations and their mapping in mammalian cells remain to be determined.

Drug Activation by One- and Two-Electron Reduction

During DNA intercalation and binding to topoisomerase II, the anthracyclines act as chemically inert compounds that owe their activity to their ability to bind to key macromolecules and distort the three-dimensional geometry of these targets. The anthracyclines are chemically reactive, however, with an extraordinarily rich chemistry that even now has not been fully documented.[98,99]

One-Electron Reduction

The one-electron reduction of the anthracyclines was initially described in hepatic microsomal systems[100–102] but was later shown to play a central role in the cardiac toxicity of this class of drugs[103–105] and may be involved in antitumor activity as well.[106–108] All of the clinically active anthracyclines are anthraquinones. As is true of quinones in general,[109,110] the anthracyclines are able to undergo one- and two-electron reduction to reactive compounds that cause widespread damage to intracellular macromolecules, including lipid membranes, DNA bases, and thiol-containing transport proteins (Fig. 18-3).[111–114] As outlined in Figure 18-4, the one-electron reduction of doxorubicin or daunorubicin may occur in essentially all intracellular compartments, including the nuclear membrane, and is catalyzed by flavin-centered dehydrogenases or reductases including cytochrome P-450 reductase, nicotinamide adenine dinucleotide (reduced form) dehydrogenase (complex I of the mitochondrial electron transport chain), xanthine oxidase, and cytochrome b_5 reductase.[115–117] In addition, studies demonstrate that all three isoforms of nitric oxide synthase (at their flavoprotein domains) are capable of catalyzing the one-electron reduction of doxorubicin with the subsequent production of superoxide and a decrease in nitric oxide.[118,119] Furthermore, doxorubicin can directly inhibit nitric oxide synthase activity,[119,120] which could produce significant alterations in vascular tone both in the heart and in tumors.[121,122] All of these flavoenzymes are widely distributed in mammalian tissues, and anthracycline-mediated free-radical formation has been demon-

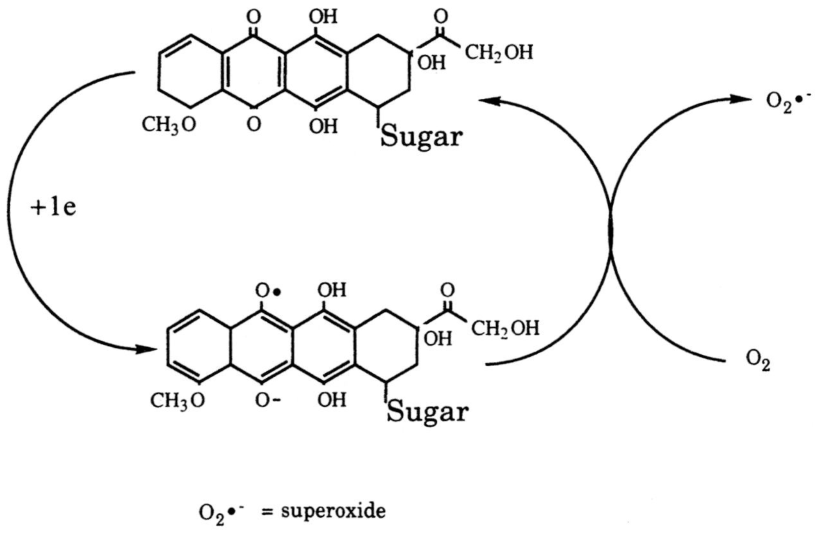

FIGURE 18-3. One-electron reduction of doxorubicin. This reduction occurs at the quinone oxygens of the chromophore. The semiquinones react rapidly with oxygen, when it is available, to yield the one-electron reduction product of oxygen, superoxide.

$O_2^{•-}$ = superoxide

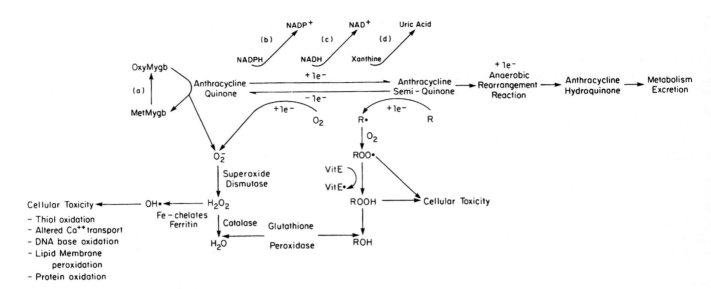

FIGURE 18-4. Schematic overview of anthracycline-induced oxyradical metabolism and detoxification. (a) Metmyoglobin reductase. (b) Reduced nicotinamide adenine dinucleotide phosphate (NADPH) cytochrome P-450 reductase. (c) Reduced nicotinamide adenine dinucleotide (NADH) dehydrogenase. (d) Xanthine oxidase. [MetMygb, metmyoglobin; NAD^+, nicotinamide adenine dinucleotide (oxidized form); $NADP^+$, nicotinamide adenine dinucleotide phosphate (oxidized form); OxyMygb, oxymyoglobin; R, unsaturated lipids; VitE, vitamin E.]

strated in a wide range of organs and tumor cell lines. In addition to being reduced by flavoproteins, doxorubicin can be reduced in the heart by oxymyoglobin, which leads to the production of strong oxidant species.[123]

One-electron reduction of the anthracyclines leads to the formation of the corresponding semiquinone free radical. In the presence of oxygen, this free radical rapidly donates its electron to oxygen to generate superoxide anion $(O_2^{\bullet-})$. Although superoxide is not highly toxic itself, its dismutation yields hydrogen peroxide (H_2O_2). Under biologic conditions, the anthracycline semiquinone or reduced metal ions such as iron reductively cleave hydrogen peroxide to produce the hydroxyl radical $(OH^{\bullet})$ or a higher-oxidation-state metal with the chemical characteristics of the hydroxyl radical, one of the most reactive and destructive chemical species known.[124,125] Reduced metals are now commonly accepted to be critical components in the formation of toxic free-radical intermediates and may well contribute to the cytotoxicity of the anthracyclines.[126] However, how reduced metal species, including iron, become available for these free-radical reactions remains an area of active investigation.

Because oxygen-radical formation occurs as a result of normal metabolic processes (including mitochondrial respiration) and is a common mechanism of action for several naturally occurring toxins, most mammalian cells have elaborate defenses against oxygen-radical toxicity.[127] Superoxide dismutase, catalase, and glutathione peroxidase act in concert to reduce superoxide, hydrogen peroxide, and lipid hydroperoxides to water or nontoxic lipid alcohols without the for-

mation of the hydroxyl or peroxyl radicals (Fig. 18-4). Glutathione, a sulfur-containing tripeptide, can react with many radicals as well as function as part of the glutathione peroxidase cycle to reduce peroxides to less reactive compounds. Specific DNA repair systems also exist to handle oxidative damage to DNA.[128–130] Antioxidant defenses are not equally distributed in various tissues in the body, however. For example, glutathione concentration is higher in the liver than in most other tissues and tumors. Catalase activity is lower in the heart than in the liver.[104,131] Likewise, the activity of several flavoproteins capable of activating the anthracyclines differs from tissue to tissue. These variations in drug activation and antioxidant defense provide ample opportunity for tissue specificity in terms of toxicity and antitumor activity. For example, the unique cardiac toxicity of the anthracyclines may result, in part, from the low level of cardiac catalase coupled with the extraordinary cardiac content of mitochondria and myoglobin, which enhance drug activation, as well as the sensitivity of cardiac glutathione peroxidase to free-radical attack,[104,132] which destroys the activity of this critical enzyme at the same time that anthracycline administration stimulates cardiac hydrogen peroxide formation.[133] In contrast, although anthracyclines can easily be activated to reactive intermediates by hepatic enzymes, the liver has a more active free-radical defense system and is able actively to efflux anthracyclines and anthracycline metabolites. The importance of hepatic antioxidant systems can be seen in the fact that in rodents pretreatment with agents that significantly diminish reduced glutathione levels, such as carmustine (bischloroethylnitrosourea, BCNU) or acetaminophen, dramatically sensitizes hepatocytes to doxorubicin-induced free-radical injury.[134,135]

The role of oxygen-radical formation in tumor cell killing, rather than in cardiac toxicity, continues to be defined.[136–139] Several lines of evidence, however, support the hypothesis that oxygen radicals do play a role in this cytotoxicity. First, doxorubicin resistance in tumor cell lines can frequently be reversed by agents that decrease glutathione concentration.[140–145] This observation cannot be explained by virtue of DNA interactions. Second, anthracycline-enhanced free-radical formation has been detected in a range of tumor cell lines,[106,146,147] the best studied of which are human breast cancer cell lines, in which both intra- and extracellular reactive oxygen species were demonstrated.[107,148] Extracellular as well as intracellular antioxidants have also been demonstrated to decrease the cytotoxicity of the anthracyclines in a wide variety of cells, including human tumor cell lines.[107,108,126,149–153] In addition, some anthracycline-resistant cancer cell lines exhibit increases in various aspects of the oxygen-free-radical defense system, including increases in glutathione and the selenoprotein glutathione peroxidase.[144,154–157] Alterations in glutathione peroxidase activity produced by manipulation of selenium status significantly affect tumor cell killing by doxorubicin.[158,159] Transfection of the human cytosolic glutathione peroxidase in the sense orientation produces doxorubicin resistance,[160] whereas antisense expression sensitizes cells to doxorubicin cytotoxicity.[161] Finally, fourfold overexpression of the manganese superoxide dismutase in Chinese hamster ovary cells produces 2.5-fold resistance to doxorubicin,[162] whereas inhibition of the copper-zinc superoxide dismutase with 1,25-dihydroxyvitamin D_3 significantly enhances doxorubicin-related cytotoxicity.[163]

Reservations about the role of oxygen-radical formation in tumor cell killing arise from several observations. First, most of the studies demonstrating anthracycline-enhanced hydroxyl-radical formation have used drug concentrations in excess of that which would be clinically relevant. This limitation is in part technical in that, at present, hydroxyl radicals cannot be detected at concentrations much below 10^{-7}. However, studies using fluorescent probes to detect hydrogen peroxide production by flow cytometry after doxorubicin exposure in human colon carcinoma cells successfully demonstrated peroxide formation after treatment with 0.4 μmol per L of doxorubicin,[147] and enhanced oxidative respiration and reactive oxygen production have been observed in human breast cancer cells using chemiluminescent probes at doxorubicin levels between 0.05 and 0.1 μmol per L.[164] Second, many tumors against which doxorubicin has great clinical utility, such as breast cancer, are clearly hypoxic, and thus the applicability of the chemistry outlined in Figures 18-3 and 18-4 might be questioned. Under low partial pressures of oxygen, however, iron-mediated lipid peroxidation and DNA damage from the doxorubicin semiquinone are actually enhanced.[165] Third,

no question exists that glutathione depletion does not sensitize all tumor cell lines to the cytotoxic effect of doxorubicin,[166] and that many doxorubicin-resistant cells have no alteration in antioxidant defense enzymes.[167] Fourth, the presumption frequently has been that oxygen-radical–mediated effects on DNA were unlikely because intercalated drug could not be reduced. Doxorubicin covalently bound to oligonucleotides can still be activated by cytochrome P-450 reductase,[168] however, and daunorubicin intercalated into calf thymus DNA can be reduced by a superoxide generating system; under these circumstances the semiquinone is accessible to hydrogen peroxide for reaction, and the disproportionation of the semiquinone to the 7-deoxyaglycone may occur by intramolecular electron transfer with migration of electrons over several base pairs.[169–171] Finally, as outlined previously, studies have demonstrated the presence of oxidized DNA bases, byproducts of anthracycline redox cycling, in both the urine[89] and peripheral blood mononuclear cells of patients receiving anthracycline therapy.[90,91] These reports provide the first, albeit indirect, evidence demonstrating the products of redox cycling in human tissues after anthracycline administration using standard treatment schedules.

Role of Iron

Although free-radical formation was originally proposed as the basis for anthracycline cardiac toxicity in 1977 and various animal model studies suggested that hydroxyl-radical scavengers could blunt doxorubicin-related heart damage, free-radical scavengers were initially unsuccessful cardioprotective agents in humans.[172] These results suggested that some additional variable was involved. This variable proved to be the interaction of anthracyclines with iron. Because of the reactivity of iron, free iron concentrations in the body are in the range of approximately 10^{-13} mol per L, whereas total iron concentrations are between 10^{-4} and 10^{-5} mol per L. Most of the iron in tissues is stored in ferritin. Doxorubicin has been found to release iron from ferritin in two ways. The drug can slowly abstract iron from the ferritin shell directly[173]; a much more rapid release of iron follows conversion of the anthracycline to its semiquinone, which can release iron under hypoxic conditions or through the reducing power of the superoxide anion in air.[174,175] Doxorubicin can also release nonheme, nonferritin iron from microsomes.[176–178] The hydroxyquinone structure of doxorubicin and daunorubicin represents a powerful site for chelation of metal ions, especially ferric iron. Iron anthracycline complexes have been shown to possess a wide range of interesting biochemical properties *in vitro*.[179,180] These complexes can bind DNA by a mechanism distinct from intercalation, cause oxidative destruction of membranes, and oxidize critical sulfhydryl groups. Whether these tight-binding iron-anthracycline complexes are stable and produce toxic effects intracellularly,[181,182] however, or whether the "delocalization" of catalytic amounts of protein-bound iron by anthracycline-stimulated free-radical formation is responsible for hydroxyl-radical formation in tissues, remains unclear.

These investigations suggested that the most effective way to interfere with the generation of highly reactive oxidants after anthracycline exposure would be to pretreat with a chelating agent that might withdraw iron from free-radical reactions. This hypothesis has been confirmed, and use of an iron chelator, dexrazoxane (ICRF-187), has been shown to prevent doxorubicin-induced lipid peroxidation[183] and cardiac toxicity in a wide range of animal models.[184,185] Randomized, controlled clinical trials in humans have confirmed the ability of this agent to diminish markedly the cardiac toxicity of doxorubicin.[186,187] Dexrazoxane is a highly effective iron chelator *in vivo*; during phase I studies it caused a tenfold increase in urinary iron clearance.[188] Dexrazoxane is itself a prodrug in that it must undergo hydrolysis to become an effective iron chelator (Fig. 18-5). This hydrolysis to ICRF-198, the major iron-binding metabolite of dexrazoxane, can occur spontaneously at physiologic pH but is markedly enhanced after uptake into cardiac myocytes, with conversion of the parent drug to

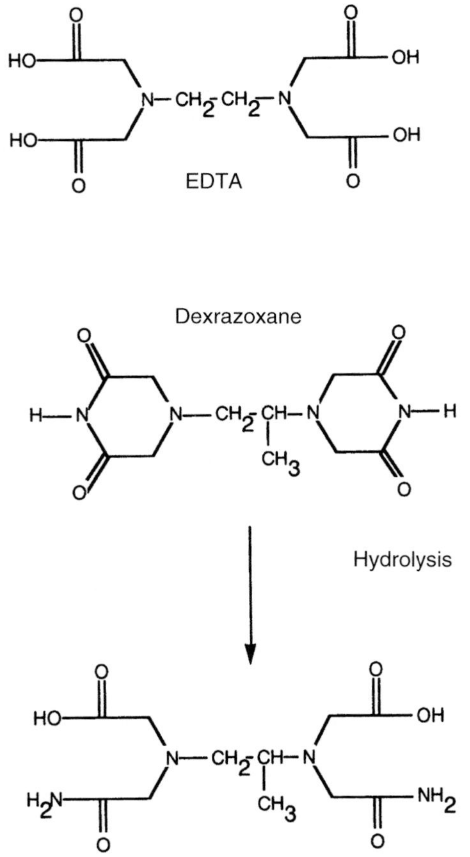

FIGURE 18-5. Dexrazoxane and its analogy to EDTA (ethylenediaminetetraacetic acid). Dexrazoxane is much more nonpolar because the carboxylic acid groups have been fused into amide rings. This allows ready entry into the cell. Dexrazoxane can undergo hydrolysis to yield a carboxylamine able to bind iron.

ICRF-198 in less than 60 seconds.[189] The parent drug is very lipid soluble and enters cells by passive diffusion. ICRF-198 has been demonstrated to efflux iron from iron-loaded myocytes. These studies suggest that the same chelating ability may be available to remove iron that has been released from cardiac iron-storage proteins.[189]

Studies have further amplified our understanding of the role of iron in anthracycline biochemistry and in the mechanism of drug-induced cardiac toxicity.[190–193] The alcohol metabolite of doxorubicin, doxorubicinol, which is produced by the two-electron reduction of the C-13 side chain carbonyl group, has been demonstrated to cause the delocalization of low-molecular-weight Fe(II) species from the iron-sulfur center of aconitase in a redox-dependent fashion. The formation of a doxorubicin-iron complex with aconitase interferes with critical interconversions of cytosolic aconitase with iron-regulatory protein 1. Iron-regulatory protein 1 plays an essential role in iron homeostasis and, hence, in the regulation of critical intracellular metabolic processes (such as the action of mitochondrial electron transport proteins, myoglobin, and various cytochromes). These effects of doxorubicin metabolites suggest that iron-dependent reactions occur that may not be directly related to the formation of reactive oxygen species. This could help to explain the utility of dexrazoxane, compared with that of free-radical scavengers that do not chelate iron, in the prevention of both acute and chronic anthracycline cardiotoxicity.

Doxorubicin is a powerful chelator of other metal ions, including Cu^{2+} and Al^{3+}. The chelation of aluminum by doxorubicin is effective enough that a doxorubicin solution left in contact with aluminum foil for only 1 hour changes from the orange-red of doxorubicin to the bright cherry red of the aluminum complex. A similar reaction occurs with iron-containing alloys; doxorubicin left within a syringe needle for any significant period of time also changes color by virtue of chelation of metal from the needle. For this reason, every effort should be made in the clinic to keep anthracyclines from prolonged contact with any metal surface.

Two-Electron Reduction
Two-electron reduction of doxorubicin (which may occur by sequential one-electron reductions or directly when strong reducing agents are applied) results in the formation of an unstable quinone methide, which rapidly undergoes a series of reactions that lead to the formation of the corresponding deoxyaglycone (Fig. 18-6).[98] Deoxyaglycones have now been established to be formed *in vivo*.[194,195] Because the deoxyaglycones exhibit far less cytotoxicity than the parent drug, the current consensus is that this is a pathway for drug inactivation. In the absence of oxygen, the one-electron reduction product, the semiquinone, probably reacts with itself to yield parent drug and the two-electron reduction product. The quinone methide intermediate in this pathway has been proposed as a potential monofunctional alkylating agent; however, little evidence exists that

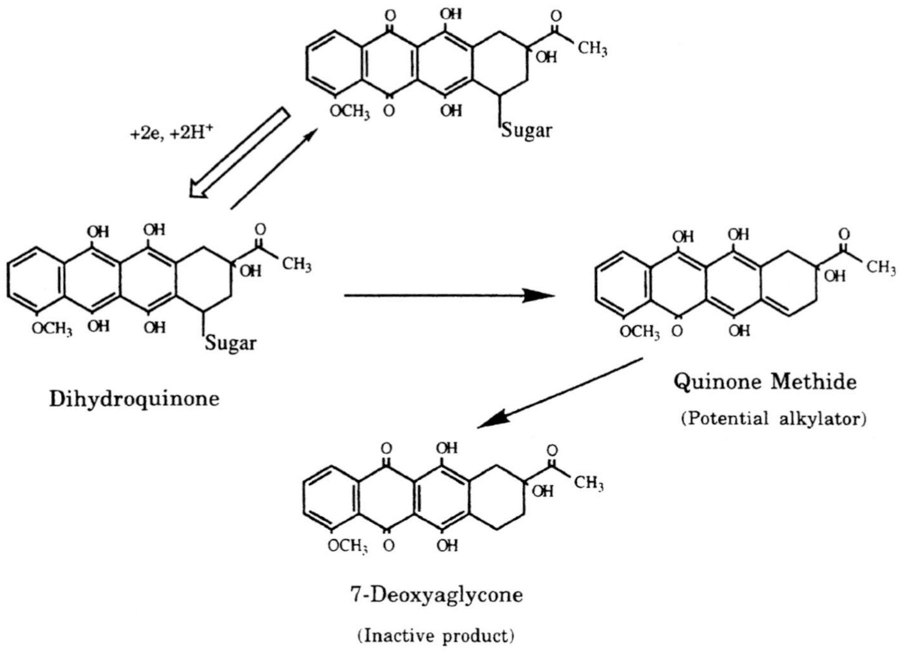

FIGURE 18-6. Two-electron reduction of anthraquinones. The immediate product is the dihydroquinone, which is not stable. This undergoes rearrangement with loss of the sugar to yield the quinone methide. This structure has activity as an alkylator in pure chemical systems. The most likely fate, however, is progression, via a second arrangement, to yield the 7-deoxyaglycone. This final product is much less active than the parent drug.

this intermediate plays an important cytotoxic role in tumor cells. Finally, two-electron reduction of the anthracyclines using powerful reducing agents to convert doxorubicin to its inactive deoxyaglycone metabolite has been advocated as a means to reduce local tissue injury after anthracycline extravasation.[196] Direct enzymatic two-electron reduction is unlikely to occur under physiologic conditions.[197]

Signal Transduction, Membrane-Related Actions of the Anthracyclines, and Apoptosis

Membrane Perturbations

For more than a decade the anthracycline antibiotics have been known to be membrane-active compounds that produce a myriad of effects at the cell surface.[198] Only in the more recent past have events that occur at the cell surface been related more clearly to anthracycline cytotoxicity and DNA damage. Doxorubicin alters the fluidity of both tumor cell plasma membranes[199,200] and cardiac mitochondria.[111] It binds avidly to phospholipids including cardiolipin,[201,202] causes an up-regulation of epidermal growth factor receptor (but not p185[HER-2/neu]),[203,204] inhibits the transferrin reductase of the plasma membrane,[205] induces iron-dependent protein oxidation in erythrocyte plasma membranes *in vivo*,[206] and can be actively cytotoxic without entering the cell.[207,208] Furthermore, studies suggest that the presence of extracellular doxorubicin is of critical importance for membrane interactions that are intimately related to the evolution of tumor cell kill[209] and that doxorubicin cytotoxicity can be manipulated by membrane phospholipid alterations[210–212] that increase drug uptake but not intracellular distribution. The confluence of these studies suggests that plasma

membrane–associated events, modulated by lipid metabolism, could be involved in the mechanism of action of the anthracyclines.

Signal Transduction and Anthracyclines

Communication between the cell surface and the nucleus plays a crucial role in growth control. Several important signal transduction pathways for mitogenic stimuli can be initiated at the plasma membrane.[213–217] If membrane interactions involving the anthracyclines are important for their mechanism of action, it should be possible to show that these compounds interact significantly with known signal transduction programs.[218]

Several laboratories have begun to provide essential pieces of evidence linking anthracycline action to effects on specific signal transduction pathways, including the protein kinase C system. Although at high concentrations (more than 100 μmol per L) anthracyclines can inhibit protein kinase C,[219,220] the doxorubicin-iron complex is more active as an inhibitor of diacylglycerol at tenfold lower concentrations.[221] At clinically relevant levels, doxorubicin increases the turnover of phosphoinositides and phosphatidylcholine in sarcoma 180 cells, which leads to the accumulation of diacylglycerol and inositol phosphates and a twofold increase in cytosolic protein kinase C activity.[222] Furthermore, activation of the protein kinase C pathway by phorbol esters enhances doxorubicin cytotoxicity and drug-related DNA-protein cross-links, whereas down-regulation of protein kinase C partially prevents cell kill.[223] Because protein kinase C can phosphorylate topoisomerase II,[224] the initiation of membrane signaling by doxorubicin could be involved in the regulation of anthracycline-mediated DNA damage.

The importance of the sphingomyelin pathway in signal transduction has become increasingly clear during the past 5 years.[213] In addition to participating in protein kinase C–related signal transduction, sphingolipid metabolites are involved in transducing signals from a wide variety of cell surface molecules, including interferon-γ, tumor necrosis factor α, and Fas/APO-1. Data suggest that the activation of sphingomyelinases by a variety of cellular stresses, including exposure to the anthracyclines, leads to the release of the critical signaling intermediate ceramide from membrane sphingomyelin.[225–227] Intracellular ceramide accumulation can produce profound effects on cell-cycle progression as well as on the effector arm of the cell death program.[228–230] Expression of glucosylceramide synthase (the enzyme that converts ceramide to glucosylceramide) in human MCF-7 cells blocks doxorubicin-induced increases in ceramide after drug exposure, which leads to an 11-fold increase in the concentration causing 50% inhibition.[231]

Signal transduction pathways involving protein kinase C and ceramide also appear to be involved in regulation of the function of the P-170 glycoprotein and the enhanced export of anthracyclines in drug-resistant cells.[232–234] Inhibition of protein kinase C has been shown to down-regulate P-170 glycoprotein function and enhance the sensitivity of myeloid leukemia cells to daunorubicin, which provides a novel strategy for overcoming multidrug resistance.[235] Furthermore, certain agents that reverse multidrug resistance, such as cyclosporin A and verapamil hydrochloride, may in part be active through an inhibition of ceramide glycosylation.[236]

Anthracyclines and Apoptosis

The explosive growth of our understanding of apoptosis (programmed cell death)[237–239] has provided crucial links between many of the pleiotropic effects of the anthracyclines that have been described previously, including anthracycline-related alterations in membrane biochemistry, signal transduction, mitochondrial metabolism, DNA damage, and free-radical formation.

Doxorubicin or daunorubicin exposure can produce the morphologic changes associated with apoptosis such as chromatin condensation, internucleosomal DNA fragmentation, reduced cell volume, and cytoplasmic blebbing in a wide variety of cell lines, including: HeLa cells,[240] the P388 murine leukemia,[241] M1 myeloid leukemia cells,[242] murine small intestinal crypt epithelium,[243] thymocytes,[244,245] and others.[139,246] In general, the degree of anthracycline-related apoptosis varies considerably between experimental model systems; in cell culture, the full expression of apoptotic morphology is often not observed until 48 to 120 hours after drug treatment. This variability is due, in part, to wide variations in the expression of both proapoptotic and anti-apoptotic molecules in cultured tumor cells, a degree of variability that has also been observed in human tumor samples.[33,247–249]

Intensive investigative efforts over the past 5 years have begun to determine the molecular mechanisms of anthracycline-related apoptosis. The picture that is starting to emerge is of a series of biochemical interactions of the anthracycline antibiotics with a wide variety of different death-initiating signaling compounds that ultimately use common effector molecules to produce apoptosis and necrotic cell kill. One of the best-described death stimuli is the interaction of the CD95 (Fas/APO-1) surface receptor with its natural ligand CD95L, or structurally related antibodies, to form a signaling complex that activates proteases of the caspase family to effect the ultimate biochemical reactions resulting in apoptotic morphology. This pathway, which plays a critical role in the regulation of lymphoid cell growth, has been shown to be active in some solid tumors and leukemias. Experiments initially suggested that doxorubicin produced apoptosis by inducing CD95L and CD95 receptor formation, and that CEM cells, Jurkat T cells, and neuroblastoma cells resistant to anti-CD95 antibody were resistant to doxorubicin-induced apoptosis.[250–252] Although doxorubicin clearly appears to up-regulate CD95L expression after doxorubicin exposure in HeLa cells transfected with a CD95L reporter construct,[253] a series of studies in different cell lines have determined that acquired resistance to CD95 by clonal selection or by treatment with other anti-CD95 antibodies that inhibit CD95-mediated apoptosis does not concomitantly engender resistance to doxorubicin-related apoptosis,[254,255] that CD95 and CD95L are frequently not up-regulated after doxorubicin exposure,[256] and that anthracycline-mediated activation of caspase 8, previously supposed to modulate CD95-induced apoptosis specifically, occurs in the absence of signaling through the CD95/CD95L pathway.[257] All of these experiments support the hypothesis that doxorubicin and CD95 use common downstream effectors of apoptosis but that the initiating death stimulus for either of these molecules may vary.

Apoptosis due to the anthracyclines has also been clearly related to ceramide generation,[225,258] which links the plasma membrane biochemistry of doxorubicin with the induction of the cell death cascade. Only recently, however, has the molecular ordering of anthracycline-induced apoptosis begun to be examined. In these studies, ceramide generation after sphingomyelinase activation leads to important effects on mitochondrial permeability, the activation of proapoptotic caspases, and serine-threonine protein phosphatases.[213,228,259] Whether ceramide production after anthracycline exposure is associated principally with the activation of cell death signals to the mitochondria or with the effector phase of apoptosis remains to be determined, however.

One of the critical steps in translating a wide variety of apoptotic stimuli into either apoptotic or necrotic cell death is the induction of cytochrome *c* release from the space between the inner and outer mitochondrial membrane.[237,260,261] Cytochrome *c* release can lead to caspase activation or to altered mitochondrial electron transport with subsequent apoptosis or necrosis. In light of the previously described extensive binding and metabolism of the anthracyclines by complex I of the mitochondrial electron transport chain,[116] the likelihood is that reactive oxygen species produced by anthracycline-treated mitochondria that can damage mitochondrial membrane integrity play an important initiating role in doxorubicin-related apoptosis. Studies indicate that various free-radical scavengers inhibit programmed cell death after anthracycline exposure.[83,139,151,152,262] Furthermore, cytokine-mediated induction of ceramide production has been found to be redox sensitive.[263] These observations link many of the known but pleiotropic biochemical effects of the anthracyclines; further studies are likely to define the order of anthracycline-related death signals at the molecular level and the relationship of these signals to intracellular anthracycline metabolism.

Two major endogenous modulators of programmed cell death, Bcl-2 and p53, as well as their associated downstream effectors, play critical roles in regulating anthracycline-related apoptosis. The Bcl-2 protein functions in the outer membranes of mitochondria, nuclei, and the endoplasmic reticulum as an inhibitor of cell death. It has been clearly shown to block apoptosis after anthracycline exposure in many experimental systems.[264,265] Furthermore, in AML blasts and HL-60 cells the cytotoxicity of daunorubicin is increased by exposure to *bcl*-2 antisense oligonucleotides.[266] The biochemical mechanisms through which Bcl-2 inhibits cell death continue to be elucidated; however, currently Bcl-2 is known to repress cytochrome *c* release from mitochondria, interfere with caspase activation, block the apoptotic effects of reactive oxygen species, and bind to transcription factors involved in doxorubicin-mediated apoptosis, such as nuclear factor-κB.[267–272] Bcl-2 has also been demonstrated to suppress p53-mediated transcriptional activation of several genes involved in the apoptotic process after doxorubicin exposure in MCF-7 cells.[267]

Programmed cell death that occurs as a consequence of doxorubicin exposure appears to be modulated by the interplay between the expression of *bcl*-2 and the *p53* tumor suppressor gene.[273] The p53 functions as a transcription factor that causes cell-cycle arrest or apoptosis after DNA damage. Among the genes activated by p53 are the cyclin-dependent kinase inhibitor *p21, cyclin G,* and the apoptosis-inducing gene *bax.* Exposure to anthracyclines leads to elevated steady-state levels of p53 in cells expressing the wild-type gene,[246,274] which produces cell-cycle arrest or apoptosis depending on the cell type studied. G_1 arrest is due to the induction of p21 in both p53-dependent and p53-independent contexts, which leads to apoptosis or cellular senescence.[274–277] Studies also suggest that p53 induction after doxorubicin treatment produces up-regulation of cyclin G expression with a consequent

increase in the accumulation of cells in the G_2-M as well as G_1 phases of the cell cycle.[278] Finally, mutations in *p53,* found in almost half of human tumors, lead to diminished apoptosis and doxorubicin resistance in many different tumor cell types.[279–281]

Mechanisms of Resistance

Enhanced Drug Efflux

P-170 Glycoprotein–Mediated Anthracycline Efflux
A majority of the doxorubicin-resistant cell lines developed in the laboratory exhibit increased expression of the P-170 glycoprotein. At present, the role of this protein in the enhancement of drug efflux and as a mechanism of experimental drug resistance has been conclusively established.[23,282,283] The evidence supporting this role includes (a) a good correlation between the presence of this protein and a pattern of broad-spectrum drug resistance that includes resistance to the anthracyclines, vinca alkaloids, actinomycin D, and the epipodophyllotoxins[284]; (b) transfer of the cloned *MDR1* gene for this protein that demonstrates the full phenotype of multidrug resistance, including resistance to doxorubicin[285]; and (c) the reversal of anthracycline resistance by a range of compounds, such as verapamil, cyclosporine A, calmodulin inhibitors, and tamoxifen, that block P-170–mediated drug efflux by binding to this protein.[286–291] The genetic mechanism behind this increased expression in selected lines *in vitro* is variable. In some cell lines demonstrating very high levels of anthracycline resistance, the notable finding has been gene amplification, either present in double minutes or integrated within the chromosome as homogeneous staining regions; other lines show only increased mRNA coding for the P-170 glycoprotein.[292,293] The nature of the resistance that develops after a single prolonged exposure to doxorubicin in a human sarcoma cell line was evaluated using classic fluctuation analysis. Induction of *MDR1* expression was not demonstrated; rather, resistance to doxorubicin arose from a spontaneous mutation with an apparent rate of approximately 2×10^{-6} per cell generation.[294] Also, the expression of the *MDR1* gene clearly may, under some circumstances, be transcriptionally modulated by doxorubicin itself, as well as by inhibitors of protein kinase C and calmodulin.[233,295,296] For resistance that develops *in vivo,* the situation is more complex, with most tumors and many normal tissues exhibiting increased expression of a single gene copy.[284]

Although the physiologic role for this protein has not been established unequivocally, its expression has been documented in a range of normal tissues. Elevated expression is seen in colon mucosa, kidney, adrenal medulla, adrenal cortex, the blood–brain barrier, and many normal bone marrow elements.[297–299] In addition, expression in liver is increased after both partial hepatectomy and exposure to carcinogens such as 2-acetylaminofluorene.[300] The combination of partial hepatectomy and carcinogen exposure is synergistic, and results in over a 100-fold increase in expression. Based on this information, some have postulated that the P-170 glycoprotein is part of an integrated system for protecting cells against toxic xenobiotics.[301,302] Other components of this system include the mixed-function oxidases, glutathione transferases, glucuronyl transferases, glutathione, and glutathione peroxidase.

A wide range of human tumors has been examined before and after treatment with anthracyclines and other drugs that participate in the multidrug resistance phenotype. Increased expression of the P-170 glycoprotein is found before treatment in renal, colon, and adrenal carcinomas, in some neuroblastomas and soft tissue sarcomas, and occasionally in tumors of lymphoid or myeloid origin. For patients with acute lymphocytic leukemia and AML, expression of P-170 glycoprotein carries an adverse prognosis.[303,304] P-170 glycoprotein expression is rarely found at significant levels either before or after therapy in small cell carcinoma of the lung, but expression is clearly increased posttreatment in some patients after failure of primary therapy for leukemia, lymphoma, or myeloma.[305,306] Expression in breast cancer is variable.[307,308] Results from clinical trials evaluating the effect of agents to reverse multidrug resistance on the efficacy of anthracycline-containing chemotherapeutic programs have begun to be available.[309-311] In general, the initial studies of this approach demonstrated that clinical strategies to overcome P-170 glycoprotein–mediated drug resistance are most likely to be effective for patients with hematologic malignancies, that better reversing agents which can be administered at the appropriate dosage with an acceptable toxicity profile are urgently needed, and that, not unexpectedly, the pharmacokinetics of the anthracyclines may be significantly altered by drugs such as cyclosporine A that markedly decrease the clearance of doxorubicin and doxorubicinol.[312] Despite these difficulties, a large randomized trial involving patients with AML demonstrated significantly improved relapse-free and overall survival when cyclosporine A was added to daunorubicin as part of a standard cytosine arabinoside and daunorubicin induction regimen.[313] Whether these results reflect reversal of P-glycoprotein–mediated acquired resistance or are due to the increased levels of daunorubicin and its alcohol metabolite found in patients treated with cyclosporine A remains to be determined.

Multidrug Resistance Protein and Other Adenosine Triphosphate–Dependent Efflux Mechanisms

In some doxorubicin-resistant cell lines that exhibit decreased drug accumulation, P-170 glycoprotein is not overexpressed, and verapamil produces quite variable alterations in resistance.[314,315] These results are explained by a unique, ATP-dependent efflux protein that was discovered in the doxorubicin-selected human small cell cancer line

H69/AR. Its mRNA encodes a 190-kd protein that is a member of the ATP-binding cassette transmembrane transporter superfamily.[27] The encoded glycoprotein has also been found in doxorubicin-resistant HL-60 leukemia cells and the doxorubicin-resistant HT1080/DR4 human sarcoma line, both of which lack P-170 glycoprotein expression.[28,316] A wide variety of other experimental tumor cell systems have also been demonstrated to overexpress the multidrug resistance protein (MRP).[317-319] The overexpression of MRP in drug-sensitive HeLa cells has been shown to produce resistance to doxorubicin, etoposide, and vincristine sulfate but not to cisplatin or traditional alkylating agents. Thus, MRP expression alone, in the absence of alterations in *MDR1* expression or levels of topoisomerase II, can produce anthracycline resistance. Furthermore, doxorubicin export by the MRP gene product is as efficient as that by the P-glycoprotein.[320] In contrast to human sarcoma cells, doxorubicin selection of leukemic cells *in vitro* leads first to the overexpression of MRP at low drug concentrations and then to the subsequent expression of the P-170 glycoprotein.[321] Furthermore, MRP may function coordinately with *MDR1* to produce anthracycline resistance in patients with acute leukemia, which suggests that MRP may play an important role in the clinic.[322,323] These studies also suggest that critical tissue specificities may be involved in the evolution of the overexpression of different transport proteins.

MRP expression occurs widely in normal tissues except the liver and small intestine, where expression is limited.[324] Studies including those using MRP knockout models[325] have suggested a variety of physiologic functions for MRP. These include transport of heavy metals, modulation of ion channels, transport of glutathione conjugates including leukotriene C_4, as well as the transport of glutathione (GSH) with and without other xenobiotics such as the anthracyclines.[30,32] Although transport of chemically prepared conjugates of doxorubicin or daunorubicin with glutathione by membrane vesicles from cells overexpressing MRP has been documented,[32] the occurrence of such conjugates has not yet been observed *in vivo*. More likely, the multidrug resistance protein plays a critical role in the cotransport of GSH with the anthracyclines as part of a series of related gene products rather than as a single glutathione-xenobiotic conjugate pump.[326]

Other ATP-dependent doxorubicin efflux pumps have been characterized.[29] Furthermore, a 110-kd lung resistance–related protein has been identified as the major vault protein, a critical component of certain subcellular organelles.[34] Overexpression of this protein has been associated with an adverse prognosis in patients with AML treated with anthracycline-containing chemotherapy.[33,35] These discoveries, taken together with the finding of an entire family of multidrug resistance genes (*MRPs*),[326] suggest the possibility that several distinct efflux mechanisms exist for the anthracyclines. This is entirely consistent with the presence of redundant mechanisms in mammalian cells to resist the toxicity of xenobiotics.

Altered Topoisomerase II Activity

Altered topoisomerase II activity has been implicated as a cause of resistance involving the anthracyclines. The resistance pattern of cells selected for topoisomerase II–mediated drug insensitivity may differ from the classic profile of *MDR1* substrates. Nonetheless, doxorubicin resistance in P388 and L1210 cells, MCF-7 breast cancer cells, and human small cell lung cancer and melanoma lines can be associated with reduced DNA topoisomerase II activity and drug-induced DNA cleavage.[54,327–332] When tumor cells are selected for anthracycline resistance in the presence of the cyclosporine A analog PSC833, which binds the P-glycoprotein, doxorubicin resistance develops in the context of significant reductions in topoisomerase IIα mRNA and protein as well as diminished catalytic activity without overexpression of *MDR1*, MRP, or the lung resistance–associated protein.[333] Tumor cells selected with an anthracycline alone relatively commonly exhibit both altered topoisomerase II activity and expression of the P-170 glycoprotein or MRP.[328,332,334] The mechanisms of decreased topoisomerase activity that have been described in *in vitro* studies include the presence of mutations in the topoisomerase IIα gene,[57] decreased topoisomerase IIα gene copy number,[55] and transcriptional down-regulation of topoisomerase gene expression.[335] Perhaps the most persuasive evidence that changes in topoisomerase II activity are causally related to doxorubicin resistance comes from studies that demonstrate reversal of resistance after transfer of a fully functional topoisomerase II gene into resistant cells.[336] The importance of these observations for the understanding of anthracycline resistance at the clinical level remains to be elucidated. In a clinical study, however, the activity of topoisomerase II in AML cells varied over a more than 20-fold range with significant cell-to-cell heterogeneity; no relationship was found between enzyme levels and drug sensitivity.[337]

Altered Free-Radical Biochemistry, Sensitivity to Apoptosis, and Other Mechanisms of Anthracycline Resistance

The relationship between changes in intracellular free-radical detoxifying species and doxorubicin resistance has been reviewed earlier. Here we need only emphasize that considerable, and probably tissue-specific, variations exist in the ability of cells to respond to a drug-induced free-radical challenge through enhanced antioxidant defense.[338,339]

In addition to changes in drug export, topoisomerase II activity, and defenses against free radicals, other resistance mechanisms are at work to prevent doxorubicin-related cell death. Clearly, overexpression of *bcl-2* can significantly

diminish the toxicity of doxorubicin, as can mutations in the *p53* gene.[264,279,281] As described earlier, however, the varied downstream effectors of anthracycline-mediated programmed cell death may individually play critical roles in drug sensitivity beyond that produced by Bcl-2 or p53 per se.[236,340–342] Furthermore, in light of the broad importance of these mediators of tumor cell killing for essentially all classes of antineoplastic agents,[343] alterations in components of the cell death cascade also likely play an important role in resistance to the anthracyclines acquired in the clinic before anthracycline administration.

Potent nuclear DNA repair systems also contribute substantially to the ability of tumor cells to withstand the cytotoxic effects of doxorubicin.[344] Attention has focused on the loss of DNA mismatch repair genes, such as *MLH1*, in the production of the doxorubicin-resistant phenotype, although the pathways to cell death that are interfered with remain unclear at present.[345–348] Mutations producing decreased levels of poly(adenosine diphosphate[ADP]–ribose)polymerase in V79 cells also dramatically decrease the efficacy of doxorubicin.[349] Because ADP-ribosylation is a well-known post-translational modification of topoisomerase II and plays an important role in utilization of nicotinamide adenine dinucleotide (oxidized form), these results suggest that critical aspects of intermediary metabolism may modify the relationship between DNA cleavage reactions and tumor cell killing.[350–352] Inhibitors of this enzyme are also capable of producing doxorubicin resistance in human tumor cells.[353,354] Resistance patterns apparently mediated by alterations in ADP-ribosylation, however, may in fact represent partial blockade of certain downstream effectors of the apoptotic cascade, because poly(ADP-ribose)polymerase is a critical substrate for the caspases.[237]

Drug Interactions

Very few drug interactions have been documented for the anthracyclines. Heparin, a large polyanion, binds to the aminosugar of doxorubicin and daunorubicin, creating insoluble aggregates. Coadministration of heparin and doxorubicin can lead to an increase in the rate of doxorubicin clearance. In rodents, phenobarbital has been shown to increase, and morphine to decrease, doxorubicin disappearance.[355,356]

Doxorubicin and daunorubicin can cause radiosensitization of normal tissues and subsequent radiation recall. The most significant aspect of this problem occurs with the heart. A cardiac radiation exposure of 2,000 cGy given in conventional 200-cGy per day fractionation results in a doubling of the rate at which cardiac toxicity develops, so that a cumulative doxorubicin dose of 250 mg per m² is equivalent to a dose of 500 mg per m² in the absence of radiation. This is not an uncommon problem in that doxorubicin is used for first-line therapy of breast cancer and Hodgkin's disease for which mediastinal or chest wall radiation therapy is also often used. Radiation techniques have reduced the cardiac radiation dose that occurs during treatment after breast-conserving surgery, which lessens this risk somewhat.

The disposition of doxorubicin was found to be significantly altered when it was administered immediately after a short intravenous infusion of paclitaxel.[357] This is due to the presence of high levels of Cremophor EL, the diluent in which paclitaxel is prepared, in the plasma after paclitaxel administration. Cremophor EL is a substrate for the P-glycoprotein, which can significantly affect the biliary excretion of doxorubicin.[358] This interaction is not observed when paclitaxel is given over 24 hours (which lowers the concentration of the diluent in plasma) or when docetaxel, rather than paclitaxel, is combined with doxorubicin, because the docetaxel is not prepared in Cremophor EL.

Clinical Pharmacology

Dose and Schedule of Administration

Doxorubicin has been successfully administered by a wide range of schedules, and at present there is little evidence that changes in schedule make any significant difference in antitumor activity. The antitumor activity of doxorubicin is proportional to the area under the concentration × time curve (AUC), not to peak drug levels. Thus, a dose of 60 mg per m² is approximately equally effective administered as a bolus or infused over 1, 2, or 4 days. Myelosuppression is also proportional to AUC and changes very little over this broad range of schedules. The most common schedule has been 45 to 60 mg per m² every 18 to 21 days. Because of evidence that peak level correlates with cardiac toxicity, weekly dosing at 20 to 30 mg per m² has also been evaluated and seems to be both less cardiotoxic and approximately as effective as bolus dosing. This trend has been extended with the administration of a 96-hour infusion that is convincingly less cardiotoxic but preserves antitumor activity.[359] As an added benefit, prolonged infusions dramatically lessen the nausea and vomiting associated with bolus administration of doxorubicin. The only major negative aspect of doxorubicin infusion is a tendency for mucositis to increase in intensity as the infusion is prolonged. Daunorubicin is usually administered as a brief intravenous infusion in dosages of 30 to 45 mg per m² daily for 3 days as induction therapy for AML.

Pharmacokinetics and Metabolism

The basic pharmacokinetic constants for doxorubicin and daunorubicin are listed in Table 18-1. The pharmacokinetics of these drugs is dominated by tissue binding. During the early distributive phase, drug levels fall rapidly as the drug gains ready access to all tissues of the body except the brain. During this phase, the bulk of the drug binds to DNA throughout the body, and in general, tissue levels of the drug are proportional to their DNA content.[360] In addition, plasma protein binding accounts for approximately 75% of the drug in the plasma.[361] In spite of this plasma protein binding, tissue/plasma ratios range from 10:1 to 500:1 by virtue of the higher affinity of the drugs for DNA than for plasma. Tumor levels have rarely been measured in humans; however, multiple myeloma patients were studied during a 96-hour infusion of doxorubicin. Doxorubicin levels of approximately 10 μmol per L were documented in myeloma cells by the end of the infusion.[362] With the extensive binding of these drugs to DNA and proteins, however, the free-drug pool probably represents a very small fraction of the drug concentrations measured in both plasma and cells. Unfortunately, no detailed studies have been done of the pharmacokinetics of this free-drug pool.

After bolus administration, or after the conclusion of a constant intravenous infusion, an initial doxorubicin half-life of 10 minutes is followed by a secondary half-life of 1 to 3 hours. The terminal half-life of 30 to 50 hours accounts for over 70% of the total drug AUC for doxorubicin. As a result of this prolonged terminal phase, plasma levels of drug remain above 10 nmol per L for the greater part of a week after a single dose of 60 mg per m² of doxorubicin.[361] In tissue culture, levels as low as 1 to 5 nmol per L are cytotoxic for sensitive tumor cells after extended exposures. Even accounting for the difference in protein content between tissue culture media and plasma, these results suggest that drug levels sufficient for tumor cell kill may persist for prolonged periods. Doxorubicinol is the primary metabolite of doxorubicin in human plasma but is present in concentrations far smaller than those of parent compound. Approximately 50% of the drug is excreted in the bile, both as parent drug and as various metabolites, including glucuronides and sulfates. Less than 10% of administered drug appears in the urine; however, this is sufficient to cause a reddish-orange discoloration of the urine in many patients. When the drug is administered at higher than standard dose levels (more than 100 mg per m²), peak plasma levels of doxorubicin may reach 6 to 7 μmol per L. When the drug is administered as a continuous intravenous infusion at high dose (150 to 165 mg per m²), steady-state doxorubicin concentrations are approximately 0.1 μmol per L.[363] The relationship of AUC to dose appears to be linear up to a doxorubicin dose level of 165 mg per m² whether the drug is administered as a bolus or as a continuous infusion.[363,364]

Pharmacokinetic studies have evaluated the effect of gender and body surface area on anthracycline pharmacokinetics.[365,366] Unexpectedly, men with normal hepatic function were found to have approximately twice the clearance of doxorubicin (administered as an intravenous bolus) than women; higher drug clearance was associated with an increased conversion rate of doxorubicin to its major alcohol metabolite. The pharmacodynamic implications of these findings remain to be explored. In related studies, the pharmacokinetics of the anthracycline analog epirubicin were shown to be independent of body surface area; normalization of epirubicin dose based on surface area on the drug's observed AUC has no effect. Although neutropenia correlated well with epirubicin AUC when the drug was administered as a single agent, the absence of an effect of body surface area normalization on systemic exposure suggests that this procedure reduces neither interpatient variability in anthracycline pharmacokinetics nor variability in hematopoietic toxicity after epirubicin treatment. Drug administration at fixed-milligram increments of this drug would appear to be rational, safe, and potentially more efficient than current standard practice.

For daunorubicin, metabolism to daunorubicinol is a major determinant of its plasma pharmacology. The parent drug is cleared rapidly from plasma, with a primary half-life of 40 minutes. The loss of parent drug from plasma correlates with the rapid appearance of C^4-O-demethyl daunorubicin, daunorubicinol, their aglycones, and various sulfate and glucuronide metabolites in bile. Within hours after a bolus dose of daunorubicin, the predominant circulating form of the drug is the alcohol metabolite,[367] which has a longer half-life (23 to 40 hours) than its parent. The opposite is the case for doxorubicin, for which doxorubicinol is typically a minor part of the total AUC.[368] The formation of either doxorubicinol or daunorubicinol is a function of the enzymatic conversion of the side-chain carbonyl to an alcohol by one or more enzymes in the hepatic aldo-ketoreductase family.[369–373]

Over the years, considerable controversy had been generated regarding the importance of the aglycone metabolites of the anthracyclines. Two families of aglycones must be considered, the 7-deoxy and 7-hydroxy aglycones. As mentioned earlier, the 7-deoxyaglycones are the result of a two-electron reduction of the parent drug to a quinone methide with subsequent elimination of the sugar. The full, two-electron reduction of the anthracyclines to the 7-deoxyaglycone stage occurs stepwise, after initial one-electron reduction by microsomal or mitochondrial flavin-containing enzymes. Thus, the demonstration of 7-deoxy by-products has been argued to be de facto evidence of anthracycline redox cycling. The 7-hydroxyaglycones result from hydrolysis of the sugar-anthraquinone bond. The latter can arise artifactually during the processing and analysis of the drug. This has especially been a problem with the older techniques that depended on thin-layer chromatography. In the past, many investigators seem to have been confused about the distinction between these two aglycone families, and thus the importance of the 7-deoxyaglycones was dismissed by some. That the 7-deoxyaglycones are indeed circulating metabolites of both daunorubicin and doxorubicin is now clear. In addition, the formation of the 7-deoxyaglycones exhibits large patient-to-patient variability. The compound 7-deoxydoxorubicin can comprise from 1% to 5% of the total drug. In contrast, 7-deoxydoxorubicinol aglycone can comprise from 0% to 20%.[194]

Doxorubicinol and daunorubicinol are cytotoxic metabolites but are considerably less active than the parent compound.[374] As mentioned earlier, deoxyaglycones are much less active than the corresponding parent drug and are currently viewed as a pathway of drug inactivation. Some information has now become available on the correlation between aglycone formation and tumor response. In one study aglycone levels in patients with AML were statistically significantly higher in nonresponders than in responders.[375]

Although the bulk of doxorubicin elimination occurs by hepatic metabolism and biliary excretion, the evidence that doses of doxorubicin or daunorubicin must be reduced in patients with compromised hepatic function is somewhat difficult to interpret.[376–379] Altered patterns of metabolism have been observed in individual patients, with prolonged terminal half-life of parent drug and decreased clearance of doxorubicinol. Patients with abnormal liver function also have a diminished capacity to clear doxorubicin when it is administered as an infusion or a bolus.[379,380] Nevertheless, no consistent pattern of increased toxicity has emerged in patients with mildly decreased drug clearance. Moderate to severe alterations in hepatic function, however, increase AUC significantly.[381] Physicians are advised to reduce dosages routinely when patients have moderate or severe hepatic dysfunction, or when marked replacement of the liver by tumor is present, in which case all forms of chemotherapy carry increased risk.

Toxicity

Table 18-1 provides a summary of the common toxicities of the anthracyclines.

Bone Marrow Suppression and Mucositis

Bone marrow suppression and mucositis are common to other anticancer drugs, and nothing is unusual about these toxic reactions after anthracycline administration. Both myelosuppression and mucositis follow an acute course, with maximal toxicity within 7 to 10 days of drug administration and rapid recovery thereafter. For daunorubicin, bone marrow suppression is more common than mucositis and is the usual dose-limiting toxicity. Doxorubicin causes these two reactions in more equal severity after bolus dose administration. With weekly dosing or continuous infusion, mucositis frequently becomes the dose-limiting toxicity.

Extravasation Injury

Extravasation of most anthracyclines leads to severe local injury that can continue to progress over weeks to months. The drug has been shown to bind locally to tissues and can still be detected in high levels at the base of a drug-induced ulcer in the soft tissues of the hand or forearm months later.[382–384] These lesions are very difficult to treat. Skin grafting is usually not successful unless preceded by extensive excision of the involved tissue. Débridement of dead tissue should be undertaken with extreme caution during the initial phases of extravasation injury, however, and local wound care to prevent infection is most important.[385] A wide range of treatments has been used immediately after extravasation in an attempt to lessen the injury. These have included ice, steroids, vitamin E, dimethyl sulfoxide, and bicarbonate.[386,387] None of these has been convincingly established, but each has adherents. The most promising preclinical studies have been with DHM_3, a powerful reductant that rapidly inactivates anthracyclines by conversion to the corresponding 7-deoxyaglycone.[196]

Cardiac Toxicity

The cardiac toxicity exhibited by doxorubicin and the other anthracyclines is unique in terms of its pathology and mechanism.[388,389] The major limiting factors in the clinical use of anthracyclines in adults are bone marrow suppression, mucositis, and drug resistance on the part of the tumor; however, in individual patients, most commonly with the use of doxorubicin to treat breast cancer, cardiac toxicity can develop while the patient's tumor is still responsive to the drug. This is a problem not only for the use of the anthracyclines alone or in combination with other chemotherapeutic agents but also for the use of the monoclonal antibody trastuzumab. Trials have demonstrated synergistic cardiac toxicity for the combination of doxorubicin and trastuzumab,[390] an antibody directed against the *HER2/neu* oncoprotein, which is itself active in the treatment of advanced breast cancer.[391] The observed potentiation of anthracycline-induced heart damage by trastuzumab has eliminated its use with doxorubicin in the population of patients whose tumors exhibit high levels of *HER2/neu* expression, a group that could benefit most from this combination.[392] Finally, children seem to be more sensitive to the cardiac toxicity of this drug, and this has become a significant problem in the use of doxorubicin in pediatric oncology.[393–395] Advances in our understanding of the impact of schedule on the cardiac toxicity of these drugs and the continued development of successful antidotal agents may reduce the importance of this problem in the future.

Clinical Presentation and Management

The anthracyclines manifest both acute and chronic cardiac toxicity. The acute toxicity is detected most commonly as a range of arrhythmias, including heart block. In its more extreme form, this acute injury can include a pericarditis-myocarditis syndrome with onset of fever, pericarditis, and congestive heart failure.[396] This syndrome can occur at low cumulative doses of doxorubicin and can have a fatal outcome. In animal models, doxorubicin administration causes significant increases in circulating catecholamines and histamine, and coadministration of α- and β-adrenergic

antagonists along with H_1 and H_2 blockers have lessened acute and subacute doxorubicin toxicity.[397] Clinical trials have not been conducted to see if such treatment might be effective in the management of the acute toxicity of doxorubicin in humans, perhaps because this syndrome is relatively uncommon and idiosyncratic. No clear correlation has been found between the manifestation of arrhythmias and the development of the chronic cardiomyopathy. Essentially no experience exists in retreating patients who have survived the pericarditis-myocarditis syndrome with doxorubicin or daunorubicin.

Cardiac toxicity has been best documented for doxorubicin administered as a bolus dose of 45 to 60 mg per m² every 21 to 28 days. With this schedule, cardiac toxicity develops as a result of cumulative injury to the myocardium. The pathology of this toxicity, determined after endomyocardial biopsy, has been described in detail; a useful grading system correlates well with the risk of clinical cardiac toxicity[398,399] (Table 18-2). These studies have shown that, with each dose of doxorubicin, progressive injury occurs to the myocardium, so that the grade increases steadily with total dose of drug administered. The major changes observed in myocytes are dilation of the sarcoplasmic reticulum and disruption of myofibrils. Early in the development of this toxicity these changes appear focally in scattered myocytes surrounded by normal-appearing cells. As the toxicity progresses, the frequency of these altered cells increases until a significant proportion of the myocardium is involved. Late in the development of this toxicity, the picture is complicated by the development of diffuse myocardial fibrosis. This pathology is unique to the anthracyclines and allows the pathologist definitely to distinguish this cardiac toxicity from other processes such as viral cardiomyopathy or ischemic heart injury. In addition, Billingham's grading system has allowed correlation of the findings among studies performed at a range of institutions and has made possible the advances that have now significantly lessened the risk of this problem.

The clinical risk of congestive heart failure is low at total doses of below 250 to 300 mg per m² of doxorubicin or 600 to 700 mg per m² of daunorubicin,[400,401] although cases of fatal congestive cardiomyopathy have been observed after a

TABLE 18-2. CRITERIA FOR GRADING ANTHRACYCLINE CARDIOMYOPATHY

Grade	Criteria
0	No change from normal
1	Scanty cells with early myofibrillar loss and/or distended sarcoplasmic reticulum
2	Groups of cells with marked myofibrillar loss and/or cytoplasmic vacuolization
3	Diffuse cell damage with total loss of contractile elements, loss of organelles and mitochondria, and nuclear degeneration

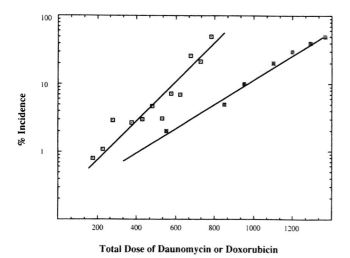

% Incidence

Total Dose of Daunomycin or Doxorubicin

FIGURE 18-7. Incidence of congestive heart failure as a function of cumulative dose (in mg/m^2) of either daunomycin (■) or doxorubicin (□). Daunomycin is a much less potent cardiotoxin than doxorubicin. (Redrawn from data presented in refs. 400 and 401.)

single dose of doxorubicin. Above these doses, the risk steadily accelerates. The total dose limit at which the risk becomes unacceptable is largely arbitrary, and as discussed earlier, the risk may in part be dependent on the treatment schedule used. For doxorubicin, the most commonly used total dose limit applied in the past has been 450 to 500 mg per m^2, at which the risk of clinically evident cardiac toxicity has generally been believed to be 1% to 10% (Fig. 18-7). The corresponding limit applied for daunorubicin has been 900 to 1,000 mg per m^2. Large trials that have prospectively evaluated heart function with radionuclide-gated cardiac blood pool scans, however, strongly suggest that subclinical, but not inconsequential, reductions in ejection fraction can be detected routinely after 250 to 300 mg per m^2 of doxorubicin.[402,403] As mentioned later, certain patients, especially those with breast cancer, may approach this total dose limit with a tumor that is still responsive to doxorubicin when few other therapeutic options exist. Changing from bolus to 96-hour infusion or adding dexrazoxane after a cumulative doxorubicin dose level of 300 mg per m^2 has been demonstrated to allow a substantial duration of additional anthracycline therapy with a significantly reduced risk of severe cardiac toxicity.[3,404,405]

Doxorubicin-induced cardiac toxicity has often been said to be difficult to treat and to be associated with a high mortality.[406] Although doxorubicin-induced congestive heart failure may have a fatal outcome, it is eminently treatable with standard measures, and many patients (probably well over half) recover or stabilize at a lower, but clinically acceptable, level of cardiac function.[406,407] One should point out, however, that congestive heart failure may occur many months after the discontinuation of doxorubicin and that patients who have been stabilized with adequate medical management are at increased risk during subsequent intercurrent ill-

nesses.[406,408] A number of techniques are now available to detect the cardiac toxicity early (Table 18-3). Endomyocardial biopsy results provide a definitive assessment of risk. However, this technique may not be available to the clinician. Ejection fraction measurement by electrocardiogram-gated radioisotopic cardiac blood pool scan has been shown to provide an accurate measure of cardiac contractility.[409,410] A significant drop in contractility measured by this technique is almost always seen before the onset of congestive heart failure. Because of the availability of these techniques, clinically significant cardiac toxicity is now detected much earlier, and this has done much to lessen the mortality of this complication. Medical management centers around afterload reduction. With conservative treatment, many patients experience gradual improvement in function, and a few patients can have rather dramatic return of exercise tolerance. This improvement can, however, take more than 1 year.

Reduction of the Risk of Cardiac Toxicity

Fortunately, much can now be done to lessen the risk of cardiac toxicity. First, patient characteristics associated with increased risk have been identified. Hypertension and pre-existing cardiac disease predisposing to diastolic dysfunction significantly increase the risk that a patient will develop clinically apparent cardiac abnormalities at a lower cumulative drug dose. Cardiac radiation exposure clearly increases the sensitivity of the heart to anthracyclines; at a radiation dose of 2,000 cGy, the slope of the curve plotting cardiac biopsy score against cumulative doxorubicin dose doubles, so that a dose of 250 mg per m^2 becomes equal to 500 mg per m^2 in the absence of radiation.[411] Modern advances in computer-based radiation treatment planning should be used to minimize cardiac radiation exposure in patients with breast cancer and lymphoma who will receive an anthracycline.

The risk of cardiac toxicity from doxorubicin has now clearly been shown to be a function of peak drug level, not AUC.[359] In contrast, both *in vitro* and in patients, the antitumor activity of doxorubicin is a function of AUC, not peak drug level. Thus, shifting from bolus drug administration to weekly dosing or prolonged infusion results in a significant reduction in the incidence of cardiac toxicity.[412] In clinical settings in which cardiac toxicity has proved to be a serious problem, such as in breast cancer or in pediatric malignancies, in which the incidence of cardiac dysfunction is higher and the late consequences more profound,[413] consideration should be given to the use of prolonged intravenous infusions or the cardioprotective agent dexrazoxane. Dexrazoxane is the first agent that has shown consistent ability to block the development of anthracycline-induced cardiac toxicity in a wide range of animal models. Randomized, controlled clinical trials have proven that this agent dramatically reduces the incidence of cardiac toxicity in patients with breast cancer without significantly altering the antitumor activity of anthracycline-containing combi-

TABLE 18-3. PHYSIOLOGIC TESTS OF CARDIAC FUNCTION

Test Used	Pertinent Measurement	Value Considered to Indicate Cardiomyopathy	Advantages	Disadvantages
Systolic time intervals	PEP/LVET	>0.42–0.45 Increase of >0.07 from control	Simple to perform; inexpensive	Large standard error; strongly affected by load factors
Echocardiography	Fractional shortening	<30%	Equipment widely available; personnel trained to perform tests widely available; moderate cost	Limited interpretability in significant proportion of adults; assumes uniformity of function and normal left ventricular geometry; measurements subject to error
	Ejection fraction	<45%		
ECG	QRS voltage	Decrease in precardial leads of ≥30%	Simple to perform; inexpensive	Large standard error of lead position; lacks adequate sensitivity; detects abnormalities associated with cardiomyopathy rather than predicting changes
Cardiac catheterization	Ejection fraction; cardiac output; pressure measurement	Ejection fraction of <45%; resting cardiac index of <2.5 L/min; exercise increase <5; pulmonary wedge pressure >12 mm Hg; resting right ventricular end-diastolic pressure >12 mm Hg	Allows comprehensive assessment of cardiac function and endomyocardial biopsy if desired	Invasive, with the risks that this entails; expensive and difficult to perform repeated measurements
Radionuclide cardiography	Ejection fraction; dV/dt during diastole and systole	Decrease of >15% from pretreatment ejection fraction, or decrease to <45%; failure to increase ejection fraction by >5% with exercise	Accurate measure of ventricular volumes; essentially noninvasive; easy to obtain values under varying conditions	Some operator-dependent variability in interpretation; moderately expensive

ECG, electrocardiogram; PEP/LVET, preejection period/left ventricular ejection time; *t*, time; *V*, volume.

nations.[186,404,405,414,415] In the first such study, 92 patients with advanced breast cancer received either 5-fluorouracil, doxorubicin, and cyclophosphamide or the same regimen plus dexrazoxane. The latter was given in doses of 1,000 mg per m² by intravenous infusion 30 minutes before the chemotherapeutic drugs. Patients receiving dexrazoxane had a response rate and duration of time to disease progression equivalent to those of patients not receiving dexrazoxane. The dexrazoxane-treated patients, however, had significantly smaller decreases in left ventricular ejection fraction at each dose level of doxorubicin, their cardiac biopsy results reflected less histologic change, and 11 patients treated with dexrazoxane tolerated doxorubicin doses above 600 mg per m², whereas only one patient not receiving dexrazoxane remained on study above this dose level. The only negative aspect of this trial was the occurrence of a modest increase in myelosuppression in the arm receiving dexrazoxane. These results have been confirmed in larger trials with both doxorubicin and its analog epirubicin and have led to the approval of dexrazoxane by the U.S. Food and Drug Administration as a cardioprotectant for patients receiving more than 300 mg per m² of doxorubicin. This approach also appears to be applicable to pediatric patients with sarcomas who are receiving doxorubicin.[395] To maintain the cardioprotective properties of dexrazoxane while reducing drug-related granulocytopenia, the currently recommended dose of dexrazoxane is ten times the doxorubicin dose on a

milligram-per-milligram basis, administered no more than 30 minutes before the anthracycline infusion is initiated.

Putative Biochemical Mechanism(s) of Anthracycline Cardiac Toxicity

In addition to accounting for the pathologic picture outlined earlier, any hypothesis that seeks to explain the cardiac toxicity of the anthracyclines must also account for the alterations in cardiac biochemistry that occur after doxorubicin exposure. The consistent changes observed involve marked alterations in calcium handling in the heart muscle and include loss of high-affinity calcium-binding sites, elevation of cardiac calcium content, and mitochondrial accumulation of calcium.[416–420] The other alteration frequently described is a diminished capacity for ATP generation. In terms of muscle physiology, these changes are critical. Calcium plays a central role in linking electrical excitation with contraction; each cycle of muscle contraction is triggered by a rapid rise in free intracellular calcium, and relaxation is dependent on a rapid drop in free calcium. In addition, calcium has been shown to play a major role in regulating the beat-to-beat force of cardiac muscle contraction. The two major sites for the beat-to-beat regulation of calcium are the sarcoplasmic reticulum and mitochondria. Sarcoplasmic reticulum avidly binds calcium, which is rapidly released when a wave of electrical depolarization sweeps through the sarcoplasmic membrane. Because extensions of the sarcoplasmic reticulum are in intimate contact with the contractile fibers, sarcoplasmic depolarization leads to rapid onset of muscle contraction. The cardiac mitochondria accumulate calcium if it is available in preference to making ATP. In general, no mechanism has been offered for a direct interaction of doxorubicin with calcium. Because anthracyclines are good metal chelators, one possibility might be that the drugs chelate calcium and, as a result, alter the distribution of this metal ion. However, doxorubicin does not chelate calcium within the physiologic concentration range for calcium. The pathology of anthracycline cardiac toxicity suggests another, more reasonable hypothesis: The major site of anatomical damage after drug exposure is the sarcoplasmic reticulum, a major site of calcium regulation. Doxorubicin injury to the sarcoplasmic reticulum leads to calcium release.[421] Calcium is then taken up by the mitochondria, which do that in preference to ATP generation. This sequence would account for the lower ATP levels and accumulation of calcium within the mitochondria.

How do the anthracyclines trigger damage to the sarcoplasmic reticulum? The hypothesis that best explains the above phenomenon is that the cardiac toxicity of the anthracyclines results from drug-induced free-radical formation (Table 18-4). Within the heart muscle are several sites where enzyme activity is capable of reducing doxorubicin to the corresponding semiquinone; doxorubicin-stimulated oxygen-radical formation by cardiac sarcoplasmic reticulum, cytosol, and mitochondria has been conclusively demonstrated.[422,423] The non–redox-active anthracycline 5-iminodaunorubicin does not generate reactive oxygen species in sarcoplasmic reticulum or mitochondria and is markedly less cardiotoxic than its parent molecule.[424] Doxorubicin can also induce peroxidation of sarcoplasmic reticulum lipid, and oxidant-related sulfhydryl loss; oxidative damage to the membrane is associated with a drop in both high-affinity calcium binding and the force of contraction.[113,416] Studies demonstrate, furthermore, that redox cycling of the doxorubicin quinone selectively inhibits critical hyperreactive sulfhydryl groups on the ryanodine-sensitive calcium channel of the sarcoplasmic reticulum, which results in enhanced channel activation and subsequent

alterations in calcium homeostasis.[425] These observations show that doxorubicin is reduced to a semiquinone at the sarcoplasmic reticulum and that this leads to oxidative damage to the sarcoplasmic membrane; the result is a subsequent loss of the capacity of this membrane to bind calcium, which thus disrupts the linkage between electrical excitation and contraction.

To confirm that oxygen radicals are indeed formed in the heart after doxorubicin exposure, isolated perfused beating rat hearts have been exposed to doxorubicin, and electron spin resonance has been used to detect hydroxyl radicals. In this setting, hydroxyl radical could easily be detected after exposure of the heart to drug levels of 1 µmol per L, attained after bolus dosing at 60 mg per m², but not at concentrations obtained during a 96-hour infusion (0.04 to 0.1 µmol per L).[133] Thus, doxorubicin can trigger the formation of reactive oxygen species *in vivo,* and this occurs at concentrations that are associated with the development of cardiac toxicity.

As outlined in Table 18-4, the anthracyclines can produce a wide variety of toxic effects in the heart, some of which may contribute to their clinical cardiac toxicity.[426,427] Unfortunately, many of the effects described occur at unrealistically high drug concentrations and do not help to explain the specificity of anthracycline cardiac damage. These considerations do not apply to studies that demonstrate specific down-regulation of cardiac α-actin and troponin I mRNAs,[428] in a fashion that is not inhibited by free-radical scavengers.[429] In light of these studies as well as studies examining the effect of doxorubicin on the activation of other cardiac-specific genes and regulatory pathways,[430,431] the likelihood is that the pathogenesis of anthracycline cardiac toxicity, and its morphologic expression, may be understood more clearly in the future at the transcriptional level.

Why is the heart, and not other tissues, a target for this free-radical damage? Several factors are probably involved. First, cardiac tissue has very low levels of catalase activity; overexpression of catalase in the hearts of transgenic mice reduces the cardiac toxicity of doxorubicin.[131] This leaves glutathione peroxidase as the only known pathway for hydrogen peroxide detoxification in the heart. Doxorubicin

TABLE 18-4. MECHANISMS OF ANTHRACYCLINE CARDIAC TOXICITY

Oxidative mechanisms	Nonoxidative mechanisms
Inhibition of calcium sequestration by sarcoplasmic reticulum; 10- to 20-fold decrease in IC_{50} by enzymatic drug activation	Inhibition of mitochondrial cytochrome oxidase; >0.5 mmol/L drug required
Inhibition of NADH dehydrogenase between its flavin and iron-sulfur center; requires low micromolar drug concentrations	Direct oxidation of ryanodine receptor sulfhydryls
Lipid membrane peroxidation	Down-regulation of cardiac β-adrenergic receptors
Oxidation of oxymyoglobin; potential for the production of "ferryl" myoglobin, a strong oxidant	Inhibition of specific cardiac mRNAs for α-actin, troponin I
Iron "delocalization"	

IC_{50}, concentration that inhibits 50%; mRNA, messenger RNA; NADH, nicotinamide adenine dinucleotide (reduced form).
Summarized in ref. 189.

administration, however, can produce a rapid drop in glutathione peroxidase activity. Thus, at a time when doxorubicin is stimulating the formation of hydrogen and lipid peroxides, it is also eliminating the major pathway for peroxide removal. This observation suggests that limitations in the ability of the heart enzymatically to detoxify oxygen radicals provide an important basis for its sensitivity to doxorubicin.[432] This hypothesis has received support from an unusual experiment. Prolonged exercise causes a marked increase in the activities of superoxide dismutase and glutathione peroxidase in rodents; these mice are then more resistant to the cardiac toxicity of doxorubicin.[433] That the robust affinity of the anthracyclines for mitochondrial lipids[434] enhances drug binding in a site-specific manner which markedly increases drug-related cardiac mitochondrial reactive oxygen production is also highly likely.[435–437] Furthermore, the heart is extraordinarily rich in iron proteins that are capable of donating their metal to catalyze strong oxidant formation.

In summary, the free-radical hypothesis has been very effective in accounting for the various characteristics of anthracycline cardiomyopathy. In addition, this hypothesis has led to the identification of an agent that is successful at dramatically reducing the cardiac toxicity of doxorubicin in humans without compromising the antitumor efficacy of this valuable anticancer agent.

DOXORUBICIN ANALOGS

A large number of doxorubicin analogs have been brought to clinical trial in the hope of finding a compound with lower cardiac toxicity and a broader spectrum of antitumor action.[438,439] The most promising of these analogs are (a) idarubicin hydrochloride, an agent with marked activity in acute nonlymphocytic leukemia and acute lymphocytic leukemia, and (b) epirubicin hydrochloride, which has activity in breast cancer. The important features of these two agents are given in Table 18-5.[74,111,315,440–457]

MITOXANTRONE

In the search for analogs of the anthracyclines, a variety of multiringed planar structures with the potential for DNA intercalation have been evaluated for antitumor activity. A promising related class of compounds, the anthracenediones, was synthesized by chemists at American Cyanamid Laboratories[458] in the late 1970s and was found to have potent antitumor activity against the P388 and L1210 leukemias. The most active of this series tested was mitoxantrone (dihydroanthracenedione), a planar tetracyclic compound having two symmetric aminoalkyl side arms but no glycosidic substituent as found in the active anthracyclines (Fig. 18-8). Against P388 it is one of the most active agents tested, yielding 500% increase in life span and a high percentage of cures.[459] Subsequent preclinical and clinical evaluation has demonstrated significant differences between mitoxantrone hydrochloride and the anthracyclines in terms of mechanism of action. The anthracenediones also cause less cardiac toxicity and show diminished potential for extravasation injury and for causing nausea and vomiting or alopecia. Their narrow spectrum of antitu-

TABLE 18-5. KEY FEATURES OF ANTHRACYCLINE ANALOGS

	Idarubicin	Epirubicin
Mechanism of action:	DNA strand breakage mediated by topoisomerase II; free radical–induced injury; induction of apoptosis	Same as for idarubicin
Mechanism of resistance:	Multidrug resistance mediated by *MDR*1 or *MRP* Topoisomerase II mutations Altered apoptotic response	Same as for idarubicin
Dosage:	10–15 mg/m² i.v. q3wk 10 mg/m² i.v. × 3 d (leukemia) 45 mg/m² p.o. q3wk	90–110 mg/m² i.v. q3wk
Pharmacokinetics:		
Elimination half-life parent compound	11.3 h	18.3 h
13-ol metabolite	40–60 h	21.1 h
Other metabolite	—	12.1 h (epiglucuronide)
Oral bioavailability	30%	—
Metabolism:	Primary metabolite, 13-idarubicinol, is cytotoxic and exceeds level of parent compound in plasma	Primary metabolites are glucuronides of parent and 13-ol
Excretion:	80% excreted in urine as 13-ol	Primarily parent compound, 13-ol, and glucuronides excreted in bile
Toxicity:	Leukopenia Thrombocytopenia Cardiotoxicity (less than doxorubicin)	Leukopenia Thrombocytopenia Cardiotoxicity (equal to doxorubicin)
Drug interactions:	None established	None established
Precautions:	None established	Possible dosage reduction in hepatic dysfunction

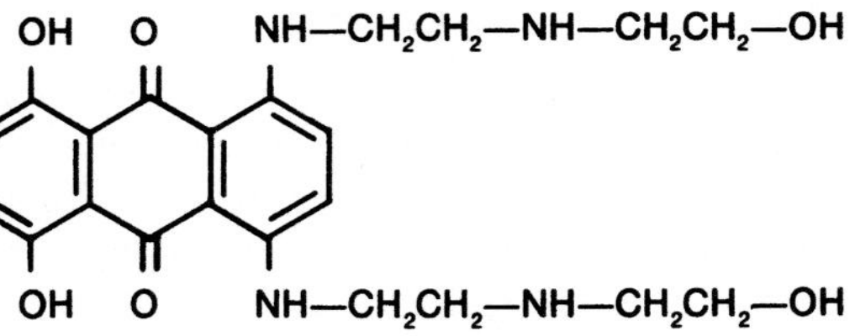

OH O NH—CH₂CH₂—NH—CH₂CH₂—OH

OH O NH—CH₂CH₂—NH—CH₂CH₂—OH

FIGURE 18-8. Structure of mitoxantrone.

mor activity, confined to breast and prostate cancer and the leukemias and lymphomas, has limited the opportunity to replace doxorubicin with mitoxantrone in clinical practice. Because of the favorable toxicity profile of mitoxantrone, however, it is an appropriate agent for use in an elderly patient population, such as in men with hormone-refractory prostate cancer, for whom treatment can provide significant palliative benefit.[460,461]

Mechanism of Action

Like the anthracyclines, mitoxantrone binds avidly to nucleic acids and inhibits DNA and RNA synthesis. Its mode of binding to DNA includes intercalation between opposing DNA strands, with preference for GC base-pairs.[462] Careful studies of the stoichiometry of binding and electron microscopic evaluation of the distortions produced *in vitro* in plasmid DNA indicate an additional type of binding that produces a compaction of chromatin[463] and, with plasmid DNA, lacelike intertwining of the DNA strands. These effects are dependent on the presence of the highly positively charged aminoalkyl side chains and probably represent electrostatic cross-linking of DNA strands. Also found are single- and double-strand breaks in DNA.[464] Because the drug has the basic quinone structure found in the anthracyclines, its ability to generate free radicals in a manner similar to that of doxorubicin has been examined. These studies revealed that the drug has a much reduced potential to undergo one-electron reduction, compared with doxorubicin,[465,466] and is less readily reduced enzymatically.[467] Because some of the single-strand breaks are protein associated, these breaks appear to result from the formation of a cleavable complex with topoisomerase II, which occurs in mitoxantrone-treated cells.[468] This possibility is heightened by the lack of evidence for lipid peroxidation in cardiac tissue, modest stimulation of oxygen consumption *in vitro*, and, indeed, inhibition of doxorubicin-induced lipid peroxidation by mitoxantrone.[469] All of these findings argue against a free-radical mechanism of tissue injury by mitoxantrone and favor enzyme-mediated DNA cleavage. The reduced potential for free-radical formation may also explain the lesser cardiotoxicity of mitoxantrone, although this drug is able to oxidize critical sulfhydryl groups on the ryanodine receptor of the sarcoplasmic reticulum.[426,427,470] As is the case for the anthracy-

clines, mitoxantrone can also readily stimulate apoptosis in a variety of cell lines.[471,472] Ceramide-dependent pathways have been implicated as part of the molecular ordering of mitoxantrone-induced programmed cell death.[227]

Mechanisms of Drug Resistance

Because mitoxantrone is a planar anthraquinone analog, the fact that it shares cross-resistance with many of the natural products, including the vinca alkaloids and doxorubicin, is not surprising.[473–475] This resistance may be mediated by amplification of the P-170 glycoprotein (classic *MDR1*); however, in some cell lines, decreased intracellular drug accumulation is related to the overexpression of MRP.[476,477] Alterations in topoisomerase II function have also been well described as a mechanism of mitoxantrone resistance.[478] In fact, clear examples are now seen in which tumor cells develop pleiotropic resistance based on both enhanced efflux and altered topoisomerase function.[479] Studies have also clarified a series of prior observations suggesting that mitoxantrone resistance *in vitro* could occur in the absence of alterations in topoisomerase II or enhanced expression of *MDR1* or MRP.[474,480–482] These investigations have identified a novel member of the ATP-binding cassette superfamily of transporters that encodes a 655–amino acid protein (termed the *breast cancer resistance protein*) that is capable of enhancing the efflux of mitoxantrone and the anthracyclines from mitoxantrone-selected tumor cell lines. Additional mechanisms of mitoxantrone resistance have been related to altered intracellular pH in tumor cells[483] and to modifications in the cellular apoptotic program.

Drug Interactions

Mitoxantrone is frequently used in combination with cytosine arabinoside in the treatment of acute nonlymphocytic leukemia, and evidence exists for biochemical synergy of the two agents. In studies of leukemic cells taken from patients during therapy, coadministration of mitoxantrone and cytosine arabinoside enhanced the accumulation of arabinosylcytidine triphosphate in leukemic blast cells.[484] In the same study, mitoxantrone alone produced no detectable single-strand breaks, but in combination with cytosine arabinoside induced easily detectable single-strand breaks as determined by alkaline elution of blast cell DNA. The molecular basis for these favorable interactions is not understood. Like doxorubicin, mitoxantrone sensitizes cells to both hyperthermia and ionizing radiation.[485]

Dose and Schedule of Administration

The recommended dosage for bolus intravenous administration of mitoxantrone is 12 mg per m² per day for 3 days for treatment of AML and 12 to 14 mg per m² per day once every 3 weeks for treatment of solid tumors. The drug has definitely established activity against breast cancer,[486] ovarian cancer,[487] non-Hodgkin's lymphoma,[488] and prostate cancer[460] in addition to its use against acute leukemia.[489] The drug is administered as a 30-minute infusion and rarely causes extravasation injury if infiltrated. Mitoxantrone should not be administered in solutions containing heparin.

Pharmacokinetics

Mitoxantrone can be measured in plasma and urine by high-pressure liquid chromatography.[490,491] The plasma disappearance of mitoxantrone is characterized by a rapid preliminary phase of clearance, with half-lives of 10 minutes and 1.1 to 1.6 hours,[490,491] followed by a long terminal half-life of 23 to 42 hours. During this final phase of drug disappearance, drug concentrations in plasma approximate 1 ng per mL or 2 nmol per L, a level at the margin of cytotoxicity. The pharmacokinetics of mitoxantrone is linear over the dose range from 8 to 14 mg per m² administered as a short infusion.[492] Less than a third of the drug can be accounted for by the fraction of drug that appears in the urine (less than 10%) and the stool (less than 20%). Like doxorubicin, the drug distributes in high concentrations into tissues (liver > bone marrow > heart > lung > kidney) and remains in these sites for weeks after therapy.[490] Although specific guidelines are not available for dose adjustment in patients with hepatic dysfunction, several authors have noted a prolongation of the terminal half-life to greater than 60 hours in patients with liver impairment.[491,493]

The specific metabolites of mitoxantrone have not been well characterized.[494] The side chains undergo oxidation, yielding the mono- and dicarboxylic acids of anthracenedione, and both have been recovered from urine.[495] Neither has antitumor activity.

As an alternative to intravenous infusion, mitoxantrone has been administered by hepatic intraarterial infusion[496] and by intraperitoneal instillation.[497,498] These trials were based on the observation that mitoxantrone has a steep dose-response curve *in vitro* and that optimal concentrations of drug (1 to 10 μg per mL) are achieved only briefly during standard intravenous therapy. Local concentrations much higher than those realized in systemic administration can be achieved by either the intraarterial or intraperitoneal routes. During intraperitoneal trials, patients with ovarian or colon cancer received 12 to 38 mg per m² as a single dose every 4 weeks in 2 L of dialysate. An advantage of 1,400-fold was found to be achieved when intraperitoneal drug concentrations were compared with simultaneous plasma levels. The terminal half-life for disappearance of drug from the intraperitoneal space was 9 hours. Toxicity was primarily leukopenia at the highest doses of drug. Abdominal discomfort and tenderness, as well as catheter dysfunction due to the formation of a fibrous sheath that reflects serositis, are not uncommon with intraperitoneal mitoxantrone.

Toxicity

The primary advantage of mitoxantrone, in comparison with doxorubicin, is its much reduced incidence of cardiac toxicity, the mildness of the nausea and vomiting that follow intravenous administration, and minimal alopecia. Early trials of mitoxantrone revealed occasional episodes of cardiac failure,[499] primarily in patients who had not been helped by prior doxorubicin therapy. No doubt exists that occasionally patients develop congestive heart failure after treatment with mitoxantrone in the absence of prior anthracycline exposure, although the incidence is less than 5%.[485,500,501] The incidence of cardiac toxicity is greatest in patients who have received prior anthracycline therapy or chest irradiation[502] and in those with underlying cardiac disease.[485,501,502]

Other toxicities include a reversible leukopenia, with recovery within 14 days of drug administration; mild thrombocytopenia; nausea and vomiting; and, rarely, abnormal liver enzyme levels in patients receiving dose levels appropriate for treatment of solid tumors.[503] One minor, and at times alarming, side effect of mitoxantrone is a bluish discoloration of the sclera, fingernails, and urine.[504]

In summary, mitoxantrone has not replaced doxorubicin in solid tumor chemotherapy, primarily because of its apparent lesser activity against breast cancer. Because of its advantageous toxicity profile, however, it is useful in the palliative treatment of hormone-resistant prostate cancer and is effective in combination therapy for the lymphomas and leukemias.

REFERENCES

1. DiMarco A, Gaetani M, Orezzi P, et al. "Daunomycin," a new antibiotic of the rhodomycin group. *Nature* 1964;201:706.
2. Arcamone F, Cassinelli G, Fantini G, et al. Adriamycin, 14-hydroxydaunomycin, a new antitumor antibiotic from *S. peucetius* var. *caesius*. *Biotechnol Bioeng* 1969;11:1101.
3. Legha SS, Benjamin RS, Mackay B, et al. Adriamycin therapy by continuous intravenous infusion in patients with metastatic breast cancer. *Cancer* 1982;49:1762.
4. Legha SS, Benjamin RS, Mackay B, et al. Role of adriamycin in breast cancer and sarcomas. In: Muggia FM, Young CW, Carter SK, eds. *Anthracycline antibiotics in cancer therapy*. The Hague: Martinus Nijhoff Publishers, 1982:432.
5. Jones RB, Holland JF, Bhardwaj S, et al. A phase I–II study of intensive-dose adriamycin for advanced breast cancer. *J Clin Oncol* 1987;5:172.
6. Bronchud MH, Howell A, Crowther D, et al. The use of granulocyte colony-stimulating factor to increase the intensity of treatment with doxorubicin in patients with advanced breast and ovarian cancer. *Br J Cancer* 1989;60:121.
7. Somlo G, Doroshow JH, Forman SJ, et al. High-dose doxorubicin, etoposide, and cyclophosphamide with autologous stem cell reinfusion in patients with responsive metastatic or high-risk primary breast cancer. *Cancer* 1994;73:1678.

8. Morgan RJ Jr, Doroshow JH, Venkataraman K, et al. High-dose infusional doxorubicin and cyclophosphamide: a feasibility study of tandem high-dose chemotherapy cycles without stem cell support. *Clin Cancer Res* 1997;3:2337.

9. Dalmark M, Johansen P. Molecular association between doxorubicin (Adriamycin) and DNA-derived bases, nucleosides, nucleotides, other aromatic compounds, and proteins in aqueous solution. *Mol Pharmacol* 1982;22:158.

10. Dalmark M, Strom HH. A fickian diffusion transport process with features of transport catalysis: doxorubicin transport in human red blood cells. *J Gen Physiol* 1981;78:349.

11. Peterson C, Trouet A. Transport and storage of daunorubicin and doxorubicin in cultured fibroblasts. *Cancer Res* 1978;38:4645.

12. Bachur NR, Steele M, Meriwether WD, et al. Cellular pharmocodynamics of several anthracycline antibiotics. *J Med Chem* 1976;19:651.

13. Gianni L, Corden B, Myers C. The biochemical basis of anthracycline toxicity and antitumor action. *Rev Biochem Toxicol* 1983;5:1.

14. Raghunand N, He X, van Sluis R, et al. Enhancement of chemotherapy by manipulation of tumour pH. *Br J Cancer* 1999;80:1005.

15. Peterson C, Baurain R, Trouet A. The mechanism for cellular uptake, storage, and release of daunorubicin: studies on fibroblasts in culture. *Biochem Pharmacol* 1980;29:1687.

16. Gerweck LE, Kozin SV, Stocks SJ. The pH partition theory predicts the accumulation and toxicity of doxorubicin in normal and low-pH-adapted cells. *Br J Cancer* 1999;79:838.

17. Schindler M, Grabski S, Hoff E, et al. Defective pH regulation of acidic compartments in human breast cancer cells (MCF-7) is normalized in adriamycin-resistant cells (MCF-7adr). *Biochemistry* 1996;35:2811.

18. Vaupel PW, Frinak S, Bicher HI. Heterogenous oxygen partial pressure and pH distribution in C3H mouse mammary adenocarcinoma. *Cancer Res* 1981;41:2008.

19. Altan N, Chen Y, Schindler M, et al. Defective acidification in human breast tumor cells and implications for chemotherapy. *J Exp Med* 1998;187:1583.

20. Simon SM, Schindler M. Cell biological mechanisms of multidrug resistance in tumors. *Proc Natl Acad Sci U S A* 1994;91:3497.

21. Johnson BA, Cheang MS, Goldenberg GJ. Comparison of adriamycin uptake in chick embryo heart and liver cells and murine L5178Y lymphoblasts in vitro: role of drug uptake in cardiotoxicity. *Cancer Res* 1986;46:218.

22. Peterson C, Paul C, Gahrton G. Studies on the cellular pharmacology of daunorubicin and doxorubicin in experimental systems and human leukemia. In: Mathe G, Maral R, De Jager R, eds. *Anthracyclines: current status and future developments.* New York: Masson Publishing USA, 1983:85.

23. Kartner N, Riordan JR, Ling V. Cell-surface P-glycoprotein associated with multidrug resistance in mammalian cell lines. *Science* 1983;221:1285.

24. Ueda K, Cardarelli C, Gottesman MM, et al. Expression of a full-length cDNA for the human "MDR1" gene confers resistance to colchicine, doxorubicin, and vinblastine. *Proc Natl Acad Sci U S A* 1987;84:3004.

25. Pastan I, Gottesman MM. Multidrug resistance. *Annu Rev Med* 1991;42:277.

26. Horio M, Chin KV, Currier SJ, et al. Transepithelial transport of drugs by the multidrug transporter in cultured Madin-Darby canine kidney cell epithelia. *J Biol Chem* 1989;264:14880.

27. Cole SPC, Bhardwaj G, Gerlach JH, et al. Overexpression of a transporter gene in a multidrug-resistant human lung cancer cell line. *Science* 1992;258:1650.

28. Slovak ML, Ho JP, Bhardwaj G, et al. Localization of a novel multidrug resistance-associated gene in the HT1080/DR4 and H69AR human tumor cell lines. *Cancer Res* 1993;53:3221.

29. Awasthi S, Singhal SS, Srivastava SK, et al. Adenosine triphosphate-dependent transport of doxorubicin, daunomycin, and vinblastine in human tissues by a mechanism distinct from the P-glycoprotein. *J Clin Invest* 1994;93:958.

30. Jedlitschky G, Leier I, Buchholz U, et al. ATP-dependent transport of glutathione S-conjugates by the multidrug resistance–associated protein. *Cancer Res* 1994;54:4833.

31. Yi J-R, Lu S, Fernandez-Checa J, et al. Expression cloning of a rat hepatic reduced glutathione transporter with canalicular characteristics. *J Clin Invest* 1994;93:1841.

32. Priebe W, Krawczyk M, Kuo MT, et al. Doxorubicin- and daunorubicin-glutathione conjugates, but not unconjugated drugs, competitively inhibit leukotriene C4 transport mediated by MRP/GS-X pump. *Biochem Biophys Res Commun* 1998;247:859.

33. Borg AG, Burgess R, Green LM, et al. Overexpression of lung-resistance protein and increased P-glycoprotein function in acute myeloid leukaemia cells predict a poor response to chemotherapy and reduced patient survival. *Br J Haematol* 1998;103:1083.

34. Schroeijers AB, Scheffer GL, Flens MJ, et al. Immunohistochemical detection of the human major vault protein LRP with two monoclonal antibodies in formalin-fixed, paraffin-embedded tissues. *Am J Pathol* 1998;152:373.

35. Michieli M, Damiani D, Ermacora A, et al. P-glycoprotein, lung resistance-related protein and multidrug resistance associated protein in de novo acute non-lymphocytic leukaemias: biological and clinical implications. *Br J Haematol* 1999;104:328.

36. Chaires JB, Fox KR, Herrera JE, et al. Site and sequence specificity of the daunomycin-DNA interaction. *Biochemistry* 1987;26:8227.

37. Bailly C, Suh D, Waring MJ, et al. Binding of daunomycin to diaminopurine- and/or inosine-substituted DNA. *Biochemistry* 1998;37:1033.

38. Trist H, Phillips DR. In vitro transcription analysis of the role of flanking sequence on the DNA sequence specificity of Adriamycin. *Nucl Acids Res* 1989;17:3673.

39. Calendi E, Marco A, Reggiani M, et al. On physicochemical interactions between daunomycin and nucleic acids. *Biochem Biophys Acta* 1965;103:25.

40. Zeman SM, Phillips DR, Crothers DM. Characterization of covalent adriamycin-DNA adducts. *Proc Natl Acad Sci U S A* 1998;95:11561.

41. Zunino F, Ganbetta R, DiMarco A, et al. A comparison of the effects of daunomycin and adriamycin on various DNA polymerases. *Cancer Res* 1975;35:754.

42. Zunino F, Gambetta R, DiMarco A. The inhibition in vitro

of DNA polymerase and RNA polymerase by daunomycin and adriamycin. *Biochem Pharmacol* 1975;24:309.

43. Siegfried JM, Sartorelli AC, Tritton TR. Evidence for the lack of relationship between inhibition of nucleic acid synthesis and cytotoxicity of adriamycin. *Cancer Biochem Biophys* 1983;6:137.

44. Ross WA, Glaubiger DL, Kohn KW. Protein-associated DNA breaks in cells treated with adriamycin and ellipticine. *Biochim Biophys Acta* 1978;519:23.

45. Zwelling LA, Michaels S, Erickson LC, et al. Protein-associated deoxyribonucleic acid strand breaks in L1210 cells treated with the deoxyribonucleic acid intercalating agents 4'-(9-acridinylamino) methanesulfon-m-anisidide and adriamycin. *Biochemistry* 1981;20:6553.

46. Kohn KW. Beyond DNA cross-linking: history and prospects of DNA-targeted cancer-treatment—fifteenth Bruce F. Cain Memorial Award Lecture. *Cancer Res* 1996;56:5533.

47. Liu LF. DNA topoisomerase poisons as antitumor drugs. *Annu Rev Biochem* 1989;58:351.

48. Tewey KM, Chen GI, Nelson EM, et al. Intercalative antitumor drugs interfere with the breakage-reunion reaction of mammalian DNA topoisomerase. *J Biol Chem* 1984;259:9182.

49. Pommier Y. DNA topoisomerase I and II in cancer chemotherapy: update and perspectives. *Cancer Chemother Pharmacol* 1993;32:103.

50. Potmesil M, Kirschenbaum S, Israel M, et al. Relationship of adriamycin concentrations to the DNA lesions induced in hypoxic and euoxic L1210 cells. *Cancer Res* 1983;43:3528.

51. Levin M, Silber R, Israel M, et al. Protein-associated DNA breaks and DNA-protein cross-links caused by DNA nonbinding derivatives of adriamycin in L1210 cells. *Cancer Res* 1981;41:1006.

52. Capranico G, Kohn KW, Pommier Y. Local sequence requirements for DNA cleavage by mammalian topoisomerase II in the presence of doxorubicin. *Nucl Acids Res* 1990;18:6611.

53. Glisson B, Gupta R, Hodges P, et al. Cross-resistance to intercalating agents in an epipodophyllotoxin-resistant Chinese hamster ovary cell line: evidence for a common intracellular target. *Cancer Res* 1986;46:1939.

54. Sinha BK, Haim N, Dusre L, et al. DNA strand breaks produced by etoposide (VP-16,213) in sensitive and resistant human breast tumor cells: implications for the mechanism of action. *Cancer Res* 1988;48:5096.

55. Withoff S, Keith WN, Knol AJ, et al. Selection of a subpopulation with fewer DNA topoisomerase II alpha gene copies in a doxorubicin-resistant cell line panel. *Br J Cancer* 1996;74:502.

56. Towatari M, Adachi K, Marunouchi T, et al. Evidence for a critical role of DNA topoisomerase II alpha in drug sensitivity revealed by inducible antisense RNA in a human leukaemia cell line. *Br J Haematol* 1998;101:548.

57. Patel S, Sprung AU, Keller BA, et al. Identification of yeast DNA topoisomerase II mutants resistant to the antitumor drug doxorubicin: implications for the mechanisms of doxorubicin action and cytotoxicity. *Mol Pharmacol* 1997;52:658.

58. Sorensen M, Sehested M, Jensen PB. Effect of cellular ATP depletion on topoisomerase II poisons. Abrogation of cleavable-complex formation by etoposide but not by amsacrine. *Mol Pharmacol* 1999;55:424.

59. Kupfer G, Bodley AL, Liu LF. Involvement of intracellular ATP in cytotoxicity of topoisomerase II-targeting antitumor drugs. *Natl Cancer Inst Monogr* 1987;4:37.

60. Ross WE, Zwelling LA, Kohn KW. Relationship between cytotoxicity and DNA strand breakage produced by adriamycin and other intercalating agents. *Int J Radiat Oncol Biol Phys* 1979;5:1221.

61. Zwelling LA, Kerrigan D, Michaels S. Cytotoxicity and DNA strand breaks by 5-iminodaunorubicin in mouse leukemia L1210 cells: comparison with adriamycin and 4'-(9-acridinylamino)methanesulfon-m-anisidide. *Cancer Res* 1982;42:2687.

62. Goldenberg GJ, Wang H, Blair GW. Resistance to Adriamycin: relationship of cytotoxicity to drug uptake and DNA single- and double-strand breakage in cloned cell lines of Adriamycin-sensitive and -resistant P388 leukemia. *Cancer Res* 1986;46:2978.

63. Munger C, Ellis A, Woods K, et al. Evidence for inhibition of growth related to compromised DNA synthesis in the interaction of daunorubicin with H-35 rat hepatoma. *Cancer Res* 1988;48:2404.

64. Fornari FA, Randolph JK, Yalowich JC, et al. Interference by doxorubicin with DNA unwinding in MCF-7 breast tumor cells. *Mol Pharmacol* 1994;45:649.

65. Binaschi M, Farinosi R, Austin CA, et al. Human DNA topoisomerase II alpha-dependent DNA cleavage and yeast cell killing by anthracycline analogues. *Cancer Res* 1998;58:1886.

66. Yamazaki K, Isobe H, Hanada T, et al. Topoisomerase II alpha content and topoisomerase II catalytic activity cannot explain drug sensitivities to topoisomerase II inhibitors in lung cancer cell lines. *Cancer Chemother Pharmacol* 1997;39:192.

67. Sandri MI, Hochhauser D, Ayton P, et al. Differential expression of the topoisomerase II alpha and beta genes in human breast cancers. *Br J Cancer* 1996;73:1518.

68. Jarvinen TA, Holli K, Kuukasjarvi T, et al. Predictive value of topoisomerase II alpha and other prognostic factors for epirubicin chemotherapy in advanced breast cancer. *Br J Cancer* 1998;77:2267.

69. Pommier Y, Leteurtre F, Fesen MR, et al. Cellular determinants of sensitivity and resistance to DNA topoisomerase inhibitors. *Cancer Invest* 1994;12:530.

70. Jensen PB, Sorensen BS, Demant EJ, et al. Antagonistic effect of aclarubicin on the cytotoxicity of etoposide and 4'-(9-acridinylamino)methanesulfon-m-anisidide in human small cell lung cancer cell lines and on topoisomerase II-mediated DNA cleavage. *Cancer Res* 1990;50:3311.

71. Sorensen BS, Sinding J, Andersen AH, et al. Mode of action of topoisomerase II–targeting agents at a specific DNA sequence. Uncoupling the DNA binding, cleavage and religation events. *J Mol Biol* 1992;228:778.

72. Jensen PB, Sorensen BS, Sehested M, et al. Different modes of anthracycline interaction with topoisomerase II. Separate structures critical for DNA-cleavage, and for overcoming topoisomerase II–related drug resistance. *Biochem Pharmacol* 1993;45:2025.

73. Nitiss JL, Pourquier P, Pommier Y. Aclacinomycin A stabilizes topoisomerase I covalent complexes. *Cancer Res* 1997;57:4564.

74. Fukushima T, Inoue H, Takemura H, et al. Idarubicin and idarubicinol are less affected by topoisomerase II–related multidrug resistance than is daunorubicin. *Leuk Res* 1998; 22:625.

75. Guano F, Pourquier P, Tinelli S, et al. Topoisomerase poisoning activity of novel disaccharide anthracyclines. *Mol Pharmacol* 1999;56:77.

76. Bachur NR, Yu F, Johnson R, et al. Helicase inhibition by anthracycline anticancer agents. *Mol Pharmacol* 1992;41:993.

77. Bachur NR, Johnson R, Yu F, et al. Anthracycline antihelicase action: new mechanism with implications for guanosine-cytidine intercalation specificity. In: Priebe W, ed. *Anthracycline antibiotics: new analogues, methods of delivery, and mechanisms of action*. Washington: American Chemical Society, 1995:204.

78. Bachur NR, Lun L, Sun PM, et al. Anthracycline antibiotic blockade of SV40 T antigen helicase action. *Biochem Pharmacol* 1998;55:1025.

79. Fornari FA Jr, Jarvis WD, Grant S, et al. Induction of differentiation and growth arrest associated with nascent (nonoligosomal) DNA fragmentation and reduced c-*myc* expression in MCF-7 human breast tumor cells after continuous exposure to a sublethal concentration of doxorubicin. *Cell Growth Differ* 1994;5:723.

80. Fornari FAJ, Jarvis DW, Grant S, et al. Growth arrest and non-apoptotic cell death associated with the suppression of c-myc expression in MCF-7 breast tumor cells following acute exposure to doxorubicin. *Biochem Pharmacol* 1996;51:931.

81. Gewirtz DA, Randolph JK, Chawla J, et al. Induction of DNA damage, inhibition of DNA synthesis and suppression of c-myc expression by the anthracycline analog, idarubicin (4-demethoxy-daunorubicin) in the MCF-7 breast tumor cell line. *Cancer Chemother Pharmacol* 1998;41:361.

82. Akman SA, Doroshow JH, Burke TG, et al. DNA base modifications induced in isolated human chromatin by NADH dehydrogenase-catalyzed reduction of doxorubicin. *Biochemistry* 1992;31:3500.

83. Muller I, Jenner A, Bruchelt G, et al. Effect of concentration on the cytotoxic mechanism of doxorubicin—apoptosis and oxidative DNA damage. *Biochem Biophys Res Commun* 1997;230:254.

84. Gajewski E, Synold TW, Akman SA, et al. Doxorubicin-induced oxidative DNA base modification and apoptosis in human MCF-10A breast cancer cells at clinically achievable drug concentrations. *Proc Am Assoc Cancer Res* 1999;40: 646(abst).

85. Lin SW, Akman SA, Chen V, et al. Comparison of doxorubicin and H_2O_2-mediated oxidative DNA damage and repair in mitochondrial and nuclear DNA of human fibroblasts by quantitative extra long PCR. *Proc Am Assoc Cancer Res* 1999;40:403(abst).

86. Palmeira CM, Serrano J, Kuehl DW, et al. Preferential oxidation of cardiac mitochondrial DNA following acute intoxication with doxorubicin. *Biochim Biophys Acta* 1997; 1321:101.

87. Serrano J, Palmeira CM, Kuehl DW, et al. Cardioselective and cumulative oxidation of mitochondrial DNA following subchronic doxorubicin administration. *Biochim Biophys Acta* 1999;1411:201.

88. Faure H, Coudray C, Mousseau M, et al. 5-Hydroxymethyl-uracil excretion, plasma TBARS and plasma antioxidant vitamins in adriamycin-treated patients. *Free Radic Biol Med* 1996;20:979.

89. Faure H, Mousseau M, Cadet J, et al. Urine 8-oxo-7,8-dihydro-2-deoxyguanosine vs. 5-(hydroxymethyl) uracil as DNA oxidation marker in adriamycin-treated patients. *Free Radic Res* 1998;28:377.

90. Olinski R, Jaruga P, Foksinski M, et al. Epirubicin-induced oxidative DNA damage and evidence for its repair in lymphocytes of cancer patients who are undergoing chemotherapy. *Mol Pharmacol* 1997;52:882.

91. Gajewski E, Synold TW, Akman SA, et al. Oxidative DNA base modification in patients (pts) treated with high dose infusional doxorubicin (DOX). *Proc Am Assoc Cancer Res* 1998;39:489(abst).

92. Breimer LH. Molecular mechanisms of oxygen radical carcinogenesis and mutagenesis: the role of DNA base damage. *Mol Carcinogenesis* 1990;3:188.

93. Hsie AW, Recio L, Katz DS, et al. Evidence for reactive oxygen species inducing mutations in mammalian cells. *Proc Natl Acad Sci U S A* 1986;83:9616.

94. Bjergaard-Pedersen J, Sigsgaard TC, Nielsen D, et al. Acute monocytic or myelomonocytic leukemia with balanced chromosome translocations to band 11q23 after therapy with 4-epi-doxorubicin and cisplatin or cyclophosphamide for breast cancer. *J Clin Oncol* 1992;10:1444.

95. Diamandidou E, Buzdar AU, Smith TL, et al. Treatment-related leukemia in breast cancer patients treated with fluorouracil-doxorubicin-cyclophosphamide combination adjuvant chemotherapy: the University of Texas M. D. Anderson Cancer Center experience. *J Clin Oncol* 1996;14:2722.

96. Hoffmann L, Moller P, Pedersen-Bjergaard J, et al. Therapy-related acute promyelocytic leukemia with t(15;17) (q22;q12) following chemotherapy with drugs targeting DNA topoisomerase II. A report of two cases and a review of the literature. *Ann Oncol* 1995;6:781.

97. Westendorf J, Marquardt HI, Marquardt H. Structure-activity relationship of anthracycline-induced genotoxicity in vitro. *Cancer Res* 1984;44:5599.

98. Abdella BRJ, Fisher J. A chemical perspective on the anthracycline antitumor antibiotics. *Environ Health Perspect* 1985;64:3.

99. Fisher J, Ramakrishnan K, Becvar JE. Direct enzyme-catalyzed reduction of anthracyclines by reduced nicotinamide adenine dinucleotide. *Biochemistry* 1983;22:1347.

100. Handa K, Sato S. Generation of free radicals of quinone group-containing anti-cancer chemicals in NADPH-microsome system as evidenced by initiation of sulfite oxidation. *Gann* 1975;66:43.

101. Goodman J, Hochstein P. Generation of free radicals and lipid peroxidation by redox cycling of adriamycin and daunomycin. *Biochem Biophys Res Commun* 1977;77:797.

102. Bachur NR, Gordon SL, Gee MV. A general mechanism for microsomal activation of quinone anticancer agents to free radicals. *Cancer Res* 1977;38:1745.

103. Myers CE, McGuire WP, Liss RH, et al. Adriamycin: the role of lipid peroxidation in cardiac toxicity and tumor response. *Science* 1977;197:165.

104. Doroshow JH, Locker GY, Myers CE. Enzymatic defenses of the mouse heart against reactive oxygen metabolites: alterations produced by doxorubicin. *J Clin Invest* 1980; 65:128.

105. Doroshow JH, Locker GY, Ifrim I, et al. Prevention of doxorubicin cardiac toxicity in the mouse by *N*-acetylcysteine. *J Clin Invest* 1981;68:1053.

106. Doroshow JH. Role of hydrogen peroxide and hydroxyl radical formation in the killing of Ehrlich tumor cells by anticancer quinones. *Proc Natl Acad Sci U S A* 1986;83:4514.

107. Sinha BK, Katki AG, Batist G, et al. Differential formation of hydroxyl radical by adriamycin in sensitive and resistant MCF-7 human breast tumor cells: implications for the mechanism of action. *Biochemistry* 1987;26:3776.

108. Doroshow JH. Glutathione peroxidase and oxidative stress. *Toxicol Lett* 1995;82/83:395.

109. Doroshow JH, Hochstein P. Redox cycling and the mechanism of action of antibiotics in neoplastic diseases. In: Autor AP, ed. *Pathology of oxygen.* New York: Academic Press, 1982:245.

110. O'Brien PJ. Molecular mechanisms of quinone cytotoxicity. *Chem Biol Interact* 1991;80:1.

111. Praet M, Laghmiche M, Pollakis G, et al. In vivo and in vitro modifications of the mitochondrial membrane induced by 4' epi-adriamycin. *Biochem Pharmacol* 1986;35:2923.

112. Carmichael AJ, Riesz P. Photoinduced reactions of anthraquinone antitumor agents with peptides and nucleic acid bases: an electron spin resonance and spin trapping study. *Arch Biochem Biophys* 1985;237:433.

113. Harris RN, Doroshow JH. Effect of doxorubicin-enhanced hydrogen peroxide and hydroxyl radical formation on calcium sequestration by cardiac sarcoplasmic reticulum. *Biochem Biophys Res Commun* 1985;130:739.

114. Vile G, Winterbourn C. Thiol oxidation and inhibition of Ca-ATPase by adriamycin in rabbit heart microsomes. *Biochem Pharmacol* 1990;39:769.

115. Pan SS, Pedersen L, Bachur NR. Comparative flavoprotein catalysis of anthracycline antibiotic reductive cleavage and oxygen consumption. *Mol Pharmacol* 1981;19:184.

116. Doroshow JH, Davies KJ. Redox cycling of anthracyclines by cardiac mitochondria. II: Formation of superoxide anion, hydrogen peroxide, and hydroxyl radical. *J Biol Chem* 1986;261:3068.

117. Thornally PJ, Bannister WH, Bannister JV. Reduction of oxygen by NADH/NADH dehydrogenase in the presence of adriamycin. *Free Radic Res Commun* 1986;2:163.

118. Vasquez-Vivar J, Martasek P, Hogg N, et al. Endothelial nitric oxide synthase-dependent superoxide generation from adriamycin. *Biochemistry* 1997;36:11293.

119. Garner AP, Paine MJ, Rodriguez-Crespo I, et al. Nitric oxide synthases catalyze the activation of redox cycling and bioreductive anticancer agents. *Cancer Res* 1999;59:1929.

120. Luo D, Vincent SR. Inhibition of nitric oxide synthase by antineoplastic anthracyclines. *Biochem Pharmacol* 1994;47:2111.

121. Ursell PC, Mayes M. Anatomic distribution of nitric oxide synthase in the heart. *Int J Cardiol* 1995;50:217.

122. Thomsen LL, Miles DW. Role of nitric oxide in tumour progression: lessons from human tumours. *Cancer Metastasis Rev* 1998;17:107.

123. Doroshow JH. Anthracycline-enhanced cardiac oxygen radical metabolism. In: Singal PK, ed. *Free radicals in the pathophysiology of heart disease* Boston: Martinus Nijhoff Publishers, 1988:31.

124. Kalyanaraman B, Sealy RC, Sinha BK. An electron spin resonance study of the reduction of peroxides by anthracycline semiquinones. *Biochim Biophys Acta* 1984;799:270.

125. Kalyanaraman B, Morehouse KM, Mason RP. An electron paramagnetic resonance study of the interactions between the adriamycin semiquinone, hydrogen peroxide, iron-chelators, and radical scavengers. *Arch Biochem Biophys* 1991;286:164.

126. Doroshow JH. Prevention of doxorubicin-induced killing of MCF-7 human breast cancer cells by oxygen radical scavengers and iron chelating agents. *Biochem Biophys Res Commun* 1986;135:330.

127. Doroshow JH, Esworthy RS. The role of antioxidant defenses in the cardiotoxicity of anthracycline. In: Muggia FM, Green MD, Speyer JL, eds. *Cancer treatment and the heart.* Baltimore: The Johns Hopkins University Press, 1992:47.

128. Breimer LH. Repair of DNA damage induced by reactive oxygen species. *Free Radic Res Commun* 1991;14:159.

129. Sancar A. DNA repair in humans. *Annu Rev Genet* 1995; 29:69.

130. Taffe BG, Larminat F, Laval J, et al. Gene-specific nuclear and mitochondrial repair of formamidopyrimidine DNA glycosylase-sensitive sites in Chinese hamster ovary cells. *Mutat Res* 1996;364:183.

131. Kang YJ, Chen Y, Epstein PN. Suppression of doxorubicin cardiotoxicity by overexpression of catalase in the heart of transgenic mice. *J Biol Chem* 1996;271:12610.

132. Tabatabaie T, Floyd RA. Susceptibility of glutathione peroxidase and glutathione reductase to oxidative damage and the protective effect of spin trapping agents. *Arch Biochem Biophys* 1994;314:112.

133. Rajagopalan S, Politi PM, Sinha BK, et al. Adriamycin-induced free radical formation in the perfused rat heart: implications for cardiotoxicity. *Cancer Res* 1988;48:4766.

134. Babson JR, Abell NS, Reed DJ. Protective role of the glutathione redox cycle against adriamycin-mediated toxicity in isolated hepatocytes. *Biochem Pharmacol* 1981;30:2299.

135. Reed DJ. Regulation of reductive processes by glutathione. *Biochem Pharmacol* 1986;35:7.

136. Keizer HG, Pinedo HM, Schuurhuis GJ, et al. Doxorubicin (adriamycin): a critical review of free radical-dependent mechanisms of cytotoxicity. *Pharmacol Ther* 1990;47:219.

137. Cervantes A, Pinedo HM, Lankelma J, et al. The role of oxygen-derived free radicals in the cytotoxicity of doxorubicin in multidrug resistant and sensitive human ovarian cancer cells. *Cancer Lett* 1988;41:169.

138. Gewirtz DA. A critical evaluation of the mechanisms of action proposed for the antitumor effects of the anthracycline antibiotics adriamycin and daunorubicin. *Biochem Pharmacol* 1999;57:727.

139. Simizu S, Takada M, Umezawa K, et al. Requirement of caspase-3(-like) protease-mediated hydrogen peroxide production for apoptosis induced by various anticancer drugs. *J Biol Chem* 1998;273:26900.

140. Hamilton TC, Winker MA, Louie KG, et al. Augmentation of adriamycin, melphalan, and cisplatin cytotoxicity in drug-resistant and -sensitive human ovarian carcinoma cell lines by buthionine sulfoximine mediated glutathione depletion. *Biochem Pharmacol* 1985;34:2583.

141. Kramer RA, Zahker J, King G. Role of glutathione redox cycle in acquired and de novo multidrug resistance. *Science* 1988;241:694.

142. Dusre L, Mimnaugh EG, Myers CE, et al. Potentiation of adriamycin cytotoxicity by buthione sulfoximine in multidrug resistant breast tumor cells. *Cancer Res* 1989;49:8.

143. Lee FY, Siemann DW, Sutherland RM. Changes in cellular glutathione content during adriamycin treatment in human ovarian cancer—a possible indicator of chemosensitivity. *Br J Cancer* 1989;60:291.

144. Samuels BL, Murray JL, Cohen MB, et al. Increased glutathione peroxidase activity in a human sarcoma cell line with inherent doxorubicin resistance. *Cancer Res* 1991;51:521.

145. Nair S, Singh SV, Samy TS, et al. Anthracycline resistance in murine leukemic P388 cells. Role of drug efflux and glutathione related enzymes. *Biochem Pharmacol* 1990;39:723.

146. Benchekroun MN, Sinha BK, Robert J. Doxorubicin-induced oxygen free radical formation in sensitive and doxorubicin-resistant variants of rat glioblastoma cell lines. *FEBS Lett* 1993;326:302.

147. Ubezio P, Civoli F. Flow cytometric detection of hydrogen peroxide production induced by doxorubicin in cancer cells. *Free Radic Biol Med* 1994;16:509.

148. Alegria AE, Samuni A, Mitchell JB, et al. Free radicals induced by Adriamycin-sensitive and Adriamycin-resistant cells. A spin-trapping study. *Biochemistry* 1989;28:8653.

149. Bredehorst R, Panneerselvam M, Vogel C-W. Doxorubicin enhances complement susceptibility of human melanoma cells by extracellular oxygen radical formation. *J Biol Chem* 1987;262:2034.

150. Kule C, Ondrejickova O, Verner K. Doxorubicin, daunorubicin, and mitoxantrone cytotoxicity in yeast. *Mol Pharmacol* 1994;46:1234.

151. Quillet-Mary A, Mansat V, Duchayne E, et al. Daunorubicin-induced internucleosomal DNA fragmentation in acute myeloid cell lines. *Leukemia* 1996;10:417.

152. Ikeda K, Kajiwara K, Tanabe E, et al. Involvement of hydrogen peroxide and hydroxyl radical in chemically induced apoptosis of HL-60 cells. *Biochem Pharmacol* 1999;57:1361.

153. Mallery SR, Clark YM, Ness GM, et al. Thiol redox modulation of doxorubicin mediated cytotoxicity in cultured AIDS-related Kaposi's sarcoma cells. *J Cell Biochem* 1999;73:259.

154. Hosking LK, Whelan RD, Shellard SA, et al. An evaluation of the role of glutathione and its associated enzymes in the expression of differential sensitivities to antitumor agents shown by a range of human tumour cell lines. *Biochem Pharmacol* 1990;40:1833.

155. Benchekroun MN, Pourquier P, Schott B, et al. Doxorubicin-induced lipid peroxidation and glutathione peroxidase activity in tumor cell lines selected for resistance to doxorubicin. *Eur J Biochem* 1993;211:141.

156. Sinha BK, Mimnaugh EG, Rajagopalan S, et al. Adriamycin activation and oxygen free radical formation in human breast tumor cells: protective role of glutathione peroxidase in adriamycin resistance. *Cancer Res* 1989;49:3844.

157. Benchekroun MN, Catroux P, Montaudon D, et al. Development of mechanisms of protection against oxidative stress in doxorubicin-resistant rat tumoral cells in culture. *Free Radic Res Commun* 1990;11:137.

158. Doroshow JH. Redox cycling and the antitumor activity of the anthracyclines. In: Davies KJA, Ursini F, eds. *The oxygen paradox*. Padova, Italy: CLEUP University Press, 1995:469.

159. Vanella A, Campisi A, di Giacomo C, et al. Enhanced resistance of adriamycin-treated MCR-5 lung fibroblasts by increased intracellular glutathione peroxidase and extracellular antioxidants. *Biochem Mol Med* 1997;62:36.

160. Doroshow JH, Esworthy RS, Chu FF, et al. Glutathione peroxidase and resistance to oxidative stress. In: Tew KD, Pickett CB, Mantle TJ, et al., eds. *Structure and function of glutathione transferases*. Boca Raton, FL: CRC Press, 1993:269.

161. Taylor SD, Davenport LD, Speranza MJ, et al. Glutathione peroxidase protects cultured mammalian cells from the toxicity of Adriamycin and paraquat. *Arch Biochem Biophys* 1993;305:600.

162. Hirose K, Longo DL, Oppenheim JJ, et al. Overexpression of mitochondrial manganese superoxide dismutase promotes the survival of tumor cells exposed to interleukin-1, tumor necrosis factor, selected anticancer drugs, and ionizing radiation. *FASEB J* 1993;7:361.

163. Ravid A, Rocker D, Machlenkin A, et al. 1,25-Dihydroxyvitamin D3 enhances the susceptibility of breast cancer cells to doxorubicin-induced oxidative damage. *Cancer Res* 1999;59:862.

164. Bustamante J, Galleano M, Medrano EE, et al. Adriamycin effects on hydroperoxide metabolism and growth of human breast tumor cells. *Breast Cancer Res Treat* 1990;17:145.

165. Winterbourn CC, Gutteridge JM, Halliwell B. Doxorubicin-dependent lipid peroxidation at low partial pressures of O_2. *J Free Radic Biol Med* 1985;1:43.

166. Bellamy WT, Dalton WS, Meltzer P, et al. Role of glutathione and its associated enzymes in multidrug-resistant human myeloma cells. *Biochem Pharmacol* 1989;38:787.

167. Crescimanno M, D'Alessandro N, Armata M-G, et al. Modulation of the antioxidant activities in dox-sensitive and -resistant Friend leukemia cells. Effect of doxorubicin. *Anticancer Res* 1991;11:901.

168. Dikalov SI, Rumyantseva GV, Weiner LM, et al. Hydroxyl radical generation by oligonucleotide derivatives of anthracycline antibiotic and synthetic quinone. *Chem Biol Interact* 1991;77:325.

169. Rouscilles A, Houee-Levin C, Gardes-Albert M, et al. τ-Radiolysis study of the reduction by COO– free radicals of daunorubicin intercalated in DNA. *Free Radic Biol Med* 1989;6:37.

170. Houee-Levin C, Gardes-Albert KB, Rouscilles A, et al. One-electron reduction of daunorubicin intercalated in DNA or in protein. A τ radiolysis study. *Free Radic Res Commun* 1990;11:127.

171. Houee-Levin C, Gardes-Albert M, Rouscilles A, et al. Intramolecular semiquinone disproportionation in DNA. Pulse radiolysis study of the one-electron reduction of daunorubicin intercalated in DNA. *Biochemistry* 1991;30:8216.

172. Myers CE, Bonow R, Palmeri S, et al. Prevention of doxorubicin cardiomyopathy by *N*-acetylcysteine. *Semin Oncol* 1983;10:53.

173. Demant EJ. Transfer of ferritin-bound iron to adriamycin. *FEBS Lett* 1984;176:97.

174. Thomas CE, Aust SD. Release of iron from ferritin by cardiotoxic anthracycline antibiotics. *Arch Biochem Biophys* 1986;248:684.

175. Monteiro HP, Vile GF, Winterbourn CC. Release of iron from ferritin by semiquinone, anthracycline, bipyridyl, and nitroaromatic radicals. *Free Radic Biol Med* 1989;6:587.

176. Minotti G. Adriamycin-dependent release of iron from microsomal membranes. *Arch Biochem Biophys* 1989;268:398.

177. Minotti G. Reactions of adriamycin with microsomal iron and lipids. *Free Radic Res Commun* 1989;7:143.

178. Minotti G. NADPH- and adriamycin-dependent microsomal release of iron and lipid peroxidation. *Arch Biochem Biophys* 1990;277:268.

179. Myers CE, Gianni L, Zweier J, et al. The role of iron in adriamycin biochemistry. *Fed Proc* 1986;45:2792.

180. Zweier JL, Gianni L, Muindi J, et al. Differences in O_2 reduction by the iron complexes of adriamycin and daunomycin: the importance of the sidechain hydroxyl group. *Biochim Biophys Acta* 1986;884:326.

181. Gelvan D, Samuni A. Reappraisal of the association between adriamycin and iron. *Cancer Res* 1988;48:5645.

182. Gelvan D, Berg E, Saltman P, et al. Time-dependent modifications of ferric-adriamycin. *Biochem Pharmacol* 1990;39:1289.

183. Vile GF, Winterbourn CC. dl-N,N'-dicarboxamidomethyl-N,N'-dicarboxymethyl-1,2-diaminopropane (ICRF-198) and d-1,2-bis(3,5-dioxopiperazine-1-yl)propane (ICRF-187) inhibition of Fe^{3+} reduction, lipid peroxidation, and CaATPase inactivation in heart microsomes exposed to adriamycin. *Cancer Res* 1990;50:2307.

184. Herman EH, Ferrans VJ, Young RS, et al. Effect of pretreatment with ICRF-187 on the total cumulative dose of doxorubicin tolerated by beagle dogs. *Cancer Res* 1988;48:6918.

185. Herman EH, Ferrans VJ. Examination of the potential long-lasting protective effect of ICRF-187 against anthracycline-induced chronic cardiomyopathy. *Cancer Treat Rev* 1990;17:155.

186. Speyer JL, Green MD, Kramer E, et al. Protective effect of the bispiperazinedione ICRF-187 against doxorubicin-induced cardiac toxicity in women with advanced breast cancer. *N Engl J Med* 1988;319:745.

187. Speyer JL, Green MD, Zeleniuch-Jacquotte A, et al. ICRF-187 permits longer treatment with doxorubicin in women with breast cancer. *J Clin Oncol* 1992;10:117.

188. Von Hoff DD, Howser D, Lewis BJ, et al. Phase I study of ICRF-187 using a daily for 3 days schedule. *Cancer Treat Rep* 1981;65:249.

189. Doroshow JH. Role of reactive-oxygen metabolism in cardiac toxicity of anthracycline antibiotics. In: Priebe W, ed. *Anthracycline antibiotics: new analogues, methods of delivery, and mechanisms of action.* Washington, DC: American Chemical Society, 1995:259.

190. Minotti G, Cairo G, Monti E. Role of iron in anthracycline cardiotoxicity: new tunes for an old song? *FASEB J* 1999;13:199.

191. Minotti G, Cavaliere AF, Mordente A, et al. Secondary alcohol metabolites mediate iron delocalization in cytosolic fractions of myocardial biopsies exposed to anticancer anthracyclines. Novel linkage between anthracycline metabolism and iron-induced cardiotoxicity. *J Clin Invest* 1995;95:1595.

192. Minotti G, Mancuso C, Frustaci A, et al. Paradoxical inhibition of cardiac lipid peroxidation in cancer patients treated with doxorubicin. Pharmacologic and molecular reappraisal of anthracycline cardiotoxicity. *J Clin Invest* 1996;98:650.

193. Minotti G, Recalcati S, Mordente A, et al. The secondary alcohol metabolite of doxorubicin irreversibly inactivates aconitase/iron regulatory protein-1 in cytosolic fractions from human myocardium. *FASEB J* 1998;12:541.

194. Cummings J, Milstead R, Cunningham D, et al. Marked inter-patient variation in Adriamycin biotransformation to 7-deoxyaglycones: evidence from metabolites identified in serum. *Eur J Cancer Clin Oncol* 1986;22:991.

195. Cummings J, Smyth JF. Pharmacology of Adriamycin: the message to the clinician. *Eur J Cancer Clin Oncol* 1988;24:579.

196. Averbuch SD, Boldt M, Gaudiano G, et al. Experimental chemotherapy-induced skin necrosis in swine. Mechanistic studies of anthracycline antibiotic toxicity and protection with a radical dimer compound. *J Clin Invest* 1988;81:142.

197. Powis G, Gasdaska PY, Gallegos A, et al. Over-expression of DT-diaphorase in transfected NIH 3T3 cells does not lead to increased anticancer quinone drug sensitivity: a questionable role for the enzyme as a target for bioreductively activated anticancer drugs. *Anticancer Res* 1995;15:1141.

198. Tritton TR. Cell surface actions of adriamycin. *Pharmacol Ther* 1991;49:293.

199. Siegfried JA, Kennedy KA, Sartorelli AC, et al. The role of membranes in the mechanism of action of the antineoplastic agent adriamycin: spin-labelling studies with chronically hypoxic and drug-resistant tumor cells. *J Biol Chem* 1983;258:339.

200. Sugiyama M, Sakanashi T, Okamoto K, et al. Membrane fluidity in Ehrlich ascites tumor cells treated with Adriamycin. *Biotechnol Appl Biochem* 1986;8:217.

201. Goormaghtigh E, Brasseur R, Huart P, et al. Study of the Adriamycin-cardiolipin complex structure using attenuated total reflection infrared spectroscopy. *Biochemistry* 1987;26:1789.

202. Heywang C, Saint-Pierre CM, Masson CM, et al. Orientation of anthracyclines in lipid monolayers and planar asymmetrical bilayers: a surface-enhanced resonance Raman scattering study. *Biophys J* 1998;75:2368.

203. Zuckier G, Tritton TR. Adriamycin causes up regulation of epidermal growth factor receptors in actively growing cells. *Exp Cell Res* 1983;148:155.

204. Pegram M, Hsu S, Lewis G, et al. Inhibitory effects of combinations of HER-2/neu antibody and chemotherapeutic agents used for treatment of human breast cancers. *Oncogene* 1999;18:2241.

205. Sun IL, Navas P, Crane FL, et al. Diferric transferrin reductase in the plasma membrane is inhibited by adriamycin. *Biochem Int* 1987;14:119.

206. DeAtley SM, Aksenov MY, Aksenova MV, et al. Adriamycin induces protein oxidation in erythrocyte membranes. *Pharmacol Toxicol* 1998;83:62.

207. Tritton TR, Yee G. The anticancer agent adriamycin can be actively cytotoxic without entering cells. *Science* 1982;217:248.

208. Rogers KE, Carr BI, Tokes ZA. Cell surface-mediated cytotoxicity of polymer-bound adriamycin against drug-resistant hepatocytes. *Cancer Res* 1983;43:2741.

209. Vichi P, Tritton TR. Adriamycin: protection from cell death by removal of extracellular drug. *Cancer Res* 1992;52:4135.

210. Burns CP, Spector AA. Membrane fatty acid modification in tumor cells: a potential therapeutic adjunct. *Lipids* 1987; 22:178.

211. Spector AA, Burns CP. Biological and therapeutic potential of membrane lipid modifications in tumors. *Cancer Res* 1987;47:4529.

212. Burns CP, North JA, Petersen ES, et al. Subcellular distribution of doxorubicin: comparison of fatty acid-modified and unmodified cells. *Proc Soc Exp Biol Med* 1988;188:455.

213. Hannun YA. Functions of ceramide in coordinating cellular responses to stress. *Science* 1996;274:1855.

214. Leevers SJ, Vanhaesebroeck B, Waterfield MD. Signalling through phosphoinositide 3-kinases: the lipids take centre stage. *Curr Opin Cell Biol* 1999;11:219.

215. Haimovitz-Friedman A. Radiation-induced signal transduction and stress response. *Radiat Res* 1998;150:S102.

216. Bredel M, Pollack IF. The p21-Ras signal transduction pathway and growth regulation in human high-grade gliomas. *Brain Res Brain Res Rev* 1999;29:232.

217. Kyriakis JM. Making the connection: coupling of stress-activated ERK/MAPK (extracellular-signal-regulated kinase/mitogen-activated protein kinase) core signalling modules to extracellular stimuli and biological responses. *Biochem Soc Symp* 1999;64:29.

218. Tritton TR, Hickman JA. How to kill cancer cells: membranes and cell signaling as targets in cancer chemotherapy. *Cancer Cells* 1990;2:95.

219. Palayoor ST, Stein JM, Hait WN. Inhibition of protein kinase C by antineoplastic agents: implications for drug resistance. *Biochem Biophys Res Commun* 1987;148:718.

220. Donella-Deana A, Monti E, Pinna LA. Inhibition of tyrosine protein kinases by the antineoplastic agent adriamycin. *Biochem Biophys Res Commun* 1989;160:1309.

221. Hannun YA, Foglesong RJ, Bell RM. The adriamycin-iron(III) complex is a potent inhibitor of protein kinase C. *J Biol Chem* 1989;264:9960.

222. Posada J, Vichi P, Tritton TR. Protein kinase C in Adriamycin action and resistance in mouse sarcoma 180 cells. *Cancer Res* 1989;49:6634.

223. Tritton TR. Cell death in cancer chemotherapy: the case of Adriamycin. In: Tomei LD, Cope FO, eds. *Apoptosis: the molecular basis of cell death*. Cold Spring Harbor, NY: Cold Spring Harbor Laboratory Press, 1991:121.

224. Sahyoun N, Wolf M, Besterman J, et al. Protein kinase C phosphorylates topoisomerase II: topoisomerase activation and its possible role in phorbol ester-induced differentiation of HL-60 cells. *Proc Natl Acad Sci U S A* 1986;83:1603.

225. Jaffrezou JP, Levade T, Bettaieb A, et al. Daunorubicin-induced apoptosis: triggering of ceramide generation through sphingomyelin hydrolysis. *EMBO J* 1996;15:2417.

226. Bose R, Verheij M, Haimovitz-Friedman A, et al. Ceramide synthase mediates daunorubicin-induced apoptosis: an alternative mechanism for generating death signals. *Cell* 1995;82:405.

227. Bettaieb A, Plo I, Mansat-De M, et al. Daunorubicin- and mitoxantrone-triggered phosphatidylcholine hydrolysis: implication in drug-induced ceramide generation and apoptosis. *Mol Pharmacol* 1999;55:118.

228. Tepper AD, de Vries E, van Blitterswijzj WJ, et al. Ordering of ceramide formation, caspase activation, and mitochondrial changes during CD95- and DNA damage-induced apoptosis. *J Clin Invest* 1999;103:971.

229. Mansat V, Bettaieb A, Levade T, et al. Serine protease inhibitors block neutral sphingomyelinase activation, ceramide generation, and apoptosis triggered by daunorubicin. *FASEB J* 1997;11:695.

230. Allouche M, Bettaieb A, Vindis C, et al. Influence of Bcl-2 overexpression on the ceramide pathway in daunorubicin-induced apoptosis of leukemic cells. *Oncogene* 1997;14:1837.

231. Liu YY, Han TY, Giuliano AE, et al. Expression of glucosylceramide synthase, converting ceramide to glucosylceramide, confers adriamycin resistance in human breast cancer cells. *J Biol Chem* 1999;274:1140.

232. Fine RL, Patel J, Chabner BA. Phorbol esters induce multidrug resistance in human breast cancer cells. *Proc Natl Acad Sci U S A* 1988;85:582.

233. Yu G, Ahmad S, Aquino A, et al. Transfection with protein kinase Cα confers increased multidrug resistance to MCF-7 cells expressing P-glycoprotein. *Cancer Commun* 1991;3:181.

234. Budworth J, Gant TW, Gescher A. Co-ordinate loss of protein kinase C and multidrug resistance gene expression in revertant MCF-7/Adr breast carcinoma cells. *Br J Cancer* 1997;75:1330.

235. Laredo J, Huynh A, Muller C, et al. Effect of the protein kinase C inhibitor staurosporine on chemosensitivity to daunorubicin of normal and leukemic fresh myeloid cells. *Blood* 1994;84:229.

236. Lavie Y, Cao H, Volner A, et al. Agents that reverse multidrug resistance, tamoxifen, verapamil, and cyclosporin A, block glycosphingolipid metabolism by inhibiting ceramide glycosylation in human cancer cells. *J Biol Chem* 1997;272:1682.

237. Reed JC. Dysregulation of apoptosis in cancer. *J Clin Oncol* 1999;17:2941.

238. Wickremasinghe RG, Hoffbrand AV. Biochemical and genetic control of apoptosis: relevance to normal hematopoiesis and hematological malignancies. *Blood* 1999;93:3587.

239. Hannun YA. Apoptosis and the dilemma of cancer chemotherapy. *Blood* 1997;89:1845.

240. Skladanowski A, Konopa J. Adriamycin and daunomycin induce programmed cell death (apoptosis) in tumour cells. *Biochem Pharmacol* 1993;46:375.

241. Ling Y-H, Priebe W, Perez-Soler R. Apoptosis induced by anthracycline antibiotics in P388 parent and multidrug-resistant cells. *Cancer Res* 1993;53:1845.

242. Lotem J, Sachs L. Hematopoietic cytokines inhibit apoptosis induced by transforming growth factor beta 1 and cancer chemotherapy compounds in myeloid leukemic cells. *Blood* 1992;80:1750.

243. Thakkar NS, Potten CS. Inhibition of doxorubicin-induced apoptosis in vivo by 2-deoxy-D-glucose. *Cancer Res* 1993; 53:2057.

244. Onishi Y, Azuma Y, Sato Y, et al. Topoisomerase inhibitors induce apoptosis in thymocytes. *Biochim Biophys Acta* 1993; 1175:147.

245. Zaleskis G, Berleth E, Verstovsek S, et al. Doxorubicin-induced DNA degradation in murine thymocytes. *Mol Pharmacol* 1994;46:901.

246. Chernov MV, Stark GR. The p53 activation and apoptosis induced by DNA damage are reversibly inhibited by salicylate. *Oncogene* 1997;14:2503.

247. Teixeira C, Reed JC, Pratt MAC. Estrogen promotes chemotherapeutic drug resistance by a mechanism involving *bcl*-2 proto-oncogene expression in human breast cancer cells. *Cancer Res* 1995;55:3902.

248. Strobel T, Swanson L, Korsmeyer S, et al. BAX enhances paclitaxel-induced apoptosis through a p53-independent pathway. *Proc Natl Acad Sci U S A* 1996;93:14094.

249. Makris A, Powles TJ, Dowsett M, et al. Prediction of response to neoadjuvant chemoendocrine therapy in primary breast carcinomas. *Clin Cancer Res* 1997;3:593.

250. Friesen C, Herr I, Krammer PH, et al. Involvement of the CD95 (APO-1/FAS) receptor/ligand system in drug-induced apoptosis in leukemia cells. *Nat Med* 1996;2:574.

251. Fulda S, Sieverts H, Friesen C, et al. The CD95 (APO-1/Fas) system mediates drug-induced apoptosis in neuroblastoma cells. *Cancer Res* 1997;57:3823.

252. Fulda S, Susin SA, Kroemer G, et al. Molecular ordering of apoptosis induced by anticancer drugs in neuroblastoma cells. *Cancer Res* 1998;58:4453.

253. Mo YY, Beck WT. DNA damage signals induction of fas ligand in tumor cells. *Mol Pharmacol* 1999;55:216.

254. Eischen CM, Kottke TJ, Martins LM, et al. Comparison of apoptosis in wild-type and Fas-resistant cells: chemotherapy-induced apoptosis is not dependent on Fas/Fas ligand interactions. *Blood* 1997;90:935.

255. Landowski TH, Shain KH, Oshiro MM, et al. Myeloma cells selected for resistance to CD95-mediated apoptosis are not cross-resistant to cytotoxic drugs: evidence for independent mechanisms of caspase activation. *Blood* 1999;94:265.

256. McGahon AJ, Costa PA, Daly L, et al. Chemotherapeutic drug-induced apoptosis in human leukaemic cells is independent of the Fas (APO-1/CD95) receptor/ligand system. *Br J Haematol* 1998;101:539.

257. Wesselborg S, Engels IH, Rossmann E, et al. Anticancer drugs induce caspase-8/FLICE activation and apoptosis in the absence of CD95 receptor/ligand interaction. *Blood* 1999;93:3053.

258. Come MG, Bettaieb A, Skladanowski A, et al. Alteration of the daunorubicin-triggered sphingomyelin-ceramide pathway and apoptosis in MDR cells: influence of drug transport abnormalities. *Int J Cancer* 1999;81:580.

259. Herr I, Wilhelm D, Bohler T, et al. Activation of CD95 (APO-1/Fas) signaling by ceramide mediates cancer therapy-induced apoptosis. *EMBO J* 1997;16:6200.

260. Garland JM, Rudin C. Cytochrome *c* induces caspase-dependent apoptosis in intact hematopoietic cells and overrides apoptosis suppression mediated by bcl-2, growth factor signaling, MAP-kinase-kinase, and malignant change. *Blood* 1999;92:1235.

261. Kroemer G, Zamzami N, Susin SA. Mitochondrial control of apoptosis. *Immunol Today* 1997;18:44.

262. Doroshow JH, Matsumoto L, van Balgooy J. Modulation of doxorubicin-induced, oxygen radical mediated apoptosis by glutathione peroxidase and free radical scavengers in human breast cancer cells. *Proc Am Assoc Cancer Res* 1999; 40:16(abst).

263. Singh I, Pahan K, Khan M, et al. Cytokine-mediated induction of ceramide production is redox-sensitive. Implications to proinflammatory cytokine-mediated apoptosis in demyelinating diseases. *J Biol Chem* 1998;273:20354.

264. Ohmori T, Podack ER, Nishio K, et al. Apoptosis of lung cancer cells caused by some anti-cancer agents (MMC, CPT-11, ADM) is inhibited by *BCL-2*. *Biochem Biophys Res Commun* 1993;192:30.

265. Reed JC. Bcl-2 and the regulation of programmed cell death. *J Cell Biol* 1994;124:1.

266. Campos L, Sabido O, Rouault J-P, et al. Effects of BCL-2 antisense oligodeoxynucleotides on in vitro proliferation and survival of normal marrow progenitors and leukemic cells. *Blood* 1994;84:595.

267. Froesch BA, Aime-Sempe C, Leber B, et al. Inhibition of p53 transcriptional activity by Bcl-2 requires its membrane-anchoring domain. *J Biol Chem* 1999;274:6469.

268. Hockenbery DM, Oltvai ZN, Yin X-M, et al. Bcl-2 functions in an antioxidant pathway to prevent apoptosis. *Cell* 1993;75:241.

269. Decaudin D, Geley S, Hirsch T, et al. Bcl-2 and Bcl-XL antagonize the mitochondrial dysfunction preceding nuclear apoptosis induced by chemotherapeutic agents. *Cancer Res* 1997;57:62.

270. Boland MP, Foster SJ, O'Neill LA. Daunorubicin activates NFkappaB and induces kappaB-dependent gene expression in HL-60 promyelocytic and Jurkat T lymphoma cells. *J Biol Chem* 1997;272:12952.

271. Wang CY, Mayo MW, Baldwin AS Jr. TNF- and cancer therapy-induced apoptosis: potentiation by inhibition of NF-kappaB. *Science* 1996;274:784.

272. Jeremias I, Kupatt C, Baumann B, et al. Inhibition of nuclear factor kappaB activation attenuates apoptosis resistance in lymphoid cells. *Blood* 1998;91:4624.

273. Haldar S, Negrini M, Monne M, et al. Down-regulation of *bcl-2* by *p53* in breast cancer cells. *Cancer Res* 1994;54:2095.

274. Bacus SS, Yarden Y, Oren M, et al. Neu differentiation factor (Heregulin) activates a p53-dependent pathway in cancer cells. *Oncogene* 1996;12:2535.

275. Gartenhaus RB, Wang P, Hoffmann P. Induction of the WAF1/CIP1 protein and apoptosis in human T-cell leukemia virus type I-transformed lymphocytes after treatment with adriamycin by using a p53-independent pathway. *Proc Natl Acad Sci U S A* 1996;93:265.

276. Michieli P, Chedid M, Lin D, et al. Induction of *WAF1/CIP1* by a p53-independent pathway. *Cancer Res* 1994;54:3391.

277. Wang Y, Blandino G, Givol D. Induced p21waf expression in H1299 cell line promotes cell senescence and protects against cytotoxic effect of radiation and doxorubicin. *Oncogene* 1999;18:2643.

278. Shimizu A, Nishida J, Ueoka Y, et al. Cyclin G contributes to G2/M arrest of cells in response to DNA damage. *Biochem Biophys Res Commun* 1998;242:529.

279. Lowe SW, Ruley HE, Jacks T, et al. p53-dependent apoptosis modulates the cytotoxicity of anticancer agents. *Cell* 1993;74:957.

280. Lowe SW, Bodis S, McClatchey A, et al. p53 status and the efficacy of cancer therapy in vivo. *Science* 1994;266:807.

281. Aas T, Borresen AL, Geisler S, et al. Specific p53 mutations are associated with de novo resistance to doxorubicin in breast cancer patients. *Nat Med* 1996;2:811.

282. Gros P, Croop J, Housman D. Mammalian multidrug resistance gene: complete cDNA sequence indicates strong homology to bacterial transport proteins. *Cell* 1986;47:371.

283. Gros P, BenNeriah Y, Croop J, et al. Isolation and expression of a complementary DNA that confers multidrug resistance. *Nature* 1986;332:728.

284. Endicott JA, Ling V. The biochemistry of P-glycoprotein-mediated multidrug resistance. *Annu Rev Biochem* 1989;58:137.

285. Sugimoto Y, Tsuruo T. DNA-mediated transfer and cloning of a human multidrug-resistant gene of adriamycin-resistant myelogenous leukemia K562. *Cancer Res* 1987;47:2620.

286. Hamada H, Hagiwara T, Nakajma T, et al. Phosphorylation of Mr 170,000 to 180,000 glycoprotein species specific to multidrug-resistant tumor cells: effects of verapamil, trifluoroperazine and phorbol esters. *Cancer Res* 1987;47:2860.

287. Chambers SK, Hait WN, Kacinski BM, et al. Enhancement of anthracycline growth inhibition in parent and multidrug-resistant Chinese hamster ovary cells by cyclosporin A and its analogues. *Cancer Res* 1989;49:6275.

288. Coley HM, Twentyman PR, Workman P. The efflux of anthracyclines in multidrug-resistant cell lines. *Biochem Pharmacol* 1993;46:1317.

289. Kang Y, Perry RR. Modulatory effects of tamoxifen and recombinant human α-interferon on doxorubicin resistance. *Cancer Res* 1993;53:3040.

290. Merlin J-L, Guerci A, Marchal S, et al. Comparative evaluation of S9788, verapamil, and cyclosporine A in K562 human leukemia cell lines and in P-glycoprotein-expressing samples from patients with hematologic malignancies. *Blood* 1994;84:262.

291. Alvarez M, Pauli K, Monks A, et al. Generation of a drug resistance profile by quantitation of mdr-1/P-glycoprotein in the cell lines of the National Cancer Institute anticancer drug screen. *J Clin Invest* 1995;95:2205.

292. Lemontt JF, Azzaria M, Gross P. Increased mdr gene expression and decreased drug accumulation in multidrug-resistant human melanoma cells. *Cancer Res* 1988;48:6348.

293. Noonan KE, Beck C, Holzmayer TA, et al. Quantitative analysis of MDR1 (multidrug resistance) gene expression in human tumors by polymerase chain reaction. *Proc Natl Acad Sci U S A* 1990;87:7160.

294. Chen G, Jaffrezou J-P, Fleming WH, et al. Prevalence of multidrug resistance related to activation of the mdr1 gene in human sarcoma mutants derived by single-step doxorubicin selection. *Cancer Res* 1994;54:4980.

295. Kato S, Nishimura J, Yufu Y, et al. Modulation of expression of multidrug resistance gene (mdr-1) by adriamycin. *FEBS Lett* 1992;308:175.

296. Chaudhary PM, Roninson IB. Induction of multidrug resistance in human cells by transient exposure to different chemotherapeutic drugs. *J Natl Cancer Inst* 1993;85:632.

297. Fojo AT, Ueda K, Siamon DJ, et al. Expression of a multidrug resistance gene in human tumors and tissues. *Proc Natl Acad Sci U S A* 1987;84:265.

298. Sparreboom A, van Asperen J, Mayer U, et al. Limited oral bioavailability and active epithelial excretion of paclitaxel (Taxol) caused by P-glycoprotein in the intestine. *Proc Natl Acad Sci U S A* 1997;94:2031.

299. Egashira M, Kawamata N, Sugimoto K, et al. P-glycoprotein expression on normal and abnormally expanded natural killer cells and inhibition of P-glycoprotein function by cyclosporin A and its analogue PSC833. *Blood* 1999;93:599.

300. Fairchild CR, Ivy SP, Rushmore T, et al. Carcinogen-induced mdr overexpression is associated with xenobiotic resistance in rat preneoplastic liver nodules and hepatocellular carcinomas. *Proc Natl Acad Sci U S A* 1987;84:7701.

301. Myers CE, Cowan K, Sinha BK, et al. The phenomenon of pleiotropic drug resistance. In: De Vita VT Jr, Hellman S, Rosenberg SA, eds. Important advances in oncology. Philadelphia: JB Lippincott, 1987:27.

302. Yeh GC, Lopaczynska J, Poore CM, et al. A new functional role for P-glycoprotein: efflux pump for benzo(a)pyrene in human breast cancer MCF-7 cells. *Cancer Res* 1992;52:6692.

303. Marie J-P, Zittoun R, Sikic BI. Multidrug resistance (*mdr1*) gene expression in adult acute leukemias: correlations with treatment outcome and in vitro drug sensitivity. *Blood* 1991;78:586.

304. Goasguen JE, Dossot J-M, Fardel O, et al. Expression of the multidrug resistance-associated P-glycoprotein (P-170) in 59 cases of de novo acute lymphoblastic leukemia: prognostic implications. *Blood* 1993;81:2394.

305. Chabner BA, Fojo A. Multidrug resistance: P-glycoprotein and its allies—the elusive foes. *J Natl Cancer Inst* 1989;81:910.

306. Grogan TM, Spier CM, Salmon SE, et al. P-glycoprotein expression in human plasma cell myeloma: correlation with prior chemotherapy. *Blood* 1993;81:490.

307. Keith WN, Stallard S, Brown R. Expression of mdr1 and gst-π in human breast tumors: comparison to in vitro chemosensitivity. *Br J Cancer* 1990;61:712.

308. Verrelle P, Meissonnier F, Fonck Y, et al. Clinical relevance of immunohistochemical detection of multidrug resistance P-glycoprotein in breast carcinoma [see comments]. *J Natl Cancer Inst* 1991;83:111.

309. Miller TP, Grogan TM, Dalton WS, et al. P-glycoprotein expression in malignant lymphoma and reversal of clinical drug resistance with chemotherapy plus high-dose verapamil. *J Clin Oncol* 1991;9:17.

310. Wishart GC, Bissett D, Paul J, et al. Quinidine as a resistance modulator of epirubicin in advanced breast cancer: mature results of a placebo-controlled randomized trial. *J Clin Oncol* 1994;12:1771.

311. Lum BL, Fisher GA, Brophy NA, et al. Clinical trials of modulation of multidrug resistance: pharmacokinetic and pharmacodynamic considerations. *Cancer* 1993;72:3502.

312. Bartlett NL, Lum BL, Fisher GA, et al. Phase I trial of doxorubicin with cyclosporine as a modulator of multidrug resistance. *J Clin Oncol* 1994;12:835.

313. List AF, Kopecky KJ, Willman CL, et al. Benefit of cyclosporine (Csa) modulation of anthracycline resistance in high-risk AML: a Southwest Oncology Group (SWOG) study. *Blood* 1998;92[Suppl 1]:312a(abst).

314. Slovak ML, Hoeltge GA, Dalton WS, et al. Pharmacological and biological evidence for differing mechanisms of doxorubicin resistance in two human tumor cell lines. *Cancer Res* 1988;48:2793.

315. Mirski SE, Gerlach JH, Cole SP. Multidrug resistance in a human small cell line selected in adriamycin. *Cancer Res* 1987;47:2594.

316. Krishnamachary N, Center MS. The MRP gene associated with a non-P-glycoprotein multidrug resistance encodes a 190-kDa membrane bound glycoprotein. *Cancer Res* 1993;53:3658.

317. Eijdems EW, Zaman GJ, de Haas M, et al. Altered MRP is associated with multidrug resistance and reduced drug accumulation in human SW-1573 cells. *Br J Cancer* 1995;72:298.

318. Welters MJ, Fichtinger-Schepman AM, Baan RA, et al. Role of glutathione, glutathione S-transferases and multidrug resistance-related proteins in cisplatin sensitivity of head and neck cancer cell lines. *Br J Cancer* 1998;77:556.

319. Moran E, Cleary I, Larkin AM, et al. Co-expression of MDR-associated markers, including P-170, MRP and LRP and cytoskeletal proteins, in three resistant variants of the human ovarian carcinoma cell line, OAW42. *Eur J Cancer* 1997;33:652.

320. Marbeuf-Gueye C, Broxterman HJ, Dubru F, et al. Kinetics of anthracycline efflux from multidrug resistance protein-expressing cancer cells compared with P-glycoprotein-expressing cancer cells. *Mol Pharmacol* 1998;53:141.

321. Slapak CA, Mizunuma N, Kufe DW. Expression of the multidrug resistance associated protein and P-glycoprotein in doxorubicin-selected human myeloid leukemia cells. *Blood* 1994;84:3113.

322. Schneider E, Cowan KH, Bader H, et al. Increased expression of the multidrug resistance-associated protein gene in relapsed acute leukemia. *Blood* 1995;85:186.

323. Legrand O, Simonin G, Beauchamp-Nicoud A, et al. Simultaneous activity of MRP1 and Pgp is correlated with in vitro resistance to daunorubicin and with in vivo resistance in adult acute myeloid leukemia. *Blood* 1999;94:1046.

324. Rappa G, Finch RA, Sartorelli AC, et al. New insights into the biology and pharmacology of the multidrug resistance protein (MRP) from gene knockout models. *Biochem Pharmacol* 1999;58:557.

325. Lorico A, Rappa G, Flavell RA, et al. Double knockout of the MRP gene leads to increased drug sensitivity in vitro. *Cancer Res* 1996;56:5351.

326. Kool M, de Haas M, Scheffer GL, et al. Analysis of expression of *cMoat* (*MRP2*), *MRP3*, *MRP4*, and *MRP5*, homologues of the multidrug resistance-associated protein (*MRP1*), in human cancer cell lines. *Cancer Res* 1997;57:3537.

327. Deffie AM, Batra JK, Goldenberg GG. Direct correlation between DNA topoisomerase II activity and cytotoxicity in adriamycin-sensitive and -resistant P388 leukemia cell lines. *Cancer Res* 1989;49:58.

328. Ganapathi R, Grabowski D, Ford J, et al. Progressive resistance to doxorubicin in mouse leukemia L1210 cells with multidrug resistance phenotype: reductions in drug-induced topoisomerase II–mediated DNA cleavage. *Cancer Commun* 1989;1:217.

329. De Jong S, Zijlstra JG, de Vries EGE, et al. Reduced DNA topoisomerase II activity and drug-induced DNA cleavage activity in an adriamycin-resistant human small cell lung carcinoma cell line. *Cancer Res* 1990;50:304.

330. Ramachandran C, Samy TS, Huang XL, et al. Doxorubicin-induced DNA breaks, topoisomerase II activity and gene expression in human melanoma cells. *Biochem Pharmacol* 1993;45:1367.

331. Son YS, Suh JM, Ahn SH, et al. Reduced activity of topoisomerase II in an Adriamycin-resistant human stomach-adenocarcinoma cell line. *Cancer Chemother Pharmacol* 1998;41:353.

332. Wyler B, Shao Y, Schneider E, et al. Intermittent exposure to doxorubicin in vitro selects for multifactorial non-P-glycoprotein-associated multidrug resistance in RPMI 8226 human myeloma cells. *Br J Haematol* 1997;97:65.

333. Beketic-Oreskovic L, Duran GE, Chen G, et al. Decreased mutation rate for cellular resistance to doxorubicin and suppression of mdr1 gene activation by the cyclosporin PSC 833 [see comments]. *J Natl Cancer Inst* 1995;87:1593.

334. Friche E, Danks MK, Schmidt CA, et al. Decreased DNA topoisomerase II in daunorubicin-resistant Ehrlich ascites tumor cells. *Cancer Res* 1991;51:4213.

335. Wang H, Jiang Z, Wong YW, et al. Decreased CP-1 (NF-Y) activity results in transcriptional down-regulation of topoisomerase II alpha in a doxorubicin-resistant variant of human multiple myeloma RPMI 8226. *Biochem Biophys Res Commun* 1997;237:217.

336. McPherson JP, Deffie AM, Jones NR, et al. Selective sensitization of adriamycin-resistant P388 murine leukemia cells to antineoplastic agents following transfection with human DNA topoisomerase II alpha. *Anticancer Res* 1997;17:4243.

337. Kaufman SH, Karp JE, Jones RJ, et al. Topoisomerase II levels and drug sensitivity in adult acute myelogenous leukemia. *Blood* 1994;83:517.

338. Lee FY, Vessey AR, Siemann DW. Glutathione as a determinant of cellular response to doxorubicin. *Natl Cancer Inst Monogr* 1988;6:211.

339. Capranico G, Babudri N, Casciarri G, et al. Lack of effect of glutathione depletion on cytotoxicity, mutagenicity and DNA damage produced by doxorubicin in cultured cells. *Chem Biol Interact* 1986;57:189.

340. Yamamoto M, Maehara Y, Oda S, et al. The p53 tumor suppressor gene in anticancer agent–induced apoptosis and chemosensitivity of human gastrointestinal cancer cell lines. *Cancer Chemother Pharmacol* 1999;43:43.

341. Meng RD, Phillips P, el-Deiry WS. p53-independent increase in E2F-1 expression enhances the cytotoxic effects of etoposide and of adriamycin. *Int J Oncol* 1999;14:5.

342. Kuhl JS, Krajewski S, Duran GE, et al. Spontaneous overexpression of the long form of the Bcl-X protein in a highly resistant P388 leukaemia. *Br J Cancer* 1997;75:268.

343. Reed JC. Bcl-2 and the regulation of programmed cell death. *J Cell Biol* 1994;124:1.

344. Nielsen D, Maare C, Skovsgaard T. Cellular resistance to anthracyclines. *Gen Pharmacol* 1996;27:251.

345. Brown R, Hirst GL, Gallagher WM, et al. hMLH1 expression and cellular responses of ovarian tumour cells to treatment with cytotoxic anticancer agents. *Oncogene* 1997;15:45.

346. Durant ST, Morris MM, Illand M, et al. Dependence on RAD52 and RAD1 for anticancer drug resistance mediated by inactivation of mismatch repair genes. *Curr Biol* 1999;9:51.

347. Belloni M, Uberti D, Rizzini C, et al. Induction of two DNA mismatch repair proteins, MSH2 and MSH6, in differentiated human neuroblastoma SH-SY5Y cells exposed to doxorubicin. *J Neurochem* 1999;72:974.

348. Fink D, Aebi S, Howell SB. The role of DNA mismatch repair in drug resistance. *Clin Cancer Res* 1998;4:1.

349. Chatterjee S, Cheng MF, Berger NA. Hypersensitivity to clinically useful alkylating agents and radiation in poly(ADP-ribose) polymerase-deficient cell lines. *Cancer Commun* 1990;2:401.

350. Darby MK, Schmitt B, Jongstra-Bilen J, et al. Inhibition of calf thymus type II DNA topoisomerase by poly(ADP-ribosylation). *EMBO J* 1985;4:2129.

351. Berger NA. Poly(ADP-ribose) in the cellular response to DNA damage. *Radiat Res* 1985;101:4.

352. Yamamoto K, Tsukidate K, Farber JL. Differing effects of the inhibition of poly(ADP-ribose) polymerase on the course of oxidative cell injury in hepatocytes and fibroblasts. *Biochem Pharmacol* 1993;46:483.

353. Tanizawa A, Kubota M, Takimoto T, et al. Prevention of adriamycin-induced interphase death by 3-aminobenzamide and nicotinamide in a human promyelocytic leukemia cell line. *Biochem Biophys Res Commun* 1987;144:1031.

354. Doroshow JH, Van Balgooy C, Akman SA. Effect of poly(ADP-ribose) polymerase inhibition on protein-associated DNA single-strand cleavage and cytotoxicity by anthracycline antibiotics. *Proc Am Assoc Cancer Res* 1995;36:444(abst).

355. Reich SD, Bachur NR. Alterations in adriamycin efficacy by phenobarbital. *Cancer Res* 1976;36:3803.

356. Innis JD, Meyer M, Hurwitz A. A novel acute toxicity resulting from the administration of morphine and adriamycin to mice. *Toxicol Appl Pharmacol* 1987;90:445.

357. Holmes FA, Madden T, Newman RA, et al. Sequence-dependent alteration of doxorubicin pharmacokinetics by paclitaxel in a phase I study of paclitaxel and doxorubicin in patients with metastatic breast cancer. *J Clin Oncol* 1996;14:2713.

358. Sparreboom A, van Tellingen O, Nooijen WJ, et al. Nonlinear pharmacokinetics of paclitaxel in mice results from the pharmaceutical vehicle Cremophor EL. *Cancer Res* 1996;56:2112.

359. Legha SS, Benjamin RS, Mackay B, et al. Reduction of doxorubicin cardiotoxicity by prolonged continuous intravenous infusion. *Ann Intern Med* 1982;96:133.

360. Terasaki T, Iga T, Sugiyama Y, et al. Experimental evidence of characteristic tissue distribution of adriamycin: tissue DNA concentration as a determinant. *Pharmacol Rev* 1989;53:496.

361. Greene R, Collins J, Jenkins J, et al. Plasma pharmacokinetics of adriamycin and adriamycinol: implications for the design of in vitro experiments and treatment protocols. *Cancer Res* 1983;43:3417.

362. Speth PAJ, Linssen PCM, Holdrinet RSG, et al. Plasma and cellular adriamycin concentrations in patients with myeloma treated with 96-hour continuous infusion. *Clin Pharmacol Ther* 1987;41:661.

363. Synold T, Doroshow JH. Anthracycline dose intensity: clinical pharmacology and pharmacokinetics of high-dose doxorubicin administered as a 96-hour continuous intravenous infusion. *J Infus Chemother* 1996;6:69.

364. Bronchud MH, Margison JM, Howell A, et al. Comparative pharmacokinetics of escalating doses of doxorubicin in patients with metastatic breast cancer. *Cancer Chemother Pharmacol* 1990;25:435.

365. Dobbs NA, Twelves CJ, Gillies H, et al. Gender affects doxorubicin pharmacokinetics in patients with normal liver biochemistry. *Cancer Chemother Pharmacol* 1995;36:473.

366. Dobbs NA, Twelves CJ. What is the effect of adjusting epirubicin doses for body surface area? *Br J Cancer* 1998;78:662.

367. Huffman DH, Bachur NR. Daunorubicin metabolism in acute myelocytic leukemia. *Blood* 1972;39:637.

368. Gill P, Favre R, Durand A, et al. Time dependency of adriamycin and adriamycinol kinetics. *Cancer Chemother Pharmacol* 1983;10:120.

369. Lovless H, Arena E, Felsted RL, et al. Comparative mammalian metabolism of adriamycin and daunorubicin. *Cancer Res* 1978;38:593.

370. Felsted RL, Gee M, Bachur NR. Rat liver daunorubicin reductase: an aldo-keto reductase. *J Biol Chem* 1974;249:3672.

371. Felsted RL, Richter DR, Bachur NR. Rat liver aldehyde reductase. *Biochem Pharmacol* 1977;26:1117.

372. Felsted RL, Bachur NR. Mammalian carbonyl reductases. *Drug Metab Rev* 1980;11:1.

373. Forrest GL, Akman S, Doroshow J, et al. Genomic sequence and expression of a cloned human carbonyl reductase gene with daunorubicin reductase activity. *Mol Pharmacol* 1991;40:502.

374. Ozols RF, Willson JKV, Weltz MD, et al. Inhibition of human ovarian cancer colony formation by adriamycin and its major metabolites. *Cancer Res* 1980;40:4109.

375. Gessner T, Preisler HD, Azarnia N, et al. Plasma levels of daunomycin metabolites and the outcome of ANLL therapy. *Med Oncol Tumor Pharmacother* 1987;4:23.

376. Benjamin RS. A practical approach to adriamycin (NSC-123127) toxicology. *Cancer Chemother Rep* 1975;6:191.

377. Brenner DE, Wiernik PH, Wesley M, et al. Acute doxorubicin toxicity: relationship to pretreatment liver function, response and pharmacokinetics in patients with acute non-lymphocytic leukemia. *Cancer* 1984;53:1042.

378. Chan KK, Chlebowski RT, Myron Tong H-S, et al. Clinical pharmacokinetics of adriamycin in hepatoma patients with cirrhosis. *Cancer Res* 1980;40:1263.

379. Ackland SP, Ratain MJ, Vogelzang NJ, et al. Pharmacokinetics and pharmacodynamics of long-term continuous-infusion doxorubicin. *Clin Pharmacol Ther* 1989;45:340.

380. Twelves CJ, Dobbs NA, Gillies HC, et al. Doxorubicin pharmacokinetics: the effect of abnormal liver biochemistry tests. *Cancer Chemother Pharmacol* 1998;42:229.

381. Doroshow J, Chan K. Relationship between doxorubicin clearance and indocyanine green dye pharmacokinetics in patients with hepatic dysfunction. *Proc Am Soc Clin Oncol* 1982;1:11(abst).

382. Sonneveld P, Wassenaar HA, Nooter K. Long persistence of doxorubicin in human skin after extravasation. *Cancer Treat Rep* 1984;68:895.

383. Dorr RT, Dordal MS, Koenig LM, et al. High levels of doxorubicin in the tissues of a patient experiencing extravasation during a 4-day infusion. *Cancer* 1989;64:2462.

384. Andersson AP, Dahlstrom KK. Clinical results after doxorubicin extravasation treated with excision guided by fluorescence microscopy. *Eur J Cancer* 1993;29A:1712.

385. Heitmann C, Durmus C, Ingianni G. Surgical management after doxorubicin and epirubicin extravasation. *J Hand Surg [Br]* 1998;23:666.

386. Bertelli G, Gozza A, Forno GB, et al. Topical dimethylsulfoxide for the prevention of soft tissue injury after extravasation of vesicant cytotoxic drugs: a prospective clinical study. *J Clin Oncol* 1995;13:2851.

387. Disa JJ, Chang RR, Mucci SJ, et al. Prevention of adriamycin-induced full-thickness skin loss using hyaluronidase infiltration. *Plast Reconstr Surg* 1998;101:370.

388. Doroshow JH. Doxorubicin-induced cardiac toxicity. *N Engl J Med* 1991;324:843.

389. Singal PK, Iliskovic N. Doxorubicin-induced cardiomyopathy. *N Engl J Med* 1998;339:900.

390. Slamon D, Leyland-Jones B, Shak S, et al. Addition of Herceptin™ (humanized anti-HER2 antibody) to first line chemotherapy for HER2 overexpressing metastatic breast

cancer (HER2+/MBC) markedly increases anticancer activity: a randomized, multinational controlled phase III trial. *Proc Am Soc Clin Oncol* 1998;17:98a(abst).

391. Cobleigh MA, Vogel CL, Tripathy D, et al. Efficacy and safety of Herceptin™ (humanized anti-HER2 antibody) as a single agent in 222 women with HER2 overexpression who relapsed following chemotherapy for metastatic breast cancer. *Proc Am Soc Clin Oncol* 1998;17:97a(abst).

392. Paik S, Bryant J, Park C, et al. erbB-2 and response to doxorubicin in patients with axillary lymph node-positive, hormone receptor-negative breast cancer. *J Natl Cancer Inst* 1998;90:1361.

393. Lipshultz SE, Colan SD, Gelber RD, et al. Late cardiac effects of doxorubicin (Adriamycin) therapy for childhood acute lymphoblastic leukemia. *N Engl J Med* 1991;324:808.

394. Schwartz CL, Hobbie WL, Truesdell S, et al. Corrected QT interval prolongation in anthracycline-treated survivors of childhood cancer. *J Clin Oncol* 1993;11:1906.

395. Wexler LH, Andrich MP, Venzon D, et al. Randomized trial of the cardioprotective agent ICRF-187 in pediatric sarcoma patients treated with doxorubicin. *J Clin Oncol* 1996;14:362.

396. Bristow MR, Thompson PD, Martin RP, et al. Early anthracycline cardiotoxicity. *Am J Med* 1978;65:823.

397. Bristow MR, Minobe WA, Billingham ME, et al. Anthracycline-associated cardiac and renal damage in rabbits. *Lab Invest* 1981;45:157.

398. Billingham ME, Mason JW, Bristow MR, et al. Anthracycline cardiomyopathy monitored by morphologic changes. *Cancer Treat Rep* 1978;62:865.

399. Bristow MR, Mason JW, Billingham ME, et al. Doxorubicin cardiomyopathy: evaluation by phonocardiography, endomyocardial biopsy, and cardiac catheterization. *Ann Intern Med* 1978;88:168.

400. Von Hoff DD, Rozencweig M, Layard M, et al. Daunomycin-induced cardiotoxicity in children and adults: a review of 110 cases. *Am J Med* 1977;62:200.

401. Von Hoff DD, Layard MW, Basa P, et al. Risk factors for doxorubicin-induced congestive heart failure. *Ann Intern Med* 1979;91:710.

402. Swain SM. Adult multicenter trials using dexrazoxane to protect against cardiac toxicity. *Semin Oncol* 1998;25:43.

403. Cottin Y, Touzery C, Dalloz F, et al. Comparison of epirubicin and doxorubicin cardiotoxicity induced by low doses: evolution of the diastolic and systolic parameters studied by radionuclide angiography. *Clin Cardiol* 1998;21:665.

404. Swain SM, Whaley FS, Gerber MC, et al. Delayed administration of dexrazoxane provides cardioprotection for patients with advanced breast cancer treated with doxorubicin-containing therapy [see comments]. *J Clin Oncol* 1997;15:1333.

405. Swain SM, Whaley FS, Gerber MC, et al. Cardioprotection with dexrazoxane for doxorubicin-containing therapy in advanced breast cancer. *J Clin Oncol* 1997;15:1318.

406. Moreb JS, Oblon DJ. Outcome of clinical congestive heart failure induced by anthracycline chemotherapy. *Cancer* 1992;70:2637.

407. Haq MM, Legha SS, Choksi J, et al. Doxorubicin-induced congestive heart failure in adults. *Cancer* 1985;56:1361.

408. Buzdar AU, Marcus C, Smith TL, et al. Early and delayed clinical cardiotoxicity of doxorubicin. *Cancer* 1985;55:2761.

409. Alexander J, Dainiak N, Berger HJ, et al. Serial assessment of doxorubicin cardiotoxicity with quantitative radionuclide angiocardiography. *N Engl J Med* 1979;300:278.

410. Dresdale A, Bonow RO, Wesley R, et al. Prospective evaluation of doxorubicin-induced cardiomyopathy resulting from postsurgical adjuvant treatment of patients with soft tissue sarcomas. *Cancer* 1983;52:51.

411. Billingham ME, Bristow MR, Glatstein E, et al. Adriamycin cardiotoxicity. Endomyocardial biopsy evidence of enhancement by irradiation. *Am J Surg Pathol* 1977;1:17.

412. Torti FM, Bristow MR, Howes AE, et al. Reduced cardiotoxicity of doxorubicin delivered on a weekly schedule: assessment by endomyocardial biopsy. *Ann Intern Med* 1983;99:745.

413. Goorin AM, Chauvenet AR, Perez-Atayde AR, et al. Initial congestive heart failure, six to ten years after doxorubicin chemotherapy for childhood cancer. *J Pediatr* 1990; 116:144.

414. Lopez M, Vici P, Di Lauro K, et al. Randomized prospective clinical trial of high-dose epirubicin and dexrazoxane in patients with advanced breast cancer and soft tissue sarcomas. *J Clin Oncol* 1998;16:86.

415. Venturini M, Michelotti A, Del Mastro L, et al. Multicenter randomized controlled clinical trial to evaluate cardioprotection of dexrazoxane versus no cardioprotection in women receiving epirubicin chemotherapy for advanced breast cancer. *J Clin Oncol* 1996;14:3112.

416. Singal PK, Pierce GN. Adriamycin stimulates low-affinity Ca^{2+} binding and lipid peroxidation but depresses myocardial function. *Am J Physiol* 1986;250:H419.

417. Singal PK, Deally CMR, Weinberg LE. Subcellular effects of adriamycin in the heart: a concise review. *J Mol Cell Cardiol* 1987;19:817.

418. Singal PK, Forbes MS, Sperelakis N. Occurrence of intramitochondrial Ca^{2+} granules in a hypertrophied heart exposed to adriamycin. *Can J Physiol Pharmacol* 1984; 62:1239.

419. Villani F, Piccinini F, Merelli P, et al. Influence of adriamycin on calcium exchangeability in cardiac muscle and its modification by ouabain. *Biochem Pharmacol* 1978; 27:985.

420. Milei J, Boveris A, Llesuy S, et al. Amelioration of adriamycin-induced cardiotoxicity in rabbits by prenylamine and vitamins A and E. *Am Heart J* 1986;111:95.

421. Keung EC, Toll L, Ellis M, et al. L-type cardiac calcium channels in doxorubicin cardiomyopathy in rats: morphological, biochemical, and functional correlations. *J Clin Invest* 1991;87:2108.

422. Doroshow JH. Effect of anthracycline antibiotics on oxygen radical formation in rat heart. *Cancer Res* 1983;43:460.

423. Davies KJ, Doroshow JH, Hochstein P. Mitochondrial NADH dehydrogenase-catalyzed oxygen radical production by adriamycin, and the relative inactivity of 5-iminodaunorubicin. *FEBS Lett* 1983;153:227.

424. Jensen RA, Acton EM, Peters JH. Electrocardiographic and transmembrane potential effects of 5-iminodaunorubicin in the rat. *Cancer Res* 1984;44:4030.

425. Feng W, Liu G, Xia R, et al. Site-selective modification of hyperreactive cysteines of ryanodine receptor complex by quinones. *Mol Pharmacol* 1999;55:821.

426. Abramson JJ, Salama G. Critical sulfhydryls regulate calcium release from sarcoplasmic reticulum. *J Bioenerg Biomembr* 1989;21:283.

427. Pessah IN, Durie EL, Schiedt MJ, et al. Anthraquinone-sensitized Ca^{2+} release channel from rat cardiac sarcoplasmic reticulum: possible receptor-mediated mechanism of doxorubicin cardiomyopathy. *Mol Pharmacol* 1990;37:503.

428. Papoian T, Lewis W. Adriamycin cardiotoxicity in vivo: selective alterations in rat cardiac mRNAs. *Am J Pathol* 1990;136:1201.

429. Torti SV, Akimoto H, Lin K, et al. Selective inhibition of muscle gene expression by oxidative stress in cardiac cells. *J Mol Cell Cardiol* 1998;30:1173.

430. Kurabayashi M, Dutta S, Jeyaseelan R, et al. Doxorubicin-induced Id2A gene transcription is targeted at an activating transcription factor/cyclic AMP response element motif through novel mechanisms involving protein kinases distinct from protein kinase C and protein kinase A. *Mol Cell Biol* 1995;15:6386.

431. Jeyaseelan R, Poizat C, Baker RK, et al. A novel cardiac-restricted target for doxorubicin. CARP, a nuclear modulator of gene expression in cardiac progenitor cells and cardiomyocytes. *J Biol Chem* 1997;272:22800.

432. Nakano E, Takeshige K, Toshima Y, et al. Oxidative damage in selenium deficient hearts on perfusion with adriamycin: protective role of glutathione peroxidase system. *Cardiovasc Res* 1989;23:498.

433. Kanter MM, Hamlin RL, Unverferth DV, et al. Effect of exercise training on antioxidant enzymes and cardiotoxicity of doxorubicin. *J Appl Physiol* 1985;59:1298.

434. Nicolay K, Fok JJ, Voorhout W, et al. Cytofluorescence detection of adriamycin-mitochondria interactions in isolated, perfused rat heart. *Biochim Biophys Acta* 1986;887:35.

435. Nohl H. Identification of the site of adriamycin-activation in the heart cell. *Biochem Pharmacol* 1988;37:2633.

436. Goormaghtigh E, Pollakis G, Ruysschaert JM. Mitochondrial membrane modifications induced by adriamycin-mediated electron transport. *Biochem Pharmacol* 1983;32:889.

437. Nohl H, Gille L, Staniek K. The exogenous NADH dehydrogenase of heart mitochondria is the key enzyme responsible for selective cardiotoxicity of anthracyclines. *Z Naturforsch [C]* 1998;53:279.

438. Weiss RB. The anthracyclines: will we ever find a better doxorubicin? *Semin Oncol* 1992;19:670.

439. Lown JW. Anthracycline and anthraquinone anticancer agents: current status and recent developments. *Pharmacol Ther* 1993;60:185.

440. LeBot MA, Begue JM, Kernaleguen D, et al. Different cytotoxicity and metabolism of doxorubicin, daunorubicin, epirubicin, esorubicin and idarubicin in cultured human and rat hepatocytes. *Biochem Pharmacol* 1988;37:3877.

441. Bertelli G, Amoroso D, Pronzato P, et al. Idarubicin: an evaluation of cardiac toxicity in 77 patients with solid tumors. *Anticancer Res* 1988;8:645.

442. Dodion P, Sanders C, Rombaut W, et al. Effect of daunorubicin, carminomycin, idarubicin, and 4-demethoxydaunorubicinol against normal myeloid stem cells and human malignant cells in vitro. *Eur J Cancer Clin Oncol* 1987;23:1909.

443. Tamassia V, Pacciarini MA, Moro E, et al. Pharmacokinetic study of intravenous and oral idarubicin in cancer patients. *Int J Clin Pharmacol Res* 1987;7:419.

444. Capranico G, Riva A, Tinelli S, et al. Markedly reduced levels of anthracycline-induced strand breaks in resistant P388 leukemia cells and isolated nuclei. *Cancer Res* 1987;47:3752.

445. Tan CT, Hancock C, Steinherz P, et al. Phase I and clinical pharmacological study of 4-demethoxydaunorubicin (idarubicin) in children with advanced cancer. *Cancer Res* 1987;47:2990.

446. Gillies HC, Herriott D, Liang R, et al. Pharmacokinetics of idarubicin (4-demethoxydaunorubicin; IMI-30; NSC 256439) following intravenous and oral administration in patients with advanced cancer. *Br J Clin Pharmacol* 1987;23:303.

447. Zwelling LA, Bales E, Altschuler E, et al. Circumvention of resistance by doxorubicin, but not by idarubicin, in a human leukemia cell line containing an intercalator-resistant form of topoisomerase II: evidence for a non-topoisomerase II–mediated mechanism of doxorubicin cytotoxicity. *Biochem Pharmacol* 1993;45:516.

448. Maessen PA, Mross KB, Pinedo HM, et al. Improved method for the determination of 4'-epidoxorubicin and seven metabolites in plasma by high-performance liquid chromatography. *J Chromatogr* 1987;417:339.

449. Hortobagyi GN, Yap HY, Kau SW, et al. A comparative study of doxorubicin and epirubicin in patients with metastatic breast cancer. *Am J Clin Oncol* 1989;12:57.

450. Havsteen H, Brynjolf I, Svahn T, et al. Prospective evaluation of chronic cardiotoxicity due to high-dose epirubicin or combination chemotherapy with cyclophosphamide, methotrexate, and 5-fluorouracil. *Cancer Chemother Pharmacol* 1989;23:101.

451. Robert J, Vrignaud P, Nguyen-Ngoc T, et al. Comparative pharmacokinetics and metabolism of doxorubicin and epirubicin in patients with metastatic breast cancer. *Cancer Treat Rep* 1985;69:633.

452. Camaggi CM, Strocchi E, Tamassia V, et al. Pharmacokinetic studies of 4'-epidoxorubicin in cancer patients with normal and impaired renal function and with hepatic metastases. *Cancer Treat Rep* 1982;66:1819.

453. Vile GF, Winterbourn CC. Microsomal lipid peroxidation induced by Adriamycin, epirubicin, daunorubicin and mitoxantrone: a comparative study. *Cancer Chemother Pharmacol* 1989;24:105.

454. Fukushima T, Yamashita T, Yoshio N, et al. Effect of PSC 833 on the cytotoxicity of idarubicin and idarubicinol in multidrug-resistant K562 cells. *Leuk Res* 1999;23:37.

455. Chan EM, Thomas MJ, Bandy B, et al. Effects of doxorubicin, 4'-epirubicin, and antioxidant enzymes on the contractility of isolated cardiomyocytes. *Can J Physiol Pharmacol* 1996;74:904.

456. Bontenbal M, Andersson M, Wildiers J, et al. Doxorubicin vs epirubicin, report of a second-line randomized phase II/III study in advanced breast cancer. EORTC Breast Cancer Cooperative Group. *Br J Cancer* 1998;77:2257.

457. Ryberg M, Nielsen D, Skovsgaard T, et al. Epirubicin cardiotoxicity: an analysis of 469 patients with metastatic breast cancer. *J Clin Oncol* 1998;16:3502.

458. Murdock KC, Wallace RE, Durr FE, et al. Antitumor agents. I. 1,4-Bis((aminoalkyl)amino)-9,10-anthracenediones. *J Med Chem* 1979;22:1024.

459. Johnson RK, Zee-Cheng RKY, Lee WW, et al. Experimental antitumor activity of aminoanthraquinones. *Cancer Treat Rep* 1979;63:425.

460. Moore MJ, Osoba D, Murphy K, et al. Use of palliative end points to evaluate the effects of mitoxantrone and low-dose prednisone in patients with hormonally resistant prostate cancer. *J Clin Oncol* 1994;12:689.

461. Bloomfield DJ, Krahn MD, Neogi T, et al. Economic evaluation of chemotherapy with mitoxantrone plus prednisone for symptomatic hormone-resistant prostate cancer: based on a Canadian randomized trial with palliative end points. *J Clin Oncol* 1998;16:2272.

462. Foye WD, Vajrargupta D, Sengupta SK. DNA binding specificity and RNA polymerase inhibitory activity of bis(aminoalkyl)anthraquinones and bis(methylthio)vinyl quinolinium iodides. *J Pharm Sci* 1982;71:253.

463. Lown JW, Hanstock CC, Bradley RD, et al. Interactions of the antitumor agents, mitoxantrone and bisantrene, with deoxyribonucleic acids studied by electron microscopy. *Mol Pharmacol* 1984;25:178.

464. Bowden GT, Roberts R, Alberts DS, et al. Comparative molecular pharmacology in leukemic L1210 cells of the anthracene anticancer drugs mitoxantrone and bisantrene. *Cancer Res* 1985;45:4915.

465. Butler J, Hoey BM. Are reduced quinones necessarily involved in the antitumor activity of quinone drugs? *Br J Cancer* 1987;55[Suppl VIII]:53.

466. Nguyen B, Gutierrez PL. Mechanism(s) for the metabolism of mitoxantrone: electron spin resonance and electrochemical studies. *Chem Biol Interact* 1990;74:139.

467. Doroshow JH, Davies KJ. Comparative cardiac oxygen radical metabolism by anthracycline antibiotics, mitoxantrone, bisantrene, 4'-(9-acridinylamino)-methanesulfon-m-anisidide, and neocarzinostatin. *Biochem Pharmacol* 1983;32:2935.

468. Crespi MO, Ivanier SE, Genovese J, et al. Mitoxantrone affects topoisomerase activities in human breast cancer cells. *Biochem Biophys Res Commun* 1986;136:521.

469. Kharasch ED, Novak RF. Inhibition of adriamycin-stimulated microsomal lipid peroxidation by mitoxantrone and ametantrone. *Biochem Biophys Res Commun* 1982;108:1346.

470. Abramson JJ, Buck E, Salama G, et al. Mechanism of anthraquinone-induced calcium release from skeletal muscle sarcoplasmic reticulum. *J Biol Chem* 1988;263:18750.

471. Bhalla K, Ibrado AM, Tourkina E, et al. High-dose mitoxantrone induces programmed cell death or apoptosis in human myeloid leukemia cells. *Blood* 1993;82:3133.

472. Bellosillo B, Colomer D, Pons G, et al. Mitoxantrone, a topoisomerase II inhibitor, induces apoptosis of B-chronic lymphocytic leukaemia cells. *Br J Haematol* 1998;100:142.

473. Inaba M, Nagashima K, Sakurai Y. Cross-resistance of vincristine-resistant sublines of P388 leukemia to mitoxantrone with special emphasis on the relationship between in vitro and in vivo cross-resistance. *Gann* 1984;75:625.

474. Dalton WS, Cress AE, Alberts DS, et al. Cytogenetic and phenotypic analysis of a human colon carcinoma cell line resistant to mitoxantrone. *Cancer Res* 1988;48:1882.

475. Bhalla K, Hindenburg A, Taub RN, et al. Isolation and characterization of an anthracycline-resistant human leukemic cell line. *Cancer Res* 1985;45:3657.

476. Nakagawa M, Schneider E, Dixon KH, et al. Reduced intracellular drug accumulation in the absence of P-glycoprotein (mdr1) overexpression in mitoxantrone-resistant human MCF-7 breast cancer cells. *Cancer Res* 1992;52:6175.

477. Satake S, Sugawara I, Watanabe M, et al. Lack of a point mutation of human DNA topoisomerase II in multidrug-resistant anaplastic thyroid carcinoma cell lines. *Cancer Lett* 1997;116:33.

478. Schneider E, Horton JK, Yang CH, et al. Multidrug resistance-associated protein gene overexpression and reduced drug sensitivity of topoisomerase II in a human breast carcinoma MCF7 cell line selected for etoposide resistance. *Cancer Res* 1994;54:152.

479. Hazlehurst LA, Foley NE, Gleason-Guzman MC, et al. Multiple mechanisms confer drug resistance to mitoxantrone in the human 8226 myeloma cell line. *Cancer Res* 1999;59:1021.

480. Miyake K, Mickley L, Litman T, et al. Molecular cloning of cDNAs which are highly overexpressed in mitoxantrone-resistant cells: demonstration of homology to ABC transport genes. *Cancer Res* 1999;59:8.

481. Doyle LA, Yang W, Abruzzo LV, et al. A multidrug resistance transporter from human MCF-7 breast cancer cells. *Proc Natl Acad Sci U S A* 1998;95:15665.

482. Ross DD, Yang W, Abruzzo LV, et al. Atypical multidrug resistance: breast cancer resistance protein messenger RNA expression in mitoxantrone-selected cell lines. *J Natl Cancer Inst* 1999;91:429.

483. Kozin SV, Gerweck LE. Cytotoxicity of weak electrolytes after the adaptation of cells to low pH: role of the transmembrane pH gradient. *Br J Cancer* 1998;77:1580.

484. Heinemann V, Murray D, Walters R, et al. Mitoxantrone-induced DNA damage in leukemia cells is enhanced by treatment with high-dose arabinosylcytosine. *Cancer Chemother Pharmacol* 1988;22:205.

485. Shenkenberg TD, VonHoff DD. Mitoxantrone: a new anticancer drug with significant clinical activity. *Ann Intern Med* 1986;105:67.

486. Neidhart JA, Gochnour D, Roach R, et al. A comparison of mitoxantrone and doxorubicin in breast cancer. *J Clin Oncol* 1986;4:672.

487. Lawton F, Blackledge G, Mould J, et al. Phase II study of mitoxantrone in epithelial ovarian cancer. *Cancer Treat Rep* 1987;71:627.

488. Coltman CAJ, McDaniel TM, Balcerzak SP, et al. Mitoxantrone hydrochloride (NSC-310739) in lymphoma. *Invest New Drugs* 1983;1:65.

489. Birot-Babapalle F, Catovsky D, Slocumbe G, et al. Phase II study of mitoxantrone and cytarabine in acute myeloid leukemia. *Cancer Treat Rep* 1987;71:161.

490. Alberts DS, Peng YM, Leigh S, et al. Disposition of mitoxantrone in cancer patients. *Cancer Res* 1985;45:1879.

491. Smyth JF, Macpherson JS, Warrington PS, et al. The clinical pharmacology of mitoxantrone. *Cancer Chemother Pharmacol* 1986;17:149.

492. Repetto L, Vannozzi MO, Balleari E, et al. Mitoxantrone in elderly patients with advanced breast cancer: pharmacokinetics, marrow and peripheral hematopoietic progenitor cells. *Anticancer Res* 1999;19:879.

493. Savaraj N, Lu K, Manuel V, et al. Pharmacology of mito-xantrone in cancer patients. *Cancer Chemother Pharmacol* 1982;8:113.

494. Wolf CR, Macpherson JS, Smyth JF. Evidence for the metabolism of mitoxantrone by microsomal glutathione transferases and 3-methylcholanthrene-inducible glucu-ronosyl transferases. *Biochem Pharmacol* 1986;35:1577.

495. Chiccarelli FS, Morrison JA, Cosulich DB, et al. Identifica-tion of human urinary mitoxantrone metabolites. *Cancer Res* 1986;46:4858.

496. Shepherd FA, Evans WK, Blackstein ME, et al. Hepatic arterial infusion of mitoxantrone in the treatment of pri-mary hepatocellular carcinoma. *J Clin Oncol* 1987;5:635.

497. Alberts DS, Surwit EA, Peng YM, et al. Phase I clinical and pharmacokinetic study of mitoxantrone given to patients by intraperitoneal administration. *Cancer Res* 1988;48:5874.

498. Husain A, Sabbatini P, Spriggs D, et al. Phase II trial of intraperitoneal cisplatin and mitoxantrone in patients with persistent ovarian cancer. *Gynecol Oncol* 1999;73:96.

499. Yap HY, Blumenschein GR, Schell FC, et al. Dihydroan-thracenedione: a promising new drug in the treatment of metastatic breast cancer. *Ann Intern Med* 1981;95:694.

500. Underferth DV, Underferth BJ, Balcerzak SP, et al. Cardiac evaluation of mitoxantrone. *Cancer Treat Rep* 1983;67:343.

501. Benjamin RS, Chawla SP, Ewer MS, et al. Evaluation of mitoxantrone cardiac toxicity by nuclear angiography and endomyocardial biopsy: an update. *Invest New Drugs* 1985;3:117.

502. Prai GR, Reed NS, Ruddell NST. A case of mitoxantrone-associated cardiomyopathy without prior anthracycline therapy. *Br J Radiol* 1987;60:1125.

503. Arlin ZA, Silver R, Cassileth P. Phase I–II trial of mito-xantrone in acute leukemia. *Cancer Treat Rep* 1985;69:61.

504. Speechly-Dick ME, Owen ERTC. Mitoxantrone-induced oncycholysis. *Lancet* 1988;1:113.

19

TOPOISOMERASE II INHIBITORS: EPIPODOPHYLLOTOXINS, ACRIDINES, ELLIPTICINES, AND BISDIOXOPIPERAZINES

YVES G. POMMIER
FRANÇOIS GOLDWASSER
DIRK STRUMBERG

DNA topoisomerase II (top2) inhibitors are the subject of considerable biochemical, pharmacologic, and clinical investigation. In addition to the epipodophyllotoxins, acridines, ellipticines, and bisdioxopiperazines that are considered in this chapter, other drugs interact with top2, including anthracyclines, mitoxantrone, and anthrapyrazoles. However, these other drugs may exhibit other mechanisms of action and are described separately in Chapter 18.

The inhibition of cellular topoisomerase(s) by antitumor agents, such as adriamycin and ellipticine, was first hypothesized by Kohn and co-workers in the late 1970s before eukaryotic top2 had been identified.[1,2] This hypothesis was based on the observations that the DNA breaks induced by adriamycin and ellipticine had unique characteristics in DNA alkaline elution assays: (a) They were only detectable after full deproteinization and therefore were called *protein-associated* (or *protein-linked*) *strand breaks,* and (b) they were associated with an equal frequency of DNA-protein cross-links. The demonstration that the drug-induced protein-associated strand breaks were mediated through inhibition of top2 took a few more years. This discovery was facilitated by the cellular pharmacology studies of Zwelling and co-workers reporting the potency of amsacrine (m-AMSA) as an inducer of protein-linked DNA breaks.[3,4] Liu and co-workers, who had isolated mammalian top2, showed that a number of inducers of protein-linked DNA breaks were acting through top2.[5] Independently, Kohn and co-workers demonstrated that the protein that was linked to DNA on m-AMSA treatment was top2.[6] The term *cleavage* (or *cleavable*) *complex* is commonly used to define the enzyme-DNA complex, because cleavage is only detectable after strong protein denaturation by sodium dodecyl sulfate (SDS). Our knowledge regarding the top2

enzyme and the mechanisms of action of and resistance to top2 poisons has considerably increased. We better understand the wide variability in the spectrum of antitumoral activity of top2 poisons as well as some of their specific toxic effects. Interference of these agents with top2 has led to a model of *myeloid-lymphoid leukemia* or *mixed-lineage leukemia (MLL)* gene translocations in which top2-mediated chromosomal breakage occasionally is resolved by translocation and may render them leukemogenic.[7]

Extracts from the mayapple or mandrake plant have long been used as a source of folk medicine.[8] The active principle in this plant, podophyllotoxin, acts as an antimitotic agent that binds to tubulin at a site distinct from that occupied by the vinca alkaloids. A number of semisynthetic derivatives of podophyllotoxin have been made. Two glycosidic derivatives, teniposide (VM-26) and etoposide (VP-16) (Fig. 19-1), are active against a number of human malignancies. VP-16 was introduced in clinical trials in 1971 and was approved by the U.S. Food and Drug Administration (FDA) for marketing by Bristol Laboratories under the trade name VePesid in 1984. VM-26 (Vumon) has been used in Europe for several years and was approved by the FDA in 1992 for refractory childhood leukemia. More recently, VP-16 phosphate (Etopophos) (Fig. 19-1) has been designed as a prodrug of VP-16 to obtain a water-soluble compound that could be activated specifically at the tumor sites using antibody alkaline–phosphatase conjugates.[9,10] In fact, VP-16 phosphate is almost immediately converted to VP-16 in the patient plasma by host endogenous phosphatase. Thus, VP-16 phosphate simplifies the formulation of VP-16 by being water soluble and readily converted to VP-16.

VP-16 is among the most commonly used drugs in cancer chemotherapy. It is active against a wide variety of neo-

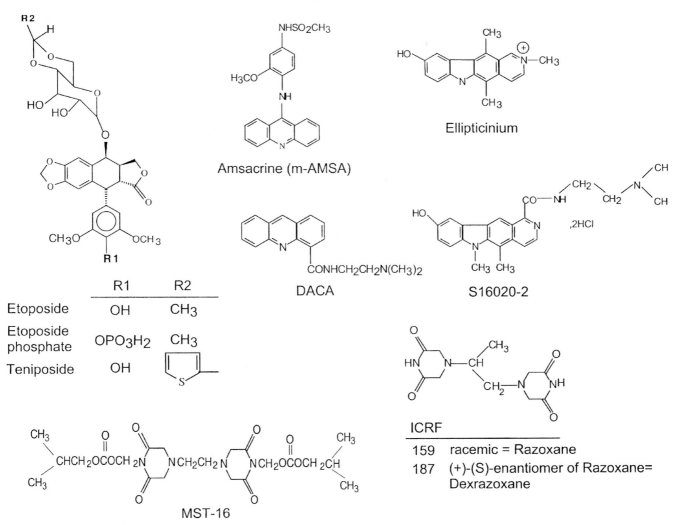

FIGURE 19-1. Chemical structures of the epipodophyllotoxins [etoposide (VP-16) and teniposide (VM-26)], the acridines [amsacrine (m-AMSA) and *N*-[2-(dimethylamino)ethyl]acridine-4-carboxamide (DACA)], and the ellipticines and olivacines (ellipticinium and S16020-2). (ICRF, bispiperazinedione; MST-16, sobuzoxane.)

plasms, including ovarian cancer, germ cell malignancies, lung cancer, non-Hodgkin's lymphomas (NHLs), leukemias, Kaposi's sarcoma, and neuroblastoma.[11] It is also one of the important agents used in preparatory regimens for bone marrow transplantation.[12,13] Use of VP-16 and cisplatin (or carboplatin) is now standard therapy for patients with small cell lung cancer (SCLC).[14] VP-16 is a component of the standard treatment regimen for advanced testicular cancer.[15] Although not part of standard initial therapy, VP-16 has high activity against Ewing's and Kaposi's sarcomas and various lymphomas.[11] VM-26 is highly active in combination in pediatric acute myelocytic leukemias.[16–18] VM-26 is a highly effective salvage therapy for initial induction failures in childhood acute lymphoblastic leukemia (ALL) and has been incorporated in salvage therapy for NHL.[19] VM-26 has shown activity against bladder cancer

(by intravenous and intravesical routes),[20,21] neuroblastoma,[22] and SCLC.[23,24] Responses have been noted in tumors of the central nervous system (CNS).[25] It is now well established that VP-16 and VM-26 exert their antineoplastic effect by inhibiting top2, and that in contrast to the parent compound podophyllotoxin, they are inactive against tubulin.

m-AMSA, or 4' (9-acridinylamino)-methanesulfon-*m*-aniside (Fig. 19-1), is the first rationally synthesized aminoacridine anticancer agent to undergo full clinical development. m-AMSA was initially described in 1974 by Cain and coworkers.[26] It first entered clinical evaluation under the U.S. National Cancer Institute's sponsorship in 1976, and its clinical profile is now established. m-AMSA is used primarily in the treatment of acute leukemias.[27] m-AMSA has substantial efficacy in acute myelogenous leukemia (AML)

TABLE 19-1. TOPOISOMERASE II INHIBITORS

	Poisons	References	Suppressors	References
Intercalators and DNA binders	Doxorubicin		Doxorubicin (high concentration)	
	Daunorubicin		Daunorubicin (high concentration)	
	Epirubicin		Epirubicin (high concentration)	
	Idarubicin	53, 55, 123, and 538	Idarubicin (high concentration)	53, 55, and 538
	Amsacrine (m-AMSA)		m-AMSA (high concentration)	
	Mitoxantrone		Mitoxantrone (high concentration)	
	Elliptinium		Elliptinium (high concentration)	
	Dactinomycin (Actinomycin D)[a]		Actinomycin D[a] (high concentration)	
	Anthrapyrazoles	539	Anthrapyrazoles (high concentration)	539
	Menogaril	540	Menogaril (high concentration)	540
	Intoplicine[a]	541,542	Intoplicine[a] (high concentration)	541, 542
	Saintopin[a]	543	Saintopin[a] (high concentration)	543
	Amonafide	544	Amonafide (high concentration)	544
	Streptonigrin	545–547	Bulgarein	548
	Makaluvamines	549	Ethidium bromide	550
	Alkylating anthraquinones	551	Ditercalinium	552, 553
	Olivacines	40	Distamycin, Hoechst 33258	554, 555
	Bisantrenes	556	Merbarone	557
Nonintercalators			Bisdioxopiperazines	114
	Etoposide, Teniposide	289,558,559	Suramin	560
	Aza IQD[a]	561	Novobiocin	562
	Flavones-flavonones	563	Chloroquine	564
	Isoflavones (Genistein)	565	Fostriecin	566
	Nitroimidazole (Ro 15-0216)	567	Aclarubicin (Aklavin, oxaunomycin, β-rhodomycinone)	568
	Terpenoids	569		
	(Terpentecin, clerocidine)	571	Quinobenoxazines	570
	Naphthoquinones	572		
	Whithangulatin	573		
	Polyaromatic quinones	574		
	Quinolones (CP-115,953)	575		
	Azatoxin	576		

Note: See Figure 19-3 and text for definition of poisons and suppressors.
[a]Dual topoisomerase I and II inhibitor.

and ALL. In AML, m-AMSA is as effective as daunorubicin when combined with cytosine arabinoside (ara-C).[28] As a single agent, m-AMSA has been reported to be as effective as high-dosage ara-C in patients with AML in relapse.[29,30] It can provide high remission rates even in patients with previous exposure to anthracyclines and in ALL and AML patients refractory to primary induction therapy.[31,32] m-AMSA is also used in intensive consolidation therapy[33] and is active in lymphomas.[34] A variety of phase II trials demonstrated no useful activity against human carcinomas.[35] More recently, a new acridine derivative, *N*-[2-(dimethylamino)ethyl]acridine-4-carboxamide (DACA) (Fig. 19-1), with high activity against solid tumors in mice[36] and a dual mode of cytotoxic action involving topoisomerases I (top1) and top2,[37,38] is entering phase I clinical trials.

Representing a third structural class of top2 inhibitor, ellipticine is an alkaloid derived from the *Apocynaceae* family, including *Ochrosia, Bleekeria vitensis,* and *Aspidosperma subincanum.*[8] Despite its promising preclinical activity, severe toxic effects observed in animal studies hampered the

progress of ellipticine toward clinical trials. The semisynthetic derivative 2-*N*-methyl-9-hydroxyellipticinium acetate, or ellipticinium (NMHE) (Fig. 19-1), can induce objective remissions in approximately 25% of patients with advanced breast cancer refractory to all other treatment. It improves the condition of patients with osteolytic breast cancer metastasis.[39] The drug S16020-2 is a new olivacine derivative that is structurally similar to NMHE (Fig. 19-1).[40] S16020-2 is highly cytotoxic *in vitro*[41] and displays remarkable antitumor activity against various experimental tumors, especially some solid tumor models.[42–44] Its activity is notably higher than that of NMHE and comparable to that of doxorubicin hydrochloride, although with a different tumor specificity. S16020-2 is being tested in phase I clinical trials.[45]

Catalytic inhibitors of top2 have recently been identified (Table 19-1). One of them, dexrazoxane, a bisdioxopiperazine derivative, has been approved as a cardioprotective agent in association with anthracyclines.[46–48] Among the bis(*N*-acyloxymethyl) dioxopiperazine derivatives, MST-16 or sobuzoxane (Fig. 19-1), has antitumoral activity in NHL and T-cell leukemia patients[49,50] and obtained official approval in Japan.

MOLECULAR AND CELLULAR PHARMACOLOGY

DNA Topoisomerase II

Enzymology and Functions

The length of eukaryotic DNA and its anchorage to nuclear matrix attachment regions limit the free rotation of one strand around the other as the two strands of the DNA double-helix are separated for DNA metabolism (transcription, replication, recombination, and repair). DNA topoisomerases catalyze the unlinking of the DNA strands by making transient DNA strand breaks and allowing the DNA to rotate around or traverse through these breaks.[51,52] There are three types of topoisomerases known in eukaryotes, which are top1, top2, and topoisomerase III (top3) (Table 19-2).[51,53–60] Eukaryotic top3 was first identified in yeast[61] in 1989, where there is only one top3 gene. This enzyme is (like top1) a single-strand specific topoisomerase and has homology to the bacterial top1 and top3 enzymes.[62,63] In contrast to yeast, human cells have two genes (like top2) encoding top3: top3α[64] and top3β.[65] Mouse top3α[66] and top3β[67,68] were identified in 1998. Mammalian DNA top3α seems to be essential in early embryogenesis.[66] Further studies revealed the existence of a second human gene (top3β) with homology to top3, which was renamed top3α.[65] DNA gyrase and topoisomerase IV (topo IV) are the bacterial equivalents of eukaryotic top2. Quinolones (nalidixic acid, ciprofloxacin, norfloxacin, and derivatives), which are widely used antibiotics, act by inhibiting DNA gyrase and topo IV with no or limited effect on the host human top2 enzymes.[69,70]

A general characteristic of the topoisomerase-mediated DNA breaks occurs through transesterification reactions, wherein a DNA-phosphoester bond is transferred to a specific enzyme tyrosine residue while the enzyme generates a break in the DNA phosphodiester backbone. In the case of top1, the enzyme becomes linked to the 3'-terminus of the cleaved DNA, whereas in the case of top3, the enzyme is linked to the 5'-DNA terminus of the DNA single-strand break. In the case of top2, each enzyme molecule of a homodimer becomes linked to the 5'-terminus of each of the cleaved DNA strands (Table 19-2 and Fig. 19-2).

Top1 and top2 can remove DNA supercoiling by catalyzing DNA relaxation. They can complement each other in this function at least in yeast, where the absence of top1 can be compensated for by the presence of the other topoisomerase for DNA relaxation. However, yeast strains deficient in top2 are not viable and die at mitosis, because top2 is essential for chromosome condensation and structure[71–74] and the proper segregation of mitotic[75–77] and meiotic[78,79] chromosomes. The reason is that in addition to its DNA-relaxing activity, top2 can separate two linked circles of duplex DNA (decatenation) as well as catalyzing the reverse reaction (catenation) by allowing one duplex to go through a double-stranded gap created in the other duplex (strand passage reaction) (see DNA Topoisomerase II Catalytic Cycle and Fig. 19-2). Decatenation is essential at the end of DNA replication for the separation of daughter DNA molecules and segregation of newly replicated chromosomes. The accumulation of top2 at the end of S phase and during G_2, and its concentration in the chromosome scaffold, are consistent with the enzyme's role in separating chromatin loops and condensing DNA at mitosis (Table 19-2).

Mammalian cells have two top2 isoenzymes, termed top2α and top2β (Table 19-2), which differ in molecular mass,[80] enzymatic properties,[81] chromosome localization, sequence,[82–84] cell-cycle regulation,[85–88] and cellular and tissue distribution.[89–92] Although top2β concentrations are relatively

TABLE 19-2. COMPARISON OF MAMMALIAN DNA TOPOISOMERASES I, II, AND III

	Topoisomerase I	Topoisomerase IIα	Topoisomerase IIβ	Topoisomerase III (top3)
Size of monomer	100 kd, acting as monomer	170 kd, acting as dimer	180 kd, acting as dimer	110 kd
Size of messenger RNA	4.2 kb	6.2 kb	6.5 kb	3.8 kb (main transcript)[535]
Chromosomal location	20q12.0–13.2	17q21–22	3p24	17p11.2–12.0 (top3α) 22q11–12 (top3β)
Catalytic intermediate	DNA single-strand breaks	DNA double-strand breaks (DSB)	DNA DSB	DNA DSB
	Covalent linkage to 3' DNA terminus	Covalent linkage to 5' DNA terminus	Covalent linkage to 5' DNA terminus	Covalent linkage to 5' DNA terminus
Adenosine triphosphate dependence	No	Yes	Yes	No
Cell-cycle expression	Throughout	G_2-M	Throughout	—
Specific inhibitors	Camptothecins, indenoisoquinolines, indolocarbazoles[59,536]	Top2 poisons and catalytic inhibitors, intercalators (see Table 19-1)	Same as topoisomerase IIα (preference for amsacrine, mitoxantrone[537])	Unknown

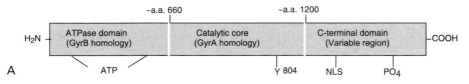

A

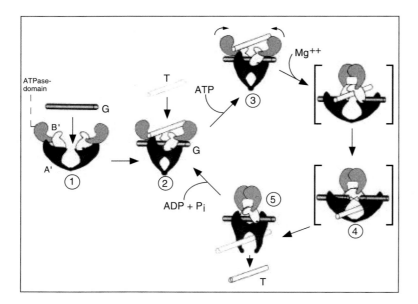

B

FIGURE 19-2. A: Domain structure of topoisomerase II. The three major domains of eukaryotic topoisomerase II are illustrated, as well as the site of adenosine triphosphate binding (ATP), the active site tyrosine (Y), the nuclear localization sequence(s) (NLS), and the sites of phosphorylation (PO₄). The N-terminal domain (homologous to the gyrase B subunit) extends from amino acid 1 to approximately 660. The catalytic core domain (homologous to A subunit of gyrase) extends from approximately residue 660 to 1,200, and the C-terminal domain (no corresponding homology with gyrase) extends from approximately residue 1,200 to the C-terminus of the enzyme. **B:** Model for the catalytic cycle of type II topoisomerases.[57] The enzyme binds to duplex DNA (G) across the A' domains (step 1). A second duplex DNA strand (T) and ATP bind to the enzyme (steps 2 and 3). Nucleotide binding promotes dimerization of the ATPase domains and closure of the clamp (*curved arrows*, step 3). Cleavage of the G-strand allows the passage of the T-strand through the cleaved G-strand (step 4 is diagrammed in brackets to indicate that the cleavage complex is a short-lived intermediate in the proposed transportation event). After G-strand religation, the T-strand is released through the dimer interface in the A' region (step 5). ATP hydrolysis completes the enzyme catalytic cycle. (ADP, adenosine diphosphate.)

constant throughout the cell cycle, top2α levels are tightly linked to the proliferative state of the cell. The concentration of the α isoform increases two- to threefold during G_2 and M[86,88,93,94] and is orders of magnitude higher in rapidly proliferating cells than it is in quiescent populations.[86,88,93,95,96]

DNA Topoisomerase II Catalytic Cycle

A description of the top2 catalytic cycle is essential for understanding how top2 poisons stabilize the cleavage complex of the DNA-strand passage reaction (Fig. 19-2).[97] In contrast to top1, top2 functions as a homodimeric molecule. Its catalytic activity requires the presence of magnesium as well as ATP, as an exogenous energy source. Hence top2 acts as a DNA-dependent ATPase. Recent structural and mechanistic studies reveal a remarkable dynamic behavior of the enzyme during its catalytic cycle.[97–101] Top2 catalyzes DNA strand passage according to the two-gate model shown in Figure 19-2.[100–102] The enzyme forms a dimer and initiates its catalytic cycle by binding to its DNA substrate with a preference for DNA crossover regions. Hence, top2 interactions with DNA are determined by DNA superstructure (e.g., DNA crossovers, bends) and local DNA sequence. Although top2 interacts with preferred sequences, its specificity is far less stringent than that of restriction endonucleases. This lack of stringency probably allows the enzyme to act at multiple sites of the genome in order to perform its vital functions. Top2 assumes two alternative conformations, open or closed clamp forms in the absence or presence of ATP, respectively.[97] The enzyme binds two seg-

ments of duplex DNA, referred to as the G and T segments. The G (*g*ate) segment is the one cleaved by the enzyme to pass the T (*t*ransported) segment through the enzyme-DNA complex (Fig. 19-2). On ATP binding, top2 undergoes a conformational change from an open to a closed clamp form (step 3). In the presence of a divalent cation (under physiologic conditions, Mg²⁺), the tyrosine active residue of each top2 monomer (tyrosine 804 for human top2α) attacks a DNA phosphodiester bond four bases apart on the G duplex and becomes covalently linked to the 5' ends of the broken DNA whereas the 3'-ends are 3'-hydroxyls. The T segment can then pass through the gap produced in the G segment (step 4). Cleavage of the G duplex is reversible in nature, and under normal conditions the cleavage complex is a short-lived intermediate. After strand passage, the T segment is released from the clamp, and the broken ends of the G segment are religated by top2 (step 5). On hydrolysis of ATP by the intrinsic ATPase activity of the enzyme, the top2-DNA complex is converted back to the open clamp form with release of the G segment. Thus, closing and opening of the top2 clamp are coupled with ATP binding and hydrolysis, respectively. Through its ability to open both strands of a DNA duplex and to catalyze strand passage in concerted reactions, top2 can perform a variety of DNA topoisomerization reactions. Whereas DNA relaxation is common to top1, conversion of circular DNA to knotted forms and removal of preexisting knots and catenanes are specific to top2. These biochemical reactions are commonly used to assay topoisomerase activities *in vitro*: relaxation of supercoiled plasmid DNA in the absence of ATP and Mg²⁺ in the case of top1, and decatenation of kinetoplast DNA and unknotting of P4 DNA in the case of top2.[53,103]

DNA Topoisomerase II Poisons

Mechanisms of Topoisomerase II Inhibition by Anticancer Drugs

The antitumor top2 inhibitors presently used in the clinic poison the enzyme by stabilizing the DNA cleavage complexes (step 4 in Fig. 19-2), preventing enzyme catalytic activity, or both.[53,55,58,104] The production of DNA cleavage complexes is due to an inhibition of DNA relegation in the case of VP-16, VM-26, and m-AMSA.[53,55,58] On the other hand, compounds, such as quinolones act by inducing the formation of cleavage complexes rather than by inhibiting relegation.[105] The cleavage complexes can be detected in cells as protein-linked DNA breaks by alkaline elution or by SDS-KCl precipitation assays.[53,55,103] Cellular topoisomerase-DNA complexes can also be detected using the *in vivo* complex of enzyme (ICE) bioassay (for Immuno Complex Topo assay).[106,107] Inhibition of top2 catalytic activity without trapping of cleavage complexes (Table 19-1; Fig. 19-3) was first demonstrated for strong DNA interca-

lating agents at drug concentrations that saturate the DNA. It is attributed to DNA structural alterations that prevent the enzyme from binding to DNA (steps 1 and 2 in Fig. 19-2) or prevent initiation of the cleavage complex.[108,109] Recently, non-DNA binders, such as merbarone and bisdioxopiperazines [ICRF 159, 187, and 193], have been found to produce the "closed clamp" type of inhibition—for example, inhibition of top2 catalytic activity without trapping of cleavage complexes (Table 19-1).[110–114] Hence, three types of curves that relate drug concentrations to cleavage complexes can be observed for top2 inhibitors (Fig. 19-3): (a) monotonal increase of cleavage complexes with drug concentration in the case of non- or weak DNA binders (VP-16, VM-26, m-AMSA, and quinolones), (b) bell-shaped curve (with initial increase in cleavage complexes with increasing drug concentrations, followed by a decrease in cleavage complexes at higher concentrations) in the case of DNA intercalators (ellipticines, anthracyclines, mitoxantrone, and anthrapyrazoles), and (c) monotonal decrease of cleavage complexes in the case of some bulky intercalators (ethidium bromide, ditercalinium, and aclarubicin) or non-DNA binders (bisdioxopiperazines) (Table 19-1) that inhibit catalytic activity without trapping cleavage complexes. It is well known that top2 inhibitors have different clinical potencies and activity spectra and that the cytotoxic potency of different compounds is not well correlated with the formation of cleavage complexes.[115–117]

Table 19-3 summarizes several factors that may account for these differences. At the biochemical level, top2 inhibitors exhibit different effects. The kinetics of cleavage complex formation and reversal in drug-treated cells vary from

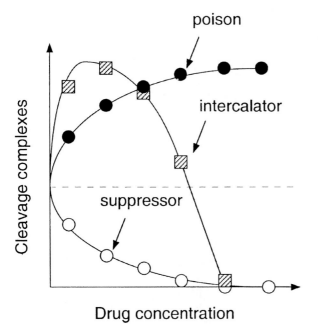

FIGURE 19-3. Different modes of drug inhibition of topoisomerase II (top2). Top2 poisons, such as the epipodophyllotoxins (etoposide or teniposide) or the azatoxins (*solid circles*), only trap the top2 cleavage complexes with increasing efficiency as their dose increases. Top2 suppressors, such as the bisdioxopiperazines (*open circles*), are pure catalytic inhibitors that only inhibit the formation of cleavage complexes. Hatched squares correspond to biphasic inhibitors, such as DNA intercalators (anthracyclines, ellipticines, and acridines; Table 19-1), which enhance top2 cleavage complexes at low concentrations and suppress cleavage complexes at higher concentrations.

TABLE 19-3. DIFFERENCES AMONG TOPOISOMERASE II (TOP2) INHIBITORS

Additional targets and effects	Free radicals: anthracyclines, mitoxantrone
	DNA intercalation (e.g., anthracyclines, mitoxantrone, and ellipticines)
Differential drug interactions with top2 DNA complexes	Base sequence preferences and location of DNA cleavage sites (Fig. 19-3)
	Ratio of DNA double- and single-strand breaks: ellipticine>anthracyclines>amsacrine (m-AMSA) and epipodophyllotoxins
	Kinetics of trapping top2 cleavage complexes (slow for anthracyclines, fast for epipodophyllotoxins and m-AMSA)
	Inhibition of cleavage complexes at higher concentrations (catalytic inhibitors, intercalators)
	Pure top2 poisons (epipodophyllotoxins)
Resistance mechanisms	Substrates for transmembrane transporters: anthracyclines and epipodophyllotoxins more than mitoxantrone, m-AMSA, and ellipticines
	Specific top2 mutations affect drug binding differentially (Table 19-4)

Note: See text for references.

slow and stable in the case of doxorubicin[3,116,118] and ellipticine[115] to very rapid and fast reversible in the case of VP-16, m-AMSA, and NMHE.[3,115,118] The higher cytotoxicity of doxorubicin versus VP-16 in experimental systems and the clinical activity of prolonged administration of oral VP-16 in patients previously exposed to VP-16 as bolus administrations may be explained by the importance of persistent cleavage complexes for cytotoxicity. Most drugs induce not only top2-mediated DNA double-strand breaks but also top2-mediated single-strand breaks, the ratio of which varies widely among drugs. Ellipticines produce almost exclusively DNA double-strand breaks, while VP-16 and m-AMSA produce ten to 20 single-strand breaks per double-strand break.[3,53,118] Anthracyclines produce a mixture of single- and double-strand breaks.[3] Hence, the higher cytotoxicity of anthracyclines compared with m-AMSA or VP-16 may be due to the higher frequency of DNA double-strand breaks that may be more cytotoxic than single-strand breaks.[53] Finally, the DNA sequence and genomic localization of top2 cleavage complexes varies among drugs.[119] Drugs that are chemically and structurally related frequently produce closely related patterns of top2 cleavage, while compounds structurally and electronically unrelated produce different patterns in purified DNA and in drug-treated cells.[53,119,120]

Base-Sequence Preference of Topoisomerase II Inhibitors and Drug-Binding Model

DNA sequencing of drug-induced cleavage sites indicates that the top2-induced breaks are not random and that each class of inhibitor tends to act at top2 cleavage sites with different base sequence preferences at the 3'- or 5'- or both, terminus of the top2-mediated DNA double-strand break[121–127] (Fig. 19-4). These drug-specific preferences for certain bases immediately flanking the cleavage sites suggest that the drugs interact directly with these bases. Because all of the top2 inhibitors, whether intercalator or not, have a planar aromatic portion that in some cases mimics a base pair (Fig. 19-1), the simplest explanation is that the drugs stack inside the cleavage sites at the enzyme-DNA interface. Depending on the drug structure, preferential base stacking would take place either at the 3'- or the 5'-terminus. This hypothesis implies that topoisomerases first cleave the DNA at many sites and that the drugs would bind specifically to some sites and prevent DNA religation.[128–130] Stud-

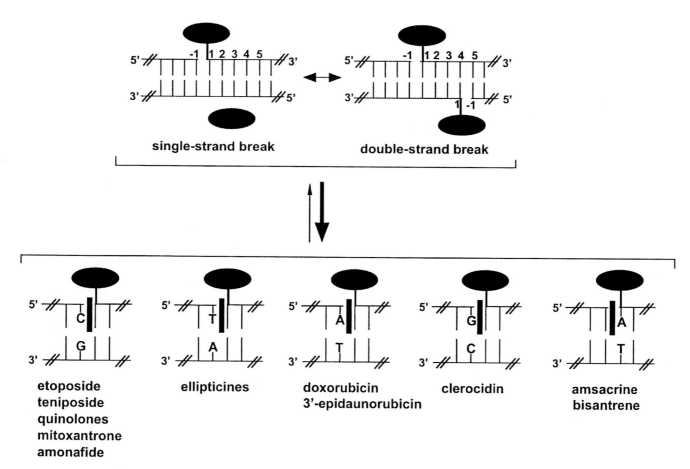

FIGURE 19-4. Topoisomerase II cleavage complexes in the absence of drug (*top*) and base-sequence preferences for topoisomerase II inhibitors. Black circles indicate topoisomerase II monomers.

ies with a photoactivable form of m-AMSA[131] or a quinolone[132] indicated that the site of drug action in the cleavage complex is near or at the site of DNA scission and support the drug-stacking model. A positional poison model proposes that the ability of drugs to stimulate the DNA cleavage reaction of top2 results from their ability to distort the double helix within the four-base overhang generated by the enzyme-mediated DNA scission.[58,133] In addition, the base sequence analysis data strongly suggest that stacking at one site is sufficient for the creation of a DNA double-strand break, a theory consistent with the concerted action of both enzyme monomers during catalysis.[121,134,135] However, cleavage reactions triggered by cooperative effects with the other monomer appear less stable than those with drug-preferred bases.[135] The enzyme sites that interact with top2 inhibitors are not well defined. Analyses of drug-resistant mutant enzymes suggest that the A' and B' regions of the enzyme reversibly bind to the drugs. Recent studies[128,135,136] indicate that the CAP homology domain determines DNA sequence recognition on the G segment of DNA and drug effects, which is consistent with drug binding at or near the DNA cleavage site and formation of a ternary complex: drug-enzyme-DNA.

Determinants of Sensitivity and Resistance to Topoisomerase II Inhibitors

Figure 19-5 summarizes the multiple factors that determine the cytotoxicity of top2 inhibitors. Before topoisomerase inhibitors reach their nuclear target, they have to be taken up by the cells and transported to the nucleus. Reduced drug accumulation, altered intracellular drug distribution, or both, are dominant features of many drug-resistant cell lines. Most clinical antitumor top2 inhibitors are substrates for the 170-kd transmembrane glycoprotein, P-glycoprotein (Pgp), which is a product of the multidrug resistance (MDR)-1 gene and responsible for the classic multidrug resistance phenotype.[137] MDR-sensitive drugs include doxorubicin and analogs, mitoxantrone, anthrapyrazoles, ellipticines, VP-16,[138] and, to a lesser extent, m-AMSA analogs.[139] Hence, cells overexpressing Pgp are generally resistant to top2 inhibitors, because the drugs are actively extruded from the cells. The amino group on the daunosamine sugar of anthracyclines is probably involved in the drug recognition by Pgp. This is probably why the deamino derivative hydroxyrubicin is less subject to drug resistance while retaining top2-inhibitory activity.[140,141] In addition to Pgp, two other proteins, multidrug resistance protein (MRP) and lung resistance–related protein (LRP), are commonly overexpressed in MDR cells. MRP is a 180-kd protein found predominantly on intracellular organelles,[142–144] while LRP is the 110-kd major vault protein found in lysosomes and other cytoplasmic particles.[145] All these membrane proteins, which belong to the same superfamily of ATP-dependent transporters, recognize many different agents with no similarities in their chemical structures (see above).[146]

Although drug metabolism is not necessary for activity of top2 inhibitors, some drugs undergo metabolic modifications that may affect the way they interact with top2, DNA, or

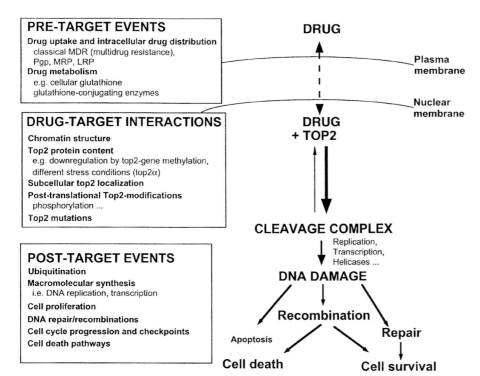

FIGURE 19-5. Determinants of sensitivity and resistance to topoisomerase II (top2) inhibitors. (LRP, lung resistance–related protein; MRP, multidrug resistance protein; Pgp, P-glycoprotein.)

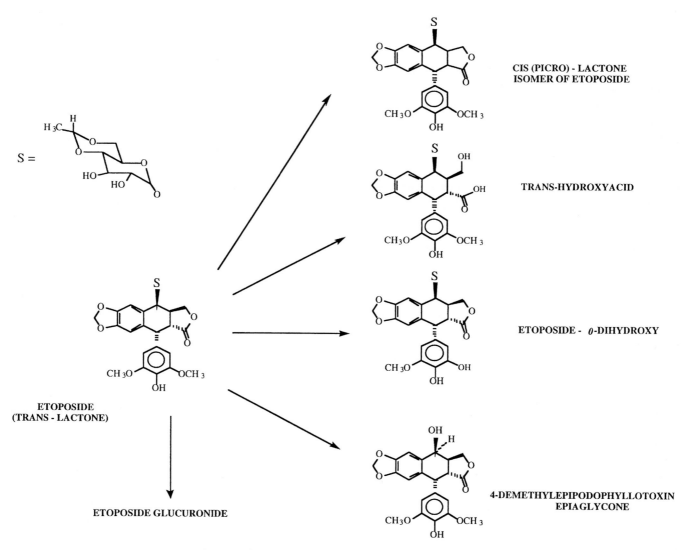

FIGURE 19-6. Metabolism of etoposide. Etoposide-o-dihydroxy and 4-demethylepipodophyllotoxin aglycone are active against topoisomerase II.

both. Anthracyclines participate in redox reactions that lead to the formation of free radicals that damage cellular lipids[147] or DNA.[148] Some adriamycin- and mitoxantrone-resistant cell lines show increased levels of cellular glutathione (GSH) or GSH-conjugating enzymes,[149] which may be a result of GSH-mediated drug inactivation with or without subsequent drug efflux mediated by the putative ATP-dependent GSH S-conjugate export pump.[150] The VP-16 metabolites demethylated on the podophyllotoxin phenyl ring and without the sugar are at least as active as VP-16 against purified top2 (Fig. 19-6).[151–154] These metabolites are more susceptible to oxidation reduction reactions and may exhibit shorter half-life ($t_{1/2}$) and higher reactivity toward other macromolecules than top2.[155–157] In the case of the ellipticines, similar oxidation reduction reactions and free radical formation have been identified and may be responsible for lesions that contribute to the drug cytotoxic effects.[39,158]

The intracellular distribution of top2 inhibitors has been well characterized for the anthracyclines. Drug-resistant cells tend to exclude doxorubicin from their nuclei.[159,160] These observations suggest that a nuclear transporter may exist. In the case of m-AMSA, cellular uptake studies suggest that the drug may be retained in some slowly exchangeable intracellular compartment.[161] An altered intracellular drug distribution with drug sequestration in cytoplasmic organelles has been described for several resistant cell lines *in vitro*[162,163] as well in patients.[164] The altered drug distribution has not been associated with any particular drug transporter.[142,145,165]

In contrast to other chemotherapeutic agents, such as antifolates, the degree of cellular sensitivity to top2 inhibitors correlates with the abundance of the target enzyme. Indeed, the higher the levels of top2, the more sensitive is the cell, because more cleavage complexes are formed and more consecutive genotoxic and cytotoxic lesions accumulate (Fig. 19-5). Cancer cells often have a higher level of top2α protein and activity at all stages of the cell cycle. In addition, the top2 content in cancer and transformed cells is less regulated by growth conditions.[95,166,167] Top2β appears to be also up-regulated in neoplastic cells compared to normal quiescent tissues.[168] Coamplification of the erbB2, top2α, and retinoid acid receptor α genes, all localized on chromosome 17q, has been observed in breast cancer cells.[169] Top2 is up-regulated by a variety of factors related to cell-cycle progression and stimulation by hormones, such as estrogens.[170,171] It has also been reported that top2α expression can be stimulated by top1 inhibitors (see section Therapeutic Interactions with the Topoisomerase II Inhibitors). Treatment of AML patients with topotecan leads to an average of threefold increase in top2α expression.[167] Furthermore, a permanent twofold increase of top2α and -β was reported for topotecan-resistant human cell lines.[172] Cloning of the top2α[173] and top2β[174] promoter regions and gene expression experiments indicate that, as in the case of top1 and housekeeping genes, the top2α and β genes lack a tumor-associated transplantation antigen box element and contain a high frequency of CpG dinucleotides. However, there is no obvious sequence homology between the 5'-flanking sequences of top2β and top2α,[174] consistent with different transcriptional control mechanisms. In addition, the top2α promoter contains elements analogous to other DNA replication–associated genes, such as thymidine kinase and DNA polymerase genes,[173] consistent with the increased accumulation of top2α during cell proliferation.[87,95,175–178] Therefore, the two main mechanisms for decreased top2 transcription are likely to involve DNA modifications (promoter mutations, gene rearrangements, and CpG methylation) and transcription factor alterations.

Many cell lines resistant to top2 inhibitors show decreased top2 protein levels.[179–182] In the cell line of Goldenberg and co-workers,[179] a rearrangement of the top2 gene was probably responsible for the seven- to eightfold reduction of top2 transcripts.[179] Methylation of the top2 gene has also been reported in association with decreased transcription.[183] Different stress conditions can lead to a decrease in expression of top2α. This is, at least in part, due to transcriptional down-regulation mediated by the tumor suppressor *p53*, which itself is activated by DNA damage.[184,185] Glucose-regulated stress, such as hypoxia and nutrient deprivation, also leads to decreased expression of top2α protein with associated resistance to VP-16 and adriamycin.[186–189] These findings may be relevant for human tumors that are drug-resistant and poorly vascularized in their center. It seems that it is mostly top2α that is altered in cell lines selected with VP-16 or VM-26,[190,191] for example, due to enhanced expression of the transcriptional suppressor.[192] Although top2α is also affected in cell lines selected with DNA intercalators, such as mitoxantrone, doxorubicin, and ellipticines, the most dramatic changes

TABLE 19-4. MUTATIONS IDENTIFIED IN HUMAN TOPOISOMERASE IIα ASSOCIATED WITH RESISTANCE TO TOPOISOMERASE II INHIBITORS

Mutation	Selecting Drug	Reference
Ala429 deleted	Etoposide (VP-16)	577
Arg449Gln	Teniposide	578
Arg486Lys	Amsacrine	579
Arg493Gln	VP-16	580
Glu494Gly	VP-16	581
Ala764Thr	Doxorubicin	582
Lys797Asn	VP-16	583
Pro802Ser	Teniposide	584
Gly851Asp	VP-16	585
Ser861Phe	VP-16	586

Ala, alanine; Arg, arginine; Asn, asparagine; Asp, aspartic acid; Gln, glutamine; Glu, glutamic acid; Gly, glycine; Lys, lysine; Phe, phenylalanine; Pro, proline; Ser, serine; Thr, threonine.

seem to concern the β-isoform, which is strongly downregulated or even missing.[193,194]

Another way to diminish drug-induced cleavage complexes is by a shift in enzyme localization from the nucleus toward the cytoplasm. This has been observed for several cell lines resistant to top2 inhibitors.[191,193,195] In such cases, the cytoplasmic top2α is still catalytically active and able to carry out its normal functions during mitosis when the nuclear membrane is disassembled.

Top2 mutations have been observed in cell lines selected *in vitro*. Table 19-4 summarizes some drug-resistant mammalian top2 mutants. Although an unambiguous etiologic role of top1 mutations in camptothecin resistance has been established,[196,197] only a few recombinant top2 mutants have been generated to demonstrate that the observed mutations are responsible for resistance.[198] The top2 mutations are clustered in two regions, one located near the ATP binding site and the other around the catalytic tyrosine (Tyr 804 for human top2) (Fig. 19-2, Table 19-4). The presence of mutations near the catalytic tyrosine is consistent with the stacking model that implies that the drugs bind at the interface of the enzyme and the DNA.[127] The existence of the second mutation cluster near the putative ATP binding site suggests that top2 folding brings this second region near the catalytic domain and that top2 inhibitors bind at the interface of these two top2 regions.[199,200] The differential resistance to epipodophyllotoxins, m-AMSA, and quinolones of some of the drug-resistant mutants is consistent with preferential interactions of each class of drugs with certain top2 amino acids[198,201–204] and with the preferred DNA bases around the top2 cleavage sites[123,127] (see above).

Changes in top2 phosphorylation may also contribute to top2-mediated drug resistance. However, in resistant cell lines, reduced cleavage complexes have been associated with hyper- and hypophosphorylation of top2. Decreased top2α protein levels were associated with hyperphosphorylation of the enzyme in VP-16–resistant cell lines.[205]

Hypophosphorylated top2α has been reported for VP-16–resistant erythroleukemia[206] and HL-60 cells,[207] and for VM-26–resistant leukemia cell lines.[208] Top2 phosphorylation increases in parallel with the cellular need for the enzyme: during the S phase of the cell cycle with a peak at the G$_2$ phase.[209,210] Casein kinase II is probably the main kinase responsible for top2 phosphorylation in cells.[211–214] Drug-induced cleavage complexes are reduced to approximately 50% after *in vitro* phosphorylation of top2α by casein kinase II and protein kinase C.[215] This finding is in contrast with top1 phosphorylation, which increases camptothecin activity.[216]

Because normal and cancer cells express top2, it is likely that drug-induced cleavage complexes are not sufficient for selective killing of cancer cells. A clear demonstration is provided by the top1 inhibition by camptothecin for which inhibition of DNA synthesis at the time of camptothecin treatment abolishes the camptothecin-induced cytotoxicity without changing the frequency of cleavage complexes.[217,218] By contrast, DNA synthesis inhibition provides only partial protection against VP-16.[217] The interaction of transcription with cleavage complexes may play a prominent role in the activity of top2 inhibitors, because VP-16 cytotoxicity is decreased by RNA synthesis inhibitors.[219,220] The dependence of top1 and top2 inhibitor cytotoxicity on ongoing replication and transcription probably explains why simultaneous treatment with camptothecin and VP-16 has been found to be antagonistic.[219–221] VP-16 may suppress camptothecin effects by inhibiting DNA replication, and camptothecin may suppress the effects of VP-16 by inhibiting RNA transcription.

Other conditions have been described in which the cytotoxicity of topoisomerase inhibitors can be abrogated without effect on cleavage complex formation. These include intracellular calcium depletion by ethylenediaminetetraacetic acid[222] and protein synthesis inhibition by cycloheximide.[53,55] Poly(adenosine diphosphoribose) synthesis also may be important for cell killing, because poly(adenosine diphosphoribose polymerase)-deficient Chinese hamster cells are resistant to VP-16 and hypersensitive to camptothecin.[223] These observations indicate that events downstream from the cleavage complexes are critical to cytotoxicity. Such events may involve the accumulation of genetic alterations, such as sister chromatid exchanges,[117,224,225] illegitimate recombinations,[226,227] and apoptosis.[228–230]

DNA repair must intervene to correct drug-induced and topoisomerase-mediated DNA damage. Yeast cells are usually resistant to topoisomerase inhibitors unless they are RAD52 mutants (e.g., deficient in DNA double-strand break repair).[231] The ubiquitin proteolysis pathway has been reported to be responsible for ubiquitination and degradation of top1 and top2 cleavage complexes.[232–234] Abnormal cell-cycle control (checkpoints) has recently emerged as a key element in possibly explaining the differ-

ential responses of normal versus neoplastic cells to DNA damage. Therefore, alterations of cell-cycle control may play a critical role in the cytotoxicity of topoisomerase inhibitors. Lack of arrest in G$_1$, as in cells with mutated or absent *p53* genes, may not provide the cell with the time required to repair damage and may lead to an accumulation of further damage. Hence, deregulation of cyclins, cell cycle–regulated kinases, and phosphatases and *p53* mutations may sensitize cells to topoisomerase inhibitors.[235–240] Furthermore, pharmacologic abrogation of drug-induced S- and G$_2$-phase checkpoints may provide a novel effective strategy for enhancing the chemotherapeutic activity of topoisomerase inhibitors.[241]

Another determinant of sensitivity to topoisomerase inhibitors is the predisposition of the cell to undergo apoptosis. Some cells, such as human leukemia HL-60 cells, are known to be hypersensitive to a variety of injuries, including DNA damage by topoisomerase inhibitors. The underlying mechanism for this hypersensitivity may be the facile induction of apoptosis.[228] Overexpression of the c-*myc* proto-oncogene and down-regulation of the *bcl*-2 gene have been involved in committing the cells to an apoptosis prone phenotype. Various reports[237,238] suggest that *p53* could play a key role in the case of VP-16 and mediate apoptosis in response to DNA damage without regulating apoptosis induced by glucocorticoids. Apoptosis also may play a role in the drug-induced side effects, such as hematopoietic or intestinal toxicity. Indeed, hematopoietic progenitors may be prone to apoptosis. Hence, studies on the pharmacologic regulation of apoptosis may prove useful. Several classes of agents can suppress topoisomerase inhibitor–induced apoptosis,[228] and *bcl*-2 overexpression renders cells resistant to VP-16.[242]

In summary, cellular response to top2 inhibitors is complex, and several mechanisms are commonly associated in laboratory cell lines: Pgp or MRP overexpression (or both), reduction of top2 protein levels, changes in subcellular localization, top2 phosphorylation, and top2 mutations. It is likely that a multiparametric approach is needed for the evaluation of clinical response to top2 inhibitors.

CLINICAL PHARMACOLOGY

Epipodophyllotoxins

Two epipodophyllotoxin derivatives are presently used in cancer chemotherapy, VP-16 and VM-26. VP-16 phosphate is an improved formulation of VP-16. VP-16 was the first drug introduced (see above). It remains one of the most active anticancer agents and is a key component for the chemotherapy of several advanced cancers and especially SCLC.[243–246] It is also used for the therapy of acute myeloid leukemias.[247,248] VM-26 is a more potent top2 inhibitor (approximately tenfold with purified top2), and it is mainly used in pediatric tumors.

Drug Assays

Quantitation of epipodophyllotoxins and their metabolites involves either high-performance liquid chromatography (HPLC) or immuno-based assays. The HPLC methods use ultraviolet (UV), fluorescence, electrochemical, or mass spectrographic detection.[249] UV spectroscopy was developed first, and, more recently, standard HPLC has been used.[249] The limit of detection by the UV spectroscopy methods is 500 ng per mL. Electrochemical detection methods can measure concentrations as low as 2 ng per mL but lose their linearity at high drug concentrations (i.e., greater than 10 μg per mL).[250,251] Two immuno-based assays have been developed more recently: radioimmunoassays and enzyme-linked immunoassay (ELISA) methods. Radioimmunoassays have been described with a sensitivity of 5 ng per mL but with poor selectivity for the parent drug, because potential metabolites may cross-react.[252] An ELISA method with a sensitivity of 0.5 ng per mL and with no cross-reactivity with the aglycone metabolite has been developed.[253]

Pharmacokinetics

Intravenous Etoposide

For both epipodophyllotoxins, there is a significant interpatient variability in pharmacokinetic parameters.[254–256] After an intravenous (IV) dose, VP-16 decay in plasma follows a two-compartment pharmacokinetic model[257] with a terminal $t_{1/2}$ of 6 to 8 hours in patients with normal renal function (Table 19-5). Inter- and intrapatient variability in pharmacokinetic parameters after IV administration is substantial and can exceed 35%.[258–260] The volume of distribution averages 4 to 10 L per m^2.[258,261,262] The peak plasma concentration and the area under the curve (AUC) are proportional to the administered dosage,[255,257,263,264] up to dosages of 800 mg per m^2, and the elimination $t_{1/2}$ is independent of dosage. Thus, based on total plasma concentrations, the pharmacokinetics are linear.[265] However, protein binding averages 96% but is nonlinear and influenced by the individual concentration of drug and albumin,[266–272] resulting in elevated free drug concentrations in patients with low serum albumin. Other conditions, including elevated serum bilirubin concentrations, which competes for albumin binding, also increase the concentration of the free or biologically active drug, resulting in greater toxicity.[273–276] Thus, the toxicity of VP-16 correlates best with the pharmacokinetics of the unbound fraction of the drug. VP-16 penetrates the cerebrospinal fluid (CSF) poorly, with CSF concentrations less than 5% of simultaneously measured plasma levels.[254,255,257,258,277] Drug levels in brain tumors have been found to be 2% to 75% of plasma concentrations.[278,279] No measurable amount of VP-16 was detected in the aqueous and vitreous humors after IV administration of 5 mg per kg, in *Macaca fascicularis* primates.[280] Pleural fluid penetration of VP-16 is poor.[255] Ascitic fluid concentrations of VP-16 are low after IV drug administration.[255,257]

VP-16 is eliminated by renal and nonrenal mechanisms.[278] Plasma clearance is approximately 22 mL per minute per m^2, and renal clearance is approximately 9.5 mL per minute per m^2.[259] Thirty-five to forty percent of administered VP-16 is cleared through the kidney unchanged.[255,257–259,264,273,281] Patients with impaired renal function have decreased VP-16 clearance rates.[261,262,273,274] Therefore, VP-16 dosage should be reduced in proportion to reductions in creatinine clearance.[261,262,273,274] Hemodialysis membranes are not permeable to VP-16, and the pharmacokinetics of VP-16 are not affected by the interval between chemotherapy and hemodialysis.[282]

Several metabolites of VP-16 have been identified in humans (Fig. 19-6).[255,274,275,281] The main metabolite is VP-16–glucuronide, which is eliminated in the urine at 8% to 20% of the administered dosage.[255,274,275,281] However, current assays may be flawed in estimating the amount of glucuronide.[283] A catechol metabolite with significant cytotoxic activity is formed after VP-16 O-demethylation in the liver.[284] Cytochrome P-450 3A metabolizes VP-16 to a catechol metabolite, which is further oxidized to a quinone. The VP-16-*o*-dihydroxy also can be converted to the *o*-quinone derivative. Both of these, as well as the 4-demethylepipodophyllotoxin, remain active against top2. Ortho and semi-quinone free radicals of VP-16 may covalently bind to DNA and induce DNA strand breakage.[285,286] Other metabolites that have been described include the *cis*-lactone (picro configuration),[255,258,273] the hydroxy acid VP-16 derivative,[261,287] VP-16-*o*-dihydroxy,[288] and epiagly-

TABLE 19-5. KEY FEATURES OF EPIPODOPHYLLOTOXIN DERIVATIVES

	Etoposide	Teniposide
Mechanism of action:	Inhibition of DNA topoisomerase II, nonintercalator	Same but approximately tenfold more potent
Pharmacokinetics:	Terminal half-life = 6–8 h	Terminal half-life = 9.5–21.0 h
Elimination:	Hepatic metabolism, renal excretion 35%–40%	Probable hepatic metabolism
Toxicities:	Neutropenia, thrombocytopenia (mild), alopecia, hypersensitivity, mucositis (high doses)	Same
Precautions:	Reduced dose proportionate to creatinine clearance	Possible increased toxicity in hepatic failure

cone(4-demethylepipodophyllotoxin).[277] However, significant conversion to the *cis*-lactone probably does not occur.[283] The *cis*-lactone and hydroxy acid metabolites are less cytotoxic than the parent VP-16.[289] The cytochrome P-450 3A4 (P-450 CYP3A4) is probably involved in VP-16 3'-demethylation.[290] A recent *in vitro* study revealed a mutual inhibition between quinine and VP-16 in human liver microsomes.[290] A correlation was found between quinine 3-hydroxylase and VP-16 3'-demethylase activities. Two inhibitors of P-450 CYP3A4, ketoconazole and troleandomycin, inhibit VP-16 3'-demethylation by 75% and 65%, respectively.[290]

Biliary excretion is a minor route of elimination. Minor alterations in liver function, such as transaminase elevations, do not require dosage reduction if renal function remains normal,[276] but elevated bilirubin may decrease the clearance of unbound VP-16[268] and increase the unbound fraction of drug, leading to a greater hematologic toxicity for any given AUC, as compared to the AUC in the presence of a normal level of serum bilirubin. Therefore, VP-16 dosage should be reduced by 50% in patients with total bilirubin levels of 1.5 to 3.0 mg per dL. No VP-16 should be given in patients with more than 5.0 mg per dL bilirubin.[291] Age-related reduction in VP-16 clearance has been suggested for VP-16.[292]

Cisplatin given before VP-16 may decrease VP-16 clearance by as much as one-third, presumably due to the effect of cisplatin on renal function.[293] Dilantin increases VP-16 clearance two- to threefold, probably through induction of microsomal metabolism.[294]

Dose Escalation Strategies with Etoposide
High-Dose Etoposide with Bone Marrow Transplantation.
VP-16 is presently used in most high-dose protocols because of the only moderate nonhematologic toxicity.[295,296] At high doses, up to 1,500 mg per m^2, bone marrow rescue is necessary, and the dose-limiting toxicities become mucositis and hepatotoxicity. The maximal tolerated dose (MTD) of VP-16 administered as a single agent is up to 2.5 g per m^2 (between 2.5 and 3.5 g per m^2). In this dose range, and in contrast to what is observed at conventional doses, the CSF concentration of VP-16 becomes significant. High-dosage VP-16 (1.6 to 2.4 g per m^2) in combination with granulocyte colony-stimulating factor (G-CSF) has been shown to be an effective strategy to mobilize peripheral blood progenitor cells, although in some patients it is associated with significant toxicity.[297] This strategy could also be effective in patients who had previously failed on high-dose cyclophosphamide with G-CSF.[297,298]

Locoregional Infusions of Etoposide. Other strategies to increase VP-16 exposure in tumors are locoregional infusions. The intraarterial route (using carotid or vertebral arteries) has been used to increase VP-16 uptake in brain tumors.[299] VP-16 has been safely combined with cisplatin,

when given at a dose of 20 to 40 mg per m^2.[300] This strategy gave better survival results in glioblastoma patients when given before the radiotherapy.[300] Intraperitoneal administrations of VP-16 have been done in ovarian cancer patients with peritoneal carcinomatosis[301–303] and for mesothelioma.[304] In ovarian cancer patients, the first clinical trials combined 100 mg per m^2 intraperitoneal cisplatin with either 200 mg per m^2 or 350 mg per m^2 VP-16.[301,302] Recently, the intraperitoneal administrations of 200 mg per m^2 VP-16 with 100 mg per m^2 cisplatin were reported to be a potentially effective treatment as consolidation therapy after negative second-look surgery.[303] Intraperitoneal administration of up to 350 mg per m^2 VP-16 has been used in combination with cisplatin.[305] Intrathecal injections of VP-16 have been reported using a 0.5-mg dose daily for 5 days, followed by a second course with two injections per day of the same dose.[306] VP-16 concentration in the central nervous fluid was 5.2 μg per mL. No toxic effect was reported.[306] The administration of intrapleural VP-16 has been proposed to prevent the recurrence of neoplastic pleural effusions.[307] Incomplete and slow systemic absorption from intrapleurally administered drug has been documented.[308]

Oral Etoposide
Oral VP-16 is formulated in a hydrophilic gelatin capsule. Peak plasma levels are obtained 0.5 to 4.0 hours after administration.[287] The mean bioavailability is 50%[264,287,309–312] with substantial inter- and intrapatient variability (range, 19% to 100%).[258,264,313–315] The bioavailability of doses lower than 100 mg (50 mg per m^2) approaches 75%,[312] whereas in doses above 100 mg per m^2 bioavailability decreases below 50%. VP-16 peak plasma concentration varies from 1.3 to 2.6 μg per mL using a schedule of 25 mg per m^2 twice a day for 7 days every 2 weeks.[316] The target plasma concentration of 1 μg per mL VP-16 can be reached for 7 to 13 hours using a single 100-mg oral dose of VP-16. The optimal oral schedule has yet to be defined, but based on the experimental relationship of response to longer durations of exposure, extended daily oral administration is preferred. VP-16 has been given orally over a prolonged 21-day schedule at a dose of 50 mg per m^2 per day. The MTD was 50 mg per m^2 and was associated with dose-limiting myelosuppression. Responses have been seen in patients resistant to standard dosages and to high-dose protocols used for bone marrow transplantation. The 50 mg per m^2 dosage has a higher bioavailability (91% to 96%) than that generally reported for VP-16, and many patients had plasma concentrations of 1 μg per mL or greater for the period of treatment. Bioavailability is not linear and decreases with doses greater than 200 mg,[314] possibly implying a saturable absorptive mechanism in the gastrointestinal tract. In addition to saturation of uptake, the very low aqueous solubility and the low stability at acid pH likely contribute to the erratic VP-16 bioavailability.[310,314,317] The intestinal Pgp mediates the efflux of VP-16, and the use of Pgp-inhibiting agents, such as

quinidine, might increase the intestinal absorption of VP-16.[318] Oral bioavailability of VP-16 is not affected by food or by concurrent IV chemotherapy.[313] A pharmacodynamic model was prospectively tested for the therapeutic monitoring of 21-day oral VP-16 (see below).[319] Of note, VP-16–related leukemias (see below) have been reported after prolonged treatments with oral VP-16.[320,321] Significant objective antitumor activity has been shown in advanced ovarian cancer patients after failure of a platinum-based first-line chemotherapy,[322] in SCLC[323–325] and non-SCLC,[319,326,327] and in AIDS-related Kaposi's sarcoma[316] with acceptable toxicity. The efficacy of these regimens could be the result of the prolonged maintenance of cytotoxic plasma concentrations during each treatment course and the absence of toxic peak levels of the drug. Oral VP-16 is well tolerated in the elderly[328] and many protocols are including oral VP-16 in elderly patients.[292] Several new regimens for NHL have included continuous administration of VP-16 at a dosage of 50 mg per m^2 per day over 3 or 4 days in combination with either doxorubicin and cyclophosphamide or doxorubicin, vincristine, prednisone, and cyclophosphamide.[329,330]

In elderly patients with aggressive NHL, chronic administration of VP-16 is feasible and active,[331] with an initial dosage of 50 mg per m^2 per day for 5 days and with two subsequent cycles given orally for 21 days. The dosage can be adjusted individually according to the fraction of the dose absorbed.[331] In elderly patients with acute myeloid leukemia, oral VP-16 has been proposed in combination with prednisone and mitoxantrone,[330] and as first-line therapy in combination with mitoxantrone.[247] A study compared the effects of oral VP-16 and IV VP-16 in advanced SCLC patients on survival and quality of life.[332] The study indicated that the oral route had a lower antitumoral activity and should not be used as first-line treatment of this disease.[332]

In conclusion, the development of oral VP-16 was emphasized because it might allow prolonged exposure to active concentrations of VP-16 and because it appeared as an interesting alternative to improve quality of life in patients treated with a palliative chemotherapy. However, the high interindividual variation in bioavailability and the results of the only study that compared oral and IV VP-16 suggest restrictions for its use as first-line therapy.

Etoposide Phosphate

VP-16 phosphate is an improved formulation of VP-16. VP-16 phosphate is a water-soluble prodrug of VP-16 and is rapidly and completely converted to VP-16 after IV dosing, regardless of the duration of administration, the dose used, or the treatment schedule.[333–337] Therefore, it does not expose the bloodstream to detergents or oils, as does the formulation of the lipid-soluble VP-16 and VM-26. VP-16 phosphate does not have to be diluted in solubilizing agents that may contribute to the toxicity of VP-16 and limit the rate at which VP-16 can be safely administered.

VP-16 phosphate can be made up to a concentration of 20 mg per mL and can be administered as an IV infusion in saline solution over 5 minutes without signs of hypotension or acute effects.[333,334] VP-16 phosphate can be substituted for VP-16 in high-dose chemotherapy regimens. Because it is not formulated with polyethylene glycol, polysorbate 80, or ethanol, VP-16 phosphate does not cause acidosis, even when given at high doses. VP-16 phosphate is completely converted to VP-16 even when high doses are used. High-dose intensity was also achieved in combination with filgrastim.[338] VP-16 phosphate can also be given as a continuous infusion in the ambulatory setting.[339] Twenty-three patients were treated with a continuous infusion of VP-16 phosphate using ambulatory pumps for 6 weeks, followed by a 2-week rest. Myelosuppression, mucositis, and fatigue were dose-limiting. Neutropenia correlated with plasma concentration of VP-16 at steady state. VP-16 phosphate was stable in pumps for at least 7 days. Cytotoxic concentrations of VP-16 were obtained at the MTD of 20 mg per m^2 per day.[339]

The pharmacokinetics of VP-16 and VP-16 phosphate were found to be comparable in a crossover trial in which patients were randomly assigned to treatment on day 1 with VP-16 and day 3 with VP-16 phosphate, or the inverse schedule.[340] The molecular weight of VP-16 and VP-16 phosphate is 558.57 and 568.55, respectively. To avoid confusion, dosages of VP-16 phosphate were expressed as molar equivalent dosages of VP-16. Toxicity of VP-16 and VP-16 phosphate were similar.[340] The MTD was 100 mg per m^2 per day of VP-16 equivalent for 5 days or 150 mg per m^2 per day for dosing on days 1, 3, and 5. A correlation was seen between VP-16 area under the concentration × time curve and leukocyte or granulocyte nadir.[337]

Clinical activity of VP-16 and VP-16 phosphate were found to be the same in combination with cisplatin in patients with SCLC.[341] VP-16 phosphate may exhibit better intestinal absorption than VP-16, with a mean bioavailability of 68%. VP-16 phosphate was proposed to overcome the inter- and intrasubject variability in absorption observed with oral VP-16.[342] A study randomized patients to receive oral VP-16 or oral VP-16 phosphate on day 1 of the first course and the alternative compound on day 1 of the second course.[343] Fifteen patients were evaluable for pharmacokinetic comparisons. The median AUC of VP-16 was 78 and 62 mg per hour per L, after VP-16 phosphate and oral VP-16, respectively. This difference in favor of VP-16 phosphate was of borderline significance. However, the same large interindividual variability of VP-16 phosphate and VP-16 AUC was observed with 42.3% and 48.4% as coefficients of variation.[343]

In conclusion, VP-16 phosphate is an improved formulation of VP-16 and is better suited for bolus administration, high-dosage treatment, and continuous infusions, provided equivalent antitumor activity is demonstrated.

Teniposide

Although VP-16 and VM-26 are similar in many respects, some pharmacokinetic parameters differ. Similar to VP-16, VM-26 demonstrates biexponential disposition after IV administration. The volume of distribution and the plasma $t_{1/2}$ of VM-26 are greater than those of VP-16, whereas plasma clearance, which also has a high interpatient variability, is lower at 16 mL per minute per m^2, as is renal clearance.[281] Only 10% to 20% of administered VM-26 is found in the urine as metabolites. The large volume of distribution is consistent with the high degree of protein binding (greater than 99%). Nonrenal clearance is similar to VP-16, as is the volume of distribution. Metabolites have not yet been identified. An inverse relationship between serum γ-glutamyl transpeptidase and VM-26 plasma clearance has been reported, suggesting an important hepatic component to clearance. A linear relationship exists between dose and AUC. To target a given exposure to VM-26 in individual patients, a Bayesian strategy with sparse sampling has been studied on an initial course to predict the dosage necessary for subsequent courses.[344] Steady-state concentrations were higher and the clearance lower in responders as compared with nonresponders in a phase I study of VM-26 given over a 72-hour continuous infusion, suggesting that dosage adjustments based on drug levels may lead to improved efficacy.[256]

In mice, VM-26 was found in highest concentrations in the liver, kidneys, and small intestine. Lowest concentrations were found in the brain. In humans, CSF levels of VM-26 are barely detectable, although VM-26 is considered clinically more effective than VP-16 in the treatment of malignant gliomas. VM-26 slowly diffuses into and is then slowly eliminated from third-space compartments, such as ascites. VM-26 is available only for IV administration but the IV formulation of VM-26 can be used orally. The bioavailability of oral VM-26 appears similar to that of oral VP-16 in that absorption is decreased at higher doses and is increased with smaller consecutive daily doses. The mean bioavailability is 41%.[315] The MTD for oral VM-26 given over 21 days was 100 mg per day, and the dose-limiting toxicity was myelosuppression.[315,345]

Pharmacodynamics

VP-16 activity shows marked schedule dependency.[258,346] The activity is concentration and time-dependent.[258,346] VP-16 clearance is not correlated with body surface area.[347] Dosing according to body surface area is a poor predictor of the peak or steady-state VP-16 concentration or AUC.[348] Several studies reproducibly found a relationship between VP-16 plasma concentration and hematotoxicity.[323,347,349–351] The extent of leukopenia is a function of plasma concentration, pretreatment white blood cell count, albumin concentration, performance status, and bone marrow function (based on transfusion requirements).[352] Plasma albumin concentration accounts for interpatient variability in protein binding of VP-16.[267,268,348] Steady-state concentration attained with continuous infusion VP-16 has been related to patient toxicity, as has the area under the VP-16 concentration versus time curve. Hematologic toxicity correlates better to the AUC of unbound VP-16 than to the AUC of total VP-16.[270] Therefore, albumin concentration and any concurrent medication that may modify the fraction of bound VP-16 should be considered to define VP-16 dosage.[347,352] Steady-state VP-16 plasma levels of more than 1 µg per mL are tumoricidal but are associated with severe myelosuppression when the VP-16 plasma levels are continuously higher than 3 µg per mL. In extensive-stage SCLC, VP-16 given orally over 5 days or intravenously over a 2-hour infusion was found to be more active than a single infusion over 24 hours.[346] Plasma concentration of VP-16 exceeded 1 µg per mL for twice as long in patients treated orally over 5 days than for those receiving a single 24-hour infusion.[346] The maintenance of a minimum plasma concentration between 2 and 3 µg per mL appears critical for efficacy. Dosage adjustments based on early steady-state measurements of plasma concentrations might allow optimal monitoring of prolonged exposure to VP-16.[353]

Modeling approaches for VP-16 interpatient variability have been attempted. Individualized dosing of VP-16 for 72-hour continuous infusion has been proposed, the main variables being the plasma albumin concentration, the starting dose, and the plasma VP-16 concentration after 24 hours of infusion.[347,352] When compared to a standard fixed-dose arm, individualized dosage adjustment led to a significant increase in the administered dosage and a substantial reduction in the variability of myelosuppression. Intrapatient pharmacokinetic variability is small (12% to 15%).[262,348] Therefore, pharmacokinetics measurements may not be necessary for each drug cycle. In the absence of measured plasma concentrations, it has been suggested to simplify VP-16 dosing to a fixed dosage independent of body surface area, 260 mg instead of 150 mg per m^2.[348] However, several studies suggested that patients with impaired renal or liver function or elderly patients are at risk with regard to increased hematologic toxicity, and, hence, it was proposed to reduce and individualize the VP-16 dosage in these patients.[354,355]

In a continuous infusion regimen, the 24-hour plasma concentration is proportional to AUC, and relationships between VP-16 AUC and toxicity have been reported.[270] Various limited-sampling methods have been proposed to estimate VP-16 AUC from one or two plasma concentration measurements.[356–358]

In patients receiving 21-day oral VP-16, VP-16 plasma concentrations are correlated with neutrophil count at the nadir.[319] Using this schedule, nadir VP-16 concentrations above 0.3 µg per mL were significantly correlated with grade 3 and 4 neutropenia.[319] Pharmacokinetically guided dosing was performed and appeared feasible in pediatric patients receiving VP-16.[359] The day 1 AUC was estimated using a limited sampling model, and day 2 target AUC defined by VP-16 dose–AUC relationship observed in 33 children. This approach may be of interest, especially in patients with renal or hepatic dysfunction or prior exposure to cisplatin.[359] Increased hematotoxicity is suggested with aging in the use of VP-16.[292]

Toxicity

Hematotoxicity

Myelosuppression is the dose-limiting toxicity of VP-16. While the single daily MTD is 300 mg per m^2, dosages of 150 mg per m^2 for 3 days and 45 mg per m^2 for 7 days have been studied. Mild leukopenia (1,000 to 3,000 per mm^3) and thrombocytopenia (less than 100,000 per mm^3) occur in fewer than 25% of patients at these doses.[360,361] Only 8% of patients treated with standard dosages have white cell nadirs below 1,000 per mm^3 occurring on day 10 (range, 8 to 14). Bone marrow toxicity is not cumulative. When given orally over 21 days, VP-16 is generally well tolerated at an MTD of 50 mg per m^2 per day. Myelosuppression is the dose-limiting toxicity, with leukocyte nadirs occurring between day 22 and 29. Hematologic toxicity is not cumulative, and most patients begin subsequent cycles on day 36. At this dosage, leukocyte nadir is less than 1,000 per mm^3 in only 4 of 20 courses, and platelet counts are less than 50,000 cells per mm^3 in only 3 of 20 courses. Myelosuppression is also the dose-limiting toxicity for VM-26. At VM-26 dosages ranging from 50 mg per m^2 per day for 5 days to 165 mg per m^2 per day twice weekly, half the patients experience white cell nadirs below 1,500 per mm^3.

Nonhematologic Toxicities

Common nonhematologic toxicities include nausea and vomiting and alopecia. Nausea and vomiting are seen in 10% to 20% of patients, and alopecia occurs in 10% to 30% of patients, depending on dosage and schedule. Rare anaphylaxis and chemical phlebitis have been reported. Peripheral neuropathy has not been associated with the epipodophyllotoxins. Hypotension, fever, bronchospasm, diarrhea, and mucositis are uncommon.[362] Hypotension has been noted in 5% to 8% of patients receiving VP-16 but is rare when the drug is given over 1 hour and is probably related to the vehicle (polysorbate 80 plus polyethylene glycol).[362] Acute hypersensitivity reactions are more common with VM-26 than with VP-16.[363] They have been estimated to occur in 6% to 7% of patients with brain tumors treated with IV epipodophyllotoxins. No hypersensitivity reactions have been reported with oral VP-16. Therefore, these reactions may be due to the excipient benzyl alcohol, Tween 80, or Cremophor EL (in the case of VM-26) used to solubilize the drugs. Most reactions consist of grade 1 or 2 urticaria, angioedema, flushing, rashes, or hypotension and are rarely dose-limiting.

After treatment with high-dose VP-16 in association with bone marrow rescue, the dose-limiting toxicity is mucositis. Mucositis may be related to metabolites of VP-16 that are excreted in the saliva. Hepatotoxicity may also become a major toxicity. Other acute toxicities can be associated with the drug infusion after high-dose regimens. They include fever, chills (in 25% of patients), and nausea and vomiting (50%). Compensated metabolic acidosis (45%) can also been observed during the week after chemotherapy. The complex solvent system has been proposed to be responsible for the acidosis. Transient and mild disorientation during drug administration has been related to the administration of ethanol included with chemotherapy. Finally, rash, transient confusion, and liver function test abnormalities are infrequent side effects.

Etoposide-Induced Secondary Leukemia

Several DNA-damaging agents, including most prominently alkylating agents, have been shown to be responsible for secondary leukemias.[364] The increased frequency of illegitimate recombination events induced by top2 reactive agents may account for their leukemogenicity.[365] VP-16 was demonstrated to be mutagenic in patients.[366] AML cases related to prior treatment with epipodophyllotoxins (VP-16 and VM-26) have been identified.[7,367–372] In contrast to alkylating agent–associated secondary AML, epipodophyllotoxin-associated AML exhibits a shorter latency period, with a median of 24 to 30 months versus 4 months.[7,370,373] Their phenotype is most often monocytic (FAB M-4 or M-5) with an acute presentation rather than with a myelodysplastic prodromal state. Acute promyelocytic leukemia after epipodophyllotoxins occurs infrequently.[371,372] Secondary myelodysplastic syndrome and chronic myelogenous leukemia have been described.[7] Therapy-related leukemia and myelodysplasia were also reported after prolonged administration of oral VP-16 in breast cancer or NHL patients.[320,321] There are no statistically significant differences in VP-16 pharmacokinetics between patients who do and do not develop secondary AML.[374] In one review done in 1991 of 37 patients, 21 of 30 patients had M-4 or M-5 acute nonlymphocytic leukemia (ANLL), with 14 of 28 patients having an 11q23 abnormality. The mean latency period was 33 months. Other studies suggest a shorter latency of 2 years.[7,368–370] Weekly or biweekly schedules of VP-16 might be associated with increased risk of secondary leukemia.[7] The administration of L-asparaginase before VP-16 might also increase the risk of leukemia.[7]

The follow-up by the National Cancer Institute Cancer Therapy Evaluation Program of patients treated with epipodophyllotoxins did not show evidence of significant variations in the incidence of secondary leukemias in patients who had received low (less than 1.5 g per m^2), moderate (between 1.50 and 2.99 g per m^2), or high (more than 3 g per m^2) cumulative dosages.[367,370] The calculated 6-year rate for development of leukemia was between 0.7% and

3.2% with the highest rate observed in the group of patients who received the lowest dosages.[367,370] The Indiana University experience with respect to VP-16–induced secondary leukemias has been reviewed.[375] In patients with germ cell malignancies treated with cisplatin, VP-16, and bleomycin (PEB) at conventional dosages, two of 538 patients developed ANLL after 22 months to 3 years. The median follow-up was 4.9 years. The VP-16 dosage is an important factor for the occurrence of ANLL after VP-16 and cisplatin combination chemotherapy for advanced non-SCLC.[376] The median VP-16 dosage was 6.8 mg per m^2 in four out of 114 patients who developed ANLL after 13, 19, 28, and 35 months after the beginning of the treatment, compared with a median VP-16 dosage of 3 mg per m^2 in the nonleukemic patients. In another report of 212 patients treated with PEB for germ cell tumors, five patients developed ANLL, for a mean cumulative risk of 4.7%.[377] All these patients had cumulative VP-16 dosages above 2,000 mg per m^2, whereas none of the 130 patients with cumulative dosage below 2,000 mg per m^2 developed leukemia. In a series of 734 children treated with epipodophyllotoxins, 21 developed secondary ANLL. Although the overall risk of developing a secondary leukemia was 3.8%, subgroup analysis revealed that the risk was substantially greater when the drug was given on a weekly or biweekly schedule (12%). The cumulative risk was substantially less (1.6%) in the children not treated with VP-16, treated with VP-16 only during remission induction, or treated every 2 weeks during continuation treatment.[370,378] Not only VP-16, but also its catechol and quinone metabolites can induce *in vitro* top2 cleavage complexes near the translocation breakpoints and are likely to also play a role in the creation of top2-mediated chromosomal breakage.[379]

These leukemias frequently involved the long arm of chromosome 11, with translocation of the *MLL* gene at chromosome band 11q23, but many less common abnormalities involved chromosomes 3, 8, 15, 16, 17, 21, or 22.[215,380–383] The *MLL* gene has recently been identified at 11q23 and is frequently involved in *de novo* leukemias. Most of the breakpoints occur in a 9-kilobase region that includes exons 5 to 11 of the *MLL* gene. This genomic region includes DNA sequences, potentially involved for illegitimate recombinations, such as Alu sequences, V(D)J recombinase recognition sites, and top2 consensus binding sequences. The *MLL* gene appears to play a role in the regulation of the differentiation of hematopoietic stem cells. Its overall sequence composition is AT rich. AT-rich sequences often correspond to nuclear matrix attachment regions, where top2 cleavage complexes are preferentially formed.[384] More than 20 different translocations involving chromosome 11q23 have been described. DNA-topoisomerase II cleavage assays have shown a correspondence between top2 cleavage sites and the translocation breakpoints.[379] The mechanism of the translocation might be a chromo-

somal breakage by top2 followed by the recombination of DNA free ends during DNA repair.

Clinical Resistance

Several studies have found an association between top2α expression and tumor cell proliferation.[385,386] Consistently, higher top2α messenger RNA (mRNA) levels were observed in high-grade than in low-grade NHLs[387] and in SCLC than in non-SCLC.[388] Increased top2α was correlated with a poor prognosis in breast cancer patients.[386,389,390] In contrast to top2α, top2β is expressed in proliferating and quiescent cells.[391] Several studies have investigated the relationship between top2 levels in leukemia cells and response to top2 inhibitors containing chemotherapy. No correlation was seen between top2α or top2β expression, as assessed by Western blot, and response to the top2 poisons in adult acute leukemias.[392,393]

One study in gastric cancer patients suggested a correlation between the MDR-1 expression and the chemoresistance of patients with gastric cancer receiving adriamycin- or VP-16–containing combinations.[394] Another study in 58 patients with squamous cell carcinoma of the esophagus compared the expression of the MRP in tumour biopsies before and after preoperative chemotherapy with cisplatin and VP-16.[395] Tumor biopsies were analyzed by either ribonuclease protection assay or by immunohistochemistry for the presence of MRP mRNA or protein.[395] MRP expression in tumors from responders to chemotherapy (partial or complete response) did not differ significantly compared to tumors from nonresponders (stable or progressive disease). However, a difference was apparent for higher MRP expression in tumors from patients with either partial response or stable disease when comparing MRP levels in paired tumor samples before and after chemotherapy, suggesting that chemotherapy selected for drug-resistant cell clones.[395] Increased LRP expression has been detected in 30 relapsed ALL samples in comparison to the 112 initial ALL samples.[396]

Neuroblastoma cell lines established at different points of VP-16 therapy progressively exhibit increased VP-16 resistance, as determined by digital image microscopy scanning (DIMSCAN) assay.[397] Hence, VP-16 resistance is probably due to stable genetic alterations occurring during therapy.[397]

Several compounds have been combined with VP-16 in an attempt to reverse MDR.[398,399] PSC833 and cyclosporin significantly increased VP-16 antitumoral activity, but cyclosporin A appears more effective than PSC833 as a modulator of VP-16 activity in L1210 leukemia–bearing BDF1 mice and Lewis lung carcinoma–bearing C57-B1 mice.[400,401] However, pharmacokinetic interactions in humans of cyclosporin and VP-16 confound the interpretation of these results. Cyclosporin, given intravenously, increases the median AUC for VP-16 from 7.2 to 12.5 mg per mL per minute in a cohort of 18 children.[399]

Cyclosporin infusion increased the normalized AUC of VP-16 by 124% and the VP-16 $t_{1/2}$ by 120% in children with AML.[402] A phase I study using the nonimmunosuppressive analog of cyclosporin A, SDZ PSC833, in combination with VP-16 and mitoxantrone[403] reported that the coadministration of PSC833 did not change the pharmacokinetics of mitoxantrone but led to increased VP-16 concentrations in serum. Clearing of leukemia cells occurred in four of six MDR-1–positive patients. Combination chemotherapy with SDZ PSC833 has been used recently with promising results for the treatment of refractory and relapsed acute myelogenous leukemia,[404,405] but the results are difficult to interpret because of the pharmacokinetic interactions. Phase III trials of PSC833 in adult AML are in progress.

Acridines

Amsacrine Pharmacokinetics

The key pharmacologic features of m-AMSA are given in Table 19-6.

Animal Data

Pharmacologic studies of ^{14}C-labeled m-AMSA have been performed in mice and rats.[406] After IV administration, plasma concentration of 9-[^{14}C]-m-AMSA exhibits a multiphasic decline, with terminal phase levels proportional to dosage. Radioactivity is well distributed to all tissues except the brain, with high concentrations in the bladder, spleen, and liver. Unchanged m-AMSA, determined after ethanol acetate extraction, has a similar pattern of plasma disappearance. Plasma concentrations of unchanged m-AMSA are 50-fold lower than total ^{14}C after 1 hour, indicating

TABLE 19-6. KEY FEATURES OF AMSACRINE

Mechanism of action:	Inhibition of DNA topoisomerase II, with possible selectivity for topoisomerase IIβ Weak intercalator
Pharmacokinetics:	Plasma disappearance Initial half-life = 30 min Terminal half-life = 7–9 h Protein binding: 50% after 2 h
Metabolism:	Conjugation with glutathione
Elimination:	Biliary route (65%, as metabolites) Urinary route (35–50%, as metabolites and parent drug)
Toxicities:	Myelosuppression Mucositis Vomiting Hepatotoxicity Ventricular arrhythmias
Precautions:	Increased toxicity if renal or liver failure: reduce dose by 30% Monitoring of serum electrolytes: avoid hypokalemia

extensive metabolism. Nearly 50% of the total radioactivity is bound to proteins after 2 hours. More than 50% of total radioactivity is excreted in the bile within 2 hours. Biliary concentration reaches 400 times the plasma concentration. The percentage of unchanged m-AMSA in the liver is low, suggesting extensive hepatic metabolism of m-AMSA. A 40% reduction in liver glutathione and a 20% reduction of glutathione transferase activity are found in mouse liver after m-AMSA administration, consistent with the importance of hepatic microsomal drug metabolism for drug elimination.[406]

m-AMSA binds covalently to plasma proteins. This binding is thought to result from the direct nucleophilic attack by protein thiols at the C-9 position of the acridine ring with consequent release of the anilino side chain 4-amino-3-methoxy-methane-sulphonanilide.[406–408]

m-AMSA is metabolized via two major routes (Fig. 19-7), both of which result in formation of conjugated thiols. The major route of metabolism and elimination of m-AMSA in the mouse and the rat is cytochrome P-450 dependent. Drug oxidation forms the reactive quinone diamine intermediate N1'-methanesulfonyl-N4'-(9-acridinyl)-3'-methoxy-2',5'-cyclohexadiene-1,4'-diimene (*m*-AQDI). This product undergoes reduction and conjugation with glutathione at the 5' and 6' positions of the anilino ring and excretion via the bile.[409–411] The second route involves nucleophilic attack at the C-9 position of the acridine ring, resulting in the formation of the 9-acridinyl thioester.[407,412]

Human Data

The pharmacokinetics of m-AMSA in humans are similar to those in rodents. The volume of distribution of m-AMSA exceeds the total water content, indicating the localization or the sequestration of the drug at some site, most likely the liver binding, protein binding, or both. m-AMSA has a biphasic plasma disappearance curve with a $t_{1/2\alpha}$ of 10 to 30 minutes and a $t_{1/2\beta}$ of 7 to 9 hours.[413,414] Approximately 50% of m-AMSA is bound to proteins after 2 hours.[413,414] In 13 adult patients with ANLL receiving 75 to 90 mg per m^2 over 1 hour, the drug had a mean clearance value of 179 mL per minute per m^2, with variation over a threefold range.[415] The mean clearance for a pediatric population was found to be similar but more variable (eightfold).[416] The interpatient variability yields a five- to eightfold difference in steady-state concentrations in patients receiving a given dosage by continuous infusion (adjusted for body size).

m-AMSA is bound to plasma proteins and is eliminated primarily by metabolism in the liver, and parent and metabolites are excreted in the bile. In the liver, the major metabolite is the m-AMSA glutathione 5'-conjugate. m-AMSA, and to a greater degree, its metabolites are also excreted in urine. There is no known *in vitro* antineoplastic activity of the glutathione metabolite of m-AMSA. The urinary excretion of m-AMSA is also a significant route of drug elimination in humans, accounting for 10% to 20%

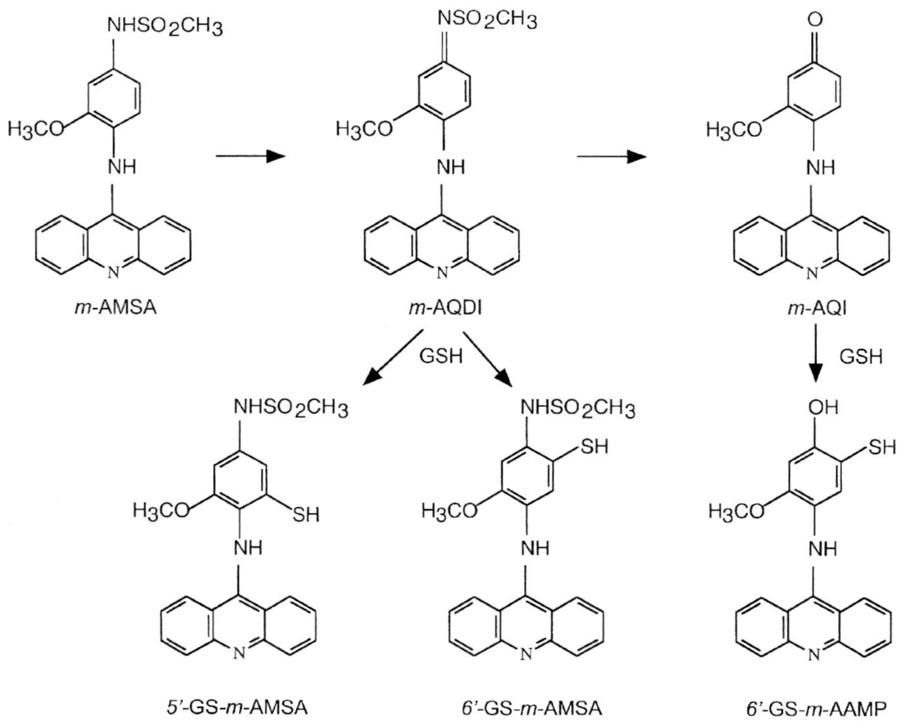

FIGURE 19-7. Metabolism of amsacrine (m-AMSA).

of parent drug elimination and an equal amount of metabolites. Urinary excretion of ^{14}C and m-AMSA increases in patients with liver disease, and a greater proportion of that excreted is unchanged m-AMSA.[414] Patients with liver disease have a reduced ability to clear m-AMSA from the plasma, although this reduction does not always correlate directly with any single measure of liver function.[414] Patients with moderate renal dysfunction but normal liver function clear m-AMSA adequately. However, in patients with severe renal impairment, m-AMSA plasma clearance is markedly reduced. The plasma clearance of total ^{14}C appears substantially more affected than that of m-AMSA in patients with renal disease, possibly because renal excretion plays a more important role in the elimination of the ^{14}C metabolites.[414] Because the m-AMSA plasma clearance in patients with severe renal disease is diminished, urinary excretion also must be an important route for the elimination of unchanged m-AMSA. Plasma $t_{1/2}$ seems to be a reasonable predictor of the toxicity of m-AMSA analogs.[417]

Cellular pharmacokinetics suggest that the cellular uptake occurs by a rapid and passive diffusion. *In vivo*, the AUC of m-AMSA in leukemic cells exhibits the same pattern as the AUC in plasma, although at higher levels. No evidence has been found that longer exposure increases *in vitro* cellular uptake.[418] Neither m-AMSA nor its metabolites penetrate the blood–brain barrier, and m-AMSA does not achieve appreciable levels in the CSF.[414] In mice, the brain uptake index values of m-AMSA were 15 plus or minus 2.2%.[419] After intracarotid administration, less than 20% of drug is extracted in its first pass through the brain.[419] The occasional occurrence of neurotoxicity, including seizures, in patients receiving systemic m-AMSA is surprising.

Toxicity of Amsacrine

Hematotoxicity of Amsacrine
A number of single- and multiple-dose schedules have been tested in phase I trials in adult patients.[420] The route of administration was oral in two trials.[421,422] In the first oral trial, single doses of from 30 to 500 mg per m^2 produced hematologic toxicity, and the MTD was not reached. In the second trial, oral m-AMSA was given on a daily schedule for 5 days. With a range of doses of from 100 to 150 mg per m^2, 120 mg per m^2 per day for five days was considered to be the MTD. The hematologic toxicity was dose-limiting. In some patients, failure to reach the MTD with doses as high as 500 mg per m^2 suggested incomplete or erratic absorption. The oral route is not used because of large and unpredictable interindividual variability in absorption. Subsequent trials have used the IV route exclusively. Although a number of schedules of administration have been tested, the optimal schedules appear to be 150 mg per m^2 per day for 5 days for adult patients with leukemia and 90 to 120 mg per m^2 given as a single dose every 21 days for patients with solid tumors. The schedules are comparable for children with leukemia and lower for pediatric solid tumor (60 mg per m^2 per day).[423] In all phase I trials, the dose-limiting toxicity was myelosuppression manifested by moderate to severe leukopenia. Antitumor activity was seen in a variety

of tumor types, especially leukemias and lymphomas.[424] The data are insufficient to evaluate whether continuous exposure to m-AMSA at conventional dosages provides any advantage. Continuous infusion of 30 to 40 mg per m² per day for 3 or 4 days in 22 patients with solid tumors or lymphoma refractory to conventional therapy produced only three objective responses.[425] Using autologous bone marrow transplantation, doses of 600 to 1,000 mg per m² were given for a period of 3 to 5 consecutive days. As expected, all the patients had severe leukopenia complicated by episodes of fever and septicemia, all the patients had nausea and vomiting, half the patients had diarrhea, and mucositis was considered the dose-limiting toxicity.[424]

Myelosuppression is the most important and dose-limiting toxicity. The degree of myelosuppression is dose dependent and is reversible at standard doses. Leukopenia, thrombocytopenia, and, to a lesser extent, anemia, occur in virtually all patients.[424] Although leukopenia is found at all dose levels and with all schedules, myelosuppression is less severe and less frequent at total doses per course of 200 mg per m² or less. The white blood cell nadir occurs around day 10 after administration, with hematologic recovery by day 25. In patients with solid tumors, thrombocytopenia is rare at conventional dose levels.

Nonhematologic Toxicities of Amsacrine

m-AMSA causes phlebitis. Consequently, it is recommended to dilute m-AMSA in 500 mL of 5% dextrose and to use a central line for continuous infusion or repeated treatments to avoid reactions at the injection site. Hearing loss and allergic reactions (anaphylaxis, urticaria and rashes, and allergic edema) are relatively rare.

Nausea and vomiting are common with m-AMSA.[426] Diarrhea is less common and occurs in 5% to 17% of patients. In a trial incorporating dose escalation, the stomatitis was dose related and relatively infrequent at doses under 120 mg per m². Stomatitis becomes dose-limiting for treatments with high doses in association with bone marrow rescue.[427]

The incidence of hepatotoxicity may reach 35%.[28] Elevation of bilirubin, the most frequent abnormality,[428] is usually dose-related and reversible.[426] Increased liver transaminases are also dose-dependent and reversible.[429] Increased alkaline phosphatases are rare.[424] However, two cases of fatal hepatotoxicity have been reported, both in heavily pretreated patients.[28,429] Because m-AMSA is conjugated in the liver and is excreted in large part via the biliary system, at least 30% dose reduction is generally recommended in patients with impaired hepatic function (elevated bilirubin).[424]

Cardiotoxicity has been reported in children and adults with high- and low-dose treatments. Although its incidence is low (less than 5% in most large series), patients may develop arrhythmia, conducting disturbances, congestive heart failure during and after m-AMSA administration, and sudden death.[430–433] More commonly, the heart rate is decreased by approximately 10%.[434] Because hypokalemia may exacerbate arrhythmias, it has been recommended that serum potassium levels be maintained at or above 4 mEq per L at the time of drug administration.[435] Normally, this value can be obtained readily with an infusion of potassium chloride at a rate of 10 mEq per hour administered over 10 hours before m-AMSA treatment. In most patients, m-AMSA produces a significant prolongation (0.050 to 0.064 seconds) of the corrected QT (QT_c) interval.[432,436] The m-AMSA–associated QT_c prolongation may persist for up to 90 minutes. Tachyarrhythmias in the setting of QT_c prolongation usually arise by triggered automaticity and may be precipitated by adrenergic hyperactivity. A prospective study suggested that this effect was present in most patients and occurred with each dose. m-AMSA also may reduce significantly the serum sodium and magnesium concentrations 20 minutes after the start of the infusion. The effect is transient and reverses by 24 hours after the infusion.[437] The decrease in magnesium levels may contribute to the m-AMSA–induced cardiac arrhythmias.[434,438] Nevertheless, m-AMSA has been administered safely to patients with myocardial dysfunction.[435]

Neurologic toxicities, such as peripheral neuropathy or seizures (grand mal), are rare. One case of peripheral neuritis of the Guillain-Barré type has been reported.[424]

The impact of m-AMSA treatments on fertility has been reported by da Cunha and co-workers,[439] who monitored the concentration, motility, and morphology of sperm in a patient during 12 courses of m-AMSA at 40 mg per m² for 3 days every 3 weeks. Sperm concentration and motility were reduced, and morphologic abnormalities were significantly increased by the third course. Azoospermia was observed by the sixth course. After interruption of the treatment, sperm concentration, motility, and morphologic abnormalities returned to normal, suggesting that m-AMSA has temporary and reversible effects on differentiating germinal cells.[439]

In summary, the optimal schedule of administration for m-AMSA appears to be a single daily dose. It seems that little advantage is gained by continuous infusion schedules. Patients with normal hepatic function or mild liver dysfunction should tolerate full drug doses. Patients with significant liver dysfunction manifested by serum bilirubin greater than 2 mg per dL should have an initial 30% dose reduction. Subsequent dose escalation may be possible based on clinical tolerance. Patients with moderate renal dysfunction (serum creatinine in the range of 1.2 to 2 mg per dL) should receive full-dose therapy; however, oliguric patients or those with more serious renal disease (serum creatinine greater than 2 mg per dL) should have an initial 30% dose reduction.

N-[2-(Dimethylamino)Ethyl] Acridine-4-Carboxamide

The acridinecarboxamide DACA (Fig. 19-1) is a lipophilic monointercalator that entered phase I clinical trials on the basis of its mixed inhibition of top1 and top2[37,38] and excellent activity in experimental solid tumors.[36] The MTD of DACA in mice is 30 mg per kg per day. At this dosage, the limiting toxicity was neurologic with sedation and seizures as main manifestations.[419] The results of a 3-hour infusion every 3 weeks in advanced cancer patients have been reported.[440] DACA demonstrated a biphasic disposition with a terminal $t_{1/2}$ of 2 hours.[441] AUC and maximum concentration (C_{max}) were linearly related to the dose between 18 and 1,000 mg per m². [441] Over 72 hours, 44% of the dose was recovered in the urine, with less than 1% occurring as intact DACA.[441] The major urinary metabolite was DACA-*N*-oxide-9-(10H)acridone, accounting for 35% of the dose.[442] Central venous lines are required to prevent local pain.[440]

Ellipticine and Olivacine Derivatives

Ellipticines and olivacines have in common the absence of dose-limiting myelosuppression and the absence of alopecia. NMHE is presently only available in Europe. However, considerable efforts are still ongoing to develop other ellipticine derivatives, and one olivacine derivative (S16020-S) (Fig. 19-1) is presently in phase I clinical trials. NMHE is primarily used to treat bone metastases from breast cancer. The objective response rates range between 15% and 25% for patients previously treated with doxorubicin.[443] Responses have also been reported in the treatment of thyroid and renal cancers and soft tissue sarcomas.[444]

Pharmacokinetics

In mice and cancer patients, the main pharmacokinetics parameters of NMHE were calculated based on plasma concentrations and urinary elimination determined by HPLC and fluorescence detection.[445,446] Plasma concentration rises quickly, and a steady state is reached by the end of a 1-hour infusion. On cessation of the infusion, NMHE plasma concentrations decrease steeply.[447] The metabolism of ellipticines has been studied in rodents and humans.[446] The hepatic extraction ratio is high. NMHE is mainly excreted by the biliary tract as glucuronide conjugates and glutathione adducts.[448,449] Oxidation of 9-hydroxyellipticine leads to the formation of phenoxy radicals and of the quinone imine 9-oxoellipticine.[448,449]

Toxicity

Initial phase I trials conducted in Europe showed responses to NMHE in advanced breast carcinoma at doses ranging between 80 and 100 mg per m² administered intravenously weekly. A high incidence of hemolytic and allergic reactions has been observed, related to oligomers of NMHE in raw material and lyophilisates. This formulation problem con-

tributed to the suspension of the clinical studies in the United States.[450]

Hematotoxicity

Myelosuppression is minimal, a particularly attractive feature of the ellipticines.[443,444,450,451] Acute intravascular hemolysis has been reported with NMHE, and approximately 20% of the patients develop detectable antiellipstinium antibodies, usually without evidence of hemolysis. Antigen-antibody complexes are found in the bloodstream, are absorbed onto the red cell membrane, and then activate complement.[452] Testing of various ellipticines for cross-reactivity suggested that the 9-hydroxyl group probably accounts for the antigenicity. Hemolysis is only observed in patients who develop antibodies with a titer greater than 1/32 (approximately 8% of patients).[453] The immunogenicity of the drug appears to be schedule dependent, and the incidence of hemolysis is high in weekly regimens but can be avoided with treatments for 3 consecutive days every 3 weeks.[454]

Nonhematologic Toxicities

Nephrotoxicity is the most severe adverse effect of NMHE. The affinity of NMHE for the kidney is high,[445] and a pitressin-resistant urinary concentrating defect has been described in NMHE-treated rats.[455] The initial lesion is an enlargement of the proximal tubular epithelial cells. Then tubular necrosis supervenes and can lead to complete denudation of the tubular basement membrane.[456] No glomerular or vascular alterations are associated. A strong affinity for membrane lipids has been shown for NMHE. Such interactions can favor fixation of NMHE on preferential sites of the brush border of proximal tubular cells, which are rich in acid phospholipids. Isolated kidney cells metabolize NMHE to *N*-acetylcysteine conjugates and to smaller amounts of glutathione and cysteine conjugates.[457] Thus, in the kidney, biooxidative activation of NMHE into an electrophilic intermediate occurs, and such a reactive metabolite may be responsible for the nephrotoxicity. Free radicals or quinones induced by oxidation of hydroxyellipticines may favor intrarenal lipid peroxidation reactions.[458] Because renal failure is dose dependent, it is recommended that the cumulative NMHE dose not exceed 2,000 mg. Because most of the drug is excreted by extrarenal routes, the dose should not be modified in case of slight to moderate renal insufficiency. Xerostomia is an additional significant, and occasionally, dose-limiting toxicity. It was initially universal at dosages greater or equal to 80 mg per m² per week.[459] Interestingly, neither alopecia nor mucositis has been reported with NMHE.

Some ellipticine derivative salts have been found to have a marked selectivity against all eight brain tumor cell lines of the United States National Cancer Institute's disease-oriented *in vitro* screen. The antitumor activity of 9-chloro-2-methylellipticinium (CME) has been recently studied *in vivo.*[460] However, in spite of its marked cytotoxicity *in vitro*, CME had a modest antitumor effect on extracranially implanted U251 glioma tumors and no beneficial effect in animals bearing U251 tumor in the brain, owing to a poor penetration into the brain parenchyma.[460] When CME was used in combination with carmustine, VP-16, or cisplatin, no synergistic activities were observed, but additive effects were demonstrated.[460]

Other ellipticine derivatives have entered in phase I clinical trials, such as datelliptium chloride.[461] Various kinds of water-soluble quaternary salts of 2-(2'-oxoalkoxy)-9-hydroxyellipticines were synthesized in a search for compounds with a potent antitumor activity and low toxicity. Some compounds exhibited more potent antitumor activities than NMHE.[462] The 9-substituted ellipticine and 2-methylellipticinium analogs appeared to be selective for central nervous tumors.[463] A series of ellipticine glycosides were also synthesized and exhibited good activity and therapeutic ratio in murine tumor systems.[464] The installation of a basic side chain on the ring nitrogen of ellipticine did improve the DNA binding properties but not their *in vivo* antitumor activity.[465]

The clinical development of the olivacine derivative S16020-2 is ongoing. This top2 inhibitor has shown a broad spectrum of antitumour activity in a large panel of *in vivo* experimental models,[44] and particularly in lung cancer models.[43] The antitumor activity of S16020-2 was investigated *in vivo* and compared with that of adriamycin and NMHE acetate in a panel of murine and human tumor models.[42] When given intravenously, S16020-2 was active against P388 leukemia implanted either intraperitoneally, subcutaneously, or intracerebrally. S16020-2 was markedly more active than NMHE acetate. Its hematologic toxicity, particularly its effects on bone marrow stem cells at pharmacologic active doses, was less pronounced than that of adriamycin.[42] Phase I clinical trials are ongoing with different administration schedules.[45,466,467] Dose-limiting toxicities thus far have been cutaneous (facial edema and acne) effects and asthenia.[45,467]

Bisdioxopiperazine Derivatives

The bisdioxopiperazines are catalytic top2 inhibitors (top2 suppressors) (Fig. 19-3 and Table 19-1). Razoxane (ICRF-159) was found to enhance the antitumor activity of anthracyclines in mice bearing L1210 leukemia.[468] The antitumor activity of ICRF-159 was found to be marginal in NHL,[469] Kaposi's sarcoma,[470] and colorectal carcinoma.[471] Dexrazoxane (ICRF-187, Zinecard) is 4,4'-(1-methyl-1,2-ethanediyl)-bis(2,6-piperazinedione) and is the (+)-(S)-enantiomer of racemic razoxane. ICRF-187 did not demonstrate any convincing antitumor activity in phase II clinical trials in patients with advanced solid tumors,[472,473] pediatric tumors, or hematologic malignancies.[474] ICRF-187 has proven to be clinically effective in reducing the car-

diotoxicity of doxorubicin and other anthracyclines.[48,475–481] On hydrolysis of the piperazinyl rings, ICRF-187 forms a double-ring opened form (ADR-925) similar to ethylenediaminetetraacetic acid, which is a strong iron chelator.[479,482–484] Iron chelation prevents or reduces site-specific oxygen radical production that damages cardiac muscle after anthracycline exposure.[479,482–484] In preclinical models, ICRF-187 could protect from the cardiotoxicity of anthracyclines[485,486] in hamsters and dogs, and ICRF-187 was developed subsequently for this use. Studies in isolated heart cells and in animals indicate that ICRF-187 is less effective in preventing the chronic cardiotoxicity of anthrapyrazoles as compared to its effects on anthracycline cardiotoxicity.[487,488]

ICRF-187 is eliminated primarily by an enzyme-catalyzed hydrolysis. Dihydropyrimidine amidohydrolase is largely responsible for metabolizing ICRF-187 in myocytes and hepatocytes.[484] In humans, the pharmacokinetics of ICRF-187 fit a two-compartment model.[46,489,490] An increased urinary excretion of iron is detectable in patients.[491]

Randomized studies have shown a reduction of doxorubicin-induced cardiotoxicity in the group of breast cancer patients receiving ICRF-187 without altering the antitumor efficacy.[47] The dose shown to be protective against adriamycin cardiotoxicity was 1,000 mg per m[2].[47] The cardioprotective effect of ICRF-187 was not associated with a change in adriamycin clearance.[490]

ICRF-187 has been given intravenously by different schedules, including weekly, daily for 3 consecutive days, and 48-hour infusion administrations. For cardioprotection, the most commonly used schedule is once every 3 weeks.[47,472,473,492–494] In this schedule, ICRF-187 is diluted in dextrose 5% and given over a 15- to 60-minute infusion 30 minutes before the administration of the anthracycline.[47]

The dose-limiting toxicity of ICRF-187 is hematologic with leukopenia and thrombocytopenia. Anemia is rare and observed at doses higher than 1,000 mg per m[2].[47,489–491] The main nonhematologic toxicity is hepatotoxicity with non–dose-dependent transaminitis, increased alkaline phosphatases, or hyperbilirubinemia.[47,489–491] Other nonhematologic toxicities included nausea and vomiting, alopecia, fever, phlebitis, and pain at injection site.[47,489–491]

The optimal ratio of ICRF-187 to doxorubicin bolus is not yet defined, although ratios of 20 to 1[47,48] to 10 to 1[475,477,478] were effective clinically. ICRF-187 was cardioprotective in patients with breast cancer who had already received a cumulative dose of 300 mg per m[2] of doxorubicin[477] before receiving the drug. ICRF-187 was later shown to reduce the risk of developing short-term subclinical cardiotoxicity in pediatric sarcoma patients treated with doxorubicin.[476] No change in antitumor efficacy has been observed in the group of patients treated with ICRF-187 in addition to the anthracycline.[476] In a phase I trial of escalating doses of paclitaxel plus doxorubicin and ICRF-187 in patients with advanced breast cancer, no decrease in left ventricular ejection fraction was observed compared with an incidence of decrease in ejection fraction in 20% to 50% of patients in other trials using this combination without ICRF-187.[495] An additional use of ICRF-187 is as a topical agent for the prevention and treatment of anthracycline-mediated tissue damage from extravasation.[496]

Combinations of agonists and antagonists have led to high-dose regimens for counteracting drug resistance. Using a similar approach to the exploitation of the folinic acid rescue for methotrexate toxicity to enable the use of high-dose methotrexate, the combination of epipodophyllotoxins with a catalytic inhibitor of top2 has been studied.[493,497] ICRF-187 protects from VP-16 and VM-26 toxicity and has been recently proposed to allow dose escalation and pharmacologic effect in sanctuaries, such as in the brain.[494] ICRF-187 protection seems optimum when ICRF-187 is given after VP-16 or VM-26. In contrast to VP-16 and VM-26, ICRF-187, because of its hydrophilicity, does not cross the blood–brain barrier. The combination with ICRF-187 allowed a 3.4-fold VM-26 dosage escalation and increased antitumor activity in CNS tumors in animal models.[494] This type of rescue by top2 suppressors might enable dose escalation for epipodophyllotoxin therapy.

More recently, a series of bis(*N*-acyloxymethyl) derivatives of ICRF-187 has been synthesized.[498] Most of them exhibited antitumoral activity in murine tumors.[498] One of these compounds, MST-16, is bis(*N*1-isobutyloxycarbonyloxymethyl-2,6-dioxopiperazine), a derivative of bis(*N*1-acyloxymethyl) ICRF-154. MST-16 is being tested clinically. It can be given orally and is metabolized to ICRF-154.[499] Its antitumor activity is dependent on the treatment schedule. Fractionated oral doses appear more effective than the same total dose given as a single dose subcutaneously or orally.[499] The dose-limiting toxicity of MST-16 is myelosuppression.[500] No activity was observed in solid tumors, but a 30% objective response rate was noted in NHL and T-cell leukemia patients.[49,50] As a result, MST-16 obtained official approval in Japan for this disease.

The dioxopiperazine derivatives, like other top2 inhibitors, appear to cause secondary AML.[501] Surprisingly, the most common cytogenetic abnormalities in these leukemias were translocations t(8;21) and t(15;17), and not mutations in the *MLL* gene. The most common FAB subtypes were M-2 and M-3.

Therapeutic Interactions with the Topoisomerase II Inhibitors

Platinum Derivatives and Bleomycin

Therapeutic synergy between VP-16 and *cis*-platinum has been demonstrated, and this combination is effective in the treatment of germ cell tumors and SCLCs.[502] In patients with testicular germ line cancers, the association PEB produces survival in 90% to 95% of all patients, including

patients with metastatic tumors.[503] This combination is also used in non-SCLCs or in locally advanced esophagus cancers in addition to irradiation.[504,505] The synergism between VP-16 and platinum derivatives has also been found in experimental systems,[506] but its mechanisms remain poorly understood. Top2 inhibition might interfere with the repair of the platinum cross-links or produce complex DNA damages that might be inefficiently repaired in tumor cells. Concomitant administration of cisplatin has also been reported to reduce the total clearance of VP-16.[293]

Topoisomerase I Inhibitors: the Camptothecins

The interactions between inhibitors of top1 and top2 are complex. In cell culture experiments, simultaneous exposure to VP-16 and to the top1 inhibitor camptothecin is antagonistic unless the two drugs are administered with a 4- to 6-hour interval.[221] This *in vitro* antagonism has been confirmed in mouse xenograft systems *in vivo* for the association of VP-16 with either of the two camptothecin derivatives, CPT-11 (irinotecan)[507] or topotecan.[508] Cell-cycle responses probably play a key role in the antagonism observed in these simultaneous exposure schedules. Top2 inhibitors deplete the S-phase cells by producing a G_2 arrest, while top1 inhibitors are most cytotoxic in S phase because of a requirement of active replication for the generation of irreversible DNA lesions.[221,509] In the sequential schedules, compensatory enzyme changes might contribute to the enhanced activity. The combination of a top1 inhibitor with a top2 inhibitor is associated with a depletion of the target topoisomerase mRNA and protein with reciprocal increases in the alternate topoisomerase mRNA and, to a lesser extent, protein.[507] A compensatory increase in top2α and increased sensitivity to VP-16 have been reported after treatment with topotecan.[508] The top2α levels declined 5 days after the last dose of topotecan and resulted in restoration of the original response of xenografts to VP-16.[508] Hence, schedule dependency plays a crucial role to optimize the effectiveness of combination chemotherapy with top1 and top2 inhibitors.

Despite these experimental findings, most clinical trials to date have explored simultaneous administration of either CPT-11 or topotecan with VP-16. A phase I combination study was conducted, starting with 30 mg per m² per day CPT-11 and 40 mg per m² per day VP-16 given simultaneously from day 1 to 3. Cytolysis and hyperbilirubinemia were observed as dose-limiting toxicities from this first dose level. The roles of the SN-38 enterohepatic circulation and of drug-drug interactions have been suggested.[510] Another phase I combination study tested 60 to 90 mg per m² per day CPT-11 at days 1, 8, and 15, with 80 mg per m² per day VP-16 from day 1 to 3, every 3 weeks, with G-CSF support.[511] Dose-limiting toxicities were diarrhea and leukopenia.[511] The concurrent administration of CPT-11 and

VP-16 for 3 days has also been evaluated.[512] The main dose-limiting toxicity was diarrhea. Granulocytopenia was also severe. The recommended dosages were 60 mg per m^2 per day in combination with 60 mg per m^2 per day CPT-11 and required prophylactic administration of G-CSF.[512] The concurrent administration of 5-day VP-16 and CPT-11 led to granulocytopenia as dose-limiting toxicity.[331] Several phase II clinical trials have combined VP-16 with either CPT-11[513] or topotecan.[514]

The sequential administration of topotecan (72-hour continuous infusion on days 1 to 3) and VP-16 (75 or 100 mg per m^2 per day as a 2-hour infusion on days 8 to 10) has been studied in patients with solid tumors.[515] Two of the six patients' tumors in which top1 was successively measured had either modest or substantial decrements in top1 levels after topotecan treatment, whereas in one of these six patients, tumor top2 levels increased.[515] Sequential administration of IV topotecan and oral VP-16 was also evaluated but not at optimum intervals.[516]

Ongoing studies will determine whether the association of top2 and top1 inhibitors is of clinical value. Tumor heterogeneity might contribute to the efficacy of concurrent administrations of top2 and top1 inhibitors. S-phase cells might be most sensitive to camptothecins, whereas the cytotoxicity of top2 inhibitors is less cell-cycle dependent. Local pharmacokinetics might also be a contributing factor. It will be interesting to evaluate clinical protocols, including sequential treatments with top2 and top1 inhibitors.

Association of Topoisomerase II Inhibitors

Top2 inhibitors are commonly combined together. VP-16 is commonly given with adriamycin in various combination protocols for the treatment of Hodgkin's lymphomas. Mitoxantrone and VP-16 or m-AMSA and VP-16 have been combined in AML.[517] Such associations may be justified because anthracyclines and mitoxantrone exhibit marked differences in the genomic location of cleavage complexes and therefore may selectively target different portions of the genome (see Base-Sequence Preference of Topoisomerase II Inhibitors and Drug-Binding Model).[119]

Antimetabolites and Nucleosides

VM-26 and VP-16 slow the efflux of methotrexate and methotrexate polyglutamates and thereby increase intracellular drug accumulation.[518] Thus, *in vitro* data suggest a synergistic effect for combination therapy of VP-16 with methotrexate,[519] but this has not been demonstrated in clinical trials.

Drug-scheduling experiments to increase the fraction of cells in S phase have been carried out to target cells with high top2 content. Using murine leukemia L1210 cells, Minford et al. have found that sublethal doses of ara-C and hydroxyurea potentiate the cytotoxicity of anthracyclines and m-AMSA.[520]

5-Azacytidine also potentiates the cytotoxicity of m-AMSA.[521] 5-Aza-2'-deoxycytidine combined with m-AMSA has been successfully applied in the treatment of patients with a relapse of AML or ALL.[522] The effect of azacitidine may be due to DNA demethylation, which increases top2-mediated DNA cleavage by m-AMSA and epipodophyllotoxins.[523]

Growth Factors, Hormones, Cytokines, and Potential New Strategies

The human colony-stimulating factors accelerate hematopoietic recovery from VP-16–induced myelosuppression. In addition, colony-stimulating factors may limit VP-16–induced myelosuppression by inhibiting apoptosis in the normal bone marrow cells. Colony-stimulating factors can also modulate the growth and drug response of tumor cells with functional receptors for these cytokines. G-CSF enhances VP-16–containing standard chemotherapy when given until 48 hours before the next chemotherapy course.[524]

Combinations of tumor necrosis factor and epipodophyllotoxins produce dose-dependent synergism.[525–528] This potentiation may be due to topoisomerase activation with increase of cleavage complexes, to enhanced apoptosis, or both. Association of top2 inhibitors and inducers of apoptosis is an exciting approach. Bcl-2 overexpression has been shown in experimental systems to increase resistance to VP-16.[529] Conversely, Bcl-2 inhibition might enhance the activity of top2 inhibitors. It might be possible to enhance apoptosis in tumor cells treated with top2 inhibitors by down-regulating the nuclear factor-κB (NF-κB) pathway[530–532] or by inhibiting the cell-surface receptor pathways that inhibit apoptosis and control cell-cycle progression.[533] A sequence-dependent synergism was recently observed between VP-16 and the cyclin kinase inhibitor flavopiridol,[534] which suggests that cell-cycle checkpoint inhibitors might potentiate the efficacy of top2 inhibitors (see *N*-[2-(Dimethylamino)Ethyl]Acridine-4-Carboxamide).

REFERENCES

1. Ross WE, Glaubiger DL, Kohn KW. Protein-associated DNA breaks in cells treated with adriamycin or ellipticine. *Biochim Biophys Acta* 1978;519:23.
2. Ross WE, Glaubiger D, Kohn KW. Qualitative and quantitative aspects of intercalator-induced DNA strand breaks. *Biochim Biophys Acta* 1979;562:41.
3. Zwelling LA, Michaels S, Erickson LC, et al. Protein-associated deoxyribonucleic acid strand breaks in L1210 cells treated with the deoxyribonucleic acid intercalating agents 4'-(9-acridinylamino) methanesulfon-m-anisidide and adriamycin. *Biochemistry* 1981;20:6553.
4. Pommier Y, Kerrigan D, Schwartz R, et al. The formation and resealing of intercalator-induced DNA strand breaks in

isolated L1210 cell nuclei. *Biochem Biophys Res Commun* 1982;107:576.

5. Nelson EM, Tewey KM, Liu LF. Mechanism of antitumor drug action: poisoning of mammalian DNA topoisomerase II on DNA by 4'-(9-acridinylamino)-methanesulfon-m-anisidide. *Proc Natl Acad Sci U S A* 1984;81:1361.

6. Minford J, Pommier Y, Filipski J, et al. Isolation of intercalator-dependent protein-linked DNA strand cleavage activity from cell nuclei and identification as topoisomerase II. *Biochemistry* 1986;25:9.

7. Felix CA. Secondary leukemias induced by topoisomerase-targeted drugs. *Biochim Biophys Acta* 1998;1400:233.

8. Cragg G, Suffness M. Metabolism of plant-derived anticancer agents. *Pharmacol Ther* 1988;37:425.

9. Senter PD, Saulnier MG, Schreiber GJ, et al. Anti-tumor effects of antibody-alkaline phosphatase conjugates in combination with etoposide phosphate. *Proc Natl Acad Sci U S A* 1988;85:4842.

10. Haisma HJ, Boven E, van Muijen M, et al. Analysis of a conjugate between anti-carcinoembryonic antigen monoclonal antibody and alkaline phosphatase for specific activation of the prodrug etoposide phosphate. *Cancer Immunol Immunother* 1992;34:343.

11. Belani CP, Doyle LA, Aisner J. Etoposide: current status and future perspectives in the management of malignant neoplasms. *Cancer Chemother Pharmacol* 1994;34:S118.

12. Armitage JO. Bone marrow transplantation [see comments]. *N Engl J Med* 1994;330:827.

13. Blume KG, Long GD, Negrin RS, et al. Role of etoposide (VP-16) in preparatory regimens for patients with leukemia or lymphoma undergoing allogeneic bone marrow transplantation. *Bone Marrow Transplant* 1994;14:S9.

14. Ihde DC. Chemotherapy of lung cancer. *N Engl J Med* 1992;327:1434.

15. Richie JP. Detection and treatment of testicular cancer. *CA Cancer J Clin* 1993;43:151.

16. Bjorkholm M. Etoposide and teniposide in the treatment of acute leukemia. *Med Oncol Tumor Phar* 1990;7:3.

17. Amylon MD, Shuster J, Pullen J, et al. Intensive high-dose asparaginase consolidation improves survival for pediatric patients with T cell acute lymphoblastic leukemia and advanced stage lymphoblastic lymphoma: a Pediatric Oncology Group study. *Leukemia* 1999;13:335.

18. Campbell M, Salgado C, Quintana J, et al. Improved outcome for acute lymphoblastic leukemia in children of a developing country: results of a Chilean trial PINDA 87. *Med Pediatr Oncol* 1999;33:88.

19. Solal-Celigny P, Lepage E, Brousse N, et al. Doxorubicin-containing regimen with or without interferon alfa-2b for advanced follicular lymphomas: final analysis of survival and toxicity in the Groupe d'Etude des Lymphomes Folliculaires 86 trial. *J Clin Oncol* 1998;16:2332.

20. Oishi N, Berenberg J, Blumenstein BA, et al. Teniposide in metastatic renal and bladder cancer—a Southwest Oncology Group Study. *Cancer Treat Rep* 1987;71:1307.

21. Lum BL, Torti FM. Adjuvant intravesicular pharmacotherapy for superficial bladder cancer. *J Natl Cancer Inst* 1991;83:682.

22. Bowman LC, Castleberry RP, Cantor A, et al. Genetic staging of unresectable or metastatic neuroblastoma in infants: a Pediatric Oncology Group Study. *J Natl Cancer Inst* 1997;89:373.

23. Grozea PN, Crowley JJ, Canfield VA, et al. Teniposide (VM-26) as a single drug treatment for patients with extensive small cell lung carcinoma—a phase II study of the Southwest Oncology Group. *Cancer* 1997;80:1029.

24. Lokich JJ. Teniposide (VM-26) as a single drug treatment for patients with extensive small cell lung carcinoma: a phase II study of the southwest oncology group. *Cancer* 1998;82:993.

25. Brandes AA, Rigon A, Zampieri P, et al. Carboplatin and teniposide concurrent with radiotherapy in patients with glioblastoma multiforme—a phase II study. *Cancer* 1998;82:355.

26. Cain BF, Atwell GJ. The experimental antitumour properties of three congeners of the acridylmethanesulphonanilide (AMSA) series. *Eur J Cancer* 1974;10:539.

27. Arlin ZA, Ahmed T, Mittelman A, et al. A new regimen of amsacrine with high-dose cytarabine is safe and effective therapy for acute leukemia. *J Clin Oncol* 1987;5:371.

28. Berman E, Arlin ZA, Gaynor J, et al. Comparative trial of cytarabine and thioguanine in combination with amsacrine or daunorubicin in patients with untreated acute nonlymphocytic leukemia: results of the L-16M protocol. *Leukemia* 1989;3:115.

29. Vogler WR, Preisler HD, Winton EF, et al. Randomized trial of high-dose cytarabine versus amsacrine in acute myelogenous leukemia in relapse: a Leukemia Intergroup Study. *Cancer Treat Rep* 1986;70:455.

30. Miller LP, Pyesmany AF, Wolff LJ, et al. Successful reinduction therapy with amsacrine and cyclocytidine in acute nonlymphoblastic leukemia in children: a report from the Childrens Cancer Study Group. *Cancer* 1991;67:2235.

31. Freund M, Giller S, Hinrichs F, et al. Five-day 4'-(9-acridinylamino)methanesulphon-m-anisidide and intermediate-dose cytosine arabinoside in high-risk relapsing or refractory acute myeloid leukemia. *J Cancer Res Clin Oncol* 1991;117:489.

32. Jehn U, Heinemann V. Phase-II study of treatment of refractory acute leukemia with intermediate-dose cytosine arabinoside and amsacrine. *Ann Hematol* 1993;66:131.

33. Harousseau JL, Milpied N, Briere J, et al. Double intensive consolidation chemotherapy in adult acute myeloid leukemia. *J Clin Oncol* 1991;9:1432.

34. Hayat M, Ostronoff M, Gilles E, et al. Salvage therapy with methyl-gag, high-dose Ara-C, M-Amsa, and ifosfamide (MAMI) for recurrent or refractory lymphoma. *Cancer Invest* 1990;8:1.

35. Cassileth PA, Gale RP. Amsacrine: a review. *Leuk Res* 1986;10:1257.

36. Baguley BC, Zhuang L, Marshall E. Experimental solid tumour activity of N-[2-(dimethylamino)ethyl]acridine-4-carboxamide. *Cancer Chemother Pharmacol* 1995;36:244.

37. Bridewell DJA, Finlay GJ, Baguley BC. Mechanism of cytotoxicity of N-[2-(dimethylamino)ethyl]acridine-4-carboxamide and of its 7-chloro derivative: the roles of topoisomerases I and II. *Cancer Chemother Pharmacol* 1999;43:302.

38. Gamage SA, Spicer JA, Atwell GJ, et al. Structure-activity relationships for substituted Bis(acridine-4-carboxamides): a new class of anticancer agents. *J Med Chem* 1999;42:2383.

39. Paoletti C, Le Pecq JB, Dat-Xuong N, et al. Antitumor activity, pharmacology, and toxicity of ellipticines, ellipti-

cinium, and 9-hydroxy derivatives: preliminary clinical trials of 2-methyl-9-hydroxy ellipticinium (NSC 264-137). *Rec Res Cancer Res* 1980;74:107.

40. Le Mee S, Pierre A, Markovits J, et al. S16020-2, a new highly cytotoxic antitumor olivacine derivative: DNA interaction and DNA topoisomerase II inhibition. *Mol Pharmacol* 1998;53:213.

41. Leonce S, Perez V, Casabianca Pignede MR, et al. In vitro cytotoxicity of S 16020-2, a new olivacine derivative. *Invest New Drugs* 1996;14:169.

42. Guilbaud N, Kraus-Berthier L, Saint-Dizier D, et al. In vivo antitumor activity of S16020-2, a new olivacine derivative. *Cancer Chemother Pharmacol* 1996;38:513.

43. Guilbaud N, Kraus-Berthier L, Saint-Dizier D, et al. Antitumor activity of S16020-2 in two orthotopic models of lung cancer. *Anticancer Drugs* 1997;8:276.

44. Kraus-Berthier L, Guilbaud N, Jan M, et al. Experimental antitumour activity of S16020-2 in a panel of human tumours. *Eur J Cancer* 1997;33:1881.

45. Awada A, Bleiberg H, Gil T, et al. Phase I study of S16020 a topoisomerase II inhibitor given q 3 w as a 3-h infusion. *Proc Am Assoc Cancer Res* 1999;40:682 (abstr. 4501).

46. Earhart RH, Tutsch KD, Koeller JM, et al. Pharmacokinetics of (+)-1,2-di(3,5-dioxopiperazin-1-yl)Propane intravenous infusions in adult cancer patients. *Cancer Res* 1982;42:5255.

47. Speyer JL, Green MD, Kramer E, et al. Protective effect of the bispiperazinedione ICRF-187 against doxorubicin induced cardiac toxicity in women with advanced breast cancer. *N Engl J Med* 1988;319:745.

48. Speyer JL, Green MD, Zeleniuch-Jacquotte A, et al. ICRF-187 permits longer treatment with doxorubicin in women with breast cancer. *J Clin Oncol* 1992;10:117.

49. Ohno R, Yamada K, Hirano M, et al. The Tokai Blood Cancer Study Group: phase II study: treatment of non-Hodgkin's lymphoma with an oral antitumor derivative of bis(2,6-dioxopiperazine). *J Natl Cancer Inst* 1992;84:435.

50. Ohno R, Masaoka T, Shirakawa S, et al. Treatment of adult T-cell leukemia/lymphoma with MST-16, a new oral antitumor drug and a derivative of bis(2,6-dioxopiperazine). *Cancer* 1993;71:2217.

51. Wang JC. DNA topoisomerases. *Annu Rev Biochem* 1996;65:635.

52. Stewart L, Redinbo MR, Qiu X, et al. A model for the mechanism of human topoisomerase I [see comments]. *Science* 1998;279:1534.

53. Pommier Y. DNA topoisomerase II inhibitors. In: Teicher BA, ed. *Cancer therapeutics: experimental and clinical agents.* Totowa, NJ: Humana Press, 1997:153.

54. Wang JC. DNA topoisomerases: why so many? *J Biol Chem* 1991;266:6659.

55. Liu L. *DNA topoisomerases: topoisomerase-targeting drugs.* New York: Academic Press, 1994.

56. Berger JM. Structure of DNA topoisomerases. *Biochim Biophys Acta* 1998;1400:3.

57. Berger JM. Type II DNA topoisomerases. *Curr Opin Struct Biol* 1998;8:26.

58. Burden DA, Osheroff N. Mechanism of action of eukaryotic topoisomerase II and drugs targeted to the enzyme. *Biochim Biophys Acta* 1998;1400:139.

59. Pommier Y, Pourquier P, Fan Y, et al. Mechanism of action of eukaryotic DNA topoisomerase I and drugs targeted to the enzyme. *Biochim Biophys Acta* 1998;1400:83.

60. Nitiss JL. Investigating the biological functions of DNA topoisomerases in eukaryotic cells. *Biochim Biophys Acta* 1998;1400:63.

61. Wallis JW, Chrebet G, Brodsky G, et al. A hyper-recombination mutation in *S. cerevisiae* identifies a novel eukaryotic topoisomerase. *Cell* 1989;58:409.

62. Kim RA, Wang JC. Identification of the yeast TOP3 gene product as a single strand-specific DNA topoisomerase. *J Biol Chem* 1992;267:17178.

63. Goulaouic H, Roulon T, Flamand O, et al. Purification and characterization of human DNA topoisomerase III[alpha] [In Process Citation]. *Nucleic Acids Res* 1999;27:2443.

64. Hanai R, Caron PR, Wang JC. Human TOP3: a single-copy gene encoding DNA topoisomerase III. *Proc Natl Acad Sci U S A* 1996;93:3653.

65. Kawasaki K, Minoshima S, Nakato E, et al. One-megabase sequence analysis of the human immunoglobulin lambda gene locus. *Genome Res* 1997;7:250.

66. Li W, Wang JC. Mammalian DNA topoisomerase IIIalpha is essential in early embryogenesis. *Proc Natl Acad Sci U S A* 1998;95:1010.

67. Seki T, Seki M, Katada T, et al. Isolation of a cDNA encoding mouse DNA topoisomerase III which is highly expressed at the mRNA level in the testis. *Biochim Biophys Acta* 1998;1396:127.

68. Seki T, Seki M, Onodera R, et al. Cloning of cDNA encoding a novel mouse DNA topoisomerase III (Topo IIIbeta) possessing negatively supercoiled DNA relaxing activity, whose message is highly expressed in the testis. *J Biol Chem* 1998;273:28553.

69. Levine C, Hiasa H, Marians KJ. DNA gyrase and topoisomerase IV: biochemical activities, physiological roles during chromosome replication, and drug sensitivities. *Biochim Biophys Acta* 1998;1400:29.

70. Hooper DC. Clinical applications of quinolones. *Biochim Biophys Acta* 1998;1400:45.

71. Adachi Y, Luke M, Laemmli UK. Chromosome assembly in vitro: topoisomerase II is required for condensation. *Cell* 1991;64:137.

72. Holm C, Goto T, Wang JC, et al. DNA topoisomerase II is required at the time of mitosis in yeast. *Cell* 1985;41:553.

73. Hirano T, Mitchison TJ. Topoisomerase II does not play a scaffolding role in the organization of mitotic chromosomes assembled in Xenopus egg extracts. *J Cell Biol* 1993;120:601.

74. Gasser SM, Laroche T, Falquet J, et al. Metaphase chromosome structure. Involvement of topoisomerase II. *J Mol Biol* 1986;188:613.

75. DiNardo S, Voelkel K, Sternglanz R. DNA topoisomerase II mutant of *Saccharomyces cerevisiae*: topoisomerase II is required for segregation of daughter molecules at the termination of DNA replication. *Proc Natl Acad Sci U S A* 1984;81:2616.

76. Holm C, Stearns T, Botstein D. DNA topoisomerase II must act at mitosis to prevent nondisjunction and chromosome breakage. *Mol Cell Biol* 1989;9:159.

77. Uemura T, Ohkura H, Adachi Y, et al. DNA topoisomerase II is required for condensation and separation of mitotic chromosomes in *S. pombe*. *Cell* 1987;50:917.

78. Moens PB. Unravelling meiotic chromosomes: topoisomerase II and other proteins. *J Cell Sci* 1990;97:1.

79. Rose D, Holm C. Meiosis-specific arrest revealed in DNA topoisomerase II mutants. *Mol Cell Biol* 1993;13:3445.

80. Drake FH, Zimmerman JP, McCabe FL, et al. Purification of topoisomerase II from amsacrine-resistant P388 leukemia cells. Evidence for two forms of the enzyme. *J Biol Chem* 1987;262:16739.

81. Drake FH, Hofmann GA, Bartus HF, et al. Biochemical and pharmacological properties of p170 and p180 forms of topoisomerase II. *Biochemistry* 1989;28:8154.

82. Tan KB, Dorman TE, Falls KM, et al. Topoisomerase II alpha and topoisomerase II beta genes: characterization and mapping to human chromosomes 17 and 3, respectively. *Cancer Res* 1992;52:231.

83. Jenkins JR, Ayton P, Jones T, et al. Isolation of cDNA clones encoding the beta isozyme of human DNA topoisomerase II and localisation of the gene to chromosome 3p24. *Nucleic Acids Res* 1992;20:5587.

84. Austin CA, Sng JH, Patel S, et al. Novel HeLa topoisomerase II is the II beta isoform: complete coding sequence and homology with other type II topoisomerases. *Biochim Biophys Acta* 1993;1172:283.

85. Tsutsui K, Okada S, Watanabe M, et al. Molecular cloning of partial cDNAs for rat DNA topoisomerase II isoforms and their differential expression in brain development. *J Biol Chem* 1993;268:19076.

86. Woessner RD, Mattern MR, Mirabelli CK, et al. Proliferation- and cell cycle-dependent differences in expression of the 170 kilodalton and 180 kilodalton forms of topoisomerase II in NIH-3T3 cells. *Cell Growth Differ* 1991;2:209.

87. Capranico G, Tinelli S, Austin CA, et al. Different patterns of gene expression of topoisomerase II isoforms in differentiated tissues during murine development. *Biochim Biophys Acta* 1992;1132:43.

88. Kimura K, Saijo M, Ui M, et al. Growth state- and cell cycle-dependent fluctuation in the expression of two forms of DNA topoisomerase II and possible specific modification of the higher molecular weight form in the M phase. *J Biol Chem* 1994;269:1173.

89. Zini N, Martelli AM, Sabatelli P, et al. The 180-kDa isoform of topoisomerase II is localized in the nucleolus and belongs to the structural elements of the nucleolar remnant. *Exp Cell Res* 1992;200:460.

90. Negri C, Scovassi AI, Braghetti A, et al. DNA topoisomerase II beta: stability and distribution in different animal cells in comparison to DNA topoisomerase I and II alpha. *Exp Cell Res* 1993;206:128.

91. Petrov P, Drake FH, Loranger A, et al Localization of DNA topoisomerase II in Chinese hamster fibroblasts by confocal and electron microscopy. *Exp Cell Res* 1993;204:73.

92. Juenke JM, Holden JA. The distribution of DNA topoisomerase II isoforms in differentiated adult mouse tissues. *Biochim Biophys Acta* 1993;216:191.

93. Saijo M, Ui M, Enomoto T. Growth state and cell cycle dependent phosphorylation of DNA topoisomerase II in Swiss 3T3 cells. *Biochemistry* 1992;31:359.

94. Burden DA, Goldsmith LJ, Sullivan DM. Cell-cycle-dependent phosphorylation and activity of Chinese-hamster ovary topoisomerase II. *Biochem J* 1993;293:297.

95. Hsiang YH, Wu HY, Liu LF. Proliferation-dependent regulation of DNA topoisomerase II in cultured human cells. *Cancer Res* 1988;48:3230.

96. Sullivan DM, Latham MD, Ross WE. Proliferation-dependent topoisomerase II content as a determinant of antineoplastic drug action in human, mouse, and Chinese hamster ovary cells. *Cancer Res* 1987;47:3973.

97. Wang JC. Moving one DNA double helix through another by a type II DNA topoisomerase: the story of a simple molecular machine. *Q Rev Biophys* 1998;31:107.

98. Osheroff N. Biochemical basis for the interactions of type I and type II topoisomerases with DNA. *Pharmacol Ther* 1989;41:223.

99. Watt PM, Hickson ID. Structure and function of type II DNA topoisomerases. *Biochem J* 1994;303:681.

100. Roca J. The mechanisms of DNA topoisomerases. *Trends Biochem Sci* 1995;20:156.

101. Berger JM, Gamblin SJ, Harrison SC, et al. Structure and mechanism of DNA topoisomerase II [published erratum appears in *Nature* 1996;380:179]. *Nature* 1996;379:225.

102. Roca J, Wang JC. DNA transport by a type II DNA topoisomerase: evidence in favor of a two-gate mechanism. *Cell* 1994;77:609.

103. Pourquier P, Kohlhagen G, Ueng L-M, et al. Topoisomerase I and II activity assays. In: Brown R, Böger-Brown U, eds. *Methods in molecular medicine: cytotoxic drug resistance mechanisms.* Totowa, NJ: Humana Press, 1999:95.

104. Andoh T, Ishida R. Catalytic inhibitors of DNA topoisomerase II. *Biochim Biophys Acta* 1998;1400:155.

105. Corbett AH, Osheroff N. When good enzymes go bad: conversion of topoisomerase II to a cellular toxin by antineoplastic drugs. *Chem Res Toxicol* 1993;6:585.

106. Shaw JL, Blanco J, Mueller GC. A simple procedure for isolation of DNA, RNA and protein fractions from cultured animal cells. *Anal Biochem* 1975;65:125.

107. Subramanian D, Kraut E, Staubus A, et al. Analysis of topoisomerase I/DNA complexes in patients administered topotecan. *Cancer Res* 1995;55:2097.

108. Pommier Y, Schwartz RE, Zwelling LA, et al. Effects of DNA intercalating agents on topoisomerase II induced DNA strand cleavage in isolated mammalian cell nuclei. *Biochemistry* 1985;24:6406.

109. Tewey KM, Chen GL, Nelson EM, et al. Intercalative antitumor drugs interfere with the breakage-reunion reaction of mammalian DNA topoisomerase II. *J Biol Chem* 1984;259:9182.

110. Drake FH, Hofmann GA, Mong SM, et al. In vitro and intracellular inhibition of topoisomerase II by the antitumor agent merbarone. *Cancer Res* 1989;49:2578.

111. Ishida R, Miki T, Narita T, et al. Inhibition of intracellular topoisomerase II by antitumor bis(2,6-dioxopiperazine) derivatives: mode of cell growth inhibition distinct from that of cleavable complex-forming type inhibitors. *Cancer Res* 1991;51:4909.

112. Tanabe K, Ikegami Y, Ishida R, et al. Inhibition of topoisomerase II by antitumor agents bis(2,6-dioxopiperazine) derivatives. *Cancer Res* 1991;51:4903.

113. Roca J, Ishida R, Berger JM, et al. Antitumor bisdioxopiperazines inhibit yeast DNA topoisomerase II by trapping the enzyme in the form of a closed protein clamp. *Proc Natl Acad Sci U S A* 1994;91:1781.

114. Andoh T. Bis(2,6-dioxopiperazines), catalytic inhibitors of DNA topoisomerase II, as molecular probes, cardioprotectors and antitumor drugs. *Biochimie* 1998;80:235.

115. Zwelling LA, Michaels S, Kerrigan D, et al. Protein-associated deoxyribonucleic acid strand breaks produced in mouse leukemia L1210 cells by ellipticine and 2-methyl-9-hydroxyellipticinium. *Biochem Pharmacol* 1982;31:3261.

116. Zwelling LA, Kerrigan D, Michaels S. Cytotoxicity and DNA strand breaks by 5-iminodaunorubicin in mouse leukemia L1210 cells: comparison with adriamycin and 4'-(9-acridinylamino)methanesulfon-m-anisidide. *Cancer Res* 1982;42:2687.

117. Pommier Y, Zwelling LA, Kao-Shan CS, et al. Correlations between intercalator-induced DNA strand breaks and sister chromatid exchanges, mutations, and cytotoxicity in Chinese hamster cells. *Cancer Res* 1985;45:3143.

118. Long BH, Musial ST, Brattain MG. Single- and double-strand DNA breakage and repair in human lung adenocarcinoma cells exposed to etoposide and teniposide. *Cancer Res* 1985;45:3106.

119. Pommier Y, Orr A, Kohn KW, et al. Differential effects of amsacrine and epipodophyllotoxins on topoisomerase II cleavage in the human c-myc protooncogene. *Cancer Res* 1992;52:3125.

120. Capranico G, Zunino F, Kohn KW, et al. Sequence-selective topoisomerase II inhibition by anthracycline derivatives in SV40 DNA: relationship with DNA binding affinity and cytotoxicity. *Biochemistry* 1990;29:562.

121. Capranico G, Kohn KW, Pommier Y. Local sequence requirements for DNA cleavage by mammalian topoisomerase II in the presence of doxorubicin. *Nucleic Acids Res* 1990;18:6611.

122. Capranico G, De Isabella P, Tinelli S, et al. Similar sequence specificity of mitoxantrone and VM-26 stimulation of in vitro DNA cleavage by mammalian DNA topoisomerase II. *Biochemistry* 1993;32:3038.

123. Capranico G, Binaschi M. DNA sequence selectivity of topoisomerases and topoisomerase poisons. *Biochim Biophys Acta* 1998;1400:185.

124. Freudenreich CH, Kreuzer KN. Mutational analysis of a type II topoisomerase cleavage site: distinct requirements for enzyme and inhibitors. *Embo J* 1993;12:2085.

125. Jaxel C, Kohn KW, Wani MC, et al. Structure-activity study of the actions of camptothecin derivatives on mammalian topoisomerase I: evidence for a specific receptor site and a relation to antitumor activity. *Cancer Res* 1989;49:1465.

126. Pommier Y, Capranico G, Orr A, et al. Local base sequence preferences for DNA cleavage by mammalian topoisomerase II in the presence of amsacrine or teniposide [published erratum appears in *Nucleic Acids Res* 1991;19:7003]. *Nucleic Acids Res* 1991;19:5973.

127. Pommier Y, Kohn KW, Capranico G, et al. Base sequence selectivity of topoisomerase inhibitors suggests a common model for drug action. In: Andoh T, Ikeda H, Oguro M, ed. *Molecular biology of DNA topoisomerases and its application to chemotherapy*. Boca Raton, FL: CRC Press, 1993: 215.

128. Strumberg D, Nitiss JL, Dong J, et al. Molecular analysis of yeast and human type II topoisomerases: enzyme-DNA and drug interactions. *J Biol Chem* 1999;274:28246.

129. Svejstrup JQ, Christiansen K, Gromova II, et al. New technique for uncoupling the cleavage and religation reactions of eukaryotic topoisomerase I. The mode of action of camptothecin at a specific recognition site. *J Mol Biol* 1991;222:669.

130. Robinson MJ, Osheroff N. Effects of antineoplastic drugs on the post-strand-passage DNA cleavage/religation equilibrium of topoisomerase II. *Biochemistry* 1991;30:1807.

131. Freudenreich CH, Kreuzer KN. Localization of an aminoacridine antitumor agent in a type II topoisomerase-DNA complex. *Proc Natl Acad Sci U S A* 1994;91:11007.

132. Kwok Y, Zeng Q, Hurley LH. Structural insight into a quinolone-topoisomerase II-DNA complex. Further evidence for a 2:2 quinobenzoxazine-mg2+ self-assembly model formed in the presence of topoisomerase ii. *J Biol Chem* 1999;274:17226.

133. Kingma PS, Osheroff N. Apurinic sites are position-specific topoisomerase II poisons. *J Biol Chem* 1997;272:1148.

134. Bigioni M, Zunino F, Capranico G. Base mutation analysis of topoisomerase II-idarubicin-DNA ternary complex formation. Evidence for enzyme subunit cooperativity in DNA cleavage. *Nucleic Acids Res* 1994;22:2274.

135. Strumberg D, Nitiss JL, Rose A, et al. Mutation of a conserved serine residue in a quinolone-resistant type II topoisomerase alters the enzyme-DNA and drug interactions. *J Biol Chem* 1999;274:7292.

136. Hsiung Y, Elsea SH, Osheroff N, et al. A mutation in yeast TOP2 homologous to a quinolone-resistant mutation in bacteria. Mutation of the amino acid homologous to Ser83 of *Escherichia coli* gyrA alters sensitivity to eukaryotic topoisomerase inhibitors. *J Biol Chem* 1995;270:20359.

137. Gottesman MM, Pastan I. The multidrug transporter, a double-edged sword. *J Biol Chem* 1988;263:12163.

138. Beck WT. Modulators of P-glycoprotein-associated multidrug resistance. *Cancer Treat Res* 1991;57:151.

139. Granzen B, Graves DE, Baguley BC, et al. Structure-activity studies of amsacrine analogs in drug resistant human leukemia cell lines expressing either altered DNA topoisomerase II or P-glycoprotein. *Oncol Res* 1992;4:489.

140. Borrel MN, Fiallo M, Priebe W, et al. P-glycoprotein-mediated efflux of hydroxyrubicin, a neutral anthracycline derivative, in resistant K562 cells. *FEBS Lett* 1994;356:287.

141. Solary E, Ling YH, Perez-Soler R, et al. Hydroxyrubicin, a deaminated derivative of doxorubicin, inhibits mammalian DNA topoisomerase II and partially circumvents multidrug resistance. *Int J Cancer* 1994;58:85.

142. Cole SP, Bhardwaj G, Gerlach JH, et al. Overexpression of a transporter gene in a multidrug-resistant human lung cancer cell line [see comments]. *Science* 1992;258:1650.

143. Barrand MA, Heppell-Parton AC, Wright KA, et al. A 190-kilodalton protein overexpressed in non-P-glycoprotein-containing multidrug-resistant cells and its relationship to the MRP gene. *J Natl Cancer Inst* 1994;86:110.

144. Schneider E, Horton JK, Yang CH, et al. Multidrug resistance-associated protein gene overexpression and reduced drug sensitivity of topoisomerase II in a human breast carcinoma MCF7 cell line selected for etoposide resistance. *Cancer Res* 1994;54:152.

145. Scheffer GL, Wijngaard PL, Flens MJ, et al. The drug resistance-related protein LRP is the human major vault protein [see comments]. *Nat Med* 1995;1:578.

146. Marquardt D, McCrone S, Center MS. Mechanisms of multidrug resistance in HL60 cells: detection of resistance-

associated proteins with antibodies against synthetic peptides that correspond to the deduced sequence of P-glycoprotein. *Cancer Res* 1990;50:1426.

147. Myers CE, Chabner BA. In: Chabner BA, Collins JM, eds. *Cancer chemotherapy: principles and practice.* Philadelphia: Lippincott Williams & Wilkins, 1990:356.

148. Taatjes DJ, Gaudiano G, Resing K, et al. Redox pathway leading to the alkylation of DNA by the anthracycline, antitumor drugs adriamycin and daunomycin. *J Med Chem* 1997;40:1276.

149. Dusre L, Mimnaugh EG, Myers CE, et al. Potentiation of doxorubicin cytotoxicity by buthionine sulfoximine in multidrug-resistant human breast tumor cells. *Cancer Res* 1989;49:511.

150. Ishikawa T. The ATP-dependent glutathione S-conjugate export pump [see comments]. *Trends Biochem Sci* 1992; 17:463.

151. Leteurtre F, Madalengoitia J, Orr A, et al. Rational design and molecular effects of a new topoisomerase II inhibitor, azatoxin [published erratum appears in *Cancer Res* 1992; 52:6136]. *Cancer Res* 52:4478, 1992.

152. Sinha BK, Politi PM, Eliot HM, et al. Structure-activity relations, cytotoxicity and topoisomerase II dependent cleavage induced by pendulum ring analogs of etoposide. *Eur J Cancer* 1990;26:590.

153. Long BH, Musial ST, Brattain MG. Comparison of cytotoxicity and DNA breakage activity of congeners of podophyllotoxin including VP16-213 and VM26: a quantitative structure-activity relationship. *Biochemistry* 1984; 23:1183.

154. Gantchev TG, Hunting DJ. The ortho-quinone metabolite of the anticancer drug etoposide (VP-16) is a potent inhibitor of the topoisomerase II/DNA cleavable complex. *Mol Pharmacol* 1998;53:422.

155. Sinha BK, Trush MA, Kalyanaraman B. Microsomal interactions and inhibition of lipid peroxidation by etoposide (VP-16, 213): implications for mode of action. *Biochem Pharmacol* 1985;34:2036.

156. Sinha BK. Free radicals in anticancer drug pharmacology. *Chem Biol Interact* 1989;69:293.

157. Sinha BK, Eliot HM. Etoposide-induced DNA damage in human tumor cells: requirement for cellular activating factors. *Biochim Biophys Acta* 1991;1097:111.

158. Auclair C. Multimodal action of antitumor agents on DNA: the ellipticine series. *Arch Biochem Biophys* 1987;259:1.

159. Schuurhuis GJ, van Heijningen TH, Cervantes A, et al. Changes in subcellular doxorubicin distribution and cellular accumulation alone can largely account for doxorubicin resistance in SW-1573 lung cancer and MCF-7 breast cancer multidrug resistant tumour cells. *Br J Cancer* 1993;68:898.

160. Takeda Y, Nishio K, Niitani H, et al. Reversal of multidrug resistance by tyrosine-kinase inhibitors in a non-P-glycoprotein-mediated multidrug-resistant cell line. *Int J Cancer* 1994;57:229.

161. Zwelling LA, Kerrigan D, Michaels S, et al. Cooperative sequestration of m-AMSA in L1210 cells. *Biochem Pharmacol* 1982;31:3269.

162. Schuurhuis GJ, Broxterman HJ, de Lange JH, et al. Early multidrug resistance, defined by changes in intracellular doxorubicin distribution, independent of P-glycoprotein. *Br J Cancer* 1991;64:857.

163. Gervasoni JE Jr, Fields SZ, Krishna S, et al. Subcellular distribution of daunorubicin in P-glycoprotein-positive and -negative drug-resistant cell lines using laser-assisted confocal microscopy. *Cancer Res* 1991;51:4955.

164. Schuurhuis GJ, Broxterman HJ, Ossenkoppele GJ, et al. Functional multidrug resistance phenotype associated with combined overexpression of Pgp/MDR1 and MRP together with 1-beta-D-arabinofuranosylcytosine sensitivity may predict clinical response in acute myeloid leukemia. *Clin Cancer Res* 1995;1:81.

165. Abbaszadegan MR, Cress AE, Futscher BW, et al. Evidence for cytoplasmic P-glycoprotein location associated with increased multidrug resistance and resistance to chemosensitizers. *Cancer Res* 1996;56:5435.

166. Nelson WG, Cho KR, Hsiang YH, et al. Growth-related elevations of DNA topoisomerase II levels found in Dunning R3327 rat prostatic adenocarcinomas. *Cancer Res* 1987;47:3246.

167. Nicklee T, Crump M, Hedley DW. Effects of topoisomerase I inhibition on the expression of topoisomerase II alpha measured with fluorescence image cytometry. *Cytometry* 1996;25:205.

168. Turley H, Comley M, Houlbrook S, et al. The distribution and expression of the two isoforms of DNA topoisomerase II in normal and neoplastic human tissues. *Br J Cancer* 1997;75:1340.

169. Keith WN, Douglas F, Wishart GC, et al. Co-amplification of erbB2, topoisomerase II alpha and retinoic acid receptor alpha genes in breast cancer and allelic loss at topoisomerase I on chromosome 20. *Eur J Cancer* 1993;10:1469.

170. Epstein RJ, Smith PJ, Watson JV, et al. Oestrogen potentiates topoisomerase-II-mediated cytotoxicity in an activated subpopulation of human breast cancer cells: implications for cytotoxic drug resistance in solid tumours. *Int J Cancer* 1989;44:501.

171. Zwelling LA, Kerrigan D, Lippman ME. Protein-associated intercalator-induced DNA scission is enhanced by estrogen stimulation in human breast cancer cells. *Proc Natl Acad Sci U S A* 1983;80:6182.

172. Sorensen M, Sehested M, Jensen PB. Characterisation of a human small-cell lung cancer cell line resistant to the DNA topoisomerase I-directed drug topotecan. *Br J Cancer* 1995;72:399.

173. Hochhauser D, Stanway CA, Harris AL, et al. Cloning and characterization of the 5'-flanking region of the human topoisomerase II alpha gene. *J Biol Chem* 1992;267:18961.

174. Ng SW, Liu Y, Schnipper LE. Cloning and characterization of the 5'-flanking sequence for the human DNA topoisomerase II beta gene. *Gene* 1997;203:113.

175. Constantinou A, Henning-Chubb C, Huberman E. Novobiocin- and phorbol-12-myristate-13-acetate-induced differentiation of human leukemia cells associated with a reduction in topoisomerase II activity. *Cancer Res* 1989;49:1110.

176. Sobczak J, Duguet M. Molecular biology of liver regeneration. *Biochimie* 1986;68:957.

177. Markovits J, Pommier Y, Kerrigan D, et al. Topoisomerase II-mediated DNA breaks and cytotoxicity in relation to cell proliferation and the cell cycle in NIH 3T3 fibroblasts and L1210 leukemia cells. *Cancer Res* 1987;47:2050.

178. Hwong CL, Wang CH, Chen YJ, et al. Induction of topoisomerase II gene expression in human lymphocytes upon phytohemagglutinin stimulation. *Cancer Res* 1990;50:5649S.

179. Deffie AM, Bosman DJ, Goldenberg GJ. Evidence for a mutant allele of the gene for DNA topoisomerase II in adriamycin-resistant P388 murine leukemia cells [published erratum appears in *Cancer Res* 1990;50:449]. *Cancer Res* 1989;49:6879.

180. Webb CD, Latham MD, Lock RB, et al. Attenuated topoisomerase II content directly correlates with a low level of drug resistance in a Chinese hamster ovary cell line. *Cancer Res* 1991;51:6543.

181. Takano H, Kohno K, Ono M, et al Increased phosphorylation of DNA topoisomerase II in etoposide-resistant mutants of human cancer KB cells. *Cancer Res* 1991;51:3951.

182. Charcosset JY, Saucier JM, Jacquemin-Sablon A. Reduced DNA topoisomerase II activity and drug-stimulated DNA cleavage in 9-hydroxyellipticine resistant cells. *Biochem Pharmacol* 1988;37:2145.

183. Tan KB, Mattern MR, Eng WK, et al. Nonproductive rearrangement of DNA topoisomerase I and II genes: correlation with resistance to topoisomerase inhibitors. *J Natl Cancer Inst* 1989;81:1732.

184. Sandri MI, Isaacs RJ, Ongkeko WM, et al. p53 regulates the minimal promoter of the human topoisomerase IIalpha gene. *Nucleic Acids Res* 1996;24:4464.

185. Wang Q, Zambetti GP, Suttle DP. Inhibition of DNA topoisomerase II alpha gene expression by the p53 tumor suppressor. *Mol Cell Biol* 1997;17:389.

186. Yun J, Tomida A, Nagata K, et al. Glucose-regulated stresses confer resistance to etoposide in human cancer cells through a decreased expression of DNA topoisomerase II. *Oncol Res* 1995;7:583.

187. Teicher BA, Holden SA, Rose CM. Effect of oxygen on the cytotoxicity and antitumor activity of etoposide. *J Natl Cancer Inst* 1985;75:1129.

188. Shen JW, Subjeck JR, Lock RB, et al. Depletion of topoisomerase II in isolated nuclei during a glucose-regulated stress response. *Mol Cell Biol* 1989;9:3284.

189. Luk CK, Veinot-Drebot L, Tjan E, et al. Effect of transient hypoxia on sensitivity to doxorubicin in human and murine cell lines. *J Natl Cancer Inst* 1990;82:684.

190. Hashimoto S, Chatterjee S, Ranjit GB, et al. Drastic reduction of topoisomerase II alpha associated with major acquired resistance to topoisomerase II active agents but minor perturbations of cell growth [published erratum appears in *Oncol Res* 1995;7:565]. *Oncol Res* 1995;7:407.

191. Feldhoff PW, Mirski SE, Cole SP, et al. Altered subcellular distribution of topoisomerase II alpha in a drug- resistant human small cell lung cancer cell line. *Cancer Res* 1994;54:756.

192. Kubo T, Kohno K, Ohga T, et al. DNA topoisomerase II alpha gene expression under transcriptional control in etoposide/teniposide-resistant human cancer cells. *Cancer Res* 1995;55:3860.

193. Harker WG, Slade DL, Parr RL, et al. Alterations in the topoisomerase II alpha gene, messenger RNA, and subcellular protein distribution as well as reduced expression of the DNA topoisomerase II beta enzyme in a mitoxantrone-resistant HL-60 human leukemia cell line. *Cancer Res* 1995;55:1707.

194. Dereuddre S, Frey S, Delaporte C, et al. Cloning and characterization of full-length cDNAs coding for the DNA topoisomerase II beta from Chinese hamster lung cells sensitive and resistant 9-OH-ellipticine. *Biochim Biophys Acta* 1995;1264:178.

195. Wessel I, Jensen PB, Falck J, et al. Loss of amino acids 1490Lys-Ser-Lys1492 in the COOH-terminal region of topoisomerase IIalpha in human small cell lung cancer cells selected for resistance to etoposide results in an extranuclear enzyme localization. *Cancer Res* 1997;57:4451.

196. Gupta M, Fujimori A, Pommier Y. Eukaryotic DNA topoisomerases I. *Biochim Biophys Acta* 1995;1262:1.

197. Pommier Y, Gupta M, Valenti M, et al. *Cellular resistance to camptothecins*. New York: The New York Academy of Sciences, 1996.

198. Liu YX, Hsiung Y, Jannatipour M, et al. Yeast topoisomerase II mutants resistant to anti-topoisomerase agents: identification and characterization of new yeast topoisomerase II mutants selected for resistance to etoposide. *Cancer Res* 1994;54:2943.

199. Liu Q, Wang JC. Similarity in the catalysis of DNA breakage and rejoining by type IA and IIA DNA topoisomerases. *Proc Natl Acad Sci U S A* 1999;96:881.

200. Fass D, Bogden CE, Berger JM. Quaternary changes in topoisomerase II may direct orthogonal movement of two DNA strands. *Nat Struct Biol* 1999;6:322.

201. Hinds M, Deisseroth K, Mayes J, et al. Identification of a point mutation in the topoisomerase II gene from a human leukemia cell line containing an amsacrine-resistant form of topoisomerase II. *Cancer Res* 1991;51:4729.

202. Nitiss JL, Liu YX, Harbury P, et al. Amsacrine and etoposide hypersensitivity of yeast cells overexpressing DNA topoisomerase II. *Cancer Res* 1992;52:4467.

203. Zwelling LA, Hinds M, Chan D, et al. Characterization of an amsacrine-resistant line of human leukemia cells. Evidence for a drug-resistant form of topoisomerase II. *J Biol Chem* 1989;264:16411.

204. Huff AC, Ward RE 4th, Kreuzer KN. Mutational alteration of the breakage/resealing subunit of bacteriophage T4 DNA topoisomerase confers resistance to antitumor agent m-AMSA. *Mol Gen Genet* 1990;221:27.

205. Matsumoto Y, Takano H, Fojo T. Cellular adaptation to drug exposure: evolution of the drug-resistant phenotype. *Cancer Res* 1997;57:5086.

206. Ritke MK, Murray NR, Allan WP, et al. Hypophosphorylation of topoisomerase II in etoposide (VP-16)-resistant human leukemia K562 cells associated with reduced levels of beta II protein kinase C. *Mol Pharmacol* 1995;48:798.

207. Ganapathi R, Constantinou A, Kamath N, et al. Resistance to etoposide in human leukemia HL-60 cells: reduction in drug-induced DNA cleavage associated with hypophosphorylation of topoisomerase II phosphopeptides. *Mol Pharmacol* 1996;50:243.

208. Chen M, Beck WT. DNA topoisomerase II expression, stability, and phosphorylation in two VM-26-resistant human leukemic CEM sublines. *Oncol Res* 1995;7:103.

209. Heck MM, Hittelman WN, Earnshaw WC. In vivo phosphorylation of the 170-kDa form of eukaryotic DNA topoisomerase II. Cell cycle analysis. *J Biol Chem* 1989;264:15161.

210. Taagepera S, Rao PN, Drake FH, et al. DNA topoisomerase II alpha is the major chromosome protein recognized by the mitotic phosphoprotein antibody MPM-2. *Proc Natl Acad Sci U S A* 1993;90:8407.

211. Cardenas ME, Dang Q, Glover CV, et al. Casein kinase II phosphorylates the eukaryote-specific C-terminal domain of topoisomerase II in vivo. *Embo J* 1992;11:1785.

212. Ackerman P, Glover CV, Osheroff N. Phosphorylation of DNA topoisomerase II by casein kinase II: modulation of eukaryotic topoisomerase II activity in vitro. *Proc Natl Acad Sci U S A* 1985;82:3164.

213. Ackerman P, Glover CV, Osheroff N. Phosphorylation of DNA topoisomerase II in vivo and in total homogenates of Drosophila Kc cells. The role of casein kinase II. *J Biol Chem* 1988;263:12653.

214. Bojanowski K, Filhol O, Cochet C, et al. DNA topoisomerase II and casein kinase II associate in a molecular complex that is catalytically active. *J Biol Chem* 1993;268:22920.

215. DeVore RF, Corbett AH, Osheroff N. Phosphorylation of topoisomerase II by casein kinase II and protein kinase C: effects on enzyme-mediated DNA cleavage/religation and sensitivity to the antineoplastic drugs etoposide and 4'-(9-acridinylamino)methane-sulfon-m-anisidide. *Cancer Res* 1992; 52:2156.

216. Pommier Y, Kerrigan D, Hartman KD, et al. Phosphorylation of mammalian DNA topoisomerase I and activation by protein kinase C. *J Biol Chem* 1990;265:9418.

217. Holm C, Covey JM, Kerrigan D, et al. Differential requirement of DNA replication for the cytotoxicity of DNA topoisomerase I and II inhibitors in Chinese hamster DC3F cells. *Cancer Res* 1989;49:6365.

218. Hsiang YH, Lihou MG, Liu LF. Arrest of replication forks by drug-stabilized topoisomerase I-DNA cleavable complexes as a mechanism of cell killing by camptothecin. *Cancer Res* 1989;49:5077.

219. D'Arpa P, Beardmore C, Liu LF. Involvement of nucleic acid synthesis in cell killing mechanisms of topoisomerase poisons. *Cancer Res* 1990;50:6919.

220. Kaufmann SH. Antagonism between camptothecin and topoisomerase II-directed chemotherapeutic agents in a human leukemia cell line. *Cancer Res* 1991;51:1129.

221. Bertrand R, O'Connor PM, Kerrigan D, et al. Sequential administration of camptothecin and etoposide circumvents the antagonistic cytotoxicity of simultaneous drug administration in slowly growing human colon carcinoma HT-29 cells. *Eur J Cancer* 1992;743.

222. Bertrand R, Kerrigan D, Sarang M, et al. Cell death induced by topoisomerase inhibitors. Role of calcium in mammalian cells. *Biochem Pharmacol* 1991;42:77.

223. Chatterjee S, Cheng MF, Berger NA. Hypersensitivity to clinically useful alkylating agents and radiation in poly(ADP-ribose) polymerase-deficient cell lines. *Cancer Commun* 1990;2:401.

224. Lim M, Liu LF, Jacobson-Kram D, et al. Induction of sister chromatid exchanges by inhibitors of topoisomerases. *Cell Biol Toxicol* 1986;2:485.

225. Singh B, Gupta RS. Mutagenic responses of thirteen anticancer drugs on mutation induction at multiple genetic loci and on sister chromatid exchanges in Chinese hamster ovary cells. *Cancer Res* 1983;43:577.

226. Pommier Y, Bertrand R. The mechanism of formation of chromosomal aberrations: role of eukaryotic DNA topoisomerases. In: Kirsch IR, ed. *The causes and consequences of chromosomal aberrations.* Boca Raton, FL: CRC Press, 1993:277.

227. Zhu J, Schiestl RH. Topoisomerase I involvement in illegitimate recombination in *Saccharomyces cerevisiae. Mol Cell Biol* 1996;16:1805.

228. Bertrand R, Solary E, Jenkins J, et al. Apoptosis and its modulation in human promyelocytic HL-60 cells treated with DNA topoisomerase I and II inhibitors. *Exp Cell Res* 1993;207:388.

229. Han YH, Austin MJ, Pommier Y, et al. Small deletion and insertion mutations induced by the topoisomerase II inhibitor teniposide in CHO cells and comparison with sites of drug-stimulated DNA cleavage in vitro. *J Mol Biol* 1993;229:52.

230. Berger NA, Chatterjee S, Schmotzer JA, et al. Etoposide (VP-16-213)-induced gene alterations: potential contribution to cell death. *Proc Natl Acad Sci U S A* 1991;88:8740.

231. Nitiss J, Wang JC. DNA topoisomerase-targeting antitumor drugs can be studied in yeast. *Proc Natl Acad Sci U S A* 1988;85:7501.

232. Desai SD, Liu LF, Vazquez-Abad D, et al. Ubiquitin-dependent destruction of topoisomerase I is stimulated by the antitumor drug camptothecin. *J Biol Chem* 1997;272:24159.

233. Nakajima T, Morita K, Ohi N, et al. Degradation of topoisomerase IIalpha during adenovirus E1A-induced apoptosis is mediated by the activation of the ubiquitin proteolysis system. *J Biol Chem* 1996;271:24842.

234. Nakajima T, Kimura M, Kuroda K, et al. Induction of ubiquitin conjugating enzyme activity for degradation of topoisomerase II alpha during adenovirus E1A-induced apoptosis. *Biochem Biophys Res Commun* 1997;239:823.

235. Goldwasser F, Shimizu T, Jackman J, et al. Correlations between S and G2 arrest and the cytotoxicity of camptothecin in human colon carcinoma cells. *Cancer Res* 1996;56:4430.

236. O'Connor PM, Kohn KW. A fundamental role for cell cycle regulation in the chemosensitivity of cancer cells? *Semin Cancer Biol* 1992;3:409.

237. Clarke AR, Purdie CA, Harrison DJ, et al. Thymocyte apoptosis induced by p53-dependent and independent pathways [see comments]. *Nature* 1993;362:849.

238. Lane DP. Cancer. A death in the life of p53 [news; comment]. *Nature* 1993;362:786.

239. Shao RG, Cao CX, Zhang H, et al. Replication-mediated DNA damage by camptothecin induces phosphorylation of RPA by DNA-dependent protein kinase and dissociates RPA:DNA-PK complexes. *Embo J* 1999;18:1397.

240. Gupta M, Fan S, Zhan Q, et al. Inactivation of p53 increases the cytotoxicity of camptothecin in human colon HCT116 and breast MCF-7 cancer cells. *Clin Cancer Res* 1997;3:1653.

241. Shao RG, Cao CX, Shimizu T, et al. Abrogation of an S-phase checkpoint and potentiation of camptothecin cytotoxicity by 7-hydroxystaurosporine (UCN-01) in human cancer cell lines, possibly influenced by p53 function. *Cancer Res* 1997;57:4029.

242. Kamesaki S, Kamesaki H, Jorgensen TJ, et al. bcl-2 Protein inhibits etoposide-induced apoptosis through its effects on

events subsequent to topoisomerase II-induced DNA strand breaks and their repair [published erratum appears in *Cancer Res* 1994;54:3074]. *Cancer Res* 1993;53:4251.

243. Fields KK, Zorsky PE, Hiemenz JW, et al. Ifosfamide, carboplatin, and etoposide: a new regimen with a broad spectrum of activity. *J Clin Oncol* 1994;12:544.

244. Felip E, Massuti B, Camps C, et al. Superiority of sequential versus concurrent administration of paclitaxel with etoposide in advanced non-small cell lung cancer: comparison of two phase II trials. *Clin Cancer Res* 1998;4:2723.

245. Giaccone G, Ardizzoni A, Kirkpatrick A, et al. Cisplatin and etoposide combination chemotherapy for locally advanced or metastatic thymoma. A phase II study of the European Organization for Research and Treatment of Cancer Lung Cancer Cooperative Group. *J Clin Oncol* 1996;14:814.

246. Paesmans M, Mascaux C, Berghmans T, et al. Etoposide and cisplatin merit their key role in chemotherapy for small cell lung cancer: a meta-analysis with a methodology assessment, by the European Lung Cancer Working Party. *Proc Annu Meet Am Soc Clin Oncol* 1999;18(Abstract 1830).

247. Bow EJ, Suntherland JA, Kilpatrick MG, et al Therapy of untreated acute myeloid leukemia in the elderly: remission-induction using a non-cytarabine-containing regimen of mitoxantrone plus etoposide. *J Clin Oncol* 1996;14:1345.

248. Bow EJ, Gallant G, Williams GJ, et al. Remission induction therapy of untreated acute myeloid leukemia using a non-cytarabine-containing regimen of idarubicin, etoposide, and carboplatin. *Cancer* 1998;83:1344.

249. Strife RJ, Jardine L, Colvin M. Analysis of the anticancer drugs VP-16-213 and VM-26 and their metabolites by high-performance liquid chromatography. *J Chromatogr* 1980;182:211.

250. Holthuis JJ, Romkens F, Pinedo H, et al. Plasma assay for the antineoplastic agent etoposide-213 (VP-16) using high-performance liquid chromatography with electrochemical detection. *J Pharm Biomed Anal* 183;1:89.

251. Sinkule J, Evans W. High-performance liquid chromatographic analysis of the semisynthetic epipodophyllotoxins teniposide and etoposide using electrochemical detection. *J Pharm Sci* 1984;73:164.

252. Aherne GW, Marks V. A radioimmunoassay for VP-16-213 in plasma. *Cancer Chemother Pharmacol* 1982;7:117.

253. Henneberry HP, Aherne GW, Marks V. An ELISA for the measurement of VP16 (etoposide) in unextracted plasma. *J Immunol Methods* 1988;107:205.

254. Creaven PJ, Allen LM. EPEG, an new anti-neoplastic epipodophyllotoxin. *Clin Pharmacol Ther* 1975;18:221.

255. Hande KR, Wedlund PJ, Noone RM, et al. Pharmacokinetics of high-dose etoposide (VP-16-213) administered to cancer patients. *Cancer Res* 1984;44:379.

256. Rodman JH, Abromowitch M, Sinkule JA, et al. Clinical pharmacodynamics of continuous infusion teniposide—systemic exposure as a determinant of response in a phase I trial. *J Clin Oncol* 1987;9:1480.

257. Holthuis JJ, Postmus PE, Van Oort WJ, et al. Pharmacokinetics of high dose etoposide (VP16-213). *Eur J Cancer Clin Oncol* 1986;22:1149.

258. D'Incalci M, Farina P, Sessa P, et al. Pharmacokinetics of VP16-213 given by different administration methods. *Cancer Chemother Pharmacol* 1982;7:141.

259. Henwood J, Brogden R. Etoposide: a review of its pharmacodynamic and pharmacokinetic properties, and therapeutic potential in combination chemotherapy of cancer. *Drugs* 1990;39:438.

260. Hande KR. Etoposide pharmacology. *Semin Oncol* 1992;19:3.

261. Sinkule JA, Hutson P, Hayes FA, et al. Pharmacokinetics of etoposide (VP-16) in children and adolescents with refractory solid tumors. *Cancer Res* 1984;44:3109.

262. Lowis SP, Pearson ADJ, Newell DR, et al. Etoposide pharmacokinetics in children: the development and prospective validation of a dosing equation. *Cancer Res* 1993;53:4881.

263. Allen L, Creaven P. Comparison of the human pharmacokinetics of VM-26 and VP-16, two antineoplastic epipodophyllotoxin glucopyranoside derivatives. *Eur J Cancer* 1975;18:697.

264. Smyth RL, Pfeffer M, Scalzo A, et al. Bioavailability and pharmacokinetics of etoposide. *Semin Oncol* 1985;12:48.

265. Rodman JH, Murry DJ, Madden T, et al. Pharmacokinetics of high doses of etoposide and the influence of anticonvulsants in pediatric cancer patients. *Clin Pharmacol Ther* 1992;51:156.

266. Fleming RA, Evans WE, Arbuck SG, et al. Factors affecting in vitro protein binding of etoposide in humans. *J Pharm Sci* 1992;81:259.

267. Stewart CF, Pieper JA, Arbuck SG, et al. Altered protein binding of etoposide in patients with cancer. *Clin Pharmacol Ther* 1989;45:49.

268. Stewart CF, Arbuck SG, Fleming RA, et al. Changes in the clearance of total and unbound etoposide in patients with liver dysfunction. *J Clin Oncol* 1990;8:1874.

269. Stewart CF, Fleming RA, Arbuck SG, et al. Prospective evaluation of a model for predicting etoposide plasma protein binding in cancer patients. *Cancer Res* 1990;50:6854.

270. Stewart CF, Arbuck SG, Fleming RA, et al. Relation of systemic exposure to unbound etoposide and hematologic toxicity. *Clin Pharmacol Ther* 1991;50:385.

271. Liliemark EK, Liliemark J, Pettersson B, et al. In vivo accumulation of etoposide in peripheral leukemic cells in patients treated for acute myeloblastic leukemia: relation to plasma concentrations and protein binding. *Leuk Lymphoma* 1993;10:323.

272. Schwinghammer TL, Fleming RA, Rosenfeld CS, et al. Disposition of total and unbound etoposide following high-dose therapy. *Cancer Chemother Pharmacol* 1993;32:273.

273. Arbuck SG, Douglass HO, Crom WR, et al. Etoposide pharmacokinetics in patients with normal and abnormal organ function. *J Clin Oncol* 4:1690, 1986.

274. D'Incalci M, Rossi C, Zucchetti M, et al. Pharmacokinetics of etoposide in patients with abnormal renal and hepatic function. *Cancer Res* 1986;46:2566.

275. Hande KR, Anthony LB, Wolff SN, et al. Etoposide clearance in patients with hepatic dysfunction. *Clin Pharmacol Ther* 1987;41:161.

276. Hande KR, Wolff SN, Greco A, et al. Etoposide kinetics in patients with obstructive jaundice. *J Clin Oncol* 1990;8:1101.

277. Postmus PE, Holthuis JJM, Haaxma-Reiche H, et al. Penetration of VP-16-213 into cerebrospinal fluid after high-dose intravenous administration. *J Clin Oncol* 1984;2:215.

278. Steward DJ, Richard MT, Hugenholtz H, et al. Penetration of etoposide (VP-16) into human intracerebral and extracerebral tumours. *J Neurooncol* 1984;2:133.

279. Zuchetti M, Rossi C, Knerich R, et al. Concentrations of VP16 and VM26 in human brain tumors. *Ann Oncol* 1991;2:63.

280. Mendelsohn ME, Abramson DH, Madden T, et al. Intraocular concentrations of chemotherapeutic agents after systemic or local administration. *Arch Ophthalmol* 1998;116:1209.

281. Clark PI, Slevin ML. The clinical pharmacology of etoposide and teniposide. *Clin Pharmacokinet* 1987;12:223.

282. Suzuki S, Koide M, Sakamoto S, et al. Pharmacokinetics of carboplatin and etoposide in a haemodialysis patient with Merckel-cell carcinoma. *Nephrol Dial Transplant* 1997;12:137.

283. Clark PI. Clinical pharmacology and schedule dependency of the podophyllotoxines derivatives. *Semin Oncol* 1992;19:20.

284. Stremetzne S, Jaehde U, Schunack W. Determination of the cytotoxic catechol metabolite of etoposide (3'O-demethyletoposide) in human plasma by high-performance liquid chromatography. *J Chromatogr B Biomed Sci Appl* 1997;703:209.

285. Mans DR, Lafleur MV, Westmijze EJ, et al. Formation of different reaction products with single- and double-strand DNA by the *ortho*-quinone and the semi-quinone free radicals of etoposide (VP-16-213). *Biochem Pharmacol* 1991;42:2131.

286. Mans DR, Lafleur MV, Westmijze EJ, et al. Reactions of glutathione with the catechol, the *ortho*-quinone and the semi-quinone free radical of etoposide. Consequences for DNA inactivation. *Biochem Pharmacol* 1992;43:1761.

287. Steward DJ, Nundy D, Maroun JA, et al. Bioavailability, pharmacokinetics, and clinical effects of an oral preparation of etoposide. *Cancer Treat Rep* 1985;69:269.

288. van Maanen JMS, Retel J, de Vries J, et al. Mechanism of action of antitumor drug etoposide: a review. *J Natl Cancer Inst* 1988;80:1526.

289. Long BH, Musial ST, Brattain MG. Comparison of cytotoxicity and DNA breakage activity of congeners of podophyllotoxin including VP16-213 and VM26: a quantitative structure-activity relationship. *Biochemistry* 1984;23:1183.

290. Zhao XJ, Kawashiro T, Ishizaki T. Mutual inhibition between quinine and etoposide by human liver microsomes. Evidence for cytochrome P450 3A4 involvement in their major metabolic pathways. *Drug Metab Dispos* 1998;26:188.

291. Perry MC. Hepatotoxicity of chemotherapeutic agents. *Semin Oncol* 1982;9:65.

292. Sekine I, Fukuda H, Kunitoh H, et al. Cancer chemotherapy in the elderly. *Jpn J Clin Oncol* 1998;28:463.

293. Relling M, McLeod H, Bowman L, et al. Etoposide pharmacokinetics and pharmacodynamics after acute and chronic exposure to cisplatin. *Clin Pharmacol Ther* 1994;56:503.

294. Mross K, Bewermeier P, Kruger W, et al. Pharmacokinetics of undiluted or diluted high-dose etoposide with or without busulfan administered to patients with hematologic malignancies. *J Clin Oncol* 1994;12:1468.

295. Beyer J, Kramar A, Mandanas R, et al. High-dose chemotherapy as salvage treatment in germ cell tumors: a multivariate analysis of prognostic variables. *J Clin Oncol* 1996;14:2638.

296. Beyer J, Kingreen D, Krause M, et al. Long-term survival of patients with recurrent or refractory germ cell tumors after high dose chemotherapy. *Cancer* 1997;79:161.

297. Kanfer EJ, McGuigan D, Samson D, et al. High-dose etoposide with granulocyte colony-stimulating factor for mobilization of peripheral blood progenitor cells: efficacy and toxicity at three dose levels. *Br J Cancer* 1998;78:928.

298. Pucci G, Irrera G, Martino M, et al. High-dose etoposide enables the collection of peripheral blood stem cells in patients who failed cyclophosphamide-induced mobilization (letter). *Br J Haematol* 1998;100:612.

299. Savaraj N, Feun LG, Lu K, et al. Clinical pharmacology of intracarotid etoposide. *Cancer Chemother Pharmacol* 1986; 16:292.

300. Tfayli A, Hentschel P, Madajewicz S, et al. Intra-arterial chemotherapy with cisplatin. *Proc Annu Meet Am Soc Clin Oncol* 1997;16:A1904.

301. Reichman B, Markman M, Hakes T, et al. Intraperitoneal cisplatin and etoposide in the treatment of refractory/recurrent ovarian carcinoma. *J Clin Oncol* 1988;7:1327.

302. Howell SB, Kirmani S, Lucas WE, et al. A phase II trial of intraperitoneal cisplatin and etoposide for primary treatment of ovarian epithelial cancer. *J Clin Oncol* 1990;8:137.

303. Barakat RR, Almadrones L, Venkatraman ES, et al. A phase II trial of intraperitoneal cisplatin and etoposide as consolidation therapy in patients with stage II-IV epithelial ovarian cancer following negative surgical assessment. *Gynecol Oncol* 1998;69:17.

304. Ito H, Imada T, Kondo J, et al. A case of malignant peritoneal mesothelioma showed complete remission with chemotherapy. *Jpn J Clin Oncol* 1998;28:145.

305. van-Rijswijk RE, Hoeckman K, Burger CW, et al. Experience of intraperitoneal cisplatin and etoposide and i.v. sodium thiosulphate protection in ovarian cancer patients with either pathologically complete response or minimal residual disease. *Ann Oncol* 1997;8:1235.

306. Gaast AV, Sonneveld P, Mans DR, et al. Intrathecal administration of etoposide in the treatment of malignant meningitis: feasibility and pharmacokinetic data. *Cancer Chemother Pharmacol* 1992;9:335.

307. Holoye PY, Jeffries DG, Dhingra HM, et al. Intrapleural etoposide for malignant effusion. *Cancer Chemother Pharmacol* 1990;26:147.

308. Jones J, Olman E, Egorin M, et al. A case report and description of the pharmacokinetic behavior of intrapleurally instilled etoposide. *Cancer Chemother Pharmacol* 1985;14:172.

309. Brunner KW, Sonntag RW, Ryssel HJ, et al. Comparison of the biologic activity of VP16-213 given IV and orally in capsules or drink ampoules. *Cancer Treat Rep* 1976;60:1377.

310. Slevin ML, Joel SP, Whomsley R, et al. The effect of dose on the bioavailability of oral etoposide: confirmation of a clinically relevant observation. *Cancer Chemother Pharmacol* 1989;24:329.

311. van der Gast A, Vlastuin M, Kok T, et al. What is the optimal dose and duration of treatment with etoposide? II. Comparative pharmacokinetic study of three schedules: 1×100 mg, 2×50 mg, and 4×25 mg of oral etoposide daily for 21 days. *Semin Oncol* 1992;19:8.

312. Hande KR, Krozely MG, Greco A, et al. Bioavailability of low-dose oral etoposide. *J Clin Oncol* 1993;11:374.

313. Harvey VJ, Slevin ML, Joel SP, et al. The effect of food and concurrent chemotherapy on the bioavailability of oral etoposide. *Br J Cancer* 1985;52:363.

314. Harvey VJ, Slevin ML, Joel SP, et al. The effect of dose on the bioavailability of oral etoposide. *Cancer Chemother Pharmacol* 1986;16:178.

315. Splinter TAW, Holthuis JJM, Kok TC, et al. Absolute bio-availability and pharmacokinetics of oral teniposide. *Semin Oncol* 1992;19:28.

316. Schwartsmann G, Sprinz E, Kromfield M, et al. Clinical and pharmacokinetic study of oral etoposide in patients with AIDS-related Kaposi's sarcoma with no prior exposure to cytotoxic therapy. *J Clin Oncol* 1997;15:2118.

317. Stahelin HF, von Wartburg A. The chemical and biological route from podophyllotoxin glucoside to etoposide: Ninth Cain Memorial Award. *Cancer Res* 1991;51:5.

318. Huang JD, Leu BL, Lai MD. Induction and inhibition of intestinal P-glycoprotein and effects on etoposide. *Proc Am Assoc Cancer Res* 1994;35:353.

319. Miller AA, Tolley EA, Niell HB. Therapeutic drug monitoring of 21-day oral etoposide in patients with advanced non-small cell lung cancer. *Clin Cancer Res* 1998;4:1705.

320. Takeda K, Shinohara K, Kameda N, et al. A case of therapy-related acute myeloblastic leukemia with t(16;21)(q24;q22) after chemotherapy with DNA-topoisomerase II inhibitors, etoposide and mitoxantrone, and the alkylating agent, cyclophosphamide. *Int J Hematol* 1998;67:179.

321. Yagita M, Ieki Y, Onishi R, et al. Therapy-related leukemia and myelodysplasia following oral administration of etoposide for recurrent breast cancer. *Int J Oncol* 1998;13:91.

322. Skarlos DV, Aravantinos G, Kosmidis P, et al. Ifosfamide plus oral etoposide for platinum resistant ovarian cancer. A Hellenic Co-Operative Oncology Group Study. *Proc Annu Meet Am Soc Clin Oncol* 1999;18(Abstr. 1484).

323. Sessa C, Zucchetti M, Torri V, et al. Chronic oral etoposide in small-cell lung cancer: clinical and pharmacokinetic results. *Ann Oncol* 1993;4:553.

324. Greco FA, Hainsworth JD. Paclitaxel, carboplatin, and oral etoposide in the treatment of small cell lung cancer. *Semin Oncol* 1996;23:7.

325. Hainsworth JD, Hopkins LG, Thomas M, et al. Paclitaxel, carboplatin, and extended-schedule oral etoposide for small-cell lung cancer. *Oncology* 1998;12:31.

326. Lee JS, Scott C, Komaki R, et al. Concurrent chemoradiation therapy with oral etoposide and cisplatin for locally advanced inoperable non-small-cell lung cancer: radiation therapy oncology group protocol 91-06. *J Clin Oncol* 1996;14:1055.

327. Frasci G, Comella P, Panza N, et al. Carboplatin-oral etoposide personalized dosing in elderly non-small cell lung cancer patients. *Eur J Cancer* 1998;34:1710.

328. Westeel V, Murray N, Gelmon K, et al. New combination of the old drugs for elderly patients with small-cell lung cancer: a phase II study of the PAVE regimen. *J Clin Oncol* 1998;16:1940.

329. Hainsworth JD, Johnson DH, Frazier SR, et al. Chronic daily administration of oral etoposide in refractory lymphoma. *Eur J Cancer* 1990;26:818.

330. Goss P, Burkes R, Rudinskas L, et al. A phase II trial of prednisone, oral etoposide, and novantrone (PEN) as initial treatment of non-Hodgkin's lymphoma in elderly patients. *Leuk Lymphoma* 1995;18:145.

331. Clark PI, Sutton P, Smith DB, et al. A phase I study of a 5 day schedule of intravenous topotecan and etoposide in untreated small cell lung cancer. *Proc Annu Meet Am Soc Clin Oncol* 1999;18:(Abstr. 1926).

332. Souhami RL, Spiro SG, Rudd RM, et al. Five-day oral etoposide treatment for advanced small-cell lung cancer: randomized comparison with intravenous chemotherapy. *J Natl Cancer Inst* 1997;89:577.

333. Budman DR, Igwemezie LN, Kaul S, et al. Phase I evaluation of a water-soluble etoposide prodrug, etoposide phosphate, given as a 5-minute infusion on days 1, 3, and 5 in patients with solid tumors. *J Clin Oncol* 1994;12:1902.

334. Brooks DJ, Srinivas N, Alberts DS, et al. Phase I and pharmacokinetic study of etoposide phosphate. *Anticancer Drugs* 1995;6:637.

335. Fields SZ, Igwemezie LN, Kaul S, et al. Phase I study of etoposide phosphate (Etopophos) as a 30-minute infusion on days 1, 3, and 5. *Clin Cancer Res* 1995;1:105.

336. Millward MJ, Newell DR, Mummaneni V, et al. Phase I and pharmacokinetic study of a water-soluble etoposide prodrug, etoposide phosphate (BMY-40481). *Eur J Cancer* 1995;31A:2409.

337. Thompson DS, Greco FA, Miller AA, et al. A phase I study of etoposide phosphate administered as a daily 30-minute infusion for 5 days. *Clin Pharmacol Ther* 1995;57:499.

338. Hainsworth JD, Utley SM, Greco FA. Phase I study of high dose etoposide phosphate with filgrastim (G-CSF) in the treatment of advanced refractory malignancies. *Invest New Drugs* 1998;15:325.

339. Soni N, Meropol NJ, Pendyala L, et al. Phase I and pharmacokinetic study of etoposide phosphate by protracted infusion in patients with advanced cancer. *J Clin Oncol* 1997;15:766.

340. Kaul S, Igwemezie LN, Steward DJ, et al. Pharmacokinetics and bioequivalence of etoposide following intravenous administration of etoposide phosphate and etoposide in patients with solid tumors. *J Clin Oncol* 1995;13:2835.

341. Hainsworth JD, Levitan N, Wampler GL, et al. Phase II randomized study of cisplatin plus etoposide phosphate or etoposide in the treatment of small-cell lung cancer. *J Clin Oncol* 1995;13:1436.

342. Sessa C, Zucchetti M, Cerny T, et al. Phase I clinical and pharmacokinetic study of oral etoposide phosphate. *J Clin Oncol* 1995;13:200.

343. de Jong RS, Mulder NH, Uges DR, et al. Randomized comparison of etoposide pharmacokinetics after oral etoposide phosphate and oral etoposide. *Br J Cancer* 1997;75:1660.

344. Rodman J, Furman W, Sunderland M, et al. Escalating teniposide systemic exposure to increase dose-intensity for pediatric cancer patients. *J Clin Oncol* 1993;11:287.

345. Smit EF, Splinter TAW, Kok TC. A phase I study of daily oral teniposide for 20 days. *Semin Oncol* 1992;19:40.

346. Slevin ML, Clark PI, Joel SP, et al. A randomised trial to evaluate the effect of schedule on the activity of etoposide in small cell lung cancer. *J Clin Oncol* 1989;7:1333.

347. Mick R, Rarain MJ. Modeling interpatient pharmacodynamic variability of etoposide. *J Natl Cancer Inst* 1991;83:1560.

348. Ratain MJ, Mick R, Schilsky RL, et al. Pharmacologically based dosing of etoposide: a means of safely increasing dose intensity. *J Clin Oncol* 1991;9:1480.

349. Miller A, Stewart C, Tolley E. Clinical pharmacodynamics of continuous-infusion etoposide. *Cancer Chemother Pharmacol* 1990;25:361.

350. Miller AA, Tolley EA, Niell HB, et al. Pharmacodynamics of three daily infusions of etoposide in patients with extensive-stage small-cell lung cancer. *Cancer Chemother Pharmacol* 1992;31:161.

351. Minami H, Shimokata K, Saka H, et al. Phase I clinical and pharmacokinetic study of a 14-day infusion of etoposide in patients with lung cancer. *J Clin Oncol* 1993;11:1602.

352. Ratain MJ, Schilsky RL, Choi KE, et al. Adaptive control of etoposide administration: impact of interpatient pharmacodynamic variability. *Clin Pharmacol Ther* 1989;45:226.

353. Slevin ML, Joel SP, Smith I, et al. Therapeutic monitoring of infusional etoposide in previously untreated small cell lung cancer. *Br J Cancer* 1994;69 (suppl. 21):23.

354. Pfuger K-H, Hahn M, Holz J-B, et al. Pharmacokinetics of etoposide: correlation of pharmacokinetic parameters with clinical conditions. *Cancer Chemother Pharmacol* 1993;31:350.

355. Joel S, Shah R, Slevin M. Etoposide dosage and pharmacodynamics. *Cancer Chemother Pharmacol* 1994;34:S69.

356. Gentili D, Zucchetti M, Torri V, et al. A limited-sampling model for the pharmacokinetics of etoposide given orally. *Cancer Chemother Pharmacol* 1993;32:482.

357. Stromgren AS, Sorensen BT, Jakobsen P, et al. A limited-sampling method for estimation of the etoposide area under the curve. *Cancer Chemother Pharmacol* 1993;32:226.

358. Lum BL, Lane KJ, Synold TW, et al. Validation of a limited sampling model to determine etoposide area under the curve. *Pharmacotherapy* 1997;17:887.

359. Lowis SP, Price L, Pearson AD, et al. A study of the feasibility and accuracy of pharmacokinetically guided etoposide dosing in children. *Br J Cancer* 77:2318, 1998.

360. Radice PA, Bunn PA, Ihde DC. Therapeutic trials of VP-16-213 and VM-26: active agents in small cell lung cancer, non-Hodgkin's lymphomas, and other malignancies. *Cancer Treat Rep* 1979;63:1231.

361. Schmoll H. Review of etoposide single-agent activity. *Cancer Treat Rev* 1982;9:21.

362. O'Dwyer P, Weus R. Hypersensitivity reactions induced by etoposide. *Cancer Treat Rep* 1984;68:959.

363. Weiss RB. Hypersensitivity reactions. *Semin Oncol* 1992;19:458.

364. Curtis RE, Boice Jr JD, Stovall M, et al. Risk of leukemia after chemotherapy and radiation treatment for breast cancer. *N Engl J Med* 1992;326:1745.

365. Pommier Y, Zwelling LA, Kao-Shan CS, et al. Correlations between intercalator-induced DNA strand breaks and sister chromatid exchanges, mutations, and cytotoxicity in Chinese hamster cells. *Cancer Research* 1985;45:3143.

366. Karnaoukhova L, Moffat J, Martins H, et al. Mutation frequency and spectrum in lymphocytes of small cell lung cancer patients receiving etoposide chemotherapy. *Cancer Res* 1997;57:4393.

367. Smith MA, Rubinstein L, Cazenave L, et al. Report of the cancer-therapy evaluation program monitoring plan for secondary acute myeloid-leukemia following treatment with epipodophyllotoxins. *J Natl Cancer Inst* 1993;85:554.

368. Smith MA, Rubinstein L, Ungerleider RS. Therapy-related acute myeloid leukemia following treatment with epipodophyllotoxins: estimating the risks. *Med Pediatr Oncol* 1994;23:86.

369. Smith MA, McCaffrey RP, Karp JE. The secondary leukemias: challenges and research directions. *J Natl Cancer Inst* 1996;88:407.

370. Smith MA, Rubinstein L, Anderson JR, et al. Secondary leukemia or myelodysplastic syndrome after treatment with epipodophyllotoxins. *J Clin Oncol* 1999;17:569.

371. Detourmignies L, Castaigne S, Stoppa AM, et al. Therapy-related acute promyelocytic leukemia—a report on 16 cases. *J Clin Oncol* 1992;10:1430.

372. Fenaux P, Lucidarme D, Lai J-L, et al. Favorable cytogenetic abnormalities in secondary leukemia. *Cancer* 1989;63:2505.

373. Kapoor G, Kadam PR, Chougule A, et al. Secondary ANLL with t(11;19)(q23;p13) following etoposide and cisplatin for ovarian germ cell tumor. *Indian J Cancer* 1997;34:84.

374. Relling MV, Yanishevski Y, Nemec J, et al. Etoposide and antimetabolite pharmacology in patients who develop secondary acute myeloid leukemia. *Leukemia* 1998;12:346.

375. Nichols CR, Breeden ES, Loehrer PJ, et al. Secondary leukemia associated with a conventional dose of etoposide-review of serial germ-cell tumor protocols. *J Natl Cancer Inst* 1993;85:36.

376. Ratain MJ, Kaminer LS, Bitran JD, et al. Acute nonlymphocytic leukemia following etoposide and cisplatin combination chemotherapy for advanced non-small-cell carcinoma of the lung. *Blood* 1987;70:1412.

377. Pedersen-Bjergaard J, Daugaard G, Hansen SW, et al. Increased risk of myelodysplasia and leukaemia after etoposide, cisplatin, and bleomycin for germ-cell tumours. *Lancet* 1991;338:359.

378. Pui CH, Ribeiro RC, Hancock ML, et al. Acute myeloid leukemia in children treated with epipodophyllotoxins for acute lymphoblastic leukemia. *N Engl J Med* 1991;325:1682.

379. Lovett BD, Strumberg D, Blair IA, et al. Etoposide metabolites enhance DNA topoisomerase II cleavage proximal to leukemia-associated *MLL* translocation breakpoints. *Biochemistry* 2001;40:1159.

380. Pedersen-Bjergaard J, Sigsgaard TC, Nielsen D, et al. Acute monocytic or myelomonoctic leukemia with balanced chromosome translocations to band 11q23 after therapy with 4-epi-doxorubicin and cisplatin or cyclophosphamide for breast cancer. *J Clin Oncol* 1992;10:1444.

381. Pedersen-Bjergaard J, Rowley JD. The balanced and unbalanced chromosome aberrations of acute myeloid leukemia may develop in different ways and may contribute differently to malignant transformation. *Blood* 1994;83:2780.

382. Pedersen-Bjergaard J, Pedersen M, Roulston D, et al. Different genetic pathways in leukemogenesis for patients presenting with therapy-related myelodysplasia and therapy-related acute myeloid leukemia. *Blood* 1995;86:3542.

383. Nasr F, Macintyre E, Venuat A-M, et al. Translocation t(4;11)(q21; q23) and MLL gene rearrangement in acute lymphoblastic leukemia secondary to anti topoisomerase II anticancer agents. *Leuk Lymphoma* 1997;25:399.

384. Pommier Y, Cockerill PN, Kohn KW, et al. Identification within the simian virus 40 genome of a chromosomal loop attachment site that contains topoisomerase II cleavage sites. *J Virol* 1990;64:419.

385. D'Andrea MR, Farber PA, Foglesong PD. Immunohistochemical detection of DNA topoisomerases IIa and IIb compared with detection of Ki-67, a marker of cellular proliferation, in human tumors. *Appl Immunohistochem* 1994;2:177.

386. Kreipe H, Alm P, Olsson H, et al. Prognostic significance of a formalin-resistant nuclear proliferation antigen in mammary carcinomas as determined by the monoclonal antibody Ki-S1. *Am J Pathol* 1993;142:651.

387. Holden JA, Perkins SL, Snow GW, et al. Immunohistochemical staining for DNA topoisomerase II in non-Hodgkin's lymphomas. *Am J Clin Pathol* 1995;104:54.

388. Guinee DG, Holden JA, Benfield JR, et al. Comparison of DNA topoisomerase IIa expression in small cell and non-small cell carcinoma of the lung; in search of a mechanism of chemotherapeutic response. *Cancer* 1996;78:729.

389. Jarvinen TA, Kononen J, Pelto-Huikko M, et al. Expression of topoisomerase IIalpha is associated with rapid cell proliferation, aneuploidy, and c-ErB2 overexpression in breast cancer. *Am J Pathol* 1996;148:2073.

390. Sandri MI, Hochhauser D, Ayton RC, et al. Differential expression of the topoisomerase IIalpha and beta genes in human breast cancers. *Br J Cancer* 1996;73:1518.

391. Turley H, Comley M, Houlbrook S, et al. The distribution and expression of the two isoforms of DNA topoisomerase II in normal and neoplastic human tissues. *Br J Cancer* 1997;75:1340.

392. Kaufmann SH, Karp JE, Jones RJ, et al. Topoisomerase II levels and drug sensitivity in adult acute myelogenous leukemia. *Blood* 1994;83:517.

393. Kaufmann SH, Karp JE, Burke PJ, et al. Addition of etoposide to initial therapy of adult acute lymphoblastic leukemia: a combined clinical and laboratory study. *Leuk Lymphoma* 1996;23:71.

394. Yeh KH, Chen CL, Shun CT, et al. Relatively low expression of multidrug resistance-1 (MDR-1) and its possible clinical implication in gastric cancers. *J Clin Gastroenterol* 1998;26:274.

395. Nooter K, Kok T, Bosman FT, et al. Expression of the multidrug resistance protein (MRP) in squamous cell carcinoma of the oesophagus and response to pre-operative chemotherapy. *Eur J Cancer* 1998;34:81.

396. den Boer ML, Pieters R, Kazemier KM, et al. Relationship between major vault protein/lung resistance protein, multidrug resistance-associated protein, P-glycoprotein expression, and drug resistance in childhood leukemia. *Blood* 1998;91:2092.

397. Keshelava N, Seegerr RC, Reynolds CP. Drug resistance in human neuroblastoma cell lines correlates with clinical therapy. *Eur J Cancer* 1997;33:2002.

398. Pein F, Pinkerton R, Rubie H, et al. A phase I trial of oral SDZ PSC-833 in combination with a rapid schedule of intravenous etoposide in children with relapsing and/or refractory solid tumors. *Proc Annu Meet Am Soc Clin Oncol* 1997;16:A1902.

399. Bisogno G, Cowie F, Boddy A, et al. High-dose cyclosporin with etoposide-toxicity and pharmacokinetic interaction in children with solid tumors. *Br J Cancer* 1998;77:2304.

400. Maia RC, Noronha H, Vasconcelos FC, et al. Interaction of cyclosporin A and etoposide. Clinical and in vitro assessment in blast phase of chronic myeloid leukaemia. *Clin Lab Haematol* 1997;19:215.

401. Slater LM, Sweet P, Stupecky M, et al. Superiority of cyclosporin A over PSC-833 in enhancement of etoposide efficacy in murine tumors in vivo. *Cancer Chemother Pharmacol* 1997;39:452.

402. Lacayo N, Lum BL, Johnson S, et al. Pharmacokinetics of etoposide and mitoxantrone in a controlled trial of cyclosporine as an MDR modulator in acute myeloid leukemia from the Pediatric Oncology Group. *Proc Annu Meet Am Soc Clin Oncol* 1997;6:A1850.

403. Kornblau SM, Estey E, Madden T, et al. Phase I study of mitoxantrone plus etoposide with multidrug blockade by SDZ PSC-833 in relapsed or refractory acute myelogenous leukemia. *J Clin Oncol* 1997;15:1796.

404. Grey M, Borg AG, Wood P, et al. Effect on cell kill of addition of multidrug resistance modifiers cyclosporin A and PSC 833 to cytotoxic agents in acute myeloid leukaemia. *Leuk Res* 1997;21:867.

405. Advani R, Saba HI, Tallman MS, et al. Treatment of refractory and relapsed acute myelogenous leukemia with combination chemotherapy plus the multidrug resistance modulator PSC 833 (Valspodar). *Blood* 1999;93:787.

406. Cysyk RL, Shoemaker DD, Adamson RH. The pharmacological disposition of 4'-(9-acridinylamino)methanesulfonanisidide in mice and rats. *Drug Metab Dispos* 1977;5:579.

407. Wilson WR, Cain BF, Baguley BC. Thiolytic cleavage of the antitumor compound 4'-(9-acridinylamino)methanesulfon-*m*-anisidide (*m*-AMSA, NSC 156303) in blood. *Chem Biol Interact* 1977;18:163.

408. Kestell P, Paxton J, Robertson I, et al. Thiolytic cleavage and binding of the antitumour agent CI-921 in blood. *Drug Metab Drug Interact* 1988;6:327.

409. Shoemaker DD, Cysyk RL, Gormley PE, et al. Metabolism of 4'-(9-acridinylamino)methanesulfon-*m*-anisidide by rat liver microsomes. *Cancer Res* 1984;44:1939.

410. Gaudich K, Przybylski M. Field desorption mass spectrometric characterization of thiol conjugates related to the oxidative metabolism of the anticancer drug 4'-(9-acridinylamino)methanesulfon-*m*-anisidide. *Biomed Mass Spectrom* 1988;10:292.

411. Lee HH, Palmer BD, Denny WA. Reactivity to nucleophiles of quinoneimine and quinonediimine metabolites of the antitumor drug m-AMSA and related compounds. *J Org Chem* 1988;53:6042.

412. Przybylski M, Cysyk RL, Shoemaker DD, et al. Identification of conjugation and cleavage products in the thiolytic metabolism of the anticancer drug 4'-(9-acridinylamino)methanesulfon-*m*-anisidide. *Biomed Mass Spectrom* 1981;8:485.

413. Van Echo DA, Chiuten DF, Gormley PE, et al. Phase I clinical and pharmacological study of 4'-(9-acridinylamino)methanesulfon-*m*-anisidide using an intermittent biweekly schedule. *Cancer Res* 1979;39:3881.

414. Hall SW, Friedman J, Legha S, et al. Human pharmacokinetics of a new acridine derivative, 4'-(9-acridinylamino)methanesulfon-*m*-anisidide (NSC 249992). *Cancer Res* 1983;43:3422.

415. Paul CY, Liliemark JO, Farmen JH, et al. Comparison of the pharmacokinetics of AMSA and AMSA-lactate in patients with acute nonlymphoblastic leukemia. *Ther Drug Monit* 1987;9:263.

416. Petros W, Rodman J, Mirro JJ, et al. Pharmacokinetics of continuous-infusion of m-AMSA and teniposide for the treatment of relapsed childhood acute nonlymphocytic leukemia. *Cancer Chemother Pharmacol* 1991;27:397.

417. Paxton JW, Kim SN, Whitfield LR. Pharmacokinetic and

toxicity scaling of the antitumor agents m-AMSA and CI-921, a new analog, in mice, rats, rabbits, dogs and humans. *Cancer Res* 1990;50:2692.

418. Linssen P, Brons P, Knops G, et al. Plasma and cellular pharmacokinetics of m-AMSA related to in vitro toxicity towards normal and leukemic clonogenic bone marrow cells (CFU-GM, CFU-L). *Eur J Haematol* 1993;50:149.

419. Cornford EM, Young D, Paxton JW. Comparison of the blood barrier and liver penetration of acridine antitumor drugs. *Cancer Chemother Pharmacol* 1992;29:439.

420. Cassileth PA, Gale RP. Amsacrine: a review. *Leuk Res* 1986;10:1257.

421. DeJager R, Body JJ, Dupont D, et al. Phase I study of oral 4'-(9-acridinylamino)-methanesulfon-*m*-anisidide (*m*-AMSA, NSC 249992). *Proc Am Soc Clin Oncol* 1979;20:429.

422. DeJager R, Dupont D, Body JJ. Phase II study of oral 4'-(9-acridinylamino)-methanesulfon-*m*-anisidide (*m*-AMSA, NSC 249992). *Proc Am Assoc Cancer Res* 1980;21:146.

423. Rivera G, Evans WE, Dahl GV, et al. Phase I clinical and pharmacokinetic study of 4'-(9-acridinylamino)-methanesulfon-*m*-anisidide in children with cancer. *Cancer Res* 1980;40:4250.

424. Louie AC, Issel BF. Amsacrine (AMSA): a clinical review. *J Clin Oncol* 1985;3:562.

425. Micetich KC, Zwelling LA, Gormley P, et al. Phase I-II study of amsacrine administered as a continuous infusion. *Cancer Treat Rep* 1982;66:1813.

426. Legha SS, Keating MJ, McCredie KB, et al. Evaluation of AMSA in previously treated patients with acute leukemia: results of therapy in 109 adults. *Blood* 1982;60:484.

427. Meloni G, De Fabritis P, Petti MC. BAVC regimen and autologous bone marrow transplantation in patients with acute myelogenous leukemia in second remission. *Blood* 1990;75:2282.

428. Arlin ZA, Sklaroff RB, Gee TS, et al. Phase I and II trial of 4'-(9-acridinylamino)-methanesulfon-*m*-anisidide in patients with acute leukemia. *Cancer Res* 1980;40:3304.

429. Applebaum F, Schulman H. Fatal hepatotoxicity associated with AMSA therapy. *Cancer Treat Rep* 1982;66:1863.

430. Legha SS, Latreille JL, McCredie KB, et al. Neurologic and cardiac rhythm abnormalities associated with 4'-(9-acridinylamino)methanesulfon-*m*-anisidide. *Cancer Treat Rep* 1979;63:2001.

431. Von Hoff DD, Elson D, Polk G, et al. Acute ventricular fibrillation and death during infusion of 4'-(9-acridinylamino)methanesulfon-*m*-anisidide (AMSA) therapy. *Cancer Treat Rep* 1980;64:356.

432. Weiss RB, Moquin D, Adams JD, et al. Electrocardiogram abnormalities induced by m-AMSA. *Cancer Chemother Pharmacol* 1983;10:133.

433. Weiss RB, Grillo-Lopez AJ, Marsoni S, et al. Amsacrine-associated cardiotoxicity: an analysis of 82 cases. *J Clin Oncol* 1986;4:918.

434. Seymour JF. Induction of hypomagnesemia during amsacrine treatment. *Am J Hematol* 1993;42:262.

435. Arlin ZA, Feldman EJ, Mittelman A, et al. M-AMSA is safe and effective therapy for patients with myocardial dysfunction and acute leukemia. *Cancer* 1991;68:1198.

436. Schwartz C, Bender K, Burke P, et al. QT interval prolongation and cardiac dysrhythmia in a patient receiving m-AMSA. *Cancer Treat Rep* 1984;68:1043.

437. Shinar E, Hasin Y. Acute electrocardiographic changes induced by m-AMSA. *Cancer Treat Rep* 1984;68:1169.

438. Tzivoni D, Keren A. Suppression of ventricular arrhythmias by magnesium. *Am J Cardiol* 1990;65:1397.

439. da Cunha MF, Meistrich MF, Haq MM, et al. Temporary effects of AMSA chemotherapy on spermatogenesis. *Cancer* 1982;49:2459.

440. McCrystal MR, Evans BD, Harvey VJ, et al. Phase I study of the cytotoxic agent N-[2-(dimethylamino)ethyl]acridine-4-carboxamide. *Cancer Chemother Pharmacol* 1999;44:39.

441. Kestell P, Dunlop IC, McCrystal MR, et al. Plasma pharmacokinetics of N-[2-(dimethylamino)ethyl]acridine-4-carboxamide in a phase I trial. *Cancer Chemother Pharmacol* 1999;44:45.

442. Schofield PC, Robertson IGC, Paxton JW, et al. Metabolism of N-[2-(dimethylamino)ethyl]acridine-4-carboxamide in cancer patients undergoing a phase I trial. *Cancer Chemother Pharmacol* 1999;44:51.

443. Rouesse J, Spielmann M, Turpin F, et al. Phase II study of elliptinium acetate salvage treatment of advanced breast cancer. *Eur J Cancer* 1993;29A:856.

444. Rouesse J, Tursz T, Le Chevalier T, et al. Intérêt de la 2N-methyl-9-hydroxyellipticine (NSC-264137) dans le traitement des cancers métastasés. *Nouv Press Med* 1981;10:1997.

445. Van Bac N, Moisand C, Gouyette A, et al. Metabolism and disposition studies of 9-hydroxyellipticine and 2-methyl-9-hydroxyellipticinium acetate in animals. *Cancer Treat Rep* 1980;64:879.

446. Monsarrat B, Maftouh M, Meunier G, et al. Human and rat urinary metabolites of the antitumor drug celiptium (N2-methyl-9-hydroxyellipticinium acetate, NSC-264137): identification of cysteine conjugates supporting the "biooxydative alkylation" hypothesis. *Biochem Pharmacol* 1983;32:3887.

447. Gouyette A, Huertas D, Droz J-P, et al. Pharmacokinetics of 2-methyl-9-hydroxyellipticinium acetate (NSC-264137) in cancer patients (Phase I study). *Eur J Clin Oncol* 1982;18:1285.

448. Bernadou J, Monsarrat B, Roche H, et al. Evidence of electrophilic properties of N2-methyl-9-hydroxyellipticinium acetate (Celiptium) from human biliary metabolites. *Cancer Chemother Pharmacol* 1985;15:63.

449. Gouyette A, Voisin E, Auclair C, et al. Isolation and characterization of the glutathione-elliptinium conjugate in human urine. *Anticancer Res* 1987;7:823.

450. Sternberg CN, Yagoda A, Casper E, et al. Phase II trial of elliptinium in advanced renal cell carcinoma and carcinoma of the breast. *Anticancer Res* 1985;5:415.

451. Kayitalire L, Thomas F, Le Chevalier T, et al. Phase II study of a combination of elliptinium and vinblastine in metastatic breast cancer. *Invest New Drugs* 1992;10:303.

452. Doll DC, Weiss RB. Hemolytic anemia associated with antineoplastic agents. *Cancer Treat Rep* 1985;69:777.

453. Criel AM, Hidajat M, Clarysse A, et al. Drug-dependent red cell antibodies and intravascular hemolysis occurring in patients treated with 9-hydroxy-methyl-ellipticinium. *Br J Haematol* 1980;46:549.

454. Piot G, Droz J-P, Theodore C, et al. Phase II trial with high-dose elliptinium acetate in metastatic renal cell carcinoma. *Oncology* 1988;45:371.

455. Thomas N, Moulin B, Raguenez-Viotte G, et al. Nephrotoxicity of an ellipticine derivative (N2-methyl-9-hydroxy-

ellipticinium acetate) in rat: a defect in urinary concentrating ability. *Renal Failure* 1991;13:243.

456. Raguenez-Viotte G, Dadoun C, Buchet P, et al. Renal toxicity of the antitumor drug N2-methyl-9-hydroxyellipticinium acetate in the Wistar rat. *Arch Toxicol* 1988;61:292.

457. Maftouh M, Amiar Y, Picard-Fraire C. Metabolism of the antitumor drug N2-methyl-9-hydroxyellipticinium acetate in isolated rat kidney cells. *Biochem Pharmacol* 1985;34:427.

458. Raguenez-Viotte G, Dieber-Rotheneder M, Dadoun C, et al. Evidence for 4-hydroxyalkenals in rat renal cortex peroxidized by N2-methyl-9-hydroxyellipticinium. *Biochim Biophys Acta* 1990;1046:294.

459. Einzig AI, Gralla RJ, Leyland-Jones BR, et al. Phase I study of elliptinium (2-N-methyl-9-hydroxyellipticinium). *Cancer Invest* 1985;3:325.

460. Arguello F, Alexander MA, Greene JFJ, et al. Preclinical evaluation of 9-chloro-2-methylellipticinium alone and in combination with conventional anticancer drugs for the treatment of human brain tumor xenografts. *J Cancer Res Clin Oncol* 1998;124:19.

461. Khayat D, Borel C, Azab M, et al. Phase I study of datelliptium chloride, hydrochloride given by 24 h continuous intravenous infusion. *Cancer Chemother Pharmacol* 1992;30:226.

462. Harada N, Kawaguchi T, Inoue I, et al. Synthesis and antitumor activity of 2-(2'-oxoalkoxy)-9-hydroxyellipticines. *Chem Pharm Bull* 1997;45:134.

463. Anderson WK, Gopalsamy A, Reddy PS. Design, synthesis, and study of 9-substituted ellipticine and 2-methylellipticinium analogs as potential CNS-selective antitumor agents. *J Med Chem* 1994;37:1955.

464. Honda T, Kato M, Inoue M, et al. Synthesis and antitumor activity of quaternary ellipticine glycosides, a series of novel and highly active antitumor agents. *J Med Chem* 1988;31:1295.

465. Werbel LM, Angelo M, Fry DW, et al. Basically substituted ellipticine analogs as potential antitumor agents. *J Med Chem* 29:1321, 1986.

466. Giacchetti S, Cornez N, Eftekhari P, et al. Phase I clinical trial of the olivacine S16020. *Proc Am Assoc Cancer Res* 1998;39:324 (abstr. 2210).

467. Di Palma M, Brain EC, Etoussami A, et al. Phase I study of Olivacine (S16020) in a weekly schedule: preliminary results. *Proc Am Assoc Cancer Res* 1999;40:83 (abstr. 555).

468. Woodman RJ, Cysyk RL, Kline I, et al. Enhancement of the effectiveness of daunorubicin (NSC-82151) or adriamycin (NSC-123127) against early mouse L1210 leukemia with ICRF-159 (NSC-129943). *Cancer Chemother Pharmacol* 1975;59:689.

469. Flannery EP, Corder MP, Sheehan WW, et al. Phase II study of ICRF-159 in non-Hodgkin's lymphomas. *Cancer Treat Rep* 1978;62:465.

470. Olweny CLM, Masara JP, Sikyewunda W, et al. Treatment of Kaposi's sarcoma with ICRF-159 (NSC-129943). *Cancer Treat Rep* 1976;60:111.

471. Bellet RE, Engstrom PF, Catalano RB, et al. Phase II study of ICRF-159 in patients with metastatic colorectal carcinoma previously exposed to systemic chemotherapy. *Cancer Treat Rep* 1976;60:1395.

472. Natale RB, Wheller RH, Liepman MK, et al. Phase II of ICRF-187 in non-small cell lung cancer. *Cancer Treat Rep* 1983;67:311.

473. Brubaker LH, Vogel CL, Einhorn LH, et al. Treatment of advanced adenocarcinoma of the kidney with ICRF-187: a Southwestern Cancer Study Group Trial. *Cancer Treat Rep* 1986;70:915.

474. Vats T, Kamen B, Krischer JP. Phase II trial of ICRF-187 in children with solid tumors and acute leukemia. *Invest New Drugs* 1991;5:187.

475. Venturini M, Michelotti A, Del Mastro L, et al. Multicenter randomized controlled clinical trial to evaluate cardioprotection of dexrazoxate versus no cardioprotection in women receiving epirubicin chemotherapy for advanced breast cancer. *J Clin Oncol* 1996;14:3112.

476. Wexler LH, Andrich MP, Venzon D, et al. Randomized trial of the cardioprotective agent ICRF-187 in pediatric sarcoma patients treated with doxorubicin. *J Clin Oncol* 1996;14:362.

477. Swain SM, Whaley FS, Gerber MC, et al. Delayed administration of dexrazoxane provides cardioprotection for patients with advanced breast cancer treated with doxorubicin-containing therapy. *J Clin Oncol* 1997;15:1333.

478. Swain SM, Whaley FS, Gerber MC, et al. Cardioprotection with dexrazoxane for doxorubicin-containing therapy in advanced breast cancer. *J Clin Oncol* 1997;15:1318.

479. Hasinoff BB, Hellmann K, Herman EH, et al. Chemical, biological and clinical aspects of dexrazoxane and other bisdioxopiperazines. *Curr Med Chem* 1998;5:1.

480. Lopez M, Vici P, Di Lauro L, et al. Randomized prospective clinical trial of high-dose epirubicin and dexrazoxane in patients with advanced breast cancer and soft tissue sarcomas. *J Clin Oncol* 1998;16:86.

481. Steinherz LJ, Wexler LH. The prevention of anthracycline cardiomyopathy. *Prog Ped Cardiol* 1998;8:97.

482. Butteridge JMC. Lipid peroxidation and possible hydroxyl radical formation stimulated by the self-reduction of doxorubicin-iron (III) complex. *Biochem Pharmacol* 1984;33:1725.

483. Hasinoff BB. The interaction of the cardioprotective agent ICRF-187; its hydrolysis product (ICRF-198) and other chelating agents with Fe (III) and CU (II) complexes of adriamycin. *Agents Actions* 1989;26:378.

484. Hasinoff BB, Reinders FX, Clark V. The enzymatic hydrolysis-activation of the adriamycin cardioprotective agent (+)-1,2-bis(3,5-dioxopiperazinyl-1-yl)propane. *Drug Metab Dispos* 1991;19:74.

485. Herman EH, Ardala B, Bier C, et al. Reduction of daunorubicin lethality and myocardial cellular alterations by pretreatment with ICRF-187 in Syrian Golden Hamsters. *Cancer Treat Rep* 1979;63:89.

486. Herman EH, Ferrans VJ. Reduction of chronic doxorubicin cardiotoxicity in dogs by treatment with (+)-1,2-bis(3,5-cardioxopiperazinyl-1-yl)propane (ICRF-187). *Cancer Res* 1981; 41:3436.

487. Alderton PM, Gross J, Green MD. Comparative study of doxorubicin, mitoxantrone, and epirubicin in combination with ICRF-187 (ADR-529) in a chronic cardiotoxicity animal model. *Cancer Res* 1992;52:194.

488. Shipp NG, Dorr RT, Alberts DS, et al. Characterization of experimental mitoxantrone cardiotoxicity and its partial inhibition by ICRF-187 in cultured neonatal rat heart cells. *Cancer Res* 1993;53:550.

489. Holcenbergh JS, Tutsch KD, Earhart RH, et al. Phase I

study of ICRF-187 in pediatric cancer patients and comparison of its pharmacokinetics in children and adults. *Cancer Treat Rep* 1986;70:703.

490. Hochster H, Liebe SL, Wadler S, et al. Pharmacokinetics of the cardioprotector ADR-529 (ICRF-187) in escalating doses combined with fixed dose doxorubicin. *J Natl Cancer Inst* 1992;84:1725.

491. Von Hoff DD, Howser D, Lewis BJ, et al. Phase I study of ICRF-187 using a daily for 3 days schedule. *Cancer Treat Res* 1981;65:249.

492. Wheeler RH, Bricker LJ, Natale RB, et al. Phase II trial of ICRF-187 in squamous cell carcinoma of the head and neck. *Cancer Treat Rep* 1984;68:427.

493. Holm B, Jensen PB, Sehested M. ICRF-187 rescue in etoposide treatment in vivo. A model targeting high-dose topoisomerase II poisons to CNS tumors. *Cancer Chemother Pharmacol* 1996;38:203.

494. Holm B, Sehested M, Jensen PB. Improved targeting of brain tumors using dexrazoxane rescue of topoisomerase II combined with supralethal doses of etoposide and teniposide. *Clin Cancer Res* 1998;4:1367.

495. Sparano JA, Speyer J, Gradishar WJ, et al. Phase I trial of escalating doses of paclitaxel plus doxorubicin and dexrazoxane in patients with advanced breast cancer. *J Clin Oncol* 1999;17:880.

496. Langer SW, Sehested M, Jensen PB. The catalytic topoisomerase II inhibitor dexrazoxane (ICRF-187) markedly reduces tissue damage from extravasation of daunorubicin in mice. *Proc Am Assoc Cancer Res* 199;40(Abstr. 4500).

497. Jensen PB, Sehested M. DNA topoisomerase II rescue by catalytic inhibitors: a new strategy to improve the antitumor selectivity of etoposide. *Biochem Pharmacol* 1997;54:755.

498. Cai JC, Shu HL, Tang CF, et al. Synthesis and antitumor properties of N1-acyloxymethyl derivatives of bis(2,6-dioxopiperazines). *Chem Pharm Bull* 1989;37:2976.

499. Narita T, Koide Y, Yaguchi S, et al. Antitumor activities and schedule dependence of orally administered MST-16, a novel derivative of bis(2,6-dioxopiperazine). *Cancer Chemother Pharmacol* 1991;28:235.

500. Furue H, Niitani H, Nakao I, et al. Phase I study of MST-16 (Sobuzoxane). *Cancer Chemother (Japanese)* 1990;17:1287.

501. Joshi R, Smith B, Phillips RH, et al. Acute myelomonocytic leukemia after rozoxane therapy. *Lancet* 1981;2:1343.

502. Matsui K, Masuda N, Fukuoka M, et al. Phase II trial of carboplatin plus oral etoposide for elderly patients with small-cell lung cancer. *Br J Cancer* 1998;77:1961.

503. Hartmann JT, Kanz L, Bokemeyer C. Diagnosis and treatment of patients with testicular germ cell cancer. *Drugs* 1999;58:257.

504. Lau DH, Crowley JJ, Gandara DR, et al. Southwest Oncology Group phase II trial of concurrent carboplatin, etoposide, and radiation for poor-risk stage III non-small-cell lung cancer. *J Clin Oncol* 1998;16:3078.

505. Stahl M, Vanhoefer U, Stuschke M, et al. Pre-operative sequential chemo- and radiochemotherapy in locally advanced carcinomas of the lower oesophagus and gastro-oesophageal junction. *Eur J Cancer* 1998;34:668.

506. Eder JP, Teicher BA, Holden SA, et al. Ability of four potential topoisomerase II inhibitors to enhance the cytotoxicity of cis-diaminedichloroplatinum (II) in Chinese hamster ovary cells and in epipodophyllotoxin-resistant subline. *Cancer Chemother Pharmacol* 1990;26:423.

507. Eder JP, Chan V, Wong J, et al. Sequence effect of irinotecan (CPT-11) and topoisomerase II inhibitors in vivo. *Cancer Chemother Pharmacol* 1998;42:327.

508. Whitacre CM, Zborowska E, Gordon NH, et al. Topotecan increases topoisomerase IIalpha levels and sensitivity to treatment with etoposide in schedule-dependent process. *Cancer Res* 1997;57:1425.

509. Pommier Y, Pourquier P, Fan Y, et al. Mechanism of action of eukaryotic DNA topoisomerase I and drugs targeted to the enzyme. *Biochim Biophys Acta* 1998;1400:83.

510. Ohtsu T, Sasaki Y, Igarashi T, et al. Unexpected hepatotoxicities in patients with non-Hodgkin's lymphoma treated with irinotecan (CPT-11) and etoposide. *Jpn J Clin Oncol* 1998;28:502.

511. Masuda N, Fukuoka M, Kudoh S, et al. Phase I and pharmacologic study of irinotecan and etoposide with recombinant human granulocyte colony-stimulating factor support for advanced lung cancer. *J Clin Oncol* 1994;9:1833.

512. Karato A, Yatsuma S, Shinkai T, et al. Phase I study of CPT-11 and etoposide in patients with refractory solid tumors. *J Clin Oncol* 1993;11:2030.

513. Nakamura S, Kudoh S, Komuta K, et al. Phase II study of irinotecan combined with etoposide for previously untreated extensive-disease small-cell lung cancer: a study of the West Japan Lung Cancer Group. *Proc Annu Meet Am Soc Clin Oncol* 1999;18(Abstr. 1815).

514. Oshita F, Noda K, Nishiwaki Y, et al. Phase II study of irinotecan and etoposide in patients with metastatic non-small-cell lung cancer. *J Clin Oncol* 1997;15:304.

515. Hammond LA, Eckardt JR, Ganapathi R, et al. A phase I and translational study of sequential administration of the topoisomerase I and II inhibitors topotecan and etoposide. *Clin Cancer Res* 1998;4:1459.

516. Herben VM, ten Bokkel Huinink WW, Dubbelman AC, et al. Phase I and pharmacological study of sequential intravenous topotecan and oral etoposide. *Br J Cancer* 1997;76:1500.

517. Wahlin A, Brinch L, Hornsten P, et al. Outcome of a multicenter treatment program including autologous or allogeneic bone marrow transplantation for de novo acute myeloid leukemia. *Eur J Haematol* 1997;58:233.

518. Yalowich J, Fry D, Goldman ID. Teniposide (VM-26) and etoposide (VP-16-213) induced augmentation of methotrexate transport and polyglutamation in Ehrlich ascites tumor cells in vitro. *Cancer Res* 1982;42:3648.

519. Lorico A, Boiocchi M, Rappa G. Increase in topoisomerase II-mediated DNA breaks and cytotoxicity of VP16 in human U937 lymphoma cells pretreated with low doses of methotrexate. *Int J Cancer* 1990;45:156.

520. Minford J, Kerrigan D, Nichols M, et al. Enhancement of the DNA breakage and cytotoxic effects of intercalating agents by treatment with sublethal doses of 1-beta-D-arabinofuranosylcytosine or hydroxyurea in L1210 cells. *Cancer Res* 1984;44:5583.

521. Zwelling LA, Minford J, Nichols M, et al. Enhancement of intercalator-induced deoxyribonucleic acid scission and cytotoxicity in murine leukemia cells treated with 5-azacytidine. *Biochem Pharmacol* 1984;33:3903.

522. Willemze R, Suciu S, Archimbaud E, et al. A randomized phase II study on the effects of 5-Aza-2'-deoxycytidine combined with either m-AMSA or idarubicin in patients with relapsed acute leukemia: an EORTC Leukemia Cooperative Group phase II study (06893). *Leukemia* 1997;11:S24.

523. Leteurtre F, Kohlhagen G, Fesen MR, et al. Effects of DNA methylation on topoisomerase I and II cleavage activities. *J Biol Chem* 1994;269:7893.

524. Tjan-Heijnen VC, Biesma B, Festen J, et al. Enhanced myelotoxicity due to granulocyte colony-stimulating factor administration until 48 hours before the next chemotherapy course in patients with small-cell lung carcinoma. *J Clin Oncol* 1998;16:2708.

525. Utsugi T, Mattern MR, Mirabelli CK, et al. Potentiation of topoisomerase inhibitor-induced DNA strand breakage and cytotoxicity by tumor necrosis factor: enhancement of topoisomerase activity as a mechanism of potentiation. *Cancer Res* 1990;50:2636.

526. Branellec D, Markovits J, Chouaib S. Potentiation of TNF-mediated cell killing by etoposide: relationship to DNA single-strand break formation. *Int J Cancer* 1990;46:1048.

527. Valenti M, Cimoli G, Parodi S, et al. Potentiation of tumour necrosis factor-mediated cell killing by VP16 on human ovarian cancer cell lines. In vitro results and clinical implications. *Eur J Cancer* 1993;29A:1157.

528. Morgavi P, Cimoli G, Ottoboni C, et al. Sensitization of human glioblastoma T98G cells to VP16 and VM26 by human tumor necrosis factor. *Anticancer Res* 1995;15:1423.

529. Kamesaki S, Kamesaki H, Jorgensen TJ, et al. Bcl-2 protein inhibits etoposide-induced apoptosis through its effects on events subsequent to topoisomerase II-induced DNA strand breaks and their repair. *Cancer Res* 1993;53:4251.

530. Barinaga M. Life-death balance within the cell. *Science* 1996;274:724.

531. Beg AA, Baltimore D. An essential role for NF-kB in preventing TNF-α-induced cell death. *Science* 1996;274:782.

532. Wang C-Y, Mayo MW, Korneluk RG, et al. NF-kB antiapoptosis: induction of TRAF1 and TRAF2 and c-IAP1 and c-IAP2 to suppress caspase-8 activation. *Science* 1998;281:1680.

533. Ciardiello F, Bianco R, Damiano V, et al. Antitumor activity of sequential treatment with topotecan and anti-epidermal growth factor receptor monoclonal antibody C225. *Clin Cancer Res* 1999;5:909.

534. Bible KC, Kaufmann SH. Cytotoxic synergy between flavopiridol (NSC 649890, L86-8275) and various antineoplastic agents: the importance of sequence of administration. *Cancer Res* 1997;57:3375.

535. Kim JC, Yoon JB, Koo HS, et al. Cloning and characterization of the 5'-flanking region for the human topoisomerase III gene [In Process Citation]. *J Biol Chem* 1998;273:26130.

536. Pommier Y. Topoisomerase inhibitors: why develop new ones. *Opinion in Oncologic, Endocrine & Metabolic Investigational Drugs* 1999;1:168.

537. Errington F, Willmore E, Tilby MJ, et al. Murine transgenic cells lacking DNA topoisomerase iibeta are resistant to acridines and mitoxantrone: analysis of cytotoxicity and cleavable complex formation. *Mol Pharmacol* 1999;56:1309.

538. Malonne H, Atassi G. DNA topoisomerase targeting drugs: mechanisms of action and perspectives. *Anticancer Drugs* 1997;8:811.

539. Gogas H, Mansi JL. New drugs. The anthrapyrazoles. *Cancer Treat Rev* 1996;21:541.

540. Taguchi T, Ohta K, Hotta T, et al. [Menogaril (TUT-7) late phase II study for malignant lymphoma, adult T-cell leukemia and lymphoma (ATLL)]. *Gan To Kagaku Ryoho* 1997;24:1263.

541. Poddevin B, Riou JF, Lavelle F, Pommier Y. Dual topoisomerase I and II inhibition by intoplicine (RP-60475), a new antitumor agent in early clinical trials. *Mol Pharmacol* 1993;44:767.

542. van Gijn R, ten Bokkel Huinink WW, Rodenhuis S, et al. Topoisomerase I/II inhibitor intoplicine administered as a 24 h infusion: phase I and pharmacologic study. *Anticancer Drugs* 1999;10:17.

543. Yamashita Y, Kawada S, Fujii N, et al. Induction of mammalian DNA topoisomerase I and II mediated DNA cleavage by saintopin, a new antitumor agent from fungus. *Biochemistry* 1991;30:5838.

544. Nitiss JL, Zhou J, Rose A, et al. The bis(naphthalimide) DMP-840 causes cytotoxicity by its action against eukaryotic topoisomerase II. *Biochemistry* 1998;37:3078.

545. Yamashita Y, Kawada S, Fujii N, et al. Induction of mammalian DNA topoisomerase II dependent DNA cleavage by antitumor antibiotic streptonigrin. *Cancer Res* 1990; 50:5841.

546. Leteurtre F, Kohlhagen G, Pommier Y. Streptonigrin-induced topoisomerase II sites exhibit base preference in the middle of the enzyme stagger. *Biochem Biophys Res Commun* 1994;203:1259.

547. Capranico G, Palumbo M, Tinelli S, et al. Unique sequence specificity of topoisomerase II DNA cleavage stimulation and DNA binding mode of streptonigrin. *J Biol Chem* 1994;40:25004.

548. Fujii N, Yamashita Y, Saitoh Y, et al. Induction of mammalian DNA topoisomerase I-mediated DNA cleavage and DNA winding by bulgarein. *J Biol Chem* 1993;268:13160.

549. Matsumoto SS, Haughey HM, Schmehl DM, et al. Makaluvamines vary in ability to induce dose-dependent DNA cleavage via topoisomerase II interaction [In Process Citation]. *Anticancer Drugs* 1999;10:39.

550. Rowe T, Kupfer G, Ross W. Inhibition of epipodophyllotoxin cytotoxicity by interference with topoisomerase-mediated DNA cleavage. *Biochem Pharmacol* 1985;34:2483.

551. Kong XB, Rubin L, Chen LI, et al. Topoisomerase II-mediated DNA cleavage activity and irreversibility of cleavable complex formation induced by DNA intercalator with alkylating capability. *Mol Pharmacol* 1992;41:237.

552. Hernandez L, Cholody WM, Hudson EA, et al. Mechanism of action of bisimidazoacridones, new drugs with potent, selective activity against colon cancer. *Cancer Res* 1995;55:2338.

553. Markovits J, Pommier Y, Mattern MR, et al. Effects of the bifunctional antitumor intercalator ditercalinium on DNA in mouse leukemia L1210 cells and DNA topoisomerase II. *Cancer Res* 1986;46:5821.

554. Cozzi P, Mongelli N. Cytotoxics derived from distamycin A and congeners [In Process Citation]. *Curr Pharm Des* 1998;4:181.

555. Fesen M, Pommier Y. Mammalian topoisomerase II activity is modulated by the DNA minor groove binder distamycin in simian virus 40 DNA. *J Biol Chem* 1989;264:11354.

556. Zagotto G, Oliva A, Guano F, et al. Synthesis, DNA-damaging and cytotoxic properties of novel topoisomerase II-directed bisantrene analogs. *Bioorg Med Chem Lett* 1998;8:121.

557. Fortune JM, Osheroff N. Merbarone inhibits the catalytic activity of human topoisomerase IIalpha by blocking DNA cleavage. *J Biol Chem* 1998;273:17643.

558. Kerrigan D, Pommier Y, Kohn KW. Protein-linked DNA strand breaks produced by etoposide and teniposide in Mouse L1210 and Human VA-13 and HT-29 cell lines: relationship to cytotoxicity. *NCI Monographs* 1987;4:117.

559. Hande KR. Etoposide: four decades of development of a topoisomerase II inhibitor. *Eur J Cancer* 1998;34:1514.

560. Bojanowski K, Lelievre S, Markovits J, et al. Suramin is an inhibitor of DNA topoisomerase II in vitro and in Chinese hamster fibrosarcoma cells. *Proc Natl Acad Sci U S A* 1992;89:3025.

561. Riou JF, Helissey P, Grondard L, et al. Inhibition of eukaryotic DNA topoisomerase I and II activities by indoloquinolinedione derivatives. *Mol Pharmacol* 1991;40:699.

562. Utsumi H, Shibuya ML, Kosaka T, et al. Abrogation by novobiocin of cytotoxicity due to the topoisomerase II inhibitor m-AMSA in Chinese hamster cells. *Cancer Res* 1990;50:2577.

563. Constantinou A, Mehta R, Runyan C, et al. Flavonoids as DNA topoisomerase antagonists and poisons: structure-activity relationships. *J Nat Prod* 1995;58:217.

564. Chen M, Beck WT. Teniposide-resistant CEM cells, which express mutant DNA topoisomerase II alpha, when treated with non-complex-stabilizing inhibitors of the enzyme, display no cross-resistance and reveal aberrant functions of the mutant enzyme. *Cancer Res* 1993;53:5946.

565. McCabe MJ Jr, Orrenius S. Genistein induces apoptosis in immature human thymocytes by inhibiting topoisomerase-II. *Biochem Biophys Res Commun* 1993;194:944.

566. Gedik CM, Collins AR. Comparison of effects of fostriecin, novobiocin, and camptothecin, inhibitors of DNA topoisomerases, on DNA replication and repair in human cells. *Nucleic Acids Res* 1990;18:1007.

567. Sorensen BS, Jensen PS, Andersen AH, et al. Stimulation of topoisomerase II mediated DNA cleavage at specific sequence elements by the 2-nitroimidazole Ro 15-0216. *Biochemistry* 1990;29:9507.

568. Holm B, Jensen PB, Sehested M, et al. In vivo inhibition of etoposide-mediated apoptosis, toxicity, and antitumor effect by the topoisomerase II-uncoupling anthracycline aclarubicin. *Cancer Chemother Pharmacol* 1994;34:503.

569. Kawada S, Yamashita Y, Fujii N, et al. Induction of a heat-stable topoisomerase II-DNA cleavable complex by nonintercalative terpenoids, terpentecin and clerocidin. *Cancer Res* 1991;51:2922.

570. Permana PA, Snapka RM, Shen LL, et al. Quinobenoxazines: a class of novel antitumor quinolones and potent mammalian DNA topoisomerase II catalytic inhibitors. *Biochemistry* 1994;33:11333.

571. Binaschi M, Zagotto G, Palumbo M, et al. Irreversible and reversible topoisomerase II DNA cleavage stimulated by clerocidin: sequence specificity and structural drug determinants. *Cancer Res* 1997;57:1710.

572. Fujii N, Yamashita Y, Arima Y, et al. Induction of topoisomerase II-mediated DNA cleavage by the plant naphthoquinones plumbagin and shikonin. *Antimicrob Agents Chemother* 1992;36:2589.

573. Juang JK, Huang HW, Chen CM, et al. A new compound, with angulatin A, promotes type II DNA topoisomerase-mediated DNA damage. *Biochem Biophys Res Commun* 1989;159:1128.

574. Fujii N, Tanaka F, Yamashita Y, et al. UCE6, a new antitumor antibiotic with topoisomerase I-mediated DNA cleavage activity produced by actinomycetes: producing organism, fermentation, isolation and biological activity. *J Antibiot (Tokyo)* 1997;50:490.

575. Robinson MJ, Martin BA, Gootz TD, et al. Effects of novel fluoroquinolones on the catalytic activities of eukaryotic topoisomerase II: influence of the C-8 fluorine group. *Antimicrob Agents Chemother* 1992;36:751.

576. Leteurtre F, Sackett DL, Madalengoitia J, et al. Azatoxin derivatives with potent and selective action on topoisomerase II. *Biochem Pharmacol* 1995;49:1283.

577. Campain JA, Gottesman MM, Pastan I. A novel mutant topoisomerase II alpha present in etoposide-resistant human melanoma cell lines has a deletion of alanine 429. *Biochemistry* 1994;33:11327.

578. Bugg BY, Danks MK, Beck WT, et al. Expression of a mutant DNA topoisomerase II in CCRF-CEM human leukemic cells selected for resistance to teniposide. *Proc Natl Acad Sci U S A* 1991;88:7654.

579. Lee MS, Wang JC, Beran M. Two independent m-AMSA-resistant human myeloid leukemia cell lines share an identical point mutation in the 170 kDa form of human topoisomerase II. *J Mol Biol* 1992;223:837.

580. Chan VT, Ng SW, Eder JP, et al. Molecular cloning and identification of a point mutation in the topoisomerase II cDNA from an etoposide-resistant Chinese hamster ovary cell line. *J Biol Chem* 1993;268:2160.

581. Kubo A, Yoshikawa A, Hirashima T, et al. Point mutations of the topoisomerase IIalpha gene in patients with small cell lung cancer treated with etoposide. *Cancer Res* 1996;56:1232.

582. Takano H, Vilalta P, Hsiung Y, et al. Characterization of intrinsic and acquired mutations in topoisomerase II (Topo II). *Proc Annu Meet Am Assoc Cancer Res* 1994;35.

583. Patel S, Fisher LM. Novel selection and genetic characterisation of an etoposide-resistant human leukaemic CCRF-CEM cell line. *Br J Cancer* 1993;67:456.

584. Danks MK, Warmoth MR, Friche E, et al. Single-strand conformational polymorphism analysis of the M(r) 170,000 isozyme of DNA topoisomerase II in human tumor cells. *Cancer Res* 1993;53:1373.

585. Hashimoto S, Danks MK, Chatterjee S, et al. A novel point mutation in the 3' flanking region of the DNA-binding domain of topoisomerase II alpha associated with acquired resistance to topoisomerase II active agents. *Oncol Res* 1995;7:21.

586. Kohno K, Danks MK, Matsuda T, et al. A novel mutation of DNA topoisomerase II alpha in an etoposide-resistant human cancer cell line. *Cellular Pharmacol* 1995;2:87.

20

TOPOISOMERASE I TARGETING AGENTS: THE CAMPTOTHECINS

CHRIS H. TAKIMOTO
SUSAN G. ARBUCK

Topoisomerase I targeting agents, such as the camptothecin analogs, are a novel class of anticancer agents with a unique molecular target, the DNA-relaxing enzyme topoisomerase I. The first compound in this class, camptothecin, is a naturally occurring alkaloid found in the bark and wood of the Chinese tree *Camptotheca acuminata*. The camptothecins have generated broad interest, both as a research tool for studying the molecular function and activity of DNA topoisomerases, and as therapeutic agents with proven activity in the treatment of human malignancies. All of the biologically active camptothecins inhibit the enzymatic activity of topoisomerase I; however, they differ from classic enzyme inhibitors, such as the antifolate methotrexate, which acts by eliminating the function of an essential enzyme, dihydrofolate reductase. Instead, the camptothecins convert an endogenous enzyme, DNA topoisomerase I, into a cellular poison by trapping it in a covalent complex bound to DNA. For this reason, the camptothecin derivatives as a clinical class of antitumor agents are best referred to as topoisomerase I poisons or targeting agents rather than inhibitors.[1]

HISTORY

As early as the 1950s, a National Cancer Institute screening program designed to identify promising new natural products discovered that extracts derived from the camptotheca tree were cytotoxic to cancer cells. Not until 1966, however, did Wall and colleagues[2] identify camptothecin as the active agent. Early biochemical studies of the pharmacology of camptothecin showed that it could damage DNA,[3] ultimately inhibiting both DNA and RNA synthesis[4–11]; however, the mechanisms underlying these drug actions remained obscure. Nonetheless, because of promising preclinical activity, the drug entered clinical trials in the early 1970s under National Cancer Institute sponsorship. Because of its insolubility in aqueous solutions, camptothecin was formulated as its sodium salt (NSC-1000880). In phase I studies, responses were observed in patients with colorectal, stomach, small

bowel, and non–small cell lung cancers, as well as in those with melanoma. Unfortunately, frequently severe toxicities, including hemorrhagic cystitis, nausea, vomiting, diarrhea, and dose-limiting myelosuppression, were also observed.[12–14] When limited phase II testing failed to demonstrate meaningful antitumor activity in gastrointestinal cancers[15] and malignant melanoma,[16] further clinical development was halted.

Important advances in the 1980s led to a resurgence of interest in the camptothecins. First was the discovery that camptothecin had a unique molecular target, DNA topoisomerase I, a key nuclear enzyme responsible for relaxing torsionally strained DNA.[17,18] Currently, the camptothecins remain the best-characterized inhibitors of topoisomerase I. The elucidation of this novel mechanism led to the successful development of more soluble and less toxic camptothecin analogs with even greater preclinical anticancer activity, such as irinotecan (CPT-11) and topotecan.[19–23] In 1996, topotecan hydrochloride (Hycamtin) was approved in the United States for use as second-line chemotherapy for patients with advanced ovarian cancer, and in that same year, irinotecan hydrochloride (Camptosar) was approved for use in patients with 5-fluorouracil (5-FU)–refractory advanced colorectal cancer. Additional camptothecin analogs in clinical testing include 9-aminocamptothecin (9-AC), 9-nitrocamptothecin, GI47211, DX8951f, and karenitecin. Several noncamptothecin agents that also interact with topoisomerase I have entered clinical trials, including NB-506, intoplicine (RP60475), TAS 101, and (*N*-[2-(dimethylamino)ethyl]acridine-4-carboxamide (DACA). The development of these new agents may further increase the importance of topoisomerase I as a target for cancer chemotherapy.

CAMPTOTHECIN STRUCTURE-ACTIVITY RELATIONSHIPS

All camptothecins contain a basic five-ring structure with a chiral center located at C-20 on the terminal lactone E

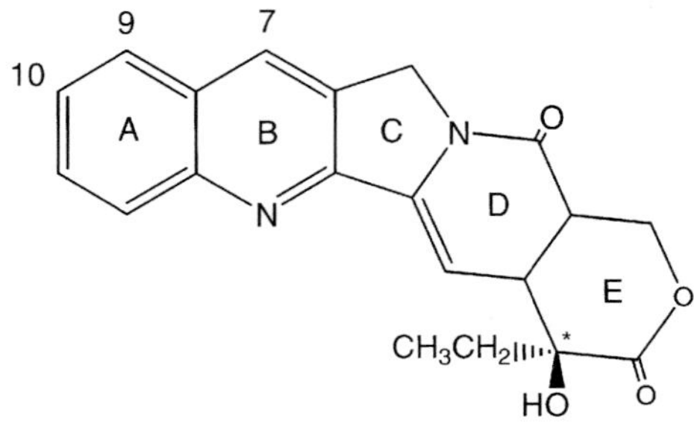

	C-10	C-9	C-7
Camptothecin	H	H	H
Topotecan	OH	$(CH_3)_2NHCH_2$	H
9-Nitrocamptothecin	H	NO_2	H
9-Aminocamptothecin	H	NH_2	H
Karenitecin	H	$(CH_3)_3SiCH_2CH_2$	H
Irinotecan	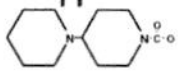	H	CH_3CH_2

* S configuration at chiral C20

FIGURE 20-1. Structure of camptothecin analogs.

ring (Fig. 20-1). The topoisomerase I–inhibitory activity of these agents is stereospecific, with the naturally occurring (S)-isomer being 10 to 100 times more biologically active than the (R)-isomer.[24,25] Substitutions at C-9 or C-10 can enhance water solubility without interfering with drug activity. Although an intact lactone ring is essential for topoisomerase I inhibition, it also confers a degree of instability to these agents. In aqueous solutions, all the camptothecins can undergo a rapid, reversible, pH-dependent, nonenzymatic hydrolysis of the lactone ring to generate an open-ring hydroxy carboxylic acid (Fig. 20-2). At neutral or physiologic pH, the equilibrium between the two species favors the less active carboxylate for all the camptothecins.[26] Although the camptothecin carboxylate is more water soluble than the lactone, it is also at least tenfold less active as an inhibitor of topoisomerase I.[27,28] An understanding of this hydrolysis reaction helps to explain the unpredictable and severe hemorrhagic cystitis observed in the early clinical development of these drugs. Because the camptothecin was initially administered as the more water-soluble sodium salt, the tumors were exposed to high systemic concentrations of the relatively inactive carboxylate species.[29] When 17% of the total administered dose was excreted in the urine,[12] however, the low pH in

the bladder favored the closure of the lactone ring, which generated the active drug species and caused severe hemorrhagic cystitis.

The presence of this unstable terminal lactone ring also complicates the accurate analytic measurement of all the camptothecins.[30–32] For example, when topotecan is in human plasma at 37°C, its half-life is only 18.2 minutes, with the majority of the drug being in the carboxylate form at equilibrium.[33] Therefore, prompt processing of blood samples and careful maintenance of low temperatures are essential for accurate camptothecin lactone measurements.[34]

Irinotecan is structurally unique among the camptothecins because of the bulky dipiperidino side chain located at the C-10 position. Enzymatic cleavage of this substituent group by a carboxylesterase-converting enzyme generates the active metabolite, SN-38 (7-ethyl-10-hydroxycamptothecin) (Fig. 20-3), which is over 1,000-fold more potent than the parent compound as a topoisomerase I poison.[35] Thus, irinotecan is a prodrug that requires enzymatic activation for its biologic activity. Converting enzyme activity has been characterized in rodent serum, liver, and small intestine; however, its activity in human tissues is less than in rats.[36–38] In patients, the plasma pharmacokinetic profile of irinotecan is complex. After intravenous administration, both the lactone and carboxylate forms of irinotecan and its active metabolite, SN-38, are detectable in plasma.[39]

In vitro structure-activity studies show a strong correlation between the ability to interact with topoisomerase I and overall cytotoxic potency.[24,27,28,40,41] In general, substitutions at C-9 and C-10 tend to increase topoisomerase I inhibition and can also increase water solubility,[41] whereas substitutions at C-12 decease activity.[24] The β-hydroxy group at C-20 appears to be important for biologic activity[27]; however, 20-chloro- and 20-bromocamptothecin derivatives with topoisomerase I–specific cytotoxic activity have been characterized.[42] Two newer camptothecins, DX8951f and karenitecin (BNP1350) are currently in clinical trials. DX8951f is a water-soluble hexacyclic camptothecin derivative with greater topoisomerase I–inhibitory activity than topotecan or SN-38.[43] Karenitecin is more lipophilic, with a lactone ring that is relatively more stable than that of other camptothecin analogs.[44]

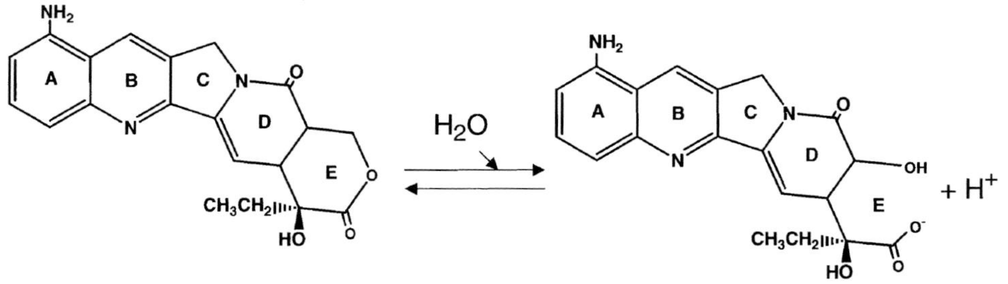

FIGURE 20-2. Hydrolysis of the lactone ring of 9-aminocamptothecin.

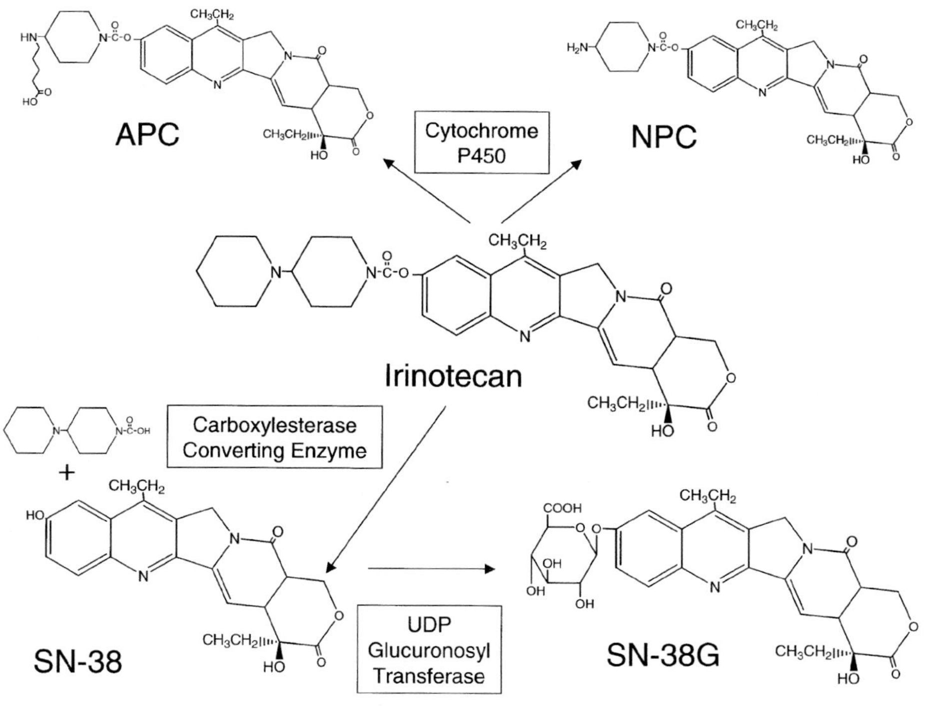

FIGURE 20-3. Metabolism of irinotecan. (UDP, uridine diphosphate.)

BIOCHEMICAL AND MOLECULAR PHARMACOLOGY

Topoisomerase I

DNA topoisomerases are important enzymes that modulate DNA topology. Human topoisomerase I is a type IB topoisomerase[45] that relaxes torsionally strained supercoiled DNA by generating a transient single-stranded nick in the DNA. The first type I DNA topoisomerase was characterized in *Escherichia coli* by James Wang in 1971.[46] Shortly thereafter, Champoux and Dulbecco characterized a eukaryotic enzyme with similar activity in mouse embryo cells.[47] Further studies revealed that these eukaryotic type I topoisomerase enzymes have relatively little sequence homology with the bacterial proteins.[48] In contrast to type I enzymes, type II DNA topoisomerases alter DNA topology by mediating the passage of a second strand of duplex DNA through a transient double-stranded break in the DNA molecule. Thus, type II enzymes catalyze the crossing of two double-stranded DNA molecules and are thought to be important in facilitating separation of daughter strands after DNA replication.[49,50]

Human DNA topoisomerase I, the target enzyme of the camptothecins, is a 100-kd protein composed of 765 amino acids.[51] The enzymatic activity of topoisomerase I is found in a 67.7-kd region located at the carboxyl-terminal end of the protein. The topoisomerase I gene is located on human chromosome 20, and it consists of 21 exons extending over 85 kilobases of DNA.[52,53] Expression of topoisomerase I is essential for mammalian cell viability,[54] and it is frequently present at estimated copy numbers as high as 10[6] per cell.[53] However, yeast mutants with a complete absence of topoisomerase I activity and a compensatory increase in topoisomerase II activity have been identified.[55,56] Human topoisomerase I may also be important in other disease states besides cancer. For example, autoantibodies against human DNA topoisomerase I have been implicated in the pathogenesis of scleroderma.[57,58]

The crystallographic structure of human topoisomerase I was characterized in a complex with DNA,[59] in which the enzyme was found to form a three-dimensional "clamp" around the DNA helix.[59,60] Human topoisomerase I can be divided into four distinct major structural domains.[61] Domain 1 spans amino acid residues 1 through 197 and is 24 kd in size. It is relatively unconserved across different species and does not appear to be essential for *in vitro* catalytic activity. It does contain several nuclear localization signals, however, and its N-terminal end is highly charged. This high density of both negatively and positively charged amino acid residues may permit elevated concentrations of the protein to exist in localized regions of the cell, such as the nucleolus.[62] Domain 2 is the proteolytically resistant, relatively conserved core of the protein, encompassing amino acid residues 198 to 651. This 54-kd domain is responsible for the enzyme's preferential binding to supercoiled DNA.[63] Clustering of positively charged lysine residues in a portion of this region may also facilitate its interaction with negatively charged DNA.[64] Mutational studies suggest a role for this domain in interacting with camptothecin and in mediating DNA cleavage and ligation steps catalyzed by the enzyme.[65] Domain 3 is a relatively unconserved, small, 5-kd, positively charged linker domain that includes residues 652 to 696. Interestingly, this region is not essential for catalytic activity, because reconstitution experiments that combine the highly conserved domains 2 and 4 as separate subunits still demonstrate catalytic activity, even in the absence of domain 3.[66] The final domain 4, defined by residues 697 to 765, is only 8 kd in size and encompasses the highly conserved C-terminal region of the protein that includes the active site tyrosine at residue 723.

Topoisomerase I Mechanism of Action

Human topoisomerase I relaxes both positively and negatively supercoiled double-stranded DNA. Unwinding of the DNA helix is essential for normal DNA function, such as DNA replication or RNA transcription.[67] This unwinding generates a torsional strain in the DNA resulting from supercoiling of the helix above and below the region of ongoing nucleic acid synthesis.[68–70] Although its exact role has not been fully elucidated, topoisomerase I is thought to relax this localized supercoiling, thereby allowing important DNA functions to proceed in an orderly fashion. In an *in vitro* SV40 system, topoisomerase I enhanced bidirectional DNA synthesis, consistent with its acting as a swivel to relax the localized supercoiling that occurs during the elongation phase of DNA replication.[71,72] Another postulated role for topoisomerase I is to facilitate RNA transcription.[73,74] Supporting evidence comes from immunohistochemical studies demonstrating high levels of topoisomerase I in the nucleolus, which is actively involved in RNA synthesis.[75] Furthermore, topoisomerase I has been found to associate intracellularly with RNA polymerase II[76,77] and other transcriptionally active proteins.[78–80] When RNA synthesis is inhibited by agents such as 5,6-dichloro-1-β-D-ribofurano-

sylbenzimidazole (DRB), these interactions are disrupted, which results in relocation of the topoisomerase I to nonnucleolar regions of the nucleus.[81] Camptothecin treatment also causes nucleolar redistribution of topoisomerase I and this drug-induced translocation may be useful as a potential marker for drug sensitivity.[82]

Many of the steps involved in the topoisomerase I–mediated reaction that relaxes supercoiled DNA have been characterized at the molecular level.[49,50,67] Human DNA topoisomerase I preferentially binds to supercoiled double-stranded DNA and cleaves the phosphodiester bond, which results in a single-stranded DNA nick (Fig. 20-4). During this process, the topoisomerase I enzyme is temporarily bound by a covalent bond between the tyrosine residue at position 723 and the 3' end of the single-stranded break in the DNA.[83,84] Once formed, this normally short-lived intermediate, called the cleavable complex,[17] allows for relaxation of the DNA torsional strain. This may occur either by passage of the intact single strand through the gap in the nicked DNA, which decreases the DNA linking number by one, or by free rotation of the DNA about the noncleaved strand.[85] Finally, re-ligation of the strand break restores the integrity of the double-stranded DNA and is followed by enzyme dissociation from the newly relaxed double helix. Unlike with type II topoisomerases, no energy-dependent cofactors are required. Typically, topoisomerase I catalysis is rapid, and DNA-bound enzyme cannot be isolated under normal conditions. Topoisomerase I cleavage sites are not random; instead, they occur at weak consensus sequences throughout the DNA, with preferential covalent binding of the protein to thymidine nucleotides.[86,87]

Topoisomerase I is expressed throughout the cell cycle, even in cells that are not actively dividing.[22,88] Increased topoisomerase I messenger RNA (mRNA) has been detected in human fibroblasts after stimulation with phorbol esters[89]

Topoisomerase I Mechanism of Action

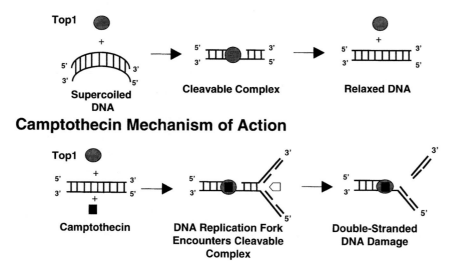

FIGURE 20-4. Mechanism of action of topoisomerase I (TopI) and the camptothecins.

and during increased proliferation states in hepatocytes[90] and fibroblasts.[91] In comparative studies, higher levels of topoisomerase I protein and mRNA were found in malignant ovarian,[92] colon,[93,94] and prostate tumors[94] than in their normal tissue counterparts. This finding may explain some of the selective cytotoxicity of the camptothecins for tumor cells compared with normal tissues. Within specific tumor types, topoisomerase I enzyme activity appears to be quite variable. In a series of solid tumor biopsy specimens from 12 patients with colon cancer and 21 patients with cervical cancer, topoisomerase I activity varied by 64-fold and 16-fold, respectively.[95] In this study, 19% of all tumor biopsy specimens had undetectable topoisomerase I enzyme activity. Whether or not these measurements relate to clinical drug sensitivity to camptothecins, however, is unknown.

Little is known about the specific regulation of topoisomerase I activity. In tumor cell lines, alterations in topoisomerase I enzyme activity have not always correlated with changes in topoisomerase I mRNA levels as measured by Northern blot testing, or with topoisomerase I protein levels, as measured by Western immunoblot testing.[96,97] This has led some investigators to hypothesize that posttranscriptional events may be important in the regulation of this enzyme.[97] Phosphorylation of topoisomerase I may be an important mechanism for enhancing enzyme activity. In a cell-free system, phosphorylation of topoisomerase I by protein kinase C enhanced catalytic activity, whereas exposure to calf intestine alkaline phosphatase abolished this effect.[98] Furthermore, in intact mouse fibroblasts stimulated by phorbol esters, the topoisomerase I phosphorylation state directly correlated with activation of the topoisomerase I enzyme.[99,100] These and other observations suggest that topoisomerase I phosphorylation may regulate topoisomerase I activity. This may also have clinical relevance, because down-regulation of topoisomerase I enzyme activity by dephosphorylation may reduce cellular sensitivity to camptothecins.[101] In contrast to phosphorylation, poly(adenosine diphosphate[ADP]-ribosyl)ation of DNA topoisomerase I by the poly(ADP-ribose) polymerase (PARP), a component of the multiprotein DNA replication complex, decreases topoisomerase I activity. Activation of PARP increases in response to DNA damage and appears to be responsible for the decrease in topoisomerase I activity seen after exposure to ionizing radiation.[102–104] The complex interplay between these potential topoisomerase I regulatory mechanisms must still be defined.

Mechanism of Action of the Camptothecins

In the presence of camptothecins, the topoisomerase I enzymatic reaction is altered, which results in a drug-induced stabilization of the cleavable complex.[17,18] Camptothecins interact noncovalently with the DNA-bound topoisomerase I and inhibit the re-ligation step of the reaction (Fig. 20-4). Consequently, stabilized cleavable complexes accumulate and single-stranded DNA breaks persist. This DNA damage alone is not toxic to the cell, however, because these lesions are highly reversible and rapidly disappear once the drug is removed.[17,105] Instead, ongoing DNA synthesis is required to convert these stabilized cleavable complexes into more lethal DNA damage.[106,107] According to the "fork collision model,"[108] lethal damage to the DNA occurs only when a DNA replication fork encounters a cleavable complex, which results in a cytotoxic double-stranded break in the DNA.[107,109,110] Thus, cleavable complex formation is necessary but not sufficient for typical camptothecin-induced cytotoxicity. In support of this theory are observations that inhibitors of DNA synthesis, such as aphidicolin[106–108] or hydroxyurea,[106] protect cells from camptothecin-induced cytotoxicity. Based on this model, camptothecins should be cytotoxic agents relatively specific to the S phase of the cell cycle, and this has been confirmed in most experimental studies.[1,3,7,108,111] This mechanism has important implications for the design of clinical therapeutic regimens, because S-phase–specific cytotoxic agents generally require prolonged exposures to drug concentrations above a minimum threshold to maximize the fractional cell kill.[112] Furthermore, the presence of topoisomerase I is absolutely essential for the generation of camptothecin-induced cytotoxicity. For example, mutant yeast cells that lack functional topoisomerase I are completely resistant to the camptothecins[113]; however, when topoisomerase I is transfected into these mutants, drug sensitivity is restored.[114]

At the molecular level, all of the camptothecins in clinical use are potent inhibitors of mammalian DNA topoisomerase I. The *in vitro* inhibitory potencies of some of the commonly used camptothecins are shown in Table 20-1. The only compound lacking direct activity is irinotecan, which is a prodrug that must be enzymatically converted to SN-38 for biologic activity. Differences in the spectrum of clinical activity of the various camptothecins are not explained by differences in drug potency in interacting with DNA topoisomerase I. Even when the inhibitory activity of the different camptothecins is similar, however, the stability

TABLE 20-1. DRUG CONCENTRATIONS NECESSARY TO INHIBIT MAMMALIAN DNA TOPOISOMERASE I ACTIVITY BY 50% *IN VITRO* (CC_{50})

Drug	CC_{50} (µmol/L)
Camptothecin	0.82 ± 0.7
Topotecan	3.2 ± 0.33
9-Aminocamptothecin	0.9
SN-38	0.8
Irinotecan	>100

From Kingsbury WD, Boehm JC, Jakas DR, et al. Synthesis of water-soluble (aminoalkyl)camptothecin analogues: inhibition of topoisomerase I and antitumor activity. *J Med Chem* 1991;34:98–107.

of the resulting drug-induced DNA–topoisomerase I cleavable complexes may differ. For example, when increased sodium chloride concentrations were used to dissociate drug-stabilized cleavable complexes, SN-38–induced lesions were much more stable than those induced by camptothecin, topotecan, or 9-AC.[41,115] The relevance of these differences to clinical activity of the various camptothecins must still be determined.

Camptothecins do not stabilize all topoisomerase I cleavable complexes equally; instead, they enhance stabilization of a subset of topoisomerase I cleavage sites. In the presence of camptothecin, topoisomerase I cleavable complexes are preferentially stabilized when a guanine residue is immediately 3' to the phosphodiester bond normally cleaved by the enzyme (position +1).[116–120] In the absence of drug, topoisomerase I has no strong base preference at this location. This has led to proposal of a camptothecin stacking model in which the drug specifically interacts with guanine residues at the topoisomerase I–DNA cleavage site.[119,121] Interestingly, different camptothecin derivatives may also stabilize different subsets of topoisomerase I cleavage sites; whether this affects clinical drug activity is also unknown.[41]

Persistence of cleavable complexes within the cell may sometimes occur, even in the absence of camptothecins. For example, abasic sites and DNA mismatches occurring downstream but in close proximity to a known topoisomerase I cleavage site can lead to stabilization of a DNA–topoisomerase I cleavable complex.[122–124] This type of DNA damage arising from radiation exposure or from DNA–alkylating agents may theoretically generate topoisomerase I–dependent cytotoxic effects in a way that is similar to that of the camptothecin mechanism. Recently, a mutant yeast topoisomerase I enzyme was identified that was also lethal to cells in a manner analogous to camptothecin-induced cytotoxicity.[125] A single amino acid substitution at residue 517 was found that interfered with the DNA re-ligation step and decreased the *in vitro* catalytic activity by 1,000-fold. This caused an accumulation of stabilized topoisomerase I–cleavable complexes, which led to eventual G_2 checkpoint arrest and cell death. Expression of this mutant was conditionally lethal to cells. Although the proposal is unproven, the idea has been put forward that DNA damage in the form of stabilization of cleavable complexes can occur endogenously in cells at low levels but may be compensated for by as yet unidentified DNA repair enzymes.[125] Exposure to camptothecin derivatives or mutations in the topoisomerase I enzyme, however, can overwhelm these repair processes and eventually lead to cell death.

Potential pathways for the removal of topoisomerase I covalently bound to DNA in the cleavable complex have been identified recently. In human tumor cell lines, degradation of topoisomerase I bound to DNA was mediated by the ubiquitin-proteasome 26S pathway.[126] Preliminary evidence suggests that some resistant cells may degrade topoisomerase I by this mechanism as a way to repair camptothecin-induced DNA damage and to avoid drug toxicity.[126] Downregulation of topoisomerase I and decreased cleavable complex formation after camptothecin treatment have also been observed in other *in vitro* cell systems.[127–129] In clinical studies, decreases in total cellular topoisomerase I have been observed in peripheral blood cells obtained from patients after treatment with camptothecin-based chemotherapy.[130–132] Further studies must confirm whether these dynamic changes in topoisomerase I expression correlate at all with drug response. In other studies, a eucaryotic protein with tyrosine–DNA phosphodiesterase activity was recently isolated from yeast cells.[133] This 55-kd protein could cleave DNA topoisomerase I that was covalently bound to DNA by hydrolyzing the 3'-phosphodiester-tyrosine bond. It was active over a pH range of 5.0 to 9.5 and at temperatures ranging from 25°C to 45°C. No energy-dependent cofactors were required for its activity, and the estimated K_m (Michaelis-Menten constant) for the tyrosine-phosphodiester substrate was in the nanomolar range. The precise function of this enzyme is not known, but speculating a role for this protein in the repair of stabilized DNA–topoisomerase I cleavable complexes is tempting. Whether the expression of this enzyme changes during treatment with topoisomerase I poisons is not known.

Camptothecins also can also induce DNA mutations and chromosomal damage, manifested by increased sister chromatid exchanges, gene deletions, and chromosomal rearrangements.[134,135] Dose-dependent increases in sister chromatid exchanges and chromatid breaks were detected in peripheral blood lymphocytes obtained from patients after irinotecan treatment,[136] and increased mutation frequencies were detected at the hypoxanthine phosphoribosyl transferase locus of V79 Chinese hamster fibroblast cells treated with camptothecin and topotecan.[135] These lesions may be caused by increased illegitimate DNA recombination that occurs after camptothecin-induced stabilization of topoisomerase I cleavable complexes.[137] This type of chromosomal damage is similar to that generated by other DNA-damaging agents, such as alkylating agents and topoisomerase II inhibitors. Thus, camptothecins possibly also could increase the potential risk of secondary malignancies.[135] Additional studies are required to assess the longterm risks associated with camptothecin chemotherapy.

Although the camptothecins produce cytotoxic DNA damage in the presence of ongoing DNA synthesis, the later-occurring events responsible for the ensuing cell death have not been fully elucidated. Like other DNA-damaging agents, the camptothecins can cause cell-cycle arrest in tumor cells.[110] The molecular mechanisms responsible for regulating this block in the cell cycle have been examined only recently. Camptothecin-induced DNA damage abolishes p34[cdc2]/cyclin B complex activity, which regulates the G_2 to M phase transition in the cell cycle.[138] Failure of cells to arrest at the G_2 checkpoint after drug treatment has been associated with increased sensitivity to camptothecins.[139]

Other downstream effects of the camptothecins include the induction of differentiation in human leukemia cells[140-142] and the increased expression of the c-*fos*[76] and c-*jun* early-response genes.[143] Finally, camptothecin cytotoxicity also has been associated with the endonucleolytic degradation of DNA, which results in an apoptotic pattern of DNA fragmentation consistent with programmed cell death.[143,144] Some investigators, however, have cautioned against assuming that all tumor cell killing in the clinical use of these agents is mediated by classic apoptosis.[145] Clearly, a better understanding of the nature of the cellular events resulting from camptothecin-induced DNA damage is required.

Finally, the camptothecins may have other potential mechanisms of cytotoxicity in some cell systems. Non–S-phase specific camptothecin-induced cytotoxicity has been described in human colon cancer cells.[146] Additional studies have also described the induction of apoptosis by camptothecin in postmitotic, cultured rat central nervous system (CNS) neurons that were not actively synthesizing DNA.[147,148] Exposure to camptothecins induced apoptosis even in the presence of DNA synthesis inhibitors, such as aphidicolin. When RNA or protein synthesis was inhibited by dactinomycin (actinomycin D or DACT) or cycloheximide, however, camptothecin-induced cytotoxicity was prevented. The (S)-camptothecin stereoisomer was inactive in these experiments, which suggests, but does not prove, that this toxicity was mediated by a specific drug interaction with topoisomerase I. Whether or not these observations can be generalized to non-neuronal tissues is not yet clear, but they do suggest that the DNA replication fork collision model of drug action may not explain all of camptothecin's cytotoxic effects.

Mechanisms of Drug Resistance

Although little is known about the mechanisms of camptothecin resistance in human tumors, *in vitro* camptothecin resistance has been characterized in several different cell lines. Several different topoisomerase I amino acid substitutions have been characterized *in vitro* that confer a relative resistance to the camptothecins without abolishing the enzyme's catalytic activity.[149] These substitutions span a large portion of the protein, and they include changing phenylalanine 301 to serine,[150] glycine 363 to cysteine,[151] aspartic acid 533 to glycine[152] or to asparagine,[153] aspartic acid 583 to glycine,[152] asparagine 722 to serine,[154] or threonine 729 to alanine.[155] Double mutations replacing glycine 717 with valine and threonine 729 with isoleucine were synergistic in decreasing camptothecin sensitivity.[156] Surprisingly, this doubly mutant resistant enzyme had normal catalytic activity, which suggests that drug resistance to camptothecins can occur with relatively little change in the enzyme's metabolic efficiency. Further research is likely to identify additional topoisomerase I mutants with relative camptothecin resistance. Unfortunately, the clinical applicability of these studies may be limited, because no topoisomerase I mutations have been identified to date in a clinical setting.[157,158]

Insensitivity to the camptothecins also can result from decreased expression of topoisomerase I.[159] A resistant subline of P388 leukemia cells with less than 4% of the topoisomerase I activity of normal cells was 1,000-fold less sensitive to camptothecin.[160] The decreased expression of topoisomerase I in this cell line was compensated for by a corresponding increase in topoisomerase II expression. Postulated mechanisms responsible for decreasing the expression of topoisomerase I in resistant cells include chromosomal deletions or hypermethylation of the topoisomerase I gene.[161]

The role of the P-glycoprotein–associated multidrug resistance (MDR) phenotype in camptothecin resistance has not been clearly defined. Irinotecan and SN-38 do not appear to be substrates for the MDR drug efflux pump,[162] and cross-resistance to irinotecan is not seen in P388 leukemia cells expressing pleiotropic drug resistance to vincristine sulfate and doxorubicin hydrochloride.[163] In recent comparison studies, MDR-expressing sublines were ninefold more resistant to topotecan and twofold more resistant to 9-AC than were parental wild-type cells.[164] No increase in resistance to camptothecin or 10,11-methylenedioxycamptothecin was observed. Although other investigators have confirmed these findings for topotecan, this degree of MDR-associated resistance is much less than the 200-fold change in sensitivity typically described for classic MDR substrates, such as doxorubicin or etoposide.[165-167] Topotecan may also be a substrate for other transport systems, such as the MDR-associated protein,[168] but the clinical relevance of all these studies is still uncertain. In human colon cancer xenografts that highly express MDR, irinotecan was still quite effective, even against a cell line resistant to topotecan.[169] Thus, different mechanisms of camptothecin resistance may be specific for certain camptothecin analogs. Further characterization of these specific mechanisms of resistance is required.

In two different cell lines, decreased drug accumulation was responsible for cross-resistance between mitoxantrone hydrochloride and a number of different camptothecins, including topotecan, SN-38, and 9-AC. A mitoxantrone-resistant breast[170] and gastric[171] cancer cell line were both characterized and found to be 101-fold and 331-fold cross-resistant to SN-38, respectively. Although decreased topotecan accumulation was observed, no change in levels of P-glycoprotein or MDR-associated protein was detected. However, a novel new mitoxantrone transporter was characterized in the resistant breast cancer cell line that may be responsible for camptothecin resistance.[172,173] The extent to which this newly identified protein alters camptothecin uptake and efflux must still be determined, but it represents a possible marker for camptothecin resistance. This line of research may improve our currently poor understanding of camptothecin transport in malignant cells.

Other potential mechanisms of decreased sensitivity to camptothecins include a reduction in the number of cells in

S phase[49] and the decreased intratumoral production of SN-38 by the irinotecan carboxylesterase–converting enzyme.[174] A preliminary association between the measured converting-enzyme activity in different tumor cell lines and their relative sensitivity to irinotecan has been reported in some cells[175,176] but not in others.[177] Finally, double-stranded DNA break repair activity may also modulate camptothecin–induced cytotoxicity. For example, yeast mutants defective in the RAD52 double-stranded DNA break repair gene are hypersensitive to camptothecin.[113,178]

Determinants of Clinical Response

The key biochemical or molecular determinants of tumor response to clinical camptothecin therapy have not yet been identified. Because of the complex, stepwise pattern of drug-induced perturbations in cellular metabolism, no single parameter may be able to identify sensitive or resistant tumors completely. Although the overall topoisomerase I activity may be important,[177,179] other factors are also relevant, including topoisomerase I enzyme mutations, the amount of cleavable complexes formed, and the extent of ongoing DNA synthesis. Total topoisomerase I protein levels in tissues as measured by Western immunoblotting correlate poorly with sensitivity to camptothecins in experimental studies.[180] Likewise, total topoisomerase I mRNA does not predict drug sensitivity when different cell lines are compared.[180,181] This poor correlation between total topoisomerase I expression and drug effects may be due either to posttranslational regulation of the enzyme, to subcellular localization of topoisomerase I away from DNA, or to other, as yet unidentified factors. Preliminary studies suggest that camptothecin sensitivity may be predicted by changes in topoisomerase I immunofluorescence patterns indicative of translocation of the protein away from the nucleus that occurs during drug treatment.[81,82,182] Newer methods of purifying topoisomerase I from human tumor tissues have been developed[183] and may help to further define our understanding of the important determinants of clinical response to topoisomerase I poisons.

Although the DNA-cleavable complex formation is necessary but not sufficient for drug toxicity, measurement of these lesions as a predictor of drug effects is an attractive approach.[180] The cleavable complex is the specific lesion in the DNA that accumulates within the cell during drug exposure. Clinical measurement of the amount of cleavable complexes formed has been hampered, however, by the lack of sufficiently sensitive tests that can be easily applied to patient tissues.[184–186] Further technologic developments are needed that allow for more sensitive methods to assay the amount of cleavable complex formation in clinical specimens. One potentially promising approach is the use of ligase-mediated polymerase chain reaction, which does not require radioactive prelabeling of cells to monitor cleavable complex formation.[187]

Also important, but even less well understood, is the role of events occurring downstream from the formation of cleavable complexes, such as DNA damage repair,[188] the triggering of apoptosis,[189–191] and alterations in the integrity of the G_2 cell-cycle checkpoint.[139,192,193] For example, two different colon cancer cell lines with different sensitivity to camptothecin were found to differ in their cell-cycle response.[139] The more resistant cells arrested in the G_2 phase of the cell cycle after camptothecin exposure, whereas the more sensitive cells passed through the G_2 checkpoint after experiencing camptothecin-induced damage. The more sensitive cells also showed a greater capacity to arrest in S phase, and they failed to down-regulate cyclin B-cdc kinase activity after camptothecin exposure. Thus, cell-cycle checkpoint integrity may also be an important determinant of camptothecin sensitivity. Despite the extensive ongoing research in this complex area, however, no single method or molecular marker can as yet reliably predict tumor responsiveness to camptothecins.

Antiviral Activity

Because camptothecins have potential antiviral activity,[194,195] examination of their effects on human immunodeficiency virus (HIV) replication has been of interest.[196] In acutely infected human peripheral blood monocytes, topotecan decreased HIV-1 replication, as assessed by a fall in p24 antigen production.[197] A similar effect was observed in chronically infected cells without evidence of substantial changes in cell viability. The mechanism for the inhibition of viral replication is under investigation; however, it may be related to the inhibition of HIV-1 long-terminal repeat-directed gene expression.[197–199] In *in vivo* murine studies, camptothecin inhibited the production of retrovirus-induced diseases, including Maloney murine leukemia and Friend erythroleukemia, without apparent systemic toxicity.[200] Preliminary studies also suggested that the orally administered drug 9-nitrocamptothecin may have anti-HIV activity.[201,202] Topotecan was effective in inhibiting HIV-1 RNA production, even in cells containing mutant topoisomerase I resistant to camptothecins.[203] Thus, camptothecins may inhibit HIV-1 replication through a mechanism independent of their interaction with topoisomerase I. Further studies are necessary to define exactly what these mechanisms might be; however, these encouraging results support further evaluation of the antiviral properties of the camptothecins.

Radiation Sensitization

Synergistic interactions between ionizing radiation and topoisomerase I poisons have been observed in a number of *in vitro* systems.[204–210] Both camptothecin- and topotecan-enhanced radiation-induced cytotoxicity in cell lines resulted in the reduction or elimination of the shoulder of the cell survival curves.[211] This interaction, however, was highly schedule dependent.[208,209] When topotecan was administered either immediately before radiation,[209] concurrently with it,[208,209] or immediately after it,[208] a synergistic interaction was observed. However, delaying drug treatment for 30 or 120 minutes after radiation exposure failed to illicit radiosensitization.[211] Thus, the timing of topoisomerase I poison administration in association with radiotherapy is very important.

The mechanism of this synergistic interaction still requires further characterization. One early hypothesis was that camptothecins interfered with topoisomerase I during the repair of radiation-induced DNA damage.[204,212] Convincing evidence that topoisomerase I is directly involved in DNA repair activity is lacking, however, and caution is warranted in correlating topoisomerase I activity with DNA repair in the absence of more definitive data.[104,213] More recently, radiation and DNA damage were found paradoxically to lead to the rapid down-regulation of topoisomerase I enzyme activity.[104,208] This led to the hypothesis that topoisomerase I protein may compete with DNA repair enzymes after DNA damage due to radiation exposure. As previously mentioned, abasic sites and DNA mismatches that may be induced by radiation exposure can also lead to further stabilization of DNA–topoisomerase I cleavable complexes[122–124] and thus may enhance camptothecin's cytotoxicity. This hypothesis is further supported by the correlation between the amount of cleavable complexes stabilized by topotecan

after radiation exposure and cell survival seen in radioresistant U1-Mel melanoma cells.[208] In addition, this mechanism may also explain the synergistic cytotoxicity seen with combinations of topoisomerase I poisons and DNA-damaging agents such as alkylators or cisplatin.[214,215] Other explanations for camptothecin-induced radiosensitization include enhanced cell killing arising from cell-cycle synchronization or from an increased S-phase cell fraction.[216–218] Regardless of the mechanism of interaction, a growing number of *in vivo* animal studies[219–222] also support the promise of this combined-modality approach. Clinical studies of topoisomerase I poisons and radiation therapy are in progress.[223]

TOPOTECAN

Topotecan is a water-soluble camptothecin derivative containing a stable basic side chain at position 9 of the A ring of 10-hydroxycamptothecin (Fig. 20-1).[19] Clinical trials of topotecan were initiated in 1989 by SmithKline Beecham in collaboration with the National Cancer Institute. In 1996, topotecan was approved in the United States for use as second-line chemotherapy in patients with advanced ovarian cancer, and in 1998 it was approved for the treatment of small cell lung cancer after failure of first-line chemotherapy. Key features of topotecan are listed in Table 20-2.

TABLE 20-2. KEY FEATURES OF TOPOTECAN

Mechanism of action:	Topoisomerase I poison. Stabilizes the cleavable complex in which topoisomerase I is covalently bound to DNA at a single-stranded break site. Conversion into lethal DNA damage follows when a DNA replication fork encounters these cleavable complexes ("fork collision model").
Metabolism:	Nonenzymatic hydrolysis of the lactone ring generates the less active open-ring hydroxy carboxylic acid. *N*-desmethyl metabolite recently characterized in plasma, urine, and feces.
Elimination:	About 26% to 41% excreted unchanged in urine over 24 h. Concentrated in the bile at levels that are 1.5 times higher than the simultaneous plasma levels.
Pharmacokinetics:	Approximate terminal half-life of topotecan lactone is 2.9 h (range, 1.6–5.5 h); approximate clearance of 62 L/h/m² (range, 14–155 L/h/m²) reported for 30-min topotecan infusions.
Toxicity:	Myelosuppression, predominantly noncumulative neutropenia, with thrombocytopenia and anemia less common Nausea and vomiting (mild) Diarrhea (mild) Fatigue Alopecia Skin rash Elevated liver function test results Mucositis
Modifications for organ dysfunction:	In minimally pretreated patients, no dosage adjustments appear to be necessary for patients with mild renal impairment (creatinine clearance 40–60 mL/min), but dosage adjustment to 0.75 mg/m²/d is recommended for patients with moderate renal impairment (20–39 mL/min). Further dosage adjustments may be necessary for patients with extensive prior chemotherapy or radiation therapy. Studies of small numbers of patients suggest that dosage adjustments are not required for hyperbilirubinemia up to 10 mg/dL.
Precautions:	For febrile or severe grade 4 neutropenia lasting >3 d, the dosage for subsequent courses should be reduced by 0.25 mg/m²/d. Monitoring of blood counts is essential.

Preclinical Activity

Topotecan was superior to camptothecin in several murine tumor models, including L1210 leukemia, Lewis lung carcinoma, and B16 melanoma tumors.[28,224] In human tumor xenograft studies, substantial activity was found in colon and ovarian adenocarcinoma,[225] CNS tumors,[226] rhabdomyosarcoma,[227] osteosarcoma,[227] and medulloblastoma tumors.[128] In addition to its enhanced solubility and excellent preclinical anticancer activity profile, topotecan had other characteristics making it a strong candidate for further clinical development. In animal studies, it had greater antitumor efficacy than the parent compound (camptothecin) at the maximally tolerated dose.[28] In addition, preclinical toxicology experiments revealed a favorable side effect profile with predictable dose-limiting neutropenia and minimal nonhematologic toxicities at the maximally tolerated dose.

Dosages and Routes of Administration

The most common dose and schedule of topotecan administration is a 30-minute intravenous infusion of 1.5 mg per m^2 daily for 5 days every 3 weeks.[32,228,229] This regimen has undergone the most widespread clinical testing, and it is currently the dosage of topotecan approved by the U.S. Food and Drug Administration (FDA) for treating ovarian and lung cancer patients. Five-day continuous infusions of topotecan at 2.0 mg per m^2 per day have been tested in patients with hematologic malignancies, although in these studies, gastrointestinal toxicities such as mucositis and diarrhea became more problematic.[230] Although based on a promising theoretical rationale,[112] prolonged 21-day infusion schedules at 0.5 to 0.6 mg per m^2 per day[231] have been disappointing in phase II studies.[232,233] Other schedules tested in phase I studies include a single 30-minute infusion every 3 weeks,[234] 24-hour infusions,[235–237] and 3-day[238,239] and 5-day continuous infusions.[238,240] Oral administration has also been tested clinically[241–243] and is currently being compared with intravenous administration in a randomized study. Finally, an intraperitoneal topotecan study also has been completed.[244]

Toxicity

Noncumulative, reversible neutropenia is the most common dose-limiting toxicity for all schedules of topotecan administration. On the daily × 5 schedule, the mean time of onset of grade 3 or 4 neutropenia is approximately 9 days after the start of topotecan administration, and the neutropenia persists until day 14, which permits retreatment of most patients by day 21.[31,228] In a combined analysis of 452 patients with advanced ovarian cancer treated at the recommended phase II dosage of 1.5 mg per m^2 per day for 5 days every 3 weeks, the overall incidence of grade 4 neutropenia (nadir neutrophil count of less than 500 per μL)

was 81%, and febrile neutropenia occurred in 26%.[245–249] Grade 4 thrombocytopenia and anemia were less common, occurring in 26% and 40% of patients, respectively. Blood product support was also quite common, with 13% of patients undergoing platelet transfusions and 56% given blood transfusions. In a phase III study of ovarian cancer patients previously treated with platinum-containing regimens, the death rate due to sepsis was 1.8% in 112 patients. The risk of myelosuppressive toxicity was increased in patients extensively pretreated with multiple prior chemotherapeutic regimens or with prior radiation therapy.[228,245] Prior carboplatin chemotherapy specifically increased the risk of thrombocytopenia and was associated with a higher number of platelet transfusions.[245]

Other less common and usually mild toxicities include nausea, vomiting, diarrhea, fever on the day of administration, fatigue, alopecia, skin rash, and elevated liver function test results. Most of these toxicities are easily managed clinically with supportive measures. Hemorrhagic cystitis and severe, life-threatening diarrhea are generally not seen with standard topotecan therapy. In phase I studies of leukemia patients treated with a 5-day continuous infusion of topotecan, other toxicities such as mucositis and diarrhea were dose limiting.[250]

Dosage Adjustment for Severe Toxicity or Abnormal Organ Function

Dosage reductions of 0.25 mg per m^2 per day from the recommended starting dosage of 1.5 mg per m^2 per day for 5 days for grade 4 neutropenia or thrombocytopenia lasting longer than 3 days have been recommended.[245] Heavily pretreated patients or those with a poor performance status may be started at topotecan dosages of 1.25 or 1.0 mg per m^2 per day. Shortening the duration of treatment to less than 5 days of therapy has not been tested and, therefore, is not recommended. Use of colony-stimulating factors such as granulocyte colony-stimulating factor (G-CSF) has been studied clinically,[246,247] and this strategy may permit some increase in dose intensity during later cycles of therapy.[251] The addition of G-CSF generally does not permit the further escalation of the starting dose of topotecan, however, because of persistent neutropenia, thrombocytopenia, and fatigue[228]; thus, its routine use is not recommended. If severe or prolonged neutropenia occurs during topotecan chemotherapy, secondary prophylactic administration of G-CSF may be considered as an alternative to dosage reduction.[252] As with other myelosuppressive agents, however, the clinical benefit of adding G-CSF as an alternative to reducing the dosage of topotecan in the face of severe myelosuppressive toxicity has not been demonstrated. Thus, in keeping with guidelines proposed by the American Society of Clinical Oncology, physicians should consider chemotherapy dosage reduction as an alternative to the use of G-CSF with topotecan.[253,254]

Renal excretion is a major route of systemic topotecan elimination. Increased topotecan-related toxicity has been observed in patients with moderate renal dysfunction.[245] Guidelines have been proposed for reducing the starting dose of topotecan in patients with impaired renal function.[245,255] For patients with normal renal function, defined as a creatinine clearance (Cl_{cr}) of more than 60 mL per minute, a standard starting dosage of 1.5 mg per m² per day is recommended, regardless of prior treatment history. For minimally pretreated patients with mildly impaired renal function and a Cl_{cr} of 40 to 59 mL per minute, the standard dosage of 1.5 mg per m² per day may still be used. For minimally pretreated patients with moderately impaired renal function, however, defined as a Cl_{cr} of 20 to 39 mL per minute, the dosage of topotecan should be reduced to 0.75 mg per m² per day. For heavily pretreated patients with a history of extensive prior chemotherapy or radiation therapy, the standard starting dosage of 1.5 mg per m² per day may still be used if the Cl_{cr} is more than 60 mL per minute. The topotecan dosage should be reduced further in these heavily pretreated patients, however, to 1.0 mg per m² per day for a Cl_{cr} of 40 to 59 mL per minute, and to 0.5 mg per m² per day for a Cl_{cr} of 20 to 39 mL per minute.[245] Guidelines for topotecan dosing for a Cl_{cr} of less than 20 mL per minute have not been established for any group of patients. Formal algorithms for pharmacokinetic dosing of topotecan based on renal function have not been defined, and given the high interpatient pharmacodynamic variability seen with this drug, these may be difficult to derive. In patients with hepatic dysfunction, defined as elevated total serum bilirubin levels greater than 1.2 mg per dL, no dosage adjustments were recommended; however, only a limited number of patients with more than a moderate increase in total bilirubin level were studied.[256] A small group of three patients with serum bilirubin concentrations ranging from 3.5 to 6.9 mg per dL tolerated topotecan dosages of 1.5 mg per m² per day as well as control patients with normal liver function.[256]

Clinical Pharmacology

Analytic Methodology

Most analytic assays for topotecan in biologic matrices use reversed-phase high-pressure liquid chromatography (HPLC) with fluorescence detection.[34,257] Deproteinization by rapid precipitation of samples with cold methanol (−30°C) can stabilize the topotecan lactone for later analysis.[257] The lactone concentration can then be determined by direct HPLC injection to separate the lactone from the carboxylate forms. In addition, preinjection acidification of plasma samples allows for total plasma topotecan (carboxylate and lactone) to be determined by the same methodology. The plasma carboxylate concentrations are then calculated by subtracting the lactone concentrations from the total drug measurement. A newer validated method for simultaneously measuring both the lactone and carboxylate forms of topotecan in plasma as a single HPLC injection has also been developed,[258] and an assay for measuring topotecan and its *N*-desmethyl metabolite in plasma, urine, and feces was also reported.[259]

General Pharmacokinetics

After intravenous topotecan administration, the lactone ring undergoes rapid hydrolysis to generate the carboxylate species.[31,32] Less than 1 hour after the start of an infusion, the majority of the circulating drug in plasma is in the carboxylate form, and this species predominates for the duration of the monitoring period.[31,32] In most studies, the ratio of the lactone to total topotecan area under the concentration × time curve (AUC) ranged from 20% to 35% (Table 20-3).[31,228,229,234–236,260] Interindividual variation in the AUC and the total-body clearance was quite large for both lactone[31] and total topotecan (lactone plus carboxylate).[236] In general, plasma concentrations and AUC levels tended to increase with increasing dose levels, consistent with linear pharmacokinetics, although in some studies, nonlinearity in drug clearance at higher dose levels was seen.[234,261]

The kinetics of topotecan were analyzed using a linear, two-compartment, open model in most studies.[31,32,237] Table 20-3 summarizes the reported pharmacokinetic parameters for topotecan from several pharmacologic trials. For topotecan lactone, the terminal half-life ranged from 2.0 to 3.5 hours, which is relatively short compared with that of other camptothecin analogs. Consequently, no accumulation of drug was observed when it was administered daily for 5 consecutive days.[32] The total-body clearance of topotecan lactone after a 30-minute infusion ranged from 25.7 to 155.0 L per hour per m², and the volume of distribution at steady state ranged from 23 to 25 L per m². No evidence exists that topotecan kinetics changes with repeated dosing cycles.[32,228,229] Limited sampling models for topotecan pharmacokinetics have been developed[262] and applied to clinical pharmacodynamic studies of topotecan in patients in phase II studies.[263] The pharmacokinetics of topotecan has also been studied in a pediatric population (Table 20-3), and no substantial difference from kinetics in adults has been observed.[236,239,264,265]

Careful analytic modeling of an early topotecan pharmacokinetic study identified inconsistencies in the data that could only be explained by degradation of the topotecan lactone ring before intravenous infusion.[32] Dilution of topotecan into 5% dextrose (pH 4.5) resulted in hydrolysis of up to 10% of the topotecan lactone with a half-life of 30 minutes.[31] In a follow-up examination of four patients, the amount of open-ring topotecan carboxylate in the infusate ranged from 6% to 16%.[32] Furthermore, greater degradation is possible when topotecan is administered in normal saline, which has an even higher pH than dextrose.[266] Administration of partially hydrolyzed topotecan solutions

TABLE 20-3. TOPOTECAN PHARMACOKINETICS

Dose & Schedule	No. of Patients	Drug	C_{max} (nmol/L)	AUC (nmol/L × h)	CL (L/h/m²)	V_{ss} (L/m²)	Terminal Half-Life (h)	Urinary Excretion (% of Dose)	Lactone/Total Drug AUC (%)	Reference
0.5–2.5 mg/m²/d over 30 min	28	Lactone	20.6–81.7	—	132 ± 25 L/h[a]	25.6 ± 3.8	3.01 ± 0.54	38.8 ± 5.6 over 24 h[b]	16–20	31
0.5–2.5 mg/m²/d over 30 min	12	Total[b]	—	—	29.6 ± 10.8	25 ± 19	1.83[c]	30 ± 18	—	32
1.25 mg/m²/d over 30 min[d]	4	Lactone	109 (range, 64–192)	55.6 (range, 36.0–154.0)	100 (range, 29–154)	161 (range, 122–283)	1.72 (range, 1.50–3.52)	—	22.3	228
	4	Total	164 (range, 97–182)	248 (range, 214–600)	22.5 (range, 8.1–26.4)	71 (range, 56–94)	2.88 (range, 2.17–5.37)	—	—	
1.5 mg/m²/d over 30 min	6	Lactone	83.0 (range, 71.1–116.1)	47.5 (range, 40.6–94.1)	155 (range, 68–165)	207 (range, 111–374)	1.62 (range, 1.15–2.38)	—	—	228
	6	Total	154 (range, 128–192)	376 (range, 223–997)	18.8 (range, 6.8–32.9)	98 (range, 51–195)	3.82 (range, 2.55–10.9)	—	—	
0.5–1.5 mg/m² over 30 min	19	Lactone	24.8–169.8	31.8–157.5	34.2 (range, 15–59)	72.7 (range, 28.5–123.5)	2.2 (range, 0.8–4.8)	25.8 (range, 7.0–58.6) over 24 h	35[e]	260
		Carboxylate	8.0–69.7	11.5–285	24 (range, 10.2–90)	15.3 (range, 1.9–64.5)	2.05 (range, 0.53–4.42)	—	—	
0.6–0.75 mg/m²/d over 30 min[f,g]	25	Lactone	—	—	19.6 ± 7.9	69.9 ± 7.9	5.0 ± 7.0	—	29.6	344
		Total	—	—	9.2 ± 3.9	33.1 ± 15.6	3.8 ± 2.7	—	—	
1.4–2.4 mg/m² over 30 min[f]	35	Lactone	164–211[h]	85–1149[h]	16.7 ± 6.5	79.5 ± 76.2	5.5 ± 3.3	—	—	264
		Total	—	—	7.5 ± 2.7	32.5 ± 11.3	4.5 ± 1.7	—	—	
0.5–1.25 mg/m² over 30 min	24	Total	48.9–104	80.3–199.8	13.8 ± 2.7	36.7 ± 6.2	2.1 ± 0.3	41 ± 10 over 5 days	—	339
		N-desmethyl-topotecan	0.23–0.53	1.04–2.60	—	—	—	1.4 ± 0.6 over 5 d	—	
2.0 mg/m² over 30 min	33	Total	118 ± 43	341 ± 14	—	—	—	—	—	283
2.0–4.2 mg/m² over 30 min	34	Lactone	23–142	15–2,300	133 ± 16	231 ± 35	2.58 ± 0.65	—	—	251
2.5–22.5 mg/m² over 30 min	17	Total	65–224	68.3–650	34.8 ± 3.0	99 ± 6	2.5 ± 0.1	—	—	234
		Lactone	308–1,377	523–2,779	25.7 ± 6.7	76.4 ± 18.5	3.4 ± 1.1[c]	—	33 ± 44	
		Total	438–1,844	1,520–8,029	8.0 ± 3.1	39.5 ± 9.8	4.3 ± 1.8[c]	40 (range, 22–60) over 24 h	—	
1.5 mg/m² c.i.v. over 24 h	7	Lactone	5.8 ± 1.2	139.7 ± 29.0	26.5 ± 5.8	—	3.2 (range, 2.2–4.8)	—	53.2	235
		Total	10.7 ± 2.7	262.7 ± 65.8	14.4 ± 3.9	—	3.7 (range, 2.4–5.8)	—	—	
2.5–10.5 mg/m² c.i.v. over 24 h	19	Lactone	6.7–41.6	147–963	35.0 (range, 21.3–55.8)	563 (range, 332–935)	4.4 (range, 1.7–7.5)	—	—	261
		Carboxylate	9.8–89.5	222–2,008	19.9 (range, 10.4–38.8)	344 (range, 175–717)	4.4 (range, 1.0–13.2)	44–64 over 48 h	—	

Dose/schedule	N	Form	Cmax	AUC	CL	Vss	t½		Reference
12.5 mg/m² c.i.v. over 24 h	7	Lactone	72.3 ± 40.3	1,491 ± 761	25 ± 14	90 ± 35	3.8 ± 1.2	—	237
15.0 mg/m² c.i.v. over 24 h	5	Lactone	95.3 ± 42.9	2,361 ± 1,275	23.2 ± 20.4	95 ± 68	5.0 ± 1.6	—	237
1.0 mg/m² c.i.v. over 72 h[f]	14	Lactone	7.3 ± 3.3	—	16.2 ± 5.2	21.8 ± 19.2[i]	2.9 ± 1.0	—	239
2.0–7.5 mg/m² c.i.v. over 24 h[f]	14	Lactone	4.1–30.7	—	28.3 ± 6.5	—	2.9 ± 1.1[i]	—	236
0.5–3.3 mg/m²/d c.i.v. over 120 h[f]	18	Total	11.8–88.7	—	9.8 ± 3.9	—	2.3 ± 0.5[j]	88–99[k]	
		Lactone	—	—	18.28 (range, 8.65–24.78)	61.9 (range, 19.1–141.0)	3.77 (range, 1.76–6.39)	71.6 (range, 30.1–107.3) over 144 h	275
		Total	—	—	8.7 (range, 3.5–13.2)	36.7 (range, 16.6–118.5)	3.5 (range, 1.38–11.83)	—	
2.3 mg orally[l]	18	Lactone	14.9 ± 9.0	53.8 ± 22.5	—	—	3.49 ± 0.87	—	241
		Total	24.2 ± 12.3	66.8 ± 29.4	—	—	3.91 ± 1.00	22.2 ± 11.0	
1.5 mg/m² orally[m]	12	Lactone	13.9 ± 1.8	36.0 ± 13.1	—	—	2.82 ± 0.85	—	268
0.15–0.60 mg/m² orally	14	Lactone	—	9.2 ± 5.6	—	—	2.35 ± 1.05	—	242
		Carboxylate	—	15.7 ± 8.7	—	—	3.61 ± 1.04	—	

AUC, area under concentration × time curve; C_{max}, maximal plasma concentration; CL, clearance; V_{ss}, volume of distribution at steady state.

Values are ranges or arithmetic means ± standard deviation unless otherwise stated. Pharmacokinetic parameters have been converted to uniform units whenever possible for ease of comparison, unless otherwise stated.

[a] L/h, not L/h/m².
[b] Total = lactone + carboxylate.
[c] Harmonic mean and pseudo–standard deviations.
[d] Median values.
[e] At the recommended phase II dose of 1.5 mg/m².
[f] Pediatric study.
[g] Combination study with cyclophosphamide, but no pharmacokinetic interaction detected.
[h] At the recommended phase II dose of 1.4 mg/m².
[i] Volume of distribution of the central compartment.
[j] At the maximally tolerated dose of 5.5 mg/m² for this study.
[k] In two patients, duration of urine collection not specified.
[l] Oral bioavailability to total topotecan 42 ± 13%.
[m] Oral bioavailability to total topotecan 30 ± 8%.

could result in clinical exposures to the active drug that are quite different than expected. More recently, a new preparation of topotecan stabilized with tartaric acid has been used clinically. Stability testing of this preparation in standard intravenous fluids suggests that the lactone stability of the drug is much improved over that of early versions.[263]

Absorption

The most common route for topotecan administration has been intravenous; however, oral formulations using prolonged administration schedules have undergone preclinical[267] and clinical testing.[242,268] Animal studies demonstrated an oral bioavailability of approximately 28% and antitumor efficacy equivalent to that with parenteral treatment in four of the five murine models studied.[267] In humans, the reported oral bioavailability ranged from 30% to 42%.[241,268] Plasma concentrations peaked approximately 47 minutes after oral ingestion, and no difference in the lactone to carboxylate ratio was observed when oral dosing was compared with intravenous administration (Table 20-3). Coadministration of food slightly deceased the rate of absorption, but it did not affect the amount of drug absorbed.[241]

Other routes of topotecan administration have been tested in preclinical models. The pharmacokinetics of intrathecally administered topotecan was studied in nonhuman primates.[269] Intraventricularly administered topotecan showed a 450-fold relative pharmacologic advantage compared with systemic administration. No clinically significant acute or chronic neurologic toxicities were associated with intrathecal drug administration, which suggests that this may be a promising means of delivering this agent to patients with CNS tumors. Intraperitoneal topotecan administration was studied in nude mice bearing peritoneally implanted human ovarian cancer xenografts.[225] Excellent antitumor efficacy and modest systemic toxicity were observed, but pharmacokinetic monitoring was not performed, so a rigorous assessment of the relative pharmacokinetic advantage for this regional drug delivery approach could not be made. In a phase I clinical study of intraperitoneal topotecan, the peritoneal to plasma AUC ratio was 31.2, which suggests a pharmacologic advantage for regional delivery to the peritoneal cavity. Systemic toxicities, consisting predominantly of neutropenia, limited dose escalation beyond 3 mg per m^2 given as a continuous intraperitoneal infusion over 24 hours every 3 weeks.[244] Further efficacy testing of regional topotecan delivery for patients with ovarian cancer was recommended. Currently, oral dosing of topotecan is being compared with intravenous dosing in patients with small cell lung cancer in a phase III trial.

Distribution

In experiments in rhesus monkeys, cerebrospinal fluid (CSF) topotecan lactone concentrations were approxi-

mately 32% of simultaneous plasma levels, and these concentrations tended to decline in parallel over time.[270,271] A physiologic pharmacokinetic model based on these primate experiments was developed and may help guide future investigations of topotecan's activity against CNS tumors.[271] The pharmacokinetic findings were confirmed in children who received topotecan by 24- or 72-hour continuous intravenous infusions.[272] The median CNS penetration of topotecan lactone and total drug was 29% (range, 10% to 59%) and 50% (range, 11% to 97%), respectively. Topotecan's penetration into the CNS is relatively higher than that of most other camptothecins. For example, the parent compound, camptothecin, has negligible penetration into the CSF in primates.[270] This difference may be due, in part, to the lower degree of protein binding exhibited by topotecan relative to other highly protein-bound camptothecins, such as camptothecin, SN-38, irinotecan, and 9-AC.[12,234,270] Unlike these other camptothecin derivatives, topotecan does not extensively interact with or bind to human serum albumin.[273] This property could have important benefits in treating tumors that metastasize to the CNS, such as acute leukemia or small cell lung cancer.

Metabolism

Recently, an *N*-desmethyl metabolite of topotecan was characterized[274] and found to be present at relatively low concentrations in human plasma, urine, and feces after intravenous administration of topotecan.[259] Further studies defining the clinical pharmacology of this metabolite are in progress. Although a specific interaction with drug metabolism enzymes has not been established, preliminary clinical data suggest enhanced topotecan clearance in pediatric patients simultaneously receiving treatment with agents that induce hepatic cytochrome P-450 enzymes, such as dexamethasone, phenobarbital, and phenytoin.[265] Furthermore, a very low topotecan clearance was described in another patient who was taking terfenadine simultaneously.[265] These observations are consistent with a potential drug interaction at the level of CYP3A; however, additional studies on the metabolism of topotecan and its potential for serious drug interactions are warranted.

Elimination

Elimination of the lactone is thought to result from the rapid hydrolysis to the carboxylate species followed by renal excretion of the open-ring metabolite.[32] Overall, 25% to 40% of the dose administered is excreted as total drug (lactone plus carboxylate) in the urine over a 24-hour period,[32,228,229] with a few studies reporting recovery of over 90% of the administered drug during more prolonged urinary collection periods (Table 20-3).[275,276] Because altered clearance of topotecan has been observed in patients with impaired renal function,[255] dosage adjustments for this special population have been recommended (see earlier section). Topotecan was concentrated in the bile at levels 1.5 times higher than simultaneous plasma concentrations in one patient with an external biliary drainage catheter, which suggests that excretion through this route may also be important.[234] As previously mentioned, no change in topotecan kinetics was observed in a limited clinical study of patients with moderately impaired hepatic function.[256] In a clinical study examining sequences of topotecan and cisplatin, the prior administration of cisplatin resulted in substantially greater hematologic toxicity.[277] A pharmacokinetic interaction causing a transient reduction in topotecan clearance when this agent was administered after intravenous cisplatin was thought to be related to subclinical renal tubular toxicity induced by the platinum analog.[277]

Pharmacodynamics

Pharmacodynamic correlations between parameters of systemic drug exposure and topotecan drug effects have been observed inconsistently.[31,228] In a pediatric study, the topotecan total (lactone plus carboxylate) AUC and lactone plasma AUC correlated with the percentage change in the platelet count and the granulocyte count after a 72-hour drug infusion.[265] Similar correlations between leucocyte or granulocyte counts and total topotecan AUC or topotecan dose have been reported after a 30-minute infusion of topotecan given daily for 5 days,[31,32] after 20-minute infusions every 3 weeks,[234] and after 24-hour continuous infusions.[235,261] In each case, measurement of the total topotecan plasma concentration was as informative about drug effects as the lactone drug levels. Thus, the need to measure lactone drug concentrations has been questioned by some investigators.[228] Finally, although interpatient variability in topotecan plasma concentrations is high, the total variability in hematologic toxicity in patients is relatively low when the drug is administered according to standard dosing guidelines.[260,263] Thus, therapeutic drug monitoring is not useful for this agent.

Single-Agent Anticancer Activity of Topotecan

Ovarian Cancer

In May 1996, the FDA approved topotecan for use in previously treated patients with ovarian cancer. The efficacy of topotecan was established in a randomized phase III study in advanced epithelial ovarian cancer patients who had progressed after treatment with prior platinum-based regimens (Table 20-4).[249] Patients were randomized to receive topotecan 1.5 mg per m^2 per day for 5 days every 3 weeks or paclitaxel 175 mg per m^2 over 3 hours every 3 weeks. Administration of G-CSF was allowed after the initial cycle if any of the following was observed: grade 3 neutropenia

that delayed therapy, grade 4 neutropenia that lasted for longer than 7 days, or febrile neutropenia. Overall, 226 patients were evaluable for response, with 112 receiving topotecan and 114 receiving paclitaxel. No significant difference in the overall response rate was observed ($p = .138$). Five complete and 18 partial responses were seen on the topotecan arm for an overall response rate of 20.5% [95% confidence interval (CI), 12.0% to 28.3%], and 3 complete and 12 partial responses were seen on the paclitaxel arm for a response rate of 15% (95% CI, 7.0% to 19.4%). The median time to progression was longer for those receiving topotecan than for those given paclitaxel—23.1 weeks versus 14 weeks ($p = .002$). The overall median survival was not significantly different ($p = .515$)—61 weeks for the group given topotecan and 43 weeks for those given paclitaxel—however, some patients did cross over to the other therapy after their original treatment failed. Toxicities were significantly greater ($p <.01$) in the topotecan arm than in the paclitaxel arm, with more grade 4 neutropenia (79% versus 25%, respectively) and more grade 4 thrombocytopenia (23% versus 2%, respectively). Documented sepsis occurred in 5% of patients receiving topotecan and 2% of patients receiving paclitaxel; two toxic deaths were reported, both on the topotecan arm. Other toxicities were mild to moderate and were generally easily managed. The overall planned dose was successfully administered in 90% of the topotecan and 98% of the paclitaxel courses. Although topotecan caused substantially greater myelosuppression, this study does demonstrate the utility of topotecan in patients with advanced ovarian cancer.

The response rates to topotecan therapy among patients with advanced ovarian cancer are influenced by the responsiveness to prior cisplatin-based chemotherapy. In a phase II study of 28 evaluable patients with advanced ovarian cancer refractory to cisplatin, four partial responses were seen for an overall response rate of 14% (95% CI, 4% to 34%) and a median survival time of 10.0 months (95% CI, 8.1 to 13.5 months).[246] A single-institution trial[278] and a separate multicenter trial[279] of topotecan also reported response rates of 14% for similar populations of patients. Another study of topotecan therapy for ovarian cancer stratified 111 patients into three subgroups based on their prior response to cisplatin chemotherapy[247]: (a) patients with cisplatin-sensitive disease who responded to cisplatin chemotherapy but experienced relapse more than 6 months after its discontinuance, (b) patients with cisplatin-resistant disease who responded initially but experienced relapse within 6 months, and (c) patients with cisplatin-refractory disease who either experienced disease progression or had stable disease as their best response while on their initial cisplatin-based regimen. Among the 92 evaluable patients, the overall response rate was 16.3%, with subgroup response rates of 5.9% for the cisplatin-refractory group (n = 34 patients), 17.8% for the cisplatin-resistant patients (n = 28 patients), and 26.7% for the cisplatin-sensitive patients (n = 30 patients). Thus, the likelihood of

TABLE 20-4. TOPOTECAN SINGLE-AGENT PHASE III STUDIES

Disease	Dose & Schedule	No. Patients Entered/No. Evaluable	No. Patients with Prior Chemotherapy	Overall Response Rate, % (95% CI)	Response Type	Median Duration of Response (mo)	Median Duration of Survival (mo)	Reference
Ovarian cancer	Topotecan 1.5 mg/m² /d × 5 d every 3 wk	112/112	112	20.5 (13.0–28.3)	5 CR, 18 PR	8.0 (range, 1.4–13.3)	15.3 (range, 0.2–15.5)	249
	versus							
	Paclitaxel 175 mg/m² over 3 h every 3 wk	114/114	114	13.2 (7.0–19.4) (p = .138)	3 CR, 12 PR	5.0 (range, 1.6–6.1) (p = .222)	10.8 (range, 0.03–18.8) (p = .515)	
Small cell lung cancer	Topotecan 1.5 mg/m² /d × 5 d every 3 wk	107/107	107	24.3 (16.2–32.4)	26 PR	3.3 (range, 2.4–12.5)	6.3 (range, 0.1–22.7)	281
	versus							
	Cyclophosphamide 1 g/m², doxorubicin hydrochloride 45 mg/m², vincristine sulfate 2 mg on d 1 every 3 wk	104/104	104	18.3 (10.8–25.7) (p = .285)	1 CR, 18 PR	3.1 (range, 2.2–17.5) (p = .552)	6.2 (range, 0.3–25.3) (p = .795)	

CI, confidence interval; CR, complete response; PR, partial response.

response to topotecan was influenced by the prior response to cisplatin chemotherapy.

A randomized phase II study compared a standard dosage of 1.5 mg per m² per day for 5 days with a weekly 24-hour infusion of 1.75 mg per m² of topotecan given for 4 out of every 6 weeks and included previously treated patients with advanced ovarian cancer.[280] Among 63 evaluable patients, the overall response rate for the daily × 5 regimen was 22.6% (95% CI, 9.6% to 41.2%) compared with a response rate of only 3.1% (95% CI, 0.1% to 16.0%) for the weekly regimen (*p* = .026). Thus, treatment on the standard dosage arm was clearly more active; however, myelosuppressive toxicity was significantly worse on this arm, with an 85% incidence of grade 4 neutropenia compared with an incidence of 21% for the weekly schedule.

Lung Cancer

In November 1998, the FDA approved topotecan for the treatment of patients with recurrent small cell lung cancer for whom initial front-line chemotherapy had failed. Supporting data came from a randomized phase III study comparing topotecan with cyclophosphamide, doxorubicin, and vincristine (CAV) in 211 patients with recurrent small cell lung cancer (Table 20-4).[281] For most of these patients, the initial chemotherapy regimen was etoposide plus cisplatin or CAV or both, and all had documented disease progression occurring at least 60 days after completion of front-line chemotherapy. The response rate was 24.3% (95% CI, 16.2% to 32.4%) for patients receiving topotecan and 18.3% (95% CI, 10.8% to 25.7%) for patients receiving CAV (*p* = .285). The median time to progression was 13.3 weeks (range, 0.4 to 55.1 weeks) for those on the topotecan arm and 12.3 weeks (range, 0.1 to 75.3 weeks) for those on the CAV arm, and the median survival was 25.0 weeks (range, 0.4 to 90.7 weeks) and 24.7 weeks (range, 1.3 to 101.3 weeks) for the topotecan and CAV groups, respectively. None of these end points was significantly different in the two groups. However, symptomatic improvement in dyspnea, cough, chest pain, hemoptysis, anorexia, insomnia, hoarseness, and fatigue, and the level of daily activity appeared to be better on the topotecan arm (*p* = .043). The number of patients with grade 4 neutropenia was similar in both topotecan and CAV groups, 70.2% and 71.7%, respectively, but the incidence of grade 4 thrombocytopenia was higher for those receiving topotecan (28.8%) than for those given CAV (5.0%). Seven toxic deaths, including four on the topotecan arm and three on the CAV arm, were associated with drug-induced myelosuppression. These findings support the similar efficacy of single-agent topotecan and the three-drug combination of CAV in treatment of recurrent small cell lung cancer.

As with ovarian cancer, the degree of refractoriness to initial front-line chemotherapy influences the response rate to second-line topotecan chemotherapy in patients with small cell lung cancer. In a single-arm phase II study, 101 previously treated patients received topotecan 1.5 mg per m² per day for 5 days.[282] Patients were divided into two groups consisting of those whose tumors progressed within 3 months of front-line treatment (refractory group) and those who initially responded (sensitive group). Among the 92 evaluable patients, the overall response rate was 21.7% (95% CI, 12.8% to 31.6%), with only 6.4% (95% CI, 1.3% to 17.6%) responding in the refractory group (n = 47) and 38% (95% CI, 23.8% to 53.5%) responding in the sensitive group (n = 45). In another study of topotecan as initial chemotherapy for untreated patients with extensive-stage small cell lung cancer, topotecan was administered to 48 patients at the slightly higher dosage of 2.0 mg per m² per day for 5 days every 3 weeks with G-CSF support in most patients.[283] The overall response in these chemotherapy-naive patients was 39% (95% CI, 25.2% to 53.0%), and the median survival time was 10.0 months (95% CI, 8.2 to 12.7 months). Thus, the activity of this nonstandard dosage of topotecan in combination with G-CSF in appears to be higher in untreated patients with small cell lung cancer than in previously treated patients. Finally, a randomized phase III trial is comparing oral administration of topotecan with standard intravenous administration in patients with small cell lung cancer.

In patients with non–small cell lung cancer, phase II studies have demonstrated objective response rates in untreated patients of 0% to 15%.[284] In a study of 45 evaluable patients with stage IIIB or stage IV non–small cell lung cancer, the overall response rate after topotecan administration at 1.5 mg per m² per day for 5 days was 15% (95% CI, 5% to 30%). Of interest, however, is that 5 of 14 patients with squamous cell cancer responded, for an overall response rate in this specific histologic lung cancer subtype of 36% (95% CI, 13.1% to 65%).[284] Despite these preliminary encouraging results, these findings have not been confirmed. Two additional studies have examined the activity of 21-day infusions of topotecan in untreated patients with non–small cell lung cancer; however, the resulting response rates of 8% (95% CI, 0% to 39%) in a group of 38 patients[232] and 4% (95% CI, 0.1% to 19.6%) in another group of 23 patients[233] did not demonstrate any advantage for longer infusion schedules in treating this disease.

Hematologic Malignancies

In studies of hematologic malignancies, 30 patients with myelodysplastic syndromes and 30 patients with chronic myelomonocytic leukemia were treated with topotecan at 2 mg per m² per day for 5 days given as a continuous infusion.[230,250] Complete responses were achieved in 37% and 27% of patients, respectively, with an overall median remission duration of 7.5 months. Remarkably, eight patients with karyotype abnormalities who subsequently achieved complete responses became cytogenetically normal while in remission. In addition to complete responses, hematologic improvement was also observed in 7 of the 60 patients entered on this trial. Unfortunately, the toxicity of this regimen was high, with 20% of patients dying during the initial 4 weeks of therapy from myelosuppression-associated complications. Gastrointestinal side effects were also common, with 23% of patients experiencing grade 3 or 4 mucositis and 17% experiencing grade 3 or 4 diarrhea. Whether similar efficacy can be achieved in these patients using less toxic schedules and doses of topotecan is not known. Nonetheless, because single-agent studies of other drugs, such as idarubicin hydrochloride[285] and cytarabine[286] show overall remission rates in myelodysplasia of only 0% to 12%, these results support further clinical investigation in this area. Such studies are ongoing.

Recent studies also suggest that topotecan has activity in acute leukemia. In a phase I study of continuous infusions of topotecan at 0.7 to 3.5 mg per m^2 per day for 5 days every 3 to 4 weeks, three complete and two partial responses were observed among 27 patients with refractory or relapsed acute leukemia, for an overall response rate of 18%.[287] Responses occurred in patients with acute myelocytic leukemia and acute undifferentiated leukemia. One of 3 patients with chronic myelocytic leukemia in blast phase also responded. At the recommended dosage of 2 mg per m^2 per day, 1 of 12 patients had severe mucositis and 5 had mild to moderate mucositis; however, other toxicities were mild. In a second phase I trial of 17 patients with acute leukemia, the recommended phase II dosage of topotecan was 2.1 mg per m^2 per day administered as a continuous intravenous infusion daily for 5 days.[240] In this study, one complete response occurred in a patient with chronic myelocytic leukemia in blast crisis and one partial response was seen in a patient with acute myelocytic leukemia. Furthermore, significant reductions in circulating blast cell numbers occurred in all courses, and transient complete clearance of leukemic blasts from the peripheral blood was described in 11 courses. In a phase II study of patients with acute lymphoblastic leukemia, single-agent topotecan was administered as a continuous intravenous infusion at 2.1 mg per m^2 per day to untreated patients using a unique window-of-opportunity design.[288] Thirteen patients with untreated acute lymphoblastic leukemia and one with relapsed acute lymphoblastic leukemia were treated; however, only one of these 14 evaluable patients experienced a complete response, for an overall response rate of 7% (95% CI, 2% to 34%). Finally, in a novel pharmacokinetically guided phase I trial in patients with acute childhood leukemia, the amount of topotecan administered was escalated to define a precise amount of drug exposure corresponding to dose-limiting toxicity.[275] For a 5-day continuous infusion of topotecan, the maximum-tolerated systemic exposure corresponded to a steady-state plasma concentration of 4.0 ng per mL (9.5 nmol per L).[275] In 18 patients, one complete and one partial response were recorded, which

occurred in patients with Burkitt's lymphoma and B-cell acute lymphoblastic leukemia, respectively. Although the peripheral blast count cleared completely in six patients, progressive disease usually occurred before or soon after the scheduled time for retreatment.

In another study of hematologic malignancy, 43 multiple myeloma patients with resistant or relapsing disease were treated with topotecan 1.5 mg per m^2 per day for 5 days; response rate was 16% (95% CI, 7% to 31%).[289] In a single study of patients with chronic lymphocytic leukemia, a disease in which the majority of malignant cells are not actively dividing, no responses were seen 12 patients.[290] Further trials of topotecan in combination with other agents active in hematologic malignancies, such as cytarabine and etoposide, are ongoing.[291]

Pediatric Malignancies

Promising preliminary activity with topotecan therapy has been reported in pediatric neuroblastoma patients.[292] In an up-front phase II window design, 63 previously untreated patients were randomized to receive either two courses of topotecan at 2 mg per m^2 per day for 5 days or paclitaxel at 350 mg per m^2 over 24 hours. Among the 32 patients randomized to receive topotecan, a response rate of 37% was observed compared with 16% for the paclitaxel arm (31 patients). In several other pediatric phase II studies of patients with a variety of different tumors, including refractory neuroblastoma, retinoblastoma, soft tissue sarcomas, and bone sarcomas, response rates ranging from 4% to 20% were seen when topotecan was administered as a 72-hour continuous infusion[276] or as a short infusion on the daily × 5 schedule.[264,293] These results are encouraging enough to warrant further clinical testing in pediatric malignancies.

Other Tumors

Because of its penetration into the CSF fluid, topotecan has also undergone testing in treatment of CNS tumors. In adults with recurrent malignant gliomas, administration of topotecan on the daily × 5 schedule resulted in responses in 3 of 22 patients with newly diagnosed malignant glioma and in 3 of 38 patients with recurrent disease.[294] In a separate study of 31 patients with malignant gliomas, all of whom had had prior radiation therapy and 48% of whom had had prior chemotherapy, the objective response rate was only 6% (95% CI, 0.8% to 21.4%).[295] In two separate pediatric CNS studies, no responses were observed in a combined total of 133 patients.[276,296] Thus, despite studies showing excellent penetration of topotecan into the CSF, its activity against CNS solid tumors is disappointing. The possibility still exists, however, that high CSF penetration might be important in other clinical settings, such as in the treatment of acute leukemia or small cell lung cancer.

In colorectal cancer, topotecan appears to be less active than irinotecan, with reported response rates ranging from 0% to 10%, whether the drug was given daily for 5 days at 1.5 mg per m² per day,[297,298] at a higher dosage of 3.5 mg per m² per day daily for 5 days with G-CSF,[299] or for 21 days as a continuous infusion.[300] Other phase II studies have also reported limited activity of topotecan against other gastrointestinal tumors such as pancreatic,[301–303] hepatocellular,[304] and gastric cancers.[305,306] The reasons why some camptothecins such as irinotecan appear to be more active than topotecan against gastrointestinal malignancies must still be determined. Results of published single-agent phase II trials with topotecan are summarized in Table 20-5.[232,307–316]

Combination Therapy

Topotecan's single-agent activity in ovarian cancer and small cell lung cancer has provided the rationale for developing combination regimens of topotecan and other agents active in these diseases, such as cisplatin. In laboratory experiments, marked synergy was observed for the combination of cisplatin and topotecan.[317,318] The molecular basis for this synergistic interaction has not been completely defined, but one hypothesis is that topotecan may interfere with topoisomerase I activity during repair of platinum-induced DNA cross-links. Camptothecin derivatives can impair the removal of platinum-DNA adducts formed after cisplatin exposure.[319,320] As discussed earlier, however, a direct role for DNA topoisomerase I in mammalian DNA repair pathways has not been defined. In the absence of such evidence, this mechanism of drug synergy is speculative. Another possible mechanism is the induction of unscheduled DNA synthesis by DNA-damaging agents, which increases the probability that a DNA replication fork will encounter a camptothecin-stabilized cleavable complex. Cisplatin-DNA adduct formation may also further stabilize topoisomerase I–DNA cleavable complexes and thereby enhance camptothecin drug effects.[317] Thus, multiple mechanisms may be responsible for the synergistic interaction between topotecan and cisplatin.

Another factor that supports the clinical use of topotecan and cisplatin in combination is their nonoverlapping clinical toxicities. Topotecan's major dose-limiting toxicity is neutropenia, whereas cisplatin dose escalation is generally limited by nephrotoxicity and neurotoxicity. Clinical trials have established recommended dosages of topotecan in combination with cisplatin.[277,321] A phase I trial of topotecan combined with cisplatin, with and without G-CSF, was conducted in patients with advanced solid tumors who had not previously received platinum compounds.[321] Topotecan was administered intravenously on days 1 through 5, and cisplatin was administered intravenously on day 1 of a 21-day cycle. The principal dose-limiting toxicity was non-cumulative neutropenia, with thrombocytopenia being somewhat less common. Nonhematologic toxicities were generally mild, although one patient experienced grade 3 renal toxicity and one developed grade 3 hepatic toxicity. Topotecan and cisplatin in combination appeared to cause more neutropenia than expected from either drug given alone. The initial recommended dosages in phase II studies were topotecan 1.0 mg per m² per day for 5 days in combination with cisplatin 50 mg per m² on day 1 without G-CSF. Cisplatin could be increased to 75 mg per m² when G-CSF was added. Fatal myelosuppressive toxicity was later seen with this regimen, however, and lower doses are now recommended.[322] Three patients with non–small cell lung cancer achieved a partial response and one patient with breast cancer had a complete response.

The importance of sequencing of drug administration for this combination was demonstrated in a phase I trial.[277] In 17 cisplatin-naive patients with solid tumors, topotecan was infused over 30 minutes daily for 5 days and cisplatin was administered either immediately before topotecan on day 1 or immediately after the last dose of topotecan on day 5. Each patient was shifted to the opposite sequence on alternating cycles of therapy, which were administered every 3 weeks. In new patients, the order of drug administration was alternated, and not randomized. The occurrence of neutropenia and thrombocytopenia precluded further dose escalation, with the recommended phase II dose being cisplatin 50 mg per m² on day 1 followed by topotecan 0.75 mg per m² per day for 5 days. Substantially more neutropenia and thrombocytopenia were observed when cisplatin was given before topotecan than with the reverse sequence. As described previously, topotecan AUCs were higher when the drug was administered after cisplatin, which suggests that subclinical renal tubular toxicity induced by cisplatin decreased topotecan clearance. Although cisplatin administration followed by topotecan administration generated more myelosuppression, this sequence was recommended for further study largely because of the synergistic antitumor activity observed in earlier mechanistic studies conducted *in vitro*. These findings highlight the importance of examining the sequence of drug administration when developing new combination chemotherapy regimens.

The difficulty in developing clinically well tolerated topotecan chemotherapy combinations was further demonstrated in two additional phase I clinical studies. The starting dosage of topotecan at 0.75 mg per m² per day for 5 days and cisplatin at 75 mg per m² administered 90 minutes after topotecan on day 1 to previously untreated patients with non–small cell lung cancer was highly myelosuppressive (grade 4 neutropenia occurred in 100% of patients).[323] Because of this toxicity, dose escalation was not possible, and no definite phase II dose recommendations were made. Another dose-escalation study analyzed response to topotecan administered as a 21-day continuous infusion every 28 days in combination with weekly cisplatin infusion on days 1 and 8.[324] Once again, however,

TABLE 20-5. TOPOTECAN SINGLE-AGENT PHASE II STUDIES

Disease	Dose & Schedule	No. Patients Entered/No. Evaluable	No. Patients with Prior Chemotherapy	Overall Response Rate, % (95% CI)	Response Type	Median Duration of Response (mo)	Median Duration of Survival (mo)	Reference
Ovarian cancer								
Ovarian cancer	1.5 mg/m²/d × 5 d every 3 wk	139/130	139	14 (8–19)	1 CR, 18 PR	4.5 (range, 2.9–16.6)	11.8 (range, 0.5–33.2)	279
Ovarian cancer	1.5 mg/m²/d × 5 d every 3 wk	30/28	30	14 (4–34)	4 PR	8.9 (range, 1.3–3.0)	10 (range, 2.1–32)	246
Ovarian cancer	1.25–1.5 mg/m²/d × 5 d every 3 wk	36/28	36	14 (4–34)	4 PR	4.5 (range, 3.0–6.0)	6.0 (range, 3–23+)	278
Ovarian cancer	1.5 mg/m²/d × 5 d every 3 wk	111/92	111	16 (9–24)	1 CR, 14 PR	5.4 (range, 1.2–10.5)	NA	247
Ovarian cancer	1.5 mg/m²/d × 5 d every 3 wk	34/31	34	23 (10–41)	7 PR	NA	11.0	280
Ovarian cancer	1.75 mg/m² c.i.v. over 24 h weekly for 4 wk every 6 wk	34/32	34	3 (0–16)	1 PR	NA	12.4	280
Lung cancer								
Small cell lung cancer	1.5 mg/m²/d × 5 d every 3 wk	101/92	101	22 (14–32)	7 CR, 13 PR	7.6 (95% CI, 5.1–12.2)	5.4 (95% CI, 4.8–6.3)	282
Small cell lung cancer	2.0 mg/m²/d × 5 d every 3 wk	48/48, all extensive stage	0	39 (25–53)	19 PR	4.8 (95% CI, 3.0–7.3)	10.0 (95% CI, 8.2–12.7)	283
Small cell lung cancer	1.25 mg/m²/d × 5 d every 3 wk	32/28	32	11 (2–28)	3 PR	1.75–47.5	5 (range, 1.5–13.5)	566
Non-small cell lung cancer	2.0 mg/m²/d × 5 d every 3 wk	20/20	0	0	0 PR	NA	7.6	266
Non-small cell lung cancer	1.5 mg/m²/d × 5 d every 3 wk	48/40	0	15 (6–30)	6 PR	25.8 (range, 2.0–15.3)	NA	284
Non-small cell lung cancer	0.5–0.6 mg/m²/d c.i.v. × 21 d every 4 wk	26/26	0	4 (0–20)	1 PR	NA	9.0	233
Non-small cell lung cancer	0.6 mg/m²/d c.i.v. × 21 d every 4 wk	12/12	0	8 (0–39)	1 PR	NA	10.25 (range, 4.25–15+)	232
Hematologic malignancies								
Acute lymphoblastic leukemia	2.1 mg/m²/d c.i.v. over 24 h for 5 d every 4 wk	14/14	0	7 (2–34)	1 CR	NA	NA	288
Multiple myeloma	1.25 mg/m²/d × 5 d every 3 wk	46/43	0	16 (7–31)	7 PR	NA	28	289
Chronic myelomonocytic leukemia	2.0 mg/m²/d c.i.v. over 24 h for 5 d every 3–4 wk	30	14	27 (12–46)	8 CR	NA	NA	250
Myelodysplastic syndrome	2.0 mg/m²/d c.i.v. over 24 h for 5 d every 3–4 wk	30	7	37 (20–56)	11 CR	NA	NA	250
Chronic lymphocytic leukemia	2.0 mg/m²/d × 5 d every 3 wk	12/12	0	0 (0–27)	6 CR	NA	NA	290

Gastrointestinal malignancies

Tumor	Dose/schedule	No.		Response (%)	CR/PR			Ref.
Colorectal cancer	1.5 mg/m²/d × 5 d every 3 wk	48/48	0	4 (1–14)	2 PR	NA	9 (95% CI, 7–16)	298
Colorectal cancer	1.5 mg/m²/d × 5 d every 3 wk	59/57	4	7 (2–17)	4 PR	11.0 (range, 9.3–12.2)	NA	297
Colorectal cancer	3.5 mg/m²/d × 5 d every 3 wk	17/16	17	0	0 PR	NA	4.0	299
Colorectal cancer	0.6 mg/m²/d c.i.v. over 24 h daily for 21 d every 4 wk	42/41	5	10 (3–23)	1 CR, 3 PR	7.0 (range, 4–11)	NA	300
Pancreatic cancer	1.5 mg/m²/d × 5 d every 3 wk	28/27	0	0	0 PR	NA	4.4	303
Pancreatic cancer	1.5 mg/m²/d × 5 d every 3 wk	35/30	0	10 (0–27)	3 PR	NA	4.8 (95% CI, 2.8–6.5)	302
Pancreatic cancer	0.5–0.6 mg/m²/d c.i.v. over 24 h daily for 21 d every 4 wk	26/26	0	8 (1–25)	2 PR	7.8 (range, 4.3–11.3)	5.0	301
Gastric cancer	1.5 mg/m²/d × 5 d every 3 wk	13/13	0	0 (0–22)	0 PR	NA	NA	305
Gastric cancer	1.5 mg/m²/d × 5 d every 3 wk	20/20	0	10 (1–32)	2 PR	NA	5.0	306

Central nervous system

Tumor	Dose/schedule	No.		Response (%)	CR/PR			Ref.
Adult malignant glioma, recurrent	1.5 mg/m²/d × 5 d every 3 wk	31/31	15	6 (1–21)	1 PR	NA	NA	295
Adult malignant glioma, recurrent	2.6 mg/m² c.i.v. over 72 h weekly	38/38	18	8 (2–21)	3 PR	4.3	NA	294
Adult malignant glioma, newly diagnosed	2.6 mg/m² c.i.v. over 72 h weekly	25/25	0	12 (3–31)	3 PR	NA	NA	294

Other adult tumors

Tumor	Dose/schedule	No.		Response (%)	CR/PR			Ref.
Head & neck cancer	1.5 mg/m²/d × 5 d every 3 wk	29/21	4	0 (0–12)	0 PR	NA	6.0	567
Head & neck cancer	1.5 mg/m²/d × 5 d every 3 wk	26/22	0	14 (3–25)	1 CR, 2 PR	4.0 (range, 2–9)	5 (range, 0.5–16+)	312
Soft tissue sarcoma	1.5 mg/m²/d × 5 d every 3 wk	32/29	0	10 (2–27)	3 PR	2.1 (range, 1.6–13.8)	NA	307
Breast cancer	1.5 mg/m²/d × 5 d every 3 wk	53/40	0	10 (3–24)	4 PR	5.0	12	313
Breast cancer	0.5 mg/m²/d c.i.v. × 21 d every 4 wk	13/13	0	15 (2–45)	2 PR	NA	13 (range, 6–15)	232
Urothelial cancer	1.5 mg/m²/d × 5 d every 3 wk	44/44	44	9 (2–26)	4 PR	4.0 (range, 3.5–14.8)	6.8	314
Prostate cancer	1.1–1.5 mg/m²/d × 5 d every 3 wk	37/34	3	3 (0–15)	1 PR	NA	17.3	309
Mesothelioma	1.5 mg/m²/d × 5 d every 3 wk	22/22	0	0	0 CR, 0 PR	NA	7.6	315
Malignant melanoma	1.5 mg/m²/d × 5 d every 3 wk	17/16	0	0	0 PR	NA	NA	310

(continued)

TABLE 20-5. (*continued*)

Disease	Dose & Schedule	No. Patients Entered/No. Evaluable	No. Patients with Prior Chemotherapy	Overall Response Rate, % (95% CI)	Response Type	Median Duration of Response (mo)	Median Duration of Survival (mo)	Reference
Germ cell tumors	1.5 mg/m²/d × 5 d every 3 wk	15/14	15	0	1 PR	NA	NA	308
Renal cell carcinoma	1.5 mg/m²/d × 5 d every 3 wk	15/14	0	0	0 PR	NA	NA	316
Pediatric tumors								
Pediatric sarcomas	1.0–1.3 mg/m²/d c.i.v. over 72 h every 3 wk	34/34	NA	0	0 PR	NA	NA	568
Pediatric solid tumors	2.0 mg/m²/d × 5 d every 3 wk	141	NA	4 (1–8)	3 CR, 2 PR	NA	NA	293
Pediatric neuroblastoma tumors	1.0–1.3 mg/m²/d c.i.v. over 72 h every 3 wk	26/26	NA	4 (0–20)	1 CR, 0 PR	NA	NA	568
Pediatric Ewing's sarcoma/peripheral neuroectodermal tumor	1.0–1.3 mg/m²/d c.i.v. over 72 h every 3 wk	25/25	NA	4 (0–20)	1 PR	NA	NA	568
Pediatric central nervous system tumors	5.5–7.5 mg/m²/d c.i.v. over 24 h every 3 wk	45/44	33	2 (0–12)	1 PR	NA	NA	276
Pediatric central nervous system tumors	1.0–1.25 mg/m²/d c.i.v. over 72 h every 3 wk	88	NA	0	0 PR	NA	NA	296

CI, confidence interval; CR, complete response; NA, data not available; PR, partial response.

because of substantial myelosuppression, the use of topotecan as a continuous intravenous infusion in combination with cisplatin was not recommended.

The combination of cisplatin and topotecan is currently undergoing phase III evaluation in previously untreated patients with advanced cervical cancer. In an ongoing three-arm study, patients are being randomized to receive either cisplatin alone, cisplatin and topotecan, or a four-drug combination of methotrexate sodium, vinblastine, doxorubicin, and cisplatin (MVAC). In this study, cisplatin 50 mg per m^2 is administered on day 1, followed by topotecan 0.75 mg per m^2 per day on days 1, 2, and 3, with treatments repeated every 3 weeks for six cycles.

Another agent with activity in both ovarian cancer and lung cancer, paclitaxel, was studied in combination with topotecan in 46 minimally pretreated adult patients with advanced solid tumors.[325] *In vitro* studies of this combination demonstrated both additive[215] and synergistic cytotoxicity.[326] The principal dose-limiting toxicity of this combination was febrile neutropenia.[325] The recommended phase II dose was paclitaxel 230 mg per m^2 infused over 3 hours on day 1 followed by topotecan at 1.0 mg per m^2 per day for 5 days given in combination with G-CSF support. Dose-limiting toxicities were febrile neutropenia seen in one patient and disabling myalgias and lower-extremity weakness, which developed in a second patient after cycle 1, with full recovery over the ensuing week. Two patients died of myelosuppressive toxicity after one cycle. Partial responses were seen in patients with head and neck cancer, non–small cell lung cancer, and colon cancer. A single phase II study of this topotecan and paclitaxel regimen has been reported involving 17 breast cancer patients, most previously treated.[327] The overall response rate of 6% (95% CI, 0.1% to 28.7%) was disappointing and was less than expected from the use of paclitaxel alone in this clinical setting.

The impact of drug sequencing on the combination of topotecan and paclitaxel was studied in a phase I trial of 22 patients with epithelial ovarian cancer or extraovarian papillary serous tumors, all of whom had had prior first-line therapy with platinum-containing regimens (Table 20-6).[328] The effect of sequencing was examined by combining topotecan given daily for 5 days and the now less commonly used paclitaxel 24-hour infusion given on either day 1 or day 5. Myelosuppression was the major dose-limiting toxicity, with thrombocytopenia and anemia being somewhat less common. Mucositis and severe diarrhea were also observed. Unlike with the topotecan-cisplatin combination, no evidence of sequence-related differences in clinical toxicity or pharmacokinetic parameters was noted. The recommended phase II doses were topotecan 0.75 mg per m^2 per day × 5 days followed by paclitaxel 135 mg per m^2 over 24 hours on day 5 repeated every 3 weeks with G-CSF support. Major antitumor responses were observed in 40% of the 22 evaluable ovarian cancer patients, with responses

seen in patients with both cisplatin-sensitive and cisplatin-resistant disease. Because of the severe myelosuppressive side effects, however, the amount of either drug administered in this combination is substantially lower than the single-agent dose.

Caution must be used when combining the camptothecin topoisomerase I inhibitors with other agents with overlapping toxicities. Substantial dose reductions of both drugs are generally required. A three-arm randomized phase II study that included two different topotecan combination regimens demonstrated severe myelosuppressive toxicity and an unanticipated number of toxic deaths when topotecan was combined with cisplatin or paclitaxel.[322] Fatal treatment-related sepsis occurred in 3 of 12 patients receiving topotecan and cisplatin and in 3 of 12 patients receiving topotecan and paclitaxel, which resulted in temporary suspension of the trial. In retrospect, the definition of dose-limiting toxicity in the phase I studies that established the phase II dosages used in this study was too aggressive. In the earlier phase I studies, the dose-limiting toxicities were defined as neutrophil counts of less than 500 per m^3 lasting for longer than 7 days or the occurrence of febrile neutropenia.[321,325] This experience highlights the issues that must be carefully considered when developing drug combinations with topoisomerase I poisons. Lower doses of both of these topotecan combinations were subsequently evaluated.

A dose-escalation study of a three-drug combination of paclitaxel, cisplatin, and topotecan was conducted involving 21 patients with previously untreated advanced ovarian cancer.[329] The recommended phase II dosages were paclitaxel 110 mg per m^2 on day 1 followed by cisplatin 75 mg per m^2 on day 2 and topotecan 0.3 mg per m^2 per day on days 2 through 6 given with G-CSF support every 3 weeks. Decreased clearance of topotecan lasting 2 to 5 days after cisplatin administration was noted in this study. Neutropenia was dose limiting and necessitated the use of reduced dosages of topotecan and paclitaxel that were well below their standard single-agent levels. At the recommended phase II dosage, however, no grade 4 neutropenia or thrombocytopenia was observed. Although this was a dose-escalation study, the overall response rate in the 15 evaluable patients with untreated advanced ovarian cancer was 87%, with nine complete responses and four partial responses. Three patients with stage III disease were pathologically free of disease at a second-look laparotomy. Currently, the combination of paclitaxel and cisplatin is a commonly used front-line chemotherapy regimen for patients with advanced ovarian cancer. Whether the addition of topotecan to this regimen represents a therapeutic advance requires further testing. Similar strategies combining weekly infusions of topotecan with cisplatin and paclitaxel,[330] or 3 days of topotecan infusions with carboplatin and paclitaxel, have also been studied in phase I clinical trials.[331]

TABLE 20-6. TOPOTECAN COMBINATION PHASE I STUDIES

Regimen and Recommended Phase II Dosages	Dose-Limiting Toxicities	Comments	Reference
Platinum derivative combinations			
Cisplatin 75 mg/m² on d 1, followed by topotecan 1.0 mg/m²/d on d 1–5. Repeat every 3 wk with G-CSF.	Neutropenia Thrombocytopenia	Fatal myelosuppressive toxicity seen with this regimen in phase II testing.[322]	321
Cisplatin 50 mg/m² on d 1, followed by topotecan 0.75 mg/m²/d on d 1–5. Repeat every 3 wk.	Neutropenia Thrombocytopenia	Pharmacokinetic interaction with reduced topotecan clearance seen when cisplatin precedes topotecan. Addition of G-CSF did not allow further dose escalation.	277
Cisplatin on d 1, followed by topotecan on d 1–5. Repeat every 3 wk.	Neutropenia	Severe toxicity at the starting dose of cisplatin 75 mg/m² on d 1, followed by topotecan 0.75 mg/m²/d on d 1–5 precluded any recommended phase II dose.	323
Cisplatin 75 mg/m² on d 1 plus topotecan 0.4 mg/m²/d c.i.v. for 14 d. Repeat every 4 wk.	Neutropenia Thrombocytopenia	Advantage of infusional combination regimen over conventional daily bolus schedule is unproven.	324
Cisplatin 40 mg/m² on d 1, plus paclitaxel 85 mg/m² over 1 h on d 1, plus topotecan 2.25 mg/m² over 30 min on d 1. Repeat weekly with G-CSF.	Neutropenia Thrombocytopenia		330
Paclitaxel 110 mg/m² on d 1, plus cisplatin 75 mg/m² on d 2, plus topotecan 0.3 mg/m²/d on d 2–6 every 3 wk with G-CSF.	Neutropenia		329
Carboplatin AUC 5.0 on d 1, plus paclitaxel 135 mg/m² on d 1, plus topotecan 0.75 mg/m² on d 1–3. Repeat every 3 wk.	Thrombocytopenia Neutropenia	Addition of G-CSF did not allow further dose escalation.	331
Paclitaxel combinations			
Paclitaxel 230 mg/m² over 3 h on d 1, plus topotecan 1.0 mg/m²/d for 5 d. Repeat every 3 wk with G-CSF.	Neutropenia Thrombocytopenia Severe myalgias and muscle weakness	Fatal myelosuppressive toxicity seen with this regimen in phase II testing.[322]	325
Topotecan 0.75 mg/m²/d on d 1–5, plus paclitaxel 135 mg/m² over 24 h on d 5. Repeat every 3 wk with G-CSF.	Neutropenia Thrombocytopenia	No sequence-related pharmacokinetic or toxic effects noted.	328
Topoisomerase II poison combinations			
Topotecan 1.5 mg/m²/d c.i.v. over 5 d, d 1–5, plus etoposide 100 mg/m²/d for 3 d on d 6–8. Repeat every 4 wk.	Mucositis	Dose-escalation study in adults with myeloid leukemia	341
Topotecan 1.0 mg/m² on d 1–5, plus oral etoposide 40 mg b.i.d. on d 6–12. Repeat every 4 wk.	Neutropenia		339
Topotecan 0.68 mg/m²/d c.i.v. over 72 h on d 1–3, plus etoposide 75 mg/m²/d over 2 h on d 8–10. Repeat every 3–4 wk.	Neutropenia Thrombocytopenia	Benefit of sequential topotecan and etoposide administration over simultaneous administration schedules is not clear.	340
Topotecan 0.75 mg/m²/d c.i.v. over 72 h on d 1–3, plus doxorubicin hydrochloride 45 mg/m² on d 5. Repeat every 3–4 wk with G-CSF.	Neutropenia Fatigue Thrombocytopenia		342
Other combinations			
Cyclophosphamide 250 mg/m² on d 1, plus topotecan 0.75 mg/m²/d for 5 d. Repeat every 3–4 weeks with G-CSF.	Neutropenia	Pediatric phase I study. No evidence for a pharmacokinetic interaction when topotecan pharmacokinetics for d 1 and d 5 were compared.	344
Cyclophosphamide 600 mg/m² on d 1, plus topotecan 1.0 mg/m²/d on d 1–5. Repeat every 3 wk with G-CSF.	Neutropenia		132
Cytarabine 1 g/m²/d on d 1–5, followed by topotecan 4.75 mg/m²/d for high-risk patients or 7.75 mg/m²/d for low-risk leukemia patients 12 h later daily on d 1–5.	Mucositis		291

AUC, area under concentration × time curve; G-CSF, granulocyte colony-stimulating factor.

Another attractive strategy is to combine the topoisomerase I poison topotecan with topoisomerase II poisons such as doxorubicin or etoposide, which have broad ranges of clinical activity. The potential of these combinations is further enhanced by the knowledge that certain yeast mutants with low topoisomerase I activity and decreased sensitivity to camptothecins can compensate by increasing their expression of topoisomerase II enzyme.[113] Thus, on purely theoretical grounds, consideration of sequential topoisomerase I and topoisomerase II poisoning strategies is attractive. Laboratory experiments examining the combination of topoisomerase I and II poisons suggests that the timing of drug administration is very important. Simultaneous administration of topoisomerase I and II poisons is antagonistic in some cell lines.[332–335] Similar findings were observed *in vivo* in human tumor xenograft models.[336] The mechanism is probably related to the interference of the topoisomerase II poison with DNA replication, which decreases the cytotoxicity of the camptothecins.[214] In contrast, sequential administration of a topoisomerase I poison followed by a topoisomerase II poison synergistically enhanced cytotoxicity.[335–337] The mechanism for synergy may be the transient elevation in topoisomerase IIα after treatment with a camptothecin, which enhances cellular sensitivity to subsequent topoisomerase II–targeting agents.[335] *In vivo* elevation of topoisomerase IIα protein levels may persist for as long as 5 days after treatment with a camptothecin.[335,338] Thus, extensive preclinical data suggest that a sequential administration schedule may be optimal. Pharmacologic synergy is not a critical end point, however. Instead, improving the therapeutic index by increasing the relative tumor cell kill while sparing normal tissues is key to improving current clinical treatment strategies. Nonetheless, these types of preclinical studies are helpful in the rational design of combination chemotherapy regimens.

A phase I study of a sequential regimen of topotecan and etoposide recommended a phase II dosage of topotecan 1.0 mg per m² per day on days 1 to 5 and etoposide 40 mg orally twice daily on days 6 to 12 every 4 weeks.[339] Myelosuppression was the dose-limiting toxicity. In another study of this combination, topotecan at 0.68 mg per m² per day was given as a 72-hour continuous infusion on days 1 to 3, followed by etoposide 100 mg per m² per day given as a 2-hour intravenous infusion daily on days 8 to 10. This regimen also produced dose-limiting myelosuppression manifested as severe neutropenia and thrombocytopenia.[340] The preclinical rationale for dual sequential topoisomerase I and II targeting was tested by performing sequential tumor biopsies in several patients. Tumor tissues from only two of six patients, however, had decreased topoisomerase I levels after treatment with topotecan, and only one tumor had an increased expression of topoisomerase II. While this experience is limited and does not permit definitive conclusions, it does highlight the current difficulty in extrapolating to the clinic a pharmacologic rationale based on laboratory findings.

This same drug combination was examined in a phase I trial in adults with acute myeloid leukemia using a sequential regimen consisting of topotecan given as a continuous infusion for 5 days followed by daily intravenous bolus etoposide for 3 days.[341] The recommended phase II dosage was topotecan 1.5 mg per m² per day as a continuous infusion on days 1 to 5 followed by etoposide 100 mg per m² per day for 3 days.[341] In nine patients, the topoisomerase IIα levels in peripheral blood leukemic blasts increased during the first 72 hours of topotecan infusion, returning to baseline by day 5. Dose-limiting mucositis was frequent and prevented further dose escalation. One complete response was seen in a patient with chronic myelocytic leukemia in blast crisis. Phase II testing of this regimen is ongoing. Sequential topoisomerase-targeting strategy was also tested in a clinical study involving adult cancer patients in which topotecan was given as a 72-hour continuous intravenous infusion on days 1 to 3 followed by intravenous bolus doxorubicin.[342] The recommended phase II doses for this combination are summarized in Table 20-6.

This same strategy was examined in a phase I study in which oral camptothecin, instead of topotecan, was administered in combination with intravenous etoposide to 33 adult patients with solid tumors.[343] The recommended phase II dose was oral camptothecin lactone given at 6 mg per m² per day for 14 days followed by intravenous etoposide at 334 mg per m². Essentially full doses of both drugs were administered in a sequential fashion. Topoisomerase I protein levels in peripheral blood mononuclear cells decreased in proportion to the plasma concentration of camptothecin, which is consistent with observations made in other studies. However, an increase in topoisomerase IIα in peripheral blood cells did not correlate with camptothecin drug exposure. Further studies are required to determine if peripheral blood mononuclear cells are an adequate surrogate tissue for predicting clinically useful changes in tumor topoisomerase I and II levels in patients.

Topotecan has also been studied in combination with cyclophosphamide, based on the rationale that alkylating agents and topotecan are synergistic *in vitro*.[214,215] In a phase I study of adult patients with refractory cancer,[132] the recommended phase II dosage for this combination was cyclophosphamide 600 mg per m² on day 1 followed immediately by topotecan 0.75 mg per m² per day × 5 days without growth factor support, and topotecan at 1.0 mg per m² per day with G-CSF support. When results were compared with previously published parameters, no effect of cyclophosphamide on topotecan pharmacokinetics was suggested. Interestingly, biochemical monitoring of peripheral blood cells revealed that peripheral blood mononuclear cell topoisomerase I decreased significantly by day 5 of therapy ($p < .1$). Furthermore, DNA fragmentation as measured by pulse field electrophoresis was demonstrated in peripheral blood mononuclear cells on day 1 of chemotherapy in 62% of patients analyzed. This measurement, however, did not correlate with the degree of myelosuppression or with efficacy seen in these patients. Further clinical studies of these molecular parameters of drug action may better define their relevance to drug toxicity or efficacy. Another phase I study of this regimen in pediatric patients determined that the recommended phase II dose was cyclophosphamide 250 mg per m² per day followed by topotecan 0.75 mg per m² per day, with each drug given daily × 5 days with G-CSF support.[344] Responses were seen for Wilms' tumor, neuroblastoma, rhabdomyosarcoma, and osteosarcoma. In the studies of topotecan and cyclophosphamide in both pediatric and adult patients, neutropenia was the dose-limiting toxicity. Finally, a randomized phase III trial in untreated patients with rhabdomyosarcoma is comparing topotecan, vincristine, and cyclophosphamide with vincristine, dactinomycin, and cyclophosphamide.

Topotecan combinations with antimetabolites have generally resulted in less than additive or antagonistic cytotoxic effects.[215] This has been attributed to the inhibition of DNA synthesis induced by most antimetabolites. Because of this interaction, a sequential rather than simultaneous administration regimen of topotecan and cytarabine was studied in patients with hematologic malignancies.[291] The recommended dosage was topotecan 4.75 mg per m² per day for 5 days plus cytarabine 1 g per m² per day for 5 days for patients at high risk and topotecan 7.0 mg per m² per day for patients at low risk. Mucositis was the dose-limiting toxicity. Clinical responses were seen in 4 of 39 patients with acute leukemia, 3 of 6 with acute lymphoblastic leukemia, and 1 of 8 patients with blast-phase chronic myelogenous leukemia. Overall, 74% of these 53 patients had previously received high-dose cytarabine chemotherapy. Interestingly, patients with bone marrow cells with high S-phase fractions were more likely to have bone marrow aplasia than those with lower S-phase fractions. Because of topotecan's excellent single-agent activity in myelodysplastic syndromes, the combination of cytarabine and topotecan is highly promising and is currently undergoing randomized testing in comparison with cytarabine and idarubicin for treatment of this disease.

Synergistic interactions between topotecan and radiation have been described *in vitro* as previously mentioned.[206,208,211,212,222] Clinical studies of topotecan in combination with radiation therapy are ongoing. One small study examined administration of topotecan as a radiation sensitizer in 12 patients with advanced non–small cell lung cancer.[345] Topotecan was tolerated when administered at 0.5 mg per m² per day over 30 minutes daily on days 1 to 5 and days 22 to 26 in combination with 60 Gy of external-beam radiation therapy. Neutropenia and gastrointestinal toxicity including esophagitis, nausea, vomiting, and anorexia precluded further escalation of the topotecan dose. Overall, these toxicities were felt to be greater than expected from either agent used alone.

In summary, a number of combinations of topotecan have been tested clinically. Most have required substantial topotecan dosage reductions, and myelosuppression has remained the major dose-limiting toxicity. The recommended phase II dosages and the major dose-limiting toxicities of these combination regimens are summarized in Table 20-6. Clear efficacy data from phase II studies for most of these combinations are still pending, and further data are needed in promising areas such as treatment of hematologic and pediatric malignancies. Currently, randomized phase III studies are evaluating topotecan combinations in treatment of ovarian cancer, small cell lung cancer, and myelodysplastic syndromes. Conclusive evidence of any increased clinical efficacy of any of these combinations depends on the outcome of these randomized trials. Clinical trials of new topotecan combinations must closely monitor potential pharmacokinetic interactions, such as those observed for cisplatin and topotecan. Incorporation of molecular and biochemical end points such as changes in topoisomerase I or II levels, cleavable complex formation, or cell-cycle checkpoint integrity may also allow for a better understanding of how these drugs are interacting at the molecular level. Because of the single-agent activity of topotecan in diseases such as ovarian and lung cancer, however, the potential exists for further improvement in clinical outcomes through the use of combination therapies with this agent.

IRINOTECAN

Irinotecan (7-ethyl-10-[4-(1-piperidino)-1-piperidino]carbonyloxycamptothecin, or CPT-11) (Fig. 20-1) was the first camptothecin derivative with increased aqueous solubility to enter clinical trials.[346] These began in the 1980s in Japan, where the drug was developed by the Daiichi Pharmaceutical and Yakult Honsha companies. Irinotecan hydrochloride became commercially available in Japan for treatment of lung cancer (small cell and non–small cell), cervical cancer, and ovarian cancer in 1994. In 1996, irinotecan was approved in the United States for use in patients with advanced colorectal cancer refractory to 5-FU. Irinotecan is unique in that it is a prodrug that must first be converted by a carboxylesterase-converting enzyme to the active metabolite SN-38 (Fig. 20-3).[35,36] SN-38 is the major metabolite believed to be responsible for irinotecan's biologic effects. Key features of irinotecan are listed in Table 20-7.

Preclinical Activity

Irinotecan has significant antitumor activity against a broad spectrum of murine tumors, including S-180, Meth A fibrosarcoma, Lewis lung carcinoma, Ehrlich carcinoma, C3H/HeN mammary carcinoma, L1210 and P388 leuke-

TABLE 20-7. KEY FEATURES OF IRINOTECAN

Mechanism of action:	After metabolic activation to 7-ethyl-10-hydroxycamptothecin (SN-38), the mechanism of action is the same as for topotecan.
Metabolism:	Irinotecan is a prodrug that requires enzymatic cleavage of the C-10 side chain by an irinotecan carboxylesterase–converting enzyme to generate the biologically active metabolite, SN-38. Both irinotecan and SN-38 can undergo nonenzymatic hydrolysis of the lactone ring to the open-ring carboxylate species. Irinotecan can also undergo hepatic oxidation of its dipiperidino side chain to form the inactive metabolite 7-ethyl-10-[4-*N*-(5-aminopentanoic acid)-1-piperidino]carbonyloxycamptothecin (APC).
Elimination:	Elimination of irinotecan occurs by urinary excretion, biliary excretion, and hepatic metabolism. About 16.1% (range, 11.1–20.9%) of an administered dose of irinotecan is excreted unchanged in the urine. SN-38 is glucuronidated, and both the conjugated and unconjugated forms are excreted in the bile. SN-38 glucuronide can also be detected in plasma.
Pharmacokinetics:	Approximate terminal half-life of irinotecan lactone is 6.8 h (range, 5.0–9.6 h) and approximate clearance is 46.9 L/h/m² (range, 39.0–53.5 L/h/m²). Approximate terminal half-life of SN-38 lactone is 11.05 h (range, 9.1–13.0 h).
Toxicity:	Early-onset diarrhea within hours or during the infusion associated with cramping, vomiting, flushing, and diaphoresis. Consider atropine 0.25–1.0 mg s.c. or i.v. in patients experiencing cholinergic symptoms. Late-onset diarrhea can occur later than 12 h after drug administration.
	Myelosuppression, predominantly neutropenia and less commonly thrombocytopenia.
	Alopecia
	Nausea and vomiting
	Mucositis
	Fatigue
	Elevated hepatic transaminases
	Pulmonary toxicity (uncommon) associated with a reticulonodular infiltrate, fever, dyspnea, and eosinophilia.
Modifications for organ dysfunction:	No definite recommendations are available for patients with impaired renal or hepatic dysfunction. Extreme caution is warranted in patients with liver dysfunction or Gilbert's disease.
Precautions:	Severe delayed-onset diarrhea may be controlled by high-dose loperamide given in an initial oral dose of 4 mg followed by 2 mg every 2 h during the day and 4 mg every 4 h during the night. High-dose loperamide should be started at the first sign of any loose stool and continued until no bowel movements occur for a 12-h period. Particular caution is also warranted in monitoring and managing toxicities in elderly patients (>64 yr) or those who have previously received pelvic/abdominal irradiation.

mias,[347] and rat Walker carcinoma.[348] It also has activity against a number of human tumor xenografts, including Co-4 colon adenocarcinoma, MX-1 mammary carcinoma, St-15 and SC-6 gastric adenocarcinomas, and QG-56 squamous cell lung carcinoma.[35] More recently, human tumor xenograft studies have demonstrated irinotecan's activity against CNS tumors,[349] testicular tumors,[350] medulloblastoma,[351] neuroblastoma,[352,353] and peripheral primitive neuroectodermal tumors.[353] Activity has also been seen in rat prostate cancers *in vivo*.[354] Irinotecan is also effective in MDR-expressing pleiotropic drug-resistant tumors both *in vivo* and *in vitro*.[163]

In preclinical studies with L1210 leukemia and in several human tumor xenograft models, repeated intermittent treatment schedules were superior to single injections of the same total drug doses.[35,355] Likewise, in human tumor xenograft studies with colon, brain, and pediatric tumors, prolonged administration of irinotecan (5 days each week for 2 of every 3 weeks) was less toxic than and at least as effective as shorter treatment schedules using higher doses.[356]

Dosages and Routes of Administration

The most commonly used schedules of irinotecan administration are a 90-minute intravenous infusion of 125 mg per m² given weekly for 4 of every 6 weeks or 350 mg per m² given every 3 weeks. In Japan, regimens of 100 mg per m² every week or 150 mg per m² every other week also have been used. The weekly × 4 schedule is more popular in North America, and the every-3-week schedule was developed predominantly in Europe. None of these regimens shows clear superiority with regard to toxicity or antitumor efficacy in nonrandomized clinical studies. Other short infusion schedules tested clinically include daily infusions for 3 days[357] and infusions every 2 weeks.[358]

Because of the schedule-dependent activity of irinotecan seen in preclinical studies, protracted or repeated irinotecan dosing schedules have been tested in phase I trials. These included short 1-hour infusions of 20 mg per m² per day daily for 5 days,[359] 10 mg per m² per day as a continuous infusion over 4 days given weekly for 2 of 3 weeks,[360] or 12.5 mg per m² per day given continuously over 14 days every 3 weeks.[361] The dose-limiting toxicity for all of these protracted administration schedules is diarrhea, with myelosuppression being less common than with the weekly or every-3-weeks short infusion schedules. Despite the somewhat low recommended dosages associated with these protracted administration schedules, the conversion of irinotecan to the active metabolite SN-38 is relatively more efficient. The AUC proportions of SN-38 relative to irinotecan range from 16% to 28%.[359,360,362] These values are much greater than the 3% to 4% proportional AUC values of SN-38 to irinotecan seen during weekly or every-3-weeks short infusion schedules, and they are consistent with an increased efficiency of irinotecan enzymatic activation. These data suggest that protracted administration schedules are worthy of further study. Oral dosing of irinotecan is also under investigation and represents a potential strategy for the more convenient delivery of protracted low doses of irinotecan to patients.[363]

Toxicity

Delayed-onset diarrhea is the most common dose-limiting toxicity of irinotecan with any of the commonly used schedules of drug administration. Delayed-onset diarrhea occurs more than several hours after the end of a drug infusion. On the weekly schedule, it is generally seen during the second or third week of treatment and lasts for approximately 2 days.[39] When irinotecan is administered every 3 weeks, the delayed diarrhea has a median time of onset of day 5 and a median duration of approximately 5 days.[364] This delayed diarrhea can be ameliorated by intensive oral loperamide hydrochloride therapy started at the onset of any loose stools beginning more than a few hours after receiving therapy (4 mg of loperamide initially, followed by 2 mg every 2 hours while the patient is awake and 4 mg every 4 hours at night).[365,366] In the initial studies, 31% of patients with colorectal cancer, most previously treated, who received irinotecan weekly experienced grade 3 or grade 4 diarrhea.[365,366] Adoption of the intensive loperamide regimen reduced this incidence by more than half.[365,367,368] Once severe delayed diarrhea does occur, standard doses of antidiarrheal agents tend to be ineffective; however, irinotecan-induced diarrhea generally resolves in 5 to 7 days and is rarely fatal.[39] Use of aggressive loperamide therapy in clinical studies has led to the escalation of irinotecan to doses as high as 500 mg per m² every 3 weeks[369] with both neutropenia and delayed diarrhea being dose limiting. Further escalation of the dosage of irinotecan beyond that recom-

mended above, however, cannot be considered for routine clinical use in the absence of further studies showing an improved therapeutic outcome for high-dose regimens.

The mechanism of irinotecan-associated delayed diarrhea has not been fully defined. In mice, diarrhea was associated with extensive vacuolation and increased apoptosis in the intestinal epithelium of the ileum, and goblet cell hyperplasia in the cecum.[370] These lesions were thought to cause malabsorption of water and electrolytes in the ileum, and hypersecretion of mucus in the cecum. Irinotecan or its metabolites were hypothesized to generate these changes by inducing apoptosis proximally and by promoting cell differentiation distally in the intestine. These changes differ from those associated with other cytotoxic agents such as cisplatin. In clinical studies, the irinotecan-associated delayed diarrhea appears to be mediated by both a secretory and an exudative mechanism.[371] Clinical testing of acetorphan, a purely antisecretory antidiarrheal agent available in Europe, showed some degree of efficacy for this agent in decreasing the irinotecan-induced delayed diarrhea.[371] Improved symptom control was seen when acetorphan was combined with loperamide, which acts by delaying gut transit times and also has an intrinsic antisecretory effect of it own. Further testing of this combination is in progress. Other experimental efforts to ameliorate irinotecan-associated diarrhea using β-glucuronidase inhibitors or antibiotics are discussed later.

Factors that appear to predispose to severe diarrhea include prior pelvic radiation therapy, poor performance status,[364] and age 65 years or older.[364,372] Prior chemotherapy did not appear to predispose patients to either diarrhea or neutropenia, and neither toxicity was cumulative in nature.[364] As discussed later, patients with Gilbert's syndrome may be at risk for more severe diarrhea due to the impaired elimination of the active metabolite SN-38. Caution is warranted in treating such patients, who may represent over 5% of the population.

The most common irinotecan-associated hematologic toxicity is neutropenia, which is noncumulative. On the weekly regimen, granulocyte counts typically reach nadir on days 21 to 29 and recover over the next 5 to 6 days.[39,373] In 304 previously treated patients with colorectal cancer given weekly irinotecan, the incidence of grade 4 neutropenia was approximately 12%,[372] with a twofold increased incidence in patients with prior pelvic or abdominal radiation. Grade 3 or 4 diarrhea was seen in 31% of patients. In a European phase II study in which irinotecan was given every 3 weeks to 213 patients with advanced colorectal cancer, the incidence of grade 3 or 4 neutropenia was 47%.[364] The median time to granulocyte nadir was 8 days, and full recovery typically occurred by day 22 in most patients. Febrile neutropenia was seen in 15% of patients, and the treatment-related death rate was 1.9%.[364] Fatalities most commonly occurred in the setting of febrile neutropenia with concomitant diarrhea. Severe thrombocytopenia and anemia were less common. Irinotecan-induced immune thrombocytopenia was reported in one patient.[374] Other nonhematologic toxicities are generally manageable and include nausea and vomiting, mucositis, elevated hepatic transaminase levels, fatigue, and alopecia. Acute diarrhea associated with irinotecan administration has been reported, most commonly in association with other cholinergic effects including abdominal cramping, vomiting, flushing, diaphoresis, visual accommodation disturbances, lacrimation, nasal congestions, salivation, and, less often, asymptomatic bradycardia.[375,376] This syndrome may be more common when higher doses of irinotecan above 240 mg per m² are administered.[366,375] These cholinergic effects have been attributed to the inhibition of acetylcholinesterase by irinotecan.[377] Interestingly, the active metabolite SN-38 does not have this effect. Administration of atropine sulfate tended to alleviate most of these symptoms, and typically this constellation of symptoms does not interfere with the ability to administer irinotecan therapy. An uncommon pulmonary syndrome described in Japanese lung cancer patients is manifested by fever, dyspnea, eosinophilia, and a reticulonodular infiltrative pattern on chest radiographs.[378] Corticosteroid administration may result in some improvement in respiratory symptoms, but fatalities have been reported.[379] In North American studies, vasodilatation or skin flushing were seen in approximately 11% of patients, but true hypersensitivity reactions were rare.[380] A case report described irinotecan-induced tumor lysis syndrome in a 42-year-old patient with colon cancer metastatic to the liver.[381] The patient had previously received 5-FU and leucovorin chemotherapy but was switched to irinotecan 300 mg per m² every 3 weeks. Eight days after her first dose, she was admitted to the hospital with hyperuricemia, hyperphosphatemia, elevated serum lactate dehydrogenase levels, and a metabolic acidosis leading to the presumptive diagnosis of tumor lysis syndrome. She ultimately died from renal failure and anuria. Finally, a single case report described two recurrent episodes of irinotecan-associated CNS toxicity manifested as a transient dysarthria lasting for approximately 2 hours shortly after each infusion of irinotecan. The patient fully recovered without any other sequelae or associated neurologic findings.[382]

Dosage Adjustments for Excessive Toxicity or Abnormal Organ Function

When grade 3 neutropenia or delayed diarrhea occurs, the dose of irinotecan should be reduced by 25 mg per m² on the weekly schedule or by 50 mg per m² on the every-3-weeks schedule. If grade 4 neutropenia or diarrhea occurred during the previous cycle, the dose of irinotecan should be reduced by 50 mg per m² on either schedule. A new course of therapy should not be initiated until any prior neutropenia or diarrhea have resolved. Patients at increased risk for severe diarrhea include those with prior

pelvic radiation, poor performance status, age 65 years or older, or Gilbert's syndrome.[364,372]

No formal guidelines exist for treating patients with impaired renal or hepatic function. In pharmacokinetic studies, modest changes in renal function do not appear to affect irinotecan plasma concentrations.[383] In contrast, a population study suggests that elevated bilirubin levels are associated with a decrease in irinotecan clearance and an elevated AUC ratio of SN-38 to irinotecan on the every-3-weeks schedule.[383] Therefore, until more formal dosing guidelines are available, extreme caution is warranted in administering irinotecan to patients with impaired hepatic function and hyperbilirubinemia. Studies are ongoing to try to better define appropriate dosages of irinotecan for these patients.

Clinical Pharmacology

Analytic Methodology

Both irinotecan and its active metabolite SN-38 circulate in plasma after drug administration. Like all camptothecins, irinotecan and SN-38 both contain a terminal α-hydroxy lactone ring that is unstable in aqueous solutions and undergoes rapid nonenzymatic hydrolysis to the open-ring carboxylate (Fig. 20-2). The early pharmacokinetic studies of irinotecan used assays that measured only total (lactone and carboxylate) concentrations of irinotecan and SN-38[36,384,385]; however, more recent assays have been validated that can separate both lactone and carboxylate forms.[386–389] Virtually all of these assays use reversed-phase HPLC with fluorescence detection.[36,384,385] Rapid precipitation of plasma samples with ice cold methanol or acetonitrile (or both) is used to trap the camptothecins in their relative lactone and carboxylate forms, which are later resolved on a reversed-phase HPLC column.[386–389] Careful attention to sample storage conditions is important for preventing interconversion of the lactone and carboxylate drug species.[388] Newer assays have also been developed for the determination of more recently recognized irinotecan metabolites, including β-glucuronidated SN-38[390,391] and 7-ethyl-10-[4-N-(5-aminopentanoic acid)-1-piperidino]carbonyloxycamptothecin (RPR121056A; APC) (Fig. 20-3).[390] Recently an assay for measuring irinotecan and SN-38 in saliva was shown to correlate with plasma drug concentrations.[392]

General Pharmacokinetics

After short intravenous infusions of irinotecan, both the parent drug and SN-38 are measurable in plasma as the lactone and open-ring carboxylate species (Fig. 20-3). After approximately 1 hour, however, the levels of SN-38 tend to be 50 to 100 times lower than the irinotecan plasma levels, and the overall AUC proportion of SN-38 relative to irinotecan is only approximately 4%.[19,23,39] In most[39,357,366,375,393] but not all[394,395] reports, irinotecan plasma concentrations and AUC increased proportionally with increasing dose, which suggests linear pharmacokinetics. In contrast, the SN-38 AUC and plasma concentrations did not correlate as well with increasing dose, which is consistent with nonlinear, saturable kinetics for the conversion of irinotecan to SN-38 by the carboxylesterase-converting enzyme.[39,357,373,375,393] Peak plasma levels of irinotecan occurred immediately after the end of the infusion period, whereas SN-38 peak levels tended to occur approximately 2.2 ± 0.1 hours later (range, 1.6 to 2.8 hours).[375] Extremely high interpatient variability in the plasma concentrations of irinotecan and SN-38 is common, although the reasons for this are only partially defined.

The kinetics of irinotecan and SN-38 has been fitted to a biexponential or triexponential model in most studies.[357,366,373,375] For short intravenous infusions, the mean terminal elimination half-life for irinotecan lactone was 6.8 hours (range, 5.0 to 9.6 hours). The plasma half-life of the active metabolite, SN-38 lactone, however, was relatively long compared with that of the other camptothecins; the terminal half-life was approximately 10.4 hours (range, 9.1 to 11.5 hours) for SN-38 lactone (Table 20-8). The prolonged duration of exposure to SN-38 is probably a function of its sustained production from irinotecan in tissues, because direct injection of SN-38 into rats resulted in extremely rapid plasma clearance with a half-life of only 7 minutes.[396,397] Race, gender, and renal function do not appear to alter the clinical pharmacology of irinotecan.[383,398] However, decreased total irinotecan clearance has been modestly correlated with abnormalities in liver function such as increased serum bilirubin and γ-glutamyl transpeptidase levels in population pharmacokinetic studies.[383] These same hepatic abnormalities also correlated with an increased ratio of SN-38 to irinotecan AUC (metabolic ratio), an observation that could potentially be explained by increased conversion of irinotecan to SN-38 or decreased clearance of the SN-38 metabolite, or both.

Several groups have attempted to use population pharmacokinetic modeling and bayesian analysis to estimate irinotecan pharmacokinetics and to develop limited sampling strategies. Most have recommended two[399–401] or three[402] sampling times to reliably predict irinotecan or SN-38 AUC values. All have attempted to estimate total irinotecan and SN-38 pharmacokinetic parameters, and none have distinguished between the lactone and carboxylate drug species. A few of these limited sampling methods have been applied to clinical studies of the pharmacokinetics of irinotecan in larger patient populations.[402,403]

Compared with topotecan, relatively large amounts of both irinotecan and SN-38 in plasma are present in the lactone form. The irinotecan lactone AUC ranged from 33% to 44% of the total irinotecan AUC, and for SN-38, the lactone percentage was even greater, ranging from 30% to 74% in most studies (Table 20-8). Thus, compared with other camptothecins, relatively large amounts of the SN-38

circulate in plasma as the biologically active lactone, which may be related to irinotecan's clinical activity.

One potential explanation for variation in the lactone to carboxylate ratios for different camptothecins is their differential protein binding. Burke and Mi showed that the equilibrium ratio in plasma between the carboxylate and lactone forms of different camptothecin derivatives was greatly affected by their relative degree of albumin binding.[404] For drugs such as camptothecin or 9-AC, the albumin-binding affinity of the open-ring carboxylate was over 200 times greater than the lactone affinity.[404] This carboxylate protein binding tends to shift the equilibrium ratio in plasma toward the less active, open-ring form of the drug. In contrast, for SN-38, the lactone and not the carboxylate preferentially binds to human albumin, which thus shifts the equilibrium in the opposite direction. Overall, the amount of drug present as lactone at equilibrium in plasma closely paralleled the relative albumin-binding affinity of the lactone species for a variety of different camptothecin analogs.[404] In the absence of any proteins, the lactone hydrolysis of a number of different camptothecins occurs at a very similar rate.[26] Thus, relatively modest structural differences in the camptothecin molecule can dramatically alter the clinical pharmacology and biologic activity of these drugs. Marked species-specific differences in camptothecin binding to murine, bovine, and human albumin have also been described,[405] which further highlights the difficulty in extrapolating from pharmacokinetic and pharmacodynamic relationships observed in animal experiments to human studies. The overall plasma protein binding for SN-38 is higher than that for irinotecan, with 92% to 96% of total SN-38 being protein bound in laboratory plasma incubation experiments compared with 30% to 43% for irinotecan.[406] Serum albumin was the major protein to which both SN-38 and irinotecan were bound.

Thus, several factors in the clinical pharmacology of irinotecan may contribute to its greater antitumor activity relative to other camptothecin derivatives. One is the longer half-life of the active metabolite SN-38, which ranges from 6 to 24 hours, after short infusion of irinotecan. As discussed earlier, this may be due to the slow conversion of irinotecan to SN-38. The second factor is the relatively large amount of circulating SN-38 that is present as the active lactone form. Finally, as discussed previously, the topoisomerase I–DNA cleavable complexes induced by SN-38 are extremely stable compared with those of other camptothecin analogs.[41] All of these factors probably contribute to the clinical antitumor activity of irinotecan.

Because of the greater difficulty in analytic determination of the unstable lactone species in plasma, several investigators have questioned the value of measuring lactone versus total (lactone plus carboxylate) plasma concentrations for pharmacokinetic studies.[397,407] Within any individual, the ratio of lactone to total drug is relatively constant; however, variation between different individuals

TABLE 20-8. IRINOTECAN PHARMACOKINETICS

Dose & Schedule	No. Patients	Compound	C_{max} (μmol/L)	AUC (μmol/L × h)	CL (L/h/m²)	V_{ss} (L/m²)	Terminal Half-Life (h)	Urinary Excretion	Lactone/Total Drug AUC (%)	Reference
100 mg/m² over 90 min	3	Irinotecan total[a]	2.43 ± 0.48	10.9 ± 2.7	17.6 ± 4.0	—	1.5 ± 0.4	—	—	394
		SN-38 total	0.046 ± 0.006	0.303 ± 0.092	—	—	3.0 ± 0.6	—	—	
125 mg/m² over 90 min	7	Irinotecan total	2.70 ± 0.51	15.7 ± 2.8	14.6 ± 1.7	—	4.3 ± 1.5	—	—	394
		SN-38 total	0.082 ± 0.029	0.643 ± 0.209	—	—	7.8 ± 2.4	—	—	
50–180 mg/m² over 90 min	32	Irinotecan total	—	—	15.3 ± 3.5	—	7.9 ± 2.8	13.9 ± 6.5 over 48 h	33.3[b]	39
		Irinotecan lactone	—	—	45.6 ± 10.8	—	6.3 ± 2.2	—	—	
		SN-38 total	—	—	—	—	13.0 ± 5.8	0.26 ± 0.19 over 48 h	30.1[b]	
		SN-38 lactone	—	—	—	—	11.5 ± 3.8	—	—	
50–145 mg/m² over 30–90 min	26	Irinotecan total	1.14–4.41	4.54–18.71	15.0 ± 0.8	142 ± 8	9.3 ± 0.5	11.1 ± 1.2 over 24 h	—	373
		SN-38 total	0.026–0.191	0.092–1.130	—	—	—	0.18 ± 0.03 over 24 h	—	
100 mg/m² over 90 min	36	Irinotecan total	2.31 ± 0.62	10.96 ± 2.84	—	—	—	—	—	416
		SN-38 total	0.067 ± 0.029	0.602 ± 0.234	—	—	—	—	—	
100 mg/m² over 90 min	12	Irinotecan total	2.11 ± 0.27	9.30 ± 0.8	18.8 ± 1.6	—	6.8 ± 0.4	—	—	407
		Irinotecan lactone	1.35 ± 0.19	3.48 ± 0.25	49.5 ± 4.2	—	6.4 ± 0.3	—	—	
		SN-38 total	0.059 ± 0.006	0.510 ± 0.058	—	—	11.3 ± 1.6	—	—	
		SN-38 lactone	0.037 ± 0.004	0.274 ± 0.027	—	—	9.1 ± 1.5	—	—	
125 mg/m² over 90 min[c]	18	Irinotecan total	2.38	3.08	—	—	—	—	—	367
		SN-38 total	0.045	0.175	—	—	—	—	—	
125 mg/m² over 90 min	26	Irinotecan total	2.36 ± 0.51	23.1 ± 6.3	—	—	—	—	—	368
		SN-38 total	0.088	1.17 ± 0.56	—	—	—	—	—	
145 mg/m² over 90 min	40	Irinotecan total	3.17 ± 1.00	20.3 ± 9.05	14.6 ± 6.4	136 ± 73.9		14.1 ± 10.3 over 24 h	—	398
		SN-38 total	0.077 ± 0.032	0.949 ± 0.950	—	—		0.22 ± 0.24 over 24 h		
		SN-38G total	0.154 ± 0.080	2.10 ± 1.91	—	—		1.09 ± 0.97 over 24 h		
100–345 mg/m² over 90 min	31	Irinotecan total	1.8–4.5	6.93–36.05	21.1 ± 34	148 ± 2.0	5.2 h[d]	37 ± 4 over 48 h	44.4 ± 4	375
		Irinotecan lactone[e]	2.0–2.3	10.1–11.4	53.5 ± 1.2	—	5.0 h[d]	—	—	

(continued)

TABLE 20-8. (continued)

Dose & Schedule	No. Patients	Compound	C_{max} (μmol/L)	AUC (μmol/L × h)	CL (L/h/m²)	V_{ss} (L/m²)	Terminal Half-Life (h)	Urinary Excretion	Lactone/Total Drug AUC (%)	Reference
		SN-38 total	0.047–0.191	0.25–1.62	—	—	5.9 h[d]	—	51 ± 3	—
		SN-38 lactone	0.021–0.089	0.157–0.933	—	—	—	—	—	—
100–750 mg/m² over 30 min	60	Irinotecan total	3.93–29.58	9.58–115.8	15 ± 1	157 ± 8	14.2 ± 0.9	19.9 ± 1.4 over 24 h	—	366
		SN-38 total	0.082–0.762	0.408–4.05	—	—	13.8 ± 1.4	0.25 ± 0.03 over 24 h	—	—
33–115 mg/m² over 30 min	21	Irinotecan total	1.90–4.86	19.4–48.1	14.3 ± 6.9	141 ± 74	8.3 ± 4.3	9.9–11.4 over 24 h	—	357
		SN-38 total	0.014–0.109	0.44–2.46	—	—	10.2 ± 6.0	0.15–0.18 over 24 h	—	—
200 mg/m² over 90 min	10	Irinotecan total	3.90 ± 0.48	25.6 ± 5.71	14.0 ± 3.2	138 ± 24.0	13.5 ± 2.1	20.9 ± 7.4 over 56 h	—	446
		SN-38 total	0.090 ± 0.023	1.14 ± 0.357	49.5 ± 4.2	—	23.8 ± 7.7	0.389 ± 0.26 over 56 h	—	—
		SN-38G	0.475 ± 0.265	8.01 ± 2.95	—	—	23.5 ± 10.6	3.39 ± 2.31 over 56 h	—	—
		APC	0.52 ± 0.29	5.90 ± 1.2	—	—	15.1 ± 2.3	2.80 ± 1.68 over 56 h	—	—
		NPC	0.057 ± 0.019	0.731 ± 0.329	—	—	9.67 ± 5.12	0.908 ± 0.198 over 56 h	—	—
300–500 mg/m² over 30–90 min	5	Irinotecan lactone	—	12.3–19.7	39.0 ± 9.6	263 ± 102	9.6 ± 3.9 h	—	36.8 ± 3.5	569
		SN-38 lactone	—	0.81–1.65	—	—	—	—	64.0 ± 3.4	—
33–750 mg/m² over 30 min	107	Irinotecan total	—	—	14.3 ± 4	150 ± 49	10.8 ± 0.5	16.7 ± 1.0 over 24 h	—	383
		SN-38 total	—	—	—	—	10.6 ± 0.8	0.23 ± 0.02 over 24 h	—	—
350 mg/m² over 30 min	47	Irinotecan total	—	42.4 ± 12.0	15.20 ± 4.3	—	—	—	—	403
		SN-38 total	—	1.43 ± 1.25	—	—	—	—	—	—
		SN-38G total	—	4.04 ± 3.07	—	—	—	—	—	—
300–350 mg/m² over 90 min	7	Irinotecan total	13.3 ± 6.0	42.7 ± 12.6	12.9 ± 3.9	76 ± 19	6.1 ± 2.2	—	—	415
		SN-38 total	0.12 (range, 0.04–0.25)	1.2 (range, 0.51–2.3)	—	—	17 (range, 3.8–33)	—	—	—
		SN-38G total	0.57 (range, 0.17–2.3)	5.0 (range, 1.9–13)	—	—	12 (range, 4.8–26)	—	—	—
		APC	2.7 (range, 0.80–10)	26 (7.0–83)	—	—	6.7 (range, 3.9–12)	—	—	—
35 mg/m²/d c.i.v. over 5 d	6	Irinotecan total	0.263 ± 0.107	35.1 ± 11.1	101.6 ± 94.1 L/h[f]	—	26.5 ± 19.2	—	—	393
		SN-38 total	0.017 ± 0.014	2.32 ± 1.40	—	—	39.0 ± 19.5	—	—	—
7.5–17.5 mg/m²/d c.i.v. over 24 h for 14–21 d	29	Irinotecan total	—	12.8 ± 3.99[g]	36.1 ± 16.0	—	2.9 ± 6.1	76 ± 3.8 over 24 h	33 ± 9	362

Dose	n	Analyte								
		SN-38 total	—	1.4 ± 0.3[g]	—	—	7.5–11.1	0.68 ± 0.56 over 24 h	63 ± 6	
		SN-38G	—	7.2 ± 5.2[g]	—	—	5.8–11.3	4.4 ± 2.1 over 24 h	—	
20–100 mg/m² orally	25	Irinotecan lactone	0.013–0.393	0.038–1.50[h]	322 ± 172	—	9.9 ± 6.5[d]	—	38 ± 7	363
		SN-38 lactone	0.006–0.090	0.033–0.291[h]	—	—	13.45 ± 7.12[d]	—	74 ± 5	
		SN-38G	0.012–0.167	0.154–1.804[h]	—	—	13.54 ± 3.17[d]	—	—	

APC, 7-ethyl-10-[4-N-(5-aminopentanoic acid)-1-piperidino]carbonyloxycamptothecin; AUC, area under concentration × time curve; C_{max}, maximal plasma concentration; CL, clearance; NPC, 7-ethyl-10-(4-amino-1-piperidino)carbonyloxycamptothecin; SN-38, 7-ethyl-10-hydroxycamptothecin; SN-38G, SN-38 glucuronide; V_{ss}, volume of distribution at steady state. Pharmacokinetic parameters have been converted to uniform units whenever possible for ease of comparison, unless otherwise stated.

[a]Total = lactone + carboxylate.
[b]At the recommended phase II dose of 150 mg/m².
[c]Median values.
[d]Harmonic mean and pseudo–standard deviations.
[e]At doses of 240–345 mg/m² only.
[f]L/h not L/h/m².
[g]At the recommended phase II dosage of 10 mg/m² i.v. over 24 h for 14 days in 6 patients.
[h]AUC from zero to 24 h.

may be quite high. Nonetheless, pharmacodynamic studies performed to date have not shown a superiority for lactone compared to total plasma drug measurements in predicting clinical drug effects.[39,375]

Absorption

Although the most common route of irinotecan administration is intravenous, oral formulations have been tested in preclinical[408] and clinical studies.[363] In nude mice, oral administration of irinotecan is active and well tolerated, with a low overall bioavailability of 12% to 21%.[35,347,408–410] The amount of SN-38 generated from oral administration of irinotecan, however, was threefold higher than that from intravenous administration when the molar AUC ratios of SN-38 to irinotecan were compared.[410] Extensive first-pass metabolism of irinotecan to SN-38 in the intestine and liver was proposed as a potential explanation. In a clinical phase I study, oral irinotecan at 20 to 100 mg per m^2 per day for 5 days every 3 weeks was well tolerated.[363] Because of the occurrence of dose-limiting age-related delayed diarrhea, the recommended phase II oral dosage was 66 mg per m^2 per day for patients younger than 65 years, and 50 mg per m^2 per day for older patients. As seen in earlier animal studies, higher molar AUC ratios of SN-38 to irinotecan were generated by the oral route, consistent with greater metabolic conversion of irinotecan to SN-38. Bioavailability was not determined. Intraperitoneal administration has also been examined in a mouse model, and preliminary evidence suggests that it may result in more efficient activation of irinotecan to SN-38 than intravenous routes of administration.[347,409,411]

Distribution

Little is known about the tissue penetration and distribution of irinotecan, although the volume of distribution at steady state is large, with mean values ranging from 76 to 157 L per m^2 for total irinotecan (Table 20-8). In rhesus monkeys, the CSF penetration of irinotecan was only 14 ± 3% of the plasma exposure, which is less than observed for topotecan,[412] and SN-38 was not detectable in the CSF. In nude mice, repeated daily intraperitoneal administration of irinotecan resulted in high prolonged irinotecan and SN-38 concentrations in the intestine[413]; however, penetration into other tissue compartments was not measured. Interestingly, when SN-38 instead of irinotecan was directly administered intravenously to rats, very little tissue accumulation was observed, which suggests that peripheral tissue conversion of irinotecan to the active metabolite may be potentially important for generating its clinical activity.[396]

In a phase II clinical study, intravenous irinotecan at 60 mg per m^2 combined with cisplatin was given to patients with malignant pleural mesothelioma, and pleural fluid pharmacokinetics was monitored in three patients.[414] Irino-tecan was detectable in pleural fluid as early as 1 hour after an intravenous infusion, with peak levels occurring after 6 hours. The active metabolite SN-38 was also detected within 1 hour after the end of an infusion; by 6 hours the SN-38 pleural fluid concentrations mirrored plasma concentrations and continued to do so for the remainder of the monitoring period, which lasted 24 to 48 hours. The maximal pleural concentrations of irinotecan and SN-38 were 37% and 76% of the plasma concentrations of drug, respectively. Thus, excellent penetration into the pleural fluid compartment was observed in this study. Dosing guidelines for patients with large third-space fluid collections such as pleural effusions and ascites are not available; however, no clinical reports have been published of excessive irinotecan toxicity in these patients.[414]

Metabolism

Irinotecan is extensively metabolized to a number of active and inactive metabolites (Fig. 20-3). This creates the potential for clinically important pharmacogenetic variability in the kinetics of this agent. Irinotecan carboxylesterase–converting enzyme metabolizes irinotecan to SN-38, which, in turn, is conjugated by liver uridine diphosphate glucuronosyl transferases to form the inactive β-glucuronidated derivative, SN-38G. The total amount of SN-38 generated in individual patients is highly variable,[39,375,403] which suggests that variations in carboxylesterase-converting enzyme activity may be important in determining irinotecan response and toxicity. The relative AUC value of the active metabolite SN-38 to irinotecan varied from 0.9% to 11% in a pharmacokinetic study of different dosages of irinotecan (dose range, 115 to 600 mg per m^2).[415] Furthermore, this ratio was highest at the lowest doses of irinotecan examined (115 mg per m^2), which suggests that less efficient conversion of irinotecan to SN-38 occurred at higher drug concentrations. Alternatively, variations in the clearance of SN-38 via the uridine diphosphate glucuronidation pathway provides another potential mechanism for variability in irinotecan pharmacokinetics. Irinotecan is also a substrate for metabolism by the cytochrome P-450 system, which creates an additional potential for drug interactions. However, no adverse drug interactions have been well characterized in clinical studies to date. Nonetheless, these studies demonstrate that the metabolic pharmacokinetics of irinotecan is complex and may be mediated by several different families of enzymes, including carboxylesterases, cytochrome P-450 enzymes, and glucuronosyl transferases.

Carboxylesterase-Converting Enzyme

In rodents, an irinotecan carboxylesterase–converting enzyme (Fig. 20-3) that can hydrolyze irinotecan to SN-38 has been purified from rat serum, and high activity is also found in rat and mouse liver, intestinal mucosa, and other tissues.[37] Carboxylesterase-converting enzyme specific activity is much lower in human serum,[416] however, and in comparable human tissues.[417] The precise carboxylesterase(s) responsible for the clinical activation of irinotecan in humans has not been characterized, although human liver carboxylesterase has been studied as the most likely candidate.[417] Human liver carboxylesterase activity is found in hepatic microsomal fractions, and this enzyme has been cloned and characterized.[418] The high interindividual variation observed in human liver microsomal carboxylesterase activity could potentially cause clinically important differences in drug metabolism.[419] In human and animal studies, no evidence exists that irinotecan induces hepatic or serum carboxylesterase activity.[420]

Carboxylesterase activity and irinotecan metabolism have been studied in detail in human liver microsomes.[421] Rate-limiting deacylation kinetics was observed, with an initial fast "burst" rate of SN-38 release occurring during the first 10 to 15 minutes of incubation followed by a slower steady-state production of SN-38. The overall activity of irinotecan carboxylesterase–converting enzyme was lower in human liver than in rats, with an apparent K_m in humans of 52.9 μmol per L and a V_{max} (maximum reaction velocity) of 0.145 nmol per L per hour. A slight inhibition of irinotecan activation by loperamide suggested that a potential drug interaction could occur when this drug was given concomitantly; however, this finding has not been evaluated further in clinical studies.

The difference between irinotecan lactone and carboxylate forms as substrates for carboxylesterase activation was studied further in human liver microsomes.[422] Irinotecan lactone was more rapidly metabolized than the carboxylate by approximately twofold, with observed K_m values of 23.3 ± 5.3 μmol per L and 48.9 ± 5.5 μmol per L for irinotecan lactone and carboxylate, respectively. Additional studies using the enzyme inhibitor phenylmethyl sulfonyl fluoride suggested that the liver carboxylesterase responsible for SN-38 formation was a serine-dependent hydrolase. Although irinotecan carboxylesterase activity correlated with the carboxylesterase-mediated hydrolysis of *para*-nitrophenol acetate, this later reaction was over 1 million times more efficient. Thus, irinotecan is a relatively poor substrate for human liver carboxylesterase. High interindividual variability in carboxylesterase-specific activity was seen in 12 different human liver microsomal preparations, with a 5- to 45-fold range of activity depending on the carboxylesterase substrate used.[419] This finding suggests that interindividual variation in this enzyme activity may be an important source of pharmacokinetic and pharmacodynamic variability.

Additional detailed studies of human liver microsomes from seven different donors identified two different isoforms with irinotecan-activating activity.[423] A high-affinity isoform with a mean K_m value of 2.3 ± 1.4 μmol per L (range, 1.4 to 3.9 μmol per L) with a V_{max} of 2.11 ± 0.82 pmol per mg per minute and a low-affinity isoform with a

K_m of 149 ± 154 μmol per L (range, 129 to 164 μmol per L) and a V_{max} of 10.8 ± 45.8 pmol per mg per minute. The hypothesis was that, at physiologically relevant concentrations of irinotecan, more than one carboxylesterase isoform may be contributing to the bioactivation of this agent. A slight inhibition of irinotecan metabolism *in vitro* by loperamide was observed in this study also, but the overall effect was small. Recently, another group has demonstrated that the human serum enzyme butyrylcholinesterase has irinotecan-activating activity.[424] The normal substrate for this enzyme is unknown, but it is clinically important for mediating the metabolic clearance of the anesthetic adjuvant succinylcholine. Pharmacogenetic deficiencies in this enzyme cause prolonged muscle paralysis in susceptible individuals after surgical procedures.[425] Because butyrylcholinesterase represents a large proportion of the total cholinesterase activity in human plasma,[424] this enzyme may be important in the clinical conversion of irinotecan to SN-38. Additional studies to characterize the precise enzyme(s) responsible for irinotecan activation in humans are necessary.

An unresolved issue is whether actual irinotecan carboxylesterase–converting enzyme activity within the tumor itself is an important determinant of irinotecan sensitivity. In general, human irinotecan carboxylesterase–activating activity is difficult to measure in human tissues and in plasma because of its low overall activity.[175,426] In a study of irinotecan-converting enzyme carboxylesterase activity in 53 human colon tumors, the enzyme-specific activity varied by 146-fold.[427] Some[175,176,428] but not all[35,177] studies have found a modest correlation between tumor carboxylesterase-converting enzyme activity and sensitivity to irinotecan. Additional correlative studies are necessary to characterize the importance of tumor carboxylesterase-converting enzyme activity as a predictor of clinical response to irinotecan chemotherapy. Despite this uncertainty, efforts to use the mammalian liver carboxylesterase gene to sensitize tumors selectively to irinotecan as a gene therapy approach are under investigation in laboratory model systems.[418,429,430]

Hepatic Metabolism

Under most circumstances, only a small amount of the total irinotecan metabolized is converted into SN-38. Recently, several additional metabolites of irinotecan have been identified and characterized in human plasma.[421] Oxidation of the terminal piperidino ring by hepatic cytochrome P-450 enzymes is thought to be responsible for the formation of 7-ethyl-10-[4-*N*-(5-aminopentanoic acid)-1-piperidino]carbonyloxycamptothecin, or APC (Fig. 20-3). Based on human hepatic microsomal experiments, the formation of APC from irinotecan appears to be principally mediated by cytochrome P-450 CYP3A isoforms.[431] Supporting evidence comes from multiple approaches, including the selective inhibition of APC formation by CYP3A inhibitors such as ketoconazole, recombinant-expressed CYP3A4 studies, and the use of anti-CYP3A antibodies.[431]

Overall, the APC metabolite was at least 100-fold less active than SN-38 as an inhibitor of topoisomerase I,[421] and it was a poor substrate for conversion to SN-38 by human liver carboxylesterases. In cytotoxicity experiments, APC was also a poor inhibitor of human nasopharyngeal KB cell growth; the concentration showing 50% growth inhibition was comparable to that of irinotecan.[421] Unlike irinotecan, APC did not interfere with acetylcholinesterase activity. Although the APC metabolite does not appear to be responsible for any of irinotecan's clinical toxicities or antitumor effects, its formation may represent an important metabolic pathway for irinotecan clearance.

The pharmacokinetics of irinotecan, including the newly identified APC metabolite, was studied in detail in 19 patients.[415] Most were treated with intravenous irinotecan at dosages ranging from 115 to 600 mg per m[2] every 3 weeks. The APC metabolite peak plasma concentrations occurred approximately 2 hours after the end of the infusion, and the metabolite was cleared with a terminal elimination half-life of 7.1 ± 2.6 hours. The AUC of APC relative to irinotecan ranged from 23% to 273%, which demonstrated that a significant amount of the parent compound was converted to the APC metabolite after an intravenous infusion. No dose dependence was observed for the conversion of irinotecan to APC or for the glucuronidation of SN-38 to SN-38G. No clear correlation between APC pharmacokinetics and drug pharmacodynamic effects was observed.

Another piperidine ring metabolite of irinotecan is 7-ethyl-10-(4-amino-1-piperidino)carbonyloxycamptothecin or NPC, which was characterized in plasma and urine of patients on irinotecan therapy (Fig. 20-3).[432] Like APC, this derivative is a poor inducer of topoisomerase I–cleavable complexes, but unlike APC, this new metabolite is a weak substrate for carboxylesterase-converting enzyme and can be enzymatically converted into SN-38.[432] Thus, NPC may contribute to the clinical activity of irinotecan. In plasma, the concentration of NPC is less than that of irinotecan or APC. The CYP3A isoform appears to be principally responsible for the production of NPC from irinotecan in human hepatic microsomes, and the lactone form of irinotecan is a better substrate for NPC formation than is the carboxylate.[38] Interconversion of APC to NPC was not observed in these experiments.

Additional hepatic metabolites of irinotecan were also found in an analysis of human bile obtained from a patient undergoing irinotecan therapy. At least 16 different irinotecan metabolites were partially identified using highly sensitive liquid chromatography/mass spectroscopy and liquid chromatography/tandem mass spectroscopy techniques.[433] These included irinotecan oxidation products involving the C-10 piperidinopiperidine side chain and a decarboxylated camptothecin derivative that lacked the terminal carboxylate group. Alkylated and *N*-oxidized species were also detected. The exact chemical structure of most of these metabolites and their clinical importance are not yet known.

Because human hepatic CYP3A appears to be important in the metabolism of irinotecan, the potential exists for serious drug-drug interactions. This enzyme is principally responsible for the metabolism of a large number of drugs, including ketoconazole, erythromycin, and cyclosporin. Further careful clinical pharmacologic studies are required to determine if clinically relevant pharmacokinetic drug interactions result from the simultaneous use of these agents in combination with irinotecan.

SN-38 Glucuronidation

The major metabolite of SN-38 is the glucuronidated derivative, 10-O-glucuronyl-SN-38 (SN-38G),[396] which is present in the plasma and bile of patients receiving irinotecan chemotherapy (Fig. 20-3).[395] This is the major detoxifying reaction responsible for the clearance of SN-38. In pharmacokinetic studies, the peak SN-38G concentrations were seen 10 to 20 minutes after the end of a 90-minute irinotecan infusion (Table 20-8).[434] The amount of SN-38G increased from time zero up to 1 hour postinfusion; this was followed by a gradual decline so that by 5 to 6 hours postinfusion, the ratio of SN-38G to SN-38 stabilized at a level of 4:1 or 5:1. The decrease in plasma concentrations of SN-38G tended to parallel the decrease in SN-38 over time. These data are consistent with the view that the enzyme uridine diphosphate glucuronosyl transferase (UGT) is the rate-limiting step responsible for the elimination of the SN-38 active metabolite.[434] Ethnic differences in glucuronidation have been reported; therefore, pharmacogenetic variations in this enzyme may also contribute to clinically significant differences in SN-38 clearance.

Incubation of SN-38 with human hepatic microsomes in the presence of the glucuronidation cofactor uridine diphosphate β-D-glucuronic acid resulted in the formation of SN-38G *in vitro*.[422] When five different liver donors were studied, the interindividual difference in the specific activity of SN-38 glucuronidation was relatively modest, showing only twofold variation. In a larger study of SN-38 glucuronidating activity in microsomes obtained from 25 different human donor livers, however, a higher degree of interpatient variability was observed, with differences of over 50-fold.[435] Coincubation with other drugs such as acetaminophen, 5-FU, loperamide, and the antiemetics metoclopramide and ondansetron hydrochloride caused only minimal changes in the reaction velocity, which suggests that interactions between these drugs were unlikely.[422] UGT may also represent a potentially exploitable target for modulating SN-38 pharmacokinetics. In mice, coadministration of irinotecan with valproic acid, an inhibitor of glucuronidation, markedly decreased the amount of SN-38G formed and increased the systemic exposure to SN-38 by 2.7-fold.[436] In contrast, coadministration with phenobarbital, which enhances hepatic glucuronidation, increased the plasma AUC for SN-38G and decreased that for SN-38.[436] If these same drug interactions occur in humans as well as in mice, then a potential strategy for using such agents is suggested, such as administering phenobarbital to decrease gastrointestinal toxicity by increasing SN-38 detoxification.

The uridine diphosphate glycosyltransferase 1 (UGT1) isoform was implicated in the glucuronidation of SN-38 in *in vitro* studies using hepatic liver microsomes from Gunn rats and from human patients with Crigler-Najjar type I syndrome, who lack this specific UGT subtype. Hepatic microsomes from these sources showed a loss of SN-38 glucuronidation activity.[435] Further studies with recombinant isoforms of UGT suggested that the specific isoform responsible is UGT1A1. Furthermore, SN-38 glucuronidation paralleled bilirubin glucuronidation, which is also a UGT1A1 substrate. Glucuronidation of acetaminophen and *para*-nitrophenol, which are not UGT1A1 substrates, did not correlate with SN-38 glucuronidation. This finding also explains the lack of utility of using acetaminophen as a probe for predicting the interindividual variation in SN-38 glucuronidating activity in an earlier clinical study.[398] These observations are important. For example, patients with Gilbert's syndrome, who are genetically deficient in UGT1A1 and have impaired bilirubin conjugating activity, may be at risk for severe irinotecan-induced diarrhea, because of an inability to conjugate and detoxify SN-38. Preliminary reports of severe diarrhea in two patients with Gilbert's syndrome who received standard doses of irinotecan have been published.[437] Genetic deficiencies in UGT1A1 activity are also common in the Inuit Indian population in northern Canada.[435]

The genetic defect in Gilbert's syndrome, which can occur in up to 15% of the population and may be clinically silent, is the presence of an additional TA repeat [(TA)$_7$TAA] in the promoter region of UGT1A1.[438] A polymerase chain reaction–based assay to detect this sequence polymorphism was used to genotype a panel of human liver microsomes from 44 different donors, and this genotypic measurement was correlated with a phenotypic assessment of SN-38 and bilirubin glucuronidation. A significant decrease in glucuronidating activity was associated with either the heterozygous or homozygous presence of the (TA)$_7$TAA genotype. The clinical significance of these findings is undergoing prospective evaluation.

In summary, much of the variability in irinotecan pharmacokinetics appears to be related to variations in its enzymatic metabolism. The existence of multiple metabolic pathways for irinotecan and its metabolites makes this a complex area to study, but ongoing research may provide a better understanding of the clinical impact of these pathways in irinotecan chemotherapy.

Elimination

In addition to hepatic metabolism, elimination of irinotecan and its metabolites also occurs by urinary and biliary excretion. Fourteen percent to 37% of the administered irinotecan dose was excreted unchanged in the urine over 48 hours after a short 90-minute infusion.[39,375] Only approximately 0.26% of the administered dose, however, was excreted as SN-38.[39] Biliary excretion of irinotecan, unconjugated SN-38, and conjugated SN-38G also appears to be a substantial mechanism of drug elimination. Biliary drug concentrations were measured in two patients; the total irinotecan concentration was 10 to 113 times higher and the SN-38 biliary concentration was 2 to 40 times higher than the simultaneous plasma drug concentrations.[39,373] For two other patients, quantitative collection of bile from percutaneous catheters was performed for up to 48 hours after a single dose of irinotecan.[439] The percentage of the total dose administered that was excreted into the bile as either irinotecan, SN-38, or SN-38G ranged from 24% to 50%. Biliary transport of irinotecan and its metabolites by the canalicular multispecific organic anion transporter (cMOAT) has been extensively studied using isolated canalicular membrane vesicles obtained from rat liver.[440,441] The cMOAT system is believed to be responsible for the biliary excretion of irinotecan carboxylate, SN-38 carboxylate, and the carboxylate and lactone forms of SN-38G, but other transport systems in the bile canaliculi may also exist.[440,441] Interestingly, the carboxylate form of SN-38G is transported more avidly in rat liver vesicles than is the lactone form.[441] Extension of these studies to human biliary transport systems would improve our understanding of the kinetics of irinotecan and SN-38 elimination. Pharmacokinetic clinical studies show indirect evidence for enterohepatic circulation of SN-38 as manifested by slight elevation in plasma concentrations observed several hours after the end of the drug infusion.[357,366,395]

Because hepatic glucuronidation followed by biliary excretion of SN-38G is a major route of drug elimination, the presence of bacterial β-glucuronidase in the intestinal lumen can potentially contribute to irinotecan's gastrointestinal toxicity. Hydrolysis of the inactive glucuronidated SN-38G by bacterial enzymes can release unconjugated SN-38, which results in prolonged exposure of the gastrointestinal mucosa to the active metabolite. This process can also enhance reabsorption of the unconjugated SN-38 from the intestinal lumen via enterohepatic circulation. Inhibition of bacterial β-glucuronidase, however, might prevent deconjugation of SN-38G and promote fecal elimination of drug, thereby lessening gastrointestinal toxicity. Consistent with this hypothesis was the finding that the Chinese herbal medicine Kampo, which contains baicalin, a β-glucuronidase inhibitor, substantially reduced the severity of irinotecan-induced diarrhea in rats.[442] In animal studies, antibiotic administration also protected against drug-associated diarrhea, presumably by altering the gut microbial flora and decreasing intestinal β-glucuronidase activity.[443] Coadministration of penicillin and streptomycin sulfate with irinotecan to rats markedly reduced drug-induced diarrhea and cecal damage. Pharmacodynamic studies in these rats receiving both irinotecan and antibiotics showed no difference in blood pharmacokinetics but demonstrated an 85% reduction in SN-38 concentrations within the large intestine.[444] Whether or not a similar approach in humans could safely alleviate irinotecan-associated diarrhea without diminishing clinical efficacy requires further evaluation.

Activity by β-glucuronidase is also present in the blood, and some carboxylic acid esters, such as organophosphates and carbamate insecticides, can increase the blood activity of this enzyme by enhancing its release from the liver.[420] Irinotecan was found to increase blood β-glucuronidase activity in rats by approximately 60-fold, with peak levels occurring 2 to 3 hours later.[420] No changes in plasma or liver carboxylesterase activity were observed. These findings may have clinical importance, because β-glucuronidase activity can convert inactivated plasma SN-38G back into the active metabolite SN-38. Because plasma SN-38G concentrations are severalfold higher than levels of free SN-38 in humans (Table 20-8), deconjugation of SN-38G could contribute to the prolonged plasma half-life of SN-38 observed after irinotecan administration. Determining if these same effects occur in humans is important.

Another intervention that could theoretically reduce gastrointestinal toxicity is reducing the amount of free SN-38 in bile by blocking biliary excretion of SN-38 and SN-38G. Cyclosporin A can reduce bile flow and inhibit bile canalicular active transport and, thus, may be a potential modulator of SN-38-induced toxicity. Coadministration of cyclosporin A with irinotecan in rats was found to increase the AUCs of irinotecan, SN-38, and SN-38G by 3.4-fold, 3.6-fold, and 1.9-fold, respectively.[445] Overall, nonrenal clearance of irinotecan decreased by 81% with no change in the calculated volume of distribution, and the terminal half-life of SN-38 increased by approximately twofold. The AUC ratio of SN-38 to irinotecan in plasma was not altered, but the AUC ratio of SN-38 to SN-38G did increase. All of these observations are consistent with cyclosporin-induced inhibition of biliary canalicular transport of irinotecan, SN-38, and SN-38G; however, the precise transport systems affected by this modulation have not been fully characterized. Nonetheless, these observations suggest another possible strategy for reducing the gastrointestinal toxicities of irinotecan.

Fecal loss also contributes to the elimination of irinotecan and its metabolites from the body. In the most complete study of irinotecan metabolite pharmacokinetics to date, which included 10 patients, the total excretion of irinotecan, SN-38, SN-38G, APC, and NPC in urine accounted for 28.1 ± 10.6% of the administered dose, whereas recovery from feces accounted for 24.4 ± 13.3%.[446] Thus, the total mass balance of known metabolites accounted for only approximately 50% of the total admin-istered dose, which indicates the likely existence of other as yet unidentified metabolites of irinotecan.

Pharmacodynamics

The major clinical toxicity of irinotecan is delayed diarrhea, which is believed to result from direct effects of the active metabolite SN-38 on the intestinal epithelium. As previously described, glucuronidation of SN-38 may prevent this toxicity by decreasing the relative amount of biologically active unconjugated SN-38 in the bile and small intestine. In an attempt to identify patients at risk for severe delayed diarrhea during irinotecan therapy, a biliary index was developed to estimate the relative amount of free and unconjugated SN-38 in the biliary system using measured plasma drug concentrations.[395] The biliary index was defined as the product of the AUC of irinotecan and the ratio of the AUC of SN-38 to that of SN-38G. In the original study, nine patients with grade 3 to 4 diarrhea had higher biliary indices (which indicated relatively more unconjugated SN-38 in the bile) than 12 patients with grade 0 to 2 diarrhea.[395] Estimation of the biliary index initially required substantial numbers of pharmacokinetic blood samples to determine the AUCs of irinotecan, SN-38, and SN-38G. However, a limited sampling strategy for estimating the biliary index was recently developed that requires only two blood samples obtained at 3.5 and 7.5 hours after a 90-minute infusion of irinotecan.[447] Thus, the biliary index may be able to be estimated during week 1 of therapy, and, if it is highly elevated, immediate dosage adjustments can be instituted to decrease the incidence of severe diarrhea. Nevertheless, other studies using a variety of different schedules of administration have yet to confirm the utility of the biliary index in predicting clinically significant diarrhea.[367,403] Therefore, further prospective validation of the usefulness of this index is necessary.

Other pharmacodynamic studies have attempted to correlate the AUC of irinotecan or SN-38 with clinical drug toxicities, with varying results. In early studies of irinotecan in Japan, no correlation between irinotecan or SN-38 AUCs and myelosuppression or diarrhea was noted.[394] In later studies, Sasaki et al. reported a strong correlation between the degree of leukopenia and the AUC of irinotecan, whereas the severity of diarrhea correlated better with SN-38 kinetics.[416] Other studies have also found pharmacodynamic correlations between the irinotecan AUC and myelosuppression,[366,373,383,403] and between the SN-38 AUC and myelosuppression.[366,373,375,383,393,403] For severe diarrhea, associations with the irinotecan AUC[357,366,373,393] and with the SN-38 AUC[366,368,373] have also been reported, but these have been observed less consistently.[357,366,373,383] Similarly, no clear relationship between pharmacokinetic parameters and tumor responses have been characterized. Finally, although SN-38 lactone is believed to the biologically active species, measurement of SN-38 lactone kinetics has not been superior to total drug (lactone and carboxylate) measurements in predicting pharmacodynamic end points.[39,375]

Single-Agent Anticancer Activity of Irinotecan

Colorectal Cancer

In 1996, irinotecan was approved in the United States for treating patients with advanced colorectal cancer who had previously been treated with 5-FU–based chemotherapy. Supporting evidence for this approval came from a series of phase II trials demonstrating activity in previously treated patients who received 125 mg per m² of irinotecan weekly for 4 of 6 weeks (Table 20-9)[367,368,448,449] Response rates in previously treated and untreated patients ranged from 25% to 32%. More recently compiled data, however, suggest that the response rate in previously treated patients is lower, ranging from 10% to 15%.[372,450,451] In all studies, complete responses were rare, and the median duration of response ranged from 6 to 9 months. A large European study examined the activity of 350 mg per m² of irinotecan infused over 30 minutes every 3 weeks in 178 evaluable patients with advanced colorectal cancer.[452] One-hundred and thirty patients had received 5-FU previously and 48 were chemotherapy naive. Twenty-three patients in the pretreated group responded (18%), with 2 complete and 21 partial responses. In the chemotherapy-naive group, nine patients responded (19%), with two complete responses. The median response duration of 9.1 months was the same in both groups, and the median survival in pretreated and chemotherapy-naive patients was not significantly different, at 10 months and 12 months, respectively. These studies led to the more widespread use of irinotecan as second-line therapy for metastatic colorectal cancer.

The efficacy of irinotecan as second-line therapy for colorectal cancer was confirmed in two randomized European trials.[453,454] In the first study, patients with advanced colorectal cancer (who had previously received 5-FU chemotherapy) were randomly assigned, in a 2:1 ratio, to receive either irinotecan at 300 to 350 mg per m² every 3 weeks or supportive care.[453] The 1-year survival was significantly better among the 189 patients treated on the chemotherapy arm than among the 90 patients in the supportive care group, 36.1% versus 13.8%, respectively (*p* = .0001). Tumor-related symptoms of fatigue, pain, dyspnea, and anorexia were all improved on the chemotherapy arm, although the incidence of diarrhea was worse. Formal quality-of-life assessment scales were also improved on the chemotherapy arm. On the irinotecan arm, grade 3 and 4 leukopenia/neutropenia was seen in 22% of patients, and grade 3 and 4 diarrhea occurred in 22%. Fourteen percent of patients developed grade 3 or 4 nausea and vomiting. Another randomized trial compared the every-3-weeks

irinotecan schedule with three different continuous infusion regimens of 5-FU in previously treated patients with advanced colorectal cancer.[454] The 1-year survival was again better in the 133 irinotecan-treated patients than in the 134 patients on the 5-FU arm, 45% versus 32%, respectively (*p* = .035). Median progression-free survival was also prolonged, 4.2 versus 2.9 months, respectively (*p* = .030). In this study, results of formal quality-of-life assessments were not significantly different in the two arms. On the irinotecan arm, grade 3 and 4 diarrhea occurred in 22% of patients, whereas grade 3 and 4 neutropenia was seen in 14% of patients. In contrast, in the groups receiving 5-FU, grade 3 or 4 diarrhea occurred in only 11% of patients and no grade 3 or 4 neutropenia was reported. These two studies confirm the utility of irinotecan as second-line therapy for advanced colorectal cancer.

Lung Cancer and Other Malignancies

Many of the early phase II trials of irinotecan were conducted in Japan. Currently, irinotecan is approved for use in that country for the treatment of a variety of malignancies, including gastric, ovarian, and lung cancers. In single-agent phase II studies of irinotecan therapy for treatment of non–small cell lung cancer, response rates ranging from 0% to 32% were reported,[378,394,455–457] and in small cell lung cancer, response rates of up to 37% to 50% have been seen.[379,456,458] Single-agent activity has also been reported against other solid tumors: Objective response rates were 0% to 24% for cervical cancer,[459–461] 24% for ovarian cancer,[459,460] 16% to 23% for breast cancer,[462,463] 15% for malignant gliomas,[464] and 23% for gastric cancer.[465] In hematologic malignancies, irinotecan has shown modest activity, including response rates of 42% of short duration in a single study of patients with non-Hodgkin's lymphoma who had previously been treated.[466] A small but encouraging experience in Japan with the use of irinotecan to treat adult T-cell leukemia-lymphoma was reported.[467] In 13 patients with refractory or relapsed disease, one complete and four partial remissions were achieved, for an overall response rate of 38%. The median duration of response was brief, however, lasting only 31 days. The single-agent activity of irinotecan is summarized in Table 20-9.

Combination Therapy

Fluoropyrimidine Combinations

Because of its single-agent activity against colorectal cancer, 5-FU has been studied extensively in preclinical experiments in combination with irinotecan. As mentioned previously, antimetabolites that decrease DNA synthesis are generally antagonistic when combined with camptothecins.[215] As with topotecan, however, this interaction is highly dependent on sequence and cell line. *In vitro* studies

TABLE 20-9. IRINOTECAN SINGLE-AGENT PHASE II STUDIES

Disease	Dose & Schedule	No. Patients Entered/No. Evaluable	No. Patients with Prior Chemotherapy	Overall Response Rate, % (95% CI)	Response Type	Median Duration of Response (mo)	Median Duration of Survival (mo)	Reference
Colorectal cancer	100 mg/m² weekly or 150 mg/m² every 2 wk	67/63	46	27 (16–38)	17 PR	6.9 (range, 3.3–12.7)	9.4	448
Colorectal cancer	125 mg/m² weekly for 4 of 6 wk	41/41	0	Prior 5-FU: 22% 32 (18–46)	13 PR	8.1 (range, 4.0–16.0)	12.1 (range, 2.1–21.7)	367
Colorectal cancer	125–150 mg/m² weekly for 4 of 6 wk	48/43	43	23 (9–32)	1 CR, 9 PR	6 (range, 2–13)	10.4 (range, 1–24±)	368
Colorectal cancer	125 mg/m² weekly for 4 of 6 wk	90/90	90	13 (7–22)	12 PR	7.7 (range, 5.3–20)	8.3 (range, 0.36–34.8)	449
Colorectal cancer	125 mg/m² weekly for 4 of 6 wk	31/31	0	26 (12–45)	8 PR	7.6 (range, 2.8–31.7)	11.8 (range, 2.1–37.4)	449
Colorectal cancer	350 mg/m² every 3 wk	130/115	115	20 (13–28)	2 CR, 21 PR	9.1	12	452
Colorectal cancer	350 mg/m² every 3 wk	48/41	0	22 (11–38)	2 CR, 7 PR	9.1	10	452
Colorectal cancer	100–125 mg/m² weekly for 4 of 6 wk	166/166	166	11 (6–16)	1 CR, 17 PR	6.4 (range, 2.8–12.8)	9.9 (range, 0.3–36.8)	450
Colorectal cancer	350 mg/m² every 3 wk	107/95	95	14 (8–22)	13 PR	8.5 (range, 4.5–13.3)	10.4 (range, 0.75–16.5)	451
Gastric cancer	100 mg/m² weekly or 150 mg/m² every 2 wk	77/60	45	23 (13–36)	NA	NA	NA	465
Pancreatic cancer	350 mg/m² every 3 wk	34/32	0	9 (3–25)	3 PR	7.5 (range, 7.2–7.8)	5.2 (range, 0.4–22)	570
Non–small cell lung cancer	100 mg/m² over 90 min weekly	NA/67	0	34 (22–47)	23 PR	NA	NA	456
Non–small cell lung cancer	100 mg/m² over 90 min weekly	NA/26	26	0	NA	NA	NA	456
Non–small cell lung cancer	100 mg/m² over 90 min weekly	NA/11	1	0	NA	NA	NA	456
Non–small cell lung cancer	100 mg/m² over 90 min weekly	73/72	0	32 (20–44)	23 PR	3.75 (range, 1.75–7.75)	10.5	378
Small cell lung cancer	100 mg/m² over 90 min weekly	NA/35	27	37 (19–55)	2 CR, 11 PR	NA	NA	456
Small cell lung cancer	100 mg/m² over 90 min weekly	16/16	16	50 (25–75)	8 PR	1.5	NA	458
Small cell lung cancer	100 mg/m² over 90 min weekly	16/15	15	47 (21–72)	7 PR	1.9 (range, 0.9–5.2)	6.2	379
Prostate cancer	125 mg/m² weekly for 4 of 6 wk	15/15	0	0	0 PR	NA	NA	571
Ovarian cancer	100 mg/m² or 150 mg/m² every 2 wk	NA/55	52	24 (12–35)	13 PR	NA	NA	460
Cervical cancer	100 mg/m² or 150 mg/m² every 2 wk	NA/55	NA	24 (12–35)	5 CR, 8 PR	NA	NA	460
Cervical cancer	125 mg/m² weekly for 4 of 6 wk	42/42	42	21 (10–35)	1 CR, 8 PR	3.0 (range, 1.5–5.25)	6.4 (range, 1.4–21.7)	461
Cervical cancer	125 mg/m² weekly for 4 of 6 wk	16/14	14	0	0 PR	NA	NA	572
Cervical cancer	125 mg/m² weekly for 4 of 6 wk	54/49	0	12 (5–25)	1 CR, 5 PR	NA	NA	573
Breast cancer	100 mg/m² weekly[a]	NA/25	NA	16 (5–36)	4 PR	NA	NA	463
Breast cancer	100 mg/m² weekly	79/65	NA	23 (14–35)	1 CR, 14 PR	NA	NA	462

Malignant glioma	125 mg/m² weekly for 4 of 6 wk	60/60	41	15 (6–24)	9 PR	NA	10.8 (range, 1.5–18.2)	464
Non-Hodgkin's and Hodgkin's lymphoma	40 mg/m²/d for 3 d weekly	NA/29	29	24 (10–44)	4 CR, 3 PR	NA	NA	574
Non-Hodgkin's and Hodgkin's lymphoma	40 mg/m²/d for 3 d weekly	79/62	62	42 (30–54)	9 CR, 17 PR	NA	5.1	466
Adult T-cell leukemia/lymphoma	40 mg/m²/d × 3 every 3–4 wk[a]	14/13	13	38 (14–68)	1 CR, 4 PR	1.03	NA	467
Acute leukemia	40 mg/m²/d for 3 d weekly	NA/26	26	12 (2–30)	1 CR, 2 PR	NA	NA	574
Acute leukemia	15–20 mg/m² twice daily for 7 d every 2–4 wk	50/41	41	5 (1–14)	2 PR	NA	NA	466

5-FU, 5-fluorouracil; CI, confidence interval; CR, complete response; NA, data not available; PR, partial response.
[a]Other schedules used include 150 mg/m² every 2 wk and 200 mg/m² every 3–4 wk.

of simultaneous administration of irinotecan or SN-38 in combination with 5-FU show generally antagonistic or subadditive cytotoxic effects; however, synergistic or supraadditive interactions are observed with the sequential administration of this combination.[468–471] For example, when SN-38 was administered before 5-FU in a panel of six human colon cancer cell lines, an enhanced cytotoxic interaction was found.[471] An examination of the molecular determinants of response in these studies revealed that colon cancer cell lines with lower thymidylate synthase activity had relatively higher levels of cleavable complex formation after treatment with SN-38. Low thymidylate synthase activity in tumors is correlated with an increased responsiveness to 5-FU–based therapy,[472] and high cleavable complex formation may correlate with optimal response to camptothecins.[180] If this observation is confirmed in tumor biopsy specimens, it would further explain the activity of the 5-FU–irinotecan combination in clinical practice. In another *in vitro* study of this combination in human colon carcinoma HT-29 cells, supraadditive toxicity was observed when a 24-hour exposure to irinotecan was immediately followed by a 24-hour exposure to 5-FU or when the order was reversed; however, simultaneous drug exposures were antagonistic.[469] The molecular mechanism of this enhanced drug effect appeared to differ for each sequence. When 5-FU was administered first, increased irinotecan and SN-38 uptake into the cells was found. When irinotecan or SN-38 was given first, however, the inhibition of thymidylate synthase by 5-FU metabolites was prolonged, and relatively greater amounts of topoisomerase I–DNA cleavable complexes were formed. SN-38–induced decreases in thymidylate synthase activity have also been observed by others.[470] Finally, when raltitrexed, a quinazoline antifolate inhibitor of thymidylate synthase, was combined with SN-38, sequential rather than simultaneous short-term exposures were optimal for maximizing *in vitro* cell kill.[473] All of these studies support the use of sequential, but not simultaneous, combination therapy with irinotecan and 5-FU.

In a mouse xenograft study, the coadministration of irinotecan with 5-FU did not produce any evidence of synergy.[474] Furthermore, a reduction in the dosages of both drugs was required for the combination regimen to be tolerated by the animals. When leucovorin calcium was added to the combination, however, the overall antitumor activity was greater than with either agent alone, which was consistent with an improved therapeutic index.[474]

Phase I and II Trials of Irinotecan and 5-Fluorouracil

Different combinations of irinotecan and 5-FU have been explored in phase I trials. The pharmacokinetics of this combination was initially studied in 12 patients with colorectal cancer who received irinotecan at 100 to 150 mg per m^2 infused over 90 minutes followed immediately by a 7-

day continuous infusion of 5-FU at 400 mg per m^2.[475] The reported AUC of irinotecan was significantly higher and the AUC of SN-38 was lower than those for historical controls, which leads to the hypothesis that 5-FU contributed to the decreased enzymatic activation of irinotecan to SN-38. More recent reports, however, failed to confirm this finding.[476,477] Given the high interpatient variability in camptothecin pharmacokinetics summarized previously, caution is warranted in comparing kinetic findings for small groups of patients to those for historical controls.

Another early attempt to combine irinotecan and 5-FU highlights the potential difficulty in developing clinical combination regimens. The maximal dose of irinotecan that could be administered was 50 mg per m^2 every 4 weeks in combination with weekly bolus 5-FU and leucovorin at doses of 500 mg per m^2 each.[478] Further dose escalation of irinotecan was limited because of the occurrence of grade 4 diarrhea. During weeks in which all drugs were given, 5-FU was administered 48 hours after irinotecan in an attempt to avoid simultaneous drug exposures. Because only very low doses of irinotecan could be tolerated on this schedule (50 mg per m^2), further testing was not recommended. Greater success was achieved by Saltz and colleagues, however, who developed a patient-tolerated combination regimen of 125 mg per m^2 of irinotecan and 500 mg per m^2 of 5-FU plus leucovorin at 20 mg per m^2 given weekly for 4 of 6 weeks.[476] Neutropenia was the major dose-limiting toxicity, and diarrhea was common. With the use of high-dose loperamide supportive therapy, however, diarrhea was less of a problem. Among 17 patients treated at the recommended phase II dosage, 5 (29%) experienced dose-limiting grade 4 or febrile neutropenia, and 3 (18%) experienced grade 3 or 4 diarrhea. The better tolerability of this 5-FU combination may also be due to that fact that a lower dose of leucovorin was used than in the earlier study. Pharmacokinetic and sequential drug administration effects were studied in the following manner. During cycle 1, a 90-minute infusion of irinotecan was given on day 1 to facilitate pharmacokinetic monitoring, followed by intravenous bolus administration of 5-FU and leucovorin on day 2. During all subsequent weeks of cycle 1, 5-FU and leucovorin were given immediately after irinotecan on the same day. During cycle 2, the order was reversed and additional pharmacokinetic sampling was performed. Finally, in cycle 3 and in all remaining cycles, the sequence of irinotecan followed immediately by 5-FU and leucovorin was used. Unlike in the earlier Japanese study, no evidence for a pharmacokinetic interaction was observed, and no clear clinical advantage was seen for any particular sequence. Thirty-five of the patients in this phase I study who had metastatic colorectal cancer were evaluable for response. Twenty-three patients had received prior chemotherapy. Overall, six patients achieved a partial response, for an overall response rate of 17%; four were previously treated and two had not been untreated. The clinical activity and tolerable side-effect profile of this combination regimen were felt to be sufficiently promising to justify its inclusion as a treatment arm in a randomized phase III trial.

Another phase I trial recommended the combination of weekly irinotecan at 80 mg per m² followed immediately by a 2-hour infusion of 500 mg per m² of leucovorin and then a 24-hour continuous infusion of 5-FU at 2.6 g per m², with the combination given weekly for 6 of 7 weeks.[477] Diarrhea was the major dose-limiting toxicity, but grade 2 vomiting was also common. This regimen represents essentially full doses of 5-FU and leucovorin on this schedule, to which a reduced dose of irinotecan has been added. Although it was a small phase I dose-escalation study, a number of tumor responses were seen in these patients with advanced colorectal cancer; all were previously untreated for metastatic disease, although 46% had received prior adjuvant chemotherapy. Fifteen of the 25 assessable patients had a partial response and 1 showed a complete response, for an overall response rate of 64% (95% CI, 45% to 83%). No major difference in response rates were seen for patients who had previously received adjuvant chemotherapy and those who had not.

Alternation of irinotecan and 5-FU was examined in a phase II trial involving previously untreated patients with advanced colorectal cancer (Table 20-10).[479] Irinotecan was administered at 350 mg per m² on day 1 followed 3 weeks later by 5-FU at 425 mg per m² per day plus leucovorin at 20 mg per m² per day daily for 5 days on days 22 through 26; cycles were repeated every 6 weeks. Diarrhea and neutropenia were the most common toxicities, but the regimen was well tolerated. The response rate for 33 patients, 28 of whom had had no previous chemotherapy, was 30% (95% CI, 16% to 49%), with nine partial and one complete response and an overall median survival of 16 months. Other phase II studies of this combination have yet to be published in complete form.

Phase III Trials of Irinotecan and 5-Fluorouracil

Preliminary results of two phase III trials involving patients with advanced colorectal cancer with no prior chemotherapy for metastatic disease have examined the utility of combining 5-FU and irinotecan together as initial therapy for this disease (Table 20-11).[480,481] Significant improvements were seen in response rates and in the time to tumor progression. One phase III trial randomly assigned 666 untreated patients with advanced colorectal cancer to one of three treatment arms.[481] Patients in arm 1 received the combination of irinotecan at 125 mg per m² followed immediately by 5-FU at 500 mg per m² and leucovorin at 20 mg per m², given weekly. Patients in arm 2 were given irinotecan alone at 125 mg per m² weekly for 4 of 6 weeks. Those in arm 3 received 5-FU alone at 425 mg per m² per day for 5 days with leucovorin at 20 mg per m² per day every 4 weeks. The overall response rate of 33% in the combination arm (n = 222) was significantly better than the rate of 18% in the 5-FU alone arm (n = 221) and of

17% in the irinotecan alone arm (n = 223) (*p* <.001). The median time to treatment failure was also significantly better for the combination group (*p* <.05), with durations of 5.0, 3.8, and 3.1 months for the groups receiving the combination of drugs, 5-FU alone, and irinotecan alone, respectively. The incidence of grade 3 or 4 diarrhea was no worse for the combination arm (22%) than for the irinotecan alone arm (30%), although it was greater than for the 5-FU alone arm (13%). Neutropenia was higher for the group receiving only 5-FU, which probably reflects the different toxicities seen with the weekly schedule versus daily × 5 days schedule for 5-FU administration.

Another study for which preliminary results were reported used a different design to randomly assign 387 patients with previously untreated colorectal cancer to receive either irinotecan plus 5-FU and leucovorin or the same schedule of 5-FU and leucovorin alone (Table 20-11).[480] On arm A, patients were given one of two different combinations of irinotecan and 5-FU with leucovorin. One combination included irinotecan at 180 mg per m² on day 1 and 5-FU at 400 mg per m² as an intravenous bolus, followed by 600 mg per m² per day as a 22-hour continuous intravenous infusion on days 1 and 2, plus leucovorin at 200 mg per m² on days 1 and 2, with the combination repeated every 2 weeks. The other combination regimen was irinotecan at 80 mg per m² plus 5-FU at 2.3 mg per m² as a 24-hour continuous infusion plus leucovorin at 500 mg per m², with the combination given weekly for 6 weeks every 7 weeks. Patients on arm B received the same dosages of 5-FU and leucovorin without irinotecan. As expected, rates of grade 3 and 4 toxicities were higher among patients on the combination arm than among those not receiving irinotecan, with diarrhea occurring in 20% versus 10% of patients, and neutropenia in 40% versus 13%, respectively. Overall, however, the combination regimens were judged to be tolerable. Antitumor efficacy was again better for the combination of 5-FU and irinotecan, with patients on the combination arm showing a response rate of 39% versus 22% for those not receiving irinotecan; progression-free survival was also longer, 35.1 weeks for the combination arm versus 18.6 weeks for the noncombination arm. Although these are preliminary reports, both studies suggest that the combination of irinotecan and 5-FU may be more effective than either drug alone for the treatment of newly diagnosed advanced colorectal cancer. The extension of these studies to provide adjuvant chemotherapy to patients with earlier stages of colorectal cancer is an appropriate next step, because increased antitumor efficacy in this setting might increase cure rates for this common disease. Such trials are now being planned. In addition, randomized phase III studies comparing 5-FU and irinotecan with other promising combinations, such as oxaliplatin plus 5-FU, in treatment of recurrent metastatic colorectal cancer are in progress. One phase III trial has also incorporated an oxaliplatin and irinotecan combination arm. Finally, because of

TABLE 20-10. IRINOTECAN COMBINATION PHASE II STUDIES

Disease	Regimen	No. Patients Enrolled/No. Evaluable	No. Patients with Prior Chemotherapy	Overall Response Rate, % (95% CI)	Response Type	Median Duration of Response (mo)	Median Duration of Survival (mo)	Reference
Platinum combinations								
Non–small cell lung cancer	Cisplatin 80 mg/m² on d 1, plus irinotecan 60 mg/m² on d 1, 8, 15. Repeat every 4 wk.	52/52	0	29 (17–41)	2 CR, 13 PR	5.9 (range, 1.0–10.6)	9.9 (range, 1.0–30.8)	494
Non–small cell lung cancer	Cisplatin 30 mg/m² on d, 1, 8, 15, plus irinotecan 60 mg/m² on d 1, 8, 15. Repeat every 4 wk.	16/16	16	31 (15–65)	5 PR	NA	NA	575
Non–small cell lung cancer	Cisplatin 20 mg/m² over 24 h on d 1–5, plus irinotecan 160 mg/m² on d 1. Repeat every 4 wk with G-CSF.	41/41	0	59 (42–75)	24 PR	8.0 (range, 1.5–30)	11.2 (range, 3.5–44)	492
Non–small cell lung cancer	Cisplatin 80 mg/m² on d 1, plus irinotecan 60 mg/m² on d 1, 8, 15. Repeat every 4 wk.	70/70	0	52 (39–64)	1 CR, 32 PR	4.8	11	491
Small cell lung cancer, extensive stage	Cisplatin 60 mg/m² on d 1, plus irinotecan 60 mg/m² on d 1, 8, 15. Repeat every 4 wk for 6 cycles.	35/35	0	86 (70–95)	10 CR, 20 PR	6.6	13.0	493
Small cell lung cancer, limited stage	Cisplatin 60 mg/m² on d 1, plus irinotecan 60 mg/m² on d 1, 8, 15. Repeat every 4 wk for 4 cycles followed by radiation therapy.	40/40	0	83 (67–93)	12 CR, 21 PR	8.0	14.3	493
Pleural mesothelioma	Cisplatin 60 mg/m² on d 1, plus irinotecan 60 mg/m² on d 1, 8, 15. Repeated every 4 wk.	15/15	0	27 (8–55)	4 PR	6.5	7.1 (range, 4.7–23.5)	414
Clear cell and mucinous ovarian carcinoma	Mitomycin C 7 mg/m² on d 1 and 15, plus irinotecan 120 mg/m² over 4 h on d 1 and 15. Repeat every 4 wk.	25/25	25	52 (32–72)	5 CR, 8 PR	31.8 (range, 12.9–34.4)	15.3 (range, 3.5–38.0)	576
Cervical cancer, locally advanced	Cisplatin 60 mg/m² on d 1, plus irinotecan 60 mg/m² on d 1, 8, 15. Repeated every 4 wk (neoadjuvant).	23/23	0	78 (58–90)	3 CR, 15 PR	NA	NA	500
Ovarian cancer	Cisplatin 50–60 mg/m² on d 1, irinotecan 50–60 mg/m² on d 1, 8, 15. Repeated every 4 wk.	25/25	25	40 (23.0–59.0)	2 CR, 8 PR	5.5 (range, 2–27)	12 (range, 3–39)	499
Gastric cancer	Irinotecan 70 mg/m² on d 1 and 15, plus cisplatin 80 mg/m² on d 1. Repeated every 4 wk.	44/44	15	48 (33–63)	1 CR, 10 PR	5.9 (range, 1.4–9.1)	9.1	498
Fluorouracil combinations								
Colorectal cancer	Irinotecan 350 mg/m² on d 1 plus 5-FU 425 mg/m²/d × 5 d on d 22–26 and leucovorin 20 mg/m²/d calcium × 5 d on d 22–26. Repeated every 6 wk.	33	28	30 (16–49)	1 CR, 9 PR	NA	16	479
Etoposide combinations								
Non–small cell lung cancer	Etoposide 60 mg/m²/d on d 1–3, plus irinotecan 60 mg/m²/d on d 1–3. Repeat every 3 wk with G-CSF.	61/59	0	21 (13–33)	13 PR	4.7 (range, 2.1–10.0)	10.0	508

CI, confidence interval; CR, complete response; 5-FU, 5-fluorouracil; G-CSF, granulocyte colony-stimulating factor; NA, data not available; PR, partial response.

TABLE 20-11. IRINOTECAN PHASE III STUDIES

Disease	Regimen	No. Patients Enrolled/No. Evaluable	No. Patients with Prior Chemotherapy	Overall Response rate, % (95% CI)	Duration of Response or Survival	Reference
Single-agent irinotecan versus supportive care or infusional 5-FU						
Metastatic colorectal cancer	Irinotecan 300–350 mg/m² every week	189/189	189	NA	Median duration of survival (mo): 9.2 (range, 0–18.9)	453
	versus					
	Supportive care only	90/90	90	NA	6.5 (range, 0.7–19.3) (*p* = .0001)	
Metastatic colorectal cancer	Irinotecan 300–350 mg/m² every 3 wk	127/127	127	NA	Median duration of survival (mo): 10.8 (range, 1.2–18.7)	454
	versus					
	Leucovorin calcium 200 mg/m² over 2 h followed by 5-FU 400 mg/m² bolus, then 5-FU 600 mg/m² c.i.v. over 22 h/d on the first 2 d of every 2 wk, or 5-FU 250–300 mg/m² prolonged c.i.v., or 5-FU 2.6–3.0 g/m²/d c.i.v. over 24 h with or without leucovorin 20–500 mg/m² per d weekly for 6 wk repeated every 8 wk	129/129	129	NA	8.5 (range, 0.8–20.9) (*p* = .035)	
Irinotecan and 5-FU versus 5-FU alone or irinotecan alone						
Colorectal cancer, untreated for metastatic disease	Irinotecan 125 mg/m², plus leucovorin 20 mg/m² bolus, plus 5-FU 500 mg/m² bolus, weekly for 4 of 6 wk	222	0 (for metastatic disease)	33 (27–39)	Time to treatment failure (mo): 5.0	481
	versus					
	5-FU 425 mg/m²/d, plus leucovorin 20 mg/m²/d, daily × 5 d every 4 wk	221	0	18 (13–24)	3.8	
	versus					
	Irinotecan 125 mg/m² weekly × 4, every 6 wk	223	0	29 (23–36) (*p* <.001)	3.1 (*p* <.05)	
Colorectal cancer, untreated for metastatic disease	Irinotecan 180 mg/m² on d 1, plus 5-FU 400 mg/m² bolus and 600 mg/m²/d c.i.v. over 22 h with leucovorin at 200 mg/m², repeated every 2 wk, or Irinotecan 80 mg/m², plus 5-FU 2.3 g/m² c.i.v. over 24 h with leucovorin at 500 mg/m², repeated weekly × 6 every 7 wk	199	0 (for metastatic disease)	39 (32–46)	Progression-free survival (mo): 8.8	480
	versus					
	Same regimen without irinotecan	188	0	22 (16–28)	4.7	

CI, confidence interval; 5-FU, 5-fluorouracil.

the developing use of oral fluoropyrimidine regimens, additional trials examining how best to combine irinotecan with oral fluoropyrimidines such as capecitabine or tegafur-uracil are necessary.

Gemcitabine Combinations

Use of the combination of gemcitabine hydrochloride and irinotecan to treat solid tumors was examined in a phase I trial.[482] The dose-limiting toxicity was diarrhea, which resulted in a recommended phase II dosage of gemcitabine 1,000 mg per m^2 over 30 minutes followed by irinotecan 100 mg per m^2 over 90 minutes on days 1 and 8, repeated every 3 weeks. In this dose-escalation phase I trial, three partial responses were observed in 18 evaluable patients (two with pancreatic cancer and one with a tumor of unknown primary). None had received prior chemotherapy. This regimen was considered of interest for treatment of pancreatic cancer.

Platinum Combinations

Because of the early clinical development of irinotecan for use in treating lung cancer in Japan, it has been studied extensively in that country in combination with other agents active against this disease, such as cisplatin. Much of the preclinical rationale for the synergistic interaction between cisplatin and the camptothecins[320,483] has already been discussed in the section on topotecan. Because of the pharmacokinetic interaction between topotecan and cisplatin, a recent clinical study examined the effect of cisplatin on the complex pharmacokinetics of irinotecan.[484] Eleven patients with solid tumors were randomized to receive either irinotecan 200 mg per m^2 over 90 minutes immediately followed by cisplatin 80 mg per m^2 intravenously over 3 hours, or the reverse sequence. The sequence of drug administration was alternated in cycle 2. No differences in toxicity or in irinotecan and cisplatin pharmacokinetics were observed. Characterization of irinotecan metabolism included pharmacokinetic monitoring of SN-38, SN-38G, APC, and NPC. Thus, cisplatin does not appear to alter irinotecan clearance, which is mediated principally by metabolism and biliary excretion. This differs from the case with topotecan, which is predominantly cleared by the kidneys.

A number of different phase I trials of this combination have been completed in Japan and the recommended phase II doses determined (Table 20-10).[485–490] In all of these studies, the major dose-limiting toxicities have been myelosuppression and diarrhea. In some cases the addition of G-CSF has allowed for slightly higher drug dosages to be administered, but in general the dosages of irinotecan and cisplatin used are well below their single-agent dosages.

The combination of irinotecan and cisplatin appears to be promising in the treatment of patients with lung cancer. In a Japanese phase II study, 70 patients with stage IIIB or IV non–small cell lung cancer were given irinotecan at 60 mg per m^2 on days 1, 8, and 15 and cisplatin 80 mg per m^2 on day 1 every 4 weeks.[491] Among 70 evaluable patients, 32 showed a partial response and one showed a complete response for an overall response rate of 52% (95% CI, 39% to 64%). The median response duration was 19 weeks, and the overall median survival was 44 weeks. As expected, the principal toxicities were grade 3 and 4 leukopenia and diarrhea, which occurred in 80% and 19% of patients, respectively. In another phase II trial, 41 patients with previously untreated non–small cell lung cancer were treated with irinotecan 160 mg per m^2 on day 1 plus cisplatin 20 mg per m^2 continuous infusion for 5 days every 4 weeks with G-CSF support.[492] The overall response rate was 58.5% (95% CI, 42.2% to 74.8%) with a median response duration of 32.1 weeks (range, 6 to 120 weeks). The median survival time was 44.8 weeks (range, 14 to 176 weeks). In this study, diarrhea was the most common major toxicity, but the overall regimen was well tolerated. These response rates confirm the activity of this combination regimen in non–small cell lung cancer.

In a study of combination therapy for small cell lung cancer, previously untreated patients were treated with irinotecan 60 mg per m^2 on days 1, 8, and 15 plus cisplatin 60 mg per m^2 on day 1 every 4 weeks.[493] Among the 40 patients with limited-stage disease, the overall response rate was 83%, including a 29% complete response rate; the median response duration was 8.0 months (95% CI, 5.2 to 11.4 months), and the median survival was 14.3 months (95% CI, 11.8 to 17.9 months). In 35 patients with extensive-stage disease, the overall response rate of 86% was similar, with a 29% complete response rate; the median response duration was 6.6 months (95% CI, 5.2 to 9.7 months), and the median survival was 13.0 months (95% CI, 9.1 to 17.4 months). Grade 3 or 4 neutropenia and diarrhea occurred in 77% and 19% of patients, respectively, and two patients died from toxic effects of combined neutropenia and diarrhea. A randomized phase III trial of irinotecan and cisplatin versus etoposide and cisplatin as front-line therapy for patients with small cell lung cancer is planned.

All of these phase II clinical studies of the use of cisplatin and irinotecan to treat lung cancer, mostly conducted in Japan, have reported encouraging response rates despite the frequent occurrence of severe myelosuppression and diarrhea that necessitated dose adjustments or missed treatments. Sequence-dependent effects were examined in only one clinical study to date, but the results suggest that such interactions are not as clinically important as in combinations of topotecan and cisplatin. In a preliminary report, a North American multicenter trial[494] in patients with untreated non–small cell lung cancer used an administration regimen of irinotecan 60 mg per m^2 on days 1, 8, and 15 and cisplatin 80 mg per m^2 on day 1 every 4 weeks, similar to that used by Masuda et al.[491] This study recorded a response rate of 29% (95% CI, 2% to 41%), lower than the rate of 52%

(95% CI, 39% to 64%) seen in the Japanese study described earlier.[491] If the activity of this combination is confirmed in additional phase II trials, a randomized phase III trial would be of interest. Finally, a number of promising three-drug combinations using irinotecan and cisplatin have been tested in phase I studies in Japan. These combinations include irinotecan, cisplatin, and vindesine,[495] and irinotecan, cisplatin, and ifosfamide.[496]

The combination of irinotecan and cisplatin has also undergone phase II testing for treatment of a small number of other tumor types, in addition to lung cancer. For treatment of advanced gastric cancer, a common tumor in Japan, a regimen of irinotecan at a dose of 70 mg per m[2] on days 1 and 15 and cisplatin 80 mg per m[2] on day 1, repeated every 4 weeks, was studied in a multicenter trial including 44 patients with metastatic gastric cancer, 29 of whom had previously been treated with chemotherapy.[497,498] The overall response rate was 48% (95% CI, 33% to 63%), with 20 partial responses and 1 complete response. The median duration of response was 5.9 months (range, 1.4 to 10.8 months), and median survival time was 9.1 months. Grade 4 neutropenia was the most common severe toxicity, occurring in 57% of patients; grade 3 or 4 diarrhea occurred in 20%. This response rate was considered promising enough to warrant further testing in phase III trials in Japan. In other phase II trials summarized in Table 20-10, anticancer activity of irinotecan and cisplatin was reported against refractory or recurrent ovarian cancer,[499] and malignant pleural mesothelioma,[414] and as neoadjuvant therapy in treatment of locally advanced cervical cancer.[500] Again, the majority of these phase II trials of irinotecan and cisplatin have been performed in Japan, and further data from North American and European trials are still pending (Table 20-10).

Irinotecan combinations using platinum analogs such as carboplatin and oxaliplatin rather than cisplatin have been less extensively studied.[501,502] One published study has examined the combination of irinotecan and the promising new dicycloamino platinum analog, oxaliplatin.[503] A recommended regimen is oxaliplatin 85 mg per m[2] infused over 30 minutes followed by irinotecan 200 mg per m[2], with the combination given every 3 weeks. Dose-limiting toxicities are diarrhea and febrile neutropenia. This dosage represents an approximately 40% dose reduction for each agent from their single-agent dosages. No evidence for a pharmacokinetic interaction was seen in this study. Although not a primary end point in this dose-escalation study, among 24 patients with mostly 5-FU–resistant metastatic colorectal cancer, the response rate was 29%, with 7 partial responses, and the median survival was 15.8 months. Further testing of this combination in treatment of advanced colorectal cancer is ongoing in randomized phase III trials comparing it to the combinations of oxaliplatin plus 5-FU, irinotecan plus 5-FU, and 5-FU plus leucovorin. The oxaliplatin and irinotecan combination is an important regimen because it

represents the first promising combination chemotherapy for advanced colorectal cancer that does not target thymidylate synthase. Currently, a randomized phase II trial comparing oxaliplatin and irinotecan with two different regimens of irinotecan and 5-FU is in progress.

Etoposide Combinations

Preclinical studies of irinotecan and the topoisomerase II inhibitor etoposide have demonstrated synergistic or supraadditive interactions.[468] In an *in vivo* rhabdomyosarcoma model, however, marked sequence-specific antagonism occurred when irinotecan was administered 2 hours before etoposide on a daily × 5 schedule for both drugs.[474] In contrast, in mice bearing a EMT-6 mammary tumor, no evidence of sequence-dependent antagonism was observed for this combination either when the drugs were given simultaneously as daily intraperitoneal injections for 5 days or when irinotecan was administered for 5 days followed by 5 days of intraperitoneal etoposide or vice versa.[504] Thus, sequence-dependent effects on antitumor activity may depend on the tumor system and schedule studied. As with topotecan and topoisomerase II inhibitors, a rationale exists for attempting to use these types of agents in sequential rather than simultaneous drug combinations. Nonetheless, the majority of clinical studies performed to date with irinotecan and topoisomerase II–targeting agents administered the drugs concurrently (Table 20-10). In phase I studies of this combination in Japan, the dose-limiting toxicities have been granulocytopenia and diarrhea.[505–507] Transient hepatic transaminase elevation has also been reported.[507] Substantially lower dosages of both drugs are required when they are used in combination than when they are used as single agents. In these dose-escalation studies, partial responses have been reported in the treatment of non–small cell lung cancer, small cell lung cancer, adenocarcinoma of unknown primary, and head and neck cancers.

In a Japanese phase II trial in 61 chemotherapy-naive patients with advanced non–small cell lung cancer, irinotecan at 60 mg per m[2] per day and etoposide at 60 mg per m[2] per day were administered simultaneously on days 1 to 3 every 3 weeks, with G-CSF support on days 4 through 17.[508] Severe neutropenia occurred in 39% of patients, and severe diarrhea occurred in 16%. Interstitial pneumonitis was seen in three patients (5%), and one toxic death related to severe diarrhea and hematemesis occurred. Partial responses were observed in 13 of 59 evaluable patients for a response rate of 21.3% (95% CI, 12.9% to 33.1%). The median duration of response was 4.7 months (range, 2.1 to 10 months), and the median survival time was 10 months. Unfortunately, as the authors point out, this response rate is not substantially different from those seen with irinotecan alone or with cisplatin-based drug combinations. One explanation for these poor clinical results and low antitumor activity is that drug antagonism may be occurring due to the simultaneous administration of both drugs. Therefore, trials were initiated in Japan to examine sequential administration of irinotecan and etoposide. In a two-arm phase I trial involving 27 patients with untreated non–small cell lung cancer, patients on one arm received irinotecan at 60 mg per m^2 per day given on days 1 to 3 followed by etoposide at 60 mg per m^2 per day given on days 3 to 6, every 3 weeks.[509] The sequence was reversed for patients on the other arm. G-CSF was administered to all patients on both regimens. Granulocytopenia and diarrhea were judged to be severe on both arms and did not appear to be sequence related. Transient elevation of liver transaminase levels was also seen on both arms. Pharmacokinetic monitoring suggested that plasma concentrations of irinotecan and SN-38 were somewhat prolonged when irinotecan was administered after etoposide, but the variability and small sample size precluded any definite conclusions. Although responses were observed on both treatment arms, the degree of severe toxicity did not support further development of these particular sequential regimens of irinotecan and etoposide.

Overall, clinical combination trials with irinotecan have mostly been limited to combination with 5-FU, cisplatin, and etoposide. Promising clinically active regimens have been established for irinotecan plus cisplatin or 5-FU. Further phase II and III testing of these regimens is ongoing. Developing patient-tolerated regimens of irinotecan and etoposide has been more problematic due to increased clinical toxicities. Additional *in vitro* synergistic interactions between irinotecan and paclitaxel,[510] and irinotecan and vinorelbine tartrate[511] have been reported. Human xenograft studies suggest that synergistic interactions may be seen when irinotecan is combined with interleukin 1,[512] interferon-α, interferon-β, and interferon-γ,[513,514] and alkylating agents such as busulfan and cyclosphosmamide.[515] Additional active and clinically useful irinotecan drug combinations are highly likely to be developed in the near future.

9-AMINOCAMPTOTHECIN

The compound 9-aminocamptothecin (9-AC) is a water-insoluble camptothecin derivative (Fig. 20-2) with impressive preclinical activity in human xenograft models of colon cancer,[93,516] malignant melanoma,[517] prostate cancer,[518] breast cancer,[519] ovarian cancer,[520] acute leukemia,[521] bladder cancer,[522] and CNS metastatic tumors.[516] In three human colon cancer xenografts, 9-AC was highly active with minimal systemic toxicity and produced the best antitumor response when compared with a panel of nine anticancer agents including 5-FU, doxorubicin, melphalan, methotrexate, vincristine, vinblastine, and several nitrosourea compounds.

Clinical testing of 9-AC began in 1993 with initial phase I trials of the drug administered as a 72-hour infusion every 2 weeks[523] or 3 weeks.[130,524] This schedule was selected because of the preclinical studies demonstrating that prolonged drug exposures were needed to see any biologic effect and that short intravenous infusions had no activity in animal models.[93] More recently, other schedules of 9-AC administration have been developed, including a prolonged 120-hour infusion weekly,[525] a 24-hour infusion weekly for 4 of 5 weeks,[526] and a short intravenous infusion daily for 5 days every 3 weeks.[527] On all of these schedules, the major dose-limiting toxicities are neutropenia and, to a lesser extent, thrombocytopenia. Other common toxicities included anemia, fatigue, nausea and vomiting, diarrhea, alopecia, and mucositis. The compound 9-AC is not associated with pulmonary toxicity or hemorrhagic cystitis, and the diarrhea is much less severe than that seen with irinotecan. Phase I trials involving pediatric patients[528] and acute leukemia patients[529] have also been completed. Oral administration schedules for 9-AC have also been studied.[530,531]

The pharmacokinetics of 9-AC has been examined using analytic assays that can measure both the lactone and carboxylate forms of the drug.[532–534] In pharmacokinetic studies, the amount of 9-AC that is present in plasma relative to the total drug levels (lactone plus carboxylate) is quite low, with most reported values below 10%.[526,528,531,535] This observation is consistent with earlier studies demonstrating greater instability of 9-AC lactone in human plasma than of other camptothecin derivatives such as topotecan or irinotecan.[273] Most of the reported terminal elimination half-lives for total 9-AC in plasma have been in the range of 7 to 10 hours[526–528,535]; volume of distribution at steady-state has been reported to be 23.6 ± 10.6 L per m^2; and systemic clearance is 2.39 ± 0.94 L per hour per m^2.[535] Urinary clearance accounts for 32.1 ± 8.3% of the total dose administered.[535] Preliminary reports suggest that patients receiving anticonvulsant medications may have increased clearance and lower plasma drug levels of 9-AC.[536] This may be due to increased metabolic clearance of 9-AC in patients receiving hepatic enzyme–inducing antiepileptic agents, such as phenytoin, carbamazepine, phenobarbital, primidone, felbamate, and valproic acid. Hepatic metabolites of 9-AC have not been identified, however.[537] An alternative explanation may be the induction of transport proteins by these same agents that could lead to increased 9-AC clearance and biliary secretion in these patients.[538] As with other camptothecins, large interpatient variability in 9-AC kinetics was observed in all pharmacokinetic studies done to date. In human studies, steady-state 9-AC plasma lactone concentrations of 2 to 10 nmol per L were achievable using a 72-hour infusion schedule.[535] In pharmacodynamic studies, 9-AC steady-state plasma concentrations[535,538] and AUC[526,527,539] correlated with the dose-limiting toxicity of neutropenia.

In phase II studies of 72-hour infusions of 9-AC administered at 50 to 59 μg per m^2 per hour every 2 weeks to 16 previously treated patients with metastatic colorectal cancer, no responses were observed, and the myelosuppressive toxicity was substantial.[540] Grade 4 neutropenia occurred in 56% of patients, and febrile neutropenia occurred in 31%. In another trial in which 17 previously untreated patients with this disease were given a lower dose of 35 μg per m[2] per hour for 72 hours every 2 weeks, no responses were observed.[541] In heavily pretreated patients with relapsed or refractory lymphoma administered 9-AC at 40 μg per m[2] per hour over 72 hours every 3 weeks with G-CSF support,[542] the response rate was 25% (95% CI, 13% to 41%), with 10 partial responses seen in 40 evaluable patients. The median duration of response was 5 months (range, 1 to 10 months), and the median survival time was 12.5 months. In 58 untreated patients with advanced non–small cell lung cancer treated with 46 to 59 μg per m[2] per hour over 72 hours every 2 weeks, the overall response rate was 8.6% (95% CI, 2.9% to 19%),[543] and the median survival was 5.4 months. Again, myelosuppressive toxicity was substantial, with grade 4 neutropenia seen in 31% of patients overall. Thus, in phase II trials, the antitumor activity of 9-AC on the 72-hour infusion schedule has been disappointing. Efforts to improve its activity include the development of longer infusion schedules.[525] Seventeen previously untreated patients with metastatic colorectal cancer were given 9-AC as a 120-hour infusion at 20 μg per m[2] per hour for 120 hours every week for 3 of 4 weeks; however, no responses occurred.[544] Phase II testing of longer infusion schedules is nearing completion.

Thus, despite its impressive preclinical activity in human colon cancer xenograft models, 9-AC has not shown effective antitumor activity in the clinical studies completed to date. One potential explanation for this discrepancy may be the inability to achieve the necessary plasma drug concentrations needed for antitumor efficacy. Because human bone marrow stem cells are more sensitive to 9-AC than is murine bone marrow, dose-limiting myelosuppression made it impossible to achieve the same plasma drug concentrations in humans that were associated with optimal antitumor efficacy in the preclinical animal models.[545]

9-NITROCAMPTOTHECIN

The compound 9-nitrocamptothecin (9-NC) is a camptothecin analog (Fig. 20-1) that is metabolically converted *in vivo* to 9-AC.[546,547] In preclinical studies, it has shown excellent anticancer activity in nude mice bearing human tumor xenografts including breast cancer,[519,548] ovarian cancer,[520] and melanoma.[517,549] It is predominantly being developed clinically as an oral agent, and in phase I testing the principal toxicities of 9-NC were myelosuppression, alopecia, and hemorrhagic cystitis.[550] The recommended dose of 9-NC is 1.5 mg per m[2] per day for 5 days each week.[551] Interestingly, after oral dosing of 9-NC in a single human subject, plasma concentrations of 9-AC above 200 nmol per L were achieved and sustained for several hours, which suggests a promising pharmacokinetic profile.[552]

Whether this will improve the therapeutic index of 9-NC relative to that of 9-AC must still be determined.

In phase II trials of 9-NC at a dosage of 1.5 mg per m[2] per day daily for 5 days each week, a response rate of 32% (95% CI, 20% to 45%) was seen in 60 evaluable patients with advanced pancreatic cancer.[553] Some of these patients had previously received gemcitabine therapy. Results of one other phase II trial have been published to date, examining treatment of patients with very refractory ovarian, tubal, or peritoneal cancers. In 29 patients treated with 9-NC at 1.5 mg per m[2] per day orally for 4 days a week, the response rate was 7%; median survival was 8 months.[554] Additional evaluation of 9-NC in treatment of pancreatic cancer is in progress.

GI47211

The compound GI47211 [7-(methylpiperazinomethylene)-10,11-ethylene-dioxy-20(S)] camptothecin dihydrochloride is a water-soluble synthetic analog of camptothecin that has also undergone clinical testing. In preclinical models, antitumor activity was documented in human colon cancer xenografts.[555] In phase I trials, the drug has been administered as a 30-minute infusion daily × 5 days every 3 weeks,[556,557] as a 72-hour continuous infusion,[558] and as a 21-day prolonged continuous infusion.[559] The schedule of GI47211 administration most widely clinically tested has been 1.2 mg per m[2] per day for 5 days every 3 weeks. The principal dose-limiting toxicities of GI47211 are neutropenia and thrombocytopenia; most other associated toxicities, such as nausea and vomiting, headaches, alopecia, and fatigue, are mild.

Validated analytic assays for the lactone form and for total plasma GI47211 have been reported.[560,561] In pharmacokinetic studies, reported terminal half-lives of total GI47211 ranged from 3.7 to 15 hours, with linear kinetics and moderate interpatient variability.[556,557] Overall, the AUC ratio of lactone to total drug was approximately 0.27, which is similar to that of topotecan; however, renal excretion of GI47211 accounted for only 11% to 12% of the administered drug.[557,558] Preliminary tests of orally administered GI47211 demonstrate a low overall bioavailability of 11.3%.[562] In pharmacodynamic studies, drug AUC significantly correlates with the nadir neutrophil counts.[556] Formal reporting of phase II studies is still pending.

NEW AGENTS

Several newer camptothecin derivatives are currently in clinical testing. These include DX-8951f[43] and kareniticin. In addition, a growing number of noncamptothecin compounds are being discovered that are believed to target topoisomerase I. These agents include the indolocarbazole NB506[563] and intoplicine.[564] Several of these agents are more stable at physiologic pH than the camptothecins and act via different mechanisms to inhibit topoisomerase I. Preclinical and early clinical evaluation of these agents is under way.[565]

CONCLUSION

Over the past several years, the camptothecins have evolved from an experimental class of antitumor agents into established agents with documented clinical utility in the treatment of human malignancies. Despite these significant advances, much more clinical research on these agents is necessary. For example, in North America, the single-agent activity of irinotecan has established it as the current treatment of choice for advanced colorectal cancer after 5-FU–based chemotherapy. Emerging evidence of its excellent activity in combination with 5-FU and leucovorin, however, suggests that it may have utility as initial therapy for this disease. Furthermore, if this increased activity is observed in the adjuvant setting, irinotecan may prove to increase cure rates in colorectal cancer. Likewise, its broad spectrum of activity, both as a single agent and in combination with cisplatin, suggests that irinotecan may have an increasing role in the treatment of other common solid tumors such as lung cancer and gastric cancer. The established activity of topotecan against previously treated ovarian and small cell lung cancer suggests a modest but still useful role for this agent in these diseases. Ongoing clinical trials to establish the utility of topotecan in treating hematologic malignancies such as chronic myelomonocytic leukemia and myelodysplastic syndromes as well as pediatric tumors such as neuroblastoma and rhabdomyosarcomas are also of interest. Additional studies should help define the evolving role both of these camptothecin analogs in the treatment of human cancers.

Despite our growing understanding of the pharmacology of the topoisomerase I poisons, several important issues must still be resolved. One is to determine the optimal method of combining these agents with other active drugs or treatment modalities such as radiation and biologic agents. Current laboratory and clinical investigations of camptothecin drug combinations may help guide further clinical development in this area. A more difficult question is why marked differences exist in the clinical activity of different camptothecin derivatives. Agents such as camptothecin and 9-AC are potent inhibitors of topoisomerase I at the molecular level, yet their clinical utility appears to be much less than that of topotecan or irinotecan. Some of this variation may be related to the clinical pharmacology of these agents, but pharmacologic differences do not fully explain the differences in clinical efficacy. Further studies of their molecular pharmacology and a clearer understanding of the relevant molecular determinants of response to the topoisomerase I

poisons may help to clarify these issues and to aid development of even more effective topoisomerase I poisons.

Almost 40 years after they first showed promising anticancer activity in a National Cancer Institute screening program, the camptothecins are established agents for the treatment of human cancer. Nonetheless, we are still learning how to optimally incorporate these agents into effective cancer treatments. The development of the camptothecins has also helped to elucidate the basic function of the topoisomerase I protein at the molecular level, and these agents have provided investigators with a valuable research tool for studying this important enzyme. The documented clinical activity of the camptothecins has highlighted topoisomerase I as a key target for cancer chemotherapy and has thereby allowed the development of completely new pharmacologic strategies for the treatment of human cancer.

REFERENCES

1. Nitiss JL, Wang JC. Mechanisms of cell killing by drugs that trap covalent complexes between DNA topoisomerases and DNA. *Mol Pharmacol* 1996;50:1095–1102.
2. Wall ME, Wani MC, Cook CE, et al. Plant antitumor agents. I. The isolation and structure of camptothecin, a novel alkaloidal leukemia and tumor inhibitor from *Camptotheca acuminata. J Am Chem Soc* 1966;88:3888–3890.
3. Horwitz SB, Horwitz MS. Effects of camptothecin on the breakage and repair of DNA during the cell cycle. *Cancer Res* 1973;33:2834–2836.
4. Bosmann HB. Camptothecin inhibits macromolecular synthesis in mammalian cells but not in isolated mitochondria of *E. coli. Biochem Biophys Res Commun* 1970;41:1412–1420.
5. Horwitz SB, Chang CK, Grollman AP. Studies on camptothecin. I. Effects of nucleic acid and protein synthesis. *Mol Pharmacol* 1971;7:632–644.
6. Wu RS, Kumar A, Warner JR. Ribosome formation is blocked by camptothecin, a reversible inhibitor of RNA synthesis. *Proc Natl Acad Sci U S A* 1971;68:3009–3014.
7. Gallo RC, Whang-Peng J, Adamson RH. Studies on the antitumor activity, mechanism of action, and cell cycle effects of camptothecin. *J Natl Cancer Inst* 1971;46:789–795.
8. Kessel D. Effects of camptothecin on RNA synthesis in leukemia L1210 cells. *Biochim Biophys Acta* 1971;246:225–232.
9. Kessel D, Bosmann HB, Lohr K. Camptothecin effects on DNA synthesis in murine leukemia cells. *Biochim Biophys Acta* 1972;269:210–216.
10. Abelson HT, Penman S. Selective interruption of high molecular weight RNA synthesis in HeLa cells by camptothecin. *Nat New Biol* 1972;237:144–146.
11. Kessel D, Dysard R. Effects of camptothecin on RNA synthesis in L-1210 cells. *Biochim Biophys Acta* 1973;312:716–721.
12. Gottlieb JA, Guarino AM, Call JB, et al. Preliminary pharmacologic and clinical evaluation of camptothecin sodium (NSC-100880). *Cancer Chemother Rep* 1970;54:461–470.
13. Creaven PJ, Allen LM, Muggia FM. Plasma camptothecin (NSC-100880) levels during a 5-day course of treatment: relation to dose and toxicity. *Cancer Chemother Rep* 1972;56:573–578.

14. Muggia FM, Creaven PJ, Hansen HH, et al. Phase I clinical trial of weekly and daily treatment with camptothecin (NSC-100880): correlation with preclinical studies. *Cancer Chemother Rep* 1972;56:515–521.

15. Moertel CG, Schutt AJ, Reitemeier RJ, et al. Phase II study of camptothecin (NSC-100880) in the treatment of advanced gastrointestinal cancer. *Cancer Chemother Rep* 1972;56:95–101.

16. Gottlieb JA, Luce JK. Treatment of malignant melanoma with camptothecin (NSC-100880). *Cancer Chemother Rep* 1972;56:103–105.

17. Hsiang YH, Hertzberg R, Hecht S, et al. Camptothecin induces protein-linked DNA breaks via mammalian DNA topoisomerase I. *J Biol Chem* 1985;260:14873–14878.

18. Hsiang YH, Liu LF. Identification of mammalian DNA topoisomerase I as an intracellular target of the anticancer drug camptothecin. *Cancer Res* 1988;48:1722–1726.

19. Creemers GJ, Lund B, Verweij J. Topoisomerase I inhibitors: topotecan and irinotecan. *Cancer Treat Rev* 1994;20:73–96.

20. Slichenmyer WJ, Donehower RC. Recent clinical advances with camptothecin analogues. *Cancer Treat Res* 1995;78:29–43.

21. Takimoto CH, Wright J, Arbuck SG. Clinical applications of the camptothecins. *Biochim Biophys Acta* 1998;1400:107–119.

22. Potmesil M. Camptothecins: from bench research to hospital wards. *Cancer Res* 1994;54:1431–1439.

23. Iyer L, Ratain MJ. Clinical pharmacology of camptothecins. *Cancer Chemother Pharmacol* 1998;42:S31–43.

24. Jaxel C, Kohn KW, Wani MC, et al. Structure-activity study of the actions of camptothecin derivatives on mammalian topoisomerase I: evidence for a specific receptor site and a relation to antitumor activity. *Cancer Res* 1989;49:1465–1469.

25. Wani MC, Nicholas AW, Wall ME. Plant antitumor agents. 28. Resolution of a key tricyclic synthon, 5'(RS)-1,5-dioxo-5'-ethyl-5'-hydroxy-2'H,5'H,6'H-6'-oxopyrano[3',4'-f]delta 6,8-tetrahydro-indolizine: total synthesis and antitumor activity of 20(S)- and 20(R)-camptothecin. *J Med Chem* 1987;30:2317–2319.

26. Fassberg J, Stella VJ. A kinetic and mechanistic study of the hydrolysis of camptothecin and some analogues. *J Pharm Sci* 1992;81:676–684.

27. Hertzberg RP, Caranfa MJ, Holden KG, et al. Modification of the hydroxy lactone ring of camptothecin: inhibition of mammalian topoisomerase I and biological activity. *J Med Chem* 1989;32:715–720.

28. Kingsbury WD, Boehm JC, Jakas DR, et al. Synthesis of water-soluble (aminoalkyl)camptothecin analogues: inhibition of topoisomerase I and antitumor activity. *J Med Chem* 1991;34:98–107.

29. Scott DO, Bindra DS, Stella VJ. Plasma pharmacokinetics of lactone and carboxylate forms of 20(S)-camptothecin in anesthetized rats. *Pharm Res* 1993;10:1451–1457.

30. Underberg WJ, Goossen RM, Smith BR, et al. Equilibrium kinetics of the new experimental anti-tumour compound SK&F 104864-A in aqueous solution. *J Pharm Biomed Anal* 1990;8:681–683.

31. Rowinsky EK, Grochow LB, Hendricks CB, et al. Phase I and pharmacologic study of topotecan: a novel topoisomerase I inhibitor. *J Clin Oncol* 1992;10:647–656.

32. Grochow LB, Rowinsky EK, Johnson R, et al. Pharmacoki-netics and pharmacodynamics of topotecan in patients with advanced cancer. *Drug Metab Dispos* 1992;20:706–713.

33. Burke TG, Munshi CB, Mi Z, et al. The important role of albumin in determining the relative human blood stabilities of the camptothecin anticancer drugs [Letter]. *J Pharm Sci* 1995;84:518–519.

34. Rosing H, Doyle E, Davies BE, et al. High-performance liquid chromatographic determination of the novel antitumour drug topotecan and topotecan as the total of the lactone plus carboxylate forms, in human plasma. *J Chromatogr B Biomed Sci Appl* 1995;668:107–115.

35. Kawato Y, Furuta T, Aonuma M, et al. Antitumor activity of a camptothecin derivative, CPT-11, against human tumor xenografts in nude mice. *Cancer Chemother Pharmacol* 1991;28:192–198.

36. Kaneda N, Nagata H, Furuta T, et al. Metabolism and pharmacokinetics of the camptothecin analogue CPT-11 in the mouse. *Cancer Res* 1990;50:1715–1720.

37. Tsuji T, Kaneda N, Kado K, et al. CPT-11 converting enzyme from rat serum: purification and some properties. *J Pharmacobiodyn* 1991;14:341–349.

38. Haaz MC, Riche C, Rivory LP, et al. Biosynthesis of an aminopiperidino metabolite of irinotecan [7-ethyl-10-[4-(1-piperidino)-1-piperidino]carbonyloxycamptothecin] by human hepatic microsomes. *Drug Metab Dispos* 1998;26:769–774.

39. Rothenberg ML, Kuhn JG, Burris HA, et al. Phase I and pharmacokinetic trial of weekly CPT-11. *J Clin Oncol* 1993;11:2194–2204.

40. Hsiang YH, Liu LF, Wall ME, et al. DNA topoisomerase I–mediated DNA cleavage and cytotoxicity of camptothecin analogues [published erratum appears in *Cancer Res* 1989;49(23):6868]. *Cancer Res* 1989;49:4385–4389.

41. Tanizawa A, Fujimori A, Fujimori Y, et al. Comparison of topoisomerase I inhibition, DNA damage, and cytotoxicity of camptothecin derivatives presently in clinical trials. *J Natl Cancer Inst* 1994;86:836–842.

42. Wang X, Zhou X, Hecht SM. Role of the 20-hydroxyl group in camptothecin binding by the topoisomerase I–DNA binary complex. *Biochemistry* 1999;38:4374–4381.

43. Joto N, Ishii M, Minami M, et al. DX-8951f, a water-soluble camptothecin analog, exhibits potent antitumor activity against a human lung cancer cell line and its SN-38-resistant variant. *Int J Cancer* 1997;72:680–686.

44. Hausheer FH, Haridas K, Murali D, et al. Discovery and development of two novel oncology drugs: BNP7787 and karenitecins. *Ann Oncol* 1998;9[Suppl 2]:21.

45. Berger JM. Structure of DNA topoisomerases. *Biochim Biophys Acta* 1998;1400:3–18.

46. Wang JC. Interaction between DNA and an *Escherichia coli* protein omega. *J Mol Biol* 1971;55:523–533.

47. Champoux JJ, Dulbecco R. An activity from mammalian cells that untwists superhelical DNA—a possible swivel for DNA replication (polyoma-ethidium bromide-mouse-embryo cells-dye binding assay). *Proc Natl Acad Sci U S A* 1972;69:143–146.

48. Tse-Dinh YC, Wang JC. Complete nucleotide sequence of the topA gene encoding *Escherichia coli* DNA topoisomerase I. *J Mol Biol* 1986;191:321–331.

49. Chen AY, Liu LF. DNA topoisomerases: essential enzymes and lethal targets. *Annu Rev Pharmacol Toxicol* 1994;34:191–218.

50. Gupta M, Fujimori A, Pommier Y. Eukaryotic DNA topoisomerases I. *Biochim Biophys Acta* 1995;1262:1–14.

51. D'Arpa P, Machlin PS, Ratrie HD, et al. cDNA cloning of human DNA topoisomerase I: catalytic activity of a 67.7-kDa carboxyl-terminal fragment. *Proc Natl Acad Sci U S A* 1988;85:2543–2547.

52. Juan CC, Hwang JL, Liu AA, et al. Human DNA topoisomerase I is encoded by a single-copy gene that maps to chromosome region 20q12-13.2. *Proc Natl Acad Sci U S A* 1988;85:8910–8913.

53. Kunze N, Yang GC, Dolberg M, et al. Structure of the human type I DNA topoisomerase gene. *J Biol Chem* 1991;266:9610–9616.

54. Morham SG, Kluckman KD, Voulomanos N, et al. Targeted disruption of the mouse topoisomerase I gene by camptothecin selection. *Mol Cell Biol* 1996;16:6804–6809.

55. Thrash C, Voelkel K, DiNardo S, et al. Identification of *Saccharomyces cerevisiae* mutants deficient in DNA topoisomerase I activity. *J Biol Chem* 1984;259:1375–1377.

56. Uemura T, Yanagida M. Isolation of type I and II DNA topoisomerase mutants from fission yeast: single and double mutants show different phenotypes in cell growth and chromatin organization. *EMBO J* 1984;3:1737–1744.

57. Shero JH, Bordwell B, Rothfield NF, et al. High titers of autoantibodies to topoisomerase I (Scl-70) in sera from scleroderma patients. *Science* 1986;231:737–740.

58. Shero JH, Bordwell B, Rothfield NF, et al. Antibodies to topoisomerase I in sera from patients with scleroderma. *J Rheumatol* 1987;14[Suppl 13]:138–140.

59. Redinbo MR, Stewart L, Kuhn P, et al. Crystal structures of human topoisomerase I in covalent and noncovalent complexes with DNA [see comments]. *Science* 1998;279:1504–1513.

60. Redinbo MR, Champoux JJ, Hol WG. Structural insights into the function of type IB topoisomerases. *Curr Opin Struct Biol* 1999;9:29–36.

61. Stewart L, Ireton GC, Champoux JJ. The domain organization of human topoisomerase I. *J Biol Chem* 1996;271:7602–7608.

62. Stewart L, Ireton GC, Parker LH, et al. Biochemical and biophysical analyses of recombinant forms of human topoisomerase I. *J Biol Chem* 1996;271:7593–7601.

63. Madden KR, Stewart L, Champoux JJ. Preferential binding of human topoisomerase I to superhelical DNA. *EMBO J* 1995;14:5399–5409.

64. Lue N, Sharma A, Mondragon A, et al. A 26 kDa yeast DNA topoisomerase I fragment: crystallographic structure and mechanistic implications. *Structure* 1995;3:1315–1322.

65. Li XG, Haluska P Jr, Hsiang YH, et al. Involvement of amino acids 361 to 364 of human topoisomerase I in camptothecin resistance and enzyme catalysis. *Biochem Pharmacol* 1997;53:1019–1027.

66. Stewart L, Ireton GC, Champoux JJ. Reconstitution of human topoisomerase I by fragment complementation. *J Mol Biol* 1997;269:355–372.

67. Liu LF. DNA topoisomerase poisons as antitumor drugs. *Annu Rev Biochem* 1989;58:351–375.

68. Liu LF, Wang JC. Supercoiling of the DNA template during transcription. *Proc Natl Acad Sci U S A* 1987;84:7024–7027.

69. Wu HY, Shyy SH, Wang JC, et al. Transcription generates positively and negatively supercoiled domains in the template. *Cell* 1988;53:433–440.

70. Tsao YP, Wu HY, Liu LF. Transcription-driven supercoiling of DNA: direct biochemical evidence from in vitro studies. *Cell* 1989;56:111–118.

71. Ishimi Y, Nishizawa M, Andoh T. Characterization of a camptothecin-resistant human DNA topoisomerase I in an in vitro system for Simian virus 40 DNA replication. *Eur J Biochem* 1991;202:835–839.

72. Yang L, Wold MS, Li JJ, et al. Roles of DNA topoisomerases in simian virus 40 DNA replication in vitro. *Proc Natl Acad Sci U S A* 1987;84:950–954.

73. Zhang H, Wang JC, Liu LF. Involvement of DNA topoisomerase I in transcription of human ribosomal RNA genes. *Proc Natl Acad Sci U S A* 1988;85:1060–1064.

74. Fleischmann G, Pflugfelder G, Steiner EK, et al. Drosophila DNA topoisomerase I is associated with transcriptionally active regions of the genome. *Proc Natl Acad Sci U S A* 1984;81:6958–6962.

75. Muller MT, Pfund WP, Mehta VB, et al. Eukaryotic type I topoisomerase is enriched in the nucleolus and catalytically active on ribosomal DNA. *EMBO J* 1985;4:1237–1243.

76. Stewart AF, Herrera RE, Nordheim A. Rapid induction of c-fos transcription reveals quantitative linkage of RNA polymerase II and DNA topoisomerase I enzyme activities. *Cell* 1990;60:141–149.

77. Kretzschmar M, Meisterernst M, Roeder RG. Identification of human DNA topoisomerase I as a cofactor for activator-dependent transcription by RNA polymerase II. *Proc Natl Acad Sci U S A* 1993;90:11508–11512.

78. Merino A, Madden KR, Lane WS, et al. DNA topoisomerase I is involved in both repression and activation of transcription. *Nature* 1993;365:227–232.

79. Bharti AK, Olson MO, Kufe DW, et al. Identification of a nucleolin binding site in human topoisomerase I. *J Biol Chem* 1996;271:1993–1997.

80. Shykind BM, Kim J, Stewart L, et al. Topoisomerase I enhances TFIID-TFIIA complex assembly during activation of transcription. *Genes Dev* 1997;11:397–407.

81. Buckwalter CA, Lin AH, Tanizawa A, et al. RNA synthesis inhibitors alter the subnuclear distribution of DNA topoisomerase I. *Cancer Res* 1996;56:1674–1681.

82. Baker SD, Wadkins RM, Stewart CF, et al. Cell cycle analysis of amount and distribution of nuclear DNA topoisomerase I as determined by fluorescence digital imaging microscopy. *Cytometry* 1995;19:134–145.

83. Champoux JJ. Strand breakage by the DNA untwisting enzyme results in covalent attachment of the enzyme to DNA. *Proc Natl Acad Sci U S A* 1977;74:3800–3804.

84. Champoux JJ. Mechanism of the reaction catalyzed by the DNA untwisting enzyme: attachment of the enzyme to 3'-terminus of the nicked DNA. *J Mol Biol* 1978;118:441–446.

85. Stivers JT, Harris TK, Mildvan AS. Vaccinia DNA topoisomerase I: evidence supporting a free rotation mechanism for DNA supercoil relaxation. *Biochemistry* 1997;36:5212–5222.

86. Edwards KA, Halligan BD, Davis JL, et al. Recognition sites of eukaryotic DNA topoisomerase I: DNA nucleotide sequencing analysis of topo I cleavage sites on SV40 DNA. *Nucleic Acids Res* 1982;10:2565–2576.

87. Been MD, Burgess RR, Champoux JJ. Nucleotide sequence preference at rat liver and wheat germ type 1 DNA topoi-

somerase breakage sites in duplex SV40 DNA. *Nucleic Acids Res* 1984;12:3097–3114.

88. Hwang JL, Shyy SH, Chen AY, et al. Studies of topoisomerase-specific antitumor drugs in human lymphocytes using rabbit antisera against recombinant human topoisomerase II polypeptide. *Cancer Res* 1989;49:958–962.

89. Hwong CL, Chen MS, Hwang JL. Phorbol ester transiently increases topoisomerase I mRNA levels in human skin fibroblasts. *J Biol Chem* 1989;264:14923–14926.

90. Sobczak J, Tournier MF, Lotti AM, et al. Gene expression in regenerating liver in relation to cell proliferation and stress. *Eur J Biochem* 1989;180:49–53.

91. Romig H, Richter A. Expression of the topoisomerase I gene in serum stimulated human fibroblasts. *Biochim Biophys Acta* 1990;1048:274–280.

92. Van der Zee AG, Hollema H, de Jong S, et al. P-glycoprotein expression and DNA topoisomerase I and II activity in benign tumors of the ovary and in malignant tumors of the ovary, before and after platinum/cyclophosphamide chemotherapy. *Cancer Res* 1991;51:5915–5920.

93. Giovanella BC, Stehlin JS, Wall ME, et al. DNA topoisomerase I–targeted chemotherapy of human colon cancer in xenografts. *Science* 1989;246:1046–1048.

94. Husain I, Mohler JL, Seigler HF, et al. Elevation of topoisomerase I messenger RNA, protein, and catalytic activity in human tumors: demonstration of tumor-type specificity and implications for cancer chemotherapy. *Cancer Res* 1994;54:539–546.

95. McLeod HL, Douglas F, Oates M, et al. Topoisomerase I and II activity in human breast, cervix, lung and colon cancer. *Int J Cancer* 1994;59:607–611.

96. Kaufmann SH, Charron M, Burke PJ, et al. Changes in topoisomerase I levels and localization during myeloid maturation in vitro and in vivo. *Cancer Res* 1995;55:1255–1260.

97. Shayo CC, Mladovan AG, Baldi A, et al. Differentiating agents modulate topoisomerase I activity in U-937 promonocytic cells: reconstitution of human topoisomerase I by fragment complementation. *Eur J Pharmacol* 1997;324:129–133.

98. Pommier Y, Kerrigan D, Hartman KD, et al. Phosphorylation of mammalian DNA topoisomerase I and activation by protein kinase C. *J Biol Chem* 1990;265:9418–9422.

99. Samuels DS, Shimizu N. DNA topoisomerase I phosphorylation in murine fibroblasts treated with 12-O-tetradecanoylphorbol-13-acetate and in vitro by protein kinase. *J Biol Chem* 1992;267:11156–11162.

100. Samuels DS, Shimizu Y, Nakabayashi T, et al. Phosphorylation of DNA topoisomerase I is increased during the response of mammalian cells to mitogenic stimuli. *Biochim Biophys Acta* 1994;1223:77–83.

101. Staron K, Kowalska-Loth B, Zabek J, et al. Topoisomerase I is differently phosphorylated in two sublines of L5178Y mouse lymphoma cells. *Biochim Biophys Acta* 1995;1260:35–42.

102. Kasid UN, Halligan B, Liu LF, et al. Poly(ADP-ribose)-mediated post-translational modification of chromatin-associated human topoisomerase I. Inhibitory effects on catalytic activity. *J Biol Chem* 1989;264:18687–18692.

103. Park JK, Kim WJ, Park YS, et al. Inhibition of topoisomerase I by NAD and enhancement of cytotoxicity of MMS by inhibitors of poly(ADP-ribose) polymerase in *Saccharomyces cerevisiae*. *Cell Mol Biol* 1991;37:739–744.

104. Boothman DA, Fukunaga N, Wang M. Down-regulation of topoisomerase I in mammalian cells following ionizing radiation. *Cancer Res* 1994;54:4618–4626.

105. Covey JM, Jaxel C, Kohn KW, et al. Protein-linked DNA strand breaks induced in mammalian cells by camptothecin, an inhibitor of topoisomerase I. *Cancer Res* 1989;49:5016–5022.

106. Holm C, Covey JM, Kerrigan D, et al. Differential requirement of DNA replication for the cytotoxicity of DNA topoisomerase I and II inhibitors in Chinese hamster DC3F cells. *Cancer Res* 1989;49:6365–6368.

107. D'Arpa P, Beardmore C, Liu LF. Involvement of nucleic acid synthesis in cell killing mechanisms of topoisomerase poisons. *Cancer Res* 1990;50:6919–6924.

108. Hsiang YH, Lihou MG, Liu LF. Arrest of replication forks by drug-stabilized topoisomerase I–DNA cleavable complexes as a mechanism of cell killing by camptothecin. *Cancer Res* 1989;49:5077–5082.

109. Ryan AJ, Squires S, Strutt HL, et al. Camptothecin cytotoxicity in mammalian cells is associated with the induction of persistent double strand breaks in replicating DNA. *Nucleic Acids Res* 1991;19:3295–3300.

110. Tsao YP, Russo A, Nyamuswa G, et al. Interaction between replication forks and topoisomerase I–DNA cleavable complexes: studies in a cell-free SV40 DNA replication system. *Cancer Res* 1993;53:5908–5914.

111. Li LH, Fraser TJ, Olin EJ, et al. Action of camptothecin on mammalian cells in culture. *Cancer Res* 1972;32:2643–2650.

112. Gerrits CJ, de Jonge MJ, Schellens JH, et al. Topoisomerase I inhibitors: the relevance of prolonged exposure for present clinical development. *Br J Cancer* 1997;76:952–962.

113. Nitiss J, Wang JC. DNA topoisomerase-targeting antitumor drugs can be studied in yeast. *Proc Natl Acad Sci U S A* 1988;85:7501–7505.

114. Bjornsti MA, Benedetti P, Viglianti GA, et al. Expression of human DNA topoisomerase I in yeast cells lacking yeast DNA topoisomerase I: restoration of sensitivity of the cells to the antitumor drug camptothecin. *Cancer Res* 1989;49:6318–6323.

115. Tanizawa A, Kohn KW, Kohlhagen G, et al. Differential stabilization of eukaryotic DNA topoisomerase I cleavable complexes by camptothecin derivatives. *Biochemistry* 1995;34:7200–7206.

116. Thomsen B, Mollerup S, Bonven BJ, et al. Sequence specificity of DNA topoisomerase I in the presence and absence of camptothecin. *EMBO J* 1987;6:1817–1823.

117. Jaxel C, Kohn KW, Pommier Y. Topoisomerase I interaction with SV40 DNA in the presence and absence of camptothecin. *Nucleic Acids Res* 1988;16:11157–11170.

118. Porter SE, Champoux JJ. Mapping in vivo topoisomerase I sites on simian virus 40 DNA: asymmetric distribution of sites on replicating molecules. *Mol Cell Biol* 1989;9:541–550.

119. Jaxel C, Capranico G, Kerrigan D, et al. Effect of local DNA sequence on topoisomerase I cleavage in the presence or absence of camptothecin. *J Biol Chem* 1991;266:20418–20423.

120. Tanizawa A, Kohn KW, Pommier Y. Induction of cleavage in topoisomerase I c-DNA by topoisomerase I enzymes from calf thymus and wheat germ in the presence and absence of camptothecin. *Nucleic Acids Res* 1993;21:5157–5166.

121. Leteurtre F, Fesen M, Kohlhagen G, et al. Specific interaction of camptothecin, a topoisomerase I inhibitor, with guanine residues of DNA detected by photoactivation at 365 nm. *Biochemistry* 1993;32:8955–8962.

122. Lanza A, Tornaletti S, Rodolfo C, et al. Human DNA topoisomerase I–mediated cleavages stimulated by ultraviolet light–induced DNA damage. *J Biol Chem* 1996;271:6978–6986.

123. Pourquier P, Pilon AA, Kohlhagen G, et al. Trapping of mammalian topoisomerase I and recombinations induced by damaged DNA containing nicks or gaps. Importance of DNA end phosphorylation and camptothecin effects. *J Biol Chem* 1997;272:26441–26447.

124. Pourquier P, Ueng LM, Kohlhagen G, et al. Effects of uracil incorporation, DNA mismatches, and abasic sites on cleavage and religation activities of mammalian topoisomerase I. *J Biol Chem* 1997;272:7792–7796.

125. Megonigal MD, Fertala J, Bjornsti MA. Alterations in the catalytic activity of yeast DNA topoisomerase I result in cell cycle arrest and cell death. *J Biol Chem* 1997;272:12801–12808.

126. Desai SD, Liu LF, Vazquez-Abad D, et al. Ubiquitin-dependent destruction of topoisomerase I is stimulated by the antitumor drug camptothecin. *J Biol Chem* 1997;272:24159–24164.

127. Beidler DR, Cheng YC. Camptothecin induction of a time- and concentration-dependent decrease of topoisomerase I and its implication in camptothecin activity. *Mol Pharmacol* 1995;47:907–914.

128. Danks MK, Pawlik CA, Whipple DO, et al. Intermittent exposure of medulloblastoma cells to topotecan produces growth inhibition equivalent to continuous exposure. *Clin Cancer Res* 1997;3:1731–1738.

129. Pawlik CA, Houghton PJ, Stewart CF, et al. Effective schedules of exposure to topotecan determined by cellular markers of drug activity in medulloblastoma and rhabdomyosarcoma cell lines and xenografts. *Proc Annu Meet Am Assoc Cancer Res* 1997;38(abst).

130. Rubin E, Wood V, Bharti A, et al. A phase I and pharmacokinetic study of a new camptothecin derivative, 9-aminocamptothecin. *Clin Cancer Res* 1995;1:269–276.

131. Hochster H, Liebes L, Speyer J, et al. Effect of prolonged topotecan infusion on topoisomerase 1 levels: a phase I and pharmacodynamic study. *Clin Cancer Res* 1997;3:1245–1252.

132. Murren JR, Anderson S, Fedele J, et al. Dose-escalation and pharmacodynamic study of topotecan in combination with cyclophosphamide in patients with refractory cancer. *J Clin Oncol* 1997;15:148–157.

133. Yang SW, Burgin AB Jr, Huizenga BN, et al. A eukaryotic enzyme that can disjoin dead-end covalent complexes between DNA and type I topoisomerases. *Proc Natl Acad Sci U S A* 1996;93:11534–11539.

134. Chatterjee S, Cheng MF, Trivedi D, et al. Camptothecin hypersensitivity in poly(adenosine diphosphate-ribose) polymerase-deficient cell lines. *Cancer Commun* 1989;1:389–394.

135. Hashimoto H, Chatterjee S, Berger NA. Mutagenic activity of topoisomerase I inhibitors. *Clin Cancer Res* 1995;1:369–376.

136. Kojima A, Shinkai T, Saijo N. Cytogenetic effects of CPT-11 and its active metabolite, SN-38 on human lymphocytes. *Jpn J Clin Oncol* 1993;23:116–122.

137. Pommier Y, Jenkins J, Kohlhagen G, et al. DNA recombinase activity of eukaryotic DNA topoisomerase I: effects of camptothecin and other inhibitors. *Mutat Res* 1995;337:135–145.

138. Tsao YP, D'Arpa P, Liu LF. The involvement of active DNA synthesis in camptothecin-induced G2 arrest: altered regulation of p34cdc2/cyclin B. *Cancer Res* 1992;52:1823–1829.

139. Goldwasser F, Shimizu T, Jackman J, et al. Correlations between S and G2 arrest and the cytotoxicity of camptothecin in human colon carcinoma cells. *Cancer Res* 1996;56:4430–4437.

140. Ling YH, Tseng MT, Nelson JA. Differentiation induction of human promyelocytic leukemia cells by 10-hydroxycamptothecin, a DNA topoisomerase I inhibitor. *Differentiation* 1991;46:135–141.

141. McSheehy PM, Gervasoni M, Lampasona V, et al. Studies of the differentiation properties of camptothecin in the human leukaemic cells K562. *Eur J Cancer* 1991;27:1406–1411.

142. Aller P, Rius C, Mata F, et al. Camptothecin induces differentiation and stimulates the expression of differentiation-related genes in U-937 human promonocytic leukemia cells. *Cancer Res* 1992;52:1245–1251.

143. Kharbanda S, Rubin E, Gunji H, et al. Camptothecin and its derivatives induce expression of the c-jun protooncogene in human myeloid leukemia cells. *Cancer Res* 1991;51:6636–6642.

144. Traganos F, Kapuscinski J, Gong J, et al. Caffeine prevents apoptosis and cell cycle effects induced by camptothecin or topotecan in HL-60 cells. *Cancer Res* 1993;53:4613–4618.

145. Kaufmann SH. Induction of endonucleolytic DNA cleavage in human acute myelogenous leukemia cells by etoposide, camptothecin, and other cytotoxic anticancer drugs: a cautionary note. *Cancer Res* 1989;49:5870–5878.

146. O'Connor PM, Nieves-Neira W, Kerrigan D, et al. S-phase population analysis does not correlate with the cytotoxicity of camptothecin and 10,11-methylenedioxycamptothecin in human colon carcinoma HT-29 cells. *Cancer Commun* 1991;3:233–240.

147. Morris EJ, Geller HM. Induction of neuronal apoptosis by camptothecin, an inhibitor of DNA topoisomerase-I: evidence for cell cycle-independent toxicity. *J Cell Biol* 1996;134:757–770.

148. Park DS, Morris EJ, Greene LA, et al. G1/S cell cycle blockers and inhibitors of cyclin-dependent kinases suppress camptothecin-induced neuronal apoptosis. *J Neurosci* 1997;17:1256–1270.

149. Gromova II, Kjeldsen E, Svejstrup JQ, et al. Characterization of an altered DNA catalysis of a camptothecin-resistant eukaryotic topoisomerase I. *Nucleic Acids Res* 1993;21:593–600.

150. Rubin E, Pantazis P, Bharti A, et al. Identification of a mutant human topoisomerase I with intact catalytic activity and resistance to 9-nitro-camptothecin. *J Biol Chem* 1994;269:2433–2439.

151. Benedetti P, Fiorani P, Capuani L, et al. Camptothecin resistance from a single mutation changing glycine 363 of human DNA topoisomerase I to cysteine. *Cancer Res* 1993;53:4343–4348.

152. Tamura H, Kohchi C, Yamada R, et al. Molecular cloning of a cDNA of a camptothecin-resistant human DNA topoisomerase I and identification of mutation sites. *Nucleic Acids Res* 1991;19:69–75.

153. Saleem A, Ibrahim N, Patel M, et al. Mechanisms of resistance in a human cell line exposed to sequential topoisomerase poisoning. *Cancer Res* 1997;57:5100–5106.

154. Fujimori A, Harker WG, Kohlhagen G, et al. Mutation at the catalytic site of topoisomerase I in CEM/C2, a human leukemia cell line resistant to camptothecin. *Cancer Res* 1995;55:1339–1346.

155. Kubota N, Kanzawa F, Nishio K, et al. Detection of topoisomerase I gene point mutation in CPT-11 resistant lung cancer cell line. *Biochem Biophys Res Commun* 1992;188:571–577.

156. Wang LF, Ting CY, Lo CK, et al. Identification of mutations at DNA topoisomerase I responsible for camptothecin resistance. *Cancer Res* 1997;57:1516–1522.

157. Ohashi N, Fujiwara Y, Yamaoka N, et al. No alteration in DNA topoisomerase I gene related to CPT-11 resistance in human lung cancer. *Jpn J Cancer Res* 1996;87:1280–1287.

158. Takatani H, Oka M, Fukuda M, et al. Gene mutation analysis and quantitation of DNA topoisomerase I in previously untreated non-small cell lung carcinomas. *Jpn J Cancer Res* 1997;88:160–165.

159. Kijima T, Kubota N, Nishio K. Establishment of a CPT-11-resistant human ovarian cancer cell line. *Anticancer Res* 1994;14:799–803.

160. Woessner RD, Eng WK, Hofmann GA, et al. Camptothecin hyper-resistant P388 cells: drug-dependent reduction in topoisomerase I content. *Oncol Res* 1992;4:481–488.

161. Tan KB, Mattern MR, Eng WK, et al. Nonproductive rearrangement of DNA topoisomerase I and II genes: correlation with resistance to topoisomerase inhibitors. *J Natl Cancer Inst* 1989;81:1732–1735.

162. Jansen WJ, Hulscher TM, van Ark-Otte J, et al. CPT-11 sensitivity in relation to the expression of P170-glycoprotein and multidrug resistance–associated protein. *Br J Cancer* 1998;77:359–365.

163. Tsuruo T, Matsuzaki T, Matsushita M, et al. Antitumor effect of CPT-11, a new derivative of camptothecin, against pleiotropic drug-resistant tumors in vitro and in vivo. *Cancer Chemother Pharmacol* 1988;21:71–74.

164. Chen AY, Yu C, Potmesil M, et al. Camptothecin overcomes MDR1-mediated resistance in human KB carcinoma cells. *Cancer Res* 1991;51:6039–6044.

165. Hendricks CB, Rowinsky EK, Grochow LB, et al. Effect of P-glycoprotein expression on the accumulation and cytotoxicity of topotecan (SK&F 104864), a new camptothecin analogue. *Cancer Res* 1992;52:2268–2278.

166. Mattern MR, Hofmann GA, Polsky RM, et al. In vitro and in vivo effects of clinically important camptothecin analogues on multidrug-resistant cells. *Oncol Res* 1993;5:467–474.

167. Hoki Y, Fujimori A, Pommier Y. Differential cytotoxicity of clinically important camptothecin derivatives in P-glycoprotein-overexpressing cell lines. *Cancer Chemother Pharmacol* 1997;40:433–438.

168. Jonsson E, Fridborg H, Csoka K, et al. Cytotoxic activity of topotecan in human tumour cell lines and primary cultures of human tumour cells from patients. *Br J Cancer* 1997;76:211–219.

169. Houghton PJ, Cheshire PJ, Hallman JC, et al. Therapeutic efficacy of the topoisomerase I inhibitor 7-ethyl-10-(4-[1-piperidino]-1-piperidino)-carbonyloxy-camptothecin against

170. human tumor xenografts: lack of cross-resistance in vivo in tumors with acquired resistance to the topoisomerase I inhibitor 9-dimethylaminomethyl-10-hydroxycamptothecin. *Cancer Res* 1993;53:2823–2829.

170. Yang CJ, Horton JK, Cowan KH, et al. Cross-resistance to camptothecin analogues in a mitoxantrone-resistant human breast carcinoma cell line is not due to DNA topoisomerase I alterations. *Cancer Res* 1995;55:4004–4009.

171. Kellner U, Hutchinson L, Seidel A, et al. Decreased drug accumulation in a mitoxantrone-resistant gastric carcinoma cell line in the absence of P-glycoprotein. *Int J Cancer* 1997;71:817–824.

172. Doyle LA, Yang W, Abruzzo LV, et al. A multidrug resistance transporter from human MCF-7 breast cancer cells. *Proc Natl Acad Sci U S A* 1998;95:15665–15670.

173. Miyake K, Mickley L, Litman T, et al. Molecular cloning of cDNAs which are highly overexpressed in mitoxantrone-resistant cells: demonstration of homology to ABC transport genes. *Cancer Res* 1999;59:8–13.

174. Saijo N, Nishio K, Kubota N, et al. 7-Ethyl-10-[4-(1-piperidino)-1-piperidino] carbonyloxy camptothecin: mechanism of resistance and clinical trials. *Cancer Chemother Pharmacol* 1994;34[Suppl]:S112–117.

175. Chen SF, Rothenberg ML, Clark G, et al. Human tumor carboxylesterase activity correlates with CPT-11 cytotoxicity in vitro. *Proc Am Assoc Cancer Res* 1994;35:365.

176. Ogasawara H, Nishio K, Kanzawa F, et al. Intracellular carboxyl esterase activity is a determinant of cellular sensitivity to the antineoplastic agent KW-2189 in cell lines resistant to cisplatin and CPT-11. *Jpn J Cancer Res* 1995;86:124–129.

177. Jansen WJ, Zwart B, Hulscher ST, et al. CPT-11 in human colon-cancer cell lines and xenografts: characterization of cellular sensitivity determinants. *Int J Cancer* 1997;70:335–340.

178. Eng WK, Faucette L, Johnson RK, et al. Evidence that DNA topoisomerase I is necessary for the cytotoxic effects of camptothecin. *Mol Pharmacol* 1988;34:755–760.

179. Matsumoto Y, Fujiwara T, Honjo Y, et al. Quantitative analysis of DNA topoisomerase I activity in human and rat glioma: characterization and mechanism of resistance to antitopoisomerase chemical, camptothecin-11. *J Surg Oncol* 1993;53:97–103.

180. Goldwasser F, Bae I, Valenti M, et al. Topoisomerase I–related parameters and camptothecin activity in the colon carcinoma cell lines from the National Cancer Institute anticancer screen. *Cancer Res* 1995;55:2116–2121.

181. Perego P, Capranico G, Supino R, et al. Topoisomerase I gene expression and cell sensitivity to camptothecin in human cell lines of different tumor types. *Anticancer Drugs* 1994;5:645–649.

182. Danks MK, Garrett KE, Marion RC, et al. Subcellular redistribution of DNA topoisomerase I in anaplastic astrocytoma cells treated with topotecan. *Cancer Res* 1996;56:1664–1673.

183. Florell SR, Martinchick JF, Holden JA. Purification of DNA topoisomerase I from the spleen of a patient with non-Hodgkin's lymphoma. *Anticancer Res* 1996;16:3467–3474.

184. Subramanian D, Kraut E, Staubus A, et al. Analysis of topoisomerase I/DNA complexes in patients administered topotecan. *Cancer Res* 1995;55:2097–2103.

185. Kaufmann SH, Svingen PA, Gore SD, et al. Altered formation of topotecan-stabilized topoisomerase I–DNA adducts in human leukemia cells. *Blood* 1997;89:2098–2104.

186. Boege F. Analysis of eukaryotic DNA topoisomerases and topoisomerase-directed drug effects. *Eur J Clin Chem Clin Biochem* 1996;34:873–888.

187. Pondarre C, Strumberg D, Fujimori A, et al. In vivo sequencing of camptothecin-induced topoisomerase I cleavage sites in human colon carcinoma cells. *Nucleic Acids Res* 1997;25:4111–4116.

188. Fujimori A, Gupta M, Hoki Y, et al. Acquired camptothecin resistance of human breast cancer MCF-7/C4 cells with normal topoisomerase I and elevated DNA repair. *Mol Pharmacol* 1996;50:1472–1478.

189. Adjei PN, Kaufmann SH, Leung WY, et al. Selective induction of apoptosis in Hep 3B cells by topoisomerase I inhibitors: evidence for a protease-dependent pathway that does not activate cysteine protease P32. *J Clin Invest* 1996;98:2588–2596.

190. Shimizu T, Pommier Y. DNA fragmentation induced by protease activation in p53-null human leukemia HL60 cells undergoing apoptosis following treatment with the topoisomerase I inhibitor camptothecin: cell-free system studies. *Exp Cell Res* 1996;226:292–301.

191. Gupta M, Fan S, Zhan Q, et al. Inactivation of p53 increases the cytotoxicity of camptothecin in human colon CHT116 and breast MCF-7 cancer cells. *Clin Cancer Res* 1997;3:1653–1660.

192. Dubrez L, Goldwasser F, Genne P, et al. The role of cell cycle regulation and apoptosis triggering in determining the sensitivity of leukemic cells to topoisomerase I and II inhibitors. *Leukemia* 1995;9:1013–1024.

193. Gradzka I, Szumiel I. Discrepancy between the initial DNA damage and cell survival after camptothecin treatment in two murine lymphoma L5178Y sublines. *Cell Biochem Funct* 1996;14:163–171.

194. Horwitz SB, Chang CK, Grollman AP. Antiviral action of camptothecin. *Antimicrob Agents Chemother* 1972;2:395–401.

195. Pantazis P, Han Z, Chatterjee D, et al. Water-insoluble camptothecin analogues as potential antiviral drugs. *J Biomed Sci* 1999;6:1–7.

196. Priel E, Showalter SD, Blair DG. Inhibition of human immunodeficiency virus (HIV-1) replication in vitro by noncytotoxic doses of camptothecin, a topoisomerase I inhibitor. *AIDS Res Hum Retroviruses* 1991;7:65–72.

197. Li CJ, Zhang LJ, Dezube BJ, et al. Three inhibitors of type 1 human immunodeficiency virus long terminal repeat-directed gene expression and virus replication. *Proc Natl Acad Sci U S A* 1993;90:1839–1842.

198. Li CJ, Wang C, Pardee AB. Camptothecin inhibits Tat-mediated transactivation of type 1 human immunodeficiency virus. *J Biol Chem* 1994;269:7051–7054.

199. Carteau S, Mouscadet JF, Goulaouic H, et al. Effect of topoisomerase inhibitors on the in vitro HIV DNA integration reaction. *Biochem Biophys Res Commun* 1993;192:1409–1414.

200. Priel E, Aflalo E, Chechelnitsky G, et al. Inhibition of retrovirus-induced disease in mice by camptothecin. *J Virol* 1993;67:3624–3629.

201. Sadaie MR, Doniger J, Hung CL, et al. 9-nitrocamptothecin selectively inhibits human immunodeficiency virus type 1 replication in freshly infected parental but not 9-nitro-camptothecin-resistant U937 monocytoid cells. *AIDS Res Hum Retroviruses* 1999;15:239–245.

202. Moulton S, Pantazis P, Epstein JS, et al. 9-Nitrocamptothecin inhibits tumor necrosis factor–mediated activation of human immunodeficiency virus type 1 and enhances apoptosis in a latently infected T cell clone. *AIDS Res Hum Retroviruses* 1998;14:39–49.

203. Zhang JL, Sharma PL, Li CJ, et al. Topotecan inhibits human immunodeficiency virus type 1 infection through a topoisomerase-independent mechanism in a cell line with altered topoisomerase I. *Antimicrob Agents Chemother* 1997;41:977–981.

204. Boothman DA, Trask DK, Pardee AB. Inhibition of potentially lethal DNA damage repair in human tumor cells by beta-lapachone, an activator of topoisomerase I. *Cancer Res* 1989;49:605–612.

205. Boothman DA, Wang M, Schea RA, et al. Posttreatment exposure to camptothecin enhances the lethal effects of x-rays on radioresistant human malignant melanoma cells. *Int J Radiat Oncol Biol Phys* 1992;24:939–948.

206. Lamond JP, Mehta MP, Boothman DA. The potential of topoisomerase I inhibitors in the treatment of CNS malignancies: report of a synergistic effect between topotecan and radiation. *J Neurooncol* 1996;30:1–6.

207. Lamond JP, Wang M, Kinsella TJ, et al. Radiation lethality enhancement with 9-aminocamptothecin: comparison to other topoisomerase I inhibitors. *Int J Radiat Oncol Biol Phys* 1996;36:369–376.

208. Lamond JP, Wang M, Kinsella TJ, et al. Concentration and timing dependence of lethality enhancement between topotecan, a topoisomerase I inhibitor, and ionizing radiation. *Int J Radiat Oncol Biol Phys* 1996;36:361–368.

209. Chen AY, Okunieff P, Pommier Y, et al. Mammalian DNA topoisomerase I mediates the enhancement of radiation cytotoxicity by camptothecin derivatives. *Cancer Res* 1997;57:1529–1536.

210. Omura M, Torigoe S, Kubota N. SN-38, a metabolite of the camptothecin derivative CPT-11, potentiates the cytotoxic effect of radiation in human colon adenocarcinoma cells grown as spheroids. *Radiother Oncol* 1997;43:197–201.

211. Mattern MR, Hofmann GA, McCabe FL, et al. Synergistic cell killing by ionizing radiation and topoisomerase I inhibitor topotecan (SK&F 104864). *Cancer Res* 1991;51:5813–5816.

212. Marchesini R, Colombo A, Caserini C, et al. Interaction of ionizing radiation with topotecan in two human tumor cell lines. *Int J Cancer* 1996;66:342–346.

213. Wang JC. DNA topoisomerases. *Annu Rev Biochem* 1996;65:635–692.

214. Cheng MF, Chatterjee S, Berger NA. Schedule-dependent cytotoxicity of topotecan alone and in combination chemotherapy regimens. *Oncol Res* 1994;6:269–279.

215. Kaufmann SH, Peereboom D, Buckwalter CA, et al. Cytotoxic effects of topotecan combined with various anticancer agents in human cancer cell lines [see comments]. *J Natl Cancer Inst* 1996;88:734–741.

216. Falk SJ, Smith PJ. DNA damaging and cell cycle effects of the topoisomerase I poison camptothecin in irradiated human cells. *Int J Radiat Biol* 1992;61:749–757.

217. Del Bino G, Bruno S, Yi PN, et al. Apoptotic cell death triggered by camptothecin or teniposide. The cell cycle

specificity and effects of ionizing radiation. *Cell Prolif* 1992;25:537–548.

218. Hennequin C, Giocanti N, Balosso J, et al. Interaction of ionizing radiation with the topoisomerase I poison camptothecin in growing V-79 and HeLa cells. *Cancer Res* 1994;54:1720–1728.

219. Kirichenko AV, Travis EL, Rich TA. Radiation enhancement by 9-aminocamptothecin. Evidence for improved therapeutic ratio with a multiple dose schedule. *Ann N Y Acad Sci* 1996;803:312–314.

220. Kirichenko AV, Rich TA, Newman RA, et al. Potentiation of murine MCa-4 carcinoma radioresponse by 9-amino-20(S)-camptothecin. *Cancer Res* 1997;57:1929–1933.

221. Tamura K, Takada M, Kawase I, et al. Enhancement of tumor radio-response by irinotecan in human lung tumor xenografts. *Jpn J Cancer Res* 1997;88:218–223.

222. Kim JH, Kim SH, Kolozsvary A, et al. Potentiation of radiation response in human carcinoma cells in vitro and murine fibrosarcoma in vivo by topotecan, an inhibitor of DNA topoisomerase I. *Int J Radiat Oncol Biol Phys* 1992;22:515–518.

223. Rich TA, Kirichenko AV. Camptothecin radiation sensitization: mechanisms, schedules, and timing. *Oncology (Hungtingt)* 1998;12:114–120.

224. Johnson RK. Preclinical profile of SK&F 104864, a water-soluble camptothecin analogue. *Cancer Invest* 1991;9:346.

225. Pratesi G, Tortoreto M, Corti C, et al. Successful local regional therapy with topotecan of intraperitoneally growing human ovarian carcinoma xenografts. *Br J Cancer* 1995;71:525–528.

226. Friedman HS, Houghton PJ, Schold SC, et al. Activity of 9-dimethylaminomethyl-10-hydroxycamptothecin against pediatric and adult central nervous system tumor xenografts. *Cancer Chemother Pharmacol* 1994;34:171–174.

227. Houghton PJ, Cheshire PJ, Myers L, et al. Evaluation of 9-dimethylaminomethyl-10-hydroxycamptothecin against xenografts derived from adult and childhood solid tumors. *Cancer Chemother Pharmacol* 1992;31:229–239.

228. Saltz L, Sirott M, Young C, et al. Phase I clinical and pharmacology study of topotecan given daily for 5 consecutive days to patients with advanced solid tumors, with attempt at dose intensification using recombinant granulocyte colony-stimulating factor [published erratum appears in *J Natl Cancer Inst* 1993;85(21):1777]. *J Natl Cancer Inst* 1993;85:1499–1507.

229. Verweij J, Lund B, Beijnen J, et al. Phase I and pharmacokinetics study of topotecan, a new topoisomerase I inhibitor. *Ann Oncol* 1993;4:673–678.

230. Beran M, Kantarjian H. Topotecan in the treatment of hematologic malignancies. *Semin Hematol* 1998;35:26–31.

231. Hochster H, Liebes L, Speyer J, et al. Phase I trial of low-dose continuous topotecan infusion in patients with cancer: an active and well-tolerated regimen. *J Clin Oncol* 1994;12:553–559.

232. Mainwaring PN, Nicolson MC, Hickish T, et al. Continuous infusional topotecan in advanced breast and non–small-cell lung cancer: no evidence of increased efficacy. *Br J Cancer* 1997;76:1636–1639.

233. Kindler HL, Kris MG, Smith IE, et al. Phase II trial of topotecan administered as a 21-day continuous infusion in previously untreated patients with stage IIIB and IV non–small-cell lung cancer. *Am J Clin Oncol* 1998;21:438–441.

234. Wall JG, Burris HA, Von Hoff DD, et al. A phase I clinical and pharmacokinetic study of the topoisomerase I inhibitor topotecan (SK&F 104864) given as an intravenous bolus every 21 days. *Anticancer Drugs* 1992;3:337–345.

235. Haas NB, LaCreta FP, Walczak J, et al. Phase I/pharmacokinetic study of topotecan by 24-hour continuous infusion weekly. *Cancer Res* 1994;54:1220–1226.

236. Blaney SM, Balis FM, Cole DE, et al. Pediatric phase I trial and pharmacokinetic study of topotecan administered as a 24-hour continuous infusion. *Cancer Res* 1993;53:1032–1036.

237. Abbruzzese JL, Madden T, Sugarman SM, et al. Phase I clinical and plasma and cellular pharmacological study of topotecan without and with granulocyte colony-stimulating factor. *Clin Cancer Res* 1996;2:1489–1497.

238. Burris HA 3rd, Awada A, Kuhn JG, et al. Phase I and pharmacokinetic studies of topotecan administered as a 72 or 120 h continuous infusion. *Anticancer Drugs* 1994;5:394–402.

239. Pratt CB, Stewart C, Santana VM, et al. Phase I study of topotecan for pediatric patients with malignant solid tumors. *J Clin Oncol* 1994;12:539–543.

240. Rowinsky EK, Adjei A, Donehower RC, et al. Phase I and pharmacodynamic study of the topoisomerase I–inhibitor topotecan in patients with refractory acute leukemia. *J Clin Oncol* 1994;12:2193–2203.

241. Herben VM, Rosing H, ten Bokkel Huinink WW, et al. Oral topotecan: bioavailability and effect of food co-administration. *Br J Cancer* 1999;80:1380–1386.

242. Creemers GJ, Gerrits CJ, Eckardt JR, et al. Phase I and pharmacologic study of oral topotecan administered twice daily for 21 days to adult patients with solid tumors. *J Clin Oncol* 1997;15:1087–1093.

243. Creemers GJ, Schellens JHM, Beijnen JH, et al. Bioavailability of oral topotecan, a new topoisomerase I inhibitor. *Proc Am Soc Clin Oncol* 1995;13:132.

244. Plaxe SC, Christen RD, O'Quigley J, et al. Phase I and pharmacokinetic study of intraperitoneal topotecan. *Invest New Drugs* 1998;16:147–153.

245. Armstrong D, O'Reilly S. Clinical guidelines for managing topotecan-related hematologic toxicity. *Oncologist* 1998;3:4–10.

246. Kudelka AP, Tresukosol D, Edwards CL, et al. Phase II study of intravenous topotecan as a 5-day infusion for refractory epithelial ovarian carcinoma. *J Clin Oncol* 1996;14:1552–1557.

247. Creemers GJ, Bolis G, Gore M, et al. Topotecan, an active drug in the second-line treatment of epithelial ovarian cancer: results of a large European phase II study [see comments]. *J Clin Oncol* 1996;14:3056–3061.

248. Gordon A, Bookman M, Malmstrom H. Efficacy of topotecan in advanced epithelial ovarian cancer after failure of platinum and paclitaxel: International Topotecan Study Group trial. *Proc Am Soc Clin Oncol* 1996;15:282.

249. ten Bokkel Huinink W, Gore M, Carmichael J, et al. Topotecan versus paclitaxel for the treatment of recurrent epithelial ovarian cancer. *J Clin Oncol* 1997;15:2183–2193.

250. Beran M, Kantarjian H, O'Brien S, et al. Topotecan, a topoisomerase I inhibitor, is active in the treatment of myelodysplastic syndrome and chronic myelomonocytic leukemia. *Blood* 1996;88:2473–2479.

251. Rowinsky EK, Grochow LB, Sartorius SE, et al. Phase I and pharmacologic study of high doses of the topoisomerase I inhibitor topotecan with granulocyte colony-stimulating factor in patients with solid tumors. *J Clin Oncol* 1996;14:1224–1235.

252. Saltz L, Janik JE. Topotecan and the treatment of recurrent ovarian cancer: is there a role for granulocyte colony-stimulating factor? *Semin Oncol* 1997;24:S5-26–S5-30.

253. American Society of Clinical Oncology. Update of recommendations for the use of hematopoietic colony-stimulating factors: evidence-based clinical practice guidelines. *J Clin Oncol* 1996;14:1957–1960.

254. American Society of Clinical Oncology. Recommendations for the use of hematopoietic colony-stimulating factors: evidence-based, clinical practice guidelines. *J Clin Oncol* 1994;12:2471–2508.

255. O'Reilly S, Rowinsky EK, Slichenmyer W, et al. Phase I and pharmacologic study of topotecan in patients with impaired renal function [see comments]. *J Clin Oncol* 1996;14:3062–3073.

256. O'Reilly S, Rowinsky E, Slichenmyer W, et al. Phase I and pharmacologic studies of topotecan in patients with impaired hepatic function. *J Natl Cancer Inst* 1996;88:817–824.

257. Beijnen JH, Smith BR, Keijer WJ, et al. High-performance liquid chromatographic analysis of the new antitumour drug SK&F 104864-A (NSC 609699) in plasma. *J Pharm Biomed Anal* 1990;8:789–794.

258. Loos WJ, Stoter G, Verweij J, et al. Sensitive high-performance liquid chromatographic fluorescence assay for the quantitation of topotecan (SKF 104864-A) and its lactone ring-opened product (hydroxy acid) in human plasma and urine. *J Chromatogr B Biomed Sci Appl* 1996;678:309–315.

259. Rosing H, van Zomeren DM, Doyle E, et al. Quantification of topotecan and its metabolite *N*-desmethyltopotecan in human plasma, urine and faeces by high-performance liquid chromatographic methods. *J Chromatogr B Biomed Sci Appl* 1999;727:191–203.

260. Van Warmerdam LJ, Verweij J, Schellens JH, et al. Pharmacokinetics and pharmacodynamics of topotecan administered daily for 5 days every 3 weeks. *Cancer Chemother Pharmacol* 1995;35:237–245.

261. Van Warmerdam LJ, ten Bokkel Huinink WW, Rodenhuis S, et al. Phase I clinical and pharmacokinetic study of topotecan administered by a 24-hour continuous infusion. *J Clin Oncol* 1995;13:1768–1776.

262. Van Warmerdam LJ, Verweij J, Rosing H, et al. Limited sampling models for topotecan pharmacokinetics. *Ann Oncol* 1994;5:259–264.

263. Van Warmerdam LJ, Creemers GJ, Rodenhuis S, et al. Pharmacokinetics and pharmacodynamics of topotecan given on a daily-times-five schedule in phase II clinical trials using a limited-sampling procedure. *Cancer Chemother Pharmacol* 1996;38:254–260.

264. Tubergen DG, Stewart CF, Pratt CB, et al. Phase I trial and pharmacokinetic (PK) and pharmacodynamics (PD) study of topotecan using a five-day course in children with refractory solid tumors: a Pediatric Oncology Group study. *J Pediatr Hematol Oncol* 1996;18:352–361.

265. Stewart CF, Baker SD, Heideman RL, et al. Clinical pharmacodynamics of continuous infusion topotecan in children: systemic exposure predicts hematologic toxicity. *J Clin Oncol* 1994;12:1946–1954.

266. Lynch TJ Jr, Kalish L, Strauss G, et al. Phase II study of topotecan in metastatic non–small-cell lung cancer. *J Clin Oncol* 1994;12:347–352.

267. McCabe FL, Johnson RK. Comparative activity of oral and parenteral topotecan in murine tumor models: efficacy of oral topotecan. *Cancer Invest* 1994;12:308–313.

268. Schellens JH, Creemers GJ, Beijnen JH, et al. Bioavailability and pharmacokinetics of oral topotecan: a new topoisomerase I inhibitor. *Br J Cancer* 1996;73:1268–1271.

269. Blaney SM, Cole DE, Godwin K, et al. Intrathecal administration of topotecan in nonhuman primates. *Cancer Chemother Pharmacol* 1995;36:121–124.

270. Blaney SM, Cole DE, Balis FM, et al. Plasma and cerebrospinal fluid pharmacokinetic study of topotecan in nonhuman primates. *Cancer Res* 1993;53:725–727.

271. Sung C, Blaney SM, Cole DE, et al. A pharmacokinetic model of topotecan clearance from plasma and cerebrospinal fluid. *Cancer Res* 1994;54:5118–5122.

272. Baker SD, Heideman RL, Crom WR, et al. Cerebrospinal fluid pharmacokinetics and penetration of continuous infusion topotecan in children with central nervous system tumors. *Cancer Chemother Pharmacol* 1996;37:195–202.

273. Mi Z, Malak H, Burke TG. Reduced albumin binding promotes the stability and activity of topotecan in human blood. *Biochemistry* 1995;34:13722–13728.

274. Rosing H, Herben VM, van Gortel-van Zomeren DM, et al. Isolation and structural confirmation of N-desmethyl topotecan, a metabolite of topotecan. *Cancer Chemother Pharmacol* 1997;39:498–504.

275. Furman WL, Baker SD, Pratt CB, et al. Escalating systemic exposure of continuous infusion topotecan in children with recurrent acute leukemia. *J Clin Oncol* 1996;14:1504–1511.

276. Blaney SM, Phillips PC, Packer RJ, et al. Phase II evaluation of topotecan for pediatric central nervous system tumors. *Cancer* 1996;78:527–531.

277. Rowinsky EK, Kaufmann SH, Baker SD, et al. Sequences of topotecan and cisplatin: phase I, pharmacologic, and in vitro studies to examine sequence dependence [see comments]. *J Clin Oncol* 1996;14:3074–3084.

278. Swisher EM, Mutch DG, Rader JS, et al. Topotecan in platinum- and paclitaxel-resistant ovarian cancer. *Gynecol Oncol* 1997;66:480–486.

279. Bookman MA, Malmstrom H, Bolis G, et al. Topotecan for the treatment of advanced epithelial ovarian cancer: an open-label phase II study in patients treated after prior chemotherapy that contained cisplatin or carboplatin and paclitaxel. *J Clin Oncol* 1998;16:3345–3352.

280. Hoskins P, Eisenhauer E, Beare S, et al. Randomized phase II study of two schedules of topotecan in previously treated patients with ovarian cancer: a National Cancer Institute of Canada Clinical Trials Group study. *J Clin Oncol* 1998;16:2233–2237.

281. Von Pawel J, Schiller JH, Shepherd FA, et al. Topotecan versus cyclophosphamide, doxorubicin, and vincristine for the treatment of recurrent small-cell lung cancer. *J Clin Oncol* 1999;17:658–667.

282. Ardizzoni A, Hansen H, Dombernowsky P, et al. Topotecan, a new active drug in the second-line treatment of small-

cell lung cancer: a phase II study in patients with refractory and sensitive disease. The European Organization for Research and Treatment of Cancer Early Clinical Studies Group and New Drug Development Office, and the Lung Cancer Cooperative Group. *J Clin Oncol* 1997;15:2090–2096.

283. Schiller JH, Kim K, Hutson P, et al. Phase II study of topotecan in patients with extensive-stage small-cell carcinoma of the lung: an Eastern Cooperative Oncology Group Trial. *J Clin Oncol* 1996;14:2345–2352.

284. Perez-Soler R, Fossella FV, Glisson BS, et al. Phase II study of topotecan in patients with advanced non–small-cell lung cancer previously untreated with chemotherapy. *J Clin Oncol* 1996;14:503–513.

285. Greenberg BR, Reynolds RD, Charron CB, et al. Treatment of myelodysplastic syndromes with daily oral idarubicin. A phase I–II study. *Cancer* 1993;71:1989–1992.

286. Tricot G, De Bock R, Dekker AW, et al. Low dose cytosine arabinoside (Ara C) in myelodysplastic syndromes. *Br J Haematol* 1984;58:231–240.

287. Kantarjian HM, Beran M, Ellis A, et al. Phase I study of topotecan, a new topoisomerase I inhibitor, in patients with refractory or relapsed acute leukemia. *Blood* 1993;81:1146–1151.

288. Gore SD, Rowinsky EK, Miller CB, et al. A phase II "window" study of topotecan in untreated patients with high risk adult acute lymphoblastic leukemia [see comments]. *Clin Cancer Res* 1998;4:2677–2689.

289. Kraut EH, Crowley JJ, Wade JL, et al. Evaluation of topotecan in resistant and relapsing multiple myeloma: a Southwest Oncology Group study. *J Clin Oncol* 1998;16:589–592.

290. O'Brien S, Kantarjian H, Ellis A, et al. Topotecan in chronic lymphocytic leukemia. *Cancer* 1995;75:1104–1108.

291. Seiter K, Feldman EJ, Halicka HD, et al. Phase I clinical and laboratory evaluation of topotecan and cytarabine in patients with acute leukemia. *J Clin Oncol* 1997;15:44–51.

292. Kretschmar C, Kletzel M, Murray K, et al. Upfront phase II therapy with Taxol (Txl) and topotecan in untreated children (>365 days) with disseminated (INSS stage 4) neuroblastoma. *Med Pediat Oncol* 1995;25:243.

293. Nitschke R, Parkhurst J, Sullivan J, et al. Topotecan in pediatric patients with recurrent and progressive solid tumors: a Pediatric Oncology Group phase II study. *J Pediatr Hematol Oncol* 1998;20:315–318.

294. Friedman HS, Kerby T, Fields S, et al. Topotecan treatment of adults with primary malignant glioma. The Brain Tumor Center at Duke. *Cancer* 1999;85:1160–1165.

295. Macdonald D, Cairncross G, Stewart D, et al. Phase II study of topotecan in patients with recurrent malignant glioma. National Clinical Institute of Canada Clinical Trials Group. *Ann Oncol* 1996;7:205–207.

296. Kadota RP, Stewart CF, Horn M, et al. Topotecan for the treatment of recurrent or progressive central nervous system tumors—a pediatric oncology group phase II study. *J Neurooncol* 1999;43:43–47.

297. Creemers GJ, Wanders J, Gamucci T, et al. Topotecan in colorectal cancer: a phase II study of the EORTC early clinical trials group. *Ann Oncol* 1995;6:844–846.

298. Macdonald JS, Benedetti JK, Modiano M, et al. Phase II evaluation of topotecan in patients with advanced colorectal

cancer. A Southwest Oncology Group trial (SWOG 9241). *Invest New Drugs* 1997;15:357–359.

299. Rowinsky EK, Baker SD, Burks K, et al. High-dose topotecan with granulocyte-colony stimulating factor in fluoropyrimidine-refractory colorectal cancer: a phase II and pharmacodynamic study. *Ann Oncol* 1998;9:173–180.

300. Creemers GJ, Gerrits CJ, Schellens JH, et al. Phase II and pharmacologic study of topotecan administered as a 21-day continuous infusion to patients with colorectal cancer. *J Clin Oncol* 1996;14:2540–2545.

301. Stevenson JP, Scher RM, Kosierowski R, et al. Phase II trial of topotecan as a 21-day continuous infusion in patients with advanced or metastatic adenocarcinoma of the pancreas. *Eur J Cancer* 1998;34:1358–1362.

302. Scher RM, Kosierowski R, Lusch C, et al. Phase II trial of topotecan in advanced or metastatic adenocarcinoma of the pancreas. *Invest New Drugs* 1996;13:347–354.

303. O'Reilly S, Donehower RC, Rowinsky EK, et al. A phase II trial of topotecan in patients with previously untreated pancreatic cancer. *Anticancer Drugs* 1996;7:410–414.

304. Wall JG, Benedetti JK, O'Rourke MA, et al. Phase II trial to topotecan in hepatocellular carcinoma: a Southwest Oncology Group study. *Invest New Drugs* 1997;15:257–260.

305. Saltz LB, Schwartz GK, Ilson DH, et al. A phase II study of topotecan administered five times daily in patients with advanced gastric cancer. *Am J Clin Oncol* 1997;20:621–625.

306. Benedetti JK, Burris HA 3rd, Balcerzak SP, et al. Phase II trial of topotecan in advanced gastric cancer: a Southwest Oncology Group study. *Invest New Drugs* 1997;15:261–264.

307. Bramwell VH, Eisenhauer EA, Blackstein M, et al. Phase II study of topotecan (NSC 609 699) in patients with recurrent or metastatic soft tissue sarcoma. *Ann Oncol* 1995;6:847–849.

308. Puc HS, Bajorin DF, Bosl GJ, et al. Phase II trial of topotecan in patients with cisplatin-refractory germ cell tumors. *Invest New Drugs* 1995;13:163–165.

309. Hudes GR, Kosierowski R, Greenberg R, et al. Phase II study of topotecan in metastatic hormone-refractory prostate cancer. *Invest New Drugs* 1995;13:235–240.

310. Kraut EH, Walker MJ, Staubus A, et al. Phase II trial of topotecan in malignant melanoma. *Cancer Invest* 1997;15:318–320.

311. Smith RE, Lew D, Rodriguez GI, et al. Evaluation of topotecan in patients with recurrent or metastatic squamous cell carcinoma of the head and neck. A phase II Southwest Oncology Group study. *Invest New Drugs* 1996;14:403–407.

312. Robert F, Soong SJ, Wheeler RH. A phase II study of topotecan in patients with recurrent head and neck cancer. Identification of an active new agent. *Am J Clin Oncol* 1997;20:298–302.

313. Levine EG, Cirrincione CT, Szatrowski TP, et al. Phase II trial of topotecan in advanced breast cancer: a Cancer and Leukemia Group B study. *Am J Clin Oncol* 1999;22:218–222.

314. Witte RS, Manola J, Burch PA, et al. Topotecan in previously treated advanced urothelial carcinoma: an ECOG phase II trial. *Invest New Drugs* 1998;16:191–195.

315. Maksymiuk AW, Marschke RF Jr, Tazelaar HD, et al. Phase II trial of topotecan for the treatment of mesothelioma. *Am J Clin Oncol* 1998;21:610–613.

316. Law TM, Ilson DH, Motzer RJ. Phase II trial of topotecan in patients with advanced renal cell carcinoma. *Invest New Drugs* 1994;12:143–145.

317. Fukuda M, Nishio K, Kanzawa F, et al. Synergism between cisplatin and topoisomerase I inhibitors, NB-506 and SN-38, in human small cell lung cancer cells. *Cancer Res* 1996; 56:789–793.

318. Romanelli S, Perego P, Pratesi G, et al. In vitro and in vivo interaction between cisplatin and topotecan in ovarian carcinoma systems. *Cancer Chemother Pharmacol* 1998;41:385–390.

319. Matsumoto N, Nakano S, Esaki T, et al. Inhibition of cis-diamminedichloroplatinum (II)-induced DNA interstrand cross-link removal by 7-ethyl-10-hydroxy-camptothecin in HST-1 human squamous-carcinoma cells. *Int J Cancer* 1995;62:70–75.

320. Ma J, Maliepaard M, Nooter K, et al. Synergistic cytotoxicity of cisplatin and topotecan or SN-38 in a panel of eight solid-tumor cell lines in vitro. *Cancer Chemother Pharmacol* 1998;41:307–316.

321. Miller AA, Hargis JB, Lilenbaum RC, et al. Phase I study of topotecan and cisplatin in patients with advanced solid tumors: a cancer and leukemia group B study. *J Clin Oncol* 1994;12:2743–2750.

322. Miller AA, Lilenbaum RC, Lynch TJ, et al. Treatment-related fatal sepsis from topotecan/cisplatin and topotecan/paclitaxel [Letter]. *J Clin Oncol* 1996;14:1964–1965.

323. Raymond E, Burris HA, Rowinsky EK, et al. Phase I study of daily times five topotecan and single injection of cisplatin in patients with previously untreated non–small-cell lung carcinoma. *Ann Oncol* 1997;8:1003–1008.

324. Lilenbaum RC, Miller AA, Batist G, et al. Phase I and pharmacologic study of continuous infusion topotecan in combination with cisplatin in patients with advanced cancer: a Cancer and Leukemia Group B study. *J Clin Oncol* 1998;16:3302–3309.

325. Lilenbaum RC, Ratain MJ, Miller AA, et al. Phase I study of paclitaxel and topotecan in patients with advanced tumors: a cancer and leukemia group B study. *J Clin Oncol* 1995;13:2230–2237.

326. Chou TC, Motzer RJ, Tong Y, et al. Computerized quantitation of synergism and antagonism of Taxol, topotecan, and cisplatin against human teratocarcinoma cell growth: a rational approach to clinical protocol design [see comments]. *J Natl Cancer Inst* 1994;86:1517–1524.

327. Fleming GF, Kugler JW, Hoffman PC, et al. Phase II trial of paclitaxel and topotecan with granulocyte colony-stimulating factor support in stage IV breast cancer. *J Clin Oncol* 1998;16:2032–2037.

328. O'Reilly S, Fleming GF, Barker SD, et al. Phase I trial and pharmacologic trial of sequences of paclitaxel and topotecan in previously treated ovarian epithelial malignancies: a Gynecologic Oncology Group study. *J Clin Oncol* 1997;15:177–186.

329. Herben VM, Panday VR, Richel DJ, et al. Phase I and pharmacologic study of the combination of paclitaxel, cisplatin, and topotecan administered intravenously every 21 days as first-line therapy in patients with advanced ovarian cancer [see comments]. *J Clin Oncol* 1999;17:747–755.

330. Frasci G, Panza N, Comella P, et al. Cisplatin-topotecan-paclitaxel weekly administration with G-CSF support for ovarian and small-cell lung cancer patients: a dose-finding study. *Ann Oncol* 1999;10:355–358.

331. Hainsworth JD, Burris HA 3rd, Morrissey LH, et al. Phase I trial of paclitaxel, carboplatin, and topotecan with or without filgrastim (granulocyte-colony stimulating factor) in the treatment of patients with advanced, refractory cancer. *Cancer* 1999;85:1179–1185.

332. Kaufmann SH. Antagonism between camptothecin and topoisomerase II–directed chemotherapeutic agents in a human leukemia cell line. *Cancer Res* 1991;51:1129–1136.

333. Bertrand R, O'Connor PM, Kerrigan D, et al. Sequential administration of camptothecin and etoposide circumvents the antagonistic cytotoxicity of simultaneous drug administration in slowly growing human colon carcinoma HT-29 cells. *Eur J Cancer* 1992;28A:743–748.

334. Masumoto N, Nakano S, Esaki T, et al. Sequence-dependent modulation of anticancer drug activities by 7-ethyl-10-hydroxycamptothecin in an HST-1 human squamous carcinoma cell line. *Anticancer Res* 1995;15:405–409.

335. Whitacre CM, Zborowska E, Gordon NH, et al. Topotecan increases topoisomerase IIalpha levels and sensitivity to treatment with etoposide in schedule-dependent process. *Cancer Res* 1997;57:1425–1428.

336. Kim R, Hirabayashi N, Nishiyama M, et al. Experimental studies on biochemical modulation targeting topoisomerase I and II in human tumor xenografts in nude mice. *Int J Cancer* 1992;50:760–766.

337. Bonner JA, Kozelsky TF. The significance of the sequence of administration of topotecan and etoposide. *Cancer Chemother Pharmacol* 1996;39:109–112.

338. Nicklee T, Crump M, Hedley DW. Effects of topoisomerase I inhibition on the expression of topoisomerase II alpha measured with fluorescence image cytometry. *Cytometry* 1996;25:205–210.

339. Herben VM, ten Bokkel Huinink WW, Dubbelman AC, et al. Phase I and pharmacological study of sequential intravenous topotecan and oral etoposide [see comments]. *Br J Cancer* 1997;76:1500–1508.

340. Hammond LA, Eckardt JR, Ganapathi R, et al. A phase I and translational study of sequential administration of the topoisomerase I and II inhibitors topotecan and etoposide. *Clin Cancer Res* 1998;4:1459–1467.

341. Crump M, Lipton J, Hedley D, et al. Phase I trial of sequential topotecan followed by etoposide in adults with myeloid leukemia: a National Cancer Institute of Canada Clinical Trials Group Study. *Leukemia* 1999;13:343–347.

342. Tolcher AW, O'Shaughnessy JA, Weiss RB, et al. A phase I study of topotecan followed sequentially by doxorubicin in patients with advanced malignancies. *Clin Cancer Res* 1997;3:755–760.

343. Gupta E, Toppmeyer D, Zamek R, et al. Clinical evaluation of sequential topoisomerase targeting in the treatment of advanced malignancy. *Cancer Ther* 1998;1:292–301.

344. Saylors RL 3rd, Stewart CF, Zamboni WC, et al. Phase I study of topotecan in combination with cyclophosphamide in pediatric patients with malignant solid tumors: a Pediatric Oncology Group study. *J Clin Oncol* 1998;16:945–952.

345. Graham MV, Jahanzeb M, Dresler CM, et al. Results of a trial with topotecan dose escalation and concurrent thoracic radiation therapy for locally advanced, inoperable nonsmall cell lung cancer. *Int J Radiat Oncol Biol Phys* 1996;36:1215–1220.

346. Wani MC, Ronman PE, Lindley JT, et al. Plant antitumor agents. 18. Synthesis and biological activity of camptothecin analogues. *J Med Chem* 1980;23:554–560.

347. Kunimoto T, Nitta K, Tanaka T, et al. Antitumor activity of 7-ethyl-10-[4-(1-piperidino)-1-piperidino]carbonyloxy-camptothecin, a novel water-soluble derivative of camptothecin, against murine tumors. *Cancer Res* 1987;47:5944–5947.

348. Furuta T, Yokokura T, Mutai M. Antitumor activity of CPT-11 against rat Walker 256 carcinoma. *Gan To Kagaku Ryoho* 1988;15:2757–2760.

349. Hare CB, Elion GB, Houghton PJ, et al. Therapeutic efficacy of the topoisomerase I inhibitor 7-ethyl-10-(4-[1-piperidino]-1-piperidino)-carbonyloxy-camptothecin against pediatric and adult central nervous system tumor xenografts. *Cancer Chemother Pharmacol* 1997;39:187–191.

350. Miki T, Sawada M, Nonomura N, et al. Antitumor effect of CPT-11, a camptothecin derivative, on human testicular tumor xenografts in nude mice. *Eur Urol* 1997;31:92–96.

351. Vassal G, Boland I, Santos A, et al. Potent therapeutic activity of irinotecan (CPT-11) and its schedule dependency in medulloblastoma xenografts in nude mice. *Int J Cancer* 1997;73:156–163.

352. Thompson J, Zamboni WC, Cheshire PJ, et al. Efficacy of systemic administration of irinotecan against neuroblastoma xenografts. *Clin Cancer Res* 1997;3:423–431.

353. Vassal G, Terrier-Lacombe MJ, Bissery MC, et al. Therapeutic activity of CPT-11, a DNA-topoisomerase I inhibitor, against peripheral primitive neuroectodermal tumour and neuroblastoma xenografts. *Br J Cancer* 1996;74:537–545.

354. Lievano G, Mirochnik Y, Rubenstein M, et al. Antitumor effect of CPT-11, a new derivative of camptothecin, against human prostate cancer (PC-3) in vitro and prostate rat tumor (AT-3) in vivo. *Methods Find Exp Clin Pharmacol* 1996;18:659–662.

355. Furuta T, Yokokura T. Effect of administration schedules on the antitumor activity of CPT-11, a camptothecin derivative. *Gan To Kagaku Ryoho* 1990;17:121–130.

356. Houghton PJ, Cheshire PJ, Hallman JD 2nd, et al. Efficacy of topoisomerase I inhibitors, topotecan and irinotecan, administered at low dose levels in protracted schedules to mice bearing xenografts of human tumors. *Cancer Chemother Pharmacol* 1995;36:393–403.

357. Catimel G, Chabot GG, Guastalla JP, et al. Phase I and pharmacokinetic study of irinotecan (CPT-11) administered daily for three consecutive days every three weeks in patients with advanced solid tumors [see comments]. *Ann Oncol* 1995;6:133–140.

358. Rothenberg ML, Kuhn JG, Schaaf LJ, et al. Alternative dosing schedules for irinotecan. *Oncology (Huntingt)* 1998;12:68–71.

359. Furman WL, Stewart CF, Poquette CA, et al. Direct translation of a protracted irinotecan schedule from a xenograft model to a phase I trial in children. *J Clin Oncol* 1999;17:1815–1824.

360. Takimoto CH, Morrison G, Harold N, et al. A phase I and pharmacologic study of irinotecan administered as a 96-hour infusion weekly to adult cancer patients. *J Clin Oncol* 2000;18(3):659–667.

361. Herben VM, Schellens JH, Swart M, et al. Phase I and pharmacokinetic study of irinotecan administered as a low-dose, continuous intravenous infusion over 14 days in patients with malignant solid tumors. *J Clin Oncol* 1999;17:1897–1905.

362. Herben VMM, Schellens JHM, Swart M, et al. Phase I and pharmacokinetic study of irinotecan administered as a low-dose, continuous intravenous infusion over 14 days in patients with malignant solid tumors. *J Clin Oncol* 1999;17:1897–1905.

363. Drengler RL, Kuhn JG, Schaaf LJ, et al. Phase I and pharmacokinetic trial of oral irinotecan administered daily for 5 days every 3 weeks in patients with solid tumors. *J Clin Oncol* 1999;17:685–696.

364. Rougier P, Bugat R. CPT-11 in the treatment of colorectal cancer: clinical efficacy and safety profile. *Semin Oncol* 1996;23:34–41.

365. Abigerges D, Armand JP, Chabot GG, et al. Irinotecan (CPT-11) high-dose escalation using intensive high-dose loperamide to control diarrhea. *J Natl Cancer Inst* 1994;86:446–449.

366. Abigerges D, Chabot GG, Armand JP, et al. Phase I and pharmacologic studies of the camptothecin analog irinotecan administered every 3 weeks in cancer patients. *J Clin Oncol* 1995;13:210–221.

367. Conti JA, Kemeny NE, Saltz LB, et al. Irinotecan is an active agent in untreated patients with metastatic colorectal cancer. *J Clin Oncol* 1996;14:709–715.

368. Rothenberg ML, Eckardt JR, Kuhn JG, et al. Phase II trial of irinotecan in patients with progressive or rapidly recurrent colorectal cancer. *J Clin Oncol* 1996;14:1128–1135.

369. Merrouche Y, Extra JM, Abigerges D, et al. High dose-intensity of irinotecan administered every 3 weeks in advanced cancer patients: a feasibility study. *J Clin Oncol* 1997;15:1080–1086.

370. Ikuno N, Soda H, Watanabe M, et al. Irinotecan (CPT-11) and characteristic mucosal changes in the mouse ileum and cecum [see comments]. *J Natl Cancer Inst* 1995;87:1876–1883.

371. Saliba F, Hagipantelli R, Misset JL, et al. Pathophysiology and therapy of irinotecan-induced delayed-onset diarrhea in patients with advanced colorectal cancer: a prospective assessment. *J Clin Oncol* 1998;16:2745–2751.

372. Von Hoff DD, Rothenberg ML, Pitot HC, et al. Irinotecan (CPT-11) therapy for patients with previously treated metastatic colorectal cancer (CRC): overall results of FDA-reviewed pivotal US clinical trials. *Proc Am Soc Clin Oncol* 1997;16:228a.

373. De Forni M, Bugat R, Chabot GG, et al. Phase I and pharmacokinetic study of the camptothecin derivative irinotecan, administered on a weekly schedule in cancer patients. *Cancer Res* 1994;54:4347–4354.

374. Bozec L, Bierling P, Fromont P, et al. Irinotecan-induced immune thrombocytopenia. *Ann Oncol* 1998;9:453–455.

375. Rowinsky EK, Grochow LB, Ettinger DS, et al. Phase I and pharmacological study of the novel topoisomerase I inhibitor 7-ethyl-10-[4-(1-piperidino)-1-piperidino]carbonyloxy-camptothecin (CPT-11) administered as a ninety-minute infusion every 3 weeks. *Cancer Res* 1994;54:427–436.

376. Miya T, Fujikawa R, Fukushima J, et al. Bradycardia induced by irinotecan: a case report. *Jpn J Clin Oncol* 1998;28:709–711.

377. Kawato Y, Sekiguchi M, Akahane K, et al. Inhibitory activity of camptothecin derivatives against acetylcholinesterase in dogs and their binding activity to acetylcholine receptors in rats. *J Pharm Pharmacol* 1993;45:444–448.

378. Fukuoka M, Niitani H, Suzuki A, et al. A phase II study of CPT-11, a new derivative of camptothecin, for previously untreated non-small-cell lung cancer [see comments]. *J Clin Oncol* 1992;10:16–20.

379. Masuda N, Fukuoka M, Kusunoki Y, et al. CPT-11: a new derivative of camptothecin for the treatment of refractory or relapsed small-cell lung cancer. *J Clin Oncol* 1992;10:1225–1229.

380. Camptosar [package insert]. Peapack, NJ: Pharmacia & Upjohn, 1996.

381. Boisseau M, Bugat R, Mahjoubi M. Rapid tumour lysis syndrome in a metastatic colorectal cancer increased by treatment (CPT-11) [Letter]. *Eur J Cancer* 1996;32A:737–738.

382. Sevilla Garcia I, Rueda A, Alba E. Irinotecan-induced central nervous system toxicity: a case report [Letter]. *J Natl Cancer Inst* 1999;91:647.

383. Chabot GG, Abigerges D, Catimel G, et al. Population pharmacokinetics and pharmacodynamics of irinotecan (CPT-11) and active metabolite SN-38 during phase I trials. *Ann Oncol* 1995;6:141–151.

384. Barilero I, Gandia D, Armand JP, et al. Simultaneous determination of the camptothecin analogue CPT-11 and its active metabolite SN-38 by high-performance liquid chromatography: application to plasma pharmacokinetic studies in cancer patients. *J Chromatogr* 1992;575:275–280.

385. Sumiyoshi H, Fujiwara Y, Ohune T, et al. High-performance liquid chromatographic determination of irinotecan (CPT-11) and its active metabolite (SN-38) in human plasma. *J Chromatogr B Biomed Sci Appl* 1995;670:309–316.

386. Rivory LP, Robert J. Reversed-phase high-performance liquid chromatographic method for the simultaneous quantitation of the carboxylate and lactone forms of the camptothecin derivative irinotecan, CPT-11, and its metabolite SN-38 in plasma. *J Chromatogr B Biomed Sci Appl* 1994;661:133–141.

387. Kaneda N, Hosokawa Y, Yokokura T. Simultaneous determination of the lactone and carboxylate forms of 7-ethyl-10-hydroxycamptothecin (SN-38), the active metabolite of irinotecan (CPT-11), in rat plasma by high performance liquid chromatography. *Biol Pharm Bull* 1997;20:815–819.

388. De Bruijn P, Verweij J, Loos WJ, et al. Determination of irinotecan (CPT-11) and its active metabolite SN-38 in human plasma by reversed-phase high-performance liquid chromatography with fluorescence detection. *J Chromatogr B Biomed Sci Appl* 1997;698:277–285.

389. Chollet DF, Goumaz L, Renard A, et al. Simultaneous determination of the lactone and carboxylate forms of the camptothecin derivative CPT-11 and its metabolite SN-38 in plasma by high-performance liquid chromatography. *J Chromatogr B Biomed Sci Appl* 1998;718:163–175.

390. Sparreboom A, de Bruijn P, de Jonge MJ, et al. Liquid chromatographic determination of irinotecan and three major metabolites in human plasma, urine and feces. *J Chromatogr B Biomed Sci Appl* 1998;712:225–235.

391. Kurita A, Kaneda N. High-performance liquid chromatographic method for the simultaneous determination of the camptothecin derivative irinotecan hydrochloride, CPT-11, and its metabolites SN-38 and SN-38 glucuronide in rat plasma with a fully automated on-line solid-phase extraction system, PROSPEKT. *J Chromatogr B Biomed Sci Appl* 1999;724:335–344.

392. Takahashi T, Fujiwara Y, Sumiyoshi H, et al. Salivary drug monitoring of irinotecan and its active metabolite in cancer patients. *Cancer Chemother Pharmacol* 1997;40:449–452.

393. Ohe Y, Sasaki Y, Shinkai T, et al. Phase I study and pharmacokinetics of CPT-11 with 5-day continuous infusion. *J Natl Cancer Inst* 1992;84:972–974.

394. Negoro S, Fukuoka M, Masuda N, et al. Phase I study of weekly intravenous infusions of CPT-11, a new derivative of camptothecin, in the treatment of advanced non-small-cell lung cancer. *J Natl Cancer Inst* 1991;83:1164–1168.

395. Gupta E, Lestingi TM, Mick R, et al. Metabolic fate of irinotecan in humans: correlation of glucuronidation with diarrhea. *Cancer Res* 1994;54:3723–3725.

396. Atsumi R, Okazaki O, Hakusui H. Pharmacokinetics of SN-38 [(+)-(4S)-4,11-diethyl-4,9-dihydroxy-1H-pyrano[3′,4′:6,7]-indolizino[1,2-b]quinoline-3,14(4H,12H)-dione], an active metabolite of irinotecan, after a single intravenous dosing of 14C-SN-38 to rats. *Biol Pharm Bull* 1995;18:1114–1119.

397. Kaneda N, Hosokawa Y, Yokokura T, et al. Plasma pharmacokinetics of 7-ethyl-10-hydroxycamptothecin (SN-38) after intravenous administration of SN-38 and irinotecan (CPT-11) to rats. *Biol Pharm Bull* 1997;20:992–996.

398. Gupta E, Mick R, Ramirez J, et al. Pharmacokinetic and pharmacodynamic evaluation of the topoisomerase inhibitor irinotecan in cancer patients. *J Clin Oncol* 1997;15:1502–1510.

399. Yamamoto N, Tamura T, Karato A, et al. CPT-11: population pharmacokinetic model and estimation of pharmacokinetics using the Bayesian method in patients with lung cancer. *Jpn J Cancer Res* 1994;85:972–977.

400. Nakashima H, Lieberman R, Karato A, et al. Efficient sampling strategies for forecasting pharmacokinetic parameters of irinotecan (CPT-11): implication for area under the concentration-time curve monitoring. *Ther Drug Monit* 1995;17:221–229.

401. Sasaki Y, Mizuno S, Fujii H, et al. A limited sampling model for estimating pharmacokinetics of CPT-11 and its metabolite SN-38. *Jpn J Cancer Res* 1995;86:117–123.

402. Chabot GG. Limited sampling models for simultaneous estimation of the pharmacokinetics of irinotecan and its active metabolite SN-38. *Cancer Chemother Pharmacol* 1995;36:463–472.

403. Canal P, Gay C, Dezeuze A, et al. Pharmacokinetics and pharmacodynamics of irinotecan during a phase II clinical trial in colorectal cancer. Pharmacology and Molecular Mechanisms Group of the European Organization for Research and Treatment of Cancer. *J Clin Oncol* 1996;14:2688–2695.

404. Burke TG, Mi Z. The structural basis of camptothecin interactions with human serum albumin: impact on drug stability. *J Med Chem* 1994;37:40–46.

405. Mi Z, Burke TG. Marked interspecies variations concerning the interactions of camptothecin with serum albumins: a frequency-domain fluorescence spectroscopic study. *Biochemistry* 1994;33:12540–12545.

406. Irinotecan hydrochloride trihydrate [investigator brochure]. Kalamazoo, MI: Upjohn Company, 1994.

407. Sasaki Y, Yoshida Y, Sudoh K, et al. Pharmacological correlation between total drug concentration and lactones of CPT-11 and SN-38 in patients treated with CPT-11. *Jpn J Cancer Res* 1995;86:111–116.

408. Thompson J, Zamboni WC, Cheshire PJ, et al. Efficacy of oral irinotecan against neuroblastoma xenografts. *Anticancer Drugs* 1997;8:313–322.

409. Choi SH, Tsuchida Y, Yang HW. Oral versus intraperitoneal administration of irinotecan in the treatment of human neuroblastoma in nude mice. *Cancer Lett* 1998;124:15–21.

410. Stewart CF, Zamboni WC, Crom WR, et al. Disposition of irinotecan and SN-38 following oral and intravenous irinotecan dosing in mice. *Cancer Chemother Pharmacol* 1997; 40:259–265.

411. Guichard S, Chatelut E, Lochon I, et al. Comparison of the pharmacokinetics and efficacy of irinotecan after administration by the intravenous versus intraperitoneal route in mice. *Cancer Chemother Pharmacol* 1998;42:165–170.

412. Blaney SM, Takimoto C, Murry DJ, et al. Plasma and cerebrospinal fluid pharmacokinetics of 9-aminocamptothecin (9-AC), irinotecan (CPT-11), and SN-38 in nonhuman primates. *Cancer Chemother Pharmacol* 1998;41:464–468.

413. Araki E, Ishikawa M, Iigo M, et al. Relationship between development of diarrhea and the concentration of SN-38, an active metabolite of CPT-11, in the intestine and the blood plasma of athymic mice following intraperitoneal administration of CPT-11. *Jpn J Cancer Res* 1993;84:697–702.

414. Nakano T, Chahinian AP, Shinjo M, et al. Cisplatin in combination with irinotecan in the treatment of patients with malignant pleural mesothelioma: a pilot phase II clinical trial and pharmacokinetic profile. *Cancer* 1999;85:2375–2384.

415. Rivory LP, Haaz MC, Canal P, et al. Pharmacokinetic inter-relationships of irinotecan (CPT-11) and its three major plasma metabolites in patients enrolled in phase I/II trials. *Clin Cancer Res* 1997;3:1261–1266.

416. Sasaki Y, Hakusui H, Mizuno S, et al. A pharmacokinetic and pharmacodynamic analysis of CPT-11 and its active metabolite SN-38. *Jpn J Cancer Res* 1995;86:101–110.

417. Satoh T, Hosokawa M, Atsumi R, et al. Metabolic activation of CPT-11, 7-ethyl-10-[4-(1-piperidino)-1-piperidino]carbonyloxycamptothecin, a novel antitumor agent, by carboxylesterase. *Biol Pharm Bull* 1994;17:662–664.

418. Danks MK, Morton CL, Krull EJ, et al. Comparison of activation of CPT-11 by rabbit and human carboxylesterases for use in enzyme/prodrug therapy. *Clin Cancer Res* 1999;5:917–924.

419. Hosokawa M, Endo T, Fujisawa M, et al. Interindividual variation in carboxylesterase levels in human liver microsomes. *Drug Metab Dispos* 1995;23:1022–1027.

420. Kaneda N, Kurita A, Hosokawa Y, et al. Intravenous administration of irinotecan elevates the blood beta-glucuronidase activity in rats. *Cancer Res* 1997;57:5305–5308.

421. Rivory LP, Riou JF, Haaz MC, et al. Identification and properties of a major plasma metabolite of irinotecan (CPT-11) isolated from the plasma of patients. *Cancer Res* 1996;56:3689–3694.

422. Haaz MC, Rivory L, Jantet S, et al. Glucuronidation of SN-38, the active metabolite of irinotecan, by human hepatic microsomes. *Pharmacol Toxicol* 1997;80:91–96.

423. Slatter JG, Su P, Sams JP, et al. Bioactivation of the anticancer agent CPT-11 to SN-38 by human hepatic microsomal carboxylesterases and the in vitro assessment of potential drug interactions. *Drug Metab Dispos* 1997;25:1157–1164.

424. Morton CL, Wadkins RM, Danks MK, et al. The anticancer prodrug CPT-11 is a potent inhibitor of acetylcholinesterase but is rapidly catalyzed to SN-38 by butyrylcholinesterase. *Cancer Res* 1999;59:1458–1463.

425. Lockridge O. Genetic variants of human serum cholinesterase influence metabolism of the muscle relaxant succinylcholine. *Pharmacol Ther* 1990;47:35–60.

426. Atsumi R, Okazaki O, Hakusui H. Metabolism of irinotecan to SN-38 in a tissue-isolated tumor model. *Biol Pharm Bull* 1995;18:1024–1026.

427. Guichard S, Terret C, Hennebelle I, et al. CPT-11 converting carboxylesterase and topoisomerase activities in tumour and normal colon and liver tissues. *Br J Cancer* 1999;80: 364–370.

428. Van Ark-Otte J, Kedde MA, van der Vijgh WJ, et al. Determinants of CPT-11 and SN-38 activities in human lung cancer cells. *Br J Cancer* 1998;77:2171–2176.

429. Danks MK, Morton CL, Pawlik CA, et al. Overexpression of a rabbit liver carboxylesterase sensitizes human tumor cells to CPT-11. *Cancer Res* 1998;58:20–22.

430. Kojima A, Hackett NR, Crystal RG. Reversal of CPT-11 resistance of lung cancer cells by adenovirus-mediated gene transfer of the human carboxylesterase cDNA. *Cancer Res* 1998;58:4368–4374.

431. Haaz MC, Rivory L, Riche C, et al. Metabolism of irinotecan (CPT-11) by human hepatic microsomes: participation of cytochrome P-450 3A and drug interactions. *Cancer Res* 1998;58:468–472.

432. Dodds HM, Haaz MC, Riou JF, et al. Identification of a new metabolite of CPT-11 (irinotecan): pharmacological properties and activation to SN-38. *J Pharmacol Exp Ther* 1998;286:578–583.

433. Lokiec F, du Sorbier BM, Sanderink GJ. Irinotecan (CPT-11) metabolites in human bile and urine. *Clin Cancer Res* 1996;2:1943–1949.

434. Rivory LP, Robert J. Identification and kinetics of a beta-glucuronide metabolite of SN-38 in human plasma after administration of the camptothecin derivative irinotecan. *Cancer Chemother Pharmacol* 1995;36:176–179.

435. Iyer L, King CD, Whitington PF, et al. Genetic predisposition to the metabolism of irinotecan (CPT-11). Role of uridine diphosphate glucuronosyltransferase isoform 1A1 in the glucuronidation of its active metabolite (SN-38) in human liver microsomes. *J Clin Invest* 1998;101:847–854.

436. Gupta E, Wang X, Ramirez J, et al. Modulation of glucuronidation of SN-38, the active metabolite of irinotecan, by valproic acid and phenobarbital. *Cancer Chemother Pharmacol* 1997;39:440–444.

437. Wasserman E, Myara A, Lokiec F, et al. Severe CPT-11 toxicity in patients with Gilbert's syndrome: two case reports. *Ann Oncol* 1997;8:1049–1051.

438. Iyer L, Hall D, Das S, et al. Phenotype-genotype correlation of in vitro SN-38 (active metabolite of irinotecan) and bilirubin glucuronidation in human liver tissue with UGT1A1 promoter polymorphism. *Clin Pharmacol Ther* 1999;65:576–582.

439. Lokiec F, Canal P, Gay C, et al. Pharmacokinetics of irinotecan and its metabolites in human blood, bile, and urine. *Cancer Chemother Pharmacol* 1995;36:79–82.

440. Chu XY, Kato Y, Niinuma K, et al. Multispecific organic anion transporter is responsible for the biliary excretion of the camptothecin derivative irinotecan and its metabolites in rats. *J Pharmacol Exp Ther* 1997;281:304–314.

441. Chu XY, Kato Y, Sugiyama Y. Multiplicity of biliary excre-

tion mechanisms for irinotecan, CPT-11, and its metabolites in rats. *Cancer Res* 1997;57:1934–1938.

442. Takasuna K, Kasai Y, Kitano Y, et al. Protective effects of kampo medicines and baicalin against intestinal toxicity of a new anticancer camptothecin derivative, irinotecan hydrochloride (CPT-11), in rats. *Jpn J Cancer Res* 1995;86:978–984.

443. Takasuna K, Hagiwara T, Hirohashi M, et al. Involvement of beta-glucuronidase in intestinal microflora in the intestinal toxicity of the antitumor camptothecin derivative irinotecan hydrochloride (CPT-11) in rats. *Cancer Res* 1996; 56:3752–3757.

444. Takasuna K, Hagiwara T, Hirohashi M, et al. Inhibition of intestinal microflora beta-glucuronidase modifies the distribution of the active metabolite of the antitumor agent, irinotecan hydrochloride (CPT-11) in rats. *Cancer Chemother Pharmacol* 1998;42:280–286.

445. Gupta E, Safa AR, Wang X, et al. Pharmacokinetic modulation of irinotecan and metabolites by cyclosporin A. *Cancer Res* 1996;56:1309–1314.

446. Sparreboom A, de Jonge MJ, de Bruijn P, et al. Irinotecan (CPT-11) metabolism and disposition in cancer patients. *Clin Cancer Res* 1998;4:2747–2754.

447. Mick R, Gupta E, Vokes EE, et al. Limited-sampling models for irinotecan pharmacokinetics-pharmacodynamics: prediction of biliary index and intestinal toxicity. *J Clin Oncol* 1996;14:2012–2019.

448. Shimada Y, Yoshino M, Wakui A, et al. Phase II study of CPT-11, a new camptothecin derivative, in metastatic colorectal cancer. CPT-11 Gastrointestinal Cancer Study Group. *J Clin Oncol* 1993;11:909–913.

449. Pitot HC, Wender DB, O'Connell MJ, et al. Phase II trial of irinotecan in patients with metastatic colorectal carcinoma. *J Clin Oncol* 1997;15:2910–2919.

450. Rothenberg ML, Cox JV, DeVore RF, et al. A multicenter, phase II trial of weekly irinotecan (CPT-11) in patients with previously treated colorectal carcinoma. *Cancer* 1999;85: 786–795.

451. Van Cutsem E, Cunningham D, Ten Bokkel Huinink WW, et al. Clinical activity and benefit of irinotecan (CPT-11) in patients with colorectal cancer truly resistant to 5-fluorouracil (5-FU). *Eur J Cancer* 1999;35:54–59.

452. Rougier P, Bugat R, Douillard JY, et al. Phase II study of irinotecan in the treatment of advanced colorectal cancer in chemotherapy-naive patients and patients pretreated with fluorouracil-based chemotherapy. *J Clin Oncol* 1997;15: 251–260.

453. Cunningham D, Pyrhonen S, James RD, et al. Randomised trial of irinotecan plus supportive care versus supportive care alone after fluorouracil failure for patients with metastatic colorectal cancer [see comments]. *Lancet* 1998;352:1413–1418.

454. Rougier P, Van Cutsem E, Bajetta E, et al. Randomised trial of irinotecan versus fluorouracil by continuous infusion after fluorouracil failure in patients with metastatic colorectal cancer [see comments] [published erratum appears in *Lancet* 1998;352(9140):1634]. *Lancet* 1998;352:1407–1412.

455. Fukuoka M, Negoro S, Niitani H, et al. A phase I study of weekly administration of CPT-11 in lung cancer [in Japanese]. *Gan To Kagaku Ryoho* 1990;17:993–997.

456. Negoro S, Fukuoka M, Niitani H, et al. A phase II study of CPT-11, a camptothecin derivative, in patients with pri-

457. Nakai H, Fukuoka M, Furuse K, et al. An early phase II study of CPT-11 in primary lung cancer [in Japanese]. *Gan To Kagaku Ryoho* 1991;18:607–612.

458. Fujita A, Takabatake H, Tagaki S, et al. Pilot study of irinotecan in refractory small cell lung cancer [in Japanese]. *Gan To Kagaku Ryoho* 1995;22:889–893.

459. Takeuchi S, Takamizawa H, Takeda Y, et al. An early phase II study of CPT-11 in gynecologic cancers. Research Group of CPT-11 in Gynecologic Cancers [in Japanese]. *Gan To Kagaku Ryoho* 1991;18:579–584.

460. Takeuchi S, Dobashi K, Fujimoto S, et al. A late phase II study of CPT-11 on uterine cervical cancer and ovarian cancer. Research Groups of CPT-11 in Gynecologic Cancers [in Japanese]. *Gan To Kagaku Ryoho* 1991;18:1681–1689.

461. Verschraegen CF, Levy T, Kudelka AP, et al. Phase II study of irinotecan in prior chemotherapy-treated squamous cell carcinoma of the cervix. *J Clin Oncol* 1997;15:625–631.

462. Taguchi T, Tominaga T, Ogawa M, et al. A late phase II study of CPT-11 (irinotecan) in advanced breast cancer. CPT-11 Study Group on Breast Cancer [in Japanese]. *Gan To Kagaku Ryoho* 1994;21:1017–1024.

463. Taguchi T, Yoshida Y, Izuo M, et al. An early phase II study of CPT-11 (irinotecan hydrochloride) in patients with advanced breast cancer [in Japanese]. *Gan To Kagaku Ryoho* 1994;21:83–90.

464. Friedman HS, Petros WP, Friedman AH, et al. Irinotecan therapy in adults with recurrent or progressive malignant glioma. *J Clin Oncol* 1999;17:1516–1525.

465. Futatsuki K, Wakui A, Nakao I, et al. Late phase II study of irinotecan hydrochloride (CPT-11) in advanced gastric cancer. CPT-11 Gastrointestinal Cancer Study Group [in Japanese]. *Gan To Kagaku Ryoho* 1994;21:1033–1038.

466. Ota K, Ohno R, Shirakawa S, et al. Late phase II clinical study of irinotecan hydrochloride (CPT-11) in the treatment of malignant lymphoma and acute leukemia. The CPT-11 Research Group for Hematological Malignancies [in Japanese]. *Gan To Kagaku Ryoho* 1994;21:1047–1055.

467. Tsuda H, Takatsuki K, Ohno R, et al. Treatment of adult T-cell leukaemia-lymphoma with irinotecan hydrochloride (CPT-11). CPT-11 Study Group on Hematological Malignancy. *Br J Cancer* 1994;70:771–774.

468. Pei XH, Nakanishi Y, Takayama K, et al. Effect of CPT-11 in combination with other anticancer agents in lung cancer cells. *Anticancer Drugs* 1997;8:231–237.

469. Guichard S, Hennebelle I, Bugat R, et al. Cellular interactions of 5-fluorouracil and the camptothecin analogue CPT-11 (irinotecan) in a human colorectal carcinoma cell line. *Biochem Pharmacol* 1998;55:667–676.

470. Mullany S, Svingen PA, Kaufmann SH, et al. Effect of adding the topoisomerase I poison 7-ethyl-10-hydroxycamptothecin (SN-38) to 5-fluorouracil and folinic acid in HCT-8 cells: elevated dTTP pools and enhanced cytotoxicity. *Cancer Chemother Pharmacol* 1998;42:391–399.

471. Pavillard V, Formento P, Rostagno P, et al. Combination of irinotecan (CPT11) and 5-fluorouracil with an analysis of cellular determinants of drug activity. *Biochem Pharmacol* 1998;56:1315–1322.

472. Johnston PG, Lenz HJ, Leichman CG, et al. Thymidylate

synthase gene and protein expression correlate and are associated with response to 5-fluorouracil in human colorectal and gastric tumors. *Cancer Res* 1995;55:1407–1412.

473. Aschele C, Baldo C, Sobrero AF, et al. Schedule-dependent synergism between raltitrexed and irinotecan in human colon cancer cells in vitro. *Clin Cancer Res* 1998;4:1323–1330.

474. Houghton JA, Cheshire PJ, Hallman JD 2nd, et al. Evaluation of irinotecan in combination with 5-fluorouracil or etoposide in xenograft models of colon adenocarcinoma and rhabdomyosarcoma. *Clin Cancer Res* 1996;2:107–118.

475. Sasaki Y, Ohtsu A, Shimada Y, et al. Simultaneous administration of CPT-11 and fluorouracil: alteration of the pharmacokinetics of CPT-11 and SN-38 in patients with advanced colorectal cancer [Letter]. *J Natl Cancer Inst* 1994;86:1096–1098.

476. Saltz L, Shimada Y, Khayat D. CPT-11 (irinotecan) and 5-fluorouracil: a promising combination for therapy of colorectal cancer. *Eur J Cancer* 1996;32A:S24–31.

477. Vanhoefer U, Harstrick A, Kohne CH, et al. Phase I study of a weekly schedule of irinotecan, high-dose leucovorin, and infusional fluorouracil as first-line chemotherapy in patients with advanced colorectal cancer. *J Clin Oncol* 1999;17:907–913.

478. Parnes HL, Tait N, Conley B, et al. A phase I study of CPT-11, weekly bolus 5-FU and leucovorin in patients with metastatic cancer. *Oncol Rep* 1995;2:1131–1134.

479. Van Cutsem E, Pozzo C, Starkhammar H, et al. A phase II study of irinotecan alternated with five days bolus of 5-fluorouracil and leucovorin in first-line chemotherapy of metastatic colorectal cancer. *Ann Oncol* 1998;9:1199–1204.

480. Douillard JY, Cunningham D, Roth AD, et al. A randomized phase III trial comparing irinotecan (IRI) + 5FU/folinic acid (FA) to the same schedule of 5FU/FA in patients (pts) with metastatic colorectal cancer (MCRC) as front line chemotherapy (CT). *Proc Am Soc Clin Oncol* 1999;18:233a.

481. Saltz LB, Locker PK, Pirotta N, et al. Weekly irinotecan (CPT-11), leucovorin (LV), and fluorouracil (FU) is superior to daily ×5 LV/FU in patients (PTS) with previously untreated metastatic colorectal cancer (CRC). *Proc Am Soc Clin Oncol* 1999;18:233a.

482. Rocha-Lima CMS, Leong SS, Sherman CA, et al. Phase I study of CPT-11 and gemcitabine in patients with solid tumors. *Cancer Ther* 1999;199:58–66.

483. Kano Y, Suzuki K, Akutsu M, et al. Effects of CPT-11 in combination with other anti-cancer agents in culture. *Int J Cancer* 1992;50:604–610.

484. De Jonge MJ, Verweij J, Planting AS, et al. Drug-administration sequence does not change pharmacodynamics and kinetics of irinotecan and cisplatin. *Clin Cancer Res* 1999;5:2012–2017.

485. Masuda N, Fukuoka M, Kudoh S, et al. Phase I and pharmacologic study of irinotecan in combination with cisplatin for advanced lung cancer. *Br J Cancer* 1993;68:777–782.

486. Masuda N, Fukuoka M, Kudoh S, et al. Phase I study of irinotecan and cisplatin with granulocyte colony-stimulating factor support for advanced non-small-cell lung cancer. *J Clin Oncol* 1994;12:90–96.

487. Mori K, Ohnishi T, Yokoyama K, et al. A phase I study of irinotecan and infusional cisplatin for advanced non-small-cell lung cancer. *Cancer Chemother Pharmacol* 1997;39:327–332.

488. Mori K, Hirose T, Machida S, et al. A phase I study of irinotecan and infusional cisplatin with recombinant human granulocyte colony-stimulating factor support in the treatment of advanced non-small cell lung cancer. *Eur J Cancer* 1997;33:503–505.

489. Kobayashi K, Shinbara A, Kamimura M, et al. Irinotecan (CPT-11) in combination with weekly administration of cisplatin (CDDP) for non-small-cell lung cancer. *Cancer Chemother Pharmacol* 1998;42:53–58.

490. Ueoka H, Tabata M, Kiura K, et al. Fractionated administration of irinotecan and cisplatin for treatment of lung cancer: a phase I study. *Br J Cancer* 1999;79:984–990.

491. Masuda N, Fukuoka M, Fujita A, et al. A phase II trial of combination of CPT-11 and cisplatin for advanced non-small-cell lung cancer. CPT-11 Lung Cancer Study Group [see comments]. *Br J Cancer* 1998;78:251–256.

492. Mori K, Machida S, Yoshida T, et al. A phase II study of irinotecan and infusional cisplatin with recombinant human granulocyte colony-stimulating factor support for advanced non-small-cell lung cancer. *Cancer Chemother Pharmacol* 1999;43:467–470.

493. Kudoh S, Fujiwara Y, Takada Y, et al. Phase II study of irinotecan combined with cisplatin in patients with previously untreated small-cell lung cancer. West Japan Lung Cancer Group. *J Clin Oncol* 1998;16:1068–1074.

494. Devore R 3rd, Johnson D, Crawford J, et al. Irinotecan plus cisplatin in patients with advanced non-small-cell lung cancer. *Oncology (Huntingt)* 1998;12:79–83.

495. Shinkai T, Arioka H, Kunikane H, et al. Phase I clinical trial of irinotecan (CPT-11), 7-ethyl-10-[4-(1-piperidino)-1-piperidino]carbonyloxy-camptothecin, and cisplatin in combination with fixed dose of vindesine in advanced non-small cell lung cancer. *Cancer Res* 1994;54:2636–2642.

496. Fujita A, Igami Y, Takabatake H, et al. Period of time patients with advanced non-small cell lung cancer could remain at home during CIC—therapy (cisplatin + ifosfamide + CPT-11) [in Japanese]. *Gan To Kagaku Ryoho* 1999;26:805–811.

497. Shirao K, Shimada Y, Kondo H, et al. Phase I–II study of irinotecan hydrochloride combined with cisplatin in patients with advanced gastric cancer. *J Clin Oncol* 1997;15:921–927.

498. Boku N, Ohtsu A, Shimada Y, et al. Phase II study of a combination of irinotecan and cisplatin against metastatic gastric cancer. *J Clin Oncol* 1999;17:319–323.

499. Sugiyama T, Yakushiji M, Nishida T, et al. Irinotecan (CPT-11) combined with cisplatin in patients with refractory or recurrent ovarian cancer. *Cancer Lett* 1998;128:211–218.

500. Sugiyama T, Nishida T, Kumagai S, et al. Combination therapy with irinotecan and cisplatin as neoadjuvant chemotherapy in locally advanced cervical cancer. *Br J Cancer* 1999;81:95–98.

501. Okamoto H, Nagatomo A, Kunitoh H, et al. A phase I clinical and pharmacologic study of a carboplatin and irinotecan regimen combined with recombinant human granulocyte-colony stimulating factor in the treatment of patients with advanced nonsmall cell lung carcinoma. *Cancer* 1998;82:2166–2172.

502. Tobinai K, Hotta T, Saito H, et al. Combination phase I/II study of irinotecan hydrochloride (CPT-11) and carbo-

platin in relapsed or refractory non-Hodgkin's lymphoma. CPT-11/Lymphoma Study Group. *Jpn J Clin Oncol* 1996;26:455–460.

503. Wasserman E, Cuvier C, Lokiec F, et al. Combination of oxaliplatin plus irinotecan in patients with gastrointestinal tumors: results of two independent phase I studies with pharmacokinetics. *J Clin Oncol* 1999;17:1751–1759.

504. Eder JP, Chan V, Wong J, et al. Sequence effect of irinotecan (CPT-11) and topoisomerase II inhibitors in vivo. *Cancer Chemother Pharmacol* 1998;42:327–335.

505. Karato A, Sasaki Y, Shinkai T, et al. Phase I study of CPT-11 and etoposide in patients with refractory solid tumors. *J Clin Oncol* 1993;11:2030–2035.

506. Masuda N, Fukuoka M, Kudoh S, et al. Phase I and pharmacologic study of irinotecan and etoposide with recombinant human granulocyte colony-stimulating factor support for advanced lung cancer. *J Clin Oncol* 1994;12:1833–1841.

507. Ohtsu T, Sasaki Y, Igarashi T, et al. Unexpected hepatotoxicities in patients with non-Hodgkin's lymphoma treated with irinotecan (CPT-11) and etoposide. *Jpn J Clin Oncol* 1998;28:502–506.

508. Oshita F, Noda K, Nishiwaki Y, et al. Phase II study of irinotecan and etoposide in patients with metastatic non-small-cell lung cancer. *J Clin Oncol* 1997;15:304–309.

509. Ando M, Eguchi K, Shinkai T, et al. Phase I study of sequentially administered topoisomerase I inhibitor (irinotecan) and topoisomerase II inhibitor (etoposide) for metastatic non-small-cell lung cancer [see comments]. *Br J Cancer* 1997;76:1494–1499.

510. Kano Y, Akutsu M, Tsunoda S, et al. In vitro schedule-dependent interaction between paclitaxel and SN-38 (the active metabolite of irinotecan) in human carcinoma cell lines. *Cancer Chemother Pharmacol* 1998;42:91–98.

511. Mogi H, Hasegawa Y, Watanabe A, et al. Combination effects of cisplatin, vinorelbine and irinotecan in non-small-cell lung cancer cell lines in vitro. *Cancer Chemother Pharmacol* 1997;39:199–204.

512. Wang Z, Sinha BK. Interleukin-1 alpha-induced modulation of topoisomerase I activity and DNA damage: implications in the mechanisms of synergy with camptothecins in vitro and in vivo. *Mol Pharmacol* 1996;49:269–275.

513. Ohwada S, Kobayashi I, Maemura M, et al. Interferon potentiates antiproliferative activity of CPT-11 against human colon cancer xenografts. *Cancer Lett* 1996;110:149–154.

514. Kobayashi I, Ohwada S, Maemura M. Interferon-alpha potentiates the antiproliferative activity of CPT-11 against human colon cancer xenografts in nude mice. *Anticancer Res* 1996;16:2677–2680.

515. Coggins CA, Elion GB, Houghton PJ, et al. Enhancement of irinotecan (CPT-11) activity against central nervous system tumor xenografts by alkylating agents. *Cancer Chemother Pharmacol* 1998;41:485–490.

516. Potmesil M, Vardeman D, Kozielski AJ, et al. Growth inhibition of human cancer metastases by camptothecins in newly developed xenograft models. *Cancer Res* 1995;55:5637–5641.

517. Pantazis P, Hinz HR, Mendoza JT, et al. Complete inhibition of growth followed by death of human malignant melanoma cells in vitro and regression of human melanoma

xenografts in immunodeficient mice induced by camptothecins. *Cancer Res* 1992;52:3980–3987.

518. De Sousa PL, Cooper MR, Imondi AR, et al. 9-Aminocamptothecin: a topoisomerase I inhibitor with preclinical activity in prostate cancer. *Clin Cancer Res* 1997;3:287–294.

519. Pantazis P, Kozielski AJ, Vardeman DM, et al. Efficacy of camptothecin congeners in the treatment of human breast carcinoma xenografts. *Oncol Res* 1993;5:273–281.

520. Pantazis P, Kozielski AJ, Mendoza JT, et al. Camptothecin derivatives induce regression of human ovarian carcinomas grown in nude mice and distinguish between non-tumorigenic and tumorigenic cells in vitro. *Int J Cancer* 1993;53:863–871.

521. Jeha S, Kantarjian H, O'Brien S, et al. Activity of oral and intravenous 9-aminocamptothecin in SCID mice engrafted with human leukemia. *Leuk Lymphoma* 1998;32:159–164.

522. Keane TE, El-Galley RE, Sun C, et al. Camptothecin analogues/cisplatin: an effective treatment of advanced bladder cancer in a preclinical in vivo model system. *J Urol* 1998;160:252–256.

523. Dahut W, Harold N, Takimoto C, et al. Phase I and pharmacologic study of 9-aminocamptothecin given by 72-hour infusion in adult cancer patients. *J Clin Oncol* 1996;14:1236–1244.

524. Eder JP Jr, Supko JG, Lynch T, et al. Phase I trial of the colloidal dispersion formulation of 9-amino-20(S)-camptothecin administered as a 72-hour continuous intravenous infusion. *Clin Cancer Res* 1998;4:317–324.

525. Takimoto C, Dahut W, Harold H, et al. A phase I trial of a prolonged infusion of 9-aminocamptothecin (9-AC) in adult patients with solid tumors. *Proc Am Soc Clin Oncol* 1996;14:471.

526. Siu LL, Oza AM, Eisenhauer EA, et al. Phase I and pharmacologic study of 9-aminocamptothecin colloidal dispersion formulation given as a 24-hour continuous infusion weekly times four every 5 weeks. *J Clin Oncol* 1998;16:1122–1130.

527. Herben VMM, van Gijn R, Schellens JHM, et al. Phase I and pharmacokinetic study of a daily times 5 short intravenous infusion schedule of 9-aminocamptothecin in a colloidal dispersion formulation in patients with advanced solid tumors. *J Clin Oncol* 1999;17:1906–1914.

528. Langevin AM, Casto DT, Thomas PJ, et al. Phase I trial of 9-aminocamptothecin in children with refractory solid tumors: a Pediatric Oncology Group study. *J Clin Oncol* 1998;16:2494–2499.

529. Vey N, Kantarjian H, Tran H, et al. Phase I and pharmacologic study of 9-aminocamptothecin colloidal dispersion formulation in patients with refractory or relapsed acute leukemia. *Ann Oncol* 1999;10:577–583.

530. Mani S, Iyer L, Janisch L, et al. Phase I clinical and pharmacokinetic study of oral 9-aminocamptothecin (NSC-603071). *Cancer Chemother Pharmacol* 1998;42:84–87.

531. Sparreboom A, de Jonge MJ, Punt CJ, et al. Pharmacokinetics and bioavailability of oral 9-aminocamptothecin capsules in adult patients with solid tumors. *Clin Cancer Res* 1998;4:1915–1919.

532. Takimoto CH, Klecker RW, Dahut WL, et al. Analysis of the active lactone form of 9-aminocamptothecin in plasma using solid-phase extraction and high-performance liquid chromatography. *J Chromatogr B Biomed Sci Appl* 1994;655:97–104.

533. Van Gijn R, Herben VM, Hillebrand MJ, et al. High-performance liquid chromatographic analysis of the investigational anticancer drug 9-aminocamptothecin, as the lactone form and as the total of the lactone and the hydroxycarboxylate forms, in micro-volumes of human plasma. *J Pharm Biomed Anal* 1998;17:1257–1265.

534. Loos WJ, Sparreboom A, Verweij J, et al. Determination of the lactone and lactone plus carboxylate forms of 9-aminocamptothecin in human plasma by sensitive high-performance liquid chromatography with fluorescence detection. *J Chromatogr B Biomed Sci Appl* 1997;694:435–441.

535. Takimoto CH, Dahut W, Marino MT, et al. Pharmacodynamics and pharmacokinetics of a 72-hour infusion of 9-aminocamptothecin in adult cancer patients. *J Clin Oncol* 1997;15:1492–1501.

536. Grossman SA, Hochberg F, Fisher J, et al. Increased 9-aminocamptothecin dose requirements in patients on anticonvulsants. NABTT CNS Consortium. The new approaches to brain tumor therapy. *Cancer Chemother Pharmacol* 1998;42:118–126.

537. Takimoto CH, Dahut W, Harold N, et al. Clinical pharmacology of 9-aminocamptothecin. *Ann N Y Acad Sci* 1996;803:324–326.

538. Minami H, Lad TE, Nicholas MK, et al. Pharmacokinetics and pharmacodynamics of 9-aminocamptothecin infused over 72 hours in phase II studies. *Clin Cancer Res* 1999;5:1325–1330.

539. De Jonge MJ, Verweij J, Loos WJ, et al. Clinical pharmacokinetics of encapsulated oral 9-aminocamptothecin in plasma and saliva. *Clin Pharmacol Ther* 1999;65:491–499.

540. Saltz LB, Kemeny NE, Tong W, et al. 9-Aminocamptothecin by 72-hour continuous intravenous infusion is inactive in the treatment of patients with 5-fluorouracil-refractory colorectal carcinoma. *Cancer* 1997;80:1727–1732.

541. Pazdur R, Diaz-Canton E, Ballard WP, et al. Phase II trial of 9-aminocamptothecin administered as a 72-hour continuous infusion in metastatic colorectal carcinoma. *J Clin Oncol* 1997;15:2905–2909.

542. Wilson WH, Little R, Pearson D, et al. Phase II and dose-escalation with or without granulocyte colony-stimulating factor study of 9-aminocamptothecin in relapsed and refractory lymphomas [published erratum appears in *J Clin Oncol* 1998;16(8):2895]. *J Clin Oncol* 1998;16:2345–2351.

543. Vokes EE, Ansari RH, Masters GA, et al. A phase II study of 9-aminocamptothecin in advanced non-small-cell lung cancer [see comments]. *Ann Oncol* 1998;9:1085–1090.

544. Pazdur R, Medgyesy DC, Winn RJ, et al. Phase II trial of 9-aminocamptothecin (NSC 603071) administered as a 120-hr continuous infusion weekly for three weeks in metastatic colorectal carcinoma. *Invest New Drugs* 1998;16:341–346.

545. Erickson-Miller CL, May RD, Tomaszewski J, et al. Differential toxicity of camptothecin, topotecan and 9-aminocamptothecin to human, canine, and murine myeloid progenitors (CFU-GM) in vitro. *Cancer Chemother Pharmacol* 1997;39:467–472.

546. Pantazis P, Harris N, Mendoza J, et al. Conversion of 9-nitrocamptothecin to 9-amino-camptothecin by human blood cells in vitro [Letter]. *Eur J Haematol* 1994;53:246–248.

547. Pantazis P, Harris N, Mendoza J, et al. The role of pH and serum albumin in the metabolic conversion of 9-nitrocamptothecin to 9-aminocamptothecin by human hematopoietic and other cells [Letter]. *Eur J Haematol* 1995;55:211–213.

548. Pantazis P, Early JA, Kozielski AJ, et al. Regression of human breast carcinoma tumors in immunodeficient mice treated with 9-nitrocamptothecin: differential response of nontumorigenic and tumorigenic human breast cells in vitro. *Cancer Res* 1993;53:1577–1582.

549. Pantazis P, Early JA, Mendoza JT, et al. Cytotoxic efficacy of 9-nitrocamptothecin in the treatment of human malignant melanoma cells in vitro. *Cancer Res* 1994;54:771–776.

550. Natelson EA, Giovanella BC, Verschraegen CF, et al. Phase I clinical and pharmacological studies of 20-(S)-camptothecin and 20-(S)-9-nitrocamptothecin as anticancer agents. *Ann N Y Acad Sci* 1996;803:224–230.

551. Verschraegen CF, Natelson EA, Giovanella BC, et al. A phase I clinical and pharmacological study of oral 9-nitrocamptothecin, a novel water-insoluble topoisomerase I inhibitor. *Anticancer Drugs* 1998;9:36–44.

552. Hinz HR, Harris NJ, Natelson EA, et al. Pharmacokinetics of the in vivo and in vitro conversion of 9-nitro-20(S)-camptothecin to 9-amino-20(S)-camptothecin in humans, dogs, and mice. *Cancer Res* 1994;54:3096–3100.

553. Stehlin JS, Giovanella BC, Natelson EA, et al. A study of 9-nitrocamptothecin (RFS-2000) in patients with advanced pancreatic cancer. *Int J Oncol* 1999;14:821–831.

554. Verschraegen CF, Gupta E, Loyer E, et al. A phase II clinical and pharmacological study of oral 9-nitrocamptothecin in patients with refractory epithelial ovarian, tubal or peritoneal cancer. *Anticancer Drugs* 1999;10:375–383.

555. Emerson DL, Besterman JM, Brown HR, et al. In vivo antitumor activity of two new seven-substituted water-soluble camptothecin analogues. *Cancer Res* 1995;55:603–609.

556. Gerrits CJ, Creemers GJ, Schellens JH, et al. Phase I and pharmacological study of the new topoisomerase I inhibitor GI147211, using a daily ×5 intravenous administration. *Br J Cancer* 1996;73:744–750.

557. Eckhardt SG, Baker SD, Eckardt JR, et al. Phase I and pharmacokinetic study of GI147211, a water-soluble camptothecin analogue, administered for five consecutive days every three weeks. *Clin Cancer Res* 1998;4:595–604.

558. Paz-Ares L, Kunka R, DeMaria D, et al. A phase I clinical and pharmacokinetic study of the new topoisomerase inhibitor GI147211 given as a 72-h continuous infusion. *Br J Cancer* 1998;78:1329–1336.

559. Stevenson JP, DeMaria D, Sludden J, et al. Phase I/pharmacokinetic study of the topoisomerase I inhibitor GG211 administered as a 21-day continuous infusion. *Ann Oncol* 1999;10:339–344.

560. Selinger K, Smith G, Depee S, et al. Determination of GI147211 in human blood by HPLC with fluorescence detection. *J Pharm Biomed Anal* 1995;13:1521–1530.

561. Stafford CG, St. Claire RL 3rd. High-performance liquid chromatographic analysis of the lactone and carboxylate forms of a topoisomerase I inhibitor (the antitumor drug GI147211) in plasma. *J Chromatogr B Biomed Sci Appl* 1995;663:119–126.

562. Gerrits CJ, Schellens JH, Creemers GJ, et al. The bioavailability of oral GI147211 (GG211), a new topoisomerase I inhibitor. *Br J Cancer* 1997;76:946–951.

563. Kanzawa F, Nishio K, Kubota N, et al. Antitumor activities

of a new indolocarbazole substance, NB-506, and establishment of NB-506-resistant cell lines, SBC-3/NB. *Cancer Res* 1995;55:2806–2813.

564. Poddevin B, Riou JF, Lavelle F, et al. Dual topoisomerase I and II inhibition by intoplicine (RP-60475), a new antitumor agent in early clinical trials. *Mol Pharmacol* 1993;44:767–774.

565. Ohe Y, Tanigawara Y, Fuji H, et al. Phase I and pharmacology study of 5-day infusion of NB-506. *Proc Am Soc Clin Oncol* 1997;16:199a.

566. Perez-Soler R, Glisson BS, Lee JS, et al. Treatment of patients with small-cell lung cancer refractory to etoposide and cisplatin with the topoisomerase I poison topotecan. *J Clin Oncol* 1996;14:2785–2790.

567. Smith MA, Rubinstein L, Cazenave L, et al. Report of the Cancer Therapy Evaluation Program monitoring plan for secondary acute myeloid leukemia following treatment with epipodophyllotoxins. *J Natl Cancer Inst* 1993;85:554–558.

568. Blaney SM, Needle MN, Gillespie A, et al. Phase II trial of topotecan administered as 72-hour continuous infusion in children with refractory solid tumors: a collaborative Pediatric Branch, National Cancer Institute, and Children's Cancer Group Study. *Clin Cancer Res* 1998;4:357–360.

569. Rivory LP, Chatelut E, Canal P, et al. Kinetics of the in vivo interconversion of the carboxylate and lactone forms of irinotecan (CPT-11) and of its metabolite SN-38 in patients. *Cancer Res* 1994;54:6330–6333.

570. Wagener DJ, Verdonk HE, Dirix LY, et al. Phase II trial of CPT-11 in patients with advanced pancreatic cancer, an EORTC early clinical trials group study [see comments]. *Ann Oncol* 1995;6:129–132.

571. Reese DM, Tchekmedyian S, Chapman Y, et al. A phase II trial of irinotecan in hormone-refractory prostate cancer. *Invest New Drugs* 1998;16:353–359.

572. Irvin WP, Price FV, Bailey H, et al. A phase II study of irinotecan (CPT-11) in patients with advanced squamous cell carcinoma of the cervix. *Cancer* 1998;82:328–333.

573. Look KY, Blessing JA, Levenback C, et al. A phase II trial of CPT-11 in recurrent squamous carcinoma of the cervix: a gynecologic oncology group study. *Gynecol Oncol* 1998;70:334–338.

574. Ohno R, Okada K, Masaoka T, et al. An early phase II study of CPT-11: a new derivative of camptothecin, for the treatment of leukemia and lymphoma. *J Clin Oncol* 1990;8:1907–1912.

575. Nakanishi Y, Takayama K, Takano K, et al. Second-line chemotherapy with weekly cisplatin and irinotecan in patients with refractory lung cancer. *Am J Clin Oncol* 1999;22:399–402.

576. Shimizu Y, Umezawa S, Hasumi K. A phase II study of combined CPT-11 and mitomycin-C in platinum refractory clear cell and mucinous ovarian carcinoma. *Ann Acad Med Singapore* 1998;27:650–656.

21

ENZYME THERAPY: L-ASPARAGINASE

BRUCE A. CHABNER
STEPHEN E. SALLAN*

The growth of malignant as well as normal cells depends on the availability of specific nutrients and cofactors used in protein synthesis. Some of these nutrients can be synthesized within the cell, but others such as essential amino acids are required from external sources. Nutritional therapy for cancer has been directed at identifying differences between the host and malignant cells that might be exploited in treatment; these attempts have been largely unsuccessful because of difficulties in producing a deficiency state by dietary means and a lack of clear differences in the nutritional requirements of rapidly proliferating host cells and the tumor. The only exception has been the use of L-asparaginase in the treatment of childhood acute leukemia.

L-Asparagine is a nonessential amino acid synthesized by transamination of L-aspartic acid (Fig. 21-1). The amine group is donated by glutamine, and the reaction is catalyzed by the enzyme L-asparagine synthetase. This enzyme is constitutive in many tissues, which accounts for the modest toxicity of asparagine depletion from the plasma, but the capacity to synthesize asparagine is lacking in certain human malignancies, particularly those of lymphocytic derivation. In tumor cells lacking L-asparagine synthetase, such as L5178Y murine leukemia cells,[1] the amino acid can be obtained only from a culture medium or, *in vivo*, from plasma.

The enzyme L-asparaginase (L-asparagine amidohydrolase, EC 3.5.1.1), which catalyzes the hydrolysis of asparagine to aspartic acid and ammonia as end products, is found in many plants and microorganisms and in the plasma of certain animals. General interest in L-asparaginase as a therapeutic agent was the result of an unexplained observation by Kidd,[2] who in 1953 reported that the growth of transplantable lymphomas in rodents was inhibited by guinea pig serum but not by rabbit, horse, or human serum. Ten years later, Broome[3] demonstrated that

the responsible factor was the enzyme L-asparaginase. Subsequently, highly purified preparations of enzyme from *Escherichia coli*[4] and *Erwinia carotovora* (also known as *Erwinia chrysanthemi*)[5] showed significant activity against childhood acute lymphocytic leukemia (ALL) and have become standard components of remission induction, consolidation, and reinduction therapy in this disease and in adult ALL, contributing to the 80% or greater 5-year disease-free survival in childhood ALL and 35% to 50% 5-year disease-free survival in adult ALL.[6,7] The clinical and biochemical features of L-asparaginase chemotherapy have been summarized in several comprehensive reviews.[8–10] The key features of L-asparaginase pharmacology are listed in Table 21-1.

PROPERTIES AND MECHANISM OF ACTION

L-Asparaginase purified from *E. coli*[11] has been used most widely in both basic and clinical research, although L-asparaginase obtained from other sources, including *E. chrysanthemi, Serratia marcescens*, guinea pig serum, and the serum of other members of the species *Caviodea* also possesses antitumor activity. The purified bacterial enzyme has a molecular weight of 133,000 to 141,000 d and is composed of four subunits, each with one active site.[12,13] The gene coding for the *E. chrysanthemi*[14] enzyme has been cloned and sequenced and expressed in *E. coli*.[15] Preparations of enzyme from different bacterial strains and by different purification methods show slight differences in enzyme characteristics. For the bacterial enzymes, the specific activity of purified enzyme is usually 300 to 400 µmol of substrate cleaved per minute per mg of protein; the isoelectric point lies between pH 4.6 and 5.5 for the *E. coli* enzyme and is 8.6 for the *Erwinia* protein; and the K_m (Michaelis-Menten constant) for asparagine is usually 1×10^{-5} mol per L.[12,13,16] The *E. coli* enzyme contains 321 amino acids in each subunit (molecular weight 34,080[13]), and the *Erwinia* subunit has a molecular weight of

*In a previous edition of this chapter, Dr. Ti Li Loo, formerly of M. D. Anderson Cancer Center and the National Cancer Institute, contributed significant portions of the manuscript.

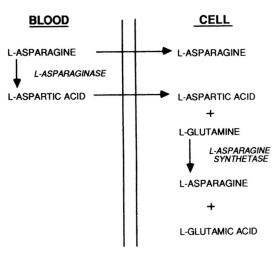

FIGURE 21-1. Sources of L-asparagine for peripheral tissues. The amino acid may be obtained directly from the circulating blood pool of L-asparagine or may be synthesized by transamination of L-aspartic acid, with L-glutamine acting as the NH$_2$ donor in a reaction catalyzed by L-asparagine synthetase.

32,000.[14] (See ref. 13 for the amino acid sequence of the *E. coli* enzyme.) The crystal structure of the *E. coli* enzyme has been solved.[17] It has only a 46% homology with the *E. chrysanthemi* enzyme; the two enzymes lack antigenic cross-reactivity and differ in biochemical properties. For example, ammonia activates *E. coli* asparaginase, whereas oxygen represses its synthesis; neither affects the *Erwinia* enzyme.[18]

TABLE 21-1. KEY FEATURES OF *ESCHERICHIA COLI* L-ASPARAGINASE PHARMACOLOGY

Mechanism of action:	Depletion of the essential amino acid asparagine leads to inhibition of protein synthesis.
Pharmacokinetics:	Plasma half-life: 30 h Blood levels proportional to dose
Dosage:	1,000–20,000 IU/m²/dose
Elimination:	Metabolic degradation

Toxicities:	Decreased protein synthesis
	    Decreased vitamin K–dependent clotting factors leading to hemorrhage or clotting
	    Hypoalbuminemia
	    Hyperglycemia
	    Hypersensitivity reactions
	        Anaphylaxis
	        Serum sickness
	    Cerebral dysfunction
	    Pancreatitis
	    Elevated hepatic enzymes

Drug interactions:	Asparaginase blocks methotrexate action, "rescues" from methotrexate toxicity.
Precautions:	Use with caution in patients with hepatic dysfunction or pancreatitis. If history of hypersensitivity to the drug, switch to *Erwinia* asparaginase.

The *E. coli* and *Erwinia* enzymes are highly specific for L-asparagine as substrates and have less than 10% activity for the D-isomer, for *N*-acylated derivatives, or for L-asparagine in peptide linkage. In contrast, the enzyme from *Saccharomyces cerevisiae* has equal or greater activity with D-asparagine and with *N*-substituted substrates.[19]

The hydrolysis of L-asparagine proceeds according to a reaction mechanism that involves an initial displacement of the amino acid NH$_2$ group during the formation of an enzyme-aspartyl intermediate, followed by hydrolytic cleavage of the latter bond to generate free L-aspartate and active enzyme. The reaction may be summarized

$$\text{E} + \text{Asn} \underset{+\text{NH}_3}{\overset{-\text{NH}_3}{\rightleftharpoons}} \text{E} \cdot \text{Asp} \rightarrow \text{E} + \text{Asp}$$

where E · Asp represents the enzyme-aspartyl intermediate.[19,20] The reaction is irreversibly inhibited by the L-asparagine analog 5-diazo-4-oxo-L-norvaline, which binds covalently to the enzyme's active site.[21]

CELLULAR PHARMACOLOGY AND RESISTANCE

The enzyme L-asparaginase owes its antitumor effects to the rapid and complete depletion of circulating pools of L-asparagine, and resistance to treatment arises through an increase in L-asparagine synthetase activity in tumor cells.[22,23] The mechanism by which L-asparagine synthetase is induced is uncertain. The most likely possibilities are the selection of a subpopulation of cells containing the synthetase or derepression of the synthetase as a result of a fall in intracellular L-asparagine levels. Plasma L-asparagine levels (usually in the range of 4×10^{-5} mol per L) are more than sufficient for L-asparagine–requiring tumor cells, which can grow at a normal rate in tissue culture medium containing 1×10^{-6} mol per L asparagine.[24] Because the K_m of the *E. coli* enzyme for L-asparagine is 1×10^{-5} mol per L, the hydrolysis of L-asparagine proceeds at less than maximal velocity once plasma levels fall below this concentration, and considerable excess L-asparaginase is required in plasma to degrade L-asparagine to sufficiently low concentrations to halt tumor growth.

The cellular effects of L-asparaginase result from inhibition of protein synthesis. Cytotoxicity correlates well with inhibition of protein synthesis. Inhibition of nucleic acid synthesis is also observed in sensitive cells but is believed to be secondary to the block in protein synthesis. Cells insensitive to asparagine depletion from growth medium *in vitro* are also insensitive to L-asparaginase and show little inhibition of protein synthesis in the presence of the enzyme. These resistant cells have high endogenous activity of asparagine synthetase.[22,23] The dependence on asparagine exhibited by sensitive cells may be related not only to the requirement for the amino acid itself as a constituent of protein but also to its role as a donor of the NH_2 group in the synthesis of glycine.[25] The mechanism of cell death may be the activation of programmed cell death, or apoptosis, as suggested by both *in vitro* and *in vivo* experiments.[26]

CHEMICAL MODIFICATION

In an attempt to reduce the immunogenicity of L-asparaginase, to eliminate L-glutaminase activity from the molecule, and to prolong the enzyme's plasma half-life, the *E. coli* asparaginase has been subjected to various modifications. Most bacterial L-asparaginase preparations contain significant L-glutaminase activity (3% to 5% of the L-asparaginase activity). Enzymes from mammalian sources or from certain bacteria (*Vibrio succinogenes* in particular) lack L-glutaminase activity but unfortunately have lesser affinity for L-asparagine[27] and thus are less desirable for clinical purposes. Evidence is found that the immunosuppressive properties of *E. coli* enzyme may result from L-glutamine depletion[28,29] and that cerebral dysfunction observed clinically may be the result of L-glutamine degradation. Attempts have been made to modify the *E. coli* enzyme to eliminate the L-glutaminase activity[30] but have met with limited success; the nitrated enzyme has little L-glutaminase but also has reduced L-asparaginase action.

A second objective has been to reduce immunogenicity. The addition of multiple poly-DL-alanine side chains varying in length from 14 to 34 amino acids markedly decreases the ability of the *E. coli* enzyme to elicit an antibody response in mice and produces a 3,000-fold decrease in reactivity with anti–L-asparaginase antibody without substantially changing the enzymatic activity or its affinity for L-asparagine.[31] The modified enzyme is markedly resistant to tryptic degradation and has a plasma half-life that is seven times longer than the native preparation. Conjugation of the *Erwinia* enzyme to dextran similarly reduces immunogenicity, extends plasma half-life, and reduces activity by only 50%.[32] The *E. coli* enzyme, modified by conjugation with monomethoxypolyethylene glycol (PEG), displays a similar decrease in immunogenicity and a dramatic increase in plasma half-life and retains 50% of its initial activity.[33,34] The PEG-asparaginase is active and nonimmunogenic in patients hypersensitive to the native enzyme.[35] A copolymer of asparaginase with albumin has markedly reduced immunoreactivity and "satisfactory" activity in mice.[36] PEG-asparaginase is available for clinical use in patients hypersensitive to the *E. coli* enzyme.

In addition to being modified chemically, the enzyme has been attached to the external surface of hollow fiber dialysis tubing[37,38] or to acrylamide microspheres[39] with the aim of hydrolyzing the filtered amino acid during hemodialysis, so that patient exposure to the immunogenic enzyme is avoided. The approach has the significant drawback of requiring prolonged periods of dialysis and is likely to achieve only temporary depletion of plasma L-asparaginase, because the amino acid levels are rapidly repleted by release of L-asparagine from the liver.[40] Enzyme incorporated into red cell ghosts is effective in lowering plasma asparagine levels in mice[41] but has not been tested in humans.

PHARMACOLOGIC CONSIDERATIONS

The *in vivo* clearance rate of the enzyme and its K_m are two important factors that may play roles in determining the efficacy of asparaginase as an antitumor agent. L-Asparaginases isolated from *Bacillus coagulans*, *Fusarium tricinctum*, and *Candida albicans* are devoid of antitumor activity and are almost completely cleared from the circulation in 30 minutes to 1 hour after intravenous administration into mice. On the other hand, enzymes derived from guinea pig serum and from *E. coli* and *Erwinia* exhibit antitumor activity and have a much longer half-life.[42,43]

The affinity of the enzyme for L-asparagine is another important factor that affects the antitumor activity of L-asparaginase.[44] Serum concentrations of L-asparagine are 60 to 75 µmol per L, which exceeds the K_m of the bacterial enzymes used in clinical chemotherapy and thus provides a high velocity of substrate hydrolysis. As serum levels of the amino acid fall, they approach and then fall below the K_m, which slows the rate of hydrolysis. *E. coli* and *Erwinia* L-asparaginase, which possess strong antitumor activity, have K_m values of 1 to 1.25×10^{-5} mol per L,[16] whereas L-asparaginases derived from agouti or guinea pig serum have only moderate antitumor activity and K_m values of 4.1 and 7.2×10^{-5} mol per L, respectively.[45] In addition, enzymes from *Erwinia aroideae* ($K_m = 3 \times 10^{-3}$ mol per L)[46] or *B. coagulans* ($K_m = 4.7 \times 10^{-3}$ mol per L)[47] have low substrate affinity and have no tumor-inhibitory activity.

CLINICAL PHARMACOLOGY

Drug Assay and Pharmacokinetics

L-Asparaginase is easily measured in biologic fluids by assays that detect ammonia release[48] or by a coupled enzymatic assay.[49] The drug is given intravenously or intramuscularly; the latter route produces peak blood levels 50% lower than the former but may be less immunogenic. For the *E. coli* enzyme, the usual dosages are a single dose of up to 25,000 IU per m² weekly, 5,000 to 10,000 IU per m² every other day or every third day for 2 to 4 weeks, or daily doses of 1,000 to 10,000 IU per m² for 10 to 20 days. A comparison of the clinical effectiveness of various doses of L-asparaginase given three times per week demonstrated a higher complete remission rate for doses of 6,000 IU per m² or higher than for doses 3,000 IU per m² or less[49a] (Fig. 21-2). L-Asparaginase activity is detectable in the blood-

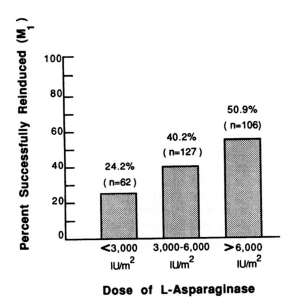

FIGURE 21-2. Relationship between dose of L-asparaginase and response in the treatment of acute lymphoblastic leukemia. Patients received the indicated doses every other day, three doses per week, for a maximum of 6 weeks. Successful induction is judged by achievement of an M_1 bone marrow status. (From Ertel IJ, Nesbit ME, Hammond D, et al. Effective dose of L-asparaginase for induction of remission in previously treated children with acute lymphocytic leukemia: a report from Children's Cancer Study Group. *Cancer Res* 1979;39:3893.

stream for 2 to 3 weeks after large single doses of the *E. coli* enzyme (25,000 IU per m^2) but depletion of asparagine lasts for only 1 week or less.[50–52] Thus asparagine levels return toward normal even in the presence of low levels of the enzyme. The threshold at which recovery takes place appears to be 0.2 to 0.3 IU per mL of plasma. Accurate measurement of serum asparagine levels requires that blood be collected and stored in the presence of an L-asparaginase inhibitor, such as 5-diazo-4-oxo-L-nor valine.[52] The enzyme distributes primarily within the intravascular space. The cerebrospinal fluid (CSF) concentration of asparagine falls rapidly, however, and an antileukemic effect is exerted in this sanctuary, despite the poor penetration of enzyme into the CSF. The drug can be given directly into the CSF but exits rapidly from this site, and use of this route seems to have no clear therapeutic advantage.

The concentration of L-asparaginase in plasma is proportional to dose for doses up to 200,000 IU per m^2 and falls with a primary half-life of 30 hours.[53] The Merck and Kyawa Hacco preparations of *E. coli* L-asparaginase have a longer half-life than the Bayer preparation. Thus, the Kyawa Hacco preparation caused excessive toxicity when given at a dosage of 10,000 U per m^2 every 3 days for eight doses, a schedule and dose well tolerated when the Bayer preparation was used.[54] The *Erwinia* enzyme, although preserving activity in patients hypersensitive to the *E. coli* preparation, has the disadvantage of a shorter half-life in plasma of 16 hours[53] and did not give equivalent therapeutic results when

used in the same dose and schedule as the *E. coli* enzyme[55] (5,000 U per m^2 three times per week). A doubling of the dosage of *Erwinia* enzyme (10,000 U per m^2 per day or 20,000 IU per m^2 3 days per week) is recommended to maintain continuous asparagine depletion and equivalent antitumor effects.[55] In patients who develop hypersensitivity to the enzyme, plasma clearance is greatly accelerated and enzyme activity may be undetectable in plasma as soon as 4 hours after administration.[56]

Covalent linkage of L-asparaginase with PEG has succeeded in markedly reducing the clearance of the enzyme, whereas the volume of distribution remains equivalent to the average plasma volume in humans. PEG-asparaginase disappears more slowly from plasma, with a half-life of 14.9 ± 10.1 days, considerably longer than that of the native enzyme; the total clearance is 5.3 ± 3.1 mL per hour per m^2 or 0.13 ± 0.08 mL per hour per kg, and the apparent volume of distribution is 2.1 ± 0.6 L per m^2 or 52.3 ± 16.1 mL per kg.[57,58] These findings were confirmed in another study[58] in which a somewhat different enzymatic assay for asparaginase was used. The recommended dosage of PEG-asparaginase is 2,500 U per m^2 every other week for 2 weeks. In patients showing hypersensitivity to *E. coli* asparaginase, both native and PEG-linked enzyme may have a shorter half-life, although the PEG enzyme remains active in hypersensitive patients.

Toxicity

The primary toxicities of L-asparaginase, listed in Table 21-2, fall into two main groups: those related to immunologic sensitization to the foreign protein and those resulting from depletion of asparagine pools and inhibition of protein synthesis. Hypersensitivity reactions to L-asparaginase are of great concern because they are a common and potentially fatal complication of therapy, particularly when the drug is used as a single agent.[56] Up to 40% of patients receiving single-agent treatment develop some evidence of sensitization.[59,60] Possibly because of the immunosuppressive effect of corticosteroids, 6-mercaptopurine, and other antileukemic agents, the incidence of hypersensitivity reactions falls to less than 20% in patients receiving combination chemotherapy.[59,61] Other factors that increase the incidence of reactions include the use of dosages above 6,000 IU per m^2 per day,[59,62] intravenous as opposed to intramuscular administration,[62] and repeated courses of treatment. Reactions to an initial dose rarely occur; more commonly, hypersensitivity phenomena appear during the second week of treatment or later.[63]

The clinical manifestations of hypersensitivity vary from urticaria (approximately two-thirds of reported reactions)[59] to true anaphylactic reactions (hypotension, laryngospasm, cardiac arrest). Rarely, serum sickness–type responses—with arthralgias, proteinuria, and fever—may develop several weeks after an extended course of treatment.[59,63] Fatal reac-

TABLE 21-2. TOXICITY OF L-ASPARAGINASE

Reaction	%
Immediate reaction	70
Nausea, vomiting, fever, chills	
Hypersensitivity reactions	<10
Urticaria	
Bronchospasm	
Hypotension	
Decreased protein synthesis	100
Albumin	
Insulin	
Clotting factors II, V, VII, VIII, IX, X	
Serum lipoproteins	
Antithrombin III	
Cerebral dysfunction	33
Disorientation	
Coma	
Seizures	
Organ toxicities	
Pancreatitis	15
Liver function test abnormalities	100
Azotemia (? increased nitrogen load)	68

From Ohnuma T, Holland JF, Sinks LF. Biochemical and pharmacological studies with L-asparaginase in man. *Cancer Res* 1970;30:2297.

tions occur in less than 1% of patients treated,[63] but evidence of hypersensitivity should prompt a change in treatment to L-asparaginase derived from *Erwinia*,[5] which does not share antigenic cross-reactivity with the *E. coli* preparation and thus can safely be given to patients hypersensitive to the latter agent. (The *Erwinia* drug is not sold commercially, but for treatment of ALL it can be obtained from Ogden BioServices Corp., 25-C Lofstrand Lane, Rockville, MD 20850; phone 301-762-0069.) Allergic reactions to *Erwinia* L-asparaginase may occur as an independent phenomenon in patients who have not previously received *E. coli* enzyme[64] and ultimately develop in 5% to 20% of patients receiving multiple courses of this enzyme.[60] PEG-asparaginase can also be used in hypersensitive patients, among whom a 30% incidence of allergy to the new drug can be expected.

Because of the frequency and severity of allergic reactions to L-asparaginase, Merck has recommended routine skin testing for prediction of allergy before the first dose of drug. Allergic reactions may occur in patients with negative skin tests,[65] however, and positive skin tests are not invariably predictive of reactions. Hypersensitive patients usually have both immunoglobulin E and immunoglobulin G antibodies to L-asparaginase in serum,[66,67] but more than half the patients with such antibodies do not display an allergic reaction to the drug clinically. Thus the antibody tests have limited value for predicting which patients will have an allergic reaction. Routine skin testing is not recommended for PEG-asparaginase.

Other toxic effects result from inhibition of protein synthesis and include hypoalbuminemia, decrease in clotting factors, decreased serum insulin with hyperglycemia, and decreased serum lipoproteins. Abnormalities in clotting function are regularly observed in association with L-asparaginase therapy and most frequently lead to thromboembolism in 2% to 11% of ALL patients during induction therapy.[68] Hemorrhagic events occur less frequently, and are probably secondary to decreased synthesis of vitamin K–dependent factors, with prolongation of the prothrombin time, partial thromboplastin time, and thrombin time[59,64,69] and decrease in factors IX and X.[70] Platelets from L-asparaginase–treated subjects display deficient aggregation in response to collagen but not to adenosine diphosphate, arachidonic acid, or epinephrine.[71] Two instances have been reported of a spontaneous intracranial hemorrhage in a child with marked hypofibrinogenemia.[72]

Inhibition of the synthesis of anticoagulant proteins is responsible for thrombotic events. L-Asparaginase decreases the synthesis of antithrombin III, a physiologic anticoagulant and protease inhibitor. Circulating levels of this factor fall to 50% or less compared with levels in controls after single large doses of L-asparaginase.[73] Also inhibited are the syntheses of vitamin K–dependent inhibitors of clotting, protein C, and its cofactor protein S, as well as the vitamin K–dependent procoagulants, factors IX and X.[73,74]

Other toxicities are not as easily explained by the drug's mode of action. In 25% of patients, cerebral dysfunction with confusion, stupor, or frank coma may develop.[51] The latter syndrome resembles ammonia toxicity and has, in some cases, been associated with elevated serum ammonia levels.[75] Alternatively, neurotoxicity may be the result of low concentrations of either L-asparagine or L-glutamine in the brain. Probable or definite improvement of cerebral dysfunction has been observed in three patients treated with infusions of L-asparagine, 1 to 2 mmol per kg per day for up to 44 days.[51] Some of these events probably represent incompletely evaluated episodes of cortical sinus thrombosis.[76]

Thrombosis typically involves the transverse on sagittal sinus circulation of the brain, where it causes seizures, headache, confusion, and stroke symptoms. Subclinical sinus occlusions can be detected by magnetic resonance imaging in patients with modest complaints of headache and undoubtedly occur more frequently than recognized clinically. Catheter-related venous thrombosis may give rise to superior vena cava or internal jugular vein thrombosis.[68]

Remarkably, the majority of L-asparaginase–associated thromboses appear to occur in patients with underlying inherited disorders of clotting.[67] A survey of 289 children with ALL treated in a German cooperative group (Bonn, Frankfurt, Munster group) trial disclosed events in 32 patients, of whom 27 (85%) had one or more defects predisposing to thrombosis (Table 21-3). These defects included the TT677 mutation in methylene tetrahydrofolate reductase (which causes homocysteine elevation in plasma), factor V Leyden, deficiency in protein C or protein S, elevated lipoprotein (a), and the 620210A variant of prothrombin. In this study 27 of 58 patients (47%) with

TABLE 21-3. PROTHROMBOTIC ABNORMALITIES IN 32 PATIENTS WITH ACUTE LYMPHOCYTIC LEUKEMIA EXPERIENCING A THROMBOTIC EVENT DURING INDUCTION THERAPY

Abnormality	Total patients (%)	Associated Abnormality						
		Methylene THF reductase TT677	Prothrombin G20210A	FVL	Lipoprotein (a)↑	Protein C↓	Protein S↓	AT-III↓
None	5 (16)	—	—	—	—	—	—	—
Methylene THF reductase TT677	7 (22)	4[a]	0	1	2	0	0	0
Prothrombin G20210A	1 (3)	0	1[a]	0	0	0	0	0
FVL	7 (22)	1	0	3[a]	2	1	0	0
Lipoprotein (a)↑	8 (25)	2	0	2	2[a]	2	0	0
Protein C↓	6 (19)	0	0	1	2	3[a]	0	0
Protein S↓	4 (13)	0	0	0	0	0	4[a]	0
AT-III↓	2 (6)	0	0	0	0	0	0	2[a]

↑, increased; ↓, reduced; AT-III, antithrombin III; FVL, factor V Leyden; THF, tetrahydrofolate.

[a]Patients with a single abnormality.

From Nowak-Gottl U, Wermes C, Junker R, et al. Prospective evaluation of the thrombotic risk in children with acute lymphoblastic leukemia carrying the MTHFR TT 677 genotype, the prothrombin G20210A variant, and further prothrombotic risk factors. *Blood* 1999;93(5):1595.

one or more of these defects experienced a thrombotic event, compared with only 5 of 231 patients (2%) with no prothrombotic defect. The overall incidence of prothrombotic abnormalities in a white population is approximately 20%. Prophylactic anticoagulation for patients at high risk may be effective but requires more extensive study.[68]

In an attempt to prevent thrombosis, pilot trials have used prophylactic replacement of antithrombin III in children undergoing L-asparaginase treatment[77] and have observed no thrombotic episodes in the small numbers of children thus treated. Definitive studies of factor monitoring and replacement during therapy have not yet been published.

Acute pancreatitis is an infrequent complication that occurs in fewer than 15% of patients, but it may progress to severe hemorrhagic pancreatitis. In most of the affected individuals, a transient increase in serum amylase concentration may coincide with mild nausea, vomiting, and abdominal pain, and these signs of pancreatitis quickly resolve with discontinuation of the drug.[61] L-Asparaginase is frequently the cause of abnormal liver function test results, including increased serum levels of bilirubin, serum glutamic-oxaloacetic transaminase, and alkaline phosphatase. Liver biopsy reveals fatty metamorphosis that is probably due to decreased mobilization of lipids.

Approximately two-thirds of patients receiving L-asparaginase experience nausea, vomiting, and chills as an immediate reaction, but these side effects can be mitigated by administration of antiemetics, antihistamines, or, in extreme cases, corticosteroids. L-Asparaginase has no known toxicity to gastrointestinal mucosa or bone marrow and is thus a favorable agent for use in combination chemotherapy.

The only well-established drug interaction is its ability to terminate the action of methotrexate.[78] The antagonism of L-asparaginase when given before methotrexate is possibly the result of inhibition of protein synthesis, with consequent prevention of cell entry into the vulnerable S phase of the cell cycle. An alternative explanation for antagonism is derived

from the inhibition of methotrexate polyglutamylation by L-asparaginase pretreatment,[79] with decreased retention of methotrexate by tumor cells.[80] After a single intravenous dose of L-asparaginase, inhibition of DNA synthesis lasts for approximately 10 days, a period during which cells are refractory to methotrexate. This interval is followed by a period of increased DNA synthetic activity as cells recover from the block in protein synthesis; during this recovery period, cells are thought to be particularly vulnerable to methotrexate.[81] These considerations form the rationale for the clinical trials that use an initial dose of L-asparaginase, followed in 10 to 14 days by methotrexate.

A second feature of L-asparaginase–methotrexate interaction is important in combination chemotherapy. If the enzyme is given 24 hours after methotrexate, the action of the antifolate is abbreviated at that point. Thus, large doses of methotrexate are well tolerated if followed in 24 hours by L-asparaginase. Lobel et al.[81] devised a regimen, shown in Table 21-4, that begins with L-asparaginase, followed in 10 days by methotrexate and 24 hours later by L-asparaginase rescue. Cycles of methotrexate and L-asparaginase are repeated thereafter at 14-day intervals. The combination seems to be particularly effective against acute leukemia

TABLE 21-4. REGIMEN FOR COMBINED METHOTREXATE-L-ASPARAGINASE TREATMENT OF REFRACTORY ACUTE LEUKEMIA

Rx	Day				
	0	13	14	27	28
L-Asparaginase 500 IU/kg	x		x		x
Methotrexate 100 mg/m²		x		x[a]	

[a]Increase or decrease depending on toxicity.

From Lobel JS, O'Brien RT, McIntosh S, et al. Methotrexate and asparaginase combination chemotherapy in refractory acute leukemia of childhood. *Cancer* 1979;43:1089.

refractory to conventional methotrexate doses, producing complete remission rates of between 33% and 67% in ALL of childhood and 35% in acute nonlymphocytic leukemia.[82,83] The complete response rate is highest in patients who have not been treated previously with L-asparaginase,[81] which indicates that the success of the regimen depends at least in part on the antitumor effects of the enzyme.

The immunosuppressive properties of L-asparaginase have been demonstrated in animals and may contribute to high rates of infection with bacteria and fungal organisms, as reported in certain ALL trials in which patients were randomized to receive, or not receive, high doses of *E. coli* L-asparaginase.[84] Hyperglycemia, hypoalbuminemia, and catheter-related thrombosis in patients treated with the drug may also contribute to the risk of infection.

OTHER FORMS OF ENZYME THERAPY AND AMINO ACID ANTAGONISTS

A number of other enzymes, primarily of bacterial origin, have antitumor activity in animal systems and may undergo clinical trial in the future. The most prominent of these are listed in Table 21-5. The reader is referred to reviews for a more detailed consideration of this subject.[8,9,10]

The enzyme L-glutaminase-L-asparaginase from *Acinetobacter glutaminasificans*[85] and a succinylated derivative of the same enzyme that has a longer plasma half-life have both received preliminary trials in acute leukemia.[86] With the nonsuccinylated enzyme, a dosage of more than 10,000 IU per m^2 per day is required to produce continuous depletion of serum L-glutamine and L-asparagine. The succinylated enzyme used in dosages of less than 1,000 IU per m^2 per day produces rapid depletion of L-glutamine that lasts for at least 24 hours.[87,88] A lowering of peripheral lymphoblast count was reported in 7 of 14 patients resistant to L-asparaginase,[87] but severe neurotoxicity with coma was observed in 5 patients in association with a marked anomalous elevation of CSF L-glutamine levels in all patients tested. The more common toxic reactions associated with L-asparaginase are also seen in patients treated with L-glutaminase, including decreases in various serum proteins, hyperglycemia, fever, and allergic reactions.

L-Glutamine analogs (Table 21-5) also have received limited clinical trial but with little success. The strong activity of 6-diazo-5-oxo-L-norleucine, an L-glutamine antagonist, against human xenografts in nude mice has prompted a reexamination of this drug. Inhibitors of the L-asparagine synthetase reaction also have been described and may have use in combination with L-asparaginase.

TABLE 21-5. AMINO ACID–DIRECTED ANTITUMOR THERAPY

Amino Acid–Degrading Enzymes with Antitumor Activity

Enzyme	Source	Substrate	Comment	Ref.
L-Glutaminase	*Acinetobacter glutaminasificans*	L-Glutamine L-Asparagine	Antitumor activity in humans	85–89
L-Threonine deaminase	Sheep liver	L-Threonine	Active versus murine leukemia	89
L-Methionase	*Clostridium sporogenes*	L-Methionine	Active versus cultured human lymphoblasts	90
Tyrosine phenol-lyase	*Erwinia herbicola*	L-TyrosineL-Phenylalanine	Active versus murine B$_{16}$ melanoma	91
L-Phenylalanine ammonia-lyase	*Rhodotorula glutinis*	L-Phenylalanine	Active versus murine leukemia	92
L-Tryptophan hydroxylase	*Rhodotorula glutinis*	L-Tryptophan	Active versus murine leukemia	93

Amino Acid Analogs

	Compound	Mechanism of Action	Antitumor Activity in Humans	Ref.
L-Glutamine analogs	6-Diazo-5-oxo-L-norleucine (DON)	Inhibits glutamine-dependent transaminases	Breast, lung, choriocarcinoma	94
	Azaserine	Inhibits glutamine-dependent transaminases	Childhood acute leukemia, Hodgkin's disease	94
	Azotomycin	Precursor of DON	Colorectal carcinomas; soft tissue sarcoma	94
L-Aspartate analogs	L-Alanosine	Inhibits purine biosynthesis	Unknown	95–97
	N-Phosphonoacetyl-L-aspartic acid	Inhibits *de novo* pyrimidine synthesis	Breast, colon carcinoma; soft tissue sarcoma	95–97

From Uren R, Handschumacher RE. Enzyme therapy. In: Becker FF, ed. *Cancer: a comprehensive treatise.* New York: Plenum Press, 1977:457.

REFERENCES

1. Haley EE, Fischer GA, Welch AD. The requirement for L-asparagine of mouse leukemic cells L5178Y in culture. *Cancer Res* 1961;21:532.

2. Kidd JG. Regression of transplanted lymphomas induced in vivo by means of normal guinea pig serum: I. Course of transplanted cancers of various kinds in mice and rats given guinea pig serum, horse serum, or rabbit serum. *J Exp Med* 1953;98:565.

3. Broome JD. Evidence that the L-asparaginase of guinea pig serum is responsible for its antilymphoma effects: I. Properties of the L-asparaginase of guinea pig serum in relation to those of the antilymphoma substance. *J Exp Med* 1963;118:99.

4. Hill JM, Loeb E, MacLellan A, et al. Response to highly purified L-asparaginase during therapy of acute leukemia. *Cancer Res* 1969;29:1574.

5. Ohnuma T, Holland JF, Meyer P. *Erwinia carotovora* asparaginase in patients with prior anaphylaxis to asparaginase from *E. coli. Cancer* 1972;30:376.

6. Todeschini G, Tecchio C, Meneghini V, et al. Estimated 6-year event-free survival of 55% in 60 consecutive adult acute lymphoblastic leukemia patients treated with an intensive phase II protocol based on a high induction dose of daunorubicin. *Leukemia* 1998;12:144.

7. Daenen S, van Imhoff GW, van den Berg E, et al. Improved outcome of adult acute lymphoblastic leukaemia by moderately intensified chemotherapy which includes a pre-induction course for rapid tumour reduction: preliminary results on 66 patients. *Br J Haematol* 1998;100:273.

8. Holcenberg JS, Roberts J. Enzymes as drugs. *Annu Rev Pharmacol* 1977;17:97.

9. Cooney DA, Rosenbluth RJ. Enzymes as therapeutic agents. *Adv Pharmacol Chemother* 1975;12:185.

10. Capizzi RL, Bertino JR, Handschumacher RE. L-Asparaginase. *Annu Rev Med* 1970;21:433.

11. Ho PK, Milikin EB, Bobbitt JL, et al. Crystalline L-asparaginase from *E. coli* B: purification and chemical characterization. *J Biol Chem* 1970;245:3703.

12. Jackson RC, Handschumacher RE. *Escherichia coli* L-asparaginase: catalytic activity and subunit nature. *Biochemistry* 1970;9:3585.

13. Maita T, Matsuda G. The primary structure of L-asparaginase from *Escherichia coli. Hoppe Seylers Z Physiol Chem* 1980;361:105.

14. Gilbert HJ, Blazek R, Bullman HMS, et al. Cloning and expression of the *Erwinia chrysanthemi* asparaginase gene in *Escherichia coli* and *Erwinia carotovora. J Gen Microbiol* 1986;132:151.

15. Minton NP, Bullman HMS, Scawen MD, et al. Nucleotide sequence of the *Erwinia chrysanthemi* NCPPB 1066 L-asparaginase gene. *Gene* 1986;46:25.

16. Howard JB, Carpenter FH. L-Asparaginase from *Erwinia carotovora*: substrate specificity and enzymatic properties. *J Biol Chem* 1972;247:1020.

17. Swain AL, Jaskolski M, Housset D, et al. Crystal structure of *Escherichia coli* L-asparaginase, an enzyme used in cancer therapy. *Proc Natl Acad Sci U S A* 1993;90:1474.

18. Wade HE, Robinson HK, Phillips BW. L-Asparaginase and glutaminase activities of bacteria. *J Gen Microbiol* 1971;69:249.

19. Dunlop PC, Meyer GM, Roon RJ. Reactions of asparaginase II of *Saccharomyces cerevisiae*: a mechanistic analysis of hydrolysis and hydroxylaminolysis. *J Biol Chem* 1980;255:1542.

20. Ehrman M, Cedar H, Schwartz JH. L-Asparaginase II of *E. coli*: studies on the enzymatic mechanism of action. *J Biol Chem* 1971;246:88.

21. Lachman LB, Handschumacher RE. The active site of L-asparaginase: dimethylsulfoxide effect of 5-diazo-4-oxo-L-norvaline interactions. *Biochem Biophys Res Commun* 1976;73:1094.

22. Haskell CM, Canellos GP. L-Asparaginase resistance in human leukemia-asparagine synthetase. *Biochem Pharmacol* 1969;18:2578.

23. Horowitz B, Madras BK, Meister A, et al. Asparagine synthetase activity of mouse leukemia. *Science* 1968;160:533.

24. Haley EE, Fischer GA, Welch AD. The requirement for L-asparagine of mouse leukemia cells L5178Y in culture. *Cancer Res* 1961;21:532.

25. Keefer JF, Moraga DA, Schuster SM. Comparison of glycine metabolism in mouse lymphoma cells either sensitive or resistant to L-asparaginase. *Biochem Pharmacol* 1985;34:559.

26. Story MD, Voehringer DW, Stephens LC, et al. L-Asparaginase kills lymphoma cells by apoptosis. *Cancer Chemother Pharmacol* 1993;32:129.

27. Distasio JA, Niederman RA, Kafkewitz D, et al. Purification and characterization of L-asparaginase with antilymphoma activity from *Vibrio succinogenes. J Biol Chem* 1976;251:6929.

28. Han T, Ohnuma T. L-Asparaginase: in vitro inhibition of blastogenesis by enzyme from *Erwinia carotovora. Nature New Biol* 1972;239:50.

29. Durden DL, Distasio JA. Comparison of the immunosuppressive effects of asparaginases from *Escherichia coli* and *Vibrio succinogenes. Cancer Res* 1980;40:1125.

30. Liu YP, Handschumacher RE. Nitroasparaginase: subunit cross-linkage and altered substrate specificity. *J Biol Chem* 1972;247:66.

31. Uren JR, Ragin RC. Improvement in the therapeutic, immunological, and clearance properties of *E. coli* and *Erwinia carotovora* L-asparaginase by attachment of poly-DL-alanyl peptides. *Cancer Res* 1979;39:1927.

32. Wileman TE, Foster RL, Elliott PNC. Soluble asparaginase-dextran conjugates show increased circulatory persistence and lowered antigen reactivity. *J Pharm Pharmacol* 1986;38:264.

33. Abuchowski A, Kago G, Verhoest C, et al. Cancer therapy with chemically modified properties of polyethylene glycol-asparaginase conjugates. *Cancer Biochem Biophys* 1984;7:175.

34. Keating MJ, Holmes R, Lerner S, et al. L-Asparaginase and PEG asparaginase—past present and future. *Leuk Lymphoma* 1993;10[Suppl]:153.

35. Yoshimoto T, Nishimura H, Saito Y, et al. Characterization of polyethylene glycol-modified L-asparaginase from *Escherichia coli* and its application to therapy of leukemia. *Jpn J Cancer Res* 1986;77:1264.

36. Yasura T, Kamisaki Y, Wada H, et al. Immunological studies on modified enzymes: I. Soluble L-asparaginase/mouse albumin copolymer with enzyme activity and substantial loss of immunosensitivity. *Int Arch Allergy Appl Immunol* 1981;64:11.

37. Mazzola G, Vecchio G. Immobilization and characterization of L-asparaginase on hollow fibers. *Int J Artif Organs* 1980;3:120.

38. Gombotz WR, Hoffman AS, Schmer G, et al. The immobilization of L-asparaginase on porous hollow fiber plasma filters. *J Controlled Release* 1985;2:375.

39. Edman P, Artursson P, Bjork E, et al. Immobilized L-asparaginase-L-glutaminase from *Acinetobacter glutaminasificans* in microspheres: some properties in vivo and in an extracorporeal system. *Int J Pharmaceut* 1987;34:225.

40. Woods JS, Handschumacher RE. Hepatic regulation of plasma L-asparaginase. *Am J Physiol* 1973;224:740.

41. Alpar HO, Lewis DA. Therapeutic efficacy of asparaginase encapsulated in intact erythrocytes. *Biochem Pharmacol* 1985;34:257.

42. Campbell HA, Mashburn LT, Boyse SE, et al. Two L-asparaginases from *E. coli* B: their separation, purification, and antitumor activity. *Biochemistry* 1967;6:721.

43. Mashburn LT, Landin LM. Some physiochemical aspects of L-asparaginase therapy. *Recent Results Cancer Res* 1970;33:48.

44. Broome JD. Factors which may influence the effectiveness of L-asparaginases as tumor inhibitors. *Br J Cancer* 1968;22:595.

45. Yellin TO, Wriston JC Jr. Purification and properties of guinea pig serum asparaginase. *Biochemistry* 1966;5:1605.

46. Peterson RE, Ciegler A. L-Asparaginase production by *Erwinia aroideae*. *Appl Microbiol* 1969;18:64.

47. Law AS, Wriston JC Jr. Purification and properties of *Bacillus coagulans* L-asparaginase. *Arch Biochem Biophys* 1971;147:744.

48. Roberts J, Holcenberg JS, Dolowy WC. Isolation, crystallization, and properties of Achromobacteraceae glutaminase-asparaginase with antitumor activity. *J Biol Chem* 1972;247:84.

49. Cooney DA, Capizzi RI, Handschumacher RE. Evaluation of L-asparagine metabolism in animals and man. *Cancer Res* 1970;30:929.

49a. Ertel IJ, Nesbit ME, Hammond D, et al. Effective dose of L-asparaginase for induction of remission in previously treated children with acute lymphocytic leukemia: a report from Children's Cancer Study Group. *Cancer Res* 1979;39:3893.

50. Nesbitt M, Chard R, Evans A, et al. Intermittent L-asparaginase therapy for acute childhood leukemia. In: *Proceedings of the 10th International Cancer Congress*. Houston, TX: Yearbook 1970:477.

51. Ohnuma T, Holland JF, Sinks LF. Biochemical and pharmacological studies with L-asparaginase in man. *Cancer Res* 1970;30:2297.

52. Asselin BL, Lorenson MY, Whitin JC, et al. Measurement of serum L-asparagine in the presence of L-asparaginase requires the presence of an L-asparaginase inhibitor. *Cancer Res* 1991;51:6568.

53. Asselin BL, Whitin JC, Coppola DJ, et al. Comparative pharmacokinetic studies of three asparaginase preparations. *J Clin Oncol* 1993;11(9):1780.

54. Sutor AH, Niemeyer C, Sauter S, et al. Gerinnungs veranderungen bei Behandlung mit den Protokollen ALL-BFM-90 und NHL-BFM-90. *Klin Padiatr* 1992;204:264.

55. Otten J, Suciu S, Lutz P, et al. The importance of L-asparaginase (A'ASE) in the treatment of acute lymphoblastic leukemia in children: results of the EORTC 58881 randomized phase trial showing greater efficiency of *Escherichia coli* as compared to *Erwinia* A'ASE. *Blood* 1996;88[Suppl 1]:669(abstr 2663).

56. Peterson RC, Handschumacher RF, Mitchell MS. Immunological responses to L-asparaginase. *J Clin Invest* 1971;50:1080.

57. Ho DH, Brown NS, Yen A, et al. Clinical pharmacology of polyethylene glycol-L-asparaginase. *Drug Metab Disp* 1986;14:349.

58. Oettgen HF, Stephenson PA, Schwartz MK, et al. Toxicity of *E. coli* L-asparaginase in man. *Cancer* 1970;25:253.

59. Capizzi RL, Bertino JR, Skeel RT, et al. L-Asparaginase: clinical, biochemical, pharmacological and immunological studies. *Ann Intern Med* 1971;74:893.

60. Clavell LA, Gelber RD, Cohen HJ, et al. Four-agent induction and intensive asparaginase therapy for treatment of childhood acute lymphoblastic leukemia. *N Engl J Med* 1986;315:657.

61. Nesbit ME, Ertel I, Hammond GD. L-Asparaginase as a single agent in acute lymphocytic leukemia: survey of studies from Children's Cancer Study Group. *Cancer Treat Rep* 1981;65[Suppl 4]:101.

62. Jones B, Holland JF, Glidewell O, et al. Optimal use of L-asparaginase (NSC-109229) in acute lymphocytic leukemia. *Med Pediatr Oncol* 1977;3:387.

63. Rutter DA. Toxicity of asparaginases. *Lancet* 1975;1:1293.

64. Land VJ, Sutow WW, Fernbach DJ, et al. Toxicity of L-asparaginase in children with advanced leukemia. *Cancer* 1972;40:339.

65. Khan A, Hill JM. Atopic hypersensitivity to L-asparaginase. *Int Arch Allergy* 1971;40:463.

66. Killander D, Dohlwitz A, Engstedt L, et al. Hypersensitive reactions and antibody formation during L-asparaginase treatment of children and adults with acute leukemia. *Cancer* 1976;37:220.

67. Nowak-Gottl U, Wermes C, Junker R, et al. Prospective evaluation of the thrombotic risk in children with acute lymphoblastic leukemia carrying the MTHFR TT 677 genotype, the prothrombin G20210A variant, and further prothrombotic risk factors. *Blood* 1999;93(5):1595.

68. Sills RH, Nelson DA, Stockman JA III. L-Asparaginase-induced coagulopathy during therapy of acute lymphocytic leukemia. *Med Pediatr Oncol* 1978;4:311.

69. Gralnick HR, Henderson E. Hypofibrinogenemia and coagulation factor deficiencies with L-asparaginase treatment. *Cancer* 1970;27:1313.

70. Ramsay NKC, Coccia PF, Krivit W, et al. The effect of L-asparaginase on plasma coagulation factors in acute lymphoblastic leukemia. *Cancer* 1977;40:1398.

71. Shapiro RS, Gerrard JM, Ramsay NK, et al. Selective deficiency in collagen-induced platelet aggregation during L-asparaginase therapy. *Am J Pediatr Hematol Oncol* 1980;2:207.

72. Cairo MS, Lazarus K, Gilmore RL, et al. Intracranial hemorrhage and focal seizures secondary to use of L-asparaginase during induction therapy of acute lymphocytic leukemia. *J Pediatr* 1980;97:829.

73. Mitchell L, Hoogendoorn H, Giles AR, et al. Increased endogenous thrombin generation in children with acute lymphoblastic leukemia: risk of thrombotic complications in L-asparaginase-induced antithrombin III deficiency. *Blood* 1994;83:386.

74. Bezeaud A, Drouet L, Leverger G, et al. Effect of L-asparaginase therapy for acute lymphoblastic leukemia on plasma vitamin K–dependent coagulation factors and inhibitors. *J Pediatr* 1986;108:698.

75. Leonard JV, Kay JDS. Acute encephalopathy and hyperammonaemia complicating treatment of acute lymphoblastic leukaemia with asparaginase. *Lancet* 1986;1:162.

76. Bushara KO, Rust RS. Reversible MRI lesions due to pegaspargase treatment of non-Hodgkin's lymphoma. *Pediatr Neurol* 1997;17:185.

77. Alberts SR, Bretscher M, Wiltsie JC, et al. Thrombosis related to the use of L-asparaginase in adults with acute lymphoblastic leukemia: a need to consider coagulation monitoring and clotting factor replacement. *Leuk Lymphoma* 1999;32(5–6):489.

78. Capizzi RL. Schedule-dependent synergism and antagonism between methotrexate and L-asparaginase. *Biochem Pharmacol* 1974; 23:151.

79. Jolivet J, Cole DE, Holcenberg JS, et al. Prevention of methotrexate polyglutamate formation. *Cancer Res* 1985;45:217.

80. Sur P, Fernandes DJ, Kute TE, et al. L-Asparaginase-induced modulation of methotrexate polyglutamylation in murine leukemia L5178Y. *Cancer Res* 1987;47:1313.

81. Lobel JS, O'Brien RT, McIntosh S, et al. Methotrexate and asparaginase combination chemotherapy in refractory acute lymphoblastic leukemia of childhood. *Cancer* 1979;43:1089.

82. Amadori S, Tribalto M, Pacilli L, et al. Sequential combination of methotrexate and L-asparaginase in the treatment of refractory acute leukemia. *Cancer Treat Rep* 1980;64:939.

83. Harris RE, McCallister JA, Provisor DS, et al. Methotrexate/L-asparaginase combination chemotherapy for patients with acute leukemia in relapse: a study of 36 children. *Cancer* 1980;46:2004.

84. Liang DC, Hung IJ, Yang CP, et al. Unexpected mortality from the use of *E. coli* L-asparaginase during remission induction therapy for childhood acute lymphoblastic leukemia: a report from the Taiwan Pediatric Oncology Group. *Leukemia* 1999;13:155.

85. Spiers ASD, Wade HE. *Achromobacter* L-glutaminase-L-asparaginase: human pharmacology, toxicology, and activity in acute leukemia. *Cancer Treat Rep* 1979;63:1019.

86. Holcenberg JS, Camitta BM, Borella LD, et al. Phase I study of succinylated *Acinetobacter* L-glutaminase-L-asparaginase. *Cancer Treat Rep* 1979;63:1025.

87. Holcenberg JS, Borella LD, Camitta BM, et al. Human pharmacology and toxicology of succinylated *Acinetobacter* glutaminase-asparaginase. *Cancer Res* 1979;39:3145.

88. Warrell RP Jr, Chou TC, Gordon C, et al. Phase I evaluation of succinylated *Acinetobacter* glutaminase-asparaginase in adults. *Cancer Res* 1980;40:4546.

89. Tan YY, Sun XH, Xu MX, et al. Efficacy of recombinant methioninase in combination with cisplatin on human colon tumors in nude mice. *Clin Cancer Res* 1999;5(8):2157.

90. Kreis W. Tumor therapy by deprivation of L-methionine: rationale and results. *Cancer Treat Rep* 1979;63:1069.

91. Elmer GW, Linden C, Meadows GG. Influence of L-tyrosine phenol-lyase on the growth and metabolism of B$_{16}$ melanoma. *Cancer Treat Rep* 1979;63:1055.

92. Abell CW, Smith WJ, Hodgkins DS. An in vivo evaluation of the chemotherapeutic potency of phenylalanine ammonia-lyase. *Cancer Res* 1973;33:2529.

93. Schmer G, Roberts J. Molecular engineering of the L-tryptophan-depleting enzyme indolyl-3 alkane alpha-hydroxylase. *Cancer Treat Rep* 1979;63:1123.

94. Catane R, Von Hoff DD, Glaubiger DL, et al. Azaserine, DON, and azotomycin: three diazo analogs of L-glutamine with clinical antitumor activity. *Cancer Treat Rep* 1979; 63:1033.

95. Jayaram HN, Cooney DA. Analogues of L-aspartic acid in chemotherapy for cancer. *Cancer Treat Rep* 1979;63:1095.

96. Royce ME, McGarry W, Bready B, et al. Sequential biochemical modulation of fluorouracil with folinic acid, N-phosphonoacetyl-L-aspartic acid, and interferon alfa-2a in advanced colorectal cancer. *J Clin Oncol* 1999;17(10):3276.

97. Uren R, Handschumacher RE. Enzyme therapy. In: Becker FF, ed. *Cancer: a comprehensive treatise*. New York: Plenum Press, 1977:457. [Contains a detailed discussion of therapies directed at amino acid depletion and analog development.]

22

PHARMACOLOGIC CONSIDERATIONS IN CHEMOTHERAPY FOR BRAIN TUMORS

TRACY T. BATCHELOR
MICHEL P. GATINEAU
JEFFREY G. SUPKO

The treatment of malignant brain tumors represents a unique challenge for oncologists due to the presence of a physiologic barrier between the circulatory system of the brain and that of the body. The existence of this blood–brain barrier (BBB) impedes the delivery of adequate concentrations of chemotherapeutic drug to the tumor. Methods of overcoming this barrier and measuring levels of chemotherapeutic agents in the brain have become a major area of research. In addition, the use of multiple ancillary agents in the medical management of brain tumor patients presents a high potential for drug interactions that may impact the efficacy of chemotherapy. This unique set of pharmacologic challenges must be addressed to improve the treatment of malignant brain tumors with chemical agents and represents the focus of this chapter.

Approximately 35,000 new primary brain tumors are diagnosed in the United States each year. Anaplastic astrocytoma and glioblastoma multiforme are the most common malignant brain tumors and represent the most frequent indication for cytotoxic chemotherapy in neuro-oncology.[1] Glioblastoma multiforme is the most common type of malignant glioma and has a median survival of less than 1 year despite treatment with surgery, radiation, and chemotherapy.[2] The goal of adjuvant chemotherapy for malignant glioma is eradication of the residual macroscopic and microscopic tumor felt to be the reason for surgical and radiation failure. Experience with adjuvant chemotherapy for malignant gliomas has been disappointing, however. Although some early randomized studies indicated a modest improvement in survival for patients treated with adjuvant 1,3-bis-(2-chloroethyl)-L-nitrosourea (BCNU, carmustine)[3,4] and the PCV combination regimen [procarbazine hydrochloride, 1-(2-chloroethyl)-3-cyclohexyl-L-nitrosourea (CCNU), vincristine sulfate],[5] other studies found no benefit. Moreover, the conclusion derived from a meta-analysis that adjuvant chemotherapy significantly increased the survival time of patients with glioblastoma multiforme[6] has been questioned.[7–10] At best, the addition of systemic chemotherapy has resulted in a very modest improvement in survival, on the order of several weeks, for adult patients with glioblastoma multiforme.[6] Nevertheless, chloroethylnitrosourea-based adjuvant chemotherapy is considered the standard of care for patients with malignant glioma after surgery and radiotherapy, despite the lack of definitive evidence of therapeutic benefit.[8]

Although malignant gliomas rarely spread beyond the central nervous system (CNS), local treatments, which include surgical debulking and radiotherapy, almost always fail. Recurrence is usually found within 2 cm of the original tumor margin after surgery and radiotherapy.[11] One of the primary reasons for failure is incomplete surgical resection due to poor definition of tumor margins. Typically, neoplastic cellular infiltration extends well beyond the tumor margin as defined by computed tomography (CT) or magnetic resonance imaging (MRI).[12] Microscopic extensions at the periphery of the tumor allow infiltration along white matter fibers and along perivascular spaces. Malignant glioma cells have been cultured from histologically normal brain tissue excised 4 cm away from the visible tumor margin.[13] This microscopic extension beyond radiographic borders prevents surgical achievement of tumor-free margins. Other potential reasons for treatment failure include the multifocal nature of gliomas, reinvasion by cells that have spread into the cerebrospinal fluid (CSF), and the intrinsic resistance of tumor cells to chemotherapy and radiation.

Mechanisms of chemotherapy resistance of brain tumors include factors common to other tumors such as multidrug resistance and increased efficiency of DNA damage-repair systems.[9,14] In addition, the difficulty in achieving adequate and sufficiently sustained levels of the cytotoxic moiety at the tumor site is considered to be one of the principal factors contributing to the failure of systemic chemotherapy for malignant brain tumors.[15–19] Preclinical studies have shown that the survival of glioma-bearing animal models is directly related to drug concentrations within the tumor.[20,21] Specifically, the higher the drug concentration achieved, the longer the survival. The accessibility of many anticancer drugs to brain tumors is at least partially constrained by the existence of the BBB, a physiologic impediment between the systemic circulation and the circulation of the CNS. Accordingly, the development of treatment strategies for brain tumors has emphasized techniques that are intended to overcome this barrier and improve drug delivery to these tumors. This chapter reviews the current state of approaches for delivering anticancer drugs to brain tumors, the various techniques that are available for assessing the extent of drug distribution to brain tumors, and important pharmacologic interactions that may affect both the accessibility of anticancer drugs to the CNS and the systemic pharmacokinetics of the anticancer agent.

BLOOD–BRAIN BARRIER

Three main factors influence the extent to which a systemically administered anticancer agent is distributed into the brain and brain tumors: (a) the plasma concentration × time profile of the drug, (b) regional blood flow, and (c) transport of the agent through the BBB and blood–tumor barrier (BTB). The two former considerations are common to all solid tumors, whereas the latter is specific to brain tumors.[15]

Erhlich was the first to propose the concept of the BBB at the beginning of this century. On administering the dye trypan blue to rats by intravenous injection, he observed that all body organs were stained except for the brain and spinal cord.[16,22,23] The anatomic basis of the BBB was determined three decades ago with the introduction of the electron microscope. It is a modified tight epithelium that consists of a sheet of cells connected by tight junctions on a basement membrane. The exchange surface is 12 m^2 in area,[24] and the physiologic role of the BBB is assumed to include maintenance of a constant biochemical content of the interstitial milieu and protection of the brain from foreign and undesirable molecules. Low hydraulic conductance, low ionic permeability, and high electrical resistance contribute to the very low permeability for hydrophilic nonelectrolytes in the absence of a membrane carrier.[25] These properties, together with the lack of intracellular fenestrations, pinocytotic vesicles, and a thicker basal lamina, create a physiologic barrier that renders the BBB relatively impermeable to many water-soluble compounds.[26,27]

Some drugs can use specific transport mechanisms of the endothelial cell to traverse the BBB.[28] Most cytotoxic drugs that gain access to the CNS, however, cross the BBB by passive diffusion. Aside from pharmacokinetic properties, the main factors that influence the extent to which these compounds distribute into the CNS include lipid solubility, molecular mass, charge, and plasma-protein binding. Drugs that are lipid soluble—that is, they have an octanol-

water partition coefficient greater than unity, are neutral at physiologic pH, are not highly bound to plasma proteins, and have a molecular weight less than 200—readily cross the BBB.[16,29] Indeed, correlations between BBB permeability and octanol-water partition coefficients have been established.[29] Only a few cytotoxic drugs fulfill these criteria, as most have molecular weights between 200 and 1,200. These properties are fulfilled by the chloroethylnitrosoureas, and they have become the most commonly used class of cytotoxic drugs for the treatment of malignant gliomas.[23]

The normal BBB has also been shown to express P-glycoprotein on the luminal surface of brain capillary endothelial cells. Expression of P-glycoprotein has been reported in malignant gliomas and may serve as another mechanism of chemotherapy resistance.[30–32] This structure has been implicated in the active efflux from the brain of many chemotherapeutic agents, including the vinca alkaloids and doxorubicin. Agents that reverse the function of P-glycoprotein, such as verapamil, may increase passage of doxorubicin across the BBB.

The normal physiologic structure of the BBB is disrupted in vasculature within and adjacent to brain tumors. Figure 22-1 contrasts the normal BBB with BBB disrupted by a brain tumor. Vick and colleagues identified junctional clefts in the endothelial cells of capillaries adjacent to brain tumors.[33] These clefts correlated with the density of infiltrating tumor cells and were present in brain capillaries not in direct contact with the tumor. Evidence also exists that the microvasculature of these tumors lacks the properties of a normal BBB and has greater permeability as a result. Morphologic studies have demonstrated that the BTB differs anatomically from the normal BBB, with open tight junctions, gap junctions, fenestrations, and numerous intracellular vesicles.[15,34] The increased permeability of these blood vessels forms the basis of contrast enhancement of brain tumors on CT and MRI scans. Iodinated, water-soluble contrast agents do not penetrate areas of the brain with an intact BBB but are able to penetrate brain tumors.[35] These alterations in permeability are highly variable between tumors and within the same tumor.[36] For example, low-grade gliomas and proliferating edges of malignant gliomas seem to have a normally functioning, selective BBB and, consequently, do not typically show contrast enhancement in CT and MRI studies. A large variation in the enhancement patterns of malignant brain tumors on CT scans is common.[37,38] Approximately 30% of patients with a type of malignant glioma, anaplastic astrocytoma, are reported to have nonenhancing lesions.[37] Finally, positron emission tomography (PET) studies have shown that alterations in permeability usually occur in the central part of large tumors, whereas the periphery is intact.[39] The presence of a selective, normal BBB near the proliferating edge of a brain tumor may result in variable delivery of water-soluble drugs in this region and account for the high local failure rate of conventional anticancer drugs.[11]

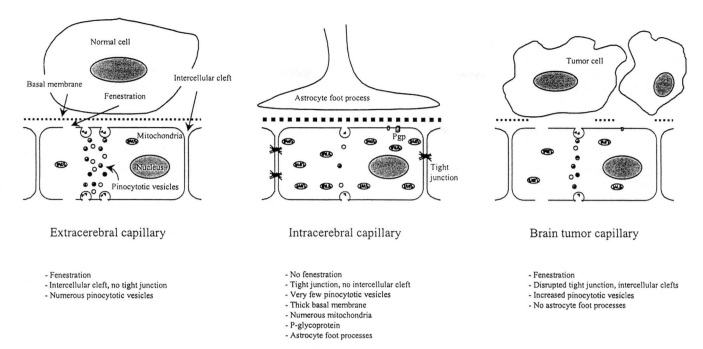

FIGURE 22-1. Schematic representation of the normal extracerebral, normal intracerebral, and brain tumor capillary. (Pgp, P-glycoprotein.)

The central role hypothesized for the BBB in the resistance of brain tumors to chemotherapy has been questioned by some authorities. These sources contend that, because the BBB adjacent to tumors and the BTB lack the normal properties of an intact BBB, drug delivery should not be compromised to these areas.[33] Indirect support for this argument comes from the observation that brain tumors occasionally respond to cytotoxic drugs that would not be expected to cross the BBB due to their physicochemical properties. A more consistent observation, however, has been that the most effective classes of antineoplastic drugs against malignant brain tumors are lipid-soluble molecules that can easily penetrate an intact BBB. Moreover, in addition to the existence of normal BBB at the proliferating edge of brain tumors, PET studies have demonstrated that, whereas the BBB and BTB may be abnormal at the time of diagnosis, these structures may become normalized on subsequent treatment.[40] These latter observations support a pivotal role for the BBB and BTB in the resistance of brain tumors to systemically administered chemotherapy. Therefore, considerable effort has been expended to develop strategies to circumvent the BBB and BTB. These include (a) intraarterial administration, (b) BBB disruption by hyperosmolar solutions[41] and biomolecules, (c) high-dose chemotherapy, (d) intrathecal injection, and (e) local delivery by direct intratumoral injection of free drug or implantation of drug embedded in a controlled-release biodegradable matrix delivery system. Even when drugs have crossed the BBB, however, their migration to tumor cells may be hindered by increased intercapillary distances, greater interstitial pressure, lower microvascular pressure, and the sink effect exerted by normal brain tissue.[42] Furthermore, intrinsic cellular resistance to specific classes of cytotoxic drugs is not addressed by drug delivery strategies. These latter obstacles, however, are common to many forms of cancer, and this chapter focuses on the unique aspects associated with drug delivery to brain tumors.

DRUG DELIVERY METHODS

Intraarterial Administration

The theoretical advantage for delivering anticancer drugs by the intraarterial route is related to the ratio of systemic to regional blood flow, so that a higher local drug concentration is achieved than with intravenous administration, and as a result the amount of the agent driven across the BBB is increased.[43] This has been confirmed by several observations, including the report of a threefold increase in tumor concentration of a chloroethylnitrosourea in the brains of several animal models after intraarterial administration compared with delivery by an intravenous route.[44,45] Another study documented a twofold increase of cisplatin in the tumors of patients with brain metastases with intraarterial administration.[46] With this technique, sufficient local drug concentrations can be achieved with smaller-than-conventional doses, so that systemic side effects are minimized.[47] Intraarterial administration of chemotherapy requires cannulation of the appropriate artery to introduce a catheter into the vessel that supplies the tumor. The pharmacokinetic advantages of intraarterial administration occur only during the first passage to the CNS, however, because the drug then enters venous circulation and the plasma profile is indistinguishable from that afforded by intravenous administration. On the basis of one pharmacologic model, the inference was that drugs that are good candidates for intraarterial delivery should possess the following properties: lipophilicity, small size, and rapid systemic inactivation to avoid systemic toxicities.[36] The chloroethylnitrosoureas exhibit these properties, and they have been used in a number of trials undertaken to evaluate intraarterial chemotherapy for brain tumors.[23]

Several studies have tested this approach in different settings, including neoadjuvant and adjuvant therapy and recurrent malignant glioma trials.[6,48–54] Thus far, clinical trials of intraarterial chemotherapy for malignant gliomas have not demonstrated clear improvement in survival over conventional intravenous therapy. A large phase III study including 315 evaluable patients with malignant gliomas failed to show any advantages of adjuvant intraarterial BCNU over an intravenous infusion of the same drug.[55] Moreover, subjects in the intraarterial BCNU arm of this trial experienced significant treatment-related toxicities, with 10% developing leukoencephalopathy and 15% developing ipsilateral blindness.

Potential disadvantages of the intraarterial route include local complications related to catheterization (thrombosis, bleeding, infection); neurotoxicity, including orbital and cranial pain, retinal toxicity, leukoencephalopathy, or cortical necrosis[6,55,56]; and inapplicability to drugs requiring systemic activation, such as cyclophosphamide and irinotecan (CPT-11). One factor that partly explains the unique toxicities associated with intraarterial administration is the "streaming" effect.[57,58] This is a consequence of infusing drug into a high-pressure and rapidly moving bloodstream, which results in heterogeneous mixing of the drug and high variability in the amount of drug reaching different regions of the vascular territory. Possibly, higher concentrations of drug might be achieved in normal brain, whereas lower amounts reach the tumor, which thus minimizes efficacy and maximizes neurotoxicity. Different strategies have been attempted to minimize the streaming effect, including rapid infusion,[57,59] superselective cannulation of the feeding artery,[46,56,60] diastole-phased pulsatile infusion,[61] and local blood flow–adjusted dosage.[60] All of these techniques were combined in a phase I trial involving 21 brain tumor patients treated with intraarterial carboplatin. The neurologic side effects were minor, and a twofold escalation of the dose beyond the conventional intraarterial dose was achieved with promising results.[60] However, toxicity, pharmacologic limitations, technical difficulty, and lack of treatment of the contralateral hemisphere[62] currently limit the applicability of this technique in the management of patients with brain tumors.

Blood–Brain Barrier Disruption

BBB disruption involves the use of hyperosmolar solutions or biomolecules to increase the permeability of the BBB and improve drug delivery to brain tumors. The specific mechanisms underlying osmotic opening of the BBB and BTB are not entirely understood. Preliminary explanations emphasized endothelial cell shrinkage with resultant tight junction separation after exposure to a hyperosmotic environment.[63] In addition to cellular shrinkage, osmotic stress results in the release of several biologically active compounds from endothelial cells, including serine proteases, that could potentially result in degradation of the collagen matrix of the basement membrane and BBB.[63] Finally, cellular shrinkage may also trigger second messenger signals and calcium influx, which could affect the integrity of tight junctions.[24]

Methods for disrupting the BBB involving both intravenous and intraarterial administration have been developed for use in brain tumor patients.[63] The results of nonrandomized studies have been encouraging for certain brain tumor subtypes, especially primary CNS lymphoma. Potential advantages of this method include increased tumor delivery of drug and lack of systemic toxicity from cytotoxic chemotherapy. Another possible advantage of this technique is avoidance of the sink effect seen with other procedures used for delivering chemotherapy to brain tumors. The *sink effect* refers to the selective achievement of higher concentrations of a drug to areas of disrupted BBB in the tumor than to the rest of the brain. As a result of this concentration gradient, the drug rapidly diffuses out of the tumor into the surrounding brain and compromises tumor exposure time. Because BBB disruption theoretically affects the endothelium of both normal brain and brain tumor, a nonselective increase in drug delivery into both areas occurs, and no concentration gradient is established. Despite these potential advantages, the technique of BBB disruption is complex and requires transfemoral angiography and general anesthesia. Moreover, an attendant risk of stroke as well as a high frequency of seizures are associated with this method. These factors have limited the application of this technique.[64,65]

Tumor location and vascular supply determine the arterial circulation that is catheterized and infused. Most commonly, one major artery (left carotid, right carotid, left or right vertebral) is cannulated and treated. Tumors located in the border zone between two arteries may be treated with successive catheterizations over 2 days. Developments have included superselective cannulations and infusions of intracranial arterial branches.[64] Some have advocated that documentation of BBB disruption with iodinated contrast agents be obtained before chemotherapy infusion. Given the technical requirements of this procedure, it has not been widely adopted, and no definitive conclusions about the efficacy of the technique can be derived from the results of nonrandomized trials that have been published to date.

Interest has been shown in the development of biologic agents to increase permeability of the BBB. Experimental data have demonstrated the efficacy of several such vasoactive compounds, including histamine, leukotriene C4, interferon-β, tumor necrosis factor α, and bradykinin. The bradykinin analog RMP-7 has been shown to selectively increase delivery of radiolabeled carboplatin to brain tumor in animal xenograft models as well as improve survival in these animals. Small, nonrandomized phase I and II human studies of intraarterial and intravenous RMP-7 have been inconclusive.[66,67]

High-Dose Chemotherapy

Considering that the BBB is a major factor in brain tumor resistance to chemotherapy and that diffusion across this barrier depends on the concentration × time profile of the free fraction of drug (i.e., drug that is not bound to plasma proteins), the assumption has been that increasing the administered dose would drive more drug across the BBB.[15,68] The rationale for high-dose chemotherapy was derived from the relatively linear *in vitro* dose-response curve exhibited by the classic alkylating agents and the assumption that intrinsic cellular resistance could be overcome by increasing the dose. In the context of treating brain tumors, the argument has been made that high-dose chemotherapy could overcome the previously mentioned sink effect and provide higher drug concentrations in the tumor for sustained periods. A number of phase I and II studies have been undertaken to evaluate this approach.[68,69]

Despite the theoretical advantages, high-dose chemotherapy for recurrent malignant glioma has not made a significant impact on patient survival, although cases of long-term survival have been observed anecdotally. Among patients with newly diagnosed tumors, the median survival achieved using high-dose chemotherapy with bone marrow or stem cell rescue is comparable to that with conventional-dose chemotherapy (12 to 26 months versus 10 to 12 months, respectively). Treatment-related morbidity and mortality have been high, however, with a mortality rate as high as 27% in one study.[70] At the present time, drawing firm conclusions regarding the potential of the technique for the treatment of malignant gliomas is difficult, because local tumor concentrations of the drugs were not measured in any of these trials. The strategy of high-dose chemotherapy followed by stem cell rescue may become an effective treatment strategy for potentially chemosensitive brain tumors such as anaplastic oligodendroglioma and primary CNS lymphoma.

Intrathecal Administration

Intrathecal chemotherapy involves the direct injection of drug into the CSF and is an obvious way to bypass the BBB. It is accomplished by injecting drug into the lumbar subarachnoid space, the cerebral ventricles, or the basal cisterns, with or without the use of catheters, pumps, or ventricular reservoirs.[71] The rationale is that the cells lining the fluid spaces of the brain are permeable, which results in a

free exchange of molecules from extracellular fluid (ECF) to CSF and vice versa. Relatively small doses of a drug given by intrathecal injection can achieve high local concentrations, due to the low volume of CSF (approximately 150 mL), which thereby minimizes systemic toxicity. Furthermore, because of the intrinsically low levels of enzymes in the CSF, some potentially useful agents that are subject to rapid metabolism in blood may avoid degradation. For example, one of the principal mechanisms of inactivation of cytosine arabinoside (ara-C) in the bloodstream is deamination catalyzed by cytidine deaminase. Cytidine deaminase is present at much lower concentrations in CSF, however, which results in an eightfold longer half-life of the drug in CSF than in plasma.[15] Finally, more unbound drug is available and free to diffuse from CSF to brain tissue because of the very low protein content of this fluid. Thus, intrathecal injection is a theoretical way to bypass the BBB and BTB while at the same time avoiding problems related to systemic toxicity, peripheral drug inactivation, and plasma protein binding.[72] The three drugs used most commonly in this manner are methotrexate sodium, ara-C, and thiotepa (thiotriethylene phosphoramide). These agents have been used mainly for the treatment of leptomeningeal metastases from systemic cancer.[73]

Intrathecal drug administration has several disadvantages, including the necessity to establish access to the CSF compartment. A ventricular access device is usually implanted in the frontal horn of the lateral ventricle to facilitate the administration of drug and minimize patient discomfort. This entails a small surgical risk of hemorrhage and infection. Moreover, the catheter may malfunction over time and require replacement.[74] Intrathecal drug administration also has numerous pharmacokinetic limitations. Among these, the drug must overcome bulk flow of CSF to penetrate the cisterns and ventricles (Fig. 22-2). In addition, the flow of interstitial fluid produced by brain cells and microvessels from ECF to CSF counteracts the diffusion of drug from CSF to ECF. Estimates are that CSF is completely renewed every 6 to 8 hours; thus, the concentration of a drug injected into the CSF decreases continuously as a consequence of this process, which can only be overcome by a continuous infusion or sustained-release system to maintain a clinically relevant concentration. Development of a liposomal form of ara-C allows sustained release of this drug into CSF and increases the effective half-life of the agent in the CSF by almost 50-fold.[75] Another pharmacologic disadvantage of the intrathecal route is the fact that production of CSF by the choroid plexus and its elimination into the venous circulation may be altered by the tumor itself, which disturbs bulk flow and modifies drug distribution and diffusion. For example, the clearance of methotrexate from CSF is decreased in the presence of leukemic meningitis.[76,77] Moreover, diffusion in the ventricular space is heterogeneous[78] and may result in uncertain and potentially toxic local concentrations in CSF,

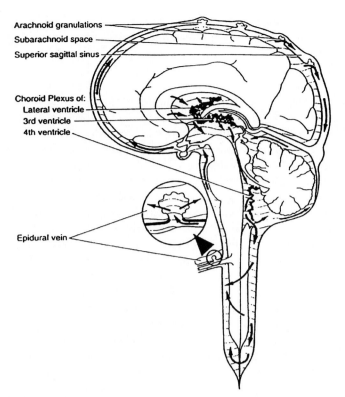

Arachnoid granulations
Subarachnoid space
Superior sagittal sinus

Choroid Plexus of:
Lateral ventricle
3rd ventricle
4th ventricle

Epidural vein

FIGURE 22-2. Cerebrospinal fluid pathways. (From Fishman RA, ed. *Cerebrospinal fluid in diseases of the nervous system*. Philadelphia: Saunders, 1992:8, with permission.)

even if continuous-infusion devices are used.[71] Finally, and most important, brain tumors are often in locations not adjacent to the ventricular system and may require diffusion of drug from CSF to tumor over a distance of several centimeters, which impairs the ability to achieve cytotoxic concentrations of the drug at the site of the tumor. In the case of methotrexate, the concentration of drug has been calculated to be no more than 0.1% of the CSF concentration 1 cm from the ependymal edge 48 hours after intrathecal administration.[79] However, the relationship is quite complex. Whereas compounds with greater lipophilicity will access the ECF more effectively, they will also be subject to a higher rate of removal by the vascular and cellular compartments, thereby limiting the extent of drug penetration into brain tissue.[80] Therefore, intrathecal chemotherapy is not feasible for brain tumors and is restricted to the treatment and prevention of leptomeningeal metastases.[81]

Intratumoral Administration

The simplest and most direct way to guarantee that a cytotoxic drug reaches its target is to deliver it directly into the tumor or into the cavity left after tumor resection.[19,82] As with intrathecal injection, this bypasses most of the previously mentioned obstacles pertaining to systemic drug administration for treating brain tumors. Systemic toxicity

may also be reduced because substantially lower doses of drug may be given, and only a relatively small amount of drug distributes from the CNS to the bloodstream, which further decreases peak plasma concentrations compared to those with intravenous dosing. A particularly attractive advantage of this strategy is that anticancer drugs that are normally impeded by the BBB may be used. Conceptually, the low permeability of the BBB to such compounds should promote their retention within the CNS by inhibiting distribution into the bloodstream. Characteristics of a drug that make it ideal for local instillation include lack of any requirement for systemic activation; amenability to local degradation, which minimizes systemic toxicity; limited toxicity to normal brain tissue; a high diffusion coefficient; and high solubility in parenteral vehicles to minimize the injection volume. Due to the high local drug concentrations that can be achieved, better distribution of drug may be provided within the tumor by diffusion and convection driven by the hydrostatic pressure of the tumor. The two techniques that have been most commonly used for directly introducing chemotherapeutic agents into brain tumors are parenteral delivery as either a bolus injection or continuous infusion through a cannula, and implantation of drug embedded in a slow-release carrier system.

The feasibility of intratumoral infusion has been demonstrated in a number of clinical trials involving approximately ten different anticancer agents.[83] These studies, however, have not shown a clear survival advantage or direct evidence of increased drug delivery within the tumor. Furthermore, toxicity has been observed with this technique, including nervous system injury and infection.[83] Even if intratumoral infusion does avoid some obstacles to drug delivery, it does not circumvent the sink effect or problems associated with drug stability. Indeed, drug molecules released into the ECF must penetrate the brain interstitial tissue to reach tumor cells.[42] Before reaching its target, the compound could be inactivated by protein binding, metabolism, chemical degradation, or elimination by the microvascular circulation.[84] Finally, obstruction of the catheter by tissue debris can occur.[83,84]

Controlled-release methods using polymer, microsphere, and liposomal carriers have been studied extensively *in vitro* and *in vivo*.[19] The goal of this strategy is to provide constant delivery of a cytotoxic drug into the tumor using a matrix that also protects the unreleased drug from hydrolysis and metabolism. Use of a solid polymeric matrix to facilitate the delivery of chemotherapeutic agents directly to brain tumors has several potential advantages. Biodegradable carriers have been developed that are unaffected by interstitial pH and provide near-zero-order release of drug, with minimal inflammatory response.[85,86] Potential disadvantages include the fact that drug release cannot be controlled once the device has been implanted without physically removing it. Other potential problems include unpredictable diffusion, stability of the device and drug in the aqueous milieu, and the possibility that the polymer may not release the drug as intended.

A biodegradable polyanhydride solid matrix, poly[bis(*p*-carboxyphenoxy)propane-sebacic acid] or p(CPP-SA), has been developed that releases drug by a combination of diffusion and hydrolytic polymer degradation.[87] Preclinical studies have demonstrated that this system is biocompatible and results in reproducible and sustained continuous release of BCNU.[88–90] Pharmacokinetic studies in animals have demonstrated higher brain concentrations of BCNU in the ipsilateral cerebral hemisphere than in blood (50-fold) or in contralateral brain (15-fold).[91,92] Finally, rodent studies have shown improved survival[21] with the use of polymers containing BCNU, paclitaxel,[93] 4-hydroperoxycyclophosphouride (4-HC),[94] carboplatin,[95] camptothecin,[96] 5-fluorouracil,[97] and cisplatin.[98,99] A primate study undertaken to address the mechanisms involved in the distribution of drugs when delivered by implanted polymers into the brain showed that convection was the most important factor for the compounds evaluated, which included BCNU, 4-HC, and paclitaxel.[98] Drug levels in the tissue surrounding the polymer were very high and were sustained for as long as 7 days at a distance of 7 mm. The animals did not have brain tumors, however, and the depth of tissue penetration was on the order of millimeters, whereas some tumors in humans may extend several centimeters from the site of surgery.[13]

These preclinical studies led to phase I–II and phase III placebo-controlled studies of the BCNU polymer to treat recurrent[100,101] and newly diagnosed[102,103] malignant gliomas, involving more than 300 patients. The phase III study demonstrated that intratumoral implantation of a 3.85% BCNU polymer was safe and resulted in minimal systemic side effects from BCNU. Doses as high as 62 mg BCNU were placed into the tumor cavity. Necrotic tissue, a probable indication of drug activity, was found up to 1 cm away from the tumor resection edge at autopsy.[102] Prior radiation therapy did not enhance neurotoxicity,[100] consistent with earlier primate studies.[90] Median survival was longer in subjects with glioblastoma multiforme who received the active polymer than in those who did not (31 weeks versus 23 weeks, *p* = .006), even after adjustment for known prognostic factors.[100] A phase I study designed to increase the amount of BCNU in the polymer (up to 20%) demonstrated that BCNU plasma levels at the highest dose were 500 times lower than those associated with systemic BCNU toxicity. As a result, no BCNU-related systemic toxicity was seen.[104] At higher polymer concentrations of BCNU, however, risk of local neurotoxicity may be increased. Other studies of this delivery strategy are ongoing and include assessment of higher polymer concentrations of BCNU, combinations of BCNU polymer and intravenous chemotherapy, and different chemotherapy agents delivered in polymer form.[105,106] The BCNU polymers currently available for clinical application provide, at best, a modest improvement in outcome for patients with recurrent glioblastoma multiforme.

Convection-Enhanced Delivery

Experimental evidence has demonstrated that properties of brain parenchyma may impede delivery of drugs to the site of a brain tumor. Therefore, the BBB may not be the only obstacle that must be overcome for successful delivery of a cytotoxic drug to a brain tumor. Diffusion barriers intrinsic to brain tissue may also be important in limiting drug delivery to tumors. The hydrostatic pressure of brain tissue and the solubility of the drug are important factors that determine the diffusion of drug into surrounding tissue. Convection-enhanced delivery (CED) is a method developed to overcome these potential barriers and consists of a direct infusion of drug solution through a catheter surgically implanted in the brain tumor. Experimental studies of CED have demonstrated that drug delivery with this method is dependent on the anatomic site of the catheter. Infusion into gray matter results in spherical distribution of the drug, whereas infusion into white matter results in distribution along white matter fiber pathways. Therefore, the specific anatomic location of the brain tumor may be an important determinant of drug delivery. CED has two principal advantages. First, concentration of the drug in the extracellular fluid can be increased or decreased by changing the infusion concentration. Second, selective placement of the catheter allows delivery of the drug to the site of the brain tumor.[107]

Studies of the delivery of ara-C to rat brain after intravenous, intrathecal, and intraventricular administration and CED have been conducted.[108] Using quantitative autoradiographic analysis, investigators demonstrated that drug concentration in brain tissue after CED was 4,000-fold higher than after intravenous administration. Moreover, the volume of distribution was tenfold higher after CED than after intrathecal or intraventricular administration. The use of CED in the treatment of patients with brain tumors has been limited. In a phase I study involving 18 patients with recurrent malignant gliomas, a high-flow interstitial microinfusion of a conjugated form of diphtheria toxin was conducted.[109] In 9 of 15 evaluable patients, at least a 50% regression of tumor was apparent on MRI, and two complete responses were observed. The treatment was well tolerated, and no treatment-related deaths or systemic toxicity occurred. The dose-limiting toxicity was local brain injury, which may have been the result of endothelial damage of cerebral capillaries.

Investigational Strategies

Other carrier systems are in development that do not require intratumoral implantation. Lipid-coated microbubbles are vesicles with a gaseous interior and thin lipid monolayer surface with entrapped drug. Two advantages of this technique identified in preclinical studies are the use of the intravenous route and the specific tumor-targeting ability of lipid-coated microbubbles.[110] Another technique is the colloid cationic delivery system, which uses magnetic aminodextran microspheres, neutral magnetic dextran microspheres, or liposomes.[111] These microspheres have an affinity for brain tumor tissue, are administered systemically, and release drug in a controlled manner. The small size of magnetic aminodextran microspheres and magnetic dextran microspheres protect them from the immune system,[112] and their electrostatic interaction with endothelial cells within the tumor results in retention of these particles inside the tumor.[113,114]

ASSESSMENT OF DRUG DELIVERY TO THE BRAIN

Pharmacokinetic studies are a fundamental component of the initial clinical trials to evaluate investigational chemotherapeutic agents. Defining the plasma concentration × time profile of a new drug provides valuable information that can significantly impact the course of its clinical development. A compound is considered unlikely to be clinically effective unless the maximum tolerated dose (MTD) achieved in cancer patients provides sufficiently long exposure to plasma concentrations comparable to those required for activity against preclinical tumor models. Furthermore, establishing relationships between pharmacokinetic data and the severity of dose-limiting toxicities may facilitate the design of an administration schedule affording a potentially effective pattern of systemic exposure to the agent with an acceptable toxicity profile. However, demonstrating that a seemingly desirable plasma profile of a chemotherapeutic agent can be achieved in patients does not necessarily predict clinical activity.

Therapeutic response ultimately depends on the distribution of drug from the bloodstream to the tumor such that biologically effective concentrations of the active form of the agent are achieved and maintained for an adequate duration within the lesion. The rate processes associated with drug distribution and elimination are dependent on the physicochemical properties of the drug and numerous physiologic factors. The situation is far more complex for agents targeted against brain tumors than for those targeted against extraneural solid malignancies because the drug must traverse the BBB or BTB with reasonable efficiency.[15,42,115] As is the case with any specific organ or tissue, the time course of the concentration of a drug or active metabolite within a tumor cannot be defined from experimental data restricted to measurements made in plasma, serum, or whole blood. Although some temporal relationship undoubtedly exists between drug concentrations in plasma and those in tumor, elucidating the tumor concen-

tration × time profile requires the measurement of drug levels within the tumor itself. Thus, although it is extremely useful when considered in proper context, the information derived from a traditional pharmacokinetic study is limited, as it provides no inferences about the distribution and accumulation of drug within a tumor, particularly those in the CNS.[116]

Until recently, evaluating the distribution of an experimental drug to a tumor depended on the acquisition of biopsy specimens. Incorporating provisions to acquire tumor biopsies into clinical studies as a routine practice has been extremely difficult, however, for several reasons. Practical limitations include exposing the patient to the risks of a surgical procedure with little or no direct benefit to the treatment of their disease. Moreover, single or serial biopsy procedures are very expensive. The most appropriate time to obtain a single biopsy specimen is also unknown, because the time of peak drug concentration within the tumor cannot be predicted from plasma pharmacokinetic data. Consequently, the presence or absence of a measurable drug concentration in a single biopsy specimen obtained after systemic administration of the agent has little interpretive value. Acquiring serial tumor specimens from the same patient presents even greater practical constraints than conducting a single biopsy, and the effect of prior procedures on altering the transport of drug to and from the tumor represents a significant confounding factor. Alternatively, as part of a phase II study in which a moderately sized cohort of patients with comparable disease characteristics is treated with the same dose of drug, single biopsies of the tumor and adjacent peritumoral tissue could be performed in different patients over a range of times, so that a composite or pooled time course could be constructed. The concurrent collection of blood specimens during the surgical procedure could permit the establishment of the temporal relationship between the plasma concentration of drug and its levels in brain tissue. Although conceptually feasible, examples of studies using an experimental protocol of this type have not been reported.

Despite the practical limitations to obtaining the most meaningful data, endeavors to determine whether adequate concentrations of the active form of a drug reach the target tissue are extremely important in the context of phase I trials to evaluate the efficacy of new anticancer drugs for treating brain tumors. Because objective antitumor responses occur infrequently in phase I studies, the availability of data regarding the extent to which a chemotherapeutic agent reaches a brain tumor would provide a rational basis for selecting drugs that warrant further clinical evaluation. As described in this section, the principal techniques that are less invasive and potentially more informative than biopsy studies for assessing the pharmacokinetics of anticancer drugs in the CNS and brain tumors include CSF sampling, microdialysis, and noninvasive imaging. Although no single method can be uniformly applied for monitoring drugs in human tissues *in vivo*, these techniques are nevertheless becoming increasingly important to the clinical development of anticancer drugs for the treatment of brain tumors.

Cerebrospinal Fluid Sampling

Pharmacologic studies of anticancer agents directed against brain tumors often include the determination of drug or drug metabolite concentrations in the CSF as a surrogate for tumor levels and as a measure of drug delivery beyond the BBB (Fig. 22-3).[116] An understanding of the composition and normal physiology of CSF is important to discern the significance of drug level monitoring in this compartment. The most distinctive difference between CSF and plasma is the substantially lower concentration of proteins in CSF. Because of this, the total concentration of compounds that are poorly soluble in water or bind avidly to protein would be expected to be lower in CSF than in plasma or brain tissue, whereas the free concentration would be measurably increased. In addition, CSF is slightly more acidic than plasma (pH of 7.32 versus 7.40), and this differential could conceivably influence the transport and retention of a drug in CSF, as well as its chemical stability relative to that in plasma, for compounds that have a functional group with a pKa in the 7 to 8 range. With regard to agents such as the camptothecins, in which the active form of the drug has an intact lactone ring that is in equilibrium with the inactive opened-ring species, the lower pH shifts the equilibrium in favor of the active moiety.[117,118]

Figure 22-2 depicts the normal process involved in CSF formation and flow. The volume of CSF contained within the ventricles, cisterns, and subarachnoid space of a normal adult is approximately 150 mL.[119] Because approximately 500 mL of CSF is produced each day, most of which is formed by the choroid plexus within the cerebral ventricles, the entire CSF volume is replenished approximately three times during the course of a day. CSF formed in the lateral ventricles flows into the third ventricle and then to the fourth ventricle. On exiting from the fourth ventricle, it passes into the basal cisterns and the cerebral and spinal subarachnoid spaces, descending through the posterior aspect of the spinal cord and returning through the anterior aspect. Ascending CSF passes over the cerebral hemispheres toward the major dural sinuses, where absorption of CSF into the venous system occurs at the arachnoid villi. The formation and flow of CSF may be perturbed in the presence of a brain tumor. The presence of increased intracranial pressure reduces CSF formation in the unusual situation in which it is high enough to reduce cerebral blood flow. Brain tumors that obstruct CSF flow may result in persistent hydrocephalus, which may reduce CSF formation and disrupt CSF flow pathways.[120]

Concentration gradients between the ventricular and lumbar regions exist for endogenous constituents of CSF as well as for xenobiotics that have gained access to the CSF. The concentration of systemically administered drugs is generally higher in CSF collected from the ventricles than from the lumbar region, as drug distribution in the CNS follows CSF flow.[121] Because drug levels are often determined in CSF acquired by lumbar puncture, one should recognize that this may significantly underestimate the concentrations in the ventricular region. Similarly, drug

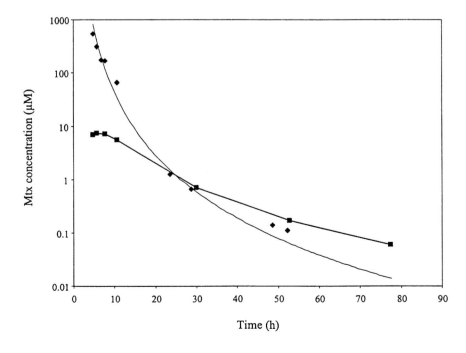

FIGURE 22-3. Plasma (♦) and cerebrospinal fluid (CSF) (■) concentration of methotrexate (Mtx) in a cancer patient treated with a dose of 8 g/m², given as a 4-hour continuous intravenous infusion. The CSF profile demonstrates that peak CSF drug concentration was approximately 100-fold lower than the plasma concentration at the end of infusion, and the elimination of drug from the CSF was at approximately the same rate as the terminal phase in plasma.

administered directly into lumbar CSF is poorly distributed to the ventricles.[78,122] Although patients cannot be subjected to frequently repeated lumbar punctures, ventricular access devices may be used to facilitate the serial acquisition of CSF specimens for drug level monitoring in the brain. Therefore, the specific space from which CSF samples were collected must be taken into account whenever drug concentrations reported in different studies are compared. Furthermore, in the process of collecting CSF specimens, the fluid balance or bulk volume of CSF could be significantly altered, which thereby affects pressure equilibrium and flow between the various CSF compartments, as well as the concentration gradients between CSF and plasma.

Although it is more informative than data based on determinations made in plasma alone, elucidating the CSF concentration × time course of an anticancer agent provides limited knowledge about the characteristics of its distribution to a brain tumor. The presence of drug in the CSF represents a strong, but not definitive, indication that the compound has gained access to brain tissue, inclusive of tumors. Some level of uncertainty exists because the vascular supply to the choroid plexus, hypophysis, and pineal gland is not protected by the BBB. Although it comprises a comparably small exchange surface, this does provide a direct pathway for the transport of compounds into the CSF. To further complicate matters, the absence of measurable drug or metabolite levels in the CSF does not absolutely imply that the agent has failed to reach a brain tumor. Conceivably, the majority of a compound reaching brain tissue could be trapped in the intracellular space, extensively bound to tissue protein, subject to chemical or enzymatic conversion to unknown products, or effluxed back into the bloodstream before migrating from interstitial spaces to the CSF. Accordingly, many drugs have been found to achieve higher concentrations in a brain tumor than would have been predicted from plasma and CSF data.[123,124] Despite the limitations of CSF as an indirect measure of drug delivery to a brain tumor, it is an accessible compartment, and CSF sampling remains an important method for screening drug access to the CNS.

Microdialysis

As previously indicated, inadequate transport of drug from systemic circulation to the interstitial space surrounding tumor cells is one of the primary reasons for the failure of chemotherapy for malignant gliomas.[42,125] Accordingly, the time course of the concentration of free drug in the interstitial fluid within a tumor provides a better indication of the potential for efficacy than data derived from plasma. Moreover, the area under the curve for this compartment is more comparable to the concentration–exposure time product that elicits *in vitro* growth-inhibitory activity against human tumor cells.[115,125] Microdialysis is a technique that enables the concentration of a compound with appropriate physico-chemical characteristics to be continuously measured in ECF within a tumor or normal tissues in a living subject.

The miniature dialysis probe consists of a chamber that is less than 1 mm in diameter and is composed of a semipermeable membrane into which two sections of microcatheter are fused.[126] Membranes with molecular weight cutoffs in the 20- to 100-kd range are commercially available. This device is stereotactically implanted so that the probe resides within the desired area of the brain or tumor and the microcatheters are externalized. One of the microcatheters is connected to a syringe pump capable of continuously delivering perfusion fluid at flow rates in the microliter-per-minute range, while dialysate is collected from the other microcatheter. The composition of the perfusion solution is prepared to approximate the matrix of interest as closely as possible, which in the case of normal or malignant brain tissue would be CSF. In theory, microdialysis mimics the passive function of a capillary blood vessel. Water, inorganic ions, and small organic molecules freely diffuse across the membrane of the probe, which is impermeable to proteins and protein-bound compounds.[126] Lipophilic compounds are also poorly recovered.[127,128]

Considerable experience has been gained with the use of microdialysis, in both animal models and human subjects, since the technique was first introduced some three decades ago.[129] The greatest advantages of the technique for pharmacodynamic and pharmacokinetic studies is the facilitation of direct, serial sampling of ECF from a highly localized area of intact tissue (approximately 1 mm^3 or less) with minimal perturbation of the preexisting conditions or functional alteration of the tissue.[115,125,126] Application of the technique for neurologic patients has been thoroughly evaluated.[115,126] The procedures involved in the insertion and removal of the dialysis probe can be performed with minimal injury to normal brain tissue or alteration of fluid balance. Although insertion of the microdialysis probe could conceivably disrupt the BBB, this has not proven to be problematic,[130,131] as demonstrated by the absence of intravenously administered markers around the probe[132] or in the dialysate.[115,133] Although it can be performed safely, microdialysis is nevertheless an invasive surgical procedure with a small risk of bleeding at the site of insertion and discomfort for the patient.

Due to the low flow rate at which the perfusion solution is delivered, the perfusate must generally be collected over intervals of 5 to 10 minutes to obtain a sufficient volume for chemical analysis. Consequently, microdialysis is not suitable for studying systems in which the concentration of the compound of interest is changing rapidly relative to this time frame. This would not be anticipated to preclude studying the rate processes describing the time course of a systemically administered anticancer agent in a brain tumor. The perfusate obtained by microdialysis can be analyzed directly by methods such as reversed-phase high-performance liquid chromatography, liquid chromatography/mass spectrometry, or capillary electrophoresis without the need for any preliminary sample preparation to remove macromolecules, as is generally required for assays performed on plasma.[115,134,135] Due to the dynamic nature of the system, in which the concentration of compounds in the ECF may be constantly changing while the perfusion fluid within the dialysis probe is continually flowing, steady-state conditions between the sampled fluid and dialysis fluid are not achieved. Nevertheless, it has been conclusively established that the *in vivo* recovery of an analyte, defined as its concentration in the dialysate relative to that in the sampled fluid, is independent of the concentration in the sampled fluid. Because the drug concentration in the dialysate is generally much lower than in ECF, however, the diluting effect of the technique demands a very sensitive analytical method to enable the detection of low concentrations of an analyte in small sample volumes.[115,136–138]

Microdialysis was first used to facilitate the measurement of dopamine levels in the brains of living rats.[129] The initial preclinical application of the technique to monitor the distribution of an anticancer drug to a brain tumor was described by de Lange, who measured the concentration of methotrexate in a rodent brain tumor model.[139] The results obtained with microdialysis were comparable to those in previous studies of methotrexate distribution to tumors based on the classic methods of autoradiography and tissue excision.[139,140] Subsequently, the technique has been used to define the concentration × time profile of camptothecin[141] and topotecan in rodent brain tumor models,[141,142] as well as of other antineoplastic agents in various preclinical tumor models.[126,127,143,144]

Microdialysis has been used extensively in head injury patients for monitoring a variety of biochemical parameters, including levels of lactic acid, glucose, glutamic acid, and γ-aminobutyric acid, partial pressure of oxygen, and pH, for the purpose of detecting complications and assessing the effect of therapeutic interventions.[145–152] Despite the common application of this technique in head injury patients, not a single report of its use for measuring levels of an anticancer agent in brain tumor patients has been published. The feasibility of using the technique in the reverse application, however—that is, for intratumoral drug delivery—has been demonstrated in a small cohort of patients with glioblastoma multiforme.[153] Moreover, only two reports have been published describing the use of microdialysis to study the intratumoral disposition of anticancer agents in patients with extraneural solid malignancies. Specifically, microdialysis has been used successfully to monitor carboplatin levels in melanomas[154] and 5-fluorouracil delivery in breast tumors.[125] In the latter study, a relationship between the area under the interstitial concentration-time curve of 5-fluorouracil and therapeutic response was established.

In summary, microdialysis represents a promising technique for assessing the disposition of anticancer agents in human brain tumors. The increasing availability of extremely sensitive and specific mass spectrometry–based detection methods coupled with improved surgical technique and monitoring will undoubtedly lead to the application of this method for studying drug distribution to brain tumors in the near future.

Noninvasive Imaging

With continual improvements in spatial resolution, temporal resolution, and sensitivity, imaging techniques such as magnetic resonance spectroscopy (MRS) and PET offer the ability to noninvasively monitor the concentration of a drug or its metabolites within brain tumors and surrounding normal tissue. MRS involves the application of a strong magnetic field to the brain, which induces the absorption of energy in the radiofrequency range by atomic nuclei with appropriate spin characteristics. The frequencies of energy required to effect a transition between nuclear spin states are characteristic for each different nucleus and can be readily distinguished by a spectrometer. The isotopes of atoms amenable to detection by MRS that are of greatest interest with regard to drug level monitoring include hydrogen 1 (^{1}H), hydrogen 2 (deuterium), boron 11, carbon 13 (^{13}C), nitrogen 15, fluorine 19, and phosphorus 31 (^{31}P). These are stable isotopes, although not always the most abundant isotopic form of an atom, such as ^{13}C, for example. The spatial location and connectivity of atoms in the immediate vicinity of any given nucleus within a molecule influence the effective magnetic field experienced by the nucleus; this results in small but distinctive shifts in the resonance energy, which convey structural information. The physical configuration of the instrumentation used for *in vivo* MRS results in a very substantial reduction in the resolution that can be achieved with analytical spectrometers. Whereas *in vivo* MRS can readily distinguish different atomic nuclei, the amount of detail pertaining to the type of molecule or functional group to which similar nuclei are bound is limited.

The intense signals associated with ^{1}H and ^{31}P, which result from the ubiquitous presence of these nuclei in bio-organic molecules, are used advantageously for diagnostic MRI. However, ^{1}H and ^{31}P MRS cannot generally be used to monitor xenobiotics *in vivo*, due to the intensity of the natural background signals, unless a compound has nuclei with chemical shifts that differ substantially from the resonance frequencies arising from endogenous molecules. Examples of the latter situation include the detection of iproplatin by ^{1}H MRS and ifosfamide by ^{31}P MRS.[155,156] Aside from these considerations, the relatively poor sensitivity of MRS is perhaps the single factor that most severely limits its utilization for *in vivo* drug level monitoring. A molecule must generally be present at concentrations in the low millimolar range to produce a detectable signal. Relatively few cytotoxic drugs, however, achieve these concentrations in plasma or tissues. Furthermore, the anticancer agents that are currently being advanced into clinical trials tend to be increasingly potent, with MTDs that provide peak plasma concentrations in the nanomolar to low micromolar range in patients. The detection limits of MRS can be improved to some degree by increasing the data acquisition time. This sacrifices temporal resolution, however, which may be extremely important for pharmacokinetic studies. MRS does not permit the determination of the absolute concentration of a drug *in vivo*, although changes in relative concentration during the course of a single experiment can be readily followed. Another important consideration in using MRS to study the time course of a drug in brain tumors is that the spatial resolution is not particularly good—only approximately 1 cm^2 with current instrumentation.[115,157]

Despite these limitations, MRS has proven to be extremely valuable for studying the tissue pharmacokinetics of some fluorinated drugs, such as 5-fluorouracil.[157–160] The ^{19}F nucleus represents an ideal object for *in vivo* MRS studies. Spectra acquired from MRS scans of the human body show no background signals in the region where ^{19}F resonates due to the lack of endogenous fluorinated organic compounds. Moreover, the nuclear spin characteristics of ^{19}F provide an excellent signal.[157] An MRS study involving 103 patients with extraneural malignancies demonstrated that therapeutic response to 5-fluorouracil was significantly correlated with the half-life of the drug within tumors.[157,159,161] Gemcitabine hydrochloride is another fluorinated anticancer agent for which ^{19}F MRS has been successfully used for *in vivo* pharmacokinetic studies.[162,163] Although the feasibility of the approach has been demonstrated, very little clinical experience has been gained with the use of MRS for studying the distribution of anticancer drugs to brain tumors.

Dynamic PET imaging is an established technique for defining the time course of radiolabeled anticancer drugs within brain tumors and surrounding normal tissue in patients. In comparison with MRS, PET enables radiolabeled compounds to be detected with 10^6 to 10^9 times greater sensitivity and superior temporal resolution due to shorter data acquisition time.[164] Furthermore, whereas MRS is effectively limited to monitoring the relative change in concentration of a compound during the course of a study, PET provides a quantitative measurement of radioactivity.[164] In addition, excellent spatial resolution, on the order of 6 mm or better, can be achieved with the current generation of detectors in whole-body PET scanners.[165]

The ability to use this methodology ultimately depends on developing a suitable procedure to introduce a positron-emitting radionuclide into the drug molecule. The fact that substituting a stable atom with a radioisotope of the same element does not affect the physicochemical, pharmacokinetic, or biologic properties of a drug has been well established. The radionuclides that have been most commonly used for PET pharmacokinetic studies are carbon 11 (^{11}C),

fluorine 18 (^{18}F), and nitrogen 13 (^{13}N).[165] Because these radionuclides have very short half-lives—10 minutes for ^{13}N, 20 minutes for ^{11}C, and 110 minutes for ^{18}F—a cyclotron and remote-controlled radiochemical synthesis facility are required for on-site generation of the radionuclide and immediate preparation of the labeled drug.[165,166] As a consequence, the technique is expensive, and relatively few institutions in the United States have assembled the physical facilities required to undertake PET pharmacokinetic studies.[115]

The most informative application of PET to pharmacokinetic studies entails the simultaneous acquisition of two sets of data as follows. A series of tomographic images are acquired for a total period of 1 to 2 hours after bolus intravenous administration of a tracer dose of the radiolabeled drug, which typically ranges from 100 to 1,000 MBq, together with the usual dose of unlabeled drug. The time over which individual images are measured generally increases during the course of the experiment and can range from 5 seconds to 10 minutes, as dictated by the combined rates of radioactive decay of the tracer and elimination of the drug from the body. The time-averaged concentration of radiotracer in discrete regions of interest within the image are used to construct time-activity curves. Arterial blood is also serially collected from the patient throughout the experiment for independent measurement of the radiotracer concentration in whole blood or plasma by solid scintillation counting. The empirical kinetic model that best relates the time course of radiotracer in tissue to its concentration in plasma is then identified.[167]

In addition to its inherent expense and technical complexities, PET has a number of other distinct limitations when applied to study of the tissue pharmacokinetics of a drug. The time period over which a radiolabeled drug can be monitored after administration of a tracer dose is effectively limited to three to four times the half-life of radioactive decay. The maximum duration of an experiment is therefore only 90 minutes for a ^{11}C-labeled drug and 6 to 8 hours when ^{18}F is used as the radiotracer. For some drugs, this may not be enough time to adequately define the time course of the uptake or decline of radiotracer in the tumor. Furthermore, expecting patients to remain within the confines of the PET camera for more than 60 to 90 minutes is unreasonable, and demands on the instrument for routine diagnostic use may also represent a significant factor that limits the duration of an experiment.

Another important deficiency is that PET measures total radioactivity without distinguishing alterations in the chemical structure of the labeled molecule. Because PET cannot distinguish the parent drug from metabolites that retain the label, or free from protein-bound drug, it may not be suitable for studying the distribution of drugs that are extensively metabolized or highly protein bound. These factors need to be taken into consideration for each individual agent when analyzing and interpreting kinetic data from PET studies.[167] Nevertheless, PET can provide highly informative insights and answer the critical question of whether radiotracer originating from the drug accumulates within a tumor.

Dynamic PET imaging has been used to study the distribution of the radiolabeled forms of several clinically approved and investigational anticancer agents to human brain tumors, including [11C]-BCNU,[168,169] [13N]-cisplatin,[170] 5-[18F]-fluorouracil,[164] and [11C]-temozolomide.[167] Temozolomide is a nonclassic alkylating agent that has been approved for clinical use in the treatment of anaplastic astrocytoma.[171] PET has been used to demonstrate that the initial uptake of radioactivity originating from [11C]-temozolomide in plasma was seven times greater in brain tumors than in normal brain tissue, with the kinetic behavior in these two regions becoming almost indistinguishable by 30 minutes after dosing.[167] In consideration of these results, the markedly greater accumulation of radiolabeled agent in the tumor than in normal brain tissue, clearly evident in the PET images, was attributed to increased drug delivery due to a breakdown of the BBB within the tumor. The suggestion that the initial uptake of temozolomide from plasma could be an important determinant of its efficacy against human brain tumors has potential clinical significance.

An excellent example of the use of PET during the preliminary clinical evaluation of drug congeners of BCNU has been described. After development of a procedure to synthesize 11C-labeled 2-chloroethyl-3-sarcosinamide-1-nitrosourea (SarCNU),[172] the sarcosinamide analog of BCNU, a pilot study involving patients with glioblastoma multiforme demonstrated that the distribution of radioactivity into the brain after intravenous administration of [11C]-BCNU closely paralleled blood flow, as measured by gallium 68–labeled ethylenediaminetetraacetic acid PET scanning.[173] Intravenous treatment with [11C]-SarCNU, however, resulted in greater accumulation of radioactivity in the tumor than in surrounding normal brain tissue. These findings were consistent with *in vitro* evidence that the uptake of SarCNU by human glioma cells was augmented by an active transport mechanism.[174] SarCNU has been advanced into phase I clinical trials due to the suggestion that it has the potential to be more effective against gliomas than BCNU, which accesses tumors only by passive diffusion.

DRUG INTERACTIONS AFFECTING BRAIN TUMOR THERAPY

The two principal objectives of most phase I clinical studies of an investigational anticancer agent are to identify the dose-limiting toxicities and to establish the MTD of the drug. According to current guidelines developed by the U.S. National Cancer Institute, the MTD for a given administration schedule determined in a phase I study is intended to be the dose used in phase II studies undertaken to identify evidence of therapeutic response in cohorts of patients with similar disease characteristics. The initial phase I trials of new compounds that are being evaluated for the treatment of solid malignancies are typically performed in adult cancer patients with advanced disease that has failed to respond to standard therapeutic modalities. Patients with hematologic malignancies or evidence of a primary or metastatic lesion in the CNS are usually excluded from these studies. The rationale for excluding patients with CNS disease from initial phase I studies is that difficulties are presented in determining whether potential indications of neurotoxicity are drug-related or a complication associated with the tumor. Furthermore, the additional supporting medications used in the clinical management of patients with brain tumors, such as anticonvulsant drugs and corticosteroids, could suppress the presentation of symptoms indicative of drug-related neurotoxicity. Nevertheless, the MTD of an anticancer agent determined in studies involving patients with systemic solid tumors is typically used for phase II trials to assess activity against brain tumors, without provisions to further refine the dose. This practice was recognized possibly to lead to significant undertreatment of patients with CNS malignancies due to pharmacokinetic interactions resulting from the medications administered concurrently to these patients, which can enhance the elimination of anticancer agents from systemic circulation as well as impede their access to the CNS.[175,176]

Interactions Affecting the Elimination of Anticancer Agents

Metabolism represents a quantitatively significant pathway of elimination for many chemotherapeutic agents that are either used or have been evaluated for the treatment of brain tumors. Xenobiotic biotransformation reactions may be broadly categorized into two classes depending on whether or not they are conjugative in nature. Oxidation, reduction, and hydrolysis are the principal nonconjugative reactions. Conjugative reactions involve the coupling of endogenous molecules, including glucuronate, glucose, sulfate, acetate, amino acid, methyl, or glutathione groups to the parent drug or a precursory metabolite. Among these reactions, hepatic oxidative metabolism probably has the greatest overall involvement in the biotransformation of anticancer drugs. This pathway is particularly susceptible to modulation by other drugs, however, which often results in clinically significant pharmacokinetic interactions.

Oxidative reactions are predominantly mediated by a large family of heme-containing isozymes known as cytochrome P-450 enzymes (CYP450).[177] The CYP450 enzymes are most abundantly expressed in the smooth endoplasmic reticulum of the liver, but they are also present in the kidney, lung, and gastrointestinal epithelium at significant levels. CYP3A4 is the predominant isozyme involved in drug metabolism, as it acts on a multitude of structurally diverse compounds, although a number of other isozymes catalyze the oxidation of some clinically important antineoplastic agents.[178] With regard to the anticancer drugs that are more commonly used for treating CNS malignancies, CYP3A4 mediates the biotransformation of ifosfamide and vincristine, whereas CYP2B6 catalyzes the initial hydroxylation reaction in the conversion of cyclophosphamide to alkylating and cytotoxic species.[179,180]

That certain classes of compounds can induce or suppress the expression of CYP450 and thereby alter the extent to which other drugs are metabolized by these pathways is well known.[175,176] In addition, competitive inhibition could result from the concurrent administration of two or more drugs that are substrates for the same CYP450 isozyme. These situations may not result in detectable effects on the pharmacokinetic behavior of most drugs. Anticancer agents are typically administered at their MTDs, however, and thus use a greater capacity of the elimination pathways than drugs given for other indications. Accordingly, the potential for clinically significant pharmacokinetic interactions may be greater for chemotherapeutic agents than for other classes of drugs.

Anticonvulsant drugs such as phenytoin, carbamazepine, and phenobarbital, which are commonly administered on a long-term basis to brain tumor patients, are potent inducers of CYP3A4.[181] Patients treated with these medications exhibit increased systemic clearance of epipodophyllotoxins[182] and vinca alkaloids.[183] In consideration of the potential for pharmacokinetic interactions such as these, several phase I studies have been designed to independently establish the MTD of new chemotherapeutic agents in brain tumor patients stratified according to whether or not they are receiving enzyme-inducing antiepileptic drugs.[184,185] The concomitant administration of enzyme-inducing anticonvulsants was found to alter the pharmacokinetics of paclitaxel when given as a 96-hour continuous intravenous infusion to patients with newly diagnosed glioblastoma multiforme, which resulted in lower steady-state plasma concentrations, reduced systemic toxicity, and higher dose requirements.[184] Similarly, the clearance of 9-aminocamptothecin, an investigational topoisomerase I inhibitor, proved to be significantly greater in patients with malignant gliomas who were receiving antiepileptic drugs than in those who were not.[185] These findings serve to demonstrate that pharmacokinetic drug interactions of this type cannot be reliably predicted on the basis of preclinical data. The probability of enhanced clearance of the epipodophyllotoxins, vinca alkaloids, and paclitaxel would have been considered high, as the importance of CYP3A4-mediated hepatic metabolism was well documented for each of these drugs. In contrast, no evidence from prior preclinical or clinical studies with 9-aminocamptothecin indicated that hepatic metabolism played a significant role in the elimination of this compound.[186,187]

Another type of interaction with potential clinical importance involves valproic acid and irinotecan. Irinotecan is a prodrug for the camptothecin analog designated SN-38, which, unlike the parent molecule, is susceptible to conjugation with glucuronic acid. The relative extent to which SN-38 is glucuronidated appears to be related to the severity of gastrointestinal toxicity, which can be dose limiting.[188] Preclinical pharmacokinetic studies in the rat have shown that valproic acid, an antiepileptic drug that does not induce CYP450 and that is frequently used in brain tumor patients, significantly decreased plasma concentrations of SN-38 glucuronide, presumably due to competitive inhibition of uridine diphosphate–glucuronyltransferase.[189] These preclinical data have led to the exclusion of brain tumor patients taking valproic acid from clinical trials of irinotecan.

Corticosteroids are widely used for the treatment of vasogenic brain edema and increased intracranial pressure in patients with brain tumors. They also induce CYP3A4 by a pretranslational mechanism involving a glucocorticoid-responsive sequence in the promoter of the gene encoding the enzyme.[190] Preclinical studies have shown that the pharmacokinetic behavior of cyclophosphamide and ifosfamide were markedly affected by pretreatment with corticosteroids.[191–193] Docetaxel metabolism was shown to be induced by dexamethasone *in vitro,* and decreased plasma concentrations of the drug have been demonstrated in a rodent model.[194,195] Corticosteroids appear to have little or no effect on the pharmacokinetics of the chloroethylnitrosourea alkylating agents.[196]

Many other supporting medications are used in the management of patients with brain tumors that can potentially affect the pharmacokinetics of anticancer agents. Drugs such as omeprazole[197] and certain antidepressants, including fluoxetine hydrochloride, are substrates or inhibitors of CYP3A4,[198] and their use may delay the elimination of anticancer drugs that are also metabolized by the enzyme; this delay could result in increased plasma concentrations that could be potentially dangerous. The potential also exists for pharmacokinetic interactions involving analgesics. Salicylates can reduce the renal tubular secretion of methotrexate.[199] Morphine and its derivatives may alter the rate and extent of absorption of orally administered cytotoxic drugs by reducing gastrointestinal motility. Because antiepileptic drugs are commonly used in brain tumor patients and may impact the metabolism of certain anticancer drugs in different ways, pharmacokinetic studies assume a crucial role in the clinical evaluation of new agents in this patient population.

Therapies That Modulate Drug Distribution to the Brain

Corticosteroids have a well-established effect on decreasing the permeability of the BBB and BTB to a wide variety of molecules. Preclinical studies have shown that dexamethasone significantly reduces the transport through the BBB of water,[200] small organic molecules with molecular weights in the 100 to 350 range,[201,202] and macromolecules such as horseradish peroxidase.[203] Treatment with corticosteroids diminishes the permeability of experimental brain tumors, brain tissue immediately adjacent to tumor, and normal brain tissue distant to tumor, but the effect is most pronounced within the tumor itself.[204] These findings have been corroborated in studies of brain tumor patients. A marked reduction in the permeability of tumor and normal brain tissue to rubidium 82 [^{82}Rb], as measured by PET imaging, was evident within 6 hours after the administration of dexamethasone by bolus injection to patients, and the effect persisted for at least 24 hours.[205] The magnitude of the decreased uptake of ^{82}Rb ranged from 6% to 48%.[206] Similar results have been observed in other studies using CT scanning[207] and MRI.[208,209] The effect of corticosteroids on the uptake of systemically administered chemotherapeutic agents has been evaluated in nude mice bearing intracranially implanted xenografts of human glioma. Steroid administration decreased the amount of carboplatin,[210] cisplatin,[211] and methotrexate[212] in the tumor and surrounding brain tissue by 20% to 40%. The extent to which the distribution of an anticancer agent to brain tumors is affected by corticosteroids in humans, however, remains to be determined.

The effect of radiotherapy on the integrity of the BBB and consequent penetration of drug into brain tumors remains an open area of investigation. Conflicting observations have been reported and may be attributed to marked differences in radiation treatment protocols, the methods used to assess the impact of the treatments on the function of the BBB, and the time course of changes in vascular physiology.[213] Consideration of the evidence derived from preclinical investigations indicates that the BBB in normal tissue becomes more permeable shortly after delivery of radiation according to the standard regimen of 5 days per week for 6 weeks.[214] This is entirely consistent with the finding that P-glycoprotein labeling decreased by 60% in the endothelial cells of brain vessels in a rodent after irradiation.[215] Slowly progressive alterations in the microvasculature of the irradiated tissue eventually result in decreased permeability.[214]

The optimal schedule for delivering chemotherapy when used in combination with radiotherapy for treating brain tumors has not been conclusively established. The accumulation of methotrexate in a brain tumor model in mice was impaired by delivering radiation either before or concurrently with the systemically administered drug and resulted in shorter survival times; this suggests that chemotherapy should be given before radiation treatments.[216] In contrast, clinical observations indicating that a 30- to 40-Gy dose of radiation increased the permeability of the BBB within the irradiated tumor by 74% but only by 24% in normal surrounding tissue, as assessed by scintigraphy, were the basis for advocating the administration of anticancer drugs after radiotherapy.[217] Another study involving pediatric leukemia patients found no difference in the CSF-to–plasma concentration ratio of chemotherapeutic agents when given before, during, or after radiotherapy.[218] Because clinical trials for many new anticancer agents in brain tumor patients are now conducted in both the preradiation and postradiation periods, comparison of drug distribution into the CNS and brain tumors for these settings may be warranted.

SUMMARY

Treatment strategies for the most common type of primary brain tumor, malignant glioma, are rapidly expanding. The persistence of normal BBB near the proliferating edge of the tumor coupled with normalization of other areas of the BBB with treatment emphasize the importance of strategies aimed at improving drug delivery across the BBB and to the tumor. In addition to the methods discussed in this review, cytotoxic drugs specifically designed for BBB penetration represent an important class of therapies to be assessed in the future. Methods for evaluating the success of these strategies are under development. Pharmacokinetic studies have assumed great importance in the development of antineoplastic therapy for hematologic and solid malignancies. Although application of the same principles to studies of brain tumor therapies is a relatively recent development and represents a unique set of challenges, these correlative studies add invaluable information in the assessment of new brain tumor therapies. Moreover, with the emergence of cytostatic therapies for cancer, the traditional radiographic end points are insufficient, and these evaluative methods are likely to become surrogate end points in future clinical trials of these therapies. Finally, drug interactions have assumed great importance in brain tumor clinical trials with the recognition that many common supporting medications used in this patient population affect the metabolism of cytotoxic drugs through induction of the CYP450 enzyme family. The development of noninvasive methods that more readily facilitate evaluation of drug distribution and accumulation in local tissue and tumor is a fundamental challenge for the future. The availability of such techniques will allow efficient assessment of promising agents for the treatment of malignant gliomas.

REFERENCES

1. CBTRUS. *Statistical report: Primary brain tumors in the United States, 1992–1997.* Central Brain Tumor Registry of the United States, 2000.
2. Landis SH, Murray T, Bolden S, et al. Cancer statistics, 1999. *CA Cancer J Clin* 1999;49:8.
3. Walker MD, Green SB, Byar DP, et al. Randomized comparisons of radiotherapy and nitrosoureas for the treatment

of malignant glioma after surgery. *N Engl J Med* 1980; 303:1323.

4. Green SB, Byar DP, Walker MD, et al. Comparisons of carmustine, procarbazine, and high-dose methylprednisolone as additions to surgery and radiotherapy for the treatment of malignant glioma. *Cancer Treat Rep* 1983;67:121.

5. Levin VA, Silver P, Hannigan J, et al. Superiority of postradiotherapy adjuvant chemotherapy with CCNU, procarbazine, and vincristine (PCV) over BCNU for anaplastic gliomas: NCOG 6G61 final report. *Int J Radiat Oncol Biol Phys* 1990;18:321.

6. Fine HA, Dear KB, Loeffler JS, et al. Meta-analysis of radiation therapy with and without adjuvant chemotherapy for malignant gliomas in adults. *Cancer* 1993;71:2585.

7. Forsyth PA, Cairncross JG. Treatment of malignant glioma in adults. *Curr Opin Neurol* 1995;8:414.

8. Prados MD, Russo C. Chemotherapy of brain tumors. *Semin Surg Oncol* 1998;14:88.

9. Prados MD, Berger MS, Wilson CB. Primary central nervous system tumors: advances in knowledge and treatment. *CA Cancer J Clin* 1998;48:331.

10. Hildebrand J, Sahmoud T, Mignolet F, et al. Adjuvant therapy with dibromodulcitol and BCNU increases survival of adults with malignant gliomas. EORTC Brain Tumor Group. *Neurology* 1994;44:1479.

11. Hochberg FH, Pruitt A. Assumptions in the radiotherapy of glioblastoma. *Neurology* 1980;30:907.

12. Kelly PJ, Daumas-Duport C, Scheithauer BW, et al. Stereotactic histologic correlations of computed tomography- and magnetic resonance imaging-defined abnormalities in patients with glial neoplasms. *Mayo Clin Proc* 1987;62:450.

13. Silbergeld DL, Chicoine MR. Isolation and characterization of human malignant glioma cells from histologically normal brain. *J Neurosurg* 1997;86:525.

14. Wiestler O, Kleihues P, Pegg AE. O[6]-alkylguanine-DNA alkyltransferase activity in human brain and brain tumors. *Carcinogenesis* 1984;5:121.

15. Greig NH. Optimizing drug delivery to brain tumors. *Cancer Treat Rev* 1987;14:1.

16. Kroll RA, Pagel MA, Muldoon LL, et al. Improving drug delivery to intracerebral tumor and surrounding brain in a rodent model: a comparison of osmotic versus bradykinin modification of the blood-brain and/or blood-tumor barriers. *Neurosurgery* 1998;43:879.

17. Levin VA, Landahl HD, Patlak CS. Drug delivery to CNS tumors. *Cancer Treat Rep* 1981;65:19.

18. Phillips PC. Antineoplastic drug resistance in brain tumors. *Neurol Clin* 1991;9:383.

19. Sipos EP, Brem H. New delivery systems for brain tumor therapy. *Neurol Clin* 1995;13:813.

20. Matsukado K, Inamura T, Nakano S, et al. Enhanced tumor uptake of carboplatin and survival in glioma-bearing rats by intracarotid infusion of bradykinin analog, RMP-7. *Neurosurgery* 1996;39:125.

21. Tamargo RJ, Myseros JS, Epstein JI, et al. Interstitial chemotherapy of the 9L gliosarcoma: controlled release polymers for drug delivery in the brain. *Cancer Res* 1993;53:329.

22. Pardridge WM, Oldendorf WH, Cancilla P, et al. Blood-brain barrier: interface between internal medicine and the brain. *Ann Intern Med* 1986;105:82.

23. Vassal G. Pharmacologic basis of chemotherapy of brain tumors in children. *Bull Cancer* 1990;77:699.

24. Zlokovic BV, Apuzzo ML. Strategies to circumvent vascular barriers of the central nervous system. *Neurosurgery* 1998;43:877.

25. Crone C. The blood-brain barrier: a modified tight epithelium. In: Succkling AJ, Rumsby MG, Bradbury MWB, eds. *The blood-brain barrier in health and disease.* Chichester, England: Ellis Horwood, 1986:17.

26. Muldoon LL, Pagel MA, Kroll RA, et al. A physiological barrier distal to the anatomic blood-brain barrier in a model of transvascular delivery. *AJNR Am J Neuroradiol* 1999;20:217.

27. Fishman RA. *Cerebrospinal fluid in diseases of the nervous system.* Philadelphia: WB Saunders, 1992:43.

28. Gouyette A, Hartmann O, Pico JL. Pharmacokinetics of high-dose melphalan in children and adults. *Cancer Chemother Pharmacol* 1986;16:184.

29. Greig NH, Momma S, Sweeney DJ, et al. Facilitated transport of melphalan at the rat blood-brain barrier by the large neutral amino acid carrier system. *Cancer Res* 1987;47:1571.

30. Henson JW, Cordon-Cardo C, Posner JB. P-glycoprotein expression in brain tumors. *J Neurooncol* 1992;14:37.

31. Fenart L, Buee-Scherrer V, Descamps L, et al. Inhibition of P-glycoprotein: rapid assessment of its implication in blood-brain barrier integrity and drug transport to the brain by an in vitro model of the blood-brain barrier. *Pharm Res* 1998;15:993.

32. Tsuji A. P-glycoprotein-mediated efflux transport of anticancer drugs at the blood-brain barrier. *Ther Drug Monit* 1998;20:588.

33. Vick NA, Khandekar JD, Bigner DD. Chemotherapy of brain tumors. The "blood brain barrier" is not a factor. *Arch Neurol* 1977;34:523.

34. Waggener JD, Beggs JL. Vasculature of neural neoplasms. *Adv Neurol* 1976;15:27.

35. Steinhoff H, Grumme T, Kazner E, et al. Axial transverse computerized tomography in 73 glioblastomas. *Acta Neurochir* 1978;42:45.

36. Blasberg RG, Groothuis DR. Chemotherapy of brain tumors: physiological and pharmacokinetic considerations. *Semin Oncol* 1986;13:70.

37. Chamberlain MC, Murovic JA, Levin VA. Absence of contrast enhancement on CT brain scans of patients with supratentorial malignant gliomas. *Neurology* 1988;38:1371.

38. DeAngelis LM. Cerebral lymphoma presenting as a nonenhancing lesion on computed tomographic/magnetic resonance scan. *Ann Neurol* 1993;33:308.

39. Brooks DJ, Beaney RP, Thomas DG. The role of positron emission tomography in the study of cerebral tumors. *Semin Oncol* 1986;13:83.

40. Orr RJ, Brada M, Flower MA, et al. Measurements of blood-brain barrier permeability in patients undergoing radiotherapy and chemotherapy for primary cerebral lymphoma. *Eur J Cancer.* 1991;27:1356.

41. Rapoport SI, Fredericks WR, Ohno K, et al. Quantitative aspects of reversible osmotic opening of the blood-brain barrier. *Am J Physiol* 1980;238:R421.

42. Jain RK. Transport of molecules in the tumor interstitium: a review. *Cancer Res* 1987;47:3039.

43. Greenberg HS, Chandler WF, Sandler HM. Brain tumor chemotherapy and chemotherapy. In: Greenberg HS, Chan-

dler WF, Sandler HM, eds. *Brain tumors*. New York: Oxford University Press, 1999:100.

44. Levin VA, Kabra PM, Freeman-Dove MA. Pharmacokinetics of intracarotid artery 14C-BCNU in the squirrel monkey. *J Neurosurg* 1978;48:587.

45. Yamada K, Ushio Y, Hayakawa T, et al. Distribution of radiolabeled 1-(4-amino-2-methyl-5-pyrimidinyl)methyl-3-(2-chloroethyl)-3-nitrosourea hydrochloride in rat brain tumor: intraarterial versus intravenous administration. *Cancer Res* 1987;47:2123.

46. Nakagawa H, Fujita T, Izumoto S, et al. *cis*-diamminedichloroplatinum (CDDP) therapy for brain metastasis of lung cancer. I. Distribution within the central nervous system after intravenous and intracarotid infusion. *J Neurooncol* 1993;16:61.

47. Bullard DE, Bigner SH, Bigner DD. Comparison of intravenous versus intracarotid therapy with 1,3-bis(2-chloroethyl)-1-nitrosourea in a rat brain tumor model. *Cancer Res* 1985;45:5240.

48. Greenberg HS, Ensminger WD, Chandler WF, et al. Intraarterial BCNU chemotherapy for treatment of malignant gliomas of the central nervous system. *J Neurosurg* 1984;61:423.

49. Kleinschmidt-DeMasters BK, Geier JM. Pathology of high-dose intraarterial BCNU. *Surg Neurol* 1989;31:435.

50. Larner JM, Phillips CD, Dion JE, et al. A phase 1-2 trial of superselective carboplatin, low-dose infusional 5-fluorouracil and concurrent radiation for high-grade gliomas. *Am J Clin Oncol* 1995;18:1.

51. Lesser GJ, Grossman S. The chemotherapy of high-grade astrocytomas. *Semin Oncol* 1994;21:220.

52. Madajewicz S, West CR, Park HC, et al. Phase II study—intra-arterial BCNU therapy for metastatic brain tumors. *Cancer* 1981;47:653.

53. Stewart DJ, Grahovac Z, Hugenholtz H, et al. Combined intraarterial and systemic chemotherapy for intracerebral tumors. *Neurosurgery* 1987;21:207.

54. West CR, Avellanosa AM, Barua NR, et al. Intraarterial 1,3-bis(2-chloroethyl)-1-nitrosourea (BCNU) and systemic chemotherapy for malignant gliomas: a follow-up study. *Neurosurgery* 1983;13:420.

55. Shapiro WR, Green SB, Burger PC, et al. A randomized comparison of intra-arterial versus intravenous BCNU, with or without intravenous 5-fluorouracil, for newly diagnosed patients with malignant glioma. *J Neurosurg* 1992; 76:772.

56. Tamaki M, Ohno K, Niimi Y, et al. Parenchymal damage in the territory of the anterior choroidal artery following supraophthalmic intracarotid administration of CDDP for treatment of malignant gliomas. *J Neurooncol* 1997;35:65.

57. Blacklock JB, Wright DC, Dedrick RL, et al. Drug streaming during intra-arterial chemotherapy. *J Neurosurg* 1986; 64:284.

58. Lutz RJ, Dedrick RL, Boretos JW, et al. Mixing studies during intracarotid artery infusions in an in vitro model. *J Neurosurg* 1986;64:277.

59. Takeda N, Diksic M. Relationship between drug delivery and the intra-arterial infusion rate of SarCNU in C6 rat brain tumor model. *J Neurooncol* 1999;41:235.

60. Cloughesy TF, Gobin YP, Black KL, et al. Intra-arterial carboplatin chemotherapy for brain tumors: a dose escalation

study based on cerebral blood flow. *J Neurooncol* 1997; 35:121.

61. Saris SC, Blasberg RG, Carson RE, et al. Intravascular streaming during carotid artery infusions. Demonstration in humans and reduction using diastole-phased pulsatile administration. *J Neurosurg* 1991;74:763.

62. Loeffler JS, Alexander Ed, Hochberg FH, et al. Clinical patterns of failure following stereotactic interstitial irradiation for malignant gliomas. *Int J Radiat Oncol Biol Phys* 1990; 19:1455.

63. Kroll RA, Neuwelt EA. Outwitting the blood-brain barrier for therapeutic purposes: osmotic opening and other means. *Neurosurgery* 1998;42:1083.

64. Gumerlock MK, Neuwelt EA. Chemotherapy of brain tumors: innovative approaches. In: Morantz RA, Walsh JW, eds. *Brain tumors*. New York: Marcel Dekker, 1994:763.

65. Neuwelt EA, Howieson J, Frenkel EP, et al. Therapeutic efficacy of multiagent chemotherapy with drug delivery enhancement by blood-brain barrier modification in glioblastoma. *Neurosurgery* 1986;19:573.

66. Ford J, Osborn C, Barton T, et al. A phase I study of intravenous RMP-7 with carboplatin in patients with progression of malignant glioma. *Eur J Cancer* 1998;34:1807.

67. Cloughesy TF, Black KL, Gobin YP, et al. Intra-arterial Cereport (RMP-7) and carboplatin: a dose escalation study for recurrent malignant gliomas. *Neurosurgery* 1999;44:270.

68. Fine HA, Antman KH. High-dose chemotherapy with autologous bone marrow transplantation in the treatment of high grade astrocytomas in adults: therapeutic rationale and clinical experience. *Bone Marrow Transplant* 1992;10:315.

69. Fernandez-Hidalgo OA, Vanaclocha V, Vieitez JM, et al. High-dose BCNU and autologous progenitor cell transplantation given with intra-arterial cisplatinum and simultaneous radiotherapy in the treatment of high-grade gliomas: benefit for selected patients. *Bone Marrow Transplant* 1996;18:143.

70. Mbidde EK, Selby PJ, Perren TJ, et al. High dose BCNU chemotherapy with autologous bone marrow transplantation and full dose radiotherapy for grade IV astrocytoma. *Br J Cancer* 1988;58:779.

71. Bakhshi S, North RB. Implantable pumps for drug delivery to the brain. *J Neurooncol* 1995;26:133.

72. Harbaugh RE. Novel CNS-directed drug delivery systems in Alzheimer's disease and other neurological disorders. *Neurobiol Aging* 1989;10:623.

73. Pinkel D, Woo S. Prevention and treatment of meningeal leukemia in children. *Blood* 1994;84:355.

74. Chamberlain MC, Kormanik PA, Barba D. Complications associated with intraventricular chemotherapy in patients with leptomeningeal metastases. *J Neurosurg* 1997;87:694.

75. Chamberlain MC, Kormanik P, Howell SB, et al. Pharmacokinetics of intralumbar DTC-101 for the treatment of leptomeningeal metastases. *Arch Neurol* 1995;52:912.

76. Ettinger LJ, Chervinsky DS, Freeman AI, et al. Pharmacokinetics of methotrexate following intravenous and intraventricular administration in acute lymphocytic leukemia and non-Hodgkin's lymphoma. *Cancer* 1982;50:1676.

77. Bleyer WA, Drake JC, Chabner BA. Neurotoxicity and elevated cerebrospinal-fluid methotrexate concentration in meningeal leukemia. *N Engl J Med* 1973;289:770.

78. Shapiro WR, Young DF, Mehta BM. Methotrexate: distribution in cerebrospinal fluid after intravenous, ventricular and lumbar injections. *N Engl J Med* 1975;293:161.

79. Blasberg RG, Patlak C, Fenstermacher JD. Intrathecal chemotherapy: brain tissue profiles after ventriculocisternal perfusion. *J Pharmacol Exp Ther* 1975;195:73.

80. Blasberg RG. Methotrexate, cytosine arabinoside, and BCNU concentration in brain after ventriculocisternal perfusion. *Cancer Treat Rep* 1977;61:625.

81. Chamberlain MC. Leptomeningeal metastases: a review of evaluation and treatment. *J Neurooncol* 1998;37:271.

82. Walker WL, Cook J. Drug delivery to brain tumors. *Bull Math Biol* 1996;58:1047.

83. Walter KA, Tamargo RJ, Olivi A, et al. Intratumoral chemotherapy. *Neurosurgery* 1995;37:1128.

84. Mak M, Fung L, Strasser JF, et al. Distribution of drugs following controlled delivery to the brain interstitium. *J Neurooncol* 1995;26:91.

85. Wu MP, Tamada JA, Brem H, et al. In vivo versus in vitro degradation of controlled release polymers for intracranial surgical therapy. *J Biomed Mater Res* 1994;28:387.

86. Leong KW, Brott BC, Langer R. Bioerodible polyanhydrides as drug-carrier matrices. I: Characterization, degradation, and release characteristics. *J Biomed Mater Res* 1985;19:941.

87. Leong KW, D'Amore PD, Marletta M, et al. Bioerodible polyanhydrides as drug-carrier matrices. II. Biocompatibility and chemical reactivity. *J Biomed Mater Res* 1986;20:51.

88. Brem H, Kader A, Epstein JI, et al. Biocompatibility of a biodegradable, controlled-release polymer in the rabbit brain. *Sel Cancer Ther* 1989;5:55.

89. Tamargo RJ, Epstein JI, Reinhard CS, et al. Brain biocompatibility of a biodegradable, controlled-release polymer in rats. *J Biomed Mater Res* 1989;23:253.

90. Brem H, Tamargo RJ, Olivi A, et al. Biodegradable polymers for controlled delivery of chemotherapy with and without radiation therapy in the monkey brain. *J Neurosurg* 1994;80:283.

91. Grossman SA, Reinhard C, Colvin OM, et al. The intracerebral distribution of BCNU delivered by surgically implanted biodegradable polymers. *J Neurosurg* 1992;76:640.

92. Yang MB, Tamargo RJ, Brem H. Controlled delivery of 1,3-bis(2-chloroethyl)-1-nitrosourea from ethylene-vinyl acetate copolymer. *Cancer Res* 1989;49:5103.

93. Walter KA, Cahan MA, Gur A, et al. Interstitial Taxol delivered from a biodegradable polymer implant against experimental malignant glioma. *Cancer Res* 1994;54:2207.

94. Judy KD, Olivi A, Buahin KG, et al. Effectiveness of controlled release of a cyclophosphamide derivative with polymers against rat gliomas. *J Neurosurg* 1995;82:481.

95. Olivi A, Ewend MG, Utsuki T, et al. Interstitial delivery of carboplatin via biodegradable polymers is effective against experimental glioma in the rat. *Cancer Chemother Pharmacol* 1996;39:90.

96. Weingart JD, Thompson RC, Tyler B, et al. Local delivery of the topoisomerase I inhibitor camptothecin sodium prolongs survival in the rat intracranial 9L gliosarcoma model. *Int J Cancer* 1995;62:605.

97. Menei P, Boisdron-Celle M, Croue A, et al. Effect of stereotactic implantation of biodegradable 5-fluorouracil-loaded microspheres in healthy and C6 glioma-bearing rats. *Neurosurgery* 1996;39:117.

98. Kong Q, Kleinschmidt-DeMasters BK, Lillehei KO. Intralesionally implanted cisplatin plus systemic carmustine for the treatment of brain tumor in rats. *J Surg Oncol* 1998;69:76.

99. Kong Q, Kleinschmidt-DeMasters BK, Lillehei KO. Intralesionally implanted cisplatin cures primary brain tumor in rats. *J Surg Oncol* 1997;64:268.

100. Brem H, Piantadosi S, Burger PC, et al. Placebo-controlled trial of safety and efficacy of intraoperative controlled delivery by biodegradable polymers of chemotherapy for recurrent gliomas. The Polymer-Brain Tumor Treatment Group. *Lancet* 1995;345:1008.

101. Brem H, Mahaley MS Jr, Vick NA, et al. Interstitial chemotherapy with drug polymer implants for the treatment of recurrent gliomas. *J Neurosurg* 1991;74:441.

102. Brem H, Ewend MG, Piantadosi S, et al. The safety of interstitial chemotherapy with BCNU-loaded polymer followed by radiation therapy in the treatment of newly diagnosed malignant gliomas: phase I trial. *J Neurooncol* 1995;26:111.

103. Valtonen S, Timonen U, Toivanen P, et al. Interstitial chemotherapy with carmustine-loaded polymers for high-grade gliomas: a randomized double-blind study. *Neurosurgery* 1997;41:44.

104. Olivi A, Barker F, Tatter S, et al. Toxicities and pharmacokinetics of interstitial BCNU administered via wafers: results of a phase I study in patients with recurrent malignant glioma. *Proc Am Soc Clin Oncol* 1999;18:142a.

105. Westphal P, Daumas-Duport C, Thoron L, et al. Gliadel (polifeprosan 20 with carmustine 3.85% implant); a multinational phase III randomized double-blind trial in newly diagnosed malignant glioma. *Proc Am Soc Clin Oncol* 1999;18:155a.

106. Limentani S, Asher A, Fraser R, et al. A phase I trial of surgery, Gliadel and carboplatin in combination radiation therapy for anaplastic astrocytoma (AA) or glioblastoma multiforme (GBM). *Proc Am Soc Clin Oncol* 1999;18:151a.

107. Groothius DR. The blood-brain and blood tumor barriers: a review of strategies for increasing drug delivery. *Neurooncology* 2000;2:45.

108. Groothuis DR, Benalcazar H, Allen CV, et al. Comparison of cytosine arabinoside delivery to rat brain by intravenous, intrathecal, intraventricular and intraparenchymal routes of administration. *Brain Res* 2000;856:281.

109. Laske DW, Youle RJ, Oldfield EH. Tumor regression with regional distribution of the targeted toxin TF-CRM107 in patients with malignant brain tumors [see comments]. *Nat Med* 1997;3:1362.

110. Ho SY, Barbarese E, D'Arrigo JS, et al. Evaluation of lipid-coated microbubbles as a delivery vehicle for Taxol in brain tumor therapy. *Neurosurgery* 1997;40:1260.

111. Khalifa A, Dodds D, Rampling R, et al. Liposomal distribution in malignant glioma: possibilities for therapy. *Nucl Med Commun* 1997;18:17.

112. Devineni D, Klein-Szanto A, Gallo JM. Tissue distribution of methotrexate following administration as a solution and as a magnetic microsphere conjugate in rats bearing brain tumors. *J Neurooncol* 1995;24:143.

113. Pulfer SK, Ciccotto SL, Gallo JM. Distribution of small magnetic particles in brain tumor–bearing rats. *J Neurooncol* 1999;41:99.

114. Pulfer SK, Gallo JM. Enhanced brain tumor selectivity of cationic magnetic polysaccharide microspheres. *J Drug Target* 1998;6:215.

115. De Lange EC, Danhof M, de Boer AG, et al. Methodological considerations of intracerebral microdialysis in pharmacokinetic studies on drug transport across the blood-brain barrier. *Brain Res Brain Res Rev* 1997;25:27.

116. Greig NH. Drug delivery to the brain. In: Neuwelt A, ed. *Blood-brain barrier.* New York: Plenum Publishing, 1988:322.

117. Supko JG, Malspeis L. A reversed-phase HPLC method for determining camptothecin in plasma with specificity for the intact lactone form of the drug. *J Liq Chromatogr* 1991;14:1779.

118. Fassberg J, Stella VJ. A kinetic and mechanistic study of the hydrolysis of camptothecin and some analogues. *J Pharm Sci* 1992;81:676.

119. Cserr HF. Physiology of the choroid plexus. *Physiol Rev* 1971;51:273.

120. Fishman RA. *Cerebrospinal fluid in diseases of the nervous system.* Philadelphia: WB Saunders, 1992:23.

121. Zamboni WC, Gajjar AJ, Mandrell TD, et al. A four-hour topotecan infusion achieves cytotoxic exposure throughout the neuraxis in the nonhuman primate model: implications for treatment of children with metastatic medulloblastoma. *Clin Cancer Res* 1998;4:2537.

122. Blaney SM, Poplack DG, Godwin K, et al. Effect of body position on ventricular CSF methotrexate concentration following intralumbar administration. *J Clin Oncol* 1995;13:177.

123. Donelli MG, Zucchetti M, D'Incalci M. Do anticancer agents reach the tumor target in the human brain? *Cancer Chemother Pharmacol* 1992;30:251.

124. Stewart DJ. A critique of the role of the blood-brain barrier in the chemotherapy of human brain tumors. *J Neurooncol* 1994;20:121.

125. Muller M, Mader RM, Steiner B, et al. 5-Fluorouracil kinetics in the interstitial tumor space: clinical response in breast cancer patients. *Cancer Res* 1997;57:2598.

126. Johansen MJ, Newman RA, Madden T. The use of microdialysis in pharmacokinetics and pharmacodynamics. *Pharmacotherapy* 1997;17:464.

127. Mary S, Muret P, Makki S, et al. A new technique for study of cutaneous biology, microdialysis. *Ann Dermatol Venereol* 1999;126:66.

128. Groth L. Cutaneous microdialysis. Methodology and validation. *Acta Derm Venereol* 1996;197[Suppl]:1.

129. Ungerstedt U, Pycock C. Functional correlates of dopamine neurotransmission. *Bull Schweiz Akad Med Wiss* 1974;30:44.

130. Major O, Shdanova T, Duffek L, et al. Continuous monitoring of blood-brain barrier opening to Cr51-EDTA by microdialysis following probe injury. *Acta Neurochir Suppl (Wien)* 1990;51:46.

131. Westergren I, Nystrom B, Hamberger A, et al. Intracerebral dialysis and the blood-brain barrier. *J Neurochem* 1995;64:229.

132. Benveniste H, Hansen AJ, Ottosen NS. Determination of brain interstitial concentrations by microdialysis. *J Neurochem* 1989;52:1741.

133. Tossman U, Ungerstedt U. Microdialysis in the study of extracellular levels of amino acids in the rat brain. *Acta Physiol Scand* 1986;128:9.

134. Hogan BL, Lunte SM, Stobaugh JF, et al. On-line coupling of in vivo microdialysis sampling with capillary electrophoresis. *Anal Chem* 1994;66:596.

135. Chen A, Lunte CE. Microdialysis sampling coupled on-line to fast microbore liquid chromatography. *J Chromatogr A* 1995;691:29.

136. Ault JM, Lunte CE, Meltzer NM, et al. Microdialysis sampling for the investigation of dermal drug transport. *Pharm Res* 1992;9:1256.

137. Sabol KE, Freed CR. Brain acetaminophen measurement by in vivo dialysis, in vivo electrochemistry and tissue assay: a study of the dialysis technique in the rat. *J Neurosci Methods* 1988;24:163.

138. Wang Y, Wong SL, Sawchuk RJ. Microdialysis calibration using retrodialysis and zero-net flux: application to a study of the distribution of zidovudine to rabbit cerebrospinal fluid and thalamus. *Pharm Res* 1993;10:1411.

139. De Lange EC, Bouw MR, Mandema JW, et al. Application of intracerebral microdialysis to study regional distribution kinetics of drugs in rat brain. *Br J Pharmacol* 1995;116:2538.

140. Devineni D, Klein-Szanto A, Gallo JM. In vivo microdialysis to characterize drug transport in brain tumors: analysis of methotrexate uptake in rat glioma-2 (RG-2)-bearing rats. *Cancer Chemother Pharmacol* 1996;38:499.

141. El-Gizawy SA, Hedaya MA. Comparative brain tissue distribution of camptothecin and topotecan in the rat. *Cancer Chemother Pharmacol* 1999;43:364.

142. Zamboni WC, Houghton PJ, Hulstein JL, et al. Relationship between tumor extracellular fluid exposure to topotecan and tumor response in human neuroblastoma xenograft and cell lines. *Cancer Chemother Pharmacol* 1999;43:269.

143. Palsmeier RK, Lunte CE. Microdialysis sampling in tumor and muscle: study of the disposition of 3-amino-1,2,4-benzotriazine-1,4-di-N-oxide (SR 4233). *Life Sci* 1994;55:815.

144. Ekstrom O, Andersen A, Warren DJ, et al. Evaluation of methotrexate tissue exposure by in situ microdialysis in a rat model. *Cancer Chemother Pharmacol* 1994;34:297.

145. Baunach S, Meixensberger J, Gerlach M, et al. Intraoperative microdialysis and tissue-pO_2 measurement in human glioma. *Acta Neurochir Suppl (Wien)* 1998;71:241.

146. Hamani C, Luer MS, Dujovny M. Microdialysis in the human brain: review of its applications. *Neurol Res* 1997;19:281.

147. Landolt H, Langemann H. Cerebral microdialysis as a diagnostic tool in acute brain injury. *Eur J Anaesthesiol* 1996;13:269.

148. Mattson RH, Scheyer RD, Petroff OA, et al. Novel methods for studying new antiepileptic drug pharmacology. *Adv Neurol* 1998;76:105.

149. Mendelowitsch A, Sekhar LN, Caputy AJ, et al. Intraoperative on-line monitoring of cerebral pH by microdialysis in neurosurgical procedures. *Neurol Res* 1998;20:142.

150. Persson L, Valtysson J, Enblad P, et al. Neurochemical monitoring using intracerebral microdialysis in patients with subarachnoid hemorrhage. *J Neurosurg* 1996;84:606.

151. Sarrafzadeh AS, Unterberg AW, Lanksch WR. Bedside-microdialysis for early detection of vasospasm after subarachnoid hemorrhage. Case report and review of the literature. *Zentralbl Neurochir* 1998;59:269.

152. Bachli H, Langemann H, Mendelowitsch A, et al. Microdialytic monitoring during cerebrovascular surgery. *Neurol Res* 1996;18:370.

153. Ronquist G, Hugosson R, Sjolander U, et al. Treatment of malignant glioma by a new therapeutic principle. *Acta Neurochir* 1992;114:8.

154. Blochl-Daum B, Muller M, Meisinger V, et al. Measurement of extracellular fluid carboplatin kinetics in melanoma metastases with microdialysis. *Br J Cancer* 1996;73:920.

155. He Q, Bhujwalla ZM, Maxwell RJ, et al. Proton NMR observation of the antineoplastic agent iproplatin in vivo by selective multiple quantum coherence transfer (Sel-MQC). *Magn Reson Med* 1995;33:414.

156. Rodrigues LM, Maxwell RJ, McSheehy PM, et al. In vivo detection of ifosfamide by ^{31}P-MRS in rat tumours: increased uptake and cytotoxicity induced by carbogen breathing in GH3 prolactinomas. *Br J Cancer* 1997;75:62.

157. Wolf W, Waluch V, Presant CA. Non-invasive ^{19}F-NMRS of 5-fluorouracil in pharmacokinetics and pharmacodynamic studies. *NMR Biomed* 1998;11:380.

158. Findlay MP, Leach MO. In vivo monitoring of fluoropyrimidine metabolites: magnetic resonance spectroscopy in the evaluation of 5-fluorouracil. *Anticancer Drugs* 1994;5:260.

159. Presant CA, Wolf W, Waluch V, et al. Association of intratumoral pharmacokinetics of fluorouracil with clinical response. *Lancet* 1994;343:1184.

160. Maxwell RJ. New techniques in the pharmacokinetic analysis of cancer drugs. III. Nuclear magnetic resonance. *Cancer Surv* 1993;17:415.

161. Presant CA, Wolf W, Albright MJ, et al. Human tumor fluorouracil trapping: clinical correlations of in vivo ^{19}F-nuclear magnetic resonance spectroscopy pharmacokinetics. *J Clin Oncol* 1990;8:1868.

162. Kristjansen PE, Quistorff B, Spang-Thomsen M, et al. Intratumoral pharmacokinetic analysis by ^{19}F-magnetic resonance spectroscopy and cytostatic in vivo activity of gemcitabine (dFdC) in two small cell lung cancer xenografts. *Ann Oncol* 1993;4:157.

163. Wolf W, Waluch V, Presant CA, et al. Pharmacokinetic imaging of gemcitabine in human tumors using non invasive ^{19}F-MRS. *Proc Am Assoc Cancer Res* 1999;40:384.

164. Kissel J, Brix G, Bellemann ME, et al. Pharmacokinetic analysis of 5-[^{18}F]fluorouracil tissue concentrations measured with positron emission tomography in patients with liver metastases from colorectal adenocarcinoma. *Cancer Res* 1997;57:3415.

165. Tilsley DW, Harte RJ, Jones T, et al. New techniques in the pharmacokinetic analysis of cancer drugs. IV. Positron emission tomography. *Cancer Surv* 1993;17:425.

166. Rubin RH, Fischman AJ. Positron emission tomography in drug development. *Q J Nucl Med* 1997;41:171.

167. Meikle SR, Matthews JC, Brock CS, et al. Pharmacokinetic assessment of novel anti-cancer drugs using spectral analysis and positron emission tomography: a feasibility study. *Cancer Chemother Pharmacol* 1998;42:183.

168. Tyler JL, Yamamoto YL, Diksic M, et al. Pharmacokinetics of superselective intra-arterial and intravenous ^{11}C-BCNU evaluated by PET. *J Nucl Med* 1986;27:775.

169. Diksic M, Sako K, Feindel W, et al. Pharmacokinetics of positron-labeled 1,3-bis(2-chloroethyl)nitrosourea in human brain tumors using positron emission tomography. *Cancer Res* 1984;44:3120.

170. Ginos JZ, Cooper AJ, Dhawan V, et al. [^{13}N]-cisplatin PET to assess pharmacokinetics of intra-arterial versus intravenous chemotherapy for malignant brain tumors. *J Nucl Med* 1987;28:1844.

171. Yung WK, Prados MD, Yaya-Tur R, et al. Multicenter phase II trial of temozolomide in patients with anaplastic astrocytoma or anaplastic oligoastrocytoma at first relapse. Temodal Brain Tumor Group. *J Clin Oncol* 1999;17:2762.

172. Conway T, Diksic M. Synthesis of "no-carrier added" carbon-11 SarCNU: the sarcosinamide analog of the chemotherapeutic agent BCNU. *J Nucl Med* 1988;29:1957.

173. Mitsuki S, Diksic M, Conway T, et al. Pharmacokinetics of ^{11}C-labelled BCNU and SarCNU in gliomas studied by PET. *J Neurooncol* 1991;10:47.

174. Skalski V, Feindel W, Panasci LC. Transport of amino acid amide sarcosinamide and sarcosinamide chloroethylnitrosourea in human glioma SK-MG-1 cells. *Cancer Res* 1990;50:3062.

175. Van Meerten E, Verweij J, Schellens JH. Antineoplastic agents. Drug interactions of clinical significance. *Drug Saf* 1995;12:168.

176. McLeod HL. Clinically relevant drug-drug interactions in oncology. *Br J Clin Pharmacol* 1998;45:539.

177. Glue P, Clement RP. Cytochrome P450 enzymes and drug metabolism—basic concepts and methods of assessment. *Cell Mol Neurobiol* 1999;19:309.

178. Kivisto KT, Kroemer HK, Eichelbaum M. The role of human cytochrome P450 enzymes in the metabolism of anticancer agents: implications for drug interactions. *Br J Clin Pharmacol* 1995;40:523.

179. Chang TK, Weber GF, Crespi CL, et al. Differential activation of cyclophosphamide and ifosphamide by cytochromes P-450 2B and 3A in human liver microsomes. *Cancer Res* 1993;53:5629.

180. Rahmani R, Zhou XJ. Pharmacokinetics and metabolism of vinca alkaloids. *Cancer Surv* 1993;17:269.

181. Tanaka E. Clinically significant pharmacokinetic drug interactions between antiepileptic drugs. *J Clin Pharm Ther* 1999;24:87.

182. Baker DK, Relling MV, Pui CH, et al. Increased teniposide clearance with concomitant anticonvulsant therapy. *J Clin Oncol* 1992;10:311.

183. Villikka K, Kivisto KT, Maenpaa H, et al. Cytochrome P450-inducing antiepileptics increase the clearance of vincristine in patients with brain tumors. *Clin Pharmacol Ther* 1999;66:589.

184. Fetell MR, Grossman SA, Fisher JD, et al. Preirradiation paclitaxel in glioblastoma multiforme: efficacy, pharmacology, and drug interactions. *J Clin Oncol* 1997;15:3121.

185. Grossman SA, Hochberg F, Fisher J, et al. Increased 9-aminocamptothecin dose requirements in patients on anticonvulsants. *Cancer Chemother Pharmacol* 1998;42:118.

186. Takimoto CH, Dahut W, Marino MT, et al. Pharmacodynamics and pharmacokinetics of a 72-hour infusion of 9-aminocamptothecin in adult cancer patients. *J Clin Oncol* 1997;15:1492.

187. Supko JG, Malspeis L. Pharmacokinetics of the 9-amino and 10,11-methylenedioxy derivatives of camptothecin in mice. *Cancer Res* 1993;53:3062.

188. Gupta E, Lestingi TM, Mick R, et al. Metabolic fate of irinotecan in humans: correlation of glucuronidation with diarrhea. *Cancer Res* 1994;54:3723.

189. Gupta E, Wang X, Ramirez J, et al. Modulation of glucuronidation of SN-38, the active metabolite of irinotecan, by valproic acid and phenobarbital. *Cancer Chemother Pharmacol* 1997;39:440.

190. Liddle C, Goodwin BJ, George J, et al. Separate and interactive regulation of cytochrome P450 3A4 by triiodothyronine, dexamethasone, and growth hormone in cultured hepatocytes. *J Clin Endocrinol Metab* 1998;83:2411.

191. Chang TK, Yu L, Maurel P, et al. Enhanced cyclophosphamide and ifosfamide activation in primary human hepatocyte cultures: response to cytochrome P-450 inducers and autoinduction by oxazaphosphorines. *Cancer Res* 1997;57:1946.

192. Brain EG, Yu LJ, Gustafsson K, et al. Modulation of P450-dependent ifosfamide pharmacokinetics: a better understanding of drug activation in vivo. *Br J Cancer* 1998; 77:1768.

193. Yu LJ, Drewes P, Gustafsson K, et al. In vivo modulation of alternative pathways of P-450-catalyzed cyclophosphamide metabolism: impact on pharmacokinetics and antitumor activity. *J Pharmacol Exp Ther* 1999;288:928.

194. Marre F, Sanderink GJ, de Sousa G, et al. Hepatic biotransformation of docetaxel (Taxotere) in vitro: involvement of the CYP3A subfamily in humans. *Cancer Res* 1996;56:1296.

195. Kamataki T, Yokoi T, Fujita K, et al. Preclinical approach for identifying drug interactions. *Cancer Chemother Pharmacol* 1998;42:S50.

196. Levin VA, Stearns J, Byrd A, et al. The effect of phenobarbital pretreatment on the antitumor activity of 1,3-bis (2-chloroethyl)-1-nitrosourea (BCNU), 1-(2-chloroethyl)-3-cyclohexyl-1-nitrosourea (CCNU) and 1-(2-chloroethyl)-3-(2,6-dioxo-3-piperidyl)-1-nitrosourea (PCNU), and on the plasma pharmacokinetics and biotransformation of BCNU. *J Pharmacol Exp Ther* 1979;208:1.

197. Yamazaki H, Inoue K, Shaw PM, et al. Different contributions of cytochrome P450 2C19 and 3A4 in the oxidation of omeprazole by human liver microsomes: effects of contents of these two forms in individual human samples. *J Pharmacol Exp Ther* 1997;283:434.

198. Nemeroff CB, DeVane CL, Pollock BG. Newer antidepressants and the cytochrome P450 system. *Am J Psychiatry* 1996;153:311.

199. Evans WE, Christensen ML. Drug interactions with methotrexate. *J Rheumatol* 1985;12[12 Suppl]:15.

200. Reid AC, Teasdale GM, McCulloch J. The effects of dexamethasone administration and withdrawal on water permeability across the blood-brain barrier. *Ann Neurol* 1983;13:28.

201. Ziylan YZ, LeFauconnier JM, Bernard G, et al. Effect of dexamethasone on transport of alpha-aminoisobutyric acid and sucrose across the blood-brain barrier. *J Neurochem* 1988;51:1338.

202. Ziylan YZ, Lefauconnier JM, Bernard G, et al. Regional alterations in blood-to-brain transfer of alpha-aminoisobutyric acid and sucrose, after chronic administration and withdrawal of dexamethasone. *J Neurochem* 1989;52:684.

203. Hedley-Whyte ET, Hsu DW. Effect of dexamethasone on blood-brain barrier in the normal mouse. *Ann Neurol* 1986; 19:373.

204. Shapiro WR, Hiesiger EM, Cooney GA, et al. Temporal effects of dexamethasone on blood-to-brain and blood-to-tumor transport of ^{14}C-alpha-aminoisobutyric acid in rat C6 glioma. *J Neurooncol* 1990;8:197.

205. Jarden JO, Dhawan V, Moeller JR, et al. The time course of steroid action on blood-to-brain and blood-to-tumor transport of +^{82}Rb: a positron emission tomographic study. *Ann Neurol* 1989;25:239.

206. Jarden JO, Dhawan V, Poltorak A, et al. Positron emission tomographic measurement of blood-to-brain and blood-to-tumor transport of +^{82}Rb: the effect of dexamethasone and whole-brain radiation therapy. *Ann Neurol* 1985;18:636.

207. Yeung WT, Lee TY, Del Maestro RF, et al. Effect of steroids on iopamidol blood-brain transfer constant and plasma volume in brain tumors measured with X-ray computed tomography. *J Neurooncol* 1994;18:53.

208. Andersen C, Astrup J, Gyldensted C. Quantitation of peritumoural oedema and the effect of steroids using NMR-relaxation time imaging and blood-brain barrier analysis. *Acta Neurochir Suppl (Wien)* 1994;60:413.

209. Ostergaard L, Hochberg FH, Rabinov JD, et al. Early changes measured by magnetic resonance imaging in cerebral blood flow, blood volume, and blood-brain barrier permeability following dexamethasone treatment in patients with brain tumors. *J Neurosurg* 1999;90:300.

210. Matsukado K, Nakano S, Bartus RT, et al. Steroids decrease uptake of carboplatin in rat gliomas—uptake improved by intracarotid infusion of bradykinin analog, RMP-7. *J Neurooncol* 1997;34:131.

211. Straathof CS, van den Bent MJ, Ma J, et al. The effect of dexamethasone on the uptake of cisplatin in 9L glioma and the area of brain around tumor. *J Neurooncol* 1998;37:1.

212. Neuwelt EA, Barnett PA, Bigner DD, et al. Effects of adrenal cortical steroids and osmotic blood-brain barrier opening on methotrexate delivery to gliomas in the rodent: the factor of the blood-brain barrier. *Proc Natl Acad Sci U S A* 1982;79:4420.

213. Trnovec T, Kallay Z, Bezek S. Effects of ionizing radiation on the blood brain barrier permeability to pharmacologically active substances. *Int J Radiat Oncol Biol Phys* 1990; 19:1581.

214. d'Avella D, Cicciarello R, Angileri FF, et al. Radiation-induced blood-brain barrier changes: pathophysiological mechanisms and clinical implications. *Acta Neurochir Suppl (Wien)* 1998;71:282.

215. Mima T, Toyonaga S, Mori K, et al. Early decrease of P-glycoprotein in the endothelium of the rat brain capillaries after moderate dose of irradiation. *Neurol Res* 1999;21:209.

216. Remsen LG, McCormick CI, Sexton G, et al. Decreased delivery and acute toxicity of cranial irradiation and chemotherapy given with osmotic blood-brain barrier disruption in a rodent model: the issue of sequence. *Clin Cancer Res* 1995;1:731.

217. Qin DX, Zheng R, Tang J, et al. Influence of radiation on the blood-brain barrier and optimum time of chemotherapy. *Int J Radiat Oncol Biol Phys* 1990;19:1507.

218. Riccardi R, Riccardi A, Lasorella A, et al. Cranial irradiation and permeability of blood-brain barrier to cytosine arabinoside in children with acute leukemia. *Clin Cancer Res* 1998;4:69.

23

RETINOIDS AND OTHER DIFFERENTIATING AGENTS

JOSEPH A. FONTANA
ARUN K. RISHI

Numerous studies have indicated that the transformation process that results in the eventual development of frank malignancy represents, in the majority of situations, a block in the normal differentiation process, with the development of malignant precursor cells. An intellectually appealing and rational approach to the treatment of malignancy has been the addition of agents that would theoretically induce the normal differentiation and maturation of these malignant cells. Numerous compounds have been synthesized with this approach in mind. The most intensively studied and characterized have been the polar-planar compounds and retinoids.

POLAR COMPOUNDS

Polar Compounds as Antitumor and Differentiating Agents

A number of polar-planar compounds have been described that possess antitumor as well as differentiating properties.[1–3] The observation that the polar solvent dimethyl sulfoxide could induce terminal differentiation in mouse erythroid leukemia cells created a significant amount of interest in this class of compounds.[4] This in turn has led to the development of other polar-apolar compounds such as hexamethylene bisacetamide (HMBA) and N-methyl formamide (NMF), both of which demonstrate broader in vitro activity (Fig. 23-1).[5,6] Although a number of solid tumor cell lines demonstrated growth inhibition when exposed to HMBA, regrowth occurred on its removal, with only a minority of the cells continuing to display differentiation markers.[7] This was in marked contrast to the terminal differentiation noted in the murine erythroid-leukemia cell lines and the human HL-60 leukemia cell line.

Clinical trials using HMBA in solid tumors have generally been disappointing; although potentially therapeutic plasma levels of 1.5 to 2.0 mmol per L HMBA were achieved, no clinical responses were noted. Neurotoxicity, renal toxicity, and thrombocytopenia were dose limiting in these trials.[8] Alkalinization of plasma along with adaptive-feedback control resulted in higher plasma levels (more than 2 mmol per L) in patients and decreased toxicity, but no significant clinical responses were noted in patients with solid tumors.[9] Phase II clinical trials involving patients with myelodysplastic syndrome have produced differing results.[10,11] Andreeff et al. examined the effect of HMBA and reported complete remission in three patients and partial remission in six patients.[10] In this trial, HMBA was given by a 10-day infusion (24 g per m² per day); this schedule achieved a mean plasma level of 0.87 mmol per L with no decrease in plasma levels noted after repeated courses. The mean duration of remission was 6.0 months for complete response and 3.7 months for partial response.[10] The most common side effect was thrombocytopenia, with grade IV thrombocytopenia noted in 11 patients and grade III in 2 patients. Rowinsky et al.[11] achieved steady-state plasma concentrations of 1 to 2 mmol per L in at least two 5-day courses using a 5-day continuous infusion schedule but found no clinical responses in 15 patients with myelodysplastic syndrome.

The mechanism(s) by which HMBA induces differentiation in the various cell types is not clear. Numerous in vitro effects have been described, including inhibition of DNA topoisomerase I activity, down-regulation of the antiapoptotic protein Bcl-2, alteration of topoisomerase II phosphorylation with subsequent alteration of nuclear architecture, and suppression of cyclin-dependent kinase 4 activity with the accumulation of unphosphorylated retinoblastoma protein and subsequent G_1 cell-cycle arrest.[12–15] Whether any of these are operative in vivo remains to be discerned.

The polar solvent NMF (Fig. 23-1) has also been shown to inhibit proliferation and induce differentiation in a number of cell types, including tumor cells displaying high levels of P-glycoprotein and thus resistance to standard concentrations of many chemotherapeutic drugs.[16] NMF

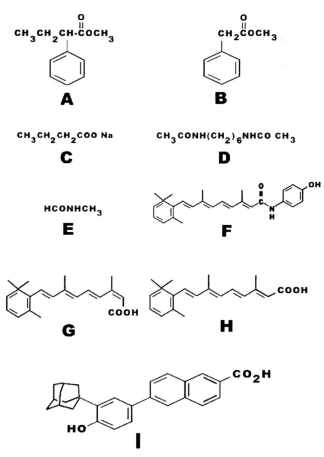

FIGURE 23-1. Chemical structures of polar-planar compounds and retinoids. **A:** Phenyl butyrate. **B:** Phenylacetate. **C:** Sodium butyrate. **D:** Hexamethylene bisacetamide (1,6-bis acetamide) hexane. **E:** *N*-methyl formamide. **F:** *N*-(4-hydroxyphenyl) retinamide. **G:** 13-*cis*-retinoic acid. **H:** *Trans*-retinoic acid. **I:** 6-[3-(1-adamantyl 4 hydroxyphenyl]-2 naphthalene carboxylic acid.

demonstrated antiproliferative activity against human colon, mammary, and lung xenografts. However, NMF did not display clinical activity in a phase II study involving patients with metastatic melanoma and was found to have significant toxicity.[17–19]

Phenylacetate and Phenylbutyrate

Phenylacetate and phenylbutyrate (Fig. 23-1) have been found to affect the growth and differentiation state of a wide variety of tumor cells *in vitro*. These effects have been found in both malignant hematopoietic as well as solid tumor cell lines. Exposure of the human leukemia cell line HL-60 to phenylacetate resulted in the rapid decline in *myc* oncogene expression, which was then followed by growth arrest and differentiation along the myelocyte pathway.[20] Similar inhibition of growth was noted in malignant melanoma, prostatic carcinoma, glioblastoma, and breast and ovarian carcinoma cell lines.[21–23] Phenylacetate down-regulated the expression of a number of positive regulators of growth, including cyclin D1 and Ras, in these cells.[22] The

cytostatic activity of phenylacetate and its derivatives appeared to correlate with their lipophilicity and ability to inhibit protein prenylation with significant inhibition of *p21* Ras activation.[21,24] In addition to showing cytostatic effects, sodium phenylbutyrate has been found to induce programmed cell death (apoptosis) in both prostate carcinoma and leukemia cells.[25,26] Studies suggest that phenylacetate-mediated cell-cycle arrest may be related to the ability of phenylacetate to enhance expression of the cyclin-dependent kinase inhibitor p21/WAF1/CIP1 through a p53-independent process.[27] In addition to enhancing expression of p21/WAF1/CIP1, phenylacetate has been found to enhance expression of the tumor suppressor gene RARβ, which appears to be an important negative regulator of growth, and to activate the human peroxisome proliferator–activated receptor, which has been shown to play a role in cellular differentiation[28,29]; whether activation of these important nuclear transcription factors is necessary for the growth inhibition and cellular differentiation induced by phenylacetate remains to be determined.

Phenylacetate also displayed antitumor activity *in vivo*. Administration of phenylacetate to rats bearing experimental brain tumors resulted in inhibition of tumor growth with evidence of tumor cell differentiation as well as extended survival of the tumor-bearing animals.[30] Mice bearing the highly tumorigenic MCF-7 human breast cancer cells transfected with the *Ha-Ras* oncogene and treated with phenylacetate demonstrated tumor growth arrest but without tumor regression.[31] Pharmacokinetic studies in both normal human volunteers and patients with cancer demonstrated that therapeutic plasma levels of phenylacetate and phenylbutyrate could be achieved with minimal toxicity.[32,33] Although both agents demonstrated significant protein binding, they also possessed significant free fractions.[33] A phase I trial of phenylacetate involving 17 patients with advanced solid tumors revealed nonlinear pharmacokinetics; reversible central nervous system depression was dose limiting.[34] Three of nine patients with metastatic hormone-refractory prostate cancer maintained stable prostate-specific antigen levels for more than 2 months; in addition, one of six patients with glioblastoma multiforme displayed functional improvement for more than 9 months.[34,35]

Histone Deacetylase and DNA Methylase Inhibitors

The ability of oncogenes to silence the expression of a wide variety of tumor suppressor genes has been well documented.[36,37] This is achieved in part by the enhanced regional hypermethylation of crucial CpG islands in genes and deacetylation of specific histones with subsequent chromatin remodeling and inhibition of messenger RNA (mRNA) transcription.[36,37] The ability of agents to inhibit and/or reverse this process has opened a unique avenue in the treatment of malignancy. Interestingly, the first agents to demonstrate the capability to inhibit or reverse CpG methylation and histone deacetylation were butyric acid and phenylbutyrate.[38,39] The ability of phenylbutyrate to inhibit histone deacetylation *in vivo* was demonstrated in a patient with acute promyelocytic leukemia (APL) that was resistant to *trans*-retinoic acid (tRA).[39] Data from several laboratories demonstrated that the oncoprotein encoded by the fusion gene *PML-RARα* found in the majority of APL patients suppresses transcription of the RARα gene, despite physiologic concentrations of tRA, through its recruitment of a histone deacetylase (see Samid[39] and references within). Pharmacologic concentrations of tRA (1 mmol per L) have been found to dissociate the *PML-RARα*/corepressor/deacetylase complex, resulting in transcription of the RARα gene.[40] In most patients with APL, however, resistance developed, and retinoic acid failed to dissociate this complex, which resulted in continued silencing of the RARα gene. The addition of phenylbutyrate given as a 2-hour infusion at a dosage of 140 mg per kg twice per day along with tRA (45 mg per m² per day in two divided doses) to a patient with tRA-refractory disease resulted in a complete clinical and cytologic remission.[39] Immunofluorescence and Western blot analysis demonstrated that phenylbutyrate caused a time-dependent increase in histone acetylation in blood and bone marrow cells.[39] In micromolar concentrations, butyrate demonstrates a broad number of effects and is not a specific inhibitor of histone deacetylase activity.[41] More specific histone acetylase inhibitors have now been found. These include the natural agents trichostatin A (TSA), depudecin, and trapoxin (TPX) as well as the synthetic benzamide derivatives, which inhibit the growth of a number of tumors *in vitro* and *in vivo* and will soon enter clinical trial.[42–45] TSA and TPX are potent inhibitors of histone deacetylation. TSA reversibly inhibits histone deacetylation with an inhibition constant (K_i) of 3.4 nmol per L, approximately 1,000-fold less than butyrate, whereas TPX is an irreversible inhibitor and is even more active than TSA.[41]

The silencing of numerous tumor suppressor genes has also been found to be the result of methylation of critical CpG islands in the promoters of genes.[37,46] The ability of demethylation agents such as 5-aza-2′deoxycytidine to significantly decrease the degree of hypermethylation of these promoters with subsequent reexpression of the gene products has been demonstrated *in vitro* using tumor cells in culture.[46,47] Whether this approach can be used in patients remains to be determined. Studies suggest that the combination of 5-aza-2′deoxycytidine followed by the histone deacetylase inhibitor TSA results in a synergistic response in terms of reexpression of tumor suppressor genes such as *p16*, *p15*, and the tissue metalloproteinase inhibitor *TIMP-3*, which are often silenced in tumor cells.[46] Thus, oncogenes may silence critical tumor suppressor genes through both methylation and histone deacetylation, and the combined use of inhibitors of both of these processes

may offer an exciting and fruitful approach to inhibiting tumor growth.

RETINOIDS

Natural retinoids and their synthetic analogs play a vital role in vertebrate development and have been shown to induce the normal differentiation of a number of tissues. Their ability to function as important agents in the prevention of many malignancies[48] and as a therapeutic agent in the treatment of APL has been well established (see later).

Biosynthesis and Metabolism

Dietary vitamin A derived from provitamin carotenoids found in vegetables and retinyl esters obtained from animal sources or dietary supplements serve as the major sources from which all retinoids are eventually synthesized. The retinoid tRA (Fig. 23-1), a polyene carboxylic acid, is derived from metabolic oxidation of vitamin A (retinol). Cleavage of carotenoids such as β-carotene by the enzyme β-carotenoid-15,15-dioxygenase yields two molecules of retinal.[49,50] A cellular retinol-binding protein type II binds this retinal and enhances its reduction to retinol.[51] Retinyl esters are hydrolyzed by lipases or esterases in the intestinal lumen before adsorption. Enterocytes then absorb the free retinol, which is reesterified by lecithin retinol acyltransferase or acylcoenzyme A:retinol acyltransferase to form retinyl palmitate and stearate, and is packaged into chylomicrons. After uptake of the retinyl esters into the liver hepatocytes and cleavage of the esters to free retinol, the retinol is bound to the retinol-binding protein (RBP), which then transports the insoluble ligand in plasma. In the case of vitamin A, excess retinol in its esterified forms is stored in the stellate or fat-bearing cells.

Retinol bound to RPB is transported in the plasma and taken up by vitamin A–dependent target tissues. The mechanism by which retinol is transported into tissues is not clear. In retinol pigmented epithelium, an RBP receptor appears to be involved[52]; in other tissues, research suggests that retinol uptake into cells is driven by the intracellular concentration of apolipoprotein cellular retinol-binding protein.[53] The pathways through which tRA is generated remain relatively unclear. Although some tRA is provided through dietary sources, this amount is probably not sufficient to account for the serum tRA that circulates bound to serum albumin.[54] Most evidence indicates that tRA is produced by oxidation of retinol, although the enzyme systems involved are unclear. Observation suggests that retinol bound to cellular retinol-binding protein is the preferred substrate for oxidation to retinal by a nicotinamide adenine dinucleotide phosphate–dependent dehydrogenase, whereas the conversion of retinal to tRA may be accomplished by a nicotinamide adenine dinucleotide–

requiring dehydrogenase.[55] Other evidence indicates that in certain tissues, β-carotene may be converted directly to tRA without the generation of a retinal intermediate.[56]

Retinoic acid has been demonstrated to have a short biologic half-life. A large number of studies have demonstrated that tRA is readily metabolized, which results in extensive changes in the polyene side chain as well as oxidations of the trimethyl-cyclohexanol ring.[57,58] A detailed discussion of retinoic acid metabolism is beyond the scope of this chapter, and reviews with detailed discussion of retinoic acid metabolism have been published (Curley and Robarge[59] and references within). In general, tRA metabolism involves a number of major metabolic steps. Conversion of tRA to its 13-*cis* or 9-*cis* isomers markedly affects retinoid biologic activity. The 9-*cis* isomer of tRA is the natural ligand for the retinoid X nuclear receptors (RXRs) (see later), and this isomer also binds extremely well to the retinoic acid nuclear receptors (RARs) with subsequent transactivation after binding to the appropriate DNA consensus sequences.[60–63] 13-*cis*-retinoic acid (Fig. 23-1) displays minimal binding to the RARs and none to the RXRs, which implies that the biologic activity seen with 13-*cis*-retinoic acid is due to its isomerization to tRA. Whether 13-*cis*-retinoic acid possesses any biologic activity is still controversial.[64,65] No specific isomerases responsible for the conversion of tRA to 13-*cis* or 9-*cis* isomers have been identified.

A prominent pathway for tRA metabolism is oxidation processes, many of which seem to involve cytochrome P-450 monooxygenases.[66,67] These oxidative processes play important biologic roles in terms of tRA metabolism, because agents such as liarozole and ketoconazole, which inhibit retinoic acid 4-hydroxylase, or the P-450 system markedly enhance the antiproliferative actions of tRA[68] (see later). Conjugation of tRA has been found *in vivo*. An *O*-acyl glucuronide of tRA, retinoyl-β-glucuronide, has been identified and is an important component of retinoid metabolites in the bile.[69,70] Observations suggest that the metabolism of tRA results in the generation of unique tRA derivatives that may indeed be responsible for the antiproliferative activity of tRA. Takatsuka et al.[71] have made the interesting observation that only the growth of those cells that display an ability to metabolize tRA to as yet unidentified metabolites is inhibited by retinoids.

Specific cytosolic binding proteins for tRA, cellular retinoic acid–binding proteins (CRABPs) types I and II, have been identified. The role of these binding proteins is unclear. The hypothesis has been presented that CRABP-bound tRA is an important substrate for metabolism.[72] Alternatively, the suggestion has also been made that these binding proteins sequester tRA from metabolic degradation or prevent exposure to high toxic concentrations of ligand in the cell; however, other studies have suggested that these proteins enhance delivery of ligand (tRA) to nuclear binding sites.[73] F9 teratocarcinoma stem cells transfected with a CRABP expression vector, which thus express high levels of CRABP I, require higher concentrations of tRA to induce differentiation into primitive endoderm; this suggests that CRABP I does indeed sequester tRA.[74] In subsequent studies, Boylan and Gudas[75] have shown that the levels of CRABP I directly influence the half-life of tRA and the types of metabolites detected in F9 cells. Higher concentrations of CRABP I result in enhanced metabolism and a shorter half-life.[76]

A number of synthetic retinoids have been synthesized in which the retinoid side chain stereochemistry has been fixed with respect to rotation about the single bond.[77,78] This class of compounds has been reviewed in terms of their structures and biologic activities.[59] Not only do a number of these derivatives display enhanced biologic activities, these compounds have also demonstrated selectivity in terms of their activation of either the RARs or RXRs through which these analogs modulate gene expression.[79] A number of these retinoid derivatives have now been synthesized that also display selectivity in terms of their binding and activation of the three RAR subtypes.[80,81] This property has allowed these compounds to serve as powerful tools in defining the role of the various RAR subtypes in modulation of gene expression or the antiproliferative activity of retinoids in a number of tissue types.[82–84] Many of these derivatives have demonstrated significant antiproliferative activity when tested against a number of malignant cell types,[85,86] and one of these analogs has been entered into clinical trials involving patients with a variety of malignancies.

In Vitro Effects of Retinoic Acid

Several comprehensive reviews have been published delineating retinoic acid modulation of cellular function, structure, and proliferation of both normal and malignant cells.[87,88] Retinoids have been demonstrated to induce terminal differentiation in a number of cells, including mouse teratocarcinoma cells, melanoma cells, human promyelocytic leukemia cells, and neuroblastoma cells.[89–91] The tRA increases the expression of a number of genes, such as those for fibronectin, laminin, and collagens III and IV, which are part of the extracellular matrix.[92–95] Modulation of these genes may be involved in tRA suppression of cancer invasion and metastasis. Differentiation of F9 embryonal carcinoma induced by tRA is associated with reduced adhesiveness, which is most likely due to decreased expression of the $\alpha_6\beta_1$ integrin in F9 cells.[96] Other investigators have found that tRA increases the expression of integrins.[97] tRA has been found to modulate the expression of a number of cellular adhesion molecules, including thrombospondins, vascular cell adhesion 1, and intercellular adhesion molecule 1.[98–100] Gap junctions are essential for the communication between normal cells, and they are not found or are significantly diminished in transformed cells. Retinoic acid increases gap junction formation as part of its reversal of the transformed state of the tumor cell, and this may be through its modulation of adhesion molecules as well as of connexin 43.[101,102]

The ability of retinoids to inhibit cellular proliferation may be subsequent to retinoid regulation of growth factor–stimulated proliferation. Expression of the epidermal growth factor receptor promoter is negatively regulated by tRA.[103] Retinoids have also been shown to down-regulate the expression of c-*erb*β receptors in breast cancer cells and inhibit both serum and insulin-like growth factor I (IGF-I) stimulation of growth in a number of systems.[104–106] In the MCF-7 breast carcinoma cell line, tRA blocks IGF-I stimulation of c-*fos* mRNA levels by decreasing c-*fos* mRNA stability.[94] The tRA-mediated inhibition of IGF-I–stimulated growth also appears to involve the induction of IGF-binding protein 3.[107] Serum stimulation of c-*fos* expression is also inhibited by tRA, perhaps through the serum response element or inhibition of the Jun N-terminal kinase (JNK)–dependent signaling pathway.[108–110]

Tumor cell invasion and metastasis have also been shown to be inhibited by retinoids. tRA has been shown to down-regulate the S100 family gene *18 A2/mts I*, which plays an important role in tumor cell invasion.[111] Tumor cell invasion into basement membranes has been correlated with type IV collagenase expression. Type IV collagenase induction is blocked by tRA, perhaps through its anti–AP-1 activity.[112] In addition, tRA up-regulates the expression of tissue inhibitors of metalloproteinase, which have a significant function in inhibiting metalloproteinase activity.[113] Metalloproteinases appear to play an important role in tumor cell invasion.

Retinoid Receptors

Retinoid modulation of tumor cell growth is mediated through binding to the nuclear receptors, which in turn act as transcription factors to regulate expression of the target genes. RARs and RXRs have been identified.[114] RARs are activated by both tRA and 9-*cis*-retinoic acid, whereas RXRs are activated by 9-*cis*-retinoic acid only. Three distinct RAR genes are found in humans, termed RARα,[115] RARβ,[116] and RARγ, as well as three RXR genes, termed RXRα, RXRβ, and RXRγ.[117,118] Highly conserved homologs of all the RAR and RXR genes have also been identified in other mammals, chickens, and amphibians.[119] Each RAR subtype has been demonstrated to have at least two isoforms that arise due to differential splicing and promoter usage. As noted previously, most cell types express more than one nuclear receptor. Although homologous recombination studies have suggested that functional redundancy exists among the RARs, other studies have indicated that the various receptor subtypes may possess separate functions.[120,121] Additional support for the concept that these RAR subtypes modulate the transcription of unique genes is found in the results of Boylan and colleagues.[122] These investigators have demonstrated that the inducibility of a number of target genes is differentially affected by disruption of either the RARα or RARγ gene, which suggests that these receptors perform specific functions in these cells.[120,121] Interestingly, the loss of one receptor in cells with a subsequent defect in retinoid-mediated phenotype can often be overcome by the expression of another RAR.[123,124]

The retinoid nuclear receptors belong to the steroid/thyroid hormone nuclear receptor superfamily. Each of the receptors has a modular structure of six domains designated A to F (Fig. 23-2). Binding of tRA to the E domain causes a conformational change leading to dimerization of the activated receptors. The ligand-bound dimeric receptors, in turn, regulate transcription from target gene promoters containing specific nucleotide sequences termed retinoic acid response elements (RAREs) or retinoid X response elements (RXREs). The dimerized receptors bind to response elements via their C domains (Fig. 23-2). RAR binding to RAREs preferentially occurs through heterodimer formation between the RAR and RXR,[125,126] whereas RXRs can modulate gene transcription through both homodimer formations as well as by heterodimer formation with the RARs, depending on the specific consensus sequence involved.[125–127] The RXRs are also known to modulate expression of a number of other genes through their ability to form heterodimers with thyroid hormone receptors, 1,25-dihydroxy vitamin D_3 receptor, eicosanoid receptors, ecdysone receptors, farnesol receptors, as well as a number of orphan nuclear receptors, including NGFI-B (nurr77) and LXRα.[128,129] The retinoid response elements for a number of the target genes have been delineated and have been found to consist of direct repeats (RARE, 5' AGTTCA 3'; RXRE, 5' AGGTCA 3') in which half-sites are separated by a certain number of base-pair spacers (Fig. 23-2). RARs generally bind to consensus sequences in which direct repeat elements are separated by five or two base-pair spacers. RXR homodimers, on the other hand, bind to consensus sequences in which direct repeat elements are separated by a one–base-pair spacer.

RARs and RXRs have also been shown to mediate negative regulation of certain genes without binding to their response elements. Such negative gene regulation is mediated via cross-modulation (crosstalk) involving AP-1 activation of promoters of target genes, including collagenase and stromelysin.[130] This crosstalk between the retinoid and AP-1 signaling pathways thus introduces an additional level of complexity in the retinoid-mediated signal transduction. This negative regulation of AP-1 transcriptional activity is due to the ability of the ligand portion of the RAR to sequester the cyclic adenosine monophosphate response element binding protein (CBP) in a ligand-dependent fashion.[131] CBP must bind to its consensus sequence for AP-1–mediated gene transcription[131]; thus, CBP sequestration by the RAR results in inhibition of AP-1–mediated transcription.

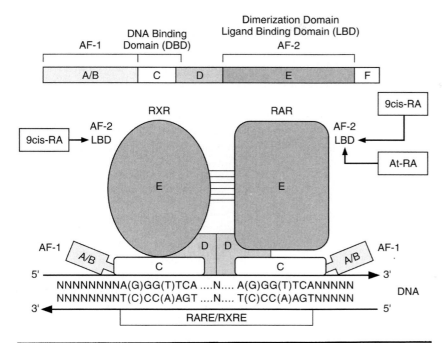

FIGURE 23-2. Schematic diagram of the modular organization of the retinoic acid receptors is shown in the upper panel. Various functional regions of the receptor are marked as A to F. Region C constitutes the DNA-binding domain (DBD), and region E serves as the ligand-binding domain. Retinoid X nuclear receptors (RXRs) bind only to 9-*cis*-retinoic acid (9-*cis*-RA), whereas retinoic acid nuclear receptors (RARs) bind both 9-*cis*-RA and all-*trans*-retinoic acid (At-RA). The E region of the receptor also contains a dimerization surface (multiple lines) and serves a receptor-type-specific, ligand-dependent transactivation function (AF-2). The A/B region located at the amino terminal possesses isoform-specific, ligand-independent transactivation function AF-1. The preferential binding of RXR/RAR heterodimers to different retinoic acid response elements (RAREs) and retinoid X response elements (RXREs) is dictated by the different asymmetric dimerization interfaces present in the DNA-binding domains (DBDs) of each receptor type. The middle panel shows a diagram of heterodimeric assembly of RARs on RARE/RXRE consisting of direct repeats (DRs) of hexanucleotide motif (5' A/GGG/TTCA 3') with varying spacer nucleotides (N) between the two DRs. The chart in the lower panel shows some of the naturally occurring polymorphic RAREs/RXREs in selected mammalian genes.

RARE/RXRE Polymorphisms and their nucleotide sequence in selected genes

Type	Gene	Sequence
Direct Repeat (DR)-1	Mouse CRABP-II	GAAGGGCAGAGGGTCACA
	Human ApoA1	GCAGGGCAGGGGTCAAG
	Mouse HHC1	TGAGGTCAGGGGTGGGG
	HBV	CGGGGTAAAGGTTCAGG
	Chicken Ovalbumin	TGGTGTCAAAGGTCAAA
	Rat ACO	CCAGGACAAAGGTCACG
	Rat PEPCK	CACGGCCAAAGGTCATG
Direct Repeat (DR)-2	Mouse CRBP-I	GTAGGTCAAAAGGTCAGA
	Mouse CRABP-II	CCAGTTCACCAGGTCAGG
	Mouse VL30-1	AAAGTTCATGTTTTCACA
	Mouse VL-30-2	TGGGGTGAAAAGTTTAGG
	Human ApoA1	AGGGGTCAAGGGTTCAGT
Direct Repeat (DR)-5	Human and mouse RARβ2	AGGGTTCACCGAAAGTTCACT
	Human RARα2	GAGGTTCAGCGAGAGTTCAGC
	Human RARγ2	CCGGGTCAGGAGGAGGTGAGC
	Mouse Hoxa-1	CAGGTTCACCGAAAGTTCAAG
	Mouse Hoxd-4	TAAGGTGAAATGCAGGTCACA
	Human MGP	AAGGTTCACCTTTTGTTCACC
	Human ADH3	AGGGGTCATTCAGAGTTCAGT
	Human Gα1	CAAGGGCAGGAGAAGGTCAGA

Additional levels of complexity in the retinoid-dependent signaling pathways have been unraveled by the discoveries of multiple putative coactivators (transcriptional mediators) and corepressors that have been found to interact directly with RXRs and RARs in the transcriptional modulation of the retinoid target genes. Using the yeast two-hybrid and the Far-Western methodologies, several proteins interacting with ligand-bound RAR and RXR were identified and cloned. A group of putative mediators of transcription (coactivators) include Trip1/Sug1, TIF1, RIP140, SRC-1, and TIF2, which specifically interact *in vitro* with the ligand (agonist)–bound ligand-binding domains, but generally not with the antagonist-bound ligand-binding domains of a variety of nuclear receptors, including RARs and RXRs.[129] RXRs interact much more efficiently with TIF1, whereas RARs interact with both Sug1 and TIF1. These coactivators are expressed ubiqui-

tously in different human tissues and cell lines. A second group of putative silencing mediators (corepressors) include the proteins N-Cor (nuclear receptor corepressor) and SMRT (silencing mediator for RAR and thyroid hormone receptors), which bind to unliganded RARs and thyroid hormone receptors and strongly transrepress the basal-level promoter activity of target genes. These corepressors are found complexed to histone deacetylases that play an important role in silencing gene expression. Both N-cor and SMRT interact with the unliganded ligand-binding domain of the receptors and are released on tRA binding.[129] The mechanisms responsible for the ligand-induced release of the corepressors from RARs remain to be elucidated. Thus, tRA-mediated transcriptional modulation of target genes involves several levels of complexity, including the polymorphic nature of the RAREs and RXREs, dimerization of ligand-activated different RARs and RXRs, and ligand-induced dissociation of corepressors and association of coactivators.

Retinoid Receptors in Cancer

RARα, RARβ, and RARγ are expressed by normal epithelial cells. Although the genes for the $RAR\alpha_2$, $RAR\beta_2$, and $RAR\gamma_2$ isoforms are known to have RAREs in their promoters, it is often the expression of RARβ that is strongly induced in many tissues by treatment with tRA. The human RARβ gene, which is located on chromosome 3, is normally expressed as two transcripts of 3.1 kilobases (kb) and 2.8 kb, differing at their 5' ends.[132] Loss of RARβ expression has been frequently observed in lung and breast carcinomas.[133] Cell lines derived from lung tumors as well as breast carcinomas expressed minimal to undetectable levels of RARβ,[134–136] whereas expression of RARα and RARγ was easily detectable in both the normal and malignant lung tissue.[137] Examination of RARβ expression in normal lung tissue samples, 33 lung carcinoma lines, and 9 primary lung tumors revealed altered RARβ levels in approximately 50% of the carcinoma lines and 30% of the tumor samples; similar results were found in breast carcinoma. Many of the carcinoma cell lines and tumor samples showed the specific loss of one transcript.[135] Possibly, mutations in the RARβ gene or alterations in the levels of *trans*-acting factors required for transcription of RARβ gene are involved in the reduced expression of RARβ in lung and breast carcinoma cells. Although chromosome region 3p is known to be commonly deleted in lung cancer,[133] interestingly, only a minority (10%) of the lung carcinoma cell lines and none of the tumor samples were shown to harbor gross changes in the RARβ gene.[135] Taken together, these findings indicate that alterations in the expression of RARβ may involve aberrations in required *trans* factors necessary for transcriptional regulation of RARβ gene or may be due to methylation of CpG islands in the RARβ promoter, with subsequent silencing of gene expression (see earlier).

Most often, tRA-dependent expression of RARβ involves the RARE present in the promoter of isoform β_2.[138] The inability to detect RARβ expression both in the presence and in the absence of tRA suggests the possibility of a defect in the regulation of transcription of the $RAR\beta_2$ promoter. To examine this issue, $RAR\beta_2$ promoter sequences were ligated to the CAT reporter gene, and the chimeric plasmids were transfected into human lung carcinoma cells displaying varying degrees of RARβ mRNA expression in the presence of tRA. The cells that had lost expression of RARβ mRNA did not show activation of transfected RARβ promoter–driven CAT activity in the presence of tRA, which suggests that failure of the RARβ gene to respond to tRA may be due to a defect in its promoter elements.[139] Further, the possibility of a defect in $RAR\beta_2$ RARE sequences was investigated in a study in which a plasmid containing $RAR\beta_2$ RARE sequences

located upstream of a heterologous thymidine kinase promoter–driven CAT gene was transfected into a variety of lung carcinoma cells possessing either tRA-responsive or tRA-nonresponsive RARβ genes. Strong activation of tRA-dependent CAT gene was observed in all the lung carcinoma cells, which suggests that the loss of RARβ expression was due to a defect in the RARβ promoter.[139]

Because $RAR\beta_2$ is the most prominent isoform of RARβ expressed in human lung carcinoma cells,[137] the possibility of a defect in promoter sequences was further investigated by using a plasmid in which an approximately 5-kb sequence upstream of the $RAR\beta_2$ transcription start site was fused to a luciferase reporter gene.[140] To evaluate the role of *cis* and *trans* mechanisms in the loss of RARβ expression, the $RAR\beta_2$ promoter–luciferase reporter plasmid construct was transfected into RARβ-positive and RARβ-negative cell lines. tRA failed to activate transcription of the luciferase gene in a number of cell lines, which indicates a potential defect in the *trans*-acting factors involved in regulation of RARβ expression.[140] In contrast to Zhang et al.,[139] however, these investigators further demonstrated a lack of tRA responsiveness of a plasmid containing $RAR\beta_2$ RARE linked to a luciferase reporter when transfected into lung carcinoma cells displaying loss of RARβ expression.[140] Using different constructs that were chimeras of the DNA and ligand-binding regions of RARβ and thyroid nuclear receptor, these investigators found that the loss of transactivation factors that interact specifically with the ligand-binding portion of the chimeric receptors may explain the loss of RARβ expression.[140]

The loss of RARβ expression is thought to play an important role in the development of lung carcinoma. Overexpression of RARβ inhibits the growth and proliferation of several of the lung carcinoma cell lines, including H157 and Calu I, both *in vitro* and in nude mice.[141] In addition, expression of RARβ causes increased sensitivity of HeLa cells to tRA-dependent growth inhibition,[142] which suggests a possible role of RARβ as a tumor suppressor gene.

A majority of the estrogen receptor (ER)–negative human breast carcinoma (HBC) cells have been found to express low to minimal levels of RARα and are generally refractory to growth-inhibitory effects of tRA.[143–145] The ER-positive breast carcinoma cells (for example, MCF-7), on the other hand, showed elevated levels of $RAR\alpha_1$ mRNA compared with a majority of their ER-negative counterparts and are sensitive to growth inhibition by tRA. Further, in breast tumor biopsy samples, the status of ER was found to be correlated with expression of $RAR\alpha_1$.[144] The ability of ER to regulate RARα expression in ER-positive HBC cells was demonstrated by the addition of estradiol to the cells growing in estradiol-depleted medium and the subsequent two- to threefold increase in $RAR\alpha_1$ mRNA levels. The physiologic relevance of ER-estradiol complex in elevated expression of $RAR\alpha_1$ mRNA was demonstrated by stable transfection of ER complementary DNA (cDNA) in ER-

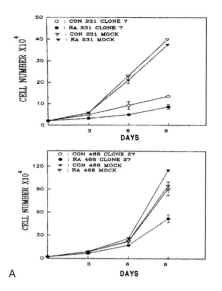

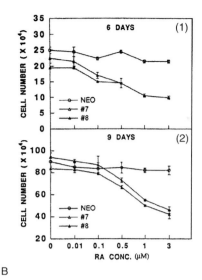

FIGURE 23-3. Retinoic acid (RA) growth inhibition of RA nuclear receptor–transfected estrogen receptor (ER)–negative human breast carcinoma (HBC) cells. **A:** MDA-MB-231 (*top panel*) and MDA-MB-468 (*bottom panel*) were stably transfected with an expression plasmid containing RA receptor α (RARα) complementary DNA. The sublines stably expressing vector only (CON) or RARα (RA 231 or RA 468) were treated with 1 μmol per L of RA. **B:** MDA-MB-231 cells stably transfected with expression plasmid containing RA receptor β (RARβ) complementary DNA. The sublines stably expressing vector only (NEO) or RARβ (#7 and #8) were treated with varying concentrations of RA. In both cases, the stable expression of either RARα or RARβ leads to significant growth inhibition of ER-negative HBC cells in the presence of RA.

negative MDA-MB-231 HBC cells. The ER-transfected MDA-MB-231 HBC cells not only showed significant increase in expression of RARα mRNA compared with their wild-type counterparts but also displayed enhanced sensitivity to tRA-dependent growth inhibition. Further, stable transfection of RARα cDNA in ER-negative MDA-MB-231 HBC cells caused their enhanced sensitivity to tRA-dependent growth inhibition[146] (Fig. 23-3), which suggests that RARα is a mediator of the antiproliferative effects of tRA in the HBC cells. When various plasmid clones containing approximately 5-kb promoter and several promoter deletion fragments fused with luciferase reporter gene were used, an estradiol-responsive 42–base-pair (bp) $RAR\alpha_1$ promoter subfragment from positions −102 to −59 relative to the transcription start was identified.[147] The ligand-bound ER up-regulates expression of RARα through a weak interaction with the Sp1 transcription factor via an imperfect half-palindromic estrogen response element (5' GGTGA 5') located ten nucleotides from the Sp1 site in the above 42-bp $RAR\alpha_1$ promoter subfragment. The similar weak interactions of ligand-bound ER and the transcription factor Sp1 have also been implicated in the estradiol-dependent up-regulation of several estradiol-responsive genes, including cathepsin D, rat brain creatine kinase, and c-myc (Fig. 23-4). The role of RARα in tRA-dependent growth inhibition of HBC cells was further highlighted by the discovery of certain ER-negative HBC cells (SKBR-3, and MDA-MB-435) that were sensitive to growth inhibition by retinoic acid.[148,149] Indeed, both of the above cell lines were found to express significantly higher levels of $RAR\alpha_1$ than their other ER-negative counterparts and were sensitive to growth-inhibitory effects of tRA as well as RARα-selective synthetic retinoids. When deletional analysis was used, a 72-bp subfragment of $RAR\alpha_1$ promoter from positions −132 to −59 relative to the transcription start site was found to participate in the estradiol-independent increased expression of RARα in ER-negative SKBR-3 cells.[149]

Retinoids and Acute Promyelocytic Leukemia

Although confirmation is still lacking that tRA or other retinoids induce differentiation of solid tumors when given *in vivo*, significant evidence exists that tRA induces differentiation of APL cells.

As noted previously, tRA has been shown to induce complete remissions and increase the survival of over 90% of patients with APL.[150] APL cells have been found to possess a t(15:17)(q22:q12-21) translocation that results in the fusion of RARα to the nuclear protein PML.[151,152] RARα has been demonstrated to play an important role in normal myeloid

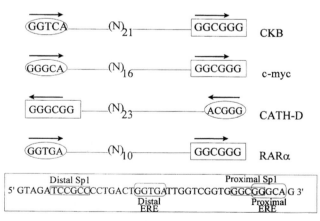

FIGURE 23-4. The estradiol-responsive regions of the rat creatine kinase B (CKB), human c-myc, human cathepsin D (CATH-D), and human retinoic acid receptor α isoform 1 gene (RARα) promoters contain common estrogen-response element (ERE) half-site/Sp1-binding site sequences. The ERE half-site and Sp1 site are indicated by an oval and a box, respectively. The nucleotide sequence in the box at the bottom is the 42 bases of the sense strand of human RARα promoter showing the locations and sequences of the distal and proximal ERE half-sites and Sp1 motifs.

lineage differentiation.[153–155] Formation of the PML-RARα fusion protein markedly prevents normal RARα-mediated differentiation of myeloid precursors in the presence of physiologic concentrations of tRA. Whether this inhibition occurs because the PML-RARα fusion product functions as a dominant negative protein, blocks RAR activation of promoters, reverses RAR inhibition of AP-1–mediated transcription, inhibits the formation of novel macromolecular organelles termed PML oncogenic domains, or tightly binds histone deacetylases (see earlier) is still not clear.[156–162] The addition of pharmacologic concentrations (1 μmol per L) of tRA results in reversal of this inhibition, with enhanced RAR activation of promoters, RAR inhibition of AP-1–mediated promoter activation, normal formation of PML oncogenic domains, and differentiation of the promyelocytes, along the

myeloid lineage as evidenced by the acquisition of normal neutrophil phenotype (Fig. 23-5).[160]

The initial study examining the clinical efficacy of tRA in APL, conducted in China, demonstrated a dramatic response; 23 of 24 patients (eight of whom had been previously treated) achieved either a partial or a complete remission after administration of an oral daily tRA dose of 45 to 100 mg per m². [150] A subsequent French study in which 22 APL patients were treated with tRA demonstrated a 64% complete remission rate and 38% partial remission rate with three early deaths.[163] Patients were given tRA 45 mg per m² per day in two oral doses. Most complete remissions were obtained within 60 days of treatment. Similar results were demonstrated in a study by Warrell et al.,[163a] in which 11 patients were treated with 45 mg per m² per day; 9

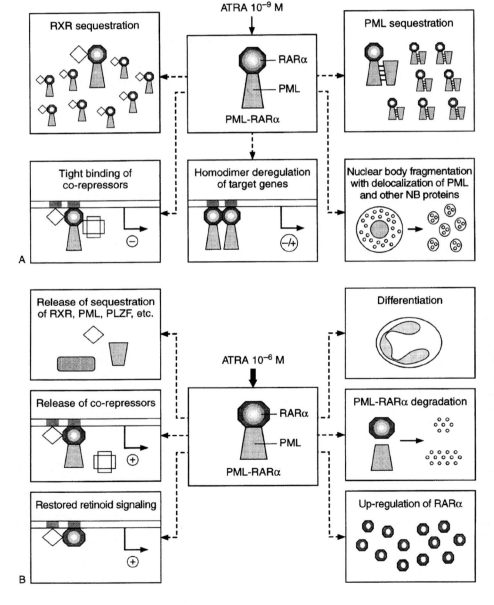

FIGURE 23-5. Retinoic acid differentiation of acute promyelocytic leukemia (APL) cells. **A:** promyelocytic leukemia–retinoic acid receptor (PML-RAR) inhibition of differentiation at physiologic concentration (1 × 10⁻⁹ mol per L) *trans*-retinoic acid (tRA). PML-RARα inhibits corepressor release, sequesters retinoid X nuclear receptors (RXRs), and prevents normal location of PML bodies in APL cells. **B:** Differentiation induced by 10⁻⁶ mol per L tRA. The addition of pharmacologic concentrations of tRA results in release of RXR and corepressors, restoration of retinoid signaling, degradation of PML-RARα, and normal differentiation of APL cells. (ATRA, all-*trans*-retinoic acid; NB, nuclear bodies.) (Adapted from Melnick A, Licht JD. Deconstructing a disease: RARα, its fusion partners and their roles in the pathogenesis of acute promyelocytic leukemia. *Blood* 1999;93:3167.)

patients achieved a complete remission, with a median time to remission of 41 days.

Unfortunately, the duration of the complete remissions obtained with tRA is brief, with an average duration of 3 to 6 months.[150,163,164] Relapse after treatment with tRA is usually accompanied by the acquisition of resistance to tRA-mediated differentiation.[163–166] A number of potential explanations have been offered for this acquired resistance to tRA-mediated differentiation. Marked reduction in the maximal achievable plasma concentrations of tRA is noted within 1 to 2 weeks after the initiation of tRA therapy.[167,168] This has been found to be partly due to increased tRA oxidation by cytochrome P-450 and lipoxygenase enzymes[167,168] (see later). Although this enhanced metabolism of tRA may explain some of the tRA resistance noted in APL patients, it does not account for the decreased sensitivity of APL cells to tRA-induced differentiation *in vitro* after relapse from tRA therapy[158,166,169,170]; this would suggest an acquired cellular mechanism for the tRA resistance. The PML-RARα fusion protein is the major site of tRA action. Missense mutations in the RARα region of the PML-RARα fusion gene have been found in 3 of 11 APL patients who relapsed after tRA therapy.[170] These missense mutations may result in the inability of tRA to appropriately interact with PML-RARα and reverse its inhibitory effects on myeloid differentiation. Other investigators have implicated enhanced expression and levels of CRABP II as a cause for the intrinsic APL cell resistance to tRA-mediated differentiation.[169,171,172] Enhanced CRABP II would result in elevated levels of tRA binding, with sequestration of tRA in the cytoplasm, and enhanced metabolism of tRA by cytoplasmic oxidative enzymes and decreased transport of the ligand to the nuclear PML-RARα receptor. However, a study examining CRABP II mRNA levels and binding activity in APL cells found that CRABP II was constitutively expressed in these cells, and no significant increases were seen in either CRABP II mRNA levels or CRABP II binding activity after the development of clinical tRA resistance.[173]

Retinoids and Solid Tumors

When used as the sole agent, tRA displayed minimal efficacy in patients with solid tumors. Combination of tRA with chemotherapy agents, although enhancing toxicity, did not appear to add significantly to therapeutic efficacy in patients with small cell carcinoma of the lung.[174] A phase II trial of tRA in combination with cisplatin–VP-16 chemotherapy in patients with advanced non–small cell lung cancer resulted in a 53% partial response rate as well as minor responses in 20% of the patients.[175] Whether tRA adds significantly to the efficacy of the cisplatin–VP-16 chemotherapy must be tested in a randomized trial. *In vitro* studies using ER-positive breast carcinoma cell lines have demonstrated that exposure to tRA results in the inhibition of growth of these cells. In a small phase I–II trial involving patients with advanced breast can-

cer, treatment with tRA and tamoxifen resulted in response in 2 of 7 patients with measurable disease and disease stability for more than 6 months and in 7 of 18 patients with evaluable, nonmeasurable disease.[176] Interestingly, responses were observed in patients whose disease had previously progressed on tamoxifen.

Pharmacology

Pharmacokinetic and pharmacodynamic studies of tRA have been conducted in patients with both leukemia and solid tumors. In patients with APL, the peak plasma level (346 ± 266 ng per mL) after an oral dose of 45 mg per m² was achieved 1 to 2 hours after dosing. The plasma level then decreased rapidly in a monoexponential fashion with a half-life of 0.8 ± 0.1 hours and was less than 10 ng per mL at 8 hours, with an area under the concentration × time curve (AUC) at 8 hours of 682 ± 500 ng per mL per hour.[167] In seven patients, after 2 to 6 weeks of continuous oral treatment, a significant decrease was noted in the peak plasma concentration achieved, which fell from 249 ± 89 ng per mL on day 1 to 138 ± 139 ng per mL, with a corresponding decrease in AUC. Increasing the oral dose to 90 mg per m² did not correct the fall in peak plasma concentration.[167] Similar decreases in peak plasma concentrations of tRA were noted in patients with solid tumors[177,178] (Fig. 23-6). The pharmacokinetic parameters of 13-*cis*-retinoic acid were significantly different from those of tRA; half-life was significantly longer (27 hours versus 1 hour) and no evidence was seen of decreased plasma concentration after continuous dosing (Table 23-1).

In APL patients receiving their initial dose of tRA, 4-oxo-all-tRA was the only metabolite detected in plasma.

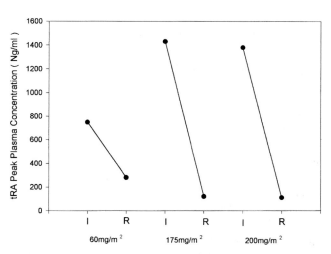

FIGURE 23-6. Fall in peak plasma *trans*-retinoic acid (tRA) concentration after continuous dosing of tRA. Patients were initially treated with tRA at either 60, 175, or 200 mg per m², and plasma levels were determined after initial dose or after repeated dosing. (From Lee JS, Newman RA, Lippman SM, et al. Phase 1 evaluation of all-*trans*-retinoic acid in adult with solid tumors. *J Clin Oncol* 1993;11:959.)

TABLE 23-1. PHARMACOLOGIC PARAMETERS OF 13-*CIS*-RETINOIC ACID (13-*CIS*-RA) AND *TRANS*-RETINOIC ACID (tRA)

Retinoid	Peak Plasma Concentration (mg/mL)	Peak Time (h)	$t_{1/2}$ (h)
13-*cis*-RA (3 mg/kg)	0.2–1.10	2.0–5.0	20.0–34.0
tRA (45 mg/m²)	0.38–1.9	1.5–3.7	0.9–1.4

$t_{1/2}$, half-life.

Only trace amounts of 13-*cis*-retinoic acid could be identified. In APL patients who underwent repeat pharmacokinetic studies after 2 to 4 weeks of continuous dosing, the 24-hour urinary excretion of 4-oxo-tRA glucuronide increased from 32 ± 12 ng after the first dose to 318 ± 116 ng.[167] In a phase I trial involving patients with solid tumors, no correlation was found between the formation of 4-oxo-tRA or its glucuronide and decreased peak plasma levels of tRA and decreased AUC.[178]

The explanation for the marked decrease in plasma tRA levels after continuous dosing remains unclear. Rapid metabolism of tRA by the cytochrome P-450 enzymes has been shown.[179] Therefore, studies were conducted to assess whether the addition of ketoconazole during continuous treatment with tRA would result in elevated tRA plasma levels in patients with APL and non–small cell lung carcinoma.[179] The addition of ketoconazole (400 mg) resulted in an increase in mean plasma AUC (218 ± 224 ng per mL per hour) on day 28 to 375 ± 285 ng per mL per hour on day 29. These results suggested that perhaps elevated P-450 levels played a role in the enhanced metabolism of tRA during continuous treatment with the drug. No evidence exists, however, that the elevated tRA plasma concentrations noted in the presence of ketoconazole result in a decreased relapse rate in APL patients receiving tRA.

Retinoids and Interferon

Studies both *in vitro* and *in vivo* have demonstrated that the combination of retinoids and interferons demonstrates marked antitumor activity. Numerous investigators showed synergistic interactions between retinoids and interferons in inhibiting a number of malignant cell types.[180–184] Marth and his coinvestigators demonstrated that the combination of either tRA or 9-*cis*-retinoic acid with interferon resulted in the synergistic inhibition of breast carcinoma proliferation.[181,185] Similarly, the combination of retinoids and interferon-α showed a synergistic antiangiogenic effect in tumor cell lines harboring human papillomavirus.[183] The interferons enhance the expression of a number of genes that appear to play important roles in their antiproliferative activity. A number of interferon-stimulated genes and their products have been identified. Protein kinase R (PKR), an interferon-regulated gene, requires double-stranded RNA

(dsRNA) for its activity; on binding to dsRNA, PKR undergoes autophosphorylation, which results in its activation. Activated PKR phosphorylates a number of substrates, including eukaryotic initiation factor 2α (eIF-2α), which results in cessation of polypeptide chain initiation.[186,187] In addition, interferons stimulate the expression of 2,5-oligoadenylate synthetase, a family of enzyme isoforms that, when dsRNA is used as a cofactor, polymerize adenosine triphosphate into 2',5'-linked oligoadenylates; this activates a latent endonuclease ribonuclease, which then cleaves single-stranded RNAs.[188,189] A potential mechanism by which retinoids can increase the cytotoxic effects of interferons is through the enhancement of interferon-mediated gene induction. This appears to be the case. Pretreatment of the human leukemia cell line HL-60 and murine embryonal carcinoma cell lines with tRA followed by interferon-α-1, interferon-β, or interferon-γ resulted in higher levels of induction of 2,5-oligoadenylate synthetase, PKR, and interferon gene–regulating factor 1.[190–193] In the squamous cell carcinoma cell line ME-180, the synergistic antiproliferative actions of interferon-α in the presence of tRA correlated with the increased expression of 2,5-oligoadenylate synthetase and transcriptional factor interferon gene–regulating factor 1 genes.[193]

The mechanism by which retinoids enhance interferon-induced gene expression has been deduced. Interferon-α and interferon-β induce cellular genes by means of an interferon response element that binds a number of transactivation factors.[194] Interferon-stimulating gene factor 3 binds this site and consists of a 48-kd DNA-binding protein and three tyrosine phosphorylated proteins, signal transducers and activators of transcription (STAT)-1α, STAT-1β, and STAT-2.[189] Cells lacking STAT-1 fail to respond to interferon-α and interferon-β as well as interferon-γ.[194–196] Numerous investigators have now found that pretreatment of a number of malignant cell types with tRA results in the enhanced expression of STAT-1[162,197–199]; tRA-mediated induction of STAT-1 gene expression is a result of increased gene transcription.[197] Weihua et al.[197] have found that the STAT-1 gene promoter contains the direct repeat sequence (GGGTCAGGG TCA) located 467 base-pairs from the transcriptional start site, which functions as a RARE. Gel shift mobility and transactivation studies have demonstrated preferential binding for the retinoic acid nuclear receptor RARβ.[197] Other genes have now been identified that play a role in interferon-β and retinoic acid–mediated cell death.[200]

Clinical trials using the combination of 13-*cis*-retinoic acid and interferon-α have been conducted, and several have demonstrated remarkable efficacy.[201,202] Thirty-two patients with heavily pretreated advanced inoperable squamous cell carcinoma of the skin were treated with a combination of oral 13-*cis*-retinoic acid (1 mg per kg per day) and subcutaneous recombinant human interferon-α-2a (3 MU per day) for at least 2 months.[201] Seven complete responses

(25%) were observed, and nineteen (68%) of the 28 assessable patients responded to the therapy. The median duration of response was longer than 5 months. A relationship appeared to exist between decreased response rate and extent of disease that was highly statistically significant. Response rates were 93% (13 of 14) in patients with advanced local disease and 25% (two of eight) in patients with distant metastases. The major limiting toxicity was fatigue. Twenty-six patients with untreated locally advanced squamous cell carcinoma of the cervix (stages IB, IIA, IIB, IIIB, and IVA) were treated with a similar regimen of 13-*cis*-retinoic acid (1 mg per kg per day) and interferon-α-2a (6 MU per day).[202] Thirteen patients showed major responses (tumor regression of 50% or more); 1 patient achieved a complete response, and 12 experienced partial responses.[198] A multicenter phase II trial examined the efficacy of interleukin 2 (IL-2), interferon-α, and 13-*cis*-retinoic acid in patients with metastatic renal cell carcinoma. Therapy consisted of IL-2 (11 MIU 4 days per week for 4 weeks), interferon-α (9 MIU 2 days per week for 4 weeks), and oral 13-*cis*-retinoic acid (1 mg per kg per day) on a 6-week cycle.[203] Eight of 47 patients responded (one complete response, seven partial responses); three of the patients showing partial response were rendered disease free by subsequent surgical resection.[203] The median duration of response was 42 weeks. Significant toxicities included hyperlipidemia (4 of 18 patients) and cardiomyopathy (1 of 18 patients). These results were significantly better than those reported in a study in which 13 patients with metastatic renal cell carcinoma were treated with interferon-α-2a (3 MU per day) and 13-*cis*-retinoic acid (1 mg per kg per day); on this regimen, two patients experienced a partial response.[204] These patients had all been previously treated with immunotherapy in association with chemotherapy, which may explain the significant difference in response rate.[205] No clinical efficacy was noted in a phase II clinical trial that used similar regimens of interferon-α (5 MU per m² three times weekly) and 13-*cis*-retinoic acid (1 mg per kg per day) in patients with metastatic melanoma.[200] Patients in the stable phase of chronic myelogenous leukemia who were treated with 13-*cis*-retinoic acid (3-day course) in combination with interferon-α experienced a significant fall in white count accompanied by a fall in the percentage of S-phase cells.[206] Two-thirds of the 43 patients studied demonstrated an increase in marrow apoptosis with suppression of expression of the antiapoptotic protein Bcl-2 as well as myc expression.

Predominately nonhematologic toxicities have been found during the oral administration of tRA.[177–179] The most common nonhematologic toxicities are cheilitis and skin manifestation such as erythema, rash, and desquamation. Other toxicities include headache, commonly occurring during the first several days of therapy; hypercalcemia; and hypertriglyceridemia, which was dose limiting in one phase I trial.[177–179] Nausea and vomiting were also frequently found with higher dosages (more than 100 mg per m² per day).[177]

Novel Retinoids Using Retinoid Receptor–Independent Mechanisms

The compound *N*-(4-hydroxyphenyl) retinamide (4-HPR) (Fig. 23-1) has been shown to have significant ability to modulate tumor growth in a variety of animal systems.[207] This compound has been used in both cancer chemoprevention and cancer therapy.[208–213] The incidence of carcinogen-induced bladder, lung, mammary, and skin tumors in animals has been reduced after treatment with 4-HPR.[214,215] *In vivo* studies have demonstrated that 4-HPR treatment inhibits prostate cancer in rats, and it is active against human ovarian carcinoma transplanted in mice and potentiates the tumoricidal effects of *cis*-platinum.[216,217] *In vitro* 4-HPR demonstrates a broad spectrum of activity, inhibiting the growth of leukemia and lymphoma, mammary, and small cell lung carcinoma cell lines.[218–220] Clinical trials using 4-HPR in patients with a variety of malignancies have been disappointing, but 4-HPR has been shown to protect against the development of ovarian carcinoma in humans.[221] In many cell lines, 4-HPR, in contrast to tRA, has been a potent inducer of apoptosis. The mechanism by which 4-HPR induces cell death is not clear. Hultin et al. reported the metabolic conversion of 4-HPR to tRA *in vivo* as well as in cultured rat bladder carcinoma cells and proposed that the biologic actions of 4-HPR could be mediated by tRA in bladder carcinoma cells.[221a] Both tRA and 4-HPR have been shown to enhance RARβ mRNA levels in normal human mammary epithelial cells, perhaps through the RARE located in the RARβ promoter.[222] Thus, the suggestion has been made that 4-HPR, like tRA, may mediate its effects via nuclear retinoid receptors.[222] In addition, 4-HPR has been found to be a weak but highly selective binder of RARγ, but only when incubated in the presence of the RAR DNA consensus sequence.[223]

Other evidence strongly suggests that 4-HPR may exert its actions independent of the classical RAR/RXR pathway. Delia et al.[218] have found a significant difference in the antiproliferative effects of 4-HPR and tRA, with 4-HPR a markedly more potent antiproliferative agent in a majority of the cell lines tested. In addition, 4-HPR also induced programmed cell death in hematopoietic cell lines that were resistant to the antiproliferative action of tRA. Also, 4-HPR inhibited the growth of tRA-resistant MDA-MB-231, MDA-MB-468, and MDA-MB-453 breast cancer cell lines (Table 23-2). It induced apoptosis in 40% of the tRA-resistant MDA-MB-231 cells and in 80% of the tRA-sensitive MCF-7 HBC cell line, whereas minimal apoptosis (less than 10%) was induced in these cells by tRA.[224] tRA strongly transactivates the RARE-mediated genes by activation of the endogenous RAR receptors in breast carcinoma

TABLE 23-2. INHIBITION OF *TRANS*-RETINOIC ACID (tRA)–RESISTANT BREAST CANCER CELL LINES BY *N*-(4-HYDROXYPHENYL) RETINAMIDE (4-HPR)

Cell Line	tRA Inhibition (%)	4-HPR Inhibition (%)
MDA-MB-231	7 ± 3	39 ± 8
MDA-MB-468	9 ± 4	50 ± 6
MDA-MB-453	9 ± 3	56 ± 7

Cells were exposed to 1 µmol per L of tRA or 4-HPR for 9 days.

cells.[145,224–226] If 4-HPR mediates its enhanced effects through the retinoid receptors, then it should also bind and activate these receptors better than tRA. Study has found 4-HPR to be an extremely poor binder to the RARs and an extremely poor transactivator of a number of RAREs and RXREs compared with tRA (Table 23-3).[224] Also, 4-HPR was shown to display minimal anti–AP-1 activity, which ruled this out as a potential mechanism of action.[224] Oridate et al.[227] have demonstrated that exposure of the human cervical carcinoma cell line C33A to 4-HPR results in a 1.85- to 4.5-fold increase in radical oxygen species, depending on the concentration of 4-HPR used; that this generation of radical oxygen species may indeed play a major role in 4-HPR–mediated apoptosis was substantiated by the ability of pyrrolidine dithiocarbamate, an oxygen radical scavenger, to suppress the rate of generation of reactive oxygen species and inhibit 4-HPR–induced apoptosis.[227]

The novel retinoid 6-[3-(1-adamantyl 4 hydroxyphenyl]-2-naphthalene carboxylic acid (AHPN, CD437) (Fig. 23-1) was initially synthesized to be RARγ selective; it displays

TABLE 23-3. DOSE-DEPENDENT EFFECTS OF RETINOIC ACID, 4-HPR, AND 4-MPR ON β_2RARE-CONTROLLED CAT ACTIVITY

Dose (mol/L)	Retinoid	Relative CAT Activity
0	4-HPR	1
	4-MPR	1
	tRA	1
10^{-8}	4-HPR	1
	4-MPR	1
	tRA	5
10^{-7}	4-HPR	1
	4-MPR	1
	tRA	11
10^{-6}	4-HPR	3
	4-MPR	2.8
	tRA	24

CAT, chloramphenicol acetyl transferase; 4-HPR, *N*-(4-hydroxyphenyl) retinamide; 4-MPR, *N*-(4-methoxyphenyl) retinamide; β_2RARE, β_2 retinoic acid response element; tRA, *trans*-retinoic acid.
Note: Cells were transiently transfected with the indicated reported vector and treated with the indicated concentrations of retinoids for 24 hours after transfection. CAT assays were performed. Results are quantitation of two independent experiments. The values are expressed relative to respective controls (cells not treated with retinoids), which were given an arbitrary value of 1.

TABLE 23-4. COMPARISON OF THE GROWTH-INHIBITORY EFFECTS OF *TRANS*-RETINOIC ACID (tRA) AND AHPN IN BREAST CANCER CELL LINES

Cell line	tRA ED$_{50}$ (µmol/L)	AHPN ED$_{50}$ (nmol/L)	AHPN-mediated apoptosis
MCF-7	1.0	300	+
T-47D	1.3	350	+
ZR-75	1.0	300	+
MDA-MB-231	>10	150	+
MDA-MB-468	>10	100	+
MDA-MB-453	>10	100	+

AHPN, 6-[3-(1-adamantyl 4 hydroxyphenyl]-2-naphthalene carboxylic acid (CD437); ED$_{50}$, median effective inhibitory dose.

poor binding and transactivation of RARβ and RARα and no binding to the RXRs.[81] AHPN has been found to induce cell-cycle arrest and apoptosis in a number of cell lines, several of which are totally resistant to the antiproliferative effects of tRA at concentrations tenfold less than those required with 4-HPR (Table 23-4).[228] In addition, AHPN is a potent inducer of G$_1$ cell-cycle arrest in both the tRA-sensitive and tRA-resistant HBC cell lines.[229] As noted previously for 4-HPR, AHPN is an extremely poor transactivator of the endogenous RARs or RXRs in breast carcinoma cell compared with tRA.[229] Thus, AHPN may exert its actions through a RAR/RXR-independent mechanism. Induction of G$_1$ cell-cycle arrest in HBC cells appeared to occur via the p53-independent induction of the cyclin-dependent kinase inhibitor p21/WAF1/CIP1.[228] The enhancement of p21/WAF1/CIP1 mRNA and protein levels occurs through AHPN-mediated p21/WAF1/CIP1 message stability.[229] AHPN-mediated G$_1$ cell-cycle arrest in breast carcinoma cells is followed by apoptosis.[228]

To further investigate the possibility that AHPN may function through an RAR/RXR-independent mechanism, the ability of this novel retinoid to inhibit the proliferation of and induce apoptosis in the human leukemia cell line HL-60R was examined.[230] HL-60R, derived from the HL-60 leukemia cell line, does not express RARβ or RARγ mRNA as demonstrated by ribonuclease protection assays and has a deletion of the last 50 amino acids of the RARα ligand-binding domain, which prevents tRA binding by the truncated RARα.[231,232] Despite the absence of functioning RARs, HL-60R is extremely sensitive to the induction of growth arrest and apoptosis mediated by AHPN.[230] Exposure of HL-60R cells to this retinoid results in activation of caspase 3 (CPP-32) and cleavage of poly–adenosine diphosphate–ribosyl polymerase (PARP), both indicators of an apoptotic process[230]; this is followed by internucleosomal fragmentation of the DNA. In addition, the antiapoptotic protein Bcl-2 is cleaved during AHPN-mediated apoptosis of HL-60R cells[230]; data would suggest that cleavage of Bcl-2 results in the generation of a proapoptotic protein.[233] Apoptosis in HL-60R is preceded by the induction of p21/WAF1/CIP1 mRNA, with a tenfold increase in p21/WAF1/CIP1 mRNA levels noted within 30 minutes of exposure to AHPN.[230] Exposure to AHPN of primary cultures of leukemia cells obtained from patients with acute myelogenous leukemia also resulted in PARP cleavage and apoptotic morphology of the cells as indicated by nuclear blebbing.[230]

Overexpression of *bcl-2* or *bcl-X*$_L$ has been found to inhibit the induction of apoptosis in malignant cells by a large number of agents.[234–236] AHPN was found to downregulate the expression of Bcl-X$_L$ protein and mRNA levels in HBC cells.[237] The overexpression of either *bcl-2* or *bcl-X*$_L$ in HL-60 cells resulted in only a 3-hour delay in apoptosis as indicated by activation of caspase 3 and cleavage of protein kinase C and PARP.[238] Although 50 and 300 nmol per L AHPN were required to induce PARP cleavage in HL-60/NEO cells and in HL-60/bcl-2 and HL-60/bcl-X$_L$ cells, respectively, maximal apoptosis in all three cell lines was achieved using 300 nmol per L AHPN. All three cell lines, however, share identical dose-response curves in terms of their growth inhibition and induction of p21/WAF1/CIP1, which suggests that AHPN-mediated inhibition of growth and induction of apoptosis represent two distinct and separable processes.[238] The signaling mechanism by which AHPN trigger apoptosis remains to be clarified. AHPN induction of apoptosis in lung carcinoma cells appears to require enhanced expression of C-Jun and NUR 77.[239] Constitutive expression of a dominant negative of C-Jun inhibits AHPN-mediated increases in NUR 77 expression and apoptosis in these cells.[239] AHPN activates both the p38 and JNK/SAPK mitogen-activated protein kinases in HL-60R cells.[240] Although activation of p38 appears to be the result of caspase activation and subsequent apoptosis in HL-60R cells, induction of JNK/SAPK kinase activity is not a result of the apoptotic process.[240] Whether activation of JNK/SAPK is required for the apoptotic process remains to be determined.

Retinoids and Immune Function

The ability of vitamin A to reduce infectious disease mortality has been documented by numerous studies over the last seven decades.[241,242] Research has strongly suggested that the ability of vitamin A and retinoids to reduce infectious disease morbidity as well as display antitumor activity may be due to their ability to enhance immune function (see Semba[243] and references within). The role of vitamin A and other retinoids in modulating many aspects of immune function has been substantiated by a number of investigators (see Semba[243] and references within). Monocytes and macrophages are important participants in the immune cascade in their role as antigen-presenting cells and as generators of oxygen and nitrogen radicals.[244] The ability of retinoids to modulate the differentiation of monocytes and the number and *in vitro* activity of mac-

rophages has been demonstrated.[90,245–248] Breitman and colleagues[245] showed that the addition of tRA resulted in the rapid differentiation of the leukemic cell line THP-1 along the monocyte pathway. Retinoid-mediated differentiation of the U937 leukemia cell line was associated with the acquisition of those phenotypic markers necessary for monocyte function.[247]

Exposure to retinoic acid results in a twofold increase in murine macrophage phagocytosis as well as increased production of the important immune cytokine IL-1 by human peripheral blood mononuclear cells, murine macrophage cell lines, and murine macrophages.[249,250] IL-1 enhances the proliferation of both T and B cells. The retinoid tRA appears to increase IL-1 expression at the transcriptional level.[251] Immunoglobulin production requires the presence of B lymphocytes, and the growth and activation of these cells appears to require retinol.[248,252] Chun et al.[253] have found that tRA is 100-fold more active than retinol in enhancing immunoglobulin G (IgG) responses in vitamin A–deficient mice.[253] The addition of tRA to *Staphylococcus aureus*–stimulated cord blood mononuclear cells resulted in a 2- to 47-fold increase in immunoglobulin M synthesis.[254] The tRA-induced enhancement in immunoglobulin synthesis appeared to be due to the recruitment of more B cells to differentiate into immunoglobulin-secreting cells. Interestingly, tRA induced immunoglobulin M synthesis in cord blood mononuclear cells and IgG synthesis in adult peripheral blood mononuclear cells. The ability of tRA to enhance B lymphocyte function may be multifactorial. tRA appears to regulate the production of factors that modulate B-cell synthesis as well as to act directly on B cells, as evidenced by the augmentation of IgG synthesis in B-cell lines transformed by Epstein-Barr virus.[254] Additional studies suggested that tRA-induced augmentation in IgG and immunoglobulin A synthesis in the Epstein-Barr virus–transformed cell lines was due to increased IL-6 production by these cells.[255] Vitamin A deficiency in mice results in a decreased ability to stimulate B lymphocyte for antigen-specific secondary IgG1 responses *in vivo* and *in vitro*. This appears to be due to an overproduction of interferon-γ by CD4+ T cells.[256] Supplementation with tRA *in vitro* decreased interferon-γ secretion from vitamin A–deficient T cells. The addition of interferon-γ–neutralizing antibodies to cultures established with immune cells from vitamin A–deficient mice resulted in markedly increased IgG1 production. Transient transfection assays in the human T lymphoblastoid cell line Jurkat revealed that the activation of the interferon-γ promoter was down-regulated in the presence of tRA, and that tRA-mediated inhibition of transcription involved a USF/EGR–1 binding element.[257]

T lymphocytes serve as major regulatory cells of the immune system; the numerous subsets of T lymphocytes include helper T (CD4+) and cytotoxic T (CD8+) lymphocytes. CD4+ lymphocytes recognize antigen in the presence of major histocompatibility complex class II complexes, whereas CD8[+] lymphocytes recognize cells bearing major histocompatibility complex class I complexes. Activation of T cells appears to require retinol, whereas tRA has been shown to increase antigen-specific T-lymphocyte proliferation.[258,259] The maintenance of normal T-cell populations requires the presence of retinoids.[260] tRA has been shown to augment IL-2 mRNA production by T cells, with a possible paracrine effect on IL-2Rα expression.[261] These effects appear to be mediated by RARα. In addition, 9-*cis*-retinoic acid, through its binding and transactivation of both RAR and RXR, inhibits activation-induced apoptosis.[262,263] Activation-induced T-cell apoptosis appears to require Fas ligand up-regulation; 9-*cis*-retinoic acid prevents up-regulation of Fas ligand and thus blocks T-cell death.[262,263]

ACKNOWLEDGMENTS

The authors were supported by a grant from the National Cancer Institute (PO1 CA51993) and a merit review grant from the Medical Research Services of the Department of Veteran Affairs. They would like to thank Donna Bennett for her excellent secretarial assistance.

REFERENCES

1. Sartorelli AC. Malignant cell differentiation as a potential therapeutic approach. *Br J Cancer* 1985;52:293.

2. Chun HG, Leyland Jones B, Hoth D, et al. Hexamethylene bisacetamide: a polar-planar compound entering clinical trials as a differentiating agent. *Cancer Treat Rep* 1986;70:991.

3. Spremuli EN, Dexter DL. Polar solvents, a novel class of antineoplastic agents. *J Clin Oncol* 1984;2:227.

4. Friend C, Sher W, Holland JG, et al. Hemoglobin synthesis in murine Erythro leukemia cells *in vitro*: stimulation of erythroid differentiation by dimethyl sulfoxide. *Proc Natl Acad Sci U S A* 1971;68:378.

5. Breslow R, Jursic B, Yan ZF, et al. Potent cytodifferentiating agents related to hexamethylene bis acetamide. *Proc Natl Acad Sci U S A* 1991;88:5542.

6. Marus PA, Richon VM, Kiyokawa H, et al. Inducing differentiation of transformed cells with hybrid polar compounds: a cell-cycle–dependent process. *Proc Natl Acad Sci U S A* 1994;91:10251.

7. Dempsey P, Winawer S, Friedman E. Twenty day treatment of HT-29 colon carcinoma cells with HMBA induces cells permanently differentiated at different stages in colonocyte differentiation, some with response to TGFβ 1. *Proc Am Assoc Cancer Res* 1989;30:47(abst).

8. Conley BA, Forrest A, Egorin MJ, et al. Phase I trial using adaptive control dosing of hexamethylene bisacetamide (NSC 95580). *Cancer Res* 1989;49:3436.

9. Conley BA, Egorin MJ, Sinibaldi V, et al. Approaches to optimal dosing of hexamethylene bisacetamide. *Cancer Chemother Pharmacol* 1992;31:37.

10. Andreeff M, Stone R, Michaeli J, et al. Hexamethylene bisacetamide in myelodysplastic syndrome and acute myelogenous leukemia: a phase II clinical trial with a differentiation inducing agent. *Blood* 1992;80:2604.

11. Rowinsky EK, Conley BA, Jones RJ, et al. Hexamethylene bisacetamide in myelodysplastic syndrome: effect of five-day exposure to maximal therapeutic concentrations. *Leukemia* 1992;6:526.

12. Shayo CC, Mladovan AG, Baldi A. Differentiating agents modulate topoisomerase I activity in U937 promonocytic cells. *Eur J Pharmacol* 1997;324:129.

13. Siegel DS, Zhang X, Feinman R, et al. Hexamethylene bisacetamide induces program cell death apoptosis and down regulates BCL-2 expression in human myeloma cells. *Proc Natl Acad Sci U S A* 1998;95:162.

14. Constantinou AI, Vaughn AT, Yamasaki H, et al. Commitment to erythroid differentiation in mouse erythroleukemia cells is controlled by alterations in topoisomerase II alpha phosphorylation. *Cancer Res* 1996;56:4192.

15. Kiyokawa H, Richon VM, Rifkind RA, et al. Suppression of cyclin-dependent kinase 4 during induced differentiation of erythroleukemia cells. *Mol Cell Biol* 1994;14:7195.

16. Scotlandi K, Serra M, Manara MC, et al. Pretreatment of human osteosarcoma cells with *N*-methylformamide enhances P-glycoprotein expression and resistance to doxorubicin. *Int J Cancer* 1994;58:95.

17. Clagett-Car K, Sarosy G, Plowman J, et al. *N*-methylformamide: cytotoxic, radiosensitizer or chemosensitizer. *J Clin Oncol* 1988;6:906.

18. Iwakawa M, Tofilon PJ, Hunter N, et al. Antitumor and antimetastatic activity of the differentiating agent *N*-methylformamide in murine tumor systems. *Clin Exp Metastasis* 1981;5:289.

19. Eton O, Bajorin DF, Casper ES, et al. Phase II trial of *N*-methylformamide in patients with metastatic melanoma. *Invest New Drugs* 1991;9:97.

20. Samid D, Shack S, Sherman LT. Phenylacetate: a novel nontoxic inducer of tumor cell differentiation. *Cancer Res* 1992;52:1988.

21. Hudgins WR, Shack S, Myers CE, et al. Cytostatic activity of phenylacetate and derivatives against tumor cells: correlation with lipophilicity and inhibition of protein prenylation. *Biochem Pharmacol* 1995;50:1273.

22. Ferrandina G, Melichar B, Loercher A, et al. Growth inhibitory effects of sodium phenylacetate (NSC 3039) on ovarian cells in vitro. *Cancer Res* 1997;57:4309.

23. Adam L, Crepin M, Israel L. Tumor growth inhibition, apoptosis and Bcl-2 down-regulation of MCF-7 RAS tumors by sodium phenylacetate and tamoxifen combination. *Cancer Res* 1997;57:1023.

24. Danesi R, Nardini D, Basolo F, et al. Phenylacetate inhibits protein isoprenylation and growth of the androgen-independent LNCaP prostate cancer cells transfected with the T24 Ha-RAS oncogene. *Mol Pharmacol* 1996;49:972.

25. Carducci MA, Nelson JB, Chan-Tack KM, et al. Phenylbutyrate induces apoptosis in human prostate cancer and is more potent than phenylacetate. *Clin Cancer Res* 1996;2:379.

26. Gore SD, Samid D, Weng LJ. Impact of the putative differentiating agents sodium phenylbutyrate and sodium phenylacetate on proliferation, differentiation and apoptosis of primary neoplastic myeloid cells. *Clin Cancer Res* 1997;10:1755.

27. Gorospe M, Shack S, Guyton KZ, et al. Up-regulation and functional role of p21 WaF1/Cip1 during growth arrest of

human breast carcinoma MCF-7 cells by phenylacetate. *Cell Growth Differ* 1996;7:1609.

28. Sidell N, Chang B, Yamashiro JM, et al. Transcriptional upregulation of retinoic acid receptor beta (RAR beta) expression by phenylacetate in human neuroblastoma cells. *Exp Cell Res* 1998;239:169.

29. Pineua T, Hudgins WR, Liu L, et al. Activation of a human peroxisome proliferator-activated receptor by the antitumor agent phenylacetate and its analogs. *Biochem Pharmacol* 1996;52:659.

30. Ram Z, Samid D, Walbridge S, et al. Growth inhibition, tumor maturation and extended survival in experimental brain tumors in rats treated with phenylacetate. *Cancer Res* 1994;54:2923.

31. Adam L, Crepin M, Savin C, et al. Sodium phenylacetate induces growth inhibition and Bcl-2 down-regulation and apoptosis in MCF7 RAS cells in vitro and in nude mice. *Cancer Res* 1995;55:5156.

32. Samid D, Hudgins WR, Shack S, et al. Phenylacetate and phenylbutyrate as novel, nontoxic differentiation inducers. *Adv Exp Med Biol* 1997;400A:501.

33. Boudoulas S, Lush RM, McCall NA, et al. Plasma protein binding of phenylacetate and phenylbutyrate, two novel antineoplastic agents. *Ther Drug Monit* 1996;18:714.

34. Thibault A, Cooper MR, Figg WD, et al. A phase I and pharmacokinetic study of intravenous phenylacetate in patients with cancer. *Cancer Res* 1994;54:1690.

35. Thibault A, Samid D, Cooper MR, et al. Phase I study of phenylacetate administered twice daily to patients with cancer. *Cancer* 1995;75:2932.

36. Knoepfler PS, Eisenman RN. Sin meets NURD and other tails of repression. *Cell* 1999;99:447.

37. Bird AP, Wolfe AP. Methylation-induced repression—bolts, braces and chromatin. *Cell* 1999;99:451.

38. Warrell RP, Li-Zhen H, Richon V, et al. Therapeutic targeting of transcription in acute promyelocytic leukemia by use of an inhibitor of histone deacetylase. *J Natl Cancer Inst* 1998;90:1621.

39. Samid D. Re: Therapeutic targeting transcription in acute promyelocytic leukemia by use of an inhibitor of histone deacetylase. *J Natl Cancer Inst* 1999;91:475.

40. Melnick A, Licht JD. Deconstructing a disease: RARα, its fusion partners and their roles in the pathogenesis of acute promyelocytic leukemia. *Blood* 1999;93:3167.

41. Redner RL, Wang J, Liu JM. Chromatin remodeling and leukemia: new therapeutic paradigms. *Blood* 1999;94:417.

42. Yoshida M, Kijima M, Akita M, et al. Potent and specific inhibition of mammalian histone deacetylase both *in vivo* and *in vitro* by Trichostatin A. *J Biol Chem* 1990;265:17174.

43. Kijima M, Yoshida M, Sugita K, et al. Trapoxin, an antitumor cyclic tetrapeptide, is an irreversible inhibitor of mammalian histone deacetylase. *J Biol Chem* 1993;268:22429.

44. Kwon HJ, Owa T, Hassig CA, et al. Depudecin induces morphological reversion of transformed fibroblasts via the inhibition of histone deacetylase. *Proc Natl Acad Sci U S A* 1998;95:3356.

45. Saito A, Yamashita T, Mariko Y, et al. A synthetic inhibitor of histone acetylase MS-27-275 with marked *in vivo* antitumor activity against human tumors. *Proc Natl Acad Sci U S A* 1999;96:4592.

46. Cameron EE, Bachman KE, Myohanen S, et al. Synergy of demethylation and histone deacetylase inhibition in the re-expression of genes silenced in cancer. *Nat Genet* 1999;21:103.

47. Izbicka E, Davidson KK, Lawrence RA, et al. 5, 6-dehydro-5'-azacytidine (DHAC) affects estrogen sensitivity in estrogen-refractory human breast carcinoma cell lines. *Anticancer Res* 1999;19(2A):1293.

48. Kelloff GJ. Perspectives on cancer chemoprevention research and drug development. *Adv Cancer Res* 2000;78:199.

49. Olson JA. Provitamin A function of carotenoids: the conversion of β-carotenes into vitamin A. *J Nutr* 1989;119:105.

50. Ganguly J. *Biochemistry of vitamin A.* Boca Raton, FL: CRC Press, 1989.

51. Kakkad BP, Ong DE. Reduction of retinaldehyde bound to cellular retinol-binding protein (type II) by microsomes from rat small intestine. *J Biol Chem* 1988;263:12916.

52. Bauik CO, Erickson U, Allen RA, et al. Identification and partial characterization of retinol pigment epithelial membrane receptor for plasma retinol-binding protein. *J Biol Chem* 1991;266:14978.

53. Noy N, Blaner WS. Interactions of retinol with binding proteins. Studies with rat cellular retinol-binding protein and with rat retinol–binding protein. *Biochemistry* 1991;30:6380.

54. De Leenheer AP, Lambert WE, Claeys I. All trans-retinoic acid: measurement of reference values in human serum by high performance liquid chromatography. *J Lipid Res* 1991;23:1362.

55. Connor MJ, Smit MH. Terminal group oxidation of retinol by mouse epidermis. *Biochem J* 1987;244:489.

56. Napoli JL, Race KR. Biogenesis of retinoic acid from β-carotene. *J Biol Chem* 1988;263:17372.

57. Rietz P, Wiss O, Weber F. Metabolism of vitamin A and the determination of vitamin A status. *Vitam Horm* 1974;32:237.

58. Hanni R, Bigler, F, Meister W, et al. Isolation and identification of three urinary metabolites of retinoic acid in the rat. *Helv Chim Acta* 1976;59:2221.

59. Curley RW, Robarge MJ. Retinoid structure, chemistry and biologically active derivatives. In: Bittar EE, Sherbet GV, eds. *Retinoids: their physiological function and therapeutic potential.* Vol 3, *Advances in organ biology.* Greenwich, CT: JAI Press, 1997:1–34.

60. Levin AA, Sturzenbecker LJ, Kazmer S, et al. 9-*cis*-retinoic acid stereoisomer binds and activates the nuclear receptor RXRα. *Nature* 1992;355:359.

61. Heyman RA, Mangelsdorf DJ, Kyck JA, et al. 9-*cis* retinoic acid is a high affinity ligand for the retinoid X receptor. *Cell* 1992;66:397.

62. Mangelsdorf DJ, Umesona K, Evans RM. The retinoid receptors. In: Sporn MB, Roberts AB, Goodman DS, eds. *The retinoids: biology, chemistry and medicine,* 2nd ed. New York: John Wiley and Sons, 1994:319–349.

63. Giguere V. Retinoic receptors and cellular retinoid binding proteins: complex interplay in retinoid signaling. *Endocr Rev* 1994;15:61.

64. Zile MH, Emerick RJ, De Luca HF. Identification of 13-*cis* retinoic acid in tissue extracts and its biological activity in rats. *Biochem Biophys Acta* 1967;141:639.

65. Newton DL, Henderson WR, Sporn MB. Structure activity relationships of retinoids in hamster tracheal organ culture. *Cancer Res* 1980;40:3413.

66. Roberts AB, Frolik CA. Recent advances in the *in vivo* and *in vitro* metabolism of retinoic acid. *Fed Proc Am Soc Exp Biol* 1979;38:2524.

67. Leo MA, Lida S, Lieber CS. Retinoic acid metabolism by a system reconstituted with cytochrome P-450. *Arch Biochem Biophys* 1984;234:305.

68. Wouters W, Van Dun J, Dillen A, et al. Effects of liarozole, a new antitumoral compound on retinoic acid-induced inhibition of cell growth and on retinoic acid metabolism in MCF-7 human breast cancer cells. *Cancer Res* 1992;52:2841.

69. Lippel K, Olson JA. Biosynthesis of β-glucuronides and of retinoic acid *in vivo* and *in vitro*. *J Lipid Res* 1968;9:168.

70. Zile MH, Cullum ME, Simpson RV, et al. Induction of differentiation of human promyelocytic leukemia cell line HL-60 by retinyl glucuronide, a biologically active metabolite of vitamin A. *Proc Natl Acad Sci U S A* 1987;84:2208.

71. Takatsuka J, Takahaski N, De Luca LM. Retinoic acid metabolism and inhibition of cell proliferation: an unexpected liaison. *Cancer Res* 1996;56:675.

72. Fiorella PD, Napoli JL. Expression of cellular retinoic acid binding protein (CRABP) in *Escherichia coli*. *J Biol Chem* 1991;266:16572.

73. Blaner WS, Olson JA. Retinol and retinoic acid metabolism. In: Sporn MB, Roberts AB, Goodman DS, eds. *The retinoids: biology, chemistry and medicine*, 2nd ed. New York: John Wiley and Sons, 1994:229–255.

74. Boylan JF, Gudas LJ. Overexpression of the cellular retinoic acid binding protein-I (CRABP-I) results in a reduction in differentiation-specific gene expression in F9 teratocarcinoma cells. *J Cell Biol* 1991;112:965.

75. Boylan JF, Gudas LJ. The level of CRABP-I expression influences the amounts and types of all-trans-retinoic acid metabolites in F9 teratocarcinoma stem cells. *J Biol Chem* 1993;267:21486.

76. Eckoff C, Collins MD, Nau H. Human plasma all trans 13-cis and 13-cis-4-oxoretinoic acid profiles during subchronic vitamin A supplementation. Comparison to retinol and retinyl ester plasma levels. *J Nutr* 1991;121:1016.

77. Loeliger P, Bollag W, Mayer H. Arotinoids, a new class of highly active retinoids. *Eur J Med Chem* 1980;15:168.

78. Dawson MI, Hobbs PD, Chan RL, et al. Aromatic retinoic acid analogues. Synthesis and pharmacological activity. *J Med Chem* 1981;24:583.

79. Dawson MI, Jong L, Hobbs PD, et al. Conformational effects on retinoid receptor selectivity. Effects of retinoid bridging group on retinoid X receptor activity and selectivity. *J Med Chem* 1995;23:1013.

80. Lehmann JM, Dawson MI, Hobbs PD, et al. Identification of retinoids with nuclear receptor subtype-selective activities. *Cancer Res* 1991;61:4804.

81. Charpentier B, Bernardon JM, Eustache J, et al. Synthesis, structure-affinity relationships and biological activities of ligands binding to retinoic acid receptor subtypes. *J Med Chem* 1995;38:4993.

82. Dawson MI, Chao WR, Pine P, et al. Correlation of retinoid binding affinity to RARα with retinoid inhibition of growth of estrogen receptor-positive MCF mammary carcinoma cells. *Cancer Res* 1995;55:4446.

83. Sun SY, Yue P, Dawson MI, et al. Differential effects of synthetic nuclear retinoid receptor-selective retinoids on the growth of human non–small cell lung carcinoma. *Cancer Res* 1997;57:4931.

84. Wu S, Zhang D, Donigan A, et al. Effects of conformationally restricted synthetic retinoids on ovarian tumor cell growth. *J Cell Biochem* 1998;68:378.

85. Shalinsky DR, Bischoff ED, Lamph WW, et al. A novel retinoic acid receptor-selective retinoid ALRT1550 has potent antitumor activity against human oral squamous carcinoma xenografts in nude mice. *Cancer Res* 1997;57:162.

86. Gottardis MM, Bischoff ED, Shirley MA, et al. Chemoprevention of mammary carcinoma by LGD 1069 (Targretin): an RXR-selective ligand. *Cancer Res* 1996;56:5566.

87. Gudas LJ, Sporn MB, Roberts AB. Cellular biology and biochemistry of the retinoids. In: Sporn MB, Roberts AB, Goodman DS, eds. *The retinoids: biology, chemistry and medicine*. New York: Raven Press, 1994:444.

88. Bittar EE, Sherbet GV, eds. *Retinoids: their physiological function and therapeutic potential*. Vol 3, *Advances in organ biology*. Greenwich, CT: JAI Press, 1997.

89. Strickland S, Smith KK, Marotti KR. Hormonal induction of differentiation in teratocarcinoma stem cells. Generation of parietal endoderm by retinoic acid. *Cell* 1980;21:347.

90. Breitman TR, Selonick S, Collins SJ. Induction of differentiation of the human promyelocytic leukemia cell line HL-60 by retinoic acid. *Proc Natl Acad Sci U S A* 1980;77:2936.

91. Haussler M, Sidell N, Kelley M, et al. Specific high affinity binding and biologic action of retinoic acid in human neuroblastoma cell lines. *Proc Natl Acad Sci U S A* 1983;80:5525.

92. Wang SY, LaRosa GJ, Gudas LJ. Molecular cloning of gene sequences transcriptionally regulated by retinoic acid and dibutyryl cyclic AMP in cultured mouse teratocarcinoma cells. *Dev Biol* 1985;197:75.

93. Horton WE, Yamanda Y, Hassel JR. Retinoic acid rapidly reduces cartilage matrix synthesis by altering gene transcription in chondrocytes. *Dev Biol* 1987;123:508.

94. Chiocca EA, Davis PJA, Stein JP. The molecular gain of retinoic acid action. Transcriptional regulation of tissue transglutaminase gene expression in macrophages. *J Biol Chem* 1988;203:11584.

95. La Rosa GJ, Gudas LJ. Early retinoic acid induced F9 teratocarcinoma stem cell gene ERA-1. Alternate splicing creates transcripts for a homeobox-containing protein and one lacking the homeobox. *Mol Cell Biol* 1988;8:3906.

96. Elias MCQB, Chammas R, Giogi RR, et al. Adhesion to laminin is down regulated upon retinoic acid-induced F9 cell differentiation. A role for alpha GI beta 1 integrin Brazilian. *J Med Biol Res* 1994;27:21181.

97. Ross SA, Ahren RA, De Luca LM. Retinoic acid enhances adhesiveness, laminin and integrin beta synthesis and retinoic acid receptor expression in F9 teratocarcinoma cells. *J Cell Physiol* 1994;159:263.

98. Liska DJ, Hawkins R, Wikstrom K, et al. Modulation of thrombospondin expression during differentiation of embryonal carcinoma cells. *J Cell Physiol* 1994;158:495.

99. Dinoto R, Schivvone EM, Ferrara F, et al. All trans retinoic acid promotes a differential regulation of adhesion molecules on acute myeloid leukemia cell blasts. *Br J Haematol* 1994;88:247.

100. Weber C, Calzadawack JC, Goretzki M, et al. Retinoic acid inhibits basal and interferon gamma induced expression of

intercellular adhesion molecule-1 in monocytic cells. *J Leukoc Biol* 1995;57:401.

101. Mehta P, Lowenstein WR. Differential regulation of communication by retinoic acid in homologous and heterologous junction between normal and transformed cells. *J Cell Biol* 1991;113:371.

102. Bex V, Mercier T, Chavmontet C, et al. Retinoic acid enhances connexin 43 expression at the post-transcriptional level in rat liver epithelial cells. *Cell Biochem Funct* 1993;13:69.

103. Hudson LG, Sunton JB, Glass CK, et al. Ligand-activated thyroid hormone and retinoic acid receptors inhibit growth factor receptor promoter expression. *Cell* 1990;62:1165.

104. Offterdinger M, Schneider SM, Huber H, et al. Retinoids control the expression of c-erb β receptors in breast cancer cells. *Biochem Biophys Res Commun* 1998;251:907.

105. Bentel JM, Lebwohl DE, Cullen KJ, et al. Insulin-like growth factors modulate the growth inhibitory effects of retinoic acid on MCF-7 breast cancer cells. *J Cell Physiol* 1995;165:212.

106. Li X-S, Chen J-C, Sheikh MS, et al. Retinoic acid inhibition of insulin-like growth factor I stimulation of c-Fos mRNA levels in a breast carcinoma cell line. *Exp Cell Res* 1994;211:68.

107. Han GR, Dohi DF, Lee HY, et al. All trans-retinoic acid increases transforming growth factor beta 2 and insulin-like growth factor binding protein-3 expression through a retinoic acid receptor-alpha dependent signaling pathway. *J Biol Chem* 1997;272:13711.

108. Jaffey P, Chan LN, Shao J, et al. Retinoic acid inhibition of serum induced c-Fos transcription in a fibrosarcoma cell line. *Cancer Res* 1992;52:2384.

109. Busan KJ, Roberts AB, Sporn MB. Inhibition of mitogen induced c-Fos expression in melanoma cells by retinoic acid involves the serum response element. *J Biol Chem* 1992; 267:19971.

110. Lee HA, Walson GL, Dawson MI, et al. All trans retinoic acid inhibits Jun N-terminal kinase dependent signaling pathways. *J Biol Chem* 1998;273:7066.

111. Sherbet GV, Lakhmi MS. Retinoid and growth factor signal transduction. In: Bittar EE, Sherbet GV, eds. *The retinoids: their physiological function and therapeutic potential.* Vol 3, *Advances in organ biology.* Greenwich, CT: JAI Press, 1997:141.

112. Hendrix MJC, Wood R, Seftor EA, et al. Retinoic acid inhibition of human melanoma cell invasion through a reconstituted basement membrane and its relation to decreases in the expression of proteolytic enzymes and motility factor receptor. *Cancer Res* 1990;50:4121.

113. Bigg HF, Cawston TE. All trans retinoic acid interacts synergistically with basic fibroblast growth factor and epidermal growth factor to stimulate the production of tissue inhibitor of metalloproteinases from fibroblasts. *Arch Biochem Biophys* 1995;319:74.

114. Gudas LJ. Retinoids, retinoid responsive genes, cell differentiation, and cancer. *Cell Growth Differ* 1992;3:655.

115. Petkovich M, Brand NJ, Krust A, et al. A human retinoic acid receptor which belongs to the family of nuclear receptors. *Nature* 1987;330:444.

116. Brand NJ, Petkovich M, Krust A, et al. Identification of a second human retinoic acid receptor. *Nature* 1988;332:850.

117. Krust A, Kastner, P, Petkovich, et al. A third human retinoic acid receptor hRARγ. *Proc Natl Acad Sci U S A* 1989;86:5310.

118. Mangelsdorf DJ, Borgmeyer U, Heyman RA. Characterization of three RXR genes that mediate the action of 9-*cis* retinoic acid. *Genes Dev* 1992;6:329.

119. Rowe A, Brickell PM. The retinoid nuclear receptors. *Int J Exp Pathol* 1993;74:117.

120. Nagpal S, Saunders M, Kastner P, et al. Promoter context- and response element-dependent specificity of the transcriptional activation and modulating function of the retinoic acid receptor. *Cell* 1992;70:1007.

121. Boylan JF, Luftkin T, Achkar CL, et al. Targeted disruption of retinoic acid receptor α (RARα) and RARγ results in receptor specific alterations in retinoic acid mediated differentiation and retinoic acid metabolism. *Mol Cell Biol* 1995; 15:843.

122. Boylan JF, Lohnes D, Taneja R, et al. Loss of retinoic acid receptor γ function in F9 cells by gene disruption in aberrant Huxo 1 expression and differentiation upon retinoic acid treatment. *Proc Natl Acad Sci U S A* 1993;90:9061.

123. Robertson KA, Emmami B, Mueller L, et al. Multiple members of the retinoic acid receptor family are capable of mediating the granulocytic differentiation of HL-60 cells. *Mol Cell Biol* 1992;12:3743.

124. Taneja R, Bouillet P, Boylan JF, et al. Re-expression of retinoic acid receptor (RAR) γ or overexpression of RARα or RARβ in RAR γ-null F9 cells reveals a partial functional redundancy between the three RAR types. *Proc Natl Acad Sci U S A* 1995;92:7854.

125. Leid M, Kastner P, Lyons R, et al. Purification cloning and RXR identity of the HeLa cell factor with which RAR or TR heterodimerizes to bind target sequences efficiently. *Cell* 1992;68:377.

126. Zhang X, Hoffman B, Tran B-V. Retinoid X receptor is an auxiliary protein for thyroid hormone and retinoic acid receptors. *Nature* 1992;335:441.

127. Kliewer SA, Umesono K, Mangelsdorf DJ, et al. Retinoid X receptor interacts with nuclear receptors in retinoic acid, thyroid hormone, and vitamin D_3 signaling. *Nature* 1992;355:446.

128. Mangelsdorf DJ, Thummel C, Beato M. The nuclear receptor superfamily: the second decade. *Cell* 1995;83:835.

129. Chambon P. A decade of molecular biology of retinoic acid receptors. *FASEB J* 1996;10:940.

130. Pfahl M. Nuclear receptor/AP-1 interaction. *Endocr Rev* 1993;14:651.

131. Kamei Y, Xu L, Heinzel T, et al. A CBP integrator complex mediates transcriptional activation and AP-1 inhibition by nuclear receptors. *Cell* 1996;85:403.

132. Mattei M-G, de The H, Mattei J-F. Assignment of the human hap retinoic acid receptor RARβ gene to the p24 band of chromosome 3. *Hum Genet* 1988;80:189.

133. Stanbridge E. Human tumor suppressor genes. *Annu Rev Genet* 1990;24:615.

134. Houle BC, Leduc F, Bradley WEC. Implication of RARβ in epidermoid (squamous) lung cancer. *Genes Chromosomes Cancer* 1991;3:358.

135. Gerbert JF, Moghal N, Frangioni JV, et al. High frequency of retinoic acid receptor β abnormalities in human lung cancer. *Oncogene* 1991;6:1859.

136. Nervi C, Voolberg TM, George MD, et al. Expression of

nuclear retinoic acid receptors in normal tracheobronchial cells and in lung carcinoma cells. *Exp Cell Res* 1991;195:163.

137. Houle BC, Pelletier M, Wu J. Fetal isoform of human retinoic acid receptor β expressed in small cell lung cancer lines. *Cancer Res* 1994;54:365.

138. Sukov HM, Murakami KK, Evans RM. Characterization of an autoregulated response element in the mouse retinoic acid receptor β gene. *Proc Natl Acad Sci U S A* 1996;87:5392.

139. Zhang X-K, Liu Y, Lee M-O, et al. A specific defect in the retinoic acid response associated with human lung cancer cell lines. *Cancer Res* 1994;54:5663.

140. Moghal N, Neel BG. Evidence for impaired retinoic acid receptor-thyroid hormone receptor AF-2 cofactor activity in human lung cancer. *Mol Cell Biol* 1995;15:3945.

141. Houle BC, Rochette-Egly C, Bradley WEC. Tumor suppressive effect of the retinoic acid receptor β in human epidermoid lung cancer cells. *Proc Natl Acad Sci U S A* 1993;90:985.

142. Frangioni JV, Moghal N, Stuart-Tilley A, et al. The DNA binding domain of the retinoic acid receptor β is required for ligand-dependent suppression of proliferation. *J Cell Sci* 1994;107:827.

143. Shao Z-M, Sheikh MS, Chen J-C, et al. Expression of the retinoic acid nuclear receptors (RARs) and retinoid X receptor (RXR) genes in estrogen receptor positive and negative breast cancer. *Int J Oncol* 1994;4:859.

144. Roman SD, Ormandy CJ, Manning DL, et al. Estradiol induction of retinoic acid receptors in human breast cancer cells. *Cancer Res* 1993;53:5940.

145. Sheikh MS, Shao Z-M, Chen J-C, et al. Estrogen receptor-negative breast cancer cells transfected with estrogen receptor exhibit increased RARα gene expression and sensitivity to growth inhibition by retinoic acid. *J Cell Biochem* 1993;53:394.

146. Sheikh MS, Shao Z-M, Li X-S, et al. Retinoid-resistant estrogen receptor negative human breast carcinoma cells transfected with retinoic acid receptor α acquire sensitivity to growth inhibition by retinoic acid. *J Biol Chem* 1994;269:21440.

147. Rishi AK, Shao Z-M, Baumann RG, et al. Estradiol regulation of the human retinoic acid receptor α gene in human breast carcinoma cells is mediated via an imperfect half-palindromic estrogen response element and Sp 1 motifs. *Cancer Res* 1995;55:4999.

148. Fitzgerald P, Teng M, Chandraratna RAS, et al. Retinoic acid receptor α expression correlates with retinoid-induced growth inhibition of human breast cancer cells regardless of estrogen receptor status. *Cancer Res* 1997;57:2642.

149. Rishi AK, Gerald TM, Shao Z-M, et al. Regulation of the human retinoic acid receptor α gene in the estrogen receptor negative breast carcinoma cell lines SKBR-3 and MDA-MB-435. *Cancer Res* 1996;56:5246.

150. Menger H, Ye YC, Chen SR, et al. Use of all-trans retinoic acid in the treatment of acute leukemia. *Blood* 1988;72:567.

151. De The H, Lavau C, Marchio A, et al. The PML-RARα fusion mRNA generated by the τ(15;17) trans location in acute promyelocytic leukemia encodes a functionally altered RAR. *Cell* 1991;66:673.

152. Kakizuka A, Miller WH Jr, Umesono K, et al. Chromosomal translocation τ(15;17) in human acute promyelocytic leukemia fuses RARα with a novel putative transcription factor, PML. *Cell* 1991;66:663.

153. Collins SJ, Robertson KA, Mueller L. Retinoic acid induced granulocytic differentiation of HL-60 myeloid leukemia cells is mediated directly through the retinoic acid receptor (RARα). *Mol Cell Biol* 1990;10:2154.

154. Onodera M, Kunisada T, Nishikawa S, et al. Overexpression of retinoic acid receptor α suppresses myeloid cell differentiation at the promyelocyte stage. *Oncogene* 1995;11:1291.

155. Tsai S, Collins SJ. A dominant negative retinoic acid receptor blocks neutrophil differentiation at the promyelocyte stage. *Proc Natl Acad Sci U S A* 1993;90:7153.

156. Rousselot P, Hardas B, Patel A, et al. The PML-RARα gene product of the τ(15;17) translocation inhibits retinoic acid-induced granulocytic differentiation and mediated transactivation in human myeloid cells. *Oncogene* 1994;9:545.

157. Early E, Moore MAS, Kakizuka A, et al. Transgenic expression of PML/RARα impairs myelopoiesis. *Proc Natl Acad Sci U S A* 1996;93:7900.

158. Kastner P, Perez A, Lutz Y, et al. Structure, localization and transcriptional properties of two classes of retinoic acid receptor α fusion proteins in acute promyelocytic leukemia (APL): structural similarities with a new family of oncoproteins. *EMBO J* 1992;11:629.

159. Doucas V, Brocues JP, Yaniv M, et al. The PML-retinoic acid receptor α translocation converts the receptor from an inhibitor to a retinoic acid-dependent activator of transcription factor AP-1. *Proc Natl Acad Sci U S A* 1993;90:9345.

160. Dyck JA, Maul GG, Miller WH Jr, et al. A novel macromolecular structure is a target of the promyelocyte-retinoic acid receptor oncoprotein. *Cell* 1994;76:345.

161. Weiss K, Rambaud S, Lavau K, et al. Retinoic acid regulates aberrant nuclear localization of PML-RARα in acute promyelocytic leukemia cells. *Cell* 1994;76:345.

162. Gianni M, Tera M, Fortino I, et al. STAT 1 is induced and activated by all-trans retinoic acid and in acute promyelocytic leukemia cells. *Blood* 1997;89:1001.

163. Castaigne S, Chomienne C, Daniel MT, et al. All trans retinoic acid as a differentiation therapy for acute promyelocytic leukemia patients. *Blood* 1990;76:1704.

163a. Warrell RP, Frankel SR, Miller WH Jr, et al. Differentiation therapy of acute promyelocytic leukemia with tretinoin (all trans-retinoic acid). *N Engl J Med* 1991;324:1385.

164. Chen Z-X, Xue Y-Q, Zhang R, et al. A clinical and experimental study on all trans retinoic acid-treated acute promyelocytic leukemia patients. *Blood* 1991;78:1413.

165. Frankel SR, Eardley A, Heller G, et al. All-trans retinoic acid for acute promyelocytic leukemia—results of the New York study. *Ann Intern Med* 1994;120:278.

166. Miller W Jr, Jakubowski A, Tong W, et al. 9 *cis* retinoic acid induces complete remission but does not reverse clinically acquired retinoid resistance in acute promyelocytic leukemia. *Blood* 1995;85:3021.

167. Muindi J, Frankel S, Huselton C, et al. Clinical pharmacology of oral all trans retinoic acid with acute promyelocytic leukemia. *Cancer Res* 1992;52:2138.

168. Muindi J, Young C. Lipid hydroperoxides greatly increase the rate of oxidative catabolism of all-trans-retinoic acid by human microsomes genetically enriched in specified cytochrome p450 isoforms. *Cancer Res* 1993;53:1226.

169. Delva L, Cornic M, Balitrand N, et al. Resistance to all-*trans* retinoic acid (ATRA) therapy in relapsing acute pro-

myelocytic leukemia: a study of in vitro sensitivity and cellular retinoic acid binding protein levels in leukemic cells. *Blood* 1993;82:2175.

170. Ding W, Li YP, Nobile LM, et al. Leukemic cellular retinoic acid resistance and missense mutations in the PML-RARα fusion gene after relapse of acute promyelocytic leukemia from treatment with all-trans retinoic acid and intensive chemotherapy. *Blood* 1998;92:1172.

171. Cornic M, Delva L, Guidez F, et al. Induction of retinoic acid-binding protein in normal and malignant human myeloid cells by retinoic acid in acute promyelocytic leukemia patients. *Cancer Res* 1992;52:3329.

172. Degos L, Dombret H, Chomienne C, et al. All-trans-retinoic acid as a differentiating agent in the treatment of acute promyelocytic leukemia. *Blood* 1995;85:2643.

173. Zhou D-C, Hallam SJ, Lee SJ, et al. Constitutive expression of cellular retinoic binding protein II and lack of correlation with sensitivity to all-trans retinoic acid in acute promyelocytic leukemia cells. *Cancer Res* 1998;58:5770.

174. Kalemkerian GP, Jiroutek M, Ettinger DS, et al. A phase II study of all-trans-retinoic acid plus cisplatin and etoposide in patients with extensive stage small lung carcinoma: an Eastern Cooperative Oncology Group Study. *Cancer* 1998;83:1102.

175. Thiruvengadam R, Atiba JO, Azawi SH. A phase II trial of a differentiating agent (tRA) with cisplatin-VP-16 chemotherapy in advanced non–small cell lung cancer. *Invest New Drugs* 1996;14:395.

176. Budd GT, Adamson PC, Gupta M, et al. Phase I/II trial of all-trans retinoic acid and tamoxifen in patients with advanced breast cancer. *Clin Cancer Res* 1998;4:635.

177. Lee JS, Newman RA, Lippman SM, et al. Phase 1 evaluation of all-trans-retinoic acid in adult with solid tumors. *J Clin Oncol* 1993;11:959.

178. Conley BA, Egorin MJ, Shridhara R, et al. Phase I clinical trial of all-trans-retinoic acid with correlation of its pharmacokinetics and pharmacodynamic. *Cancer Chemother Pharmacol* 1993;39:291.

179. Rigas JR, Francis PA, Muindi JRF, et al. Constitutive variability in the pharmacokinetics of the natural retinoid all trans retinoic acid and its modulation by ketoconazole. *J Natl Cancer Inst* 1993;85:1921.

180. Marth C, Widschwendter M, Daxenbichler G. Mechanism of synergistic action of all-trans or 9-*cis*-retinoic acid and interferon in breast cancer cells. *J Steroid Biochem Mol Biol* 1993;47:123.

181. Marth CH, Zech J, Bock G, et al. Effects of retinoids and interferon gamma on cultured breast cancer cells in comparison with tumor necrosis factor alpha. *Int J Cancer* 1987;40:840.

182. Agarwal C, Hembree JR, Rorue EA, et al. Interferon and retinoic acid suppress the growth of human papillomavirus type 16 immortalized cervical epithelial cells but only interferon suppresses the level of the human papillomavirus transforming oncogenes. *Cancer Res* 1994;54:2018.

183. Majewski S, Szmurlo A, Marczak M, et al. Synergistic effect of retinoids and interferon-α on tumor-induced angiogenesis: anti-angiogenic effect on HPV-harboring tumor cell lines. *Int J Cancer* 1994;37:81.

184. Lippman SM, Glisson BM, Kavanaugh JJ, et al. Retinoic acid and interferon combination studies in human cancer. *Eur J Cancer* 1993;29A[Suppl 5]:S9.

185. Marth CH, Daxenbichler G, Dapunt O. Synergistic antiproliferative effect of human recombinant interferons and retinoic acid in cultured breast cancer cells. *J Natl Cancer Inst* 1986;77:1197.

186. Moore DM, Kalvakolanu DV, Lippman SM, et al. Retinoic acid and interferon in human cancer. Mechanistic and clinical studies. *Semin Hematol* 1994;31:31.

187. Hovanessian AG. The double-stranded RNA-activated protein kinase induced by interferon: ds RNA-PK. *J Interferon Res* 1989;9:641.

188. Hovanessian A. Interferon-induced and double stranded RNA-activating enzymes. A specific protein kinase and 2'-5' oligoadenylate synthetase. *J Interferon Res* 1991;11:199.

189. Meurs EF, Watanabe Y, Kadereit S, et al. Constitutive expression of double-stranded RNA-activated p68 kinase in murine cells mediates phosphorylation of eukaryotic initiation factor 2 and partial resistance to encephalomyocarditis virus growth. *J Virol* 1992;66:5804.

190. Bandyopadhuay SK, Kumor R, Rubin BY, et al. Interferon-inducible gene expression in HL-60 cells. Effects of the state of differentiation. *Cell Growth Differ* 1992;3:369.

191. Schwartz E, Nilson L. Activation of 2'-5' oligoadenylate synthetase activity on induction of HL-60 leukemia cell differentiation. *Mol Cell Biol* 1989;9:3897.

192. Kalvakolanu DVR, Sen GC. Differentiation-dependent activation of interferon-stimulated gene factors and transcription factor: NF-kappa B. *Proc Natl Acad Sci U S A* 1993;90:3167.

193. Pelicano L, Li F, Schindler C, et al. Retinoic acid enhances the expression of interferon-induced proteins: evidence for multiple mechanisms of action. *Oncogene* 1997;15:2349.

194. Schindler C, Darnell JE Jr. Transcriptional responses to polypeptide ligands: the JAK-STAT pathway. *Annu Rev Biochem* 1995;64:621.

195. Muller M, Briscoe J, Laxton C, et al. The protein tyrosine kinase JAK 1 complements defects in interferon-alpha/beta and -gamma signal transduction. *Nature* 1993;366:129.

196. Muller M, Laxton C, Briscoe J. Complementation of a mutant cell line: central role of the 91 kDa polypeptide ISGF3 in the interferon-alpha and -gamma signal transduction pathway. *EMBO J* 1993;12:4221.

197. Weihua X, Kolla V, Kalvakolanu DV. Modulation of interferon action by retinoids: induction of murine STAT 1 gene expression by retinoic acid. *J Biol Chem* 1997;272:9742.

198. Matikainen S, Lehtonen A, Sareneva T, et al. Regulation of IRF and STAT gene expression by retinoic acid. *Leuk Lymphoma* 1998;30:67.

199. Matikainen S, Ronni T, Lehtonen A, et al. Retinoic acid induces signal transducer and activator of transcription (STAT) 1, STAT 2 and p48 expression in myeloid leukemia cells and enhances their responsiveness to interferons. *Cell Growth Differ* 1997;8:687.

200. Hofman ER, Boyanapalli M, Lindner J, et al. Thioredoxin reductase mediates cell death effects of the combination of beta interferon and retinoic acid. *Mol Cell Biol* 1998;18:6493.

201. Lippman SM, Parkinson D, Itri LM, et al. 13-*cis*-retinoic acid plus interferon α-2a: effective combination therapy for advanced squamous cell carcinoma of the skin. *J Natl Cancer Inst* 1992;84:235.

202. Lippman SM, Kavanagh JJ, Paredes-Espinoza M, et al. 13-*cis*-retinoic acid plus interferon α-2a. Highly active systemic

therapy for squamous cell carcinoma of the cervix. *J Natl Cancer Inst* 1992;84:241.

203. Stadler WM, Kuzel T, Dumas M, et al. Multicenter phase II trial of interleukin-2 interferon-alpha and 13-*cis*-retinoic acid in patients with metastatic renal-cell carcinoma. *J Clin Oncol* 1998;16:1820.

204. Casali A, Sega FM, Casali M, et al. 13-*cis*-retinoic acid and interferon alpha-2a in the treatment of metastatic renal cell carcinoma. *J Exp Clin Cancer Res* 1998;17:227.

205. Rosenthal MA, Ortaz R. Phase II clinical trial of recombinant alpha 2b interferon and 13 *cis* retinoic acid in patients with metastatic melanoma. *Am J Clin Oncol* 1998;21:252.

206. Handa H, Hegde UP, Kotelnikov VM, et al. The effects of 13-*cis* retinoic acid and interferon-alpha in chronic myelogenous leukemia cells in vivo in patients. *Leuk Res* 1997;21:1087.

207. Ohsima M, Ward JM, Wenk ML. Preventive and enhancing effects of retinoid on the development of naturally occurring tumors of skin, prostate gland and endocrine pancreas in aged male ACI/seg Hap BR rats. *J Natl Cancer Inst* 1985;74:517.

208. Pollard M, Lukert PH, Sporn MB. Prevention of primary prostate cancer by 4-(hydroxyphenyl) retinamide. *Cancer Res* 1991;51:3610.

209. Veronesi V, DePalo G, Costa A, et al. Chemoprevention of breast cancer with retinoids. *J Natl Cancer Inst Monogr* 1992;12:93.

210. Chiesa F, Tradati N, Marazza M, et al. Prevention of relapses and new localization of oral leukoplakias with the synthetic retinoid Fenretimide (4-HPR). Preliminary results oral. *Eur J Cancer B Oral Oncol* 1992;28B:97.

211. Moon RC, Mehta RG, Roo KVN. Retinoids and cancer in experimental animals. In: Sporn MB, Roberts AB, Goodman DS, eds. *The retinoids: biology, chemistry and medicine*, 2nd ed. New York: Raven Press, 1994:573.

212. Oridate N, Loton D, Mitchel MF, et al. Inhibition of proliferation and induction of apoptosis in cervical carcinoma cells by retinoids: implications for chemoprevention. *J Cell Biochem Suppl* 1995;23:80.

213. Oridate N, Lotan D, Xu XC, et al. Differential induction of apoptosis by all-trans-RA and *N*-(4-hydroxyphenyl) retinamide in human head and neck squamous cell carcinoma cell lines. *Clin Cancer Res* 1996;2:855.

214. Welsch CW, DeHoog JV, Moon RC. Inhibition of mammary tumorigenesis in nulliparous C3H mice by chronic feeding of the synthetic retinoid *N*-(4-hydroxyphenyl) retinamide. *Carcinogenesis* 1983;4:1185.

215. Moon RC, Mehta RG. Chemoprevention of experimental carcinogenesis in animals. *Prev Med* 1989;18:576.

216. Pienta KJ, Nguyen NM, Lehr JE. Treatment of prostate cancer in the rat with the synthetic retinoid fenretinide. *Cancer Res* 1993;53:224.

217. Formelli F, Cleris L. Synthetic retinoid phenetidin is effective against human ovarian carcinoma xenograft and potentiates *cis*-platinic activity. *Cancer Res* 1993;53:5374.

218. Delia D, Aiello A, Lombordi L, et al. *N*-(4-hydroxyphenyl) retinamide induces apoptosis of malignant hemopoietic cell lines including those unresponsive to RA. *Cancer Res* 1993;53:6036.

219. Bhatnagar R, Abou-Issa H, Curley RW, et al. Growth suppression of human carcinoma cells in culture by *N*-(4-hydroxy-phenyl) retinamide and its glucuronide and through synergism with glucuronate. *Biochem Pharmacol* 1991;41:1471.

220. Kalemkerian GP, Slusher R, Sakkaraiappan R, et al. Growth inhibition and induction of apoptosis by Fenretinide in small-cell lung cancer cell lines. *J Natl Cancer Inst* 1995;87:1674.

221. De Palo G, Veronesi U, Camerini T, et al. Can Fenretinide protect women against ovarian cancer? *J Natl Cancer Inst* 1995;87:146.

221a. Hultin TA, Filla MS, McCormick DL. Distribution and metabolism of the retinoid, N-(4-methoxyphenyl)-all-trans-retinamide, the major metabolite of N-(4-hydroxyphenyl)-all-trans-retinamide, in female mice. *Drug Metab Dispos* 1990;18:175.

222. Swisshelm K, Rayn K, Lee X, et al. Down-regulation of retinoic acid receptor β in mammary carcinoma cell lines and its up-regulation in senescing normal mammary epithelial cells. *Cell Growth Differ* 1994;5:133.

223. Fanjul AN, Delia D, Pierotti MA, et al. 4-Hydroxyphenyl retinamide is a highly selective activator of retinoid receptors. *J Biol Chem* 1996;271:22441.

224. Sheikh MS, Shao Z-M, Li X-S, et al. *N*-(4-hydroxyphenyl) retinamide (4-HPR)-mediated biological actions involve retinoid receptor-independent pathways in human breast cancer. *Carcinogenesis* 1995;16:2477.

225. Van der Burg B, van der Leede BM, Kwakkenbos-Isbrucker L, et al. Retinoic acid resistance of estradiol-independent breast cancer cell coincides with diminished retinoic acid receptor function. *Mol Cell Endocrinol* 1993;91:149.

226. Allenby G, Bocquel MT, Saunders M, et al. Retinoic acid receptors and retinoid X receptors: interactions with endogenous retinoic acids. *Proc Natl Acad Sci U S A* 1993;90:30.

227. Oridate N, Suzuki S, Higuchi M, et al. Involvement of reactive oxygen species in *N*-(4-hydroxyphenyl) retinamide induced apoptosis in cervical carcinoma cells. *J Natl Cancer Inst* 1997;89:1191.

228. Shao ZM, Dawson MI, LiX-S, et al. p53 independent G_0/G_1 arrest and apoptosis induced by a novel retinoid in human breast cancer cells. *Oncogene* 1993;11:493.

229. Li X-S, Rishi AK, Shao ZM, et al. Posttranscriptional regulation of p21$^{WAF1/CIP1}$ expression in human breast carcinoma cells. *Cancer Res* 1996;56:5055.

230. Hsu CA, Rishi AK, Li X-S, et al. Retinoid induced apoptosis in leukemia cells through a retinoic acid nuclear receptor-independent pathway. *Blood* 1997;89:4470.

231. Robertson KA, Emami B, Collins SJ. Retinoic acid resistant HL-60R cells harbor a point mutation in the retinoic acid receptor ligand binding domain that confers dominant negative activity. *Blood* 1992;80:1881.

232. Nagy L, Thomazy VA, Shipley GL, et al. Activation of retinoid X receptors induces apoptosis in HL-60 cell lines. *Mol Cell Biol* 1995;15:3570.

233. Cheng EH-Y, Kirsch DG, Clem RJ, et al. Conversion of Bcl-2 to a Bax-like death effector by caspases. *Science* 1997;278:1966.

234. Yang E, Korsmeyer SJ. Molecular thanatopsis: a discourse on the bcl-2 family and cell death. *Blood* 1996;88:386.

235. Igrado AM, Huang Y, Fang G, et al. Overexpression of bcl-2 or bcl-X$_L$ inhibits AraC-induced CPP32/YAMA protease activity and apoptosis of human acute myelogenous leukemia HL-60. *Cancer Res* 1996;56:4743.

236. Boise LH, Gonzales M, Garcia M, et al. Bcl-X, a bcl-2 related gene that functions as a dominant regulator of cell death. *Cell* 1993;74:597.

237. Hsu CKA, Rishi AK, Li X-S, et al. Bcl-X$_L$ expression and its down regulation by a novel retinoid in breast carcinoma cells. *Exp Cell Res* 1997;232:17.

238. Fontana JA, Sun R-J, Rishi AK, et al. Overexpression of bcl-2 or bcl-X$_L$ fails to inhibit apoptosis by a novel retinoid. *Oncol Res* 1998;10:313.

239. Li Y, Lin B, Agadir A, et al. Molecular determinants of AHPN (CD437)-induced growth arrest and apoptosis in human lung cancer cell lines. *Mol Cell Biol* 1998;18:4719.

240. Zhang Y, Hang Y, Rishi AK, et al. Activation of the p38 and JNK/SAPK mitogen activated protein kinase pathways during apoptosis is mediated by a novel retinoid. *Exp Cell Res* 1999;247:233.

241. Green HN, Mellanby E. Vitamin A as an anti-infective agent. *BMJ* 1928;2:691.

242. Scrimshaw NS, Taylor CE, Gordon JE. *Interactions of nutrition and infection.* Geneva: World Health Organization.

243. Semba RD. The role of vitamin A and related retinoids in immune function. *Nutr Rev* 1998;56:538.

244. Guzman JJ, Marus JF, Caren LD. In vivo and in vitro studies on the effects of vitamin A on the chemiluminescent response of murine peritoneal exudate cells. *Toxicol Lett* 1991;57:125.

245. Hemmi H, Breitman TR. Induction of functional differentiation of a human monocytic leukemia cell line (THP-1) by retinoic acid and choleratoxin. *Jpn J Cancer Res* 1985;76:345.

246. Katz DR, Drzymala M, Turton JA, et al. Regulation of accessory cell function in delayed-type hypersensitivity responses. *Br J Exp Pathol* 1987;60:343.

247. Oberg F, Botling J, Nillson K. Functional antagonism between vitamin D$_3$ and retinoic acid in the regulation of CD14 and CD23 expression during monocytic differentiation of U-937 cells. *J Immunol* 1993;150:3487.

248. Buck J, Ritter G, Dannecker L, et al. Retinol is essential for growth of activated human B cells. *J Exp Med* 1990;171:1613.

249. Dillehay DL, Walia AS, Lamon EW. Effects of retinoids on macrophage function and IL-1 activity. *J Leuk Biol* 1988;44:353.

250. Trechsel U, Evequoz V, Fleisch H. Stimulation of interleukin 1 and 3 production by retinoic acid in vitro. *Biochem J* 1985;230:339.

251. Matikainen S, Serkkola E, Hurme M. Retinoic acid enhances IL-1β expression in myeloid leukemia cells and in human monocytes. *J Immunol* 1991;147:162.

252. Blomhoff HK, Smeland EB, Erikstein B, et al. Vitamin A is a key regulator for cell growth, cytosine production and differentiation in normal B cells. *J Biol Chem* 1992;267:23988.

253. Chun TY, Carman JA, Hayes CE. Retinoid repletion of vitamin A-deficient mice restores IgG responses. *J Nutr* 1992;122:1062.

254. Ballow M, Wang W, Xiang S. Modulation of B-cell immunoglobulin synthesis by retinoic acid. *Clin Immunol Immunopathol* 1996;90:573.

255. Ballow M, Ziang S, Wang W, et al. The effects of retinoic acid on immunoglobulin synthesis: role of interleukin 6. *J Clin Immunol* 1996;16:171.

256. Carman JA, Hayes CE. Abnormal regulation of IFN-gamma secretion in vitamin A deficiency. *J Immunol* 1991;147:1247.

257. Cippitelli M, Ye J, Viggiano V, et al. Retinoic acid-induced transcriptional modulation of the human interferon-gamma promoter. *J Biol Chem* 1996;271:26783.

258. Garber A, Buck J, Hammerling U. Retinoids are important cofactors in T cell activation. *J Exp Med* 1992;176:109.

259. Friedman A, Halevy O, Schrift M, et al. Retinoic acid promotes proliferation and induces expression of retinoic acid receptor α gene in murine T lymphocytes. *Cell Immunol* 1993;152:240.

260. Zhao Z, Ross AC. Retinoic acid repletion restores the number of leukocytes and their subsets and stimulates natural cytotoxicity in vitamin A deficient rats. *J Nutr* 1995;125:2064.

261. Ballow M, Xiang S, Greenberg SJ, et al. Retinoic acid induced modulation of IL-2 mRNA production and IL-2 receptor expression on T cells. *Int Arch Allergy Immunol* 1997;113:167.

262. Yang Y, Minucci S, Ozato K, et al. Efficient inhibition of activation-induced Fas ligand upregulation and T cell apoptosis by retinoids requires occupancy of both retinoid X receptors and retinoic acid receptors. *J Biol Chem* 1995;270:18672.

263. Yang Y, Mercep M, Ware CF, et al. Fas and activation induced Fas ligand mediate apoptosis of T cell hybridomas: inhibition of Fas ligand expression by retinoic acid and glucocorticoids. *J Exp Med* 1995;181:1673.

24

BISPHOSPHONATES

MATTHEW R. SMITH

Bone metastases are a major cause of morbidity for patients with advanced cancers. The complications of bone metastases include hypercalcemia, pain, fracture, and spinal cord compression. Most complications of bone metastases result from tumor-mediated osteoclast activation.

Bisphosphonates are potent inhibitors of bone resorption. These agents are used to treat benign diseases associated with excessive bone resorption, including Paget's disease and osteoporosis. Bisphosphonates have become increasingly important in the management of cancer patients. Bisphosphonates are the treatment of choice for hypercalcemia of malignancy and reduce the rate of skeletal events in patients with multiple myeloma and breast cancer metastatic to bone. In addition, bisphosphonates may prevent or delay development of bone metastases in women with high-risk primary breast cancer.

PHARMACOLOGY

Bisphosphonates are synthetic analogs of pyrophosphate characterized by a phosphorus-carbon-phosphorus backbone that renders them resistant to hydrolysis (Fig. 24-1). The properties of bisphosphonates are determined by the R_1 and R_2 carbon side chains.[1] Most bisphosphonates contain a hydroxyl group at the R_1 position that confers high-affinity binding to calcium phosphate. The R_2 side chain is the critical determinant of antiresorptive potency (Table 24-1). Bisphosphonates that contain a primary amino group (pamidronate and alendronate) are approximately 100-fold more potent than first-generation bisphosphonates that do not contain an amino group (etidronate and clodronate). Bisphosphonates that contain a secondary or tertiary amino group (ibandronate, risedronate, and zoledronate) are among the most potent bisphosphonates, with approximately 10,000-fold more activity than the first-generation bisphosphonates.

Bisphosphonates are poorly absorbed after oral administration, and their bioavailability is less than 1%.[2] Bisphosphonates bind calcium, and drug absorption is altered by calcium-containing foods, beverages, and medications. Oral administration is also complicated by gastrointestinal toxicity.

Bisphosphonates are not metabolized and are eliminated by renal excretion. Bisphosphonates have potential renal toxicity related to total drug dose and rate of administration. Renal toxicity results from the R_1 carbon side chain. Because most bisphosphonates share the same R_1 carbon side chain, newer, more potent bisphosphonates have an improved therapeutic index. Third-generation bisphosphonates (zoledronate and ibandronate) can be safely administered by rapid intravenous infusion.

Bisphosphonates are adsorbed to calcium phosphate (hydroxyapatite) crystals in bone. Approximately one-half of an intravenously administered dose accumulates in the skeleton. Bisphosphonates preferentially bind to sites of active bone remodeling. Bisphosphonates become biologically inactive after they are incorporated into quiescent bone, and repetitive administration is required to maintain inhibition of bone resorption.

MECHANISM OF ACTION

Bisphosphonates inhibit bone resorption by multiple mechanisms. They directly inhibit osteoclast activity by cellular mechanisms that affect osteoclast attachment to bone, osteoclast precursor differentiation, and osteoclast survival.[1] Bisphosphonates also reduce osteoclast activity indirectly through effects on osteoblasts. Bisphosphonates increase osteoblast secretion of an inhibitor of osteoclast recruitment.[3] They also increase osteoblast secretion of transforming growth factor β (TGF-β), a signal for osteoclast apoptosis.[4]

The growth of bone metastases involves reciprocal interactions between tumor cells and metabolically active bone.[5] Remodeling bone produces growth factors that promote tumor growth, including TGF-β, insulin-like growth factor I (IGF-I), and interleukin 6. Tumor-derived growth factors, including parathyroid hormone–related protein (PTHrP),

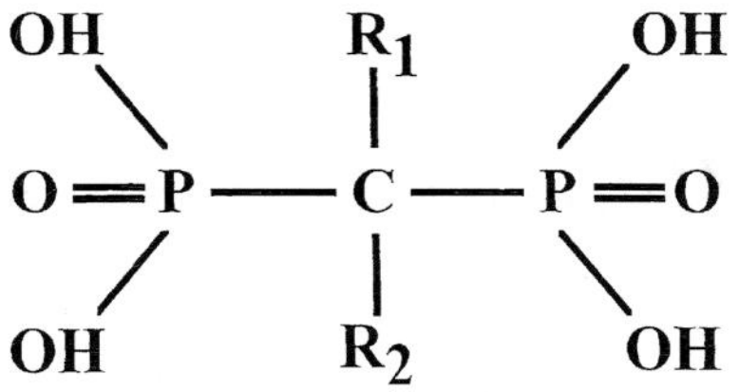

OH   R₁   OH

O = P — C — P = O

OH   R₂   OH

FIGURE 24-1. General chemical structure of bisphosphonates.

increase bone resorption. Bisphosphonates may interrupt this cycle by inhibiting local production of bone-derived growth factors. The anticancer activity of bisphosphonates may also involve modification of the bone surface, inhibition of specific enzymatic pathways, and induction of tumor cell apoptosis.[6]

HYPERCALCEMIA

Hypercalcemia of malignancy results primarily from increased release of calcium from bone. In the presence of bone metastases, calcium is released from the skeleton by local osteolytic bone destruction. In addition, hypercalcemia of malignancy may result from tumor secretion of PTHrP.[7] PTHrP causes hypercalcemia by increasing bone resorption and decreasing renal calcium excretion. Many malignancies produce PTHrP, including breast cancer, squamous cell carcinoma, renal cell carcinoma, multiple myeloma, and some types of lymphoma.

Bisphosphonates are the treatment of choice for hypercalcemia of malignancy. In a double-blind study, 40 breast cancer patients with hypercalcemia were randomized to receive hydration plus intravenous clodronate (300 mg daily for 7 days) or hydration plus placebo.[8] Seventeen of 21 evaluable patients treated with clodronate achieved normocalcemia compared with only 4 of 19 patients treated with placebo ($p = .003$). Other studies of intravenous clodronate therapy have reported similar results.[9,10]

Treatment with intravenous pamidronate disodium (90 mg) results in normocalcemia in more than 90% of patients with hypercalcemia of malignancy.[11] Treatment appears to be effective independent of the tumor type or presence of bone metastases. Among patients with humoral hypercalcemia of malignancy, treatment with lower doses of pamidronate results in inferior response rates and longer times to normocalcemia.[12–14]

Treatment with pamidronate appears to result in more complete and long-lasting responses than clodronate. In a double-blind study, 41 patients with hypercalcemia of malignancy persisting after 48 hours of saline rehydration were randomly assigned to receive intravenous pamidronate (90 mg) or intravenous clodronate (1,500 mg).[15] Nineteen of 19 patients (100%) treated with pamidronate achieved normocalcemia compared with 16 of 20 patients (80%) given clodronate. The median duration of normocalcemia was 28 days after pamidronate therapy compared with 14 days after clodronate treatment ($p < .01$).

Several studies have evaluated newer and more potent bisphosphonates for the treatment of hypercalcemia. In a randomized phase II trial encompassing 174 cancer patients who experienced hypercalcemia after rehydration, treatment with 0.6, 1.1, or 2.0 mg of ibandronate achieved normocalcemia in 44%, 52%, and 67% of patients, respectively.[16] Only the initial serum calcium level ($p < .0001$; odds ratio, 0.083) and dose of ibandronate ($p = .016$; odds ratio, 2.09) correlated with response. In another dose-response study, the response rates for patients taking 4 mg (76% response) or 6 mg (77% response) of ibandronate were significantly higher than for patients taking the 2-mg dose (50% response; $p < .05$).[17] Response duration was not affected by dose. In a multicenter phase I trial, 33 patients with hypercalcemia after rehydration were treated with intravenous zoledronate (0.002, 0.005, 0.01, 0.02, or 0.04 mg per kg).[18] Five of five patients became normocalcemic after receiving 0.02 mg per kg of zoledronate. Fourteen of 15 (93%) became normocalcemic after receiving 0.04 mg per kg of zoledronate. The median time to reach normal serum calcium was 2 days. The median duration of normocalcemia was 33 days.

Bisphosphonates should be administered to all patients with hypercalcemia of malignancy and serum calcium levels of 3.0 mmol per L (12 mg per dL) or greater.[19] Bisphosphonates should also be administered to symptomatic patients with more moderate hypercalcemia. Recommended treatment schedules include clodronate 1,500 mg intravenously over 2 hours, pamidronate 90 mg intravenously over 2 hours, and ibandronate 4 mg over 2 hours. Clodronate and ibandronate are not commercially available in the United States.

TABLE 24-1. PROPERTIES OF SELECTED BISPHOSPHONATES

Drug	Trade Name	R₁ Side Chain	R₂ Side Chain	Relative Potency
Etidronate disodium	Didronel	–OH	–CH₃	1
Clodronate	Ostac	–Cl₂	–Cl₂	10
Pamidronate disodium	Aredia	–OH	–(CH₂)₂NH₂	100
Ibandronate	—	–OH	–(CH₂)₂NCH₃(CH₂)₄CH₃	10,000
Zoledronate	—	–OH	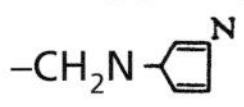 –CH₂N⟨N⟩ (imidazole ring)	10,000

MULTIPLE MYELOMA

Multiple myeloma is a malignancy characterized by osteolytic bone lesions and accumulation of mature plasma cells in the bone marrow. Osteoclasts are activated through local release of osteoclast-stimulating factors by myeloma and stromal cells. The growth of myeloma cells in the skeleton is promoted by bone production of interleukin 6 and other growth factors.

Six large randomized trials of bisphosphonate administration for multiple myeloma have been reported. These trials are summarized in Table 24-2.

In a Canadian study, 166 patients with previously untreated multiple myeloma were randomly assigned to receive either daily oral etidronate disodium (5 mg per kg) or placebo indefinitely.[20] All patients were treated with intermittent oral melphalan and prednisone. No significant differences were seen in skeletal outcomes (fracture, hypercalcemia, bone pain) between the two groups.

Three randomized studies of oral clodronate use for multiple myeloma have been reported. In a Finnish study, 336 patients with previously untreated disease were randomly assigned to receive oral daily clodronate (2,400 mg) or placebo for 2 years.[21] All patients were treated with intermittent oral melphalan and prednisolone. No significant differences were noted between the two groups in rates of fracture or hypercalcemia. Bone pain and analgesic usage were also similar in both groups. The proportion of patients with progression of osteolytic bone lesions was lower in the clodronate-treated group than in the control group (12% versus 24%; $p = .026$).

In an open-label German study, 170 previously untreated patients were randomly assigned to receive oral daily clodronate (1,600 mg) or no bisphosphonate for 1 year.[22] All patients were treated with intravenous melphalan and oral prednisone. Less than one-half of participants completed the 1-year study. No difference was observed in rate of radiographically apparent disease progression in bone. A trend was seen toward fewer new sites of bone involvement in the clodronate-treated group.

In a Medical Research Council study, 536 patients with previously untreated multiple myeloma were randomly assigned to receive either daily oral clodronate (1,600 mg) or placebo.[23] All patients were treated with primary chemotherapy. Overall survival, time to first skeletal event, hypercalcemia, and need for radiation therapy to bone were no different in the two groups. The proportion of patients with vertebral and nonvertebral fractures was significantly lower in the clodronate-treated group than in the placebo-treated group.

Two randomized studies of pamidronate for multiple myeloma have been reported. In a Danish-Swedish cooperative group study, 300 previously untreated patients were randomly assigned to receive daily *oral* pamidronate (300 mg) or placebo.[24] All patients were treated with intermittent melphalan and prednisone. Fewer episodes of severe pain were observed in the pamidronate-treated group. After a median of 18 months, the two groups showed no significant differences in skeleton-related morbidity, incidence of hypercalcemia, or survival.

In a Myeloma Aredia Study Group trial, 392 patients with Durie-Salmon stage III multiple myeloma and at least one lytic lesion were treated with antimyeloma therapy and either placebo or pamidronate (90 mg intravenously every month for 9 months).[25] The proportion of patients who had any skeletal events (pathologic fracture, irradiation of or surgery on bone, or spinal cord compression) was significantly lower in the pamidronate group than in the placebo group (24% versus 41%, $p < .001$). The patients who received pamidronate had significant decreases in bone pain and improved quality of life. Survival was similar for the two treatment groups overall. Among patients receiving second-line chemotherapy at study entry, median survival was significantly longer in the pamidronate-treated group than in the placebo-treated group (21 versus 14 months, $p = .041$).[26]

The results of these randomized trials indicate that treatment with bisphosphonates plus chemotherapy results in lower skeletal morbidity than chemotherapy alone for myeloma patients and osteolytic lesions. Based on these observations, bisphosphonates should be administered with chemotherapy to patients with multiple myeloma and osteolytic

TABLE 24-2. SELECTED RANDOMIZED TRIALS OF BISPHOSPHONATE THERAPY FOR MULTIPLE MYELOMA

Study (Reference)	Patient Population	No. of Evaluable Patients	Treatment	Result
Canadian (Belch et al.[20])	No prior treatment	166	Etidronate disodium, 5 mg/kg p.o. qd	No difference in skeletal morbidity
Finnish (Lahtinen et al.[21])	No prior treatment	336	Clodronate, 2,400 mg p.o. qd	No difference in skeletal morbidity
German (Heim et al.[22])	No prior treatment	170	Clodronate, 1,600 mg p.o. qd	Trend toward fewer new bone lesions
Medical Research Council (McCloskey et al.[23])	No prior treatment	536	Clodronate, 1,600 mg p.o. qd	Reduced proportion of patients with fracture
Danish-Swedish (Brincker et al.[24])	No prior treatment	300	Pamidronate disodium, 300 mg p.o. qd	No difference in skeletal morbidity; improved pain
Myeloma Aredia Study (Berenson et al.[25])	On stable chemotherapy	377	Pamidronate disodium, 90 mg i.v. q4wk	38% decrease in skeletal morbidity rate

TABLE 24-3. SELECTED RANDOMIZED TRIALS OF BISPHOSPHONATE THERAPY FOR BREAST CANCER

Study (Reference)	Patient Population	No. of Evaluable Patients	Treatment	Result
Canadian (Paterson et al.[27])	Bone metastases	173	Clodronate, 1,600 mg p.o. qd	28% decrease in skeletal events
Netherlands (van Holten-Verzantvoort et al.[28])	Bone metastases	161	Pamidronate disodium, 300/600 mg p.o. qd	38% reduction is skeletal morbidity rate
Aredia Multinational (Conte et al.[29])	Bone metastases; chemotherapy	224	Pamidronate disodium, 45 mg i.v. q3-4wk	48% increase in median time to skeletal progression
Aredia Protocol 18 (Theriault et al.[30])	Bone metastases; chemotherapy	380	Pamidronate disodium, 90 mg i.v. q4wk	37% reduction in skeletal morbidity rate
Aredia Protocol 19 (Hortobagyi et al.[31])	Bone metastases; hormonal therapy	371	Pamidronate disodium, 90 mg i.v. q4wk	42% reduction in skeletal morbidity rate
Heidelberg (Diel et al.[32])	High-risk primary disease	302	Clodronate, 1,600 mg p.o. qd	50% decrease in rate of distant metastases

lesions. The optimal dose, schedule, and duration of therapy are undefined. Additional studies are needed to evaluate the value of bisphosphonate monotherapy and the role of bisphosphonates for patients without osteolytic lesions.

BREAST CANCER

Several large randomized trials have evaluated the effect of bisphosphonate therapy on skeletal events in women with breast cancer metastatic to bone. The results of these studies are summarized in Table 24-3.

In a double-blind Canadian study, 173 women with breast cancer metastatic to bone were randomly assigned to receive either daily oral clodronate (1,600 mg) or placebo.[27] No significant difference in survival was found between the two groups. The combined rate of skeletal events was 28% lower in the clodronate-treated group ($p <.001$). Treatment with clodronate resulted in significant reduction in the incidence of hypercalcemia, number of vertebral fractures, and number of vertebral deformities.

In an open-label study in the Netherlands, 161 women with predominantly osteolytic metastases were randomly assigned to receive daily oral pamidronate (300 to 600 mg) or no bisphosphonate.[28] Treatment with pamidronate resulted in a statistically significant 38% reduction in skeletal morbidity. The benefit of treatment appeared to be dose-dependent, although significant gastrointestinal toxicity was observed at the higher dose.

Three randomized studies of intravenous pamidronate therapy have been reported. In an open-label Aredia Multinational Cooperative Group Study, 295 women with progressive bone metastases were randomly assigned to receive either pamidronate (45 mg intravenously every 3 or 4 weeks) or no bisphosphonate until skeletal disease progression.[29] All women were treated with standard chemotherapy. Among 224 evaluable patients, treatment with pamidronate resulted in a statistically significant 48% increase in time to skeletal disease progression. Decreases in

other skeleton-related events were not significant. The lack of significant improvements in other skeletal events may reflect the low dose of pamidronate used and discontinuation of treatment at skeletal disease progression.

In the Protocol 18 Aredia Breast Cancer Study, 372 women with metastatic breast cancer and at least one lytic bone lesion who were receiving hormonal therapy were randomly assigned to receive either placebo or pamidronate (90 mg intravenously every 4 weeks) for 24 cycles.[30] The skeletal morbidity rate (ratio of number of skeletal events to time on study) was significantly reduced at 12, 18, and 24 cycles in women treated with pamidronate ($p = .028, .023,$ and $.008$, respectively). At 24 cycles, the proportion of patients with any skeletal complication was 56% in the pamidronate group and 67% in the placebo group ($p = .027$). The time to first skeletal complication was longer in patients treated with pamidronate than in those receiving placebo ($p = .049$). No significant difference in survival was seen.

In the Protocol 19 Aredia Breast Cancer Study, 380 women with metastatic breast cancer and at least one lytic bone lesion were treated with cytotoxic chemotherapy and either placebo or pamidronate (90 mg intravenously every month for 12 months).[31] The median time to the occurrence of the first skeletal complication (pathologic fractures, need for radiation to bone or bone surgery, spinal cord compression, and hypercalcemia requiring treatment) was greater in the pamidronate group than in the placebo group (13.1 versus 7.0 months, $p = .005$). In addition, the proportion of patients in whom any skeletal complication occurred was lower in the pamidronate treatment group (43% versus 56%, $p = .008$). The pamidronate group showed significantly less increase in bone pain ($p = .046$) and deterioration of performance status ($p = .027$) than the placebo group.

The results of these randomized trials indicate that treatment with bisphosphonates reduces skeletal morbidity in breast cancer patients with osteolytic metastases. The optimal dose, schedule, and duration of therapy are undefined.

In addition to reducing skeletal morbidity in patients with osteolytic bone metastases, bisphosphonates appear to reduce the incidence and number of new bony and visceral metastases in women with high-risk primary breast cancer. In a randomized trial involving 302 patients with primary breast cancer and tumor cells in the bone marrow (a risk factor for the development of distant metastases), administration of clodronate (1,600 mg by mouth daily for 2 years) reduced the incidence of distant metastases by 50% (p <.001).[32] The incidence of both osseous and visceral metastases was significantly lower in the clodronate-treated group than in the control group (p = .003). The mean number of bony metastases per patient in the clodronate group was roughly half that in the control group (3.1 versus 6.3). Two open-label studies of women with breast cancer have reported decreased incidence of bone metastases with adjuvant clodronate.[33,34] Additional studies are required to evaluate the potential role of bisphosphonates as adjuvant therapy for breast cancer.

PROSTATE CANCER

Prostate cancer is the only malignancy to develop predominantly osteoblastic metastases, although biochemical and histomorphometric studies also demonstrate increased osteoclast activity.[35–41] Limited data are available on the use of bisphosphonates in men with prostate cancer. Several small nonrandomized clinical studies suggest a palliative benefit of bisphosphonates in men with symptomatic metastatic disease.[41–44] The effects of bisphosphonates on skeletal morbidity have not been prospectively evaluated. Two large randomized studies of pamidronate and zoledronate therapy in men with androgen-independent prostate cancer and bone metastases are ongoing.

OTHER NEOPLASMS

Limited data are available regarding the use of bisphosphonates in patients with osteolytic bone metastases from other malignancies. Several studies have evaluated the effect of bisphosphonate treatment on bone pain. In a short-term crossover study, 24 patients with symptomatic bone metastases from breast, lung, or prostate cancer were treated once with intravenous clodronate (600 mg) or placebo.[45] Treatment with clodronate was associated with improvements in pain and analgesic requirements, but these were not statistically significant.

In a British study, patients with symptomatic bone metastases from multiple myeloma, breast, lung, or prostate cancer were randomly assigned to oral daily clodronate (1,600 mg) or placebo.[46] Treatment with clodronate resulted in significant improvements in pain scores (p = .03). No difference in analgesic requirements was seen in the two groups.

In another British study, 52 pretreated patients with painful progressive bone metastases were randomly

assigned to receive either intravenous pamidronate (120 mg) or placebo.[47] After the first 4 weeks, all patients were treated with intravenous pamidronate (120 mg every 4 weeks). During the first 4 weeks, significant differences were found in symptomatic response (p <.05) and quality of life (p <.05) in favor of the pamidronate-treated group. Symptomatic response was correlated closely with the rate of bone resorption. Symptomatic responses were frequent in patients with lower baseline elevation in bone resorption markers and in those in whom bone resorption markers returned to the normal range after treatment.

CONCLUSION

Bisphosphonate therapy has become an important part of supportive care for patients with advanced malignancies. High-potency bisphosphonates administered by the intravenous route are the treatment of choice for patients with hypercalcemia of malignancy. Bisphosphonates reduce the skeletal morbidity associated with multiple myeloma and breast cancer with osteolytic bone metastases. Treatment with bisphosphonates reduces pain in patients with symptomatic bone metastases from other primary sites.

In addition to having an established role in supportive care, bisphosphonates show the potential to change the natural history of some cancers. Several studies suggest that adjuvant treatment with bisphosphonates may prevent or delay new bone metastases in women with breast cancer. Ongoing studies are evaluating newer and more potent bisphosphonates as potential anticancer agents.

REFERENCES

1. Rogers MJ, Watts DJ, Russell RG. Overview of bisphosphonates. *Cancer* 1997;80(8[Suppl]):1652–1660.
2. Compston JE. The therapeutic use of bisphosphonates. *BMJ* 1994;309(6956):711–715.
3. Vitte C, Fleisch H, Guenther HL. Bisphosphonates induce osteoblasts to secrete an inhibitor of osteoclast-mediated resorption. *Endocrinology* 1996;137(6):2324–2333.
4. Hughes DE, Wright KR, Uy HL, et al. Bisphosphonates promote apoptosis in murine osteoclasts in vitro and in vivo. *J Bone Miner Res* 1995;10(10):1478–1487.
5. Mundy GR. Mechanisms of bone metastasis. *Cancer* 1997;80(8[Suppl]):1546–1556.
6. Mundy GR, Yoneda T. Bisphosphonates as anticancer drugs. *N Engl J Med* 339:398–400.
7. Rankin W, Grill V, Martin TJ. Parathyroid hormone-related protein and hypercalcemia. *Cancer* 1997;80(8[Suppl]):1564–1571.
8. Rotstein S, Glas U, Eriksson M, et al. Intravenous clodronate for the treatment of hypercalcaemia in breast cancer patients with bone metastases—a prospective randomised

placebo-controlled multicentre study. *Eur J Cancer* 1992;28A(4–5):890–893.

9. Bonjour JP, Philippe J, Guelpa G, et al. Bone and renal components in hypercalcemia of malignancy and responses to a single infusion of clodronate. *Bone* 1988;9(3):123–130.

10. O'Rourke NP, McCloskey EV, Vasikaran S, et al. Effective treatment of malignant hypercalcaemia with a single intravenous infusion of clodronate. *Br J Cancer* 1993;67(3):560–563.

11. Body JJ, Dumon JC. Treatment of tumour-induced hypercalcaemia with the bisphosphonate pamidronate: dose-response relationship and influence of tumour type. *Ann Oncol* 1994;5(4):359–563.

12. Gurney H, Grill V, Martin TJ. Parathyroid hormone-related protein and response to pamidronate in tumour-induced hypercalcaemia. *Lancet* 1993;341(8861):1611–1613.

13. Walls J, Ratcliffe WA, Howell A, et al. Response to intravenous bisphosphonate therapy in hypercalcaemic patients with and without bone metastases: the role of parathyroid hormone-related protein. *Br J Cancer* 1994;70(1):169–172.

14. Dodwell DJ, Abbas SK, Morton AR, et al. Parathyroid hormone-related protein(50-69) and response to pamidronate therapy for tumour-induced hypercalcaemia. *Eur J Cancer* 1991;27(12):1629–1633.

15. Purohit OP, Radstone CR, Anthony C, et al. A randomised double-blind comparison of intravenous pamidronate and clodronate in the hypercalcaemia of malignancy. *Br J Cancer* 1995;72(5):1289–1293.

16. Pecherstorfer M, Herrmann Z, Body JJ, et al. Randomized phase II trial comparing different doses of the bisphosphonate ibandronate in the treatment of hypercalcemia of malignancy. *J Clin Oncol* 1996;14(1):268–276.

17. Ralston SH, Thiebaud D, Herrmann Z, et al. Dose-response study of ibandronate in the treatment of cancer-associated hypercalcaemia. *Br J Cancer* 1997;75(2):295–300.

18. Body JJ. Clinical research update: zoledronate. *Cancer* 1997;80(8[Suppl]):1699–1701.

19. Body JJ, Bartl P, Burckhardt P, et al. Current use of bisphosphonates in oncology. *J Clin Oncol* 1998;16(12):3890–3899.

20. Belch AR, Bergsagel DE, Wilson K, et al. Effect of daily etidronate on the osteolysis of multiple myeloma. *J Clin Oncol* 1991;9(8):1397–1402.

21. Lahtinen R, Laakso M, Palva I, et al. Randomised, placebo-controlled multicentre trial of clodronate in multiple myeloma. Finnish Leukaemia Group. *Lancet* 1992;340(8827):1049–1052.

22. Heim ME, Clemens MR, Queisser W, et al. Prospective randomized trial of dichloromethylene bisphosphonate (clodronate) in patients with multiple myeloma requiring treatment—a multicenter study. *Onkologie* 1995;18:439–448.

23. McCloskey EV, MacLennan IC, Drayson MT, et al. A randomized trial of the effect of clodronate on skeletal morbidity in multiple myeloma. Medial Research Council Working Party on Leukaemia in Adults. *Br J Haematol* 1998;100(2):317–325.

24. Brincker H, Westin J, Abildgaard N, et al. Failure of oral pamidronate to reduce skeletal morbidity in multiple myeloma: a double-blind placebo-controlled trial. Danish-

Swedish co-operative study group. *Br J Haematol* 1998;101(2):280–286.

25. Berenson JR, Lichtenstein A, Porter L, et al. Efficacy of pamidronate in reducing skeletal events in patients with advanced multiple myeloma. Myeloma Aredia Study Group. *N Engl J Med* 1996;334(8):488–493.

26. Berenson JR, Lichtenstein A, Porter L, et al. Long-term pamidronate treatment of advanced multiple myeloma patients reduces skeletal events. Myeloma Aredia Study Group. *J Clin Oncol* 1998;16(2):593–602.

27. Paterson AH, Powles TJ, Kanis JA, et al. Double-blind controlled trial of oral clodronate in patients with bone metastases from breast cancer. *J Clin Oncol* 1993;11(1):59–65.

28. Van Holten-Verzantvoort AT, Kroon HM, Bijvoet OL, et al. Palliative pamidronate treatment in patients with bone metastases from breast cancer. *J Clin Oncol* 1993;11(3):491–498.

29. Conte PF, Latreille J, Mauriac L, et al. Delay in progression of bone metastases in breast cancer patients treated with intravenous pamidronate: results from a multinational randomized controlled trial. The Aredia Multinational Cooperative Group. *J Clin Oncol* 1996;14(9):2552–2559.

30. Theriault RL, Lipton A, Hortobagyi GN, et al. Pamidronate reduces skeletal morbidity in women with advanced breast cancer and lytic bone lesions: a randomized, placebo-controlled trial. *J Clin Oncol* 1999;17(3):846–854.

31. Hortobagyi GN, Theriault RL, Porter L, et al. Efficacy of pamidronate in reducing skeletal complications in patients with breast cancer and lytic bone metastases. Protocol 19 Aredia Breast Cancer Study Group. *N Engl J Med* 1996;335(24):1785–1791.

32. Diel IJ, Solomayer EF, Costa SD, et al. Reduction in new metastases in breast cancer with adjuvant clodronate treatment. *N Engl J Med* 1998;339(6):357–363.

33. Kanis JA, Powles T, Paterson AHG, et al. Clodronate decreases the frequency of skeletal metastases in women with breast cancer. *Bone* 1996;16:663–667.

34. Powles TJ, Patterson AHG, Nevantaus A, et al. Adjuvant clodronate reduces the incidence of bone metastases in patients with primary operable breast cancer. *Prog Proc Am Soc Clin Oncol* 1998;17:123a(abst).

35. Percival RC, Urwin GH, Watson ME. Biochemical and histological evidence that carcinoma of the prostate is associated with increased bone resorption. *Eur J Surg Oncol* 1987;113:41–49.

36. Clarke NW, McClure J, George NJR. Morphometric evidence for bone resorption and replacement in prostate cancer. *Br J Urol* 1991;68:74–80.

37. Coleman RE, Houston S, James I, et al. Preliminary results of use of urinary excretion of pyridium cross-links for monitoring bone disease. *Br J Cancer* 1992;73:1089–1095.

38. Ikeda I, Miura T, Konde I. Pyridium cross-links as urinary markers of bone metastases in patients with prostate cancer. *Br J Urol* 1996;77:102–106.

39. Takeuchi SI, Arai K, Saitoh H, et al. Urinary pyridinoline and deoxypyridinoline as potential markers of bone metastases in patients with prostate cancer. *J Urol* 1996;156:1691–1695.

40. Vinholes J, Guo CY, Purohit OP, et al. Metabolic effects of pamidronate in patients with metastatic bone disease. *Br J Cancer* 1996;73:1089–1095.

41. Clarke NW, McClure J, George NJR. Disodium pamidronate identifies differential osteoclastic bone resorption in metastatic prostate cancer. *Br J Urol* 1992;69:64–70.

42. Adami S, Salvagno G, Guarrera G, et al. Dichloromethylene-diphosphonate in patients with prostatic carcinoma metastatic to the skeleton. *J Urol* 1985;134(6):1152–1154.

43. Masud T, Slevin ML. Pamidronate to reduce bone pain in normocalcaemic patient with disseminated prostatic carcinoma. *Lancet* 1989;1(8645):1021–1022.

44. Pelger RC, Lycklama a Nijeholt AA, Papapoulos SE. Short-term metabolic effects of pamidronate in patients with prostatic carcinoma and bone metastases. *Lancet* 1989; 2(8667):865.

45. Ernst DS, MacDonald RN, Paterson AH, et al. A double-blind, crossover trial of intravenous clodronate in metastatic bone pain. *J Pain Symptom Manage* 1992;7(1):4–11.

46. Robertson AG, Reed NS, Ralston SH. Effect of oral clodronate on metastatic bone pain: a double-blind, placebo-controlled study. *J Clin Oncol* 1995;13(9):2427–2430.

47. Vinholes JJ, Purohit OP, Abbey ME, et al. Relationships between biochemical and symptomatic response in a double-blind randomised trial of pamidronate for metastatic bone disease. *Ann Oncol* 1997;8(12):1243–1250.

25

RADIATION MODIFIERS

C. NORMAN COLEMAN
JAMES B. MITCHELL

This chapter has undergone extensive revision since the last edition of this text. The previous chapter, entitled Radiation and Chemotherapy Sensitizers and Protectors, emphasized the approaches toward hypoxic cells, the use of thiol-based radioprotectors, and S-phase–specific halopyrimidines. Although these areas are updated, they represent only part of the potential clinical combinations of radiation with a "drug." With the rapid advances in cellular and molecular biology, the range of agents that might be used in conjunction with radiation therapy has grown substantially. However, most of the agents are in developmental stages.

Anticipating a dynamic future for radiation modifiers, this chapter emphasizes the scope of emerging therapies, including focused discussions of the more classic radiation sensitizers and protectors, principles of combined modality therapy using cytotoxic agents, the microenvironment and how it can be assessed, and the innovative molecular therapeutic approaches that are likely to reach the clinic before the next edition of this book.

There are two radiation and chemotherapy modifiers either approved for clinical use (amifostine) or for which confirmatory clinical trials are necessary before U.S. Food and Drug Administration (FDA) approval (tirapazamine). Figure 25-1 and Tables 25-1 and 25-2 summarize the pharmacologic and clinical properties of these compounds.

GENERAL CONSIDERATIONS

Radiation Dose

To most oncologists, radiation dose is envisioned as a prescribed dose within an isodose curve. The dosage selected for a patient's treatment varies based on the tumor burden, tumor type, particular normal tissues at risk, and therapeutic intent (curative versus palliative). For the purpose of treatment planning, computer models are used to calculate the dose administered by the various beams. Dosage is prescribed in gray (Gy) or centigray (cGy), where the dosage is based on the measured deposition of energy in water in joules per kilogram. Isodose plots are made that, like isotherms or isobars on a weather map or contour lines on a topographic map, designate a volume that receives a certain dose in Gy. In biologic terms, however, the dose to tissue is far more complex than the dose displayed in a treatment plan. This is an important consideration that is especially relevant to the field of radiation modifiers.

The "pharmacokinetics" of radiation are different than those of drugs. Radiation will penetrate tissue and cellular boundaries unlike drugs, which require distribution from the site of administration to the blood, tissue, interstitial space, cell, and subcellular target. The concentration at the target determines the drug action. Although radiation will freely penetrate tissue, on a nanometer scale the radiation is not homogeneously delivered. Track structure studies indicate that low–linear energy transfer radiation, such as x-rays or electrons, deposits energy heterogeneously along its path with more dense clustering toward the end. Goodhead and Nikjoo estimated the number of biochemical changes for an x-ray dosage of 1 Gy, which leaves 70% of the cells surviving.[1,2] There are many millions of lesions produced within the nucleus and, although not measured, there are likely millions created within the cytoplasm, membranes, and organelles. In essence, there are many biochemical perturbations that do not lead directly to cell killing.

What might this mean for combined modality treatment and radiation modifiers? Recent work looking at the radiation survival curve that relates log survival versus dose indicates that in the low-dose region (0.5 Gy), there is an adaptive response. That is, if cells are preexposed to a low dose of radiation before the second low dose, they have an *increased* surviving fraction compared to cells that have not been preexposed.[3] The precise mechanism remains to be fully determined, but the information to date indicates that it is not due to a sensitized subpopulation of cells, but to another biochemical perturbation, possibly a difference in repair at low doses.[3] Recent studies using DNA microarrays by Amundson and Fornace demonstrate that cells irradiated

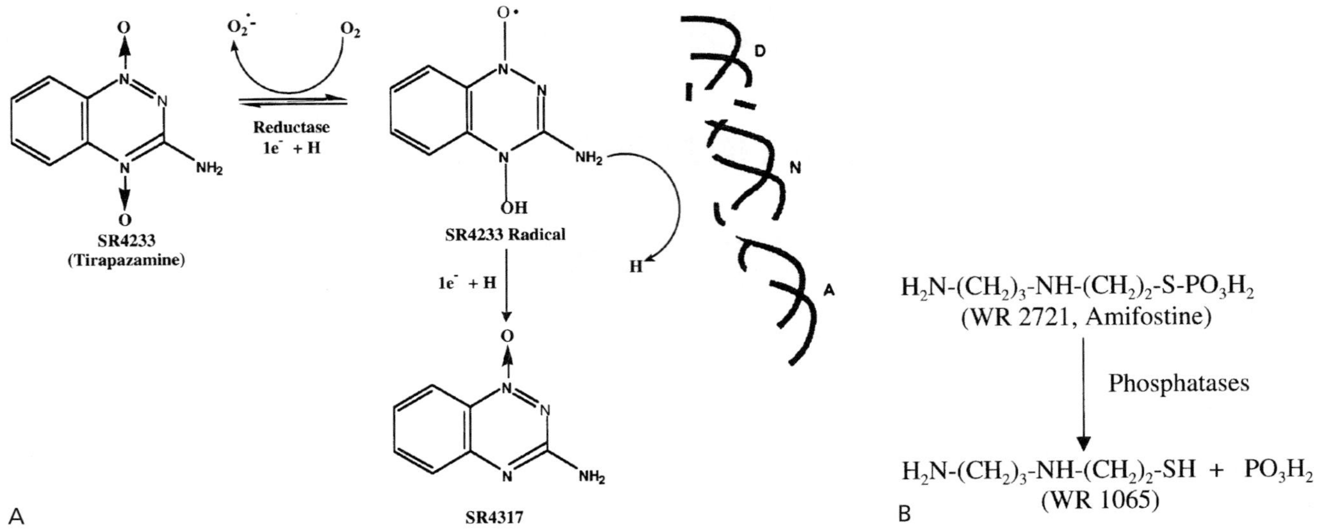

FIGURE 25-1. A: Structure and activation of tirapazamine (SR 4233). By sequential single electron reduction, reactive intermediates are formed. The active compounds are formed before the 2-electron reduction product of tirapazamine (SR 4317), which is inactive. [Reprinted with permission from Brown JM. SR 4233 (tirapazamine): a new anticancer drug exploiting hypoxia in solid tumors. *Br J Cancer* 1993;67:1163.] **B:** Structure of WR 2721 (amifostine) and activation to free sulfhydryl (WR 1065).

in vitro at low doses of 2 to 50 cGy (remember that the usual radiation fraction size is 200 cGy, so this is 1% to 25% of a single radiation treatment) can induce stress genes, such as GADD 45 and CDKN1A.[4] The stress genes were activated at radiation dosages that produced minimal cell killing, and they remained active for a number of hours.

Radiation Physics and Biophysics Are Focused Biologies

Is there a different way to consider radiation therapy? Rather than conceptualizing radiation just as a series of iso-dose curves superimposed on an anatomic structure, radiation can be described as an amalgamation of biologic perturbations. Newer linear accelerators linked with newer treatment planning systems have the ability to vary the intensity of radiation within the target (called *intensity modulated radiation therapy*, IMRT), and brachytherapy can also deliver a large local dose, although the complexity of dose inhomogeneity and dose rate of delivery remains to be fully understood. Figure 25-2 (prepared in collaboration with Dr. Mary Ann Stevenson) indicates that there are conceptually two non–mutually exclusive pathways for radiation-induced cell killing.[5] On the left is the most

TABLE 25-1. KEY FEATURES OF THE HYPOXIC CYTOTOXIC AGENT TIRAPAZAMINE (TIRAZONE)

Mechanism of action:	Bioreductive activation by 1-electron addition produces DNA double-strand breaks.
	Preferentially activated under hypoxic conditions.
	Can enhance radiotherapy and chemotherapy if given in close proximity (best if given 15–30 min before).
Metabolism and elimination:	Rapidly cleared from the plasma. The metabolites SR-4317 (2-electron reduction product) and SR-4330 (4-electron reduction product) are detectable in plasma but are not active.
Pharmacokinetics:	Half-life is approximately 45 min.
Drug interactions:	None known.
Toxicity:	Common: muscle cramps, nausea, and fatigue.
Dose of 260 mg/m²	Less common: blood count depression and abnormal liver function tests.
Dose greater than 330 mg/m²	Reversible ototoxicity.
Precautions:	May alter pharmacokinetics of carboplatin.
	Caution needed with other myelosuppressive agents.
	Caution must be used in combined modality regimens.

TABLE 25-2. KEY FEATURES OF THE PROTECTOR AMIFOSTINE (WR-2721, ETHYOL)

Proposed mechanisms of action:	Scavenging free radicals, hydrogen donation, binding to critical biologic targets, and mixed disulfide formation.
	Antimutagenic activity may involve binding to DNA.
	FDA approved for reducing the cumulative renal toxicity associated with cisplatin (single dose, 910 mg/m^2). Recent trials indicate radioprotection of parotid gland.
Metabolism:	Alkaline phosphatase catalyzes the hydrolysis of amifostine into the active thiol form, WR-1065.
	WR-1065 is the major non–protein-bound metabolite produced in normal tissues soon after administration of amifostine.
Pharmacokinetics:	Half-life α = 0.87 min, half-life β = 8.76 min; plasma clearance, 2.17 L/min.
Urinary excretion:	Within 1 h of administration, 1.05% of the total amifostine dose is excreted.
Drug interactions:	Avoid drugs that might cause decreases in blood pressure before amifostine.
Toxicity:	Nausea, emesis, sneezing, decrease in systolic blood pressure, somnolence (rare), allergic reaction or rash (rare), hypocalcemia (decrease parathyroid hormone level).
Precautions:	Monitor blood pressure every 2 min during amifostine infusion. Interrupt schedule with a fall in blood pressure. Drug may be resumed with transient decline. For more prolonged decline, reduce dosage.
	Oral calcium and calcitriol supplements useful for hypocalcemia.
	Administer amifostine within 30 min of reconstitution.

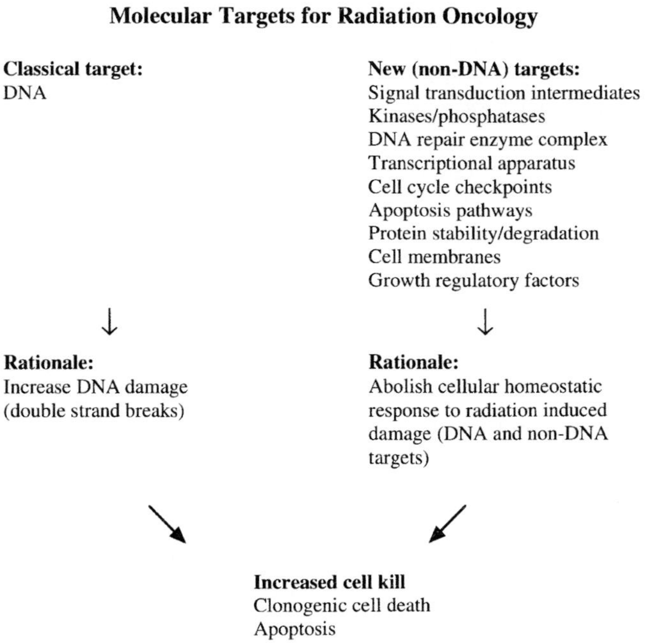

Molecular Targets for Radiation Oncology

Classical target:
DNA

New (non-DNA) targets:
Signal transduction intermediates
Kinases/phosphatases
DNA repair enzyme complex
Transcriptional apparatus
Cell cycle checkpoints
Apoptosis pathways
Protein stability/degradation
Cell membranes
Growth regulatory factors

$\downarrow$ $\downarrow$

Rationale:
Increase DNA damage
(double strand breaks)

Rationale:
Abolish cellular homeostatic response to radiation induced damage (DNA and non-DNA targets)

Increased cell kill
Clonogenic cell death
Apoptosis

FIGURE 25-2. There are two non–mutually exclusive approaches to radiation modification. Alteration in DNA damage is the classic concept on the left-hand side. The right-hand side indicates that it may be possible to alter cellular homeostasis by agents that do not kill the cell but set the cell up for killing by ionizing radiation. It may be possible to use agents in much lower concentrations than needed for direct cell killing. Many treatments that are cytostatic would require a second modality (e.g., radiation, cytotoxic drug, and immunologic directed cell killing) to be effective. Furthermore, the efficacy of an agent that targets a novel molecular target might be most easily demonstrated in a clinical trial with the "focused biology" obtainable with radiation. [Concept in this figure generated in conjunction with Dr. Mary Ann Stevenson. Adapted with permission from Coleman CN, Harris JR. Current scientific issues related to clinical radiation oncology (comment). *Radiat Res* 1998;150:125.]

important, direct damage to the DNA that results in sufficient DNA damage to induce cell killing. How the cell dies, a mitotic or apoptotic death, may vary with tissue type and other factors. In the left-hand side of the figure, radiation modifiers would alter the DNA damage or its repair to enhance cell killing. On the right-hand side is a second conceptual model for radiation modification. This takes advantage of the processes that are induced by radiation so that the cell might be perturbed by a drug, but not to the extent that the cell is killed. Rather, the cell is killed only when exposed to radiation. Thus, by conceptualizing radiation as *focused biology*, one can envision a range of biologically based therapies that might improve the outcome with radiation, taking advantage of the new imaging and treatment techniques that will allow the radiation to be better focused. The use of this approach is not limited to external beam radiation. It might be possible to use this conceptual approach with systemically administered radiation, as with radiolabeled antibodies or ligands. Additionally, this approach might be applied to other sources of energy, such as hyperthermia and phototherapy.[6]

THEORETICAL AND PRACTICAL CONSIDERATIONS FOR RADIATION MODIFIERS

Radiation and chemotherapy modifiers differ substantially from "standard" anticancer agents in that they are not designed to be cytotoxic. The characteristics of an "ideal" sensitizer are included in Table 25-3. An essential component is that of selectivity for the tumor with a sensitizer and for normal tissue with a protector. An agent that enhances

TABLE 25-3. CHARACTERISTICS OF AN IDEAL RADIATION MODIFIER

Radiation sensitizer
Acts selectively in tumor compared to normal tissues
Reaches tumor in adequate concentration
Predictable pharmacokinetics for timing with radiation therapy
Able to be administered with every radiation treatment in a standard regimen
Minimal toxicity of the drug itself
Minimal or manageable enhancement of radiation toxicity
Range of potential mechanism of action includes:
    Directly enhances DNA damage
    Alters cell biochemical and molecular response to radiation
    Decreases repair of radiation damage
    Causes cell death by novel mechanism (e.g., apoptosis)
Radiation protector
Acts selectively in normal tissue compared to tumor
Reaches normal tissue in adequate concentration
Excluded from tumor
Predictable pharmacokinetics for timing with radiation therapy
Able to be administered with every radiation treatment
Minimal toxicity of the drug itself
Result may be decreased acute or late effect
Range of potential mechanism of action includes:
    Prevents DNA damage
    Alters cellular biochemical response to radiation
    Enhances repair of radiation damage
    Enhances repopulation of normal tissue
    Alters late effect

Adapted from Herscher LL, Cook JA, Pacelli R, et al. Principles of chemoradiation: theoretical and practical considerations. *Oncology Suppl* 1999;5:11.

the normal tissue and tumor effect equally is theoretically no better than simply administering a higher dose of radiation. This point is often not given sufficient consideration. Specifically, radiation modifiers or combined modality therapy should *not* substitute for an adequate dose of radiation. In the current era of three-dimensional conformal radiation therapy, including IMRT and particle treatment, to obtain the best result one needs to optimize radiation dose delivery and then apply the appropriate modifier. A lesson learned from past studies[7] is that one should not use a less-effective radiation schedule simply to optimize the radiation modifier. In general, the modifier should be used with the "best" radiation schedule, recognizing that in many instances there is a range of acceptable schedules. For drugs that produce toxicity such that a limited number of doses can be administered, fractionation that includes more than one fraction per day may be preferable (e.g., twice-daily radiation therapy).

PRINCIPLES OF COMBINED MODALITY THERAPY

Although radiation modifiers are not designed to be cytotoxic, the principles behind the development of radiation modifiers are similar to those of combined modality ther-

apy with radiation and standard chemotherapeutic agents.[8] Agents that target the microenvironment are discussed later in the chapter.

Historical Considerations

The genesis of concurrent chemoradiation dates back to the 1950s, when investigators began searching for chemical agents that might enhance the effects of radiation.[9,10] "Potentiation of activity" by combining 5-fluorouracil (5-FU) with radiation was obtained by Heidelberger et al. in 1958 in a preclinical study[11] that was later translated into clinical trials, often with contradictory results, as seen in the treatment of lung cancer.[12,13] However, a major breakthrough was achieved in the early 1970s when, encouraged by the results obtained with chemoradiotherapy at the Mayo Clinic on gastrointestinal (GI) cancers,[14,15] Nigro and colleagues used a combination of 5-FU and mitomycin C concurrent with radiation as neoadjuvant treatment in patients with cancer of the anal canal.[16] They reported that all three patients achieved complete responses, confirmed on histologic examination of surgical tissue specimens. Despite the small numbers of patients, the results of this initial pilot study (and subsequent clinical trials) were so dramatic as to prompt a paradigm shift from exenterative surgery for anal cancer to organ preservation. Since the 1970s, numerous chemoradiation trials have been done with differing levels of success in a variety of cancer histologies.

Why, then, is a particular chemoradiation regimen successful in the treatment of one cancer histology and not in others? What are the limitations of chemoradiation? The major limitation of combining two modalities has been cumulative normal tissue toxicity.[17,18] The radiosensitivities of tumor and normal tissues are often similar, or, unfortunately, in many cases the tumor cells may be more resistant than surrounding normal tissues. Thus, a major barrier in the use of radiation or chemotherapy to treat cancer, either alone or in combination, is lack of specificity. A radiation beam, no matter how well shaped or conformed to the dimensions of the tumor, will undoubtedly expose some normal tissue, although dose escalation may be possible using the newer conformal and intensity-modulated radiation approaches. Radiation alone can and does damage normal tissue if threshold doses are exceeded. Acute toxicity may be ameliorated with supportive care or usually will resolve; however, long-term late effects are generally not reversible and are the true dose-limiting toxicity. Systemic drug therapy theoretically exposes all tissues, normal and tumor, and a toxicity not related to the radiation field, such as myelosuppression, may compromise the rate of delivery and administered dose of radiation and drug. Prolonging treatment may have an adverse impact on local tumor control, owing to tumor repopulation.[19] During chemotherapy patients frequently relapse after initial treatment and become progressively less responsive to second- or third-line treatments.[20] Combination modality therapies may complicate these issues further.

We focus on several aspects of combined modality therapy that should be considered as new combinations are explored. Space does not permit the review of each radiation dose–modifying agent in current use; the reader is directed to several reviews that provide more detail, particularly with respect to specific drugs and radiosensitization.[21–23] This information is also contained in other chapters in this text that discuss the specific drugs. The properties of an ideal radiation modifier are listed in Table 25-3. In reality, an ideal radiation modifier does not presently exist, but we can use the characteristics of an ideal radiation modifier as a standard as new agents for radiation modification become available.

Radiation Sensitizers

In general, the mechanisms by which agents sensitize cells to radiation can be categorized into three broad areas.

Increase in Initial Damage

Radiation-induced cellular effects result from the production of free-radical species, direct ionization of target molecules, or both. The exact identification of critical cellular structures or molecules and the specific type of damage rendered by radiation are not completely known. However, there is considerable evidence pointing to DNA as the critical target for radiation damage,[24] with DNA double-strand breaks (DSB) as the lethal lesion.[25] After radiation treatment, cells die by mitotic-linked death, programmed cell death (apoptosis), or both. An agent that causes more initial damage to critical cellular targets would be expected to enhance the cytotoxic effects of radiation if repair systems become saturated. A class of modifiers that, in part, enhance the radiation response by increasing damage are the halogenated pyrimidines. Incorporation of halogenated pyrimidines into cellular DNA has been shown to increase the amount of DNA damage[26] and compromise repair systems[27] as discussed below.

Repair Inhibition

The ability to repair radiation damage is a vital and necessary cellular function. Repair in this context is the "undoing" of damage to a structure or molecule necessary for viability and function. There are most likely several ways cells could accomplish this objective. First, molecules that can "chemically" restore damaged molecules may be present in cells. An example might be a reducing species that could donate electrons to oxidized (damaged) substrates. Second, a variety of molecules and enzymatic systems recognize and repair damaged substrates through a set of complex and ordered reactions. Last, in a loose sense regarding repair, there may be cellular systems that prevent damage before it

occurs. Such systems would involve detoxification of toxic species by chemical or enzymatic means.[28,29] Much is being learned about the specific enzyme(s) responsible for the recognition and repair of radiation damage; undoubtedly, specifically targeting these enzymes will afford another avenue for radiation modification.

The radiation dose-response curve plotting log surviving fraction versus radiation dose for most human tumor cell lines derived from solid tumors is characterized by a shoulder in the low-dose region of the curve.[30] The implication of the shoulder region of the curve is that cells have the capacity to repair radiation damage, particularly for radiation doses delivered in radiotherapy (approximately 2 Gy), a phenomenon called *sublethal damage repair*. Extensive studies reveal that the time required for maximal radiation damage repair varies between 3 and 6 hours.[31] The extent of repair is dependent on the particular cell type and can be quite significant, particularly in tumors that do not respond well to radiation, such as melanoma and glioblastoma. Normal tissues can also repair radiation damage to different extents. Time-dependent repair of normal tissue is the major reason radiation dose is fractionated. Thus, cells and tissue treated with 2 Gy on Monday morning will have repaired all of the damage they are capable of repairing by the time the next fraction is given on Tuesday, and so forth. However, attention to interfraction interval is important in twice-daily radiation regimens, in which 6 hours is usually the interfraction interval. Ideally, agents that inhibit radiation damage repair (in the tumor) would need to be present daily as the radiation is administered. Because of the lack of specificity of most agents used presently, normal tissue may also be radiosensitized.

Cell-Cycle Redistribution

Tumor growth is governed by (a) the fraction of cells within the tumor that are actively dividing (cycling versus quiescent cells), (b) the duration of the cell cycle, and (c) the cell loss factor.[32] It has been known for more than 30 years that cells vary in their response to radiation as a function of their position in the cell cycle[33]; cells in G_2-M phase at the time of irradiation are approximately threefold more sensitive than cells in late S phase or early G_1. The exact reason(s) for the variation in sensitivity to ionizing radiation throughout the cell cycle is not known. An agent that selectively blocks tumor cells in a radiosensitive phase might provide a means for significant radiosensitization.

A number of chemotherapeutic agents are capable of imposing cell-cycle blocks with subsequent radiosensitization.[34] As an example, preclinical studies have shown that paclitaxel, a drug that is presently being evaluated in clinical chemoradiation trials, imposes a significant G_2-M block and radiosensitizes many human tumor cell lines[35,36] and murine tumor models.[37] Figure 25-3 demonstrates the dependency of the G_2-M block for radiosensitization of

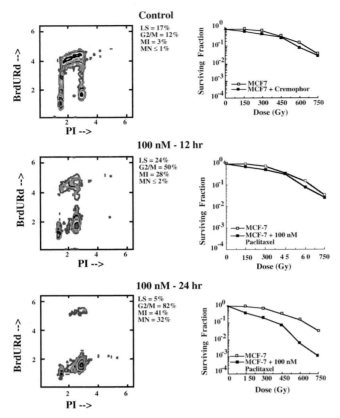

FIGURE 25-3. Two-dimensional DNA and bromodeoxyuridine (BrdUrd) flow histograms and cell survival for MCF-7 cells treated with paclitaxel for 0 to 24 hours. MCF-7 cells were incubated with 100 nmol/L paclitaxel for 0, 12, and 24 hours, and the cells were pulsed for 1 hour with 10 μmol/L BrdUrd, fixed for DNA flow-cytometry analysis (using the BrdUrd antibody technique) (*left panels*), or irradiated and plated for clonogenic survival (*right panels*). (LS, late S phase; MI, mitotic index; MN, multinucleated; PI, propidium iodide.) (Reprinted with permission from Herscher LL, Cook JA, Pacelli R, et al. Principles of chemoradiation: theoretical and practical considerations. *Oncology Suppl* 1999;5:11.)

MCF-7 breast cancer cells. Note that radiosensitization did not occur until cells were emptied from S phase into G_2-M.

Armed with encouraging preclinical results, a number of institutions are evaluating the combination of paclitaxel and radiation in a variety of tumor types. Will the preclinical information and enthusiasm be translated into benefits for cancer patients? The answer to this question must await the results of the trials; however, are the studies combining paclitaxel and radiation designed properly for success, and if the trials fail, will we know why? These are difficult questions to answer.[38] Clinical trials are begun with the minimal assumption that the results, and possibly the mechanisms observed using laboratory *in vitro* and *in vivo* models, will translate into the human model. Unfortunately, few clinical studies are designed to actually determine whether expected mechanisms are operational in the human model.[38] In preclinical studies it has been shown that for paclitaxel to behave as a radiosensitizer, cells must be moving in the cell

cycle to block in G_2-M.[36] Cells in plateau phase (G_0) are not radiosensitized by paclitaxel.[36] Therefore, tumors with a low growth fraction (few cells cycling) would not be expected to be radiosensitized to the same extent as tumors with high growth fractions, although it is likely that the pretreatment state of the tumor may change during the course of treatment such that the growth fraction might increase. Considerable data are available regarding the growth kinetics of human tumors[39]; thus, phase II trials should be initially done to treat those tumors that have the best chance to respond. Obtaining tumor samples during the course of treatment is difficult but may provide useful information.

Dose-Effect Factor and Therapeutic Gain

For an agent to be considered for use as a radiation modifier, preclinical studies are usually (although not always) conducted. Radiation dose-response curves are generated for a variety of tumor cell types in the absence and presence of the drug. Depending on what is known about the mechanism of action of the drug, various concentrations and durations of exposure either before, during, or after radiation treatment are examined. After the cytotoxicity of the drug treatment alone is normalized, the effect of the drug on radiosensitivity can be assessed for a given end point. In the case of cell-survival curves, the dose-effect factor (DEF) is calculated at a given survival level. The dose of radiation alone required to yield a given survival level is divided by the dose to yield the same survival level for the radiation and drug combination. If the ratio yields a number greater than one, the agent "enhances" the radiation response; likewise, if the agent yields a ratio less than one, the agent "protects." DEFs may be determined not only for cells in culture, but also for tumor and normal tissues in animal models.[23] Determining DEFs in animal models provides the option of determining the therapeutic gain (TG), which is calculated by dividing the DEF of the tumor by the DEF of the normal tissues. For radiation modification to be successful, a TG of greater than one is the goal.

In reality, however, determination of a meaningful TG in experimental models is laborious and difficult to interpret. These experiments are laborious in the sense that combined chemoradiation studies in animals are time consuming; costly, because they involve numerous permutations of drug concentrations and timings; and often difficult to interpret, in that most rodent tumor models are not thought to be reflective of human tumors because of their rapid growth kinetics. An alternative to rodent tumors is experimentation with human tumor xenografts in immune-compromised mice; however, these are human tumors growing under the control of the mouse physiology. On the other hand, the radiation response of normal tissues in mice closely matches the response in humans[23] and, at a minimum, provides the clinician some measure of the vulnerability of various normal tissues.

Because of the issues discussed above, new agents are frequently brought to radiation modifier clinical trials without preclinical TG information. Commonly, DEFs are determined for cell lines (human tumor) and perhaps a few studies are conducted regarding efficacy of tumor response to the combination in mice. Rarely are murine normal tissue DEFs determined. Perhaps the rationalization is made that most new agents considered for chemoradiation have already undergone clinical trials as single agents and much is already known about toxicity profiles. What is not known, however, is the extent to which radiation will enhance these toxicities. Given these realities, what DEF value, derived primarily from *in vitro* studies, warrants the introduction of a new agent to chemoradiation evaluation (e.g., 1.1, 1.5, or 2.0)? This question is indeed difficult to answer. A DEF of 1.1 means that a radiation dose will be enhanced by 10%, a seemingly modest amount. However, if one assumes that the radiation response will be enhanced by the agent for *each* radiation fraction, over the course of 30 fractions this could amount to a significant enhancement even for a DEF of 1.1 (1.1^{30} = 17.5-fold increase, 1.3^{30} = 2,600-fold increase, and 1.5^{30} = 191,751-fold increase). Whether a tumor DEF of 1.3 to 1.5 for a particular agent can be achieved in the clinic depends on numerous factors, including inherent radiosensitivity and a variety of factors as discussed below.

Potential Barriers and Solutions to the Effective Use of Radiation Modifiers and Chemoradiation

Normal Tissue Toxicity

The use of three-dimensional conformal treatment can reduce the dose and volume to normal tissue treated, with the challenge of not compromising dose to microscopic tumor at the margin of the field. The use of radiation protectors, such as amifostine,[40] is described below, as is the recent observation that late effects may be partially reversible, even years later.[41] Another new class of radioprotective agents, known as *nitroxides*, are currently being studied preclinically.[42] Preclinical studies have demonstrated that nitroxides exhibit selective normal tissue radioprotection.[43] The additional feature of these agents is that they can be imaged *in vivo,* noninvasively, using electron paramagnetic resonance (EPR) imaging approaches.[44]

Effective Drug Delivery

On the scale of the tumor cell, radiation is delivered to the tumor without any pharmacokinetic barriers, and the dose delivered can be preplanned with external beam radiation and brachytherapy. Unlike radiation, a drug administered systemically to a patient may encounter various barriers or impediments that reduce the drug concentration before it reaches its final destination: the tumor cell, and more precisely, the target within the cell. Although drug pharmacokinetic profiles in the blood are helpful, such studies do not directly measure the effective concentration reaching the tumor cells. As a chemotherapeutic drug traverses the vascular system, it can be metabolized and detoxified by various organs. Likewise, given the altered and compromised vascularization that often accompanies cancerous masses, uniform drug delivery within a tumor can be difficult to obtain. Other factors, such as tumor interstitial fluid pressure and compromised blood flow, can also influence drug delivery.[45] In addition to compromised drug delivery to the tumor, there may be inherent or evolved drug resistance[46] that may result from an overabundance of specific intracellular detoxifying enzymes.[47]

For example, a recent study compared the plasma level of methotrexate (MTX) in nine breast cancer patients versus the level of MTX in the tumor interstitial space (as determined by insertion of a microdialysis probe into the tumor).[48] In none of the patients did the plasma-MTX level agree with the tumor interstitial level; mean area under the concentration versus time curve (AUC) values for the tumor interstitial space were approximately 50% of AUC values for the drug in the plasma. Therefore, to say that achievable plasma levels of a particular drug are in the range necessary to kill tumor cells (based on preclinical *in vitro* data) may be entirely misleading, as the actual level at and within the tumor cell is critical.

Imposed on the complicated issue of drug delivery is the impact of daily radiation doses delivered to the tumor and their possible effects on tumor vasculature. Radiation treatment may result in damage to tumor vasculature; the consequences might be compromised drug delivery developing and increasing as the radiation dose accumulates (often called the *tumor bed effect*). On the other hand, cell killing with a decrease in interstitial tumor pressure may enhance tumor perfusion.

Considering such points, an important question to ask regarding radiation modifier clinical trials is Does the drug actually get to the tumor cells in adequate concentration to kill the tumor cell or enhance the radiation response? Although this is a reasonable question, there are few studies conducted to obtain the answer because measuring drug concentration in tumor is a difficult task. Taking multiple tumor biopsies is inconvenient, adds cost to the study, and can pose certain risks to the patient. The location of the tumor for biopsies is often problematic, and there is the concern of increased tissue injury from multiple biopsies in an irradiated field. The interpretation of drug concentration in tumor biopsies can be complicated because of the infiltration of host cells into the tumor mass, as discussed below. Last, the availability of suitable assays for the drug and its metabolites is not always straightforward. These concerns can be partially addressed for agents whose mechanism of action are known with functional biologic assays. As an example, pacli-

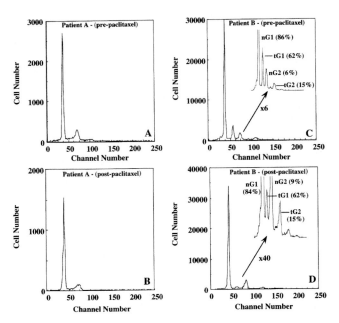

FIGURE 25-4. DNA flow cytometry histograms of biopsy specimens taken from head and neck patients treated with paclitaxel for 48 hours. **A** and **C**: Pre-paclitaxel samples (120 mg/m²). **B** and **D**: Forty-eight–hour paclitaxel infusion samples (105 mg/m²). The percent of cells in G_1 and G_2 are listed in parentheses. (nG1, normal cells in G_1; nG2, normal cells in G_2; tG1, tumor cells in G_1; tG2, tumor cells in G_2.) (Reprinted with permission from Herscher LL, Cook JA, Pacelli R, et al. Principles of chemoradiation: theoretical and practical considerations. *Oncology Suppl* 1999;5:11.)

taxel treatment results in a G_2-M arrest in cells in culture. If arrest of cells in G_2-M is required for paclitaxel-mediated enhancement of radiation toxicity, then determining cell-cycle parameters from biopsy material taken from the patient's tumor as a function of time after paclitaxel administration should reveal whether the drug is reaching the tumor cells in adequate concentration to achieve the goal.

In a National Cancer Institute pilot clinical trial evaluating continuous infusion of paclitaxel with concomitant radiation therapy for head and neck cancer, tumor biopsies are taken before and 48 to 96 hours after paclitaxel infusion. The tumor samples were analyzed by flow cytometry, as shown in Figure 25-4. Seven out of nine patients showed no cell-cycle blocks as a result of the 48- to 96-hour continuous infusion of paclitaxel (started at 105 mg per m² to 120 mg per m²). Figure 25-4A and B shows pre- and post-paclitaxel treatment DNA flow-cytometry profiles from a patient's tumor that did not show a treatment-related cell-cycle block in G_2-M. One patient's tumor did show some modest cell-cycle redistribution as a result of the paclitaxel treatment (Fig. 25-4C and D). The reasons for the failure of paclitaxel in this study to arrest cells in G_2-M are most likely multiple. First, the concentration of paclitaxel infused may not be adequate. Second, should drug-resistant phenotypes be present or result from the continuous paclitaxel treatment, one would not expect to see cell-cycle redistribution. Third, the biopsy taken represents only a

small fraction of the total tumor mass; perhaps the biopsies were taken from areas where cells are quiescent and not cycling. Fourth, 48 to 96 hours of continuous drug infusion may not be long enough to detect significant changes in cell-cycle distribution. Last, yet-to-be-identified factors could contribute to the lack of the G_2-M arrest. This example serves to highlight the complexity of asking the simple question of whether a drug reaches and affects a tumor; nonetheless, attempts should be made to obtain this type of important information. The functional parameters will be correlated with ultimate treatment outcome. If a drug fails to be an effective radiation modifier, it is important to know why so that a good concept is given a fair trial.

Knowledge of Optimal Timing of Agents

Preclinical *in vitro* studies can contribute considerable information toward defining the optimal timing of a drug and radiation in clinical protocols. In practice, timing considerations in chemoradiation clinical trials are often based, in part, on scheduling data derived from preclinical *in vitro* studies. There can, however, be a vast difference between controlled *in vitro* studies and the *in vivo* situation. Most *in vitro* chemoradiation studies are conducted using a single radiation dose, and drug treatment occurs either before, during, or after the radiation treatment. Radiation is delivered to patients by daily fractions (often twice per day). If the drug is administered as a weekly bolus, will sufficient concentrations of the drug be present to enhance radiation doses given by the end of the week? Moreover, will the radiation doses given the first week impact the ability of the drug given on subsequent weeks of treatment to enhance radiation effects? In the case of cell-cycle–specific drugs, does radiation treatment (which alone can induce cell-cycle blocks) retard the ability of the drug to influence the cell-cycle distribution? As an example, numerous investigators have shown that paclitaxel given before radiation results in radiation enhancement of cytotoxicity.[35,36] However, treatment of cells first with radiation was shown to antagonize the cytotoxic effects of paclitaxel.[49] One wonders if this is an issue in the present clinical protocols combining paclitaxel and radiation.

There is considerable data presently available for certain tumor types to suggest that, after the first 3 to 4 weeks of fractionated radiotherapy, the surviving tumor cell clonogens have an increased growth rate.[19] To compensate for this accelerated tumor cell growth and repopulation, additional radiation dose would be required if the radiation course is protracted beyond the scheduled time. For oropharyngeal tumors, it is estimated that an additional 0.6 Gy per day would have to be added to compensate for repopulation.[19] If this is true, perhaps the use of cell-cycle–specific radiation enhancement agents might be more effective given at the end of the normally scheduled radiation protocol, rather than at the beginning. Similarly, it might be more interesting and efficacious to use halogenated pyrimidines toward the end of radiation treatment, when tumor cell growth is accelerated. The downside of this approach is that radiation treatment may stimulate the repopulation of certain normal tissues and enhance their susceptibility to the drug.

It is not entirely obvious how the issue of timing should be approached in clinical trials. This is why knowing the mechanism of action of an agent brought into clinical trials is so important and, likewise, how, at least at the cellular level, the agent interacts with radiation. With this information, one is able to biopsy tumor material while the trial is ongoing to determine whether the basic mechanisms presumed to be operational are indeed working in the patient's tumor. If they are not, then alternate timing protocols should be considered. Without such information, a range of schedules is usually employed and phase I trials determine the maximum tolerated dose that is then used empirically in phase II and III trials.

Physiologic Considerations

A variety of physiologic factors, some unique to the tumor, can influence a tumor's response to drugs and radiation. Such factors include tumor blood flow,[50] oxygen transport,[51] hypoxia,[52] interstitial fluid pressure,[45,53] and tumor pH.[54] In radiobiology, significant research has gone into determining the impact that hypoxia has on the radiation response and is further detailed later in this chapter. The existence of hypoxic regions in human tumors was hypothesized in the mid 1950s,[52] and, over the past several years its presence in human tumors has been verified by oxygen electrode studies.[55] Because a great deal of the radiation modifier field has focused on hypoxia, it is covered in greater depth in a subsequent section. Briefly, the importance of hypoxic regions (both chronic and acute or intermittent) in tumors to oncology is that (a) hypoxic cells can be viable and capable of proliferation if oxygen becomes available, (b) hypoxic cells are approximately two- to threefold more resistant to radiation than aerobic cells, and (c) the presence of hypoxic cells in a tumor is an unfavorable prognostic indicator for local control of tumors treated with radiotherapy or surgery.[55] In the context of chemoradiation and delivery of radiation modifiers, the presence of hypoxic regions in tumors could mean that drug delivery to these areas is compromised: If oxygen cannot readily reach these areas, how can a low-molecular-weight drug and even more so, how can a high-molecular-weight agent, such as an antibody or gene therapy vector? Antihypoxic therapies are discussed below.

Drug Resistance

The development of drug resistance during the course of chemotherapy is a formidable problem. Although much has been learned about the cellular and molecular mechanisms of drug resistance, effective approaches to circumvent this problem have yet to be identified. Drug resistance in tumor cells might, in effect, decrease the dose of drug available for radiosensitization. Several studies have convincingly shown that drug-resistant cells are not necessarily radioresistant[56]; however, to our knowledge, there is no information as to whether drug-resistant cells can be radiosensitized by the drug(s) that they are resistant to. Stated differently, does a cell's mechanism for detoxication of cytotoxic agents result in loss of radiosensitization? As a corollary, a drug need not be effective in inducing a tumor response by itself for it to be an effective radiosensitizer. Such is clearly the case with a drug that targets only a small portion of the tumor, as with agents toxic to hypoxic cells (discussed below).

Host Cell Infiltration of Tumor

As early as 1863, tumor infiltration by leukocytes was noted, and based on this observation, Virchow concluded that tumors arise in areas of chronic inflammation.[57] More recently, the presence of leukocytes has been linked to the concept of "immune surveillance," which proposed that tumor cells are recognized as antigenically different from normal host cells and, thus, they incite an immune reaction.[58] Pathologists seldom mention in their reports the presence of reactive cellular infiltration.[59] In an analysis of breast carcinoma, Underwood found that the mean total tumor cell volume of two medullary carcinomas was 64.5%, although in ten scirrhous carcinomas the tumor cell volume was only 21.5%.[60] Thus, it is possible that a significant portion of the tumor cell mass may be composed of cells other than malignant cells. In the National Cancer Institute Radiation Biology Branch, we have evaluated the extent of tumor infiltration by normal host leukocytes from biopsies of 26 human tumors from the lung, including primary and metastatic lesions. Delineation of leukocyte infiltration was accomplished by double staining tumor sections with a pan antileukocyte monoclonal antibody (HLE-1) and propidium iodide (PI). Images of the staining patterns of the total nuclei (stained by PI) and leukocytes (labeled with a biotinylated anti-mouse secondary antibody and fluorescein isothiocyanate-streptavidin) examined under low magnification were acquired and stored using a laser scanning microscope and computer-based image analysis system. The staining pattern of individual leukocytes varied markedly throughout all tumor sections examined. In general, the leukocytes were seen in either "clumps" of varying sizes or as individual leukocytes scattered through the entire tumor section. The percentage of tumor leukocyte infiltration was quantitated by taking the ratio of leukocyte staining to the nuclei staining for each section. The proportion of leukocytes in the individual tumors ranged from 4% to 90% with a mean of 40%, as shown in Figure 25-5. In 15 out of 26 specimens, the leukocyte fraction was equal to or greater than 40% of the entire tumor sample. In addition,

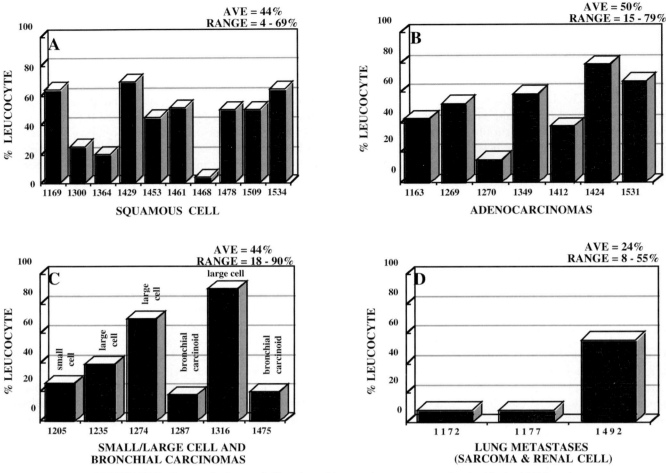

FIGURE 25-5. Percent leukocyte infiltration of human lung tumors stained with the HLE-1 antibody and quantitated with the computer-assisted image analysis method (patient sample number on ordinate). **A:** Squamous cell lung carcinomas. **B:** Adenocarcinomas of the lung. **C:** A group of lung tumors, including one small cell carcinoma, two large cell carcinomas, and two bronchial carcinoids. **D:** Lung metastasis from two soft tissue sarcomas (1172 and 1177) and one renal cell carcinoma (1492). (AVE, average.) (Reprinted with permission from Herscher LL, Cook JA, Pacelli R, et al. Principles of chemoradiation: theoretical and practical considerations. *Oncology Suppl* 1999;5:11.)

we attempted to classify the types of leukocytes present in 15 of 26 patients, using antibodies specific for monocytes and macrophages, granulocytes, and T- and B-cell lymphocytes. A majority of the specimens analyzed contained macrophages and granulocytes (12 of 15 samples), although only two samples had T cells in excess of 19%.

The reason(s) for the extensive infiltration of host cells in these tumor samples and whether their presence poses a barrier to effective chemoradiation (or chemotherapy alone) are not known. Without question, the presence of these cells within a tumor biopsy complicates precise determination of tumor cell drug uptake and functional cellular and molecular assays specific to drug treatment and to new complementary DNA microarray analysis. Are these cells "activated and inactivated" for tumoricidal activity? Do these cells represent a means of drug detoxification that would, in effect, decrease the drug concentration delivered

ultimately to tumor cells? Does the response of these hematopoietic cells to various treatment protocols have important influences on what is perceived as a partial or complete tumor response to cytotoxic therapies? The answers to these questions will require additional confirmation and an understanding of their importance to tumor growth behavior and response to therapeutic modalities. Furthermore, they demonstrate the importance of correlation between histology and molecular studies of a tumor biopsy. Techniques such as laser capture microscopy are important in this regard.[61,62]

Summary

This section has posed more questions than answers. The use of chemotherapeutic agents or specific radiation modifiers to effectively enhance the radiation response is indeed

TABLE 25-4. CONSIDERATIONS FOR CHEMORADIATION CLINICAL TRIALS

Does the drug to be used have antitumor activity and any selectivity for tumor?

What is known about the mechanism of action?

Does the drug enhance the radiation response?

    Preclinical *in vitro* data? Have dose effect factor values been determined?

    Preclinical *in vivo* data? Have dose effect factor values been determined (tumor and normal tissues)?

    What is known about optimal timing and administration of the drug for radiation enhancement?

Is there a quantitative chemical assay for the drug?

Is there a cellular and molecular assay for the drug that reveals or reports on the drug's mechanism and action?

Is there a way to image the drug's distribution and its biologic effects in humans?

Can the drug's mechanism of action be demonstrated from biopsies taken from the tumor?

Does the drug, when administered to the patient, get to the tumor cells, the target in the tumor cell, or both, in sufficient concentrations for radiation enhancement?

Have plans been included in the protocol to biopsy the tumor to obtain mechanistic information?

Adapted from Herscher LL, Cook JA, Pacelli R, et al. Principles of chemoradiation: theoretical and practical considerations. *Oncology Suppl* 1999;5:11.

complex. What must be kept in mind is that, despite the myriad of problems and concerns regarding concurrent chemoradiation under an increasing number of clinical circumstances, including head and neck, lung, rectal, and cervical cancer, the approach works, in that better local control can be achieved with acceptable normal tissue toxicity. Chemoradiation trials can be designed not only to study possible efficacy for the cancer patient, but to gain more information regarding mechanisms of action (in the patient) and pharmacokinetics and pharmacodynamics of drug uptake and action in the tumor and tumor cell. Based on concepts brought forth in this section, Table 25-4 lists several possible considerations for chemoradiation trials. Although it is realized that designing clinical trials to address specific basic science questions is a more difficult task than is encountered in the research laboratory, to not do so consigns the trial to empiric permutations. There is nothing particularly wrong with empiric approaches; however, teamwork between basic scientists and clinicians can add a new dimension of scientific information that will undoubtedly advance the area.[38] For example, if the drug(s) are not reaching the target in the patient's tumor in sufficient concentrations to enhance the radiation response, then research needs to be focused on means of enhancing drug delivery.

SPECIFIC RADIATION MODIFIERS

The following sections cover the radiation sensitizers and protectors. The more commonly used radiation-chemotherapy combinations are included in the chapters on the specific drugs. A number of the agents emphasized in the previous edition of this chapter have had "null" clinical trials—that is, the sensitizer was neither better nor worse than the control. Therefore, they will be covered in much less detail, and the reader is referred to the previous edition for many of the historical and theoretical details.[63] Likewise, there are numerous chemotherapy drugs used concurrently with radiation and it is beyond the scope of this chapter to cover each of them in detail. The reader is directed to several excellent reviews on this topic[21–23,64] and elsewhere in this book. Some of the newer agents that are currently being evaluated include taxanes,[35,36,65–67] gemcitabine,[68] and topoisomerase inhibitors.[69–71]

Halopyrimidine Radiation Sensitizers

Halopyrimidines, Bromodeoxyuridine, and Iododeoxyuridine

A clinical approach toward radiosensitization is the use of halogenated pyrimidines, bromodeoxyuridine (BUdR), and iododeoxyuridine (IUdR). A preclinical approach under development uses chlorodeoxycytidine (CldC) plus tetrahydrouridine.[72] BUdR and IUdR were designed as thymidine analogs that would be incorporated into the DNA of cycling cells and make them more sensitive to radiation. The rationale for the use of the halopyrimidine 5-FU and related thymidylate synthase modulators with radiation therapy appears in a recent review[73] and elsewhere in this book.

Structure

In the halogenated pyrimidines, the methyl group in the 5-position of thymidine is replaced by the halogen. The substitution of the halogenated pyrimidine into the DNA in place of thymidine is believed to be due to the stereochemical similarity between the methyl group of thymidine (2.0 Å), bromide (1.95 Å), and iodine (2.15 Å) atoms of the halogenated pyrimidines.[74,75]

Mechanism of Action

The mechanism of sensitization includes an influence on the radiation-induced strand breaks and effects on repair.[26,75,76] The degree of radiosensitization increases as the percentage of thymidine replacement increases. Kinsella et al. demonstrated *in vitro* a direct correlation between percent thymidine replacement, reduction of radiation survival parameters, and the production of DNA strand breaks using drug concentrations clinically achievable.[26] For example, the enhancement factor for the production of DSB formation was approximately 1.3 to 1.6. Because incorporation into DNA is critical for sensitization, the cells must be exposed to the sensitizer for a sufficient period of time so the halogenated pyrimidine will be incorporated during DNA synthesis.

Assessment of tumor cell incorporation is an important aspect of the clinical trial, as it will indicate optimal drug schedules and appropriate tumor types for treatment with this approach.[77]

Clinical Pharmacology

The scheduling of drug administration is designed such that tumor incorporation is maximized while the dose-limiting myelosuppression is kept at an acceptable level. The earliest clinical trials with BUdR showed little efficacy and excessive normal tissue toxicity, the latter due in part to the disease site selected. Patients treated for head and neck cancer had increased mucosal reactions due to the rapid cell cycling of the normal mucosa, which incorporated more of the BUdR than the tumor.[78] This serves as a clear example of the importance of understanding the tumor and normal tissue biology. In a phase I trial of BUdR using a daily 12-hour infusion for 14 days, the final dose achieved was 850 mg per m^2 per 12 hours; pharmacokinetic data were available for seven patients.[79] The mean steady-state arterial plasma concentrations were 7.0×10^{-7} mol per L for an infusion of 350 mg per m^2 and 2.1×10^{-6} mol per L, for an infusion of 700 mg per m^2. At the dose range of 650 to 700 mg per m^2 per 12 hours, the arterial plasma levels were in the range of 2 to 3×10^{-6} mol per L, which produced a sensivity enhancement ratio (SER) greater than 1.5 using the human bone marrow colony-forming units in culture assay.[79,80] There was a trend toward increasing SER with increasing dose of BUdR.[80]

IUdR later replaced BUdR owing to the photosensitivity seen with the latter compound,[76,81,82] although it is not certain which is the superior agent.[83] In a phase I study with IUdR, a dose range of 250 to 1,200 mg per m^2 per 12 hours was studied for 14 consecutive days. Two 14-day courses were administered. The arterial plasma levels achieved ranged from 1 to 8×10^{-6} mol per L, with no suggestion of saturation of the drug metabolism pathways.[84,85] The steady-state arterial concentration by dose was, at a dose of 500 mg per m^2, 2.9 μmol per L; at a dose of 1,000 mg per m^2, 5.6 μmol per L; and at a dose of 1,200 mg per m^2, a concentration of 7.4 μmol per L. Total body clearance was the same for all drug dose levels.[85] Studies of IUdR incorporation, using an anti-IUdR monoclonal antibody, disclosed that 50% to 70% of the sarcoma cells had incorporated IUdR; a smaller proportion of glioblastoma cells incorporated the sensitizer in a single patient studied.[84]

BUdR is still under investigation. Eisbruch et al. used an innovative treatment scheme and performed tumor plus normal tissue biopsies in a phase I study for patients with advanced uterine-cervix cancer.[86] BUdR was administered for 4 days in 1 week followed by radiation therapy, 1.5 Gy twice a day, for 15 Gy in the second week. This cycle was repeated three times, for a total radiation dose of 45 Gy followed by a brachytherapy procedure. The maximum toler-ated dose of BUdR was 1,000 mg per m^2 per day, with the dose-limiting toxicity being myelosuppression. The percentage of DNA deoxythymidine replaced by BUdR was similar in the tumor and rectal mucosa (4% to 7%), as was the percentage of cells that had nuclear staining for BUdR (50% to 70%). However, as the time from the end of the 4-day infusion progressed (day 10 compared to day 5), the pattern of BUdR staining in the mucosa demonstrated migration of the BUdR away from the crypts toward the surface—that is, to a cell population that is not likely to be sensitized (nondividing cells). This "wash out" of the crypt stem cells may improve the therapeutic index. In this limited phase I study, the response and local control rates were similar to historical controls.

The Michigan group has also piloted the use of BUdR by hepatic arterial infusion in patients with primary hepatobiliary cancers or colorectal liver metastases, using conformal radiotherapy to a dose ranging from 24 (whole liver) to 66 Gy (cone down).[87] Toxicities included those from the hepatic artery catheter with a dose-limiting hematologic toxicity above 25 mg per kg per day (the length of the infusions varied somewhat). There was no clinical evidence of sensitization of liver parenchyma or GI mucosa, although biopsies were not performed.

It has been proposed that other halogenated pyrimidines, such as CldC, may be good radiation sensitizers, particularly when used with agents such as tetrahydrouridine (an inhibitor of cytidine deaminase) and other biomodulators that alter the normal metabolic pathways of the halopyrimidine.[72,88,89] Clinical trials with CldC plus tetrahydrouridine are under development.

Toxicity and Efficacy

The skin toxicity encountered with BUdR was not observed with IUdR.[84] The dose-limiting toxicity for both sensitizers was myelosuppression—in particular, thrombocytopenia. Phase II trials for sarcomas, gliomas, and liver metastases produced encouraging early results[84,90–95]; however, a recent phase III Radiation Therapy Oncology Group (RTOG) randomized trial for patients with anaplastic astrocytoma demonstrated no benefit to the addition of BUdR to treatment with radiation therapy and procarbazine, CCNU, and vincristine.[95] A number of groups have demonstrated in the laboratory the potential for using the halopyrimidines with continuous low-dose rate radiation[96–98] and with an implantable biodegradable polymer tested in murine–human glioma xenografts.[99] Pilot data indicate some potential utility in colorectal cancer metastatic to the liver[83] and in head and neck cancer,[100] although this latter study suggested that an intermittent drug schedule might be less toxic. The prodrug 5-iodo-2-pyrimidone-2'-deoxyribose, which is metabolized to IUdR, is being investigated, as it can be orally administered.[101] It is possible that IUdR may increase chromosomal aberrations after radiation.[102]

Therefore, although there is no proven clinical benefit, increased understanding of the mechanism of action, maneuvers to increase incorporation in tumors relative to surrounding normal tissue, and understanding of the need for cell proliferation to ensure adequate uptake have sustained a continued interest in this class of agents.

Hypoxic Cell Sensitizers and Enhancers

The most studied approach to clinical radiosensitization has been targeting the hypoxic tumor cells. The importance of the oxygen effect in cell killing by ionizing irradiation has been known for more than 70 years. To kill the same proportion of hypoxic cells compared to oxygenated cells requires approximately two to three times the radiation dose. Thus, the oxygen enhancement ratio (OER) is two to three. Although the term *hypoxia* is commonly used, *nutritional deprivation* is a better descriptor, as it indicates that in poorly perfused tumor cells there is a limitation in the availability of nutrients in addition to oxygen. The molecular response to hypoxia via the hypoxia-inducible factor (HIF)-1α transcription factor and the phenotypic consequences resulting from nutrient gradients, dynamic alteration, or both, in nutrient concentration are now being defined and have greatly increased the potential to understand and exploit hypoxia in the clinic.

"Seven Percent Solution" ("a la Sherlock Holmes")—Realistic Expectations from Hypoxic Modifiers

Hypoxia is but one potential cause of radiation resistance[103–105]; other causes include intrinsic cell radiosensitivity, cellular response and adaptation to radiation, tumor cell proliferation, and other epigenetic effects. As is described below, it has now been demonstrated that hypoxia exists in human tumors and, therefore, it provides a relatively tumor-specific therapeutic target for modulation. The ability to overcome the clinical radiation resistance of tumor hypoxia and nutrient deprivation should be expected to only partially overcome the problem of incomplete local tumor control after irradiation.[106] To illustrate this point, for advanced head and neck tumors, the local control rate with standard radiotherapy is roughly 60%. If half the local failures are due to hypoxia (20%), and if the sensitizer could help radiation control as many as three-fourths of the group of failures, then the overall local control rate would improve by only 15%. Furthermore, assuming that half of these patients eventually develop distant metastases, the overall survival would increase by only 7%. Therefore, even a successful approach toward hypoxia-related radiation resistance would be expected to bring only modest local control and survival benefits. To demonstrate such a modest but clinically important success rate would require a large trial or a meta-analysis of many trials. Indeed, a meta-analysis conducted by Overgaard et al. that analyzed a wide variety of approaches to overcome the radioresistance of hypoxia demonstrated a benefit in local tumor control by antihypoxia treatment compared to control.[107]

MEASURING HYPOXIA IN TUMORS

Techniques to assess hypoxia are presented next. Although these are of great interest, it is necessary to understand how the assays correlate with one another. It is not clear that any one is a solid-gold standard, although the one most frequently used is the oxygen electrode. Another key issue is resolution—what volume of hypoxia can be detected as a small proportion may impact outcome. The ultimate technique would be a noninvasive, nontoxic assessment that could be repeated before, during, and after a course of therapy to prognosticate tumor biology, predict response to therapy, and guide therapeutic strategy. Oxygen may well be one of the first molecules that can be measured as a prognostic and predictive factor. In that molecular and functional imaging are of intense interest, this section is covered in detail, as it is likely that these and other techniques will be introduced into clinical oncology relatively soon.[108–110]

Oxygen Electrodes

In the mid-1950s, Thomlinson and Gray examined tissue specimens and hypothesized that hypoxic cells exist in human tumors.[52] The relative radioresistance of hypoxic cells[111] represents a potential barrier to effective tumor treatment with radiation. Likewise, hypoxia could present a problem for systemic forms of therapy, such as chemotherapy, because of compromised delivery of the drug to the tumor cells.[112] Although the presence of hypoxic cells has been demonstrated in rodent tumors and human tumor xenografts,[113–115] it was not until the late 1980s that the presence of hypoxic regions in human tumors was documented.[116] The proof required inserting glass oxygen electrodes directly into accessible head and neck tumors and recording partial pressure of oxygen (pO_2) measurements. A significant relationship between the low-mean intratumoral pO_2 values and failure to respond to fractionated radiotherapy was reported.[116] Subsequent studies using oxygen electrodes inserted into a variety of human tumors have demonstrated significant levels of hypoxia.[117–122] Hockel et al. measured pO_2 levels in locally advanced tumors of the uterine cervix and found that 50% of the patients had tumors with median pO_2 readings of less than 10 mm Hg.[55] After these measurements were made, patients received either radiotherapy or surgery. As predicted from previous studies, patients receiving radiotherapy, and whose tumors had pO_2 readings less than 10 mm Hg, had significantly worse disease-free and overall survival probabilities than patients with nonhypoxic tumors.[55] Interestingly, histopathologic examination of tumors taken from patients receiving surgery showed a clear relationship between tumors with low pO_2 levels and greater tumor extensions, more frequent parametrial spread, and more extensive lymph–vascular space involvement compared to well-oxygenated tumors. The poorer outcome of patients with tumors with low pO_2 levels was due to locoregional failures (with or without distant metastases), irrespective of whether surgery or radiotherapy was performed. Thus, not only did the presence of hypoxic cells in tumor compromise therapy, their presence also denoted a more aggressive disease.[55,123]

Immunohistochemical Techniques

During the course of developing nitroimidazole hypoxic radiosensitizing agents, it was observed that these agents could selectively bind to hypoxic cells.[124–127] Under hypoxic conditions, adducts are formed between the nitroimidazole and cellular proteins (sulfhydryl containing) in hypoxic cells. These adducts may be detected using the specific monoclonal antibody conjugated to a fluorochrome, and the number of hypoxic cells can then be quantified by flow cytometry. Additionally, spatial information of hypoxia in tumor samples may be microscopically examined. Recent studies have demonstrated the efficacy of this approach.[128–130] The technique involves pretreating the patient with the nitroimidazole and obtaining tumor biopsies.

Comet Assay

The comet assay is a microelectrophoretic technique for the direct visualization and quantification of DNA damage in individual cells.[131] Irradiated cells are embedded in agarose, lysed, subjected to an electric field, stained with a fluorescent DNA stain, and viewed microscopically. Because DNA, which has been broken by radiation, migrates further in the electric field, the cell appears as a "comet" with a head and tail region. The length of the tail region (tail moment) increases with increasing radiation dosage.[132] Because of the differential radiation-induced damage that occurs between aerobic and hypoxic cells, this technique can be used to estimate the hypoxic fraction in tumors.[133–136] The technique does require obtaining biopsy material promptly after treatment with radiation.

Noninvasive Techniques

The use of the invasive techniques described previously demonstrates that hypoxia does exist in human tumors and points to the importance of *a priori* knowledge of pO_2 levels in tumors to select the most appropriate and effective treatment option. Preferably, noninvasive means of making pO_2 measurements would be desirable. There are several noninvasive techniques under development that have the potential to provide tissue oxygen information. Clinical

imaging techniques, such as magnetic resonance spectroscopy,[137–141] gradient-recalled echo magnetic resonance imaging,[142] Overhauser magnetic resonance imaging,[143,144] electron paramagnetic resonance imaging (EPRI),[44,145] and positron emission tomography (PET) scanning,[146–149] are under development and may permit the serial evaluation of tumor oxygenation and energy state during a course of treatment. PET scanning is accomplished using fluorine-labeled agents (nitroimidazoles) that selectively bind to hypoxic cells, as discussed previously.

Of all the noninvasive techniques for oxygen assessment in tissue, the most direct method is that of EPRI. Tissue oxygen information can be extracted from EPRI studies as a result of a physical interaction of molecular oxygen, which is paramagnetic, and the spin probe (nitroxide or carbon-centered free radical probe), thereby modifying the spectral characteristics of the spin probe. The extent of spectral broadening can, by appropriate calibrations, be directly correlated to oxygen concentration. Because the sensitivity of EPRI is inversely related to the spectral broadening, EPRI becomes more sensitive as the pO_2 decreases. Figure 25-6A shows EPRI spectra of a free-radical probe in normal muscle tissue of a rat. On application of a tourniquet with subsequent hypoxia induction to the leg, the spectra become more narrow and signal intensity increases, indicating greater sensitivity under low oxygen conditions. Figure 25-6B shows an example of EPRI evaluation of oxygenation status in normal versus tumor tissue in a mouse. The well-oxygenated normal tissue (muscle) was found to have pO_2 levels of approximately 40 mm Hg, whereas the tumor (RIF-1) had values of approximately 10 to 12 mm Hg as measured by EPRI. Closing off the blood supply by tourniquet application to the leg clearly shows that EPRI can readily distinguish changes in oxygenation in normal and tumor tissue.[44] These results show the potential usefulness of EPRI in noninvasively obtaining valuable information regarding oxygen status in tissue. For each of the noninvasive techniques, serial imaging will be complex due to the limit of tissue volume that can be imaged and the difficulties in registration of the patient such that the tumor is imaged in the proper position each time. Nevertheless, these emerging techniques should be useful in the understanding of the effects of treatment on tumor physiology and biochemistry, as well as being a guide for radiation therapy treatment options.

Do Hypoxic Cells Exist in Tumors, and What Is the Implication for Therapy?

Surveys of rodent tumors and human tumor xenografts indicate that almost all solid tumors contain hypoxic cells.[114,115] The presence of hypoxic cells within human tumors has been identified from studies using microelectrode techniques that measure oxygen content directly and from autoradiography studies using agents that selectively

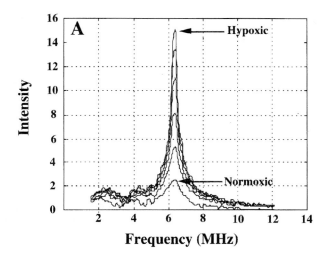

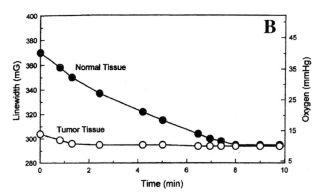

FIGURE 25-6. A: Electron paramagnetic resonance spectra of a lithium phthalocyanine spin probe implanted in the thigh muscle of a rat. The signals were detected using a 300-MHz Fourier transform electron paramagnetic resonance imaging spectrometer and a surface coil resonator. The broad signal corresponds to normoxic tissue, and the narrow and intense signal was obtained after induction of hypoxia by applying a tourniquet. (Reprinted with permission from Krishna MC, Kuppusamy P, Afeworki M, et al. Development of functional electron paramagnetic resonance imaging. *Breast Dis* 1998;10:209.) **B:** Measurement of oxygen concentration in normal and tumor tissue using electron paramagnetic resonance spin label oximetry. After infusion of the spin probe, either the tumor-bearing leg or the normal leg was clamped to restrict tissue blood flow. The figure shows a significant difference between oxygenation status initially, the tumor being much more hypoxic. Both tissues showed a drop in tissue oxygen to approximately 8 mm Hg in 10 minutes. (Reprinted with permission from Kuppusamy P, Afeworki M, Shankar RA, et al. In vivo electron paramagnetic resonance imaging of tumor heterogeneity and oxygenation in a murine model. *Cancer Res* 1998;58:1562.)

bind to hypoxic cells.[109,110] The most commonly used technique to quantify hypoxia has been the Eppendorf oxygen electrode.[55,117,118,150,151] Representative results (Fig. 25-7) are presented in a histogram that shows the number of measurements within a certain range of oxygen content. The two bars on the left, with pO_2 from 0.0 to 2.5 mm Hg [hypoxic fraction $(HF)_{2.5}$] and 2.5 to 5.0 mm Hg $(HF_{5.0})$, contain radiobiologically hypoxic cells.

Although there is still much to be learned, the following are some of the observations reported in a recent sympo-

sium on tumor hypoxia,[151] along with a few other recent articles that help to summarize the current state of the field:

1. Approximately 40% of breast cancers contain hypoxic cells.[152] The impact of advancing stage on lower pO_2 was not found consistently, and no clinical parameters predicted tumor oxygenation.[152]

2. Approximately 25% of head and neck cancers and 15% of sarcomas studied by Nordsmark had detectable hypoxic cells. Hypoxia did not correlate with other tumor parameters or with serum hemoglobin. The patients who had locoregional failure had a higher percentage of tumors with $HF_{2.5}$ (22% versus 6%), indicating that hypoxia is important in prognosis, but other factors are obviously relevant.[153]

3. The change in hypoxia with treatment has been measured in patients with head and neck cancers and sarcomas with two interesting findings. The median tumor pO_2

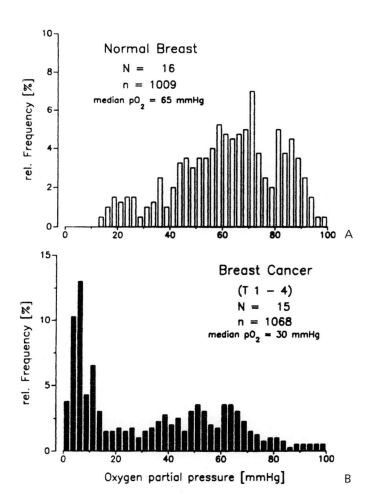

FIGURE 25-7. Oxygen content histogram. The oxygen electrode measurements for normal breast tissue (**A**) and breast cancers (**B**) are plotted. The two bars on the left represent radiobiologically hypoxic cells, which are seen in the tumor and not in the normal tissues. (rel., relative.) (Reprinted with permission from Vaupel P, Schlenger K, Knoop C, et al. Oxygenation of human tumors: evaluation of tissue oxygen distribution in breast cancers by computerized O_2 tension measurements. *Cancer Res* 1991;51:3316.)

before and after 10 to 15 Gy of fractionated radiation was 8 mm Hg and 10 mm Hg, respectively, indicating that reoxygenation does occur[154]—that is, the proportion of hypoxic cells does not increase as the more sensitive aerobic cells are killed. Whether reoxygenation can eliminate hypoxia is an open and critical issue. Hyperthermia increased the pO_2, which may partially explain its therapeutic efficacy. The patients with a pretreatment median pO_2 below 10 mm Hg had more viable tumor in the neck dissection specimen, as well as statistically inferior locoregional control, disease-free survival, and survival compared to patients with pO_2 above 10 mm Hg. For each of the parameters of "survival," the percentage was approximately 30% for the low-oxygen group compared, to 70% for the patients with median pO_2 above 10 mm Hg. This research group from Duke had previously shown an adverse impact of hypoxia on outcome, including an increased incidence of distant metastases.[155] Measuring oxygen consumption with ^{15}O PET, there was a correlation between oxygen delivery and consumption, suggesting that methods that overcome hypoxia through increased oxygen delivery might, in a sense, be self-defeating, because the increased oxygen delivery would increase oxygen consumption.

4. For patients with head and neck cancer, the pretreatment median pO_2 correlated with hemoglobin concentration (less than 11, 11 to 13, and greater than 13 g per dL) and the median pO_2 increased while the percentage of pO_2 values below 5 mm Hg decreased in patients who underwent blood transfusion (increase from 9.7 to 11.6 g per dL). This would favor the use of blood transfusion or erythropoietin. These investigators also found a lower concentration of plasma vascular endothelial growth factor in patients with hemoglobin levels above 13 g per dL.[156,157]

5. Carbogen breathing was able to increase the pooled median pO_2 from 20 to 61 mm Hg.[158]

6. The relationship between the extent of hypoxia and tumor response during treatment is complex. Molls reported that the percentage of measurements with $HF_{2.5}$ and $HF_{5.0}$ increased during radiation after a reduction in tumor volume, indicating that hypoxia persists despite tumor regression, yet, because of tumor regression, the total number of cells in the hypoxic subfraction decreased. A trend in decrease in median pO_2 also occurred.[159] These findings suggest that the need for antihypoxia therapy persists during a course of treatment, even in the face of an ongoing partial response—that is, reoxygenation may not necessarily be sufficient to eliminate the resistant hypoxic subpopulation.

7. Hockel's studies in patients with cervical cancer indicate that hypoxia by itself is an indicator of worse histopathologic features (lymph–vascular space invasion or occult regional spread) and prognosis, the worse prognosis with radiation or with surgery. This supports the concept that hypoxia is among the features of a "worse" cancer.[55] The role of hypoxia in treatment failure will be answered by the use of treatments to overcome hypoxia, such as erythropoietin.[160,161]

8. A recent report[161a] measured tumor hypoxia with the Eppendorf pO_2 histograph and cell proliferation with BUdR in 43 patients with cervical cancer and found no correlation between labeling index and hypoxia. Clinical outcome is not yet available for clinical correlation with the oxygen and labeling index assays.

9. Fyles correlated pretreatment and posttreatment pO_2 in patients with cervical cancer and found that the percentage of reading below 5 mm Hg was more or less similar before and after a course of radiation therapy, and the values did not correlate with outcome with limited follow-up available.[162]

Thus, it can be concluded that radiobiologic hypoxia exists; hypoxia may persist during the course of radiation therapy; anemic patients tend to have more hypoxic measurements; hypoxia correlates with poor histologic features and worse treatment outcome (with radiation or surgery), and the impact of antihypoxic therapies on hypoxia; and outcome of local and regional and distant disease remains to be determined. These findings certainly encourage future efforts to image hypoxia, understand the biologic properties that create and maintain tumor hypoxia, elucidate the molecular consequences of hypoxia, and develop treatments that overcome its presence, effects, or both. Although the studies of hypoxic sensitizers to date have been disappointing, they are not entirely negative. Undue negativism would be inappropriate and possibly detrimental to important progress in clinical oncology.

CHRONIC AND INTERMITTENT NUTRIENT DEPRIVATION AND REOXYGENATION

The initial model of hypoxia was developed by Thomlinson and Gray, who noted the pathologic appearance in lung cancer specimens of small necrotic foci approximately 150 μm from the capillaries.[52] This "diffusion-limited," or chronic, hypoxia is one type of hypoxia, the other being "perfusion-limited," or intermittent. Figure 25-8 is a schematic illustration of the two types of tissue nutrient deprivation.[163] Chronic hypoxia is illustrated in the left-hand side of the figure. The assumption is made that the nutrient vessel remains open and blood flow is constant. In this setting, the hypoxic cells would be confined to the area surrounding the necrosis (the cross-hatched cells). Of note, cells deprived of glucose and oxygen will not survive as long as cells that are only oxygen deprived,[164] so the size of the necrotic zone would depend on which nutrients are available. Intermittent hypoxia, illustrated on the right-hand side of the diagram, has been demonstrated using flow cytometric and fluorescence microscopic techniques.[165–168] Intermittent perfusion is the result of dysfunctional opening and closing of tumor vessels, which may be due to a combination of intratumoral pressure[169,170] and other humoral factors.

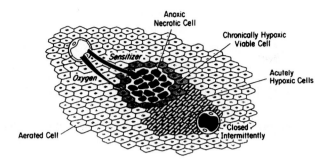

Approaches to Chronic Hypoxia

- Increase Oxygen Delivery
  Transfusion
  Hyperbaric Oxygen
  Perfluorochemical
  Altered Hgb Affinity for oxygen
- Hypoxic Cell Sensitizers
  ± Thiol Modification
- Bioreductive Agents
  Mitomycin-C
- ?Hyperthermia

Approaches to Acute Hypoxia

- Altered Oxygen Delivery
  Likely to have minimal impact
- Hypoxic Cell Sensitizers
  ± Thiol modification
- Bioreductive Agents
  Would need rapid action under hypoxia
- ?Hyperthermia
- ?Chemotherapy

FIGURE 25-8. Chronic and intermittent hypoxia. Chronically hypoxic cells (*left*) are "diffusion limited." Intermittently hypoxic cells (*right*) are "perfusion limited," in that they are hypoxic only when blood flow stops in their nutrient vessel. Possible methods of overcoming acute and chronic hypoxia are suggested. The clinical importance of the different types of hypoxia and the efficacy of the approaches listed remains to be established. (Hgb, hemoglobin.) (Reprinted with permission from Coleman CN, Beard CJ, Kinsella TJ. Radiation sensitizers. In: DeVita VT, Hellman S, Rosenberg SA, eds. *Cancer: principles and practices of oncology.* Philadelphia: JB Lippincott Co, 1993:2701.)

Cells irradiated when effective blood flow is present will behave radiobiologically as oxygenated cells. However, when blood flow transiently stops, existing oxygen and nutrients can be rapidly exhausted, leaving previously well-perfused cells in a temporary state of nutritional deprivation. If radiation is given when these cells are not perfused, they will respond as hypoxic cells. The different forms of hypoxia may require different types of modulators, analogous to the need for combination rather than single-agent chemotherapy.

An important concept of tumor biology is tumor reoxygenation.[112,171–173] Immediately after a large single dose of radiation, essentially all the remaining cells are those that were most hypoxic at the time of radiation exposure. However, within a few hours, the percentage of hypoxic cells returns toward the preradiation level. After a single high dose of irradiation, magnetic resonance spectroscopic studies have detected a rapid improvement in metabolic parameters (high-energy phosphates) that indicate a reduction in the hypoxic fraction.[174] The time course for reoxygenation is much faster than that for the process of tumor cell death and removal or for major vascular remodeling. A likely explanation for reoxygenation is the presence of intermittent perfusion, as the restitution of blood flow within tumor vessels could rapidly restore the oxygenated cell compartment within the tumor.[175] Reoxygenation is con-

sidered to be a major reason for the success of fractionated irradiation, as the relative radioresistance of hypoxia can be overcome. The degree to which reoxygenation occurs during clinical radiation therapy awaits the further development of methods to identify and quantify hypoxic cells. Results shown above from the Mainz symposium (discussed above) indicate that reoxygenation does occur to some extent, and its efficiency in eliminating the hypoxic fraction is not yet known.

WHAT IS MEANT BY HYPOXIC FRACTION?

When the percentage of hypoxic cells is stated, it is derived from the result of a radiobiologic assay that indicates the proportion of cells that were hypoxic *at the specific time* of irradiation. For rodent tumors, this is approximately 20% to 30%. However, given the presence of intermittent nutrient deprivation, it may be possible that, although 20% to 30% of cells are hypoxic at any given point in time, the percentage of cells that are hypoxic at some point over an extended duration of observation may be much higher. Furthermore, although the percentage of hypoxia is usually defined as the fully hypoxic cells (i.e., less than 2.5 mm Hg with the Eppendorf electrode), Wouters and Brown have recently modeled that with the diffusion-limited hypoxia, the tumor response is highly dependent on the cells at intermediate oxygen concentration (5 to 20 mm Hg).[176] The presence of intermittent hypoxia and the importance of intermediate hypoxic cells have important implications in the effects of hypoxia on tumor progression and transiently induced processes due to the cellular and molecular stress response and on the target for hypoxic cells. The intermediate hypoxic cells are a prime target for the bioreductive agent tirapazamine.

TRANSIENTLY INDUCED CELLULAR PHENOTYPE

Previously, it had been demonstrated that intermittent nutrient deprivation could alter the overall cellular phenotype, so radiation resistance, drug resistance, metastatic potential, and so forth may be transiently inducible.[177–185] There has been an explosion in the knowledge of hypoxia biology in the last few years. Given the rapidity of change and the extent and complexity of the field, it is not possible to include more than a few salient features of hypoxia biology in this chapter.

Among the major findings in hypoxia biology in the last decade has been the discovery by Wang and Semenza[186] of HIF-1.[187] HIF-1 has two subunits, HIF-1α and HIF-1β, the latter being identical to the arylhydrocarbon nuclear translocator protein, a component of the xenobiotic response pathway.[188] The major impact of hypoxia appears to be the posttranslational stabilization of the HIF-1α protein that complexes with the constitutively expressed HIF-1β and arylhydrocarbon nuclear translocator to activate genes that include a hypoxia-response element (HRE). This transactivates a range of genes, including those involved in angiogenesis (vascular endothelial growth factor), erythropoietin, the shift in glucose metabolism from aerobic to anaerobic, wound healing and inflammation (tumor growth factor β, inducible nitric oxide synthase), and others.[188] The cell may have a range of sensors for oxygen and reactive oxygen species.[189] The expression of HIF-1α may play an important role in tumor progression.[190] Hypoxia and the stress response may not only lead to a change in phenotype, and possibly an increased ability of the cell to withstand cancer treatment and a poor environment, but Giaccia has shown that hypoxia itself may enhance tumor progression by selectively killing cells with normal p53 protein and allowing those with mutant p53 to survive.[187]

Because hypoxia has been demonstrated in so many tumors, and because it correlates with a worse response to treatment, understanding the interrelationship between hypoxia development and tumor progression is a critical challenge to cancer researchers. In parallel with this has been the approach of exploiting hypoxia by the use of bioreductively activated drugs (see below), as well as the potential use of bacteria, genes, or both, activated by hypoxia to kill cancer cells or to help activate agents by the use of enzyme-directed prodrug therapy. Such therapies are under development.[191–194]

COMPETITION MODEL

The most important cellular effect of ionizing radiation is *clonogenic cell death*, defined as the inability of a cell to generate a colony of more than 50 cells.[195] This end point appears to be a consequence of DNA damage, because irradiation of the cell nucleus is approximately 100 times more cytotoxic than irradiation of the cell membrane or cytoplasm.[196] The critical DNA lesions appear to be those that consist of multiple structural alterations within a short segment of the DNA molecule.[197] A simplified characterization of these lesions is that they are DSB in the DNA molecule. In general, the number of such lesions correlates well with the probability of clonogenic cell killing under a variety of conditions.[25,198,199] Similarly, chromosome aberrations[200] and chromosome breaks visualized by premature chromosome condensation[201] correlate well with clonogenic cell killing, and it is reasonable to presume that DSB are the precursors to chromosome breaks. Approximately 40 initial DSB correspond to one unrepaired or misrepaired chromosome break, a lesion sufficient to result in clonogenic cell death. In contrast, approximately 10^6 single-strand DNA lesions are required to kill a cell,[197] indicating the relative lack of importance of single-strand breaks as compared to DSB.

The principal strategy used to date for chemical modification of radiation sensitivity has been to interfere with the rapid reactions of DNA radicals, which are the precursors to DSB. Oxygen, for example, must be present within 10 milliseconds before irradiation to enhance clonogenic cell killing. If oxygen is added 1 millisecond after irradiation, much of the oxygen enhancing effect is lost.[202] If the concentration of thiols (-SH groups) is increased, the lifetime of radicals produced by photons is shortened. The latter is called *protection* or *chemical restitution*.

The set of reactions just described forms the basis for the competition model for modification of radiation sensitivity—that is, that sensitizers and protectors compete for reaction with radiation-induced DNA radicals (Fig. 25-9).[203] Reaction with protectors results in restoration of the original DNA structure,[204,205] although reaction with sensitizers renders the lesion nonrestorable. The rationale for the development of the major classes of radiation modifiers used to date is illustrated in Figure 25-9. Antihypoxia approaches include strategies to increase oxygen delivery, such as hyperbaric oxygen, perfluorochemicals, carbogen, nicotinamide, oxygen-mimetic electron-affinic sensitizers

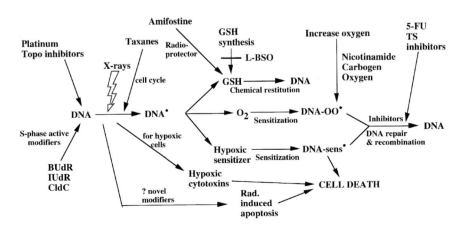

FIGURE 25-9. Radiation modifiers for clinical use. Embedded within the figure is the competition model in which the DNA radical (DNA·) may undergo either chemical restitution by reducing species (SH-) or damage "fixation" by O_2. This figure also includes other agents in clinical use or development. (BUdR, bromodeoxyuridine; CldC, chlorodeoxycytidine; 5-FU, 5-fluorouracil; GSH, gonadotropin-stimulating hormone; IUdR, iododeoxyuridine; L-BSO, L-buthionine sulfoximine; TS, thymidylate synthase.) (Adapted from Coleman CN. Of what use is molecular biology to the practicing radiation oncologist? *Radiother Oncol* 1998;46:117.)

(nitroimidazoles), and agents that are selectively toxic to hypoxic cells. This effect can be augmented by depletion of intracellular thiols, using agents such as L-buthionine sulfoximine.[206–208] On the other hand, cellular radioresistance is enhanced by increasing thiol concentration with radioprotectors (e.g., amifostine) now approved for clinical use (discussed below).[209]

Oxygen and Sensitizer Enhancement Ratios

The potency of a sensitizer is described by the ratio of the radiation dose required for a given level of cell killing under hypoxic conditions compared with the radiation dose needed in air [the oxygen enhancement ratio (OER)] or in the presence of sensitizer (SER). The OER will depend on the oxygen concentration as the SER will depend on the sensitizer concentration at the time of irradiation. The *therapeutic index* for sensitizers can be defined as the SER for the tumor divided by the SER for the normal tissues. Because radiobiologic hypoxia is limited to tumors, the SER for normal tissues is 1.0 for the electron-affinic, oxygen-mimetic radiosensitizers, as there is no radiosensitization of normal tissues. Also, because oxygen is the best "oxygen-like" sensitizer, the SER of an oxygen-mimetic compound should, at best, equal the OER, unless the sensitizer has inherent cytotoxic properties or provides sensitization by mechanisms beyond the oxygen effect.[210] The latter can theoretically occur if there is bioreductive metabolism of the sensitizer that has cell-killing properties in addition to the oxygen-mimetic effect.[210–213]

HYPOXIC CELL RADIOSENSITIZERS

Because the role of oxygen-mimetic hypoxic cell sensitizers in clinical oncology remains investigational with a positive meta-analysis,[107] but null trials with etanidazole (RTOG), this section is greatly shortened from the previous edition of this chapter. The background for the 2-nitroimidazole radiation sensitizers and the rationale for analog development has been described previously.[63]

Nitroimidazole Sensitizers

Metronidazole

The first compound tested was the 5-nitroimidazole metronidazole. Urtasun et al. conducted the classic randomized study for patients with glioblastoma multiforme using a nonstandard radiation fractionation scheme of 330 cGy, 3 times a week for 3 weeks with or without metronidazole.[7] The radiation scheme was chosen to synchronize with drug delivery. The trial was positive in that the median survival of the sensitizer group, 7 months, was superior to the 3-month median survival of the controls (p = .02). However,

almost all the patients died by 1 year and the outcome of the sensitizer group was not superior to historical controls given standard radiation therapy. This study indicated that an oxygen-mimetic sensitizer could demonstrate clinical activity, but that it should be added to the most effective radiation schema to provide the maximum clinical benefit.

Misonidazole

Misonidazole was the first in a series of 2-nitroimidazole compounds to be used in the clinic. It was available as an oral and intravenous (i.v.) preparation. The maximum tolerated single dose was limited by nausea and vomiting, and the cumulative total dose was limited by peripheral and central neuropathy.[214,215] Given the toxicity profile, it was possible to use either a modest drug dose (2 g per m²) with only a few radiation fractions, yielding a reasonable SER but leaving most of the radiation fractions unsensitized, or a low dose (0.5 g per m²) with multiple radiation fractions. The latter dose produced a low SER for each individual treatment. Therefore, in either case the overall SER for the entire regimen would be low. When Dische reviewed the results of 33 clinical trials with misonidazole, only five showed some possible benefit.[216] Four of these five positive trials were from 12 head and neck cancer studies. In a large randomized trial in Denmark conducted from 1979 to 1985, Overgaard showed that misonidazole was of benefit for male patients with pharyngeal cancer, with an overall disease-free survival of 46% for the misonidazole group versus 26% for controls. The misonidazole group had a statistically superior 3-year survival rate, 59% versus 39% for controls.[217] This finding was not confirmed in a retrospective analysis of the RTOG phase III trial.[218] Long-term follow-up from a misonidazole cervical cancer trial showed no benefit.[219] However, a meta-analysis of misonidazole for high-grade astrocytoma provided evidence of efficacy,[220] which is consistent with some phase I data with etanidazole (see following section). Desmethylmisonidazole, a metabolite of misonidazole, had lower lipophilicity and was expected to be less neurotoxic than misonidazole. Desmethylmisonidazole was not sufficiently superior and did not proceed beyond its phase I trial.[221]

Etanidazole

Using pharmacokinetic principles, Brown and co-workers developed etanidazole, a less lipophilic analog of misonidazole.[222–225] As predicted from the preclinical testing, etanidazole produced significantly less neurotoxicity than misonidazole. Using a single dose size of 1.8 to 2.0 g per m², total doses of up to 36 to 40 g per m² can be given over 4 to 6 weeks.[126,127] In the RTOG phase I trial, one-third of the patients experienced a peripheral neuropathy when receiving a total of 34 to 36 g per m².[226] A retrospective analysis of the phase I data indicated that the risk of neuropathy for any given patient could be predicted from the patient's individual pharmacokinetic profile.[227] The single-dose AUC was calculated from a series of plasma drug concentrations measured at several specific time points after administration of a single dose.[227,228] Because the AUC remains constant throughout a course of treatment, the predicted cumulative exposure is the product of the AUC × the number of doses.[226,227,229] For a single dose of 2 g per m^2, a typical single-dose AUC is approximately 2.2 mmol per L per hour, but can be less than 5 mmol per L per hour. In this retrospective analysis, the risk of neurotoxicity increased with increasing cumulative AUC, although slightly more drug could be tolerated as the overall duration of the treatment course lengthened.[227]

The ability of this model to predict neurotoxicity was prospectively validated in a phase II trial for patients with locally advanced adenocarcinoma of the prostate.[230] Subsequent trials have incorporated the principles of pharmacokinetic monitoring and dose and demonstrated that pharmacologically derived dosing is successful in preventing serious drug-related neuropathy for etanidazole.

Clinical Efficacy of Etanidazole

Two randomized trials for patients with head and neck cancer did not demonstrate a benefit to the use of etanidazole.[231–234] Positive aspects of these trials were the ability to use pharmacokinetic monitoring and dose modification to optimize the use of etanidazole[234a] and the observation of the adverse impact of anemia on treatment outcome.[235] There were a number of phase I and II trials, which are referenced for completeness, including continuous infusion, intraoperative radiotherapy, accelerated fractionation, and chemomodification.[230,235–247] Although there are no current plans for clinical trials with etanidazole, it is conceivable that the drug may be of use when a large single dose of radiation is used, such as intraoperative radiotherapy or stereotactic radiosurgery, as hypoxic cells may be relevant in such a setting, or with fractionated radiotherapy if hypoxia can be imaged and patients selected for antihypoxia therapy. The latter may well include a combination of antihypoxic agents,[234] possibly including hyperthermia and chemotherapy.[6]

Etanidazole has also been evaluated as a chemosensitizer with alkylating agents with suggestion of benefit in some studies[242–244] but no definitive evidence of efficacy.

Pimonidazole, Ro-03-8799

Pimonidazole is a lipophilic 2-nitroimidazole that, because of the basicity of its side group, tends to concentrate in the acidic environment within tumors.[245–247] It is also a more efficient hypoxic cell sensitizer than etanidazole due to its higher electron affinity. In a phase III trial for patients with cervical cancer treated with external beam irradiation (50 Gy in 5 weeks) with or without pimonidazole, followed by

intracavitary treatment, the patients who received pimonidazole had a lower incidence of clinical complete regression and statistically significantly lower local control, freedom from distant metastases, disease-free survival, and overall survival.[248] Known prognosticators seemed to be balanced between the two arms of the trial. The reason for the poor outcome in the sensitizer patients is not known with certainty, although there was speculation that the pimonidazole may have decreased tumor perfusion, a finding seen in murine systems.[249] This change in perfusion would exacerbate tumor hypoxia. Pimonidazole is being used in much lower doses as a marker for hypoxic cells.

A Second 5-Nitroimidazole: Nimorazole

Nimorazole,[250] a 5-nitroimidazole similar to metronidazole, is a less potent sensitizer than the 2-nitroimidazole compounds. However, it does not have the cumulative neurotoxicity seen with misonidazole or etanidazole. Rather, the dose-limiting toxicity of nimorazole is nausea and vomiting. Thus, although not as electron affinic as the 2-nitroimidazole compounds, nimorazole can be administered with each radiation treatment.

The Danish Head and Neck Cancer Group conducted a phase III trial of nimorazole with 422 patients with squamous cell cancer of the larynx and pharynx.[251–253] Patients were randomized to nimorazole, 1.2 g per m^2, or placebo with each of the 30 fractions of radiotherapy. The results demonstrated a statistically significant improvement in locoregional control and cancer-related, but not overall, survival (and these are consistent with the Danish Head and Neck Cancer Group trial using misonidazole for head and neck cancers).[217] A pilot study demonstrated that nimorazole can be safely administered with continuous hyperfractionated accelerated radiation therapy and that tumor responses were encouraging.[254]

Dual-Function Hypoxic Cell Sensitizers

A number of other oxygen mimetic sensitizers are under consideration, including a fluorinated 2-nitroimidazole, KU-2285[255,256] and a 3-nitrotriazole, AK-2123.[257] Because many of the other 2-nitroimidazole sensitizers evaluated in the laboratory were not sufficiently superior to etanidazole to progress to the clinic, attention turned toward taking advantage of the reductive metabolism of the 2-nitroimidazole ring.[212,213] The reductive metabolism produces an SER greater than the OER[210–213]—that is, there is a hypoxic cytotoxic effect. Dual-functional 2-nitroimidazole compounds use two properties of the nitrogroup in the nitroimidazole ring: the electron-affinic oxygen mimetic properties and the reductive metabolism properties. The dual-functional molecules contain an active moiety in the side chain, one that is preferentially activated to a toxic species in the presence of hypoxia. For example, a monofunctional alkylating agent, such as an aziridine ring, is added to the side chain. The added potency of such a compound is based on DNA cross-linking, which could occur using the bioreductive activation of *both* the nitro-group and the side chain. This would augment the oxygen-mimetic sensitization produced by the nonmetabolized nitro group.

The prototype for this type of agent is RSU-1069, a 2-nitroimidazole containing a monofunctional, alkylating aziridine ring. RSU-1069 induced a dose-dependent loss of up to 50% of the clonogenic KHT cells in the absence of radiation and greater hypoxic cell sensitization activity than misonidazole in experimental systems.[258–263] Phase I testing revealed severe nausea,[263] limiting its use in the clinic at the present time. A less toxic analog, RB-6145, was next developed[264,265] as a prodrug of RB-1069.[266] Preclinical testing of this compound, which was renamed CI-1010, produced the unexpected finding of retinal degeneration in rats and further development was discontinued.[267] The dual-function compounds form a link between the classic nitroimidazole sensitizers and the novel bioreductive agents, such as tirapazamine (SR 4233), to be discussed next.

In summary, after extensive development and testing of the nitroimidazole radiosensitizers, there are hints of utility and evidence of inefficacy. One clinical trial demonstrated that nimorazole is effective as a radiosensitizer. Etanidazole can be used safely either with radiation alone or in combined modality regimens if dosing is based on pharmacokinetic guidance. It is possible that these agents will be of some limited use in the clinic as hypoxia is better understood.

Increasing the Oxygen Content of the Blood

To date, the clinical investigations designed to overcome hypoxic cell radioresistance have been largely of two types: either an increase in oxygen delivery or the use of oxymimetic radiosensitizers. Methods to increase oxygen delivery have included the use of hyperbaric oxygen,[268–271] carbogen,[272,273] red cell transfusions,[274,275] and perfluorocarbons, such as Fluosol-DA.[276–278] The hyperbaric oxygen chamber was the first widely explored approach. Of nine prospective randomized trials, three gave statistically significant positive results for hyperbaric oxygen.[279] Because of the technical difficulty in hyperbaric oxygen administration, radiation therapy was often administered in regimens that had only a few high-dose fractions. This fractionation is disadvantageous, as it does not take full advantage of reoxygenation and can lead to increased normal tissue injury.[270,279] Nevertheless, because some trials suggested benefit, the results were of biologic interest.

In an attempt to improve oxygen delivery, red blood cell transfusions have been administered before treatment. This strategy was based on retrospective studies that suggested low initial hemoglobin values adversely affected local tumor control and overall survival.[274,275] These findings did not prove a cause-and-effect relationship between anemia and a

decrease in tumor control, as other important prognosticators, such as stage, size of tumors, and poorer performance status, may have coexisted with low hemoglobin.[280] However, a prospective randomized trial using red blood cell transfusion did improve the results of treatment of cervical cancer.[275] Additionally, a phase I and II study of the perfluorochemical oxygen-carrying emulsion Fluosol-DA and 100% O_2 as adjunct to radiotherapy in the treatment of advanced malignancies of the head and neck was sufficiently promising[276,277] to suggest that a phase III trial would be appropriate. As an alternative to transfusion, recombinant human erythropoietin is now under investigation to correct anemia without the need for blood transfusion.[281] Rhesus erythropoietin has been shown to correct anemia.[282]

APPROACHES USING HYPOXIC CYTOTOXIC AGENTS

In an effort to develop sensitizers superior to the hypoxic cell sensitizers, a novel approach was investigated using drugs that kill the hypoxic cells rather than sensitize them to ionizing radiation. The compounds included three different classes of drugs: the benzotriazine dioxides, such as tirapazamine; the quinones, such as EO9, which are analogs of mitomycin C; and the alkylaminoanthraquinone N-oxides, AQ4N.

The hypoxic cytotoxic approach has been under investigation for a number of years. Mitomycin C and its analog porfiromycin[283] had been developed as bioreductive chemotherapeutic agents that would be activated in the hypoxic state. Trials using mitomycin C in conjunction with radiation therapy were conducted to see if treatment of the resistant hypoxic fraction of tumors with a chemotherapeutic agent could enhance the efficacy of irradiation. One positive phase III trial indicated a superior local control rate in the mitomycin C plus radiation group compared to the control of radiation alone.[284] The interpretation of this trial is complex in that some patients had surgery, whereas others did not. Nevertheless, it provided further impetus to the development of the bioreductive therapies as radiation enhancers.

At the time of this writing, tirapazamine is close to approval by the FDA as a chemotherapy enhancer with cisplatin awaiting the necessary confirmatory study.

Novel Bioreductive Agent: Benzotriazine Dioxide

Tirapazamine (also known as SR 4233, WIN 59075) (3-amino-1,2,4-benzotriazine 1,4-dioxide) is a bioreductive agent developed by Zeman, Brown, and co-workers.[285–291] It is preferentially cytotoxic to hypoxic cells *in vitro*, with 25 to 100 times more drug required to produce a given level of cell killing in aerobic as compared to anaerobic conditions.[286–288] For a comprehensive review of the development of this agent, the readers are referred to the Cain Memorial Lecture by Brown.[191–194,292]

The mechanism of action has not been fully defined, but the drug appears to induce DNA strand scission resulting from oxidative damage to pyrimidines[293]; a free-radical 1-electron reduction product, formed rapidly under hypoxic conditions, is believed to be the toxic species,[289–291] as indicated in Figure 25-1.[286] Analysis of DNA and chromosomal breaks after hypoxic exposure to SR 4233 suggests that DNA DSBs are the primary lesion causing cell death.[293] The enzyme system that metabolizes SR 4233 can lead to bioactivation if single electrons are added sequentially, or to bioprotection if two electrons are added simultaneously, as with the enzyme DT-diaphorase.[294] Recent studies suggest that the reductive metabolism of tirapazamine occurs on the nuclear matrix, thereby producing a sufficient number of lesions to create the DSB. The breaks may involve the reduced activity of topoisomerase II after tirapazamine treatment.[292]

The bioreductive agents differ from the oxymimetic sensitizers in that they require metabolic activation. The oxygen dependency of drug activation[295] will influence the activity of bioreductive drugs in the clinic. The profile of oxygen concentration that produces radiation resistance and that which activates tirapazamine make this drug attractive—that is, the drug will be particularly active against cells that are most difficult to kill with radiation.[176,295] However, the rate of activation of the molecule influences its ability to penetrate spheroids.[290] Excessively rapid bioreduction leads to a limited drug delivery to deeper parts of tumor spheroids. It is unknown whether the same phenomenon occurs in tumor tissue. As noted earlier, the different types of hypoxia might be differentially affected by the bioreductive agents. Tirapazamine is well suited for low and intermediate levels of hypoxia.

Tirapazamine markedly enhances radiation-induced tumor killing *in vitro*[296] and *in vivo*.[292,297–300] This enhancement is seen when drug is given before or after radiation.[291] Postradiation sensitization indicates that this compound does not act as an electron-affinic oxymimetic sensitizer. In fractionated radiotherapy of murine tumors, tirapazamine is at least as effective as, if not superior to, etanidazole.[298]

The theoretical benefit to the use of an effective bioreductive agent is indicated in Figure 25-10A from Brown,[299] which shows the surviving fraction of cells after radiation doses with sensitizers and enhancers of different properties. Hypothetical survival curves were mathematically simulated under a variety of scenarios of radiation fractionation and tumor reoxygenation, thereby demonstrating the theoretical benefit to the use of a hypoxic cell toxin. In this figure, it is

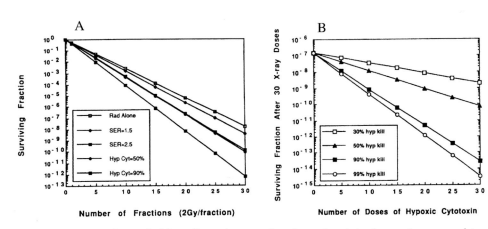

FIGURE 25-10. A: Theoretical benefit to the use of an hypoxic cytotoxic agent compared to a dose-modifying agent. In this mathematical model, an agent such as tirapazamine would be superior to an oxymimetic sensitizer, such as etanidazole. However, many assumptions are made that are not yet known, such as the rate of reestablishment of the hypoxic fraction after tirapazamine (rehypoxiation) and the relative efficacy of the hypoxic cytotoxic agent to kill the hypoxic cells. In this figure, either 50% or 90% of the hypoxic cells are killed each time the drug is used. The curves are in the same order as in the legend. (Hyp cyt, hypoxic cytotoxicity; SER, sensivity enhancement ratio.) [Reprinted with permission from Brown JM, Koong A. Therapeutic advantage of hypoxic cells in tumors: a theoretical study (see comments). *J Natl Cancer Inst* 1991;83:178.] **B:** Theoretical calculation of the efficacy of tirapazamine in the clinic based on its efficacy in killing hypoxic cells and number of times it can be used during a 30-fraction radiotherapy treatment. Ninety-percent Hyp cyt indicates that 90% of hypoxic cells are killed each time the drug is used. The more frequently that a drug can be given in an effective dose, the better the clinical result will be. However, in reality, there is usually a compromise between the single-dose size and the number of doses that can be given. Models such as this are helpful in determining the optimal dose for the phase II and III trials. [Reprinted with permission from Doherty N, Hancock SL, Kaye S, et al. Muscle cramping in phase I clinical trials of tirapazamine (SR 4233) with and without radiation. *Int J Radiat Oncol Biol Phys* 1994;29:379.]

assumed that a tumor has 20% hypoxic cells and that complete reoxygenation occurs between two Gy fractions. Thus, each time a treatment is given the tumor has 20% hypoxic cells. The curves for SER 1.5 and 2.5 indicate the impact of a dose-modifying hypoxic cell radiosensitizer (e.g., etanidazole) of varying potency. Similarly, "Hyp Cyt" indicates the impact of a hypoxic cytotoxic agent that is given with each treatment of irradiation and that kills either 50% or 90% of the hypoxic cells. In this model, the hypoxic cytotoxic agent is at least as good as a hypoxic cell sensitizer.

An important caveat is that the efficacy of a radiation modifier depends on the number of effective doses that can be administered during a course of radiation therapy. Figure 25-10B indicates that the additional cell killing by a hypoxic cell cytotoxin depends on the number of times it can be administered, the latter depending on drug toxicity to normal tissues in conjunction with radiation.[299]

These laboratory and theoretical modeling results have led Brown to propose the concept of "rehypoxiation," the ability of a tumor to regenerate its *anoxic fraction* after cell killing by a hypoxic cytotoxin. This concept resembles the concept of reoxygenation conventional radiation therapy in which the oxygenated cells are killed and the surviving hypoxic component becomes oxygenated. This information is of more than theoretical interest. The initial clinical trials indicate that it may not be possible to administer SR 4233 with every radiation fraction.[301] Therefore, knowing when the hypoxic fraction is restored will help to develop an optimal schedule for the clinical use of SR 4233. It is worth noting that agents that selectively kill a certain population of tumor cells may not need to be given with every fraction of radiation to be effective in the clinic. Kapp has demonstrated that, using hyperthermia, which is also toxic to the poorly nourished areas of the tumor, two treatments were as effective as six during a course of fractionated radiotherapy and hyperthermia.[302] Therefore, if a bioreductive agent can be given in a limited number of effective doses, it may have a important role in the clinic.

Because poorly perfused tumor cells may be more difficult to reach by chemotherapeutic drugs and nutrients, experiments were conducted that evaluated tirapazamine as a chemomodifier. Dorie and Brown demonstrated potentiation of carboplatin, cyclophosphamide, doxorubicin, etoposide, and paclitaxel (Taxol) in mice.[303] Other groups have demonstrated potentiation of cisplatin.[304]

The efficacy of tirapazamine as a radiation and chemotherapy modifier may depend on the drug exposure rather than on peak concentration,[295,305] and the AUC achieved in the clinical trials is in the range that would be predicted to be effective based on the laboratory experiments, an encouraging observation. The muscle toxicity of tirapazamine may be related to redox cycling of the drug.[306] Iron chelators reduced tirapazamine toxicity in tissue culture,[307] although the muscle cramping observed in the clinic does not imply any muscle cell death, as there has been no indication of direct muscle cell damage in the clin-

ical trials based on creatine phosphokinase assay and clinical observation (see below).[308]

Preclinical Pharmacology

Murine data demonstrated that three metabolites can be detected in plasma: the parent compound (SR 4233), the 2-electron reduction product (SR 4317), and the 4-electron reduction product (SR 4330).[309,310] A SR 4233 radical produced by the addition of one electron is the reactive active molecule (Fig. 25-1). In mice, the tumor to plasma ratio was 32% for SR 4233 and almost 200% for the two metabolites. The concentration of SR 4233 in brain was similar to that in tumors. Oral dosing produced a bioavailability of 75%, with a lower peak plasma level compared to i.v. administration. The latter two points suggest that it is reasonable to test this compound in all tumor sites and, if peak plasma concentration is not critical, an oral preparation might be used.

Clinical Trials

Phase I trials[305,308] indicated that the maximum tolerated single dose was 260 mg per m², administered 3 times per week. Five-day-per-week schedules produced muscle cramping, which was the dose-limiting toxicity. Additional toxicities were nausea and vomiting (that were controllable with ondansetron), fatigue, leukopenia, skin rash, and abnormal liver function tests; however, few of these reached the level of grade III. There was no ocular toxicity,[311] which was a concern based on the results from CI-1010 noted above. At a dose of greater than 330 mg per m², reversible ototoxicity was encountered.[305] A phase I trial of tirapazamine plus cisplatin demonstrated that the dose of 260 mg per m² could be administered along with full-dose platinum and with no alteration in cisplatin pharmacokinetics.[312]

The phase II development included a radiation therapy trial for head and neck cancer using standard radiation therapy with tirapazamine, 159 mg per m² 3 times per week for 12 doses,[313] and a similar dose schedule for brain tumors. After a few phase II trials of tirapazamine and cisplatin in non–small cell lung cancer and melanoma suggested increased activity of the combination compared to historical results,[314,315] a randomized trial was conducted. For patients with non–small cell lung cancer, with approximately 220 patients per arm, the overall response rate and survival were superior in the combination group, with an overall response of 27.5% versus 13.7% (*p* <.001) and median survival of 34.6 weeks versus 27.7 weeks (*p* = .0078). By personal communication (CN Coleman), confirmatory randomized trial did not produce a significant advantage, so additional randomized chemomodifier trials are in progress.

Pharmacokinetic Data

Pharmacokinetic data from three phase I trials are included in Table 25-5. Because the rate of drug administration (mg

TABLE 25-5. TIRAPAZAMINE PHARMACOKINETIC PARAMETERS: SHORT INFUSION[a] (260 mg/m²)

Dosage (mg/m²)	AUC (µg/mL × min)	Maximum Concentration (µg/mL)	Constant Infusion (L/min)	Half-Life (min)	Vd$_{ss}$ (L)
260 (Shulman)[308]	453.6 ± 28.6	2.88 ± 0.30	1.11 ± 0.41	19–58	—
260 (Johnson)[312]	811.4 ± 311.9	3.38 ± 0.43	0.64 ± 0.074	48.33 ± 14.6	41.97 ± 5.4
330[b] (Senan)[305]	1,026.5	—	0.624 ± 0.157	46.6 ± 9.53	39 ± 12.5

AUC, area under the concentration × time curve.
[a]Drug infusion rate was often constant mg/min so that infusion duration increased with increasing doses.
[b]Half-life increased with dose.

per min) was held constant, the infusion duration increased with increasing dose, so that C_{max} did not increase much over the higher dose ranges.[305,308] The AUC increased with dose[305,308]; however, within a given patient, the AUC was relatively constant.[308] Ototoxicity was seen at the higher AUCs,[305] with none below 1,252 µg per mL per minute (doses greater than 330 mg per m²), which is a reason for the dosage selected for clinical studies.

Other Bioreductive Agents under Development: EO9, Alkylaminoanthraquinone N-oxides, and Others

There are other bioreductive agents under investigation. EO9 is an indoloquinone, akin to mitomycin C.[284,316,317] In a phase I trial, the dose-limiting toxicity was reversible renal dysfunction with the MTD of 27 mg per m².[318] NLCQ-1 (4-[3-(2-nitroimidazolyl)-propylamino]-7-chloroquinoline hydrochloride) is a DNA affinic molecule that is being developed as a chemosensitizer.[319]

There is interest in another DNA binding agent, an anthraquinone (AQ4N), which has activity as a radiation modifier[320,321] and as a chemomodifier.[322] This agent is activated by the human cytochrome P-450 enzyme CYP3A, which is highly expressed in a wide array of human tumors, making this an attractive agent for further study.[323] The success of tirapazamine in one randomized trial has helped sustain the interest in developing other bioreductive drugs, such as AQ4N, that have different characteristics than tirapazamine (i.e., DNA binding), yet are activated under hypoxia. It remains to be seen how toxic such agents will be to normal tissues, to the surrounding oxygenated cells, or both, once the drug is activated. There is likely to be substantial further investigation of the bioreductive drug concept.

For a look well down the road, it is worth mentioning (see also the section Transiently Induced Cellular Phenotype) other approaches under investigation for hypoxia, specifically hypoxia-related gene therapy, which includes exploiting the HRE (see Transiently Induced Cellular Phenotype).[188,189] The HRE may be linked to an enzyme that activates a prodrug, or the HRE could be used to activate a toxic molecule. A number of bacterial species are activated under hypoxic conditions and these are being considered for antihypoxia-related therapy.

MODULATING TUMOR BLOOD FLOW

Modulation of tumor blood flow offers the theoretical advantages of increasing tumor blood flow to reduce hypoxia and, on the other hand, decreasing blood flow and tumor oxygenation to enhance the efficacy of the bioreductive agents.[324]

The microcirculation of tumors has been studied extensively and is characterized by low internal pressure, intermittent stasis, spontaneous hemorrhage, bidirectional flow, and regions of hypoxia.[173,249,325–327] Because tumors already have compromised blood flow, a minor change in systemic blood pressure should increase their proportion of hypoxic cells. Systemically administered agents, such as hydralazine,[328–336] nicotinamide,[337,338] calcium-channel blockers,[339,340] and pentoxyfylline,[341,342] had been investigated to alter tumor blood flow and secondarily modulate hypoxia. Another general approach was to alter the hemoglobin affinity for oxygen. These included maneuvers to increase the red blood cell concentration of 2,3-diphosphoglycerate (2,3-DPG),[343] which will decrease red blood cell affinity for oxygen, thereby increasing tissue oxygenation. Agents that increase hemoglobin affinity for oxygen and increase tumor hypoxia, such as BW12C,[332,344] were explored.

The approach investigated in the clinic over the last few years has been the use of nicotinamide with carbogen (95% O_2, 5% CO_2, the latter being added to prevent the vasoconstrictive effects of pure oxygen breathing). Normobaric and hyperbaric oxygen have also been investigated. For a group of patients with cervix cancer, normobaric oxygen did not affect outcome, although the subset of patients with stage IIB disease had improved locoregional control.[345] Long-term follow-up from a hyperbaric (4 atm) oxygen plus hypofractionated radiotherapy[346] reaffirmed the detrimental normal tissue impact of the hypofractionation (few large-sized fractions) and produced tumor control no better than more protracted radiation therapy.

Stern compared a number of antihypoxia therapies in mice using fractionated radiotherapy.[347] The agents tested were nicotinamide, perflubron emulsion, tirapazamine, and carbogen breathing and found the best results with the combination of nicotinamide and carbogen, with or without tirapazamine. Brizel et al. conducted a similar study with hyperbaric oxygen, carbogen, and nicotinamide, and hyperbaric oxygen and nicotinamide, carbogen, and air, using a single dose of radiation. Hyperbaric oxygen produced the best result.[348] The effect of these agents and fractionated radiation is complex.[349]

The hypothesis that increasing oxygenation to the tumor will improve local control and overall outcome is being investigated in the clinic using regimens with accelerated radiotherapy (often hyperfractionated as well), carbogen, and nicotinamide (ARCON). Although ARCON was deemed to be feasible in glioblastoma,[350,351] head and neck cancer,[352] lung cancer,[353] and bladder cancer,[354] the nicotinamide was not well tolerated due to GI toxicity,[351,353] leading to the conclusion that the dosage of 6 g per day may be too high. Bernier reported on pharmacokinetic studies and indicated that the target plasma concentration of 700 nmol per mL was easily obtainable and that a dosage lower than 6 g per day could produce the necessary concentration.[353] The available data from these phase I and II studies did not indicate any major changes in local control, although some studies had encouraging data. Some increased mucositis was reported in the glioblastoma study by Miralbell,[351] but not in the other studies.

In correlative studies, for patients with glioblastoma there was no change in normal tissue or tumor perfusion by 99-mTc hexamethylpropyleneamine oxime single-photon emission computed tomography,[355] and in xenograft studies, the oxygenation was variable with ARCON-like therapy.[356,357] A xenograft study showed that tirapazamine, nicotinamide, and carbogen produced radiosensitization with tirapazamine being slightly better, but the best results required frequent administration, which may not be a limiting factor in the efficacy of the combination in the clinic due to drug toxicity.[358] In summary, the toxicity and tolerance of ARCON and related regimens have been established. Coupling such therapeutic maneuvers with oxygen assessment may provide improvements in outcome, but definitive studies remain to be done.

Radiation Protectors

Since the previous edition of this book, amifostine has been approved for clinical use, culminating a long gestation period initiated with the U.S. Army radioprotector program. This section focuses on two drugs that are chemical radioprotectors, amifostine and tempol, recognizing that growth factors and colony-stimulating factors are used to abrogate myelosuppression, particularly with chemotherapy and combined modality therapy regimens. These growth factors are discussed elsewhere in this book. Cytokines, such as interleukin 1,[359] and others, such as keratinocyte[360] and basic fibroblast growth factor,[361] have been shown to be

radioprotectors in murine systems. This unique and interesting approach of using cytokines for radiation modification[362] is beyond the scope of this chapter.

Amifostine (WR-2721)

The Armed Forces Radiological Research Institute undertook a systematic search for compounds that could protect humans against radiation damage. Since Patt[363] reported that cysteine markedly reduced radiation-induced lethality in animals, sulfhydryl compounds have been the primary candidates. The *protection factor* (PF) of a compound is defined as the radiation dose needed to produce an effect in the presence of protector, divided by the radiation dose required to produce the same effect in the absence of protector. It is similar in concept to that of the sensitizer enhancement ratio. Amifostine [S-2-(3-aminopropylamino) ethyl-phosphorothioic acid] was the most effective and least toxic of more than 1,000 sulfhydryl radioprotectors tested.[364,365]

Yuhas and Storer[366] first reported that systemic administration of amifostine preferentially increased the radiation resistance of murine skin and bone marrow by PFs of 2.4 and 2.7, respectively, without increasing the radiation resistance of a mammary tumor. Since then, additional data have been obtained for multiple animal species and normal tissues and for transplanted and spontaneous tumors.[367] Although amifostine protects some experimental tumors,[368–370] differential protection of normal tissues has been observed in most experimental tumor and normal tissue model systems.[366,371,372] Because it penetrates the blood–brain barrier poorly, amifostine does not protect the brain[373] or the spinal cord[374] from radiation injury. Among its other effects, intraluminal administration of amifostine diminished duodenal toxicity in experimental intraoperative radiotherapy[375] and protected animals against secondary malignancies induced by irradiation.[376,377]

In animal models, amifostine selectively protects normal tissues against the cytotoxicities of cisplatin, cyclophosphamide, nitrogen mustard, and L-phenylalanine mustard.[367,378] Amifostine improves renal tolerance to cisplatin by a factor of 1.3 to 1.7.[374] Bone marrow tolerance to cyclophosphamide and nitrogen mustard is improved by factors of 1.5 to 2.0 and 2 to 4, respectively.[367,378]

Mechanisms of Action

Amifostine has been shown to be anticytotoxic and antimutagenic.[379,380] The anticytotoxic effect for radiation is felt to be due to scavenging of free radicals and reactive drug derivatives[379,380] by the free thiol compound, WR-1065. The free thiol structurally resembles endogenous nuclear polyamines and may stabilize DNA and enhance normal cellular antimutagenic biochemical pathways.[379,380] There are a number of other proposed biochemical mechanism(s) by which sulfhydryl compounds protect against radiation and chemotherapy toxicity including: (a) scavenging of free radicals, (b) hydrogen atom transfer to DNA radicals, (c) depletion of oxygen near DNA, (d) enhancement of biochemical repair processes,[367,381] (e) alteration in c-*myc* gene expression,[382] and (f) others.[383] The cytotoxicity of cisplatin complexes can be reduced by thiol compounds, which inhibit platinum binding. Thiols may react with either the chloride or aquo-platinum species to prevent DNA cross-linking.[384] Studies of the reactivity of amifostine and its metabolites combined with clinical pharmacologic data indicate that inactivation of the platinum drugs by amifostine and its metabolites is not expected to occur in the circulation.[385]

In the aminophosphorothioate amifostine, the phosphate group covers the sulfhydryl portion of the molecule, reducing the potential systemic toxicity of a free thiol group. The phosphate charge and hydrophilicity render intact amifostine poorly transmissible through membranes. Intact amifostine is unable to protect various cultured cell lines.[386–388] The dephosphorylated metabolite WR-1065 is believed to be the active protecting agent.[389]

Amifostine is also unique in that *in vivo* it preferentially protects normal tissues compared to solid tumors. Alkaline phosphatase is the primary enzyme responsible for the dephosphorylation of amifostine. This plasma membrane enzyme[390] is responsible for the hydrolysis of amifostine to WR-1065 and the subsequent uptake of WR-1065 by cells *in vivo*. A high concentration of alkaline phosphatase is found in the plasma membrane of endothelial cells in small blood vessels[391] and the brush border of the kidney proximal tubules.[392] The lower uptake in tumors than in normal tissues, as seen in animals, is the result of a combination of decreased uptake of amifostine and a slower intracellular conversion of amifostine to WR-1065 in tumors that have a lower inherent level of alkaline phosphatase and more acidic pH than normal tissues.[389]

Shortly after amifostine is administered, the reactive free sulfhydryl compound, WR-1065, appears as the major non–protein-bound metabolite. It is probable that WR-1065 is rapidly converted into other metabolites that can contribute to protection or toxicity, including cysteamine, sulfonate, and sulfonate oxidation products, and rapidly reacts to form mixed disulfides with low-molecular-weight substances, such as cysteine and glutathione, and with proteins containing reactive sulfhydryl groups.[393]

The biodistribution properties of amifostine are important for its protective properties. In animals, intraperitoneal amifostine provides significant radioprotection to most normal tissues, except for the brain and spinal cord, which do not contain measurable amounts of the drug.[367] Normal tissues are protected against radiation toxicity to a varying degree. For example, the radiation PF ranges from 1.2 for lung to 2.7 for bone marrow.[368,394,395] The differential tissue protection by amifostine of normal cells as compared to tumor may be related to several pharmacologic as well as biochemical factors. Data from Yuhas indicated that ami-

fostine is actively transported into normal tissues by facilitated diffusion, but solid tumors absorb the drug slowly by passive diffusion.[396] Selective normal tissue protection may also be due, in part, to the reduced delivery of amifostine to the tumor due to deficient tumor vasculature,[397] and to decreased protection of hypoxic tumor cells. Yuhas et al. reported that hydrophilicity was a major factor underlying the selective uptake of WR-2721 into normal tissues as less hydrophilic sulfhydryl compounds (e.g., cysteine and dephosphorylated disulfide and thiol derivatives of amifostine) more readily crossed tumor cell membranes.[398]

Although one would expect that the protection provided by amifostine is, in part, related to the concentration of the parent compound and its active metabolite WR-1065 achieved in various tissues, there is not a direct correlation between concentration of radiolabeled amifostine and radioprotection.[399,400] This discrepancy is due, in part, to the fact that the concentration of oxygen and endogenous thiols influences the degree to which a tissue can *express* protection.

Clinical Pharmacology

Several pharmacokinetic assay systems have been developed to measure amifostine and its metabolites, including (a) an electrochemical detection system using high-pressure liquid chromatography for the detection and measurement of WR-2721, WR-1065, and the symmetric disulfide of WR-1065, WR-33278, in urine, blood, and tissues[386,393,401]; (b) high-pressure liquid chromatography with fluorescence detection[402]; and (c) cation exchange chromatography and fluorescence detection of monobromobimane derivatives.[403] The development of a reliable assay system had been impeded by the instability of amifostine and its metabolites. Amifostine undergoes rapid hydrolysis that is pH and temperature dependent.[398,404]

Table 25-6 shows the pharmacokinetic parameters of amifostine given as 150 mg per m² i.v. bolus in patients with advanced malignancy.[380,393,401] Less than 10% of WR-2721 is in the plasma compartment 6 minutes after the injection. Pharmacokinetic analysis after the administration of 740 mg per m² and 910 mg per m² amifostine given as 15-minute infusions produced parameters similar to those after a bolus injection, although there is a suggestion of saturation of clearance at the higher dose. The average percent of the total administered amifostine excreted in the urine during a 1-hour pharmacologic study period was 1.05%, 1.38%, and 4.20% for amifostine, WR-1065, and WR-33278, respectively. These excretion data suggest that amifostine is rapidly dephosphorylated and enters normal tissues as WR-1065, the active thiol metabolite.

Utley measured the tissue concentrations of WR-1065 after a 500 mg per kg i.v. dose of amifostine to mice.[403] Maximal tissue concentrations of WR-1065 were achieved 5 to 15 minutes after injection. Fifteen minutes after injection, WR-1065 accounted for half the total drug in all normal tissues. However, in the tumor, the concentration of

TABLE 25-6. AMIFOSTINE PHARMACOKINETIC PARAMETERS: BOLUS DOSE[381,394,402]

Dose (mg/m²)	V_c (L)	AUC (mmol/L × h)	Clearance (L/min)	$t_{1/2\alpha}$ (min)	$t_{1/2\beta}$ (min)	C_{max} (mmol/L)	V_{ss} (L)	V_d (L)
150	3.50	—	2.17	0.88	8.76	—	6.44	—
	SE = 0.90		SE = 0.39	SE = 0.12	SE = 2.03		SE = 1.46	
740	—	90.36	4.3	1.5	—	0.100	—	8.7
910	—	231.12	2.1	2.7	—	0.235	—	7.4

AUC, area under the concentration × time curve; C_{max}, maximum concentration; SE, standard error; $t_{1/2}$, half-life; V_c volume of central compartment; V_d, apparent volume of distribution; V_{ss}, volume of distribution, steady state.

WR-1065 was only one-third of the total drug concentration. The rate of decline in the concentration of WR-1065 varied among tissues. Thirty minutes after maximal WR-1065 levels were achieved, there was an 18-fold drop in WR-1065 tissue concentration in the kidney and a sixfold drop in the lung. However, 1 hour after administration, WR-1065 tissue levels only decreased by 17% in salivary gland and by 29% in cardiac muscle.

Shaw et al. studied the distribution of WR-1065 in tumor-bearing mice after a 365 mg per kg intraperitoneal injection of amifostine.[393] Within 10 minutes of injection, maximal concentrations of WR-1065 were achieved in blood, liver, and kidney. WR-1065 concentrations continued to increase in cardiac muscle and in two solid tumors for 30 minutes after injection.

Toxicity

In the phase I trial of amifostine, the single dose was escalated from 25 to 1,330 mg per m². The drug was generally well tolerated, with transient side effects including nausea, vomiting, sneezing, a warm or flushed feeling, mild somnolence, hypocalcemia, and, rarely, allergic reactions. Amifostine can produce transient hypocalcemia due to inhibition of parathyroid hormone secretion and direct inhibition of bone resorption,[405–408] but these can be managed by the use of oral calcium and calcitriol supplements.[408]

The most serious toxicity of amifostine is hypotension, which in the phase I studies was defined as a decrease in systolic blood pressure of at least 20 mm Hg lasting at least 5 minutes. Only 5% of patients required drug interruption because of a decrease in blood pressure. Hypotension occurs more often when the drug is given at slower infusion rates. The incidence of hypotension appears to be increased among patients with cancers of the head and neck, esophagus, or lung, and among patients with prior neck irradiation, carotid artery disease, or hypercalcemia.[395] The single dose of amifostine chosen for phase II studies with chemotherapy was 910 mg per m² for low-risk patients and 740 mg per m² for patients at high risk for hypotension. For fractionated radiotherapy trials, a daily dose ranging from 100 mg per m² to 340 mg per m² four times per week for 5 weeks is being used.[401,409,410] The drug is given by an infusion approximately 15 minutes before treatment. Based on data from Ben-Josef et al., a phase I trial is in progress using rectal administration for patients with prostate cancer.[411]

Amifostine and Radiotherapy

At the writing of the previous chapter, there had been a number of trials that suggested clinical efficacy for amifostine, and some of the trials have been reported.[410] Recently, a number of phase III trials have demonstrated efficacy, and the drug is now approved by the FDA.

A phase III trial for patients with advanced rectal cancer used a radiation dose of 225 cGy, 4 days per week, with or without 340 mg per m² of amifostine, to a total dose of 4,500 cGy followed, in both arms, by a boost of 720 cGy. One hundred patients were entered with no difference in acute toxicity, but a statistically significant difference in moderate and severe late toxicity (0 of 34 versus 5 of 37, p = .03).[409]

A pivotal phase III head and neck cancer trial was conducted by Brizel et al.[412,413] In this trial, patients received amifostine (200 mg per m² daily) 15 to 30 minutes before radiation. The radiation was to include at least 40 Gy to bilateral salivary glands (greater than 75% of both glands). Total tumor doses ranged from 66 to 70 Gy. The incidence of acute grade 2 xerostomia was reduced from 78% to 51% (p <.0001); the median dose to produce this side effect was higher in the amifostine group, 60 Gy versus 42 Gy (p = .0001); the incidence of chronic grade 2 xerostomia was reduced from 57% to 34% (p = .002), and unstimulated saliva production was better in the amifostine group (p = .008). There was no statistically significant difference in acute mucositis, disease-free survival, and survival (marginally better in the amifostine group, p = .11). Future studies will include higher doses of amifostine and the use of conformal, intensity modulated radiotherapy, which may add further salivary gland protection. Of note is a study indicating that amifostine protects against salivary gland toxicity for radioiodine treatment.[414]

Amifostine and Chemotherapy: Combined Modality Therapy

The data from the initial phase I and II chemoprotector trials suggested that amifostine may provide some protection against cisplatin-induced nephrotoxicity, neurotoxicity, ototoxicity,[415,416] and cyclophosphamide-induced granulocytopenia.[416,417] A number of single-arm studies have been conducted that used amifostine with chemotherapy alone, using cisplatin,[418] carboplatin,[419] or both,[420] or as part of a combined modality regimen with radiation and chemotherapy.[421] The efficacy results of these phase I and II trials had been variable, with some producing evidence of normal tissue protection.[419,420] As well, studies of interaction of amifostine with the pharmacokinetics of the platinum compounds has indicated minimal interaction with cisplatin[422] and some increase in plasma level of ultrafilterable platinum with carboplatin.[423] Such findings should be taken into consideration in chemomodifier studies with amifostine.

A randomized trial of 242 women with ovarian cancer treated with cisplatin and cyclophosphamide, with or without amifostine, demonstrated a statistically significant decrease in bone marrow toxicity and decreased incidence of neuro- and nephrotoxicity.[424] There was no loss of antitumor efficacy and survival. A phase II trial of amifostine with combined chemotherapy and radiation for unresectable stage III lung cancer produced normal tissue protection with no patients having esophagitis,[425] and in other lung cancer trials there was no evidence of tumor protection.[426,427] Thus, it appears that amifostine can produce selective normal tissue protection, representing a triumph of a prolonged effort to develop radiation protectors. Not all agents are protected from toxicity, as amifostine was shown not to reduce the incidence of neurotoxicity or hematologic toxicity of paclitaxel.[428]

The recent American Society of Clinical Oncology Clinical Practice Guidelines for the Use of Chemotherapy and Radiotherapy Protectants[429] indicates that amifostine may be considered for the reduction of nephrotoxicity for cisplatin-based chemotherapy, and xerostomia for radiotherapy. Amifostine is among the agents for reduction of neutropenia; however, the preferred agents were the growth factors. Insufficient data were available for its use in thrombocytopenia, neurotoxicity, ototoxicity, or paclitaxel-associated neurotoxicity. The Hensley et al. article is strongly recommended for the methodology and the results of the analysis for amifostine and other agents, including mesna and dexrazoxane.

Nitroxides

Preclinical studies have shown that the stable free-radical nitroxide, tempol, protects cells against the aerobic lethal damage induced by ionizing radiation in a concentration-dependent manner as shown in Figure 25-11A.[430] Nitroxides could provide biologic radioprotection by inhibiting the damage mediated by radiation-induced reactive species (X·) to biologically important molecules (BIM), such as DNA, by at least two modes.

Damage:

$$X\cdot + BIM\text{-}H \rightarrow XH + BIM\cdot \qquad [25\text{-}1]$$

Protection by radical scavenging:

$$H^+ + X\cdot + RR'NO\cdot \rightarrow HX + RR'NO^+ \qquad [25\text{-}2]$$

$$X\cdot + RR'NO\cdot \rightarrow RR'NO\text{-}X \qquad [25\text{-}3]$$

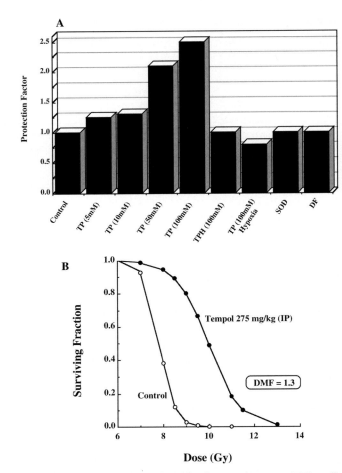

FIGURE 25-11. A: Protection of Chinese hamster V79 cells treated with tempol (TP) at concentrations of 5, 10, 50, and 100 mmol/L (aerobic and hypoxic), tempol-H (TPH) at 100 mmol/L, sodium (SOD) at 100 µg/mL, and desferrioxamine mesylate (Desferal) (DF) at 500 µmol/L, and those exposed to x-rays. Protection factors were calculated at the 10% survival by dividing the radiation dose of control cells by the radiation dose of treated cells. (Adapted with permission from Mitchell JB, DeGraff W, Kaufman D, et al. Inhibition of oxygen-dependent radiation-induced damage by the nitroxide superoxide dismutase mimic, Tempol. *Arch Biochem Biophys* 1991;289:62.) **B:** Survival of mice 30 days after whole-body radiation. Control mice received saline intraperitoneally, and treated mice received 275 mg per kg of tempol intraperitoneally 10 minutes before radiation. The dose modification factor (DMF) is 1.3. (Adapted with permission from Hahn SM, Tochner Z, Krishna CM, et al. Tempol, a stable free radical, is a novel murine radiation protector. *Cancer Res* 1992;52:1750.)

Protection by repair:

$$X\cdot + BIM\text{-}H \rightarrow XH + BIM\cdot \qquad [25\text{-}4]$$

$$H^+ + BIM\cdot + RR'NO\cdot \rightarrow BIM\text{-}H + RR'NO^+ \qquad [25\text{-}5]$$

Radiation exposure can result in the formation of carbon-centered radicals on BIM (in the case of radiation, the most likely critical intracellular target is the DNA), as shown in Equation 25-1. As proposed in Equations 25-2 and 25-3, nitroxides could scavenge radiation-induced reactive species. Likewise, Equations 25-4 and 25-5 demonstrate that nitroxides have the capability to restore a carbon-centered radical on BIM to normal by donating an electron (BIM-H). It is possible that a combination of Equations 25-2 to 25-5 operate to provide radioprotection. Radiation-induced, unrepaired, DNA DSB and subsequent production of chromosome aberrations have been closely linked with radiation-induced cell killing.[431–433] A recent study[434] showed a direct correlation between tempol-mediated *in vitro* radioprotection (cell survival) and reduced DNA DSB. Johnstone et al. showed that tempol significantly reduced the frequency of radiation-induced chromosome aberrations in human peripheral blood lymphocytes.[435] Both of these studies strongly suggest that tempol-mediated radioprotection is accompanied by a reduction in DNA damage.

The protective effects of nitroxides in *in vitro* experiments prompted the study of nitroxides using *in vivo* models. To screen stable nitroxides as *in vivo* radioprotectors, the toxicity, pharmacology, and *in vivo* radioprotective effects of tempol were studied in C3H mice.[436] Tempol administered 10 minutes before whole-body irradiation provided a PF of 1.3 at the $LD_{50/30}$ level as shown in Figure

25-11B. The primary tissue protected in this particular assay is the bone marrow. *In vivo*, tempol is rapidly reduced to the hydroxylamine, a form shown not to be radioprotective *in vitro* (see Fig. 25-11A). Despite the rapid reduction of tempol *in vivo*, significant radioprotection was observed. It is expected that *in vivo* radioprotection would be increased if higher concentrations of the oxidized form of the nitroxide were available at the time of irradiation.

The ability to selectively protect normal tissues in cancer patients receiving radiation treatment would be most advantageous. If selective protection of normal tissues were possible, higher radiation doses could be delivered to the tumor, accompanied with higher local control rates. The key, however, is *selective* normal tissue protection, because if a systemic radioprotector also protects the tumor, no advantage would be realized. To test whether systemic administration of tempol would protect against local irradiation delivered to a tumor, Hahn et al. used a RIF-1 transplantable rodent tumor to evaluate the effect of tempol on local tumor control by radiation.[43] As shown in Figures 25-11B and 25-12A, the administration of tempol to tumor-bearing mice at the same concentration and timing

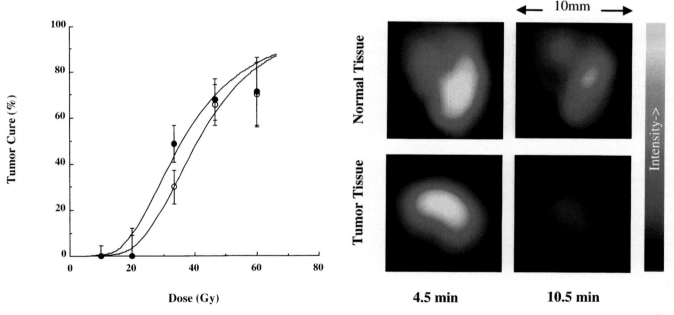

FIGURE 25-12. A: Radiation tumor control curves for animals treated in the absence or presence of tempol. The closed circles indicate tempol-treated mice and the open circles indicate phosphate-buffered saline (PBS)-treated mice. There was no statistical difference between the two curves (p = .54). The calculated tumor control dose ($TCD_{50/30}$) values for tempol-treated and PBS-treated mice were 36.7 and 41.8 grays (Gy), respectively. There was no statistical difference between these values (p = .32). (Adapted with permission from Hahn SM, Sullivan FJ, DeLuca AM, et al. Evaluation of tempol radioprotection in a murine tumor model. *Free Radic Biol Med* 1997;22:1211.) **B:** Spatially resolved clearance of nitroxide in normal and tumor tissue. After a tail vein infusion of the nitroxide, a series of two-dimensional images of the nitroxide from normal muscle (*top*) and tumor (*bottom*) were measured using L-band electron paramagnetic resonance imaging instrumentation. The nitroxide was cleared and metabolized faster in tumor compared to normal tissue. The yellow areas represent maximum uptake of the nitroxide probe. (Adapted with permission from Kuppusamy P, Afeworki M, Shankar RA, et al. In vivo electron paramagnetic resonance imaging of tumor heterogeneity and oxygenation in a murine model. *Cancer Res* 1998;58:1562.)

as used for whole-body irradiation, resulted in no protection of tumor. To identify a mechanism for the apparent differential protection of the hematopoietic system and tumor tissue, pharmacologic and EPRI studies were carried out. Pharmacologic studies showed that the percentage of oxidized tempol (the radioprotective form) was approximately twofold greater in the bone marrow compartment compared to RIF-1 tumor at the time of irradiation. Greater bioreduction of tempol occurred in the RIF-1 tumor. To further study the differential metabolism of nitroxides in normal versus tumor tissue, mice bearing approximately 1-cm-diameter tumors were administered the nitroxide, and EPRI was performed. Either the right leg with tumor or the left leg with normal tissue (muscle and skin) was used for the imaging studies. The presence of nitroxide in normal and tumor tissue was readily detected by using EPRI. A two-dimensional spatial image of the distribution of the nitroxide in normal muscle and RIF-1 tumor as a function of time is shown in Figure 25-12B. The panels in the top row show the clearance of the nitroxide in normal muscle as a function of time after administration, and the corresponding images in the bottom row show clearance from tumors. The data from the images indicate that the rate of clearance of nitroxide in tumors is faster than in normal tissue. These preliminary data imply that a potential difference exists between normal and tumor tissues with respect to bioreduction. Such a result may provide at least a partial explanation for the absence of tumor radioprotection, because it previously had been demonstrated that the oxidized form of tempol is the active radioprotector. These observations agree with earlier studies that suggest hypoxic cells within tumors reduce nitroxides more efficiently than well-oxygenated normal tissue.[437] Estimates of oxygen concentration in the tissues shown in Figure 25-2B using EPRI and oximetry indeed confirmed that the tumor tissue was much lower in oxygen concentration than normal tissue.[44] As the technique evolves and becomes more sensitive, EPRI may play a useful role in advancing functional imaging in clinical medicine and providing a means to determine whether nitroxides might be useful as selective normal tissue radioprotectors.

Another application of nitroxides as radioprotectors, which may have benefit in a clinical setting, would be to protect against radiation-induced alopecia, a common radiotherapeutic problem. Hair loss as a result of irradiation, especially from whole-brain irradiation, often leads to cosmetic, social, and psychological problems for the radiotherapy patient. Clinically, no successful interventions are available. Topical application of tempol was evaluated for possible protective effects against radiation-induced alopecia, using guinea pig skin as a model. For single acute doses up to 30 Gy, tempol, when topically applied 15 minutes before irradiation, provided a marked increase in the rate and extent of new hair recovery when compared to untreated irradiated skin.[437] Using EPR spectroscopy, tem-

pol was detected in treated skin specimens. EPR measurements of blood samples and brain tissue failed to show any systemic nitroxide signal resulting from topical application to skin or scalp. These studies have been extended to evaluate fractionated radiation delivery with multiple applications of tempol or tempo.[438] Topical administration of tempol or Tempo 15 minutes before each radiation treatment (daily fractions of 7 Gy, for a total of eight treatments over 10 days) resulted in statistically significant radioprotection with respect to hair loss and regrowth of hair in the treatment field.[438] Histologic evaluation showed that radiation treatment without nitroxide resulted in a marked decrease in the number of hair follicles, and poor development of remaining follicles; however, nitroxide pretreatment resulted in no appreciable decrease in hair follicles and hair follicles appeared mature, similar to unirradiated controls.[438] These studies suggest that the topical application of nitroxides may be useful clinically to reduce the undesirable toxicity of radiation-induced alopecia. Likewise, topical application of nitroxides may have utility in other sites, such as rectum and bladder, two normal tissues at risk from radiation treatment of prostate or cervix cancer, or both. The advantage of topical application is that high concentrations of the nitroxide could be used directly on the tissue at risk. The resulting systemic levels of the drug after topical administration would hopefully be inadequate to protect the tumor or cause systemic toxicity. The use of nitroxides to protect against radiation-induced alopecia is presently being evaluated in the clinic.

Prostaglandin Analogs as Radiation Protectors

Hanson and co-workers have shown that the prostaglandin E_1 analog, misoprostol [(16RS)-15-deoxy-16-hydroxy-16-methyl prostaglandin E_1 methyl ester], is a most effective radioprotector of a variety of normal tissues, including gut,[439] hematopoietic stem cells,[439] oral muscosa,[440] and hair follicles.[441–443] Preclinical studies have shown that administration of misoprostol to tumor-bearing animals does not protect against radiation-induced tumor regrowth or cure.[444] The mechanism of radioprotection is poorly understood but apparently does not involve free-radical scavenging.[445] It has recently been suggested that misoprostol-mediated radioprotection occurs by changes in chromatin structure and DNA repair.[446] A phase II clinical trial was recently completed evaluating misoprostol as a protector against oral and pharyngeal mucositis in head and neck cancer patients receiving fractionated radiotherapy, and results of the trial are pending.

Other Protectors

There is interest in the novel protectors from mucosal tissue injury, including potential uses of keratinocyte growth factor, as noted above,[412] and other unique approaches, such as the somatostatin analog octreotide.[447] Analogous to the success with hematologic growth factors, these represent novel areas of investigation likely to be in clinical trials over the next few years. One interesting observation that has important implications for the mechanism of late radiation injury is the report of the reversal of chronic radiotherapy damage in a clinical trial of the combination of pentoxifylline and tocopherol.[41] This finding implies that "chronic" injury may have a substantial ongoing inflammatory and biochemical process that can be reversed, at least in part.

FUTURE APPROACHES

The explosion in new knowledge of cancer, tumor, cellular, molecular, and structural biology along with highly innovative techniques, such as complementary DNA microarrays, combinatorial chemistry, and sequencing, have produced an almost innumerable number of potential new therapeutic targets. In this section, some of the possibilities are illustrated in "cartoon" fashion, as it is well beyond the scope of any single chapter to cover all the new molecular findings in radiation oncology and biology. We apologize to the many investigators for not specifically referencing their work.

Figure 25-13 is an updated illustration of the many potential targets for radiation modification. It also illustrates the importance of the tumor cell environment. The molecular targets for radiation therapy exist in a number of levels or environments. Figure 25-14 is an attempt at a cartoon to illustrate the different dimensions at which radiation therapy "works." Some poetic license is taken in subdividing the environments.

The "macro" environment includes the surrounding normal tissue. This is approached through improved radiation technology, such as three-dimensional conformal therapy, IMRT, improved brachytherapy techniques, and new imaging modalities. Biologically, there are the normal tissue radioprotectors. The *normo* environment is defined as the circulation and perfusion. This includes not only oxygen and nutrients, but also drugs and biologics, such as pharmacokinetic consideration. As new therapies are developed, they must reach the tumor in adequate concentration. Pharmacokinetic-derived therapy is becoming more and more common as the relationship between drug concentration and efficacy and toxicity is better understood. Furthermore, using techniques, such as PET, MRI, and EPRI, it might be possible to image drug delivery and time therapy accordingly. The *micro* environment includes all of the cells, stroma, growth factors, cytokines, and so forth. The tumor is a complex structure and the response of a tumor cell to treatment depends on its neighbors and neighborhood. The microenvironment is not only complex in composition but also in dynamism. Intermittent blood flow produces an ischemia reperfusion situation in which any measure is only indicative of the environment at the time of

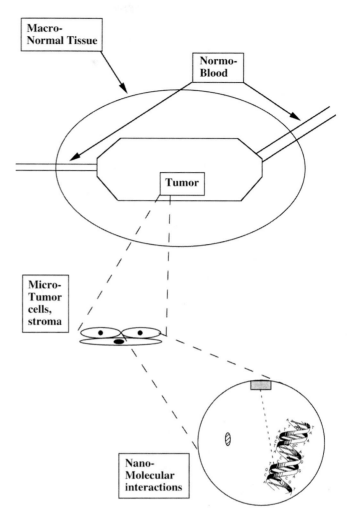

FIGURE 25-13. Radiation targets are illustrated by environments in the "powers of 1,000." Imaging and technical delivery improve results at the macroenvironmental level by reducing dose to normal tissue and increasing dose to tumor tissue. The normoenvironment includes blood flow, drug delivery, and prognostic factors, such as secreted factors, that can be measured in the clinical laboratory. The microenvironment includes what can be seen under the microscope, such as tumor cells, stroma, and inflammatory cells, and that which can be measured with instruments, such as the oxygen electrode or pressure transducers for interstitial pressure. The nanoenvironment is where physics and biology begin to meet (at the subcellular and molecular targets). To optimize the use of radiation and radiation modifiers, it is useful to conceptualize radiation as working in all of its "environments."

the measurement. For that reason, functional and molecular imaging are critical to understanding tumor biology. The *nano* environment refers to molecular interaction and pharmacology. For radiation, there is a heterogeneous distribution at the end of the energy deposition track. Similarly, it is becoming clear that the cell is an organized structure, so that the relationship among molecules is such that many exist in multimolecular complexes.

The range of molecular targets is enumerated in Figure 25-13. As described earlier, there are two general types of

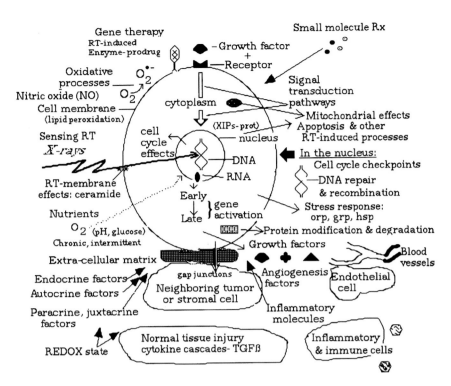

FIGURE 25-14. Radiation biology—year 2000 (Y2K) compliant. This "cartoon figure" has evolved over the years to include the complexity of radiation biology. Taken in conjunction with Figure 25-13, it contains some of the new cellular, subcellular, and molecular targets that will be the focus of the new biology that is rapidly emerging with the sequencing of the human genome, the new techniques to study gene expression (e.g., complementary DNA and tissue microarrays), and the new approaches to drug development (targeting specific molecular targets using structural biology and developing an enormous range of structures through combinatorial chemistry). Although Y2K compliant, this figure will undoubtedly be out of date almost as soon as it is published. (grp, glucose-regulated protein; hsp, heat-shock protein; orp, oxygen-regulated protein; REDOX, oxidation-reduction; RT, radiation therapy; TGFβ, transforming growth factor β; XIP, x-ray–inducible protein.)

targets. DNA damage is a critical lesion, so that processes that increase DNA damage and decrease DNA repair would be effective strategies. The other group of targets is the many molecular processes that are induced by irradiation, the modification of which might lead to cell death. These include, but are not limited to, cell membrane, receptors, signal transduction, cell-cycle checkpoints, gene transcription, posttranslational modification, protein degradation, apoptosis, growth factor and cytokine production, cell motility, immunologic response, angiogenesis, and cell-cell interaction.

CONCLUSIONS

In the same chapter from the previous edition, the conclusion noted that there has been steady and logical progress in the chemical modifiers field in understanding the basic biology of radiation resistance and in developing improved therapies. In the year 2000, there was a phenomenal increase in new knowledge, but limited introduction of new therapies. Amifostine was approved, and tirapazamine may soon be approved, opening up a new approach toward the hypoxic cell. The hypoxic cell–sensitizer etanidazole did not provide a therapeutic benefit, yet there are studies indicating that hypoxia is important in clinical radiation therapy. The next few years will bring exciting changes in cancer biology. Conceptualizing radiation and other forms of energy, such as heat, light, and sound, as focused biologies makes it easy to see the important role that the fields radiation oncology and radiation biology will have in

improving the quality and duration of life, and how the clinical use of radiation may be critical to the clinical "proof of principle" of many of the molecular therapeutics that are rapidly emerging.

REFERENCES

1. Goodhead DT. Initial events in the cellular effects of ionizing radiations: clustered damage in DNA. *Int J Radiat Biol* 1994;65:7.
2. Nikjoo H, Uehara S, Wilson WE, et al. Track structure in radiation biology: theory and applications. *Int J Radiat Biol* 1998;73:355.
3. Wouters BG, Skarsgard LD. Low-dose radiation sensitivity and induced radioresistance to cell killing in HT-29 cells is distinct from the adaptive response and cannot be explained by a subpopulation of sensitive cells [see comments]. *Radiat Res* 1997;148:435.
4. Amundson SA, Do KT, Fornace AJJ. Induction of stress genes by low doses of gamma rays. *Radiat Res* 1999;152:225.
5. Coleman CN, Harris JR. Current scientific issues related to clinical radiation oncology [comment]. *Radiat Res* 1998;150:125.
6. Bornstein BA, Herman TS, Hansen JL, et al. Pilot study of local hyperthermia, radiation therapy, etanidazole, and cisplatin for advanced superficial tumours. *Int J Hyperthermia* 1995;11:489.
7. Urtasun R, Band P, Chapman JD, et al. Radiation and high-dose metronidazole in supratentorial glioblastomas. *N Engl J Med* 1976;294:1364.
8. Herscher LL, Cook JA, Pacelli R, et al. Principles of chemoradiation: theoretical and practical considerations. *Oncology Suppl* 1999;5:11.

9. Levine M. The action of colchicine on cell division in human cancer, animal, and plant tissues. *Ann N Y Acad Sci* 1951;51:1365.

10. Skipper HG, Chapman JB, Bell M. The antileukemic action of combinations of certain known antileukemic agents. *Cancer Res* 1951;11:109.

11. Heidelberger C, Griesbach L, Montag BJ, et al. Studies of fluorinated pyrimidines. II. Effects of transplanted tumors. *Cancer Res* 1958;18:305.

12. Gollin FF, Ansfield FJ, Curreri AR, et al. Combined chemotherapy and irradiation in inoperable bronchogenic carcinoma. *Cancer* 1962;15:1209.

13. Hall TG, Dederick MM, Chalmers TC, et al. A clinical pharmacologic study of chemotherapy and x-ray therapy in lung cancer. *Am J Med* 1967;43:186.

14. Childs DS, Moertel CG, Holbrook MA. Treatment of unresectable adenocarcinomas of the stomach with a combination of 5-fluorouracil and radiation. *Am J Roentgenol Radium Ther Nucl Med* 1968;102:541.

15. Moertel CG, Childs DS, Reitemeier RJ, et al. Combined 5-fluorouracil and supervoltage radiation therapy of locally unresectable gastrointestional cancer. *Lancet* 1969;2:865.

16. Nigro ND, Vaitkevicus VK, Considine B. Combined therapy for cancer of the anal canal: a preliminary report. *Dis Col Rect* 1974;17:354.

17. Phillips TL, Fu KK. Quantification of combined radiation therapy and chemotherapy effects on critical normal tissues. *Cancer* 1976;37:1186.

18. Tubiana M. The combination of radiotherapy and chemotherapy: a review. *Int J Radiat Biol* 1989;55:497.

19. Withers HR, Taylor JMG, Maciejewski B. The hazard of accelerated tumor clonogen repopulation during radiotherapy. *Acta Oncologica* 1988;27:131.

20. Young RC. *Drug resistance in cancer therapy*. Boston: Kluwer Academic Publishers, 1989:1.

21. Hill BT, Bellamy AS. *Antitumor drug-radiation interactions*. Boca Raton, FL: CRC Press, 1990.

22. Phillips TL. Terminology for chemoradiation effects. In: Flam MS, Legha SS, Phillips TL, eds. *Chemoradiation: an integrated approach to cancer treatment*. Philadelphia: Lea & Febiger, 1993:11.

23. Phillips TL. Radiation-chemotherapy interactions. In: Pass HI, Mitchell JB, Johnson DH, et al., eds. *Lung cancer: principles and practice*. Philadelphia: Lippincott–Raven Publishers, 1996:251.

24. Munro TR. The relative radiosensitivity of the nucleus and cytoplasm of the Chinese hamster fibroblasts. *Radiat Res* 1970;42:451.

25. Radford IR. Evidence for a general relationship between the induced level of DNA double-strand breakage and cell-killing after X-irradiation of mammalian cells. *Int J Radiat Biol* 1986;49:611.

26. Kinsella TJ, Dobson PP, Mitchell JB, et al. Enhancement of X ray induced DNA damage by pre-treatment with halogenated pyrimidine analogs. *Int J Radiat Oncol Biol Phys* 1987;13:733.

27. Wang Y, Pantelias GE, Iliakis G. Mechanism of radiosensitization by halogenated pyrimidines: the contribution of excess DNA and chromosome damage in BrdU radiosensitization may be minimal in plateau-phase cells. *Int J Radiat Biol* 1994;66:133.

28. Utsumi H, Elkind MM. Potentially lethal damage versus sublethal damage: independent repair processes in actively growing Chinese hamster cells. *Radiat Res* 1979;77:346.

29. Elkind MM, Whitmore GF. Chromosome damage and other cytological effects. In: Elkind MM, ed. *The radiobiology of cultured mammalian cells*. New York: Gordon & Breach, 1967:383.

30. Puck TT, Markus PI. Action of x-rays on mammalian cells. *J Exp Med* 1956;103:653.

31. Steel GG, Deacon JM, Duchesne GM, et al. The dose-rate effect in human tumour cells. *Radiother Oncol* 1987;9:299.

32. Steel GG. *Growth kinetics of tumours*. Oxford, UK: Clarendon, 1977:191.

33. Terasima R, Tolmach LJ. X-ray sensitivity and DNA synthesis in synchronous populations of HeLa cells. *Science* 1963;140:490.

34. Sinclair WK. Hydroxyurea revisited: a decade of clinical effects studies. *Int J Radiat Oncol Biol Phys* 1981;7:631.

35. Tishler RB, Geard CR, Hall EJ, et al. Taxol sensitizers human astrocytoma cells to radiation. *Cancer Res* 1992;52:3495.

36. Liebmann JE, Cook JA, Fisher J, et al. In vitro studies of paclitaxel (Taxol) as a radiation sensitizer in human tumor cells. *J Natl Cancer Inst* 1994;86:441.

37. Milas L, Saito Y, Hunter N, et al. Therapeutic potential of paclitaxel-radiation treatment of a murine ovarian carcinoma. *Radiother Oncol* 1996;40:163.

38. Coleman CN, Mitchell JB. Clinical radiosensitization: why it does and does not work. *J Clin Oncol* 1999;17:1.

39. Wilson GD. Assessment of human tumour proliferation using bromodeoxyuridine—current status. *Acta Oncologica* 1991;30:903.

40. Rojas A, Steward FA, Soranson JA, et al. Fractionation studies with WR-2721: normal tissues and tumour. *Radiother Oncol* 1986;6:51.

41. Delanian S, Balla-Mekias S, Lefaiz JL. Striking regression of chronic radiotherapy damage in a clinical trial of combined pentoxifylline and tocopherol. *J Clin Oncol* 1999;17:3283.

42. Hahn SM, Krishna MC, Samuni A, et al. Potential use of nitroxides in radiation oncology. *Cancer Res* 1994;54:2006.

43. Hahn SM, Sullivan FJ, DeLuca AM, et al. Evaluation of tempol radioprotection in a murine tumor model. *Free Radic Biol Med* 1997;22:1211.

44. Kuppusamy P, Afeworki M, Shankar RA, et al. In vivo electron paramagnetic resonance imaging of tumor heterogeneity and oxygenation in a murine model. *Cancer Res* 1998;58:1562.

45. Jain RK. Barriers to drug delivery in solid tumors. *Sci Am* 1994;271:58.

46. Kartner N, Ling V. Multidrug resistance in cancer. *Sci Am* 1989;260:44.

47. Batist G, Tulpule A, Sinha B, et al. Overexpression of a novel anionic glutathione transferase in multidrug-resistant human breast cancer cells. *J Biol Chem* 1986;261:15544.

48. Muller M, Brunner M, Schmid R, et al. Interstitial methotrexate kinetics in primary breast cancer lesions. *Cancer Res* 1998;58:2982.

49. Liebmann J, Herscher L, Fisher J, et al. Antagonism of paclitaxel cytotoxicity by x-rays: implications for the sequence of combined modality therapy. *Int J Oncol* 1996;8:991.

50. Chaplin DJ, Hill SA, Bell KM, et al. Modification of tumour blood flow: current status and future directions. *Semin Radiat Oncol* 1998;8:151.

51. Dewhirst MW. Concepts of oxygen transport at the microcirculatory level. *Semin Radiat Oncol* 1998;8:143.

52. Thomlinson RH, Gray LH. The histological structure of some human lung cancers and the possible implications for radiotherapy. *Br J Cancer* 1995;9:539.

53. Yuan F. Transvascular drug delivery in solid tumors. *Semin Radiat Oncol* 1998;8:164.

54. Gerweck L. Tumor pH: implications for treatment and novel drug design. *Semin Radiat Oncol* 1998;8:176.

55. Hockel M, Schlenger K, Aral B, et al. Association between tumor hypoxia and malignant progression in advanced cancer of the uterine cervix. *Cancer Res* 1996;56:4509.

56. Mitchell JB, Gamson J, Russo A, et al. Chinese hamster pleiotropic multidrug-resistant cells are not radioresistant. *NCI Monogr* 1988;6:187.

57. Virchow R. *Krankhaften geschwulste*. Berlin, 1863.

58. Burnet FM. The concept of immunological surveillance. *Prog Exp Tumor Res* 1970;13:1.

59. Ioachim HL. The stromal reaction of tumors: an expression of immune surveillance. *J Natl Cancer Inst* 1976;57:465.

60. Underwood JC. A morphometric analysis of human breast carcinoma. *Br J Cancer* 1972;26:234.

61. Simone NL, Bonner RF, Gillespie JW, et al. Laser-capture microdissection: opening the microscopic frontier to molecular analysis. *Trends Genet* 1998;14:272.

62. Pappalardo PA, Bonner R, Krizman DB, et al. Microdissection, microchip arrays, and molecular analysis of tumor cells (primary and metastases). *Semin Radiat Oncol* 1998;8:217.

63. Coleman CN. Radiation and chemotherapy sensitizers and protectors. In: Chabner BA, Longo DL, eds. *Cancer chemotherapy and biotherapy*. Philadelphia: Lippincott–Raven Publishers, 1996:553.

64. Hall EJ. Chemotherapeutic agents from the perspective of the radiation biologist. In: Hall EJ, ed. *Radiobiology for the radiologist*. Philadelphia: JB Lippincott Co, 1994:289.

65. Milas L, Milas MM, Mason KA. Combination of taxanes with radiation: preclinical studies. *Semin Radiat Oncol* 1999;9:12.

66. Choy H. Concurrent paclitaxel and radiation therapy in the treatment of solid tumors. *Semin Radiat Oncol* 1999;9:1.

67. Ornstein DL, Nervi AM, Rigas JR. Docetaxel (Taxotere) in combination chemotherapy and in association with thoracic radiotherapy for the treatment of non-small-cell lung cancer. Thoracic Oncology Program. *Am Oncol* 1999;10(Suppl 5):S35.

68. Lawrence TS, Eisbruch A, McGinn CJ, et al. Radiosensitization by gemcitabine. *Oncology* 1999;10(Suppl 5):55.

69. Chen AY, Okunieff P, Pommier Y, et al. Mammalian DNA topoisomerase I mediates the enhancement of radiation cytotoxicity by camptothecin derivatives. *Cancer Res* 1997;57:1529.

70. Rothenberg ML, Blanke CD. Topoisomerase I inhibitors in the treatment of colorectal cancer. *Semin Radiat Oncol* 1999;6:632.

71. Chen AY, Choy H, Rothenberg ML. DNA topoisomerase I-targeting drugs as radiation sensitizers. *Oncology* 1999;13:39.

72. Perez LM, Greer S. Sensitization to X ray by 5-chloro-2'-deoxycytidine co-administered with tetrahydrouridine in several mammalian cell lines and studies of 2'-chloro derivatives. *Int J Radiat Oncol Biol Phys* 1986;12:1523.

73. McGinn CJ, Shewach DS, Lawrence TS. Radiosensitizing nucleosides. *J Natl Cancer Inst* 1996;88:1193.

74. Szybalski W. X-ray sensitization by halopyrimidines. *Cancer Chemother Rep* 1974;58:539.

75. Kinsella TJ, Mitchell JB, Russo A, et al. The use of halogenated thymidine analogs as clinical radiosensitizers: rationale, current status, and future prospects: non-hypoxic cell sensitizers. *Int J Radiat Oncol Biol Phys* 1984;10:1399.

76. Mitchell JB, Russo A, Kinsella TJ, et al. The use of non-hypoxic cell sensitizers in radiobiology and radiotherapy. *Int J Radiat Oncol Biol Phys* 1986;12:1513.

77. Cook JA, Glass J, Lebovics R, et al. Measurement of thymidine replacement in patients with high grade gliomas, head and neck tumors, and high grade sarcomas after continuous intravenous infusions of 5-iododeoxyuridine. *Cancer Res* 1992;52:719.

78. Bagshaw MA, Doggett RL, Smith KC, et al. Intra-arterial 5-bromodeoxyuridine and x-ray therapy. *Am J Roentgenol Radium Ther Nucl Med* 1967;99:886.

79. Kinsella TJ, Russo A, Mitchell JB, et al. A Phase I study of intermittent intravenous bromodeoxyuridine (BUdR) with conventional fractionated irradiation. *Int J Radiat Oncol Biol Phys* 1984;10:69.

80. Mitchell JB, Kinsella TJ, Russo A, et al. Radiosensitization of hematopoietic precursor cells (CFUc) in glioblastoma patients receiving intermittent intravenous infusions of bromodeoxyuridine (BUdR). *Int J Radiat Oncol Biol Phys* 1983;9:457.

81. Mitchell JB, Morstyn G, Russo A, et al. Differing sensitivity to fluorescent light in Chinese hamster cells containing equally incorporated quantities of BUdR versus IUdR. *Int J Radiat Oncol Biol Phys* 1984;10:1447.

82. Kinsella TJ, Glatstein E. Clinical experience with intravenous radiosensitizers in unresectable sarcomas. *Cancer* 1987;59:908.

83. Lawrence TS, Davis MA, Maybaum J, et al. The potential superiority of bromodeoxyuridine to iododeoxyuridine as a radiation sensitizer in the treatment of colorectal cancer. *Cancer Res* 1992;52:3698.

84. Kinsella TJ, Russo A, Mitchell JB, et al. A phase I study of intravenous iododeoxyuridine as a clinical radiosensitizer. *Int J Radiat Oncol Biol Phys* 1985;11:1941.

85. Klecker RWJ, Jenkins JF, Kinsella TJ, et al. Clinical pharmacology of 5-iodo-2'-deoxyuridine and 5-iodouracil and endogenous pyrimidine modulation. *Clin Pharmacol Ther* 1985;38:45.

86. Eisbruch A, Robertson JM, Johnston CM, et al. Bromodeoxyuridine alternating with radiation for advanced uterine cervix cancer: a phase I and drug incorporation study [see comments]. *J Clin Oncol* 1999;17:31.

87. Robertson JM, McGinn CJ, Walker S, et al. A phase I trial of hepatic arterial bromodeoxyuridine and conformal radiation therapy for patients with primary hepatobiliary cancers or colorectal liver metastases. *Int J Radiat Oncol Biol Phys* 1997;39:1087.

88. Greer S, Schwade J, Marion HS. Five-chlorodeoxycytidine and biomodulators of its metabolism result in fifty to eighty

percent cures of advanced EMT-6 tumors when used with fractionated radiation. *Int J Radiat Oncol Biol Phys* 1995;32:1059.

89. Russell KJ, Rice GC, Brown JM. In vitro and in vivo radiation sensitization by the halogenated pyrimidine 5-chloro-2'-deoxycytidine. *Cancer Res* 1986;46:2883.

90. Tochner Z, Kinsella TJ, Rowland J, et al. *BIR Report 19.* London: British Institute of Radiology, 1989:107.

91. Chang AE, Collins JM, Speth PA, et al. A phase I study of intraarterial iododeoxyuridine in patients with colorectal liver metastases. *J Clin Oncol* 1989;7:662.

92. Rodriguez R, Kinsella TJ. Halogenated pyrimidines as radiosensitizers for high grade glioma: revisited [editorial; comment]. *Int J Radiat Oncol Biol Phys* 1991;21:859.

93. Phillips TL, Levin VA, Ahn DK, et al. Evaluation of bromodeoxyuridine in glioblastoma multiforme: a Northern California Cancer Center Phase II study [see comments]. *Int J Radiat Oncol Biol Phys* 1991;21:709.

94. Urtasun RC, Kinsella TJ, Farnan N, et al. Survival improvement in anaplastic astrocytoma, combining external radiation with halogenated pyrimidines: final report of RTOG 86-12, Phase I–II study [see comments]. *Int J Radiat Oncol Biol Phys* 1996;36:1163.

95. Prados MD, Scott CB, Rotman M, et al. Influence of bromodeoxyuridine radiosensitization on malignant glioma patient survival: a retrospective comparison of survival data from the Northern California Oncology Group (NCOG) and Radiation Therapy Oncology Group trials (RTOG) for glioblastoma multiforme and anaplastic astrocytoma. *Int J Radiat Oncol Biol Phys* 1998;40:653.

96. Nath R, Bongiorni P, Rockwell S. Iododeoxyuridine radiosensitization by low- and high-energy photons for brachytherapy dose rates. *Radiat Res* 1990;124:249.

97. Tishler RB, Geard CR. Low dose rate irradiation and halogenated pyrimidine effects on human cervical carcinoma cells. *Int J Radiat Oncol Biol Phys* 1991;21:975.

98. McLaughlin PW, Mancini WR, Stetson PL, et al. Halogenated pyrimidine sensitization of low dose rate irradiation in human malignant glioma. *Int J Radiat Oncol Biol Phys* 1993;26:637.

99. Williams JA, Dillehay LE, Tabassi K, et al. Implantable biodegradable polymers for IUdR radiosensitization of experimental human malignant glioma. *J Neurooncol* 1997;32:181.

100. Epstein AH, Lebovics RS, Van Waes C, et al. Intravenous delivery of 5'-iododeoxyuridine during hyperfractionated radiotherapy for locally advanced head and neck cancers: results of a pilot study. *Laryngoscope* 1998;108:1090.

101. Kinsella TJ, Kunugi KA, Vielhuber KA, et al. Preclinical evaluation of 5-iodo-2-pyrimidinone-2'-deoxyribose as a prodrug for 5-iodo-2'-deoxyuridine-mediated radiosensitization in mouse and human tissues. *Clin Cancer Res* 1998;4:99.

102. Franken NA, van Bree C, Veltmaat MA, et al. Increased chromosome exchange frequencies in iodo-deoxyuridine-sensitized human SW-1573 cells after gamma-irradiation. *Oncol Rep* 1999;6:59.

103. Peters LJ, Withers HR, Thames HDJ, et al. Tumor radioresistance in clinical radiotherapy. *Int J Radiat Oncol Biol Phys* 1982;8:101.

104. Fertil B, Malaise EP. Intrinsic radiosensitivity of human cell lines is correlated with radioresponsiveness of human tumors: analysis of 101 published survival curves. *Int J Radiat Oncol Biol Phys* 1985;11:1699.

105. Coleman CN. Hypoxic cell radiosensitizers: expectations and progress in drug development. *Int J Radiat Oncol Biol Phys* 1985;11:323.

106. *Seminars in radiation oncology.* Philadelphia: WB Saunders, 1996:1.

107. Overgaard J, Horsman MR. Modification of hypoxia-induced radioresistance in tumors by the use of oxygen and sensitizers. *Semin Radiat Oncol* 1996;6:10.

108. Stone HB, Brown JM, Phillips TL, et al. Oxygen in human tumors: correlations between methods of measurement and response to therapy. Summary of a workshop held November 19–20, 1992, at the National Cancer Institute, Bethesda, Maryland. *Radiat Res* 1993;136:422.

109. Horsman MR. Measurement of tumor oxygenation. *Int J Radiat Oncol Biol Phys* 1998;42:701.

110. Siemann DW. The tumor microenvironment: a double-edged sword. *Int J Radiat Oncol Biol Phys* 1998;42:697.

111. Hall EJ. The oxygen effect and reoxygenation. In: Hall EJ, ed. *Radiobiology for the radiologist.* Philadelphia: JB Lippincott Co, 1994:133.

112. Teicher BA, Holden SA, al-Achi A, et al. Classification of antineoplastic treatments by their differential toxicity toward putative oxygenated and hypoxic tumor subpopulations in vivo in the FSaIIC murine fibrosarcoma. *Cancer Res* 1990;50:3339.

113. Powers WE, Tolmach LJ. A multicomponent x ray survival curve for mouse lymphosarcoma cells irradiated in vivo. *Nature* 1963;197:710.

114. Moulder JE, Rockwell S. Hypoxic fractions of solid tumors: experimental techniques, methods of analysis, and a survey of existing data. *Int J Radiat Oncol Biol Phys* 1984;10:695.

115. Rockwell S, Moulder JE. Hypoxic fractions of human tumors xenografted into mice: a review. *Int J Radiat Oncol Biol Phys* 1990;19:197.

116. Gatenby RA, Kessler HB, Rosenblum JS, et al. Oxygen distribution in squamous cell carcinoma metastases and its relationship to outcome of radiation therapy. *Int J Radiat Oncol Biol Phys* 1988;14:831.

117. Vaupel P, Schlenger K, Knoop C, et al. Oxygenation of human tumors: evaluation of tissue oxygen distribution in breast cancers by computerized O2 tension measurements. *Cancer Res* 1991;51:3316.

118. Hockel M, Knoop C, Schlenger K, et al. Intratumoral pO2 predicts survival in advanced cancer of the uterine cervix. *Radiother Oncol* 1993;26:45.

119. Brizel DM, Sibley GS, Prosnitz LR, et al. Tumor hypoxia adversely affects the prognosis of carcinoma of the head and neck. *Int J Radiat Oncol Biol Phys* 1997;38:285.

120. Horsman MR, Nordsmark M, Overgaard J. Techniques to assess the oxygenation of human tumors: state of the art. *Strahlenther Onkol* 1998;174(Suppl 4):2.

121. Fyles AW, Milosevic M, Wong R, et al. Oxygenation predicts radiation response and survival in patients with cervix cancer. *Radiother Oncol* 1998;48:149.

122. Movsas B, Chapman JD, Horwitz EM, et al. Hypoxic regions exist in human prostate carcinoma. *Urology* 1999; 53:11.

123. Vaupel P, Thews O, Kelleher DK, et al. Oxygenation of

human tumors: the Mainz experience. *Strahlenther Onkol* 1998;174(Suppl 4):6.

124. Chapman JD, Franko AJ, Sharplin J. A marker for hypoxic cells in tumours with potential clinical applicability. *Br J Cancer* 1981;43:546.

125. Franko AJ, Chapman JD, Koch CJ. Binding of misonidazole to EMt6 and V79 spheroids. *Int J Radiat Oncol Biol Phys* 1982;8:737.

126. Horowitz M, Blasberg R, Molnar P, et al. Regional [14C]misonidazole distribution in experimental RT-9 brain tumors. *Cancer Res* 1983;43:3800.

127. Urtasun RC, Chapman JD, Raleigh JA, et al. Binding of 3H-misonidazole to solid human tumors as a measure of tumor hypoxia. *Int J Radiat Oncol Biol Phys* 1986;12:1263.

128. Evans SM, Jenkins WT, Joiner B, et al. 2-Nitroimidazole (EF5) binding predicts radiation resistance in individual 9L s.c. tumors. *Cancer Res* 1996;56:405.

129. Lee J, Siemann DW, Koch CJ, et al. Direct relationship between radiobiologic hypoxia in tumors and monoclonal antibody detection of EF5 cellular adducts. *Int J Cancer* 1996;67:372.

130. Varia MA, Calkins-Adams DP, Rinker LH, et al. Pimonidazole: a novel hypoxia marker for complementary study of tumor hypoxia and cell proliferation in cervical carcinoma. *Gynecol Oncol* 1998;71:270.

131. Ostling O, Johanson KJ. Microelectrophoretic study of radiation-induced DNA damages in individual mammalian cells. *Biochem Biophys Res Commun* 1984;123:291.

132. Olive PL, Banath JP, Durand RE. Heterogeneity in radiation-induced DNA damage and repair in tumor and normal cells measured using the "Comet" assay. *Radiat Res* 1990;122:86.

133. Olive PL, Horsman MR, Grau C, et al. Detection of hypoxic cells in a C3H mouse mammary carcinoma using the comet assay. *Br J Cancer* 1997;76:694.

134. McLaren DB, Pickles T, Thomson T, et al. Impact of nicotinamide on human tumour hypoxic fraction measured using the comet assay. *Radiother Oncol* 1997;45:175.

135. Banath JP, Wallace SS, Thompson J, et al. Radiation-induced DNA base damage detected in individual aerobic and hypoxic cells with endonuclease III and formamidopyrimidine-glycosylase. *Radiat Res* 1999;151:550.

136. Aquino-Parsons C, Luo C, Vikse CM, et al. Comparison between the comet assay and the oxygen microelectrode for measurement of tumor hypoxia. *Radiother Oncol* 1999;51:179.

137. Fu KK, Wendland MF, Iyer SB, et al. Correlations between in vivo 31P NMR spectroscopy measurements, tumor size, hypoxic fraction and cell survival after radiotherapy. *Int J Radiat Oncol Biol Phys* 1990;18:1341.

138. Thomas C, Counsell C, Wood P, et al. Use of fluorine-19 nuclear magnetic resonance spectroscopy and hydralazine for measuring dynamic changes in blood perfusion volume in tumors in mice. *J Natl Cancer Inst* 1992;84:174.

139. McCoy CL, McIntyre DJ, Robinson SP, et al. Magnetic resonance spectroscopy and imaging methods for measuring tumour and tissue oxygenation. *Br J Cancer Suppl* 1996;27:S226.

140. Aboagye EO, Maxwell RJ, Kelson AB, et al. Preclinical evaluation of the fluorinated 2-nitroimidazole N-(2-hydroxy-3,3,3-trifluoropropyl)-2-(2-nitro-1-imidazolyl) ace-

tamide (SR-4554) as a probe for the measurement of tumor hypoxia. *Cancer Res* 1997;57:3314.

141. Robinson SP, Howe FA, Rodrigues LM, et al. Magnetic resonance imaging techniques for monitoring changes in tumor oxygenation and blood flow. *Semin Radiat Oncol* 1998;8:197.

142. Griffiths JR, Taylor NJ, Howe FA, et al. The response of human tumors to carbogen breathing, monitored by Gradient-Recalled Echo Magnetic Resonance Imaging. *Int J Radiat Oncol Biol Phys* 1997;39:697.

143. Leunbach I. On a novel MRI technique (OMRI) for the determination of tissue parameters. *Acta Anaesthesiol Scand Suppl* 1997;110:121.

144. Golman K, Leunbach I, Ardenkjaer-Larsen JH, et al. Overhauser-enhanced MR imaging (OMRI). *Acta Radiol* 1998;39:10.

145. Afeworki M, van Dam GM, Devasahayam N, et al. Three-dimensional whole body imaging of spin probes in mice by time-domain radiofrequency electron paramagnetic resonance. *Magnet Res Med* 2000;43:375.

146. Koh WJ, Rasey JS, Evans ML, et al. Imaging of hypoxia in human tumors with [F-18]fluoromisonidazole. *Int J Radiat Oncol Biol Phys* 1992;22:199.

147. Rasey JS, Koh WJ, Evans ML, et al. Quantifying regional hypoxia in human tumors with positron emission tomography of [18F]fluoromisonidazole: a pretherapy study of 37 patients. *Int J Radiat Oncol Biol Phys* 1996;36:417.

148. Chapman JD, Engelhardt EL, Stobbe CC, et al. Measuring hypoxia and predicting tumor radioresistance with nuclear medicine assays. *Radiother Oncol* 1998;46:229.

149. Rasey JS, Hofstrand PD, Chin LK, et al. Characterization of [18F]fluoroetanidazole, a new radiopharmaceutical for detecting tumor hypoxia. *J Nucl Med* 1999;40:1072.

150. Hockel M, Schlenger K, Knoop C, et al. Oxygenation of carcinomas of the uterine cervix: evaluation by computerized O2 tension measurements. *Cancer Res* 1991;51:6098.

151. Vaupel P, Kelleher DK. Tumor hypoxia: pathophysiology, clinical significance, and therapeutic perspectives. Stuttgart, Germany, Germany: Wissenchaftliche Verlagsgesellschaft, 1999:1.

152. Vaupel P, Hockel M. Oxygenation status of breast cancers: the Mainz experience. In: Vaupel P, Kelleher DK, eds. *Tumor hypoxia: pathophysiology, clinical significance, and therapeutic perspectives*. Stuttgart, Germany: Wissenchaftliche Verlagsgesellschaft, 1999:1.

153. Nordsmark M, Overgaard J. Oxygenation of human tumors: the Aarhus experience. In: Vaupel P, Kelleher DK, eds. *Tumor hypoxia: pathophysiology, clinical significance, and therapeutic perspectives*. Stuttgart, Germany: Wissenchaftliche Verlagsgesellschaft, 1999:19.

154. Brizel DM. Human tumor oxygenation: the Duke University Medical Center experience. In: Vaupel P, Kelleher DK, eds. *Tumor hypoxia: pathophysiology, clinical significance, and therapeutic perspectives*. Stuttgart, Germany: Wissenchaftliche Verlagsgesellschaft, 1999:29.

155. Brizel DM, Scully SP, Harrelson JM, et al. Radiation therapy and hyperthermia improve the oxygenation of human soft tissue sarcomas. *Cancer Res* 1996;56:5347.

156. Dunst J, Feldmann J, Becker A, et al. Oxygenation of human tumors: the Munich/Halle experience. In: Vaupel P,

Kelleher DK, eds. *Tumor hypoxia: pathophysiology, clinical significance, and therapeutic perspectives.* Stuttgart, Germany: Wissenchaftliche Verlagsgesellschaft, 1999:39.

157. Becker A, Stadler P, Lavey RS, et al. Severe anemia is associated with poor tumor oxygenation in head and neck squamous cell carcinomas. *Int J Radiat Oncol Biol Phys* 2000;46:459.

158. Lartigau E, Lusinchi A, Eschwege F, et al. Tumor oxygenation: the Institut Gustave Roussy experience. In: Vaupel P, Kelleher DK, eds. *Tumor hypoxia: pathophysiology, clinical significance, and therapeutic perspectives.* Stuttgart, Germany: Wissenchaftliche Verlagsgesellschaft, 1999:47.

159. Molls M, Adam JF, Stadler P, et al. The impact of tumor oxygenation on clinical radiation oncology. In: Vaupel P, Kelleher DK, eds. *Tumor hypoxia: pathophysiology, clinical significance, and therapeutic perspectives.* Stuttgart, Germany: Wissenchaftliche Verlagsgesellschaft, 1999:53.

160. Kelleher DK, Thews O, Vaupel P. Modulation of tumor oxygenation and radiosensitivity by erythropoietin. In: Vaupel P, Kelleher DK, eds. *Tumor hypoxia: pathophysiology, clinical significance, and therapeutic perspectives.* Stuttgart, Germany: Wissenchaftliche Verlagsgesellschaft, 1999:83.

161. Lavey RS. Clinical trial experience using erythropoietin during radiation therapy. In: Vaupel P, Kelleher DK, eds. *Tumor hypoxia: pathophysiology, clinical significance, and therapeutic perspectives.* Stuttgart, Germany: Wissenchaftliche Verlagsgesellschaft, 1999:99.

161a. Tsang RW, Fyles AW, Milosevic M, et al. Interrelationship of proliferation and hypoxia in carcinoma of the cervix. *Int J Radiat Oncol Biol Phys* 2000;46:95.

162. Fyles AW, Milosevic M, Pintilie M, et al. Cervix cancer oxygenation measured following external radiation therapy. *Int J Radiat Oncol Biol Phys* 1998;42:751.

163. Coleman CN, Bump EA, Kramer RA. Chemical modifiers of cancer treatment. *J Clin Oncol* 1988;6:709.

164. Hlatky L, Sachs RK, Alpen EL. Joint oxygen-glucose deprivation as the cause of necrosis in a tumor analog. *J Cell Physiol* 1988;134:167.

165. Olive PL, Chaplin DJ, Durand RE. Pharmacokinetics, binding and distribution of Hoechst 33342 in spheroids and murine tumours. *Br J Cancer* 1985;52:739.

166. Trotter MJ, Chaplin DJ, Durand RE, et al. The use of fluorescent probes to identify regions of transient perfusion in murine tumors. *Int J Radiat Oncol Biol Phys* 1989;16:931.

167. Chaplin DJ, Durand RE, Olive PL. Acute hypoxia in tumors: implications for modifiers of radiation effects. *Int J Radiat Oncol Biol Phys* 1986;12:1279.

168. Chaplin DJ, Olive PL, Durand RE. Intermittent blood flow in a murine tumor: radiobiologic effects. *Cancer Res* 1987;47:597.

169. Roh HD, Boucher Y, Kalnicki S, et al. Interstitial hypertension in carcinoma of uterine cervix in patients: possible correlation with tumor oxygenation and radiation response. *Cancer Res* 1991;51:6695.

170. Boucher Y, Jain RK. Microvascular pressure is the principal driving force for interstitial hypertension in solid tumors: implications for vascular collapse. *Cancer Res* 1992;52:5110.

171. Howes AE. An estimation of changes in the proportions and absolute numbers of hypoxic cells after irradiation of transplanted C3H mouse mammary tumours. *Br J Radiol* 1969;42:441.

172. Van Putten LM, Kallman RF. Oxygenation status of a transplantable tumor during fractionated radiation therapy. *J Natl Cancer Inst* 1968;40:441.

173. Vaupel P, Frinak S, O'Hara M. Direct measurement of reoxygenation in malignant mammary tumors after a single large dose of irradiation. *Adv Exp Med Biol* 1984;180:773.

174. Koutcher JA, Alfieri AA, Devitt ML, et al. Quantitative changes in tumor metabolism, partial pressure of oxygen, and radiobiologic oxygenation status postradiation. *Cancer Res* 1992;52:4620.

175. Dewhirst MW, Braun RD, Lanzen JL. Temporal changes in pO$_2$ of R3230AC tumors in Fischer-344 rats. *Int J Radiat Oncol Biol Phys* 1998;42:723.

176. Wouters BG, Brown JM. Cells at intermediate oxygen levels can be more important than the "hypoxic fraction" in determining tumor response to fractionated radiotherapy. *Radiat Res* 1997;147:541.

177. Koch CJ, Meneses JJ, Harris JW. The effect of extreme hypoxia and glucose on the repair of potentially lethal and sublethal radiation damage by mammalian cells. *Radiat Res* 1977;70:542.

178. Varnes ME, Dethlefsen LA, Biaglow JE. The effect of pH on potentially lethal damage recovery in A549 cells. *Radiat Res* 1986;108:80.

179. Young SD, Hill RP. Effects of reoxygenation on cells from hypoxic regions of solid tumors: anticancer drug sensitivity and metastatic potential [see comments]. *J Natl Cancer Inst* 1990;82:371.

180. Luk CK, Veinot-Drebot L, Tjan E, et al. Effect of transient hypoxia on sensitivity to doxorubicin in human and murine cell lines. *J Natl Cancer Inst* 1990;82:684.

181. Wilson RE, Keng PC, Sutherland RM. Drug resistance in Chinese hamster ovary cells during recovery from severe hypoxia [published erratum appears in *J Natl Cancer Inst* 1990;82:239]. *J Natl Cancer Inst* 1989;81:1235.

182. Kwok TT, Sutherland RM. The radiation response of cells recovering after chronic hypoxia. *Radiat Res* 1989;119:261.

183. Gupta V, Belli JA. Enhancement of radiation sensitivity by postirradiation hypoxia: time course and oxygen concentration dependency. *Radiat Res* 1988;116:124.

184. Young SD, Marshall RS, Hill RP. Hypoxia induces DNA overreplication and enhances metastatic potential of murine tumor cells. *Proc Natl Acad Sci U S A* 1988;85:9533.

185. Young SD, Hill RP. Effects of reoxygenation on cells from hypoxic regions of solid tumors: analysis of transplanted murine tumors for evidence of DNA overreplication. *Cancer Res* 1990;50:5031.

186. Wang GL, Semenza GL. Characterization of hypoxia-inducible factor1 and regulation of DNA binding activity by hypoxia. *J Biol Chem* 1993;268:21513.

187. Giaccia AJ, Koumensi C, Denko N. The influence of tumor hypoxia on malignant progression. In: Vaupel P, Kelleher DK, eds. *Tumor hypoxia: pathophysiology, clinical significance, and therapeutic perspectives.* Stuttgart, Germany: Wissenchaftliche Verlagsgesellschaft, 1999:115.

188. Stratford IJ, Patterson AV, Dachs GU, et al. Hypoxia-mediated gene expression. In: Vaupel P, Kelleher DK, eds. *Tumor hypoxia: pathophysiology, clinical significance, and therapeutic perspectives.* Stuttgart, Germany: Wissenchaftliche Verlagsgesellschaft, 1999:107.

189. Semenza GL. Perspectives on oxygen sensing. *Cell* 1999;98:281.

190. Zhong H, DeMarzo AM, Laughner E, et al. Overexpression of hypoxia-inducible factor 1a in common human cancers and their metastases. *Cancer Res* 1999;59:5830.

191. Blancher C, Harris AL. The molecular basis of the hypoxia response pathway: tumour hypoxia as a therapy target. *Cancer Metastasis Rev* 1998;17:187.

192. Shibata T, Akiyama N, Noda M, et al. Enhancement of gene expression under hypoxic conditions using fragments of the human vascular endothelial growth factor and the erythropoietin genes. *Int J Radiat Oncol Biol Phys* 1998;42:913.

193. Brown JM, Giaccia AJ. The unique physiology of solid tumors: opportunities (and problems) for cancer therapy. *Cancer Res* 1998;58:1408.

194. Gazit G, Hung G, Chen X, et al. Use of the glucose starvation-inducible glucose-regulated protein 78 promoter in suicide gene therapy of murine fibrosarcoma. *Cancer Res* 1999;59:3100.

195. Bristow RG, Hardy PA, Hill RP. Comparison between in vitro radiosensitivity and in vivo radioresponse of murine tumor cell lines. I: Parameters of in vitro radiosensitivity and endogenous cellular glutathione levels. *Int J Radiat Oncol Biol Phys* 1990;18:133.

196. Warters RL, Hofer KG. Radionuclide toxicity in cultured mammalian cells. Elucidation of the primary site for radiation-induced division delay. *Radiat Res* 1977;69:348.

197. Brenner DJ, Ward JF. Constraints on energy deposition and target size of multiply damaged sites associated with DNA double-strand breaks. *Int J Radiat Biol* 1992;61:737.

198. Murray D, Prager A, Vanankeren SC, et al. Comparative effect of the thiols dithiothreitol, cysteamine and WR-151326 on survival and on the induction of DNA damage in cultured Chinese hamster ovary cells exposed to gamma-radiation. *Int J Radiat Biol* 1990;58:71.

199. Wlodek D, Hittelman WN. The relationship of DNA and chromosome damage to survival of synchronized X-irradiated L5178Y cells. II. Repair. *Radiat Res* 1988;115:566.

200. Nagasawa H, Robertson J, Little JB. Induction of chromosomal aberrations and sister chromatid exchanges by alpha particles in density-inhibited cultures of mouse 10T1/2 and 3T3 cells. *Int J Radiat Biol* 1990;57:35.

201. Cornforth MN, Bedford JS. X-ray–induced breakage and rejoining of human interphase chromosomes. *Science* 1983;222:1141.

202. Prise KM, Davies S, Michael BD. A comparison of the chemical repair rates of free radical precursors of DNA damage and cell killing in Chinese hamster V79 cells. *Int J Radiat Biol* 1992;61:721.

203. Coleman CN. Of what use is molecular biology to the practicing radiation oncologist? *Radiother Oncol* 1998;46:117.

204. Wilson RL. Free radical repair mechanisms and the interaction of glutathione and vitamins C and E. In: Nygaard OF, Simic MG, eds. *Radioprotectors and anticarcinogens*. New York: Academic Press, 1983:1.

205. Raleigh JA, Fuciarelli AF, Kulatunga CR. Potential limitation to hydrogen atom donation as a mechanism of repair in chemical models of radiation damage. In: Cerutti PA, Nygaard OF, Simic MG, eds. *Anticarcinogens and radiation protection*. New York: Plenum Publishing, 1987:33.

206. Liebmann JE, Hahn SM, Cook JA, et al. Glutathione depletion by L-buthionine sulfoximine antagonizes taxol cytotoxicity. *Cancer Res* 1993;53:2066.

207. Lacreta FP, Brennan JM, Hamilton TC, et al. Stereoselective pharmacokinetics of L-buthionine SR-sulfoximine in patients with cancer. *Drug Metab Dispos* 1994;22:835.

208. Vanhoefer U, Cao S, Minderman H, et al. D,L-buthionine-(S,R)-sulfoximine potentiates in vivo the therapeutic efficacy of doxorubicin against multidrug resistance protein-expressing tumors. *Clin Cancer Res* 1996;2:1961.

209. Kligerman MM, Liu T, Liu Y, et al. Interim analysis of a randomized trial of radiation therapy of rectal cancer with/without WR-2721. *Int J Radiat Oncol Biol Phys* 1992;22:799.

210. Taylor YC, Brown JM. Radiosensitization in multifraction schedules. II. Greater sensitization by 2-nitroimidazoles than by oxygen. *Radiat Res* 1987;112:134.

211. Fu K, Hurst A, Brown JM. The effects of misonidazole and continuous low dose irradiation. In: Brady LW, ed. *Radiation sensitizers, their use in the clinical management of cancer*. New York: Masson, 1980:167.

212. Laderoute KR, Eryavec E, McClelland RA, et al. The production of strand breaks in DNA in the presence of the hydroxylamine of SR-2508 (1-[N-(2-hydroxyethyl)acetamido]-2-nitroimidazole) at neutral pH. *Int J Radiat Oncol Biol Phys* 1986;12:1215.

213. Berube LR, Farah S, McClelland RA, et al. Depletion of intracellular glutathione by 1-methyl-2-nitrosoimidazole. *Int J Radiat Oncol Biol Phys* 1992;22:817.

214. Dische S, Saunders MI, Flockhart IR, et al. Misonidazole—a drug for trial in radiotherapy and oncology. *Int J Radiat Oncol Biol Phys* 1979;5:851.

215. Wasserman TH, Phillips TL, Johnson RJ, et al. Initial United States clinical and pharmacologic evaluation of misonidazole (Ro-07-0582), an hypoxic cell radiosensitizer. *Int J Radiat Oncol Biol Phys* 1979;5:775.

216. Dische S. Chemical sensitizers for hypoxic cells: a decade of experience in clinical radiotherapy. *Radiother Oncol* 1985;3:97.

217. Overgaard J, Hansen HS, Andersen AP, et al. Misonidazole combined with split-course radiotherapy in the treatment of invasive carcinoma of larynx and pharynx: report from the DAHANCA 2 study. *Int J Radiat Oncol Biol Phys* 1989;16:1065.

218. Fazekas J, Pajak TF, Wasserman T, et al. Failure of misonidazole-sensitized radiotherapy to impact upon outcome among stage III–IV squamous cancers of the head and neck. *Int J Radiat Oncol Biol Phys* 1987;13:1155.

219. Grigsby PW, Winter K, Wasserman TH, et al. Irradiation with or without misonidazole for patients with stages IIIB and IVA carcinoma of the cervix: final results of RTOG 80-05. Radiation Therapy Oncology Group. *Int J Radiat Oncol Biol Phys* 1999;44:513.

220. Huncharek M. Meta-analytic re-evaluation of misonidazole in the treatment of high grade astrocytoma. *Anticancer Res* 1998;18:1935.

221. Coleman CN, Wasserman TH, Phillips TL, et al. Initial pharmacology and toxicology of intravenous desmethylmisonidazole. *Int J Radiat Oncol Biol Phys* 1982;8:371.

222. Brown JM, Lee WW. Pharmacokinetic considerations in radiosensitizer development. In: Brady LW, ed. *Radiation*

sensitizers, their use in the clinical management of cancer. New York: Masson, 1980:2.

223. Brown JM, Yu NY. The optimum time for irradiation relative to tumour concentration of hypoxic cell sensitizers. *Br J Radiol* 1980;53:915.

224. Brown JM, Yu NY, Brown DM, et al. SR-2508: a 2-nitroimidazole amide which should be superior to misonidazole as a radiosensitizer for clinical use. *Int J Radiat Oncol Biol Phys* 1981;7:695.

225. Brown JM. Clinical perspectives for the use of new hypoxic cell sensitizers. *Int J Radiat Oncol Biol Phys* 1982;8:1491.

226. Coleman CN, Wasserman TH, Urtasun RC, et al. Phase I trial of the hypoxic cell radiosensitizer SR-2508: the results of the five to six week drug schedule. *Int J Radiat Oncol Biol Phys* 1986;12:1105.

227. Coleman CN, Halsey J, Cox RS, et al. Relationship between the neurotoxicity of the hypoxic cell radiosensitizer SR 2508 and the pharmacokinetic profile. *Cancer Res* 1987;47:319.

228. Workman P, Ward R, Maughan TS, et al. Estimation of plasma area under the curve for etanidazole (SR 2508) in toxicity prediction and dose adjustment. *Int J Radiat Oncol Biol Phys* 1989;17:177.

229. Coleman CN, Buswell L, Noll L, et al. The efficacy of pharmacokinetic monitoring and dose modification of etanidazole on the incidence of neurotoxicity: results from a phase II trial of etanidazole and radiation therapy in locally advanced prostate cancer. *Int J Radiat Oncol Biol Phys* 1992;22:565.

230. Beard C, Buswell L, Rose MA, et al. Phase II trial of external beam radiation with etanidazole (SR 2508) for the treatment of locally advanced prostate cancer. *Int J Radiat Oncol Biol Phys* 1994;29:611.

231. Lee DJ, Cosmatos D, Marcial VA, et al. Results of an RTOG phase III trial (RTOG 85-27) comparing radiotherapy plus etanidazole with radiotherapy alone for locally advanced head and neck carcinomas [see comments]. *Int J Radiat Oncol Biol Phys* 1995;32:567.

232. Eschwege F, Sancho-Garnier H, Chassagne D, et al. Results of a European randomized trial of Etanidazole combined with radiotherapy in head and neck carcinomas [see comments]. *Int J Radiat Oncol Biol Phys* 1997;39:275.

233. Brown JM. Hypoxic cell radiosensitizers: the end of an era? Regarding Lee et al., *Int J Radiat Oncol Biol Phys* 32:567–576; 1995 [editorial; comment] [see comments]. *Int J Radiat Oncol Biol Phys* 1995;32:883.

234. Coleman CN. Reports of my death [may be] greatly exaggerated (adapted from Mark Twain)—in response to Dr. J. M. Brown, *Int J Radiat Oncol Biol Phys* 32:883–885; 1995 [letter; comment]. *Int J Radiat Oncol Biol Phys* 1995;32:1264.

234a. Riese NE, Buswell L, Noll L, et al. Pharmacokinetic monitoring and dose modification of etanidazole in the RTOG 85-27 phase III head and neck trial. *Int J Radiat Oncol Biol Phys* 1997;39:855–858.

235. Lee WR, Berkey B, Marcial V, et al. Anemia is associated with decreased survival and increased locoregional failure in patients with locally advanced head and neck carcinoma: a secondary analysis of RTOG 85-27. *Int J Radiat Oncol Biol Phys* 1998;42:1069.

236. Coleman CN, Noll L, Riese N, et al. Final report of the phase I trial of continuous infusion etanidazole (SR 2508): a

Radiation Therapy Oncology Group study. *Int J Radiat Oncol Biol Phys* 1992;22:577.

237. Newman HF, Bleehen NM, Ward R, et al. Hypoxic cell radiosensitizers in the treatment of high grade gliomas: a new direction using combined Ro 03-8799 (pimonidazole) and SR 2508 (etanidazole). *Int J Radiat Oncol Biol Phys* 1988;15:677.

238. Hurwitz SJ, Coleman CN, Riese N, et al. Distribution of etanidazole into human brain tumors: implications for treating high grade gliomas. *Int J Radiat Oncol Biol Phys* 1992;22:573.

239. Coleman CN, Riese N, Buswell L, et al. Clinical trials of etanidazole (SR 2508): RTOG and Joint Center for Radiation Therapy trials. In: Dewey WC, ed. *Radiation research: a twentieth century perspective.* San Diego: Academic Press, 1992:595.

240. Lawton CA, Coleman CN, Buzydlowski JW, et al. Results of a phase II trial of external beam radiation with etanidazole (SR 2508) for the treatment of locally advanced prostate cancer (RTOG Protocol 90-20). *Int J Radiat Oncol Biol Phys* 1996;36:673.

241. Chang EL, Loeffler JS, Riese NE, et al. Survival results from a phase I study of etanidazole (SR2508) and radiotherapy in patients with malignant glioma. *Int J Radiat Oncol Biol Phys* 1998;40:65.

242. Urtasun RC, Palmer M, Kinney B, et al. Intervention with the hypoxic tumor cell sensitizer etanidazole in the combined modality treatment of limited stage small-cell lung cancer. A one-institution study. *Int J Radiat Oncol Biol Phys* 1998;40:337.

243. Shulman LN, Buswell L, Goodman H, et al. Phase I pharmacokinetic study of the hypoxic cell sensitizer etanidazole with carboplatin and cyclophosphamide in the treatment of advanced ovarian cancer. *Int J Radiat Oncol Biol Phys* 1994;29:545.

244. Elias AD, Wheeler C, Ayash LJ, et al. Dose escalation of the hypoxic cell sensitizer etanidazole combined with ifosfamide, carboplatin, etoposide, and autologous hematopoietic stem cell support. *Clin Cancer Res* 1998;4:1443.

245. Dische S, Bennett MH, Orchard R, et al. The uptake of the radiosensitizing compound Ro 03-8799 (Pimonidazole) in human tumors. *Int J Radiat Oncol Biol Phys* 1989;16:1089.

246. Lespinasse F, Thomas C, Bonnay M, et al. Ro 03-8799: preferential relative uptake in human tumor xenografts compared to a murine tumor: comparison with SR-2508. *Int J Radiat Oncol Biol Phys* 1989;16:1105.

247. Cobb LM, Nolan J, Butler SA. Distribution of pimonidazole and RSU 1069 in tumour and normal tissues. *Br J Cancer* 1990;62:915.

248. Dische S. Radiotherapy, carcinoma of cervix, and the radiosensitizer Ro-03-8799 (pimonidazole). In: Dewey WC, ed. *Radiation research, a twentieth-century perspective.* San Diego: Academic Press, 1992:584.

249. Chaplin DJ, Horsman MR. Tumor blood flow changes induced by chemical modifiers of radiation response. *Int J Radiat Oncol Biol Phys* 1992;22:459.

250. Overgaard J, Overgaard M, Nielsen OS, et al. A comparative investigation of nimorazole and misonidazole as hypoxic radiosensitizers in a C3H mammary carcinoma in vivo. *Br J Cancer* 1982;46:904.

251. Overgaard J, Sand Hansen H, Lindeløv B, et al. Nimorazole as a hypoxic radiosensitizer in the treatment of supraglottic larynx and pharynx carcinoma. First report from the Danish Head and Neck Cancer Study (DAHANCA) protocol 5-85. *Radiother Oncol* 1991;20(Suppl 1):143.

252. Overgaard J, Sand Hansen H, Overgaard M. The Danish Head and Neck Cancer Study Group (DAHANCA) randomized trials with hypoxic radiosensitizers in carcinoma of the larynx and pharynx. In: Dewey WC, ed. *Radiation research, a twentieth-century perspective.* San Diego: Academic Press, 1992:573.

253. Overgaard J, Sand Hansen H, Overgaard M, et al. A randomized double-blind phase II study of nimorazole as a hypoxic radiosensitizer of primary radiotherapy in supraglottic larynx and pharynx carcinoma. Results of the Danish Head and Neck Cancer Study (DAHANCA) Protocol 5-85. *Radiother Oncol* 1998;46:135.

254. Cottrill CP, Bishop K, Walton MI, et al. Pilot study of nimorazole as a hypoxic-cell-sensitizer with the "chart" regimen in head and neck cancer. *Int J Radiat Oncol Biol Phys* 1998;42:807.

255. Shibamoto Y, Takahashi M, Abe M. A phase I study of a hypoxic cell sensitizer KU-2285 in combination with conventional radiotherapy. *Radiother Oncol* 1996;40:55.

256. Shibamoto Y, Ohshio G, Hosotani R, et al. A phase I/II study of a hypoxic cell radiosensitizer KU-2285 in combination with intraoperative radiotherapy. *Br J Cancer* 1997;76:1474.

257. Garcia-Angulo AH, Kagiya VT. Intratumoral and parametrial infusion of a 3-nitrotriazole (AK-2123) in the radiotherapy of the uterine cervix cancer: stage II–III—preliminary positive results. *Int J Radiat Oncol Biol Phys* 1992;22:589.

258. Adams GE, Ahmed I, Sheldon PW, et al. Radiation sensitization and chemopotentiation: RSU 1069, a compound more efficient than misonidazole in vitro and in vivo. *Br J Cancer* 1984;49:571.

259. Ahmed I, Jenkins TC, Walling JM, et al. Analogues of RSU-1069: radiosensitization and toxicity in vitro and in vivo. *Int J Radiat Oncol Biol Phys* 1986;12:1079.

260. Chaplin DJ, Durand RE, Stratford IJ, et al. The radiosensitizing and toxic effects of RSU-1069 on hypoxic cells in a murine tumor. *Int J Radiat Oncol Biol Phys* 1986;12:1091.

261. Deacon JM, Holliday SB, Ahmed I, et al. Experimental pharmacokinetics of RSU-1069 and its analogues: high tumor/plasma ratios. *Int J Radiat Oncol Biol Phys* 1986;12:1087.

262. Stratford IJ, O'Neill P, Sheldon PW, et al. RSU 1069, a nitroimidazole containing an aziridine group. Bioreduction greatly increases cytotoxicity under hypoxic conditions. *Biochem Pharmacol* 1986;35:105.

263. Horwich A, Holliday SB, Deacon JM, et al. A toxicity and pharmacokinetic study in man of the hypoxic-cell radiosensitizer RSU-1069. *Br J Radiol* 1986;59:1238.

264. Cole S, Stratford IJ, Fielden EM, et al. Dual function nitroimidazoles less toxic than RSU 1069: selection of candidate drugs for clinical trial (RB 6145 and/or PD 130908. *Int J Radiat Oncol Biol Phys* 1992;22:545.

265. Sebolt-Leopold JS, Vincent PW, Beningo KA, et al. Pharmacologic/pharmacokinetic evaluation of emesis induced by analogs of RSU 1069 and its control by antiemetic agents. *Int J Radiat Oncol Biol Phys* 1992;22:549.

266. Wood PJ, Horsman MR, Khalil AA, et al. A comparison of the physiologic effects of RSU1069 and RB6145 in the SCCVII murine tumour. *Acta Oncol* 1996;35:989.

267. Breider MA, Pilcher GD, Graziano MJ, et al. Retinal degeneration in rats induced by CI-1010, a 2-nitroimidazole radiosensitizer. *Toxicol Pathol* 1998;26:234.

268. Churchill-Davidson I, Sanger C. High-pressure oxygen and radiotherapy. *Lancet* 1955;10:1091.

269. Dische S. Hyperbaric oxygen: the Medical Research Council trials and their clinical significance. *Br J Radiol* 1978;51:888.

270. Henk JM. Does hyperbaric oxygen have a future in radiation therapy? *Int J Radiat Oncol Biol Phys* 1981;7:1125.

271. Brady LW, Plenk HP, Hanley JA, et al. Hyperbaric oxygen therapy for carcinoma of the cervix—stages IIB, IIIA, IIIB and IVA: results of a randomized study by the Radiation Therapy Oncology Group. *Int J Radiat Oncol Biol Phys* 1981;7:991.

272. Rubin P, Hanley J, Keys HM, et al. Carbogen breathing during radiation therapy—the Radiation Therapy Oncology Group Study. *Int J Radiat Oncol Biol Phys* 1979;5:1963.

273. Martin L, Lartigau E, Weeger P, et al. Changes in the oxygenation of head and neck tumors during carbogen breathing. *Radiother Oncol* 1993;27:123.

274. Bush RS. The significance of anemia in clinical radiation therapy. *Int J Radiat Oncol Biol Phys* 1986;12:2047.

275. Dische S, Saunders MI, Warburton MF. Hemoglobin, radiation, morbidity and survival. *Int J Radiat Oncol Biol Phys* 1986;12:1335.

276. Rose C, Lustig R, McIntosh N, et al. A clinical trial of Fluosol DA 20% in advanced squamous cell carcinoma of the head and neck. *Int J Radiat Oncol Biol Phys* 1986;12:1325.

277. Lustig R, McIntosh-Lowe N, Rose C, et al. Phase I/II study of Fluosol-DA and 100% oxygen as an adjuvant to radiation in the treatment of advanced squamous cell tumors of the head and neck. *Int J Radiat Oncol Biol Phys* 1989;16:1587.

278. Evans RG, Kimler BF, Morantz RA, et al. Lack of complications in long-term survivors after treatment with Fluosol and oxygen as an adjuvant to radiation therapy for high-grade brain tumors. *Int J Radiat Oncol Biol Phys* 1993;26:649.

279. Dische S. Hypoxia and local tumour control. Part 2. *Radiother Oncol* 1991;20(Suppl 1):9.

280. Dische S. Radiotherapy and anaemia—the clinical experience. *Radiother Oncol* 1991;20(Suppl 1):35.

281. Lavey RS, Dempsey WH. Erythropoietin increases hemoglobin in cancer patients during radiation therapy. *Int J Radiat Oncol Biol Phys* 1993;27:1147.

282. Henke M, Guttenberger R, Barke A, et al. Erythropoietin for patients undergoing radiotherapy: a pilot study. *Radiother Oncol* 1999;50:185.

283. Sartorelli AC. Therapeutic attack of hypoxic cells of solid tumors: presidential address. *Cancer Res* 1988;48:775.

284. Adams GE, Stratford IJ, Edwards HS, et al. Bioreductive drugs as post-irradiation sensitizers: comparison of dual function agents with SR 4233 and the mitomycin C analogue EO9. *Int J Radiat Oncol Biol Phys* 1992;22:717.

285. Brown JM. Keynote address: hypoxic cell radiosensitizers: where next? *Int J Radiat Oncol Biol Phys* 1989;16:987.

286. Brown JM. SR 4233 (tirapazamine): a new anticancer drug exploiting hypoxia in solid tumors. *Br J Cancer* 1993;67:1163.

287. Zeman EM, Hirst VK, Lemmon MJ, et al. Enhancement of

radiation-induced tumor cell killing by the hypoxic cell toxin SR 4233. *Radiother Oncol* 1988;12:209.

288. Baker MA, Zeman EM, Hirst VK, et al. Metabolism of SR 4233 by Chinese hamster ovary cells: basis of selective hypoxic cytotoxicity. *Cancer Res* 1988;48:5947.

289. Edwards DI, Virk NS. Repair of damage induced by SR 4233. *Int J Radiat Oncol Biol Phys* 1992;22:677.

290. Durand RE, Olive PL. Evaluation of bioreductive drugs in multicell spheroids. *Int J Radiat Oncol Biol Phys* 1992;22:689.

291. Zeman EM, Brown JM. Pre- and post-irradiation radiosensitization by SR 4233. *Int J Radiat Oncol Biol Phys* 1989;16:967.

292. Brown JM. The hypoxic cell: a target for selective cancer therapy—Eighteenth Bruce F. Cain Memorial Award Lecture. *Cancer Res* 1999;59:5863.

293. Wang J, Biedermann KA, Brown JM. Repair of DNA and chromosome breaks in cells exposed to SR 4233 under hypoxia or to ionizing radiation. *Cancer Res* 1992;52:4473.

294. Walton MI, Sugget N, Workman P. The role of human and rodent DT-diaphorase in the reductive metabolism of hypoxic cell cytotoxins. *Int J Radiat Oncol Biol Phys* 1992;22:643.

295. Koch CJ. Unusual oxygen concentration dependence of toxicity of SR-4233, a hypoxic cell toxin. *Cancer Res* 1993;53:3992.

296. Bailey SM, Sugget N, Walton MI, et al. Structure-activity relationships for DT-diaphorase reduction of hypoxic cell directed agents: indoloquinones and diaziridinyl benzoquinones. *Int J Radiat Oncol Biol Phys* 1992;22:649.

297. Brown JM, Lemmon MJ. Potentiation by the hypoxic cytotoxin SR 4233 of cell killing produced by fractionated irradiation of mouse tumors. *Cancer Res* 1990;50:7745.

298. Brown JM, Lemmon MJ. SR 4233: a tumor specific radiosensitizer active in fractionated radiation regimes. *Radiother Oncol* 1991;20(Suppl 1):151.

299. Brown JM, Koong A. Therapeutic advantage of hypoxic cells in tumors: a theoretical study [see comments]. *J Natl Cancer Inst* 1991;83:178.

300. Brown JM, Lemmon MJ. Tumor hypoxia can be exploited to preferentially sensitize tumors to fractionated irradiation [see comments]. *Int J Radiat Oncol Biol Phys* 1991;20:457.

301. Doherty N, Hancock SL, Kaye S, et al. Muscle cramping in phase I clinical trials of tirapazamine (SR 4233) with and without radiation. *Int J Radiat Oncol Biol Phys* 1994;29:379.

302. Kapp DS, Petersen IA, Cox RS, et al. Two or six hyperthermia treatments as an adjunct to radiation therapy yield similar tumor responses: results of a randomized trial. *Int J Radiat Oncol Biol Phys* 1990;19:1481.

303. Dorie MJ, Brown JM. Modification of the antitumor activity of chemotherapeutic drugs by the hypoxic cytotoxic agent tirapazamine. *Cancer Chemother Pharmacol* 1997;39:361.

304. Siemann DW, Hinchman CA. Potentiation of cisplatin activity by the bioreductive agent tirapazamine. *Radiother Oncol* 1998;47:215.

305. Senan S, Rampling R, Graham MA, et al. Phase I and pharmacokinetic study of tirapazamine (SR 4233) administered every three weeks. *Clin Cancer Res* 1997;3:31.

306. Tuttle SW, Hazard L, Koch CJ, et al. Bioreductive metabolism of SR-4233 (WIN 59075) by whole cell suspensions under aerobic and hypoxic conditions: role of the pentose

307. cycle and implications for the mechanism of cytotoxicity observed in air. *Int J Radiat Oncol Biol Phys* 1994;29:357.

307. Herscher LL, Krishna MC, Cook JA, et al. Protection against SR 4233 (Tirapazamine) aerobic cytotoxicity by the metal chelators desferrioxamine and tiron. *Int J Radiat Oncol Biol Phys* 1994;30:879.

308. Shulman LN, Buswell L, Riese N, et al. Phase I trial of the hypoxic cell cytotoxin tirapazamine with concurrent radiation therapy in the treatment of refractory solid tumors. *Int J Radiat Oncol Biol Phys* 1999;44:349.

309. Minchinton AI, Lemmon MJ, Tracy M, et al. Second-generation 1,2,4-benzotriazine 1,4-di-N-oxide bioreductive anti-tumor agents: pharmacology and activity in vitro and in vivo. *Int J Radiat Oncol Biol Phys* 1992;22:701.

310. Walton MI, Workman P. Pharmacokinetics and bioreductive metabolism of the novel benzotriazine di-N-oxide hypoxic cell cytotoxin tirapazamine (WIN 59075; SR 4233; NSC 130181) in mice. *J Pharmacol Exp Ther* 1993;265:938.

311. Prager TC, Kellaway J, Zou Y, et al. Evaluation of ocular safety: tirapazamine plus cisplatin in patients with metastatic melanomas. *Anticancer Drugs* 1998;9:515.

312. Johnson CA, Kilpatrick D, von Roemeling R, et al. Phase I trial of tirapazamine in combination with cisplatin in a single dose every 3 weeks in patients with solid tumors. *J Clin Oncol* 1997;15:773.

313. Lee DJ, Trotti A, Spencer S, et al. Concurrent tirapazamine and radiotherapy for advanced head and neck carcinomas: a Phase II study. *Int J Radiat Oncol Biol Phys* 1998;42:811.

314. Treat J, Johnson E, Langer C, et al. Tirapazamine with cisplatin in patients with advanced non-small-cell lung cancer: a phase II study. *J Clin Oncol* 1998;16:3524.

315. Bedikian AY, Legha SS, Eton O, et al. Phase II trial of escalated dose of tirapazamine with cisplatin in advanced malignant melanoma. *Anticancer Drugs* 1999;10:735.

316. Workman P. Bioreductive mechanisms. *Int J Radiat Oncol Biol Phys* 1992;22:631.

317. Workman P, Binger M, Kooistra KL. Pharmacokinetics, distribution, and metabolism of the novel bioreductive alkylating indoloquinone EO9 in rodents. *Int J Radiat Oncol Biol Phys* 1992;22:713.

318. Schellens JH, Planting AS, van Acker BA, et al. Phase I and pharmacologic study of the novel indoloquinone bioreductive alkylating cytotoxic drug EO9. *J Natl Cancer Inst* 1994;86:906–912.

319. Papadopoulou MV, Ming JI, Bloomer WD. NLCQ-1, a novel hypoxic cytotoxin: potentiation of melphalan, cis-DDP, and cyclophosphamide in vivo. *Int J Radiat Oncol Biol Phys* 1998;42:775.

320. McKeown SR, Friery OP, McIntyre IA, et al. Evidence for a therapeutic gain when AQ4N or tirapazamine is combined with radiation. *Br J Cancer* 1996;27:S39.

321. Rauth AM, Melo T, Misra V. Bioreductive therapies: an overview of drugs and their mechanisms of action. *Int J Radiat Oncol Biol Phys* 1998;42:755.

322. Friery OP, Gallagher R, Murray MM, et al. Enhancement of the antitumor effect of cyclophosphamide by the bioreductive drugs AQ4N and tirapazamine. *Br J Cancer* 2000;82:1469.

323. Raleigh SM, Wanogho E, Burke MD, et al. Involvement of human cytochromes P450 (CYP) in the reductive metabo-

lism of AQ4N, a hypoxia activated anthraquinone di-n-oxide prodrug. *Int J Radiat Oncol Biol Phys* 1998;42:763.

324. Coleman CN, Beard CJ, Hlatky L. Biochemical modifiers: hypoxic cell sensitizers. In: Mauch P, Loeffler JS, eds. *Radiation oncology*. Philadelphia: WB Saunders, 1994:56.

325. Siemann DW. Tissue oxygen manipulation and tumor blood flow. *Int J Radiat Oncol Biol Phys* 1992;22:393.

326. Dewhirst MW, Oliver R, Tso CY, et al. Heterogeneity in tumor microvascular response to radiation. *Int J Radiat Oncol Biol Phys* 1990;18:559.

327. Dewhirst MW, Ong ET, Klitzman B, et al. Perivascular oxygen tensions in a transplantable mammary tumor growing in a dorsal flap window chamber. *Radiat Res* 1992;130:171.

328. Chaplin DJ, Peters CE, Horsman MR, et al. Drug induced perturbations in tumor blood flow: therapeutic potential and possible limitations. *Radiother Oncol* 1991;20(Suppl 1):93.

329. Okunieff P, Walsh CS, Vaupel P, et al. Effects of hydralazine on in vivo tumor energy metabolism, hematopoietic radiation sensitivity, and cardiovascular parameters. *Int J Radiat Oncol Biol Phys* 1989;16:1145.

330. Horsman MR, Overgaard J, Chaplin DJ. The interaction between RSU-1069, hydralazine and hyperthermia in a C3H mammary carcinoma as assessed by tumour growth delay [letter]. *Acta Oncol* 1988;27:861.

331. Okunieff P, Kallinowski F, Vaupel P, et al. Effects of hydralazine-induced vasodilation on the energy metabolism of murine tumors studied by in vivo 3IP-nuclear magnetic resonance spectroscopy. *J Natl Cancer Inst* 1988;80:745.

332. Cole S, Robbins L. Manipulation of oxygenation in a human tumour xenograft with BW12C or hydralazine: effects on responses to radiation and to the bioreductive cytotoxicity of misonidazole or RSU-1069. *Radiother Oncol* 1989;16:235.

333. Guichard M, Lespinasse F, Trotter M, et al. The effect of hydralazine on blood flow and misonidazole toxicity in human tumour xenografts. *Radiother Oncol* 1991;20:117.

334. Horsman MR, Christensen KL, Overgaard J. Relationship between the hydralazine-induced changes in murine tumor blood supply and mouse blood pressure. *Int J Radiat Oncol Biol Phys* 1992;22:455.

335. Lemmon MJ, Brown JM. Hydralazine does not increase hypoxia in tumors growing in preirradiated tissue. *Int J Radiat Oncol Biol Phys* 1991;21:1435.

336. Rowell NP, Flower MA, McCready VR, et al. The effects of single dose oral hydralazine on blood flow through human lung tumours. *Radiother Oncol* 1990;18:283.

337. Jonsson GG, Kjellén E, Pero RW. Nicotinamide as a radiosensitizer of a C3H mouse mammary adenocarcinoma. *Radiother Oncol* 1984;1:349.

338. Horsman MR, Høyer M, Honess DJ, et al. Nicotinamide pharmacokinetics in humans and mice: a comparative assessment and the implications for radiotherapy. *Radiother Oncol* 1993;27:131.

339. Wood PJ, Hirst DG. Calcium antagonists as radiation modifiers: site specificity in relation to tumor response. *Int J Radiat Oncol Biol Phys* 1989;16:1141.

340. Fenton BM, Sutherland RM. Effect of flunarizine on microregional distributions of intravascular HbO2 saturations in RIF-1 and KHT sarcomas. *Int J Radiat Oncol Biol Phys* 1992;22:447.

341. Song CW, Hasegawa T, Kwon HC, et al. Increase in tumor oxygenation and radiosensitivity caused by pentoxifylline. *Radiat Res* 1992;130:205.

342. Lee I, Kim JH, Levitt SH, et al. Increases in tumor response by pentoxifylline alone or in combination with nicotinamide. *Int J Radiat Oncol Biol Phys* 1992;22:425.

343. Siemann DW, Alliet KL, Macler LM. Manipulations in the oxygen transport capacity of blood as a means of sensitizing tumors to radiation therapy. *Int J Radiat Oncol Biol Phys* 1989;16:1169.

344. Ramsay JR, Bleehen NM, Dennis I, et al. Phase I study of BW12C in combination with mitomycin C in patients with advanced gastrointestinal cancer. *Int J Radiat Oncol Biol Phys* 1992;22:721.

345. Sundfor K, Trope C, Suo Z, et al. Normobaric oxygen treatment during radiotherapy for carcinoma of the uterine cervix. Results from a prospective controlled randomized trial. *Radiother Oncol* 1999;50:157.

346. Haffty BG, Hurley RA, Peters LG. Carcinoma of the larynx treated with hypofractionated radiation and hyperbaric oxygen: long-term tumor control and complications. *Int J Radiat Oncol Biol Phys* 1999;45:13.

347. Stern S, Guichard M. Efficacy of agents counteracting hypoxia in fractionated radiation regimes. *Radiother Oncol* 1996;41:143.

348. Brizel DM, Hage WD, Dodge RK, et al. Hyperbaric oxygen improves tumor radiation response significantly more than carbogen/nicotinamide. *Radiat Res* 1997;147:715.

349. Fenton BM, Lord EM, Paoni SF. Enhancement of tumor perfusion and oxygenation by carbogen and nicotinamide during single- and multifraction irradiation. *Radiat Res* 2000;153:75.

350. Fatigante L, Ducci F, Cartei F, et al. Carbogen and nicotinamide combined with unconventional radiotherapy in glioblastoma multiforme: a new modality treatment. *Int J Radiat Oncol Biol Phys* 1997;37:499.

351. Miralbell R, Mornex F, Greiner R, et al. Accelerated radiotherapy, carbogen, and nicotinamide in glioblastoma multiforme: report of European Organization for Research and Treatment of Cancer Trial 22933. *J Clin Oncol* 1999;17:3143.

352. Saunders MI, Hoskin PJ, Pigott K, et al. Accelerated radiotherapy, carbogen and nicotinamide (ARCON) in locally advanced head and neck cancer: a feasibility study. *Radiother Oncol* 1997;45:159.

353. Bernier J, Stratford MR, Denekamp J, et al. Pharmacokinetics of nicotinamide in cancer patients treated with accelerated radiotherapy: the experience of the Co-operative Group of Radiotherapy of the European Organization for Research and Treatment of Cancer. *Radiother Oncol* 1998; 48:123.

354. Hoskin PJ, Saunders MI, Dische S. Hypoxic radiosensitizers in radical radiotherapy for patients with bladder carcinoma: hyperbaric oxygen, misonidazole, and accelerated radiotherapy, carbogen, and nicotinamide. *Cancer* 1999;86:1322.

355. Hulshof MC, Rehmann CJ, Booij J, et al. Lack of perfusion enhancement after administration of nicotinamide and carbogen in patients with glioblastoma: a 99mTc-HMPAO SPECT study. *Radiother Oncol* 1998;48:135.

356. Bussink J, Kaanders JH, Van der Kogel AJ. Clinical outcome and tumour microenvironmental effects of accelerated

radiotherapy with carbogen and nicotinamide. *Acta Oncol* 1999;38:875.

357. Stuben G, Stuschke M, Knühmann K, et al. The effect of combined nicotinamide and carbogen treatments in human tumour xenografts: oxygenation and tumour control studies. *Radiother Oncol* 1998;48:143.

358. el-Said A, Menke D, Dorie MJ, et al. Comparison of the effectiveness of tirapazamine and carbogen with nicotinamide in enhancing the response of a human tumor xenograft to fractionated irradiation. *Radiat Oncol Investig* 1999;7:163.

359. Neta R, Oppenheim JJ, Douches SD. Interdependence of the radioprotective effects of human recombinant interleukin 1 alpha, tumor necrosis factor alpha, granulocyte colony-stimulating factor, and murine recombinant granulocyte-macrophage colony-stimulating factor. *J Immunol* 1988;140:108.

360. Farrell CL, Bready JV, Rex KL, et al. Keratinocyte growth factor protects mice from chemotherapy and radiation-induced gastrointestinal injury and mortality. *Cancer Res* 1998;58:933.

361. Okunieff P, Abraham EH, Moini M, et al. Basic fibroblast growth factor radioprotects bone marrow and not RIF1 tumor. *Acta Oncol* 1995;34:435.

362. Herskind C, Bamberg M, Rodemann HP. The role of cytokines in the development of normal-tissue reactions after radiotherapy. *Strahlenther Onkol* 1998;174(Suppl 3):12.

363. Patt HM, Tyree EB, Staube RL, et al. Cysteine protection against X-irradiation. *Science* 1949;110:213.

364. Brown DQ, Graham WJD, MacKenzie LJ, et al. Can WR-2721 be improved upon? *Pharmacol Ther* 1988;39:157.

365. Grdina DJ, Sigdestad CP. Radiation protectors: the unexpected benefits. *Drug Metab Rev* 1989;20:13.

366. Yuhas JM, Storer VB. Differential chemoprotection of normal and malignant tissues. *J Natl Cancer Inst* 1969;42:331.

367. Yuhas JM. On the potential application of radioprotective drugs in radiotherapy. In: Sokol GH, eds. *Radiation-drug interaction in cancer management.* New York: Wiley-Liss, 1980:114.

368. Harris JW, Phillips TL. Radiobiological and biochemical studies of thiophosphate radioprotective compounds related to cysteamine. *Radiat Res* 1971;46:362.

369. Stewart FA, Rojas A, Denekamp J. Radioprotection of two mouse tumors by WR-2721 in single and fractionated treatments. *Int J Radiat Oncol Biol Phys* 1983;9:507.

370. Milas L, Hunter N, Ito H, et al. Effect of tumor type, size, and endpoint on tumor radioprotection by WR-2721. *Int J Radiat Oncol Biol Phys* 1984;10:41.

371. Phillips TL, Kane L, Utley JF. Radioprotection of tumor and normal tissues by thiophosphate compounds. *Cancer* 1973;32:528.

372. Yuhas JM. Efficacy testing of WR-2721 in Great Britain everything is black and white at the gray lab. *Int J Radiat Oncol Biol Phys* 1983;9:595.

373. Washburn LC, Rafter JJ, Hayes RL. Prediction of the effective radioprotective dose of WR-2721 in humans through an interspecies tissue distribution study. *Radiat Res* 1976;66:100.

374. Yuhas JM, Culo F. Selective inhibition of the nephrotoxicity of cis-dichlorodiammineplatinum(II) by WR-2721 without altering its antitumor properties. *Cancer Treat Rep* 1980;64:57.

375. Halberg FE, LaRue SM, Rayner AA, et al. Intraoperative radiotherapy with localized radioprotection: diminished duodenal toxicity with intraluminal WR2721. *Int J Radiat Oncol Biol Phys* 1991;21:1241.

376. Milas L, Hunter N, Stephens LC, et al. Inhibition of radiation carcinogenesis in mice by S-2-(3-aminopropylamino)-ethylphosphorothioic acid. *Cancer Res* 1984;44:5567.

377. Grdina DJ, Carnes BA, Grahn D, et al. Protection against late effects of radiation by S-2-(3-aminopropylamino)-ethylphosphorothioic acid. *Cancer Res* 1991;51:4125.

378. Wasserman TH, Phillips TL, Ross G, et al. Differential protection against cytotoxic chemotherapeutic effects on bone marrow CFUs by WR-2721. *Cancer Clin Trials* 1981;4:3.

379. Grdina DJ, Shigematsu N, Dale P, et al. Thiol and disulfide metabolites of the radiation protector and potential chemopreventive agent WR-2721 are linked to its anti-cytotoxic and anti-mutagenic mechanisms of action. *Carcinogenesis* 1995;16:767.

380. Dorr RT. Radioprotectants: pharmacology and clinical applications of amifostine. *Semin Radiat Oncol* 1998;8:10.

381. Smoluk GD, Fahey RC, Calabro-Jones PM, et al. Radioprotection of cells in culture by WR-2721 and derivatives: form of the drug responsible for protection. *Cancer Res* 1988;48:3641.

382. Liu SC, Murley JS, Woloschak G, et al. Repression of c-myc gene expression by the thiol and disulfide forms of the cytoprotector amifostine. *Carcinogenesis* 1997;18:2457.

383. Woloschak GE, Paunesku T, Chang-Liu CM, et al. Expression of thymidine kinase messenger RNA and a related transcript is modulated by radioprotector WR1065. *Cancer Res* 1995;55:4788.

384. Chabner BA. *Pharmacologic principles of cancer treatment.* Philadelphia: WB Saunders, 1982:309.

385. Treskes M, Holwerda U, Klein I, et al. The chemical reactivity of the modulating agent WR2721 (ethiofos) and its main metabolites with the antitumor agents cisplatin and carboplatin. *Biochem Pharmacol* 1991;42:2125.

386. Vos O, Budke L, Grant GA. Modification of the radiation response of the mouse kidney by misonidazole and WR-2721. *Int J Radiat Oncol Biol Phys* 1976;9:1731.

387. Purdie JW. A comparative study of the radioprotective effects of cysteamine, WR-2721, and WR-1065 in cultured human cells. *Radiat Res* 1979;77:303.

388. Mori T, Nikaido O, Sugahara T. Dephosphorylation of WR-2721 with mouse tissue homogenates. *Int J Radiat Oncol Biol Phys* 1984;10:1529.

389. Calabro-Jones PM, Aguilera JA, Ward JF, et al. Uptake of WR-2721 derivatives by cells in culture: identification of the transported form of the drug. *Cancer Res* 1988;48:3634.

390. Nakamura J, Shaw LM, Brown DQ. Hydrolysis of WR2721 by mouse liver cell fractions. *Radiat Res* 1987;109:143.

391. Hatoff DE, Toyota N, Wong C, et al. Rat liver alkaline phosphatases. Evidence hepatocyte and portal triad enzymes differ. *Dig Dis Sci* 1985;30:564.

392. McComb RB, Bowers GN, Posen S. *Alkaline phosphatase.* New York: Plenum Publishing, 1979.

393. Shaw LM, Glover D, Turrisi A, et al. Pharmacokinetics of WR-2721. *Pharmacol Ther* 1988;39:195.

394. Williams MV, Denekamp J. Modification of the radiation response of the mouse kidney by misonidazole and WR-2721. *Int J Radiat Oncol Biol Phys* 1983;9:1731.

395. Denekamp J, Michael BD, Rojas A, et al. Radioprotection of mouse skin by WR-2721: the critical influence of oxygen tension. *Int J Radiat Oncol Biol Phys* 1982;8:531.

396. Yuhas JM. Active versus passive absorption kinetics as the basis for selective protection of normal tissues by S-2-(3-aminopropylamino)-ethylphosphorothioic acid. *Cancer Res* 1980;40:1519.

397. Turrisi AT, Glover DJ, Hurwitz S, et al. Final report of the phase I trial of single-dose WR-2721 [S-2-(3-aminopropyl-amino)ethylphosphorothioic acid]. *Cancer Treat Rep* 1986; 70:1389.

398. Yuhas JM, Davis ME, Glover D, et al. Circumvention of the tumor membrane barrier to WR-2721 absorption by reduction of drug hydrophilicity. *Int J Radiat Oncol Biol Phys* 1982;8:519.

399. Rasey JS, Krohn KA, Grunbaum Z, et al. Synthesis, biodistribution, and autoradiography of radiolabeled S-2-(3-methylaminopropylamino)ethylphosphorothioic acid (WR-3689). *Radiat Res* 1986;106:366.

400. Rasey JS, Spence AM, Badger CC, et al. Specific protection of different normal tissues. *Pharmacol Ther* 1988;39:33.

401. Shaw LM, Turrisi AT, Glover DJ, et al. Human pharmacokinetics of WR-2721. *Int J Radiat Oncol Biol Phys* 1986;12:1501.

402. Swynnerton NF, McGovern EP, Niño JA, et al. An improved HPLC assay for S-2-(3-aminopropylamino)ethyl phosphorothioate (WR-2721) in plasma. *Int J Radiat Oncol Biol Phys* 1984;10:1521.

403. Utley JF, Seaver N, Newton GL, et al. Pharmacokinetics of WR-1065 in mouse tissue following treatment with WR-2721. *Int J Radiat Oncol Biol Phys* 1984;10:1525.

404. Risley JM, Van Etten RL, Shaw LM, et al. Hydrolysis of S-2-(3-aminopropylamino)ethylphosphorothioate (WR-2721). *Biochem Pharmacol* 1986;35:1453.

405. Glover D, Riley L, Carmichael K, et al. Hypocalcemia and inhibition of parathyroid hormone secretion after administration of WR-2721 (a radioprotective and chemoprotective agent). *N Engl J Med* 1983;309:1137.

406. Glover DJ, Shaw L, Glick JH, et al. Treatment of hypercalcemia in parathyroid cancer with WR-2721, S-2-(3-amino-propylamino)ethyl-phosphorothioic acid. *Ann Intern Med* 1985;103:55.

407. Kligerman MM, Turrisi AT, Urtasun RC, et al. Final report on phase I trial of WR-2721 before protracted fractionated radiation therapy. *Int J Radiat Oncol Biol Phys* 1988;14:1119.

408. Wadler S, Haynes H, Beitler JJ, et al. Management of hypocalcemic effects of WR2721 administered on a daily times five schedule with cisplatin and radiation therapy. The New York Gynecologic Oncology Group [see comments]. *J Clin Oncol* 1993;11:1517.

409. Liu T, Liu Y, He S, et al. Use of radiation with or without WR-2721 in advanced rectal cancer. *Cancer* 1992;69:2820.

410. Mehta MP. Protection of normal tissues from the cytotoxic effects of radiation therapy: focus on amifostine. *Semin Radiat Oncol* 1998;8:14.

411. Ben-Josef E, Mesina J, Shaw LM, et al. Topical application of WR-2721 achieves high concentrations in the rectal wall. *Radiat Res* 1995;143:107.

412. Brizel DM. Future directions in toxicity prevention. *Semin Radiat Oncol* 1998;8:17.

413. Brizel DM, Wasserman TH, Strnad V, et al. Final report of a phase III randomized trial of amifostine as a radioprotectant in head and neck cancer. *Int J Radiat Oncol Biol Phys* 1999;45:147.

414. Bohuslavizki KH, Klutmann S, Brenner W, et al. Salivary gland protection by amifostine in high-dose radioiodine treatment: results of a double-blind placebo-controlled study. *J Clin Oncol* 1998;16:3542.

415. Glover D, Glick JH, Weiler C, et al. Phase I/II trials of WR-2721 and cis-platinum. *Int J Radiat Oncol Biol Phys* 1986;12:1509.

416. Glover D, Glick JH, Weiler C, et al. WR-2721 protects against the hematologic toxicity of cyclophosphamide: a controlled phase II trial. *J Clin Oncol* 1986;4:584.

417. Glick JH, Glover D, Weiler C, et al. Phase I controlled trials of WR-2721 and cyclophosphamide. *Int J Radiat Oncol Biol Phys* 1984;10:1777.

418. Buzaid AC, Murren J, Durivage HJ. High-dose cisplatin plus WR-2721 in a split course in metastatic malignant melanoma. A phase II study. *Am J Clin Oncol* 1991;14:203.

419. Budd GT, Ganapathi R, Bauer L, et al. Phase I study of WR-2721 and carboplatin. *Eur J Cancer* 1993;29A:1122.

420. Gill I, Muggia R, Parker R. WR-2721 pretreatment protects against the marrow toxicity of carboplatin and cisplatin [Abstract]. *Proc Am Soc Clin Oncol* 1992;11:132.

421. Wadler S, Beitler JJ, Rubin JS, et al. Pilot trial of cisplatin, radiation, and WR2721 in carcinoma of the uterine cervix: a New York Gynecologic Oncology Group study. *J Clin Oncol* 1993;11:1511.

422. Korst AE, van der Sterre ML, Gall HE, et al. Influence of amifostine on the pharmacokinetics of cisplatin in cancer patients. *Clin Cancer Res* 1998;4:331.

423. Korst AE, van der Sterre ML, Eeltink CM, et al. Pharmacokinetics of carboplatin with and without amifostine in patients with solid tumors. *Clin Cancer Res* 1997;3:697.

424. Kemp G, Rose P, Lurain J, et al. Amifostine pretreatment for protection against cyclophosphamide-induced and cisplatin-induced toxicities: results of a randomized control trial in patients with advanced ovarian cancer. *J Clin Oncol* 1996;14:2101.

425. Mehta MP. Protection of normal tissues from the cytotoxic effects of radiation therapy: focus on amifostine. *Semin Radiat Oncol* 1998;8:14.

426. Schiller JH, Storer B, Berlin J, et al. Amifostine, cisplatin, and vinblastine in metastatic non-small-cell lung cancer: a report of high response rates and prolonged survival. *J Clin Oncol* 1996;14:1913.

427. Tannehill SP, Mehta MP, Larson M, et al. Effect of amifostine on toxicities associated with sequential chemotherapy and radiation therapy for unresectable non-small-cell lung cancer: results of a phase II trial. *J Clin Oncol* 1997;15:2850.

428. Gelman K, Eisenhauer E, Bryce C, et al. Randomized phase II study of high-dose paclitaxel with or without amifostine in patients with metastatic breast cancer. *J Clin Oncol* 1999;17:3038.

429. Hensley ML, Schuchter LM, Lindley C, et al. American Society of Clinical Oncology Clinical Practice Guidelines for the use of chemotherapy and radiotherapy protectants. *J Clin Oncol* 1999;17:3333.

430. Mitchell JB, DeGraff W, Kaufman D, et al. Inhibition of oxygen-dependent radiation-induced damage by the nitroxide superoxide dismutase mimic, Tempol. *Arch Biochem Biophys* 1991;289:62.

431. Puck TT. Action of radiation on mammalian cells: III. Relationships between reproductive death and induction of chromosome anomalies by X-irradiation of euploid human cells in vitro. *Proc Natl Acad Sci U S A* 1958;44:772.

432. Carrano AV. Chromosome aberrations and radiation-induced cell death: II. Predicted and observed cell survival. *Mutat Res* 1973;17:355.

433. Bedford JS, Mitchell JB, Griggs HG, et al. Radiation-induced cellular reproductive death and chromosome aberrations. *Radiat Res* 1978;76:573.

434. DeGraff WG, Krishna MC, Kaufman D, et al. Nitroxide-mediated protection against x-ray- and neocarzinostatin-induced DNA damage. *Free Radic Biol Med* 1992;13:479.

435. Johnstone PAS, DeGraff WG, Mitchell JB. Protection of radiation-induced chromosomal aberrations by the nitroxide Tempol. *Cancer* 1995;75:2323.

436. Hahn SM, Tochner Z, Krishna CM, et al. Tempol, a stable free radical, is a novel murine radiation protector. *Cancer Res* 1992;52:1750.

437. Goffman T, Cuscela D, Glass J, et al. Topical application of nitroxide protects radiation induced alopecia in guinea pigs. *Int J Radiat Oncol Biol Phys* 1992;22:803.

438. Cuscela D, Coffin D, Lupton G, et al. Protection from radiation-induced alopecia with topical application of nitroxides: fractionated studies. *Cancer J Sci Am* 1996;2:273.

439. Hanson WR, Ainsworth EJ. 16,16-Dimethyl prostaglandin E2 induces radioprotection in murine intestinal and hematopoietic stem cells. *Radiat Res* 1985;103:196.

440. Hanson WR, Marks JE, Reddy SP, et al. Protection from radiation-induced oral mucositis by a mouth rinse containing the prostaglandin E1 analog, misoprostol: a placebo controlled double blind clinical trial. *Adv Exp Med Biol* 1997;400B:811.

441. Hanson WR, Pelka AE, Nelson AK, et al. Subcutaneous or topical administration of 16,16 dimethyl prostaglandin E2 protects from radiation-induced alopecia in mice. *Int J Radiat Oncol Biol Phys* 1992;23:333.

442. Geng L, Hanson WR, Malkinson FD. Topical or systemic 16, 16 dm prostaglandin E2 or WR-2721 (WR-1065) protects mice from alopecia after fractionated irradiation. *Int J Radiat Biol* 1992;61:533.

443. Malkinson FD, Geng L, Hanson WR. Prostaglandins protect against murine hair injury produced by ionizing radiation or doxorubicin. *J Invest Dermatol* 1993;101:135S.

444. Hanson WR, Zhen W, Geng L, et al. The prostaglandin E1 analog, misoprostol, a normal tissue protector, does not protect four murine tumors in vivo from radiation injury. *Radiat Res* 1995;142:281.

445. Hanson WR. Eicosanoid-induced radioprotection and chemoprotection of normal tissue during cancer treatment. In: Harris JE, Braun DP, Anderson KM, eds. *Prostaglandin inhibitors in tumor immunology and immunotherapy*. Boca Raton, FL: CRC Press, 1994:171.

446. Van Buul PPW, Van Duyn-Goedhart A, De Rooij DG, et al. Differential radioprotective effects of misoprostol in DNA repair-proficient and -deficient or radiosensitive cell systems. *Int J Radiat Biol* 1997;71:259.

447. Wang J, Zheng H, Sung CC, et al. The synthetic somatostatin analogue, octreotide, ameliorates acute and delayed intestinal radiation injury. *Int J Radiat Oncol Biol Phys* 1999;45:1289.

26

PHARMACOLOGY OF INTERFERONS: INDUCED PROTEINS, CELL ACTIVATION, AND ANTITUMOR ACTIVITY

DEBORAH J. VESTAL
TAOLIN YI
ERNEST C. BORDEN

Interferon-α (IFN-α) was the first human protein effective for cancer treatment. As the first economically important clinical product for cancer from recombinant DNA technology, IFNs have been prototypes for the clinical development of other immunomodulatory and growth-regulatory cytokines. IFN-α-2, one IFN-α family member, has proven effective not only as an antitumor protein, but also for antiviral therapy. IFNs are now serving as paradigms to begin to dissect the mechanisms of therapeutic resistance to cytokines.

Potent modulation of gene expression, which is reviewed below, must underlie the clinical activities of IFNs. One significant regulatory pathway for gene induction, the Janus kinase/signal transducers and activators of transcription (Jak-STAT) pathway, was originally elucidated by the study of IFNs but has proven to be critical for signaling by other cytokines and growth factors. The complex biologic and therapeutic activities of IFNs include virus inhibition, immunomodulation, slowing of cell proliferation, oncogene suppression, angiogenesis inhibition, alterations in differentiation, and induction of other cytokines (Table 26-1). The IFN-induced proteins that mediate these activities have only been partially identified.[1]

Like many other cytokines, the IFNs are a family of proteins that include more than a dozen different members encoded on human chromosome 9p (except IFN-γ, which is encoded on human chromosome 12q). The biologic and clinical significance of the individual proteins encoded by the approximately 15 distinct nonallelic IFN-α genes has barely been studied. These individual proteins differ over a 50× range in their potency in eliciting antiproliferative, immunomodulatory, and antiviral cellular effects.[2] Other than IFN-α-2, the only IFN-α gene product generated for clinical research trial has been IFN-α-1, which has proven to be better tolerated than was IFN-α-2.[3]

IFN-β has therapeutic usefulness in some stages of multiple sclerosis[4,5] and, potentially, for cancer and hyperlipidemias.[6,7] IFN-γ decreases the frequency of bacterial infections in chronic granulomatous disease and may be efficacious, either alone or in combination with antimicrobial agents, at inhibiting the replication of intracellular microbial pathogens.[8,9] IFNs-α, IFN-β, and IFN-γ are now licensed for clinical use by regulatory authorities in more than 50 countries. Second-generation IFN molecules, bioengineered for potentially desirable effects, have now entered clinical trials in oncology. One of these has been approved for use in chronic active hepatitis.[10–12]

In at least six to eight malignancies, IFN-α-2 results in regression or control of disease processes (Table 26-2). The spectrum of single-agent activity of IFNs compares favorably with other systemic cancer treatment modalities. The antitumor effects of IFNs can be enhanced in experimental tumor models by cytotoxic compounds, radiation, and other biologics. Greater clinical benefit will undoubtedly result through the use of IFNs in combination with other treatments, a topic beyond the scope of this chapter, but dependent on understanding IFNs effects as a single agent.

INTERFERONS: THEIR STRUCTURE AND INDUCERS

IFNs are a family of proteins, each residing at a specific genetic locus retained through evolution (Table 26-3). The three major classes of IFNs (α, β, γ) were initially defined on the basis of their chemical, antigenic, and biologic variation. These variations result from differences in their primary amino acid sequences. Complete nucleotide sequences have been obtained for almost 20 human IFNs.[13–16] IFN-α and IFN-β have approximately 45% homology of nucle-

TABLE 26-1. BIOLOGIC EFFECTS OF INTERFERONS

Microbial inhibition
RNA viruses
DNA viruses
Intracellular pathogens
Immunomodulatory
T cell (major histocompatibility complex restricted)
Natural killer/lymphokine-activated killer cell (non–major histo-
　compatibility complex restricted)
Monocytes
Dendritic cells
Antiproliferative effects and apoptosis
Oncogene depression
Slow mitotic cycle
Differentiation
Protein induction
Cell surface proteins
Enzymes
Cytokines
Apoptosis
Antigen processing
Vascular
Angiogenesis inhibition
Lipoprotein reduction
Antitumor
Mouse
Human

TABLE 26-3. FAMILY OF INTERFERON (IFN) MOLECULES: IFN FAMILIES

Family	Chromosome (human)	Types (n)	Amino Acids	Homology[a] (%)
Alpha	9	≥12	166	75–85
Beta	9	1	166	30
Gamma	12	1	143	1
Omega	9	>1	173	50

[a]Compared to IFN-α.
Note: The IFN licensed for clinical use and produced by recombinant DNA technology is IFN-α. IFN-α-2a (Hoffmann LaRoche) differs from IFN-α-2b (Schering-Plough) by a single amino acid at position 23 (lysine in IFN-α-2a; arginine in IFN-α-2b). IFN-α-2 is 165 amino acids, with a deletion of an aspartate residue at amino acid 44 when compared to other members of the IFN-α family.

otides and 29% homology of amino acids. Each of the non-allelic human IFN-α genes differs by approximately 10% in nucleotide sequence and 15% to 25% in amino acid sequence (Table 26-3). IFN-γ, 143 amino acids in length, is located on chromosome 12[16,17] and has only minimal sequence homology with IFNs-α or IFN-β. Two additional IFN classes, ω and τ, have been defined. IFN-ω binds to the same receptor as IFNs-α and IFN-β and mediates similar biologic effects.[18,19] IFN-τ is a novel class of IFN, identified in domestic ruminants but not humans, that maintains the

TABLE 26-2. INTERFERONS: INTERNATIONALLY APPROVED INDICATIONS

Malignancies
Hairy cell leukemia
Chronic myelogenous leukemia
Myeloma
Follicular lymphoma
Renal cell carcinoma
Kaposi's sarcoma
Melanoma
Viral diseases
Hepatitis C
Hepatitis B
Herpetic keratitis
Papillomas
　Genital
　Laryngeal
Immunomodulation
Multiple sclerosis
Chronic granulomatous disease

appropriate milieu in the endometrium for trophoblastic implantation.[20,21] Despite the glycosylation of endogenous IFN-β and IFN-γ, the biologic effects of the unglycosylated proteins produced in *Escherichia coli* have been similar.[22] The glycosylated and unglycosylated IFNs inhibit the replication of RNA and DNA viruses.

In addition to the direct administration of IFNs, chemically defined IFN inducers may have several therapeutic applications. They may possess advantageous pharmacokinetics of IFN induction, directly induce additional cytokines, activate immune effector cells, and, if administered orally, be more convenient. In some clinical settings, they might prove more effective as therapeutic agents, in addition to potentially being chemopreventive. The first chemically defined inducers of IFNs were double-stranded polyribonucleotides, such as polyriboinosinic-polyribocytidilic acid (poly I:poly C). Although potent IFN inducers and immunomodulators in mice, poly I:poly C, or various modifications do not consistently induce IFN or have any antitumor activity in humans at clinically tolerable doses.[23] Subsequently, low-molecular-weight organic compounds, such as tilorone, halopyrimidinones, acridines, substituted quinolones, and flavone acetic acid, were identified as inducers of IFNs in different animal species. Several IFN inducers have been introduced into human clinical trials, and some induce substantial amounts of IFN and activate the IFN system. The induction of IFN is associated with the cytokine symptomatology of chills, fever, and fatigue. These symptoms confirm the *in vivo* physiologic activity of the inducers and demonstrate the need to better define biologically and clinically effective dosage.[24–28]

SIGNAL TRANSDUCTION AND CONTROL OF INTERFERON-STIMULATED GENE EXPRESSION

Cellular responses to IFNs are initiated by the binding to a specific cell surface receptor that transduces signals to the

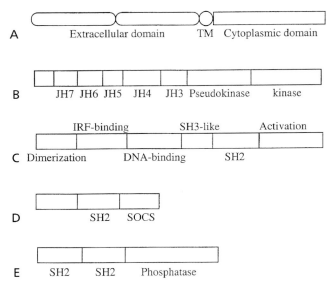

FIGURE 26-1. Protein components of interferon (IFN) signaling pathway. **A:** Structure of IFN receptor subunits. *TM* denotes a transmembrane domain. **B:** Structure of Janus kinases (Jak). *JH* denotes a Jak-homology domain. **C:** Structure of signal transducers and activators of transcription (STAT) proteins. **D:** Structure of suppressor of cytokine signaling (SOCS) proteins. *SOCS* denotes a SOCS box domain. **E:** Structure of src-homology 2 domain–containing protein tyrosine phosphatase (SHP)-1.

cytoplasm and nucleus.[29] These receptors have been characterized using genetic, biochemical, and molecular biologic approaches.[30] Exploration of the IFN signal transduction and gene regulation pathways has enhanced the understanding of biologic responses to IFNs as well as other cytokines. The following sections focus on IFN receptors, the mechanisms by which IFN-stimulated genes (ISGs) are induced, and the genes regulated by IFNs.

Unlike many other cell surface receptors, IFN receptors lack intrinsic enzymatic activity[29] but instead are specifically associated with intracellular tyrosine kinases belonging to the Jak family (Jak kinases, including Jak1, Jak2, Jak3, and Tyk2).[29,31] IFN binding to an IFN receptor activates the preassociated Jak kinases to phosphorylate tyrosine residues on multiple latent cytoplasmic transcriptional factors, designated *STATs*, which then migrate to the nucleus and control transcription of IFN-modulated genes (Figs. 26-1 and 26-2).[29,32]

Interferon Receptors

IFN-α, IFN-β, and IFN-ω bind to a common type of IFN receptor (type I IFN receptor), whereas IFN-γ binds to a distinct type of receptor (type II IFN receptor).[33] The two types of IFN receptors are found on all normal and malignant tissues, as demonstrated by binding of iodine 125 (^{125}I)–labeled IFNs.[34] Binding constants between 10^{-11} and

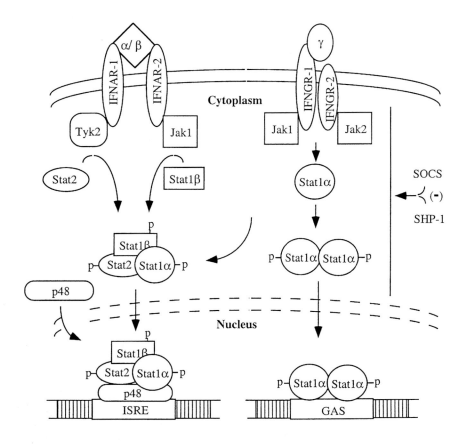

FIGURE 26-2. Components of the interferon (IFN) signaling pathways. The major components responsible for relaying IFN-mediated signals from the cell surface to the regulatory elements of IFN-stimulated genes are represented. (GAS, IFN-γ activation site; IFNAR, IFN-α receptor; IFNGR, IFN-γ receptor; ISRE, IFN-stimulated response element; Jak, Janus kinase; p, phosphotyrosine; SHP, src-homology 2 domain–containing protein tyrosine phosphatase; SOCS, suppressor of cytokine signaling; STAT, signal transducers and activators of transcription; Tyk, Jak family kinase.)

10^{-9} have been calculated, and the number of receptors is between 100 and 2,000 per cell. The receptors for type I and type II IFNs are transmembrane glycoproteins (Figs. 26-1 and 26-2). The extracellular domains of the receptor proteins form IFN binding sites, whereas the cytoplasmic domains of the receptor proteins associate with the Jak family kinases.

Two subunits of the type I IFN receptor, IFNAR-1[35] and IFNAR-2,[36,37] have been cloned. They associate with Tyk2 (tyrosine kinase 2) and Jak1 kinases, respectively.[38,39] The genes encoding the two subunits are clustered in the q22.1 region of human chromosome 21.[38–40] The functional importance of the two receptor subunits has been highlighted by the capacity of the human IFNAR-1 and IFNAR-2, when expressed in mouse cells, to activate intracellular signaling events and elicit an antiviral state in response to type I human IFNs.[41] Accessory factors for the type I IFN receptor are suggested by studies that cross-linked IFN-α to membrane proteins of molecular weights of 110 kd, 130 kd, and 210 kd and showed that these same proteins communoprecipitated with antibodies specific to the IFN-α receptor.[42] In addition, the failure of human IFNAR-1 and IFNAR-2 to confer to mouse cells the antiproliferative activity of human type I IFNs also suggested the involvement of additional molecules in the receptor complex.[41]

The IFN-γ receptor has two subunits, IFNGR-1 and IFNGR-2,[43–45] which are associated with the Jak1 and Jak2 kinases, respectively.[46,47] In humans, IFNGR-1 has 486 amino acids and is located on chromosome 6q.[43] IFN-γ binds to IFNGR-1, inducing IFNGR-1 dimerization and association with IFNGR-2 to activate the receptor-coupled Jak1 and Jak2 kinases in transducing signals.[46]

Signal Transduction

IFNs, like many other cytokines, activate protein tyrosine kinases to transduce signals into the cells. This was first suggested by the observations that binding of IFNs to membrane receptors induces a rapid increase in the tyrosine phosphorylation of various cellular proteins. The lack of protein tyrosine kinase domains in the IFN-α, IFN-β, or IFN-γ receptors indicated that additional receptor or nonreceptor protein tyrosine kinases must be involved.[36,37,43–45] Complementation of IFN-resistant mutant cell lines by genes for members of the Jak family of nonreceptor protein kinases provides direct evidence for involvement of these proteins: Jak1, Jak2, and Tyk2. A mutant cell line that completely lacked the ability to respond to IFN-α or IFN-γ became responsive to IFNs when the Jak1 tyrosine kinase was expressed in the mutant,[48] indicating the central role of Jak1 in IFN-α and IFN-γ signaling pathways. Complementation of an IFN-γ nonresponsive mutant (IFN-α and β response intact) with the gene for Jak2 demonstrated the requirement for Jak2 in the IFN-γ response.[49] Complementation of an IFN-α nonresponsive mutant (IFN-γ response

intact) with the gene for Tyk2 demonstrated that Tyk2 is essential for the IFN-α response.[50] Biochemical studies have demonstrated that each subunit of the IFN receptors associates specifically with a Jak family kinase (Figs. 26-1 and 26-2), which is activated by IFN's binding to the receptors to phosphorylate tyrosine residues in cellular protein substrates, including STATs.

STATs are a family of cellular proteins that transduce signals from a variety of cell surface receptors to the nucleus and activate transcription by binding to regulatory DNA elements.[29] Each of the STATs has a dimerization domain at its N-terminal region, an IFN-regulatory factor (IRF)–binding domain, a DNA-binding domain, SH2 and SH3 domains, and a C-terminal transcription activation domain.[32] The Jak kinases, when activated by IFN binding to the receptors, undergo autophosphorylation, cross-phosphorylate each other, and phosphorylate the receptor subunits.[31] The phosphorylated tyrosine residues in these proteins provide binding sites for the SH2 domains of STATs, resulting in the recruitment of the STATs to the receptor and Jak complexes and the phosphorylation of tyrosine residues in the STAT proteins.[29] This leads to STAT dimerization, translocation into the nucleus, and binding to regulatory DNA elements to control the transcription of IFN-regulated genes.[29,31,32]

So far, six STAT proteins (STAT1 through 6) have been cloned and characterized.[32] Two isoforms of STAT1 (STAT1a and STAT1b) are produced through alternative splicing and differ at their C-termini.[51] Unlike STAT1a, STAT1b lacks the transcriptional activation domain and, thus, functions as a signal transducer but not a transcriptional activator. Complementation of mutant cell lines lacking endogenous STAT expression demonstrates that STAT1 is essential for IFN-α, β, and γ signal transduction, whereas STAT2 is required for IFN-α and β signaling only.[52,53] The functional importance of STAT1 in IFN signaling has been further supported by the failure of STAT1-deficient mice to respond to IFNs and by the markedly heightened susceptibility of these mice to viral and other microbial infections.[54,55]

Two types of regulatory DNA elements have been identified that are recognized by IFN-activated STATs to control the transcription of IFN-regulated genes. The IFN-stimulated response element (ISRE) is an enhancer element, conserved among all species that respond to IFN-α and β.[29] Genes stimulated by IFN-γ contain a cis-acting element called the *IFN-γ activation site* (GAS).[32]

The core sequence of the ISRE is a direct repeat of GAAA spaced by one or two nucleotides [GAAAN(N)GAAA]. Mutational analysis of ISRE reporter constructs defined the ISRE necessary and sufficient for IFN responsiveness.[56] The ISRE is recognized by three DNA-binding complexes designated IFN-stimulated gene factor 1 (ISGF-1), IRF-1, and ISGF-3. Unlike ISGF-1, which is constitutively expressed, IRF-1 and ISGF-3 are induced by IFNs.[57] Initial studies demonstrated that ISGF-3 is composed of two biochemically distinct species. The ISGF-3α component is a cytoplasmic complex of three proteins (STAT1a, STAT1b, and STAT2), all activated via tyrosine phosphorylation to associate and translocate to the nucleus.[58] The ISGF-3γ component is a 48-kd protein (p48) found in the cytoplasm and nucleus and having intrinsic DNA-binding activity.[57] Activated ISGF-3α binds the ISGF-3γ component in the nucleus, forming the ISGF-3 complex. This complex then binds to the ISRE to activate transcription.[58]

The consensus sequence of a GAS element is AANNNNNTT.[29] The GAS element is sometimes contained within the ISRE element and is conserved between species. IFN-γ stimulation induces tyrosine phosphorylation of STAT1a, which forms homodimers (also called *GAF*) and binds to GAS to activate transcription.[30]

In light of the pivotal role of the Jak-STAT pathway in IFN signaling, it is not surprising that molecules that interact with and regulate the Jak and STAT proteins also affect IFN signaling. Src-homology 2 domain–containing protein tyrosine phosphatase (SHP)-1 and SHP-2 are protein tyrosine phosphatases that contain SH2 domains.[59] SHP-1 can associate with and dephosphorylate the Jak family kinases to inactivate the kinases and terminate signaling.[60] Its negative regulatory role in IFN signaling is demonstrated by a heightened response to IFNs in SHP-1–deficient cells.[61] Similarly, SHP-2–deficient cells show augmented STAT activation and reduction of cell viability in response to IFNs, suggesting that SHP-2 also down-regulates IFN signaling.[62] Additional protein tyrosine phosphatases regulating Jak and STAT proteins have been indicated by a number of studies and may be involved in the control of IFN signaling.[41,63–65]

Recently, a family of suppressor of cytokine signaling (SOCS, also known as *CIS-cytokine-inducible SH2*) proteins has been identified.[66,67] These proteins have a central SH2 domain and a C-terminal SOCS box (also known as *CIS-homology* or *CH domain*) that is conserved among all family members. Most SOCS are induced by several different cytokines, and some of them have been shown to negatively regulate cytokine signaling through binding to Jak kinases or STATs to inhibit their activities,[68] targeting the protein for degradation, or both.[69] Importantly, the expression of SOCS1 (also termed *Jak-binding protein*), SOCS2, and SOCS3 is strongly induced by IFN-γ.[70,71] Stable expression of SOCS1 or SOCS3 blocks IFN-mediated antiviral effects and IFN-induced growth arrest.[70,71] Thus, these SOCS may be the effectors of a negative feedback mechanism that shuts down IFN response after IFN stimulation (Figs. 26-1 and 26-2).

Although the Jak-STAT pathway plays an essential role in IFN signaling, it is clear that other kinases and transcriptional factors are also involved in IFN signaling. The antiproliferative activity of IFN-α in T cells has been shown to require components of the T-cell receptor signaling pathway, including the Lck and ZAP-70 protein tyrosine kinases.[72] IRF-1 and IRF-2 are also involved in regulating ISGs by binding to ISREs.[73,74] IRF-1 and IRF-2 are transcriptional factors related to p48.[75] Complementary DNA expression studies showed that IRF-1 acts as a positive regulator of IFN-α–, IFN-β–, and IFN-γ–induced genes, whereas IRF-2 represses the effects of IRF-1.[76,77] These antagonistic factors may play a role in oncogenesis, because experimental expression of IRF-2 resulted in the transformation and enhanced tumorigenicity of NIH-IIIT3 cells, which was then reversed by expression of IRF-1.[78] Transgenic mice deficient in IRF-1 or IRF-2 confirm the important roles of these regulatory proteins.[79] Fibroblasts from IRF-1–deficient mice lack the normally observed IFN induction by poly I:poly C, although they induce IFN to normal levels when challenged with Newcastle disease virus. A substantial reduction in T cell population of antigen receptor (TCR) αβ+ CD4⁻ CD8⁺ T cells is also observed in the IRF-1–deficient mice, demonstrating the critical role of IRF-1 in T-cell development. In contrast, fibroblasts from IRF-2–deficient mice show an enhanced type I IFN induction when challenged with Newcastle disease virus.

The IFN consensus sequence-binding protein (ICSBP) is another negative regulatory factor that binds to the ISRE of many IFN-regulated genes, including the major histocompatibility complex (MHC) class I genes.[80] The DNA-binding domain of ICSBP is approximately 50% identical to that of IRF-1 and IRF-2.[81] Expression of ICSBP is restricted to cells of the hematopoietic lineage and is induced by IFN-γ, but not by IFN-α and β.[82] ICSBP represses IFN-induced promoter activity of MHC class I and of the 2',5'-oligoadenylate synthetase (2-5A synthetase), guanylate binding protein (GBP), and ISG-15 gene in embryonal carcinoma cells.[81]

Mechanism of Interferon Resistance

Despite the successful application of IFNs to the treatment of several malignancies, the potential of the IFNs in antitumor therapies has not yet been fully realized. So far, the mechanism of IFN resistance in human cancer patients has been little studied. Some fresh tumor cells from untreated patients are completely resistant to the antiproliferative effects of IFNs, demonstrating primary IFN resistance in these tumor cells.[83] Although IFN-α results in a good response in 75% of patients with chronic myelogenous leukemia (CML), it induces complete cytogenetic remission in fewer than 20%. This suggests the presence of partial or complete primary IFN resistance in the nonresponding patients.[84] On the other hand, development of acquired IFN resistance *in vivo* appears to be common and is indicated by the eventual loss of IFN responsiveness in some of the patients who were initially responsive to IFNs. This is illustrated by a patient with a T-cell lymphoma whose initial positive response to IFN therapy was followed by rapid progression, due to the appearance of a subpopulation of IFN-resistant malignant cells.[85]

Interferon Signaling Molecules in Interferon Resistance

Cell lines unresponsive to IFNs have been generated by mutagenesis, and these lack distinct IFN signaling molecules, including components of IFN receptors, Jak kinases, or STATs.[30] Complementation of the mutant cell lines with the corresponding signaling molecules restores the response to IFNs.[30] Defects of signaling molecules in human tumor cells have also been reported. The association of IFN resistance with the lack of expression of a component of an IFN receptor was found in a human leukemia cell line.[86] *In vivo* sensitivity and resistance of CML cells to IFN-α correlates with reduced receptor binding.[87] Characterization of an IFN-resistant tumor cell variant (Hut78R) from a human CTLL cell line Hut78 reveals a lack of STAT1 expression, which was required for the growth-inhibitory effects of IFNs.[88] These observations indicate that defects of the IFN receptor and STAT1 may be present in certain IFN-resistant human tumor cells and may block IFN antitumor activity. Interestingly, in contrast to the antiproliferative effect of IFN-α on the parental cells, increased concentrations of IFN-α caused a marked stimulation of growth in the IFN-resistant Hut78R cells.[88] Thus, STAT defects might also be involved in tumor progression.

SHP-1 involvement in human leukemia is suggested by the localization of the SHP-1 gene at chromosome 12p13,[89] a region frequently affected in acute lymphoblastic leukemia (ALL), and by the deletion of the SHP-1 gene in some of the ALL cases with 12p abnormalities.[90] Given the negative regulatory role of SHP-1 in IFN signaling,[61] ALL cases with reduced or absent SHP-1 expression could be predicted to be more sensitive to IFNs and are potential clinical candidates for IFN therapies. Because increased expression of SOCS family members can block IFN signaling,[67] potential involvement of these signaling molecules in IFN resistance is also a topic that warrants future studies.

The biologic activity of IFNs depends on the induction of specific genes that affect cell morphology, cell viability, cell-cycle progression, differentiation, and intercellular interactions. Defects in IFN-induced gene expression are also detected in IFN-resistant primary leukemia cells.[91] The recent identification of a large number of novel ISGs using the DNA-chip technique will help to further assess the involvement of ISGs in IFN resistance.[92]

Besides proteins that are intrinsic components of the IFN-signaling pathways, a number of other cellular factors may also participate in IFN resistance. A recent study demonstrated a correlation between IFN resistance and heightened expression of the *bcl*-2 proto-oncogene in primary myeloma cells.[93] As induction of apoptosis is likely important in IFN-mediated antitumor activity,[94] overexpression

of bcl-2 protein may protect the tumor cells from IFN-induced apoptosis and confer IFN resistance. A number of viruses can also produce factors that block IFN responses. Adenovirus, Epstein-Barr virus, and hepatitis B virus have all been implicated in the pathogenesis of human malignancies. The E1A and virus-associated (VA) I RNA of adenovirus, the EBNA-2 protein of Epstein-Barr virus and the terminal protein of hepatitis B virus inhibit the cellular response to IFN.[91,95,96] Therefore, IFN resistance in virus-associated human tumors may be mediated, at least in part, by the expression of specific viral proteins.

CELLULAR MECHANISMS OF ANTITUMOR ACTION

The antitumor effects of IFN can be divided into two broad categories: (a) direct antiproliferative or proapoptotic effects on the tumor cells themselves, and (b) indirect induction of host antitumor mechanisms (via enhancement of immune function, inhibition of angiogenesis, enhancement of tumor–surface antigen expression, or a combination of all three). Human tumor cells are sensitive to the antiproliferative and apoptotic effects of IFNs,[97–99] but the molecular details of how IFNs mediate these responses have only been partially elucidated. However, underlying the antitumor effects must be a plethora of genes that are regulated in expression (Table 26-4). Specific genetic mutation of the tumor cell, its surrounding environment, or both may determine which of these mechanisms plays a more significant role in mediating the antitumor effects of IFN.

Direct Mechanisms

The influence of IFNs on cell proliferation and cell death or apoptosis is cell type specific and influenced by the environment and state of differentiation of the cells.[98,100–103] Indeed, signals for proliferation and apoptosis are linked and overlapping.[104] Proliferation of normal cells is rigidly regulated by proteins that serve as checkpoints for the control of cell-cycle progression.[105] As a prerequisite to unregulated growth, cancer cells develop defects in one or more proteins in these pathways. Probably the best studied of these is the tumor suppressor p53, a transcription factor that, when activated by phosphorylation, promotes either growth arrest, apoptosis, or both. Many tumors have inactivating mutations in p53 itself or in proteins that influence p53 activation. p53 probably promotes apoptosis by inducing the expression of proapoptotic genes, such as Bax, and blocks cell-cycle progression primarily by inducing the cdk inhibitor p21/WAF1 (Fig. 26-3). The response of p53 is influenced positively and negatively by the expression of a number of oncogenes. IFNs regulate a number of these proto-oncogenes and tumor suppressors, such as c-*myc*,[106–108] *bcl*-2,[99,109,110] c-Ha-ras,[111] and c-*src*.[111]

TABLE 26-4. INTERFERON (IFN)-REGULATED GENE PRODUCTS AND THEIR FUNCTIONS

Genes	Function	Reference
Antiviral		
Guanylate binding protein (GBP)-1	Guanosine triphosphatase (GTPase), antiviral	211
MxA	GTPase, antiviral (neg. strand RNA viruses)	202
TGTP	GTPase, antiviral	218, 221
Antigen processing and presentation		
β_2-microglobulin	Component of major histocompatibility complex (MHC) class I	149, 189, 222
Cathepsins B, H, and S	Lysosomal proteases	233, 234
CIITA	Transcription factor	232
Invariant chain	MHC class II assembly	231
Low-molecular-weight protein (LMP)-2, LMP-7, LMP-10	Proteasome subunits	224, 225
MHC class I	Antigen presentation	149
MHC class II	Antigen presentation	189
Proteasome accelerator 28	Proteasome regulator	222
Cytokines and chemokines		
β-R1/TAC	Chemokine	253, 254
IP-10	Chemokine	181, 250
RANTES	Chemokine	249
ISG-15	Chemokine	248
Signal transduction		
IFN consensus sequence-binding protein	DNA binding protein	81, 82
IFI 16	DNA binding protein	265
INF-regulatory factor (IRF)-1	Transacting factor	73
IRF-2	Transacting factor	74
Protein synthesis inhibition		
2',5'-oligoA synthetase	2-5A synthesis	30, 191, 193
PKR	Protein kinase	192, 194–196
Tryptophan metabolism		
Tryptophanyl–transfer RNA synthetase	Aminoacylation of transfer RNA trp	240
Indoleamine 2,3-dioxygenase	Tryptophan metabolism	236, 237
Respiratory burst/nitric oxide metabolism		
gp91-phox	Reduced form of nicotinamide adenine dinucleotide phosphate (NADPH) oxidase subunit	243, 245
GTP-cyclohydroxylase	Converts GTP to tetrahydrobiopterin	246
Nitric oxide synthetase	Produces nitric oxide	246, 247
p47-phox	NADPH oxidase subunit	243–245
GTPases		
GBP-2	GTPase	211
MxB	GTPase	203
Miscellaneous		
Carcinoembryonic antigen	Tumor-associated antigen	151, 276
Fc-γ receptor	Binds Fc of IgG	155, 189
ISG-20	Nuclear protein	274
Myeloid cell nuclear differentiation antigen	DNA binding protein	263, 264
Promyelocytic leukemia	Nuclear protein	106
SP-100	Nuclear protein	272
TAG-72	Tumor-associated antigen	151, 276

Another important checkpoint protein mutated in many cancers is the retinoblastoma protein (RB). RB is a tumor-suppressive transcription factor regulated by phosphorylation.[112,113] RB becomes hyperphosphorylated with entry into late G_1 and S phases and then is dephosphorylated after mitosis.[114–117] The underphosphorylated RB (the active form) specifically binds and inhibits the transcription factor E2F,[118] thus inhibiting cell-cycle progression. Although IFN-α up-regulates expression of the RB gene in Burkitt's lymphoma cells,[112] the primary regulation of RB by IFN-α is the inhibition of its hyperphosphorylation by

IFN treatment.[112,113] The inhibition of RB hyperphosphorylation by IFN may result from rapid reduction of the expression of cyclin D3, which in turn, results in a reduction in the formation of cyclin D-cdk4 and cyclin D-cdk6 kinase complexes.[119]

E2F is a heterodimeric transcription factor that controls a number of cell-cycle related genes, such as c-*myc* and cdc2.[120] IFN-α treatment of Burkitt's cells results in the reduction of one of the E2F proteins, E2F-1.[121] Free E2F is composed of E2F-1 and E2F-4, and the reduction in E2F-1 results in lower DNA-binding capacity. In addition, IFN-α converts

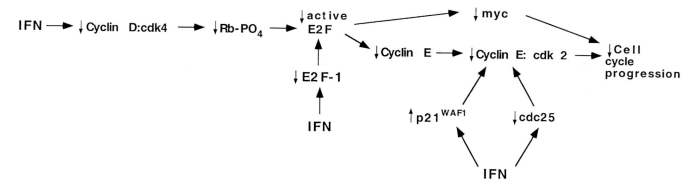

FIGURE 26-3. Interferon (IFN) mediation of cell cycle. The antiproliferative actions of IFNs are, at least in part, the consequence of IFN perturbation of cell cycle through the mechanisms represented here.

the E2F-RB complex into a transcription repressor by inducing the dephosphorylation of RB.[121] IFN-α reduction of transcription of the c-*myc* oncogene is, at least in part, a consequence of IFN reduction in DNA binding of the transcription factor E2F, which binds to the c-*myc* promoter.[122] Down-regulation of c-*myc* can be further amplified by activation of a negative regulatory element by IFN-γ.[108]

Downstream of RB and E2F, IFN-α rapidly reduces the amount of the cdc25 tyrosine phosphatase, resulting in the loss of activation of cyclin E-cdk2 and cyclin A-cdk2 kinase complexes, which require dephosphorylation by cdc25 for activation.[119] Also, the cdk-inhibitor p21/WAF1 is induced,[123] which negatively regulates cyclin E-cdk2. In addition, IFN-γ directly induces p21/WAF1 through STAT1.[124–126]

Another key pathway for the induction of apoptosis involves the Fas surface glycoprotein (CD95) and its ligand (FasL). Binding of Fas to FasL or an anti-Fas antibody triggers apoptosis by recruitment of the death domain–containing protein FADD, and the subsequent activation of caspases, such as caspase-8, which begin to destroy the cell. IFN-γ up-regulates the expression of Fas and FasL on the human colon adenocarcinoma cell line HT-29.[127] IFNs up-regulate Fas expression and, therefore, may work through the Fas-mediated apoptotic pathway in other cells as well.[110,128–132]

In addition, IFN-mediated apoptosis may involve novel mechanisms. The prostate cancer cell line, DU-145, has multiple defects in tumor suppressor genes having mutations in RB, p53, and KAI1.[133–135] Despite this, IFN-α treatment inhibits the progression of DU-145 cells from G_1 through S phase, suggesting involvement of an as-yet unidentified pathway. Along with the reduction in cdk2 activity, the cdk2 kinase inhibitor p21 is induced.[136] Recently, these same cells were shown to be responsive to IFN-γ.[137] IFN-γ induces the expression of p21/WAF1 and blocks cell cycle but, unlike IFN-α, it also induces phenotypic changes that result in a reduction in invasive potential.[137] In Burkitt's cells, which are induced to differentiate and undergo apoptosis with type I IFNs, IFN-γ does not inhibit cell proliferation and, as might be expected, does not induce p21/WAF1 expression.[123]

Using a functional genetic approach, several novel proteins have been identified as being involved in IFN-γ–induced apoptosis in HeLA epithelial carcinoma cells. These novel death associated proteins (DAPs) were identified as antisense complementary DNAs that are capable of suppressing IFN-γ–induced apoptosis in HeLA cells but that do not interfere with the inhibition of proliferation (cytostatic). DAP-1 is a novel 15-kd protein that is highly proline rich and contains a potential SH3 site and RGD sequence.[138] DAP-2 is a 160-kd calmodulin-dependent serine and threonine kinase that contains a death domain and a series of ankyrin repeats, and binds to the cytoskeleton.[138,139] DAP-3 is a 46-kd protein containing a putative P-loop, which suggests adenosine triphosphate and guanosine triphosphate (GTP) binding.[140] DAP-5 is a 97-kd homolog of the eukaryotic-initiation factor 4G.[141] DAP-5 appears to have a concentration-dependent effect on apoptosis. Expression at high levels stops cell proliferation and promotes cell death, but expression at low levels protected cells from death. In addition to the novel DAPs, this method also identified thioredoxin[142] and cathepsin D[143] as mediating IFN-γ–induced apoptosis. A similar antisense strategy identified thioredoxin reductase, which uses thioredoxin as a substrate as a mediator of cell death induced by the combination of IFN-β and retinoic acid.[144]

Finally, the inability to respond, or to respond only partially, to the antiproliferative effects of IFNs may play a role in transformation. For chronic B-cell lymphocytic leukemia cells, IFN-γ appears to promote cell survival by inhibiting apoptosis. Patients with this disease have higher than normal serum levels of IFN-γ, which may explain the enhanced survival of the BCLL cells *in vivo*.[145] Conversely, in murine models IFNs can inhibit chemical carcinogenesis, suggesting a possible role in chemoprevention.[146–148]

Indirect Mechanisms

The *in vivo* antitumor activity of IFN may also involve enhancement of host-mediated defenses. IFN may make tumor cells better targets for recognition by the immune system by increasing the expression of MHC I and II[149,150] tumor-associated antigens (TAAs),[151–154] Fc-γ receptors,[155] and intercellular adhesion molecules[156] on tumor cells. IFNs also directly alter the immune response by enhancing the activity of cytotoxic and helper T cells (CTLs),[157,158] natural killer (NK) cells,[159,160] macrophages,[161,162] and dendritic cells.[163,164]

The development and function of CTLs are influenced by IFN-γ. In addition to promoting CTL maturation,[165] IFN-γ promotes CTL expansion by increasing interleukin (IL)-2 receptor expression.[166] CTLs are thought to be the primary tumor-specific cytotoxic effector cells, based on observations such as CTL reactivity of patients toward autologous tumor cells.[167] In addition, in animals, tumor-specific lytic activity toward melanoma cells has been demonstrated; this was augmented by IFN-γ and could induce tumor regression.[168]

Direct injection of IFN-α and IFN-γ into skin recurrences of breast cancer results in tumor regression in more than 50% of patients.[156] While regressing, these tumors show evidence of enhanced intercellular adhesion molecule 1, increased human leukocyte antigen–DR (HLA-DR), and infiltration of the tumor with activated T cells.

IFN-γ enhances macrophage involvement in MHC-restricted and MHC-nonrestricted responses. As mentioned previously, IFN-γ up-regulates MHC class II expression, which displays antigens to CD4+ T-helper cells. These T-helper cells respond by proliferation and secretion of IFN-γ, creating a feedback loop. IFN-γ also enhances non–MHC-restricted cytotoxicity. Although CTL lysis of tumor targets *in vitro* is relatively rapid (approximately 6 hours), tumors that express low levels of surface MHC are poor targets for CTLs. These tumors are still capable of recognition by macrophages through a poorly understood mechanism that does not involve MHC. This macrophage-tumoricidal activity is also enhanced by IFN-γ that, in addition to up-regulating components of the oxidative burst and inducible nitric oxide synthetase (NOS) pathway, primes macrophages to heightened responses to bacterial lipopolysaccharide and other mitogens.[161,162] These fully activated macrophages secrete IFN-α and compounds believed responsible for the tumor cytotoxicity, such as tumor necrosis factor α, superoxides, and free-radical compounds.[161,162]

The importance of IFN in promoting NK activity has been suggested by studies in immunocompetent and athymic-nude mice. That IFN exposure enhances the activity of these cells is demonstrated by the observation that treatment of nude mice with anti–Mu-IFN-α and β antibody results in accelerated growth of transplanted human prostate carcinomas.[169] Similarly, treatment of immunocompetent mice with anti–Mu-IFN-α and β antibody enhances the growth of several different murine-derived tumors,[170] suggesting the role of host components in influencing IFN antitumor activity.

Neovascularization must accompany the growth of any solid tumor beyond the microscopic stage. Another important component of IFN-mediated tumor inhibition is the ability to inhibit angiogenesis. After IFN treatment, tumor endothelial cells exhibit microvascular injury and a pattern of coagulation necrosis.[171] Studies of the growth of related IFN-sensitive and -insensitive human bladder carcinomas show that systemic administration of IFN-α reduces tumor cell growth in the IFN-sensitive cells by directly regulating the expression of the angiogenic protein, b–fibroblast growth factor (FGF).[172] IFN-α and IFN-β also down-regulate bFGF in other human carcinomas.[173] IFN-γ also inhibited signals generated by potent angiogenic proteins, such as FGF[174,175] and platelet-derived growth factor.[175] Interruption of the angiogenic signal by IFNs precedes the antiproliferative effect and is detectable between 24 and 48 hours after tumor inoculation.[176] IFN down-regulation of bFGF correlates with reduced vascularization and reduced growth of the tumors in nude mice.[172] IFN-γ may also inhibit angiogenesis by blocking proliferation of endothelial cells[174] and by inhibiting collagen synthesis.

IL-8 has also been shown to be a potent mediator of angiogenesis[177,178] and, consequently, tumorigenesis.[179] IL-8 is also one of the angiogenic proteins whose production is inhibited by IFN-α.[180] In addition to inhibiting angiogenic proteins, IFN-γ up-regulates the expression of an angiostatic chemokine, IP-10.[181] IP-10 is an IFN-γ–induced C-X-C chemokine with the ability to repress the angiogenic activities of bFGF and IL-8.[181]

Clinically, IFN-α treatment has been successful in inducing regression of bulky hemangiomas, tumors consisting of abnormal endothelial cells.[182–184] Kaposi's sarcoma, a neoplastic disease of endothelial origin, also responds to treatment with IFN-α.[185–188]

INTERFERON-INDUCED PROTEINS

The pleiotropic cellular effects observed on exposure of cells to IFNs is mediated primarily through the transcriptional regulation of gene expression. In the last few years, the magnitude of the number of IFN-regulated genes has become more apparent (Table 26-4). A recent review, which can be found at http://www.annurev.org, documents more than 200 proteins regulated by IFN-γ.[189] More recently, use of oligonucleotide arrays identified a list of candidate genes that may be regulated by IFN-α, IFN-β, or IFN-γ[190]; the list can be found at http://www.lerner.ccf.org/labs/williams/der.html. Although type I and type II IFNs regulate a number of unique genes, there is also significant overlap in the genes regulated by both classes of IFNs.[30,189,191,192] Because many of the genes regulated by IFNs have functions that remain elusive, a complete understanding of how IFNs cause many biologic effects is not yet possible. However, those for which at least one function has been identified can be grouped into several categories.

Some of the best studied of the IFN-induced genes were first associated with antiviral activity but have now been implicated in the direct antiproliferative and immunomodulatory effects of IFNs.[191,193] One of these is the double-stranded RNA-dependent protein kinase (dsRNA-PKR).[192,194–196] PKR is induced by type I and type II IFNs, and, on activation, it slows cellular and viral proliferation by phosphorylating the eukaryotic initiation factor–2, an event that inhibits protein synthesis. PKR can be activated by dsRNA heparin or the newly identified protein PACT.[197] In the absence of viral infection, PKR has been implicated in cell growth control and apoptosis.[107,195,198]

The 2',5'-oligoadenylate synthetases (2-5A synthetase) have also been shown to be antiviral.[30,191,193,199] There are three size classes of 2-5A synthetase (small, medium, and large synthetases), and these are induced by all three types of IFNs. On activation by dsRNAs, these enzymes polymerize ATP into a series of 2',5'-oligoadenylates. These 2',5'-oligoadenylates activate the enzyme RNase-L, which degrades single-stranded RNAs, thereby inhibiting protein synthesis.

A third IFN-induced protein that binds dsRNA is the dsRNA-specific adenosine deaminase.[200,201] This enzyme uses dsRNA as a substrate to produce inositol from the deamination of adenosine and is believed to be involved in RNA editing.

There are at least three families of GTPases that are induced by IFNs. The best characterized is the Mx family.[191,192] Two human Mx proteins, MxA and MxB,[202,203] are induced primarily by type I IFNs. Human MxA has been shown to have antiviral activity against negative-strand RNA viruses, but no function has been identified for MxB.[204] Homologs of the human Mx proteins have been identified in a number of species.[205] The Mx proteins belong to the dynamin superfamily of large GTPases, proteins involved in endocytosis and vesicle transport,[206] and may have functions other than viral protection.[207,208]

Two other families of GTPases are some of the most abundant proteins in IFN-treated murine[209] or human[210] cells. One of these is the GBPs.[210] To date, two human GBPs have been cloned, and these are induced by type I and type II IFNs.[211] In the mouse, in addition to the two GBPs homologous to the human GBPs,[209,211–213] there are two more distantly related GBP members that differ in size and structural features,[209,212,214] suggesting two subgroups within the family. These are GTPases with unusual GTP hydrolysis profiles; recent studies have suggested an antiviral function for human GBP-1.[215]

The other abundant family of GTPases includes IRG-47,[216] LRG-47,[217] TGTP[218]/Mg-21,[219] and IGTP.[220] These proteins share a size of approximately 47 kd, GTPase motifs, and induction by IFN-γ. Although little is known about the function of this family of proteins, TGTP has been shown to have antiviral activity.[221]

Type I and type II IFNs increase the surface expression of MHC class I proteins, thereby facilitating activation of CD8⁺ cytotoxic T cells.[149,189] IFNs not only up-regulate the transcription of MHC class I genes themselves, but also coordinately stimulate the expression of other proteins required for surface expression of mature MHC class I complex.[149,189,222] This complex contains the MHC class I polypeptide, β_2-microglobulin, and an 8– to 10–amino acid–proteolytic antigenic peptide bound to the MHC polypeptide. As nascent class I molecules are synthesized, they associate with the cofactor, β_2-microglobulin, in the endoplasmic reticulum (ER) to be transported to the cell surface. IFN regulates β_2-microglobulin expression. The generation of antigenic peptides for loading onto class I molecules occurs predominantly in the proteasome.[223] IFNs up-regulate three proteasome subunits, low-molecular-weight protein (LMP)–2, LMP-7, and multicatalytic endopeptidase complex–like 1 (MECL-1/LMP-10).[224,225] Expression of these subunits and their incorporation into proteasomes changes the cleavage products generated for loading onto the class I protein.[226–228] In addition, the proteasome accelerator, PA28, and the heterodimeric transporter associated with antigen processing (TAP) are up-regulated by IFN-γ.[222,229] TAP transports the peptides generated by the proteasome from the cytosol into the ER to be loaded onto the class I protein. Without TAP, class I proteins remain empty, and class I surface expression is greatly reduced. Two additional proteins thought to be involved in MHC class I antigen presentation, tapasin (or gp48) and the ER protein gp96, are also IFN-γ induced.[189]

IFN-γ also induces the MHC class II response,[150,189,230] which activates CD4⁺ T cells. The MHC class II receptor is a heterodimeric protein that associates with the single polypeptide invariant (Ii) chain during its transport to a special endosomal compartment, where it receives its antigenic peptide. Here, the Ii chain is degraded, and with the assistance of two DM proteins, the class II heterodimer is loaded with antigenic peptide and transported to the cell surface. IFN-γ up-regulates the MHC class II heterodimer, the Ii chain,[231] DM proteins, and the transcription factor CIITA required for the expression of these proteins.[232] In addition, three of the cathepsins, proteolytic enzymes located in the lysosomes and thought to be at least partly responsible for the cleavage of exogenous proteins into peptides for loading onto the class II protein,[230] are also regulated by IFN-γ.[233,234]

Two additional components of the immune response up-regulated by IFN-γ are the high-affinity Fc-γ receptor[155,189] and components of the complement system.[189,235] Both have the capacity to increase host tumoricidal activity.

At least two enzymes involved in tryptophan metabolism are induced by IFNs. The first is indoleamine 2,3-dioxygenase, a 42-kd enzyme that converts indoleamine derivatives, such as tryptophan or serotonin, to N-formylkynurenine.[236,237] It has been proposed that the subsequent tryptophan depletion is growth inhibitory to tumor cells and cells infected with intracellular pathogens.[238,239] The second is tryptophanyl–transfer RNA synthetase.[240] This enzyme is responsible for the aminoacylation of transfer RNA Trp, required for protein synthesis.

IFN-γ–mediated microbial and tumor cell killing is believed to be augmented by the respiratory burst and nitric oxide (NO) responses. These are observed most robustly in neutrophils and monocyte macrophages, and have been included together here because their products can synergize to enhance tumor cell killing. The oxidative, or respiratory, burst results in the production of superoxide anion (O_2^-) and other toxic oxidants through activation of a large multiprotein complex, the reduced form of nicotinamide adenine dinucleotide phosphate (NADPH)–dependent oxidase.[241,242] IFN-γ activation of NADPH oxidase involves regulation of the expression of two of the components of this complex, gp91-phox and p47-phox.[243–245] NO production is enhanced by IFN-γ through the induction of the enzyme NOS, which converts L-arginine to NO.[246,247] In addition, IFN-γ coordinately regulated the enzymes GTP-cyclohydroxylase, which converts GTP to the NOS cofactor tetrahydrobiopterin (BH4), and arginosuccinate synthetase, which is necessary for arginine synthesis. The exact molecular mechanism by which superoxide anion or NO mediates microbial or tumor cell killing is still under investigation.

IFNs induce the production of a number of growth factors and cytokines. ISG-15, a secreted protein induced by IFN-α and IFN-β, results in IFN-γ synthesis by T cells and proliferation of NK and lymphokine-activated killer cells.[248] A number of these fall into the category of chemokines, small-molecular-weight secreted proteins that are chemoattractants. IFN-induced chemokines include RANTES,[249] IP-10,[250] MCP-1,[251] MIP-1α, MIG,[252] and β-R1/I-TAC.[253,254] These proteins, selectively chemoattractive to primarily lymphocytes and monocytes, are believed to play a crucial role in the recruitment of these cells out of the circulation into the surrounding tissues.

Overexpression of the mouse *p202* gene, a member of the Ifi 200 family of IFN-induced proteins, has been shown to inhibit cell proliferation, probably due to binding to and negative regulation of a number of transcription factors, including the retinoblastoma protein (pRB),[255] the tumor suppressor p53,[256] E2F,[257,258] nuclear factor-κB (NF-κB),[259] c-fos,[259] and c-jun.[259] In mice, the Ifi 200 or gene 200 cluster is a genetic locus suggested to contain at least six linked IFN-regulated genes.[260,261] These proteins each contain at least one representative of a conserved domain of approximately 200 amino acids.[260] Recently, the p204 protein was shown to inhibit ribosomal RNA transcription and cell proliferation.[262] Genes from the homologous locus in humans have been identified and include the myeloid cell–nuclear differentiation antigen,[263,264] Ifi 16,[265] and absent in melanoma.[266] Ifi 16 and myeloid cell–nuclear differentiation antigen are DNA-binding nuclear proteins that have expression patterns consistent with myeloid cell differentiation.[265] Whether they also modulate transcription and inhibit cell growth remains to be determined.

Several IFN-induced proteins have been localized to small domains having a speckled appearance in the nucleus, called *nuclear bodies* (NBs). The function of NBs is unknown. The best studied of these NB proteins is the promyelocytic leukemia (PML) protein that was originally identified in acute PMLs, where the t(15:17) translocation creates a fusion protein containing PML fused to the retinoic acid receptor α.[106] The resulting fusion protein, while remaining nuclear, fails to localize into NBs. Treatment of these leukemias with retinoic acid results in differentiation and the return of the fusion protein to the NBs. PML has been shown to suppress tumor cell growth.[267,268] Recently, PML knockout mice were used to demonstrate that PML is necessary for programmed cell death induced by a number of factors, including type I and II IFNs, ceramide, tumor necrosis factor α, and Fas.[269] Conversely, overexpression of PML induces cell death.[270] Furthermore, PML is critical for expression of antigen-processing proteins and regulates MHC expression.[271] SP-100, originally identified as an autoantigen in primary biliary cirrhosis, is also an IFN-induced protein that localizes to the NBs.[272] The same is true for the human nuclear dot protein 52[273] and ISG-20.[274] Functions have not been ascribed to these proteins.

Using oligonucleotide arrays, a number of new candidates for IFN-regulated genes have been identified.[190] One of these, phospholipid scramblase, flips phosphatidylserine from the inner layer of the plasma membrane to the outer layer.[275] The appearance of phosphatidylserine on the outer layer of the cell membrane has been observed in apoptotic cells.

IFNs also up-regulate specific TAAs, such as TAG-72 and carcinoembryonic antigen.[151,276] Carcinoembryonic antigen is closely related and genetically linked to two other cell surface glycoproteins, biliary glycoprotein and nonspecific cross-reacting antigen.[277] As discussed previously, the up-regulation of TAAs by IFNs may increase host-mediated antitumor responses.

IFNs also down-regulate some proteins. IFN-γ down-regulates the expression of the multidrug resistance gene in human colon carcinoma cells,[278] which may serve as a means of making chemotherapy more effective. Nucleotide arrays showed that the breakpoint cluster region gene may also be down-regulated by IFN-α and IFN-γ.[190]

CLINICAL PHARMACOLOGY OF INTERFERONS

Pharmacokinetics of Interferon in Humans

A number of studies have described the pharmacokinetics of natural or recombinant IFNs after bolus or continuous administration (Table 26-5). Substantial individual differences in serum IFN concentration, time to peak serum concentration, and half-life have been observed.[279–292] In general, however, IFNs are detected in serum within 30 minutes after a single intramuscular (i.m.) or subcutaneous (s.c.)

TABLE 26-5. PHARMACOKINETICS OF INTERFERONS (IFNs)

Route of Administration	Dose (mU)	Serum Concentration (U/mL)	Peak Time	Duration (from–to)	IFN Type	Reference
IFN-α						
i.m.	72	300	2–8 h	0.5 to >48 h	α2a	28
	3,108	400	8 h	0.5 to >48 h		
	198	1,000	2 h	0.5 to >48 h		
	3–36	20–200	2–8 h	<0.5–24 h		
i.m.	50	2,000 pg/mL	6 h	<0.5 to >24 h	r	279
	36	1,000 pg/mL	6 h	<0.5–24 h		
	18	500 pg/mL	6 h	<0.5–24 h		
i.m.	3	60	6 h	<24 h	Cantell buffy coat	282
	9	230	2 h	>24 h		
i.m.	1	80	6 h		α Lymphoblastoid	280
	3	400	6 h			
	10	1,200	6 h			
i.m.	9–18	100	6–8 h	<0.5–12 h	α 2a	281
	36–50	200	6–8 h	<0.5–24 h		
	68	500	6–8 h	<0.5 to >4 h		
	86	600	6–8 h			
Continuous i.v. infusion	5–10 mU/m^2	100–800	<24 h	Continuous	α n	283
	10–50	10^3	<24 h	Continuous		
	100–200	10^3–10^4	<24 h	Continuous		
Continuous s.c. infusion	2–5	20–60	Steady state	24–72 h	α 2b	284
IFN-β						
i.v.	4–10	10–300	30 min		Fibroblast β	285
	40–80	200–10,000	30 min			
	160–320	2,000–20,000	30 min			
s.c.	90	10^2		1–8 h	β 1b	286
i.v.	90	10^3	5 min	5 min–12 h		
i.v. 4-h infusion	0.01–1.00	<10			β 1b	287
	10	25–30	6 h	0.5–24 h		
	30	140	4 h	0.05–24 h		
i.v.	45	350	5 min		β 1b	288
	180	1,800	5 min			
s.c.	45	0				
	180	25				
IFN-γ						
i.v. 10-min infusion	0.01–20.00	0			γ	292
	30		15 min	<0.5–12 h		
	75		15 min	<0.5–24 h		
i.v. 6-h infusion	0.5 mg/m^2	3 ng/mL	6 h	2–8 h	γ	289
	1 mg/m^2	6 ng/mL	6 h	<1–8 h		
s.c.	1 mU	4 mg/mL	13 h		γ	290

injection and remain detectable for hours. Typically, an injection of 5 to 50 × 10^6 U of IFN-α resulted in peak serum concentrations of 10^2 to 10^3 U per mL at 4 to 6 hours. After intravenous (i.v.) bolus injection, IFN-α is detectable in serum immediately and remains detectable for 12 to 48 hours. In contrast, after a single s.c. injection, IFN-β is usually undetectable in serum.

The proteins induced by a single IFN dose follow a similar but delayed time course compared to serum levels of IFN. Comparing single and multiple administrations of IFN-β in the same subjects, the increase in serum neopterin and β$_2$-microglobulin levels, and reduction in tryptophan, all peak at 48 hours. In contrast, the 2-5A synthetase activity in peripheral blood mononuclear cells peaks at 24 hours, the earliest time point measured. These biologic responses remain significantly altered between 24 and 72 hours after a single dose but return to baseline levels within 7 days.[293] The magnitude of response at 24 and 48 hours after multiple administrations is not different from the response to the first administration at any dose, suggesting that the immune system of healthy individuals is not refractory to IFNs, at least for short durations.[293]

Effects of Route, Dose, and Schedule of Administration

Many of the IFN-mediated gene modulatory and cellular effects, first identified in preclinical studies and reviewed

TABLE 26-6. GENE MODULATION BY INTERFERONS IN HUMAN CLINICAL TRIALS

Induced proteins
2-5A synthetase
Indoleamine 2,3 dioxygenase (product: tryptophan)
Guanosine triphosphate cyclohydrolase (product: neopterin)
Guanylate binding protein 1
Mx protein (p78)
β_2-microglobulin: on cell surface and shed into serum
Fc receptor (CD64)
Major histocompatibility complex class I
Major histocompatibility complex class II
Interleukin-1 receptor antagonist
Tumor necrosis factor–soluble receptor
Cell activation
Natural killer cell cytotoxicity
Monocyte
   Nonspecific cytotoxicity
   Antibody-dependent cell-mediated cytotoxicity
   Peroxide generation
   Growth inhibition

above, have been confirmed in patients (Table 26-6). Pharmacodynamic changes in these proteins have been studied to evaluate the biologic effectiveness of different routes of administration. In melanoma patients, no significant differences in monocyte activation (Fc receptor expression, H_2O_2 generation) are found when s.c. and i.m. routes of administration of IFN-γ are compared.[294] Increases in 2-5A synthetase, NK cell activity, and CD4 and CD8 ratios are similar after IFN-γ is administered by daily bolus injection or by continuous infusion for 14 days.[295] IFN-β administered s.c. is as effective as i.v. in increasing a number of IFN-induced biologic responses.[292] Serum IFN-β concentration, however, is only marginally detectable after s.c. administration, showing that biologic response can occur in the absence of detectable IFN in serum.

Studies in mice suggest that oral administration of IFNs results in antitumor, antiviral, and immunomodulatory effects.[296–298] Although beneficial clinical effects have been reported, particularly with low doses of oral IFN-α,[299–301] these effects have not been confirmed in all studies.[302–304] Additional phase III multiinstitutional studies will be required for confirmation. Regional and systemic immune effects not yet defined mechanistically may explain some of these findings.[297,298,305]

These biologic response parameters have also been evaluated to define an effective dose range of IFNs. A bell-shaped curve of biologic response is supported by some studies.[306] NK cell cytotoxicity is greater after lower doses of IFN-α than after higher doses.[307,308] MHC-nonrestricted monocyte cytotoxicity is enhanced as well as by low-dose IFN-γ (21×10^6 units) as high-dose (71×10^6 units), and antibody-dependent cell-mediated cytotoxicity is increased by the low but not the high dose.[309] Other studies found more direct correlations between dose and biologic response as measured by IFN-induced

proteins. The human Mx protein shows a significant correlation to the IFN-α dose given.[310] IFN-β treatment of renal cancer patients leads to a dose response in 2-5A synthetase activity, but not NK cell cytotoxicity.[311] A dose-dependent increase in β_2-microglobulin, but not in neopterin, is observed after i.v. administration of a purified fibroblast IFN-β in the range of 1 to 46 MU.[312] A dose-dependent increase is measured in 2-5A synthetase 24 hours after administration of 3 to 300 MU i.v. bolus of IFN-β or 3 to 3,000 μg per m^2 of IFN-γ.[295] Greater increases in 2-5A synthetase activity and neopterin, but not β_2-microglobulin, are observed after higher, compared to lower, doses of IFN-β.[293] However, no dose-dependent increase is detectable in patients with advanced malignancy after i.v. IFN-β.[7] A significant correlation with dose of more than approximately a 500-fold range of IFN-β in 2-5A synthetase, neopterin, and β_2-microglobulin is observed in healthy volunteers.[293]

Increases in monocyte surface expression and serum concentration of β_2-microglobulin correlates with a dose of IFN-γ over the range of 3 to 300 MU; however, increases in HLA class II, 2-5A synthetase, and H_2O_2 generation by monocytes, a measure of their metabolic activity, did not correlate.[313] A dose-dependent increase in β_2-microglobulin was seen over the range of 0.1 to 1.0 mg per m^2 of IFN-γ.[290] Dose-dependent increases in HLA-DR and FcR on monocytes, monocyte H_2O_2 production, and NK-cell cytotoxicity are observed after 0.0001 to 0.2500 mg per m^2 i.m. IFN-γ over 15 days.[294] In patients with metastatic malignant melanoma, at higher doses (0.10 and 0.25 compared to 0.01 mg per m^2), IFN-γ–induced immunologic effects are heightened, including neopterin and surface expression of β_2-microglobulin, HLA-ABC, CD64 (=FcR), and CD14.[314] A dose-dependent decrease in HLA-DR on monocytes and Leu7 on lymphocytes is measured at 4 hours after IFN-γ in advanced renal cell cancer patients.[315]

The quantification of proteins induced in patients has facilitated comparison of IFN types, combinations of cytokines, or combinations of cytokines and other therapies. Recombinant and natural IFN-β are biologically equivalent in their ability to induce 2-5A synthetase, neopterin, and Mx protein.[22] Direct comparisons of IFN-β and IFN-γ in the same patients suggest IFN-β was more effective in increasing 2-5A synthetase activity and IFN-γ was more effective in increasing serum β_2-microglobulin or indoleamine 2,3-dioxygenase activity.[316]

Increases in IFN-stimulated genes, particularly 2-5A synthetase, has been correlated with therapeutic response to IFN (Table 26-7). Response has also been correlated with an increase in T-cell infiltration.[317] Individuals who have greater gene induction and cellular effects may have the best therapeutic responses.[87,317–322] However, it has not yet been established which of these proteins are essential for antitumor activity. In two other studies, no correlation was found between induction of ten different IFN-induced

TABLE 26-7. CORRELATIONS OF 2-5A SYNTHETASE INCREASE WITH CLINICAL RESPONSE IN CANCER

Positive Correlation		Reference
Carcinoid	Clinical response in 43% (some measured as in 5-hydroxyindoleacetic acid) (n = 22)	318
	6.7× increase in responder group, 1.8× in nonresponder (p <.01)	
Lymphoma	5 complete or partial responses, 1 minor response, 5 no response (n = 11)	319
	No correlation of response with peripheral blood mononuclear cell; 2-5A increase in lymph node B cells *in vitro*	
CML	Response measured as hematologic remission (n = 14)	87
	2-5A increase in responders, not in nonresponders (p <.04)	
CLL, CGL, ET	Greater 2-5A messenger RNA (mRNA) induction in responders (n = 35, p <.05)	320
CLL	2-5A increase and blast transformation (n = 24, p <.05)	321
Breast	24 primary human breast carcinoma extracts contained 2-5A synthetase but at 1,000× range with no correlation to estrogen or progesterone receptor expression	322

Lack of Correlation		Reference
CML	2 responders, 3 resistant, 5 healthy controls	323
	No increase in 2-5A mRNA or other interferon-induced protein (MT11, HLA-1, 15K, 56K, 78K, IF14, 8, or 6–16). All 10 induced *in vivo* and *in vitro* the same	
CML	n = 27 patients; 10 sensitive (responders) and 17 resistant	324
	No correlation of mRNA of 2-5A, ISG-54 and 6–16 with clinical response	

CGL, chronic granulocytic leukemia; CLL, chronic lymphocytic leukemia; CML, chronic myelogenous leukemia; ET, essential thrombocytopenia.

mRNAs, including 2-5A synthetase and β_2-microglobulin and clinical response, or between NK cell increases *in vivo* or *in vitro* and clinical response.[323,324] Thus, it is possible that although these increases may predict responsiveness to IFN, undefined proteins or a combination of these activities may contribute to antitumor activity.

An example of a more specific correlation of gene expression with response comes from studies of CML. Loss of expression of the ICSBP gene in mice results in a myelo-proliferative syndrome phenotypically similar to CML.[325] ICSBP expression was found to be low in patients with acute and CMLs.[326] Treatment with IFN-α-2 over several months resulted in normalization of ICSBP expression. Interestingly, *in vitro* IFN-α-2 did not result in ICSBP induction in CML cells, whereas IFN-γ did.[326]

TOXICITIES

IFNs have toxicities when administered at pharmacologic doses (Table 26-8). The side effects with the initial dose are predominantly constitutional.[327,328] Beginning a few hours after the first s.c. injection, influenza-like symptoms occur uniformly and last for 2 to 8 hours. This acute syndrome disappears with subsequent daily injections. The rapidity of the appearance of tachyphylaxis is dependent on type of IFN, dose, route, and schedule of administration. Flu-like symptoms, which occur despite increases in endogenous glucocorticoids,[329] can be partially controlled with acetaminophen. Any nausea and vomiting are usually mild and of short duration.

Fatigue and anorexia are the dose-limiting toxicities with chronic administration; weight loss may be significant with IFN-α-2 (greater than 10%).[327] In general, older patients tolerate these symptoms less well than younger patients. IFN-β is better tolerated with chronic dosing; weight loss and fatigue are uncommon.[7,330] The most frequent neurologic side effect of IFN-α-2 (other than the possible relationship of the fatigue) is somnolence, confusion, depression, and decreased cognitive function. However, neurologic symptoms have not prevented IFN-β administration in multiple sclerosis patients. The fatigue and anorexia likely result from the peripheral and central nervous system release of cytokines by IFNs.[331,332]

The hematologic effects of IFN administration include mild granulocytopenia, with a reduction in counts of 40%

TABLE 26-8. INTERFERON SIDE EFFECTS

Initial injections
Chills and rigors
Fevers
Malaise
Myalgias
Mild neutropenia
Chronic administration
Fatigue
Anorexia
Mild neutropenia
Transaminase elevations
Weight loss
Depression
General
At least partly result from receptor-triggered effects
Individual patient variability
Correlated with dose and duration
Chronic anorexia and fatigue most limiting
Reversible-side effects resolve off treatment

to 60%. This is followed by a rapid rebound to normal 3 to 10 days after discontinuation of therapy.[333] No increase in infectious sequelae has occurred during IFN-induced leukopenia, and granulocytopenia is rarely dose-limiting. Anemia occurred with chronic therapy but was rarely severe. Mild thrombocytopenia was reported in 5% to 50% of patients; this may be influenced by marrow infiltration with tumor.[333]

The elevation of transaminases, usually mild, occurs more commonly in the presence of pretreatment hepatic abnormalities and is reversible and dose-related.[333] Cholesterol levels decrease, often accompanied by a rise in triglycerides. Although low-density lipoprotein commonly declines, high-density lipoprotein either increases or decreases, depending on dose and type of IFN.[334,335] Creatinine levels do not change. The most common renal toxicity described is mild proteinuria, but nephrotic syndrome and acute renal insufficiency have been rarely reported.[336,337] Although little or no IFN can be identified in urine, nephrectomy in the rat reduces, but does not eliminate, clearance, suggesting that catabolism by renal tubular cells is one degradative pathway for IFN.[338,339] This preclinical finding was confirmed when patients with impaired renal function had a twofold decrease in serum clearance, with persisting IFN-α-2 levels at 24 hours.[340] Although occasional patients may develop alterations in thyroid function,[341] in general, no residual toxicities in parenchymal organ function have been identified.[333]

With chronic administration, a minority of patients develop neutralizing antibody to the administered IFN.[342–344] Antibody development is a function of dose, schedule, route, duration, and, possibly, underlying disease. Antibodies have rarely been identified with less than 4 months of IFN administration and are not clearly related to IFN type or preparation. Particularly when antibodies are present in high titer, they may be correlated with disease progression.[345] However, patients with multiple sclerosis treated with IFN-β had a significant frequency of neutralizing antibody, which usually correlates with a loss of therapeutic effects. Such IFN resistance can sometimes be overcome by using alternative IFN preparation.[346–348] Although potentially a problem in a minority of patients treated for extended periods, antibodies are probably not a major mechanism of resistance to IFN for most cancer patients.[344,345]

CONCLUSION

IFNs have become increasingly important in treating hematologic malignancies. In CML, IFN-α-2 has demonstrated sustained clinical and cytogenetic responses.[349] With continued treatment, approximately 25% of patients develop complete cytogenetic response, with disappearance of the Ph1 chromosome. The median survival for responding patients who show some, although not complete, evidence of cytogenetic

response is approximately 6 years. More than 90% of cytogenetic complete responders will be in remission at 10 years.[350] The superiority of IFN-α-2 to hydroxyurea has been demonstrated; survival for IFN-treated patients exceeded 5 years, whereas that of hydroxyurea-treated patients was approximately 4 years.[350,351] Addition of cytosine arabinoside to IFN-α-2 has resulted in an increase in major cytogenetic responses and further prolongation of survival.[352,353]

For B-cell neoplasms, the significant single-agent activity of IFN-α-2 is being integrated with effective chemotherapy for low and intermediate grade non-Hodgkin's lymphoma.[354,355] Combination with chemotherapy regimens has prolonged disease-free survival and overall survival in two of the prospectively randomized trials in follicular lymphoma. In one, even though only a maximum of 8 cycles of 5 days of IFN-α-2 was administered, a positive therapeutic impact was evident and has been maintained with 10 years of observation.[356] In the other trial, although 11% of patients developed toxicity, IFN-α-2 resulted in significant gains in event-free survival ($p <.001$) and overall survival ($p = .02$) for follicular lymphoma.[355] For myeloma, some, but not all, phase II and III studies in melanoma have suggested that either for induction or maintenance, IFN-2 may add to effectiveness.[357–359]

Prolongation of disease-free survival has emerged from use of IFN-α-2 as an adjuvant to surgery for high-risk patients with primary melanoma and metastatic renal cell carcinoma.[360–363] In conjunction with radiation, IFN-β has been suggested as a radiosensitizer.[364,365] The combination of IFNs with other biologic response modifiers remains an active area of investigation. Use with IL-2 has not yet yielded any substantial advance over the activity of each cytokine individually in renal carcinoma or melanoma.[366,367] In combination with retinoids, substantial regressions have been observed in squamous carcinomas of the skin and cervix.[368–370] These effects may result partly from induction of STAT1 leading to novel and augmented induction of ISGs.[371,372]

Clinical trials have thus defined therapeutic effectiveness in hematologic malignancies and solid tumors. Although many challenges remain (Table 26-9), therapeutic applications are likely to substantially broaden. During the past decade, a

TABLE 26-9. INTERFERON SYSTEM: 2000 TO 2010 CHALLENGES

Expand therapeutic usefulness
Individual types
Inducers
Combinations
Define mechanism(s) of action
Gene modulation
Cellular
Immunologic
Cause of limiting toxicities
Significance of antibody

combination of biochemical and genetic approaches has led to the identification of a new cellular signal transduction pathway and more than 200 genes that are transcriptionally activated. Further exploration of signal transduction and the genes induced should enhance the understanding of the biologic and pharmacologic effects of IFNs, the focus of this chapter. In the next decade, the clinical benefits of this potent and pleiotropic family of cytokines for the treatment of malignancy will be even more completely realized.

ACKNOWLEDGMENTS

The authors would like to thank Pamela McKenzie for secretarial assistance and to acknowledge the support of Ares Serano and the National Institutes of Health (1RO1CA089344.01A1) (E.C.B), the National Institutes of Health (1RO1CA79891-01 and 1RO1GM58893 to T.L.Y.), and the American Cancer Society (RPG-98-034-01-CIM to D.J.V.).

REFERENCES

1. Pfeffer LM, Dinarello CA, Herberman RB, et al. Biologic properties of recombinant alfa interferons: 40th anniversary of the discovery of interferons. *Cancer Res* 1998;58:2489–2499.

2. Pestka S. The human interferon-alpha species and hybrid proteins. *Semin Oncol* 1997;24:9–17.

3. Hawkins MJ, Borden EC, Merritt JA, et al. Comparison of the biologic effects of two recombinant human interferons alpha (rA and rD) in humans. *J Clin Oncol* 1984;2:221–226.

4. PRISMS (Prevention of Relapses and Disability by Interferon beta-1a Subcutaneously in Multiple Sclerosis) Study Group. Randomised double-blind placebo-controlled study of interferon beta-1a in relapsing/remitting multiple sclerosis. *Lancet* 1998;352:1498–1504.

5. European Study Group on Interferon beta-1b in Secondary Progressive MS. Placebo-controlled multicentre randomised trial of interferon beta-1b in secondary progressive multiple sclerosis. *Lancet* 1998;352:1491–1497.

6. Dixon RM, Borden EC, Spennetta T, et al. Decreases in serum high density lipoprotein cholesterol and total cholesterol resulting from naturally produced and recombinant DNA derived leukocyte interferons. *Metabolism* 1984;33:400–404.

7. Borden EC, Rinehart J, Storer BM, et al. Biological and clinical effects of interferon beta ser at two doses. *J Interferon Res* 1990;10:559–570.

8. The International Chronic Granulomatous Disease Cooperative Study Group. A controlled trial of interferon gamma to prevent infection in chronic granulomatous disease. *N Engl J Med* 1991;324:509–516.

9. Badaro R, Falcoff E, Badaro FS, et al. Treatment of visceral leishmaniasis with pentavalent antimony and interferon gamma. *N Engl J Med* 1990;322:15–21.

10. Lee WM, Reddy KR, Tong MJ, et al. Early hepatitis C virus-RNA responses predict interferon treatment outcomes in chronic hepatitis C. The Consensus Interferon Study Group. *Hepatology* 1998;28:1411–1415.

11. Pockros PJ, Tong M, Lee WM, et al. Relationship between biochemical and virological responses to interferon therapy in chronic hepatitis C infection. Consensus Interferon Study Group. *J Viral Hepat* 1998;5:271–276.

12. Tong MJ, Blatt LM, Resser KJ, et al. Treatment of chronic hepatitis C virus infection with recombinant consensus interferon. *J Interferon Cytokine Res* 1998;18:81–86.

13. Nagata S, Mantei N, Weissmann C. The structure of one of the eight or more distinct chromosomal genes for human interferon α. *Nature* 1980;287:401–408.

14. Goeddel DV, Leung DW, Dull TJ, et al. The structure of eight distinct cloned human leukocyte interferon cDNAs. *Nature* 1981;290:20–26.

15. Streuli M, Nagata S, Weissman C. At least three human type alpha interferons: structure of alpha 2. *Science* 1980; 209:1343–1357.

16. Jay E, MacKnight D, Lutze-Wallace C, et al. Chemical synthesis of a biologically active gene for human immune interferon-gamma. Prospect for site-specific mutagenesis and structure-function studies. *J Biol Chem* 1984;259:6311–6317.

17. Gray PW, Goeddel DV. Structure of the human immune interferon gene. *Nature* 1982;298:859–863.

18. Adolf GR. Antigenic structure of human interferon omega (interferon alpha II): comparison with other human interferons. *J Gen Virol* 1987;68:1669–1676.

19. Capon DJ, Shepard HM, Goeddel DV. Two distinct families of human and bovine interferon-alpha genes are coordinately expressed and encode functional polypeptides. *Mol Cell Biol* 1985;5:768–779.

20. Roberts RM, Cross JC, Leaman DW. Unique features of the trophoblast interferons. *Pharmacol Ther* 1991;51:329–345.

21. Leaman DW, Cross JC, Roberts RM. Multiple regulatory elements are required to direct trophoblast interferon gene expression in choriocarcinoma cells and trophectoderm. *Mol Endocrinol* 1994;8:456–468.

22. Liberati AM, Garofani P, DeAngelis V, et al. Double-blind randomized phase I study on the clinical tolerance and pharmacodynamics of natural and recombinant interferon-beta given intravenously. *J Interferon Res* 1994;14:61–69.

23. Hawkins MJ, Levin M, Borden EC. An ECOG Phase I-II pilot study of polyriboinosinic-polyribocytidylic acid poly-L-Lysine complex (Poly ICLC) in patients with metastatic malignant melanoma. *J Biol Resp Mod* 1985;4:664–668.

24. Litton G, Hong R, Grossberg SE, et al. Biological and clinical effects of the oral immunomodulator 3,6-bis (2-piperidinoethoxy)acridine trihydrochloride in patients with advanced malignancy. *J Biol Resp Mod* 1990;9:61–70.

25. Rios A, Stringfellow DA, Fitzpatrick FA, et al. Phase I study of 2-amino-5bromo-6-phenyl-4 (3H)-pyrimidinone (ABPP), an oral interferon inducer, in cancer patients. *J Biol Resp Mod* 1986;5:330–338.

26. Urba WJ, Longo DL, Weiss RB. Enhancement of natural killer activity in human peripheral blood by flavone acetic acid. *J Natl Cancer Inst* 1988;80:521–525.

27. Goldstein D, Hertzog P, Tomkinson E, et al. Administration of imiquimod, an interferon inducer, in asymptomatic human immunodeficiency virus-infected persons to determine safety and biologic response modification. *J Infect Disease* 1998;178:858–861.

28. Witt PL, Ritch PS, Reding D, et al. Phase I trials of an oral

immunomodulator and interferon inducer in cancer patients. *Cancer Res* 1993;53:5176–5180.

29. Darnell J Jr, Kerr IM, Stark GR. Jak-STAT pathways and transcriptional activation in response to IFNs and other extracellular signaling proteins. *Science* 1994;264:1415–1421.

30. Stark GR, Kerr IA, Williams BRG, et al. How cells respond to interferons. *Annu Rev Biochem* 1998;67:227–264.

31. Ihle JN. Cytokine receptor signalling. *Nature* 1995;377:591–594.

32. Ihle JN. STATs: signal transducers and activators of transcription. *Cell* 1996;84:331–334.

33. Branca AA, Baglioni C. Evidence that types I and II interferons have different receptors. *Nature* 1981;294:768–770.

34. Merlin G, Falcoff E, Aguet M. 125I-labelled human interferons alpha, beta and gamma: comparative receptor-binding data. *J Gen Virol* 1985;66:1149–1152.

35. Uze G, Lutfalla G, Gresser I. Genetic transfer of a functional human interferon alpha receptor into mouse cells: cloning and expression of its cDNA. *Cell* 1990;60:225–234.

36. Novick D, Cohen B, Rubinstein M. The human interferon alpha/beta receptor: characterization and molecular cloning. *Cell* 1994;77:391–400.

37. Domanski P, Witte M, Kellum M, et al. Cloning and expression of a long form of the beta subunit of the interferon alpha beta receptor that is required for signaling. *J Biol Chem* 1995;270:21606–21611.

38. Lutfalla G, Gardiner K, Proudhon D, et al. The structure of the human interferon alpha/beta receptor gene. *J Biol Chem* 1992;267:2802–2809.

39. Colamonici OR, Domanski P. Identification of a novel subunit of the type I interferon receptor localized to human chromosome 21. *J Biol Chem* 1993;268:10895–10899.

40. Cleary CM, Donnelly RJ, Soh J, et al. Knockout and reconstitution of a functional human type I interferon receptor complex. *J Biol Chem* 1994;269:18747–18749.

41. Platanias LC, Domanski P, Nadeau OW, et al. Identification of a domain in the beta subunit of the type I interferon (IFN) receptor that exhibits a negative regulatory effect in the growth inhibitory action of type I IFNs. *J Biol Chem* 1998;273:5577–5581.

42. Colamonici OR, Pfeffer LM, D'Alessandro F, et al. Multichain structure of the IFN-alpha receptor on hematopoietic cells. *J Immunol* 1992;148:2126–2132.

43. Aguet M, Dembic Z, Merlin G. Molecular cloning and expression of the human interferon-gamma receptor. *Cell* 1988;55:273–280.

44. Soh J, Donnelly RJ, Kotenko S, et al. Identification and sequence of an accessory factor required for activation of the human interferon gamma receptor. *Cell* 1994;76:793–802.

45. Hemmi S, Bohni R, Stark G, et al. A novel member of the interferon receptor family complements functionality of the murine interferon gamma receptor in human cells. *Cell* 1994;76:803–810.

46. Greenlund AC, Farrar MA, Viviano BL, et al. Ligand-induced IFN gamma receptor tyrosine phosphorylation couples the receptor to its signal transduction system (p91). *Embo J* 1994;13:1591–1600.

47. Igarashi K, Garotta G, Ozmen L, et al. Interferon-gamma induces tyrosine phosphorylation of interferon-gamma receptor and regulated association of protein tyrosine kinases, Jak1 and Jak2, with its receptor. *J Biol Chem* 1994;269:14333–14336.

48. Muller M, Briscoe J, Laxton C, et al. The protein tyrosine kinase JAK1 complements defects in interferon-alpha/beta and -gamma signal transduction. *Nature* 1993;366:129–135.

49. Watling D, Guschin D, Muller M, et al. Complementation by the protein tyrosine kinase JAK2 of a mutant cell line defective in the interferon-gamma signal transduction pathway. *Nature* 1993;366:166–170.

50. Velazquez L, Fellous M, Stark GR, et al. A protein tyrosine kinase in the interferon alpha/beta signaling pathway. *Cell* 1992;70:313–322.

51. Schindler C, Fu XY, Improta T, et al. Proteins of transcription factor ISGF-3: one gene encodes the 91- and 84-kDa ISGF-3 proteins that are activated by interferon alpha. *Proc Natl Acad Sci U S A* 1992;89:7836–7839.

52. Muller M, Laxton C, Briscoe J, et al. Complementation of a mutant cell line: central role of the 91 kDa polypeptide of ISGF3 in the interferon-alpha and -gamma signal transduction pathways. *Embo J* 1993;12:4221–4228.

53. Leung S, Qureshi SA, Kerr IM, et al. Role of STAT2 in the alpha interferon signaling pathway. *Mol Cell Biol* 1995;15:1312–1317.

54. Meraz MA, White JM, Sheehan KC, et al. Targeted disruption of the Stat1 gene in mice reveals unexpected physiologic specificity in the JAK-STAT signaling pathway. *Cell* 1996;84:431–442.

55. Durbin JE, Hackenmiller R, Simon MC, et al. Targeted disruption of the mouse Stat1 gene results in compromised innate immunity to viral disease. *Cell* 1996;84:443–450.

56. Williams BR. Transcriptional regulation of interferon-stimulated genes. *Eur J Biochem* 1991;200:1–11.

57. Levy DE, Kessler DS, Pine R, et al. Interferon-induced nuclear factors that bind a shared promoter element correlate with positive and negative transcriptional control. *Genes Dev* 1988;2:383–393.

58. Schindler C, Shuai K, Prezioso VR, et al. Interferon-dependent tyrosine phosphorylation of a latent cytoplasmic transcription factor. *Science* 1992;257:809–813.

59. Adachi M, Fishcher EH, Ihle J, et al. Mammaliam SH2-containing protein tyrosine phosphatases. *Cell* 1996;85:15.

60. Jiao H, Berrada K, Yang W, et al. Direct association and dephosphorylation of Jak2 kinase by SH2 domain-containing protein tyrosine phosphatase SHP-1. *Mol Cell Biol* 1996;16:6985–6992.

61. David M, Chen HE, Goelz S, et al. Differential regulation of the alpha/beta interferon-stimulated Jak-Stat pathway by the SH2 domain-containing tyrosine phosphatase SHPTP1. *Mol Cell Biol* 1995;15:7050–7058.

62. You M, Yu DH, Feng GS. SHP-2 tyrosine phosphatase functions as a negative regulator of the interferon-stimulated Jak-Stat pathway. *Mol Cell Biol* 1999;19:2416–2424.

63. Igarashi K, David M, Finbloom DS, et al. In vitro activation of the transcription factor gamma interferon activation factor by gamma interferon: evidence for a tyrosine phosphatase/kinase signaling cascade. *Mol Cell Biol* 1993;13:1634–1640.

64. Wang D, Stravopodis D, Teglund S, et al. Naturally occurring dominant negative variants of Stat5. *Mol Cell Biol* 1996;16:6141–6148.

65. Haque SJ, Wu Q, Kammer W, et al. Receptor-associated constitutive protein tyrosine phosphatase activity controls the kinase function of JAK1. *Proc Natl Acad Sci U S A* 1997;94:8563–8568.

66. Yoshimura A. The CIS/JAB family: novel negative regulators of JAK signaling pathways. *Leukemia* 1998;12:1851–1857.

67. Nicholson SE, Hilton DJ. The SOCS proteins: a new family of negative regulators of signal transduction. *J Leukoc Biol* 1998;63:665–668.

68. Yasukawa H, Misawa H, Sakamoto H, et al. The JAK-binding protein JAB inhibits Janus tyrosine kinase activity through binding in the activation loop. *Embo J* 1999; 18:1309–1320.

69. Zhang JG, Farley A, Nicholson SE, et al. The conserved SOCS box motif in suppressors of cytokine signaling binds to elongins B and C and may couple bound proteins to proteasomal degradation. *Proc Natl Acad Sci U S A* 1999;96: 2071–2076.

70. Sakamoto H, Yasukawa H, Masuhara M, et al. A *Janus* kinase inhibitor, JAB, is an interferon-γ-inducible gene and confers resistance to interferon. *Blood* 1998;92:1668–1676.

71. Song MM, Shuai K. The suppressor of cytokine signaling (SOCS) 1 and SOCS3 but not SOCS2 proteins inhibit interferon-mediated antiviral and antiproliferative activities. *J Biol Chem* 1998;273:35056–35062.

72. Petricoin ER, Ito S, Williams BL, et al. Antiproliferative action of interferon-alpha requires components of T-cell-receptor signalling. *Nature* 1997;390:629–632.

73. Miyamoto M, Fujita T, Kimura Y, et al. Regulated expression of a gene encoding a nuclear factor, IRF-1, that specifically binds to IFN-beta gene regulatory elements. *Cell* 1988; 54:903–913.

74. Harada H, Fujita T, Miyamoto M, et al. Structurally similar but functionally distinct factors, IRF-1 and IRF-2, bind to the same regulatory elements of IFN and IFN-inducible genes. *Cell* 1989;58:729–739.

75. Veals SA, Schindler C, Leonard D, et al. Subunit of an alpha-interferon-responsive transcription factor is related to interferon regulatory factor and Myb families of DNA-binding proteins. *Mol Cell Biol* 1992;12:3315–3324.

76. Fujita T, Kimura Y, Miyamoto M, et al. Induction of endogenous IFN-alpha and IFN-beta genes by a regulatory transcription factor, IRF-1. *Nature* 1989;337:270–272.

77. Harada H, Willison K, Sakakibara J, et al. Absence of the type I IFN system in EC cells: transcriptional activator (IRF-1) and repressor (IRF-2) genes are developmentally regulated. *Cell* 1990;63:303–312.

78. Harada H, Kitagawa M, Tanaka N, et al. Anti-oncogenic and oncogenic potentials of interferon regulatory factors-1 and -2. *Science* 1993;259:971–974.

79. Matsuyama T, Kimura T, Kitagawa M, et al. Targeted disruption of IRF-1 or IRF-2 results in abnormal type I IFN gene induction and aberrant lymphocyte development. *Cell* 1993;75:83–97.

80. Driggers PH, Ennist DL, Gleason SL, et al. An interferon gamma-regulated protein that binds the interferon-inducible enhancer element of major histocompatibility complex class I genes. *Proc Natl Acad Sci U S A* 1990;87:3743–3747.

81. Nelson N, Marks MS, Driggers PH, et al. Interferon consensus sequence-binding protein, a member of the interferon regulatory factor family, suppresses interferon-induced gene transcription. *Mol Cell Biol* 1993;13:588–599.

82. Politis AD, Sivo J, Driggers PH, et al. Modulation of interferon consensus sequence binding protein mRNA in murine peritoneal macrophages. Induction by IFN-gamma and down-regulation by IFN-alpha, dexamethasone, and protein kinase inhibitors. *J Immunol* 1992;148:801–807.

83. Einhorn S, Vanky F, Grander D, et al. Induction of 2',5'-oligoadenylate synthetase in freshly separated malignant cells from solid tumors. Variability in the susceptibility of interferon. *Eur J Cancer Clin Oncol* 1987;23:1607–1613.

84. Gutterman JU. Cytokine therapeutics: lessons from interferon alpha. *Proc Natl Acad Sci U S A* 1994;91:1198–1205.

85. Heyman M, Nordgren A, Jeddi-Tehrani M, et al. A T cell lymphoblastic lymphoma patient with two malignant cell populations carrying different 9p deletions including the p16INK4 and p15INK4B genes: clinical response to interferon-alpha therapy in one of the subclones. *Leukemia* 1996;10:909–917.

86. Colamonici OR, Uyttendaele H, Domanski P, Yan H, Krolewski JJ. p135tyk2, an interferon-alpha-activated tyrosine kinase, is physically associated with an interferon-alpha receptor. *J Biol Chem* 1994;269:3518–3522.

87. Rosenblum MG, Maxwell BL, Talpaz M, et al. In vivo sensitivity and resistance of chronic myelogenous leukemia cells to alpha-interferon: correlation with receptor binding and induction of 2',5'-oligoadenylate synthetase. *Cancer Res* 1986;46:4848–4852.

88. Sun WH, Pabon C, Alsayed Y, et al. Interferon-alpha resistance in a cutaneous T-cell lymphoma cell line is associated with lack of STAT1 expression. *Blood* 1998;91:570–576.

89. Yi TL, Cleveland JL, Ihle JN. Protein tyrosine phosphatase containing SH2 domains: characterization, preferential expression in hematopoietic cells, and localization to human chromosome 12p12-p13. *Mol Cell Biol* 1992;12:836–846.

90. Komuro H, Valentine MB, Rubnitz JE, et al. p27kip1 deletions in childhood acute lymphoblastic leukemia. *Neoplasia* 1999;1(3):253–261.

91. Kanda K, Decker T, Aman P, et al. The EBNA2-related resistance towards alpha interferon (IFN-alpha) in Burkitt's lymphoma cells effects induction of IFN-induced genes but not the activation of transcription factor ISGF-3. *Mol Cell Biol* 1992;12:4930–4936.

92. Der SD, Zhou A, Williams BR, et al. Identification of genes differentially regulated by interferon alpha, beta, or gamma using oligonucleotide arrays. *Proc Natl Acad Sci U S A* 1998;95:15623–15628.

93. Sangfelt O, Osterborg A, Grander D, et al. Response to interferon therapy in patients with multiple myeloma correlates with expression of the Bcl-2 oncoprotein. *Int J Cancer* 1995;63:190–192.

94. Sangfelt O, Erickson S, Castro J, et al. Induction of apoptosis and inhibition of cell growth are independent responses to interferon-alpha in hematopoietic cell lines. *Cell Growth Differ* 1997;8:343–352.

95. Foster GR, Ackrill AM, Goldin RD, et al. Expression of the terminal protein region of hepatitis B virus inhibits cellular responses to interferons alpha and gamma and double-stranded RNA. *Proc Natl Acad Sci U S A* 1991;88:2888–2892.

96. Reich N, Pine R, Levy D, et al. Transcription of interferon-stimulated genes is induced by adenovirus particles but is suppressed by E1A gene products. *J Virol* 1988;62:114–119.

97. Luchetti F, Gregorini A, Papa S, et al. The K562 chronic myeloid leukemia cell line undergoes apoptosis in response to interferon-α. *Haematologica* 1998;83:974–980.

98. Otsuki T, Yamada O, Sakaguchi H, et al. Human myeloma cell apoptosis induced by interferon-α. *Br J Haematol* 1998;103:518–529.

99. Sgonc R, Fuerhapter C, Boeck G, et al. Induction of apoptosis in human dermal microvascular endothelial cells and infantile hemangiomas by interferon-α. *Int Arch Allergy Immunol* 1998;117:209–214.

100. Rojas R, Roman J, Torres A, et al. Inhibition of apoptotic cell death in B-CLL by interferon gamma correlates with clinical stage. *Leukemia* 1996;10:1782–1788.

101. Novelli F, Di Pierro F, di Celle PF, et al. Environmental signals influencing expression of the IFN-γ receptor on human T cells control whether IFN-γ promotes proliferation or apoptosis. *J Immunol* 1994;152:496–504.

102. Sekiya M, Adachi M, Takayama S, et al. IFN-γ upregulates anti-apoptotic gene expression and inhibits apoptosis in IL-3-dependent hematopoietic cells. *Biochem Biophys Res Commun* 1997;239:401–406.

103. Grawunder U, Melchers F, Rolink A. Interferon-γ arrests proliferation and causes apoptosis in stromal cell/interleukin-7-dependent normal murine pre-B cell lines and clones *in vitro*, but does not induce differentiation to surface immunoglobulin-positive B cells. *Eur J Immunol* 1993;23:544–551.

104. Evan G, Littlewood T. A matter of life and cell death. *Science* 1989;281:1317–1322.

105. Morgan DO. Cyclin-dependent kinases: engines, clocks, and microprocessors. *Annu Rev Cell Dev Biol* 1997;13:261–291.

106. Kakizuka A, Miller WH, Umesono K, et al. Chromosomal translocation t(15;17) in human acute promyelocytic leukemia fuses RARα with a novel putative transcription factor, PML. *Cell* 1991;66:663–674.

107. Raveh T, Hovanessian AG, Meurs EF, et al. Double-stranded RNA-dependent protein kinase mediates c-Myc suppression induced by type I interferons. *J Biol Chem* 1996;271:25479–25484.

108. Romana CV, Grammatikakis N, Chernov M, et al. Regulation of c-myc expression by IFN-gamma through Stat1-dependent and -independent pathways. *EMBO J* 2000;19:263–272.

109. Imam H, Gobl A, Eriksson B, et al. Interferon-alpha induced bcl-2 proto-oncogene in patients with neuroendocrine gut tumor responding to its antitumor action. *Anticancer Res* 1997;17:4659–4666.

110. Koshiji M, Adachi Y, Sogo S, et al. Apoptosis of colorectal adenocarcinoma (COLO 201) by tumour necrosis factor-alpha (TNF-α) and/or interferon-gamma (IFN-γ), resulting from down-regulation of Bcl-2 expression. *Clin Exp Immunol* 1998;111:211–218.

111. Samid D, Chang EH, Friedman RM. Biochemical correlates of phenotypic reversion in interferon-treated mouse cells transformed by a human oncogene. *Biochem Biophys Res Commun* 1984;119:21–28.

112. Kumar R, Atlad I. Interferon α induces the expression of retinoblastoma gene product in human Burkitt lymphoma

113. Daudi cells: role in growth regulation. *Proc Natl Acad Sci U S A* 1992;89:6599–6603.

113. Resnitzky D, Tiefenbrun N, Berissi H, et al. Interferons and interleukin 6 suppress phosphorylation of the retinoblastoma protein in growth-sensitive hematopoietic cells. *Proc Natl Acad Sci U S A* 1992;89:402–406.

114. Buchkovich K, Duffy LA, Harlow E. The retinoblastoma protein is phosphorylated during specific phases of the cell cycle. *Cell* 1989;58:1097–1105.

115. DeCaprio JA, Ludlow JW, Lynch D, et al. The product of the retinoblastoma susceptibility gene has properties of a cell cycle regulatory element. *Cell* 1989;58:1085–1198.

116. Chen P-L, Scully P, Shew J-Y, et al. Phosphorylation of the retinoblastoma gene product is modulated during the cell cycle and cellular differentiation. *Cell* 1989;58:1193–1198.

117. Mihara K, Cao X-R, Yen A, et al. Cell cycle-dependent regulation of phosphorylation of the human retinoblastoma gene product. *Science* 1989;246:1300–1303.

118. Chellappan SP, Hiebert S, Mudryj M, et al. The E2F transcription factor is a cellular target for the RB protein. *Cell* 1991;65:1053–1061.

119. Tiefenbrun N, Melamed D, Levy N, et al. Alpha interferon suppresses the cyclin D3 and *cdc25A* genes, leading to a reversible G_0-like arrest. *Mol Cell Biol* 1996;16:3934–3944.

120. Nevins JR. E2F: a link between the Rb tumor suppressor protein and viral oncoproteins. *Science* 1992;258:424–429.

121. Iwase S, Furukawa Y, Kikushi J, et al. Modulation of E2F activity is linked to interferon-induced growth suppression of hematopoietic cells. *J Biol Chem* 1997;272:12406–12414.

122. Melamed D, Tiefenbrun H, Yarden A, et al. Interferons and interleukin-6 suppress the DNA-binding activity of E2F in growth-sensitive hematopoietic cells. *Mol Cell Biol* 1993;13:5255–5265.

123. Subramaniam PS, Cruz PE, Hobeika AC, et al. Type I interferon induction of the Cdk-inhibitor p21^WAF1 is accompanied by order G1 arrest, differentiation and apoptosis of the Daudi B-cell line. *Oncogene* 1998;16:1885–1890.

124. Chin YE, Kitagawa M, Su W-CS, et al. Cell growth arrest and induction of cyclin-dependent kinase inhibitor p21WAF1/CIP1 mediated by STAT1. *Science* 1996;272:719–722.

125. Chin YE, Kitagawa M, Kuida K, et al. Activation of the stat signaling pathway can cause expression of caspase 1 and apoptosis. *Mol Cell Biol* 1997;17:5328–5337.

126. Nguyen H, Lin R, Hiscott J. Activation of multiple growth regulatory genes following inducible expression of IRF-1 or IRF/RelA fusion proteins. *Oncogene* 1997;15:1425–1435.

127. Xu X, Fu X-Y, Plate J, et al. IFN-γ induces cells growth inhibition by Fas-mediated apoptosis: requirement of STAT1 protein for up-regulation of Fas and FasL expression. *Cancer Res* 1998;58:2832–2837.

128. Weller M, Frei K, Groscurth P, et al. Anti-Fas/APO-1 antibody-mediated apoptosis of cultured human glioma cells. Induction and modulation of sensitivity by cytokines. *J Clin Invest* 1994;94:954–964.

129. Matsue H, Kobayashi H, Hosokawa T, et al. Keratinocytes constitutively express the Fas antigen that mediates apoptosis in IFN-γ-treated keratinocytes. *Arch Dermatol Res* 1995;287:315–320.

130. Leithauser F, Dhein J, Mechtersheimer GK, et al. Constitutive and induced expression APO-1, a new member of the

nerve growth factor/tumor necrosis factor receptor super-family, in normal and neoplastic cells. *Lab Invest* 1993; 69:415–429.

131. Itoh N, Yonehara S, Ishii A, et al. The polypeptide encoded by the cDNA for human cell surface antigen Fas can mediate apoptosis. *Cell* 1991;88:355–365.

132. Spets H, Georgii-Hemming P, Siljason J, et al. Fas/APO-1 (CD95)-mediated apoptosis is activated by Interferon-γ and Interferon-α in Interleukin-6 (IL-6)-dependent and IL-6-independent multiple myeloma cell lines. *Blood* 1998; 92:2914–2923.

133. Bookstein R, Shew JY, Chen P-L, et al. Suppression of tumorigenicity of human prostate carcinoma cells by replacing a mutant RB gene. *Science* 1990;247:712–714.

134. Isaacs WB, Carter BS, Ewing CM. Wild-type p53 suppresses growth of human prostate cancer cells containing mutant p53 alleles. *Cancer Res* 1991;51:4716–4720.

135. Dong J-T, Lamb PW, Rinker-Schaeffer CW, et al. KAI1, a metastasis suppressor gene for prostate cancer on human chromosome 11p11.2. *Science* 1995;268:884–886.

136. Hobeika AC, Subramaniam PS, Johnson HM. IFNα induces the expression of the cyclin-dependent kinase inhibitor p21 in human prostate cancer cells. *Oncogene* 1997;14:1165–1170.

137. Hobeika AC, Etienne W, Cruz PE, et al. IFNγ induction of p21^{WAF1} in prostate cancer cells: role in cell cycle, alteration of phenotype and invasive potential. *Int J Cancer* 1998; 77:138–145.

138. Deiss LP, Feinstein E, Berissi H, et al. Identification of a novel serine/threonine kinase and a novel 15-kD protein as potential mediators of the γ interferon-induced cell death. *Genes Dev* 1995;9:15–30.

139. Cohen O, Feinstein E, Kimshi A. DAP-kinase is a Ca^{2+}/calmodulin-dependent, cytoskeletal-associated protein kinase with cell death-inducing functions that depend on its catalytic activity. *EMBO J* 1997;16:998–1008.

140. Kissil JL, Deiss LP, Bayewitch M, et al. Isolation of DAP3, a novel mediator of interferon-γ-induced cell death. *J Biol Chem* 1995;270:27932–27936.

141. Levy-Strumpf N, Deiss LP, Berissi H. DAP-5, a novel homolog of eukaryotic translation initiation factor 4G isolated as a putative modulator of gamma interferon-induced programmed cell death. *Mol Cell Biol* 1997;17:1615–1625.

142. Deiss LP, Kimchi A. A genetic tool used to identify thioredoxin as a mediator of a growth inhibitory signal. *Science* 1991;252:117–120.

143. Deiss L, Galinka H, Berissi H, et al. Cathepsin D protease mediates programmed cell death induced by interferon-γ, Fas/APO-1 and TNF-α. *EMBO J* 1996;15:3861–3870.

144. Hofman ER, Boyanapalli M, Lindner DJ, et al. Thioredoxin reductase mediates cell death effects of the combination of beta interferon and retinoic acid. *Mol Cell Biol* 1998;18:6493–6504.

145. Buschle M, Campana D, Carding SR, et al. Interferon-γ inhibits apoptotic cell death in B cell chronic lymphocytic leukemia. *J Exp Med* 1993;177:213–218.

146. Hassan Y, Huleihel M, Priel E, et al. Effect of mouse interferon on chemical carcinogenesis in normal rat kidney cells infected with Moloney murine leukemia virus. *Carcinogenesis* 1985;6:2787–2790.

147. Salerno RA, Whitmire CE, Garcia IM. Chemical carcinogenesis in mice inhibited by interferon. *Nat New Biol* 1972;239:31–32.

148. Borden EC, Sidky YA, Erturk C, et al. Protection from carcinogen-induced murine bladder carcinoma by interferons and an oral interferon-inducing pyrimidine, bropirimine. *Cancer Res* 1990;50:1071–1074.

149. Pamer E, Cresswell P. Mechanisms of MHC class I-restricted antigen processing. *Annu Rev Immunol* 1998; 16:323–358.

150. Mach B, Steimle V, Martinez-Soria E, et al. Regulation of MHC class II genes: lessons from a disease. *Annu Rev Immunol* 1996;14:310–331.

151. Greiner JW, Hand PH, Noguchi P, et al. Enhanced expression of surface tumor-associated antigens on human breast and colon tumor cells after recombinant human leukocyte α-interferon treatment. *Cancer Res* 1984;44:3208–3214.

152. Leon JA, Mesa-tejada R, Gutierrez MC, et al. Increased surface expression and shedding of tumor associated antigens by human breast carcinoma cells treated with recombinant human interferons or phorbol ester tumor promoters. *Anticancer Res* 1989;9:1639–1648.

153. Sivinski CL, Lindner DJ, Borden EC, et al. Modulation of tumor-associated antigen expression on human pancreatic and prostate carcinoma cells in vitro by α- and γ-interferons. *J Immunotherapy* 1995;18:156–165.

154. Ghosh AK, Cerny T, Wagstaff J, et al. Effect of in vivo administration of interferon gamma on expression of MHC products and tumour associated antigens in patients with metastatic melanoma. *Eur J Cancer Clin Oncol* 1989;25: 1637–1643.

155. Daeron M. Fc receptor biology. *Annu Rev Immunol* 1997;15:203–234.

156. Ozzello L, Habif DV, DeRosa CM, et al. Cellular events accompanying regression of breast carcinomas treated with intralesional injections of natural interferons α and γ. *Cancer Res* 1992;52:4571–4581.

157. von Hoegen P. Synergistic role of type I interferons in the induction of protective cytotoxic T lymphocytes. *Immunol Lett* 1995;47:157–162.

158. McAdam AJ, Pulaski BA, Storozynsky E, et al. Analysis of the effect of cytokines (interleukins 2, 3, 4, and 6, granulocyte-monocyte colony-stimulating factor, and interferon-γ) on generation of primary cytotoxic T lymphocytes against a weakly immunogenic tumor. *Cell Immunol* 1995;165:183–192.

159. Zarling JM, Eskra L, Borden EC, et al. Activation of human natural killer cells cytotoxic for human leukemia cells by purified interferon. *J Immunol* 1979;126:203–209.

160. Biron CA. Activation and function of natural killer cell responses during viral infections. *Curr Opin Immunol* 1997;9:24–34.

161. Pace JL, Russell SW, Torres BA, et al. Recombinant mouse gamma interferon induces the priming step in macrophage activation for tumor cell killing. *J Immunol* 1983;130: 2011–2013.

162. Hayes MP, Zoon KC. Priming of human monocytes for enhanced lipopolysaccharide responses: expression of alpha interferon, interferon regulatory factors, and tumor necrosis factor. *Infect Immun* 1993;61:3222–3227.

163. Luft T, Pang KC, Thomas E, et al. Type I IFNs enhance the terminal differentiation of dendritic cells. *J Immunol* 1998;161:1947–1953.

164. Kitajima T, Caceres-Dittmar G, Tapia FJ, et al. T cell-mediated terminal maturation of dendritic cells. *J Immunol* 1996;157:2340–2347.

165. Raulet DH, Bevan MH. A differentiation factor required for the expression of cytotoxic T-cell function. *Nature* 1982;296:754–757.

166. Siegel JP. Effects of interferon-gamma on the activation of human T lymphocytes. *Cell Immunol* 1988;111:461–472.

167. DeVries JE, Spits H. Cloned human cytotoxic T lymphocyte (CTL) lines reactive with autologous melanoma cells: I. In vivo generation, isolation, and analysis to phenotype and specificity. *J Immunol* 1984;132:510–519.

168. Urban JL, Schreiber H. Selections of macrophage-resistant progressor tumor variants by the normal host: requirement for concomitant T cell mediated immunity. *J Exp Med* 1983;157:642–656.

169. Reid LM, Minato N, Gresser I, et al. Influence of anti-mouse interferon serum on the growth and metastasis of tumor cells persistently infected with virus and of human prostatic tumors in athymic nude mice. *Proc Natl Acad Sci U S A* 1981;78:1171–1175.

170. Gresser I, Belardelli F, Maury C, et al. Injection of mice with antibody to interferon enhances the growth of transplantable murine tumors. *J Exp Med* 1983;158:2095–2107.

171. Dvorak HF, Gresser I. Microvascular injury in pathogenesis of interferon-induced necrosis of subcutaneous tumors in mice. *J Natl Cancer Inst* 1989;81:497–502.

172. Dinney CP, Bielenberg DR, Perrotte P, et al. Inhibition of basic fibroblast growth factor expression, angiogenesis, and growth of human bladder carcinoma in mice by systemic interferon-alpha administration. *Cancer Res* 1998;58:808–814.

173. Singh RK, Gutman M, Bucana CD, et al. Interferons α and β down-regulate the expression of basic fibroblast growth factor in human carcinomas. *Proc Natl Acad Sci U S A* 1995;92:4562–4566.

174. Wang W, Chen HJ, Schwartz A, et al. T cell lymphokines modulate bFGF-induced smooth muscle cell fibrinolysis and migration. *Am J Physiol* 1997;272:C392–398.

175. Sato N, Nariuchi H, Tsuruoka N, et al. Actions of TNF and IFN-gamma on angiogenesis in vitro. *J Invest Dermatol* 1990;95:85S–89S.

176. Sidky Y, Borden EC. Inhibition of angiogenesis by interferons: effects on tumor- and lymphocyte-induced vascular responses. *Cancer Res* 1987;47:5155–5161.

177. Koch AE, Polverini PJ, Kunkel SL, et al. Interleukin-8 as a macrophage-derived mediator of angiogenesis. *Science* 1992;258:1798–1801.

178. Yoshida S, Ono M, Shono T, et al. Involvement of interleukin-8, vascular endothelial growth factor, and basic fibroblast growth factor in tumor necrosis factor alpha-dependent angiogenesis. *Mol Cell Biol* 1997;17:4015–4023.

179. Arenberg DA, Kunkel SL, Polverini PJ, et al. Inhibition of interleukin-8 reduces tumorigenesis of human non-small cell lung cancer in SCID mice. *J Clin Invest* 1996;97:2792–2802.

180. Reznikov LL, Puren AJ, Fantuzzi G, et al. Spontaneous and inducible cytokine responses in healthy humans receiving a single dose of IFN-α2b: increased production of interleukin-1 receptor antagonist and suppression of IL-1-induced IL-8. *J Interferon Cyto Res* 1998;18:897–903.

181. Strieter RM, Kunkel SL, Arenberg DA, et al. Interferon gamma-inducible protein 10 (IP-10), a member of the C-X-C chemokine family, is an inhibitor of angiogenesis. *Biochem Biophys Res Commun* 1995;210:51–57.

182. Ezekowitz RAB, Milliken JB, Folkman J. Interferon alpha-2a therapy for life-threatening hemangiomas of infancy. *N Engl J Med* 1992;326:1456–1463.

183. Chang E, Boyd A, Nelson CC, et al. Successful treatment of infantile hemangiomas with interferon-alpha-2b. *J Pediatr Hematol Oncol* 1997;19:237–244.

184. Robenzadeh A, Don PC, Weinberg JM. Treatment of tufted angioma with interferon alfa: role of bFGF. *Pediatr Dermatol* 1998;15:482.

185. Krown SE. Interferon-α: evolving therapy for AIDS-associated Kaposi's sarcoma. *J Interferon Cytokine Res* 1998;18:209–214.

186. Tur E, Brenner S. Classic Kaposi's sarcoma: low-dose interferon alpha treatment. *Dermatology* 1997;197:37–42.

187. Deichmann M, Thome M, Jackel A, et al. Non-human immunodeficiency virus Kaposi's sarcoma can be effectively treated with low-dose interferon-alpha despite the persistence of herpesvirus-8. *Br J Dermatol* 1998;139:1052–1054.

188. Pfrommer C, Tebbe B, Tidona CA, et al. Progressive HHV-8-positive classic Kaposi's sarcoma: rapid response to interferon alpha-2a but persistence of HHV-8 DNA sequences in lesional skin. *Br J Dermatol* 1998;139:516–519.

189. Boehm U, Klamp T, Groot M, et al. Cellular responses to interferon-γ. *Annu Rev Immunol* 1997;15:749–795.

190. Der SD, Zhou A, Williams BRG, et al. Identification of genes differentially regulated by interferon α, β, or γ using oligonucleotide arrays. *Proc Natl Acad Sci U S A* 1998;95:15623–15628.

191. Sen GC, Ransohoff RM. Interferon-induced antiviral actions and their regulation. *Adv Virus Res* 1993:57–102.

192. Samuel CE. Antiviral actions of interferon: interferon-regulated cellular proteins and their surprisingly selective antiviral activities. *Virology* 1991;183:1–11.

193. Silverman RH, Cirino NM. RNA decay by the interferon-regulated 2-5A system as a host defense against viruses. In: Hartford JB, ed. *mRNA metabolism and post-translational gene regulation.* New York: Wiley-Liss, 1997:295–309.

194. Hovanessian AG. Interferon-induced dsRNA-activated protein kinase (PKR): antiproliferative, antiviral and antitumoral functions. *Semin Virol* 1993;4:237–245.

195. Clemens MJ, Elia A. The double-stranded RNA-dependent protein kinase PKR: structure and function. *J Interferon Cytokine Res* 1997;17:503–524.

196. Meurs E, Chong K, Galabru J, et al. Molecular cloning and characterization of the human double-stranded RNA-activated protein kinase induced by interferon. *Cell* 1990;62:379–390.

197. Patel RC, Sen GC. PACT, a protein activator of the interferon-induced protein kinase, PKR. *EMBO J* 1998;17:4379–4390.

198. Balachandran S, Kim CN, Yeh W-C, et al. Activation of the dsRNA-dependent protein kinase PKR, induces apoptosis through FADD-mediated death signaling. *EMBO J* 1998;17:6888–6902.

199. Hovanessian AG. Interferon-induced and double-stranded

RNA-activated enzymes: a specific protein kinase and 2',5'-oligoadenylate synthetases. *J Interferon Res* 1991;11:199–205.

200. Patterson JB, Samuel CE. Expression and regulation by interferon of a double-stranded-RNA-specific adenosine deaminase from human cells: evidence for two forms of the deaminase. *Mol Cell Biol* 1995;15:5376–5388.

201. Patterson JB, Thomis DC, Hans SL, et al. Mechanism of interferon action: double-stranded RNA-specific adenosine deaminase from human cells is inducible by alpha and gamma interferons. *Virology* 1995;210:508–511.

202. Aebi M, Fah J, Hurt N, et al. cDNA structures and regulation of two interferon-induced human Mx proteins. *Mol Cell Biol* 1989;9:5062–5072.

203. Horisberger MA, McMaster GK, Zeller H, et al. Cloning and sequence analyses of cDNAs for interferon- and virus-induced human Mx proteins reveal that they contain putative guanine nucleotide-binding sites: functional study of the corresponding gene promoter. *J Virol* 1990;64:1171–1181.

204. Haller O, Frese M, Kochs G. Mx proteins: mediators of innate resistance to RNA viruses. *Rev Sci Tech* 1998;17:220–230.

205. Staeheli P. Interferon-induced proteins and the antiviral state. *Adv Virus Res* 1990;38:147–200.

206. Obar RA, Collins CA, Hammerback JA, et al. Molecular cloning of the microtubule-associated mechanochemical enzyme dynamin reveals homology with a new family of GTP-binding protein. *Nature* 1990;347:256–261.

207. Li Y, Youssoufian H. MxA overexpression reveals a common genetic link in four Fanconi anemia complementation groups. *J Clin Invest* 1997;100:2873–2880.

208. Horisberger MA. Interferon-induced human protein MxA is a GTPase which binds transiently to cellular proteins. *J Virol* 1992;66:4705–4709.

209. Boehm U, Guethlein L, Klamp T, et al. Two families of GTPases dominate the complex cellular response to IFN-γ. *J Immunol* 1998;161:6715–6723.

210. Cheng Y-SE, Colonno RJ, Yin FH. Interferon induction of fibroblast proteins with guanylate binding activity. *J Biol Chem* 1983;258:7746–7750.

211. Cheng Y-SE, Patterson CE, Staeheli P. Interferon-induced guanylate-binding proteins lack an N(T)KXD consensus motif and bind GMP in addition to GDP and GTP. *Mol Cell Biol* 1991;11:4717–4725.

212. Wynn TA, Nicolet CM, Paulnock DM. Identification and characterization of a new gene family induced during macrophage activation. *J Immunol* 1991;147:4384–4392.

213. Vestal DJ, Buss JE, McKercher SR, et al. Murine GBP-2: a new IFN-γ-induced member of the GBP family of GTPases isolated from macrophages. *J Interferon Cytokine Res* 1998;18:977–985.

214. Han BHH, Park DJ, Lim RW, et al. Cloning, expression, and characterization of a novel guanylate-binding protein, GBP3, in murine erythroid progenitor cells. *Biochim Biophys Acta* 1998;1384:373–386.

215. Anderson SL, Carton JM, Lou J, et al. Interferon-induced guanylate binding protein-1 (GBP-1) mediates an antiviral effect against vesicular stomatitis virus and encephalomyocarditis virus. *Virology* 1999;256:8–14.

216. Gilly M, Wall R. The IRG-47 gene is IFN-gamma induced in B cells and encodes a protein with putative GTP-binding motifs. *J Immunol* 1992;148:3275–3281.

217. Sorace J, Johnson R, Howard D, et al. Identification of an endotoxin and IFN-inducible cDNA: possible identification of a novel gene family. *J Leukoc Biol* 1995;58:477–484.

218. Carlow D, Marth J, Clark-Lewis I, et al. Isolation of a gene encoding a developmentally regulated T cell specific protein with a guanine nucleotide triphosphate-binding motif. *J Immunol* 1995;154:1724–1734.

219. Lafuse W, Brown D, Castle L, et al. Cloning and characterization of a novel cDNA that is IFN-γ-induced in mouse peritoneal macrophages and encodes a putative GTP-binding protein. *J Leukoc Biol* 1995;57:477–483.

220. Taylor G, Jeffers M, Largaespada D, et al. Identification of a novel GTPase, the inducibly expressed GTPase that accumulates in response to interferon γ. *J Biol Chem* 1996;271:20399–20405.

221. Carlow DA, Teh S-J, Teh H-S. Specific antiviral activity demonstrated by TGTP, a member of a new family of interferon-induced GTPases. *J Immunol* 1998;161:2348–2355.

222. Min W, Pober JS, Johnson DR. Kinetically coordinated induction of TAP1 and HLA Class I by IFN-γ. *J Immunol* 1996;156:3174–3183.

223. Rock KL, Gramm C, Rothstein L, et al. Inhibitors of the proteasome block the degradation of most cell proteins and the generation of peptides presented on MHC class I molecules. *Cell* 1994;78:761–771.

224. Nandi D, Jiang H, Monaco JJ. Identification of MECL-1 (LMP-10) as the third IFN-γ-inducible proteasome subunit. *J Immunol* 1996;156:2361–2364.

225. Foss GS, Larsen F, Solheim J, et al. Constitutive and interferon-γ-induced expression of the human proteasome subunit multicatalytic endopeptidase complex-like 1. *Biochim Biophys Acta* 1998;1402:17–28.

226. Aki M, Shimbara N, Takasina M, et al. Interferon-γ induces different subunit organizations and functional diversity of proteasomes. *J Biochem* 1994;115:257–269.

227. Driscoll J, Brown MG, Finley D, et al. MHC-linked *LMP* gene products specifically alter peptidase activities of the proteasome. *Nature* 1993;365:262–264.

228. Gaczynska M, Rock KL, Goldberg AL. γ-Interferon and expression of *MHC* genes regulate peptide hydrolysis by proteasomes. *Nature* 1993;365:264–267.

229. Ma W, Lehner PJ, Cresswell P, et al. Interferon-γ rapidly increases peptide transporter (TAP) subunit expression and peptide transport capacity in endothelial cells. *J Biol Chem* 1997;272:16585–16590.

230. Watts C. Capture and processing of exogenous antigens for presentation on MHC molecules. *Annu Rev Immunol* 1997;15:821–850.

231. Barr CL, Saunder GF. Interferon-γ-inducible regulation of the human invariant chain gene. *J Biol Chem* 1991;266:3475–3481.

232. Chang C-H, Flavell RA. Class II transactivator regulates the expression of multiple genes involved in antigen presentation. *J Exp Med* 1995;181:765–767.

233. Lafuse WP, Brown D, Castle L, et al. IFN-γ increases cathepsin H mRNA levels in mouse macrophages. *J Leukoc Biol* 1995;57:663–669.

234. Lah TT, Hawley M, Rock KL, et al. Gamma-interferon causes a selective induction of the lysosomal proteases, cathepsin B and L, in macrophages. *FEBS Lett* 1995;363:85–89.

235. Volanakis JE. Transcriptional regulation of complement genes. *Annu Rev Immunol* 1995;13:277–305.

236. Taylor MW, Feng G. Relationship between interferon-γ, indoleamine 2,3-dioxygenase, and tryptophan catabolism. *FASEB J* 1991;5:2516–2522.

237. Carlin JM, Ozaki Y, Byrne GI, et al. Interferons and indoleamine 2,3-dioxygenase: role in antimicrobial and antitumor effects. *Experientia* 1989;45:535–541.

238. Gupta SL, Carlin JM, Pyati P, et al. Antiparasitic and antiproliferative effects of indoleamine 2,3-dioxygenase enzyme expression in human fibroblasts. *Infect Immun* 1994;62:2277–2284.

239. Pfefferkorn ER. Interferon γ blocks the growth of *Toxoplasma gondii* in human fibroblasts by inducing the host cells to degrade tryptophan. *Proc Natl Acad Sci U S A* 1984;81:908–912.

240. Seegert D, Strehlow I, Klose B, et al. A novel interferon-α-regulated, DNA-binding protein participates in the regulation of the IFP53/tryptophanyl-tRNA synthetase gene. *J Biol Chem* 1994;269:8590–8595.

241. Segal AW. The electron transport chain of the microbicidal oxidase of phagocytic cells and its involvement in the molecular pathology of chronic granulomatous disease. *J Clin Invest* 1989;83:1785–1793.

242. Rossi F. The O2-forming NADPH oxidase of the phagocytes: nature, mechanisms of activation and function. *Biochim Biophys Acta* 1986;853:65–89.

243. Cassatella MA, Bazzoni F, Flynn RM, et al. Molecular basis of interferon-γ and lipopolysaccharide enhancement of phagocyte respiratory burst capability. *J Biol Chem* 1990;265:20241–20246.

244. Cassatella MA, Bazzoni F, Calzetti F, et al. Interferon-γ transcriptionally modulates the expression of the genes for the high affinity IgG-Fc receptor and the 47-kDa cytosolic component of NADPH oxidase in human polymorphonuclear leukocytes. *J Biol Chem* 1991;266:22079–22082.

245. Gupta JW, Kubin M, Hartman L, et al. Induction of expression of genes encoding components of the respiratory burst oxidase during differentiation of human myeloid cell lines induced by tumor necrosis factor and γ-interferon. *Cancer Res* 1992;52:2530–2537.

246. MacMicking J, Xie Q, Nathan C. Nitric oxide and macrophage function. *Annu Rev Immunol* 1997;15:323–350.

247. Morris SM, Billiar TR. New insights into the regulation of inducible nitric oxide synthesis. *Am J Physiol* 1994;268:E829–E839.

248. D'Cunha J, Ramanujam S, Wagner RJ, et al. In vitro and in vivo secretion of human ISG15, an IFN-induced immunomodulatory cytokine. *J Immunol* 1996;157:4100–4108.

249. Marfaing-Koka A, Gorgone O, Devergne G, et al. Regulation of the production of the RANTES chemokine by endothelial cells. Synergistic induction by IFN-γ plus TNF-α and inhibition by IL-4 and IL-13. *J Immunol* 1995;154:1870–1878.

250. Taub DD, Lloyd AR, Conlon D, et al. Recombinant human interferon-inducible protein 10 is a chemoattractant for human monocytes and T lymphocytes and promotes T cell adhesion to endothelial cells. *J Exp Med* 1993;177:1809–1814.

251. Rollins BJ, Yoshimura T, Leonard EJ, et al. Cytokine-activated human endothelial cells synthesize and secrete a monocyte chemoattractant, MCP-1/JE. *Am J Pathol* 1990;136:1229–1233.

252. Laio R, Rabin RL, Yannelli JR, et al. Human Mig chemokine: biochemical and functional characterization. *J Exp Med* 1995;182:1301–1314.

253. Rani MRS, Foster GR, Leung S, et al. Characterization of β-R1, a gene that is selectively induced by interferon β (IFN-β) compared with IFN-α. *J Biol Chem* 1996;271:22878–22884.

254. Cole KE, Strick CA, Paradis TJ, et al. Interferon-inducible T cell alpha chemoattractant (I-TAC): a novel non-ELR CXC chemokine with potent activity on activated T cells through selective high affinity binding to CXCR3. *J Exp Med* 1998;187:2009–2021.

255. Choubey D, Lengyel P. Binding of an interferon-inducible protein (p202) to the retinoblastoma protein. *J Biol Chem* 1995;270:6134–6140.

256. Datta B, Li B, Choubey D, et al. p202, an interferon-inducible modulator of transcription, inhibits transcriptional activation by the p53 tumor suppressor protein, and a segment from the p53-binding protein 1 that binds to p202 overcomes this inhibition. *J Biol Chem* 1996;271:27544–27555.

257. Choubey D, Li S-J, Datta B, et al. Inhibition of E2F-mediated transcription by p202. *EMBO J* 1996;15:5668–5678.

258. Choubey D, Gutterman JU. Inhibition of E2F/DP-1-stimulated transcription by p202. *Oncogene* 1997;15:291–301.

259. Min W, Ghosh S, Lengyel P. The interferon-inducible p202 protein as a modulator of transcription: inhibition of NF-κB, c-Fos, and c-Jun activities. *Mol Cell Biol* 1996;16:359–368.

260. Choubey D, Snoddy J, Chaturvedi V, et al. Interferons as gene activators. Indications for repeated gene duplication during the evolution of a cluster of interferon-activatable genes on murine chromosome 1. *J Biol Chem* 1989;264:17182–17189.

261. Opdenakker G, Snoddy J, Choubey D, et al. Interferons as gene activators: a cluster of six interferon-activatable genes is linked to the erythroid α-spectrin locus on murine chromosome 1. *Virology* 1989;171:568–578.

262. Liu C-J, Wang H, Lengyel P. The interferon-inducible nucleolar p204 protein binds the ribosomal RNA-specific UBF1 transcription factor and inhibits ribosomal RNA transcription. *EMBO J* 1999;18:2845–2854.

263. Briggs JA, Burrus GR, Stickney BD, et al. Cloning and expression of the human myeloid cell nuclear differentiation antigen: regulation by interferon α. *J Cell Biochem* 1992;49:82–92.

264. Briggs RC, Briggs JA, Ozer J, et al. The human myeloid cell nuclear differentiation antigen gene is one of at least two related interferon-inducible genes located on chromosome 1q that are expressed specifically in hematopoietic cells. *Blood* 1994;83:2153–2162.

265. Dawson MJ, Trapani JA. IFI 16 gene encodes a nuclear protein whose expression is induced by interferons in human myeloid leukaemia cell lines. *J Cell Biochem* 1995;57:39–51.

266. DeYoung KL, Ray ME, Su YA, et al. Cloning a novel member of the human interferon-inducible gene family associated with control of tumorigenicity in a model of human melanoma. *Oncogene* 1997;15:453–457.

267. Mei S-M, Chin K-V, Liu J-H, et al. PML, a growth suppressor disrupted in acute promyelocytic leukemia. *Mol Cell Biol* 1994;14:6858–6867.

268. Koken MHM, Linares-Cruz G, Quignon F, et al. The PML growth-suppressor has an altered expression in human oncogenesis. *Oncogene* 1995;10:1315–1324.

269. Wang Z-G, Ruggero D, Ronchetti S, et al. PML is essential for multiple apoptotic pathways. *Nat Genet* 1998;20:266–272.

270. Quignon F, De Bels F, Koken M, et al. PML induces a novel caspase-independent death process. *Nat Genet* 1998;20:259–265.

271. Zheng P, Guo Y, Nie Q, et al. Proto-oncogene PML controls genes devoted to MHC class I antigen presentation. *Nature* 1998;396:373–376.

272. Scostecki C, Guldner HH, Netter HJ, et al. Isolation and characterization of cDNA encoding a human nuclear antigen predominantly recognized by autoantibodies from patients with primary biliary cirrhosis. *J Immunol* 1990; 145:4338–4347.

273. Koriath F, Gieffers C, Maul GG, et al. Molecular characterization of NDP52, a novel protein of the nuclear domain 10, which is redistributed on virus infection and interferon treatment. *J Cell Biol* 1995;130:1–13.

274. Gongora C, David G, Pintard L, et al. Molecular cloning of a new interferon-induced PML nuclear body-associated protein. *J Biol Chem* 1997;272:19457–19463.

275. Zhao J, Zhou Q, Wiedmer T, et al. Level of expression of phospholipid scramblase regulates induced movement of phosphatidylserine to the cell surface. *J Biol Chem* 1998; 273:6603–6606.

276. Roselli M, Guadagni F, Buonomo O, et al. Systemic administration of recombinant interferon alfa in carcinoma patients upregulates the expression of the carcinoma-associated antigens tumor-associated glycoprotein-72 and carcinoembryonic antigen. *J Clin Oncol* 1996;14:2031–2042.

277. Takahashi H, Okai Y, Paxton RJ, et al. Differential regulation of carcinoembryonic antigen and biliary glycoprotein by γ-interferon. *Cancer Res* 1993;53:1612–1619.

278. Stein U, Walther W, Shoemaker RH. Modulation of mdr1 expression by cytokines in human colon carcinoma cells: an approach for reversal of multidrug resistance. *Br J Cancer* 1996;74:1384–1391.

279. Gutterman JU, Fine S, Quesada J, et al. Recombinant leukocyte A interferon: pharmacokinetics, single-dose tolerance, and biologic effects in cancer patients. *Ann Intern Med* 1982;96:549–555.

280. Maluish AE, Reid JW, Crisp EA, et al. Immunomodulatory effects of poly(I,C)-LC in cancer patients. *J Biol Resp Mod* 1985;4:656–663.

281. Robins HI, Sielaff KM, Storer B, et al. Phase I trial of human lymphoblastoid interferon with whole body hyperthermia in advanced cancer. *Cancer Res* 1989;49:1609–1615.

282. Quesada JR, Gutterman JU. Clinical study of recombinant DNA-produced leukocyte interferon (Clone A) in an intermittent schedule in cancer patients. *J Nat Cancer Inst* 1983; 70:1041–1046.

283. Quesada JR, Hawkins M, Horning S, et al. Collaborative phase I-II study of recombinant DNA-produced leukocyte interferon (clone A) in metastatic breast cancer, malignant lymphoma, and multiple myeloma. *Am J Med* 1984;77: 427–432.

284. Rohatiner AZS, Balkwill FR, Griffin DB, et al. A phase I study of human lymphoblastoid interferon administered by continuous intravenous infusion. *Cancer Chemother Pharmacol* 1982;9:97–102.

285. Dorr RT, Salmon SE, Robertone A, et al. Phase I-II trial of interferon-alpha 2b by continuous subcutaneous infusion over 28 days. *J Interferon Res* 1988;8:717–725.

286. Abdi EA, Kamitomo VJ, McPherson TA, et al. Extended phase I study of human β-interferon in human cancer. *Clin Invest Med* 1986;9:33–40.

287. Chiang J, Gloff CA, Soike KF, et al. Pharmacokinetics and antiviral activity of recombinant human interferon-βser17 in African green monkeys. *J Interferon Res* 1993;13:111–120.

288. Grunberg SM, Kempf RA, Venturi CL, et al. Phase I study of recombinant beta-interferon given by four-hour infusion. *Cancer Res* 1987;47:1174–1178.

289. Rinehart JJ, Malspeis L, Young D, et al. Phase I/II trial of human recombinant interferon gamma in renal cell carcinoma. *J Biol Resp Mod* 1986;5:300–308.

290. Vadhan-Raj S, Al-Katib A, Bhalla R, et al. Phase I trial of recombinant interferon gamma in cancer patients. *J Clin Oncol* 1986;4:137–146.

291. Thompson JA, Cox WW, Lindgren CG, et al. Subcutaneous recombinant gamma interferon in cancer patients: toxicity, pharmacokinetics and immunomodulatory effects. *Cancer Immunol Immunother* 1987;25:47–53.

292. Goldstein D, Sielaff KM, Storer BE, et al. Human biologic response modification by interferon in the absence of measurable serum concentrations: a comparative trial of subcutaneous and intravenous interferon beta serine. *J Natl Cancer Inst* 1989;81:1061–1068.

293. Witt PL, Storer BE, Bryan GT, et al. Pharmacodynamics of biological response in vivo after single and multiple doses of interferon-β. *J Immunotherapy* 1993;13:191–200.

294. Maluish AE, Urba WJ, Longo DL, et al. The determination of an immunologically active dose of interferon-gamma in patients with melanoma. *J Clin Oncol* 1988;6:434–445.

295. Kirkwood JM, Ernstoff MS, Trautman T, et al. In vivo biological response to recombinant interferon-gamma during a phase I dose-response trial in patients with metastatic melanoma. *J Clin Oncol* 1990;8:1070–1082.

296. Fleischmann J, Masoor J, Wu TY, et al. Orally administered IFN-alpha acts alone and in synergistic combination with intraperitoneally administered IFN-gamma to exert an antitumor effect against B16 melanoma in mice. *J Interferon Cytokine Res* 1998;18:17–20.

297. Beilharz MW, McDonald W, Watson MW, et al. Low-dose oral type I interferons reduce early virus replication of murine cytomegalovirus in vivo. *J Interferon Cytokine Res* 1997;17:625–630.

298. Nagao Y, Yamashiro K, Hara N, et al. Oral-mucosal administration of IFN-alpha potentiates immune response in mice. *J Interferon Cytokine Res* 1998;18:661–666.

299. Brod SA, Kerman RH, Nelson LD, et al. Ingested IFN-alpha has biological effects in humans with relapsing-remitting multiple sclerosis. *Mult Scler* 1997;3:1–7.

300. Dhingra K, Duvic M, Hymes S, et al. A phase-I clinical study of low-dose oral interferon-α. *J Immunotherapy* 1993;14:51–55.

301. Lecciones JA, Abejar NH, Dimaano EE, et al. A pilot double-blind, randomized, and placebo-controlled study of

orally administered IFN-alpha-n1 in pediatric patients with measles. *J Interferon Cytokine Res* 1998;18.

302. Witt PL, Goldstein D, Storer BE, et al. Absence of biological effects of orally administered interferon-βser. *J Interferon Res* 1992;12:411–413.

303. Wright SE, Hutcheson DP, Cummins JM. Low dose oral interferon alpha 2a in HIV-1 seropositive patients: a double-blind, placebo-controlled trial. *Biotherapy* 1998;11:229–234.

304. Eid P, Meritet JF, Maury C, et al. Oromucosal interferon therapy: pharmacokinetics and pharmacodynamics. *J Interferon Cytokine Res* 1999;19:157–169.

305. Katabira ET, Sewankambo NK, Mugerwa RD, et al. Lack of efficacy of low dose oral interferon alpha in symptomatic HIV-1 infection: a randomised, double-blind, placebo controlled trial. *Sex Transm Infect* 1998;74:265–270.

306. Talmadge JE, Tribble HR, Pennington RW, et al. Immunomodulatory and immunotherapeutic properties of recombinant gamma-interferon and recombinant tumor necrosis factor in mice. *Cancer Res* 1987;47:2563–2570.

307. Einhorn S, Ahre A, Blomgren H, et al. Interferon and natural killer activity in multiple myeloma: lack of correlation between interferon-induced enhancement of natural killer activity and clinical response to human interferon-α. *Int J Cancer* 1982;30:167–172.

308. Edwards BS, Merritt JA, Fuhlbrigge RC, et al. Low doses of interferon alpha result in more effective clinical natural killer cell activation. *J Clin Invest* 1985;75:1908–1913.

309. Weiner LM, Steplewski Z, Koprowski H, et al. Divergent dose-related effects of gamma-interferon therapy on in vitro antibody-dependent cellular and nonspecific cytotoxicity by human peripheral blood monocytes. *Cancer Res* 1988;48:1042–1046.

310. Jakschies D, Hochkeppel H, Horisberger M, et al. Emergence and decay of the human Mx homolog in cancer patients during and after interferon-α therapy. *J Biol Resp Mod* 1990;9:305–312.

311. Rinehart JJ, Young D, Laforge J, et al. Phase I/II trial of interferon beta-serine in patients with renal cell carcinoma: immunological and biological effects. *Cancer Res* 1987;47:2481–2487.

312. Liberati AM, Fizzotti M, Proietti MG, et al. Biochemical host response to interferon-beta. *J Interferon Res* 1988;8:765–777.

313. Paulnock DM, Havlin KA, Storer BM, et al. Induced proteins in human peripheral mononuclear cells over a range of clinically tolerable doses of interferon gamma. *J Interferon Res* 1989;9:457–473.

314. Kopp WC, Smith JW II, Ewel CH, et al. Immunomodulatory effects of interferon gamma in patients with metastatic malignant melanoma. *J Immunotherapy* 1993;13:181–190.

315. Aulitzky WE, Aulitzky W, Gastl G, et al. Acute effects of single doses of recombinant interferon gamma on blood cell counts and lymphocyte subsets in patients with advanced renal cell cancer. *J Interferon Res* 1989;9:425–433.

316. Schiller JH, Storer B, Paulnock DM, et al. A direct comparison of biological response modifiers and clinical side effects by human interferon beta-serine, interferon gamma, or combination of interferons beta plus gamma in humans. *J Clin Invest* 1990;86:1211–1221.

317. Hakansson A, Gustafsson B, Krysander L, et al. Effect of IFN-alpha on tumor-infiltrating mononuclear cells and regressive changes in metastatic malignant melanoma. *J Interferon Cytokine Res* 1998;18:33–39.

318. Grander D, Oberg K, Lundquist ML, et al. Interferon-induced enhancement of 2',5'-oligoadenylate synthetase in mid-gut carcinoid tumours. *Lancet* 1990;336:337–340.

319. Ferbus D, Khosravi S, Dumont J, et al. In vivo and in vitro induction of 2'-5' oligoadenylate synthetase by interferon-alpha in nodular non-Hodgkin's lymphoma and correlations with the clinical response. *J Biol Regul Homeost Agents* 1990;4:127–134.

320. de Mel WCP, Hoffbrand AV, Giles FJ, et al. Alpha interferon therapy for haematological malignancies: correlation between in vivo induction of the 2',5' oligoadenylate system and clinical response. *Br J Haematol* 1990;74:452–456.

321. Ostlund L, Einhorn S, Robert K-H. Induction of 2',5'-oligoadenylate synthetase and blast transformation in primary chronic lymphocytic leukemia cells following exposure to interferon in vitro. *Cancer Res* 1986;46:2160–2163.

322. Liu DK, Owens GF, Feil PD. 2',5'-oligoadenylate synthetase activity in human mammary tumors and its potential correlation with tumor growth or hormonal responsiveness. *Cancer Res* 1986;46:6207–6210.

323. Clauss IM, Vandenplas B, Wathelet MG, et al. Analysis of interferon-inducible genes in cells of chronic myeloid leukemia patients responsive or resistant to an interferon-alpha treatment. *Blood* 1990;76:2337–2342.

324. Talpaz M, Chernajovsky Y, Troutman-Worden K, et al. Interferon-stimulated genes in interferon-sensitive and -resistant chronic myelogenous leukemia patients. *Cancer Res* 1992;52:1087–1090.

325. Holtschke T, Lohler J, Kanno Y, et al. Immunodeficiency and chronic myelogenous leukemia-like syndrome in mice with a targeted mutation of the ICSBP gene. *Cell* 1996;87:307–317.

326. Schmidt M, Nagel S, Proba J, et al. Lack of interferon consensus sequence binding protein (ICSBP) transcripts in human myeloid leukemias. *Blood* 1998;91:22–29.

327. Weiss K. Safety profile of interferon-alpha therapy. *Semin Oncol* 1998;25:9–13.

328. Borden EC, Parkinson D. A perspective on the clinical effectiveness and tolerance of interferon-alpha. *Semin Oncol* 1998;25:3–8.

329. Nolten WE, Goldstein D, Lindstrom M, et al. Effects of cytokines on the pituitary-adrenal axis in cancer patients. *J Interferon Res* 1993;13:349–357.

330. Hawkins M, Horning S, Konrad M, et al. Phase I evaluation of a synthetic mutant of interferon β. *Cancer Res* 1985;45:5914–5920.

331. Licinio J, Kling MA, Hauser P. Cytokines and brain function: relevance to interferon-alpha-induced mood and cognitive changes. *Semin Oncol* 1998;25:30–38.

332. Plata-Salaman CR. Cytokines and anorexia: a brief overview. *Semin Oncol* 1998;25:64–72.

333. Quesada JR, Talpaz M, Rios A, et al. Clinical toxicity of interferons in cancer patients: a review. *J Clin Oncol* 1986;4:234–243.

334. Massaro ER, Borden EC, Hawkins MJ, et al. Effects of recombinant alpha-2 interferon treatment on lipid concentrations and lipoprotein composition. *J Interferon Res* 1986;6:655–662.

335. Rosenzweig IB, Wiebe DA, Borden EC, et al. Plasma lipoprotein changes in humans induced by beta interferon. *Atherosclerosis* 1987;67:261–267.

336. Averbuch SD, Austin HA III, Sherwin SA, et al. Acute interstitial nephritis with nephrotic syndrome following recombinant leukocyte A IFN therapy for mycosis fungoides. *N Engl J Med* 1984;310:32–35.

337. Selby P, Kohn J, Raymond J, et al. Nephrotic syndrome during treatment with IFN. *BMJ* 1985;290:1180.

338. Sumpio BE, Ernstoff MS, Kirkwood JM. Urinary excretion of IFN, albumin and beta2-microglobulin during IFN treatment. *Cancer Res* 1984;44:3599–3603.

339. Tokazewski-chen SA, Marafino J, Stebbing N. Effects of nephrectomy on the pharmacokinetics of various cloned human IFNs in the rat. *J Pharmaco Exper Therapeut* 1983;227:9–15.

340. Rostaing L, Chatelut E, Payen JL, et al. Pharmacokinetics of alpha IFN-2b in chronic hepatitis C virus patients undergoing chronic hemodialysis or with normal renal function: clinical implications. *J Am Soc Nephrol* 1998;9:2344–2348.

341. Burman P, TottermanTH, Oberg K, et al. Thyroid autoimmunity in patients on long-term therapy with leukocyte-derived interferon. *J Clin Endocrinol Metab* 1986;63:1086–1090.

342. Itri LM, Sherman MI, Palleroni AV, et al. Incidence and clinical significance of neutralizing antibodies in patients receiving recombinant IFN-alpha-2a. *J Interferon Res* 1989;9:S9–15.

343. Larocca AP, Leung S, Marcus SG, et al. Evaluation of neutralizing antibodies in patients treated with recombinant interferon-beta ser. *J Interferon Res* 1989;9:S51–S60.

344. von Wussow P, Jakschies D, Freund M, et al. Humoral response to recombinant interferon-alpha 2b in patients receiving recombinant interferon-alpha 2b therapy. *J Interferon Res* 1989;9:S25–S31.

345. Steis RG, Smith JW, Urba WJ, et al. Loss of interferon antibodies during prolonged continuous interferon-alpha 2a therapy in hairy cell leukemia. *Blood* 1991;77:792–798.

346. von Wussow P, Pralle H, Hochkeppel HK, et al. Effective natural interferon-alpha therapy in recombinant interferon-alpha-resistant patients with hairy cell leukemia. *Blood* 1991;78:38–43.

347. Wussow PV, Jakschies D, Freund M, et al. Treatment of anti-recombinant interferon-alpha 2 antibody positive CML patients with natural interferon-alpha. *Br J Haematol* 1991;78:210–216.

348. Abdul-Ahad AK, Galazka AR, Revel M, et al. Incidence of antibodies to interferon-beta in patients treated with recombinant human interferon-beta 1a from mammalian cells. *Cytokines Cell Mol Ther* 1997;3:27–32.

349. Kantarjian HM, Deisseroth A, Kurzrock R, et al. Chronic myelogenous leukemia: a concise update. *Blood* 1993;82:691–703.

350. The Italian Cooperative Study Group on chronic myeloid leukemia. Long-term follow-up of the Italian trial of interferon-alpha versus conventional chemotherapy in chronic myeloid leukemia. *Blood* 1998;92:1541–1548.

351. Anonymous. A prospective comparative study of α-interferon and conventional chemotherapy in chronic myeloid leukemia. *Haematologica* 1992;77:204–214.

352. Guilhot F, Chastang C, Michallet M, et al. Interferon alpha-2b combined with cytarabine versus interferon alone in chronic myelogenous leukemia. *New Engl J Med* 1997;337:223–229.

353. Kantarjian HM, O'Brien S, Smith TL, et al. Treatment of Philadelphia chromosome-positive early chronic phase chronic myelogenous leukemia with daily doses of interferon alpha and low-dose cytarabine. *J Clin Oncol* 1999;17:284–292.

354. Smalley RV, Andersen JW, Hawkins MJ, et al. Interferon alfa combined with cytotoxic chemotherapy for patients with non-Hodgkin's lymphoma. *N Engl J Med* 1992;327:1336–1341.

355. Solal-Celigny P, Lepage E, Brousse N, et al. Recombinant interferon alpha-2b combined with a regimen containing doxorubicin in patients with advanced follicular lymphoma. Groupe d'Etude des Lymphomes de l'Adulte. *N Engl J Med* 1993;329:1608–1614.

356. Smalley RV, Weller E, Hawkins MJ, et al. Final analysis of the ECOG1-COPA trial (E6484) in patients with non-Hodgkin's lymphoma treated with IFN-α (IFN-α2a) plus an anthracycline-based induction regimen. *Leukemia* 2001:*in press*.

357. Mandelli F, Avvisati G, Amadori S, et al. Maintenance treatment with recombinant interferon alpha-2b in patients with multiple myeloma responding to conventional induction chemotherapy. *N Engl J Med* 1990;322:1430–1434.

358. Osterborg A, Bjorkholm M, Bjoreman M, et al. Natural interferon-alpha in combination with melphalan/prednisone (MP/IFN) versus melphalan/prednisone (MP) in the treatment of multiple myeloma stages II and III. A randomized study from the Myeloma Group of Central Sweden (MGCS). *Blood* 1993;81:1428–1434.

359. Oken MM. Multiple myeloma: prognosis and standard treatment. *Cancer Invest* 1997;15:57–64.

360. Kirkwood J, Ibrahim JG, Sosman JA, et al. High-dose interferon alfa-2b significantly prolongs relapse-free and overall survival compared with the gm2-klh/qs-21 vaccine in patients with resected stage iib-iii melanoma: results of intergroup trial e1694/s9512/c509801. *J Clin Oncol* 2001;19:2370–2380.

361. Pehamberger H, Soyer HP, Steiner A, et al. Adjuvant interferon alpha-2a treatment in resected primary stage II cutaneous melanoma. *J Clin Oncol* 1998;16:1425–1429.

362. Grob JJ, Dreno B, de la Salmoniere P, et al. Randomised trial of interferon alpha-2a as adjuvant therapy in resected primary melanoma thicker than 1.5 mm without clinically detectable node metastases. *Lancet* 1998;351:1905–1910.

363. Medical Research Renal Cancer Collaborators. Interferon-alpha and survival in metastatic renal carcinoma: early results of a randomised controlled trial. *Lancet* 1999;353:14–17.

364. McDonald S, Chang AY, Rubin P, et al. Combined betaseron R (recombinant human interferon beta) and radiation for inoperable non-small cell lung cancer. *Int J Radiat Oncol Biol Phys* 1993;27:613–619.

365. Byhardt R, Vaickus L, Witt P, et al. Recombinant human interferon-beta (r-HuIFN-beta) and radiation therapy for inoperable non-small cell lung cancer. *J Interferon Cytokine Res* 1996;16:891–902.

366. Figlin RA, Belldegrun A, Moldawer N, et al. Concomitant administration of recombinant human interleukin-2 and recombinant interferon alfa-2A: an active outpatient regimen in metastatic renal cell carcinoma. *J Clin Oncol* 1992;10:414–421.

367. Sparano JA, Fisher RI, Sunderland M, et al. Randomized phase III trial of treatment with high-dose interleukin-2 either alone or in combination with interferon alfa-2a in patients with advanced melanoma. *J Clin Oncol* 1993;11:1969–1977.

368. Lippman SM, Kavanagh JJ, Paredes-Espinoza M, et al. 13-cis-retinoic acid plus interferon alpha-2a: highly active systemic therapy for squamous cell carcinoma of the cervix. *J Natl Cancer Inst* 1992;84:241–245.

369. Lippman SM, Parkinson DR, Itri LM, et al. 13-cis-retinoic acid and interferon alpha-2a: effective combination therapy for advanced squamous cell carcinoma of the skin. *J Natl Cancer Inst* 1992;84:235–241.

370. Hong K. Inhibition of development of new squamous carcinomas by a combination of interferons and retinoids. *N Engl J Med* 1999;in press.

371. Lindner DJ, Borden EC, Kalvakolanu DV. Synergistic antitumor effects of a combination of interferons and retinoic acid on human tumor cells *in vitro* and *in vivo*. *Clin Cancer Res* 1997;3:931–937.

372. Kolla V, Lindner DJ, Xiao W, et al. Modulation of interferon (IFN)-inducible gene expression by retinoic acid. Upregulation of STAT1 protein in IFN-unresponsive cells. *J Biol Chem* 1996;271:10508–10514.

27

CLINICAL PHARMACOKINETICS OF INTERLEUKIN 1, INTERLEUKIN 2, INTERLEUKIN 4, TUMOR NECROSIS FACTOR, INTERLEUKIN 12, AND MACROPHAGE COLONY-STIMULATING FACTOR

RONALD M. BUKOWSKI
CHARLES S. TANNENBAUM
JAMES H. FINKE

The discovery and study of cytokines have evolved from the description of protein factors mediating particular cellular functions to studies at the molecular level using recombinant proteins that allow definitive identification of their structures and functions. The biologic activities of these molecules are complex, with pleiotropic and redundant actions common. The fact that cytokines are often part of a cascade that can then lead to synthesis and production of other mediators and result in either positive or negative regulatory effects is also clear. The antitumor activities of various cytokines have led to their use in patients with malignancy, and a large body of data now exists on their clinical effects and pharmacokinetic behavior. This chapter discusses six different factors, all of which have been used clinically and demonstrate the difficulties encountered in evaluating biologic agents with complex functions *in vivo*.

INTERLEUKIN 1

The interleukin 1 (IL-1) family consists of three related polypeptides, all of which are expressed during infections and inflammatory reactions[1] and bind to the same receptors. Interleukin 1α (IL-1α) and interleukin 1β (IL-1β) are both functional cytokines that induce a broad spectrum of immunologic,[2] hematopoietic,[3] proinflammatory,[4] cardiovascular,[5] and endocrinologic[6] effects. The third member of this family is the IL-1 receptor antagonist (IL-1ra), which acts as a competitive inhibitor of the active forms.[7] IL-1ra binds to IL-1 receptors with an affinity equal to that of IL-1α and IL-1β,[1] but the inability of IL-1ra to transduce a signal after receptor ligation renders it an important regula-

tor of IL-1 activity.[8] Physiologically, it may act to provide some protection against the effects of IL-1. Plasma concentrations of IL-1α and IL-1β are usually undetectable in normal subjects.[9,10] Polymerase chain reaction studies indicate that freshly isolated mononuclear cells from normal individuals do not synthesize IL-1 messenger RNA (mRNA).[1] Although some reports suggest that IL-1 does not play a role in normal homeostasis,[4] more recent findings indicate that keratinocytes of the skin, granulosa cells of the ovary, and hypothalamic cells in the brain contain IL-1 mRNA even in the absence of disease.[1] An association is found, however, between elevated IL-1 levels and the severity of some diseases, including sepsis,[11] inflammatory bowel disease,[12] atherosclerosis,[13] and insulin-dependent diabetes.[14] The fact that neutralizing antibodies to IL-1ra exacerbate several clinical conditions suggest that endogenous IL-1ra may play a role in modulating some of the deleterious inflammatory effects attributable to IL-1α and IL-1β.[15,16] Notwithstanding abundant data supporting the role of IL-1 in promoting tumor growth and metastatic activity, administration of IL-1 to cancer patients has also been found to reduce tumor growth via an adjuvant effect.[17] This latter observation provides the basis for using IL-1 therapeutically as an antitumor agent.

Structure and Mechanisms of Action

A significant amount of information has been published regarding the structure and function of IL-1.[1,8,17–20] The IL-1 family consists of several different polypeptides that are products of distinct genes.[21] IL-1α and IL-1β share most biologic activities but have only 27% structural homology.[1,4,17,20] The IL-1α and IL-1β gene products are first synthesized as 31-kd precursors that lack the hydrophobic leader sequence common to secreted proteins.[20,22] Pro-IL-1α has activity in this precursor form and can be cleaved to its 17-kd mature form and released from the cell by the action of membrane-associated cysteine proteases called calpains.[17] Unlike IL-1α, pro-IL-1β has little or no functional activity and is released from the cell as a mature, active molecule only after cleavage by an IL-1β convertase enzyme (ICE) between the aspartic acid–alanine amino acids at position 116–117 of the molecule.[1] Because IL-1β secretion is highly dependent on catalysis by ICE, stimuli that modulate ICE activity may account for apparent alterations in IL-1β activity.[22,23]

The expression of IL-1 is complicated due to its regulation at the transcriptional, posttranscriptional, translational, and posttranslational levels.[1,23,24] Monocytes begin to accumulate additional mRNA transcripts encoding IL-1α and IL-β within 15 minutes of lipopolysaccharide (LPS) stimulation,[1] although IL-1β mRNA levels begin to decrease after 4 hours due to an altered half-life and an induced transcriptional repressor.[23] Cells stimulated with IL-1 itself can express elevated IL-1β mRNA for longer than 24 hours,[25,26] which suggests that different stimuli differentially modulate IL-1β mRNA expression. Interestingly, a significant dissociation can be seen between mRNA expression and functional activity, as numerous stimuli that induce elevated IL-1β mRNA levels do not stimulate translation of the protein.[27] Although IL-1 or LPS can remove the translational block, in the absence of those agents the IL-1 mRNA can be rapidly degraded without appreciable protein synthesis.[1] The ability of LPS to induce both transcription and translation of IL-1 explains why endotoxin is such a potent stimulus for augmenting IL-1 activity.[1]

Two different functional forms of the IL-1 receptor (IL-1R) exist, which are transcribed from distinct, homologous genes.[17] These molecules are classified as members of the immunoglobulin superfamily, as their extracellular regions are each composed of three immunoglobulin G–like domains.[1,17,28] The type I IL-1R (IL-1RI) (80 kd) is present in low numbers, often less than 200 receptors per cell, on a variety of cell types, including keratinocytes, fibroblasts, hepatocytes, endothelial cells, and T cells.[8] The type II receptor (IL-1RII) (65 kd) is also expressed on many cell types, but mostly monocytes, neutrophils, and B cells.[1,17,28] The protein encoded by the human IL-1RI gene is predicted to have a 29% homology with IL-1RII.[1] One study demonstrated that murine helper T subset 2 lymphocytes express both type I and type II IL-1R, but only IL-1RI binding augments proliferation induced by T-cell receptor stimulation.[29] High-affinity binding to IL-1RI is now known to require the interaction of an additional receptor-like protein related to IL-1R called the IL-1 receptor accessory protein (IL-RAcP).[30] The belief is that IL-1 first binds with low affinity to IL-1RI, which then provides a docking location for the attachment of IL-1RAcP and the development of the high-affinity association.[17] Interestingly, although IL-1ra can bind IL-1RI with high affinity, it cannot complex with IL-RI/IL-1RAcP, which thus explains its inability to act as an agonist.[17] Although the IL-1RI complex transduces a signal after IL-1 binding, IL-1RII appears to be a decoy molecule, as it binds IL-1 with high affinity but has no capacity for signal transduction due to its truncated cytoplasmic region.[1,8,28,30] Indeed, up-regulation of IL-1RII reduces the activity of IL-1, and antibodies to IL-1RI but not to IL-1RII inhibit IL-1 function.[17]

The signal transduction pathways activated by the IL-1R have been elucidated. For a long time, this had been a controversial area, as several second messengers and various protein kinases had been implicated in the cascade of events.[30] IL-1 is known to mediate its effects via its ability to modulate over 90 different genes, many of which encode molecules with proinflammatory and immunologic function.[31] The induction of many of these IL-1–stimulated gene products involves nuclear factor κB (NF-κB), and at least one arm of the IL-1 signal transduction pathway leads to the generation of this factor.[30] After IL-1 binds to the IL-1RI/IL-1RAcP, the protein kinase IL-1R–associated kinase (IRAK) is now believed to join the IL-1/IL-1RI/IL-RAcP complex.[32] Tumor necrosis–associated factor 6 is now recruited to IRAK,[30] which in turn recruits and interacts with NF-κB–inducing kinase (NIK).[30] NIK is the upstream regulator of protein kinase IκB1 and IκB2,[33] which phosphorylate IκB and release active NF-κB.[34]

In addition to activating NF-κB, IL-1 signaling probably involves additional pathways. Cells transfected with IRAK induce a prolonged activation of Jun amino-terminal kinase (JNK) after IL-1 stimulation,[30] and IRAK has also been found to be involved in interleukin 2 (IL-2) production.[30] IL-1 has also been shown to activate three major mitogen-activated protein kinase (MAPK) cascades, those initiated with MAP kinase kinase 7 (MKK7), MKK3/6, and MAP/extracellular signal–related kinase (MEK).[30] These pathways are known to be variously involved in the IL-1–mediated induction of IL-2, interleukin 8 (IL-8), and prostaglandins, as well as in the expression of proteases and the glucose transporter.[30,35,36] IL-1 is also known to activate the tumor necrosis factor (TNF)/IL-1–induced protein kinase (TIP kinase), which is the only kinase known to be specifically activated by IL-1 and TNF alone.[37]

Cellular Pharmacology

Although monocytes and macrophages are the major source of IL-1α and IL-1β, a wide variety of cells are known to secrete IL-1 under the appropriate conditions.[8,20] These include endothelial cells, smooth muscle cells, and fibroblasts. IL-1 mRNA is not constitutively expressed, but is inducible in these cells.[8,20] Constitutive expression of IL-1 mRNA is, however, observed in epithelial cells, keratinocytes and Kupffer cells; IL-1 is not secreted unless these cells are stimulated, however.[8] The list of agents capable of stimulating IL-1 secretion is extensive.[8,20] Circulating levels of IL-1 can be induced by various infectious agents, traumatic injury, radiation, and stress. Cytokines such as TNF-α, granulocyte-macrophage colony-stimulating factor (GM-CSF), interferon-γ (IFN-γ), and IL-2 can also induce IL-1 production.[8,20,38] IL-1 expression can be negatively regulated by cytokines such as interleukin 10 (IL-10), transforming growth factor β (TGF-β), interleukin 4 (IL-4), and interleukin 6 (IL-6).[38] Prostaglandin E$_2$ (PGE$_2$) and glucocorticoids can also inhibit IL-1 secretion.[38]

In addition to regulators of IL-1 expression and secretion, antagonists to IL-1R binding are found.[2] Of particular importance is IL-1ra, which is a member of the IL-1 family and binds to both receptors with the same affinity as IL-1α and IL-1β.[8,39,40] The 152–amino acid protein IL-1ra has a 25–amino acid leader sequence that allows it to be secreted.[39,40] In contrast to IL-1α and IL-1β, which bind to IL-1R and transduce signals, IL-1ra does not signal cells and is not internalized.[7,40] Multiple cellular sources of IL-1ra exist, including macrophages and keratinocytes.[7,20] The complementary DNA (cDNA) for IL-1ra has been expressed in *Escherichia coli* and is an active competitor of IL-1 binding to IL-1RI. This recombinant product can inhibit IL-1 bioactivity *in vitro* and is a potent inhibitor of IL-1–induced glucocorticoid production *in vivo*.[7]

IL-1 has a wide range of biologic activities that affect a variety of different systems. It is a potent inducer of acute-phase proteins that include serum amyloid A, fibrinogen, ceruloplasmin, and metallothionein.[20,40,41] Stimulation of acute-phase protein production by IL-1 may involve the action of other cytokines, such as IL-6, that are induced by IL-1.[20,40,41] Changes in neuroendocrine function have also been documented after IL-1 administration and include fever and stimulation of the hypothalamic-pituitary-adrenal axis[19,20,42] with increases in levels of glucocorticoids, adrenocorticotropic hormone (ACTH), vasopressin, and somatostatin.[20,43]

The ability of IL-1 to potentiate the inflammatory response is well known. Systemic administration of this cytokine to animals results in inflammatory reactions that include fever, neutrophilia, and elevation of acute-phase proteins. Erythema and inflammatory cell infiltration develop when IL-1 is administered locally.[20] This inflammatory activity is in part mediated by induction and release of other cytokines such as TNF-α and IL-6, which then enhance acute-phase responses and necrosis.[20,40] IL-1 also facilitates the accumulation of macrophages, neutrophils, and lymphocytes at the site of inflammation by inducing local expression of chemoattractants, including monocyte chemotactic protein 1 (MCP-1) and IL-8.

The administration of IL-1 has significant effects on the hematopoietic system, such as the induction of neutrophilia and expansion of myeloid progenitor cells in the bone marrow.[20] It appears to function in this capacity by stimulating the production of hematopoietic growth factors from a variety of cell types.[20] In addition, IL-1 also protects against bone marrow suppression after irradiation.[2,3,44] IL-1 has also been shown to augment T- and B-cell responses.[20] IL-1 secreted by thymic epithelium appears to function to support the growth of immature thymocytes by inducing IL-2 and IL-2 receptor (IL-2R) expression.[2] The effect of IL-1 on mature T cells is unclear. Although some studies[45] suggest that IL-1 is not necessary for their activation, others[29] provide evidence that IL-1α can stimulate a signal via IL-1RI that potentiates the proliferation of helper T clones. Additional studies are needed to clarify the role of IL-1 in T-cell activation.

The proinflammatory and immunopotentiating activities of IL-1 are thought to account for many of its reported antitumor effects. Research has clearly demonstrated in murine models that systemic injection of IL-1 can promote tumor rejection and response, which can then be transferred adoptively to syngeneic animals by administration of lymphocytes from IL-1–treated donors.[46] In addition, IL-1–transfected tumors are rejected, and the animals then develop immunity to tumor rechallenge.[47] Transfection of non–IL-1–producing fibrosarcomas with an IL-1α gene converted the progressive tumor to a regressive phenotype. Therefore, IL-1 secretion appears to be able to initiate events that lead to potentiation of host antitumor immunity.

Clinical Pharmacokinetics

The various recombinant IL-1 preparations available for clinical trials are outlined in Table 27-1. The preparation rhuIL-1α (Immunex) is produced in *E. coli* by a plasmid that expresses amino acids 113–271 of natural human IL-1α.[48] The nucleotide sequences of rhuIL-1α and natural IL-1α are identical, and the molecular weight of rhuIL-1α is 18.2 + 0.75 kd. Recombinant IL-1α (rIL-1α; Immunex/Syntex) is also produced in *E. coli* and has a molecular weight of 17.5 kd.[49] An rIL-1α analog has also been produced (Otsuka Pharmaceutical Co.) in *E. coli* in an attempt to improve IL-1α stability by replacing cysteine residues.[49] Studies comparing the activities of these preparations have not been published, and their specific *in vitro* activities are variable.

Assays for serum levels of IL-1 are available and are either bioassays or enzyme-linked immunoabsorbent assays (ELISAs). Several bioassays have been described including a mouse thymocyte proliferation assay[50] and melanoma cell line inhibition assay.[55] This latter procedure may discriminate IL-1β from IL-1α and is not affected by IL-2 or PGE$_2$.

Table 27-2 summarizes some of the clinical trials with the various recombinant IL-1 preparations. Information on the pharmacokinetic behavior of this cytokine in patients is limited. In a single trial,[52] multiple serum samples were

TABLE 27-1. RECOMBINANT INTERLEUKIN 1 PREPARATIONS

Source	Type	Maximum Tolerated Dose	Specific Activity	Vector System
Syntex/Immunex[49]	rIL-1β	0.068 µg/kg/d (30-min i.v. infusion)	1×10^7 U/mg	*Escherichia coli*
Otsuka Pharmaceutical [51]	rIL-1β (OCT-43)	NS	5×10^7 U/mg	*E. coli*
Dainippon Pharmaceutical [52]	rIL-1α	0.3 µg/kg/d (15-min i.v. infusion d 1–7)	2×10^7 U/mg	*E. coli*
Hoffmann-La Roche[53]	rIL-1α	NA	2.5×10^9 U/mg	*E. coli*
Immunex[48,54]	rhuIL-1α	NA	5×10^9 U/mg	*E. coli*

NA, not available; NS, not stated; rIL-1α, recombinant interleukin 1α; rIL-1β, recombinant interleukin 1β.

obtained, and detectable IL-1α was found only at the highest dosage level of 1.0 µg per kg per day. Insufficient data were available to calculate a serum half-life. The pharmacokinetics of rhuIL-1α (Immunex) has been defined in various animal species, however.[48] In BALB/C mice, intravenous administration of iodine 125 (^{125}I)–labeled rhuIL-1α was used, and the distribution half-life was 1.3 + 0.3 minutes. The primary route of elimination was the kidneys, with the liver being a secondary route. The pharmacokinetics of rhuIL-1α was also investigated in cynomolgus monkeys, with serum levels determined using an ELISA. Intravenous and subcutaneous administration was used at a dosage of 5.0 µg per kg. For the intravenous route, the α half-life ($t_{1/2\alpha}$) ranged from 52.5 to 57.3 minutes on day 1. When the subcutaneous route was used, the $t_{1/2\alpha}$ ranged from 86.1 to 130 minutes and the β half-life ($t_{1/2\beta}$) from 134 to 203 minutes.

A recombinant form of IL-1R (rhuIL-1R) is also in clinical trials. It is a soluble truncated form of the type I full-length membrane receptor, with identical affinity for IL-1.[56] The half-life of rhIL-1R is 24 to 30 hours. Dose levels from 1.0 to 55 mg per m² have been used, and no toxicity attributed to this preparation was reported.[56] McDermott et al.[56] used rhuIL-1R before administration of high-dose recombinant IL-2 (rIL-2). No effects on recombinant IL-2–induced toxicity were noted. Bernstein et al.[57] used rhuIL-1R in patients with refractory or relapsed acute myeloid leukemia. The rhuIL-1R was administered on day 1 as an intravenous bolus (500 to 2,000 µg per m²) and then for 13 days subcutaneously (250 to 1,000 µg per m² per day). The

half-life was reported as 48 to 96 hours after subcutaneous administration.

Clinical Effects and Toxicity

The pleiotropic effects of IL-1 in preclinical studies and the expression of IL-1Rs by a wide range of cells in the body[40] predict that administration of IL-1 to patients would affect multiple organ systems. Tables 27-2 and 27-3 summarize clinical trials using IL-1α or IL-1β. The majority are phase I studies investigating the toxicity and maximum tolerated dose (MTD) of these preparations.

A phase I trial of intravenous rIL-1α (Dainippon Pharmaceutical Co.) identified fever, chills, nausea, headaches, and myalgia in most patients, with no significant differences among patients receiving various dose levels.[52] Dose-limiting toxicities included hypotension, which developed 1 to 3 hours after rIL-1α therapy and lasted up to 50 hours. Dosages of 0.3 to 1.0 µg per kg per day produced hypotension requiring fluid support and vasopressor therapy. This hypotension was associated with decreased systemic vascular resistance and compensatory increases in heart rate and cardiac output.

Worth et al.[63] conducted a phase II trial using rhuIL-1α in combination with chemotherapy. Patients with relapsed osteosarcoma were treated with rhuIL-1α immediately followed by etoposide daily for 5 days. Toxicities included myelosuppression, hypotension, edema, and weight gain. Three of nine patients had partial responses. The trial was terminated early when production of the cytokine was discontinued.

TABLE 27-2. CLINICAL TRIALS WITH RECOMBINANT INTERLEUKIN 1β (rIL-1β)

Study	Type of Trial	IL-1 Preparation	Dose Levels of rIL-1	Schedule	Maximum Tolerated Dose
Crown et al.[49]	Phase I	rhIL-1β (Immunex/Syntex)	0.002, 0.027, 0.068, 0.1 µg/kg	30 min i.v.b. d 1 & 2	0.068 µg/kg
Marumo et al.[51]	Phase I	rIL-1β (Otsuka Pharmaceutical)	1 to 4×10^4 U	s.c. d 1 × 4 wk	ND
Starnes et al.[58]	Phase I	rhIL-1β (Syntex)	0.001–0.1 µg/kg	i.v. d 1–5	NS
Iizumi et al.[59]	Phase II	rIL-1β (Otsuka Pharmaceutical)	5×10^4 U (1.1 µg)	s.c. d 1 & 2	NA
Nemunaitis et al.[60]	Phase I	rhIL-1β (Syntex)	0.01–0.02 µg/kg	30 min i.v. d 1–4	NS

i.v.b., intravenous bolus; NA, not applicable; ND, not determined; NS, not stated; rhIL-1β, recombinant human IL-1β.

TABLE 27-3. CLINICAL TRIALS WITH RECOMBINANT INTERLEUKIN 1α (rIL-1α)

Study	Type of Trial	IL-1 Preparation	Dose Levels of rIL-1α	Schedule	Maximum Tolerated Dose
Smith et al.[52]	Phase I	rIL-1α (Dainippon Pharmaceutical)	0.01, 0.03, 0.1, 0.3, 1.0 µg/kg	15 min i.v.b. d 1–7	0.3 µg/kg
Dennis et al.[54]	Phase I	rhuIL-1α (Immunex)	0.08–5.0 µg/m²	2-h i.v. infusion d 1–5	NS
Verschraegen et al.[61]	Phase I	rhuIL-1α (NS)	0.1–10 µg/m²	c.i.v. d 1–4	3.0 µg/m²/d
Rosenthal et al.[62]	Phase I	rhuIL-1α (NS)	0.08, 0.2, 0.8, 2.0, 5.0 µg/m²	2-h i.v. infusion d 1–5	2.0 µg/m²/d
Worth et al.[63]	Phase II	rhuIL-1α (NS)	—	i.v. infusion followed by VP-16 d 1–5	NA

c.i.v., continuous intravenous infusion; i.v.b., intravenous bolus; NA, not applicable; NS, not dated; rhIL-1α, recombinant human IL-1α; VP-16, etoposide.

The hematologic effects of rIL-1α therapy[52] are significant and include increases in total white blood cells, consisting predominantly of neutrophils. Platelet counts decreased at rIL-1α doses of more than 0.1 µg per kg, and bone marrow cellularity increased. Bone marrow cell colony formation in soft agar decreased in most patients. Finally, elevated levels of serum cortisol, ACTH, C-reactive protein, and thyroid stimulating hormone and decreases in serum cholesterol, triglycerides, and testosterone were reported.

Crown et al.[49] performed a slightly different phase I trial administering rIL-1α (Immunex/Syntex) to patients receiving intravenous 5-fluorouracil (5-FU) chemotherapy. The MTD of rIL-1α in this study was 0.068 µg per kg per day, and the dose-limiting toxicity was hypotension. Neutropenia and leukopenia developed transiently after intravenous injection, with subsequent neutrophilia and platelet increases. When administered after 5-FU, recombinant IL-1β (rIL-1β) appeared to decrease the days of neutropenia, but the differences were not significant. No changes in the incidence or severity of mucositis after 5-FU chemotherapy were seen when rIL-1β was administered.

Subcutaneous administration of rIL-1β (Otsuka Pharmaceutical Co.) had a similar side effect profile, including chills, fever, and fatigue. Doses were not escalated to toxicity, however, and hypotension was not reported.[51,59] Thus, the toxicity of the various IL-1 preparations appears similar, and in most reports includes dose-limiting hypotension at relatively low doses of the cytokine.

The immunologic effects of IL-1 administration have also been characterized.[49,52,64] Peripheral blood mononuclear cytolytic activities, including the activity of lymphokine-activated killer (LAK) cells and *in vitro* proliferative response to rIL-2, show an increase,[49] accompanied by significant increases in soluble IL-2R levels.[64] These data are consistent with T-cell activation, as suggested by the preclinical information. Serum cytokine levels, including levels of GM-CSF and IL-6, have also been investigated[52]; increases are seen in the latter at rIL-1α doses above 0.03 µg per kg.

Antitumor effects of IL-1 were also suggested by various preclinical studies.[46,47] During the phase I and II clinical trials, little evidence for such activity was seen, with one report

noting partial tumor regression in two of nine patients with melanoma.[58] Of more interest have been studies suggesting increases in platelet counts after rIL-1 administration[65] and amelioration of the thrombocytopenic effects of various chemotherapeutic agents such as 5-FU,[49] carboplatin[66] and of various combination regimens such as ifosfamide, carboplatin, and etoposide.[67] The secondary induction of cytokines such as GM-CSF, granulocyte colony-stimulating factor (G-CSF), and IL-6 may be responsible for some of the hematopoietic findings. Randomized trials confirming these effects have not been published.

Drug Interactions

Because IL-1 has multiple effects when administered to humans and has substantial toxicity even at low doses, information is needed on potential interactions and methods of diminishing its side effects. Use in combination with other cytokines such as GM-CSF or G-CSF should be explored, and the suggestion in preclinical models that IL-1α decreases IL-2 toxicity[53] is also being explored clinically.

IL-1ra may form a natural feedback loop that can downregulate IL-1 production or activity. The cDNA for IL-1ra was cloned and sequenced, and expressed in *E. coli*.[7] Sufficient quantities of the recombinant protein are now available, and clinical trials have been completed in normal volunteers.

In preclinical studies, IL-1ra blocks the binding of IL-1 to IL-1RI or IL-1RII and the accompanying secondary cytokine synthesis.[68] In animal models, IL-1ra prevented IL-1–induced fever and *E. coli*–induced shock in rabbits.[69] In patients with sepsis, significant elevations of IL-1ra are seen.[70] IL-1ra was administered to normal volunteers in a phase I clinical trial as a continuous 3-hour intravenous infusion at doses of 1.0 to 10.0 µg per kg.[71] Plasma IL-1ra levels produced were 3.1 µg per mL at 1.0 µg per kg and 29 µg per mL at 10.0 µg per kg. After completion of the IL-1ra infusions, a $t_{1/2\alpha}$ of 21 minutes and $t_{1/2\beta}$ of 108 minutes were found. Less than 3.2% of administered IL-1ra was found in the urine. Interestingly, no significant clinical or biochemical toxicity was seen, and immunologically only a decrease of LPS-stimulated IL-6 secretion *in vitro* by mononuclear cells from treated subjects was noted. Thus, IL-1ra appears to have minimal toxicity associated with its administration.

Interleukin 2

The recognition in 1965 that soluble mitogenic factors were present in conditioned supernatants from mixed lympho-cyte cultures[72] provided the initial observation indicating the existence of lymphokines that could stimulate cell division. In 1976, Morgan et al.[73] demonstrated that normal human T lymphocytes obtained from bone marrow could be maintained in culture for periods of up to 1 year by using media from phytohemagglutinin (PHA)–stimulated mono-nuclear cells. Shortly thereafter, this media was also found to sustain the proliferation of antigen-specific cytolytic T cells.[74] This cytokine was ultimately designated as IL-2 (Second Annual Lymphokine Workshop, 1979), and the cDNA encoding human IL-2 was isolated.[75] During the next 10 years, the molecular characteristics, biologic functions, and clinical uses of IL-2 were explored.

Structure and Mechanisms of Action

IL-2 is a 15-kd glycoprotein that varies in degree of glycosy-lation and sialylation.[76,77] It contains a carbohydrate-binding domain that is thought to be involved in the clearance and intracellular distribution of this protein.[78] The structure of the IL-2 molecule has been investigated and appears to be similar to that of GM-CSF and IL-4.[76,77] IL-2 has four major amphipathic α helices that are arranged in an anti-parallel manner[76,77] (Fig. 27-1). One disulfide bridge exists in the IL-2 protein; it provides stability of the tertiary struc-ture and is necessary for biologic activity, which is elimi-nated when this bond is disrupted.[79]

T cells are the primary source of IL-2, and among mature T cells most of the IL-2 is produced by the CD4+ subset. In murine systems, IL-2 is produced by unprimed CD4+ cells (T_H0) and by the T_H1 subset of helper cells that is involved in delayed-type hypersensitivity responses.[80]

IL-2 is not constitutively produced but is induced on T-cell activation.[81] Two signals are required for IL-2 gene expression. One is provided by stimulation through the T-cell receptor (TCR)/CD3 complex. The second signal appears to be provided by accessory cells that express the cell surface molecule B7, which is the ligand for CD28 or CTLA-4 molecules that are present on T cells.[82] The stimu-lation of T cells via the TCR in the absence of costimula-tion (B7/CD28) can induce T-cell anergy, a state of T-cell unresponsiveness, and involves a block in IL-2 gene tran-scription.[83] When both signals are provided, IL-2 gene expression develops, with peak levels of IL-2 mRNA accu-mulation within 6 hours of stimulation.[84] The induction of IL-2 gene expression is under the control of a transcrip-tional enhancer located approximately 300 base pairs upstream of the transcription site.[85] This region contains binding sites for several DNA-binding proteins that are required for the transcription of the IL-2 gene, including nuclear factor AT, activating protein 1 (AP-1), NF-κB, AP-3, and Oct.[84]

IL-2 mediates its biologic effects by binding to the IL-2 receptor (IL-2R), which is composed of three distinct chains, α (55 kd), β (75 kd), and γ (64 kd).[76,86] All three chains have external domains of similar length, whereas the cytoplasmic domains vary. The β subunit (286 residues) has the largest internal domain, and the α chain has the smallest (13 residues).[86–89] The IL-2R that binds IL-2 with high affinity [K_d (dissociation constant) = 10 pmol per L] requires the presence of all three chains.[76] Cells that express both the β and γ chains but are missing the α chain have an intermediate-affinity receptor (approximately 100-fold less than the high-affinity) that is capable of signal transduc-tion. The expression of only the α chain results in cells with a low IL-2 binding affinity and no intracellular signaling.[86]

Signaling via the IL-2R requires oligomerization of the β and γ chains.[90–92] Neither of these chains has sequences consistent with kinases; however, they appear to be sub-strates for protein tyrosine kinases (PTKs), which associate with the IL-2R after IL-2 binding (Fig. 27-2). Multiple PTKs are involved, each associated with a specific region of the intracytoplasmic tails of the γ and β chains.[92,93] This interaction results in the activation of PTKs and the phos-phorylation of multiple substrates that include the γ and β chains themselves.[93] The binding of Janus kinase 3 (Jak3) to the γ chain is critical to transducing the proliferative sig-nal via the IL-2R.[94–96] The importance of Jak3 and γ chain function is illustrated by the fact that loss of either Jak3 or

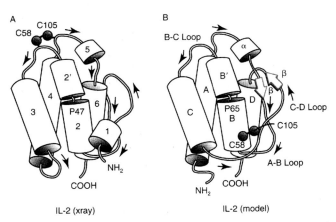

FIGURE 27-1. Comparison of x-ray–derived and model folds of interleukin 2 (IL-2). **A:** Schematic drawing of the IL-2 x-ray helix bundle (3). Cylindrical helices are marked 1 to 6. Loops are drawn as loose ribbons; Pro⁴⁷ (P47) is marked. The disulfide bond is noted by linked spheres. **B:** In the granulocyte-macrophage col-ony-stimulating factor–IL-4–like IL-2 model, the chain through the core helices is retraced and reconnected, the disulfide bridge is relocated, and the existence of a small β sheet is proposed; Pro⁶⁵ (P65) is marked. Only helix D remains fully equivalent in sequence to x-ray helix 6. (From Bazan JF. Unraveling the struc-ture of IL-2. *Science* 1992;257:410–413, with permission.)

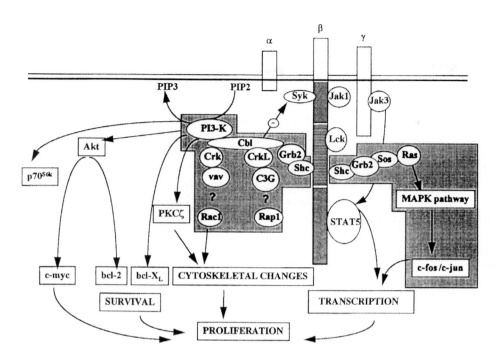

FIGURE 27-2. Schematic diagram of the interleukin 2 signal transduction cascade. (MAPK, mitogen-activated protein kinase; PI3K, phosphatidylinositol 3 kinase; PKC, protein kinase C; STAT, signal transduction and transcription-activating factor.) (From Gesbert F, Delespine-Carmagnat M, Bertoglio J. Recent advances in the understanding of interleukin-2 signal transduction. *J Clin Immunol* 1998;18:307–320, with permission.)

the γ chain results in severe combined immunodeficiency syndrome in humans.[97] The proximal region of the IL-2Rβ chain, which is rich in serine residues, is also important for proliferation and cell survival through the induction of c-myc and Bcl-2/Bcl-XL, respectively.[93] This region is required for activation of phosphatidylinositol 3 kinase (PI3K) and the downstream kinase Akt, which are likely involved in the expression of c-myc and Bcl-2.[98,99] Both the Zap-70 kinase, Syk, and Janus kinase 1 (Jak1), bind to the serine-rich region, and although Syk appears to be involved in c-myc induction, the role of Jak1 is not defined.[100,101] The acidic region of the IL-2Rβ chain appears to be responsible for the signaling pathway leading to c-fos and c-jun induction.[102,103] The src kinase p56lck constitutively associates with this region and is activated by IL-2 binding.[102,103] Evidence is growing of a linkage between p56lck and the Ras pathway, which is involved in the IL-2–dependent activation of c-fos and c-jun and T-cell proliferation.[92,104–106] The carboxy-terminal domain of the IL-2Rβ chain appears to be involved in signal transduction and transcription-activating factor 5 (STAT5) activation through a poorly defined process.[107,108] STAT5 may regulate T-cell proliferation partly through the induction of the high-affinity IL-2Rα chain.[109] Thus, the binding of IL-2 to its receptors triggers several different signal transduction pathways that lead to the induction of c-myc, Bcl-2, and c-fos/c-jun.[92,93] These and other events ultimately result in the IL-2–dependent progression from the G_1 phase of the cell cycle to the S phase, which is an important event in cellular proliferation. IL-2 signaling can also promote survival through the expression of Bcl-2 and Bcl-XL.[92,93]

Several cell types involved in inflammation and immunity express IL-2R.[76,110–112] The IL-2Rβ chain is constitutively expressed on monocytes/macrophages and certain lymphoid cells such as natural killer (NK) cells. The majority of NK cells (90%) express the intermediate-affinity IL-2R; only a subset has the high-affinity receptor.[112] Activation of T cells via the T-cell receptor complex up-regulates IL-2Rβ and induces IL-2Rα chain expression, which leads to formation of the high-affinity receptor.[113] B cells can also be induced to express IL-2R and become IL-2 responsive after cross-linking of surface immunoglobulin.[114] IL-2 stimulation also leads to activation of other kinases, including the serine/threonine-specific kinase Raf-1.[115,116] Evidence also exists that IL-2 binding to its receptor on T cells leads to the phosphorylation of the retinoblastoma-susceptibility-gene product p110Rb, a process that is important for cell-cycle progression.[117]

Cellular Pharmacology

IL-2 is a major growth factor for lymphoid cells, including T cells and NK cells.[73,76,118] IL-2 binding to IL-2R on activated T cells promotes clonal expansion of antigen-specific cells, an important component in the development of host immunity. It also plays an important role in potentiating cytotoxic activity of lymphocytes, including antigen-specific major histocompatibility complex (MHC)–restricted cytotoxic CD8+ and CD4+ T lymphocytes.[119,120] IL-2 can also enhance the cytolytic activity of NK cells, which are responsible for what has been referred to as *LAK cell activity*.[121] The potentiation of cytotoxic activity is likely due to IL-2 up-regulation of the expression of proteins involved in the lytic process. IL-2 alone or in combination with other stimuli can up-regulate mRNA levels for perforin and granzyme B in both T and NK cells.[76,122] Macrophage cytotoxicity is also potentiated by IL-2.[120] IL-2 is also known to stimulate cytokine secretion from mononuclear cells, including NK cells, T cells, and macrophages.[120] NK cells cultured with IL-2 secrete cytokines [TNF-α, IFN-γ, GM-CSF], which can facilitate inflammation and immunity by acting on monocytes and macrophages.[76,120] IL-2 can also cooperate with TCR triggering to induce IFN-γ secretion from T lymphocytes.[120]

Evidence also is found that IL-2 may have a negative regulatory effect on the immune response.[123,124] IL-2 plays an important role in regulating apoptosis in T cells, a major mechanism of controlling immune responses. This concept is supported by the observation that knock-out mice missing IL-2 or the α or β chains of the IL-2R display autoimmunity and lymphadenopathy.[125–127] Thus, mice deficient in IL-2R signaling have abnormal accumulation of activated T cells with impaired TCR-induced apoptosis. IL-2 enhances activation-induced cell death (AICD) mediated through Fas pathway.[123–127] Crossing IL-2 knockout mice with TCR transgenic mice demonstrated that activated T cells from these animals were impaired in Fas-mediated AICD.[128] IL-2 augments AICD by increasing transcription of Fas ligand in antigen-stimulated T cells, partly through the induction of STAT5.[124,129] IL-2 also inhibits transcription of the inhibitor of the Fas pathway, FLIP [FADD-like IL-1β–converting enzyme (FLICE) inhibitory protein].[129] In the potentiation of AICD, IL-2 cannot be replaced by other cytokines such as interleukin 7 (IL-7) or IL-4. Thus, although IL-2 serves as a growth signal during the early phase of an immune response, it can potentiate apoptosis in T cells after repeated antigen activation, which results in termination of an immune response. IL-2 is also important for the induction of passive apoptosis in T cells. This form of apoptosis results when there is no further antigen stimulation where the induction of IL-2 and IL-2R ceases, resulting in lymphokine withdrawal.[123,124] This pathway of apoptosis is distinct from Fas-mediated AICD. Passive apoptosis results from an increase in mito-

chondrial permeability and cytochrome *c* release and can be blocked by Bcl-2.[123,124]

Clinical Pharmacokinetics

Clinical assessment of the immunopharmacology of IL-2 has been assisted by the availability of a sensitive bioassay procedure, development of ELISAs,[130] and the use of cytolytic (NK- and LAK-cell) assays to define the biologic effects of IL-2 administration. The bioassay assesses the capacity of the sera or supernatant in question to maintain the growth of an IL-2–dependent T-cell clone.

Initial studies with IL-2 used material produced by the Jurkat T-cell tumor line and purified by affinity chromatography.[131] Doses of 14 to 2,000 μg were administered, and serum levels were measured using a bioassay.[132] The biologic half-life varied from 6 to 10 minutes after a bolus infusion. Sustained serum levels during continuous infusion were also noted.

Several recombinant preparations of IL-2 (rIL-2) have been used clinically and are outlined in Table 27-4. They are nonglycosylated and produced in *E. coli*. The Chiron preparation[133] differs from natural human IL-2, with the cysteine residue at amino acid 125 replaced by serine, and also lacks the N-terminal alanine. These alterations permit correct folding and maintain biologic activity of this agent. Amgen rIL-2[134] has a similar serine substitution at position 125, and, in addition, has an N-terminal methionine residue. The Hoffmann-La Roche rIL-2 preparation[135] lacks the amino acid substitution at position 125, has an additional N-terminal methionine residue, and has a specific activity similar to that of natural IL-2. These molecules can form only one disulfide bridge and belong to the class of proteins known as muteins, or mutationally altered and biologically active products.

Confusion has arisen because of the definitions used for units of activity and the methods used to calculate dosage (body surface area versus kg). At present, the accepted definition for a unit is based on an international standard described by the World Health Organization.[139] A unit of IL-2 is defined as the reciprocal of the dilution that produces 50% of the maximal proliferation of murine HT2 cells in a short-term tritium-labeled thymidine incorpo-

TABLE 27-4. RECOMBINANT INTERLEUKIN 2 (rIL-2) PREPARATIONS

Source	Formulation	Activity	Study
Chiron	Des-alanye, serine-125 rIL-2	16.5×10^6 IU/mg	Lotze et al.[133]
Amgen	r-met HuIL-2 (ala 125)	9.4×10^6 IU/mg	Sarna et al.[134]
Hoffmann-La Roche	r-met IL-2	12–15×10^6 IU/mg	Sosman et al.[135]
Chiron	PEG rIL-2	4×10^6 IU/mg	Zimmerman et al.[136]
Roussel-Uclaf	rIL-2	$1.2 \pm 0.6 \times 10^7$ IU/mg	Tursz et al.,[137] Tzannis et al.[138]

PEG rIL-2, polyethylene glycol interleukin 2; r-met HuIL-2, recombinant methionyl human interleukin 2; r-met IL-2, recombinant methionyl interleukin 2.

ration assay. One mg of Chiron rIL-2 contains 16.3 IU per mg of drug. In the past, a Cetus unit was commonly used to express doses of this cytokine, with 3×10^6 Cetus units equaling 1 mg of rIL-2. Hoffmann-La Roche rIL-2 contained 15.0×10^6 U per mg of protein. One Hoffmann-La Roche unit was reported as equivalent to one Biological Response Modification Program (BRMP) unit[140] and approximately 3.0 IU. This situation has produced confusion when the attempt is made to compare dosages and toxicity among studies that used the various rIL-2 preparations.

The clinical and *in vitro* activities of these two rIL-2 preparations have been compared by Hank et al.[141] Equivalent international units of each cytokine were used, and quantitative differences were noted. A dosage of 1.5×10^6 IU per m^2 per day of Roche rIL-2 was equivalent in toxicity to 4.5×10^6 IU per m^2 per day of Chiron rIL-2. Equivalent amounts also differed in the induction of proliferation by various T-cell lines and binding to IL-2 receptors. These findings suggested that 3 to 6 IU of Chiron rIL-2 are required for induction of the biologic effects produced by 1 IU of Hoffmann-La Roche rIL-2.

The only preparation currently available for clinical use in the United States is Chiron rIL-2. Findings such as these suggest that one must be cautious when using doses and schedules developed with alternative preparations. The reasons for these differences in biologic activity may be related to structural and solubility differences between these proteins. Two other IL-2 preparations used clinically are natural human IL-2 (nIL-2) and Sanofi rIL-2; however, limited information is available concerning these agents.

The various rIL-2 preparations are formulated differently. Chiron rIL-2 contains sodium dodecyl sulfate, which produces polymeric IL-2 complexes. Hoffmann-La Roche rIL-2 did not contain sodium dodecyl sulfate and yielded monomeric IL-2. The bioavailability of rIL-2 preparations has also been studied.[142] Chiron rIL-2, when dissolved in saline, appears to lose significant activity if exposed to plastic. This was not seen with the Hoffmann-La Roche and Amgen muteins. The use of dextrose or 2% albumin prevented loss of bioactivity. Thus, Chiron rIL-2 may form aggregates, which may be prevented by the addition of albumin.

The inactivation of rIL-2 in pump-based delivery systems has also been reported. Tzannis et al.[138] reported that the biologic activity of Roussel-Uclaf rIL-2 is reduced by 90% when a 24-hour infusion is given using a Panomat V-5 infusion system (Disentronic Medical Systems; Plymouth, MN). The diluent used was 10 mmol per L phosphate buffer with 150 mmol per L sodium chloride. Hank et al.[141] examined the effects on the biologic activity of Chiron and Hoffmann-La Roche rIL-2 when delivered via a portable infusion pump. They reported no significant decrease in IL-2 activity for either preparation. The differences in these results may be due to the diluents used, the pump systems used, or the rIL-2 preparation used.

The clinical pharmacokinetics of both the Chiron and Hoffmann-La Roche preparations have been studied, and the features of the latter more fully characterized. Like many other cytokines, rIL-2 has a short half-life. Various parameters for Jurkat cell–derived IL-2 and recombinant IL-2 preparations are outlined in Table 27-5. When rIL-2 is administered as an intravenous bolus, its pharmacokinetics are approximately linear, and the resulting serum levels are proportional to the dose.[143] Injection of 6×10^6 IU per m^2 produces serum levels of 1,950 IU per mL. The levels decrease with a $t_{1/2\alpha}$ of 12.9 minutes followed by a slower phase with a $t_{1/2\beta}$ of 85 minutes. Figure 27-3 illustrates the serum levels obtained after injection of an intravenous bolus of 6×10^6 IU per m^2.[144] The reported clearance rate of 117 mL per minute is consistent with renal filtration's being the major route of elimination.

The variables influencing rIL-2 pharmacokinetics have been studied in animal models.[104,145,146] The biodistribution of ^{125}I-radiolabeled rIL-2 was studied in Sprague-Dawley rats.[104] The most significant uptake was found in the kidney and liver, with the kidney cortex demonstrating the highest activity. Irradiated and splenectomized mice have been used to assess the potential role of rIL-2 binding to lymphoid cells.[146] The rIL-2 was injected intravenously, and no alterations were found. In addition, the half-life of rIL-2 in nephrectomized animals rose from 2.5 to 3.5 minutes to 84 minutes, and ureteral ligation had minimal effect on rIL-2 half-life. Finally, active IL-2 is not excreted in the urine, which implies renal tubular catabolism.

TABLE 27-5. PHARMACOKINETICS OF INTERLEUKIN 2 PREPARATIONS AFTER INTRAVENOUS BOLUS ADMINISTRATION

IL-2 preparation	Source	Serum $t_{1/2}$ (min)		AUC (U · min/mL)	Clearance (mL/min)
		$t_{1/2\alpha}$	$t_{1/2\beta}$		
Recombinant IL-2 (rIL-2)[133]	Chiron	13.8 ± 7.7	86 ± 34	18,200 ± 15,900	117
PEG IL-2[143]	Chiron	183	740	NS	4.50
Native IL-2[131]	Dupont	5–7	30	NS	NS
rIL-2[135]	Amgen	13.4 (8.5–18.8)	NS	NS	NS

AUC, area under the concentration × time curve; NS, not stated; PEG IL-2, polyethylene glycol interleukin 2; $t_{1/2}$, half-life.

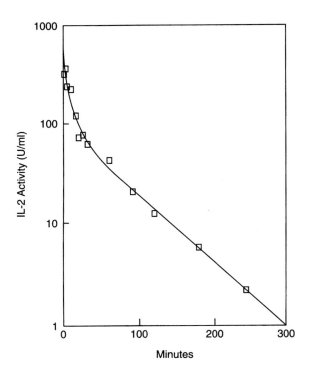

FIGURE 27-3. Interleukin 2 (IL-2) serum clearance after an intravenous bolus. A dose of 1.0 MU per m² was given as a 5-minute intravenous bolus. Serum samples were taken, and the IL-2 bioactivity was determined. A biexponential curve has been fitted to the assay values, minimizing the sum of the squares of the percentage of deviation of the curve from the data. (From Konrad MW, Hemstreet G, Hersh EM, et al. Pharmacokinetics of recombinant interleukin 2 in humans. *Cancer Res* 1990;50:2009–2017, with permission.)

Other schedules of intravenous rIL-2 administration, such as continuous infusion, have also been investigated. Infusion times have varied from 2 to 24 hours, and steady-state levels are generally achieved within 2 hours (Fig. 27-4). Median steady-state levels of 123 IU per mL are produced by infusion of 6×10^6 IU per m² over 6 hours, and the levels then fall rapidly after termination of rIL-2 infusion. The clearance rate after intravenous infusion resembles that seen with bolus administration.

The pharmacokinetics of very low doses of rIL-2 may be different than that observed with higher doses. Saturable pathways, binding to serum proteins or receptors, and internalization of the receptor-ligand complex may play significant roles in altering distribution. Continued administration of rIL-2, and the accompanying lymphocytosis with increased IL-2 receptor density, may potentially result in an increase of rIL-2 metabolism. In addition, alterations in renal function may change clearance of this cytokine.

Most frequently, rIL-2 is administered as a subcutaneous injection.[144] Time to peak concentration varies from 120 to 360 minutes, and with doses of 6×10^6 IU per m², median peak serum levels of 32.1 IU per mL and 42 IU per mL have been reported. The kinetics of lower-dose subcutaneous rIL-2 is different than that of high-dose intravenous

administration. Studies demonstrate that IL-2 serum levels are 50- to 100-fold less than with intravenous administration.[144] Some studies[147] do suggest alternative clearance mechanisms at lower doses. Interleukin-2 may be bound to proteins such as soluble IL-2R (sIL-2R), α_2-macroglobulin, and immunoglobulins with saturable processes in operation.[147] Administration to an anephric patient on dialysis produced slightly higher IL-2 concentrations, but the pharmacokinetics of subcutaneous rIL-2 appeared similar to that in patients with normal renal function.[147] Kirchner et al.[148] examined the pharmacokinetics of subcutaneously administered rIL-2. Two schedules were investigated (20 MIU per m² daily and 10 MIU per m² twice daily). For the once-daily schedule, the 24-hour area under the concentration × time curve (AUC) was 627 IU per mL × 1 hour, and for the twice-daily schedule 1,130 IU per mL × 1 hour. The highest observed concentration for both schedules was similar. By 72 hours, the levels of sIL-R increased, with some reductions in AUC seen. The authors concluded that two daily doses of rIL-2 provide superior bioavailability.

Clinical Effects and Toxicity

The variables influencing serum levels and biologic activity have led to the clinical investigation of multiple schedules

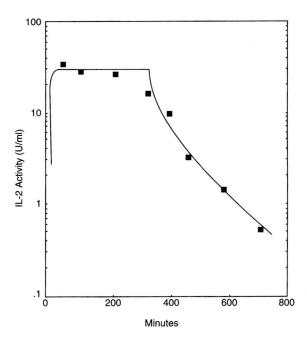

FIGURE 27-4. Serum levels during and after a 6-hour intravenous infusion of interleukin 2 (IL-2). The patient received 1 MU per m² over 6 hours, and the steady-state level of approximately 28 U per mL is close to the dose-normalized median level seen in all patients. Because the first blood sample was taken 60 minutes after the start of the infusion, the rising phase of the curve was not accurately determined, and the curve seen here is somewhat symbolic of the actual time course expected. (From Konrad MW, Hemstreet G, Hersh EM, et al. Pharmacokinetics of recombinant interleukin 2 in humans. *Cancer Res* 1990;50:2009–2017, with permission.)

TABLE 27-6. DOSES AND SCHEDULES OF RECOMBINANT INTERLEUKIN 2 (rIL-2) IN TRIALS INVOLVING PATIENTS WITH RENAL CELL CARCINOMA

Study	rIL-2 Source	Dose and Schedule of rIL-2	No. Patients	Response (CR + PR)
Fisher et al.[150]	Chiron	600,000 IU/kg q8h × 5 d, i.v.b. (repeated in 1 wk)	255	15% (17 CRs)
Bukowski et al.[151]	Chiron	60×10^6 IU/m^2 t.i.w. (i.v.b.)	41	9.7% (1 CR)
Palmer et al.[152]	Chiron	18×10^6 IU/m^2 c.i.v. d 1–5	225	15% (7 CRs)
Sleijfer et al.[153]	Chiron	18×10^6 IU/m^2 s.c. d 1–5 (wk 1) and d 1 & 2 (wk 2–6), followed by 9×10^6 IU/m^2 s.c. d 3–5 (wk 2–6).	47	19% (2 CRs)
Negrier et al.[154]	Chiron	18×10^6 IU/m^2 c.i.v. d 1–5, 12–16	138	6.5% (2 CRs)

c.i.v., continuous intravenous infusion; CR, complete response; i.v.b., intravenous bolus; PR, partial response.

and doses (Table 27-6). Among the solid tumors, malignant melanoma and renal cell carcinoma appear the most responsive to rIL-2 therapy, and in both tumor types, rIL-2 has been approved for treatment. Rosenberg et al.[149] used dosages of 1.8 to 6.0×10^5 IU per kg every 8 hours for 5 days. This approach using high doses of rIL-2 administered frequently is associated with severe and life-threatening toxicity. These doses were investigated when initial studies using lower doses or less frequent administration produced limited antitumor effects. The response and survival data for this type of schedule and dose of rIL-2 in patients with renal cancer is summarized in Table 27-7. Approximately 5% of patients experienced durable complete responses.[155]

A comparison of results reported with various schedules and routes of rIL-2 administration is provided in Table 27-8. Overall, the results appear similar. Randomized studies to detect differences are in progress.

The short half-life of intravenous bolus rIL-2 prompted investigation of continuous intravenous (c.i.v.) administration of this cytokine. The majority of reports have used 18.0 MIU per m^2 per day. Response rates between studies vary, but in a group of 922 patients reviewed (Table 27-8), the overall response rate was 13.3%. Complete regressions occur, and in some series[156] the rates are similar to those reported with high-dose bolus rIL-2.

A single randomized trial in which patients on one of the arms received c.i.v. rIL-2 has been reported. In this trial[154] patients with metastatic renal cancer were randomly assigned to receive either c.i.v. rIL-2 (18.0 MIU per m^2 per day on days 1 through 5 and 12 through 16), IFN-α, or the combination. The response rate in the 138 patients receiving c.i.v. rIL-2 was 6.5%. Sixty-nine percent of individuals developed hypotension resistant to vasopressor agents. Thus, the toxicity of single-agent rIL-2 given as a c.i.v. infusion at doses greater than 18 MIU per m^2 is substantial. At this dose level, hospitalization is required, and outcomes do not appear different from those for single-agent IFN-α. Lower doses of rIL-2 administered as a c.i.v. infusion produce less toxicity. Caligiuri et al.[157] administered 0.05 to 0.6 MIU per m^2 per day c.i.v. for up to 90 days. The clinical activity of this approach is unclear.

Subcutaneous administration of rIL-2 in patients with renal cell carcinoma has also been examined, but published experience with this route is limited. In the group of 290 patients for which data are summarized in Table 27-8, a response rate of 16.8% was noted. In the report by Buter et al.,[158] two complete responses lasting for 29 months and for longer than 35 months were seen in patients with metastatic renal cancer, which suggests that some of these responses may be durable. Yang et al.[159] are conducting a prospective randomized trial to determine the effectiveness of subcutaneous rIL-2 compared with bolus rIL-2. Regimens used include the following: high-dose bolus (720,000 IU per kg), low-dose bolus (72,000 IU per kg), and subcutaneous (250,000 IU per kg per day for 5 of 7 days in week 1, followed by 125,000 IU per kg per day for 5 of 7 days in weeks 2 to 6). One hundred and sixty-four patients have been randomly assigned to the different treatment regimens, and the preliminary response rates are 16%, 4%, and 11%, respectively. The lower-dose regimens produce less

TABLE 27-7. CLINICAL RESULTS WITH HIGH-DOSE RECOMBINANT INTERLEUKIN 2 IN PATIENTS WITH RENAL CELL CARCINOMA

No. patients	255
Median age (range)	52 (18–71)
Sex (male/female)	178/77
ECOG performance status	
0	166
1	80
≥2	9
Prior therapy	
Nephrectomy	218
Chemotherapy	8
Responses (CR + PR)	36 (14%)
CR	12
Median response duration (mo)	
CR	Not reached
PR	19.0
CR + PR	20.3

CR, complete response; ECOG, Eastern Cooperative Oncology Group; PR, partial response.
From Fisher RI, Rosenberg SA, Sznol M, et al. High-dose aldesleukin in renal cell carcinoma: long-term survival update. *Cancer J Sci Am* 1997;3[Suppl 1]:S70–S72.

TABLE 27-8. RESULTS OF SINGLE-AGENT RECOMBINANT INTERLEUKIN 2 (rIL-2) TREATMENT OF METASTATIC RENAL CELL CARCINOMA

Method of rIL-2 Administration	Number of Patients	No. CR (%)	No. PR (%)	Overall (%)
Subcutaneous[160]	290	8 (3.0)	40 (13.8)	16.8
Continuous intravenous infusion[160]	922	25 (2.7)	98 (10.6)	13.3
Intravenous bolus[161]	733	38 (5.2)	86 (11.3)	16.5
Total	1,945	71 (3.7)	221	15.0

CR, complete response; PR, partial response.

severe toxicity. Data on response frequency, duration, and median survival remain preliminary.

Administration of nebulized IL-2 via inhalation has also been investigated. Aerosol therapy produces high pulmonary drug concentrations and low systemic drug levels, which thereby enhances the therapeutic index.[162] Huland et al.[163] reported on the use of natural IL-2 administered via nebulizer. Aerosol IL-2 100,000 U was delivered five times daily and was combined with systemic IL-2 and IFN-α. The toxicity of inhaled IL-2 was reported as minimal, which allowed administration in the outpatient department. Antitumor responses were reported; however, the contribution of inhaled IL-2 is unclear in view of the concurrent administration of other cytokines.

These results have been updated in 116 patients with pulmonary or mediastinal metastatic disease (or both).[164] Three different IL-2 formulations were used and included nIL-2, glycosylated rIL-2 (Sanofi; Montpellier, France), and nonglycosylated rIL-2 (Chiron). Thirty-six, 12, and 68 patients received the respective IL-2 preparations via inhalation. Eleven percent received only inhaled IL-2; 33% received concomitant subcutaneous rIL-2; and 56% were given concomitant rIL-2 and IFN-α. In 105 patients with pulmonary metastases, 16 patients responded (15.2%), of whom three individuals showed complete responses. The median response duration was 15.5 months. The administration of inhaled rIL-2 has also been reported by Lorenz et al.[165] and Nakamoto et al.[166] In these studies 16 patients with renal cancer were treated, and four responses (including one complete response) were noted. To assess the value of this approach, randomized trials comparing results in patients receiving only inhaled cytokine with those in patients receiving systemic therapy with and without inhaled cytokine are required. The delivery of liposome-encapsulated rIL-2 as an aerosol to dogs with pulmonary metastasis has also been reported,[167] and this method may in the future provide an alternative delivery system. Other routes of delivery for rIL-2 such as intraarterial,[165] intrapleural,[168] and intraperitoneal[169] have also been examined. Results remain preliminary.

Administration of rIL-2 produces functional alterations in most organ systems. A decrease in lymphocytes occurs initially, and then resolves. Subsequently, the peripheral blood lymphocyte pool (CD3+, CD56+) expands. Soluble IL-2R levels increase in the circulation, and IL-2R positive

lymphocytes also are seen.[170,171] Cytolytic activity of peripheral blood lymphocytes may be enhanced during continuous infusion of high doses, which results in increased NK cell activity and the appearance of LAK cells in the circulation.[172] The effects of rIL-2 on lymphocytes are mediated through specific cell surface receptors on the various subsets. The expression of high-affinity receptors and their saturation by prolonged low-dose infusion of rIL-2 has been reported.[173] The possibility that these cytolytic mononuclear cells mediate the antitumor effects of systemically administered rIL-2 has been investigated. The inability to demonstrate correlations of response and development of cytolytic activity in patients treated with rIL-2, however, does not support this hypothesis.

Other effects of rIL-2 include endothelial cell activation with increased expression of adhesion molecules such as intercellular adhesion molecule 1 (ICAM-1) and endothelial-leukocyte adhesion molecule 1 (ELAM-1).[174] Secondary cytokine production (TNF-α, IFN-γ, IL-6) and increased C-reactive protein levels[175–177] also have been noted. Finally, rIL-2 may be immunosuppressive in certain circumstances, with decreased delayed hypersensitivity[178] and neutrophil chemotaxis reported.[179]

The severity and nature of rIL-2 side effects are related to the dose and schedule used. The toxicity of bolus, c.i.v., and subcutaneous rIL-2 are outlined in Table 27-9. Uniformly, patients develop chills, fever, and malaise. A vascular leak syndrome occurs with higher dosages of rIL-2 and is characterized by weight gain, oliguria, tachycardia, and hypotension.[180] When this syndrome is present, supplemental intravenous fluids, vasopressors, and diuretics may be required for management. Cardiac toxicity including arrhythmias and myocardial infarction, and pulmonary side effects such as dyspnea and pleural effusions may develop. Cardiovascular toxicity includes not only the vascular leak syndrome and hypotension but direct effects on the myocardium. Hemodynamic studies[181] have demonstrated decreased mean arterial pressure and systemic vascular resistance consistent with changes noted during septic shock. Myocardial injury with creatine phosphokinase elevations[182] and myocarditis secondary to lymphocyte infiltration[183] have also been noted.

Hematopoietic findings include anemia, thrombocytopenia, and leukopenia,[184] and an increased frequency of

TABLE 27-9. TOXICITY PRODUCED BY VARIOUS SCHEDULES AND DOSES OF RECOMBINANT INTERLEUKIN 2 (rIL-2)

	Yang et al.[159]	Buter et al.[158]	Negrier et al.[154]
rIL-2 dose level & schedule	720,000 MIU/kg i.v.b. q8h × 5 d	18 MIU/m² s.c. d 1–5 (wk 1), 9.0 MIU/m² s.c. d 1 & 2, then 18 MIU/m² d 3–5 (wk 2–6)	18 MIU/m² c.i.v. d 1–5, 12–16
Type of toxicity	% >grade 3[a]	% any grade[b]	% >grade 3[b]
Nausea/vomiting	19%	96%	34%
Diarrhea	11%	55%	27.5%
Elevated creatinine level	2% (>8 mg/dL)	9% (>200 μmol/L)	3.6%
Renal effects	21% (oliguria <80 mL/8 h)	NS	15.2%
Hypotension	43%	26% (11% <90 mm Hg)	68% (vasopressor resistant)
Neuropsychiatric effects	14%	21%	12.3%
Elevated bilirubin level	4%	2%	1%
Cardiac effects	5%	4%	12.3%
Anemia	NS	NS	17.4%
Thrombocytopenia	9%	0	3.6%

c.i.v., continuous intravenous; i.v.b., intravenous bolus; NS, not stated.
[a]Expressed as percent of courses.
[b]Expressed as percent of patients.

sepsis in patients requiring central venous lines has been reported.[185] This latter complication may relate to the previously noted granulocyte defect.[178] Finally, hepatic toxicity characterized by increases in serum bilirubin levels and minimal changes in transaminase levels are common. Fisher et al.[150] investigated this phenomenon using technetium-labeled disofenin and noted delayed excretion and uptake consistent with cholestasis. Return to baseline levels within 4 to 6 days of rIL-2 discontinuation is usual. Gastrointestinal toxicity includes nausea, vomiting, diarrhea, and mucositis. Colon dilation,[186] perforation,[187] and ischemic necrosis[188] have also been seen but represent uncommon manifestations of rIL-2 toxicity.

Neurologic and neuropsychiatric effects can develop acutely or chronically during rIL-2 administration. Patients receiving high-dose intensive therapy may become agitated, disoriented, and occasionally comatose.[189] Increases in peritumoral edema in a series of patients with gliomas receiving rIL-2[180] and increases of brain water content[190] indicate that cerebral edema may be responsible. These effects are generally transient and resolve with drug discontinuation. Neuropsychiatric effects including a decrease in cognitive function and impaired memory have been reported in patients receiving c.i.v. rIL-2.[191] These latter findings resemble the chronic central nervous system toxicity associated with IFN-α.[192]

Miscellaneous toxicities include dermatologic complications such as erythema, pruritus, and generalized erythroderma.[193] In patients with preexisting dermatologic conditions such as psoriasis, exacerbation of the underlying condition has been described.[194] Finally, hypothyroidism or hyperthyroidism has also been seen.[195] The cause of this complication is uncertain, but the development of autoimmune thyroiditis secondary to induction of class II antigens in thyroid tissue has been proposed.[196] The suggestion has also been made that patients developing this complication are more likely to respond.[197]

The etiology of rIL-2 related toxicity is uncertain but may involve interstitial lymphocyte infiltrates, vascular leaks, and secondary production of cytokines such as TNF-α.[177] The side effects are generally self-limited and resolve rapidly on discontinuation of rIL-2 therapy. Rapid resolution with use of systemic glucocorticoids has also been reported.[198] Attempts to diminish rIL-2–related toxicity by coadministration of agents such as the phosphoesterase inhibitor pentoxifylline,[199] soluble TNF-α receptor,[200] and soluble IL-1 receptor[56] have not been successful.

Drug Interactions

Initial studies with rIL-2 involved single-agent therapy with or without coadministration of *ex vivo*–activated peripheral blood lymphocytes (LAK cells)[201] or tumor-infiltrating lymphocytes.[202] These studies were based on preclinical investigations demonstrating benefit of adoptive immunotherapy.[203] Randomized trials comparing use of rIL-2 alone with administration of rIL-2 together with LAK or tumor-infiltrating lymphocytes have not, however, demonstrated significant increases in response rates or survival in patients with renal cell carcinoma or melanoma.[163,203]

Cytokine combinations involving rIL-2 and a variety of other lymphokines based on studies in animal models have also been used clinically. The cytokines combined with rIL-2 have included IFN-α, interferon-β (IFN-β), IFN-γ, IL-1, IL-4, and TNF-α.[149,204–207a] The combination of rIL-2 and IFN-α has been the most widely investigated and may produce higher response rates in patients with renal cell carcinoma[208,209] than rIL-2 alone.[154] Combinations of rIL-2 and monoclonal antibodies have also been studied. Murine antibodies such as R-24[210] and MG-22[211] have been given in combination with rIL-2 to patients with melanoma. Results are preliminary at this time.

The combination of chemotherapy and rIL-2 has also been studied. In renal cell carcinoma, administration of vinblastine sulfate and rIL-2 did not produce enhanced antitumor effects.[212] The preclinical finding of synergistic effects for doxorubicin hydrochloride and rIL-2[213] have led to a series of phase I trials investigating different schedules and doses of these two agents.[214,215] Additive toxicity and no immunomodulatory interactions were seen. Finally, cyclophosphamide has been administered before rIL-2 at doses of 350 or 1,000 mg per m².[216,217] The rationale involves the possible immunomodulatory effects of cyclophosphamide in patients.[218] No convincing evidence for enhancement of responses to rIL-2 has been seen.

Multiagent combinations including rIL-2 have been investigated in patients with renal cell carcinoma and malignant melanoma. In patients with renal cancer, the combination of rIL-2, IFN-α, and fluorouracil has been used. Atzpodien et al.[219] initially reported regression rates over 35%; however, response rates of 1.8%[168] and 8.2%[220] have been noted. The benefit of this regimen remains unclear. In patients with malignant melanoma, combinations of rIL-2, IFN-α, and chemotherapy consisting of imidazole carboximide, carmustine (bischloroethylnitrosourea, or BCNU), and tamoxifen have been used.[221] Response rates over 50% have been reported, and randomized trials are in progress.

The inhibition of hepatic cytochrome P-450 by cytokines such as IL-6 and TNF-α[222] has been reported. The induction of these cytokines by rIL-2 therefore suggests that impairment of drugs metabolized by this system may occur. Clinical studies investigating such interactions are limited. Piscitelli et al.[223] have examined the effect of c.i.v. rIL-2 (3 to 12 MIU per day) on clearance of indinavir sulfate, a protease inhibitor, in patients infected with the human immunodeficiency virus. Increases in indinavir serum concentrations and AUC (mean, 88%) and decreased clearance was found during rIL-2 administration. The authors suggest that IL-6 may be responsible. This type of study indicates that drug-cytokine interactions should be examined more closely.

Other Recombinant Interleukin 2 Preparations

The clinical antitumor effects and toxicity of rIL-2, and its immunomodulatory activities, have prompted development of different rIL-2 formulations in an attempt to diminish toxicity and enhance efficacy. Covalent binding of rIL-2 to polyethylene glycol (PEG) at amino acid sites results in an rIL-2 preparation with persistent antitumor activity in murine models.[224] Phase I[143] and phase II trials[225] have been completed. The MTD of PEG–IL-2 given as an intravenous bolus once weekly is 20×10^6 IU per m². Pharmacokinetic studies have demonstrated a prolonged $t_{1/2\alpha}$ (183 minutes) and $t_{1/2\beta}$ (740 minutes). Serum levels of 15,000 IU per mL were seen, and the clearance was 4.5 mL per minute per m². The prolonged half-life and decreased clearance were predicted by animal models[145] and may be secondary to elimination of renal clearance because of the large hydrodynamic size of PEG–IL-2. The clinical toxicity reported resembles that seen with rIL-2, and antitumor responses were noted in patients with metastatic renal cell carcinoma (2 of 31 patients). The advantage of weekly administration for an agent such as rIL-2 make the pegylated formulation attractive; however, delayed and unpredictable toxicities have been seen.

Another method to limit the toxicity of rIL-2 is to incorporate it into liposomes. This produces altered distribution, metabolism, and elimination of the cytokine. A phase I trial of liposome-encapsulated rIL-2 has been initiated and uses escalating doses given as an intravenous bolus. Mild toxicity has been noted,[226] and immunologic activity, including elevated serum IL-2R levels, NK activity, and numbers of CD16+CD56+ cells, was seen. Use of this preparation may result in a decrease in overall rIL-2–related side effects while maintaining its immunomodulatory activities.

INTERLEUKIN 4

IL-4 is a cytokine with pleiotropic actions that was first described in 1982 as a T-cell–derived factor with B-lymphocyte stimulatory activity.[227,228] Since its initial description, IL-4 has been reported to affect a wide variety of cell types[229] and to have both stimulatory and suppressive effects on various responses. The genes encoding murine and human IL-4 have been cloned[230,231] and expressed in *E. coli*. *In vivo* and *in vitro* antitumor effects have been found, and initial trials of recombinant IL-4 are under way in patients with various malignancies.

Structure and Mechanisms of Action

IL-4 is a glycoprotein with a molecular weight between 15 and 19 kd. The human and murine forms share extensive homology[230,232]; however, unlike other cytokines, they are species specific.[233] The cDNA for human IL-4 encodes a protein of 153 amino acids, which is then cleaved to yield a mature protein containing 129 amino acids.[230] The IL-4 gene is on band q23-31 of chromosome 5[234] and is located in the vicinity of the genes encoding interleukin 3 (IL-3) and GM-CSF.[235] This gene occurs as a single copy and contains four exons and three introns.[232]

The human IL-4 gene has been expressed in *E. coli* (Schering-Plough), and milligram quantities are available. Recombinant IL-4 (Schering-Plough) has a molecular weight of 14.9 kd and contains 129 amino acids. It contains two potential glycosylation sites and six cysteine residues that form three disulfide bonds.[236] The three-dimensional topology of recombinant human IL-4 (rhuIL-4) has been investigated[237] and, interestingly, is similar to that described for recombinant human GM-CSF.[238]

The Sterling preparation of rhuIL-4 also has 129 amino acid residues and differs from the natural protein at six sites.[239] It was expressed in a yeast strain (*Saccharomyces cerevisiae*), and amino acids 1 to 4 (Glu-Ala-Glu-Ala) are not in natural IL-4 but are a consequence of the expression system. Asp38 and Asp105 are substituted for asparagine to preclude glycosylation. These changes result in a recombinant molecule that has the same biologic activity as the fully glycosylated rhuIL-4. *In vitro* comparative studies of the two preparations of rhuIL-4 are not available.

IL-4 produces its effects by interaction with cell surface receptors (IL-4Rs) that are present on various hematopoietic and nonhematopoietic cells. IL-4R is up-regulated by cytokines such as IL-2, IL-4,[240,241] IFN-γ, and IL-6.[242,243] IL-4 signaling depends on binding to the IL-4R, which is composed of two chains. IL-4 actually binds the 140-kd IL-4Rα chain with high affinity (K_d 20 to 3,000 pmol per L).[244–247] The IL-4Rα chain is a member of the hematopoietin receptor superfamily and also serves a part of the interleukin 13 receptor.[244,248–250] IL-4 bound to the IL-4Rα then heterodimerizes with the common γ chain, which does not change the affinity of IL-4 for the receptor but is necessary for initiating signal transduction.[251,252] Activation of the IL-4R leads to tyrosine phosphorylation of the α chain at multiple sites.[253] Three Janus kinase members are activated by the IL-4Rα chain.[254–256] Studies using deletion mutants of the IL-4Rα chain indicate that different cytoplasmic regions have distinct functions, which include binding to Janus kinases, initiation of proliferation, and induction of gene expression.[247,257–260] The IL-4–dependent pathway leading to proliferation is initiated by the phosphorylation of insulin receptor substrate 1 (IRS-1) by Jak1 and possibly by Janus kinase 2 (Jak2) after IRS-1 interaction with the IL-4Rα chain (residues 437–557).[244,261–263] PI3K, which is composed of an 85-kd regulatory unit and a 110-kd catalytic subunit, then binds to the phosphorylated IRS-1.[262,264,265] This lipid kinase initiates the generation of the second messenger molecules phosphatidylinositol-(3,4,5)-triphosphate and phosphatidylinositol-(3,4)-bisphosphate.[266,267] These molecules are involved in the downstream activation of protein kinase C and Akt kinase.[268,269] The IL-4 stimulation of PI3K and Akt kinase is also thought to enhance the survival of hematopoietic cells.[244,268,269] The phosphorylation of IRS-1 by IL-4 is also known to activate the Ras/MAPK pathway, although not consistently in all cell lines tested.[244] The region between residues 557 and 657 of the IL-4Rα chain is responsible for IL-4–dependent gene expression through the activation of STAT6.[244,260] In IL-4–treated cells, nuclear translocation of this transcription factor results in the expression of a number of genes including, class II MHC molecules, select immunoglobulins, and CD23.[244,247,260,270,271]

Cellular Pharmacology

IL-4 is produced by activated T helper cells[272] and mast cells,[273] and has pleiotropic effects both *in vitro* and *in vivo* (Table 27-10). Stimulation of B- and T-cell functions has

TABLE 27-10. BIOLOGIC EFFECTS OF INTERLEUKIN 4 ON HUMAN CELLS

Cell Type	Responses	
	Stimulation	**Inhibition**
T and NK/LAK cells	T-cell, TIL, CTL proliferation	IL-2–induced T-cell proliferation, IL-2–induced NK/LAK cytotoxicity, T-cell IFN-γ secretion
B cells	Proliferation, IgG and IgM secretion, IgE and IgG class switch, CD23/FcR expression	Antigen-specific Ig secretion, IL-2–induced proliferation
Monocytes	Class I expression, G-CSF	IL-1, TNF, IL-6, and GM-CSF production, FcR and CD23 expression
Hematopoietic progenitors	G-CSF–supported CFU-GM	IL-3–induced CFU-GM, EPO–induced BFU-E, and M-CSF–induced CFU-M
Mast cells	Proliferation, ICAM-1 expression	
Endothelial cells	IL-6 production, T-cell adhesion, ICAM-1 and ELAM-1 expression	

BFU-E, burst-forming unit, erythroid; CFU-GM, colony-forming unit–granulocyte-macrophage; CFU-M, colony-forming unit–macrophage; CTL, cytolytic T lymphocyte; ELAM-1, endothelial-leukocyte adhesion molecule 1; EPO, erythropoietin; FcR, Fc receptor; G-CSF, granulocyte colony-stimulating factor; GM-CSF, granulocyte-macrophage colony-stimulating factor; ICAM-1, intercellular adhesion molecule 1; IFN, interferon; Ig, immunoglobulin; IL, interleukin; LAK, lymphokine-activated killer; M-CSF, macrophage colony-stimulating factor; NK, natural killer; TIL, tumor-infiltrating lymphocyte; TNF, tumor necrosis factor.
Adapted from Puri RK, Siegel JP. Interleukin-4 and cancer therapy. *Cancer Invest* 1993;11:473–486, with permission.

TABLE 27-11. RECOMBINANT INTERLEUKIN 4 PREPARATIONS

Source	Molecular Weight (kd)	Number of Amino Acids	Expression Vector	Activity	Clinical Trials
Schering-Plough[291]	14.9	129	*Escherichia coli*	NA	Phase I and II
Immunex/Sterling[290]	15.4	129	*Saccharomyces cerevisiae*	$1.8 + 0.7 \times 10^7$ µg/mg[a]	Phase I

NA, not applicable.

[a] One unit of recombinant human interleukin 4 is defined as the amount that stimulates 50% of maximum uptake of tritium-labeled thymidine in human tonsil B-cell assay.

been recognized, and a wide range of effects on diverse cell populations has also been reported. IL-4–deficient mice produced by genetic manipulation have provided some insights into its function.[274] These animals have normal T- and B-lymphocyte development, but serum levels of immunoglobulin G1 and immunoglobulin E are decreased. Transgenic mice overexpressing IL-4,[274] in contrast, have elevated levels of serum immunoglobulin G1 and immunoglobulin E.[275] Thus, IL-4 may play a critical role in the development of humoral immunity, particularly immunoglobulin E. Studies with IL-4R knockout mice and STAT6 knockout mice revealed that IL-4–producing T cells play an important role in the development of an immune response to infections with helminths and other parasites. IL-4 has other functions related to the immune system, including up-regulation of the expression of MHC class II molecules on B cells. It also functions in inflammatory responses by increasing the expression of vascular cell adhesion molecule 1 (VCAM-1) on endothelial cells.

In addition to these pleiotropic immunoregulatory activities, IL-4 is involved in the proliferation and maturation of dendritic cells. These cells represent antigen-processing cells that *in vivo* capture, process, and present foreign antigenic peptides to T lymphocytes. A variety of steps in the maturation and functioning of these cells have been identified, and *in vitro* a variety of cytokines are involved in their generation. The combination of GM-CSF and IL-4 generates functional dendritic cells that can endocytose antigens and stimulate T cells.[276] This property of IL-4 and its control of dendritic cell proliferation are being used for production of these cells for use in current vaccination approaches.

Antitumor activity has also been attributed to IL-4 and is suggested by a series of observations. Various murine epithelial tumor cells express IL-4R,[277] and *in vivo* administration to mice with fibrosarcomas or spontaneous adenocarcinomas has antitumor effects. Tepper et al.[278] demonstrated that IL-4 gene transfection into murine tumor cells resulted in their rejection. This appeared to correlate with the degree of eosinophil and macrophage infiltration. In another model, IL-4–producing tumor cells[279] induced systemic immunity against murine spontaneous renal carcinoma cells (RENCA).

Studies with human tumors have demonstrated that rhuIL-4 inhibits the *in vitro* growth of various tumor cells.[280–282] These include hematopoietic tumors as well as various solid tumors, such as breast cancer, ovarian cancer, and head and neck tumors.[283,284] Various reports indicate that the effects of IL-4 may be mediated by inhibition of autocrine growth factors such as IL-6[285] and GM-CSF.[286] IL-4 may have both direct and indirect effects on hematopoietic malignancies. Solid tumors may also contain IL-4R, and *in vitro* inhibition by IL-4 of cell growth in a wide variety of tumors has been reported.[287,288]

Clinical Pharmacokinetics

Two recombinant IL-4 preparations have been evaluated and are outlined in Table 27-11. They have been produced after expression of the IL-4 gene in either *E. coli* or yeast. The results of reported phase I trials using these preparations are summarized in Table 27-12.

Serum assays for IL-4 are performed with both biologic and ELISA methods. The traditional assay involves prolif-

TABLE 27-12. PHASE I CLINICAL TRIALS OF INTERLEUKIN 4 (IL-4)

Study	IL-4 Preparation	Dose Range	Schedule	MTD	$t_{1/2\alpha}$	$t_{1/2\beta}$
Lotze[291]	Sterling	1–30 µg/kg	i.v. q.d. or t.i.d.	20 µg/kg	8 min	48 min
Markowitz et al.[293]	Sterling	20–1,280 µg/m²/d	i.v. q.d. d 1, d 4–17	NS	NS	NS
Taylor et al.[294]	Sterling	40–1,200 µg/m²/d	s.c. d 1–5	500 µg/m²	NS	NS
Atkins et al.[295]	Sterling	10, 15 µg/kg	i.v. t.i.d. d 1–5, 15–19	10 µg/kg	NS	NS
Prendiville et al.[292]	Sterling	40, 120, 280, 400 µg/m²	i.v. q.d. d 1, 24-h c.i. d 4–5, s.c. d 8–22	400 µg/m²	15–22 min	NS
Gilleece et al.[296]	Schering-Plough	0.5, 1.0, 5.0 µg/kg	s.c. d 1, 8–17, 29–57	>1.0 and <5.0 µg/kg	NS	NS
Maher et al.[297]	Schering-Plough	0.25, 1.0, 5.0 µg/kg	s.c. d 1, 8–17, 28–57	Not reached	NS	NS

c.i., continuous infusion; MTD, maximum tolerated dose; NS, not stated; $t_{1/2}$, half-life.

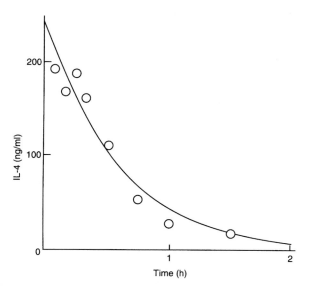

FIGURE 27-5. Concentration of interleukin 4 (IL-4) over time in the serum of a patient receiving 400 μg per m² of IL-4 as an intravenous bolus. [From Prendiville J, Thatcher N, Lind M, et al. Recombinant human interleukin-4 (rhu IL-4) administered by the intravenous and subcutaneous routes in patients with advanced cancer—a phase I toxicity study and pharmacokinetic analysis. *Eur J Cancer* 1993;29A:1700–1707, with permission.]

TABLE 27-13. PHARMACOKINETICS OF INTERLEUKIN 4 AFTER INTRAVENOUS BOLUS INJECTION

Dose rhuIL-4 (μg/m²/d)	AUC (ng· h/mL)	$t_{1/2}$ (min)	Cl_{tot} (mL/min)	V_d (L)
40	5.76	15.69	202.63	4.65
120	22.34	20.04	240.06	7.17
280	74.21	19.39	153.03	4.24
400	108.95	22.13	108.80	3.41

AUC, area under concentration × time curve; Cl_{tot}, total plasma clearance; rhuIL-4, recombinant human interleukin 4; $t_{1/2}$, elimination half-life; V_d, apparent volume of distribution.
Adapted from Prendiville J, Thatcher N, Lind M, et al. Recombinant human interleukin 4 (rhu IL-4) administered by the intravenous and subcutaneous routes in patients with advanced cancer—a phase I toxicity study and pharmacokinetic analysis. *Eur J Cancer* 1993;29A:1700–1707, with permission.

Clinical Effects and Toxicity

Preclinical evaluation of rhuIL-4 has demonstrated a wide range of pharmacologic and toxicologic effects in target organs including the cardiac system, liver, spleen, and bone marrow.[298] These effects were dose related and included death, cardiac inflammation and necrosis, and hepatitis. These were seen at doses greater than 25 μg per kg per day in cynomolgus monkeys. In human trials, rhuIL-4 was safe and well tolerated at dose levels of up to 5 μg per kg per day subcutaneously.

The toxicity of rhuIL-4 in humans is dose dependent. Subcutaneous administration at low dose produces fever, headache, sinus congestion, nausea, and elevated hepatic enzyme levels.[296] Anorexia, fatigue, and flulike symptoms also are seen and generally resolve within 24 hours of

eration of human tonsillar B lymphocytes in the presence of cross-linking antibodies to immunoglobulin M. A variation[289] involves induction of CD23 expression in various Burkitt's lymphoma and Epstein-Barr virus–transformed B-cell lines by IL-4. Serum may inhibit this assay and therefore must be used as a control. Finally, an ELISA using purified rabbit anti–IL-4 antibodies is available.[290]

The pharmacokinetic behavior of IL-4 has been investigated in a variety of studies. Lotze et al.[291] used a biologic assay and estimated an α distribution phase of 8 minutes and a β clearance phase of 48 minutes. Ghosh et al.[290] and Prendiville et al.[292] investigated the serum levels and pharmacokinetic behavior of rhuIL-4 (Sterling) after a single intravenous bolus dose, a 24-hour infusion, or subcutaneous administration. Serum IL-4 levels were determined using an ELISA. After intravenous bolus administration, serum levels of IL-4 increased with increasing doses, and the agent was rapidly cleared (Fig. 27-5 and Table 27-13). The half-life was between 15 and 22 minutes, and peak serum levels achieved after subcutaneous administration of rhuIL-4 (Fig. 27-6) were tenfold less than after comparable intravenous administration. Serum levels produced were dose dependent, and after subcutaneous administration of 400 μg per m², rhuIL-4 bioavailability was 71% ± 14.[290] A linear relationship between IL-4 dose level and AUC was found, which indicates linear pharmacokinetics for the dose ranges investigated.[292] The rapid clearance found and low distribution volume are consistent with binding to IL-4R on peripheral lymphocytes. The short half-life observed for rhuIL-4 is similar to that seen for other cytokines.

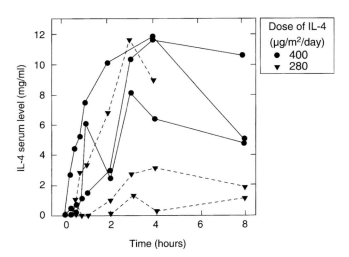

FIGURE 27-6. Serum levels of interleukin 4 (IL-4) following subcutaneous injection in patients receiving recombinant human IL-4. (From Ghosh AK, Smith NK, Prendiville J, et al. A phase I study of recombinant human interleukin-4 administered by the intravenous and subcutaneous route in patients with advanced cancer: immunological studies. *Eur Cytokine Netw* 1993;4:205–211, with permission.)

TABLE 27-14.   PHASE II TRIALS WITH RECOMBINANT HUMAN INTERLEUKIN 4 (rhuIL-4)

Study	Malignancy	Dose and Schedule of rhuIL-4	No. Patients	CR + PR
Whitehead et al.[300]	Malignant melanoma	5 μg/kg s.c. d 1–28	34	1 (CR)
Vokes et al.[301]	Non–small cell lung cancer	0.25, 1.0 μg/kg t.i.w. s.c.	22 (0.25 μg/kg); 41 (1.0 μg/kg)	1 (PR)
Tulpule et al.[302]	AIDS-related Kaposi's sarcoma	1 μg/kg/d s.c.	18	1 (PR)

AIDS, acquired immunodeficiency syndrome; CR, complete response; PR, partial response.

rhuIL-4 discontinuation.[296] Dose-limiting toxicity reported at 5 μg per kg per day includes headaches and arthralgias.

At higher dose levels and with intravenous administration,[291,295] toxicity is more severe. Nasal congestion, periorbital and peripheral edema, weight gain, diarrhea, and dyspnea have been seen.[291,295] A vascular leak syndrome resembling that produced by rIL-2 has been reported,[291] and gastritis with gastric ulceration was also seen.[299]

In a series of phase II trials involving patients with melanoma or renal cell carcinoma[295] rhuIL-4 was administered at a dose of 600 to 800 μg per m² by intravenous bolus every 8 hours on days 1 through 5. With this high-dose intensive schedule, four patients developed cardiac toxicity characterized by electrocardiographic changes consistent with infarction and elevated creatinine phosphokinase-MB fractions. One patient expired, and at autopsy myocardial infiltration by polymorphonuclear leukocytes, including eosinophils and mast cells, was observed. These findings appear to be related to frequent high-dose administration of rhuIL-4 above the recognized MTD.

The immunologic effects of rhuIL-4 are quite variable. Absolute lymphocyte counts decrease during rhuIL-4 therapy[295]; however, flow cytometry studies have not demonstrated consistent and reproducible changes in distribution of lymphocyte phenotypes.[290,295,296] Lymphocyte cytolytic activities (NK, LAK) are not augmented or induced, and occasional increases in proliferative responses produced by mitogens or rIL-2 have been reported.[290]

Administration of high doses of rhuIL-4 is not associated with increases in serum TNF-α or IL-1β levels but does produce significant elevations of IL-1ra.[295] Soluble CD23 levels also increase with rhuIL-4 therapy.[295] No alterations in serum immunoglobulin levels have been noted,[295] and antibody production to rhuIL-4 has not been seen.

In the phase I trials reported to date, no responses have been seen in patients with solid tumors. In patients with hematologic malignancies, tumor regression has been reported in individual patients with Hodgkin's disease and non-Hodgkin's lymphoma.[297] Experience to date is limited, however. Phase II studies involving patients with malignant melanoma, non–small cell lung cancer, and acquired immunodeficiency syndrome–related Kaposi's sarcoma have been reported. The results of these studies are summarized in Table 27-14. Limited activity of rhuIL-4 has been

noted, and no further investigation of its antitumor activities is planned.

TUMOR NECROSIS FACTOR

The observations of Dr. William Coley that patients who developed streptococcal infections occasionally had clinical tumor regressions and his use of bacterial extracts to treat patients with advanced malignancies[303] was one of the earliest applications of biologic therapy as a treatment for cancer. Shear et al.[304] used an extract of *Serratia marcescens* and noted hemorrhagic necrosis in mice bearing transplanted tumors. The responsible ingredient was identified as an LPS from bacterial cell walls. Carswell and colleagues[305] then identified a factor termed *tumor necrosis factor* in the sera of mice receiving LPS that produced hemorrhagic necrosis in transplanted murine Meth A sarcoma tumors. An *in vitro* bioassay using cytotoxicity of these sera for specific tumor cell lines was developed, followed by purification and cloning of human TNF, and subsequent large-scale production of recombinant TNF-α.

Coincidentally, lymphotoxin, a cytolytic protein produced by lymphocytes, was recognized.[306] It shows 30% homology with TNF-α and appears to share the same receptor.[307] This cytokine has been termed tumor necrosis factor β (TNF-β) and along with TNF-α has been implicated in monocyte- and lymphocyte-mediated tumor cell killing. Clinical trials with TNF-α have been performed, and its properties are discussed in this section. For a discussion of TNF-β, the reader is referred to reviews of lymphotoxin.[308]

Structure and Mechanisms of Action

The TNF-α gene is located on chromosome 6 in the 6p23 segment.[309] It is approximately 3 kb in length and is comprised of four exons, the last of which encodes over 80% of the secreted protein. TNF-α production is a two-step process, with gene transcription and translation tightly controlled. The basal level of TNF gene expression in human monocytes is minimal[310] and is enhanced by agents such as LPS[311] or 12-O-tetradecanoylphorbol 13-acetate. PGE₂ and cyclic nucleotides appear to be mediators of TNF gene regulation,[312] and phosphoesterase inhibitors such as pentoxifylline block TNF production.[313] Secretion of TNF-α protein is regulated by a separate process and appears to require additional signals.[314] A variety of inducers have been identified and include endotoxin, calcium ionophores, and Fc-receptor cross-linking.[315,316] Inhibitors of the secretory process have also been found and include botulinum D toxin.[317]

Secreted TNF-α contains 154 to 157 amino acids and one disulfide bridge. It is initially synthesized as a proprotein containing 230 amino acids[318] and may exist as a transmembrane surface protein that is cytotoxic to TNF-sensitive cells. Cleavage of the proprotein results in the secretion of a mature TNF protein containing 157 amino acids. Purified natural or recombinant TNF exists in solution as a trimer and under denaturing condition has a molecular weight of 17 kd.[319,320]

As with other cytokines, TNF acts through specific cell surface receptors that bind both TNF-α and TNF-β.[307] Most cells contain TNF receptors (TNFRs); however, the density varies from 200 to 7,000.[321] Once TNF binds to its receptor, the complex is internalized and degraded.[322] Studies have identified two receptor proteins (TNFR1 and TNFR2) with molecular weights of 55 kd and 75 kd[323] that are also shed into the circulation. TNFR1 (p55) can trigger either an apoptotic or an antiapoptotic pathway. The binding of TNF-α to TNFR1 causes the dimerization of receptor death domains in the cytoplasmic tail.[324] The adaptor molecule TNFR-associated death domain (TRADD) interacts with the activated receptor.[325] This interaction then leads to the recruitment of TNF-associated factor 2 (TRAF-2) and receptor-interacting protein (RIP), which results in the activation of the transcription factors NF-κB and JNK/AP-1.[325-327] The signaling pathway for the activation of NF-κB via TNFR1, in which TRAF-2 and RIP can activate the NF-κB kinase NIK, which then activates the IKKα, β, γ, has been relatively well characterized.[34,325,327] This enzyme complex is responsible for the phosphorylation of the IκBα and IκBβ inhibitors, which leads to their polyubiquitination and degradation by the 26S proteasome.[328] Activation of the death pathway results from the recruitment by TNFR1–bound TRADD of another death domain–containing protein, FADD.[325,328] FADD couples the TNFR1–TRADD complex with the activation of procaspase 8 to the active form, which in turn activates effector caspases and results in apoptosis.[328] Unlike with TNFR1, the cytoplasmic domains of TNFR2 directly bind TRAF to induce NF-κB activation and promote cell survival.[326-328] Because TNFR2 does not bind TRADD family members, it does not appear to play a major role in the induction of apoptosis.[328] The density of TNF receptors on cells is also regulated. Type I interferons and IFN-γ increase expression,[329,330] and agents such as LPS and IL-1 down-regulate this protein.[331]

The probable role of TNF-α in the pathogenesis of various disease such as rheumatoid arthritis and in the toxicity produced by cytokines such as rIL-2 led to investigation of approaches to decrease toxicity. One of these uses administration of soluble TNF receptors (sTNFR). Etanercept produced by Immunex (Seattle, WA) is a genetically engineered fusion protein consisting of two identical chains of recombinant TNFR p75 monomer fused with the Fc domain of human immunoglobulin G1.[332] This preparation binds and inactivates TNF. It has been shown to be effective therapy for rheumatoid arthritis.[333,334] In addition, it has been used unsuccessfully in patients receiving high-dose rIL-2 to ameliorate toxicity.[138]

Cellular Pharmacology

The *in vitro* activities of TNF are pleiotropic. The best recognized are antiproliferative effects on a wide range of human and murine tumor cell lines.[335] Cytolytic and cytostatic effects have both been described. The antiproliferative effects are measured *in vitro* by growth inhibition or cytotoxicity assays,[336] which are also used to define a unit of TNF activity. Cell surface receptors are required for these activities, but the receptor density does not correlate with the sensitivity of cells to TNF-α effects.[337]

In some cell types, TNF-α can induce apoptosis; however, most cells are protected from apoptosis due to the expression of NF-κB–regulated antiapoptotic genes.[338,339] The inhibition of protein synthesis of the selective inhibitors of the antiapoptotic genes makes cells susceptible to TNF-α–mediated apoptosis.[328] TNF-α also can affect differentiation of various cell types. One early observation indicated that TNF-α reversed adipocyte differentiation, which resulted in "dedifferentiation."[340] Proliferation of hematopoietic precursors such as colony-forming unit granulocyte erythroid monocyte-megakaryocyte (CFU-GEMM), colony-forming unit granulocyte-macrophage (CFU-GM) and erythroid burst-forming unit is inhibited,[341,342] and in HL-60 cells monocyte differentiation is promoted.[343] TNF also has mitogenic properties, and in normal fibroblast cultures increases DNA synthesis.[344] The growth of a wide variety of other human tumor cells is stimulated by TNF.[345]

The immunomodulatory effects of TNF-α have also been well studied and include variable effects on T and B lymphocytes, mononuclear phagocytes, and neutrophils. Table 27-15 summarizes some of the reported effects. TNF-α appears to act as an activation signal for various classes of leukocytes during the inflammatory response.

Finally, TNF-α up-regulates a variety of different molecules on the surface of endothelial cells, including class I MHC antigens[346] and leukocyte adhesion molecules (ELAM-1, ICAM-1).[347,348] Production of various inflammatory mediators such as IL-1,[349] platelet-activating factor,[350] and IL-6[351] are also enhanced by TNF-α.

Clinical Pharmacokinetics

In view of the hemorrhagic necrosis produced by TNF preparations and the multiple *in vitro* effects suggesting

TABLE 27-15. IMMUNOMODULATORY EFFECTS OF TUMOR NECROSIS FACTOR α (TNF-α)

Cell Type	Effect
Monocytes	TNF-α production, secretion of cytokines (IL-1, IL-6, G-CSF, GM-CSF)
Macrophages	Superoxide production, secretion of chemoattractants, increased HLA-DR expression, increased proliferation, secretion of PGE_2, secretion of thromboxane
Lymphocytes	Increased IL-2R, enhanced proliferation, increased production of G-CSF/GM-CSF/M-CSF, increased LAK activity, decreased NK activity, TNFR up-regulated, immunoglobulin secretion
Neutrophils	Increased H_2O_2 production, increased phagocytic activity, enhanced adherence, enhanced ADCC

ADCC, antibody-dependent cell-mediated cytotoxicity; G-CSF, granulocyte colony-stimulating factor; GM-CSF, granulocyte-macrophage colony-stimulating factor; IL, interleukin; IL-2R, interleukin 2 receptor; LAK, lymphokine-activated killer cells; M-CSF, macrophage colony-stimulating factor; NK, natural killer cells; PGE_2, prostaglandin E_2; TNFR, tumor necrosis factor receptor.
Based on Logan TF, Gooding WE, Whiteside TL, et al. Biologic response modulation by tumor necrosis factor alpha (TNF alpha) in a phase Ib trial in cancer patients. *J Immunother* 1997;20:387–398; and Spriggs DR. Tumor necrosis factor: basic principles and preclinical studies. In: DeVita VT Jr, Hellman S, Rosenberg SA, eds. *Biologic therapy of cancer*. Philadelphia: JB Lippincott, 1989:361–370.

potential antitumor properties of this agent, initial clinical trials were performed in patients with advanced malignancies. Because of endotoxin contamination of purified natural TNF-α, the various recombinant preparations listed in Table 27-16 have been used. They contain from 155 to 157 amino acid residues and have specific activities from 2.2×10^6 to 4.0×10^7 U per mg protein. Two varieties of recombinant TNF-α (rTNF-α) are found, one containing 155 and the other 157 amino acid residues. The two types are identical except for the addition of a Val-Arg sequence at the N-terminus of the smaller molecule. The biologic activities of these preparations are similar[320]; however, specific activities vary.

Phase I trials of rTNF-α preparations involving over 500 patients have been conducted and have used a variety

TABLE 27-16. RECOMBINANT TUMOR NECROSIS FACTOR α PREPARATIONS USED IN CLINICAL TRIALS

Source	Amino Acid Residues	Specific Activity (U/mg protein)	Nature of Product
Dainippon Pharmaceutical	155	3×10^6	Lyophilized
Asahi	155	2.2×10^6	Lyophilized
Genentech	157	4×10^7	Liquid
Cetus	157	25×10^6	Liquid
Knoll	157	8.2×10^6	Lyophilized

Adapted from Taguchi T, Sohmura Y. Clinical studies with TNF. *Biotherapy* 1991;3:177–186, with permission.

TABLE 27-17. PHASE I CLINICAL TRIALS OF RECOMBINANT HUMAN TUMOR NECROSIS FACTOR α

Total no. patients:	529	
Routes/schedules used:	i.v.b. × 1 d	
	0.5- to 120-h i.v. infusion over 1–5 d	
	i.m.	
	s.c.	
	Alternating s.c.–i.v. or i.m.–i.v.	
Dose ranges:	1–818 μg/m²/d	
Maximum tolerated doses:	Schedule	Dose (μg/m²)
	i.v. single bolus	227–818 μg/m²
	24-h i.v. × 1 d	200 μg/m²
	24-h i.v. × 5 d	160 μg/m²
	i.m. 3 × 1 wk	150 μg/m²
	s.c. 5 × 1 wk	150 μg/m²

i.v.b., intravenous bolus.
Adapted from Taguchi T, Sohmura Y. Clinical studies with TNF. *Biotherapy* 1991;3:177–186; and Mittelman A, Puccio C, Gafney E, et al. A phase I pharmacokinetic study of recombinant human tumor necrosis factor administered by a 5-day continuous infusion. *Invest New Drugs* 1992;10:183–190.

of administration routes and schedules. These are summarized in Table 27-17. The MTD identified in most trials is less than 200 μg per m² per day and may vary with the route of administration.

The measurement of TNF-α in bodily fluids has been performed using several different methods. Bioassays for detecting cytotoxicity in various cell lines including L-M cells,[352] L-929 cells,[353] and WEHI-164 cells[354] have been used and can detect TNF-α concentrations in sera as low as 50 pg per mL. Cell lysis is measured by either crystal violet dye uptake by residual viable cells[352] or tritium-labeled thymidine incorporation.[353] In addition, ELISA assays using polyclonal antibodies to TNF-α have been developed and can detect TNF-α at levels from 100 to 2,800 pg per mL.[354] Comparison of both methods for detection of serum levels of rTNF-α in several clinical studies[354,355] has demonstrated that they provide similar results.

Pharmacokinetic studies in rats and nonhuman primates have been performed. Pang et al.[356] administered ^{125}I-labeled and unlabeled rTNF-α (Genentech) to Sprague-Dawley rats. A biexponential clearance was found, with a $t_{1/2\alpha}$ of 5 minutes and a $t_{1/2\beta}$ of 30 minutes for unlabeled TNF-α. The ^{125}I-labeled cytokine had a prolonged β phase of 280 minutes, which suggests altered receptor binding and degradation *in vivo*. Similar results have been reported in mice.[357] In rhesus monkeys,[358] short-term infusion (0.5 hour) of rTNF-α (Genentech) at various doses was administered, and two different elimination mechanisms were found. At low doses, a saturable specific process was evident. At higher dose levels, a nonspecific nonsaturable process was found. This latter process was felt probably to represent glomerular filtration of

TABLE 27-18. PHARMACOKINETICS OF HUMAN RECOMBINANT TUMOR NECROSIS FACTOR α (rHuTNF-α) AFTER INTRAVENOUS ADMINISTRATION

Study	rHuTNF-α preparation	Schedule	Levels	$t_{1/2}$	C_{max}
Chapman et al.[363]	Genentech	i.v.b.	1–200 µg/m²	20 min	2.5–80.0 ng/mL
Feinberg et al.[364]	Genentech	30-min i.v. infusion	5–200 µg/m²	NS	20 pg/mL
Moritz et al.[355]	Knoll	10-min i.v. infusion	40–280 µg/m²	11–70 min	12 ng/mL
Blick et al.[354]	Genentech	i.v.b.	1–150 µg/m²	13.9–18.0 min	500–8,000 pg/mL
Creaven et al.[365]	Asahi	1-h i.v. infusion	1–48 × 10⁴ U/m²	0.20–0.72 h	NS
Mittelman et al.[361]	Knoll	24-h infusion	40–200 µg/m²	20–30 min	300–500 pg/mL
Spriggs et al.[362]	Asahi	24-h infusion	4.5–645 µg/m²	NS	90–900 pg/mL
Kimura et al.[360]	Asahi	30-min i.v. infusion	1–16 × 10⁵ U/m²	10–80 min	4.8–896.0 U/mL

C_{max}, highest observed concentration; i.v.b., intravenous bolus; NS, not stated; $t_{1/2}$, elimination half-life.

TNF-α. Similarly, in nephrectomized rats, clearance of rTNF-α was significantly reduced.[359]

In humans, rTNF-α has been administered by a variety of routes and schedules. Table 27-18 summarizes pharmacokinetic data for trials using intravenous administration. In the report by Blick et al.,[354] rTNF-α was given as an intravenous bolus, and the half-life did not appear to change with increasing doses. The volume of distribution decreased, however, and the AUC increased when doses were escalated (Table 27-19). These data suggest a one-compartment model as illustrated in Figure 27-7. In the reports by Moritz et al.[355] and Kimura et al.,[360] serum half-life and clearance increased with higher doses, which is consistent with a saturable receptor-mediated clearance mechanism. Administration of rTNF-α as a 24-hour continuous infusion[361] did not yield detectable serum TNF-α concentrations except at the highest dose levels (160 and 200 µg per m² per day). Serum levels were undetectable after 60 minutes. The influence of TNFR levels in serum and tissues on rTNF-α pharmacokinetics is uncertain; however, as with other cytokines, these may play a role in which clearance mechanisms are operative. Induction of TNF-α clearance mechanisms is also suggested by the observations during 24-hour continuous infusion of rTNF-α.[361,362]

The intramuscular and subcutaneous routes of administration for rTNF-α have also been investigated.[366] Blick et al.[354] administered doses from 5 to 200 µg per m². Unlike with the intravenous route, serum rTNF-α levels were not consistently detected until doses were higher than 150 µg per m². Peak serum levels were noted at 2 hours and occasionally persisted for 24 hours. Zamkoff et al.[367] administered rTNF-α (Chiron) subcutaneously at doses from 5 to 150 µg per m² per day. No serum rTNF-α levels were detected, even at the highest doses. Thus, these routes of administration produce lower or undetectable serum levels compared with the intravenous route.

Other modes of administration such as intratumoral, intraperitoneal, and regional have also been studied. These approaches were suggested by animal studies indicating

TABLE 27-19. PHARMACOKINETICS OF RECOMBINANT TUMOR NECROSIS FACTOR α (rTNF-α) AFTER INTRAVENOUS BOLUS ADMINISTRATION

rTNF-α Dose (µg/m²)	$t_{1/2}$ (min)	V_d (L)	AUC (ng · min/mL)
25	15.9 + 3.6	66 + 30	10.5 + 2.7
35	13.9 + 1.0	13.3 + 5.0	19.7 + 5.3
50	16.0 + 2.0	13.4 + 1.1	89.6 + 13.9
60	18.0 + 0.4	17.7 + 4.0	114.6 + 26.5
100	17 + 2	12 + 4	224.8 + 69.0

AUC, area under the concentration × time curve; $t_{1/2}$, elimination half-life; V_d, volume of distribution.
Values are expressed as mean + standard error of the mean.
Adapted from Saks S, Rosenblum S. Recombinant human TNF-α: preclinical studies and results from early clinical trials. *Immunol Ser* 1992;56:567–587, with permission.

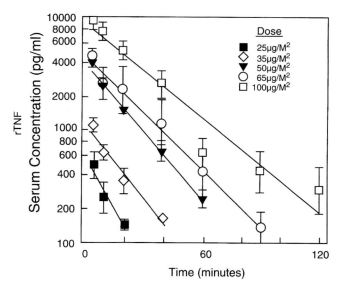

FIGURE 27-7. Serum disappearance of recombinant tumor necrosis factor (rTNF) after intravenous administration as measured by enzyme-linked immunosorbent assay. Symbols represent the mean blood levels for each dose for all patients at that dose. Standard error bars are shown unless insufficient data points were available. (From Blick M, Sherwin SA, Rosenblum M, et al. Phase I study of recombinant tumor necrosis factor in cancer patients. *Cancer Res* 1987;47:2986–2989, with permission.)

that high levels of TNF are required for antitumor effects.[368] Pfreundschuh et al.[369] administered escalating doses of rTNF-α as a single intralesional injection to cancer patients. The MTD was 391 μg per m[2], and detectable serum levels of rTNF-α were found at higher doses, consistent with systemic absorption. Intraperitoneal instillation of rTNF-α in patients with advanced gastrointestinal tumors and ovarian carcinoma has been reported.[370] Prolonged TNF-α levels in ascitic fluid without detectable serum levels were seen.

Finally, intraarterial administration of rTNF has been investigated. Hepatic artery infusion of TNF-α[371] produced tumor regressions in 14% of patients with liver metastases, but the MTD of TNF-α was not altered compared with intravenous administration. Use of TNF-α in isolated limb perfusion in an attempt to increase local TNF-α concentrations without systemic exposure has also been studied.[372] The rTNF-α was administered to three patients at doses of 2.0, 3.0, and 4.0 μg for 90 minutes via isolated extremity perfusion. Serum levels of TNF-α during perfusion never exceeded 62 ng per mL. Perfusate levels of TNF-α varied between 970 and 2,000 ng per mL (ELISA) with no apparent decay. Higher, more stable levels of TNF-α appear to be maintained using this route of administration than with systemic administration. When TNF-α is administered in this fashion, doses exceeding the MTD can be given; however, severe systemic toxicity occurs. The stable concentrations maintained in the perfusate are therefore of interest.

Clinical Effects and Toxicity

The role of TNF in homeostasis predicts that a sepsis-like clinical syndrome would result from its administration. In humans, the toxicity seen is dose related except for fever and chills, which have occurred even at low doses. The fever appears rapidly after administration and generally resolves within several hours.[354,355] Additional systemic toxicities include anorexia, fatigue, malaise, and myalgia.

The initial hemodynamic effects of intravenous TNF-α include tachycardia and hypertension, followed within several hours by hypotension. This has been the dose-limiting toxicity reported in most trials and becomes less severe with repeated administration. The mechanisms responsible for the hypotension are unclear but may include myocardial depression,[373] vascular endothelial changes,[374] and secondary secretion of IL-1 and IL-6.[375,376]

Hematologic toxicity includes thrombocytopenia, which has been dose limiting in several reports.[360,367,377] This is generally mild, and in all instances recovery occurred within 24 to 48 hours after rTNF-α discontinuation. Leukopenia has been noted at 30 to 90 minutes after injection[359,360] and quickly returns to baseline or higher (neutrophilia). These findings resemble those reported with other cytokines such as GM-CSF. The changes in leukocyte

and platelet counts have generally not been associated with either bleeding or infection. Coagulation parameters such as prothrombin time and activated partial thromboplastin time remain normal, and mild elevations of fibrin degradation products have been seen.[378]

Hepatic toxicity is also common, with increased levels of transaminase, alkaline phosphatase, and total bilirubin reported.[320] These have generally returned to normal or baseline during continued therapy. In several instances,[360,379] however, these changes were dose limiting. Mild renal toxicity in the form of slight elevation of blood urea nitrogen and creatinine may occur[355,360] but is felt to be of little clinical significance.

Other less frequent toxicities reported include confusion, somnolence, hallucinations, and speech defects.[354,380] Pulmonary toxicity is rare, with occasional reports of dyspnea[381,382] and decreased carbon monoxide diffusing capacity.[382] The metabolic changes developing during rTNF-α therapy include increases in serum triglycerides and reciprocal decreases in cholesterol.[364] Although weight loss has been noted in animal studies with rTNF-α,[383] this has not been a significant finding in human studies.

Administration of rTNF as a subcutaneous or intramuscular injection has a similar toxicity spectrum.[363,367,384,385] In contrast to intravenous injection, these routes are also associated with pain and induration at the injection sites. Subcutaneous administration also induces erythema and vesiculation associated with neutrophil and mononuclear cell infiltration.[363,367]

Regional rTNF-α administration has similar toxicity. Hepatic artery infusion produces effects resembling those seen during intravenous administration. Isolated limb perfusion with doses of rTNF-α from 2.0 to 4.0 μg also produces systemic side effects, with hypotension, tachycardia, fever, chills, and renal toxicity noted.[372] Use of hydration with prophylactic dopamine in these patients has controlled the cardiovascular complications, however.

The immunologic effects of rTNF-α administration in humans have been well characterized. Chapman et al.[363] reported mild elevation of the acute-phase reactant C-reactive protein during rTNF-α administration. Delayed hypersensitivity to various antigens has been examined in 26 patients, six of whom were anergic before rTNF-α therapy.[385] Three of these latter patients then developed positive skin tests during therapy. NK and LAK activity in peripheral blood has also been studied.[148,384,386] Significant depression at 48 hours was noted during a 120-hour continuous infusion of rTNF-α, with subsequent increases above baseline.[384,386] Decreases in IL-2–inducible LAK cells have also been reported.[387] Monocyte studies[388] have demonstrated increases in hydrogen peroxide production after intravenous therapy with rTNF-α. Studies of lymphocyte subsets demonstrate decreases in percentages of CD8[+] and CD56[+] cells, with increases in CD4[+] and CD19[+] subsets.[387] Secondary increases in IL-6,[334] G-CSF,[389] and macrophage colony-stimulating factor (M-CSF)[389] serum concentrations after TNF-α administration have also been noted. The increases in these latter two hematopoietic growth factors coincided temporally with the leukocytosis seen during TNF-α infusion.

In contrast to the hemorrhagic necrosis of tumors seen in murine tumor models, the clinical antitumor effects of systemically administered rTNF have been minimal. Responses have been reported in phase I trials in patients with non-Hodgkin's lymphoma,[390] gastric carcinoma,[320] hepatoma,[320] renal cell carcinoma,[379] breast cancer,[362] and pancreatic cancer.[390] Phase II trials of rTNF treatment of most of these malignancies,[391] however, have not demonstrated significant clinical activity. The apparent differences between the effects in murine and human tumors may be related to the tolerance of mice to much larger doses of rTNF-α than humans. Estimates are that a dose of 5 μg, which produces hemorrhagic necrosis of murine tumors, is equivalent to 1,000 μg per m² of rTNF-α in humans.[392] This represents a fivefold greater dose than the MTD of rTNF-α in humans, which is 200 μg per m². The responses seen with intratumor injection of rTNF-α appear more frequent[320] and would suggest that this differential tolerance may be an important factor in the lack of antitumor effects clinically.

The local administration of TNF-α has been investigated as a strategy to minimize systemic toxicity and serum levels, increase local concentrations, and concomitantly increase the antitumor effects of this cytokine. Intraperitoneal administration in patients with ascites and ovarian carcinoma has been evaluated in a small randomized trial.[393] The recombinant human TNF-α was given at a dose of 0.06 mg per m² intraperitoneally after paracentesis at weekly intervals (× 3) and compared with paracentesis alone. Intraperitoneal instillation was well tolerated, with pain in 42.1% of patients, fever and chills in 36.9%, and hypotension in 5.3%. Responses were not seen in either group.

TNF-α has also been used to perfuse extremities and the hepatic circulation. Limb perfusion using IFN-γ, TNF-α, and melphalan in patients with nonresectable sarcomas has been reported.[394] In a series of 55 patients, complete responses were seen in 18%, partial responses in 64%, and no change in 18%. Limb salvage was achieved in 84%. Systemic side effects were moderate. In contrast with this experience, hepatic perfusion with TNF-α with or without chemotherapy has produced significant systemic toxicity.[395] The use of TNF-α perfusion techniques has also been explored for primary renal cell carcinoma.[396] The clinical utility of this approach is uncertain.

Drug Interactions

Preclinical studies have indicated that combining rTNF-α with other cytokines or chemotherapeutic agents may enhance the results. IFN-γ produces an up-regulation of TNFR on various cells *in vitro*,[307] and therefore rTNF-α and IFN-γ have been combined in phase I studies. Dose-limiting toxicity has included hyperbilirubinemia,[397] hypotension,[398] and acute dyspnea with hypoxemia.[398] The MTD for rTNF-α in these trials is less than 156 μg per m² per day, which suggests synergistic toxicity. In murine models, the combination of rTNF-α and rIL-2 has had significant antitumor effects.[399,400] Clinical trials of this combination have been conducted to determine toxicity.[149] In addition, rTNF-α has been administered with rIL-2 and IFN-α in a phase I trial.[401] Patients received 40 to 120 μg per m² of rTNF-α on days 1 through 5, and fixed doses of rIL-2 (1 to 3 × 10⁶ IU per m² on days 1 through 5, days 8 through 12, and days 15 through 19) and IFN-α (9 × 10⁶ IU per m² three times a week). Systemic toxicity was substantial, but outpatient administration was felt to be possible.

TNF-α shows synergy with a variety of chemotherapeutic compounds *in vitro*, including doxorubicin[402] and cisplatin.[403] Synergistic *in vitro* cytotoxicity against tumor cells has also been noted with combinations of rTNF-α and topoisomerase II inhibitors such as etoposide and dactinomycin (actinomycin D or DACT).[404,405] Phase I trials of rTNF-α and etoposide have been conducted.[406] Regional administration of rTNF-α in combination with melphalan[394] has been used. Clinical results suggest that the combination has significant activity; however, randomized studies are now required.

INTERLEUKIN 12

Interleukin 12 (IL-12), originally named natural killer cell stimulatory factor (NKSF)[407] and cytotoxic lymphocyte maturation factor (CLMF)[408] by the respective groups identifying its multiple activities, was first isolated as a molecule secreted from Epstein-Barr virus–transformed B-cell lines. Early characterization revealed that this protein could act synergistically with IL-2 to augment cytotoxic lymphocyte responses,[409] could cause the proliferation of mitogen-activated peripheral blood lymphoblasts,[410] and could induce IFN-γ secretion by resting peripheral blood lymphocytes.[411]

Structure and Mechanisms of Action

On purification, IL-12 was determined to be a 70-kd disulfide-linked heterodimeric protein composed of two polypeptides with approximate molecular weights of 35 and 40 kd.[407,412,413] Characterization of the cDNAs encoding the subunits revealed that the p35 component was a 219–amino acid polypeptide containing seven cysteine residues and three potential *N*-glycosylation sites, whereas the p40 molecule was composed of 328 amino acids, ten of which are cysteines, with four possible glycosylation sites.[414–416] The mature protein encoded by the p35 cDNA has an actual molecular weight of 27,500 but appears larger on sodium dodecyl sulfate polyacrylamide gel electrophoresis (SDS-PAGE) due to its extensive glycosylation. Mature p40 has a calculated molecular weight of 34,700 and is comparatively less glycosylated than the mature p35 molecule.[414–416]

The heterodimeric structure of IL-12 is unique among the cytokines.[417] Although transfection of cell lines with cDNAs encoding either the p35 or p40 IL-12 polypeptides results in synthesis and secretion of the respective individual molecules, expression of active, secreted IL-12 requires that the same cell be cotransfected with both cDNAs.[418] Interestingly, expression studies suggest that the p35 gene is synthesized by numerous cell types of both hematopoietic and nonhematopoietic origin,[418,419] but that active IL-12 is secreted by only those cells that also transcribe p40.[418] Thus p40 likely is required for the efficient export of the p70 molecule. Reports indicate that the p40 polypeptide is produced in large excess of the IL-12 heterodimer[419] and that secreted p40 homodimers may even act as IL-12 antagonists.[420] The actual physiologic significance or importance of p40 overexpression and homodimerization, however, remain largely unknown.

The genes encoding the p40 and p35 subunits are completely unrelated and have been mapped to different chromosomes.[421] The p35 gene maps to human chromosome band 3p12-3q13.2.[421] It has a primary amino acid sequence that is suggestive of a richly α-helical protein and hence in this regard is similar to most other cytokines.[418] Indeed, many of the amino acid positions conserved between IL-6 and GM-CSF are also shared by the IL-12 p35 subunit.[422] The p40 gene has been mapped to human chromosome band 5q31-q33 and, although not homologous to any known cytokines, does strongly resemble members of the hematopoietic cytokine receptor family.[421] The p40 sequence has particularly strong homologies with the extracellular regions of receptors for IL-6 and ciliary neurotropic factor,[415,423] and is closely linked genetically to the M-CSF receptor.[421] The p70 heterodimer thus has the characteristics of a disulfide-linked complex between a cytokine and a receptor.[418]

Cellular Pharmacology

A number of different cell types are important sources of IL-12. Among normal peripheral blood mononuclear cells, monocytes and monocyte-derived macrophages are perhaps the most significant producers of the cytokine,[419,424] although the production of IL-12 by dendritic cells during antigen presentation is the crucial signal for induction of a T_H1 response pattern and effective cell-mediated immunity.[418,424–426] Some studies now also suggest that IL-12 is the requisite "third signal" that participates with class I MHC/antigen complexes and B7 to induce the proliferation and activation of naive CD8+ T cells[427] and, hence, the cytolytic component of antitumor function. Neutrophils have also been shown to make IL-12,[428] although some controversy exists as to whether non-

transformed B cells are also a physiologically relevant source of the molecule.[428,429] Langerhans cells,[430] murine mast cells,[431] and keratinocytes[432] have also been reported to produce IL-12 under some stimulatory conditions.

The most potent inducers of IL-12 are bacteria, microbial components such as LPS, and intracellular parasites.[419,425,426] IL-12 production was found to be significantly enhanced when peripheral blood mononuclear cells were stimulated with Gram-positive and Gram-negative bacteria, endotoxin, *Mycobacterium tuberculosis*, *Mycobacterium leprae*, and *Toxoplasma gondii*.[419] LPS has also been shown to induce IL-12 synthesis by polymorphonuclear leukocytes.[426]

In addition to being modulated by the components of pathogens, IL-12 synthesis is also positively and negatively regulated by various cytokines. IFN-γ and GM-CSF are both capable of stimulating IL-12 production by phagocytic cells,[433] although, interestingly, the p35 and p40 polypeptide components of IL-12 seem to be differentially induced: Although IFN-γ directly stimulates the accumulation of p35 mRNA by monocytes and neutrophils, it can only augment the LPS-induced synthesis of p40 mRNA by those same cell types.[433,434] Among the cytokines with inhibitory effects on IL-12 are IL-10, IL-4, and TGF-β.[435,436] These products mediate their effects at the level of both RNA and protein, as they inhibit the secretion of the p70 heterodimeric protein as well as the accumulation of mRNAs encoding the p35 and p40 polypeptides.[435,436] The IL-10–mediated inhibition of IFN-γ production by T and NK cells has been demonstrated to occur indirectly through its ability to prevent IL-12 synthesis by phagocytic cells.[417,435]

Membrane-bound ligands present on activated T lymphocytes also stimulate phagocytes to synthesize and secrete IL-12.[437–439] Although they are not yet fully defined, at least several receptor-ligand interactions have been characterized that mediate this induction. Perhaps most significant in this regard is the augmented production of IL-12 by antigen-presenting cells on engagement of their CD40 receptor by CD40 ligand (CD40L) expressed on antigen [phytohemagglutinin (PHA)]–stimulated T cells.[437,439] The importance of this CD40/CD40L binding in mediation of IL-12 induction has been demonstrated for both murine and human cells. In human peripheral blood mononuclear cells, CD40/CD40L interactions stimulated IFN-γ production via an IL-12–dependent mechanism when the mononuclear cells were first optimally prestimulated with PHA.[439] Direct CD28 engagement can also stimulate IFN-γ production and does so in an IL-12–dependent fashion by two different mechanisms: either by increasing CD40L expression on T cells, which then stimulate CD40 receptors and IL-12 synthesis by antigen-presenting cells, or by augmenting the levels of the IL-12 receptor β1 (IL-12Rβ1) chain on T cells and hence the capacity of IL-12 to bind to their receptors.[439] Some suggestion also exists, however, that CD28/B7 interactions can enhance IFN-γ synthesis independently of IL-12. Evidence for cooperation of the

CD40L/CD40 and B7/CD28 pathways for stimulating IL-12 expression comes from studies performed under conditions of low B7 expression (inadequate antigen or PHA concentrations), in which CD40L-stimulated IL-12 production was found to be enhanced by anti-CD28.[439]

Cells expressing IL-12 receptors (IL-12Rs) were originally identified using fluorescent anti–IL-12 antibodies to detect the cell-bound cytokine. Using this technique, IL-12R were observed on activated NK cells and T cells but not on B cells or resting T cells.[440] When IL-12 was added to peripheral blood mononuclear cells and cross-linked after binding, anti–IL-12 antibodies immunoprecipitated a single protein of approximately 110 kd that was purported to be the IL-12 receptor.[440] Subsequent expression cloning studies identified what were believed to be two distinct low-affinity IL-12 receptors, which together reportedly formed a high-affinity binding site.[441] Each was characterized as having the general composition of a β-type cytokine receptor subunit and as being a gp130-like member of the cytokine receptor family.[441] Thus originally the functional high-affinity IL-12 receptor was thought to be composed of these two subunits, each of which independently exhibited a low affinity for IL-12.[442]

Additional studies have determined that the functional IL-12 receptor is a heterodimer composed of a β1 and β2 polypeptide, and that each mediates a specific activity requisite to IL-12 responsiveness.[443,444] IL-12Rβ1 is the polypeptide that binds IL-12,[445] and the β2 chain is the component that transduces the IL-12 signal into the nucleus.[444,446,447] Normal T_H1 cells express both chains and hence are fully IL-12 responsive. T_H2 cells express only the IL-12Rβ1 chain, and although they thus bind IL-12 with high affinity, no reactivity to the cytokine is exhibited with the absence of signal transduction capacity.[444,448] Indeed, the selective loss of IL-12Rβ2 expression is an important correlate of T_H2 cell differentiation,[443] and ongoing T_H1 responses can be inhibited by immunosuppressive cytokines that act by negatively regulating that molecule.[449–451] IFN-γ and IFN-α have been shown to induce IL-12Rβ2 expression in the mouse and human, respectively.[446] Others have reported that the expression of both IL-12Rβ1 and IL-12Rβ2 mRNA is increased in the lymph nodes of naive mice after systemic administration of recombinant IL-12.[443] The notion that the IL-12 inductive effect on IL-12Rβ2 mRNA is mediated indirectly through IFN-γ was suggested by the observation that in IFN-γ receptor –/– mice, β2 mRNA levels were significantly lower than in wild-type mice after IL-12 treatment.[452] Several pathologic conditions are characterized by predominantly T_H2 cell populations, and lymphocytes from such individuals display no IL-12Rβ2 chains due to their high production of IL-4, interleukin 5 (IL-5), IL-10, and TGF-β.[444,451] Antibodies to TGF-β and IL-10 restore IL-12Rβ2 chain synthesis and IFN-γ production[451] by these peripheral blood lymphocytes *in vitro*, which supports the notion that T_H1 protective responses are highly dependent on adequate expression levels of IL-12 receptor components. It is perhaps because of its potent immunostimulatory effects that IL-12 has its activity stringently regulated at both the agonist (see earlier) and receptor levels.

The binding of IL-12 to its receptor induces dimerization of the component IL-12Rβ1 and IL-12Rβ2 chains, which leads to the interaction of their receptor-associated Jak2 tyrosine kinases.[453] These kinases mediate each other's transactivation,[454] which allows the now-functional enzymes to phosphorylate tyrosine residue 800 in the IL-12Rβ2 chain cytoplasmic region.[447] Signal transduction and transcription-activating factor 4 (STAT4) has specificity for the resulting unique phosphorylated peptide sequence on IL-12Rβ2 [GpYLPSNID, where pY represents phosphotyrosine, and the core G-pY(800)-L is the critical motif for binding][447,455] and is itself phosphorylated by Jak2 on binding by its SH2 domain to this receptor site.[455] Phosphorylated STAT4 molecules dimerize and migrate to the nucleus, where they bind specific DNA sequences and activate transcription of proinflammatory genes that stimulate T_H1 responses.[456,457] The requirement for STAT4 in IL-12–mediated responses was demonstrated by experiments indicating that IL-12–dependent increases in IFN-γ production, cellular proliferation, and NK cell cytotoxicity were abrogated in lymphocytes from STAT4-deficient mice.[458] The involvement of both Jak2 and tyrosine kinase 2 (Tyk2) in the IL-12 pathway[453,454,459,460] is circumstantially supported by the finding that TGF-β inhibits IL-12–induced phosphorylation of Jak2, Tyk2, and STAT4, and that TGF-β also inhibits IL-12–induced IFN-γ production.[460] The possibility that Jak2 or Tyk2 molecules can independently mediate STAT4 phosphorylation is suggested by data indicating that tyrosine phosphorylation of STAT4 is not abrogated when either Tyk2 alone or Jak2 alone is inhibited.[459]

As discussed briefly above, IL-12 was originally isolated as a cytokine that induced proliferation and cytolytic activity of NK cells, LAK cells, and cytolytic T lymphocytes. This stimulatory activity is now known to be specific for T cells and NK cells preactivated with either antireceptor antibody,[461] mitogens, or IL-2,[410] as freshly isolated peripheral blood T cells exhibit minimal responsiveness to IL-12.[461] The requirement for activation is related to the absence of IL-12Rs on resting cells[461] and their induction on mitogenic stimulation.[461–463] T-cell activation is also necessary to induce components of the transduction pathway (STAT4) required for IL-12 signaling.[461] Use of purified T-cell clones and PHA-stimulated T-cell subpopulations indicates that both CD4+ and CD8+ T-cell subsets are susceptible to IL-12 stimulation.[407,409,413,464–467]

IL-12 has a pivotal role in establishing the T_H1 versus T_H2 balance of a developing immune response.[468–470] Dendritic cells processing foreign antigen in peripheral tissues migrate to lymph nodes and, by secreting IL-12, induce

IFN-γ production by NK cells, and IFN-γ and IL-2 synthesis by antigen-stimulated T cells.[417,468–472] Dendritic cell–derived IL-12 is also capable of acting synergistically with the induced IFN-γ to steer naive T-cell precursors towards $T_H 1$ cellular immune responses,[428] and with IL-2 to further augment IFN-γ production and cytotoxic lymphocyte responses.[407,410,413]

In addition to stimulating $T_H 1$ activity by naive cells,[417] IL-12 also has been shown to transform preexisting $T_H 2$ responses into responses with an effective $T_H 1$ cellular component. Such activity was particularly noteworthy in a murine infectious disease model in which the characteristic detrimental $T_H 2$ response was converted into a predominantly curative cellular response after systemic administration of IL-12.[473] That IL-12 can reverse $T_H 2$ responses is somewhat paradoxical, as $T_H 2$ cells secrete large quantities of IL-4, IL-5, and IL-10,[417] cytokines known to strongly down-regulate the signaling IL-12Rβ2 chain of the IL-12 receptor. Whether this reversal is mediated by the purported capacity of IL-12 to induce transient, low-level production of IFN-γ by $T_H 2$ clones[473–475] or rather by the initiation of an overlapping $T_H 1$ immune response capable of dominating the preexisting $T_H 2$ activity is unclear. The determination that IFN-γ inhibits IL-4, IL-5, and IL-10 synthesis by $T_H 2$ cells suggests the possibility that IL-12 mediates its anti-$T_H 2$ effects indirectly via stimulation of IFN-γ production by NK cells.[476]

IL-12 has been shown to be an effective antitumor agent in a number of murine models, including the renal cell carcinoma RENCA,[477,478] CT-26 colon adenocarcinoma,[478,479] MCA-105 sarcoma,[480] M5076 reticulum cell sarcoma, B16-F10 melanoma,[477] MC38/colon carcinoma,[480] KA 31 sarcoma,[481] OV-HM ovarian carcinoma,[482] HTH-K breast carcinoma,[483] MBT-2 bladder carcinoma,[484] MB-48 transitional cell carcinoma,[484] as well as others. Numerous studies have now demonstrated that IL-12 therapy results in inhibition of tumor growth, reduction of metastatic lesions, increased survival time, and in some models regression of and resistance to secondary challenge with the same tumor.[477,484] IL-12 is distinctive among cytokines displaying antitumor activity in that it often has proven effective even when therapy is initiated weeks after establishment of a significant tumor burden.[477,478,484,485] An exception to this pattern is the HTH-K breast carcinoma model, against which IL-12 mediated measurable antitumor activity only when administered 3 days but not 7 days after tumor cell inoculation.[483]

IL-12 has no direct cytotoxicity or antiproliferative effect on cultured tumor cells, which indicates that its antitumor effect is mediated indirectly through IL-12–inducible cellular and molecular intermediates.[477] One molecule induced by and central to IL-12 activity is IFN-γ, as antibodies to that protein essentially abrogate IL-12–mediated antitumor function.[480,486,487] Interestingly, although IFN-γ is required for IL-12 activity, administration of exogenous IFN-γ does not mediate the potent antitumor function characteristic of IL-12.[488] Several factors may explain this paradox, including the differential half-lives of the two cytokines and the more limited capacity of IFN-γ to reach the tumor site: Whereas IFN-γ receptors are ubiquitously expressed on numerous cell types outside the tumor environment, IL-12 receptors are limited to NK cells and activated T cells.[488] Thus, compared with IFN-γ, systemically administered IL-12 is much less apt to be completely consumed by cells irrelevant to the antitumor immune response before reaching the specific effector cell types that will ultimately mediate function.[488]

Many investigators have shown that IL-12 enhances NK and cytolytic T-lymphocyte activity, stimulates antigen-primed T cells to proliferate and differentiate into $T_H 1$ cells, and induces NK cells and sensitized T cells to secrete IFN-γ. One study demonstrated that a preexisting CD8 and NK cell tumor infiltrate is required for maximal efficacy of IL-12–mediated antitumor therapy.[488] The suggestion was made that these IL-12–responsive cells synthesize IFN-γ within the tumor bed, which induces the local molecular events required for tumor eradication.[488] This hypothesis would explain why established tumors are often more susceptible to IL-12 administration than nascent tumors, because large immunogenic tumors are more apt than small ones to contain significant inflammatory infiltrates.

Data support at least three distinct mechanisms of IL-12–mediated antitumor activity, each of which requires IFN-γ as an induced molecular intermediate to execute the response. The authors' laboratory has demonstrated that a molecular correlate of effective IL-12 antitumor activity in the murine RENCA model is the expression of the chemokines monokine induced by IFN-γ (MIG) and IFN-γ–inducible protein 10 (IP-10) within the regressing tumor.[489] These molecules have since been determined to be chemotactic for NK and activated T cells, which correlates well with immunohistologic data indicating a tremendous influx of CD8+ and CD4+ cells into the treated tumor.[478,489] The tumors undergoing therapy were also characterized by elevated levels of the cytotoxins perforin and granzyme B, which may be among the terminal effector molecules of the infiltrating CD8 T cells in this system.[478,489,490] An integral role for the IFN-γ–inducible chemokines in IL-12–mediated antitumor activity was indicated by subsequent studies in which antibodies to MIG and IP-10 abrogated all correlates of IL-12–mediated tumor eradication: tumor shrinkage, the T-cell infiltrate, and perforin expression within the tumor bed.[478] When explants of human renal tumors were treated *in vitro* with IL-12, a sequence of molecular events similar to those observed in the murine model was observed: explanted renal cell carcinoma synthesized IFN-γ and IP-10 mRNA in response to the IL-12 treatment.[491] These results were also consistent with the authors' findings that biopsied renal tumors from patients enrolled in a phase I IL-12 trial variably expressed augmented levels of those molecules after therapy.[491] The conclusion was thus that, as in the murine system, recombinant human IL-12 treatment of patients with renal cell carcinoma has the potential to induce the expression of gene products within the tumor bed that may contribute to the development of a successful immune response.

Numerous other studies support the role of enhanced cellular immunity in the IL-12 antitumor effect. Early experiments performed with this cytokine demonstrated a strict requirement for T cells, as IL-12 antitumor function was essentially abrogated in nude mice and in mice depleted of CD8 T cells.[477] A negligible role for NK cells was suggested, however, by the finding that IL-12 antitumor function remained basically normal when therapy was performed in beige mice or wild-type mice depleted of NK cells by treatment with anti-asialo GM1.[477] Multiple laboratories also reported a rapid and significant infiltration of IL-12–treated tumors by macrophages,[489,492] and additional studies determined that tumor-infiltrating polymorphonuclear leukocytes are also an important component of the IL-12 response.[493] Perforin knockout mice have been shown to be unresponsive to IL-12 antitumor therapy,[490] a result that supports the correlation originally found between IL-12 efficacy and intratumoral perforin expression.[489]

When the antitumor activities of intratumorally and intraperitoneally administered IL-12 were compared, both therapeutic modalities were found to lead to similar immune responses at the tumor site: Both augmented IFN-γ expression, cytokine expression, chemokine expression, and inflammatory cell infiltration into the tumor bed. Systemic therapy orchestrated these responses more quickly and with greater efficacy than did local IL-12 treatment.[493] Compared with systemic therapy, which immediately activated and rendered peripheral cells responsive to chemotactic signals simultaneously induced at the target site,[493] locally administered IL-12 required additional time to diffuse and stimulate the same sequence of events. The greater rapidity and intensity of the global immune response after systemic IL-12 treatment was thus associated with a more favorable cure rate for large subcutaneous tumors.[493]

A second mechanism by which IL-12–induced IFN-γ mediates antitumor activity is through its stimulation of other molecules with cytotoxic function, including nitric oxide synthase. Nitric oxide synthase is produced by endothelial cells, neurons, epithelial cells, macrophages, and tumor cells themselves, and catalyzes the production of nitric oxide.[494] Nitric oxide is now known to be an important contributor to macrophage antitumor activity, and its central role in the protective process has been demonstrated by the ability of the nitric oxide inhibitor N^G-monomethyl-L-arginine to abrogate IL-12 antitumor efficacy.[494] IFN-γ has also been shown to induce the tryptophan degradation enzyme indolamine 2,3-dioxygenase within the tumor bed, which converts L-tryptophan to *N*-formyl L-kynurenine.[495]

RNA encoding this enzyme has been detected in IL-12–treated regressing tumor masses, and the enzyme effectively starves the tumor of that required amino acid.

A third mechanism purported to be involved in IL-12–mediated antitumor function is the IFN-γ–dependent induction of various antiangiogenic factors.[496–498] Growing tumors require ongoing neovascularization for nourishment, expansion, and metastatic spread.[499] Several molecules, including the IFN-inducible chemokines MIG, IP-10, and platelet factor 4, have been demonstrated to inhibit IL-8–stimulated angiogenic activity in the rabbit corneal pocket assay[497,500] and in several other *in vivo* models[496,501–504] and *in vitro* correlates[496,505,506] of blood vessel formation. One reported determinant of whether a specific CXC chemokine mediates angiogenic or antiangiogenic activity is the amino acid composition of its N-terminal region.[507] The presence of Glu-Leu-Arg, the ELR motif, in the N-terminus of a CXC chemokine endows the molecule with chemotactic activity for neutrophils[508] and angiogenic activity.[503,507] CXC chemokines lacking this motif, on the other hand, such as IP-10, MIG, and PF4, have been found not only to lack chemotactic function but also to inhibit neovascularization.[507] The mechanisms by which these non-ELR CXC chemokines mediate antiangiogenic function is not certain, but *in vitro* studies show that nanogram concentrations of IP-10 can inhibit endothelial cell chemotaxis,[505] proliferation,[506] and differentiation into tubelike structures.[496] The actual contribution the antiangiogenic molecules make to IL-12–mediated antitumor activity is uncertain; some workers find that IL-12 efficacy is abrogated in T-cell–depleted animals[477,493] and that IP-10 is an effective antitumor agent in euthymic but not in nude mice. Several reports have nonetheless supported a significant role for MIG and IP-10 in tumor necrosis and damage to tumor vasculature when these molecules are injected directly into the tumors of nude mice or induced in those lesions by local or systemic IL-12 therapy.[509,510]

Clinical Pharmacokinetics

IL-12 was cloned from an Epstein-Barr virus–transformed B-cell line. Recombinant human IL-12 manufactured by Genetics Institute is available for clinical trials. It is a lyophilized product and is reconstituted with sterile water. Phase I trials using either intravenous or subcutaneous administration have been performed.

Motzer et al.[511] performed a phase I trial in which IL-12 was administered subcutaneously at a fixed dose weekly for 3 weeks. An MTD of 0.5 μg per kg per week was identified, with hepatic, hematopoietic, and pulmonary toxicity being dose limiting. The toxicities seen with IL-12 are summarized in Table 27-20. A second phase of this trial involved gradual escalation of the IL-12 dose level after an initial dose of 0.1 μg per kg. In this portion, the MTD identified was 1.25 μg per kg.

TABLE 27-20. INTERLEUKIN 12 TOXICITY

Constitutional
Fever and chills
Headaches
Nausea and vomiting
Fatigue
Hematologic
Anemia
Leukopenia
Thrombocytopenia
Dose limiting
Leukopenia
Hepatic toxicity
Pulmonary toxicity
Stomatitis

TABLE 27-21. ANTITUMOR EFFECTS OF INTERLEUKIN 12 IN PHASE I AND II TRIALS

Tumor Type	No. Patients Treated	CR/PR	Comments
Renal cell cancer	118	2/2	CR durations >18 mo
Melanoma	22	0/1	Regressions of subcutaneous and liver lesions reported in 3 patients
Miscellaneous	8	0/0	5/8 had colon cancer

CR, complete response; PR, partial response.
Adapted from Motzer RJ, Rakhit A, Schwartz LH, et al. Phase I trial of subcutaneous recombinant human interleukin-12 in patients with advanced renal cell carcinoma. *Clin Cancer Res* 1998;4:1183–1191; Atkins MB, Robertson MJ, Gordon M, et al. Phase I evaluation of intravenous recombinant human interleukin 12 in patients with advanced malignancies. *Clin Cancer Res* 1997;3:409–417; and Bajetta E, Del Vecchio M, Mortarini R, et al. Pilot study of subcutaneous recombinant human interleukin 12 in metastatic melanoma. *Clin Cancer Res* 1998;4:75–85.

Intravenous IL-12 has also been investigated in a phase I trial. Forty patients, including 20 with renal cancer, 12 with melanoma, 5 with colon cancer were enrolled.[512] Two weeks after a single injection of IL-12 (3 to 1,000 ng per kg), patients received an additional 6-week course of intravenous IL-12 therapy, administered 5 consecutive days every 3 weeks. The MTD was 0.5 µg per kg per day, and toxicities include fever and chills, fatigue, nausea, and headaches. Laboratory findings included anemia, neutropenia, lymphopenia, hyperglycemia, thrombocytopenia, and hypoalbuminemia.

A phase II trial of intravenous IL-12 was then initiated using 0.5 µg per kg per day for 5 days.[513] Seventeen patients were entered, and due to unexpectedly severe toxicity, the study was abandoned. The data from both the subcutaneous and intravenous phase I trials suggest that a single predose of IL-12 may be associated with a decrease in toxicity and permits escalation to high dosages. The antitumor effects of IL-12 in early clinical trials are summarized in Table 27-21. Responses have been seen in patients with renal cancer and melanoma, but are infrequent.

Table 27-22 outlines serum IL-12 levels in patients receiving IL-12 subcutaneously.[511,514] Studies were also performed during weeks 1 and 7 of drug administration and demonstrate a decrease in IL-12 levels after prolonged administration. This has been termed an adaptive response and has been attributed to either antibody formation or an immunoregulatory feedback response. Antibody formation in response to IL-12 has not been found.[511] Rakhit et al.[514] examined this issue in murine models and noted down-regulation of serum IL-12 levels correlated with up-regulation of IL-12R expression, which was not observed in IL-12Rβ –/– mice. These observation suggest that receptor-mediated clearance is operative and that increases in IL-12R enhance clearance of IL-12.

In preclinical studies, IL-12 induces secretion of IFN-γ by a variety of lymphoid cells. After subcutaneous or intravenous administration, increases in serum levels of this cytokine are also observed. Rakhit et al.[514] reported that 0.5 µg per kg of IL-12 produces peak levels of 250 pg per mL, with the maximum concentration occurring approximately 24 hours after administration. IFN-γ levels then gradually decreased to baseline over the next 7 days and are minimally elevated with

TABLE 27-22. PHARMACOKINETICS OF INTERLEUKIN 12 AFTER SUBCUTANEOUS ADMINISTRATION: WEEK 1 VERSUS WEEK 7

Parameter	0.5 µg/kg		1.0 µg/kg	
	Week 1	Week 7	Week 1	Week 7[a]
C_{max} (pg/mL)	321 ± 46	128 ± 422	1,092 ± 275	352 ± 1,693
T_{max} (h)	13.00 ± 1.65	14.0 ± 2.7	16.0 ± 2.7	8.0 ± 0.9
AUC (pg h/mL)	7,043 ± 1,325	1,473 ± 604[b]	26,589 ± 6,633	3,597 ± 1,300[c]

AUC, area under the concentration × time curve; C_{max}, highest observed concentration; T_{max}, sampling time of C_{max}.
[a]Dose reduced to 50%; data are for 0.5 µg/kg given in weeks 2–7.
[b]$p < .001$ for week 7 versus week 1.
[c]$p < .005$ for week 7 versus week 1.
Adapted from Rakhit A, Yeon MM, Ferrante J, et al. Down-regulation of the pharmacokinetic-pharmacodynamic response to interleukin-12 during long-term administration to patients with renal cell carcinoma and evaluation of the mechanism of this "adaptive response" in mice. *Clin Pharmacol Ther* 1999;65:615–629.

TABLE 27-23. INTERFERON γ (IFN-γ) AND INTERLEUKIN 10 (IL-10) LEVELS AFTER SUBCUTANEOUS ADMINISTRATION OF INTERLEUKIN 12 (0.5 µg/kg)[a]

Cycle[b]	IFN-γ (pg/mL)		IL-10 (pg/mL)	
	1	2	1	2
C_{max} (pg/mL)	267 ± 53	34 ± 4	80 ± 13	35 ± 17
T_{max} (h)	24 (24–72)	24 (24)	24 (24–96)	24 (24–48)

[a]Patients with renal cancer (n = 5).
[b]Data for cycle 1 collected on day 1 of weekly (weeks 1–6) subcutaneous administration of IL-12; data for cycle 2 collected on week 7. Adapted from Rakhit A, Yeon MM, Ferrante J, et al. Down-regulation of the pharmacokinetic-pharmacodynamic response to interleukin-12 during long-term administration to patients with renal cell carcinoma and evaluation of the mechanism of this "adaptive response" in mice. *Clin Pharmacol Ther* 1999;65:615–629.

continuous administration of IL-12 (Table 27-23). In patients receiving escalating doses of cytokine, 1.0 µg per kg produced lower serum IFN-γ levels on day 15.[511] In patients receiving intravenous IL-12, dose-dependent increases in serum IFN-γ levels have also been reported.[515] Other surrogate markers such as neopterin also increase, with peak concentrations noted between 72 and 96 hours after administration of a single IL-12 dose.[511] In addition to these effects, administration of IL-12 increases serum levels of IL-10,[514] which results in activation of a complex immunoregulatory cytokine network (Table 27-23).

After IL-12 administration, significant lymphopenia is observed after 24 hours.[515] This involves all the major lymphocyte subsets, with NK cells the most severely affected.[515,516] Augmented NK cytolytic activity and T-cell proliferative responses have also been noted.[515]

Bukowski et al.[491] have investigated the expression of a variety of genes in peripheral blood mononuclear cells after subcutaneous administration of IL-12 to patients with renal cell carcinoma. Rapid induction of IFN-γ mRNA was found and was accompanied by subsequent induction of mRNA for IP-10 and MIG. These chemokines are IFN-γ inducible and mediate chemotaxis of T lymphocytes.[489] In addition, IP-10 appears to have antiangiogenic effects and decreases proliferation of endothelial cells. Other investigators[506] have also suggested that the antitumor effects of IL-12 may involve inhibition of angiogenesis.[503,506]

Pharmacodynamic studies in patients and preclinical models suggest that IL-12 has complex immunoregulatory effects on cytokine networks and lymphoid cell populations, and may also inhibit tumor-associated angiogenesis.

Drug Interactions

Preclinical studies suggest that combination of IL-12 with IL-2 or IFN-α may enhance the antitumor effects. Clinical investigations of these combinations are currently under study and results are preliminary.

MACROPHAGE COLONY-STIMULATING FACTOR

The description of a factor present in the supernatants of cultured mouse L cells that supported mononuclear phagocyte growth and differentiation *in vitro* provided the initial observation indicating the existence of a monocyte-macrophage lineage growth factor.[517] Subsequent *in vitro* studies also demonstrated that this factor augmented a variety of monocyte functions, including tumoricidal effects[518] and secretion of plasminogen activator,[519] prostaglandin E,[520] and cytokines.[521] This cytokine was termed *colony-stimulating factor 1* or, more recently, *macrophage colony-stimulating factor* (*M-CSF*). In 1985, the cDNA encoding M-CSF was isolated and integrated into COS-7 cells and *E. coli*.[522] Subsequently, some of the biologic and clinical effects of recombinant M-CSF (rM-CSF) have been elucidated.

Structure and Mechanisms of Action

Human M-CSF is encoded by a single gene spanning 20 kb that contains 10 exons.[523] Initially, the gene was mapped to chromosome 5 at band q33.1[524] and appeared to be one of a cluster of growth factor genes on the long arm of this chromosome. Studies using fluorescence *in situ* hybridization appear to demonstrate that the gene location is on chromosome 1 at bands p13-p21.[525]

Human M-CSF was originally isolated from urine, and purified urinary M-CSF was then used to generate cDNA probes by which the human genomic clone was isolated. Two alternately spliced messenger RNA transcripts (4.0 kb and 1.6 kb) code for precursor proteins of 61 kd and 26 kd.[522,523,526,527] The 61-kd protein is glycosylated and processed to a 45-kd subunit, which is then assembled into a 90-kd disulfide-linked homodimer and secreted. This form has been detected in serum and urine.[528] The 26-kd protein is also glycosylated, assembled into a homodimer of 40 to 50 kd, and expressed on the cell membrane.[529] Both the secreted and membrane-bound forms can stimulate M-CSF–responsive cells.

M-CSF binds to a specific high-affinity receptor (M-CSF-R) that is termed c-*fms*. The gene for this receptor is located on chromosome band 5q23.[530] M-CSF-R is homologous to v-*fms*, an oncogene in SM-*fsv* feline sarcoma virus.[531] This receptor is a 150-kd transmembrane glycoprotein with a C-terminal cytoplasmic domain having tyrosine kinase activity.[532] After M-CSF binding, the receptor-ligand complex is internalized and subsequently degraded.[533] In addition to mononuclear phagocytes, various neoplastic cells such as choriocarcinoma and myeloid leukemia[534,535] have been noted to express M-CSF-R.

After exposure to M-CSF, monocytes increase their membrane-associated guanosine triphosphatase activity[536] and proliferate. Preclinical studies with M-CSF demonstrate that it induces proliferation of mature mononuclear phagocytes *in vitro*.[536,537] Human bone marrow culture studies demonstrate that M-CSF acts on committed pro-

TABLE 27-24. MACROPHAGE COLONY-STIMULATING FACTOR PREPARATIONS USED IN CLINICAL TRIALS

Source	Nature	Activity
Alpha Therapeutic/Green Cross[561]	hM-CSF purified from urine	1.5×10^8 U/mg
Cetus[562]	rM-CSF produced in *Escherichia coli*	$>1.0 \times 10^7$ U/mg
Genetics Institute[563]	rM-CSF produced in COS cells	0.8×10^6 U/mg

hM-CSF, human macrophage colony-stimulating factor; rM-CSF, recombinant macrophage colony-stimulating factor.

genitor cells corresponding to the late colony-forming unit/granulocyte-macrophage stage to produce macrophage colonies[538,539] and, when combined with other factors such as IL-3, can influence more immature precursors.[540]

Cellular Pharmacology

M-CSF is produced by a variety of cell types, including monocytes, macrophages and fibroblasts,[541] endothelial cells,[542] lymphocytes,[543,544] and granulocytes.[545] *In vivo*, it participates in the inflammatory response, and the constitutive presence of M-CSF in human sera suggests that it also regulates normal monocyte-macrophage production.[546,547] M-CSF binds to receptors on mononuclear phagocytes and is internalized and then degraded. It appears to participate in a feedback mechanism by which M-CSF-R expression is increased and M-CSF clearance possibly increased.[548,549]

In addition to causing proliferation of macrophages, M-CSF also stimulates secondary production of a variety of cytokines, including TNF-α, IL-1, G-CSF, and GM-CSF.[521,550] M-CSF can also activate mononuclear phagocytes with subsequent development of tumor cell cytotoxicity,[551,552] enhance phagocytosis of *Candida albicans*,[553] and act as a chemotactic factor for monocytes.[554]

Clinical Pharmacokinetics

The role of macrophages in host defense and inflammation[551,555] and the possibility that tumor-associated macrophages may play a role in controlling tumor growth[556] provided a rationale for investigating the use of M-CSF to treat patients with malignancy. Table 27-24 outlines the different M-CSF preparations that have been used in clinical trials. These include purified urinary M-CSF, a full-length (90-kd) recombinant form that is glycosylated and produced in COS cells, and a truncated form expressed in *E. coli*. These preparations appear to have equivalent *in vitro* activities.[557]

M-CSF activity is expressed as units per milligram, with 1 U defined as the amount required to form one colony in a mouse colony-forming assay.[546] M-CSF serum assays have also been developed and include a bioassay,[558] a radioimmunoassay,[559] and an ELISA.[560] The bioassay involves a cell proliferation assay using M-NFS-60 cells that respond to human and murine M-CSF and IL-3.[558]

Trials in which purified natural human M-CSF (hM-CSF) had been given to patients receiving chemotherapy,[561] to patients after allogeneic or autologous bone marrow transplantation,[564] and to children with chronic neutropenia[565] have been performed. Early studies with incompletely purified material[566] produced significant fever, malaise, and rashes, but in later studies using more pure material[561] the incidence of toxicity was substantially lower. Study end points were improvement in neutropenia and a decrease in the severity and duration of granulocytopenia.[567] The rationale for this approach is the secondary cytokine production mediated by M-CSF. Pharmacokinetic data were not reported in these studies.

Trials using recombinant forms of M-CSF are summarized in Table 27-25. The majority of studies reported have been

TABLE 27-25. PHASE I TRIALS OF RECOMBINANT MACROPHAGE COLONY-STIMULATING FACTOR (rM-CSF)

Study	rM-CSF Source	Dose Levels	Schedule	Maximum Tolerated Dose	Half-Life
Zamkoff et al.[568]	Cetus	30–33,000 µg/m²/d	i.v.b. d 1–5, 5–19	Not reached	19.8–258 min
Nemunaitis et al.[573]	Cetus	100–200 µg/m²/d repeated ×3	2-h i.v. d 1–7, infusion dose escalation permitted	Not reached, intrapatient	ND
Sanda et al.[572]	Cetus	10–100,000 µg/m²/d	30-min i.v. infusion q8h d 1–7, repeated ×1	Not reached	1.9–4.1 h
Redman et al.[569]	Cetus	20–1,100 µg/m²/d	15-min i.v. infusion q8h d 1–5	Not reached	0.42–1.4 h
Bukowski et al.[570]	Cetus	100–25,600 µg/m²/d	s.c. injection d 1–5, 8–12, repeated q1mo	12,800 µg/m²/d	ND
Bajorin et al.[574]	Genetics Institute	10–120 µg/kg²/d	c.i.v. days 1–7, 22–28	Not stated	ND

c.i.v., continuous intravenous infusion; i.v.b., intravenous bolus; ND, not determined.

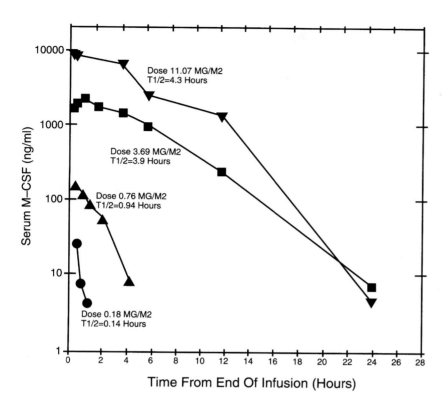

FIGURE 27-8. Representative curves for four patients receiving different doses of recombinant macrophage colony-stimulating factor (M-CSF). At the two higher doses, the curves demonstrate both the first-order clearance (renal) and the saturable clearance (cellular uptake) seen at low serum concentrations. Below a serum concentration of 1,000 ng per mL, the clearance was determined mainly by cellular uptake. ($t_{1/2}$, half-life.) (From Zamkoff KW, Hudson J, Groves ES, et al. A phase I trial of recombinant human macrophage colony-stimulating factor by rapid intravenous infusion in patients with refractory malignancy. *J Immunother* 1992;11:103–110.)

performed with the *E. coli*-derived product (Cetus), and various schedules and methods of administration have been used. The rate of clearance of intravenous rM-CSF is dose-dependent at lower doses (19.8 and 56.4 minutes at 180 µg per m² and 760 µg per m², respectively), and at higher dose levels was saturable.[568] Figure 27-8 illustrates serum concentrations of M-CSF after rapid intravenous infusion at two different dose levels, demonstrating what probably represents a saturable mechanism of clearance.[569] The mechanisms for rM-CSF clearance appear to be inducible, with more rapid clearance seen when kinetics is examined after repetitive doses.

A single trial using subcutaneous injections of rM-CSF has been reported.[570] The rM-CSF (Cetus) was administered subcutaneously on days 1 through 5 and days 8 through 12 at doses ranging from 100 to 25,600 µg per m² per day. Pharmacokinetic studies demonstrated that the systemic clearance rate of rM-CSF increased during week 1 and resulted in lower blood levels of rM-CSF during week 2 of therapy (Fig. 27-9). These findings probably represent cellular mechanisms of clearance secondary to increased numbers of M-CSF-R per cell or increased numbers of monocytes.

These findings are consistent with preclinical studies of M-CSF in mice in which more than 90% of radiolabeled M-CSF is cleared by macrophage uptake, with urinary excretion forming a minor route of elimination.[571] In primate studies, continuous intravenous administration of rM-CSF produced steady-state levels by 24 hours, which declined to undetectable levels over 3 to 4 days.[549]

The MTD of intravenous M-CSF has not been clearly defined, but doses of 30,000 and 100,000 µg per m² per

day produced unacceptable toxicity.[572] The subcutaneous route of administration is well tolerated, with the MTD determined to be 12,800 µg per m² per day.[570] Comparisons of the available clinical preparations of M-CSF have not been performed.

Clinical Effects and Toxicity

The hematologic and biologic effects of M-CSF have been variable. In the study by Bukowski et al.[570] hematologic effects included a dose-related monocytosis when rM-CSF was administered subcutaneously at doses of more than 3,200 µg per m² per day (Fig. 27-10). Changes in other peripheral blood cell populations were not seen except for thrombocytopenia, which developed at higher dose levels and was rapidly reversible when rM-CSF was discontinued. Intravenous administration also produced monocytosis when doses of more than 1,000 µg per m² were administered.[569,572]

Mononuclear phagocyte function has been extensively investigated in three clinical trials. Enhanced mRNA expression for TNF-α, IL-1β, and IL-6 in monocytes obtained from rM-CSF–treated patients[570] and secondary cytokine secretion of TNF-α and IL-1β by *in vitro* cultured monocytes was noted. No consistent effects on monocyte tumor cell cytotoxicity, NK or LAK cytotoxicity, or antibody-dependent cellular cytotoxicity have been found.[568–570] Nonhematologic effects including decreases in serum levels of cholesterol and high-density lipoproteins have also been noted.[574] Effects on alveolar macrophages and tumor-

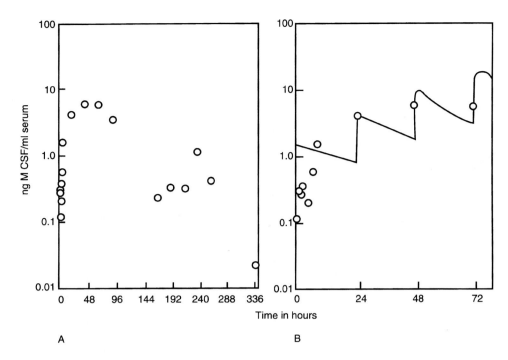

FIGURE 27-9. Serum concentration of macrophage colony-stimulating factor (M-CSF) over time in a patient receiving subcutaneous recombinant M-CSF at 3.2 µg per m² per day. **A:** M-CSF concentrations during first 350 hours of therapy. **B:** M-CSF concentrations during the first 80 hours, with curve fitting of the data. (From Bukowski RM, Budd GT, Gibbons JA, et al. Phase I trial of subcutaneous recombinant macrophage colony-stimulating factor: clinical and immunomodulatory effects. *J Clin Oncol* 1994;12:97–106, with permission.)

associated macrophages have also been studied. No consistent effects on alveolar macrophages were seen, but in one of four patients, increased tumor infiltration by CD14+ cells was reported.[570]

The toxicity of rM-CSF is mild to moderate except at very high dosages. Urinary hM-CSF[570] was reported to produce mild fever in less than 10% of patients; with rM-CSF, fever and myalgia have been noted in 0%[569] to more than 40%[570] of patients. Respiratory symptoms described as dyspnea, wheezing, or both were noted in 20% of individuals in one trial[568] but not in other studies. Dose-limiting toxicities have been thrombocytopenia and episcleritis,[570] with a particularly

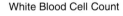

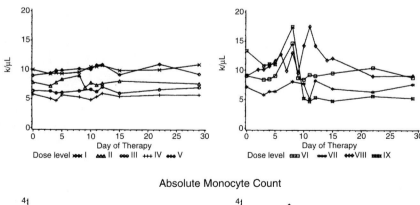

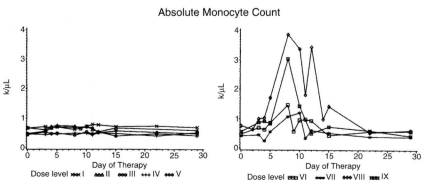

FIGURE 27-10. Absolute monocyte and white blood cell counts in patients receiving recombinant macrophage colony-stimulating factor. I, 100 µg per m²; II, 200 µg per m²; III, 400 µg per m²; IV, 800 µg per m²; V, 1,600 µg per m²; VI, 3,200 µg per m²; VII, 6,400 µg per m²; VIII, 12,800 µg per m²; IX, 25,600 µg per m². (From Bukowski RM, Budd GT, Gibbons JA, et al. Phase I trial of subcutaneous recombinant macrophage colony-stimulating factor: clinical and immunomodulatory effects. *J Clin Oncol* 1994;12:97–106, with permission.)

high incidence of ophthalmologic side effects noted in the report by Sanda et al.[572] Toxicity with rM-CSF has been self-limited and resolves rapidly with drug discontinuation.

The clinical effects of rM-CSF have also included anti-tumor responses. Patients with melanoma,[574] renal cell carcinoma,[572] and soft tissue sarcoma[569] have shown brief responses. Overall, minimal antitumor effects have been seen in the phase I trials. In a report by Nemunaitis et al.,[573] 24 bone marrow transplant recipients with fungal infections received escalating doses of rM-CSF, and 6 of 12 evaluable patients experienced resolution of invasive infections.

The effects of purified urinary hM-CSF in treatment of patients with chemotherapy-induced neutropenia, patients after bone marrow transplantation, and children with neutropenia have also been studied. In a randomized trial,[567] significant decreases in time to neutrophil recovery (more than 5×10^9 granulocytes per L) and improved survival were reported in allogeneic and syngeneic bone marrow transplant patients receiving hM-CSF compared with those given placebo. In children with neutropenia,[565] three of nine patients showed resolution of the cytopenia with administration of hM-CSF.

Drug Interactions

As a single agent, rM-CSF appears to have minimal antitumor effects. In treatment of patients with invasive fungal infections after myelosuppressive therapy, rM-CSF may be of value. Clinical combinations with other growth factors, cytokines, or monoclonal antibodies are also of interest in view of preclinical information. *In vitro*, rIL-2 enhances the expression of M-CSF-R by monocytes,[575] and therefore combinations of rM-CSF and rIL-2 may be clinically relevant. Augmentation of antibody-dependent monocyte cytotoxicity produced by various murine monoclonal antibodies in the presence of rM-CSF has been noted.[576,577] Clinical trials of combinations of various monoclonal antibodies and rM-CSF are under way. The minimal toxicity of rM-CSF make it an attractive cytokine for use in adjuvant settings in which prolonged therapy may be required.

REFERENCES

1. Dinarello CA. The interleukin-1 family: 10 years of discovery. *FASEB J* 1994;8:1314–1325.
2. Falk W, Mannel DN, Darjes H, et al. IL-1 induces high affinity IL-2 receptor expression of CD4-8-thymocytes. *J Immunol* 1989;143:513–517.
3. Oppenheim JJ, Neta R, Tiberghien P, et al. Interleukin-1 enhances survival of lethally irradiated mice treated with allogeneic bone marrow cells. *Blood* 1989;74:2257–2263.
4. Dinarello CA, Wolff SM. The role of interleukin-1 in disease [published erratum appears in *N Engl J Med* 1993;328(10):744]. *N Engl J Med* 1993;328:106–113.
5. Libby P, Warner SJ, Friedman GB. Interleukin 1: a mitogen for human vascular smooth muscle cells that induces the release of growth-inhibitory prostanoids. *J Clin Invest* 1988;81:487–498.
6. Rivier C, Chizzonite R, Vale W. In the mouse, the activation of the hypothalamic-pituitary-adrenal axis by a lipopolysaccharide (endotoxin) is mediated through interleukin-1. *Endocrinology* 1989;125:2800–2805.
7. Carter DB, Deibel MR Jr, Dunn CJ, et al. Purification, cloning, expression and biological characterization of an interleukin-1 receptor antagonist protein. *Nature* 1990;344:633–638.
8. Dinarello CA. Interleukin-1 and interleukin-1 antagonism. *Blood* 1991;77:1627–1652.
9. Eastgate JA, Symons JA, Wood NC, et al. Correlation of plasma interleukin 1 levels with disease activity in rheumatoid arthritis. *Lancet* 1988;2:706–709.
10. Cannon JG, Friedberg JS, Gelfand JA, et al. Circulating interleukin-1 beta and tumor necrosis factor-alpha concentrations after burn injury in humans. *Crit Care Med* 1992;20:1414–1419.
11. Okusawa S, Gelfand JA, Ikejima T, et al. Interleukin 1 induces a shock-like state in rabbits. Synergism with tumor necrosis factor and the effect of cyclooxygenase inhibition. *J Clin Invest* 1988;81:1162–1172.
12. Cominelli F, Nast CC, Dinarello CA, et al. Regulation of eicosanoid production in rabbit colon by interleukin-1. *Gastroenterology* 1989;97:1400–1405.
13. Endres S, Ghorbani R, Kelley VE, et al. The effect of dietary supplementation with n-3 polyunsaturated fatty acids on the synthesis of interleukin-1 and tumor necrosis factor by mononuclear cells. *N Engl J Med* 1989;320:265–271.
14. Besedovsky HO, Del Rey A. Metabolic and endocrine actions of interleukin-1. Effects on insulin-resistant animals. *Ann N Y Acad Sci* 1990;594:214–221.
15. Chensue SW, Bienkowski M, Eessalu TE, et al. Endogenous IL-1 receptor antagonist protein (IRAP) regulates schistosome egg granuloma formation and the regional lymphoid response. *J Immunol* 1993;151:3654–3662.
16. Ferretti M, Casini-Raggi V, Pizarro TT, et al. Neutralization of endogenous IL-1 receptor antagonist exacerbates and prolongs inflammation in rabbit immune colitis. *J Clin Invest* 1994;94:449–453.
17. Dinarello CA. Biologic basis for interleukin-1 in disease. *Blood* 1996;87:2095–2147.
18. Kolenko V, Bloom T, Rayman P, et al. Inhibition of NF-kappa B activity in human T lymphocytes induces caspase-dependent apoptosis without detectable activation of caspase-1 and -3. *J Immunol* 1999;163:590–598.
19. Sipe JD. The molecular biology of interleukin 1 and the acute phase response. *Adv Intern Med* 1989;34:1–20.
20. Neta R, Oppenheim JJ. Can we exploit Jekyll and subjugate Hyde? In: DeVita VT, Hellman S, Rosenberg SA, eds. *Biology therapy of cancer updates*, vol 2. Philadelphia: JB Lippincott, 1992:1–11.
21. Eisenberg SP, Brewer MT, Verderber E, et al. Interleukin 1 receptor antagonist is a member of the interleukin 1 gene family: evolution of a cytokine control mechanism. *Proc Natl Acad Sci U S A* 1991;88:5232–5236.
22. Kobayashi Y, Matsushima K, Oppenheim JJ. Differential gene expression, synthesis, processing and release of inter-

leukin-1α and interleukin-1β. In: Bomford RHR, Henderson R, eds. *Interleukin 1, inflammation and disease.* Amsterdam: Elsevier Science, 1989:47–62.

23. Fenton MJ, Vermeulen MW, Clark BD, et al. Human pro-IL-1 beta gene expression in monocytic cells is regulated by two distinct pathways. *J Immunol* 1988;140:2267–2273.

24. Schindler R, Clark BD, Dinarello CA. Dissociation between interleukin-1 beta mRNA and protein synthesis in human peripheral blood mononuclear cells. *J Biol Chem* 1990;265:10232–10237.

25. Serkkola E, Hurme M. Synergism between protein-kinase C and cAMP-dependent pathways in the expression of the interleukin-1 beta gene is mediated via the activator-protein-1 (AP-1) enhancer activity. *Eur J Biochem* 1993;213:243–249.

26. Schindler R, Ghezzi P, Dinarello CA. IL-1 induces IL-1. IV. IFN-gamma suppresses IL-1 but not lipopolysaccharide-induced transcription of IL-1. *J Immunol* 1990;144:2216–2222.

27. Schindler R, Gelfand JA, Dinarello CA. Recombinant C5a stimulates transcription rather than translation of interleukin-1 (IL-1) and tumor necrosis factor: translational signal provided by lipopolysaccharide or IL-1 itself. *Blood* 1990;76:1631–1638.

28. McMahan CJ, Slack JL, Mosley B, et al. A novel IL-1 receptor, cloned from B cells by mammalian expression, is expressed in many cell types. *EMBO J* 1991;10:2821–2832.

29. McKean DJ, Podzorski RP, Bell MP, et al. Murine T helper cell-2 lymphocytes express type I and type II IL-1 receptors, but only the type I receptor mediates costimulatory. *J Immunol* 1993;151:3500–3510.

30. O'Neill LA, Greene C. Signal transduction pathways activated by the IL-1 receptor family: ancient signaling machinery in mammals, insects, and plants. *J Leukoc Biol* 1998;63:650–657.

31. O'Neill LA. Towards an understanding of the signal transduction pathways for interleukin 1. *Biochim Biophys Acta* 1995;1266:31–44.

32. Huang J, Gao X, Li S, et al. Recruitment of IRAK to the interleukin 1 receptor complex requires interleukin 1 receptor accessory protein. *Proc Natl Acad Sci U S A* 1997;94:12829–12832.

33. Mercurio F, Zhu H, Murray BW, et al. IKK-1 and IKK-2: cytokine-activated IκB kinases essential for NF-κB activation. *Science* 1997;278:860–866.

34. Woronicz JD, Gao X, Cao Z, et al. IκB kinase-beta: NF-κB activation and complex formation with IκB kinase-α and NIK. *Science* 1997;278:866–869.

35. Ridley SH, Sarsfield SJ, Lee JC, et al. Actions of IL-1 are selectively controlled by p38 mitogen-activated protein kinase: regulation of prostaglandin H synthase-2, metalloproteinases, and IL-6 at different levels. *J Immunol* 1997;158:3165–3173.

36. Kumar S, Orsini MJ, Lee JC, et al. Activation of the HIV-1 long terminal repeat by cytokines and environmental stress requires an active CSBP/p38 MAP kinase. *J Biol Chem* 1996;271:30864–30869.

37. Guesdon F, Knight CG, Rawlinson LM, et al. Dual specificity of the interleukin 1- and tumor necrosis factor-activated beta casein kinase. *J Biol Chem* 1997;272:30017–30024.

38. Neta R, Sayers T, Oppenheim JJ. Relationship of tumor necrosis factor to interleukins. In: Vilcek J, Aggarwal B, eds. *Tumor necrosis factor: structure and mechanisms of action.* New York: Marcel Dekker, 1992:499–566.

39. Eisenberg SP, Evans RJ, Arend WP, et al. Primary structure and functional expression from complementary DNA of a human interleukin-1 receptor antagonist. *Nature* 1990;343:341–346.

40. Dinarello CA, Thompson RC. Blocking IL-1: interleukin-1 receptor antagonist in vitro. *Immunol Today* 1991;12:404–410.

41. Baumann H, Gauldie J. Regulation of hepatic acute phase plasma protein genes by hepatocyte stimulating factors and other mediators of inflammation. *Mol Biol Med* 1990;7:147–159.

42. Imura H, Fukata J, Mori T. Cytokines and endocrine function: an interaction between the immune and neuroendocrine systems. *Clin Endocrinol (Oxf)* 1991;35:107–115.

43. Whitnall MH, Perlstein RS, Mougey EH, et al. Effects of interleukin-1 on the stress-responsive and -nonresponsive subtypes of corticotropin-releasing hormone neurosecretory axons. *Endocrinology* 1992;131:37–44.

44. Neta R, Oppenheim JJ, Schreiber RD, et al. Role of cytokines (interleukin 1, tumor necrosis factor, and transforming growth factor beta) in natural and lipopolysaccharide-enhanced radioresistance. *J Exp Med* 1991;173:1177–1182.

45. Faherty DA, Claudy V, Plocinski JM, et al. Failure of IL-1 receptor antagonist and monoclonal anti-IL-1 receptor antibody to inhibit antigen-specific immune responses in vivo. *J Immunol* 1992;148:766–771.

46. North RJ, Neubauer RH, Huang JJ, et al. Interleukin 1-induced, T cell-mediated regression of immunogenic murine tumors. *J Exp Med* 1988;168:2031–2043.

47. Douvdevani A, Huleihel M, Zoller M, et al. Reduced tumorigenicity of fibrosarcomas which constitutively generate IL-1 alpha either spontaneously or following IL-1 alpha gene transfer. *Int J Cancer* 1992;51:822–830.

48. Recombinant Human Interleukin-1α (rhuIL-1α). Investigator brochure. Seattle: Immunex Corporation, June 1, 1991.

49. Crown J, Jakubowski A, Kemeny N, et al. A phase I trial of recombinant human interleukin-1 beta alone and in combination with myelosuppressive doses of 5-fluorouracil in patients with gastrointestinal cancer. *Blood* 1991;78:1420–1427.

50. Luger TA, Stadler BM, Katz SI, et al. Epidermal cell (keratinocyte)-derived thymocyte-activating factor (ETAF). *J Immunol* 1981;127:1493–1498.

51. Marumo K, Tachibana M, Deguchi N, et al. Enhancement of lymphokine-activated killer activity induction in vitro by interleukin-1 administered in patients with urological malignancies. *J Immunother* 1992;11:191–197.

52. Smith JW, Urba WJ, Curti BD, et al. The toxic and hematologic effects of interleukin-1 alpha administered in a phase I trial to patients with advanced malignancies. *J Clin Oncol* 1992;10(7):1141–1152.

53. Puri RK, Travis WD, Rosenberg SA. Decrease in interleukin 2-induced vascular leakage in the lungs of mice by administration of recombinant interleukin 1 alpha in vivo. *Cancer Res* 1989;49:969–976.

54. Dennis D, Chachoua A, Caron D. Biologic activity of interleukin-1 (IL-1) alpha in patients with refractory malignancies. *Proc Am Soc Clin Oncol* 1992;11:255(abst).

55. Nakai S, Mizuno K, Kaneta M, et al. A simple, sensitive bioassay for the detection of interleukin-1 using human melanoma A375 cell line. *Biochem Biophys Res Commun* 1988;154:1189–1196.

56. McDermott DF, Trehu EG, Mier JW, et al. A two-part phase I trial of high-dose interleukin 2 in combination with soluble (Chinese hamster ovary) interleukin 1 receptor. *Clin Cancer Res* 1998;4:1203–1213.

57. Bernstein SH, Fay J, Frankel S, et al. A phase I study of recombinant human soluble interleukin-1 receptor (rhu IL-1R) in patients with relapsed and refractory acute myeloid leukemia. *Cancer Chemother Pharmacol* 1999;43:141–144.

58. Starnes HF, Hartman G, Torti F. Recombinant human IL-1b has anti-tumor activity and acceptable toxicity in metastatic malignant melanoma. *Proc Am Soc Clin Oncol* 1991;10:292(abst).

59. Iizumi T, Sato S, Iiyama T, et al. Recombinant human interleukin-1 beta analogue as a regulator of hematopoiesis in patients receiving chemotherapy for urogenital cancers. *Cancer* 1991;68:1520–1523.

60. Nemunaitis J, Appelbaum FR, Lilleby K, et al. Phase I study of recombinant interleukin-1 beta in patients undergoing autologous bone marrow transplant for acute myelogenous leukemia. *Blood* 1994;83:3473–3479.

61. Verschraegen CF, Kudelka AP, Termrungruangert W, et al. Effects of interleukin 1 alpha on ovarian carcinoma in patients with recurrent disease. *Eur J Cancer* 1996;32A:1609–1611.

62. Rosenthal MA, Dennis D, Liebes L, et al. Biologic activity of interleukin 1 (IL-1) alpha in patients with refractory malignancies. *J Immunother* 1998;21:371–378.

63. Worth LL, Jaffe N, Benjamin RS, et al. Phase II study of recombinant interleukin 1alpha and etoposide in patients with relapsed osteosarcoma. *Clin Cancer Res* 1997;3:1721–1729.

64. Smith T, Urba W, Steis R. Interleukin-1 alpha (IL-1a): results of a phase I toxicity and immunomodulatory trial. *Proc Am Soc Clin Oncol* 1990;9:186(abst).

65. Tewari A, Buhles WC Jr, Starnes HF Jr. Preliminary report: effects of interleukin-1 on platelet counts [retracted by Buhles WC, Starnes HF, in *Lancet* 1992;340(8817):496]. *Lancet* 1990;336:712–714.

66. Smith JW, Longo DL, Alvord WG, et al. The effects of treatment with interleukin-1 alpha on platelet recovery after high-dose carboplatin. *N Engl J Med* 1993;328:756–761.

67. Wilson WH, Bryant G, Jain V. Phase I study of infusional interleukin-1a (IL-1) with ifosfamide (I), CBDCA (C), and etoposide (E) (ICE) and autologous bone marrow transplant (BMT). *Proc Am Soc Clin Oncol* 1992;11:335(abst).

68. Granowitz EV, Clark BD, Mancilla J, et al. Interleukin-1 receptor antagonist competitively inhibits the binding of interleukin-1 to the type II interleukin-1 receptor. *J Biol Chem* 1991;266:14147–14150.

69. Wakabayashi G, Gelfand JA, Burke JF, et al. A specific receptor antagonist for interleukin 1 prevents *Escherichia coli*–induced shock in rabbits. *FASEB J* 1991;5:338–343.

70. Fischer E, Van Zee KJ, Marano MA, et al. Interleukin-1 receptor antagonist circulates in experimental inflammation and in human disease. *Blood* 1992;79:2196–2200.

71. Granowitz EV, Porat R, Mier JW, et al. Pharmacokinetics, safety and immunomodulatory effects of human recombinant interleukin-1 receptor antagonist in healthy humans. *Cytokine* 1992;4:353–360.

72. Kasakura S, Lowenstein L. A factor stimulating DNA synthesis derived from the medium of leukocyte cultures. *Nature* 1965;208:794–795.

73. Morgan DA, Ruscetti FW, Gallo R. Selective in vitro growth of T lymphocytes from normal human bone marrows. *Science* 1976;193:1007–1008.

74. Gillis S, Union NA, Baker PE, et al. The in vitro generation and sustained culture of nude mouse cytolytic T-lymphocytes. *J Exp Med* 1979;149:1460–1476.

75. Taniguchi T, Matsui H, Fujita T, et al. Structure and expression of a cloned cDNA for human interleukin-2. *Nature* 1983;302:305–310.

76. Smith KA. Lowest dose interleukin-2 immunotherapy. *Blood* 1993;81:1414–1423.

77. Bazan JF. Unraveling the structure of IL-2 [Letter]. *Science* 1992;257:410–413.

78. Sherblom AP, Sathyamoorthy N, Decker JM, et al. IL-2, a lectin with specificity for high mannose glycopeptides. *J Immunol* 1989;143:939–944.

79. Landgraf BE, Williams DP, Murphy JR, et al. Conformational perturbation of interleukin-2: a strategy for the design of cytokine analogs. *Proteins* 1991;9:207–216.

80. Mosmann TR, Cherwinski H, Bond MW, et al. Two types of murine helper T cell clone. I. Definition according to profiles of lymphokine activities and secreted proteins. *J Immunol* 1986;136:2348–2357.

81. Kroemer G, Helmberg A, Bernot A, et al. Evolutionary relationship between human and mouse immunoglobulin kappa light chain variable region genes. *Immunogenetics* 1991;33:42–49.

82. Linsley PS, Clark EA, Ledbetter JA. T-cell antigen CD28 mediates adhesion with B cells by interacting with activation antigen B7/BB-1. *Proc Natl Acad Sci U S A* 1990;87:5031–5035.

83. Mueller DL, Jenkins MK, Schwartz RH. Clonal expansion versus functional clonal inactivation: a costimulatory signalling pathway determines the outcome of T cell antigen receptor occupancy. *Annu Rev Immunol* 1989;7:445–480.

84. Lindstein T, June CH, Ledbetter JA, et al. Regulation of lymphokine messenger RNA stability by a surface-mediated T cell activation pathway. *Science* 1989;244:339–343.

85. Ullman KS, Northrop JP, Verweij CL, et al. Transmission of signals from the T lymphocyte antigen receptor to the genes responsible for cell proliferation and immune function: the missing link. *Annu Rev Immunol* 1990;8:421–452.

86. Takeshita T, Asao H, Ohtani K, et al. Cloning of the gamma chain of the human IL-2 receptor. *Science* 1992;257:379–382.

87. Leonard WJ, Depper JM, Crabtree GR, et al. Molecular cloning and expression of cDNAs for the human interleukin-2 receptor. *Nature* 1984;311:626–631.

88. Nikaido T, Shimizu A, Ishida N, et al. Molecular cloning of cDNA encoding human interleukin-2 receptor. *Nature* 1984;311:631–635.

89. Hatakeyama M, Tsudo M, Minamoto S, et al. Interleukin-2 receptor beta chain gene: generation of three receptor forms by cloned human alpha and beta chain cDNA's. *Science* 1989;244:551–556.

90. Nakamura Y, Russell SM, Mess SA, et al. Heterodimerization of the IL-2 receptor beta- and gamma-chain cytoplasmic domains is required for signalling. *Nature* 1994;369:330–333.

91. Nelson BH, Lord JD, Greenberg PD. Cytoplasmic domains of the interleukin-2 receptor beta and gamma chains mediate the signal for T-cell proliferation. *Nature* 1994;369:333–336.

92. Gesbert F, Delespine-Carmagnat M, Bertoglio J. Recent advances in the understanding of interleukin-2 signal transduction. *J Clin Immunol* 1998;18:307–320.

93. Miyazaki T, Liu ZJ, Kawahara A, et al. Three distinct IL-2 signaling pathways mediated by bcl-2, c-myc, and lck cooperate in hematopoietic cell proliferation. *Cell* 1995;81(2):223–231.

94. Nosaka T, van Deursen JM, Tripp RA, et al. Defective lymphoid development in mice lacking Jak3 [published erratum appears in *Science* 1996;271(5245):17]. *Science* 1995;270:800–802.

95. Chen M, Cheng A, Chen YQ, et al. The amino terminus of JAK3 is necessary and sufficient for binding to the common gamma chain and confers the ability to transmit interleukin 2-mediated signals. *Proc Natl Acad Sci U S A* 1997;94:6910–6915.

96. Kawahara A, Minami Y, Miyazaki T, et al. Critical role of the interleukin 2 (IL-2) receptor gamma-chain-associated Jak3 in the IL-2-induced c-fos and c-myc, but not bcl-2, gene induction. *Proc Natl Acad Sci U S A* 1995;92:8724–8728.

97. Noguchi M, Yi H, Rosenblatt HM, et al. Interleukin-2 receptor gamma chain mutation results in X-linked severe combined immunodeficiency in humans. *Cell* 1993;73:147–157.

98. Kanazawa T, Keeler ML, Varticovski L. Serine-rich region of the IL-2 receptor beta-chain is required for activation of phosphatidylinositol 3-kinase. *Cell Immunol* 1994;156:378–388.

99. Ahmed NN, Grimes HL, Bellacosa A, et al. Transduction of interleukin-2 antiapoptotic and proliferative signals via Akt protein kinase. *Proc Natl Acad Sci U S A* 1997;94:3627–3632.

100. Minami Y, Nakagawa Y, Kawahara A, et al. Protein tyrosine kinase Syk is associated with and activated by the IL-2 receptor: possible link with the c-myc induction pathway. *Immunity* 1995;2:89–100.

101. Miyazaki T, Kawahara A, Fujii H, et al. Functional activation of Jak1 and Jak3 by selective association with IL-2 receptor subunits. *Science* 1994;266:1045–1047.

102. Hatakeyama M, Kono T, Kobayashi N, et al. Interaction of the IL-2 receptor with the src-family kinase p56lck: identification of novel intermolecular association. *Science* 1991;252:1523–1528.

103. Minami Y, Kono T, Yamada K, et al. Association of p56lck with IL-2 receptor beta chain is critical for the IL-2-induced activation of p56lck. *EMBO J* 1993;12:759–768.

104. Gennuso R, Spigelman MK, Vallabhajosula S, et al. Systemic biodistribution of radioiodinated interleukin-2 in the rat. *J Biol Response Mod* 1989;8:375–384.

105. Evans GA, Goldsmith MA, Johnston JA, et al. Analysis of interleukin-2-dependent signal transduction through the Shc/Grb2 adapter pathway. Interleukin-2-dependent mitogenesis does not require Shc phosphorylation or receptor association. *J Biol Chem* 1995;270:28858–28863.

106. Satoh T, Minami Y, Kono T, et al. Interleukin 2-induced activation of Ras requires two domains of interleukin 2 receptor beta subunit, the essential region for growth stimulation and Lck-binding domain. *J Biol Chem* 1992;267(35):25423–25427.

107. Gaffen SL, Lai SY, Ha M, et al. Distinct tyrosine residues within the interleukin-2 receptor beta chain drive signal transduction specificity, redundancy, and diversity. *J Biol Chem* 1996;271:21381–21390.

108. Fujii H, Nakagawa Y, Schindler U, et al. Activation of Stat5 by interleukin 2 requires a carboxyl-terminal region of the interleukin 2 receptor beta chain but is not essential for the proliferative signal transmission. *Proc Natl Acad Sci U S A* 1995;92:5482–5486.

109. Nakajima H, Liu XW, Wynshaw-Boris A, et al. An indirect effect of Stat5a in IL-2-induced proliferation: a critical role for Stat5a in IL-2-mediated IL-2 receptor alpha chain induction. *Immunity* 1997;7:691–701.

110. Siegel JP, Sharon M, Smith PL, et al. The IL-2 receptor beta chain (p70): role in mediating signals for LAK, NK, and proliferative activities. *Science* 1987;238:75–78.

111. Tsudo M, Goldman CK, Bongiovanni KF, et al. The p75 peptide is the receptor for interleukin 2 expressed on large granular lymphocytes and is responsible for the interleukin 2 activation of these cells. *Proc Natl Acad Sci U S A* 1987;84:5394–5398.

112. Caligiuri MA, Zmuidzinas A, Manley TJ, et al. Functional consequences of interleukin 2 receptor expression on resting human lymphocytes. Identification of a novel natural killer cell subset with high affinity receptors. *J Exp Med* 1990;171:1509–1526.

113. Cantrell DA, Smith KA. Transient expression of interleukin 2 receptors. Consequences for T cell growth. *J Exp Med* 1983;158:1895–1911.

114. Muraguchi A, Kehrl JH, Longo DL, et al. Interleukin 2 receptors on human B cells. Implications for the role of interleukin 2 in human B cell function. *J Exp Med* 1985;161:181–197.

115. Turner B, Rapp U, App H, et al. Interleukin 2 induces tyrosine phosphorylation and activation of p72–74 Raf-1 kinase in a T-cell line. *Proc Natl Acad Sci U S A* 1991;88:1227–1231.

116. Zmuidzinas A, Mamon HJ, Roberts TM, et al. Interleukin-2-triggered Raf-1 expression, phosphorylation, and associated kinase activity increase through G_1 and S in CD3-stimulated primary human T cells. *Mol Cell Biol* 1991;11:2794–2803.

117. Evans GA, Wahl LM, Farrar WL. Interleukin-2-dependent phosphorylation of the retinoblastoma-susceptibility-gene product p110-115RB in human T-cells. *Biochem J* 1992;282:759–764.

118. Baker PE, Gillis S, Smith KA. Monoclonal cytolytic T-cell lines. *J Exp Med* 1979;149:273–278.

119. Baker PE, Gillis S, Ferm MM, et al. The effect of T cell growth factor on the generation of cytolytic T cells. *J Immunol* 1978;121:2168–2173.

120. Kroemer G, Andreu JL, Gonzale JA, et al. Interleukin-2, autotolerance and autoimmunity. *Adv Immunol* 1991;50:147–235.

121. Grimm EA, Mazumder A, Zhang HZ, et al. Lymphokine-activated killer cell phenomenon. Lysis of natural killer-resistant fresh solid tumor cells by interleukin 2-activated autologous human peripheral blood lymphocytes. *J Exp Med* 1982;155:1823–1841.

122. Liu CC, Rafii S, Granelli-Piperno A, et al. Perforin and serine esterase gene expression in stimulated human T cells. Kinetics, mitogen requirements, and effects of cyclosporin A. *J Exp Med* 1989;170:2105–2118.

123. Lenardo M, Chan KM, Hornung F, et al. Mature T lymphocyte apoptosis—immune regulation in a dynamic and unpredictable antigenic environment. *Annu Rev Immunol* 1999;17:221–253.

124. Refaeli Y, Van Parijs L, Abbas AK. Genetic models of abnormal apoptosis in lymphocytes. *Immunol Rev* 1999;169:273–282.

125. Willerford DM, Chen J, Ferry JA, et al. Interleukin-2 receptor alpha chain regulates the size and content of the peripheral lymphoid compartment. *Immunity* 1995;3:521–530.

126. Suzuki H, Kundig TM, Furlonger C, et al. Deregulated T cell activation and autoimmunity in mice lacking interleukin-2 receptor beta. *Science* 1995;268:1472–1476.

127. Sadlack B, Merz H, Schorle H, et al. Ulcerative colitis-like disease in mice with a disrupted interleukin-2 gene. *Cell* 1993;75(2):253–261.

128. Lenardo MJ. Interleukin-2 programs mouse alpha beta T lymphocytes for apoptosis. *Nature* 1991;353:858–861.

129. Refaeli Y, Van Parijs L, London CA, et al. Biochemical mechanisms of IL-2-regulated Fas-mediated T cell apoptosis. *Immunity* 1998;8:615–623.

130. Bocci V, Carraro F, Zeuli M, et al. The lymphatic route. VIII. Distribution and plasma clearance of recombinant human interleukin-2 after SC administration with albumin in patients [published erratum appears in *Biotherapy* 1993;6(3):233]. *Biotherapy* 1993;6:73–77.

131. Lotze MT, Matory YL, Ettinghausen SE, et al. In vivo administration of purified human interleukin 2. II. Half life, immunologic effects, and expansion of peripheral lymphoid cells in vivo with recombinant IL 2. *J Immunol* 1985;135(4):2865–2875.

132. Gillis S, Ferm MM, Ou W, et al. T cell growth factor: parameters of production and a quantitative microassay for activity. *J Immunol* 1978;120:2027–2032.

133. Lotze MT, Matory YL, Rayner AA, et al. Clinical effects and toxicity of interleukin-2 in patients with cancer. *Cancer* 1986;58:2764–2772.

134. Sarna GP, Figlin RA, Pertcheck M, et al. Systemic administration of recombinant methionyl human interleukin-2 (Ala 125) to cancer patients: clinical results. *J Biol Response Mod* 1989;8:16–24.

135. Sosman JA, Kohler PC, Hank JA, et al. Repetitive weekly cycles of interleukin-2. II. Clinical and immunologic effects of dose, schedule, and addition of indomethacin. *J Natl Cancer Inst* 1988;80:1451–1461.

136. Zimmerman RJ, Aukerman SL, Katre NV, et al. Schedule dependency of the antitumor activity and toxicity of polyethylene glycol-modified interleukin 2 in murine tumor models. *Cancer Res* 1989;49:6521–6528.

137. Tursz T. Interleukin 2. Present and future role in cancerology [Editorial] [in French]. *Presse Med* 1991;20:241–243.

138. Tzannis ST, Hrushesky WJ, Wood PA, et al. Irreversible inactivation of interleukin 2 in a pump-based delivery environment. *Proc Natl Acad Sci U S A* 1996;93:5460–5465.

139. Gearing AJ, Thorpe R. The international standard for human interleukin-2. Calibration by international collaborative study. *J Immunol Methods* 1988;114:3–9.

140. Rossio JL, Thurman GB, Long C, et al. The BRMP IL-2 reference reagent. *Lymphokine Res* 1986;5[Suppl 1]:S13–S18.

141. Hank JA, Surfus J, Gan J, et al. Distinct clinical and laboratory activity of two recombinant interleukin-2 preparations. *Clin Cancer Res* 1999;5:281–289.

142. Vlasveld LT, Beijnen JH, Sein JJ, et al. Reconstitution of recombinant interleukin-2 (rIL-2): a comparative study of various rIL-2 muteins. *Eur J Cancer* 1993;29A:1977–1979.

143. Meyers FJ, Paradise C, Scudder SA, et al. A phase I study including pharmacokinetics of polyethylene glycol conjugated interleukin-2. *Clin Pharmacol Ther* 1991;49:307–313.

144. Konrad MW, Hemstreet G, Hersh EM, et al. Pharmacokinetics of recombinant interleukin 2 in humans. *Cancer Res* 1990;50:2009–2017.

145. Knauf MJ, Bell DP, Hirtzer P, et al. Relationship of effective molecular size to systemic clearance in rats of recombinant interleukin-2 chemically modified with water-soluble polymers. *J Biol Chem* 1988;263:15064–15070.

146. Donohue JH, Rosenberg SA. The fate of interleukin-2 after in vivo administration. *J Immunol* 1983;130:2203–2208.

147. Banks RE, Forbes MA, Hallam S, et al. Treatment of metastatic renal cell carcinoma with subcutaneous interleukin 2: evidence for non-renal clearance of cytokines. *Br J Cancer* 1997;75:1842–1848.

148. Kirchner GI, Franzke A, Buer J, et al. Pharmacokinetics of recombinant human interleukin-2 in advanced renal cell carcinoma patients following subcutaneous application. *Br J Clin Pharmacol* 1998;46(1):5–10.

149. Rosenberg SA, Lotze MT, Yang JC, et al. Experience with the use of high-dose interleukin-2 in the treatment of 652 cancer patients [see discussion]. *Ann Surg* 1989;210:474–484.

150. Fisher B, Keenan AM, Garra BS, et al. Interleukin-2 induces profound reversible cholestasis: a detailed analysis in treated cancer patients. *J Clin Oncol* 1989;7:1852–1862.

151. Bukowski RM, Goodman P, Crawford ED, et al. Phase II trial of high-dose intermittent interleukin-2 in metastatic renal cell carcinoma: a Southwest Oncology Group study. *J Natl Cancer Inst* 1990;82:143–146.

152. Palmer PA, Vinke J, Philip T, et al. Prognostic factors for survival in patients with advanced renal cell carcinoma treated with recombinant interleukin-2. *Ann Oncol* 1992;3:475–480.

153. Sleijfer DT, Janssen RA, Buter J, et al. Phase II study of subcutaneous interleukin-2 in unselected patients with advanced renal cell cancer on an outpatient basis. *J Clin Oncol* 1992;10:1119–1123.

154. Negrier S, Escudier B, Lasset C, et al. Recombinant human interleukin-2, recombinant human interferon alfa-2a, or both in metastatic renal-cell carcinoma. Groupe Francais d'Immunotherapie. *N Engl J Med* 1998;338:1272–1278.

155. Fisher RI, Rosenberg SA, Sznol M, et al. High-dose aldesleukin in renal cell carcinoma: long-term survival update [see comments]. *Cancer J Sci Am* 1997;3[Suppl 1]:S70-S72.

156. Escudier B, Ravaud A, Fabbro M, et al. High-dose interleukin-2 two days a week for metastatic renal cell carcinoma: a FNCLCC multicenter study. *J Immunother Emphasis Tumor Immunol* 1994;16:306–312.

157. Caligiuri MA. Low-dose recombinant interleukin-2 therapy: rationale and potential clinical applications. *Semin Oncol* 1993;20:3–10.

158. Buter J, Sleijfer DT, van der Graaf WT, et al. A progress report on the outpatient treatment of patients with advanced renal cell carcinoma using subcutaneous recombinant interleukin-2. *Semin Oncol* 1993;20:16–21.

159. Yang JC, Rosenberg SA. An ongoing prospective randomized comparison of interleukin-2 regimens for the treatment of metastatic renal cell cancer. *Cancer J Sci Am* 1997; 3[Suppl 1]:S79–S84.

160. Bukowski RM, Dutcher JD. Low dose interleukin-2: single agent and combination regimens. In: Scardino PT, Shipley W, Cobbey DS, eds. *Comprehensive textbook of genitourinary oncology*. Philadelphia: Lippincott Williams & Wilkins, 2000:218–233.

161. Bukowski RM. Natural history and therapy of metastatic renal cell carcinoma: the role of interleukin-2. *Cancer* 1997;80:1198–1220.

162. Newman SP, Clarke SW. Therapeutic aerosols 1—physical and practical considerations. *Thorax* 1983;38:881–886.

163. Huland E, Huland H, Heinzer H. Interleukin-2 by inhalation: local therapy for metastatic renal cell carcinoma. *J Urol* 1992;147:344–348.

164. Huland E, Heinzer H, Mir TS, et al. Inhaled interleukin-2 therapy in pulmonary metastatic renal cell carcinoma: six years of experience [see comments]. *Cancer J Sci Am* 1997;3[Suppl 1]:S98–S105.

165. Lorenz J, Wilhelm K, Kessler M, et al. Phase I trial of inhaled natural interleukin 2 for treatment of pulmonary malignancy: toxicity, pharmacokinetics, and biological effects. *Clin Cancer Res* 1996;2:1115–1122.

166. Nakamoto T, Kasaoka Y, Mitani S, et al. Inhalation of interleukin-2 combined with subcutaneous administration of interferon for the treatment of pulmonary metastases from renal cell carcinoma. *Int J Urol* 1997;4:343–348.

167. Khanna C, Anderson PM, Hasz DE, et al. Interleukin-2 liposome inhalation therapy is safe and effective for dogs with spontaneous pulmonary metastases. *Cancer* 1997;79:1409–1421.

168. Ravaud A, Audhuy B, Gomez F, et al. Subcutaneous interleukin-2, interferon alfa-2a, and continuous infusion of fluorouracil in metastatic renal cell carcinoma: a multicenter phase II trial. Groupe Francais d'Immunotherapie. *J Clin Oncol* 1998;16:2728–2732.

169. Freedman RS, Gibbons JA, Giedlin M, et al. Immunopharmacology and cytokine production of a low-dose schedule of intraperitoneally administered human recombinant interleukin-2 in patients with advanced epithelial ovarian carcinoma. *J Immunother Emphasis Tumor Immunol* 1996;19: 443–451.

170. Kolitz JE, Welte K, Wong GY, et al. Expansion of activated T-lymphocytes in patients treated with recombinant interleukin 2. *J Biol Response Mod* 1987;6:412–429.

171. Gambacorti-Passerini C, Radrizzani M, Marolda R, et al. In vivo activation of lymphocytes in melanoma patients receiving escalating doses of recombinant interleukin 2. *Int J Cancer* 1988;41:700–706.

172. Thompson JA, Lee DJ, Lindgren CG, et al. Influence of dose and duration of infusion of interleukin-2 on toxicity and immunomodulation. *J Clin Oncol* 1988;6:669–678.

173. Caligiuri MA, Murray C, Robertson MJ, et al. Selective modulation of human natural killer cells in vivo after prolonged infusion of low dose recombinant interleukin 2. *J Clin Invest* 1993;91:123–132.

174. Cotran RS, Pober JS, Gimbrone MA Jr, et al. Endothelial activation during interleukin 2 immunotherapy. A possible mechanism for the vascular leak syndrome. *J Immunol* 1988;140:1883–1888.

175. Gemlo BT, Palladino MA Jr, Jaffe HS, et al. Circulating cytokines in patients with metastatic cancer treated with recombinant interleukin 2 and lymphokine-activated killer cells. *Cancer Res* 1988;48:5864–5867.

176. Mier JW, Vachino G, van der Meer JW, et al. Induction of circulating tumor necrosis factor (TNF alpha) as the mechanism for the febrile response to interleukin-2 (IL-2) in cancer patients. *J Clin Immunol* 1988;8:426–436.

177. Kasid A, Director EP, Rosenberg SA. Induction of endogenous cytokine-mRNA in circulating peripheral blood mononuclear cells by IL-2 administration to cancer patients. *J Immunol* 1989;143:736–739.

178. Wiebke EA, Rosenberg SA, Lotze MT. Acute immunologic effects of interleukin-2 therapy in cancer patients: decreased delayed type hypersensitivity response and decreased proliferative response to soluble antigens. *J Clin Oncol* 1988;6:1440–1449.

179. Klempner MS, Noring R, Mier JW, et al. An acquired chemotactic defect in neutrophils from patients receiving interleukin-2 immunotherapy [see comments]. *N Engl J Med* 1990;322:959–965.

180. Parkinson DR. Interleukin-2 in cancer therapy. *Semin Oncol* 1988:15:10–26.

181. Gaynor ER, Vitek L, Sticklin L, et al. The hemodynamic effects of treatment with interleukin-2 and lymphokine-activated killer cells. *Ann Intern Med* 1988;109:953–958.

182. Nora R, Abrams JS, Tait NS, et al. Myocardial toxic effects during recombinant interleukin-2 therapy. *J Natl Cancer Inst* 1989;81:59–63.

183. Osanto S, Cluitmans FH, Franks CR, et al. Myocardial injury after interleukin-2 therapy [Letter]. *Lancet* 1988;2:48–49.

184. Ettinghausen SE, Moore JG, White DE, et al. Hematologic effects of immunotherapy with lymphokine-activated killer cells and recombinant interleukin-2 in cancer patients. *Blood* 1987;69:1654–1660.

185. Snydman DR, Sullivan B, Gill M, et al. Nosocomial sepsis associated with interleukin-2 [see comments]. *Ann Intern Med* 1990;112:102–107.

186. Post AB, Falk GW, Bukowski RM. Acute colonic pseudo-obstruction associated with interleukin-2 therapy. *Am J Gastroenterol* 1991;86:1539–1541.

187. Schwartzentruber D, Lotze MT, Rosenberg SA. Colonic perforation. An unusual complication of therapy with high-dose interleukin-2. *Cancer* 1988;62:2350–2353.

188. Rahman R, Bernstein Z, Vaickus L, et al. Unusual gastrointestinal complications of interleukin-2 therapy. *J Immunother* 1991;10:221–225.

189. Denicoff KD, Rubinow DR, Papa MZ, et al. The neuropsychiatric effects of treatment with interleukin-2 and lymphokine-activated killer cells. *Ann Intern Med* 1987;107:293–300.

190. Saris SC, Patronas NJ, Rosenberg SA, et al. The effect of intravenous interleukin-2 on brain water content. *J Neurosurg* 1989;71:169–174.

191. Caraceni A, Martini C, Belli F, et al. Neuropsychological and neurophysiological assessment of the central effects of interleukin-2 administration. *Eur J Cancer* 1993;29A:1266–1269.

192. Adams F, Quesada JR, Gutterman JU. Neuropsychiatric manifestations of human leukocyte interferon therapy in patients with cancer. *JAMA* 1984;252:938–941.

193. Gaspari AA, Lotze MT, Rosenberg SA, et al. Dermatologic changes associated with interleukin 2 administration. *JAMA* 1987;258:1624–1629.

194. Lee RE, Gaspari AA, Lotze MT, et al. Interleukin 2 and psoriasis. *Arch Dermatol* 1988;124:1811–1815.

195. Atkins MB, Mier JW, Parkinson DR, et al. Hypothyroidism after treatment with interleukin-2 and lymphokine-activated killer cells. *N Engl J Med* 1988;318:1557–1563.

196. Pichert G, Jost LM, Zobeli L, et al. Thyroiditis after treatment with interleukin-2 and interferon alpha-2a. *Br J Cancer* 1990;62:100–104.

197. Franzke A, Peest D, Probst-Kepper M, et al. Autoimmunity resulting from cytokine treatment predicts long-term survival in patients with metastatic renal cell cancer. *J Clin Oncol* 1999;17:529–533.

198. Papa MZ, Vetto JT, Ettinghausen SE, et al. Effect of corticosteroid on the antitumor activity of lymphokine-activated killer cells and interleukin 2 in mice. *Cancer Res* 1986;46:5618–5623.

199. Margolin K, Atkins M, Sparano J, et al. Prospective randomized trial of lisofylline for the prevention of toxicities of high-dose interleukin 2 therapy in advanced renal cancer and malignant melanoma. *Clin Cancer Res* 1997;3:565–572.

200. Du Bois JS, Trehu EG, Mier JW, et al. Randomized placebo-controlled clinical trial of high-dose interleukin-2 in combination with a soluble p75 tumor necrosis factor receptor immunoglobulin G chimera in patients with advanced melanoma and renal cell carcinoma. *J Clin Oncol* 1997;15:1052–1062.

201. Rosenberg SA, Lotze MT, Muul LM, et al. A progress report on the treatment of 157 patients with advanced cancer using lymphokine-activated killer cells and interleukin-2 or high-dose interleukin-2 alone. *N Engl J Med* 1987;316:889–897.

202. Bukowski RM, Sharfman W, Murthy S, et al. Clinical results and characterization of tumor-infiltrating lymphocytes with or without recombinant interleukin 2 in human metastatic renal cell carcinoma. *Cancer Res* 1991;51:4199–4205.

203. Papa MZ, Mule JJ, Rosenberg SA. Antitumor efficacy of lymphokine-activated killer cells and recombinant interleukin 2 in vivo: successful immunotherapy of established pulmonary metastases from weakly immunogenic and nonimmunogenic murine tumors of three district histological types. *Cancer Res* 1986;46:4973–4978.

204. Rosenberg SA, Lotze MT, Yang JC, et al. Combination therapy with interleukin-2 and alpha-interferon for the treatment of patients with advanced cancer. *J Clin Oncol* 1989;7:1863–1874.

205. Redman BG, Flaherty L, Chou TH, et al. A phase I trial of recombinant interleukin-2 combined with recombinant interferon-gamma in patients with cancer. *J Clin Oncol* 1990;8:1269–1276.

206. Krigel RL, Padavic-Shaller KA, Rudolph AR, et al. Renal cell carcinoma: treatment with recombinant interleukin-2 plus beta-interferon. *J Clin Oncol* 1990;8:460–467.

207. Triozzi P, Martin E, Kim J, et al. Phase 1b trial of interleukin-1β (IL-1β)/interleukin-2 (IL-2) in patients with metastatic cancer. *Proc Am Soc Clin Oncol* 1993;12:290.

207a. Olencki T, Finke J, Tubbs R, et al. Phase IA/IB trial of interleukin-2 and interleukin-4 in patients with refractory malignancy. *J Immunother* 1996;19:69–80.

208. Ilson DH, Motzer RJ, Kradin RL, et al. A phase II trial of interleukin-2 and interferon alfa-2a in patients with advanced renal cell carcinoma [published erratum appears in *J Clin Oncol* 1992;10(11):1822]. *J Clin Oncol* 1992;10:1124–1130.

209. Budd GT, Murthy S, Finke J, et al. Phase I trial of high-dose bolus interleukin-2 and interferon alfa-2a in patients with metastatic malignancy. *J Clin Oncol* 1992;10:804–809.

210. Greekmore S, Urba W, Kopp W. Phase IB/II trial of R24 antibody and interleukin-2 (IL-2) in melanoma. *Proc Am Soc Clin Oncol* 1992;11:345(abst).

211. Goodman GE, Hellstrom I, Stevenson U. Phase I trial of murine monoclonal antibody MG-22 and IL-2 in patients with disseminated melanoma. *Proc Am Soc Clin Oncol* 1992;11:346(abst).

212. Kuebler JP, Whitehead RP, Ward DL, et al. Treatment of metastatic renal cell carcinoma with recombinant interleukin-2 in combination with vinblastine or lymphokine-activated killer cells. *J Urol* 1993;150:814–820.

213. Gautam SC, Chikkala NF, Ganapathi R, et al. Combination therapy with adriamycin and interleukin 2 augments immunity against murine renal cell carcinoma. *Cancer Res* 1991;51:6133–6137.

214. Bukowski RM, Sergi JS, Budd GT, et al. Phase I trial of continuous infusion interleukin-2 and doxorubicin in patients with refractory malignancies. *J Immunother* 1991;10:432–439.

215. Paciucci PA, Bekesi JG, Ryder JS, et al. Immunotherapy with IL2 by constant infusion and weekly doxorubicin. *Am J Clin Oncol* 1991;14:341–348.

216. Dillman RO, Church C, Oldham RK, et al. Inpatient continuous-infusion interleukin-2 in 788 patients with cancer. The National Biotherapy Study Group experience. *Cancer* 1993;71:2358–2370.

217. Mitchell MS. Chemotherapy in combination with biomodulation: a 5-year experience with cyclophosphamide and interleukin-2. *Semin Oncol* 1992;19:80–87.

218. Berd D, Maguire HC Jr, Mastrangelo MJ. Potentiation of human cell-mediated and humoral immunity by low-dose cyclophosphamide. *Cancer Res* 1984;44:5439–5443.

219. Atzpodien J, Kirchner H, Hanninen EL, et al. Interleukin-2 in combination with interferon-alpha and 5-fluorouracil for metastatic renal cell cancer. *Eur J Cancer* 1993;29A[Suppl 5]:S6–S8.

220. Negrier S, Escudier B, Dovillard JY. Randomized study of interleukin 2 (IL-2) and interferon (IFN) with or without 5-FU (FUCY study) in metastatic renal cell carcinoma (MRCC). *Proc Am Soc Clin Oncol* 1997;16:326a.

221. Legha SS, Ring S, Eton O, et al. Development and results of biochemotherapy in metastatic melanoma: the University of Texas M. D. Anderson Cancer Center experience [see comments]. *Cancer J Sci Am* 1997;3[Suppl 1]:S9–S15.

222. Reiss WG, Piscitelli SC. Drug-cytokine interactions: mechanisms and clinical implications. *Bio Drugs* 1998;9:389–395.

223. Piscitelli SC, Vogel S, Figg WD, et al. Alteration in indinavir clearance during interleukin-2 infusions in patients infected with the human immunodeficiency virus. *Pharmacotherapy* 1998;18:1212–1216.

224. Katre NV, Knauf MJ, Laird WJ. Chemical modification of recombinant interleukin 2 by polyethylene glycol increases its potency in the murine Meth A sarcoma model. *Proc Natl Acad Sci U S A* 1987;84:1487–1491.

225. Bukowski RM, Young J, Goodman G, et al. Polyethylene glycol conjugated interleukin-2: clinical and immunologic effects in patients with advanced renal cell carcinoma. *Invest New Drugs* 1993;11:211–217.

226. Gause B, Longo DL, Janik J. A phase I study of liposome-encapsulated IL-2 (LE-IL-2). *Proc Am Soc Clin Oncol* 1993;12:293(abst).

227. Isakson PC, Pure E, Vitetta ES, et al. T cell-derived B cell differentiation factor(s). Effect on the isotype switch of murine B cells. *J Exp Med* 1982;155:734–748.

228. Howard M, Farrar J, Hilfiker M. Identification of a T cell-derived B cell stimulatory factor distinct from IL-2. *J Exp Med* 1982;155:914–923.

229. Puri RK, Siegel JP. Interleukin-4 and cancer therapy. *Cancer Invest* 1993;11:473–486.

230. Yokota T, Otsuka T, Mosmann T, et al. Isolation and characterization of a human interleukin cDNA clone, homologous to mouse B-cell stimulatory factor 1, that expresses B-cell- and T-cell-stimulating activities. *Proc Natl Acad Sci U S A* 1986;83:5894–5898.

231. Lee F, Yokota T, Otsuka T, et al. Isolation and characterization of a mouse interleukin cDNA clone that expresses B-cell stimulatory factor 1 activities and T-cell- and mast-cell-stimulating activities. *Proc Natl Acad Sci U S A* 1986; 83:2061–2065.

232. Arai N, Nomura D, Villaret D, et al. Complete nucleotide sequence of the chromosomal gene for human IL-4 and its expression. *J Immunol* 1989;142:274–282.

233. Ohara J, Coligan JE, Zoon K, et al. High-efficiency purification and chemical characterization of B cell stimulatory factor-1/interleukin 4. *J Immunol* 1987;139:1127–1134.

234. Le Beau MM, Lemons RS, Espinosa R, et al. Interleukin-4 and interleukin-5 map to human chromosome 5 in a region encoding growth factors and receptors and are deleted in myeloid leukemias with a del(5q). *Blood* 1989;73:647–650.

235. Van Leeuwen BH, Martinson ME, Webb GC, et al. Molecular organization of the cytokine gene cluster, involving the human IL-3, IL-4, IL-5, and GM-CSF genes, on human chromosome 5. *Blood* 1989;73:1142–1148.

236. Yokota T, Arai N, de Vries J, et al. Molecular biology of interleukin 4 and interleukin 5 genes and biology of their products that stimulate B cells, T cells and hemopoietic cells. *Immunol Rev* 1988;102:137–187.

237. Walter MR, Cook WJ, Zhao BG, et al. Crystal structure of recombinant human interleukin-4. *J Biol Chem* 1992;267: 20371–20376.

238. Walter MR, Cook WJ, Ealick SE, et al. Three-dimensional structure of recombinant human granulocyte-macrophage colony-stimulating factor. *J Mol Biol* 1992;224:1075–1085.

239. Dorr RT, Von Hoff DD. Interleukin-4 drug monograph. In: Dorr RT, Von Hoff DD, eds. *Cancer chemotherapy handbook.* East Norwalk, CT: Appleton & Lange, 1994:601–605.

240. Ohara J, Paul WE. Receptors for B-cell stimulatory factor-1 expressed on cells of haematopoietic lineage. *Nature* 1987;325:537–540.

241. Ohara J, Paul WE. Up-regulation of interleukin 4/B-cell stimulatory factor 1 receptor expression. *Proc Natl Acad Sci U S A* 1988;85:8221–8225.

242. Wagteveld AJ, van Zanten AK, Esselink MT, et al. Expression and regulation of IL-4 receptors on human monocytes and acute myeloblastic leukemic cells. *Leukemia* 1991;5:782–788.

243. Feldman GM, Finbloom DS. Induction and regulation of IL-4 receptor expression on murine macrophage cell lines and bone marrow-derived macrophages by IFN-gamma. *J Immunol* 1990;145:854–859.

244. Nelms K, Keegan AD, Zamorano J, et al. The IL-4 receptor: signaling mechanisms and biologic functions. *Annu Rev Immunol* 1999;17:701–738.

245. Lai SY, Molden J, Liu KD, et al. Interleukin-4-specific signal transduction events are driven by homotypic interactions of the interleukin-4 receptor alpha subunit. *EMBO J* 1996;15:4506–4514.

246. Fujiwara H, Hanissian SH, Tsytsykova A, et al. Homodimerization of the human interleukin 4 receptor alpha chain induces Cepsilon germline transcripts in B cells in the absence of the interleukin 2 receptor gamma chain. *Proc Natl Acad Sci U S A* 1997;94:5866–5871.

247. Reichel M, Nelson BH, Greenberg PD, et al. The IL-4 receptor alpha-chain cytoplasmic domain is sufficient for activation of JAK-1 and STAT6 and the induction of IL-4-specific gene expression. *J Immunol* 1997;158:5860–5867.

248. Obiri NI, Debinski W, Leonard WJ, et al. Receptor for interleukin 13. Interaction with interleukin 4 by a mechanism that does not involve the common gamma chain shared by receptors for interleukins 2, 4, 7, 9, and 15. *J Biol Chem* 1995;270(15):8797–8804.

249. Miloux B, Laurent P, Bonnin O, et al. Cloning of the human IL-13R alpha1 chain and reconstitution with the IL4R alpha of a functional IL-4/IL-13 receptor complex. *FEBS Lett* 1997;401:163–166.

250. Obiri NI, Leland P, Murata T, et al. The IL-13 receptor structure differs on various cell types and may share more than one component with IL-4 receptor. *J Immunol* 1997; 158:756–764.

251. Letzelter F, Wang Y, Sebald W. The interleukin-4 site-2 epitope determining binding of the common receptor gamma chain. *Eur J Biochem* 1998;257:11–20.

252. Russell SM, Keegan AD, Harada N, et al. Interleukin-2 receptor gamma chain: a functional component of the interleukin-4 receptor [see comments]. *Science* 1993;262:1880–1883.

253. Kammer W, Lischke A, Moriggl R, et al. Homodimerization of interleukin-4 receptor alpha chain can induce intracellular signaling. *J Biol Chem* 1996;271:23634–23637.

254. Witthuhn BA, Silvennoinen O, Miura O, et al. Involvement of the Jak-3 Janus kinase in signalling by interleukins

2 and 4 in lymphoid and myeloid cells. *Nature* 1994;370 (6485):153–157.

255. Murata T, Noguchi PD, Puri RK. IL-13 induces phosphorylation and activation of JAK2 Janus kinase in human colon carcinoma cell lines: similarities between IL-4 and IL-13 signaling. *J Immunol* 1996;156:2972–2978.

256. Johnston JA, Kawamura M, Kirken RA, et al. Phosphorylation and activation of the Jak-3 Janus kinase in response to interleukin-2. *Nature* 1994;370:151–153.

257. Keegan AD, Nelms K, Wang LM, et al. Interleukin 4 receptor: signaling mechanisms. *Immunol Today* 1994;15:423–432.

258. Koettnitz K, Kalthoff FS. Human interleukin-4 receptor signaling requires sequences contained within two cytoplasmic regions. *Eur J Immunol* 1993;23:988–991.

259. Seldin DC, Leder P. Mutational analysis of a critical signaling domain of the human interleukin 4 receptor. *Proc Natl Acad Sci U S A* 1994;91:2140–2144.

260. Ryan JJ, McReynolds LJ, Keegan A, et al. Growth and gene expression are predominantly controlled by distinct regions of the human IL-4 receptor. *Immunity* 1996;4(2):123–132.

261. Wang LM, Myers MG Jr, Sun XJ, et al. IRS-1: essential for insulin- and IL-4-stimulated mitogenesis in hematopoietic cells. *Science* 1993;261:1591–1594.

262. Sun XJ, Wang LM, Zhang Y, et al. Role of IRS-2 in insulin and cytokine signalling. *Nature* 1995;377:173–177.

263. Wang LM, Keegan AD, Li W, et al. Common elements in interleukin 4 and insulin signaling pathways in factor-dependent hematopoietic cells. *Proc Natl Acad Sci U S A* 1993;90:4032–4036.

264. Sun XJ, Crimmins DL, Myers MG Jr, et al. Pleiotropic insulin signals are engaged by multisite phosphorylation of IRS-1. *Mol Cell Biol* 1993;13:7418–7428.

265. Dhand R, Hiles I, Panayotou G, et al. PI 3-kinase is a dual specificity enzyme: autoregulation by an intrinsic protein-serine kinase activity. *EMBO J* 1994;13:522–533.

266. Stephens LR, Jackson TR, Hawkins PT. Agonist-stimulated synthesis of phosphatidylinositol(3,4,5)-trisphosphate: a new intracellular signalling system? *Biochim Biophys Acta* 1993;1179:27–75.

267. Auger KR, Serunian LA, Soltoff SP, et al. PDGF-dependent tyrosine phosphorylation stimulates production of novel polyphosphoinositides in intact cells. *Cell* 1989;57:167–175.

268. Franke TF, Kaplan DR, Cantley LC, et al. Direct regulation of the Akt proto-oncogene product by phosphatidylinositol-3,4-bisphosphate [see comments]. *Science* 1997;275:665–668.

269. Franke TF, Kaplan DR, Cantley LC. PI3K: downstream AKTion blocks apoptosis. *Cell* 1997;88:435–437.

270. Delphin S, Stavnezer J. Regulation of antibody class switching to IgE: characterization of an IL-4-responsive region in the immunoglobulin heavy-chain germline epsilon promoter. *Ann N Y Acad Sci* 1995;764:123–135.

271. Takeda K, Tanaka T, Shi W, et al. Essential role of Stat6 in IL-4 signalling. *Nature* 1996;380:627–630.

272. Mossmann TR, Cherwinski H, Bond MW. Two types of murine helper T cell clones. Definition according to profiles of lymphokines, activities, and secreted proteins. *J Immunol* 1986;136:2348–2357.

273. Plaut M, Pierce JH, Watson CJ, et al. Mast cell lines produce lymphokines in response to cross-linkage of Fc epsilon RI or to calcium ionophores. *Nature* 1989;339:64–67.

274. Kuhn R, Rajewsky K, Muller W. Generation and analysis of interleukin-4 deficient mice. *Science* 1991;254:707–710.

275. Tepper RI, Levinson DA, Stanger BZ, et al. IL-4 induces allergic-like inflammatory disease and alters T cell development in transgenic mice. *Cell* 1990;62:457–467.

276. Tarte K, Lu ZY, Fiol G, et al. Generation of virtually pure and potentially proliferating dendritic cells from non-CD34 apheresis cells from patients with multiple myeloma. *Blood* 1997;90:3482–3495.

277. Puri RK, Ogata M, Leland P, et al. Expression of high-affinity interleukin 4 receptors on murine sarcoma cells and receptor-mediated cytotoxicity of tumor cells to chimeric protein between interleukin 4 and *Pseudomonas* exotoxin. *Cancer Res* 1991;51:3011–3017.

278. Tepper RI, Pattengale PK, Leder P. Murine interleukin-4 displays potent anti-tumor activity in vivo. *Cell* 1989;57:503–512.

279. Golumbek PT, Lazenby AJ, Levitsky HI, et al. Treatment of established renal cancer by tumor cells engineered to secrete interleukin-4. *Science* 1991;254:713–716.

280. Karray S, DeFrance T, Merle-Beral H, et al. Interleukin 4 counteracts the interleukin 2-induced proliferation of monoclonal B cells. *J Exp Med* 1988;168:85–94.

281. DeFrance T, Fluckiger AC, Rossi JF, et al. Antiproliferative effects of interleukin-4 on freshly isolated non-Hodgkin malignant B-lymphoma cells. *Blood* 1992;79:990–996.

282. Taylor CW, Grogan TM, Salmon SE. Effects of interleukin-4 on the in vitro growth of human lymphoid and plasma cell neoplasms. *Blood* 1990;75:1114–1118.

283. Gooch JL, Lee AV, Yee D. Interleukin 4 inhibits growth and induces apoptosis in human breast cancer cells. *Cancer Res* 1998;58:4199–4205.

284. Mehrotra R, Varricchio F, Husain SR, et al. Head and neck cancers, but not benign lesions, express interleukin-4 receptors in situ. *Oncol Rep* 1998;5:45–48.

285. Herrmann F, Andreeff M, Gruss HJ, et al. Interleukin-4 inhibits growth of multiple myelomas by suppressing interleukin-6 expression. *Blood* 1991;78:2070–2074.

286. Akashi K, Shibuya T, Harada M, et al. Interleukin 4 suppresses the spontaneous growth of chronic myelomonocytic leukemia cells. *J Clin Invest* 1991;88:223–230.

287. Tungekar MF, Turley H, Dunnill MS, et al. Interleukin 4 receptor expression on human lung tumors and normal lung. *Cancer Res* 1991;51:261–264.

288. Toi M, Bicknell R, Harris AL. Inhibition of colon and breast carcinoma cell growth by interleukin-4. *Cancer Res* 1992;52:275–279.

289. Custer MC, Lotze MT. A biologic assay for IL-4. Rapid fluorescence assay for IL-4 detection in supernatants and serum. *J Immunol Methods* 1990;128:109–117.

290. Ghosh AK, Smith NK, Prendiville J, et al. A phase I study of recombinant human interleukin-4 administered by the intravenous and subcutaneous route in patients with advanced cancer: immunological studies. *Eur Cytokine Netw* 1993;4:205–211.

291. Lotze MT. Role of IL-4 in the anti-tumor response. In: Spitz H, ed. *IL-4: structure and function.* Boca Raton, FL: CRC Press, 1992:237–262.

292. Prendiville J, Thatcher N, Lind M, et al. Recombinant human interleukin-4 (rhu IL-4) administered by the intra-

venous and subcutaneous routes in patients with advanced cancer—a phase I toxicity study and pharmacokinetic analysis. *Eur J Cancer* 1993;29A:1700–1707.

293. Markowitz A, Kleinerman E, Hudson M. Phase I study of recombinant IL-4 in patients with advanced cancer. *Blood* 1989;74[Suppl]:146a(abst).

294. Taylor CW, Hultquist KE, Taylor AM. Immunopharmacology of recombinant human interleukin-4 administered by the subcutaneous route in patients with malignancy. *Blood* 1992;76[Suppl]:221a(abst).

295. Atkins MB, Vachino G, Tilg HJ, et al. Phase I evaluation of thrice-daily intravenous bolus interleukin-4 in patients with refractory malignancy. *J Clin Oncol* 1992;10:1802–1809.

296. Gilleece MH, Scarffe JH, Ghosh A, et al. Recombinant human interleukin 4 (IL-4) given as daily subcutaneous injections—a phase I dose toxicity trial. *Br J Cancer* 1992;66:204–210.

297. Maher D, Boyd A, McKendrick J. Rapid response of B cell malignancies induced by interleukin 4. *Blood* 1990;76 [Suppl]:152a(abst).

298. Leach MW, Rybak ME, Rosenblum IY. Safety evaluation of recombinant human interleukin-4. II. Clinical studies. *Clin Immunol Immunopathol* 1997;83:12–14.

299. Rubin JT, Lotze MT. Acute gastric mucosal injury associated with the systemic administration of interleukin-4. *Surgery* 1992;111:274–280.

300. Whitehead RP, Unger JM, Goodwin JW, et al. Phase II trial of recombinant human interleukin-4 in patients with disseminated malignant melanoma: a Southwest Oncology Group study. *J Immunother* 1998;21:440–446.

301. Vokes EE, Figlin R, Hochster H, et al. A phase II study of recombinant human interleukin-4 for advanced or recurrent non-small cell lung cancer. *Cancer J Sci Am* 1998;4:46–51.

302. Tulpule A, Joshi B, DeGuzman N, et al. Interleukin-4 in the treatment of AIDS-related Kaposi's sarcoma. *Ann Oncol* 1997;8:79–83.

303. Coley WB. The treatment of malignant tumors by repeated inoculations of erysipelas. With a report of ten original cases. 1893 [classical article]. *Clin Orthop* 1991;Feb(263):3–11.

304. Shear MJ, Turner FC, Perrault A. Chemical treatment of tumors. V. Isolation of the hemorrhage producing fraction from *Serratia marcescens* culture filtrates. *J Natl Cancer Inst* 1943;4:81–97.

305. Carswell EA, Old LJ, Kassel RL, et al. An endotoxin-induced serum factor that causes necrosis of tumors. *Proc Natl Acad Sci U S A* 1975;72:3666–3670.

306. Aggarwal BB, Moffat B, Harkins RN. Human lymphotoxin. Production by a lymphoblastoid cell line, purification, and initial characterization. *J Biol Chem* 1984;259:686–691.

307. Aggarwal BB, Eessalu TE, Hass PE. Characterization of receptors for human tumour necrosis factor and their regulation by gamma-interferon. *Nature* 1985;318:665–667.

308. Ruddle NH. Tumor necrosis factor (TNF-alpha) and lymphotoxin (TNF-beta). *Curr Opin Immunol* 1992;4:327–332.

309. Nedwin GE, Naylor SL, Sakaguchi AY, et al. Human lymphotoxin and tumor necrosis factor genes: structure, homology and chromosomal localization. *Nucleic Acids Res* 1985;13:6361–6373.

310. Sariban E, Imamura K, Luebbers R, et al. Transcriptional and posttranscriptional regulation of tumor necrosis factor gene expression in human monocytes. *J Clin Invest* 1988;81:1506–1510.

311. Shakhov AN, Collart MA, Vassalli P, et al. Kappa B-type enhancers are involved in lipopolysaccharide-mediated transcriptional activation of the tumor necrosis factor alpha gene in primary macrophages. *J Exp Med* 1990;171:35–47.

312. Kunkel SL, Spengler M, May MA, et al. Prostaglandin E$_2$ regulates macrophage-derived tumor necrosis factor gene expression. *J Biol Chem* 1988;263:5380–5384.

313. Strieter RM, Remick DG, Ward PA, et al. Cellular and molecular regulation of tumor necrosis factor-alpha production by pentoxifylline. *Biochem Biophys Res Commun* 1988;155:1230–1236.

314. Hibbs JB Jr, Taintor RR, Chapman HA Jr, et al. Macrophage tumor killing: influence of the local environment. *Science* 1977;197:279–282.

315. Debets JM, Van der Linden CJ, Dieteren IE, et al. Fc-receptor cross-linking induces rapid secretion of tumor necrosis factor (cachectin) by human peripheral blood monocytes. *J Immunol* 1988;141:1197–1201.

316. Kornbluth RS, Gregory SA, Edgington TS. Initial characterization of a lymphokine pathway for the immunologic induction of tumor necrosis factor-alpha release from human peripheral blood mononuclear cells. *J Immunol* 1988;141:2006–2015.

317. Imamura K, Spriggs D, Ohno T, et al. Effects of botulinum toxin type D on secretion of tumor necrosis factor from human monocytes. *Mol Cell Biol* 1989;9:2239–2243.

318. Muller R, Marmenout A, Fiers W. Synthesis and maturation of recombinant human tumor necrosis factor in eukaryotic systems. *FEBS Lett* 1986;197:99–104.

319. Smith RA, Baglioni C. The active form of tumor necrosis factor is a trimer. *J Biol Chem* 1987;262:6951–6954.

320. Taguchi T, Sohmura Y. Clinical studies with TNF. *Biotherapy* 1991;3:177–186.

321. Creasey AA, Doyle LV, Reynolds MT, et al. Biological effects of recombinant human tumor necrosis factor and its novel muteins on tumor and normal cell lines. *Cancer Res* 1987;47:145–149.

322. Watanabe N, Kuriyama H, Sone H, et al. Continuous internalization of tumor necrosis factor receptors in a human myosarcoma cell line. *J Biol Chem* 1988;263:10262–10266.

323. Hohmann HP, Remy R, Brockhaus M, et al. Two different cell types have different major receptors for human tumor necrosis factor (TNF alpha). *J Biol Chem* 1989;264:14927–14934.

324. Ware CF, VanArsdale S, VanArsdale TL. Apoptosis mediated by the TNF-related cytokine and receptor families. *J Cell Biochem* 1996;60:47–55.

325. Hsu H, Shu HB, Pan MG, et al. TRADD-TRAF2 and TRADD-FADD interactions define two distinct TNF receptor 1 signal transduction pathways. *Cell* 1996;84:299–308.

326. Rothe M, Pan MG, Henzel WJ, et al. The TNFR2-TRAF signaling complex contains two novel proteins related to baculoviral inhibitor of apoptosis proteins. *Cell* 1995;83:1243–1252.

327. Rothe M, Sarma V, Dixit VM, et al. TRAF2-mediated activation of NF-kappa B by TNF receptor 2 and CD40. *Science* 1995;269:1424–1427.

328. Wickremasinghe RG, Hoffbrand AV. Biochemical and genetic control of apoptosis: relevance to normal hematopoiesis and hematological malignancies. *Blood* 1999;93:3587–3600.

329. Tsujimoto M, Feinman R, Vilcek J. Differential effects of type I IFN and IFN-gamma on the binding of tumor necrosis factor to receptors in two human cell lines. *J Immunol* 1986;137:2272–2276.

330. Ruggiero V, Tavernier J, Fiers W, et al. Induction of the synthesis of tumor necrosis factor receptors by interferon-gamma. *J Immunol* 1986;136:2445–2450.

331. Holtmann H, Wallach D. Down regulation of the receptors for tumor necrosis factor by interleukin 1 and 4 beta-phorbol-12-myristate-13-acetate. *J Immunol* 1987;139:1161–1167.

332. Etanercept. Soluble tumour necrosis factor receptor, TNF receptor fusion protein, TNFR-Fc, TNR 001, Enbrel. *Drugs R D* 1999;1:258–261.

333. Moreland LW, Baumgartner SW, Schiff MH, et al. Treatment of rheumatoid arthritis with a recombinant human tumor necrosis factor receptor (p75)-Fc fusion protein [see comments]. *N Engl J Med* 1997;337:141–147.

334. Moreland LW, Schiff MH, Baumgartner SW, et al. Etanercept therapy in rheumatoid arthritis. A randomized, controlled trial. *Ann Intern Med* 1999;130:478–486.

335. Sugarman BJ, Aggarwal BB, Hass PE, et al. Recombinant human tumor necrosis factor-alpha: effects on proliferation of normal and transformed cells in vitro. *Science* 1985;230:943–945.

336. Dealtry GB, Balkwill FR. Cell growth inhibition by interferons and tumor necrosis factor. In: *Lymphokines and interferons, a practical approach*. Washington: IRL Press, 1987:371.

337. Tsujimoto M, Yip YK, Vilcek J. Tumor necrosis factor: specific binding and internalization in sensitive and resistant cells. *Proc Natl Acad Sci U S A* 1985;82:7626–7630.

338. Chu ZL, McKinsey TA, Liu L, et al. Suppression of tumor necrosis factor-induced cell death by inhibitor of apoptosis c-IAP2 is under NF-kappaB control. *Proc Natl Acad Sci U S A* 1997;94:10057–10062.

339. Van Antwerp DJ, Martin SJ, Kafri T, et al. Suppression of TNF-alpha-induced apoptosis by NF-kappaB [see comments]. *Science* 1996;274:787–789.

340. Torti FM, Dieckmann B, Beutler B, et al. A macrophage factor inhibits adipocyte gene expression: an in vitro model of cachexia. *Science* 1985;229:867–869.

341. Murase T, Hotta T, Saito H, et al. Effect of recombinant human tumor necrosis factor on the colony growth of human leukemia progenitor cells and normal hematopoietic progenitor cells. *Blood* 1987;69:467–472.

342. Broxmeyer HE, Williams DE, Lu L, et al. The suppressive influences of human tumor necrosis factors on bone marrow hematopoietic progenitor cells from normal donors and patients with leukemia: synergism of tumor necrosis factor and interferon-gamma. *J Immunol* 1986;136:4487–4495.

343. Peetre C, Gullberg U, Nilsson E, et al. Effects of recombinant tumor necrosis factor on proliferation and differentiation of leukemic and normal hemopoietic cells in vitro. Relationship to cell surface receptor. *J Clin Invest* 1986;78:1694–1700.

344. Vilcek J, Palombella VJ, Henriksen-DeStefano D, et al. Fibroblast growth enhancing activity of tumor necrosis fac-

tor and its relationship to other polypeptide growth factors. *J Exp Med* 1986;163:632–643.

345. Sidhu RS, Bollon AP. Tumor necrosis factor activities and cancer therapy—a perspective. *Pharmacol Ther* 1993;57:79–128.

346. Pober JS, Gimbrone MA Jr. Expression of Ia-like antigens by human vascular endothelial cells is inducible in vitro: demonstration by monoclonal antibody binding and immunoprecipitation. *Proc Natl Acad Sci U S A* 1982;79:6641–6645.

347. Collins T, Lapierre LA, Fiers W, et al. Recombinant human tumor necrosis factor increases mRNA levels and surface expression of HLA-A,B antigens in vascular endothelial cells and dermal fibroblasts in vitro. *Proc Natl Acad Sci U S A* 1986;83:446–450.

348. Bevilacqua MP, Stengelin S, Gimbrone MA Jr, et al. Endothelial leukocyte adhesion molecule 1: an inducible receptor for neutrophils related to complement regulatory proteins and lectins. *Science* 1989;243:1160–1165.

349. Kurt-Jones EA, Fiers W, Pober JS. Membrane interleukin 1 induction on human endothelial cells and dermal fibroblasts. *J Immunol* 1987;139:2317–2324.

350. Bussolino F, Camussi G, Baglioni C. Synthesis and release of platelet-activating factor by human vascular endothelial cells treated with tumor necrosis factor or interleukin 1 alpha. *J Biol Chem* 1988;263:11856–11861.

351. Lapierre LA, Fiers W, Pober JS. Three distinct classes of regulatory cytokines control endothelial cell MHC antigen expression. Interactions with immune gamma interferon differentiate the effects of tumor necrosis factor and lymphotoxin from those of leukocyte alpha and fibroblast beta interferons. *J Exp Med* 1988;167:794–804.

352. Kramer SM, Carver ME. Serum-free in vitro bioassay for the detection of tumor necrosis factor. *J Immunol Methods* 1986;93:201–206.

353. Garrelds IM, Zijlstra FJ, Tak CJ, et al. A comparison between two methods for measuring tumor necrosis factor in biological fluids. *Agents Actions* 1993;38[Spec No]:C89–C91.

354. Blick M, Sherwin SA, Rosenblum M, et al. Phase I study of recombinant tumor necrosis factor in cancer patients. *Cancer Res* 1987;47:2986–2989.

355. Moritz T, Niederle N, Baumann J, et al. Phase I study of recombinant human tumor necrosis factor alpha in advanced malignant disease. *Cancer Immunol Immunother* 1989;29:144–150.

356. Pang XP, Hershman JM, Pekary AE. Plasma disappearance and organ distribution of recombinant human tumor necrosis factor-alpha in rats. *Lymphokine Cytokine Res* 1991;10:301–306.

357. Beutler BA, Milsark IW, Cerami A. Cachectin/tumor necrosis factor: production, distribution, and metabolic fate in vivo. *J Immunol* 1985;135:3972–3977.

358. Greischel A, Zahn G. Pharmacokinetics of recombinant human tumor necrosis factor alpha in rhesus monkeys after intravenous administration. *J Pharmacol Exp Ther* 1989;251:358–361.

359. Ferraiolo BL, McCabe J, Hollenbach S, et al. Pharmacokinetics of recombinant human tumor necrosis factor-alpha in rats. Effects of size and number of doses and nephrectomy. *Drug Metab Dispos* 1989;17:369–372.

360. Kimura K, Taguchi T, Urushizaki I, et al. Phase I study of recombinant human tumor necrosis factor. *Cancer Chemother Pharmacol* 1987;20:223–229.

361. Mittelman A, Puccio C, Gafney E, et al. A phase I pharmacokinetic study of recombinant human tumor necrosis factor administered by a 5-day continuous infusion. *Invest New Drugs* 1992;10:183–190.

362. Spriggs DR, Sherman ML, Michie H, et al. Recombinant human tumor necrosis factor administered as a 24-hour intravenous infusion. A phase I and pharmacologic study. *J Natl Cancer Inst* 1988;80:1039–1044.

363. Chapman PB, Lester TJ, Casper ES, et al. Clinical pharmacology of recombinant human tumor necrosis factor in patients with advanced cancer. *J Clin Oncol* 1987;5:1942–1951.

364. Feinberg B, Kurzrock R, Talpaz M, et al. A phase I trial of intravenously-administered recombinant tumor necrosis factor-alpha in cancer patients. *J Clin Oncol* 1988;6:1328–1334.

365. Creaven PJ, Plager JE, Dupere S, et al. Phase I clinical trial of recombinant human tumor necrosis factor. *Cancer Chemother Pharmacol* 1987;20:137–144.

366. Saks S, Rosenblum S. Recombinant human TNF-α: preclinical studies and results from early clinical trials. *Immunol Ser* 1992;56:567–587.

367. Zamkoff KW, Newman NB, Rudolph AR, et al. A phase I trial of subcutaneously administered recombination tumor necrosis factor to patients with advanced malignancy. *J Biol Response Mod* 1989;8:539–552.

368. Van de Wiel PA, Bloksma N, Kuper CF, et al. Macroscopic and microscopic early effects of tumour necrosis factor on murine Meth A sarcoma, and relation to curative activity. *J Pathol* 1989;157:65–73.

369. Pfreundschuh MG, Steinmetz HT, Tuschen R, et al. Phase I study of intratumoral application of recombinant human tumor necrosis factor. *Eur J Cancer Clin Oncol* 1989;25:379–388.

370. Raeth U, Schmid H, Hofman J. Intraperitoneal application of recombinant tumor necrosis factor as an effective palliative treatment of malignant ascites from ovarian and gastroenteropancreatic carcinomas. *Proc Am Soc Clin Oncol* 1989;8:181(abst).

371. Mavligit GM, Zukiwski AA, Charnsangavej C, et al. Regional biologic therapy. Hepatic arterial infusion of recombinant human tumor necrosis factor in patients with liver metastases. *Cancer* 1992;69:557–561.

372. Lienard D, Ewalenko P, Delmotte JJ, et al. High-dose recombinant tumor necrosis factor alpha in combination with interferon gamma and melphalan in isolation perfusion of the limbs for melanoma and sarcoma. *J Clin Oncol* 1992;10:52–60.

373. Suffredini AF, Fromm RE, Parker MM, et al. The cardiovascular response of normal humans to the administration of endotoxin [see comments]. *N Engl J Med* 1989;321:280–287.

374. Bevilacqua MP, Pober JS, Majeau GR, et al. Recombinant tumor necrosis factor induces procoagulant activity in cultured human vascular endothelium: characterization and comparison with the actions of interleukin 1. *Proc Natl Acad Sci U S A* 1986;83:4533–4537.

375. Dinarello CA, Cannon JG, Wolff SM, et al. Tumor necrosis factor (cachectin) is an endogenous pyrogen and induces production of interleukin 1. *J Exp Med* 1986;163:1433–1450.

376. Jablons DM, Mule JJ, McIntosh JK, et al. IL-6/IFN-beta-2 as a circulating hormone. Induction by cytokine administration in humans. *J Immunol* 1989;142:1542–1547.

377. Sherman ML, Spriggs DR, Arthur KA, et al. Recombinant human tumor necrosis factor administered as a five-day continuous infusion in cancer patients: phase I toxicity and effects on lipid metabolism. *J Clin Oncol* 1988;6:344–350.

378. Logan TF, Bontempo FA, Kirkwood JM. Evidence for the presence of fibrin degradation products in patients on a phase 1 trial with tumor necrosis factor. *Proc Am Assoc Cancer Res* 1988;29:370(abst).

379. Creaven PJ, Brenner DE, Cowens JW, et al. A phase I clinical trial of recombinant human tumor necrosis factor given daily for five days. *Cancer Chemother Pharmacol* 1989;23:186–191.

380. Lenk H, Tanneberger S, Muller U, et al. Human pharmacological investigation of a human recombinant tumor necrosis factor preparation (PAC-4D) a phase-I trial. *Arch Geschwulstforsch* 1988;58:89–97.

381. Moldawer NP, Figlin RA. Tumor necrosis factor: current clinical status and implications for nursing management. *Semin Oncol Nurs* 1988;4:120–125.

382. Figlin R, deKernion J, Sarna G. Phase II study of recombinant tumor necrosis factor in patients with metastatic renal cell carcinoma and malignant melanoma. *Proc Am Soc Clin Oncol* 1988;7:169(abst).

383. Tracey KJ, Wei H, Manogue KR, et al. Cachectin/tumor necrosis factor induces cachexia, anemia, and inflammation. *J Exp Med* 1988;167:1211–1227.

384. Kist A, Ho AD, Rath U, et al. Decrease of natural killer cell activity and monokine production in peripheral blood of patients treated with recombinant tumor necrosis factor. *Blood* 1988;72:344–348.

385. Bartsch HH, Nagel GA, Mule R. Tumor necrosis factor in man: clinical and biologic observations. *Br J Cancer* 1987;56:803–808.

386. Charnetsky PS, Greisman RA, Salmon SE, et al. Increased peripheral blood leukocyte cytotoxic activity in cancer patients during the continuous intravenous administration of recombinant human tumor necrosis factor. *J Clin Immunol* 1989;9:34–38.

387. Logan TF, Gooding WE, Whiteside TL, et al. Biologic response modulation by tumor necrosis factor alpha (TNF alpha) in a phase Ib trial in cancer patients. *J Immunother* 1997;20:387–398.

388. Conkling PR, Chua CC, Nadler P, et al. Clinical trials with human tumor necrosis factor: in vivo and in vitro effects on human mononuclear phagocyte function. *Cancer Res* 1988;48:5604–5609.

389. Logan TF, Gooding W, Kirkwood JM, et al. Tumor necrosis factor administration is associated with increased endogenous production of M-CSF and G-CSF but not GM-CSF in human cancer patients. *Exp Hematol* 1996;24:49–53.

390. Creagan ET, Kovach JS, Moertel CG, et al. A phase I clinical trial of recombinant human tumor necrosis factor. *Cancer* 1988;62:2467–2471.

391. Hersh EM, Metch BS, Muggia FM, et al. Phase II studies of recombinant human tumor necrosis factor alpha in patients with malignant disease: a summary of the Southwest Oncology Group experience. *J Immunother* 1991;10:426–431.

392. Spriggs DR. Tumor necrosis factor: basic principles and preclinical studies. In: DeVita VT Jr, Hellman S, Rosenberg SA, eds. *Biologic therapy of cancer.* Philadelphia: JB Lippincott, 1989:361–370.

393. Hirte HW, Miller D, Tonkin K, et al. A randomized trial of paracentesis plus intraperitoneal tumor necrosis factor-alpha versus paracentesis alone in patients with symptomatic ascites from recurrent ovarian carcinoma. *Gynecol Oncol* 1997;64:80–87.

394. Eggermont AM, Schraffordt Koops H, Klausner JM, et al. Isolated limb perfusion with tumor necrosis factor and melphalan for limb salvage in 186 patients with locally advanced soft tissue extremity sarcomas. The cumulative multicenter European experience [see discussion]. *Ann Surg* 1996;224:756–764.

395. De Vries MR, Rinkes IH, van de Velde CJ, et al. Isolated hepatic perfusion with tumor necrosis factor alpha and melphalan: experimental studies in pigs and phase I data from humans. *Recent Results Cancer Res* 1998;147:107–119.

396. Walther MM, Jennings SB, Choyke PL, et al. Isolated perfusion of the kidney with tumor necrosis factor for localized renal-cell carcinoma. *World J Urol* 1996;14[Suppl 1]:S2–S7.

397. Abbruzzese JL, Levin B, Ajani JA, et al. Phase I trial of recombinant human gamma-interferon and recombinant human tumor necrosis factor in patients with advanced gastrointestinal cancer. *Cancer Res* 1989;49:4057–4061.

398. Demetri GD, Spriggs DR, Sherman ML, et al. A phase I trial of recombinant human tumor necrosis factor and interferon-gamma: effects of combination cytokine administration in vivo. *J Clin Oncol* 1989;7:1545–1553.

399. McIntosh JK, Mule JJ, Merino MJ, et al. Synergistic antitumor effects of immunotherapy with recombinant interleukin-2 and recombinant tumor necrosis factor-alpha. *Cancer Res* 1988;48:4011–4017.

400. McIntosh JK, Mule JJ, Krosnick JA, et al. Combination cytokine immunotherapy with tumor necrosis factor alpha, interleukin 2, and alpha-interferon and its synergistic antitumor effects in mice. *Cancer Res* 1989;49:1408–1414.

401. Eskander ED, Harvey HA, Givant E, et al. Phase I study combining tumor necrosis factor with interferon-alpha and interleukin-2. *Am J Clin Oncol* 1997;20:511–514.

402. Safrit JT, Belldegrun A, Bonavida B. Sensitivity of human renal cell carcinoma lines to TNF, adriamycin, and combination: role of TNF mRNA induction in overcoming resistance. *J Urol* 1993;149:1202–1208.

403. Mutch DG, Powell CB, Kao MS, et al. In vitro analysis of the anticancer potential of tumor necrosis factor in combination with cisplatin. *Gynecol Oncol* 1989;34:328–333.

404. Alexander RB, Isaacs JT, Coffey DS. Tumor necrosis factor enhances the in vitro and in vivo efficacy of chemotherapeutic drugs targeted at DNA topoisomerase II in the treatment of murine bladder cancer. *J Urol* 1987;138:427–429.

405. Alexander RB, Nelson WG, Coffey DS. Synergistic enhancement by tumor necrosis factor of in vitro cytotoxicity from chemotherapeutic drugs targeted at DNA topoisomerase II. *Cancer Res* 1987;47:2403–2406.

406. Lush R, Schwartz R, Logan T. Phase I and pharmacological evaluation of tumor necrosis factor (rHuTNF) administered in combination with etoposide. *Proc Am Soc Clin Oncol* 1993;12:158(abst).

407. Kobayashi M, Fitz L, Ryan M, et al. Identification and purification of natural killer cell stimulatory factor (NKSF), a cytokine with multiple biologic effects on human lymphocytes. *J Exp Med* 1989;170:827–845.

408. Gately MK, Wilson DE, Wong HL. Synergy between recombinant interleukin 2 (rIL 2) and IL 2-depleted lymphokine-containing supernatants in facilitating allogeneic human cytolytic T lymphocyte responses in vitro. *J Immunol* 1986;136:1274–1282.

409. Gately MK, Wolitzky AG, Quinn PM, et al. Regulation of human cytolytic lymphocyte responses by interleukin-12. *Cell Immunol* 1992;143:127–142.

410. Gately MK, Desai BB, Wolitzky AG, et al. Regulation of human lymphocyte proliferation by a heterodimeric cytokine, IL-12 (cytotoxic lymphocyte maturation factor). *J Immunol* 1991;147:874–882.

411. Chan SH, Perussia B, Gupta JW, et al. Induction of interferon gamma production by natural killer cell stimulatory factor: characterization of the responder cells and synergy with other inducers. *J Exp Med* 1991;173:869–879.

412. Podlaski FJ, Nanduri VB, Hulmes JD, et al. Molecular characterization of interleukin 12. *Arch Biochem Biophys* 1992;294:230–237.

413. Stern AS, Podlaski FJ, Hulmes JD, et al. Purification to homogeneity and partial characterization of cytotoxic lymphocyte maturation factor from human B-lymphoblastoid cells. *Proc Natl Acad Sci U S A* 1990;87:6808–6812.

414. Wolf SF, Temple PA, Kobayashi M, et al. Cloning of cDNA for natural killer cell stimulatory factor, a heterodimeric cytokine with multiple biologic effects on T and natural killer cells. *J Immunol* 1991;146:3074–3081.

415. Schoenhaut DS, Chua AO, Wolitzky AG, et al. Cloning and expression of murine IL-12. *J Immunol* 1992;148:3433–3440.

416. Gubler U, Chua AO, Schoenhaut DS, et al. Coexpression of two distinct genes is required to generate secreted bioactive cytotoxic lymphocyte maturation factor. *Proc Natl Acad Sci U S A* 1991;88:4143–4147.

417. Murphy EE, Terres G, Macatonia SE, et al. B7 and interleukin 12 cooperate for proliferation and interferon gamma production by mouse T helper clones that are unresponsive to B7 costimulation. *J Exp Med* 1994;180:223–231.

418. Trinchieri G. Interleukin-12: a cytokine produced by antigen-presenting cells with immunoregulatory functions in the generation of T-helper cells type 1 and cytotoxic lymphocytes. *Blood* 1994;84:4008–4027.

419. D'Andrea A, Rengaraju M, Valiante NM, et al. Production of natural killer cell stimulatory factor (interleukin 12) by peripheral blood mononuclear cells. *J Exp Med* 1992;176:1387–1398.

420. Mattner F, Fischer S, Guckes S, et al. The interleukin-12 subunit p40 specifically inhibits effects of the interleukin-12 heterodimer. *Eur J Immunol* 1993;23:2202–2208.

421. Sieburth D, Jabs EW, Warrington JA, et al. Assignment of genes encoding a unique cytokine (IL12) composed of two unrelated subunits to chromosomes 3 and 5. *Genomics* 1992;14:59–62.

422. Merberg DM, Wolf SF, Clark SC. Sequence similarity between NKSF and the IL-6/G-CSF family [Letter]. *Immunol Today* 1992;13:77–78.

423. Gearing DP, Cosman D. Homology of the p40 subunit of natural killer cell stimulatory factor (NKSF) with the extracellular domain of the interleukin-6 receptor [Letter]. *Cell* 1991;66:9–10.

424. Macatonia SE, Hsieh CS, Murphy KM, et al. Dendritic cells and macrophages are required for Th1 development of CD4+ T cells from alpha beta TCR transgenic mice: IL-12 substitution for macrophages to stimulate IFN-gamma production is IFN-gamma-dependent. *Int Immunol* 1993;5: 1119–1128.

425. Macatonia SE, Hosken NA, Litton M, et al. Dendritic cells produce IL-12 and direct the development of Th1 cells from naive CD4+ T cells. *J Immunol* 1995;154:5071–5079.

426. Cassatella MA, Meda L, Gasperini S, et al. Interleukin-12 production by human polymorphonuclear leukocytes. *Eur J Immunol* 1995;25:1–5.

427. Curtsinger JM, Schmidt CS, Mondino A, et al. Inflammatory cytokines provide a third signal for activation of naive CD4+ and CD8+ T cells. *J Immunol* 1999;162:3256–3262.

428. Hall SS. IL-12 at the crossroads [News] [see comments]. *Science* 1995;268:1432–1434.

429. Guery JC, Ria F, Galbiati F, et al. Normal B cells fail to secrete interleukin-12. *Eur J Immunol* 1997;27:1632–1639.

430. Kang K, Kubin M, Cooper KD, et al. IL-12 synthesis by human Langerhans cells. *J Immunol* 1996;156:1402–1407.

431. Smith TJ, Ducharme LA, Weis JH. Preferential expression of interleukin-12 or interleukin-4 by murine bone marrow mast cells derived in mast cell growth factor or interleukin-3. *Eur J Immunol* 1994;24:822–826.

432. Muller G, Saloga J, Germann T, et al. Identification and induction of human keratinocyte-derived IL-12. *J Clin Invest* 1994;94:1799–1805.

433. Kubin M, Chow JM, Trinchieri G. Differential regulation of interleukin-12 (IL-12), tumor necrosis factor alpha, and IL-1 beta production in human myeloid leukemia cell lines and peripheral blood mononuclear cells. *Blood* 1994;83: 1847–1855.

434. Snijders A, Kalinski P, Hilkens CM, et al. High-level IL-12 production by human dendritic cells requires two signals. *Int Immunol* 1998;10:1593–1598.

435. D'Andrea A, Aste-Amezaga M, Valiante NM, et al. Interleukin 10 (IL-10) inhibits human lymphocyte interferon gamma-production by suppressing natural killer cell stimulatory factor/IL-12 synthesis in accessory cells. *J Exp Med* 1993;178:1041–1048.

436. D'Andrea A, Ma X, Aste-Amezaga M, et al. Stimulatory and inhibitory effects of interleukin (IL)-4 and IL-13 on the production of cytokines by human peripheral blood mononuclear cells: priming for IL-12 and tumor necrosis factor alpha production. *J Exp Med* 1995;181:537–546.

437. Shu U, Kiniwa M, Wu CY, et al. Activated T cells induce interleukin-12 production by monocytes via CD40-CD40 ligand interaction. *Eur J Immunol* 1995;25:1125–1128.

438. Hunter CA, Ellis-Neyer L, Gabriel KE, et al. The role of the CD28/B7 interaction in the regulation of NK cell responses during infection with *Toxoplasma gondii*. *J Immunol* 1997; 158:2285–2293.

439. McDyer JF, Goletz TJ, Thomas E, et al. CD40 ligand/CD40 stimulation regulates the production of IFN-gamma from human peripheral blood mononuclear cells in an IL-12- and/or CD28-dependent manner. *J Immunol* 1998;160: 1701–1707.

440. Chizzonite R, Truitt T, Desai BB, et al. IL-12 receptor. I. Characterization of the receptor on phytohemagglutinin-activated human lymphoblasts. *J Immunol* 1992;148:3117–3124.

441. Gubler U, Presky DH. Molecular biology of interleukin-12 receptors. *Ann N Y Acad Sci* 1996;795:36–40.

442. Presky DH, Yang H, Minetti LJ, et al. A functional interleukin 12 receptor complex is composed of two beta-type cytokine receptor subunits. *Proc Natl Acad Sci U S A* 1996;93:14002–14007.

443. Thibodeaux DK, Hunter SE, Waldburger KE, et al. Autocrine regulation of IL-12 receptor expression is independent of secondary IFN-gamma secretion and not restricted to T and NK cells. *J Immunol* 1999;163:5257–5264.

444. Showe LC, Fox FE, Williams D, et al. Depressed IL-12-mediated signal transduction in T cells from patients with Sezary syndrome is associated with the absence of IL-12 receptor beta 2 mRNA and highly reduced levels of STAT4. *J Immunol* 1999;163:4073–4079.

445. Wang X, Wilkinson VL, Podlaski FJ, et al. Characterization of mouse interleukin-12 p40 homodimer binding to the interleukin-12 receptor subunits. *Eur J Immunol* 1999;29:2007–2013.

446. Murphy KM, Ouyang W, Szabo SJ, et al. T helper differentiation proceeds through Stat1-dependent, Stat4-dependent and Stat4-independent phases. *Curr Top Microbiol Immunol* 1999;238:13–26.

447. Naeger LK, McKinney J, Salvekar A, et al. Identification of a STAT4 binding site in the interleukin-12 receptor required for signaling. *J Biol Chem* 1999;274:1875–1878.

448. Rogge L, Papi A, Presky DH, et al. Antibodies to the IL-12 receptor beta 2 chain mark human Th1 but not Th2 cells in vitro and in vivo. *J Immunol* 1999;162:3926–3932.

449. Wu C, Warrier RR, Wang X, et al. Regulation of interleukin-12 receptor beta1 chain expression and interleukin-12 binding by human peripheral blood mononuclear cells. *Eur J Immunol* 1997;27:147–154.

450. Szabo SJ, Jacobson NG, Dighe AS, et al. Developmental commitment to the Th2 lineage by extinction of IL-12 signaling. *Immunity* 1995;2:665–675.

451. Zhang F, Nakamura T, Aune TM. TCR and IL-12 receptor signals cooperate to activate an individual response element in the IFN-gamma promoter in effector Th cells. *J Immunol* 1999;163:728–735.

452. Mountford AP, Coulson PS, Cheever AW, et al. Interleukin-12 can directly induce T-helper 1 responses in interferon-gamma (IFN-gamma) receptor-deficient mice, but requires IFN-gamma signalling to downregulate T-helper 2 responses. *Immunology* 1999;97:588–594.

453. Yamamoto K, Shibata F, Miura O, et al. Physical interaction between interleukin-12 receptor beta 2 subunit and Jak2 tyrosine kinase: Jak2 associates with cytoplasmic membrane-proximal region of interleukin-12 receptor beta 2 via amino-terminus. *Biochem Biophys Res Commun* 1999;257:400–404.

454. Bacon CM, Petricoin EF, Ortaldo JR, et al. Interleukin 12 induces tyrosine phosphorylation and activation of STAT4

in human lymphocytes. *Proc Natl Acad Sci U S A* 1995;92:7307–7311.

455. Yao BB, Niu P, Surowy CS, et al. Direct interaction of STAT4 with the IL-12 receptor. *Arch Biochem Biophys* 1999;368:147–155.

456. Akira S. Functional roles of STAT family proteins: lessons from knockout mice. *Stem Cells* 1999;17:138–146.

457. Ouyang W, Jacobson NG, Bhattacharya D, et al. The Ets transcription factor ERM is Th1-specific and induced by IL-12 through a Stat4-dependent pathway. *Proc Natl Acad Sci U S A* 1999;96:3888–3893.

458. Kaplan MH, Sun YL, Hoey T, et al. Impaired IL-12 responses and enhanced development of Th2 cells in Stat4-deficient mice. *Nature* 1996;382:174–177.

459. Bright JJ, Du C, Sriram S. Tyrphostin B42 inhibits IL-12-induced tyrosine phosphorylation and activation of Janus kinase-2 and prevents experimental allergic encephalomyelitis. *J Immunol* 1999;162:6255–6262.

460. Pardoux C, Ma X, Gobert S, et al. Downregulation of interleukin-12 (IL-12) responsiveness in human T cells by transforming growth factor-beta: relationship with IL-12 signaling. *Blood* 1999;93:1448–1455.

461. Gollob JA, Schnipper CP, Orsini E, et al. Characterization of a novel subset of CD8(+) T cells that expands in patients receiving interleukin-12. *J Clin Invest* 1998;102:561–575.

462. Gately MK, Renzetti LM, Magram J, et al. The interleukin-12/interleukin-12-receptor system: role in normal and pathologic immune responses. *Annu Rev Immunol* 1998;16: 495–521.

463. Adorini L. Interleukin-12, a key cytokine in Th1-mediated autoimmune diseases. *Cell Mol Life Sci* 1999;55:1610–1625.

464. Aste-Amezaga M, Ma X, Sartori A, et al. Molecular mechanisms of the induction of IL-12 and its inhibition by IL-10. *J Immunol* 1998;160:5936–5944.

465. Trinchieri G, Wysocka M, D'Andrea A, et al. Natural killer cell stimulatory factor (NKSF) or interleukin-12 is a key regulator of immune response and inflammation. *Prog Growth Factor Res* 1992;4:355–368.

466. Soiffer RJ, Robertson MJ, Murray C, et al. Interleukin-12 augments cytolytic activity of peripheral blood lymphocytes from patients with hematologic and solid malignancies. *Blood* 1993;82:2790–2796.

467. Robertson MJ, Soiffer RJ, Wolf SF, et al. Response of human natural killer (NK) cells to NK cell stimulatory factor (NKSF): cytolytic activity and proliferation of NK cells are differentially regulated by NKSF. *J Exp Med* 1992;175:779–788.

468. Mosmann TR, Coffman RL. Heterogeneity of cytokine secretion patterns and functions of helper T cells. *Adv Immunol* 1989;46:111–147.

469. Mosmann TR, Coffman RL. TH1 and TH2 cells: different patterns of lymphokine secretion lead to different functional properties. *Annu Rev Immunol* 1989;7:145–173.

470. Scott P. IL-12: initiation cytokine for cell-mediated immunity [Comment]. *Science* 1993;260:496–497.

471. Manetti R, Gerosa F, Giudizi MG, et al. Interleukin 12 induces stable priming for interferon gamma (IFN-gamma) production during differentiation of human T helper (Th) cells and transient IFN-gamma production in established Th2 cell clones. *J Exp Med* 1994;179:1273–1283.

472. Heufler C, Koch F, Stanzl U, et al. Interleukin-12 is produced by dendritic cells and mediates T helper 1 development as well as interferon-gamma production by T helper 1 cells. *Eur J Immunol* 1996;26:659–668.

473. Meyaard L, Hovenkamp E, Otto SA, et al. IL-12-induced IL-10 production by human T cells as a negative feedback for IL-12-induced immune responses. *J Immunol* 1996;156:2776–2782.

474. Yssel H, Fasler S, de Vries JE, et al. IL-12 transiently induces IFN-gamma transcription and protein synthesis in human CD4+ allergen-specific Th2 T cell clones. *Int Immunol* 1994;6:1091–1096.

475. Jung T, Witzak K, Dieckhoff K, et al. IFN-gamma is only partially restored by co-stimulation with IL-12, IL-2, IL-15, IL-18 or engagement of CD28. *Clin Exp Allergy* 1999;29:207–216.

476. Huang T, MacAry PA, Wilke T, et al. Inhibitory effects of endogenous and exogenous interferon-gamma on bronchial hyperresponsiveness, allergic inflammation and T-helper 2 cytokines in Brown-Norway rats. *Immunology* 1999;98: 280–288.

477. Brunda MJ, Luistro L, Warrier RR, et al. Antitumor and antimetastatic activity of interleukin 12 against murine tumors. *J Exp Med* 1993;178:1223–1230.

478. Tannenbaum CS, Tubbs R, Armstrong D, et al. The CXC chemokines IP-10 and Mig are necessary for IL-12-mediated regression of the mouse RENCA tumor. *J Immunol* 1998;161:927–932.

479. Martinotti A, Stoppacciaro A, Vagliani M, et al. CD4 T cells inhibit in vivo the CD8-mediated immune response against murine colon carcinoma cells transduced with interleukin-12 genes. *Eur J Immunol* 1995;25:137–146.

480. Nastala CL, Edington HD, McKinney TG, et al. Recombinant IL-12 administration induces tumor regression in association with IFN-gamma production. *J Immunol* 1994;153:1697–1706.

481. Gately MK, Gubler U, Brunda MJ, et al. Interleukin-12: a cytokine with therapeutic potential in oncology and infectious diseases. *Ther Immunol* 1994;1:187–196.

482. Mu J, Zou JP, Yamamoto N, et al. Administration of recombinant interleukin 12 prevents outgrowth of tumor cells metastasizing spontaneously to lung and lymph nodes. *Cancer Res* 1995;55:4404–4408.

483. Dias S, Thomas H, Balkwill F. Multiple molecular and cellular changes associated with tumour stasis and regression during IL-12 therapy of a murine breast cancer model. *Int J Cancer* 1998;75:151–157.

484. Brunda MJ, Luistro L, Rumennik L, et al. Antitumor activity of interleukin 12 in preclinical models. *Cancer Chemother Pharmacol* 1996;38[Suppl]:S16–S21.

485. Fujiwara H, Hamaoka T. Antitumor and antimetastatic effects of interleukin 12. *Cancer Chemother Pharmacol* 1996;38[Suppl]:S22–S26.

486. Brunda MJ, Luistro L, Hendrzak JA, et al. Role of interferon-gamma in mediating the antitumor efficacy of interleukin-12. *J Immunother Emphasis Tumor Immunol* 1995; 17:71–77.

487. Seder RA, Gazzinelli R, Sher A, et al. Interleukin 12 acts directly on CD4+ T cells to enhance priming for interferon gamma production and diminishes interleukin 4 inhibition

of such priming. *Proc Natl Acad Sci U S A* 1993;90:10188–10192.

488. Colombo MP, Vagliani M, Spreafico F, et al. Amount of interleukin 12 available at the tumor site is critical for tumor regression. *Cancer Res* 1996;56:2531–2534.

489. Tannenbaum CS, Wicker N, Armstrong D, et al. Cytokine and chemokine expression in tumors of mice receiving systemic therapy with IL-12. *J Immunol* 1996;156:693–699.

490. Hashimoto W, Osaki T, Okamura H, et al. Differential antitumor effects of administration of recombinant IL-18 or recombinant IL-12 are mediated primarily by Fas-Fas ligand- and perforin-induced tumor apoptosis, respectively. *J Immunol* 1999;163:583–589.

491. Bukowski RM, Rayman P, Molto L, et al. Interferon-gamma and CXC chemokine induction by interleukin 12 in renal cell carcinoma. *Clin Cancer Res* 1999;5(10):2780–2789.

492. Ha SJ, Lee SB, Kim CM, et al. Rapid recruitment of macrophages in interleukin-12-mediated tumour regression. *Immunology* 1998;95:156–163.

493. Cavallo F, Di Carlo E, Butera M, et al. Immune events associated with the cure of established tumors and spontaneous metastases by local and systemic interleukin 12. *Cancer Res* 1999;59:414–421.

494. Wigginton JM, Kuhns DB, Back TC, et al. Interleukin 12 primes macrophages for nitric oxide production in vivo and restores depressed nitric oxide production by macrophages from tumor-bearing mice: implications for the antitumor activity of interleukin 12 and/or interleukin 2. *Cancer Res* 1996;56:1131–1136.

495. Yu WG, Yamamoto N, Takenaka H, et al. Molecular mechanisms underlying IFN-gamma-mediated tumor growth inhibition induced during tumor immunotherapy with rIL-12. *Int Immunol* 1996;8:855–865.

496. Angiolillo AL, Sgadari C, Tosato G. A role for the interferon-inducible protein 10 in inhibition of angiogenesis by interleukin-12. *Ann N Y Acad Sci* 1996;795:158–167.

497. Kerbel RS, Hawley RG. Interleukin 12: newest member of the antiangiogenesis club [Editorial; Comment]. *J Natl Cancer Inst* 1995;87:557–559.

498. Sgadari C, Angiolillo AL, Tosato G. Inhibition of angiogenesis by interleukin-12 is mediated by the interferon-inducible protein 10. *Blood* 1996;87:3877–3882.

499. O'Reilly MS, Boehm T, Shing Y, et al. Endostatin: an endogenous inhibitor of angiogenesis and tumor growth. *Cell* 1997;88:277–285.

500. Voest EE, Kenyon BM, O'Reilly MS, et al. Inhibition of angiogenesis in vivo by interleukin 12 [see comments]. *J Natl Cancer Inst* 1995;87:581–586.

501. Sgadari C, Angiolillo AL, Cherney BW, et al. Interferon-inducible protein-10 identified as a mediator of tumor necrosis in vivo. *Proc Natl Acad Sci U S A* 1996;93:13791–13796.

502. Keane MP, Arenberg DA, Lynch JP, et al. The CXC chemokines, IL-8 and IP-10, regulate angiogenic activity in idiopathic pulmonary fibrosis. *J Immunol* 1997;159:1437–1443.

503. Arenberg DA, Kunkel SL, Polverini PJ, et al. Interferon-gamma-inducible protein 10 (IP-10) is an angiostatic factor that inhibits human non-small cell lung cancer (NSCLC)

tumorigenesis and spontaneous metastases. *J Exp Med* 1996;184:981–992.

504. Strieter RM, Polverini PJ, Arenberg DA, et al. Role of C-X-C chemokines as regulators of angiogenesis in lung cancer. *J Leukoc Biol* 1995;57:752–762.

505. Strieter RM, Kunkel SL, Arenberg DA, et al. Interferon gamma-inducible protein 10 (IP-10), a member of the C-X-C chemokine family, is an inhibitor of angiogenesis. *Biochem Biophys Res Commun* 1995;210:51–57.

506. Luster AD, Greenberg SM, Leder P. The IP-10 chemokine binds to a specific cell surface heparan sulfate site shared with platelet factor 4 and inhibits endothelial cell proliferation. *J Exp Med* 1995;182:219–231.

507. Strieter RM, Polverini PJ, Arenberg DA, et al. The role of CXC chemokines as regulators of angiogenesis. *Shock* 1995;4:155–160.

508. Clark-Lewis I, Dewald B, Geiser T, et al. Platelet factor 4 binds to interleukin 8 receptors and activates neutrophils when its N terminus is modified with Glu-Leu-Arg. *Proc Natl Acad Sci U S A* 1993;90:3574–3577.

509. Sgadari C, Farber JM, Angiolillo AL, et al. Mig, the monokine induced by interferon-gamma, promotes tumor necrosis in vivo. *Blood* 1997;89:2635–2643.

510. Kanegane C, Sgadari C, Kanegane H, et al. Contribution of the CXC chemokines IP-10 and Mig to the antitumor effects of IL-12. *J Leukoc Biol* 1998;64:384–392.

511. Motzer RJ, Rakhit A, Schwartz LH, et al. Phase I trial of subcutaneous recombinant human interleukin-12 in patients with advanced renal cell carcinoma. *Clin Cancer Res* 1998;4:1183–1191.

512. Atkins MB, Robertson MJ, Gordon M, et al. Phase I evaluation of intravenous recombinant human interleukin 12 in patients with advanced malignancies. *Clin Cancer Res* 1997;3:409–417.

513. Mier J, Dollob JA, Atkins M. Interleukin 12, a new antitumor cytokine. *Int J Immunopharmacol* 1998;11:109–115.

514. Rakhit A, Yeon MM, Ferrante J, et al. Down-regulation of the pharmacokinetic-pharmacodynamic response to interleukin-12 during long-term administration to patients with renal cell carcinoma and evaluation of the mechanism of this "adaptive response" in mice. *Clin Pharmacol Ther* 1999;65:615–629.

515. Robertson MJ, Cameron C, Atkins MB, et al. Immunological effects of interleukin 12 administered by bolus intravenous injection to patients with cancer. *Clin Cancer Res* 1999;5:9–16.

516. Bajetta E, Del Vecchio M, Mortarini R, et al. Pilot study of subcutaneous recombinant human interleukin 12 in metastatic melanoma. *Clin Cancer Res* 1998;4:75–85.

517. Stanley ER, Heard PM. Factors regulating macrophage production and growth. Purification and some properties of the colony stimulating factor from medium conditioned by mouse L cells. *J Biol Chem* 1977;252:4305–4312.

518. Wing EJ, Waheed A, Shadduck RK, et al. Effect of colony stimulating factor on murine macrophages. Induction of antitumor activity. *J Clin Invest* 1982;69:270–276.

519. Lin HS, Gordon S. Secretion of plasminogen activator by bone marrow-derived mononuclear phagocytes and its enhancement by colony-stimulating factor. *J Exp Med* 1979;150:231–245.

520. Kurland JI, Bockman RS, Broxmeyer HE, et al. Limitation of excessive myelopoiesis by the intrinsic modulation of macrophage-derived prostaglandin E. *Science* 1978;199:552–555.

521. Warren MK, Ralph P. Macrophage growth factor CSF-1 stimulates human monocyte production of interferon tumor necrosis factor, and colony stimulating activity. *J Immunol* 1986;137:2281–2285.

522. Kawasaki ES, Ladner MB, Wang AM, et al. Molecular cloning of a complementary DNA encoding human macrophage-specific colony-stimulating factor (CSF-1). *Science* 1985;230:291–296.

523. Ladner MB, Martin GA, Noble JA, et al. Human CSF-1: gene structure and alternative splicing of mRNA precursors. *EMBO J* 1987;6:2693–2698.

524. Pettenati MJ, Le Beau MM, Lemons RS, et al. Assignment of CSF-1 to 5q33.1: evidence for clustering of genes regulating hematopoiesis and for their involvement in the deletion of the long arm of chromosome 5 in myeloid disorders. *Proc Natl Acad Sci U S A* 1987;84:2970–2974.

525. Morris SW, Valentine MB, Shapiro DN, et al. Reassignment of the human CSF1 gene to chromosome 1p13-p21. *Blood* 1991;78:2013–2020.

526. Wong GG, Temple PA, Leary AC, et al. Human CSF-1: molecular cloning and expression of 4-kb cDNA encoding the human urinary protein. *Science* 1987;235:1504–1508.

527. Cerretti DP, Wignall J, Anderson D, et al. Human macrophage-colony stimulating factor: alternative RNA and protein processing from a single gene. *Mol Immunol* 1988;25:761–770.

528. Suzu S, Yanai N, Sato-Somoto Y, et al. Characterization of macrophage colony-stimulating factor in body fluids by immunoblot analysis. *Blood* 1991;77:2160–2165.

529. Rettenmier CW, Roussel MF, Ashmun RA, et al. Synthesis of membrane-bound colony-stimulating factor 1 (CSF-1) and downmodulation of CSF-1 receptors in NIH 3T3 cells transformed by cotransfection of the human CSF-1 and c-fms (CSF-1 receptor) genes. *Mol Cell Biol* 1987;7:2378–2387.

530. Guilbert LJ, Stanley ER. The interaction of 125I-colony-stimulating factor-1 with bone marrow-derived macrophages. *J Biol Chem* 1986;261:4024–4032.

531. Rettenmier CW, Jackowski S, Rock CO, et al. Transformation by the v-fms oncogene product: an analog of the CSF-1 receptor. *J Cell Biochem* 1987;33:109–115.

532. Rettenmier CW, Chen JH, Roussel MF, et al. The product of the c-fms proto-oncogene: a glycoprotein with associated tyrosine kinase activity. *Science* 1985;228:320–322.

533. Chen BD, Kuhn C, Lin HS. Receptor-mediated binding and internalization of colony-stimulating factor (CSF-1) by mouse peritoneal exudate macrophages. *J Cell Sci* 1984;70:147–166.

534. Rambaldi A, Wakamiya N, Vellenga E, et al. Expression of the macrophage colony-stimulating factor and c-fms genes in human acute myeloblastic leukemia cells. *J Clin Invest* 1988;81:1030–1035.

535. Rettenmier CW, Sacca R, Furman WL, et al. Expression of the human c-fms proto-oncogene product (colony-stimulating factor-1 receptor) on peripheral blood mononuclear cells and choriocarcinoma cell lines. *J Clin Invest* 1986;77:1740–1746.

536. Imamura K, Kufe D. Colony-stimulating factor 1-induced Na+ influx into human monocytes involves activation of a pertussis toxin-sensitive GTP-binding protein. *J Biol Chem* 1988;263:14093–14098.

537. Munn DH, Armstrong E. Coordinate regulation of M-CSF-induced anti-tumor cytotoxicity and cell cycle progression by IL-4 during human macrophage differentiation in vitro. *Proc Am Assoc Cancer Res* 1992;33:301(abst).

538. Stanley ER, Guilbert LJ, Tushinski RJ, et al. CSF-1—a mononuclear phagocyte lineage-specific hemopoietic growth factor. *J Cell Biochem* 1983;21:151–159.

539. Koike K, Stanley ER, Ihle JN, et al. Macrophage colony formation supported by purified CSF-1 and/or interleukin 3 in serum-free culture: evidence for hierarchical difference in macrophage colony-forming cells. *Blood* 1986;67:859–864.

540. Zhou YQ, Stanley ER, Clark SC, et al. Interleukin-3 and interleukin-1 alpha allow earlier bone marrow progenitors to respond to human colony-stimulating factor 1. *Blood* 1988;72:1870–1874.

541. Fibbe WE, Van Damme J, Billiau A, et al. Human fibroblasts produce granulocyte-CSF, macrophage-CSF, and granulocyte-macrophage-CSF following stimulation by interleukin-1 and poly(rI).poly(rC). *Blood* 1988;72:860–866.

542. Seelentag WK, Mermod JJ, Montesano R, et al. Additive effects of interleukin 1 and tumour necrosis factor-alpha on the accumulation of the three granulocyte and macrophage colony-stimulating factor mRNAs in human endothelial cells. *EMBO J* 1987;6:2261–2265.

543. Hallet MM, Praloran V, Vie H, et al. Macrophage colony-stimulating factor (CSF-1) gene expression in human T-lymphocyte clones. *Blood* 1991;77:780–786.

544. Reisbach G, Sindermann J, Kremer JP, et al. Macrophage colony-stimulating factor (CSF-1) is expressed by spontaneously outgrown EBV-B cell lines and activated normal B lymphocytes. *Blood* 1989;74:959–964.

545. Lindemann A, Riedel D, Oster W, et al. Granulocyte-macrophage colony-stimulating factor induces cytokine secretion by human polymorphonuclear leukocytes. *J Clin Invest* 1989;83:1308–1312.

546. Hanamura T, Motoyoshi K, Yoshida K, et al. Quantitation and identification of human monocytic colony-stimulating factor in human serum by enzyme-linked immunosorbent assay. *Blood* 1988;72:886–892.

547. Shadle PJ, Allen JI, Geier MD, et al. Detection of endogenous macrophage colony-stimulating factor (M-CSF) in human blood. *Exp Hematol* 1989;17:154–159.

548. Bartocci A, Mastrogiannis DS, Migliorati G, et al. Macrophages specifically regulate the concentration of their own growth factor in the circulation. *Proc Natl Acad Sci U S A* 1987;84:6179–6183.

549. Timothy G, Bree A, Metzger M. Pharmacokinetics of recombinant human macrophage-colony stimulating factor (rhM-CSF). *Blood* 1990;76:169a(abst).

550. Motoyoshi K, Yoshida K, Hatake K, et al. Recombinant and native human urinary colony-stimulating factor directly augments granulocytic and granulocyte-macrophage colony-stimulating factor production of human peripheral blood monocytes. *Exp Hematol* 1989;17:68–71.

551. Morahan P, Volkman A, Melnicoff M, et al. Macrophage heterogeneity. In: Heppner GH, Fulton AM, eds. *Macrophages and cancer*. Boca Raton, FL: CRC Press, 1988:1.

552. Adams DO, Hamilton TA. Activation of macrophages for tumor cell kill:effector mechanisms and regulation. In: Heppner GH, Fulton AM, eds. *Macrophages and cancer.* Boca Raton, FL: CRC Press, 1988:27.

553. Karbassi A, Becker JM, Foster JS, et al. Enhanced killing of *Candida albicans* by murine macrophages treated with macrophage colony-stimulating factor: evidence for augmented expression of mannose receptors. *J Immunol* 1987;139:417–421.

554. Wang JM, Griffin JD, Rambaldi A, et al. Induction of monocyte migration by recombinant macrophage colony-stimulating factor. *J Immunol* 1988;141:575–579.

555. Fidler IJ. Macrophages and metastasis—a biological approach to cancer therapy. *Cancer Res* 1985;45:4714–4726.

556. Hume DA, Donahue RE, Fidler IJ. The therapeutic effect of human recombinant macrophage colony stimulating factor (CSF-1) in experimental murine metastatic melanoma. *Lymphokine Res* 1989;8:69–77.

557. Munn DH, Cheung NK. Preclinical and clinical studies of macrophage colony-stimulating factor. *Semin Oncol* 1992; 9:395–407.

558. Weinstein Y, Ihle JN, Lavu S, et al. Truncation of the c-myb gene by a retroviral integration in an interleukin 3-dependent myeloid leukemia cell line. *Proc Natl Acad Sci U S A* 1986;83:5010–5014.

559. Shadduck RK, Waheed A. Development of a radioimmunoassay for human macrophage colony-stimulating factor (CSF-1). *Ann N Y Acad Sci* 1989;554:156–166.

560. Yong K, Salooja N, Donahue RE, et al. Human macrophage colony-stimulating factor levels are elevated in pregnancy and in immune thrombocytopenia [see comments]. *Blood* 1992;80:2897–2902.

561. Motoyoshi K, Takaku F, Maekawa T, et al. Protective effect of partially purified human urinary colony-stimulating factor on granulocytopenia after antitumor chemotherapy. *Exp Hematol* 1986;14:1069–1075.

562. Halenbeck R, Kawasaki E, Wrin J, et al. Renaturation and purification of biologically active recombinant human macrophage colony stimulating factor expressed in *E. coli. Biotechnology* 1989;7:710.

563. Ulich TR, del Castillo J, Watson LR, et al. In vivo hematologic effects of recombinant human macrophage colony-stimulating factor. *Blood* 1990;75:846–850.

564. Masaoka T, Motoyoshi K, Takaku F, et al. Administration of human urinary colony stimulating factor after bone marrow transplantation. *Bone Marrow Transplant* 1988;3:121–127.

565. Komiyama A, Ishiguro A, Kubo T, et al. Increases in neutrophil counts by purified human urinary colony-stimulating factor in chronic neutropenia of childhood. *Blood* 1988; 71:41–45.

566. Motoyoshi K, Takaku F, Miura Y. High serum colony-stimulating activity of leukocytopenic patients after intravenous infusions of human urinary colony-stimulating factor. *Blood* 1983;62:685–688.

567. Masaoka T, Shibata H, Ohno R, et al. Double-blind test of human urinary macrophage colony-stimulating factor for allogeneic and syngeneic bone marrow transplantation: effectiveness of treatment and 2-year follow-up for relapse of leukaemia. *Br J Haematol* 1990;76:501–505.

568. Zamkoff K, Hudson J, Groves E, et al. A phase I trial of recombinant macrophage colony stimulating factor, human (rM-CSF), by rapid intravenous infusion in patients with refractory malignancy. *Proc Am Soc Clin Oncol* 1991; 10:93(abst).

569. Redman B, Flaherty L, Chou TH, et al. Phase I trial of recombinant macrophage-colony stimulating factor by rapid intravenous (IV) infusion in patients with cancer. *Proc Am Soc Clin Oncol* 1991;10:98(abst).

570. Bukowski RM, Budd GT, Gibbons JA, et al. Phase I trial of subcutaneous recombinant macrophage colony-stimulating factor: clinical and immunomodulatory effects. *J Clin Oncol* 1994;12:97–106.

571. Shadduck RK, Waheed A, Porcellini A, et al. Physiologic distribution of colony-stimulating factor in vivo. *Blood* 1979;54:894–905.

572. Sanda MG, Yang JC, Topalian SL, et al. Intravenous administration of recombinant human macrophage colony-stimulating factor to patients with metastatic cancer: a phase I study. *J Clin Oncol* 1992;10:1643–1649.

573. Nemunaitis J, Meyers JD, Buckner CD, et al. Phase I trial of recombinant human macrophage colony-stimulating factor in patients with invasive fungal infections. *Blood* 1991;78:907–913.

574. Bajorin DF, Cheung NK, Houghton AN. Macrophage colony-stimulating factor: biological effects and potential applications for cancer therapy. *Semin Hematol* 1991;28: 42–48.

575. Espinoza-Delgado I, Longo DL, Gusella GL, et al. IL-2 enhances c-fms expression in human monocytes. *J Immunol* 1990;145:1137–1143.

576. Mufson RA, Aghajanian J, Wong G, et al. Macrophage colony-stimulating factor enhances monocyte and macrophage antibody-dependent cell-mediated cytotoxicity. *Cell Immunol* 1989;119:182–192.

577. Nakoinz I, Ralph P. Stimulation of macrophage antibody-dependent killing of tumor targets by recombinant lymphokine factors and M-CSF. *Cell Immunol* 1988;116:331–340.

28

COLONY-STIMULATING FACTORS

WILLIAM P. PETROS

The relatively short time from the initial isolation of genes that regulate hematopoiesis to clinical development of therapeutic agents using these targets is unprecedented. Furthermore, the number of dollars spent on these commercial products is phenomenal, and they often appear as one of the top five drugs at institutions with major cancer treatment programs. Despite the fact that some colony-stimulating factors (CSFs) have been used in humans for more than 10 years, we are still learning more about their basic pharmacology and clinical applications. The primary function of these acidic glycoprotein molecules appears to be augmentation of the clonal proliferation and activation of hematopoietic cells. They may also play a role in immune response and wound healing.[1]

The CSFs have multiple therapeutic and clinical laboratory uses in oncology as shown in Table 28-1. The focus of this chapter is to evaluate the cytokines with potential clinical importance for hematopoiesis in the patient with cancer. Most justification for the current role of CSFs in therapeutics is directly linked to both the degree of interpatient variability in chemotherapy-induced myelosuppression and the role of dose intensity in the treatment of a particular malignancy. At the present time these agents should not be used indiscriminately to increase chemotherapy doses without justification.

CHEMISTRY AND PHARMACEUTICS

Chemically, the CSFs are glycoproteins typically consisting of a primary chain of over 100 amino acids that are intermittently bridged by disulfide bonds. The tertiary structure of the proteins is also potentially important in their biologic activity. Some CSFs circulate as dimers. The molecular weight of these molecules (19 kd to 90 kd) is dependent on both the primary chemical structure and the extent of glycosylation. Several endogenous forms of a particular CSF may be found in the circulation varying in the degree of glycosylation. Recombinant CSFs may be glycosylated depending on the type of expression system used in their manufacture. Three expression systems have been used in CSF synthesis: bacterial, yeast, and mammalian cell lines. Bacterial systems, such as *Escherichia coli*, do not produce glycosylated products, whereas yeast cells do provide some degree of glycosylation. Mammalian cells produce glycosylation that is more similar to the human pattern. Whether differences in glycosylation translate into clinically important effects is not yet clear. *In vitro* studies suggest that glycosylation may alter the receptor binding, elimination patterns, and immunogenicity of cytokines.[2,3] Thus, individual generic names have been assigned depending on the expression vector used in the manufacturing process [e.g., see entries for granulocyte-macrophage colony-stimulating factor (GM-CSF) in Table 28-2]. The unknown clinical significance of variations in glycosylation and the use of different activity assay methods by the various manufacturers make dosage comparisons, even between different generic types of a CSF, difficult.

Several novel approaches to recombinant CSF design are being actively pursued. One approach entails development of a series of novel chimeric CSFs that are agonists for multiple receptor types; for example, leridistim (Searle/Monsanto) is an interleukin 3 (IL-3)/granulocyte colony-stimulating factor (G-CSF) agonist. Importantly, these ligands are selected from libraries containing hundreds of sequences, which thus allows for optimization of desired agonist abilities and minimizes the potential for generation of inflammatory responses.

COLONY-STIMULATING FACTOR RECEPTORS

Glycoprotein receptors for CSFs are transcribed and expressed in a variety of hematologic and nonhematologic cells, including many cancer cell lines. The clinical implications of CSF receptor expression in malignant cells are unknown; however, one study has shown that the ability of multiple malignant cell lines to transcribe genes encoding for a cytokine receptor is, by itself, insufficient to render these cells responsive to cytokine stimulation.[4]

TABLE 28-1. CURRENT AND POTENTIAL CLINICAL USES OF COLONY-STIMULATING FACTOR IN ONCOLOGY

Aid to hematopoietic reconstitution after myelosuppressive therapy
Treatment of bone marrow failure
Treatment of myelodysplastic syndromes
Treatment of neutropenic fever
Regional therapy for localized infections
Treatment of fungal infections
In vivo cellular expansion of hematopoietic stem cells
Ex vivo cellular expansion
Generation of immune effector cells, e.g., dendritic cells
Transport of toxins to treat hematologic malignancies

TABLE 28-2. PHARMACEUTICAL CHARACTERISTICS OF COLONY-STIMULATING FACTORS

Cyto-kine	Names	Generic Name of Synthesized Agent	Expression Vector	Brand Name (Manufacturer)	No. of Amino Acids	Human Chromosome Location	Normal Endogenous Sources
G-CSF	Granulocyte colony-stimulating factor	Filgrastim Lenograstim	*Escherichia coli* CHO	Neupogen (Amgen) Neutrogin (Chugai)	174	17	Monocytes/macrophages, fibroblasts, endothelial cells, keratinocytes
GM-CSF	Granulocyte-macrophage colony-stimulating factor	Sargramostim Molgramostim Regramostim	Yeast *E. coli* CHO	Leukine (Immunex) Leucomax (Schering)	127	5	T lymphocytes, monocytes/macrophages, fibroblasts, endothelial cells, osteoblasts, epithelial cells
EPO	Erythropoietin	Epoetin-α Epoetin-α	CHO CHO	Epogen (Amgen) Procrit (Ortho)	165	7	Renal cells, hepatocytes
IL-1	Interleukin 1, lymphocyte activating factor, osteoclast activating factor, hematopoietin 1, catabolin, tumor inhibitory factor 2				159 (α) 153 (β)	2	Monocytes/macrophages, neutrophils, endothelial cells, fibroblasts, keratinocytes, T and B lymphocytes, NK cells, synovial lining cells, dermal dendritic cells, astrocytes
IL-3	Interleukin 3, multi-potential CSF, T-cell stimulating factor				133	5	T lymphocytes, NK cells, mast cells, keratinocytes, thymic epithelium
IL-6	Interleukin 6, interferon-β-2, B-cell stimulating factor 2, myeloma/plasmacytoma growth factor, hepatocyte-stimulating factor, cytotoxic T-cell differentiation factor				184	7	Endothelial cells, fibroblasts, neutrophils, monocytes/macrophages, T and B lymphocytes, bone marrow stromal cells, keratinocytes
IL-11	Interleukin 11	Oprelvekin	*E. coli*	Neumega (Genetics Institute)	178	19	Stromal fibroblasts, trophoblasts
SCF	Stem cell factor, Steel factor, mast cell growth factor, c-kit ligand	Ancestim	*E. coli*	Stemgen (Amgen)	165	12	Endothelial cells, fibroblasts, circulating mononuclear cells, bone marrow stromal cells
TPO	Thrombopoietin, megakaryocyte growth and development factor				332	3	Liver, kidney

CHO, Chinese hamster ovary cells; CSF, colony-stimulating factor; NK, natural killer.

Hematopoietin receptors contain either one subunit [e.g., erythropoietin (EPO), G-CSF, thrombopoietin (TPO)] or multiple subunits [(e.g., GM-CSF, IL-3, interleukin 6 (IL-6)], and frequently subunits are shared. Most common is a unique α subunit and a shared β subunit, with the latter essential for both high-affinity binding and signal transduction. Cytokine binding to cell surface receptors results in receptor clustering (oligomerization), activation, and finally generation of intracellular signals. In general, the CSF receptors lack intrinsic tyrosine kinase domains [except for macrophage colony-stimulating factor (M-CSF), stem cell factor (SCF), and FLT3]; however, cytoplasmic tyrosine kinases have been implicated in signal transduction pathways for some of these cytokines.[5] CSF receptor density is both cell and maturation specific. The general view is that occupancy of only a small percentage of available receptors for a particular CSF is required to adequately stimulate a hematopoietic cell.[6] Exposure to exogenously administered cytokines may result in altered regulation of that cytokine's receptor or receptors for other cytokines, which thus accounts for synergistic or antagonistic effects.[7–9]

Several factors may directly determine the ultimate physiologic effect of circulating CSF. These include both the cytokine concentration in blood and the presence of receptor antagonists or inhibitors or both (Fig. 28-1). A number of studies have investigated the relevance of soluble forms of the CSF receptors. The potential biologic effects of these molecules are numerous and include ligand stabilization before binding, receptor competition with ligand, receptor down-regulation, and cell sensitization to enhance response to a ligand (Fig. 28-2).[10] Studies have shown that soluble forms of tumor necrosis factor (TNF) receptors may compete with the cell surface receptors and thus may inhibit TNF bioactivity[11,12]; conversely, soluble IL-6 receptors may enhance ligand activity.[13] Diverse biologic

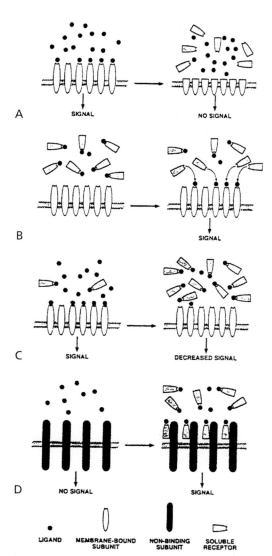

FIGURE 28-2. Some potential pharmacologic interactions of soluble colony-stimulating factor receptors. **A:** Proteolytic cleavage of soluble receptors results in a down-modulation of the membrane-bound receptor. **B:** Ligand binding to soluble receptor results in prolongation of ligand effect by stabilizing it in extracellular space. **C:** Competition between soluble and membrane-bound receptors for ligand results in decreased signal. **D:** Association of soluble receptors with ligand and nonbinding receptor subunits produces ligand sensitivity in cells without expression of membrane-bound receptor. (From Heaney ML, Golde DW. Soluble cytokine receptors. *Blood* 1996;87:847–857, with permission.)

responses to soluble receptors may be a function of their concentration. The origin of these molecules is tightly regulated and is thought to be primarily from proteolytic cleavage of the transmembrane receptor's extracellular ligand-binding domain or from alternative splicing of a truncated messenger RNA for the receptor.[14] Receptor antagonists that block cell surface receptors and compounds that down-modulate cell surface receptors may also inhibit cytokine activity. Elevated serum concentrations of various soluble receptors have been associated with inflammation or malignant diseases.

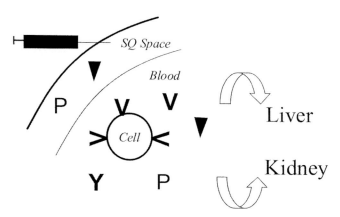

FIGURE 28-1. Potential routes of cytokine action and clearance. [▼, cytokine receptor antagonist; P, protease; V, receptors for cytokine (soluble or attached to cell membrane); Y, antibodies to cytokine.]

MECHANISM OF ACTION AND BIOLOGIC EFFECTS

Multiple biologic and biochemical effects are influenced by CSF; thus, an overall paradigm for their mechanism of action is not well established. In addition to amplifying activation and proliferation, these cytokines also aid in committing cells to a restricted differentiation pathway as well as in increasing the survival of some cells. Interpretation of biologic effects resulting from administration of a CSF is sometimes complex, because these effects may be attributable to the CSF's ability to alter the endogenous concentrations of other cytokines.

Animal models that are genetically deficient in a particular CSF have helped define their putative roles. For example, homozygous G-CSF–deficient mice are viable, fertile, and superficially healthy but display a chronic neutropenia, whereas those rendered GM-CSF deficient do not have altered hematopoiesis.[15,16]

The hematopoietic effects elicited by the various CSFs are often depicted by drawings such as the one displayed in Figure 28-3. Although such a representation is useful as a basic learning tool, the true nature of the system that produces hundreds of billions of cells per day at steady-state conditions is undoubtedly much more complex than shown here. Interactions between recombinant and endogenous cytokines may play an important role in their biologic effects.[17,18]

Best established are the interactions of CSFs such as EPO and G-CSF on the terminal differentiation of eryth-rocytes and neutrophils, respectively. Data indicate that the *in vitro* sensitivity of bone marrow cells to stimulation by G-CSF may be related to the patient's age, with a lower sensitivity noted in older subjects.[19] Other important effects include a reduction in the time taken for newly produced neutrophils to be released from the bone marrow into the circulation and increases in antibody-dependent cytotoxic capacity. The former effect occurs more strongly with G-CSF compared to GM-CSF.[20] Administration of G-CSF after chemotherapy stimulates primitive hematopoietic progenitors to appear in the peripheral blood to such a degree that they may exceed the concentrations of these cells in normal bone marrow.[21] Responses such as membrane depolarization, release of arachidonic acid, and generation of superoxide anions by neutrophils are also enhanced by G-CSF.

Therapeutic effects of EPO include maintenance of the induction, proliferation, and differentiation of erythroid progenitors from the bone marrow. Clearly the primary effects of EPO are on the erythroid lineage; however, it may also play a role in the stimulation of early multipotent progenitors.[22] Its erythropoietic activity may be at least partly attributable to induction of heme synthetic enzymes such as porphobilinogen deaminase. Other data suggest that EPO may act by suppressing apoptosis of colony-forming units.

The primary effect of GM-CSF on hematopoietic cells is to augment the survival and proliferation of cells in the granulocytic and macrophage lineages as well as megakaryocyte progenitors at high concentrations. *In vitro* studies

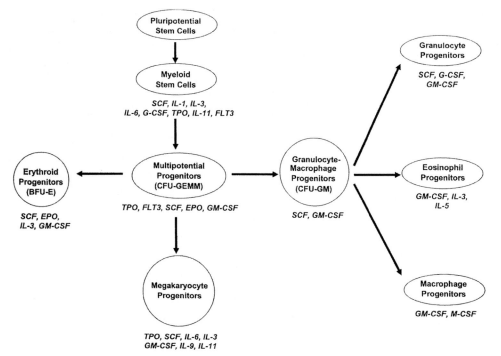

FIGURE 28-3. Representation of myeloid hematopoietic differentiation. Cytokines capable of stimulating specific cells are listed below such cells. (See Table 28-2 for other names of cytokines shown here.) (BFU-E, burst-forming unit, erythroid; CFU-GEMM, colony-forming unit granulocyte-erythrocyte-megakaryocyte macrophage; CFU-GM, colony-forming unit–granulocyte-macrophage; EPO, erythropoietin; G-CSF, granulocyte colony-stimulating factor; GM-CSF, granulocyte-macrophage colony-stimulating factor; IL, interleukin; M-CSF, macrophage colony-stimulating factor; SCF, stem cell factor; TPO, thrombopoietin.)

with GM-CSF have demonstrated an ability to increase the proportion of hematopoietic cells entering the S phase of the cell cycle and a dose-dependent shortening in the length of the cell cycle. Increases in granulocyte life span, metabolic functional activity, and antibody-dependent cellular cytotoxicity have been noted with *in vitro* incubations. These may be particularly important for the monocyte/macrophage cell lines, because production of other cytokines seems to be an important function of these cells. CSFs may display both acute and subacute effects on the peripheral blood concentrations of myeloid cells. For example, leukocyte concentrations initially decline after administration of GM-CSF, most likely as a result of Mo1 leukocyte cell surface adhesion antigen induction.[23] Other alterations of cellular function by GM-CSF for which there is clinical evidence include inhibition of neutrophil migration to sterile inflammatory fields.[24]

The glycoprotein TPO, also known as the c-mpl ligand or megakaryocyte growth and development factor (MGDF), is thought to play a very important, early, and relatively specific role in the regulation of platelet production. Mice deficient in mpl have mature, functional platelets, albeit at 15% of the normal platelet concentration.[25] TPO has been shown to stimulate blast colony formation in cells obtained from patients with acute myelogenous leukemia, but solid tumors do not routinely express the mpl receptor.[26–29]

Interleukin 11 (IL-11) is known for its properties as a stimulator of megakaryopoiesis, perhaps interacting at a later stage than TPO; however, it also has been shown to act synergistically with early and later acting cytokines in various stages of hematopoiesis. In addition, it is expressed and has activity in many other tissues, including those of the central nervous system, gastrointestinal tract, and testes.

IL-3 is thought to play a vital role in controlling the production of cells in all major blood cell types; however, it requires additional (terminally acting) cytokines for complete cell differentiation. Cells stimulated to proliferate are believed to be more primitive than those sensitive to GM-CSF. IL-3 acts synergistically with other early-acting cytokines such as IL-6 and interleukin 1 (IL-1) on blast cells. Other activities include augmentation of antibody-dependent cytotoxicity, superoxide anion production, and eosinophil complement–mediated phagocytosis.

Two types of endogenous IL-1 receptor agonists (α and β) and one endogenous receptor antagonist (IL-1ra) all appear to bind to both of the independent IL-1 receptors (types I and II). *In vitro* studies have demonstrated effects on multiple cell lines, including induction of acute-phase proteins from hepatocytes, activation of lymphocytes, and proliferation of fibroblasts, smooth muscle cells, keratinocytes, and thymocytes. Many biologic effects of IL-1 are thought to be due at least in part to its ability to induce secretion of and modulate the receptors for several other cytokines. *In vitro* IL-1 exposure confers protection of nor-mal hematopoietic progenitor cells to the effects of alkylating agents such as 4-hydroperoxycyclophosphamide.[30]

A variety of substances can induce the secretion of IL-6. Perhaps not surprisingly, it has a multitude of biologic effects, as evidenced by its assortment of names (Table 28-2). Biologic activities include regulation of immune responses, hematopoiesis, and acute-phase reactions. The hematopoietic functions of this cytokine are wide ranging and extend from stimulation of early progenitor cells to terminal differentiation of B lymphocytes into plasma cells.

SCF is a very-early-acting cytokine that is a ligand for the oncogene c-*kit*. Stimulation of *in vitro* proliferation has been demonstrated in mast cells as well as early and intermediate bone marrow progenitors. SCF can also protect hematopoietic cells from radiation-induced damage.

CLINICAL PHARMACOLOGY

Endogenous production of CSFs occurs in a wide variety of both hematopoietic and nonhematopoietic cells (Table 28-2). Some of these cytokines are found in detectable quantities in blood; however, many factors influence their concentrations, including concurrent drug therapy, disease, and cell homeostasis.[31,32] For example, concentrations of G-CSF and TPO increase during periods of neutropenia and thrombocytopenia, respectively. This has led to speculation that such cytopenias cause enhanced production of these cytokines.[33] An alternative explanation may be that during periods of neutropenia clearance mechanisms for the CSF are altered (see later). Exogenously administered cytokines or other drugs may also influence endogenous cytokine concentrations in patients with cancer. Relatively higher concentrations of M-CSF, IL-6, and tumor necrosis factor α (TNF-α) have been noted in patients receiving GM-CSF than in those receiving G-CSF after autologous bone marrow transplantation (Fig. 28-4).[34] These observations are in accordance with *in vitro* studies indicating that recombinant GM-CSF can induce neutrophil and macrophage production of multiple cytokines.[35–37] Blood obtained after administration of G-CSF to human volunteers has been shown to yield an increase in the concentrations of antiinflammatory cytokines (e.g., soluble TNF receptors and IL-1ra) on *ex vivo* stimulation.[38] Endogenous cytokine concentrations have also been helpful in evaluating the efficacy[18,34,39] and toxicity[34,40] of CSF therapy.

Assay Methodology

Most published pharmacokinetic studies of CSF use enzyme-linked immunosorbent assay (ELISA) or radioimmunoassay quantitative techniques. Use of an automated plate reader with these immunoassays allows the measurement of approximately 75 samples in several hours or less. ELISA assays provide easy and sensitive quantitative measurement of cytokine

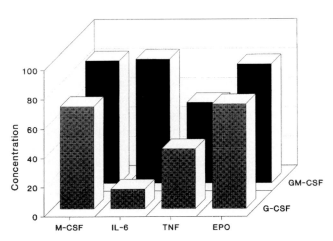

FIGURE 28-4. Median concentrations of endogenous cytokines in patients receiving either granulocyte-macrophage colony-stimulating factor (GM-CSF) (n = 20) or granulocyte colony-stimulating factor (G-CSF) (n = 17) after high-dose chemotherapy and autologous bone marrow transplantation. Units: M-CSF (macrophage colony-stimulating factor), ng/mL × 10; interleukin 6 (IL-6), pg/mL × 0.4; tumor necrosis factor (TNF), percent >7.5 pg/mL; EPO (erythropoietin), mU/mL × 2.5. (From Rabinowitz J, Petros WP, Stuart AR, et al. Characterization of endogenous cytokine concentrations after high-dose chemotherapy with autologous bone marrow support. *Blood* 1993;81:2452–2459.)

concentrations; however, they determine immunologic activity, not necessarily the biologic activity, of proteins. False-positive results are possible when a molecule that has been rendered biologically inactive remains intact at the assay's antibody-binding site. However, currently used biologic assays are often too cumbersome, too costly, and too variable for extensive studies of cytokines at multiple sample time points. Furthermore, they may be influenced by endogenous inhibitors sometimes found in clinical samples. Neither assay type can distinguish endogenous CSF from an exogenously administered recombinant form.

Pharmacokinetics

A variety of processes may influence the pharmacokinetic disposition of recombinant proteins such as the CSFs, as summarized in Figure 28-1. Some characteristics may be predictable by the molecular weight and glycosylation, whereas others may vary depending on receptor concentrations at a particular time.

Absorption

Subcutaneous administration of CSF generally has been shown to produce lower bioavailability. This effect is thought to be secondary to degradation of the recombinant protein by subcutaneous proteases. Conversely, subcutaneous administration may result in greater clinical efficacy than short intravenous infusions. One explanation for these

effects may be the low, yet prolonged, blood concentrations achieved with subcutaneous delivery. A study to evaluate this effect conducted a clinical comparison of intravenous and subcutaneous administration of GM-CSF in patients with myelodysplasia.[41] Twenty patients were randomly assigned to receive GM-CSF (yeast) either by 2-hour intravenous infusion or subcutaneously every 12 hours. Treatment lasted for 2 weeks and was followed by a 2-week washout; thereafter, patients were crossed over to the alternative administration route. Data demonstrates optimal hematopoietic stimulation with the subcutaneous route. Severe toxicity occurred at a similar rate in each group.

Distribution

CSFs typically have displayed relatively small volumes of distribution, approximating that of the volume of plasma. As expected, studies designed to evaluate multiple-compartment pharmacokinetics have described rapid distribution phases followed by more prolonged elimination. Peak concentrations generally follow a linear dose dependency.

Metabolism and Excretion

Serum CSF concentrations may be influenced by exogenous drug administration, increased endogenous CSF production, or reduced CSF elimination. Decay of CSF from the circulation may occur via a variety of possible mechanisms, including attachment of ligand to the cell surface receptor with subsequent endocytosis, metabolism by proteolytic enzymes (especially in the liver), and urinary excretion by glomerular filtration followed by reabsorption and catabolism (Fig. 28-1). The pattern and elimination pathways of exogenously administered cytokines may be affected by dose, administration route and schedule, degree of glycosylation of the recombinant protein, specific receptors available, production of antibodies, and, in some cases, renal function. Presence of other proteins, such as receptor antagonists or modulators of receptor expression, may also significantly affect receptor-mediated clearance. Attempts to modulate pharmacokinetics in preclinical trials have attached CSF molecules onto polyethylene glycol, which results in prolongation of the serum half-life and increased biologic activity.[42] Others have demonstrated dramatic reductions in the systemic clearance of a cytokine by concurrent administration of antibodies to that cytokine.[43] The mechanism of these effects may involve a substantial increase in molecular weight of the complex, which could limit its ability to be filtered by the glomerulus.

A summary of the pharmacokinetic parameters reported in published studies of selected CSFs is provided in Table 28-3. Factors that potentially contribute to the variability in the studies include assay methods, patient age, CSF dosage, receptor concentrations (e.g., white blood cell count), and expression vector of the recombinant protein.

TABLE 28-3.   SUMMARY OF PHARMACOKINETIC STUDIES OF COLONY-STIMULATING FACTORS

CSF	Route	N	Half-Life (h)	T_{max}(h)	Cl (mL/min/kg)
G-CSF	s.c.	37	2.5–5.8	4–8	19–56
G-CSF	i.v.	58	1.3–5.1 (α, 8[b]; β, 1.8)	NA	4–21
GM-CSF	s.c.	55	1.6–5.8	2.7–20.0	249–312
GM-CSF	i.v.	63	1.1–2.4 (α, 5–20[b]; β, 1.1–2.5)	NA	9.9–178
EPO	s.c.	125	9–38	12–28	NA
EPO	i.v.	135	4.0–11.2	NA	2.8–6.7
IL-3	s.c.	19	3.0–3.5	3	351
IL-3	i.v.	20	0.38–0.67	NA	282
IL-11	s.c.	18	6.9	3.2	NA[a]

Cl, systemic clearance (values are "apparent" for s.c. route); CSF, colony-stimulating factor; EPO, erythropoietin; G-CSF, granulocyte colony-stimulating factor; GM-CSF, granulocyte-macrophage colony-stimulating factor; IL, interleukin; N, number of patients; NA, not applicable; T_{max}, time of maximal concentration after s.c. injection. Data presented are ranges of mean values in the reviewed studies.[44,45,168–175]
[a]Clearance of IL-11 in infants and children is 1.2-fold to 1.6-fold higher than in adults or adolescents.
[b]Values are in minutes.

The effects of organ dysfunction on the pharmacokinetics of these proteins have not been extensively evaluated. Systemic clearance and urinary excretion of regramostim has been reported to be altered in bone marrow transplant patients with increased serum creatinine after an ablative regimen that included cisplatin.[44] The hypothesis is that the tubular toxicity produced by cisplatin alters the renal metabolism of regramostim, and this is modified further by reduced creatinine clearance. One should note that, even though the data in Table 28-3 are summarized for multiple recombinant forms (degrees of glycosylation) of each product for comparison between different CSFs, one cannot necessarily extrapolate data such as those presented above to other GM-CSF molecules with different degrees of glycosylation.

Limited clinical data are available that evaluate the effects of glycosylation on these molecules. For example, research has firmly established that EPO needs terminal sialic acid residues on the oligosaccharides to protect the molecule from immediate proteolytic attack.[3] Other CSFs, however, such as GM-CSF, do not require glycosylation to be of practical clinical use. Hovgaard et al. have published a comparison between molgramostim and regramostim in a small series of patients.[45] This noncrossover study found a significantly shorter distributional half-life, higher peak serum concentration, and lower area under the concentration × time curve in patients receiving intravenous molgramostim. Comparison of the products after subcutaneous administration yielded a quicker time to peak concentration and shorter duration of detectable levels for molgramostim (Fig. 28-5). Although a pharmacodynamic study must be completed, the data thus far suggest that differences in glycosylation may limit interchangeability in dosing data for products such as these.

CLINICAL DATA FOR INDIVIDUAL COLONY-STIMULATING FACTORS

A number of factors must be taken into consideration in interpreting the clinical results of CSF trials. Neutrophil

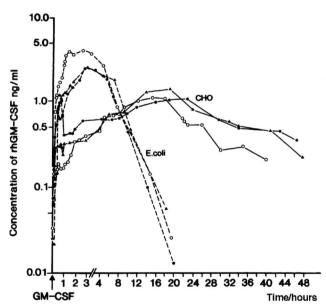

FIGURE 28-5. Serum disposition of molgramostim (derived from *Escherichia coli*) (*dashed line*) and regramostim (derived from Chinese hamster ovary cells) (*solid line*) after subcutaneous injection in patients treated with 5.5 or 8.0 μg per kg per day, respectively. GM-CSF, granulocyte-macrophage colony-stimulating factor; rhGM-CSF, recombinant human granulocyte-macrophage colony-stimulating factor. (From Hovgaard D, Mortensen BT, Schifter S, et al. Comparative pharmacokinetics of single-dose administration of mammalian and bacterially derived recombinant human granulocyte-macrophage colony-stimulating factor. *Eur J Haematol* 1993;50:32–36, with permission.)

recovery is obviously influenced by the chemotherapy regimen and dosages selected. Individual patient factors are also important, as evidenced by descriptions of reduced CSF efficacy in patients who have undergone extensive prior myelosuppressive therapy. Likewise, later-acting CSFs such as G-CSF or GM-CSF may not be very effective in patients receiving even low doses of stem cell toxins such as thiotepa.[46] Early CSF studies typically did not include concomitant administration of prophylactic antibiotics, a practice that is currently somewhat standard.

Administration of stem cell transfusions obviously influences reconstitution. The number and type of cells used—for example, CD34[+] selected peripheral blood progenitors, umbilical cord blood, etc.—can also cause sufficient heterogeneity in reconstitution to make any comparisons difficult.

Caution may need to be exercised in the use of these products, because concomitant administration of cycle-specific chemotherapy and G-CSF or GM-CSF has led to enhanced myelosuppression in some regimens.[47,48]

Erythropoietin

Many factors may account for anemia in patients with cancer, although the predominant causes are thought to be related to the cancer itself or to cytotoxic chemotherapy. The etiology is multifactorial and can be explained by both increased red cell destruction and reduced production. Erythropoiesis has been found to be correlated with disease stage in malignancies such as multiple myeloma, in which deficient red cell production is thought to be the primary mechanism.[49] Chemotherapy may obviously alter the ability of the bone marrow to produce erythrocytes while also eliciting toxic effects on the kidney. The latter is important

because almost all endogenous EPO is produced in the peritubular interstitial cells of the kidney and regulated by an oxygen sensor (Fig. 28-6). Although the cause of these effects was thought to be related partly to platinum analog toxicity, some data suggest that other mechanisms are important.[50] More specifically, investigators have noted an apparent deficiency in endogenous serum EPO associated with malignancy-related anemia that is not entirely explained by clinically apparent renal dysfunction. Platinum-associated anemia may be due to reduced EPO production secondary to toxic effects on EPO-producing renal cells or possibly to effects of platinum on cytochrome P-450 hemoproteins.[51,52] Both inappropriately low and surprisingly high EPO concentrations have been reported after chemotherapy.[53–55] One reason for such variability may be acute paradoxical elevations of endogenous EPO concentrations immediately after chemotherapy.[56–58] Measurement of endogenous concentrations of EPO may allow selection of anemic cancer patients who would show the greatest therapeutic benefit from administration of the recombinant protein.[59,60] Evaluations of patients undergoing high-dose chemotherapy with bone marrow transplantation indicate that perhaps endogenous EPO production may be a rate-limiting step in erythropoiesis after allogeneic transplantation, but not to such an important degree after autologous bone marrow transplantation.[61]

Abels summarized the results of a randomized, placebo-controlled study that used recombinant EPO to treat anemia [hematocrit (HCT) < 32%] in patients with cancer.[51,62] Recombinant EPO (100 to 150 U per kg per day) was administered three times weekly for 8 to 12 weeks or until the patient's HCT reached 38% to 40%. Patients were divided into three groups depending on whether they were

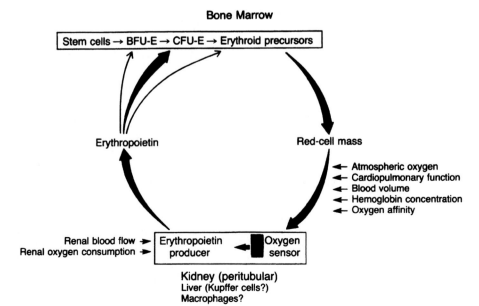

FIGURE 28-6. Feedback control of erythropoietin and erythrocyte production. (BFU-E, burst-forming unit, erythroid; CFU-E, colony-forming unit, erythroid.) (From Erslev AJ. Erythropoietin. *N Engl J Med* 1991;324:1339–1344, with permission.)

TABLE 28-4. RESULTS OF RANDOMIZED, PLACEBO-CONTROLLED TRIAL OF ERYTHROPOIETIN (EPO) THERAPY IN PATIENTS WITH MALIGNANCIES

	EPO			Placebo		
	I	II	III	I	II	III
Number of patients	63	79	64	55	74	61
Change in HCT (mg/dL)	+2.8[a]	+6.9[a]	+6.0[a]	−0.1	+1.1	+1.3
Correction of anemia (% with HCT ≥38)	20.6[a]	40.5[a]	35.9[a]	3.6	4.1	1.6
Patients receiving transfusion (%)	33.3	40.5	53.1	38.2	48.6	68.9
Mean transfusions per patient	1.52	2.03	3.56	2.19	2.75	4.01

HCT, hematocrit.
Patients in group I were not receiving chemotherapy. Patients in group II received non–platinum-based chemotherapy. Patients in group III underwent chemotherapy regimens that included cisplatin.
[a]Values significantly different from placebo group.
From Abels RI. Use of recombinant human erythropoietin in the treatment of anemia in patients who have cancer. *Semin Oncol* 1992;19[Suppl 8]:29–35.

receiving chemotherapy and whether the regimen included cisplatin. Criteria for red blood cell (RBC) transfusion were apparently not standardized but appeared similar for all groups. As shown in Table 28-4, the patients treated with EPO in each group demonstrated statistically significant increases in HCT and a higher frequency of correction of anemia; however, transfusion requirements were not significantly different for the groups. When data for the two groups receiving chemotherapy were combined, a significant reduction in the number of patients undergoing transfusion (27.8% versus 45.5%) and the number of transfusions used per patient (1.04 versus 1.81) was evident after the first month of therapy in the EPO group. Others have confirmed these findings.[63]

Randomized trials of prophylactic EPO therapy have also demonstrated efficacy in the prevention of anemia during treatment with a cyclophosphamide, epirubicin hydrochloride, and fluorouracil combination chemotherapy regimen for breast cancer and a platinum-based combination regimen for small cell lung cancer.[64,65]

A randomized (but not placebo-controlled) evaluation of EPO therapy after allogeneic bone marrow transplantation has been reported in 28 patients with leukemia.[66] EPO (100 to 150 U per kg per day) was administered for 30 days after transplant. EPO therapy significantly accelerated the appearance of reticulocytes and reduced RBC transfusion requirements (12 units in the control group versus 4 units in the treatment group); however, median hemoglobin levels were unaffected. Interestingly, patients in the EPO group also demonstrated significantly faster platelet recovery, which translated into a reduction in the number of platelet transfusions; however, more patients in the control group experienced venoocclusive disease, which complicates the interpretation. Some preclinical studies indicate that long-term administration of high-dose EPO may produce competition between erythrocytic and megakaryocytic cell lines, which results in thrombocytopenia.[67] Subsequent randomized trials in the allogeneic and autologous bone marrow transplantation

settings have failed to show a substantial benefit of prophylaxis with EPO.[68–70]

Overall, the application of data from clinical trials of EPO is not straightforward because the level of hemoglobin that would optimize functional status of a patient with cancer is not well defined.

A variety of alternative EPO dosing schedules have been evaluated. Studies conducted in healthy volunteers suggest that the thrice weekly subcutaneous regimen provides better erythropoietic response than the same total dose given once weekly[71]; however, the initial report of a large, open-label, once weekly EPO regimen in cancer patients did demonstrate efficacy.[72]

Granulocyte Colony-Stimulating Factor

An extensive review of clinical data from phase I and II studies of G-CSF or GM-CSF can be found in a publication by Lieschke and Burgess.[73] Many randomized, placebo-controlled phase III clinical trials have evaluated the efficacy of G-CSF for prophylaxis of febrile neutropenia after myelosuppressive chemotherapy (Table 28-5).[74–84] In general, these trials have demonstrated a significant acceleration of neutrophil recovery with use of the CSF, resulting in some trials to a reduction in hospitalization for neutropenic fever (Fig. 28-7). One must realize that chemotherapy regimens expected to produce substantial myelosuppression were selected for many of these studies to optimize potential differences between the groups.

Most published CSF clinical trials were not designed to evaluate differences achieved in chemotherapy dose intensity. Nonrandomized and randomized studies have demonstrated an increased ability to administer chemotherapy cycles on the planned time schedule with use of G-CSF or GM-CSF prophylaxis.[85–88] Over the past several years, some phase I studies of new cytotoxic agents that find myelosuppression to be the dose-limiting toxicity have been successful in obtaining additional escalations with the aid of prophylactic CSF.[89] A European randomized study

TABLE 28-5. RESULTS OF RANDOMIZED, PLACEBO-CONTROLLED CLINICAL TRIALS OF G-CSF OR GM-CSF PROPHYLAXIS AFTER CHEMOTHERAPY IN PATIENTS NOT RECEIVING HEMATOPOIETIC CELLULAR SUPPORT

Study	Cancer Diagnosis	Chemotherapy	CSF Given	N	N+	H+	Ab+	ID
Ohno et al.[74]	Leukemias	ME	G-CSF (*Escherichia coli*)	108	↓	NR	NR	↓
Crawford et al.[75]	SCLC	CAE	G-CSF (*E. coli*)	211	↓	↓	↓	NR
Kotake et al.[76]	Urogenital cancer	Various	G-CSF (*E. coli*)	77	↓	NR	NR	NR
Trillet-Lenoir et al.[78]	SCLC	CAE	G-CSF (*E. coli*)	130	↓	↓	↓	NC
Pettengell et al.[77]	NHL	VAPEC-B	G-CSF (*E. coli*)	80	↓	NC	NC	NC
Pui et al.[79]	Pediatric ALL	Standard + VP-16/ara-C	G-CSF (*E. coli*)	164	↓	↓	NC	↓
Hartmann et al.[80]	Solid tumors, lymphoma	Various	G-CSF (*E. coli*)[a]	138	↓	NC	NC	NC
Chevallier et al.[81]	Breast cancer	FEC	G-CSF (CHO)	120	↓	↓	↓	↓
Dombret et al.[82]	AML	DNM, ara-C	G-CSF (CHO)	173	↓	NR	NR	NC
Godwin et al.[83]	AML (>54 yr)	DNM, ara-C	G-CSF (*E. coli*)	234	↓	NC	↓	NC
Heil et al.[84]	AML	DNM, ara-C, VP-16	G-CSF (*E. coli*)	521	↓	↓	↓	NC
Gerhartz et al.[113]	NHL	COP-BLAM	GM-CSF (*E. coli*)	182	↓	↓	↓	↓
De Vries et al.[112]	Ovarian cancer	CC	GM-CSF (CHO)	15	↓	NR	NR	NR
Eguchi et al.[114]	NSCLC	MVP	GM-CSF (NR)	52	↓	NR	NR	NR
Stone et al.[115]	AML (>59 yr)	DNM, ara-C	GM-CSF (*E. coli*)	388	↓	NC	NR	NC
Rowe et al.[117]	AML (>55 yr)	DNM, ara-C	GM-CSF (yeast)	124	↓	NC	NR	↓
Jones et al.[116]	Breast cancer	FAC	GM-CSF (yeast)	142	↓	NC	NR	NR

↓, decreased; Ab+, use of antibiotics; ALL, acute lymphoblastic leukemia; AML, acute myelogenous leukemia; ara-C, cytosine arabinoside; CAE, cyclophosphamide, doxorubicin hydrochloride, and etoposide; CC, carboplatin and cyclophosphamide; COP-BLAM, cyclophosphamide, vincristine sulfate, prednisone, bleomycin sulfate, doxorubicin hydrochloride, and procarbazine; CSF, colony-stimulating factor; DNM, daunomycin; FAC, 5-fluorouracil, doxorubicin hydrochloride, and cyclophosphamide; FEC, fluorouracil, etoposide, and cisplatin; G-CSF, granulocyte colony-stimulating factor; GM-CSF, granulocyte-macrophage colony-stimulating factor; H+, duration of hospitalization; ID, frequency of infectious complications; ME, behenoylcytosine arabinoside and etoposide; MVP, mitomycin, vinblastine sulfate, and cisplatin; N, number of patients; N+, duration of neutropenia; NC, no significant change; NHL, non-Hodgkin's lymphoma; NR, not reported or no data provided regarding statistical significance; NSCLC, non–small cell lung cancer; SCLC, small cell lung cancer; VAPEC-B, vincristine, doxorubicin, prednisolone, etoposide, cyclophosphamide, bleomycin; VP-16, etoposide.
[a]CSF initiated when absolute neutrophil count was <500/mm^3.

examining the use of filgrastim with cyclophosphamide, doxorubicin hydrochloride (Adriamycin), and etoposide (CAE) therapy in patients with small cell lung cancer[78] differed from the U.S. trial[75] in that patients on the placebo arm were not allowed to receive filgrastim if they had become neutropenic and febrile on a previous cycle. This permitted evaluation of the effect of filgrastim on the dose intensity of CAE. Chemotherapy doses were reduced secondary to myelosuppression in 29% of patients treated with filgrastim compared with 61% of patients receiving placebo. Although this difference was statistically significant, the median percentage of the prescribed dose given

(mg per m^2 per week) was approximately 88% for the patients on placebo compared with 96% for patients treated with filgrastim. These results demonstrate that CSF alone probably does not allow substantial increases in dose intensity unless some type of cellular support is incorporated into the regimen.

In a randomized, open-label study in which lenograstim was administered after vincristine sulfate, ifosfamide, carboplatin, and etoposide (VICE) chemotherapy for small cell lung cancer, the CSF-treated group displayed a 6% increase in dose intensity and higher acute mortality but a trend toward better 2-year survival.[90]

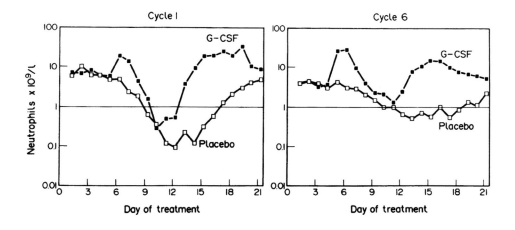

FIGURE 28-7. Neutrophil concentrations in 129 patients randomly assigned to receive either granulocyte colony-stimulating factor (G-CSF) or placebo after cyclophosphamide, doxorubicin hydrochloride, and etoposide (CAE) chemotherapy. (From Trillet-Lenoir V, Green J, Manegold C, et al. Recombinant granulocyte colony stimulating factor reduces the infectious complications of cytotoxic chemotherapy. *Eur J Cancer* 1993;29A:319–324, with permission.)

A randomized, open-label study in which filgrastim was given during part of the induction chemotherapy (cyclophosphamide, cytosine arabinoside, methotrexate sodium, 6-mercaptopurine) to 76 patients with acute lymphoblastic leukemia found substantial improvement in the duration of neutropenia, less interruptions in the chemotherapy schedule, and no change in disease-free survival at a median of 20 months follow-up.[91]

Use of G-CSF or placebo to treat febrile neutropenia was assessed in a double-blind, randomized trial involving 218 patients who were also receiving standard antibiotic therapy. Use of G-CSF was associated with an acceleration of neutrophil recovery and a shortening in the duration of neutropenic fever; however, the overall hospitalization duration was unaffected.[92]

Similarly, delay in institution of G-CSF prophylaxis for afebrile patients until the absolute neutrophil count is 500 per mm^3 or lower has been shown to shorten the period of neutropenia but not to change the rate or duration of hospitalization.[80]

G-CSF has been used in several phase I, II, and III trials for acceleration of hematopoietic recovery after stem cell transplantation (Table 28-6).[93–95] In general, these trials

indicate that G-CSF administered after high-dose chemotherapy and autologous bone marrow transplantation improves the rate of peripheral blood neutrophil recovery once it begins but has no substantial effect on the approximately 8-day period of absolute leukopenia or on platelet recovery. The proportion of patients with febrile neutropenia has not been substantially altered by treatment, although the number of days of febrile neutropenia has been reduced with G-CSF. In some studies G-CSF has also been administered for several days approximately 2 weeks before bone marrow transplantation to produce high concentrations of progenitor cells in the peripheral blood (PBPCs).[96–98] These cells are then extracted by leukapheresis and given back to the patient after high-dose chemotherapy along with G-CSF. The PBPC is thought to express receptors for terminally acting CSFs (such as G-CSF) and thus to be immediately able to proliferate, providing some neutrophils during the 8-day period of absolute leukopenia. The results from these trials support such a hypothesis, and G-CSF is the most common cytokine used to generate *in vivo* production of PBPC either alone or after administration of myelosuppressive, standard-dose chemotherapy (Table 28-6). A somewhat unexpected benefit of this ther-

TABLE 28-6. RESULTS OF RANDOMIZED CLINICAL TRIALS OF G-CSF OR GM-CSF THERAPY IN ASSOCIATION WITH HIGH-DOSE CHEMOTHERAPY AND STEM CELL TRANSPLANTATION

Study	Cancer Type	Stem Cell Source	CSF Given after Cells	N	WBC Recovery	Days ANC > 500/ mm^3 vs. Control	PLT Recovery	Fever
Powles et al.[119]	Leukemia	Allo-BM	GM-CSF (CHO)	20[a]	−	3	NC	↑
Nemunaitis et al.[120]	Lymphoma	Auto-BM	GM-CSF (Yeast)	128[a]	+	7	NC	NC
Link et al.[121]	Lymphoma/ALL	Auto-BM	GM-CSF (*Escherichia coli*)	81[a]	+	13	NC	NC
Khwaja et al.[122]	Lymphoma	Auto-BM	GM-CSF (*E. coli*)	61[a]	+	7	NC	NC
Advani et al.[123]	Lymphoma	Auto-BM	GM-CSF (*E. coli*)	69[a]	+	4	NC	NR
De Witte et al.[124]	Leukemia/etc.	Allo-BM	GM-CSF (CHO)	57[a]	+	4	NC	NC
Gorin et al.[125]	NHL	Auto-BM	GM-CSF (*E. coli*)	91[a]	+	7	NC	NC
Gulati et al.[126]	Hodgkins	Auto-BM	GM-CSF (*E. coli*)	24[a]	+	NR	+	NR
Nemunaitis et al.[127]	Various	Allo-BM	GM-CSF (yeast)	109[a]	+	4	NC	NC
Hiraoka et al.[128]	Various	Allo-BM	GM-CSF (*E. coli*)	53[a]	+	4	NC	NC
Asano et al.[93]	NR	Allo-BM	G-CSF (CHO)	53[a]	+	10	NR	NR
Stahel et al.[95]	Lymphoma	Auto-BM	G-CSF (*E. coli*)	43	+	8	NC	↓
Schmitz et al.[94]	Lymphoma	Auto-BM	G-CSF (*E. coli*)	54	+	7	NC	NC
Legros et al.[133]	Various	Auto-PBPC	GM-CSF (*E. coli*)	50[a]	NC	NR	NC	↑
Klumpp et al.[100]	Various	Auto-PBPC	G-CSF (NR)	41	+	5.5	NC	NC
Lee et al.[103]	Lymphoma	Auto-PBPC	G-CSF (*E. coli*)	23	+	3.5	NC	NC
Kawano et al.[101]	Various (pediatric)	Auto-PBPC	G-CSF (*E. coli*)	63	+	1	NC	NC
McQuaker et al.[102]	Lymphoma/ myeloma	Auto-PBPC	G-CSF (*E. coli*)	38[a]	+	4	NC	NC
Spitzer et al.[108]	Various	Auto-PBPC	G-CSF (NR) + GM-CSF (NR)	37[a]	+	6	NC	NC

+, augmented; −, worsened; ↑, increased; ↓, decreased; ALL, acute lymphoblastic leukemia; allo-BM, allogeneic bone marrow transplant; auto-BM, autologous bone marrow transplant; ANC, absolute neutrophil count; auto-PBPC, autologous peripheral blood progenitor cells; CHO, Chinese hamster ovary; CSF, colony-stimulating factor; G-CSF, granulocyte colony-stimulating factor; GM-CSF, granulocyte-macrophage colony-stimulating factor; NC, no significant change; NHL, non-Hodgkin's lymphoma; NR, not reported or no data provided regarding statistical significance; PLT, platelet; WBC, white blood cell count.
[a]Placebo-controlled.

apy is a reduction in platelet transfusion requirements. Such effects may be explained in part by a dose-dependent increase in the early peripheral blood myeloid progenitors (CD34+) noted in the PBPC product.

Data suggest that administration of G-CSF after PBPC reinfusion aids engraftment.[99–103] Most of the original investigations initiated CSF therapy immediately after administration of the bone marrow; however, some studies have suggested that a 5- to 6-day delay in G-CSF use may achieve similar efficacy.[104,105] Caution should be exercised in translating these data to situations in which progenitor cells are being administered, due to their quicker hematopoietic reconstitution and potentially different interactions with CSF; however, similar results have been found in relatively small trials.[106]

Other controversial areas being studied include the optimal timing of leukapheresis and concomitant use of other cytokines to aid trilineage engraftment. CSF-primed PBPCs have also been used to compress the schedule of multicyclic cytotoxic chemotherapy regimens such as ifosfamide, carboplatin, and etoposide (ICE).[107]

The optimal schedule, dose, and combination of G-CSF with other cytokines is an area of intense clinical research. One randomized study could not demonstrate any benefit of adding GM-CSF to an autologous G-CSF priming regimen; however, no CSFs were given after reinfusion of the transplanted cells.[108] A combination of G-CSF with cyclophosphamide is routinely used to increase the generation of CD34+ cells; however, a randomized study found greater efficacy and less toxicity with G-CSF alone in patients with multiple myeloma.[109]

A wide variety of G-CSF doses and administration techniques have been used in clinical trials. The most common dose for prophylaxis of myelosuppression after standard or high-dose chemotherapy is 5 µg per kg per day. Lower doses of lenograstim (2 mg per kg per day) appear to have similar efficacy to standard doses (5 mg per kg per day).[110] Discontinuation of G-CSF during the recovery phase after myelosuppressive chemotherapy typically results in a rebound depression of the white blood count by approximately 50% within 24 hours.

Adverse effects thought to be secondary to G-CSF administration have been fairly mild in the clinical trials reported to date. Bone pain is the most frequent complaint, often occurring near the time of maximal hematopoiesis. Concurrent administration of G-CSF with cycle-specific chemotherapy may paradoxically worsen the myelosuppressive effects of the latter.[111]

Granulocyte-Macrophage Colony-Stimulating Factor

GM-CSF has been used in numerous phase I, II, and III trials after standard doses of myelosuppressive chemotherapy; it does seem to reduce the occurrence of febrile neutro-

penia (Table 28-5).[112–116] A large phase III, placebo-controlled study of the use of sargramostim as prophylaxis for neutropenic fever was conducted in elderly patients with acute myeloblastic leukemia. In addition to the benefit of enhanced neutrophil recovery and reduction of infections, the sargramostim-treated group also displayed significantly longer survival.[117]

A randomized, placebo-controlled study that evaluated initiation of molgramostim treatment to patients at the onset of chemotherapy-induced febrile neutropenia could not demonstrate substantial clinical or monetary benefit.[118]

Randomized, placebo-controlled clinical trials involving GM-CSF have also been conducted in the setting of high-dose chemotherapy with stem cell support, as indicated in Table 28-6.[119–128] The results from these trials demonstrate an ability of GM-CSF to accelerate neutrophil recovery after a few days of absolute leukopenia when bone marrow alone is used as the sole stem cell source (Fig. 28-8). Patients who were previously exposed to drugs that deplete stem cells (e.g., carmustine or busulfan) experienced less benefit from GM-CSF.[129] Most studies could not discern an effect of the CSF on the rate of documented bacterial infections. The impact of GM-CSF on platelet recovery is inconsistent, and its use generally has not solved the problem of transfusion dependence. GM-CSF therapy had no significant effect on the incidence or severity of graft-versus-host disease in patients receiving allogeneic transplants.

As with G-CSF, a number of nonrandomized and randomized trials have found GM-CSF (given alone or after chemotherapy) useful to prime PBPCs for subsequent leukapheresis.[96,130–133] Kritz et al. randomly assigned patients to receive GM-CSF–primed PBPCs or no cellular support after cytotoxic chemotherapy, with autologous marrow rescue given if needed on day 15. The study was stopped early due to a substantial difference in myeloid and platelet recovery

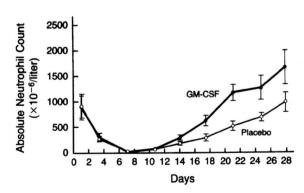

FIGURE 28-8. Neutrophil concentrations in 129 patients randomly assigned to receive either granulocyte-macrophage colony-stimulating factor (GM-CSF) or placebo after high-dose chemotherapy with autologous bone marrow transplantation. (From Nemunaitis J, Rabinowe SN, Singer JW, et al. Recombinant granulocyte-macrophage colony-stimulating factor after autologous bone marrow transplantation for lymphoid cancer. *N Engl J Med* 1991;324:1773–1778, with permission.)

between the groups that favored the PBPC-treated patients.[134] Although this study included a low number of patients and had a short follow-up, it demonstrates the potential ability to influence hematopoiesis by PBPCs alone.

Filgrastim and molgramostim appear to produce similar yields of CD34+ PBPCs when used in conjunction with chemotherapy for priming; however, use of filgrastim may shorten this process.[135,136] Some data suggest that a combination of G-CSF and GM-CSF may yield a better progenitor product for allogeneic transplantation than either cytokine alone.[137] Caballero et al. randomly assigned 42 patients with breast cancer to receive open-label filgrastim or molgramostim after cyclophosphamide/cisplatin/carmustine or cyclophosphamide/carboplatin/thiotepa high-dose chemotherapy and autologous, filgrastim-stimulated PBPC infusion.[138] All patients also received acetaminophen before CSF doses and prophylactic antibiotics. The only differences noted were slightly faster platelet recovery and 2 days' fewer hospitalization in the filgrastim arm.

Dose-related adverse effects with GM-CSF treatment include capillary leak syndrome, central vein thrombosis, and hypotension. Effects seen over a variety of dosages include fever, pleuritis, myalgia, bone pain, pulmonary infiltrates, rash, and thrombophlebitis. Some patients have experienced a syndrome of transient hypoxia and hypotension after the first dose but not subsequent doses of GM-CSF.[139] Most randomized studies that used the standard dose (250 μg per m^2 per day) have shown only mild adverse effects. GM-CSF is a known inducer of other endogenous cytokines, which are thought to account for at least some of the adverse effects. As with G-CSF, the simultaneous administration of GM-CSF and cycle-specific chemotherapy or radiation therapy has worsened myelosuppression.[140,141]

Clinical Synopsis of Granulocyte Colony-Stimulating Factor and Granulocyte-Macrophage Colony-Stimulating Factor

The intent of this chapter is to provide a description of growth-factor clinical pharmacology; however, a brief summary of how agents such as G-CSF and GM-CSF fit into current practice is presented in this section. Introduction of G-CSF and, to a lesser extent GM-CSF, into routine clinical practice has profoundly influenced the treatment of chronic neutropenias and generation of PBPCs for collection and subsequent reinfusion after high-dose chemotherapy. The most frequent use of these agents, however, has been for prophylaxis of chemotherapy-induced neutropenic fever, an indication for which the outcome data are less clear. Not much evidence yet exists that administration of a CSF influences disease-free or overall survival, even for tumor types typically thought to be chemosensitive. This suggests that routine CSF use for primary prophylaxis is not justified for most patients. Probably a majority of current CSF prescriptions are for secondary prophylaxis (i.e., written for patients who experienced

myelosuppression on a previous cycle of chemotherapy). Even less data exist to justify any impact on disease-free survival or overall survival for such an indication. Another common use of CSFs is in the treatment of neutropenic fever; data suggest no substantial benefit to such therapy.

The use of CSF for priming PBPCs does decrease toxicity, both in the priming period and after transplantation, in addition to reducing hospital stay and cost of therapy. Administration of CSF after stem cell infusion probably has some benefit; however, the degree of effect is most likely dependent on the quality and quantity of cells infused. Older studies that report differences in hospitalization should be interpreted with caution when compared with contemporary practice due to changes in outpatient treatment of neutropenic fever, even after high-dose chemotherapy.

Interleukin 11

Preclinical and *in vitro* studies indicated that IL-11 may have direct effects as a megakaryocyte potentiator. Oprelvekin (recombinant IL-11) was the first cytokine to reach the market for prevention of chemotherapy-induced thrombocytopenia, and this occurred only 3 years after the initial research application. Phase I evaluations in patients with cancer demonstrated an impressive ability to increase steady-state platelet counts by over twofold.[142]

The ability of recombinant IL-11 to prevent thrombocytopenia was evaluated in a randomized, placebo-controlled trial involving 77 patients with breast cancer who had not previously experienced severe chemotherapy-induced thrombocytopenia. Patients received two cycles of doxorubicin and cyclophosphamide followed by G-CSF and the study drug on each cycle. The transfusion criterion was 20,000 platelets per μL; 43% of patients taking the placebo required a transfusion, compared with 30% of patients treated with IL-11. The mean number of transfusions was 2.2 versus 0.8 for the two groups, respectively.[143]

A randomized, placebo-controlled trial evaluated the use of IL-11 for secondary prophylaxis of thrombocytopenia in 93 patients with cancer who had previously received platelet transfusions for chemotherapy-induced toxicity. As expected, more than 90% of patients on the placebo arm required a platelet transfusion compared with 72% of the IL-11–treated patients. The mean number of transfusions in the two arms was 3.3 and 2.2, respectively.[144]

Administration of IL-11 did not appear to substantially alter platelet recovery or transfusion requirements in 80 patients with breast cancer who were enrolled in a randomized, placebo-controlled study after high-dose chemotherapy and G-CSF–primed PBPC infusion.[145]

Approximately 60% of patients treated with IL-11 experience some degree of generalized edema, which is thought to be secondary to increased retention of sodium. In addition, atrial arrhythmias, tachycardia, conjunctival injection, and worsening of effusions can occur. Constitutional symptoms such as myalgias, arthralgias, and fatigue were dose limiting during phase I trials.

Thrombopoietin

The development of TPO exemplifies the rapid pace of CSF research—clinical trials were initiated only 9 months after publication of discovery. Murine studies suggested a nonmonotonic dose versus platelet response curve for TPO, and this may be due to inhibitory effects on platelet progenitors at high doses.[146] Murine and nonhuman primate studies have demonstrated a synergism between TPO and G-CSF in acceleration of neutrophil and platelet recovery after myelosuppressive chemotherapy, with no evidence of lineage competition.

Clinical studies of recombinant TPO have been conducted with either the full-length, glycosylated TPO molecule (rTPO, Genentech) or a truncated, polyethylene glycol–bound derivative (rMGDF, Amgen). A clinical study of rMGDF involving 17 patients with cancer (who were not currently receiving chemotherapy) demonstrated a dose-dependent increase in platelet counts. Those receiving the highest doses achieved a 51% to 584% increase in platelet counts. The effect was clinically evident after 6 days of therapy, and counts continued to rise several days after drug discontinuation.[147,148] Platelets generated in these patients appeared to have normal function based on *in vitro* assays. The rMGDF therapy increased the appearance of progenitor cells in the bloodstream, which indicated that it may be useful for priming. Similar data were found with the full-length rTPO molecule.[149]

In two other studies rMGDF was administered to a total of 94 patients with lung cancer both before and after a carboplatin and cyclophosphamide regimen. A significant shortening in the time to platelet nadir and faster platelet recovery were noted.[150,151]

The rTPO and rMGDF were generally well tolerated in these early studies, with essentially no evidence of dose-limiting adverse effects; nor were any fever or flulike symptoms discernible. A few patients did experience thrombotic events, however. The role of the study drug in such processes is unclear.

Clinical development of MGDF was halted when some patients in cancer trials and normal, healthy volunteers given the cytokine began to demonstrate neutralizing antibodies to TPO. A similar phenomenon has occurred when some other recombinant growth factors, molgramostim and PIXY321 (an IL-3/GM-CSF fusion protein), have been used, with or without immunosuppressive chemotherapy; the result is abrogation of their hematopoietic activities.[152,153]

Stem Cell Factor

SCF is thought to stimulate very immature hematopoietic progenitor cells. Preclinical studies have established its ability to mobilize early progenitor cells into the circulation and have revealed a synergistic effect with later-acting cytokines such as G-CSF.[154] Phase I evaluations of SCF in humans have demonstrated both bone marrow expansion and peripheral blood mobilization of hematopoietic progenitors.[155,156] Administration of recombinant SCF plus filgrastim was shown to result in a significantly better yield of CD43+ PBPCs than filgrastim alone in a randomized dose-finding study.[157] A follow-up phase III study of this combination found that 63% of patients achieved the target CD34+ cell count (5×10^6 cells per kg) within a median of four leukapheresis procedures, whereas 47% of those treated with filgrastim alone achieved this level after five leukapheresis procedures.[158] The design of this study was not optimal for evaluation of differences in posttransplant engraftment, and no differences in such were evident between the groups. Patients in these studies required premedication with diphenhydramine, ranitidine, pseudoephedrine, and inhaled albuterol to prevent mast cell–related reactions induced by SCF.

Interleukin 1

Human IL-1 exists in at least two forms (α and β), which have identical receptor-binding sites and similar biologic activity, despite only a 26% structural homology. Preclinical studies of IL-1 revealed its ability as a cytoprotective agent,[159,160] whereas *in vitro* studies demonstrated its ability to induce the cellular secretion of multiple cytokines, including G-CSF, GM-CSF, M-CSF, IL-3, and IL-6.[161] Phase I and II studies have also noted some evidence of cytokine induction and a delayed effect on stimulation of platelet counts, which peak approximately 2 weeks after initiation of therapy.[162] Administration of IL-1α to patients with ovarian cancer undergoing treatment with carboplatin appears to attenuate treatment-induced thrombocytopenia.[163] The future of this cytokine as a hematopoietin will probably depend on trials that combine it with a later-acting agent. Adverse effects are dose related and include supraventricular arrhythmias, fever, hypotension, chills, phlebitis, confusion, and bone pain.[164]

FLT3 Ligand

In vitro studies have shown that the FLT3 ligand increases recruitment of primitive progenitors into the cell cycle. Initial clinical trials demonstrated its ability to mobilize CD34+ cells into peripheral blood. Synergism is seen when it is combined with G-CSF, GM-CSF, or other cytokines.[165] FLT3 is also a very potent stimulator of dendritic cell production. Clinical trials using it as a priming agent for PBPC are in progress.

Combination Colony-Stimulating Factor Therapy

Preclinical and clinical data presented for the last few molecules discussed above suggest that optimal hematopoietic

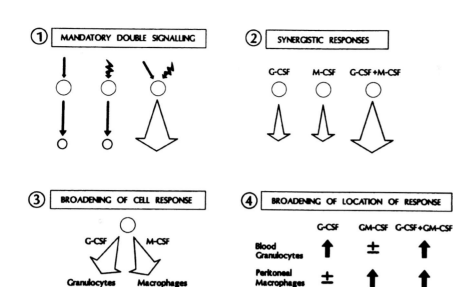

FIGURE 28-9. Examples of interactions among cytokines on hematopoiesis. (G-CSF, granulocyte colony-stimulating factor; GM-CSF, granulocyte-macrophage colony-stimulating factor; M-CSF, macrophage colony-stimulating factor.) (From Metcalf D. Hematopoietic regulators: redundancy or subtlety? *Blood* 1993;82:3515–3523, with permission.)

recovery after myelosuppressive therapy requires interaction between various cytokines; however, the sequence and intensity of cytokine production and destruction after such therapy has not been fully evaluated. Obtaining such data is critical to optimize the design of novel cytokines. In the absence of such data, one strategy is to design combination regimens that include a cytokine which may act on an early hematopoietic precursor and one which acts on a more mature progeny. Sequencing of CSFs may be an important component to such trials, because *in vitro* studies demonstrate receptor modulation after introduction of CSFs. The redundancy of cytokines at various steps in the theoretical cell maturation cascade, as shown in Figure 28-3 and reviewed by Metcalf,[166] exemplifies the potential complexity of this approach. Beyond the cascade effects of sequential cell activation, one can envision multiple alternative mechanisms of cytokine interactions as outlined in Figure 28-9.

One example of the unpredictability of interactions is the effects of adding recombinant EPO to G-CSF. A relatively small but randomized trial found that administration of this combination after a cisplatin-based chemotherapy regimen resulted in a significantly faster neutrophil recovery and higher production of CD34+ PBPCs than with G-CSF alone.[167] Such effects could be due to direct or simultaneous interactions of cytokines on a cell or, more likely, to a sequential recruitment phenomenon.

REFERENCES

1. Wolchok JD, Vilcek J. There is more to hemorrhagic necrosis than tumor necrosis factor. *J Natl Cancer Inst* 1991;83: 807–809.
2. Moonen P, Mermod JJ, Ernst JM, et al. Increased biological activity of deglycosylated recombinant human granulocyte/macrophage colony-stimulating factor produced by yeast or animal cells. *Proc Natl Acad Sci U S A* 1987;84:4428–4431.
3. Fukuda M, Sasaki H, Fukuda MN. Erythropoietin metabolism and the influence of carbohydrate structure. *Contrib Nephrol* 1989;76:78–89.
4. Guillaume T, Sekhavat M, Rubinstein DB, et al. Transcription of genes encoding granulocyte-macrophage colony-stimulating factor, interleukin 3, and interleukin 6 receptors and lack of proliferative response to exogenous cytokines in nonhematopoietic human malignant cell lines. *Cancer Res* 1993;53:3139–3144.
5. Miyajima A, Mui ALF, Ogorochi T, et al. Receptors for granulocyte-macrophage colony-stimulating factor, interleukin-3, and interleukin-5. *Blood* 1993;82:1960–1974.
6. Park LS, Urdal DL. Colony-stimulating factor receptors. *Transplant Proc* 1989;21:54–56.
7. Dubois CM, Ruscetti FW, Stern EW, et al. Hematopoietic growth factors upregulate the p65 type II interleukin-1 receptor on bone marrow progenitor cells in vitro. *Blood* 1992;80:600–608.
8. Jacobsen SEW, Ruscetti FW, Dubois CM, et al. Induction of colony-stimulating factor receptor expression on hematopoietic progenitor cells: proposed mechanism for growth factor synergism. *Blood* 1992;80:678–687.
9. Jacobsen SE, Ruscetti FW, Dubois LM, et al. TNF-α directly and indirectly regulates hematopoietic progenitor cell proliferation: role of CSF receptor modulation. *J Exp Med* 1992;175:1759–1772.
10. Heaney ML, Golde DW. Soluble hormone receptors. *Blood* 1993;82:1945–1948.
11. Engelmann H, Novick D, Wallach D. Tumor necrosis factor-binding proteins purified from human urine. Evidence for immunological cross-reactivity with cell surface tumor necrosis factor receptors. *J Biol Chem* 1990;265:1531–1536.
12. Engelmann H, Aderka D, Rubinstein M, et al. A tumor necrosis factor-binding protein purified to homogeneity from human urine protects cells from tumor necrosis factor toxicity. *J Biol Chem* 1989;264:11974–11980.
13. Yasukawa K, Saito T, Fukunaga T, et al. Purification and characterization of soluble human IL-6 receptor expressed in CHO cells. *J Biochem* 1990;108:673–676.

14. Porteu F, Nathan C. Shedding of tumor necrosis factor receptors by activated human neutrophils. *J Exp Med* 1990;172:599–607.

15. Lieschke GJ, Grail D, Hodgson G, et al. Mice lacking granulocyte colony-stimulating factor have chronic neutropenia, granulocyte and macrophage progenitor cell deficiency, and impaired neutrophil mobilization. *Blood* 1994;84;1737–1746.

16. Dranoff G, Crawford AD, Sadelain M, et al. Involvement of granulocyte-macrophage colony-stimulating factor in pulmonary homeostasis. *Science* 1994;264:713–716.

17. Gilmore GL, DePasquale DK, Fischer BC, et al. Enhancement of monocytopoiesis by granulocyte colony-stimulating factor: evidence for secondary cytokine effects in vivo. *Exp Hematol* 1995;23:1319–1323.

18. Petros WP, Rabinowitz J, Gibbs JP, et al. Effect of endogenous TNF-alpha on recombinant G-CSF stimulated hematopoiesis in mice and humans. *Pharmacotherapy* 1998;18:816–823.

19. Chatta GS, Andrews RG, Rodger E, et al. Hematopoietic progenitors and aging: alterations in granulocytic precursors and responsiveness to recombinant human G-CSF, GM-CSF, and IL-3. *J Gerontol* 1993;48:M207–M212.

20. Lord BI, Gurney H, Chang J, et al. Haemopoietic cell kinetics in humans treated with rGM-CSF. *Int J Cancer* 1992;50:26–31.

21. Pettengell R, Testa NG, Swindell R, et al. Transplantation potential of hematopoietic cells released into the circulation during routine chemotherapy for non-Hodgkin's lymphoma. *Blood* 1993;82:2239–2248.

22. Jaar B, Baillou C, Viron B, et al. Long-term effects of recombinant human erythropoietin on bone marrow progenitor cells. *Nephrol Dial Transplant* 1993;8:614–620.

23. Arnaout MA, Wang EA, Clark SC, et al. Human recombinant granulocyte-macrophage colony-stimulating factor increases cell-cell adhesion and surface expression of adhesion-promoting surface glycoproteins on mature granulocytes. *J Clin Invest* 1986;7:597–601.

24. Peters WP, Stuart A, Affronti ML, et al. Neutrophil migration is defective during recombinant human granulocyte-macrophage colony-stimulating factor infusion after autologous bone marrow transplantation in humans. *Blood* 1988;72:1310–1315.

25. Gurney AL, Carver-Moore K, de Sauvage FJ, et al. Thrombocytopenia in c-mpl-deficient mice. *Science* 1995;265:1445–1447.

26. Motoji T, Takanashi M, Motomura S, et al. Growth stimulatory effect of thrombopoietin on the blast cells of acute myelogenous leukaemia. *Br J Haematol* 1996;94:513–516.

27. Drexler HG, Quentmeier H. TPO: expression of its receptor MPL and proliferative effects on leukemic cells. *Leukemia* 1996;10:1405–1421.

28. Graf G, Dehmel U, Drexler HG. Expression of TPO and TPO receptor MPL in human leukemia-lymphoma and solid tumor cell lines. *Leuk Res* 1996;20:831–838.

29. Wetzler M, Bernstein SH, Baumann H, et al. Expression and function of the megakaryocyte growth and development factor receptor in acute myeloid leukemia blasts. *Leuk Lymphoma* 1998;30:415–431.

30. Moreb J, Zucali JR, Gross MA, et al. Protective effects of IL-1 on human hematopoietic progenitor cells treated in

vitro with 4-hydroperoxycyclophosphamide. *J Immunol* 1989;142:1937–1942.

31. Rabinowitz J, Petros WP, Peters WP. Cytokine kinetics: clinical pharmacology studies complementing recombinant growth factor trials. *Cancer Bull* 1994;46:40–47.

32. Milsits K, Beyer J, Siegert W. Serum concentrations of G-CSF during high-dose chemotherapy with autologous stem cell rescue. *Bone Marrow Transplant* 1993;11:372–377.

33. Cairo MS, Suen Y, Sender L, et al. Circulating granulocyte colony-stimulating factor levels after allogeneic and autologous bone marrow transplantation: endogenous G-CSF production correlates with myeloid engraftment. *Blood* 1992;79:1869–1873.

34. Rabinowitz J, Petros WP, Stuart AR, et al. Characterization of endogenous cytokine concentrations after high-dose chemotherapy with autologous bone marrow support. *Blood* 1993;81:2452–2459.

35. Lindemann A, Riedel D, Oster W, et al. Granulocyte-macrophage colony-stimulating factor induces cytokine secretion by human polymorphonuclear leukocytes. *J Clin Invest* 1989;83:1308–1312.

36. Cannistra SA, Vellenga E, Groshek P, et al. Human granulocyte-macrophage colony-stimulating factor and interleukin-3 stimulate monocyte cytotoxicity through a tumor necrosis factor-dependent mechanism. *Blood* 1988;71:672–676.

37. Cicco NA, Lindermann A, Content J, et al. Inducible production of interleukin-6 by human polymorphonuclear neutrophils: the role of granulocyte-macrophage colony-stimulating factor and tumor necrosis factor-alpha. *Blood* 1990;75:2049–2052.

38. Hartung T, Docke W-D, Gantner F, et al. Effect of granulocyte colony-stimulating factor treatment on ex vivo blood cytokine response in human volunteers. *Blood* 1995;85:2482–2489.

39. Elkordy M, Crump M, Vredenburgh JJ, et al. Phase I trial of recombinant human IL-1β (OCT-43) following high-dose chemotherapy and autologous bone marrow transplantation. *Bone Marrow Transplant* 1997;19:315–322.

40. Holler E, Kolb HG, Moller A, et al. Increased serum levels of tumor necrosis factor alpha precede major complications of bone marrow transplantation. *Blood* 1990;75:1011–1016.

41. Rosenfeld CS, Sulecki M, Evans C, et al. Comparison of intravenous versus subcutaneous recombinant human granulocyte-macrophage colony-stimulating factor in patients with primary myelodysplasia. *Exp Hematol* 1991;19:273–277.

42. Johnston E, Crawford J, Lackbaum P, et al. Single-dose subcutaneous, sustained-duration filgrastim versus daily filgrastim in non-small cell lung cancer patients: a randomized, controlled, dose-escalation study. *Proc Am Soc Clin Oncol* 1998;17:73a(abst 284).

43. Tomlinson-Jones A, Ziltener HJ. Enhancement of the biologic effects of interleukin-3 in vivo by anti-interleukin-3 antibodies. *Blood* 1993;82:1133–1141.

44. Petros WP, Rabinowitz J, Stuart AR, et al. Disposition of recombinant human granulocyte-macrophage colony-stimulating factor in patients receiving high-dose chemotherapy and autologous bone marrow support. *Blood* 1992;80:1135–1140.

45. Hovgaard D, Mortensen BT, Schifter S, et al. Comparative pharmacokinetics of single-dose administration of mammalian and bacterially-derived recombinant human granulocyte-macrophage colony-stimulating factor. *Eur J Haematol* 1993;50:32–36.

46. O'Dwyer PJ, LaCreta FP, Schilder R, et al. Phase I trial of thiotepa in combination with recombinant human granulocyte-macrophage colony-stimulating factor. *J Clin Oncol* 1992;10:1352–1358.

47. Petros WP, Crawford J. Safety of concomitant use of granulocyte colony-stimulating factor or granulocyte-macrophage colony-stimulating factor with cytotoxic chemotherapy agents. *Curr Opin Hematol* 1997;4:213–216.

48. Tjan-Heijnen VCG, Biesma B, Festen J, et al. Enhanced myelotoxicity due to granulocyte colony-stimulating factor administration until 48 hours before the next chemotherapy course in patients with small-cell lung carcinoma. *J Clin Oncol* 1998;16:2708–2714.

49. Beguin Y, Yerna M, Loo M, et al. Erythropoiesis in multiple myeloma: defective red cell production due to inappropriate erythropoietin production. *Br J Haematol* 1992;82:648–653.

50. Miller CB, Jones RJ, Piantadosi S, et al. Decreased erythropoietin response in patients with the anemia of cancer. *N Engl J Med* 1990;322:1689–1692.

51. Abels RI. Use of recombinant human erythropoietin in the treatment of anemia in patients who have cancer. *Semin Oncol* 1992;19[Suppl 8]:29–35.

52. Fandrey J, Seydel FP, Siegers CP, et al. Role of cytochrome P450 in the control of the production of erythropoietin. *Life Sci* 1990;47:127–134.

53. Smith DH, Goldwasser E, Volkes EE. Serum immunoerythropoietin levels in patients with cancer receiving cisplatin-based chemotherapy. *Cancer* 1991;68:1101–1105.

54. Hasegawa I, Tanaka K. Serum erythropoietin levels in gynecologic cancer patients during cisplatin combination chemotherapy. *Gynecol Oncol* 1992;46:65–68.

55. Birgegard G, Wide L, Simonsson B. Marked erythropoietin increase before fall in Hb after treatment with cytostatic drugs suggests mechanism other than anaemia for stimulation. *Br J Haematol* 1989;72:462–466.

56. Grace RJ, Kendall RG, Chapman C, et al. Changes in serum erythropoietin levels during allogeneic bone marrow transplantation. *Eur J Haematol* 1991;47:81–85.

57. Schapira M, Antin JH, Ransil BJ, et al. Serum erythropoietin levels in patients receiving intensive chemotherapy and radiotherapy. *Blood* 1990;76:2354–2359.

58. Lazarus HM, Goodnough LT, Goldwasser E, et al. Serum erythropoietin levels and blood component therapy after autologous bone marrow transplantation: implications for erythropoietin therapy in this setting. *Bone Marrow Transplant* 1992;10:71–75.

59. Osterborg A, Boogaerts MA, Cimino R, et al. Recombinant human erythropoietin in transfusion-dependent anemic patients with multiple myeloma and non-Hodgkin's lymphoma—a randomized multicenter study. *Blood* 1996;87:2675–2682.

60. Ludwig H, Fritz E, Leitgeb C, et al. Prediction of response to erythropoietin treatment in chronic anemia of cancer. *Blood* 1994;84:1056–1063.

61. Beguin Y, Oris R, Gillet G. Dynamics of erythropoietic recovery following bone marrow transplantation: role of marrow proliferative capacity and erythropoietin production in autologous versus allogeneic transplants. *Bone Marrow Transplant* 1993;11:285–292.

62. Case DC, Bukowski RM, Carey RW, et al. Recombinant human erythropoietin therapy for anemic cancer patients on combination chemotherapy. *J Natl Cancer Inst* 1993;85:801–806.

63. Cascinu S, Fedeli A, Del Ferro E, et al. Recombinant human erythropoietin treatment in cisplatin-associated anemia: a randomized, double-blind trial with placebo. *J Clin Oncol* 1994;12:1058–1062.

64. Del Mastro L, Venturini M, Lionetto R, et al. Randomized phase III trial evaluating the role of erythropoietin in the prevention of chemotherapy-induced anemia. *J Clin Oncol* 1997;15:2715–2721.

65. De Campos E, Radford J, Steward W, et al. Clinical and in vitro effects of recombinant human erythropoietin in patients receiving intensive chemotherapy for small-cell lung cancer. *J Clin Oncol* 1995;13:1623–1631.

66. Steegmann JL, Lopez J, Otero MJ, et al. Erythropoietin treatment in allogeneic BMT accelerates erythroid reconstitution: results of a prospective controlled randomized trial. *Bone Marrow Transplant* 1992;10:541–546.

67. McDonald TP, Clift RE, Cottrell MB. Large, chronic doses of erythropoietin cause thrombocytopenia in mice. *Blood* 1992;80:352–358.

68. Biggs JC, Atkinson KA, Booker V, et al. Prospective randomised double-blind trial of the in vivo use of recombinant human erythropoietin in bone marrow transplantation from HLA-identical sibling donors. *Bone Marrow Transplant* 1995;15:129–134.

69. Chao NJ, Schriber JR, Long GD, et al. A randomized study of erythropoietin and granulocyte colony-stimulating factor (G-CSF) versus placebo and G-CSF for patients with Hodgkin's and non-Hodgkin's lymphoma undergoing autologous bone marrow transplantation. *Blood* 1994;83:2823–2828.

70. Link H, Boogaerts MA, Fauser AA, et al. A controlled trial of recombinant human erythropoietin after bone marrow transplantation. *Blood* 1994;84:3327–3335.

71. Cheung WK, Goon BL, Guilfoyle MC, et al. Pharmacokinetics and pharmacodynamics of recombinant human erythropoietin after single and multiple subcutaneous doses to healthy subjects. *Clin Pharmacol Ther* 1998;64:412–423.

72. Gabrilove JL, Einhorn LH, Livingston RB, et al. Once-weekly dosing of Epoetin Alpha is similar to three-times-weekly dosing in increasing hemoglobin and quality of life. *Proc Am Soc Clin Oncol* 1999;18:574a (abst 2216).

73. Lieschke GJ, Burgess AW. Granulocyte colony-stimulating factor and granulocyte-macrophage colony-stimulating factor (second of two parts). *N Engl J Med* 1992;327:99–106.

74. Ohno R, Tomonaga M, Kobayashi T, et al. Effect of G-CSF after intensive induction therapy in relapsed or refractory acute leukemia. *N Engl J Med* 1990;323:871–877.

75. Crawford J, Ozer H, Stoller R, et al. Reduction by granulocyte colony-stimulating factor of fever and neutropenia induced by chemotherapy in patients with small-cell lung cancer. *N Engl J Med* 1991;325:164–170.

76. Kotake T, Miki T, Akaza H, et al. Effect of recombinant granulocyte colony-stimulating factor on chemotherapy-induced neutropenia in patients with urogenital cancer. *Cancer Chemother Pharmacol* 1991;27:2553–2557.

77. Pettengell R, Gurney H, Radford JA, et al. Granulocyte colony-stimulating factor to prevent dose-limiting neutropenia in non-Hodgkin's lymphoma: a randomized controlled trial. *Blood* 1992;80:1430–1436.

78. Trillet-Lenoir V, Green J, Manegold C, et al. Recombinant granulocyte colony stimulating factor reduces the infectious complications of cytotoxic chemotherapy. *Eur J Cancer* 1993;29A:319–324.

79. Pui C-H, Boyett JM, Hughes WT, et al. Human granulocyte colony-stimulating factor after induction chemotherapy in children with acute lymphoblastic leukemia. *N Engl J Med* 1997;336:1781–1787.

80. Hartmann LC, Tschetter LK, Habermann TM, et al. Granulocyte colony-stimulating factor in severe chemotherapy induced afebrile neutropenia. *N Engl J Med* 1997;336:1776–1780.

81. Chevallier B, Chollet P, Merrouche Y, et al. Lenograstim prevents morbidity from intensive induction chemotherapy in the treatment of inflammatory breast cancer. *J Clin Oncol* 1995;13:1564–1571.

82. Dombret H, Chastang C, Fenaux P, et al. A controlled study of recombinant human granulocyte colony-stimulating factor in elderly patients after treatment for acute myelogenous leukemia. *N Engl J Med* 1995;332:1678–1683.

83. Godwin JE, Kopecky KJ, Head DR, et al. A double-blind placebo-controlled trial of granulocyte colony-stimulating factor in elderly patients with previously untreated acute myeloid leukemia: a Southwest Oncology Group study (9031). *Blood* 1998;91:3607–3615.

84. Heil G, Hoelzer D, Sanz MA, et al. A randomized, double-blind, placebo-controlled, phase III study of filgrastim in remission induction and consolidation therapy for adults with de novo acute myeloid leukemia. *Blood* 1997;90:4710–4713.

85. Gabrilove JL, Jakubowski A, Scher H, et al. Effect of granulocyte colony-stimulating factor on neutropenia and associated morbidity due to chemotherapy for transitional cell carcinoma of the urothelium. *N Engl J Med* 1988;318:1414–1422.

86. Bronchud MH, Howell A, Crowther D, et al. The use of granulocyte colony-stimulating factor to increase the intensity of treatment with doxorubicin in patients with advanced breast and ovarian cancer. *Br J Cancer* 1989;60:121–125.

87. Scinto AF, Ferraresi V, Campioni N, et al. Accelerated chemotherapy with high-dose epirubicin and cyclophosphamide plus r-met-HUG-CSF in locally advanced and metastatic breast cancer. *Ann Oncol* 1995;6:665–671.

88. Piccart MJ, Bruning P, Wildiers J, et al. An EORTC pilot study of filgrastim (recombinant human granulocyte colony stimulating factor) as support to a high dose-intensive epiadriamycin-cyclophosphamide regimen in chemotherapy-naïve patients with locally advanced or metastatic breast cancer. *Ann Oncol* 1995;6:673–677.

89. Rowinsky EK, Grochow LB, Sartorius SE, et al. Phase I and pharmacologic study of high doses of the topoisomerase I inhibitor topotecan with granulocyte colony-stimulating factor in patients with solid tumors. *J Clin Oncol* 1996;14:1224–1235.

90. Woll PJ, Hodgetts J, Lomax L, et al. Can cytotoxic dose-intensity be increased by using granulocyte colony-stimulating factor? A randomized controlled trial of lenograstim in small-cell lung cancer. *J Clin Oncol* 1995;13:652–659.

91. Ottmann OG, Hoelzer D, Gracien E, et al. Concomitant granulocyte colony-stimulating factor and induction chemoradiotherapy in adult acute lymphocytic leukemia: a randomized phase III trial. *Blood* 1995;86:444–450.

92. Maher DW, Lieschke GJ, Green M, et al. Filgrastim in patients with chemotherapy-induced febrile neutropenia. *Ann Intern Med* 1994;121:492–501.

93. Asano S, Masaoka T, Takaku F. Beneficial effect of human glycosylated granulocyte colony-stimulating factor in marrow-transplanted patients: results of multicenter Phase II-III studies. *Transplant Proc* 1991;23:1701–1703.

94. Schmitz N, Dreger P, Zander AR, et al. Results of a randomized, controlled, multicentre study of recombinant human granulocyte colony-stimulating factor (filgrastim) in patients with Hodgkin's disease and non-Hodgkin's lymphoma undergoing autologous bone marrow transplantation. *Bone Marrow Transplant* 1995;15:261–266.

95. Stahel RA, Jost LM, Cerny T, et al. Randomized study of recombinant human granulocyte colony-stimulating factor after high-dose chemotherapy and autologous bone marrow transplantation for high-risk lymphoma malignancies. *J Clin Oncol* 1994;12:1931–1938.

96. Peters WP, Rosner G, Ross M, et al. Comparative effects of granulocyte-macrophage colony-stimulating factor and granulocyte colony-stimulating factor on priming peripheral blood progenitor cells for use with autologous bone marrow after high-dose chemotherapy. *Blood* 1993;81:1709–1719.

97. Chao NJ, Schriber JR, Grimes K, et al. Granulocyte colony-stimulating factor "mobilized" peripheral blood progenitor cells accelerate granulocyte and platelet recovery after high-dose chemotherapy. *Blood* 1993;81:2031–2035.

98. Sheridan WP, Begley CG, Juttner CA, et al. Effect of peripheral-blood progenitor cells mobilised by filgrastim (G-CSF) on platelet recovery after high-dose chemotherapy. *Lancet* 1992;339:640–644.

99. Shimazaki C, Oku N, Uchiyama H, et al. Effect of granulocyte colony-stimulating factor on hematopoietic recovery after peripheral blood progenitor cell transplantation. *Bone Marrow Transplant* 1994;13:271.

100. Klumpp TR, Magan KF, Goldberg SL, et al. Granulocyte colony-stimulating factor accelerates neutrophil engraftment following peripheral-blood stem-cell transplantation: a prospective, randomized trial. *J Clin Oncol* 1995;13:1323–1327.

101. Kawano Y, Takaue Y, Mimaya J, et al. Marginal benefit/disadvantage of granulocyte colony-stimulating factor therapy after autologous blood stem cell transplantation in children: results of a prospective randomized trial. *Blood* 1998;92:4040–4046.

102. McQuaker IG, Hunter AE, Pacey S, et al. Low-dose filgrastim significantly enhances neutrophil recovery following autologous peripheral-blood stem-cell transplantation in

patients with lymphoproliferative disorders: evidence for clinical and economic benefit. *J Clin Oncol* 1997;15:451–457.

103. Lee SM, Radford JA, Dobson L, et al. Recombinant human granulocyte colony-stimulating factor (filgrastim) following high-dose chemotherapy and peripheral blood progenitor cell rescue in high-grade non-Hodgkin's lymphoma: clinical benefits at no extra cost. *Br J Cancer* 1998;77:1294–1299.

104. Torres Gomez A, Jimenez MA, Alvarez MA, et al. Optimal timing of granulocyte colony-stimulating factor (G-CSF) administration after bone marrow transplantation. A prospective randomized study. *Ann Hematol* 1995;71:65–70.

105. Vey N, Molnar S, Faucher C, et al. Delayed administration of granulocyte colony-stimulating factor after autologous bone marrow transplantation: effect on granulocyte recovery. *Bone Marrow Transplant* 1994;14:779–782.

106. Faucher C, Le Corroller AG, Chabannon C, et al. Administration of G-CSF can be delayed after transplantation of autologous G-CSF-primed blood stem cells: a randomized study. *Bone Marrow Transplant* 1996;17:533–536.

107. Pettengell R, Wall P, Thatcher N, et al. Multicyclic, dose-intensive chemotherapy supported by sequential reinfusion of hematopoietic progenitors in whole blood. *J Clin Oncol* 1995;13:148–156.

108. Spitzer G, Adkins D, Mathews M, et al. Randomized comparison of G-CSF + GM-CSF vs G-CSF alone for mobilization of peripheral blood stem cells: effects on hematopoietic recovery after high-dose chemotherapy. *Bone Marrow Transplant* 1997;20:921–930.

109. Desikan KR, Barlogie B, Jagannath S, et al. Comparable engraftment kinetics following peripheral-blood stem-cell infusion mobilized with granulocyte colony-stimulating factor with or without cyclophosphamide in multiple myeloma. *J Clin Oncol* 1998;16;1547–1553.

110. Toner GC, Shapiro JD, Laidlaw CR, et al. Low-dose versus standard-dose lenograstim prophylaxis after chemotherapy: a randomized, crossover comparison. *J Clin Oncol* 1998;16;3874–3879.

111. Meropol NJ, Miller LL, Korn EL, et al. Severe myelosuppression resulting from concurrent administration of granulocyte colony-stimulating factor and cytotoxic chemotherapy. *J Natl Cancer Inst* 1992;84:1201–1203.

112. De Vries EGE, Biesma B, Willemese PHB, et al. A double-blind placebo-controlled study with granulocyte-macrophage colony-stimulating factor during chemotherapy for ovarian carcinoma. *Cancer Res* 1991;51:116–122.

113. Gerhartz HH, Engelhard M, Meusers P, et al. Randomized, double-blind, placebo-controlled, phase III study of recombinant human granulocyte-macrophage colony-stimulating factor as adjunct to induction treatment of high-grade malignant non-Hodgkin's lymphomas. *Blood* 1993;82:2329–2339.

114. Eguchi K, Kabe J, Kudo S, et al. Efficacy of recombinant human granulocyte-macrophage colony-stimulating factor for chemotherapy-induced leukemia in patients with non-small-cell lung cancer. *Cancer Chemother Pharmacol* 1994;34:37–43.

115. Stone RM, Berg DT, George SL, et al. Granulocyte-macrophage colony-stimulating factor after initial chemotherapy for elderly patients with primary acute myelogenous leukemia. *N Engl J Med* 1995;332:1671–1677.

116. Jones SE, Schottstaedt MW, Duncan LA, et al. Randomized double-blind prospective trial to evaluate the effects of sargramostim versus placebo in a moderate-dose fluorouracil, doxorubicin, and cyclophosphamide adjuvant chemotherapy program for stage II and III breast cancer. *J Clin Oncol* 1996;14:2976–2983.

117. Rowe JM, Andersen JW, Mazza JJ, et al. A randomized placebo-controlled phase III study of granulocyte-macrophage colony-stimulating factor in adult patients (>55 to 70 years of age) with acute myelogenous leukemia: a study of the Eastern Cooperative Oncology Group (E1490). *Blood* 1995;86:457–462.

118. Vellenga E, Uyl-de Groot CA, de Wit R, et al. Randomized placebo-controlled trial of granulocyte-macrophage colony-stimulating factor in patients with chemotherapy-related febrile neutropenia. *J Clin Oncol* 1996;14:619–627.

119. Powles R, Smith C, Milan S, et al. Human recombinant GM-CSF in allogeneic bone-marrow transplantation for leukemia: double-blind, placebo-controlled trial. *Lancet* 1990;336:1417–1420.

120. Nemunaitis J, Rabinowe SN, Singer JW, et al. Recombinant granulocyte-macrophage colony-stimulating factor after autologous bone marrow transplantation for lymphoid cancer. *N Engl J Med* 1991;324:1773–1778.

121. Link H, Boogaerts MA, Carella AM, et al. A controlled trial of recombinant human granulocyte-macrophage colony-stimulating factor after total body irradiation, high-dose chemotherapy, and autologous bone marrow transplantation for acute lymphoblastic leukemia or malignant lymphoma. *Blood* 1992;80:2188–2195.

122. Khwaja A, Linch DC, Goldstone AH, et al. Recombinant human granulocyte-macrophage colony-stimulating factor after autologous bone marrow transplantation for malignant lymphoma: a British National Lymphoma Investigation double-blind, placebo-controlled trial. *Br J Haematol* 1992;82:317–323.

123. Advani R, Chao NJ, Horning SJ, et al. Granulocyte-macrophage colony-stimulating factor as an adjunct to autologous hemopoietic stem cell transplantation for lymphoma. *Ann Intern Med* 1992;116:183–189.

124. De Witte T, Gratwohl A, Van Der Lely N, et al. Recombinant human granulocyte-macrophage colony-stimulating factor accelerates neutrophil and monocyte recovery after allogeneic T-cell-depleted bone marrow transplantation. *Blood* 1992;79:1359–1365.

125. Gorin NC, Coiffier B, Hayat M, et al. Recombinant human granulocyte-macrophage colony-stimulating factor after high-dose chemotherapy and autologous bone marrow transplantation with unpurged and purged marrow in non-Hodgkin's lymphoma: a double-blind placebo-controlled trial. *Blood* 1992;80:1149–1157.

126. Gulati SC, Bennett CL. Granulocyte-macrophage colony-stimulating factor as adjunctive therapy in relapsed Hodgkin disease. *Ann Intern Med* 1992;116:177–182.

127. Nemunaitis J, Rosenfeld CS, Ash R, et al. Phase III randomized, double-blind placebo-controlled trial of rhGM-CSF following allogeneic bone marrow transplantation. *Bone Marrow Transplant* 1995;15:949–954.

128. Hiraoka A, Masaoka T, Mizoguchi H, et al. Recombinant human non-glycosylated granulocyte-macrophage colony

stimulating factor in allogeneic bone marrow transplantation: double-blind placebo-controlled phase III clinical trial. *Jpn J Clin Oncol* 1994;24:205–211.

129. Rabinowe SN, Neuberg D, Bierman PJ, et al. Long-term follow-up of a phase III study of recombinant human granulocyte-macrophage colony-stimulating factor after autologous bone marrow transplantation for lymphoid malignancies. *Blood* 1993;81:1903–1908.

130. Boiron JM, Marit G, Faberes C, et al. Collection of peripheral blood stem cells in multiple myeloma following single high-dose cyclophosphamide with and without recombinant human granulocyte-macrophage colony-stimulating factor. *Bone Marrow Transplant* 1993;12:49–55.

131. Elias AD, Ayash L, Anderson KC, et al. Mobilization of peripheral blood progenitor cells by chemotherapy and granulocyte-macrophage colony-stimulating factor for hematopoietic support after high-dose intensification for breast cancer. *Blood* 1992;79:3036–3044.

132. Huan SD, Hester J, Spitzer G, et al. Influence of mobilized peripheral blood cells on the hematopoietic recovery by autologous marrow and recombinant human granulocyte-macrophage colony-stimulating factor after high-dose cyclophosphamide, etoposide, and cisplatin. *Blood* 1992;79:3388–3393.

133. Legros M, Fleury J, Bay JO, et al. RhGM-CSF vs placebo following rhGM-CSF-mobilized PBPC transplantation: a phase III double-blind randomized trial. *Bone Marrow Transplant* 1997;19:209–213.

134. Kritz A, Crown JP, Motzer RJ, et al. Beneficial impact of peripheral blood progenitor cells in patients with metastatic breast cancer treated with high-dose chemotherapy plus granulocyte-macrophage colony-stimulating factor. A randomized trial. *Cancer* 1993;71:2515–2521.

135. Hohaus S, Martin H, Wassmann B, et al. Recombinant human granulocyte and granulocyte-macrophage colony-stimulating factor administered following cytotoxic chemotherapy have a similar ability to mobilize peripheral blood stem cells. *Bone Marrow Transplant* 1998;22:625–630.

136. Ballestrero A, Ferrando F, Garuti A, et al. Comparative effects of three cytokine regimens after high-dose cyclophosphamide: granulocyte colony-stimulating factor, granulocyte-macrophage colony-stimulating factor, and sequential interleukin-3 and GM-CSF. *J Clin Oncol* 1999;17:1296–1303.

137. Ho AD, Young D, Maruyama M, et al. Pluripotent and lineage-committed CD34$^+$ subsets in leukapheresis products mobilized by G-CSF, GM-CSF vs. a combination of both. *Exp Hematol* 1996;24:1460–1468.

138. Caballero MD, Vazquez L, Barragan JM, et al. Randomized study of filgrastim versus molgramostim after peripheral stem cell transplant in breast cancer. *Haematologica* 1998;83:514–518.

139. Lieschke GJ, Cebon J, Morstyn G. Characterization of the clinical effects after the first dose of bacterially synthesized recombinant human granulocyte-macrophage colony-stimulating factor. *Blood* 1989;74:2634–2643.

140. Shaffer DW, Smith LS, Burris HA, et al. A randomized phase I trial of chronic oral etoposide with or without granulocyte-macrophage colony-stimulating factor in patients with advanced malignancies. *Cancer Res* 1993;53:5929–5933.

141. Bunn PA, Crowley J, Kelly K, et al. Chemoradiotherapy with or without granulocyte-macrophage colony-stimulating factor in the treatment of limited-stage small-cell lung cancer: a prospective phase III randomized study of the Southwest Oncology Group. *J Clin Oncol* 1995;13:1632–1641.

142. Gordon MS, McCaskill-Stevens WJ, Battiato LA, et al. A phase I trial of recombinant human interleukin-11 (Neumega rhIL-11 growth factor) in women with breast cancer receiving chemotherapy. *Blood* 1996;87:3615–3624.

143. Isaacs C, Robert NJ, Bailey A, et al. Randomized placebo-controlled study of recombinant human interleukin-11 to prevent chemotherapy-induced thrombocytopenia in patients with breast cancer receiving dose-intensive cyclophosphamide and doxorubicin. *J Clin Oncol* 1997;15:3368–3377.

144. Tepler I, Elias L, Smith JW, et al. A randomized placebo-controlled trial of recombinant human interleukin-11 in cancer patients with severe thrombocytopenia due to chemotherapy. *Blood* 1996;87:3607–3614.

145. Hussein A, Vredenburgh J, Elkordy M, et al. Randomized, placebo-controlled study of recombinant human interleukin eleven (Neumega rhIL-11 growth factor) in patients with breast cancer following high-dose chemotherapy with autologous hematopoietic progenitor cell support. *Exp Heme* 1996;24:634a.

146. Choi ES, Hokom MM, Chen JL, et al. The role of MGDF in terminal stages of thrombopoiesis. *Br J Haematol* 1996;95:227–233.

147. Basser RL, Rasko JE, Clarke K, et al. Thrombopoietic effects of pegylated recombinant human megakaryocyte growth and development factor in patients with advanced cancer. *Lancet* 1996;348;1279–1281.

148. O'Malley CJ, Rasko JEJ, Basser RL, et al. Administration of pegylated recombinant human megakaryocyte growth and development factor to humans stimulates the production of functional platelets that show no evidence of in vivo activation. *Blood* 1996;88:3288–3298.

149. Vadhan-Raj S, Murray LJ, Bueso-Ramos C, et al. Stimulation of megakaryocyte and platelet production by a single dose of recombinant human thrombopoietin in patients with cancer. *Ann Intern Med* 1997;126:673–681.

150. Fanucchi M, Glaspy J, Crawford J, et al. Effects of polyethylene glycol-conjugated recombinant human megakaryocyte growth and development factor on platelet counts after chemotherapy for lung cancer. *N Engl J Med* 1997;336:404–409.

151. Basser RL, Rasko JEJ, Clarke K, et al. Randomized, blinded, placebo-controlled phase I trial of pegylated recombinant human megakaryocyte growth and development factor with filgrastim after dose-intensive chemotherapy in patients with advanced cancer. *Blood* 1997;89:3118–3128.

152. Ragnhammar P, Friesen H-J, Frodin J-E, et al. Induction of anti-recombinant human granulocyte-macrophage colony-stimulating factor (*Escherichia coli*–derived) antibodies and clinical effects in nonimmunocompromised patients. *Blood* 1994;84:4078–4087.

153. Miller LL, Korn EL, Stevens DS, et al. Abrogation of the hematological and biological activities of the interleukin-3/

granulocyte-macrophage colony-stimulating factor fusion protein PIXY321 by neutralizing anti-PIXY321 antibodies in cancer patients receiving high-dose carboplatin. *Blood* 1999;93:3250–3258.

154. Ulich TR, del Castillo J, McNiece IK, et al. Stem cell factor in combination with granulocyte colony-stimulating factor (CSF) or granulocyte-macrophage CSF synergistically increases granulopoiesis in vivo. *Blood* 1991;78:1954–1962.

155. Tong J, Gordon MS, Srour EF, et al. In vivo administration of recombinant methionyl human stem cell factor expands the number of human marrow hematopoietic stem cells. *Blood* 1993;82:784–791.

156. Demetri GD, Gordon M, Hoffman R, et al. Effects of recombinant methionyl human stem cell factor on hematopoietic progenitor cells in vivo: preliminary results from a phase I trial. *Proc Am Assoc Cancer Res* 1993;34:217.

157. Basser RL, To LB, Begley CG, et al. Rapid hematopoietic recovery after multicycle high-dose chemotherapy: enhancement of filgrastim-induced progenitor-cell mobilization by recombinant human stem-cell factor. *J Clin Oncol* 1998;16:1899–1908.

158. Shpall EJ, Wheeler CA, Turner SA, et al. A randomized phase 3 study of peripheral blood progenitor cell mobilization with stem cell factor and filgrastim in high-risk breast cancer patients. *Blood* 1999;93:2491–2501.

159. Neta R, Douches S, Oppenheim JJ. Interleukin-1 as a radioprotector. *J Immunol* 1986;136:2483–2485.

160. Futami H, Jansen R, MacPhee MJ, et al. Chemoprotective effects of recombinant human IL-1 alpha in cyclophosphamide-treated normal and tumor-bearing mice. Protection from acute toxicity, hematologic effects, development of late mortality, and enhanced therapeutic efficacy. *J Immunol* 1990;145:4121–4130.

161. Starnes HF. Biological effects and possible clinical applications of interleukin 1. *Semin Hematol* 1991;28[Suppl 2]:34–41.

162. Smith JW, Longo DL, Alvord WG, et al. The effects of treatment with interleukin-1α on platelet recovery after high-dose carboplatin. *N Engl J Med* 1993;328:756–761.

163. Vadhan-Raj S, Kudelka AP, Garrison L, et al. Effects of interleukin-1α on carboplatin-induced thrombocytopenia in patients with recurrent ovarian cancer. *J Clin Oncol* 1994;12:707–714.

164. Smith JW, Urba WJ, Curti BD, et al. The toxic and hematologic effects of interleukin-1 alpha administered in a phase I trial to patients with advanced malignancies. *J Clin Oncol* 1992;10:1141–1152.

165. Molineux G, McCrea C, Yan XQ, et al. Flt-3 ligand synergizes with granulocyte colony-stimulating factor to increase neutrophil numbers and to mobilize peripheral blood stem cells with long-term repopulating potential. *Blood* 1997;89:3998–4004.

166. Metcalf D. Hematopoietic regulators: redundancy or subtlety? *Blood* 1993;82:3515–3523.

167. Pierelli L, Perillo A, Greggi S, et al. Erythropoietin addition to granulocyte colony-stimulating factor abrogates life-threatening neutropenia and increases peripheral-blood progenitor-cell mobilization after epirubicin, paclitaxel, and cisplatin combination chemotherapy: results of a randomized comparison. *J Clin Oncol* 1999;17:1288–1295.

168. Petros WP, Rabinowitz J, Stuart A, et al. Clinical pharmacology of filgrastim following high-dose chemotherapy and autologous bone marrow transplantation. *Clin Cancer Res* 1997;3:705–711.

169. Petros WP. Pharmacokinetics and administration of colony-stimulating factors. *Pharmacotherapy* 1992;12(2 Pt 2):32S–38S.

170. Macdougall IC, Roberts DE, Coles GA, et al. Clinical pharmacokinetics of epoetin (recombinant human erythropoietin). *Clin Pharmacokinet* 1991;20:99–113.

171. Stute N, Santana VM, Rodman JH, et al. Pharmacokinetics of subcutaneous recombinant human granulocyte colony-stimulating factor in children. *Blood* 1992;79:2849–2854.

172. Furman WL, Fairclough DL, Huhn RD, et al. Therapeutic effects and pharmacokinetics of recombinant human granulocyte-macrophage colony-stimulating factor in childhood cancer patients receiving myelosuppressive chemotherapy. *J Clin Oncol* 1991;9:1022–1028.

173. Kearns CM, Wang WC, Stute N, et al. Disposition of recombinant human granulocyte colony-stimulating factor in children with severe chronic neutropenia. *J Pediatr* 1993;123:471–479.

174. Lindemann A, Ganser A, Herrmann F, et al. Biologic effects of recombinant human interleukin-3 in vivo. *J Clin Oncol* 1991;9:2120–2127.

175. Biesma B, Pokorny R, Kovarik JM, et al. Pharmacokinetics of recombinant human interleukin 3 administered subcutaneously and by continuous intravenous infusion in patients after chemotherapy for ovarian cancer. *Cancer Res* 1993;53:5915–5919.

29

ANTIBODY-BASED IMMUNOTHERAPIES FOR CANCER

DAVID A. SCHEINBERG
GEORGE SGOUROS
RICHARD P. JUNGHANS

Monoclonal antibodies (mAbs) are remarkably versatile agents with potential therapeutic applications in a number of human diseases, including cancer. The mAbs have long promised to offer a safe, specific approach to therapy. Over more than a decade, preclinical evaluation and human clinical trials have identified new strategies for the use of mAbs, as well as a number of difficult obstacles to their effective application. Although the use of antibodies as targeting agents dates to the 1950s,[1] not until the mid-1970s, when methods for production of mAbs appeared that allowed reproducible lots of a defined molecule to be produced in quantities adequate for clinical study,[2] could the properties of antibodies as therapeutic agents for cancer be studied appropriately.

Five approaches to therapy are used in the application of mAbs in humans *in vivo*. First, mAbs can be used to focus an inflammatory response against a target cell. Binding of a mAb to a target cell can result in fixation of complement, which yields cell lysis or results in opsonization, which marks the cell for lysis by various effector cells such as natural killer (NK) cells, neutrophils, or monocytes. Second, mAbs may be used as carriers to deliver another small molecule, atom, radionuclide, peptide, or protein to a specific site *in vivo*. Third, mAbs may be directed at critical hormones, growth factors, interleukins, or other regulatory molecules or their receptors to control growth or other cell functions. Fourth, antiidiotypic mAbs may be used as vaccines to generate an active immune response. Finally, mAbs may be used to speed the clearance of other drugs or toxins or fundamentally alter the pharmacokinetic properties of other therapeutic agents. For example, mAbs may be fused to drugs or factors to increase their plasma half-life, change their biodistribution, or render them multivalent. Alternatively, mAbs may be used to clear previously infused mAbs from the circulation.

Yet despite the diversity of approaches, significant problems remain that are peculiar to mAbs. The mAbs are large, immunogenic proteins, often of rodent origin, that rapidly generate neutralizing immune responses in patients within days or weeks after their first injection. The sheer size of mAbs—150 kd for immunoglobulin G to 950 kd for immunoglobulin M, 100 times larger than that of typical drugs—makes their pharmacology (particularly diffusion into bulky tumors or other extravascular areas) problematic for effective use. Many early mAbs or mAb constructs were either poorly cytotoxic or relatively nonspecific, which rendered them ineffective. Moreover, the high degree of mAb specificity that is routinely achievable now can work against mAbs, because tumor cells that do not bear the specific antigen target may escape from cytotoxic effects.

Despite these problems, clearly mAbs still have great potential to be safe and effective anticancer agents. Recent clinical investigations have highlighted several areas in which mAbs can be effective, either alone or in combination with other, more conventional agents.

This chapter reviews the basic biochemical and biologic properties of mAbs and the most commonly used derivatives (immunotoxins, radioimmunoconjugates, mAb fragments), discusses the pharmacologic issues peculiar to mAbs, and outlines some of the important clinical results with mAbs. Potential solutions to the most difficult issues in the use of mAbs are presented. Because mAbs and conjugates of mAbs represent many different drugs with characteristics that result from their origin (rodent or human), their isotypes, their structure, or the various conjugated toxic agents, generalizations about the properties of mAbs often may not be possible. Treatment of cancer with mAbs is a new and rapidly changing field, and readers are encouraged to consult other reviews for more comprehensive discussions of individual areas.[3–6]

IMMUNOGLOBULIN CLASSES

Immunoglobulins are separated into five classes or isotypes based on structure and biologic properties: immunoglobu-

TABLE 29-1. PROPERTIES OF ANTIBODY CLASSES

Property	IgG	IgA	IgM	IgD	IgE
Usual molecular form	Monomer	Monomer, dimer, etc.	Pentamer	Monomer	Monomer
Molecular formula	$\gamma_2\kappa_2$ or $\gamma_2\lambda_2$	$(\alpha_2\kappa_2)n$ or $(\alpha_2\lambda_2)n$	$(\mu_2\kappa_2)5$ or $(\mu_2\lambda_2)5$	$\delta_2\kappa_2$ or $\delta_2\lambda_2$	$\varepsilon_2\kappa_2$ or $\varepsilon_2\lambda_2$
Heavy-chain domains	V, C_H1–3	V, C_H1–3	V, C_H1–4	V, C_H1–3	V, C_H1–4
Other chains	—	J chain, S piece	J chain	—	—
Subclasses	IgG1, IgG2, IgG3, IgG4	IgA1, IgA2	—	—	—
Heavy-chain allotypes	Gm (~30)	Am (2)	Mm (2)	—	—
Molecular weight	150,000	160,000	950,000	175,000	190,000
Sedimentation constant (S)	6.6	7, 9, 11, 14	19	7	8
Carbohydrate content (%)	3	7	10	9	13
Serum level (mg/100 mL)	1,250 ± 300	210 ± 50	125 ± 50	4	0.03
Percentage of total serum Ig	75–85	7–15	5–10	0.3	0.003
Half-life (days)	23 (IgG3, 7)	5.8	5.1	2.8	2.5
Antibody valence	2	2,4,6, . . .	10	1 or 2	2
Complement fixation (classic)	+ (Ig G1, G2, G3)	—	++	—	—
Fc receptors	FcγR-I, FcγR-II, FcγR-III				FcεR-I, FcεR-II
Binding to cells	Monocyte macrophages, neutrophils, LGLs	—	?	—	Mast cells
Other biologic properties	Secondary Ab response; placental transfer	Secretory antibody	Primary Ab response; B-cell surface Ig, rheumatoid factor	B-cell surface Ig	Homocytotropic Ab; anaphylaxis; allergy

+, active; ++, strongly active; Ab, antibody; C_H, constant region of the heavy chain; Ig, immunoglobulin; LGLs, large granular lymphocytes; V, variable region.

lin M (IgM), immunoglobulin D (IgD), immunoglobulin E (IgE), immunoglobulin A (IgA), and immunoglobulin G (IgG). For reasons discussed in the later section on ontogeny, IgM is the primordial antibody whose expression by the B cell on its surface represents the commitment of that cell to a particular but broad recognition space that subsequently narrows as part of the maturation response induced by antigen interactions.[7] IgD is normally coexpressed with IgM on B cells and may play a signaling role in B-cell development. IgE, IgA, and IgG are mature immunoglobulins that are expressed after maturation of the response and class switch have occurred. Each of these antibodies participates in specialized functions: IgE in immediate-type hypersensitivity reactions and parasite immunity, IgA in mucosal immunity, and IgG in humoral immunity. In some cases, the antibodies interact with specialized receptors that link their action to host cellular defenses; in others, the antibodies interact with the humoral complement system. IgG is further divided into four subclasses and IgA into two subclasses. Heritable deficiencies in individual immunoglobulin classes or IgG subclasses are associated with susceptibility to particular infections and autoimmune disorders.[8] Table 29-1 summarizes various features of the antibodies that are discussed in this section.

STRUCTURE

The fundamental structural elements of all antibodies are indicated by size as heavy and light chains of 55 to 75 kd and 22 kd, respectively (Fig. 29-1). Light chains are either κ or λ and are each distributed among all immunoglobulin subclasses. Overall, κ comprises 60% of light chains in humans and 95% of light chains in mice. Heavy chains are μ, δ, γ, ε, and α, corresponding to IgM, IgD, IgG, IgE, and IgA, and conferring the biologic characteristics of each antibody class. Each chain is composed of Ig-like domains of antiparallel β-pleated sheets, two such domains for light chain and four for heavy chain, except for IgM and IgE, which have five. The amino-terminal domain of each chain is the variable (V_H or V_L) region that mediates antigen recognition; the remaining domains are constant regions designated C_L for light chain and C_H1, C_H2, and C_H3 for heavy chain (and C_H4 for μ and ε). Between C_H1 and C_H2 is the hinge region, which confers flexibility on the antibody "arms" and susceptibility to proteases (see later), except in IgM and IgE in which the C_H2 domain itself serves this role.

Heavy (H) and light (L) chains are normally paired 1:1 with each other, but the smallest stable unit is a four-chain (HL)$_2$ structure (Fig. 29-1), for a nominal total mass of 150 to 160 kd for IgG and higher for other isotypes (Table 29-1). Although isolated light chain (Bence Jones protein) exists in small amounts as monomers or dimers in normal individuals, the isolated heavy chain is stable only in association with another heavy chain to mask the hydrophobic surface on the carboxy-terminal C_H3 domain (C_H4 in IgM) and to generate a high-affinity noncovalent interaction between the molecular halves.[9] Of note, the inter–heavy chain disulfides and heavy-light chain disulfides are not required for assembly, which is mediated through primary noncovalent interchain inter-

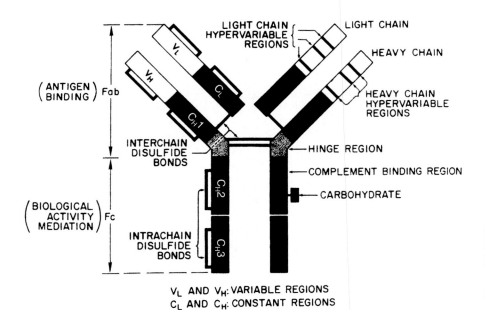

LIGHT CHAIN HYPERVARIABLE REGIONS

LIGHT CHAIN

HEAVY CHAIN

HEAVY CHAIN HYPERVARIABLE REGIONS

(ANTIGEN BINDING) Fab

INTERCHAIN DISULFIDE BONDS

HINGE REGION

COMPLEMENT BINDING REGION

CARBOHYDRATE

(BIOLOGICAL ACTIVITY MEDIATION) Fc

INTRACHAIN DISULFIDE BONDS

V_L AND V_H: VARIABLE REGIONS
C_L AND C_H: CONSTANT REGIONS

FIGURE 29-1. Antibody structure. The structural relationships and functions of domains of immunoglobulin G. (From Wasserman RL, Capra JD. Immunoglobulins. In: Horowitz MI, Pigman W, eds. *The glycoconjugates.* New York: Academic Press, 1977:323, with permission.)

actions. IgE and IgG are composed of a single $(HL)_2$ unit, whereas IgM exists as a pentamer of $(HL)_2$ units joined by disulfide bonding with a third J-chain component. IgA exists mainly as a monomer in serum but in secretions exists primarily as a dimer plus trimer and higher forms in which the oligomers are linked by J chain as well as the fragment of secretory chain (secretory piece) that is involved in the mucosal transport.

The V region itself is composed of subdomains—relatively conserved framework regions interdigitated with the complementarity-determining regions (CDRs) [also termed *hypervariable segments* (HVSs)] that make primary contact with antigen[9,10] (Fig. 29-1). Three CDRs are found in each heavy and light chain that may participate in antigen binding. The V regions should be seen as juxtaposed three-fingered gloves, with the CDRs covering the tips (Fig. 29-2), arrayed in a broad contact surface with antigen (Fig. 29-3).

Antibodies are glycoproteins. Glycosylation of proteins plays various roles related to solubility, transport, conformation, function, and stability. Carbohydrate is located mainly in antibody C domains, with a lower frequency in V regions (see data on M195 later).[11] IgG contains a major conserved glycosylation site in C_H2 that contributes to the conformation of this domain, which is crucial to the functional ability to bind to complement and to $Fc\gamma$ receptors.

The IgG antibody "unit" has been defined in terms of susceptibility to proteases that cleave in the exposed, nonfolded regions of the antibody (Fig. 29-1). A tabulation of antibody fragments and engineered or synthetic products is presented in Table 29-2. Fab contains the V region and first C domain of the heavy chain ($V_H + C_H1 = Fd$) and the entire light chain (L); Fab' includes in addition a portion of the H chain hinge region and one or more free cysteines

(Fd'); Fabc2 is a dimer of Fab' linked through hinge disulfide(s); and Fv is a semistable antibody fragment that includes only $V_H + V_L$, the smallest antigen-binding unit. Fc is the C-terminal crystallizable fragment that includes the complement and Fc receptor–binding domains (see later). Genetically engineered products include the δC_H2 constructs, which lack the second C domain of heavy chain and behave like a Fab'2, with bivalence, abbreviated survival, and lack of interaction with host effector systems, but which do not require enzymic processing.[12] Another genetically engineered product, sFv (single-chain Fv), is Fv with a peptide linkage engineered to join the C-terminus of one chain to the N-terminus of the other for improved stability. More advanced products have been designed that conceptually represent the antigen-binding domain in a single peptide product[13]; this is not related structurally to an antibody and is therefore considered an antibody mimic.

ONTOGENY

Antibodies possibly represent the most strikingly evolved, adaptive system in all of biology. This is both an ancient and an evolved system, present in mammals, birds, reptiles, amphibians, teleosts, elasmobranchs (sharks), and possibly also in cyclostomes (hagfish, lampreys). If the latter is true, then all chordates would be included.[14] Its most diverse representation of classes and functions is found in Mammalia. The power of antigen recognition begins with an inherited array of duplicated and diversified germ-line V genes, a random mutational process that creates novel CDRs, a combinatorial selection process that amplifies the germ-line capabilities, and a controlled and directed mutational process that hones the specificity and matures the antibody into a high-affinity, antigen-specific reagent.

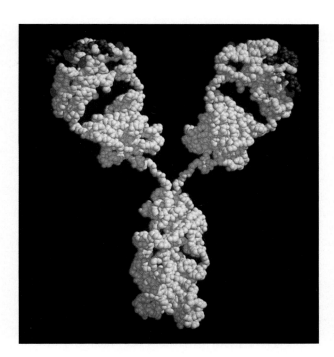

FIGURE 29-2. Space-filling model of human immunoglobulin G1 antibody with complementarity-determining regions in color representing anti–Tac-H; human myeloma protein Eu with complementarity-determining regions grafted from murine anti-Tac. (Photo provided courtesy of Dr. C. Queen.)

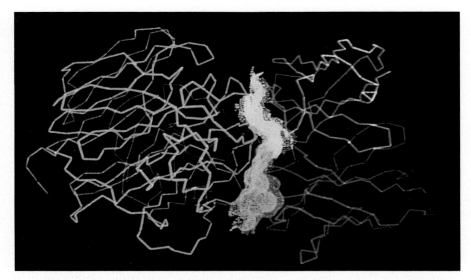

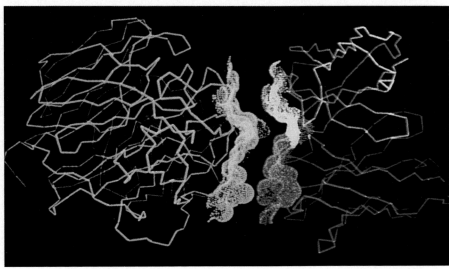

FIGURE 29-3. Antigen-antibody binding surface juxtaposition. The variable (V) region (Fv) of antibody (*right*) binds to influenza virus protein neuraminidase (*left*) in the top panel. The V$_H$ (*red*) and V$_L$ (*blue*) regions are separately colored to show their respective binding contributions. The bottom panel offsets the two molecules by 8 Å to show the complementarity of surfaces that promotes the binding interaction. The stippled surface of the neuraminidase defines the antigen "epitope." (Photo provided courtesy of Drs. P.M. Colman and W.R. Tulip, CSIRO Australia.)

TABLE 29-2. ANTIBODY FRAGMENT DEFINITIONS

Designation	Representation	Description
Fabc		Complete immunoglobulin G
Enzyme-generated products		
Fab	Fd / L	Papain digest; Fd + L
Fab'	Fd' / L	Pepsin digest monomer; Fd' + L
Fab'2	Fab'	Pepsin digest dimer
Fv	V_H / V_L	V region digestion fragment; V_H + V_L
Fc (or Fc')	CH_2 / CH_3	C region digestion fragment; crystallizable fragment
pFc (or pFc')	CH_2 / CH_3	Smaller fragments of Fc
Genetically engineered products		
$\delta C_H 2$	CH_3	Deleted $C_H 2$ domain; dimer of $V - C_H 1 - C_H 3$ + L
sFv	V_H / V_L	Single-chain Fv; V_H and V_L joined by peptide linker
Synthetic products		
ABU		Antigen-binding unit; peptide mimic

C, constant region; C_H, constant region of the heavy chain; L, light chain; V, variable; V_H, variable region of the heavy chain; V_L, variable region of the light chain.

The biologic expression of antibody begins with the B-cell progenitor, which undergoes a series of maturation steps that begins with V gene selection for heavy chain followed by light chain V selection that yields surface expression and secretion by the mature B cell. On interaction with antigen, the B cells are activated to proliferate, secrete antibody, and undergo CDR mutagenesis and affinity maturation, and finally to undergo chain switch and plasma cell conversion. Plasma cells remain in tissues, spleen, or lymph nodes and secrete large quantities of antibody, which is the sole function of this terminally differentiated cell.[7]

The genes of heavy and light chains share important features of structure and maturation. Each gene locus contains widely separated V, C, and minigene domains that are placed into juxtaposition by DNA recombination mechanisms. The minigenes—diversity (D) and joining (J) regions for heavy chain and J regions for light chain—contribute to or constitute, with modifications, the CDR3.[15] The κ and λ light chain loci are located on chromosomes 2 and 22, respectively, but all heavy chains are contained within a single massive locus on chromosome 14.

To aid in understanding the nature of the generation of the antibody repertoire, recapitulation of what is known about germ-line diversity is instructive. On the heavy chain locus are an estimated 80 functional V_H genes, 12 D regions, and 6 J regions for a potential of 6,000 combinations[16–19] (Fig. 29-4). Roughly 80 Vκ light chain and 5 Jκ domains are found, which, randomly associated, can generate 400 combinations (the λ locus contains a smaller number of distinct V genes). A simple arithmetic calculation suggests that $V_\kappa V_H$ combinations alone could generate a diversity of approximately 2×10^6. Yet even this number is

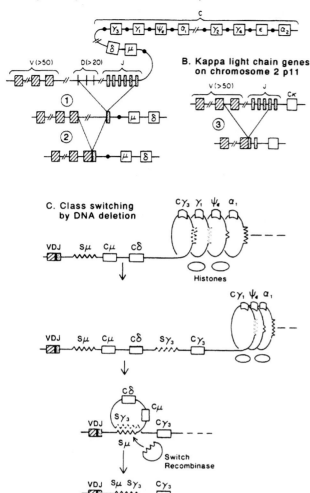

A. Heavy chain genes on chromosome 14 p32

B. Kappa light chain genes on chromosome 2 p11

C. Class switching by DNA deletion

Histones

Switch Recombinase

FIGURE 29-4. Generation of diversity. VJ and VDJ joining occur in L chain and H chain by excision of intervening DNA in the genome. Class switch involves deletion of intervening constant (C) domains (C_μ, C_δ, etc.) and transcription through the new proximal C region. C is finally joined to the V gene by splicing of the messenger RNA. (C, constant; J, joining; V, variable.) (From Cooper MD. Current concepts: B lymphocytes—normal development. *N Engl J Med* 1987;317:1452, with permission.)

conservative, because this diversity is amplified in turn by errors in recombination and processes called N and P nucleotide addition in CDR3, which add enormously to the potential complexity, in theory exceeding the total lifetime B-cell output by several orders of magnitude.[16] Many authors, however, have cautioned that the mathematical diversity does not allow for the redundancy in configurations that could provide equivalent binding domains; in terms of antigen binding, the practical diversity is probably in range of 1 to 10×10^6. The smallest "complete" immune system is that of the young tadpole with 10^6 B cells, which suggests that repertoires of 10^5 to 10^6 constitute a sufficiently complete topologic set for meaningfully diverse, if not exhaustive, antigen recognition.[20]

V gene selection is based on random expression followed by specific amplification. The argument has been made on physicochemical grounds that 10^5 different antibody molecules are sufficient to create a topologic set that recognizes any antigen surface with an affinity of 10^5 to 10^6 M^{-1},[21] a weak but biologically important number that corresponds to recognition affinities of naive antibody-antigen contacts that are often broadly polyreactive. B cells express antibody, principally IgM and IgD, on their membranes. On contacting antigen, these cells are stimulated to divide and undergo CDR mutations. Subsequent binding and stimulation are in proportion to the strength of the binding reaction; hence, an *in vivo* selection occurs for mutations that enhance the affinity of the antibody for the antigen, a process termed *affinity maturation*.[22] Simultaneous with this increased affinity is a narrowing of the specificity, with the antibody shedding its early polyreactive phenotype. The cell then undergoes "class switch" to one of the mature antibodies (IgG, IgA, IgE) by deleting out DNA between the VDJ region and the new C region of the heavy chain, which brings this new C domain in juxtaposition with the V region (Fig. 29-4). (The light chain is unchanged.) Some time after commitment to a mature antibody, the cell ceases its CDR mutagenesis, affinity maturation is completed, and the B cell undergoes morphogenesis to a tissue-resident plasma cell.[7]

ANTIGEN-ANTIBODY INTERACTIONS

Affinity is a quantitative measure of the strength of the interaction between an antibody and its cognate antigen and is intended in the same sense as the equilibrium constant in the chemical mass action equation:

$$[AB] = K_a [A] [B] \qquad [29\text{-}1]$$

The equilibrium or affinity constant (K_a) is represented in units of M^{-1}. In most instances studied by x-ray crystallography, contacts between antibody and protein antigen are dominated by noncovalent hydrogen bonds (O—H), with a lower frequency of salt bridges (COO$^-$— + H$_3$N), with a total of 15 to 20 contacts. The effect of adding a new H–bond can be estimated from the free energy gain (0.5 to 1 kcal per mole·°C) and from $\Delta G = -RT \ln K_a$ to yield affinity increases of threefold to tenfold. Therefore, the affinity maturation that takes place (or affinity that may be *lost* in antibody engineering) changes quickly with a relatively small change in the number of bonds; that is, creating as few as three new hydrogen bonds may generate an affinity enhancement of more than 100-fold. This has been borne out by affinity changes that accompanied productive amino acid substitutions in V region engineering (see later). Of note, antibody affinities are generally much higher for protein antigens than for carbohydrate antigens, which may have less opportunity for hydrogen-bonding interactions (but are also "T-independent" antigens).

Although affinity and K_a directly express the binding potential of the antibody and are the most suitable measures for comparing affinities, the inverse of the K_a, termed K_d or *dissociation constant,* is expressed in molar units and indicates the concentration that is the middle of the range for the biologic action of the antibody:

$$1 \ K_d = -1/K_a \qquad [29\text{-}2]$$

That is, the K_d is the concentration of free antibody at which antigen is 50% saturated; if the antibody is in large excess, the input antibody concentration approximates the *free concentration.* The K_d is a frequently used term, but its relationship to affinity must always be borne in mind: that is, low affinity = high K_d; high affinity = low K_d. For example, a K_a of 2×10^9 M^{-1} implies a K_d of 0.5×10^{-9} mol per L (0.5 nmol per L), or approximately 0.1 mg per mL antibody concentration for IgG. If antigen is in the picomolar (10^{-12} mol per L) range, this concentration of antibody will have half of the antigen saturated and half of antigen will remain "free." At tenfold higher antibody concentration (1 mg per mL, $10 \times K_d$), antigen will be 90% saturated and 10% free, and at 100-fold higher concentration (10 mg per mL, $100 \times K_d$), antigen will be 99% saturated and only 1% unbound. *A key point of understanding is that the ratio of antibody to antigen has very little impact on the degree of antigen saturation when antibody is in excess.* If antibody concentration is 1 nmol per L with a K_d of 1 nmol per L, it does not matter whether antigen is 0.1 nmol per L at the K_d, 0.1 pmol per L, or 0.1 fmol per L; antigen in each case is 50% bound, although the ratio of antibody to antigen is 10, 10^4, and 10^7. *Only the relation of free antibody to its* K_d *determines the degree of antigen saturation.*

The affinity constant K_a is itself composed of two terms that describe the on rate (forward; units of M$^{-1 \cdot z}$) and off rate (back; units of s^{-1}) of the reaction:

$$K_a = k_f - k_b \qquad [29\text{-}3]$$

To a first approximation, the forward rate is diffusion limited and is comparable for many antibodies reacting with macromolecules or cell-bound structures. Reactions of antibodies with haptens and other small molecules in solution are dominated by the faster linear and rotational diffusion rates of the smaller component.[23] For example, when 0.1 nmol per L of dinitrophenyl-lysine (0.1 ng per mL) or 0.1 nmol per L of cell-bound HLA-A2 (50 ng per mL) is mixed with specific IgG antibody at 10 mg per mL (65 nmol per L), 0.1 second is required for the antibody to react with 50% of the antigen for the hapten but 4 minutes is required to react with the surface protein. Yet they have virtually the same affinity constant.[23] This is due to the fact that the fast association rate is balanced by a fast dissociation rate for the hapten [clearance half-time $(t_{1/2})$ = 0.7 seconds] whereas stability is longer for the protein antigen $(t_{1/2}$ = 6 minutes).

Although exceptions exist, the on rates of antibodies to protein and cell-bound antigens are primarily in this range

and inversely proportional to antibody concentration for antibody in excess of antigen (i.e., at 1 mg per mL, the 50% time would be on the order of 0.5 to 1 hour). Accordingly, differences in affinity between antibodies to the same cellular antigen are in many instances reflective of the off rate (k_b). For most purposes, an antibody is generally considered of "good" affinity if its K_a is equal to or greater than 10^9 M^{-1}, where off rate $t_{1/2}$ values of an hour or more at 4°C are common. Association and dissociation times at 37°C are both accelerated relative to the times at 4°C, on the order of 5 or more, frequently with a net decrease in antibody affinity of twofold to tenfold. This must be explicitly tested, however, because in some instances protein-ligand affinities have been found to be enhanced by higher temperature.[24]

The foregoing expresses basic principles of binding processes. A further important feature of antibodies is their multivalent structures. Although the on rates for monovalent Fab and bivalent Fab'2 constructs are comparable, the bivalent off times may be tenfold or more longer than for the monovalent constructs, which yields affinities that are similarly enhanced.[23] To discriminate the affinity that is intrinsic to the V region antigen interaction from the effective affinity in a bi- or multivalent interaction, the latter is often referred to as *avidity.* For monovalent interactions, avidity equals affinity; for multivalent interactions, avidity is greater than or equal to affinity. Theory predicts avidity enhancements that vastly exceed observed numbers, but structural constraints undoubtedly restrain the energy advantage of multivalent binding.[25,26] In the extreme, steric factors constrain some bivalent antibodies (e.g., anti-Tac[27]) to bind only monovalently to antigens on cell surfaces although they will bind bivalently to antigen in solution. Yet even when antigen on the surface is not bivalently bound by antibody, and for all solution interactions, careful treatment of these settings will reveal the molarity of *binding site* rather than antibody in comparing Fab with higher-valence homologs. When antigens are presented multivalently on the surfaces of cells, viruses, or other pathogens, even the low-affinity IgM interactions can yield a high-avidity, stable binding to such targets *in vivo.*

PHARMACOKINETICS AND PHARMACODYNAMICS

Metabolism of immunoglobulins determines the duration of usefulness of antibodies *in vivo.* Under normal conditions, the serum levels of endogenous immunoglobulins are determined by a balance between synthetic and catabolic rates.[28] When antibodies are administered as therapeutics, these catabolic rates effectively specify the dose and schedule necessary to maintain therapeutic blood levels when steady-state exposures are targeted. Table 29-1 lists the half-lives of human antibody survival in humans.

IgG has the longest survival, 23 days (this value is for IgG1, IgG2, and IgG4; IgG3 survival is 7 days). Autologous IgG survival is correlated with animal size, with IgG survival of 4 days in mouse, 8 days in dog, 12 days in baboon, and 21 days in cow.[20] Of interest, however, is the observation of survival in heterologous systems, in which the shorter of the IgG survival times, whether that of the host or that of the donor, is dominant. In other words, murine IgG survives for the same time in humans and in mice, whereas human IgG survives for a shorter time in mice than in humans, with a survival time compatible with that of mice's own catabolism of IgG.[20] A key element in the regulation of IgG catabolism is the Brambell receptor (FcRB), named after its discoverer Professor F. W. R. Brambell, who described this receptor more than 30 years ago (see Junghans[29] for a review). This receptor is located in endosomes of endocytically active tissues, primarily vascular endothelium, which is mainly responsible for the catabolism of plasma proteins, including IgG. There, FcRB binds IgG, recycling it to the cell surface and diverting it from the pathway to lysosomes and catabolism that is the fate of other, nonprotected proteins. In this role, FcRB is also termed the IgG protection receptor (FcRp). Yet FcRB is also responsible for transmission of IgG from mother to young, via yolk sac, placenta, or newborn intestine; in this manifestation it is termed the IgG neonatal transport receptor (FcRn) for neonatal intestine, the tissue from which the receptor was initially cloned.

A substantial body of knowledge exists on the metabolism of immunoglobulins in various disease states. Conditions of protein wasting (enteropathies, vascular leak syndromes, burns), febrile states, hyperthyroidism, hypergammaglobulinemia, and inflammatory disorders are accompanied by significant acceleration of immunoglobulin catabolism.[28] This information is of importance to understanding *in vivo* survival data in various clinical applications. In fact, the controlled conditions of testing immunoglobulin metabolism are rarely duplicated in practice, with antibody survivals typically shorter than suggested by the numbers above. Typically, murine antibody survival $t_{1/2}$ values are in the range of less than 1 to 3 days, and antibodies with human gamma Fc domains (chimeric or humanized) have $t_{1/2}$ values in the range of 1 to 15 days. Some of this acceleration in clearance is clearly due to disease-associated catabolic factors and to antigen binding *in vivo*, but subtle changes in the drug structure during product preparation may have a role in this acceleration as well. Influence on antibody clearance of antigen expression *in vivo* is considered later.

Antibody fragments have been studied because of their abbreviated survival and because small size may translate into better tissue penetration. Fab and Fab'2 have survivals *in vivo* of 2 to 5 hours in mice, with comparable values in humans, and survival is dependent largely on kidney filtration mechanisms.[28] This is not based on size alone, because the Fc fragment, which is comparable in size to Fab, is not filtered and has an *in vivo* survival of 10 days in humans. These rapidly catabolized fragments, like other filtered proteins, are largely absorbed in the proximal tubule and degraded to amino acids, which are returned to circulation. No intact immunoglobulin or fragments reenter circulation once filtered.[30] In normal kidney, less than 5% of filtered light chain is excreted intact, whereas this fraction increases in the setting of renal tubular disease.[31]

A recently active area of investigation has been the role of circulating antigen in the setting of antitumor therapies. This was first encountered in antiidiotype therapies (see later) directed at the surface Ig on B-cell lymphomas, some of which secreted high levels of idiotype.[32] This prevented access of administered antibody to the idiotype on tumor cells, which effectively neutralized the drug, unless very high doses were given to overwhelm the secreted quantities of idiotype. Subsequent further studies showed that other tumor antigens, including carcinoembryonic antigen (CEA),[33] gangliosides GD2 and GD3,[34,35] and Tac[36,37] could achieve significant levels that might require adjustments to therapy. Figure 29-5 shows a simulation of the impact on the bindability (bioactivity) of antibody of increasing doses in the presence of a fixed amount of antigen as well as the impact of continued synthesis of antigen in the presence of antibody. These predictions have been verified in measurements obtained during treatment of patients with Tac-expressing tumors.[36]

Key features of these observations[36] are (a) a direct relationship between the soluble antigen levels and the dose necessary to attain 50% (or 90% or 99%) bindability of administered antibody and (b) a predictable relationship of the rate of antigen synthesis and the time to antibody saturation. The actual partitioning of antibody between soluble and cellular antigen depends on several features, including the effective avidity of antibody for antigen on cells, which may be higher, and other factors influencing tumor penetration.

A special concern in this setting is that many soluble forms of antigen have short $t_{1/2}$ values once shed from tumor cell surfaces, and the interaction with antibody may prolong their *in vivo* survival and increase their level in the whole body. When the target itself is a cytokine or cytokine receptor, adverse consequences conceivably could derive from the antibody treatment if the antigen retains activity in the antibody complex, as shown for interleukin 3, interleukin 4, and interleukin 7 complexes *in vivo*.[38] If the antigen does not retain activity in complex, then this problem causes no concern because the free concentration of antigen cannot be *increased* by the presence of antibody, even after antibody is fully saturated with excess antigen. A different potential consequence of antigen load is that it may reduce transport of radioantibody to tumor for imaging or therapy. Study has shown, however, that antibody

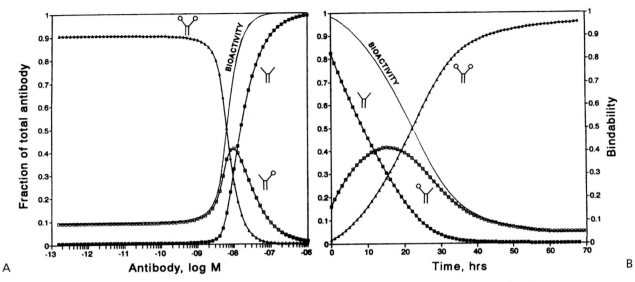

FIGURE 29-5. Simulation of bioactivity (bindability) of antibody in the presence of antigen. Antibody with one or two "arms" free is bindable. **A:** Antigen-antibody complexes and bioactivity with increasing doses of antibody in the presence of 10 nmol per L antigen and an affinity of 10^9 M^{-1}. **B:** Impact on bioactivity of antibody (10 nmol per L) with an initial antigen load of 2 nmol per L, continued antigen synthesis (0.5 nmol per L per hour), and an antibody physical half-life of 100 hours that is not affected by antigen binding. The antibody bioactivity is lost long before the clearance of antibody from the host. (R.P. Junghans, *unpublished calculations.*)

can partition sufficiently between soluble and cellular antigen to yield targeting adequate for tumor imaging purposes (CEA,[33] Tac[36]).

BIOLOGIC FUNCTIONS

Antibodies mediate several actions of potential therapeutic interest, some of which are part of the normal biologic function of antibodies and some of which are adapted in novel ways to the needs of specific settings.

Complement-Dependent Cytotoxicity

The complement (C') system is at least as primitive evolutionarily as antibodies.[14] One view is that the alternate (antibody-independent) pathway is the primordial system, which then diversified to create the classic pathway to collaborate with antibody to direct the attack complex (C5–C9) against antibody-coated targets. The most effective mediator of complement-dependent cytotoxicity (CDC) is IgM. Single IgM molecules can fix and activate complement on cell surfaces. In contrast, IgG-mediated CDC depends on the juxtaposition of pairs of IgG molecules to bind complement to cells,[39] with substantially lower complement fixation and reduced killing efficiency relative to IgM. Human IgG1 and IgG3; mouse IgG2a, IgG2b, and IgG3; rat IgG2a; and rabbit IgG all fix and activate complement, whereas human IgG2 fixes C' poorly and human IgG4 and murine IgG1 normally do not fix C'.[40] (Complement fixation depends on conserved residues in the C_H2 domain; short hinge regions are thought to hinder C1q access and binding with these latter isotypes.) Although human IgG3 fixes human C' better than IgG1, actual target lysis may be better with IgG1 due to more efficient activation of C4.[41] For the most part, human and murine antibodies function comparably well in directing CDC with rabbit C' in *in vitro* tests and in fixing human or rabbit C'. Some cases may exist, however, in which murine IgG3 is more potent due to the unique feature of Fc polymerization on cell surfaces apparently not similarly available to human IgG.[42]

Despite these considerations, the impact of C' fixation and CDC in therapeutic applications against cancer is uncertain. Cells vary greatly in susceptibility to complement *in vitro*, but, except for erythrocytes, no convincing evidence exists that human antibodies kill nucleated cellular targets *in vivo* by CDC, although the means of correlating response with the mechanisms of cell killing have not always been available. Two considerations may bear on this feature: (a) the complete first component of human complement is very large (approximately 800 kd) and, like IgM,[28] probably has limited extravascular penetration; and (b) the cells to which complement has ready access (e.g., cells of the hematopoietic system and vascular endothelium) are endowed with potent phosphoinositol-linked membrane protease activities, decay-accelerating factor, and homologous restriction factor (HRF), which act as steps subsequent to C1 fixation to inactivate the human complement cascade.[43,44] Rabbit, guinea pig, or other heterologous

TABLE 29-3. FCγ RECEPTORS: PROPERTIES AND BINDING CHARACTERISTICS

Receptor	Size (kd)	K_a	Cells	Mouse IgG	Human IgG
FcRI (CD64)	72	10^8	Mono, mac, act. PMN, eos	2a, 3	3 > 1 > 4
FcRII (CD32)	40	10^6	Mono, mac, gran, B cell, plt	2a, 2b, 1 (immune complexes or aggregates)	3, 1
FcRIII (CD16A) transmembrane (CD16B) PI-linked	50–70	5×10^5	LGL/NK, mac, few T, act. mono PMN, act. eos	3, 2a > 1	3, 1 > 2, 4

act., activated; eos, eosinophile; gran, granulocyte; LGL, large granular lymphocytes; mac, macrocytes; mono, monocytes; NK, natural killer cells; plt, platelet; PMN, polymorphonuclear leukocyte.
Adapted from Van de Winkel GJ, Capel JA. Human IgG Fc receptor heterogeneity: molecular aspect and clinical implications. *Immunol Today* 1993;14:215; Simmons D, Seed B. The Fcγ receptor of natural killer cells is a phosphoinositol-linked membrane protein [later shown not PI-linked]. *Nature* 1988;333:568; and Walker MR, Woof JM, Bruggemann M, et al. Interaction of human IgG chimeric antibodies with the human FcR1 and FcR11 receptors: requirements for antibody-mediated host cell-target cell interaction. *Mol Immunol* 1989;26:403.

sera can kill cells *in vitro* that are resistant to human C' because they bypass the human species restriction of these protease activities.

Antibody-Dependent Cellular Cytotoxicity

In antibody-dependent cellular cytotoxicity (ADCC), target cells are coated with antibody and engage effector cells equipped with Fc receptors (FcRs) that bind to the Fc region of IgG, release cytolysins, and lead to cell killing. The only classes demonstrated to mediate ADCC are IgE and IgG. Because of the dangers of anaphylaxis that would be associated with IgE use, antitumor IgE antibodies are not likely to be developed, and further discussion therefore focuses on IgG.

Classically, cells that mediated ADCC were called *K* (*killer*) *cells*, and all bear FcRs on their surfaces. Of these, at least three IgG FcRs and two IgE FcRs are found. Table 29-3 lists the FcRs for IgG and their properties.[45–47] All FcRs are capable of directing ADCC of effectors against appropriate antibody-coated targets. Cytolytic mechanisms include perforins, a system closely related to the C9 protein of the complement attack complex (C5–C9), and serine proteases (granzymes) in large granular lymphocytes (LGLs); superoxides, free radicals, proteases, and lysozymes in monocytes-macrophages and granulocytes; tumor necrosis factor; and other components. As far as is known, the lytic mechanisms of LGLs and cytotoxic lymphocytes are similar or identical, whereas the monocyte-macrophage and granulocyte mechanisms share numerous features. The monocyte-granulocyte mechanisms are probably adapted to killing and engulfment of microorganisms, whereas T cells, the closest lineage relative of LGL-NK cells, have the role of killing cells of self-origin that express foreign or neoantigens. In general, the most potent of the mediators of cellular killing in circulation have been the LGLs. These cells also perform natural killing (NK cells), which is an antibody-independent lectin-like ligand interaction system.[48] Other effectors, for example, monocytes and granulocytes, have been shown to mediate ADCC against nucleated targets,[49,50] but in most direct comparisons with LGLs, the LGLs were more potent than these other numerically more dominant cells.[51,52] Nevertheless, the most effective approaches may include a multipronged attack that enlists the collaboration of more than a single cellular system to kill antibody-coated tumor targets.

Among the features that influence the amount of killing in ADCC are (a) the species origin of the antibody, (b) IgG subclass, (c) the number of antibody molecules bound per target cell, (d) the ratio of effector cells to targets, (e) the activation state of effectors, (f) the presence of irrelevant IgG, and, perhaps, (g) the presence of tumor cell protective factors. These are discussed in turn.

1. The species origin appears to have a significant influence on the ability of an antibody to recruit human effectors to kill human tumors. Although human and rat antibodies mediate ADCC with human effectors, murine antibodies are often less potent in this role. Long ago isologous antiserum was established to be more effective with any species' effector cells,[53] which suggests that the match of antibody to effector cell Fc receptor is a significant feature of ADCC.

2. All IgG subclasses are in principle capable of ADCC. However, the IgG1 subclass of humans, the IgG2a and IgG3 subclasses of the mouse, and the IgG2b and IgG3 subclasses of the rat have been inferred to be the most active with human cells. This does not always parallel the order of FcR binding affinity, and other factors of Fc-FcR binding must be postulated that influence induction of cytolysis.[54]

3. Selection of target antigens that are highly expressed has a direct impact on the likelihood that the cell can be killed with ADCC. Control of the number of antibody molecules bound reveals that a nearly linear relationship exists with cytolysis.[55] A corollary of this phenomenon is that modulation of antigen by antibody binding (antigen-antibody complex internalization or shedding) reduces target susceptibility even when baseline antigen is highly expressed.

4. Higher effector to target ratios yield increased killing, although a plateau in efficacy typically is achieved at higher ratios.[53,56] *In vivo,* the ratio of effector cells to targets is not so readily controlled, except by stimulating proliferation or supplementing effectors, but this effect may provide a stronger rationale for treatment in adjuvant settings when the tumor burden is small, that is, after debulking surgery or induction chemotherapy.

5. The activation state of effectors has been shown in several systems, both *in vitro* and *in vivo,* to play an important role in the lysis of targets. This activation is achieved with any of several agents. Evaluation of the application of cytokines specific to the range of potential effectors is beyond the scope of this review, but in each instance cytolytic capacity has been strongly correlated with the degree of effector cell activation. Only LGLs (NK cells) appear to have significant antitumor potency in ADCC in the absence of cytokine activation, but here, too, activation with cytokines also increases ADCC killing[56] (Fig. 29-6). Interleukin 2 (IL-2) activation of LGLs has been the most widely applied in clinical trials to date (see Chapter 32).

6. The presence of circulating IgG is probably the most problematic of features for exploiting ADCC *in vivo.* Clearly, the very existence of FcRs and the presence of cytolytic granules are teleologic indications of the relevance of this capability to biology. Although one might argue that monocytes-macrophages and granulocytes are adapted to combat microorganisms, the sole role of T cells is to kill nucleated cells of self that present viral or other abnormal peptides, for which they use distinct cytolytic mechanisms. As stated above, LGLs apparently duplicate the cytolytic mechanisms of T cells but in addition possess FcRs to enable them to interact with antibodies that will direct them to these targets through non–major histocompatibility complex mechanisms.

The problem of this interaction is that monomeric Fc of IgG has an affinity of approximately 5×10^5 M^{-1} (K_d = 2 mmol per L) for the dominant FcR on LGLs (Table 29-3). At 1 g per dL *in vivo* concentration, IgG is 65 mmol per L and 30-fold above this K_d, which implies that more than 95% of the FcR on LGLs is occupied with IgG Fc. (The occupancy fraction on monocytes-macrophages with higher-affinity FcR type I is still higher.) Countering this in the biologic interaction is that affinity of specific IgG for antigen is typically much higher than this, which yields a stable multivalent surface presentation of IgG Fc on the target that in turn may interact in a multivalent manner with the effector cell FcR. In practice, however, most ADCC assays are markedly inhibited by added human serum. (Assays using fetal calf serum are not so affected because IgG is absent due to lack of placental transport in ungulates.[28]) Whether the longer-term *in vivo* incubations of days versus the brief duration (approximately 3 hours) of *in vitro* assays allows a therapeutic effect in a treatment program requires further study. However, observed clinical responses to antibody therapies (see later) suggest that ADCC may in some instances be operative *in vivo.*

7. Interest has recently focused on *tumor-based* factors that may mediate *resistance* to ADCC. One such factor is the complement regulatory protein HRF. HRF was originally defined as acting at C2 and C9 of the complement cascade. The cytolytic protein perforin I that is released by LGL-NK cells and cytotoxic lymphocytes is also referred to as *C9-related protein* and is likewise subject to proteolysis by HRF, which thereby neutralizes the lytic power of the killer cell.[57] [The observation has been made, however, that HRF-related protein Ly6 (CD59) does not protect against perforin lysis.[58]] HRF is present at high levels on activated T cells and NK cells and is thought to play a role in protecting these cells from autolysis during lysis of intended targets. Cells that are resistant to ADCC could be induced to become sensitive by blocking with anti-HRF antibodies.[44] Another factor that may contribute to cellular resistance is the secretion of mucins, which inhibit the penetration of antibodies and other macromolecules to the cell surfaces. Other issues of tumor penetration are discussed later.

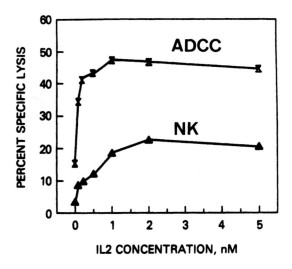

FIGURE 29-6. Impact of interleukin 2 (IL-2) on antibody-dependent cellular cytotoxicity (ADCC) after 16 hours of activation of peripheral blood lymphocytes. (NK, natural killer cells.) (From Junghans RP. A strategy for evaluating lymphokine activation and novel monoclonal antibodies in antibody-dependent cell-mediated cytotoxicity and effector cell retargeting assays. *Cancer Immunol Immunother* 1990;31:207.)

Finally, the relevance of the *in vitro* ADCC assay to *in vivo* function is much discussed. Only in a few instances has this been examined by comparing ADCC-competent and ADCC-*in*competent antibodies. In the first such study, using a complement-deficient leukemic AKR mouse model, an IgG monoclonal antibody against a leukemia antigen suppressed tumor, but an IgM antibody of the same specificity was ineffective.[58] This suggested that binding to antigen was not sufficient and that C' played no role. Two further reports of studies in mice showed that the only antibody to induce an *in vivo* response was that which showed ADCC activity *in vitro*.[59,60] Several studies have shown that antibody plus IL-2 activation of effectors was much more effective than either alone (e.g., see Honsik et al.[61] and Schulz et al.[62]), which implicates cooperation between the cellular and humoral immune systems that is the sine qua non of ADCC. Human trials in which a leukemic patient received human IgG Fc coupled to a murine antibody showed a more effective response than when the antibody was without human Fc.[63] A further human trial with class/isotype-switched CAMPATH-1 antilymphocyte antibody showed a dramatic response in patients with B-cell chronic lymphocytic leukemia only for the one isotype that mediates ADCC *in vitro*.[64] Similarly, the humanized anti-CD33 antibody that expresses ADCC *in vitro* suppresses leukemic cells *in vivo*, whereas the parental murine antibody lacks ADCC *in vitro* and is inactive *in vivo* (P. Caron and D. A. Scheinberg, *unpublished research*, 1993). Enhancements to this function are discussed later.

PHAGOCYTOSIS

Antibody-dependent phagocytosis may be performed by cells of the granulocytic and monocyte-macrophage lineages. Furthermore, these cells have receptors for C3 fragments, which enhance binding of antibody-coated targets that also activate complement leading to C3 fixation. Only *activated* macrophages, however, are capable of engulfing antibody-coated erythrocytes. The ability to engulf larger tumor cells has been uncertain, but one *in vitro* evaluation of activated monocytes demonstrated phagocytosis of melanoma and neuroblastoma targets when assays were appropriately monitored.[65] Nevertheless, phagocytic cells in the liver (i.e., Kupffer cells) and spleen probably are the primary mediators of circulatory clearance of antibody-coated platelets in alloimmune and autoimmune settings[66] and in the instances in which rapid clearance of leukemic cells was observed during antibody therapies. Whether these cells are trapped and then lysed by ADCC mechanisms rather than phagocytosis is uncertain.

RECEPTOR BLOCKADE

What antibodies do best is to bind, and sometimes very tightly, and this does not require the uncertain collabora-

tion of other elements of the immune system. By the same mechanism by which antitoxin can prevent a toxin from acting at its target site in the body, antibody also can deny access of growth factors to tumors whose proliferation is factor dependent. This approach has been applied more widely in nonmalignant settings for the suppression of immune responses in autoimmune and alloimmune settings (e.g., see Kirkman et al.[67]). This approach is limited in malignancy because most tumors appear to be autonomous. In principle, antibody to the cytokine should have the same result. The short half-lives of most cytokines and the locally high concentrations that may be achieved may make this approach more difficult, however. Such autocrine or paracrine loops may be better interrupted by antireceptor than by anticytokine antibody. One report has documented a marked *enhancement* of cytokine activity by antibody to cytokine via $t_{1/2}$ prolongation, which runs counter to the goal of suppressing cytokine activity.[38]

Design of such applications also must consider the receptor occupancy that is necessary for cell survival and proliferation. Only 10% occupancy of the receptor for granulocyte-macrophage colony-stimulating factor is sufficient to induce maximal activation of granulocytes.[68] Similarly, one must block more than 90% of the α chain of IL-2 receptor with antibody to have a significant impact on IL-2–dependent, antigen-induced T-cell proliferation.[55]

APOPTOSIS

Apoptosis is a process by which signals are transmitted through cell surface receptors to induce autoenzyme-mediated cell death, or by which downstream events are accessed to achieve the same result. This has been demonstrated most persuasively during development and in the programming of T-cell precursors in the thymus. The *fas* antigen is probably the natural membrane receptor for this process and is expressed in liver, heart, thymus, lung, and ovary, although other antigens may exert similar effects. An extraordinarily complete and rapid tissue destruction resulted from anti-Fas antibody administration.[69] One report suggests that part of the killing mechanism of T cells is to engage this receptor on target cells.[70] Some hematologic malignant cells, like their normal counterparts, are Fas positive and in principle could be targets of therapy (a) if antibodies could be found that are not cross-reactive for normal tissue, (b) if ways of engaging the receptor can be selectively achieved (i.e., bifunctional anti-Fas × antitumor antibody), or (c) if other antigens unique to tumors can be found that also access this cellular process. To date, such tumor-specific apoptosis-inducing antigens have not been described, but lineage-associated apoptosis-inducing antigens have been targeted in the treatment of lymphoma (see later).

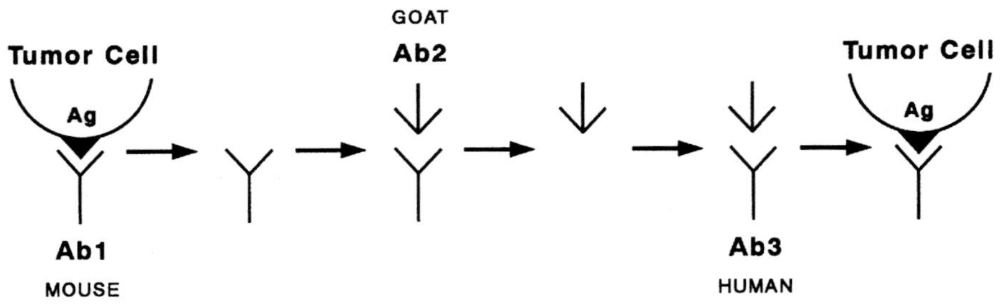

FIGURE 29-7. Idiotype network demonstrating relation of Ab2 to antigen (Ag).

INTRACELLULAR ACTION

In a still poorly understood process, cases are seen in which IgA and IgG antibodies have been deduced to be transported transmembrane to act by intracellular mechanisms against cytoplasmic targets to thwart viral infections.[71–73] Whether this process can be adapted to antitumor therapy (except in the context of toxin conjugates) is unclear, and to the authors' knowledge, no one is presently exploring such an approach.

Ab2 VACCINES

Antibody recognition of antigen entails the presentation of a molecular surface that is the complement in space of the antigen (Fig. 29-3), termed a *mirror image.* In the Jerne network nomenclature, the designation of antigen and antibody becomes arbitrary. The antigen is Ab0, the antibody is Ab1, antibody to the antibody idiotype is Ab2, and so forth. Although antibody can react with idiotype in many ways, a subset of Ab2 is still considered to exist that mimics Ab0 (antigen), and a fraction of Ab3 raised against Ab2 mimics Ab1 and reacts with Ab0 (antigen) (Fig. 29-7) (see Bona[74] for details of nomenclature). Therefore, a tumor antigen may not be immunogenic in the human host that carries it, but a murine antibody (Ab1) can be raised to this antigen, and a goat antibody (Ab2) can be raised to this. This Ab2 antibody includes epitopes that mimic antigen but presents them in a novel context in which they may be immunogenic in the original host. Such Ab2s have been used as vaccines to induce Ab3 antibody responses in the host that can cross-react with antigen (Ab0) on tumor. Antibody therapy in this sense is applied to induce an endogenous antibody and occasionally a T-cell response against tumor. Animal studies have shown that Ab2 vaccine immune responses can prevent growth on challenge with tumor.[75] Clinical trials are currently under way, with unpublished data too preliminary to judge the potential of this modality. A correlation between spontaneous induction of Ab3 during Ab1 anti–colon cancer therapy and reduced recurrence was observed,[76,77] however, although cause and effect are at present hard to deduce.

ANTIBODY MODIFICATIONS FOR THERAPY

As discussed later, for all the functions that antibodies can and do perform *in vivo,* their use as therapeutic agents against cancer has been largely unsuccessful. Two major factors have been the focus of research efforts considered in this section: (a) immunogenicity and (b) lack of therapeutic and cytolytic potency. The approaches to improve potency have themselves been twofold: (a) to improve the collaboration of antibodies with the other components of the immune system and (b) to use the antibody as a vector to deliver toxic agents (toxins or radioactivity) to tumor cells. This latter approach essentially abandons the immunologic collaboration of antibodies with the remainder of the immune system.

Reduction of Immunogenicity

Immunogenicity (see the section Clinical Studies) derives from the fact that most mAbs are of mouse origin and as such are foreign proteins in the human host. The human antiglobulin response to mouse antibodies is directed mainly against the C domains of the murine antibody, with typically lower titers against the V domains. To address this problem, two versions of the foreign protein have been prepared (Fig. 29-8): a chimeric version in which the mouse C domains are substituted by human C domains, and a "humanized" or hyperchimeric version in which the murine framework regions are in addition replaced with human framework sequences. Moreover, methods to prepare pure "human" IgG *in vitro* and *in vivo* (in transgenic mice) have been described, but the use of these products in humans as therapeutic agents is not yet known (see later). (Despite early attempts to standardize the nomenclature of these constructs using the suffixes *C* for chimeric and *H* for hyperchimeric or humanized,[55,78] a chaotic proliferation of nomenclatures exists at present. The humanized version is also referred to as "CDR-grafted.")

In practice, these two products are prepared by different methods. The simpler construct is typically prepared by linking the genomic or messenger RNA–derived human heavy and light chain C domains with the murine heavy and light chain V regions as DNA recombinants. These constructs are expressed in recipient cells that secrete the

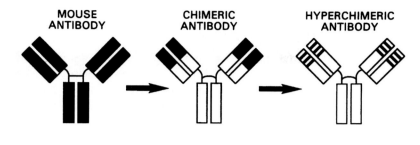

MOUSE   **CHIMERIC**   **HYPERCHIMERIC**
ANTIBODY   **ANTIBODY**   **ANTIBODY**

■ MOUSE

□ HUMAN

FIGURE 29-8. Schematic of chimeric versus hyperchimeric (humanized) antibodies. See also Figure 29-2. (From Junghans RP, Waldmann TA, Landolfi NF, et al. Anti Tac-H, a humanized antibody to the interleukin 2 receptor with new features for immunotherapy in malignant and immune disorders. *Cancer Res* 1990; 50:1495.)

recombinant protein into the medium, from which it is recovered by biochemical techniques. Preparation of humanized antibodies (Fig. 29-2) typically begins with a computer modeling of the three-dimensional structure of the V region of the murine antibody from its amino acid sequence (crystallography is rarely performed) and comparison with known crystallographic structures of V regions of human myeloma proteins (antibodies).[79] A human antibody V domain is selected that is most like the murine antibody in its three-dimensional presentation of the binding surface. The CDRs of the mouse antibody are "grafted" onto the human antibody V domain by total V gene synthesis with a series of long overlapping oligonucleotides. In anti–Tac-H, these murine segments are 6 to 19 amino acids in length, and this product is fairly representative of other antibody constructs. This synthetic V gene is then linked to C domains as indicated earlier and expressed. The resulting proteins are over 90% human, or less than 10% rodent, in origin. In contrast, the chimeric molecules are 30% to 35% rodent in origin.

The first humanized antibody for cancer therapy was the panlymphocyte antibody CAMPATH-1H.[78] Since that time, others have been prepared, including the anti–IL-2 receptor antibody anti–Tac-H for various leukemias and lymphomas,[55,79] the HER2/neu anti–breast carcinoma antibody,[80] HuM195 anti-CD33 for myeloid leukemias,[81] and more that have yet to be tested in humans. Clinical experience to date remains limited, but clearly the hyperchimeric antibodies have been much more successful in avoiding antiglobulin responses, with an incidence of 4% with CAMPATH-1H[82] and comparably low antiglobulin response rates with anti–Tac-H[83] and HuM195.[84] The less extensively substituted chimeric antibodies have been more widely applied. One chimeric antibody (Ch17.1A) appeared not to induce anti–V region antibodies despite the intact murine V domain (Fig. 29-8), whereas brisk anti-V responses were elicited in another trial with a second chimeric anticarcinoma antibody (ChB72.3) accompanied by accelerated clearances.[85,86] Lesser but significant anti-V responses were observed with a chimeric anti-CD4 mAb in mycosis fungoides[87] and with a chimeric anti-GD2 antibody (Ch14.18) in melanoma patients.[88] The structural features of proteins that are necessary for recognition and processing by T cells[89] to engender help to stimulated B cells appear to be differentially represented in different murine V regions and in different individuals. Further experience is required to ascertain the rules governing these responses.

Finally, human antibodies may be thought to represent the ultimate step in the strategy to create minimally immunogenic, biologically active molecules for therapy. Yet this approach has in some ways been the most frustrating, particularly in cases in which antitumor or self-reacting activities are sought. Individuals rarely make antibody responses to autologous tumor antigens, antibodies are frequently IgMs (less useful for *in vivo* therapies), and immortalization and identification of stable clones for mass production of clinical reagents all present significant problems.[90] Mouse-human severe combined immunodeficiency disease (SCID)–hu hybrids may permit generation of human antibodies by traditional mouse immunization techniques, but the promise of this technology is yet to be fulfilled.[91,92] Moreover, significant lacunae will exist within the SCID-hu repertoire even when this system is optimally functioning; no antigen present on human cells during hematopoiesis is antigenic. The innovation of human combinatorial phage display libraries[93] is also being applied for deriving antiself and antitumor human antibodies (R.P. Junghans and D.R. Burton, *unpublished research*).

Efforts to suppress human antimurine antibody with immunosuppressive drugs have not been successful to date. Newer approaches attempt to induce tolerance to administered antibody by manipulation of host T cells with antibody to T-cell targets and administration of cytokines that control T-cell suppression.[94] If these approaches are successful, a means may be found in the future to use rodent antibodies in human therapy without inducing antiglobulin responses and thereby also reducing the impetus to undertake the considerable effort to humanize these products.

A further impact of humanization is that human IgG C domains (specifically, C_H2) could confer a longer *in vivo* $t_{1/2}$ on the order of 23 days for human IgG in humans versus the 1- to 3-day $t_{1/2}$ of murine antibody in humans.[28] One study compared a chimeric antiidiotype antibody with the parental murine antibody, demonstrating a prolonged *in vivo* survival (with $t_{1/2}$ longer than 10 days for a nonreactive chimeric construct).[55] Other studies involving chimeric antibodies against colon carcinoma yielded survival $t_{1/2}$ values of 3 to 6 and 4 to 12 days.[85,86] The humanized CAMPATH-1H had survival $t_{1/2}$ values of 1 to 6 days,[82] and anti–Tac-H showed survival of 2 to 15 days.[83] Thus, observed survivals fall short of those expected from controlled studies in normal volunteers. Some of this acceleration in clearance is clearly due to disease-associated catabolic factors,[28] but what further contributions antigen binding *in vivo* and product preparation have in this acceleration is uncertain. Further studies are required to sort this out.

Binding Affinity of Engineered Antibodies

The affinity for substrate (antigen) is an intrinsic characteristic of an antibody conferred by the particular amino acid sequence and spatial presentation of the CDRs. In the past, the affinity that was retrieved from a given hybridoma was an immutable feature of the antibody; it could be altered only by reducing the valence of the product (i.e., Fab versus Fab'2, IgG versus IgM), which only reduced affinity. More recent efforts in the preparation of IgG dimers, however, have shown a marked increase in affinity of up to 1,000-fold,[95] which may accentuate the improvement in Fc-dependent functions with such constructs (see later).

With CDR manipulation in the humanization of antibodies, a major disturbance sometimes occurred in the affinity for antigen. Search for causes of this affinity loss revealed the importance of single, critical residues to total affinity. For example, the affinity of a humanized antilysozyme antibody was markedly lower than that of the parental antibody. Exchange of one serine for a phenylalanine generated a 15-fold improvement in affinity.[96] The anti-HER2/neu antibody CDRs were grafted into a human framework and then modified with a large number of amino acid substitutions. Many of these were neutral, but every *productive* substitution that appeared to generate a new hydrogen bond also increased affinity by a factor of 5,[80] in accordance with the calculations above. By this, creation or loss of as few as three hydrogen bonds can cause affinity changes of 100-fold or more. Yet secondary structural effects on affinity have been noted in alteration of a carbohydrate addition site at the V region framework (outside the CDRs) in HuM195.[97]

Novel procedures using phage display libraries allow a far more elegant procedure to improve affinities. Fab molecules are expressed on the surface of phage and are selected against immobilized antigen and enriched in proportion to their affinity. This observation has enabled a random CDR mutagenesis-selection procedure that recapitulates *in vitro* the *in vivo* process of affinity selection and maturation.[98]

By this procedure, the affinity for antigen of any low-affinity antibody can be enhanced by 1,000-fold or more in a simple selection procedure.

One further strategy to improve antigen binding on cell surfaces goes beyond the conceptually simple approaches of control of valence and antigen-antibody affinity. If the target molecule A is present at a concentration of 500 per cell and a second, irrelevant molecule B is present at 50,000 per cell, the net avidity for molecule A can be shown to be much greater with a bifunctional antibody (BFA) that recognizes molecules A and B with equal affinity than with bivalent recognition of A. Jacques et al.[99] prepared such a BFA, linking the highly expressed α chain with the poorly expressed β chain of the IL-2 receptor. Although the intent was to block the α and β chains, the success of their approach is more likely due to another reason. The α chains were not appreciably blocked at the concentrations of antibody used, but the blockade of β+++ chain (which is involved in IL-2 signaling) was greatly improved by this strategy because of the high concentration of α chain. Because α chain is expressed only on activated T cells, this strategy has the advantage of suppressing β chain only on cells participating in the graft rejection.

Finally, the issue of valence has been addressed to reduce the likelihood of antigen modulation during therapy by preparing *univalent* IgG that still retains the Fc effector domains and Fc-dependent functions.[100,101]

Complement-Dependent Cytotoxicity

The opportunities and problems of CDC as a means of killing tumors were outlined earlier. The humanization of antibodies has in some instances shown an improvement in cellular killing with heterologous complement, but for the most part the effect has not been dramatic and was not sufficiently more potent to kill human tumor cells with human complement when murine antibodies failed. On the other hand, the principle of the relative advantage of human over mouse antibodies has been clearly violated by occasional observations of failure to fix C' with chimeric human IgG1 and IgG3 molecules when the murine antibodies have fixed C', first noted by Junghans et al.[55] and since corroborated by others[80,102] (also, S. Morrison, *personal communications*, 1991). The implications of this result are still uncertain, but it means that nothing can be assumed in this regard without actual testing. In any case, the impact of humanization of IgG antibodies is not expected to render them as effective as IgM antibodies for CDC killing. In addition, the possibility exists that the murine IgG3 may be more potent than any human IgG with its capacity for polymerization on cell membranes with enhanced C' fixation and lysis.[42] Finally, dimeric forms of human IgG1 antibodies have been engineered that are far more effective in fixing complement than monomeric versions[103,104] but none has yet undergone *in vivo* testing.

Other approaches were developed with the observation that C3b-coupled antibodies can increase deposition of attack complex (C5–C8) on IgG-coated bacteria. If cells are resistant due to their protective activities, this strategy might overwhelm the cellular defenses.[105] Activation of C3 to C3b (C5 convertase) is late enough in the cascade to bypass the inhibitory effects of decay-accelerating factor and HRF, which inactivate C2b, but it does not escape the HRF inhibition that occurs at C9. When this procedure was adapted to a Tac+ cell line that was resistant to anti-Tac antibody plus human C' (but susceptible to rabbit C'), no increase in target lysis was seen (R.P. Junghans, L.F. Fries, and M.M. Frank, *unpublished research*).

Antibody-Dependent Cellular Cytotoxicity

Unlike with CDC, human antibodies show a fairly consistent advantage of over mouse antibodies in their efficacy of interaction with human effector cells. In several tests, a marked increase is seen in potency of cellular killing in the chimeric constructs with human Fc domains. Of the human isotypes, IgG1 has been consistently the most effective, and chimeric and humanized antibodies are equivalent when normalized to molecules bound per target cell.[55] BFAs, discussed later, appear to have the best opportunity to enhance this killing activity, although clinical data are very limited at this point. Another approach has been to apply anti-HRF antibodies to block the inhibitory effects of HRF on ADCC (see earlier), which has been demonstrated *in vitro*[44] but to date has not been not tested in *in vivo* models.

FEATURES OF SPECIFIC MODIFICATIONS

Chimeric Antibodies

The simple chimeric constructs (Fig. 29-8) were the first to be prepared, in work pioneered by Morrison and co-workers[106] and rapidly adopted by others. These constructs uniformly maintained the antigen-binding characteristics of their parental murine (or rat) antibodies, because the V regions were not altered. In addition, with human Fc domains, they generally demonstrated improved ADCC with human effector cells *in vitro*. The effect on CDC was variable, as noted previously. These constructs were mainly IgG1, based on conclusions that ADCC and CDC would be best expressed with this human isotype. As noted earlier, the antibody survivals in clinical settings were not as prolonged as anticipated with the human Fc domains for the variety of possible reasons previously discussed.

Subsequently, Winter and collaborators showed that the CDRs of antibodies could be transferred from murine to human frameworks with maintenance of binding specificity,[107,108] albeit with losses in affinity of 1.6- to 15-fold. Such

affinity losses became a recurrent concern with these constructs. Subsequently, this group humanized a rat antibody, CAMPATH-1, which is directed at a human panlymphocyte antigen, with the intention of therapeutic application in leukemias and lymphomas (see later). The second antibody to be humanized for therapy, anti–Tac-H, was derived from murine anti–human IL-2 receptor antibody anti-Tac for use in alloimmune and autoimmune settings and in Tac-expressing leukemias and lymphomas[55,79] (Fig. 29-2). The manipulations to create this antibody also had a modest impact on affinity, which was reduced from 9×10^9 to 3×10^9 M^{-1},[55] but one antibody (HuM195) actually showed increased affinity after engineering.[97] Since that time, several further antibodies have been humanized. Humanization effectively reduces immunogenicity, but the impact on therapeutic outcome has yet to be fully evaluated (see later).

Immunoadhesins

Another type of chimeric antibody genetically couples a natural ligand with an immunoglobulin Fc domain to confer *in vivo* survival characteristics of antibodies and recruitment of host effector functions. The prototypical immunoadhesin was CD4IgG, which was used to target gp120-expressing cells infected with human immunodeficiency virus[109] but may plausibly be extended to human tumor antigens for which ligands can be derived or for which effector cell antigens can be recruited (see the following section).

Bifunctional Antibodies

BFAs were devised to address two problems of ADCC. First, effector-target conjugate formation is inefficient due to competition with circulating Fc for FcR binding. Second, mouse antibodies, as noted, often fail to promote ADCC with natural human targets, even in the absence of competing IgG,[53] a difficulty partially addressed by "humanization" of antibodies.

BFAs improve conjugate formation by creating molecules that have dual specificities, one to the target cell and one to an "activator" antigen of the killer cell[110] (Fig. 29-9). BFAs direct killer cells—both K cells *and* T cells—to lyse targets dictated by the antibody specificity in a function called *effector cell retargeting*. In the case of K cells, the BFA substitutes through its anti-FcR (anti-CD16) moiety a high-affinity antigen-antibody interaction for a low-affinity, nonspecific Fc-FcR interaction, with a marked improvement in conjugate formation and target cell lysis, even in the presence of human serum. In the case of T cells, the BFA recruits an entirely new cell class into antibody-directed killing. With the binding of anti-CD3 to the CD3 antigen, the T cell is stimulated into a killing mode, bypassing the normal major histocompatibility complex and antigen-specific restrictions of T-cell killing.

1) heteroconjugate

complete immunoglobulins,
chemically cross-linked,
multimeric form,
multivalent

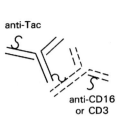
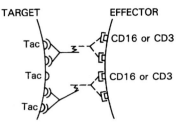

2) bispecific

hemi globulins,
native disulfide linkage,
(hybrid hybridomas or
disulfide exchange)
monomeric form,
bivalent

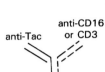
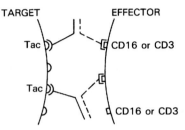

FIGURE 29-9. Schematic of bifunctional antibodies as conjugates versus quadroma (hybrid hybridoma) products.

CD16 and CD3 each involve proteins that are central to the killing mechanisms of LGLs and cytotoxic lymphocytes. The CD3 antibodies are mainly directed against the ε chain of the CD3 complex. Other surface antigens on these cells also have been used, generally to less effect,[110,111] although promising results with *tri*functional antibodies that are also anti-CD28 have been obtained.[112] Other FcRs have been targeted on monocytes-macrophages.[49]

Bifunctional constructs are generated by chemical processes, by chemical cross-linking (heteroaggregates) of complete IgG, by chain shuffling, by cross-linking of Fab' molecules, or by hybrid hybridoma (*quadroma*) technology.[113] These latter products are the most useful for therapy because they provide a continuous supply of monomeric IgG products with normal *in vivo* survivals; however, because ten combinations of heavy and light chains are predicted from the parental antibodies in the mix, of which only one is the desired BFA, purification by standard chromatographic methods may not be able to provide a pure BFA preparation.[114] On the other hand, aggregates and fragments prepared with high yield by other methods have abbreviated survivals *in vivo*. Newer genetic constructs are in preparation—single-chain BFAs, *fos-jun*–linked Fabs, immunoadhesin with antitumor antibody, and so on—whose efficacy and advantages will be determined over the near future. Bifunctional immunoadhesin antibody constructs have linked anti-CD3 antibody with hormones or cytokines to interact with receptor-bearing cells on tumor targets,[115,116] and other work is under way using B7 as an immunoadhesin in BFAs to recruit effector cells through CD28.

These constructs are typically markedly more active than the parental antibodies in net lysis of tumor cell targets, particularly when compared in the presence of human serum. BFAs can cure or prevent tumors in animal hosts in which unmodified antitumor antibodies are inactive.[117–120]

To date, clinical trials have been limited, but this is an area of great promise.

Antibody as Vector for Toxic Agents

Many of the deficiencies of antibodies in recruitment of host effector functions are being addressed by the methods described previously. Other approaches have bypassed this effort and instead have simply exploited the specificity and affinity of antibodies to direct cytotoxic agents against tumor cells. These toxic agents include chemotoxins, biotoxins, and radioisotopes. Radioimmunotherapies and diagnostics are discussed later.

Chemotoxins

Conjugates of antibody with anthracyclines and other chemotherapy agents have the potential to permit delivery of high doses of drug to antigen-expressing tumor cells while sparing nonexpressor normal cells from the toxic effects of the drug. Several studies have shown efficacy in animal models in which antibody alone and drug alone were ineffective.[121,122] As a rule, chemotoxins and biotoxins are expected to be more effective in cases in which the antigen is known to be internalized after antibody binding, as with the Lewis Y antigen targeted by BR96-doxorubicin conjugates.[122] This approach has been taken furthest with the anti-CD33 targeting of leukemia in patients using a humanized Ig conjugated to a small-molecule toxin (drug) calicheamicin (see later section on therapy).

A merging of BFA technology with chemotherapy delivery has been developed that displays an enzymatic activity which converts prodrug to active agent at the site of the tumor,[123] called *antibody-dependent enzyme-prodrug therapy* (ADEPT). The design of this therapy is dictated by a prob-

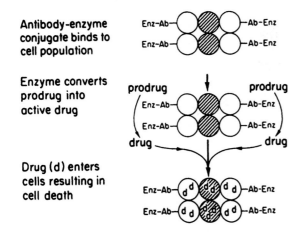

Antibody-enzyme conjugate binds to cell population

Enzyme converts prodrug into active drug

Drug (d) enters cells resulting in cell death

FIGURE 29-10. Schematic of antibody-dependent enzyme-prodrug therapy (ADEPT). (From Senter PD. Activation of prodrugs by antibody-enzyme conjugates: a new approach to cancer therapy. *FASEB J* 1990;4:188.)

lem common to all antibody-toxin/radioisotope approaches: the high body burden of toxin and nonspecific toxic effects at sites away from tumor. To circumvent this situation, antibody in the form of enzyme-conjugated antibody (ECA) is allowed to equilibrate to obtain optimal tumor penetration (Fig. 29-10). This process may take days because of issues related to tumor penetration. When antigen saturation is achieved and the tumor to normal ratio of ECA is optimal, then a low-molecular-weight prodrug is injected, which achieves rapid tumor penetration, converts to active drug, and attacks tumor. To accentuate this effect, the unbound ECA may be cleared from circulation by a second antibody to exaggerate the tumor to plasma ratio of ECA and minimize prodrug conversion except at sites of antibody binding. Optimizations of this strategy have been analyzed by Jain and co-workers.[124] Analogous approaches are under development in radiotherapies.[125]

Several animal studies have validated the principles of this approach. Clinical studies have been initiated,[126] but results are still too limited for conclusions on the potential of this method.

Biotoxins

In pioneering work by Pastan, Vitetta, and others, the application of extremely potent biotoxins to clinical cancer therapy was explored. The first-generation products were chemically cross-linked conjugates of antibody with unmodified toxins. Early studies determined that whole toxin molecules coupled with antibody were too toxic due to nonspecific uptake.[127] Molecular analysis of toxin domains ensued for the design of less nonspecifically toxic molecules. Three domains corresponded to specific functions, as exemplified by work with the *Pseudomonas* exotoxin (PE): *adherence,* causing nonspecific binding and

uptake, mainly by liver; *translocation,* responsible for moving the toxin from the endosomic vesicle to the cytoplasm; and *adenosine diphosphate ribosylation,* the enzymic activity that is responsible for inactivating elongation factor 2 and arresting protein synthesis.[128] In principle, a single molecule of toxin is sufficient to kill the cell. Studies were performed with diphtheria toxin, which acts similarly to PE, and with ricin, which inhibits protein synthesis by acting on the ribosome directly.

Modifications were made to eliminate or block the adherence domain, which led to a marked reduction in nonspecific toxicity. In addition, the discovery was made that the chemical coupling of toxins to antibody could be accompanied by a loss of specific activity of the toxin due to preferential use of key active-site lysines by the linkage. To bypass this, a genetic construct of PE was prepared that put into a single chain the antigen-recognition domain of the antibody (single-chain Fv) and a truncated version of the toxin[129] (Fig. 29-11). This construct, anti-Tac (single-chain Fv)–PE40, had high toxicity for antigen-expressing cells and no toxicity for antigen-negative cells; the concentration causing 50% inhibition (IC_{50}) was higher for lower-expressing cells, but in each case the IC_{50} corresponded to binding of approximately 100 antibody molecules per cell. A modification on this approach was to couple toxin to a receptor ligand in an IL-2–diphtheria toxin construct.[130] Several additional toxin constructs have been prepared with similar *in vitro* profiles of activity, including B4-blocked ricin[131] and CD22-ricin A for treating B-cell chronic lymphocytic leukemia and purging leukemic cells from autologous marrow grafts.[132,133] Excellent summaries of these applications are available.[127,134–136]

BFAs also have found a role in biotoxin delivery with an anti–ricin A chain × anti-CEA BFA for colon cancer[137] and an antisaporin × anti-CD22 BFA for lymphoma.[138] Unfortunately, none of these biotoxin molecular constructs has yet achieved significant clinical penetration due to persistence of hepatotoxicity in the clinical setting, despite removal or inactivation of adherence domains. The role of liver as a catabolic site for many absorbed proteins is the probable mechanism of this susceptibility. Whether other antibody-based strategies can be developed to take advantage of this potency while overcoming nonspecific effects is a subject of ongoing studies. A second major problem with these molecules is the rapid development of neutralizing antibodies directed at the toxin moiety.

Antibody as a Vector for Radioactivity

Labeling of antibodies with radioactive atoms is another major approach to antibody-based cancer treatment that has received considerable attention.[6] Although clinical results have not met the expectations generated by the initial animal studies, this approach remains promising and benefits from some inherent advantages over direct (passive) or

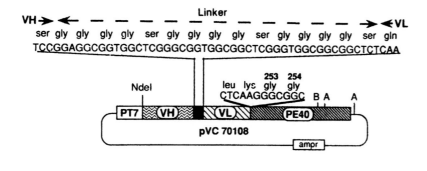

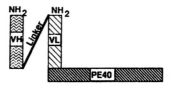

FIGURE 29-11. Single-chain Fv-PE40 toxin. (PE40, truncated version of *Pseudomonas* exotoxin; VH, variable region of the heavy chain; VL, variable region of the light chain.) (From Chaudary VK, Queen C, Junghans RP, et al. A recombinant immunotoxin consisting of two antibody variable domains fused to *Pseudomonas* exotoxin. *Nature* 1989;339:394.)

toxin-based immunotherapy. These advantages result from the use of radiation as the primary cytotoxic agent. The cytotoxic activity of radiolabeled antibodies is the result of electron or alpha-particle emissions that occur when the radionuclide decays while attached to an antibody that is attached to tumor-associated antigen. These emissions travel a distance that depends on their type (electron or alpha) and energy. As they travel, they deposit energy along their paths. If an adequate number of such emissions traverse a given tumor cell nucleus, the total energy deposited within the nucleus will kill the cell by causing an irreparable number of DNA strand breaks. A radiolabeled antibody attached to a particular tumor cell may also, because of the range and random direction of its emissions, kill adjacent tumor cells that do not express the antigen or that have not been reached by the radiolabeled antibody. Because of the range of the emissions, tumor cell kill is not necessarily dependent on internalization of the antigen-bound antibody, nor does it depend on any specific metabolic process of the tumor cell.

A further distinguishing feature of radiolabeled antibody therapy, the loss of cytotoxic activity due to the decrease in radioactivity over time arising from radioactive decay, also has important implications in comparison to passive or toxin-based immunotherapy. Depending on the clearance kinetics of the antibody and of the free radionuclide after detachment from the antibody, radionuclide loss due to decay may be either advantageous or disadvantageous. If the half-life of the radionuclide matches the uptake kinetics of the target tissue and the antibody remains tumor associated for a sufficient period of time, the decrease in radioactivity reduces normal tissue exposure once the antibody dissociates or is catabolized. Too short-lived a radionuclide will deliver the largest fraction of its decay energy to normal tissue before reaching the tumor. Too long-lived a radionuclide will deliver a small fraction of its decay energy to the tumor, because the time during which it is tumor associated is a small proportion of its total decay lifetime.

The radionuclide half-life also determines the rate at which radiation is delivered to the target cells (the dose rate). Depending on the repair rate of the target cells, this value may be more important than the total dose. A very long-lived radionuclide (i.e., one with a very low dose rate) may be incapable of eradicating tumor cells that exhibit a rapid repair capacity, because the cells may be capable of repairing the radiation-induced damage as it occurs. This phenomenon does not apply to alpha-particle emitters, because the energy deposited along each alpha-particle track and the ensuing potential damage to DNA are far greater than the repair capacity of cells.

Although it is not essential for tumor cell kill, an additional feature of some radionuclides that has permitted a detailed investigation of the *in vivo* pharmacokinetics of radiolabeled antibodies is the release of photons in addition to electron and alpha particles during decay. Relative to electron and alpha particles, photons deposit very little energy within tissue. Photon emissions of the appropriate energy (100 to 400 keV), however, can be imaged externally. Images of the spatial distribution of radiolabeled antibody within a patient at one or more times may be obtained using nuclear medicine scanners. After a low level of radioactivity is administered, such pharmacokinetic information can be used to assess antibody targeting and to determine the likelihood of tumor eradication or normal tissue morbidity before a therapeutic dose is given.

In addition to aiding in evaluation of therapeutic potential, antibodies that are labeled with an appropriate photon-emitting radionuclide also may be used for diagnosis. To avoid radiation-induced morbidity, low levels of radioactivity are used for radiolabeled antibody diagnosis (radioimmunodiagnosis). Radioimmunodiagnosis has been particularly useful in conjunction with computed tomography or magnetic resonance imaging in revealing sites of recurrent or metastatic disease in colorectal cancer patients.[139] In general, the detection efficiencies vary with cancer type, with the antibody and radionuclide used, and with the particular radioimmunodetection protocol.[6] Radiolabeled antibodies that are promising diagnostic agents for a given tumor type are also candidates for therapeutic use.

This brief introduction to the unique aspects of antibody therapy combined with radionuclides reveals some of the complexity of radioimmunotherapy. A large number of parameters must be chosen for each implementation of this treatment approach. The optimal implementation for one set of circumstances (disease type, location, radiosensitivity, patient treatment history) may not apply under a different set of conditions. The following section reviews some of the pharmacologic and dosimetric considerations associated with the implementation of radioimmunotherapy.

Pharmacology and Pharmacokinetics of Radiolabeled Monoclonal Antibodies

The pharmacokinetics of radiolabeled antibodies is difficult to describe in terms of average or typical kinetics. In general, *in vivo* behavior depends on the antibody, the target antigen, the radiolabel, and the patient's prior treatment history (i.e., exposure to mouse-derived antibody). The kinetics may change depending on whether the antibody is an intact IgG or a fragment and whether it cross-reacts with normal tissue. Antigens shed into the circulation also may affect antibody kinetics by complexing with and increasing the clearance rate of circulating antibody. Internalization of a cell-bound antibody-antigen complex may lead to catabolism of the complex followed by release of the radionuclide. Depending on the technique used to label the antibody, radionuclide also may be released while the antibody is in circulation. The kinetics of the free radionuclide reflect the pharmacokinetics of the parent element rather than that of the administered antibody. The most profound effect on antibody pharmacokinetics occurs once the administered antibody has elicited a human immune reaction. Mouse-derived antibodies elicit human antimouse activity (HAMA); humanized antibodies may elicit human antihuman activity (HAHA). The effect in both cases is usually rapid complexing with administered antibody followed by rapid clearance of the complex from the circulation. This phenomenon may eliminate the therapeutic activity of radiolabeled antibody, and thereby greatly reduce the applicability of radioimmunotherapy; the human immune reaction (HAMA or HAHA) usually precludes the use of multiple courses of radioimmunotherapy or the retreatment of patients who have undergone radioimmunotherapy.

Macroscopic Pharmacokinetics

As indicated earlier, the photon emissions of most radionuclides used in radioimmunotherapy allow for a detailed assessment of antibody pharmacokinetics. Measurement of the radioactivity in sequential blood samples is generally combined with gamma camera imaging and with whole-body or urine measurements or both. Imaging is rarely performed after a therapeutic administration, however, because the radioactivity in the patient exceeds the imaging (or counting) capacity of most nuclear medicine imaging devices. Imaging information obtained from a trace-labeled administration of antibody is used instead to project the kinetics of the therapeutic administration.

The distinction between a therapeutic and a tracer administration of antibody lies in the amount of radioactivity and type of radionuclide administered. A second parameter, the milligram amount of antibody that is administered, also may vary. These two parameters are related only to the extent that the labeling chemistry limits the number of radioactive atoms that may be attached to an antibody molecule without destroying its immunoreactivity. The radioactivity, expressed in megabecquerels (MBq) (millions of decays per second), may vary from a tracer or diagnostic administration of 20 to 200 MBq to a therapeutic administration of 2,000 to 15,000 MBq for iodine 131 (^{131}I), one of the most commonly used radionuclides in radioimmunotherapy. The very large range of values for therapy reflects the diversity of antibodies used and the range of patient responses. Doses as low as 1,000 MBq have elicited patient responses in B-cell lymphoma.[140] Alternatively, when tracer-based estimates are used to treat to the maximum normal tissue-absorbed dose (see the Dosimetry section for the definition of absorbed dose) and with a different antibody and antigen target, therapeutic administrations of as much as 22,000 MBq also have been used in the treatment of B-cell lymphoma.[141] A typical therapeutic administration of ^{131}I-labeled antibody is on the order of 5,000 MBq, administered intravenously over 20 to 60 minutes.

The milligram amount of antibody administered in either a diagnostic or therapeutic administration may range from 0.1 to 50 mg; a typical dose is 10 mg. For therapy, this value is generally chosen to ensure that the immunoreactivity of the antibody is not diminished significantly by the accompanying radioactivity. In some cases, a large excess amount of unlabeled antibody also may be administered to overcome binding to circulating antigen or cross-reactivity with normal tissue or to saturate the target antigen sites (see Therapeutic Interventions later).

Table 29-4 lists the early and late plasma clearance half-times as well as the whole-body clearance half-times, the urinary excretion rates, and the distribution volumes of a series of antibodies labeled with different radionuclides. Although the table is not exhaustive, the entries in it are representative of the various antibodies, radiolabels, and milligram amounts that have been used. Most of the studies listed are diagnostic, because such studies provide the greatest detail regarding antibody pharmacokinetics. The effect of different radionuclides on overall pharmacokinetics is illustrated in the two OC-125 F(ab')$_2$ studies[142,143] and also in the intact B72.3 studies.[144–147] In both cases the difference in plasma clearance half-time between the ^{131}I- and indium 111

TABLE 29-4. RESULTS OF STUDIES OF THE PHARMACOKINETICS OF RADIONUCLIDE-LABELED ANTIBODIES[a]

Ab, Label	Radio-nuclide	Amount (mg)	Plasma/serum $t_{1/2\alpha}$, $t_{1/2\beta}$ (h) — Intact Solid Tumor	Intact Hema. Malig.	F(ab')2 Solid Tumor	F(ab')2 Hema. Malig.	Fab' Solid Tumor	Whole Body $t_{1/2}$ (h)	Urinary Excretion (%ID/day)	V_d (L)	Comments	Ref.
48.7	^{131}I	2–10					2 ± 1	25			10 patients, no dependence on mg amount	231
OC 125	^{111}In	1			21 ± 7				7		13 patients, preinjection serum CA125 levels ranged from 0 to >500; no correlation between clearance and CA125 levels.	142
OC 125	^{131}I	0.5–1.0			30				25		5 patients; preinjection serum CA125 (the target antigen) levels ranged from 26 to 9,570 U/mL, no correlation between serum clearance and serum CA125 levels	143
19-9	^{111}In	1				5 ± 4, 27 ± 7			6		7 patients	142
ZME-018	^{111}In	2.5		1.5 ± 0.3, 18 ± 2					8.5 ± 2.5	4.6 ± 0.7	4 patients	149
ZME-018	^{111}In	5	25 ± 3						4.4 ± 0.3	4.0 ± 0.5	5 patients	149
ZME-018	^{111}In	10	3 ± 3, 28 ± 3						4.8 ± 0.4	3.6 ± 0.5	5 patients	149
ZME-018	^{111}In	20	29 ± 5						5.3 ± 0.3	4.4 ± 0.4	6 patients	149
T101	^{131}I	10			0.9 ± 0.5, 20 ± 6			43 ± 17	30 ± 12		5 patients, 200 to 480 MBq ^{131}I administered for diagnosis	232
T101	^{131}I	10–17		18 ± 7				36 ± 10			4 patients, 3,700 to 5,500 MBq ^{131}I administered for therapy	232
96.5	^{131}I	<2–20					90 ± 26				16 patients	150
96.5	^{111}In	1	27 ± 9						11.5 ± 3	8 ± 1	4 patients	151
96.5	^{111}In	2	36 ± 3						9.5 ± 1.5	7.5 ± 0.6	5 patients	151
96.5	^{111}In	5	32 ± 3						9 ± 1	4 ± 0.3	5 patients	151
96.5	^{111}In	10	31 ± 4						9 ± 2	4 ± 1	5 patients	151
96.5	^{111}In	20	31 ± 4						8 ± 1.5	3.4 ± 0.1	7 patients	151
96.5	^{111}In	20	30 ± 3						10.5 ± 4.5	3 ± 0.5	5 patients, ± SEM not SD	233
B72.3	^{131}I	0.3–20.0	65					82	14 ± 6		35 patients, no dependence on mg amount	144
B72.3	^{131}I	0.2–1.4	52 ± 10					79	16 ± 5		13 patients	145
B72.3	^{111}In	0.4–20.0	63 ± 5					283	3 ± 0.8		8 patients	145
B72.3	^{111}In	20		7 ± 5, 64 ± 14					4 ± 3		5 patients	146

Antibody	Isotope	Dose							Comments	Ref.
B72.3	^{111}In	0.2	41 ± 3				9 ± 1	4 ± 0.7	4 patients	147
B72.3	^{111}In	2	36 ± 5				6 ± 1	4 ± 0.7	6 patients	147
B72.3	^{111}In	20	33 ± 3				4.5 ± 0.5	2.4 ± 0.3	3 patients	147
ch B72.3	^{131}I	2–3		18 ± 4 230 ± 25		68			5 patients, ± SEM not SD	148
ZCE-025 (anti-CEA)	^{111}In	2.5	29 ± 8				19 ± 4	5 ± 1	4 patients, ± SEM not SD	152
ZCE-025 (anti-CEA)	^{111}In	5	27 ± 6				8 ± 1.5	5 ± 1	4 patients, ± SEM not SD	152
ZCE-025 (anti-CEA)	^{111}In	10	29 ± 6				12.5 ± 4	5 ± 2	5 patients, ± SEM not SD	152
ZCE-025 (anti-CEA)	^{111}In	20		38 ± 10			7.5 ± 2	5.5 ± 0.4	4 patients, ± SEM not SD	152
ZCE-025 (anti-CEA)	^{111}In	40	41 ± 6				5 ± 1	4.1 ± 0.4	7 patients, ± SEM not SD	152
ZCE-025 (anti-CEA)	^{111}In	80	39 ± 8				5 ± 2	4 ± 1	5 patients, ± SEM not SD	152
ZCE-025 (anti-CEA)	^{111}In	2–5			31 ± 5		6 ± 0.5	4.3 ± 0.2	8 patients, ± SEM not SD	162
ZCE-025 (anti-CEA)	^{111}In	10–20			38 ± 4		4.5 ± 0.5	3.6 ± 0.3	8 patients, ± SEM not SD	162
HMFG1	^{111}In	0.25		24 ± 3 58 ± 4	2.5 ± 1		2 ± 0.5		6 patients	234
HMFG1	^{111}In	0.25		16 ± 2 95 ± 24	48 ± 5		2 ± 0.6		7 patients	234
ch 17-1A	^{131}I	10		19 ± 3 106 ± 30					5 patients	85
ch 17-1A	^{131}I	40		16 ± 2 86 ± 7					5 patients	85
ch 17-1A	^{131}I	0.5–0.7				43			5 patients, ± SEM not SD	148
MB-1 (anti-CD37)	^{131}I	0.5 mg/kg		12–30		17–30			10 patients, ranges are shown	141
MB-1 (anti-CD37)	^{131}I	2.5 mg/kg		9–70		20–46			10 patients, ranges are shown	141
MB-1 (anti-CD37)	^{131}I	10 mg/kg		9–74		37–77			10 patients, ranges are shown	141
NP4 (Immu-4, anti-CEA)	^{123}I	1			2 ± 3 34 ± 25				11 patients, plasma CEA values ranged from 2.3 to 1,074 µg/L	235
NP4 (Immu-4, anti-CEA)	^{99m}Tc	1				0.7 ± 0.5 13 ± 5			5 patients, plasma CEA values ranged from <3.2 to 285 µg/L	235
NP4 (Immu-4, anti-CEA)	^{131}I	<1		2 ± 2 29 ± 14					24 patients	33

(continued)

TABLE 29-4. (*continued*)

Ab, Label	Radio-nuclide	Amount (mg)	Plasma/serum $t_{1/2\alpha}$, $t_{1/2\beta}$ (h)					Whole Body $t_{1/2}$ (h)	Urinary Excretion (%ID/day)	V_d (L)	Comments	Ref.
			Intact		F(ab')2		Fab'					
			Solid Tumor	Hema. Malig.	Solid Tumor	Hema. Malig.	Solid Tumor					
NP4 (Immu-4, anti-CEA)	131I	1–2.5		5 ± 4 49 ± 27								23 injections	33
NP4 (Immu-4, anti-CEA)	131I	5–16		6 ± 3 44 ± 22							33 injections (some patients were also injected with 1–2.5 mg 2 wk before the 5–16 mg injections)	33
C110 (anti-CEA)	111In	5–20		34 ± 14						3 ± 0.6	12 patients, serum CEA values ranged from 0.6 to 2,546 ng/mL; serum clearance was unaffected by Ab dose or by CEA levels. Clearance of antibody (150 MW peak on HPLC) also measured separately in serum; $t_{1/2}$ = 22 ± 8 h, V_d = 3 ± 2 L	153
C110 (anti-CEA)	111In	5–20	38 ± 9						4 ± 2	3 ± 0.6	21 patients; plasma CEA titers up to 500 ng/mL did not influence serum half-life, also no dependence on mg amount	154
OKB7 (anti-EBV)	131I	0.1–40.0			2 ± 2 27 ± 16			25 ± 9	28 ± 10		18 patients, no effect of mg amount on serum kinetics. A patient with $t_{1/2\beta}$ of 115.5 and another patient with total body $t_{1/2}$ of 227 excluded in calculating mean and SD for this table.	155
A33	131I	0.2–50		6.3, 38.5						3.6	17 patients, no effect of mg amount on serum kinetics	156
LL2	131I	0.2–3.9			2 ± 1 32 ± 13				43 ± 23		13 patients	140
LL2	131I	0.2–3.9				4 ± 3 30 ± 7			46 ± 13		6 patients	140
M195 (anti-CD33)	131I	6–76			2 ± 1 56 ± 21			57 ± 26		4 ± 2 L/m2	10 patients, no effect of mg amount on serum kinetics	157
NR-LU-10	186Re	40		5 ± 3 26 ± 5 (n = 12)					11 ± 2		12 patients; 3 patients	236
NR-CO-02	186Re	46			14 ± 7				36 ± 17		20 patients	236

Antibody	Isotope	Dose	$t_{1/2}$		Patients/comments	Ref
NR-CO-02	^{99m}Tc	46		11 ± 5	43 ± 16	20 patients	236
Lym-1	^{131}I	3–100	3 ± 3, 31 ± 11		33 ± 12	52 patients, unlabeled Ab administered 5 min before labeled Ab. No correlation between pre-dosing with cold Ab and blood kinetics observed.	161
BrE-3	^{111}In	10–100	9.5 ± 2.7, 56 ± 25		4 ± 2	15 patients, no significant difference in kinetics with increased Ab dose	158
G250	^{131}I	0.2–50	5.5, 47			16 patients, no effect of mg amount on serum kinetics	159

[a]When two values are given for $t_{1/2}$, the first refers to the α, the second, to the β. When a single value for $t_{1/2}$ is given, no definition of α or β half-lives was possible.
Ab, antibody; CA125, cancer antigen 125; CEA, carcinoembryonic antigen; EBV, Epstein-Barr virus; Hema. malig., hematologic malignancy; HPLC, high-pressure liquid chromatography; ID, injected dose; MW, molecular weight; SD, standard deviation; SEM, standard error of the mean; $t_{1/2}$, clearance half-time; V_d, volume of distribution. Values are mean ± standard deviation unless otherwise noted.

(^{111}In)–labeled antibodies is negligible, which indicates that *antibody* pharmacokinetics and catabolism are the same. The second set of B72.3 studies, however, which was specifically designed to compare the radioisotope biodistribution of B72.3 labeled with ^{111}In versus that labeled with ^{131}I in colorectal cancer patients,[145] found markedly different organ pharmacokinetics for the different isotopes and a corresponding difference in the urinary excretion rates. Hepatic clearance of ^{131}I-B72.3 followed blood pool clearance.[144] In contrast, ^{111}In-B72.3 exhibited a rapid uptake in liver with negligible clearance over the next several days.[145] In general, except for ^{131}I accumulation in the thyroid, ^{131}I catabolites clear more rapidly than ^{111}In catabolites, which exhibit a prolonged residence time in the liver. A number of radionuclides have been considered for radioimmunotherapy, and as in the case described earlier, each exhibits its own kinetics once separated from the antibody.

The fourth series of B72.3 studies examined the biodistribution of ^{111}In-B72.3 in breast cancer patients at three different antibody doses.[144] Consistent with the first set of studies,[145–147] plasma clearance half-time was found to be independent of the amount of administered antibody. The measured value, however, was found to be approximately one-half that obtained in the previous two studies of ^{111}In-B72.3 in colon cancer patients. A possible explanation for the difference in plasma antibody kinetics lies in the distribution of antigen. Specifically, the number of available antigen sites and their accessibility (e.g., the fraction in circulation) could influence antibody pharmacokinetics. Alternatively, differences in the labeling chemistry could account for the more rapid clearance.

The last B72.3 study[148] listed in Table 29-4 shows the effect of chimerizing (or humanizing) mouse-derived antibodies. The clearance half-times for chimeric B72.3 is strikingly longer than that for the mouse-derived antibody. This increased plasma clearance half-time is also seen with the chimeric version of 17-1A. Although the clearance half-times are not equal to those of human antibodies, the decreased immunogenicity of the chimeric antibodies leads to clearance half-times that begin to approach those of human antibodies. If antibody clearance kinetics is influenced primarily by binding to circulating tumor cells, as in the targeting of hematologic malignancies, the clearance half-time of a chimeric or humanized antibody may not increase to the extent observed for a solid-tumor antibody.[81]

A number of studies have examined the relationship between the amount of antibody administered and the resulting pharmacokinetics.[141,144,147,149–160] In most cases, a (non–statistically significant) trend toward longer plasma clearance half-times is observed with increasing milligram dose. In those cases in which a statistically significant effect is observed,[33,141,151,160] the results may be due to diminished binding and removal of antibody from the circulation once target antigen sites are saturated. The relationship between serum pharmacokinetics and antibody dose is

therefore likely to depend on the available antigen sites and their distribution relative to the milligram amount of administered antibody. Antibodies that exhibit such dependence generally yield improved diagnostic[6,160] and therapeutic results[141] when the dose is increased.

The plasma clearance half-times of antibodies that target hematologic malignancies are generally shorter than those of solid tumor antibodies. In hematologic malignancies, the half-time of the first component of plasma clearance is on the order of 1 to 3 hours.[140,155,157,161] This is thought to reflect rapid binding of antibody to circulating and therefore readily available target antigen sites. Except for antibodies that target antigen which is also released in circulation, the plasma clearance curves for solid tumor antibodies are generally fit by a single-exponential or double-exponential curve in which the half-time of the rapid component is on the order of 3 to 10 hours.

To improve targeting, reduce immunogenicity, and increase plasma clearance (i.e., background) kinetics, radiolabeled F(ab')$_2$ and Fab fragments have been developed. Such fragments have yielded improvements in radioimmunodiagnosis by increasing the target-to-background concentration ratio.[6,162] The anticipated reduction in immunogenicity due to the absence of a murine Fc region has been minimal.[163] In the context of radioimmunotherapy, *urinary excretion* refers to the amount of radiolabeled, not intact, antibody that is collected in the urine. The molecular weight of the labeled moiety is not usually measured. As Table 29-4 demonstrates, the urinary excretion is heavily dependent on the radionuclide used; the excretion rate for ^{131}I-labeled antibodies is three to four times greater than that for ^{111}In-labeled antibodies. This difference occurs despite the generally similar plasma clearance kinetics of antibodies labeled with these two radionuclides. Because urinary excretion reflects the fate of the radiolabel after antibody catabolism, the expectation is that this parameter should be most heavily dependent on the radionuclide.

Due to the 150-kd molecular weight of the antibody, the initial distribution of intravenously administered antibody is generally confined to the vascular space and to the extracellular space of tissues that lack a fully developed capillary basal lamina (e.g., marrow, liver, spleen, and other tissues of the reticuloendothelial system).[164,165] In a 70-kg man, this volume is approximately 4 L, that is, it modestly exceeds plasma volume. Significantly higher "apparent" distribution volumes may be observed when targeting tumor cells that are rapidly accessible to intravenously administered radiolabeled antibody.[157] In such cases, antibody binding to tumor cells provides an alternative mechanism for the rapid reduction in plasma concentration.

Alternative Administration Routes

Alternative injection routes have been examined to overcome two significant limitations of radioimmunotherapy: inade-

TABLE 29-5.   ANTIBODY PHARMACOKINETICS IN RADIOIMMUNOTHERAPY BY INJECTION ROUTE

	Intralymphatic/Subcutaneous	Intraperitoneal	Intrathecal
Clearance half-time	20–30 h (from injection site)	30–67 h (from peritoneum)	~38 h (from CSF)
Maximum blood value, time reached	12% ID at 1 d	2–30% ID at 1–3 d	21% ID at 1 d
Dose-limiting toxicity	Marrow/injection site	Marrow	Neurologic and marrow
References	171, 222, 223	47, 166, 237–240	241, 242

CSF, cerebrospinal fluid; ID, injected dose per gram.

quate antibody delivery and red marrow toxicity. The pharmacokinetic aspects of these efforts are summarized in Table 29-5. In most cases the red marrow remains a dose-limiting organ. Comparisons of antibody concentration in biopsy samples after intraperitoneal versus intravenous antibody administration have yielded mixed results.[166,167] No consequential improvement for the intraperitoneal route was observed when large nodules[166] or extraperitoneal micrometastases were targeted.[164] Intraperitoneal injection did demonstrate 4- to 70-fold improvement over intravenous administration in targeting of peritoneal implants[167] and ascites cells.[166]

Microscopic Pharmacokinetics

The molecular weight of the antibody isotype most commonly used for cancer treatment, IgG, is 150 kd. In contrast, the molecular weight of most chemotherapeutic agents is less than 1 kd. The larger molecular weight of antibodies raises issues that are not generally relevant to targeting of chemotherapeutic agents. To reach antigen-positive cells, intravenously administered antibody must cross the capillary basal lamina and then must traverse the extravascular space of solid tumor.

In most normal organs, the capillary basal lamina would present a substantial barrier to traversal of a 150-kd protein.[168] Due to the "leaky" nature of tumor vasculature,[169–172] this barrier is greatly diminished in tumors, and passage of antibodies is close to that of low-molecular-weight chemotherapeutic agents. The vascular permeability coefficient of tumor capillaries for methotrexate, for example, ranges from 1 to 10 $\times 10^{-6}$ cm per second[173]; the corresponding value for IgG is 0.6×10^{-6} cm per second.[172] Once the antibody is on the extravascular side of the capillary, it must cross the interstitial space to reach antigen-positive cells. For most chemotherapeutic agents, such transport occurs by diffusion.[173] A typical low-molecular-weight cytotoxic agent (350 d) has a diffusion coefficient in the interstitial space of tumor of approximately 6.4×10^{-6} cm^2 per second.[174] The corresponding value for IgG antibody ranges from 0.005 to 0.015×10^{-6} cm^2 per second.[175] These values translate into 4 seconds (for the low-molecular-weight cytotoxic agent) versus 0.5 to 1 hour (for the antibody) to achieve 16% of the source concentration at a 100-mm distance.[175] Antibody transport across the interstitial space is therefore primarily dependent on bulk fluid flow or convection. Such flow relies on a positive pressure difference between the periphery and the tumor center.

Measurements of the interstitial pressure in solid tumors have consistently found significantly higher levels than in normal tissues.[176,177] This pressure is thought to arise because solid tumors do not have completely developed lymphatics. In normal tissue, vascular fluid that filters into the interstitial space and is not reabsorbed into the microvascular network is taken up by lymphatic vessels. In solid tumors such vessels may not exist or may be inadequate to reabsorb excess interstitial fluid rapidly enough. Tumor cell proliferation also may diminish the available interstitial space and further increase the interstitial pressure. Eventually, such fluid may be reabsorbed by the lymphatic vessels of surrounding normal tissue.[178] Consistent with this is the finding that interstitial pressure increases with the size of the tumor.[178] Such interstitial fluid pressure presents a significant physiologic barrier to antibody penetration of large solid tumors and may help explain the highly nonuniform distribution of antibody in solid tumors as well as observations of increased antibody uptake in smaller tumor cell clusters.[179]

A further barrier to antibody penetration of a cluster of antigen-positive cells is the *binding-site barrier phenomenon*.[180,181] The binding-site barrier arises as a result of the low antibody concentration in the tumor interstitial space relative to the local antigen concentration. [The local concentration of antigen sites depends on the number of antigen sites per cell (typically 10^4 to 10^6) and the number of cells per unit volume.] The antibody is, in effect, prevented from diffusing to the interior of the solid tumor until the antigen sites in the periphery are occupied. In systems in which interstitial pressure is not of concern (e.g., *in vitro* tumor cell spheroids or micrometastases), the binding-site barrier may, depending on the concentration of antibody, yield a highly nonuniform distribution of antigen-bound, radiolabeled antibody, with very high concentrations in the periphery and negligible amounts in the center.[182,183]

CONSIDERATIONS SPECIFIC TO RADIOIMMUNOTHERAPY

Dosimetry

Dose in the context of chemotherapy is fundamentally different from the therapeutically relevant quantity in radioimmunotherapy. The quantity of a cytotoxic agent that is delivered to a patient in the chemotherapeutic context is generally the amount in milligrams or the area under a blood time × concentration curve. The latter provides a measure of the drug's residence time in the circulation. The radioimmunotherapeutic equivalents are *activity* (also often referred to as *dose*) in megabecquerels (millions of radionuclide decays per second) and cumulated activity in megabecquerels × seconds (total number of radionuclide decays). The cumulated activity need not be limited to blood circulation. For solid tumors in particular, one is interested in the cumulated activity of the tumor. Using external imaging at various times after antibody administration to obtain a time-activity curve that is then integrated over time, one may obtain the cumulated activity for tumor or other tissues. The therapeutically relevant quantity for radioimmunotherapy, however, is the *absorbed dose* (also often referred to as the *dose*) in grays (energy absorbed per unit volume of tissue). This value is obtained by multiplying the total number of decays that have occurred in a given tissue (i.e., the cumulated activity) by the total energy released per radionuclide decay and by a factor that accounts for the fraction of emitted energy that is absorbed within the tissue. This fraction depends on the tissue's geometry and the energy (or range) of each radionuclide emission. The resulting absorbed-dose estimate only accounts for emissions that occur within the given tissue. Depending on the range and type of radionuclide emissions, radioactivity in other organs also may contribute to the total absorbed dose of a given target organ. Contributions from other organs are calculated as described earlier, except that the geometric factor reflects the fraction of emitted energy in a source organ that is absorbed by the given target organ. The total target tissue absorbed dose is then obtained by adding the absorbed dose contributions from all the source organs to the target tissue self-dose. The procedure described here has been developed by the Medical Internal Radiation Dose Committee.[184] The absorbed dose to a given organ is a much more precise measure of cytotoxic potential than the administered activity or the cumulated activity, because the pharmacokinetics and the radionuclide properties are accounted for by the absorbed-dose value.

The red marrow is the dose-limiting organ in most implementations of intravenously administered radiolabeled antibody.[185,186] Marrow vasculature, unlike that of most normal organs, is fenestrated and does not present a significant barrier to antibody penetration.[162] The red marrow is composed of cells that are continuously undergoing cell division and that are therefore more radiosensitive.[187] These two factors—early accessibility and enhanced radiosensitivity—account for the marrow toxicity that is observed in almost all radiolabeled-antibody dose-escalation studies.

Studies performed with radioiodine for the treatment of thyroid cancer as well as experience gained from external-beam irradiation suggest that 2 to 4 Gy may be delivered to the marrow before significant marrow toxicity is observed.[186] Higher absorbed doses may be delivered if cytokines are used

to reduce hematopoietic suppression.[188] The marrow absorbed dose from radiolabeled antibody that does not bind to components of the marrow, blood, or bone is generally obtained by assuming that marrow kinetics is the same as that of blood and multiplying by a factor to account for the different antibody concentrations in the two volumes.[186,189] In hematologic disease, antibody binding to specific blood or marrow components occurs and must be considered in determining the red marrow absorbed dose. In this case, imaging of a marrow-rich, low-background region (e.g., head and neck of the femur), in combination with one or more bone marrow biopsies, is generally used to obtain a time-activity curve for red marrow dosimetry.[190,191] Red marrow absorbed-dose estimates are particularly important because prediction of toxicity from the amount of radioactivity administered is very difficult. In the treatment of B-cell lymphoma, for example, a 1,850-MBq dose of ^{131}I-labeled LL2 antibody led to grade IV marrow toxicity[140]; in contrast, doses of 7,400 MBq ^{131}I-labeled OKB7 antibody have been administered to patients without evidence of significant toxicity.[155]

Several of the radioimmunotherapy protocols for patients with hematologic disease include a bone marrow transplant component. In such protocols, the red marrow is no longer the dose-limiting organ, and preliminary results suggest that lung or liver morbidity may limit the total dose that can be administered.[192,193] In such cases, determination of the spatial distribution of absorbed dose and a dose-volume histogram for the actual organ volume of each patient are necessary to assess the probability of normal tissue morbidity. Although techniques for determining the spatial distribution of absorbed dose by performing three-dimensional dosimetry have been developed,[194,195] a key obstacle to their clinical implementation has been the difficulty associated with obtaining accurate, patient-specific, three-dimensional biodistribution data. Ongoing improvements in quantitative imaging with single photon emission computed tomography may eventually overcome this difficulty.

Radionuclide Choice

A unique and fundamental feature of radioimmunotherapy is the availability of a large number of radionuclides that may be used in conjunction with the antibody to deliver the cytotoxic radiation. Selection of the most appropriate radionuclide for a given implementation of radioimmunotherapy[196] is an important area of research and one that is evolving as the issues of antibody targeting and heterogeneity become better understood.[197–200] The following characteristics must be taken into consideration when deciding on the appropriate choice for radioimmunotherapy: availability (cost), labeling chemistry, *in vivo* toxicity of the free label, half-life, range, energy, and type of emissions. The first three impose constraints on the radionuclides from which one may choose. Optimization of the remaining four depends on the pharmacokinetics of a given antibody and on the characteristics of the tumor target. As indicated earlier, the distribution of radiolabeled antibody in solid tumor is generally nonuniform. To improve the spatial uniformity of the resulting absorbed-dose distribution, radionuclides that emit long-range electrons have been investigated. One such radionuclide, yttrium 90 (^{90}Y), has a 2.7-day half-life and emits electrons (beta particles) with an average energy of 935 keV (90% of the energy is deposited within 5.3 mm).[201] The long emission range is ideal for depositing energy in regions that have not been reached by the radiolabeled antibody (this is referred to as the *cross-fire* or *dose-enhancement effect*).[202] In targeting hematologic disease or small tumor cell clusters (micrometastases), however, in which the source to target distance is on the order of 6 to 100 mm (distance from cell surface to nucleus and radius of a cell cluster, respectively), use of ^{90}Y is inappropriate because only a very small fraction of its emission energy will be absorbed within the target region.[203] Under such circumstances, a radionuclide with shorter-range emissions such as iodine 123 (90% of the energy of which is deposited within a 180-mm radius) is more appropriate. The most frequently used radionuclide for radioimmunotherapy, ^{131}I, has a half-life of 8 days, and 90% of its energy is deposited within 830 mm. In practice, most of the radionuclides that have been used for radioimmunotherapy have been selected based on prior clinical experience (e.g., ^{131}I treatment of thyroid cancer) and because the chemistry of labeling the antibody had been well established (e.g., chloramine-T, iodogen methods for ^{131}I).[204,205]

Alpha Particle Emitters

Although the extensive experience with and easy availability of ^{131}I have made it the most commonly used radionuclide for antibody therapy, this agent is not ideal for targeting disseminated disease. Given the number of antigen sites per cell for most antibodies, the achievable specific activity, and the limitations on the amount of ^{131}I that may be administered due to red marrow toxicity, ^{131}I-labeled antibodies are not capable of single-cell kill.[206]

Alpha particles are effective cytotoxic agents, capable of achieving single-cell kill without causing dose-limiting morbidity.[207] Alpha particles are effective because the amount of energy deposited per unit distance traveled (linear energy transfer) is approximately 400 times greater than that of beta particles (80 keV per μm versus 0.2 keV per μm). Each traversal of an alpha particle through the nucleus results in a very highly ionizing track. Cell survival studies have shown that alpha-particle–induced killing is independent of oxygenation state or cell-cycle stage during irradiation and that a single track across the nucleus may result in cell death.[208–209a] Most studies of the use of alpha-particle-emitting radionuclides for therapy have examined either bismuth 212 (^{212}Bi) or astatine 211.[210] Both radionuclides are short-lived, with 61 minute and 7.2 hour half-lives. Both agents emit alpha particles whose range is 40 to

80 mm. In rapidly accessible, disseminated disease, these radionuclides have demonstrated a significant curative potential with minimal toxicity.

Although use of ^{212}Bi has shown promise in animal models, its use in patients has not been examined. Instead, the first human trial of an alpha particle emitter was conducted with bismuth 213 (^{213}Bi). Bismuth 213 which, like ^{212}Bi, is available in a generator system, has a half-life of 45.6 minutes and a branched decay scheme that is similar to that of ^{212}Bi but without the high frequency of energetic and potentially hazardous (2.6 MeV) photon emissions found in ^{212}Bi. The highly stable CHXA-diethylenetriamine pentaacetic acid chelate has been used for labeling the antileukemia antibody HuM195 with ^{213}Bi.[211,212] To date, 18 patients have participated in a phase I study of this agent without evidence of significant extramedullary toxicity. Dosimetry and pharmacokinetics associated with this trial have been described.[213] Astatine 211 has also entered human trials.[210]

Two radionuclides that decay with a longer half-life have been proposed for targeting tumor cells that are not rapidly accessible: radium 223 (^{223}Ra) and actinium 225 (^{225}Ac). Radium 223 has an 11.4-day half-life and may be obtained from a generator system using an actinium 227 parent (21.8-year half-life). The first three decays of ^{223}Ra yield three alpha particles in rapid succession.[214] These are then followed by the emission of another alpha particle that is delayed by approximately 40 minutes, with a beta-emitting lead intermediate that could localize to the red blood cells. Actinium 225 has a 10-day half-life, and a generator system has been described[215] that is based on the decay of thorium 229. The first three decays of ^{225}Ac also yield three alpha particles in rapid succession before ^{213}Bi is reached.

Therapeutic Interventions

Almost all interventions in radioimmunotherapy are designed either to increase the concentration of antibody in the tumor or to reduce marrow toxicity. Table 29-6 lists several of the approaches that have been considered. Most of the proposed approaches are still under preclinical evaluation. All the approaches listed have achieved their intended effect to some extent. The cold-hot-chase approaches include variations of the biotin-avidin technique in which radionuclide-free biotinylated antibody is allowed to distribute and bind to tumor-associated antigen over several days. Once the free antibody has cleared from the body, labeled avidin is administered that is smaller and therefore more rapidly localizing.[216,217] This approach reduces normal tissue exposure, because antibody binding to antigen occurs while the antibody is unlabeled. The subsequently injected labeled avidin rapidly binds to antibody-bound biotin, which thereby delivers the radionuclide to tumor cells faster than could a radiolabeled antibody. The cold-hot-chase category also includes attempts to improve antibody targeting by increasing the milligram amount that

TABLE 29-6. THERAPEUTIC INTERVENTIONS IN RADIOIMMUNOTHERAPY

Intervention	Agent/Manipulation	Ref.
Increase vascular permeability	Tumor necrosis factor	243
	Hyperthermia	244
	External radiation	245
	Interleukin 2	246
Increase tumor radiosensitivity	SR4233	247
	5-Iododeoxyuridine	248
Increase tumor delivery/reduce background	Cold-wait-hot	218
	Cold-wait-chase-hot	249
	Hot-wait-chase	250
	Immunoadsorption	251
Increase antibody expression	Interferon-γ	252
	Human interferon-α	233
Increase marrow radioresistance	Interleukin 1	188

is administered or administering unlabeled antibody before injection of the labeled agent.[203,218,219] The chaser techniques typically involve administering an antiantibody antibody a specified time after the labeled antibody has been administered. The antiantibody antibody complexes with circulating labeled antibody and increases its clearance rate, which thereby reduces background and marrow exposure.[220,221] These techniques have not been widely implemented, largely because they introduce a new series of parameters that are difficult to optimize (e.g., milligram amount of unlabeled antibody, time between the administration of labeled and unlabeled agent[203]) as well as an additional layer of complexity to an already relatively complex treatment modality. Several implementations of radioimmunotherapy have overcome the limitation imposed by red marrow toxicity by performing bone marrow transplantation when necessary.[141] This approach has allowed the administration of much larger doses of antibody.

TOXICITY OF ANTIBODY THERAPIES

Most native mAbs, whether rodent or human, are remarkably nontoxic, a fact that is perhaps not surprising, because most unconjugated mAbs are relatively nonpotent. Maximum tolerated doses are generally not reached in therapeutic trials of mAbs; their achievement may be irrelevant, because the goal of the mAb infusions is usually to saturate available target sites and deliver the maximum biologic response to the tumor. Hence, further increases in delivered doses may not improve killing and may have the theoretical adverse consequences of increased immunogenicity and more rapid modulation (loss) of cell surface protein targets.

The mAbs with the most potent activities *in vitro* (CMC or ADCC) tend to have the most prominent toxicities. Administration of R24 (anti-GD3) and CAMPATH-1H (CDW52), each a potent activator of the human immune system, result in fever, chills, and rigors in a dose-dependent manner.[82,224] Release of cytokines from targeted cells also may contribute to toxicity (see also trials section later). R24 also promotes generalized urticaria, often initiating at sites of melanoma. In principle, one would expect that toxicities of mAbs should relate to targeted tissues, neoplastic or normal. Hence, the more specific an mAb, the fewer toxic effects should be expected. The antibody 3F8, a potent activator of human complement, targets GD2 on neuroblastoma but also binds to GD2 on peripheral nerve, which results in a severe pain syndrome.[224] CAMPATH-1H is capable of killing normal as well as malignant lymphoid cells and depletes the lymphoid immune system as a consequence. This has resulted in a high rate of opportunistic infections in treated patients, including infections with herpes viruses, cytomegalovirus, and *Pneumocystis carinii*.[82]

HAMA is sometimes characterized as an adverse effect, but it is not generally a "toxicity." Treatment of patients with an active HAMA response does not appear to increase toxicity; it can lead to adverse consequences for pharmacokinetics, due to clearing of antibody.[225] Anaphylaxis has been reported in far fewer than 1% of infused patients.

Toxicities associated with conjugated mAbs are generally a consequence of the cytotoxic agent carried by the mAb. In other words, these are nonspecific toxicities. With radioconjugates, myelosuppression is prominent in all studies in which dose escalation is applied.[161,192,218,225–228] Autologous or allogeneic bone marrow transplantation is often required as a rescue in treated patients.[192,225,226] Toxin conjugates pose a special situation, and some unusual toxicities have been observed. Temporary hepatic damage, as evidenced by elevations in plasma liver enzyme function test results, and vascular leak syndromes, characterized by weight gain, edema, and hypoalbuminemia, are also seen.[127,128,131,133] Neurologic toxicity also has been observed, but this effect may be due to neural targeting.[229] The long-term consequences of therapy with mAb constructs are entirely unknown but are not expected to differ from those of the cytotoxic agent carried by the mAb.

CLINICAL TRIALS OF MONOCLONAL ANTIBODIES IN CANCER THERAPY

Dozens of different therapeutic clinical trials with mAbs or mAb constructs have been reported, in addition to numerous radioimmunodiagnostic studies. Only those of particular interest that illustrate important aspects of the different approaches to mAb therapy are addressed here.

Trials Using Native Rodent Monoclonal Antibody to Treat Solid Tumors

A number of trials have examined the use of native mAb, usually of mouse origin, for the treatment of solid tumors. Several trials have focused on the ganglioside targets GD2 and GD3, which are highly expressed on the surface of melanoma.[88,224,230,253,254] Gangliosides have served as surprisingly good targets because they are expressed in high numbers (millions of molecules per cell), do not down-regulate or mutate easily, and appear to be reliable targets for efficient CMC and ADCC. Major responses (complete and partial) were seen in these early phase I studies and have prompted additional trials. Protein antigens and high-molecular-weight sulfated antigens also have been targeted in melanoma with limited success.[255,256] Antibody therapy for colon cancers[257,258] and other carcinomas[259] has been studied extensively as well, and occasional responses have been reported in phase I studies. For the treatment of genitourinary cancers, renal-specific murine antibodies[260] and a murine antibody to prostate-specific membrane antigen[261] have entered phase I trials as well. These trials with murine mAb have demonstrated the remarkable tolerability of the drugs at a wide range of doses (up to several grams) but have been marked by high rates of HAMA (in up to 100% of patients). This fact is likely to limit the usefulness of any of these rodent mAbs.

Trials of antibody therapy for hematologic cancers began more successfully due to the accessibility of these cells to the drug.[3,4] Antitumor activity was seen in many patients but was usually incomplete and short-lived.[262] One unique approach showed early promising results. A series of trials in which low-grade lymphomas were treated using antiidiotype mAb (mouse mAb to the antigen-binding site of the patient-specific human Ig found on the surface of the B-lymphoma cells) has shown consistent response rates (40% to 60%) to the therapy, either alone or in combination with interferon-α or chemotherapy.[263,264] Some of the responses have been long-lasting, but relapse is the rule. Lymphoma escape and relapse are marked by mutations in the idiotype; the approach is also limited because a unique mAb must be prepared for each patient. The mechanism of action of these unconjugated mAbs is still unclear, because many are of murine isotypes not capable of effector activity. Most evidence suggests that the antiidiotypes induce signal transduction through the surface Ig and this leads to activation-induced cell death.

Another strategy achieving modest initial success has been to target the IL-2 receptor on tumors that require IL-2 as an autocrine or paracrine growth factor.[37,265–267] This includes adult T-cell leukemias and lymphomas. Major responses have been seen, but rapid relapse is common. Combinations of murine mAb with cytokines such as IL-2 to activate NK effector cells, or macrophage colony-stimulating factor to activate monocytes, are also under study.[65,268–270] Other novel approaches have included the targeting of the epidermal growth factor receptor,[271] which appears especially active in combination with other agents, or targeting of nontumor cell components of the cancers, such as the vasculature[272] or the stroma.[273]

Clinical Trials of Chimeric, Fully Humanized, and Human Monoclonal Antibodies

The frequent development of HAMA and its adverse effects on murine mAb pharmacokinetics have led to great efforts at producing human and part-human mAbs. To date, development of true human mAbs of appropriate specificity, isotype, and affinity has been limited due to the technical problems of their production. Much effort has therefore been directed toward the construction of partly human (chimeric) or more fully human (CDR-grafted) mAbs. Other than the ability of chimeric mAbs in some instances to mediate new effector functions by virtue of their new human Fc portions, chimeric mAbs appear to offer little advantage to murine mAbs, because a significant portion of the Ig remains of murine origin. Five CDR-grafted humanized mAbs have reached clinical trials in cancer therapy, including CAMPATH-1H against CDW52 of lymphomas, anti–Tac-H (IL-2 receptor CD25) for T-cell lymphoma and leukemias, HuM195 and CMA-676 against CD33 in myeloid leukemias, and antibodies against HER2 on the surface of breast and other carcinomas.[64,82,84,274–276] Importantly, several of the mAbs showed significant activity against their targets, minimal toxicity, and a marked reduction in HAMA compared with their murine counterparts. HuM195 has been used for up to 12 doses over 4 months without development of HAMA.[84] HuM195 has shown activity alone, at low and high doses, in patients with relapsed and refractory myeloid leukemias.[84,97,277] The responses were seen in patients with low tumor burden. In patients with acute promyelocytic leukemia, in whom residual leukemia can be assessed by reverse transcriptase–polymerase chain reaction for the t(15;17), infusions of unlabeled HuM195 into patients in "clinical" complete response were able to induce a "molecular complete response," defined as negative results by reverse transcriptase–polymerase chain reaction, in 50% of treated patients.[277] HuM195 and another anti-CD33 antibody conjugated to the chemotherapeutic agent colicheamycin, known as CMA-676,[275] are in late-stage trials for treatment of acute myeloid leukemia.

Food and Drug Administration–Approved Antibody Treatment of Cancer

Two mAbs have been approved for human use in the treatment of cancer. Rituximab is a chimeric anti-CD20 antibody now approved by the Food and Drug Administration for the treatment of B-cell non-Hodgkin's lymphoma. Multiple mechanisms of action of rituximab have been proposed, including complement fixation, ADCC, and direct cytotoxicity via apoptotic pathways activated by binding to

CD20.[278] Response rates (complete and partial) in low-grade lymphoma to the antibody alone are 48%.[279] When antibody therapy is combined with conventional chemotherapy, such as the combination of cyclophosphamide, hydroxydaunomycin, vincristine sulfate (Oncovin), and prednisone (CHOP), response rates over 90% are seen.[280] These data suggest that additive or synergistic effects, without significant toxicity, can be achieved by combination chemotherapy and immunotherapy.

The other antibody approved drug is Herceptin, a fully humanized antibody directed at the her2/neu antigen found on breast carcinomas and other cancers.[281] Like rituximab, trastuzumab (Herceptin) appears to act via multiple mechanisms, including sensitization of breast cancer cells to chemotherapy, on binding to its target.[282] Alone, it is cytostatic,[276] and it will probably be used largely in combination with other agents.[283]

Radioimmunotherapy for Hematopoietic Cancers

Hematopoietic cancers have been treated successfully with radiolabeled mAbs in a number of systems.[6] This is due to the accessibility of the cells to the vasculature, their relative radiosensitivity, and the large number of differentiation antigens available as cell surface targets. Current technology and pharmacologic issues have limited the success of this approach for the treatment of solid tumors or neuroblastoma[226] or for intraperitoneal (regional) infusions.[283,284] In general, radioimmunotherapy for solid tumors remains problematic.[285] In the early trials of radioimmunotherapeutic treatment of leukemia and lymphoma, antitumor activity was seen in the majority of patients. The isotope used most widely has been ^{131}I, not because it is the most effective but because it is inexpensive and is readily conjugated to mAbs through simple chemistry; it also provides a gamma emission for imaging and quantitative dosimetry, in addition to its cytotoxic beta emission. Trials against lymphoma antigens including CD5, CD20, HLA-DR, CD37, CD21, and idiotypes have shown variable myelosuppression but modest to absent extramedullary toxicity and objective response rates of 55% to 100%.[140–142,218,228,286–289] Nonmyeloablative use of ^{131}I anti-CD20 murine antibody is both safe and highly effective at doses below that which cause significant pancytopenia.[281] Similar data are available for an anti–HLA-DR antibody Lym-1.[289] Anti-CD20 agents labeled with ^{90}Y also appear promising.[290] One of the most promising strategies has been the use of high doses of conjugated ^{131}I, which are significantly toxic to the marrow, followed by autologous bone marrow reinfusion.[192,291] Complete responses are seen in most patients, and toxicity is limited to the marrow. These trials, however, have been limited to patients who displayed the best targeting in a pretreatment imaging study. The agent ^{131}I-BC8 (anti-CD45) appears to be effective at clearing the bone marrow of normal and leukemic cells before allogeneic bone marrow transplant.[292] Long-term survival has been seen in a significant fraction of patients treated in this manner. A high-dose approach also has been taken with ^{131}I-M195 (CD33) and HuM195[225,227] and with a similar mAb (p67)[293] in the treatment of myeloid leukemia. The agent ^{131}I-M195 mAb specifically targets the marrow and at high doses can kill 99% of leukemia cells, even with tumor burdens as high as 1 kg. Preliminary studies in which conventional allogeneic bone marrow transplant was performed after ^{131}I-M195 ablation in patients with refractory leukemia have resulted in high response rates (90%) in phase I trials with little apparent toxicity above that expected with an allogeneic transplant. At lower doses, this agent appears active against minimal disease in myeloid leukemia as well.[294]

Cancer Therapy with Immunotoxins

Although several trials of the use of immunotoxins to treat solid tumors have been conducted, pharmacologic reasons dictate that this strategy is also likely to be most effective for the hematopoietic neoplasms (reviewed in Multani and Grossbard[4] and Vitetta et al.[127]). Various forms of ricin, a plant toxin, conjugated to intact or fragmented Ig have been used extensively. Ricin is a heterodimer that is extraordinarily toxic in its native form. Removal of the binding (B) chain or chemical modification ("blocking") of its binding site has resulted in toxin constructs that are useful in humans.

A CD19-blocked ricin construct and a deglycosylated ricin A chain anti-CD22 construct have been used to treat B-cell lymphomas.[131,133,295–298] Some major responses have been seen, but the degree of success of this strategy may be limited by HAMA and antitoxin antibody, as well as by toxicities of ricin, which include vascular leak syndromes and hepatic damage (discussed earlier).

Conclusions Drawn from Clinical Studies

The mAbs are now proven to be both safe and effective anticancer therapies. In 2000, two agents are already approved for use in cancer in the United States. Although most mAbs for cancer therapy are largely still at the phase I and early phase II stages of investigation, a great deal can be learned that will direct the focus of future work. Several generalizations can be made:

First, many mAbs can be administered safely and can reach their target tissues. Most efficient delivery appears to occur with hematopoietic neoplasms and with small tumor burdens.

Second, and perhaps more important, rodent mAbs are highly immunogenic, and neutralizing human antibody responses develop in most patients except those who are very immunosuppressed (Table 29-7). This problem appears to be partly avoidable by the use of fully human-

TABLE 29-7. INCIDENCE OF HUMAN ANTIMOUSE ACTIVITY (HAMA) RESPONSES IN CLINICAL TRIALS OF MONOCLONAL ANTIBODIES (mABs)

Population of Patients	No. of Trials	No. of Patients	Incidence of HAMA (%)
Patients with solid tumors given murine mAb	9	167	74
Patients with hematopoietic tumors given rodent mAbs			
Lymphoid neoplasms	7	124	9
Myeloid neoplasms	3	32	54
Patients with solid tumors given chimeric mAbs	4	45	46
Patients with hematopoietic tumors given CDR-grafted mAbs			
Lymphoid neoplasms	1	2	0
Myeloid neoplasms	2	28	0

CDR, complementarity-determining region.
From P. Chapman, D.A. Scheinberg, *unpublished research.*

TABLE 29-8. CURRENT OBSTACLES TO MONOCLONAL ANTIBODY (mAB) TREATMENT OF CANCER

Biochemical and biologic instability
  Of the immunoglobulin
  Of the radionuclide or radiometal chelate
  Of the immunotoxin linkage
Difficulties in pharmacology
  Poor extravascular diffusion and penetration into tumors
  Rapid cell surface modulation of immune complexes
  Long half-lives (may also be an advantage with native mAb)
Immunogenicity of rodent-derived (and human?) mAb
Specificity and tumor heterogeneity
  Inadequate specificity and targeting of normal cells
  Excessive specificity and sparing of antigen-negative cells
Inadequate potency of native mAb
Toxicity
  Bystander cell kill by radioconjugates
  Normal cell kill by immunotoxins
  Allergic reactions (very rare)

ized mAbs and possibly of chimeric mAbs, but much additional study is required with longer dosing schedules to confirm this. Toxins also appear to be highly immunogenic in humans.

Third, mAbs without potent effector functions *in vitro* are not likely to be active against tumors *in vivo*. As a corollary, mAbs that are highly active either via ADCC or CMC (as with R24), via apoptosis (as with Rituximab), via ^{131}I (as with M195 or MB1), or via toxins (as with B4, blocked ricin) are active *in vivo*.

Fourth, the pharmacodynamics and kinetics of the large IgG structure are significant obstacles to the effective use of radiolabeled mAbs to treat solid tumors. Use of mAbs may be most appropriate for elimination of residual disease or in the adjuvant setting, an area in which it is difficult to confirm activity without large randomized studies. In contrast, even large numbers of leukemia and lymphoma cells are easily killed by radioimmunoconjugates, and this approach may well be the earliest effective use of mAbs.

CURRENT OBSTACLES TO MONOCLONAL ANTIBODY CANCER THERAPY

A number of significant obstacles have slowed successful therapeutic applications of mAbs (Table 29-8). Better chemical methods for attaching radionuclides or toxins to mAbs appear to be resolving some of the issues of biochemical stability. New approaches using antibody fragments or genetically engineered single-chain binding proteins may improve delivery to tumors, but the pharmacologic difficulties may still be significant. Rapid modulation of cell surface immune complexes, a phenomenon that reduces ADCC and CMC, can be used to advantage by coupling of

toxins or isotopes that require entry into the cell. Efficient delivery of the toxin to the appropriate subcellular compartment and retention of radionuclides within cells may still pose problems, however.

New methods of engineering rodent into humanized mAbs or of producing true human mAbs may resolve many of the issues related to HAMA (Table 29-7), but whether antiidiotype responses (directed to the mAb binding site, which by definition is unique and therefore a potential foreign antigen) will be seen after repeated doses is unknown.

One of the paradoxes of mAb-based therapies is that increasing the specificity of the agents may yield more avenues of tumor cell escape. Because native mAbs target and kill individual cells based on the presence of antigen, tumor cells that have little or no antigen may be spared any cytocidal effects. Antigen-negative cells are thus selected for later relapse.[299] In contrast, radioconjugates with long-range beta emissions may kill antigen-negative bystander cells[300] but will consequently have greater toxicity.

CONCLUSION

Monoclonal antibodies are versatile anticancer agents with wide-ranging potential for therapy. Two mAb-based agents have already been approved for the treatment of cancer. Most mAbs or their constructs remain in the early stages of clinical development. The mAbs are of great interest primarily because of their specificity. In addition, their long half-lives and ability to kill cells via a variety of mechanisms also make them attractive drugs. A nonimmunogenic, humanized mAb of appropriate specificity might be used repeatedly to block a receptor or to lyse tumor cells via ADCC or CMC or, when radioconjugated, to kill individual cells or a mass of cells within a large field. The likelihood is that, for the various reasons cited earlier, mAbs will not be curative alone except in the setting of residual cancer. Finally, mAbs may ultimately be most effective when integrated into combination therapeutic strategies involving chemotherapy, radiation therapy, and biologic therapy.

REFERENCES

1. Pressman D, Korngold L. The *in vivo* localization of anti-Wagner osteogenic sarcoma antibody. *Cancer* 1953;6:619.

2. Kohler G, Milstein C. Continuous culture of fused cells secreting antibody of predefined specificity. *Nature* 1975; 256:495.

3. Jurcic J, Scheinberg DA, Houghton AN. Monoclonal antibody therapy. In: Longo D, ed. *Cancer chemotherapy and biological response modifiers annual*, vol. 17. Amsterdam: Elsevier Medical Publishers, 1997.

4. Multani PS, Grossbard ML. Monoclonal antibody-based therapies for hematologic malignancies. *J Clin Oncol* 1998;15:3691.

5. Houghton AN, Scheinberg DA. Monoclonal antibodies: potential applications to the treatment of cancer. *Semin Oncol* 1986;13:165.

6. Wilder RB, DeNardo GL, De Nardo SJ. Radioimmunotherapy: recent results and future directions. *J Clin Oncol* 1996;14:1383.

7. Burrows PD, Cooper MD. B cell development in man. *Curr Opin Immunol* 1993;5:201.

8. Rosen FS, Cooper MD, Wedgwood RJP. The primary immunodeficiencies. *N Engl J Med* 1984;311:235.

9. Dorrington KJ, Petersen L. An *in vitro* system for studying the kinetics of interchain disulfide bond formation in immunoglobulin G. *J Biol Chem* 1974;249:5633.

10. Kabat EA, Wu TT, Perry HM, et al. *Sequences of proteins of immunologic interest*, 5th ed. Washington: US Government Printing Office, 1991:xiii. NIH publication 91-3242.

11. Morrison SL, Wright A. Antibody variable region glycosylation. *Semin Immunopathol* 1993;15:259.

12. Mueller BM, Reisfeld RA, Gillies SD. Serum half-life and tumor localization of a chimeric antibody deleted of the CH2 domain and directed against the disialoganglioside GD2. *Proc Natl Acad Sci U S A* 1990;87:5702.

13. Welling GW, Geurts T, van Gorkum J, et al. Synthetic antibody fragment as ligand in immunoaffinity chromatography. *J Chromatogr* 1990;512:337.

14. Travis J. Tracing the immune system's evolutionary history. *Science* 1993;261:164.

15. Gearhart PJ. Generation of immunoglobulin variable gene diversity. *Immunol Today* 1982;3:107.

16. Hunkapiller T, Hood L. Diversity of the immunoglobulin gene superfamily. *Adv Immunol* 1989;44:1.

17. Max EE. Immunoglobulins: molecular genetics. In: Paul WE, ed. *Fundamental immunology*. New York: Raven Press, 1989:235.

18. Walter MA, Surti U, Hofker MH, et al. The physical organization of the human immunoglobulin heavy chain gene complex. *EMBO J* 1990;9:3303.

19. Cooper MD. Current concepts: B lymphocytes. Normal development and function. *N Engl J Med* 1987;317:1452.

20. DuPasquier L. Ontogeny of the immune response in cold blooded vertebrates. *Curr Top Microbiol Immunol* 1973;61:37.

21. Perelson A. Immune network theory. *Immunol Rev* 1989;110:5.

22. Tonegawa S. Somatic generation of antibody diversity. *Nature* 1983;302:575.

23. Mason DW, Williams AF. Kinetics of antibody reactions and the analysis of cell surface antigens. *Handbook Exp Immunol* 1986;1:1.

24. Moore JP, McKeating JA, Haung Y, et al. Virions of primary human immunodeficiency virus type 1 isolate resistant to soluble CD4 (sCD4) neutralization differ in sCD4 binding and glycoprotein gp120 retention from sCD4-sensitive isoplates. *J Virol* 1992;66:235.

25. Dower SK, Ozato K, Segal DM. The interaction of monoclonal antibodies with MHC class I antigens on mouse spleen cells: I. Analysis of the mechanism of binding. *J Immunol* 1984;132:751.

26. Kaufman EN, Jain RK. Effect of bivalent interaction upon apparent antibody affinity: experimental confirmation of theory of using fluorescence photobleaching and implications for antibody bonding assays. *Cancer Res* 1992;52:4157.

27. Robb JR, Greene WC, Ruck CM. Low- and high-affinity cellular receptors for interleukin 2: implications at the level of Tac antigen. *J Exp Med* 1984;160:207.

28. Waldmann TA, Strober W. Metabolism: metabolism of immunoglobulins. *Prog Allergy* 1969;13:1.

29. Junghans RP. The Brambell receptor (FcRB): mediator of transmission of immunity and protection from catabolism for IgG. *Immunol Res* 1997;16:29.

30. Mogielnicki PR, Waldmann TA, Strober W. Renal handling of molecular weight proteins: I. I-chain metabolism in experimental renal disease. *J Clin Invest* 1971;50:901.

31. Waldmann TA, Strober W, Mogielnicki PR. The renal handling of low molecular weight proteins: II. Disorders of serum protein catabolism in patients with tubular proteinuria, the nephrotic syndrome, or uremia. *J Clin Invest* 1972;51:2162.

32. Meeker TC, Maloney DG, Miller RA, et al. A clinical trial of anti-idiotype therapy for B cell malignancy. *Blood* 1985;65:1349.

33. Sharkey RM, Goldenberg DM, Goldenberg H, et al. Murine monoclonal antibodies against carcinoembryonic antigen: immunological, pharmacokinetic, and targeting properties in humans. *Cancer Res* 1990;50:2823.

34. Schulz G, Cheresh DA, Varki NM, et al. Detection of ganglioside GD2 in tumor tissues and sera of neuroblastoma patients. *Cancer Res* 1984;44:5914.

35. Sela B-A, Ilipoulos D, Ghuerry D, et al. Levels of disialogangliosides in sera of melanoma patients monitored by sensitive thin layer chromatography and immunostaining. *J Natl Cancer Inst* 1989;81:1489.

36. Junghans RP, Carrasquillo JA, Waldmann TA. Impact of antigenemia on the bioactivity of infused anti-Tac antibody: implications for dose selection in antibody immunotherapies. *Proc Natl Acad Sci U S A* 1998;95:17527.

37. Waldmann TA, White DW, Goldman CK, et al. The interleukin-2 receptor: a target for monoclonal antibody treatment of human T-cell lymphotrophic virus I-induced adult T-cell leukemia. *Blood* 1993;82:1701.

38. Finkelman FD, Madden KB, Morris SC, et al. Anti-cytokine antibodies as carrier proteins. *J Immunol* 1993;151:1235.

39. Borsos T, Rapp HL. Complement fixation on cell surfaces by 19S and 7S antibodies. *Science* 1965;150:505.

40. Brown EJ, Joiner KA, Frank MM. Complement. In: Paul WE, ed. *Fundamental immunology*. New York: Raven Press, 1984:645.

41. Bindon CI, Hale G, Bruggemann M, et al. Human monoclonal IgG isotypes differ in complement activating function at the level of c4 as well as C1q. *J Exp Med* 1988; 168:127.

42. Greenspan NS, Cooper LJN. Intermolecular cooperativity: a clue to why mice have IgG3. *Immunol Today* 1992; 13:164.

43. Davitz MA. Decay-accelerating factor (DAF): a review of its function and structure. *Acta Med Scand Suppl* 1987;715:111.

44. Martin DE, Zalman LS, Muller-Eberhard HJ. Induction of expression of cell-surface homologous restriction factor upon anti-CD3 stimulation of human peripheral lymphocytes. *Proc Natl Acad Sci U S A* 1988;85:213.

45. Van de Winkel GJ, Capel JA. Human IgG Fc receptor heterogeneity: molecular aspect and clinical implications. *Immunol Today* 1993;14:215.

46. Simmons D, Seed B. The Fcγ receptor of natural killer cells is a phosphoinositol-linked membrane protein [later shown not PI-linked]. *Nature* 1988;333:568.

47. Walker MR, Woof JM, Bruggemann M, et al. Interaction of human IgG chimeric antibodies with the human FcR1 and FcR11 receptors: requirements for antibody-mediated host cell-target cell interaction. *Mol Immunol* 1989;26:403.

48. Giorda R, Rudert WA, Vavassori C, et al. NKR-P1, a signal transduction molecule on natural killer cells. *Science* 1990;249:1298.

49. Fanger MW, Shen L, Graziano RF, et al. Cytotoxicity mediated by human Fc receptors for IgG. *Immunol Today* 1989;10:92.

50. Barker E, Reisfeld RA. A mechanism for neutrophil-mediated lysis of human neuroblastoma cells. *Cancer Res* 1993; 53:362.

51. Ortaldo JR, Woodhouse C, Morgan AC, et al. Analysis of effector cells in human antibody-dependent cellular cytotoxicity with murine monoclonal antibodies. *J Immunol* 1987;138:3566.

52. Lanier LL, Ruitenberg JJ, Phillips JH. Functional biochemical analysis of CD16 antigen on natural killer cells and granulocytes. *J Immunol* 1988;141:3478.

53. Lovchick JC, Hong R. Antibody-dependent cell-mediated cytolysis (ADCC): analyses and projections. *Prog Allergy* 1977;22:1.

54. Gergely J, Sarmay G. The two binding-site models of human IgG binding Fc gamma receptors. *FASEB J* 1990; 4:3275.

55. Junghans RP, Waldmann TA, Landolfi NF, et al. Anti Tac-H, a humanized antibody to the interleukin 2 receptor with new features for immunotherapy in malignant and immune disorders. *Cancer Res* 1990;50:1495.

56. Junghans RP. A strategy for evaluating lymphokine activation and novel monoclonal antibodies in antibody-dependent cell-mediated cytotoxicity and effector cell retargeting assays. *Cancer Immunol Immunother* 1990;31:207.

57. Zalman LS, Brothers MA, Strauss KL. Inhibition of cytolytic lymphocytes by homologous restriction factor: lack of species restriction. *J Immunol* 1991;144:4278.

58. Bernstein I, Tamm M, Nowinski RC. Mouse leukemia: therapy with monoclonal antibodies against a thymus differentiation antigen. *Science* 1980;207:68.

59. Kodama K, Ghanta VK, Hiramoto NS, et al. Regression of MOPC 104E plasmacytoma with monoclonal anti-idiotype antibodies. *J Biol Response Mod* 1989;8:385.

60. Buschbaum DJ, Wahl RL, Normolle DP, et al. Therapy with unlabeled and I-131-labeled pan-B cell monoclonal antibodies in nude mice bearing Raji Burkitt's lymphoma xenografts. *Cancer Res* 1992;52:6476.

61. Honsik CJ, Jung H, Reisfeld RA. Lymphokine-activated killer cells targeted by monoclonal antibodies to the disialogangliosides GD2 and GD3 specifically lyse human tumor cells of neuroectodermal origin. *Proc Natl Acad Sci U S A* 1986;83:7893.

62. Schulz KR, Klarnet JP, Peace DJ, et al. Monoclonal antibody therapy of murine lymphoma: enhanced efficacy by concurrent administration of interleukin 2 or lymphokine-activated killer cells. *Cancer Res* 1990;50:5421.

63. Hamblin TJ, Cattan AR, Glennie MJ, et al. Initial experience in treating human lymphoma with a chimeric univalent derivative of monoclonal anti-idiotype antibody. *Blood* 1987;69:790.

64. Dyer MJ, Hale G, Hayhoe FG, et al. Effects of CAMPATH-1 antibodies *in vivo* in patients with lymphoid malignancies: influence of antibody isotype. *Blood* 1989;3:1431.

65. Munn DH, Cheung NK. Phagocytosis of tumor cells by human monocytes cultured in recombinant macrophage colony-stimulating factor. *J Exp Med* 1990;172:231.

66. Mylavaganam R, Sprinz PG, Ahn YS, et al. An animal model of alloimmune thrombocytopenia. I. The role of the mononuclear phagocytic system (MPS). *Clin Immunol Immunopathol* 1984;31:163.

67. Kirkman RL, Shapiro ME, Carpenter CB, et al. A randomized prospective trial of anti-Tac monoclonal antibody in human renal transplantation. *Transplantation* 1991;51:107.

68. Begley CG, Metcalf D, Nicola NA. Proliferation of normal human promyelocytes and myelocytes after a single pulse stimulation by purified GM-CSF or G-CSF. *Blood* 1988;71:640.

69. Ogasawara J, Watanabe-Fukanga R, Masashi A, et al. Lethal effect of the anti-Fas antibody in mice. *Nature* 1993;364:806.

70. Rouvier E, Luciani MF, Golstein P. Fas involvement in Ca 2+-independent T cell-mediated cytotoxicity. *J Exp Med* 1993;177:195.

71. Levine B, Harwick JM, Trapp BD, et al. Antibody-mediated clearance of alphavirus infection from neurons. *Science* 1991;254:856.

72. Mazanec MB, Kaetzel CS, Lamm ME, et al. Intracellular neutralization of virus by immunoglobulin A antibodies. *Proc Natl Acad Sci U S A* 1992;89:6901.

73. Dietschold B, Kao M, Zheng YM, et al. Delineation of putative mechanisms involved in antibody-mediated clearance of rabies virus from the central nervous system. *Proc Natl Acad Sci U S A* 1992;89:7252.

74. Bona CA. Idiotypic networks. In: Paul WE, ed. *Fundamental immunology*. New York: Raven Press, 1989:577.

75. Greer JM, Halliday WJ. Effects of anti-idiotype vaccine on tumor growth and on production of soluble factors modulating cell-mediated immunity *in vitro*. *Cancer Immunol Immunother* 1991;33:171.

76. Wettendorf M, Iliopoulos D, Tempero M, et al. Idiotypic cascades in cancer patients treated with monoclonal antibody CO17-1A. *Proc Natl Acad Sci U S A* 1989;86:3787.

77. Frodin JE, Faxas ME, Hagstrom B, et al. Induction of anti-idiotypic (ab2) and anti-anti-idiotypic (ab3) antibodies in patients treated with mouse monoclonal antibody 17-1A (ab1): relation to the clinical outcome—an important anti-tumoral effector function. *Hybridoma* 1991;10:421.

78. Hale G, Dyer MJ, Clark MR, et al. Remission induction in non-Hodgkin's lymphoma with reshaped human monoclonal antibody CAMPATH-1H. *Lancet* 1988;2:1394.

79. Queen C, Schneider WP, Selik HE, et al. A humanized antibody that binds to the interleukin 2 receptor. *Proc Natl Acad Sci U S A* 1989;86:10029.

80. Carter P, Presta L, Groman CM, et al. Humanization of an anti-p185HER2 antibody for human cancer therapy. *Proc Natl Acad Sci U S A* 1992;89:4285.

81. Co MS, Avdalovic NM, Caron PC, et al. Chimeric and humanized antibodies with specificity for the CD33 antigen. *J Immunol* 1992;148:1149.

82. Clendeninn NJ, Hethersell ABW, Scott JE, et al. Phase I/II trials of CAMPATH-1H, a humanized anti-lymphocyte monoclonal antibody (MoAb), in non-Hodgkin's lymphoma (NHL) and chronic lymphocytic leukemia (CLL). *Blood* 1992;80[Suppl 1]:158a.

83. Anasetti C, Hansen JA, Waldmann T, et al. Treatment of acute graft-versus-host disease with a humanized monoclonal antibody specific for the IL-2 receptor. *Blood* 1992;80[Suppl 1]:373a.

84. Caron PC, Jurcic JG, Scott AM, et al. A phase IB trial of humanized monoclonal antibody M195 (Anti-CD33) in myeloid leukemia: specific targeting without immunogenicity. *Blood* 1994;7:1760.

85. LoBuglio AF, Wheeler RH, Trang J, et al. Mouse/human chimeric monoclonal antibody in man: kinetics and immune response. *Proc Natl Acad Sci U S A* 1989;86:4220.

86. Khazaeli MB, Saleh MN, Liu TP, et al. Pharmacokinetics and immune response of 131 I-chimeric mouse/human B72.3 (human gamma 4) monoclonal antibody in humans. *Cancer Res* 1991;52:5461.

87. Knox S, Levy R, Hodgkinson S, et al. Observations on the effect of chimeric anti-CD4 monoclonal antibody in patients with mycosis fungoides. *Blood* 1991;77:20.

88. Saleh MN, Khazaeli MB, Wheeler RH, et al. Phase I trial of the chimeric anti-CD2 monoclonal antibody ch14.18 in patients with malignant melanoma. *Hum Antibodies Hybridomas* 1992;3:19.

89. Berezofsky JA. Structural basis for antigen recognition by T lymphocytes. *J Clin Invest* 1988;82:1811.

90. Carons DA, Freimark BD. Lymphocyte hybridomas and monoclonal antibodies. *Adv Immunol* 1986;38:275.

91. McCune JM, Kaneshima H, Lieberman M, et al. The Scid-hu mouse: current status and potential applications. *Curr Top Microbiol Immunol* 1989;152:183.

92. Mosier DE. Adoptive transfer of human lymphoid cells to severely immunodeficient mice: models for normal human immune function, autoimmunity, lymphomagenesis, and AIDS. *Adv Immunol* 1991;50:303.

93. Barbas CF, Kang AS, Lerner RA, et al. Assembly of combinatorial antibody libraries on phage surfaces: the gene III site. *Proc Natl Acad Sci U S A* 1991;90:7978.

94. Waldmann H, Cobbold S. The use of monoclonal antibodies to achieve immunological tolerance. *Immunol Today* 1993;14:247.

95. Wolff EA, Esselstyn J, Maloney G, et al. Human monoclonal antibody homodimers: effect of valency on *in vitro* and *in vivo* antibacterial activity. *J Immunol* 1992;148:2469.

96. Riechmann L, Clark M, Waldmann H, et al. Reshaping human antibodies for therapy. *Nature* 1988;332:323.

97. Caron PC, Co MS, Bull MK, et al. Biological and immunological features of humanized M195 (Anti-CD33) monoclonal antibodies. *Cancer Res* 1992;52:6761.

98. Gram H, Marconi LA, Barbas CF III, et al. In vitro selection and affinity maturation of antibodies from a naive combinatorial immunoglobulin library. *Proc Natl Acad Sci U S A* 1992;89:3576.

99. Jacques Y, Francois C, Boeffard F, et al. Construction of a bispecific antibody reacting with the alpha- and beta-chains of the human IL-2 receptor. *J Immunol* 1993;150:4610.

100. Cobbold SP, Waldmann H. Therapeutic potential of monovalent monoclonal antibodies. *Nature* 1984;308:460.

101. Stevenson GT, Glennie MJ, Hamblin TJ, et al. Problems and prospects in the use of lymphoma idiotypes as therapeutic targets. *Int J Cancer* 1988;3:9.

102. Sims MJ, Hassal DG, Brett S, et al. A humanized CD18 antibody can block function without cell destruction. *J Immunol* 1993;151:2296.

103. Shopes B. A genetically engineered human IgG mutant with enhanced cytolytic activity. *J Immunol* 1992;148:2918.

104. Caron PC, Class K, Laird W, et al. Enhanced biological and immunological properties of CDR-grafted multimeric human immunoglobulins. *J Exp Med* 1992;176:1191.

105. Joiner KA, Fries LF, Schmetz MA, et al. IgG bearing covalently bound C3b has enhanced bactericidal activity for *Escherichia coli* 0111. *J Exp Med* 1985;162:877.

106. Morrison SL, Johnson MJ, Herzenberg LA, et al. Chimeric human antibody molecules: mouse antigen-binding domains with human constant regions domains. *Proc Natl Acad Sci U S A* 1984;81:6851.

107. Jones PT, Dear PH, Foote J, et al. Replacing the complementarity-determining regions in a human antibody with those from a mouse. *Nature* 1986;321:522.

108. Verhoeyen M, Cesar M, Winter G. Reshaping human antibodies: grafting an antilysozyme activity. *Science* 1988;239:1534.

109. Byrn RA, Mordenti J, Lucas C, et al. Biological properties of a CD4 immunoadhesin. *Nature* 1990;334:667.

110. Segal D, Wunderlich J. Targeting of cytotoxic cells with heterocrosslinked antibodies. *Cancer Invest* 1988;6:83.

111. Scott CT, Blattler WA, Lambert JM, et al. Requirements for the construction of antibody heterodimers for the direction of lysis of tumors by human T cells. *J Clin Invest* 1988;81:1427.

112. Tutt A, Stevenson GT, Glennie MJ. Trispecific F(ab')3 derivatives that use cooperative signaling via the TCR/CD3 complex and CD2 to activate and redirect resting cytotoxic T cells. *J Immunol* 1991;147:60.

113. Lanzavecchia A, Scheidegger D. The use of hybrid hybridomas to target human cytotoxic T lymphocytes. *Eur J Immunol* 1987;17:106.

114. Tada H, Toyoda Y, Iwasa S. Bispecific antibody-producing hybrid hybridoma and its use in one-step immunoassays for human lymphotoxin. *Hybridoma* 1989;8:73.

115. Liu MA, Nussbaum SR, Eisen HN. Hormone conjugated with antibody to CD33 mediates cytotoxic T cell lysis of human melanoma cells. *Science* 1988;239:395.

116. Gillies SD, Wesolowski JS, Lo K-M. Targeting human cytotoxic T lymphocytes to kill heterologous epidermal growth factor receptor-bearing tumor cells. *J Immunol* 1991;146:1067.

117. Staerz UD, Bevan MJ. Use of anti-receptor antibodies to focus T cell activity. *Immunol Today* 1986;7:241.

118. Titus JA, Garrido MA, Hecht TT, et al. Human T cells targeted with anti-T3 cross-linked to antitumor antibody prevent tumor growth in nude mice. *J Immunol* 1987;138:4018.

119. Titus JA, Perez P, Kaubsich A, et al. Human K/natural killer cells targeted with heterocrosslinked antibodies specifically lyse tumor cells *in vitro* and prevent tumor growth *in vivo. J Immunol* 1987;139:153.

120. Garrido MA, Valdayo MJ, Winkler DF, et al. Targeting human T lymphocytes with bispecific antibodies to react against human ovarian carcinoma cells growing in nu/nu mice. *Cancer Res* 1990;50:4227.

121. Pietersz GA, McKinzie IF. Antibody conjugates for the treatment of cancer. *Immunol Rev* 1992;129:57.

122. Trail PA, Wilner D, Lasch SJ, et al. Cure of xenografted human carcinomas by BR96-doxorubicin immunoconjugates. *Science* 1993;261:212.

123. Senter PD. Activation of prodrugs by antibody-enzyme conjugates: a new approach to cancer therapy. *FASEB J* 1990;4:188.

124. Yuan F, Baxter LT, Jain RK. Pharmacokinetic analysis of two-step approaches using bifunctional and enzyme-conjugated antibodies. *Cancer Res* 1991;51:3119.

125. Stickney DR, Anderson LD, Slater JB, et al. Bifunctional antibody: a binary radiopharmaceutical delivery system for imaging colorectal carcinoma. *Cancer Res* 1991;51:6650.

126. Bagshawe KD, Shrma SK, Springer CJ, et al. Antibody directed enzyme prodrug therapy (adept): clinical report. *Dis Markers* 1991;9:233.

127. Vitetta ES, Thorpe PE, Uhr JW. Immunotoxins: magic bullets or misguided missiles. *Immunol Today* 1993;14:252.

128. Pastan I, Fitzgerald D. Recombinant toxins for cancer treatment. *Science* 1991;254:1173.

129. Chaudary VK, Queen C, Junghans RP, et al. A recombinant immunotoxin consisting of two antibody variable domains fused to *Pseudomonas* exotoxin. *Nature* 1989;339:394.

130. Williams DP, Parker K, Bacha P, et al. Diphtheria toxin receptor binding domain substitution with interleukin 2: genetic construction and properties of a diphtheria toxin related interleukin 2 fusion protein. *Cancer Res* 1991; 51:6236.

131. Grossbard ML, Lambert JM, Goldmacher VS, et al. Anti-B4-blocked ricin: a phase I trial of 7-day continuous infusion in patients with B-cell neoplasms. *J Clin Oncol* 1993;11:726.

132. Lambert JM, Goldmacher VS, Collison AR, et al. An immunotoxin prepared with blocked ricin: a natural plant toxin adapted for therapeutic use. *Cancer Res* 1991;51:6236.

133. Vitetta ES, Stone M, Amlor P, et al. Phase I immunotoxin trial in patients with B-cell lymphoma. *Cancer Res* 1991; 15:4052.

134. Ghetie M-A, Ghetie V, Vitetta ES. The use of immunoconjugates in cancer therapy. *Exp Opin Invest Drugs* 1996;5:309.

135. Kreitman RJ, Pastan I. Accumulation of a recombinant immunotoxin in a tumor *in vivo:* fewer than 1000 molecules per cell are sufficient for complete response. *Cancer Res* 1998;58:968.

136. Ghetie M-A, Tucker K, Richardson J, et al. Eradication of minimal disease in severe combined immunodeficient mice with disseminated Daudi lymphoma using chemotherapy and an immunotoxin cocktail. *Blood* 1994;84:702.

137. Robins RA, Embleton MJ, Pimm MV, et al. Bispecific antibody that binds carcinoembryonic antigen and ricin toxin A chain cytotoxic for gastrointestinal tract tumor cells. *J Natl Cancer Inst* 1990;82:1295.

138. Bonardi MA, French RR, Amlot P, et al. Delivery of saporin to human B-cell lymphoma using bispecific antibody: targeting via CD22 but not CD19, CD37, or immunoglobulin results in efficient killing. *Cancer Res* 1993;53:3015.

139. Goldenberg DM, Larson SM. Radioimmunodetection in cancer identification. *J Nucl Med* 1992;33:803.

140. Goldenberg DM, Horowitz JA, Sharkey RM, et al. Targeting, dosimetry and radioimmunotherapy of B-cell lymphomas with iodine-131-labeled LL2 monoclonal antibody. *J Clin Oncol* 1991;9:548.

141. Eary JF, Press OW, Badger CC, et al. Imaging and treatment of B-cell lymphoma. *J Nucl Med* 1990;31:1257.

142. Hnatowich DJ, Gionet M, Rusckowski M, et al. Pharmacokinetics of In-111-labeled OC-125 antibody in cancer patients compared with the 19-9 antibody. *Cancer Res* 1987;47:6111.

143. Haisma HJ, Moseley KR, Battaile A, et al. Distribution and pharmacokinetics of radiolabeled monoclonal antibody OC-125 after intravenous and intraperitoneal administration in gynecologic tumors. *Am J Obstet Gynecol* 1988; 159:843.

144. Carrasquillo JA, Sugarbaker P, Colcher D, et al. Radioimmunoscintigraphy of colon cancer with iodine-131-labeled B72.3 monoclonal antibody. *J Nucl Med* 1988;29:1022.

145. Yokoyama K, Carrasquillo JA, Chang AE, et al. Differences in biodistribution of indium-111- and iodine-131-labeled B72.3 monoclonal antibodies in patients with colorectal cancer. *J Nucl Med* 1989;30:320.

146. Harwood SJ, Carroll RG, Webster WB, et al. Human biodistribution of In-111-labeled monoclonal antibody. *Cancer Res* 1990;50[Suppl]:932s.

147. Lamki LM, Buzdar AU, Singletary SE, et al. Indium-111-labeled B72.3 monoclonal antibody in the detection and staging of breast cancer: a phase I study. *J Nucl Med* 1991;32:1326.

148. Meredith RF, Khazaeli MB, Plott WE, et al. Comparison of two mouse/human chimeric antibodies in patients with metastatic colon cancer. *Antibody Immunocon Radiopharmacol* 1992;5(1):75.

149. Murray JL, Rosenblum MG, Lamki L, et al. Clinical parameters related to optimal tumor localization of indium-111-labeled mouse antimelanoma monoclonal antibody ZME-018. *J Nucl Med* 1987;28:25.

150. Larson SM, Carrasquillo JA, Krohn KA, et al. Localization of I131-labeled p97-specific Fab fragments in human melanoma as a basis for radiotherapy. *J Clin Invest* 1983; 72:2101.

151. Rosenblum MG, Murray JL, Lamki L, et al. Comparative clinical pharmacology of [In111]-labeled murine monoclonal antibodies. *Cancer Chemother Pharmacol* 1987;20:41.

152. Patt YZ, Lamki LM, Haynie TP, et al. Improved tumor localization with increasing dose of indium-111-labeled anti-carcinoembryonic antigen monoclonal antibody ZCE-025 in metastatic colorectal cancer. *J Clin Oncol* 1988;6:1220.

153. Hnatowich DJ, Rusckowski M, Brill AB, et al. Pharmacokinetics in patients of anti-carcinoembryonic antigen antibody radiolabeled with indium-111 using a novel diethylenetriamine pentaacetic acid chelator. *Cancer Res* 1990;50:7272.

154. Griffin TW, Brill AB, Stevens S, et al. Initial clinical study of Indium-111-labeled clone 110 anticarcinoembryonic antigen antibody in patients with colorectal cancer. *J Clin Oncol* 1991;9(4):631.

155. Scheinberg DA, Straus DJ, Yeh SD, et al. A phase I toxicity, pharmacology, and dosimetry trial of monoclonal antibody OKB7 in patients with non-Hodgkin's lymphoma: effects of tumor burden and antigen expression. *J Clin Oncol* 1990;8:792.

156. Welt S, Divgi CR, Real FX, et al. Quantitative analysis of antibody localization in human metastatic colon cancer: a phase I study of monoclonal antibody A33. *J Clin Oncol* 1990;8:1894.

157. Scheinberg DA, Lovett D, Divgi CR, et al. A phase I trial of monoclonal antibody M195 in acute myelogenous leukemia: specific bone marrow targeting and internalization of radionuclide. *J Clin Oncol* 1991;9:478.

158. Kramer EL, DeNardo SJ, Liebes L, et al. Radioimmunolocalization of metastatic breast carcinoma using indium-111-methyl benzyl DTPA BrE-3 monoclonal antibody: phase I study. *J Nucl Med* 1993;34:1067.

159. Oosterwijk E, Bander NH, Divgi CR, et al. Antibody localization in human renal cell carcinoma: a phase I study of monoclonal antibody G250. *J Clin Oncol* 1993;11:738.

160. Carrasquillo JA, Abrams PG, Schroff RW, et al. Effect of antibody dose on the imaging and biodistribution of indium-111 9.2.27 anti-melanoma monoclonal antibody. *J Nucl Med* 1988;29:39.

161. DeNardo GL, Mahe MA, DeNardo SJ, et al. Body and blood clearance and marrow radiation dose of I-131-Lym-1 in patients with B-cell malignancies. *Nucl Med Commun* 1993;14:587.

162. Lamki LM, Patt YZ, Rosenblum MG, et al. Metastatic colorectal cancer: radioimmunoscintigraphy with a stabilized In-111-labeled F(ab')$_2$ fragment of an anti-CEA monoclonal antibody. *Radiology* 1990;174:147.

163. Maher VE, Drukman SJ, Kinders RJ, et al. Human antibody response to the intravenous and intraperitoneal administration of the F(ab')$_2$ fragment of the OC125 murine monoclonal antibody. *J Immunother* 1992;11:56.

164. Renkin EM. Multiple pathways of capillary permeability. *Circ Res* 1977;41:735.

165. Zamboni L, Pease DC. The vascular bed of bone marrow. *J Ultrastruct Res* 1961;5:65.

166. Ward BG, Mather SJ, Hawkins LR, et al. Localization of radioiodine conjugated to the monoclonal antibody HMFG2 in human ovarian carcinoma: assessment of intravenous and intraperitoneal routes of administration. *Cancer Res* 1987;47:4719.

167. Colcher D, Esteban JM, Carrasquillo JA, et al. Quantitative analyses of selective radiolabeled monoclonal antibody localization in metastatic lesions of colorectal cancer patients. *Cancer Res* 1987;47:1185.

168. Dewey WC. Vascular-extravascular exchange of I-131 plasma proteins in the rat. *Am J Physiol* 1959;197:423.

169. Dvorak HF, Magy JA, Dvorak JT, et al. Identification and characterization of the blood vessels of solid tumors that are leaky to circulating macromolecules. *Am J Pathol* 1988;133:95.

170. Thomas GD, Chappell MJ, Dykes PW, et al. Effect of dose, molecular size, affinity, and protein binding on tumor uptake of antibody or ligand: a biomathematical model. *Cancer Res* 1989;49:3290.

171. Keenan AM, Weinstein JN, Carrasquillo JA, et al. Immunolymphoscintigraphy and dose dependence of In-111-labeled T101 monoclonal antibody in patients with cutaneous T-cell lymphoma. *Cancer Res* 1987;47:6093.

172. Gerlowski LE, Jain RK. Microvascular permeability of normal and neoplastic tissues. *Microvasc Res* 1986;31:288.

173. Jain RK, Wei J. Dynamics of drug transport in solid tumors: distributed parameter model. *J Bioeng* 1977;1:313.

174. Nugent LJ, Jain RK. Extravascular diffusion in normal and neoplastic tissues. *Cancer Res* 1984;44:238.

175. Clauss MA, Jain RK. Interstitial transport of rabbit and sheep antibodies in normal and neoplastic tissues. *Cancer Res* 1990;50:3487.

176. Butler TP, Grantham FH, Gullino PM. Bulk transfer of fluid in the interstitial compartment of mammary tumors. *Cancer Res* 1975;35:3084.

177. Jain RK, Baxter LT. Mechanisms of heterogeneous distribution of monoclonal antibodies and other macromolecules in tumors: significance of elevated interstitial pressure. *Cancer Res* 1988;48:7022.

178. Jain RK. Transport of molecules in the tumor interstitium: a review. *Cancer Res* 1987;47:3039.

179. Williams LE, Duda RB, Proffitt RT, et al. Tumor uptake as a function of tumor mass: a mathematic model. *J Nucl Med* 1988;29:103.

180. Fujimori K, Covell DG, Fletcher JE, Weinstein JN. Modeling analysis of the global and microscopic distribution of immunoglobulin G, F(ab')$_2$, and Fab in tumors. *Cancer Res* 1989;49:5656.

181. Fujimori K, Covell DG, Fletcher JE, et al. A modeling analysis of monoclonal antibody percolation through tumors: a binding-site barrier. *J Nucl Med* 1990;31:1191.

182. Langmuir VK, Mendonca HL. The role of radionuclide distribution in the efficacy of I-131-labeled antibody as modeled in multicell spheroids. *Antibody Immunocon Radiopharmacol* 1992;5:273.

183. Juweid M, Neumann R, Paik C, et al. Micropharmacology of monoclonal antibodies in solid tumors: direct experimental evidence for a binding site barrier. *Cancer Res* 1992;52:5144.

184. Loevinger R, Budinger TF, Watson EE. *MIRD primer for absorbed dose calculations.* New York: The Society of Nuclear Medicine, 1989.

185. Bigler RE, Zanzonico PB, Leonard R, et al. Bone marrow dosimetry for monoclonal antibody therapy. In: Schlafke-Stelson AT, Watson EE, eds. *Proceedings of the Fourth International Dosimetry Symposium.* Oak Ridge, TN: Department of Energy, 1985:535. CONF-851113 (DE86010102).

186. Siegel JA, Wessels BW, Watson EE, et al. Bone marrow dosimetry and toxicity for radioimmunotherapy. *Antibody Immunocon Radiopharmacol* 1990;3:213.

187. *IAEA/WHO manual on radiation hematology.* Technical report series, no. 123. Vienna: International Atomic Energy Agency and the World Health Organization, 1971.

188. Blumenthal RD, Sharkey RM, Quinn LM, et al. Use of hematopoietic growth factors to control myelosuppression caused by radioimmunotherapy. *Cancer Res* 1990;50 [Suppl]:1003s.

189. Sgouros G. Bone marrow dosimetry for radioimmunotherapy: theoretical considerations. *J Nucl Med* 1993;34:689.

190. Siegel JA, Lee RE, Pawlyk DA, et al. Sacral scintigraphy for BM dosimetry in radioimmunotherapy. *Nucl Med Biol* 1989;16:553.

191. Sgouros G, Graham MC, Divgi CR, et al. Modeling and dosimetry of monoclonal antibody M195 (anti-CD33) in acute myelogenous leukemia. *J Nucl Med* 1993;34:422.

192. Press OW, Eary JF, Badger CC, et al. Treatment of refractory non-Hodgkin's lymphoma with radiolabeled MB-1 (Anti-CD37) antibody. *J Clin Oncol* 1989;7:1027.

193. Larson SM, Scott AM, Divgi CR, et al. I-131 M195 (anti-CD33) radioimmunotherapy trials in patients with myeloid leukemias. *J Nucl Med* 1993;34:53.

194. Sgouros G, Barest G, Thekkumthala J, et al. Treatment planning for internal radionuclide therapy: three-dimensional dosimetry for nonuniformly distributed radionuclides. *J Nucl Med* 1990;31:1884.

195. Roberson PL, Buchsbaum DJ, Heidorn DB, et al. Three-dimensional tumor dosimetry for radioimmunotherapy using serial autoradiography. *Int J Radiat Oncol Biol Phys* 1992;24:329.

196. Mausner LF, Srivastava SC. Selection of radionuclides for radioimmunotherapy. *Med Phys* 1993;20:503.

197. Yorke ED, Williams LE, Demidecki AJ, et al. Multicellular dosimetry for beta-emitting radionuclides: autoradiography, thermoluminescent dosimetry and three-dimensional dose calculations. *Med Phys* 1993;20:543.

198. Meredith RB, Johnson TK, Plott G, et al. Dosimetry of solid tumors. *Med Phys* 1993;20:583.

199. Langmuir VK, Fowler JF, Knox SJ, et al. Radiobiology of radiolabeled antibody therapy as applied to tumor dosimetry. *Med Phys* 1993;20:601.

200. Humm JL, Cobb LM. Nonuniformity of tumor dose in radioimmunotherapy. *J Nucl Med* 1990;31:75.

201. Simpkin DJ, Mackie TR. EGS4 Monte Carlo determination of the beta dose kernel in water. *Med Phys* 1993;17:179.

202. Humm JL. Dosimetric aspects of radiolabeled antibodies for tumor therapy. *J Nucl Med* 1986;27:1490.

203. Willins J, Sgouros G. Improving the therapeutic ratio in radioimmunotherapy of micrometastases: a mathematical modeling analysis of multiple antibody infusions. *Med Phys* 1993;20:865.

204. Hunter WM, Greenwood FC. Preparation of I-131-labeled human growth hormone of high specific activity. *Nature* 1962;194:495.

205. Fraker PJ, Speck JC. Protein and cell membrane iodination with a sparingly soluble chloramide, 1,3,4,6-tetrachloro-3a, 6a-diphenylglycouril. *Biochem Biophys Res Commun* 1978;80:849.

206. Willins JD, Sgouros G. Modeling analysis of Platinum-195m for targeting individual blood-borne cells in adjuvant radioimmunotherapy. *J Nucl Med* 1995;36:100.

207. McDevitt MR, Sgouros G, Finn RD, et al. Radioimmunotherapy with alpha-emitting nuclides. *Eur J Nucl Med* 1999;25:1341.

208. Humm JL. A microdosimetric model of astatine-211 labeled antibodies for radioimmunotherapy. *Int J Radiat Oncol Biol Phys* 1987;13:1767.

209. Macklis RM, Kinsey BM, Kassis AI, et al. Radioimmunotherapy with alpha-particle-emitting immunoconjugates. *Science* 1988;240:1024.

209a. Humm JL, Chin LM. A model of cell inactivation by alpha-particle internal emitters. *Radiat Res* 1993;134:143.

210. Zalutsky MR, Vaidyanathan G. Astatine-211-labeled radiotherapeutics: an emerging approach to targeted alpha-particle radiotherapy. *Curr Pharm Des.* 2000 Sep;6:1433.

211. Jurcic JG, McDevitt MR, Sgouros G, et al. Targeted alpha-particle therapy for myeloid leukemias: a phase I trial of bismuth-213-HuM195 (anti-CD33). *Blood* 1997;90[Suppl]:504a(abst).

212. McDevitt MR, Finn RD, Sgouros G, et al. An ^{225}Ac/^{213}Bi generator system for therapeutic clinical applications: construction and operation. *Appl Radiat Isot* 1999;50:895.

213. Sgouros G, Ballangrud ÅM, Humm JL, et al. Pharmacokinetics and dosimetry of an alpha-particle emitter labeled antibody: ^{213}Bi-HuM195 (anti-CD33) in patients with leukemia. *J Nucl Med* 1999;40(11):1935.

214. Fisher DR, Sgouros G. Dosimetry of radium-223 and progeny. *Proceedings of the 6th International Radiopharmaceutical Dosimetry Symposium.* Oak Ridge, TN: Department of Energy, 1996:375–391.

215. Geerlings MW, Kaspersen FM, Apostolidis C, et al. The feasibility of Ac-255 as a source of a-particles in radioimmunotherapy. *Nucl Med Comm* 1993;14:121.

216. Hnatowich DJ, Virzi F, Rusckowski M. Investigations of avidin and biotin for imaging applications. *J Nucl Med* 1984;28:1294.

217. Paganelli G, Riva P, Deleide G, et al. *In vivo* labeling of biotinylated monoclonal antibodies by radioactive avidin: a strategy to increase tumor radiolocalization. *Int J Cancer* 1988;2:121.

218. DeNardo SJ, DeNardo GL, O'Grady LF, et al. Pilot studies of radioimmunotherapy of B cell lymphoma and leukemia using I-131 Lym-1 monoclonal antibody. *Antibody Immunocon Radiopharmacol* 1988;1:17.

219. Blumenthal RD, Sharkey RM, Boerman OC, et al. The effect of antibody protein dose on the uniformity of tumor distribution of radioantibodies: an autoradiographic study. *Cancer Immunol Immunother* 1991;33:351.

220. Goodwin D, Meares C, Diamanti C, et al. Use of specific antibody for rapid clearance of circulating blood background from radiolabeled tumor imaging proteins. *Eur J Nucl Med* 1984;9:209.

221. Breitz H, Knox S, Weiden P, et al. Pretargeted radioimmunotherapy™ with antibody-streptavidin and Y-90 DOTA-

biotin (Avidicin®): result from a dose escalation study. *J Nucl Med* 1998;38[Suppl]:71P.

222. Wahl RL, Geatti O, Liebert M, et al. Kinetics of interstitially administered monoclonal antibodies for purposes of lymphoscintigraphy. *J Nucl Med* 1987;28:1736.

223. Wahl RL, Liebert M, Headington J, et al. Lymphoscintigraphy in melanoma: initial evaluation of a low protein dose monoclonal antibody cocktail. *Cancer Res* 1990;50[Suppl]:941s.

224. Cheung NV, Lazarus H, Miraldi FD, et al. Ganglioside GD2 specific monoclonal antibody 3F8: a phase I study in patients with neuroblastoma and malignant melanoma. *J Clin Oncol* 1987;5:1430.

225. Schwartz MA, Lovett DR, Redner A, et al. A dose-escalation trial of M195 labeled with iodine 131 for cytoreduction and marrow ablation in relapsed or refractory myeloid leukemias. *J Clin Oncol* 1993;11:294.

226. Cheung N-KV, Miraldi FD. Iodine-131 labeled G_{D2} monoclonal antibody in the diagnosis and therapy of human neuroblastoma. In: Evans AE, D'Angio GJ, Knudson AG, et al. *Advances in neuroblastoma research 2: proceedings of the Fourth Symposium on Advances in Neuroblastoma Research held in Philadelphia, Pennsylvania, May 14-16, 1987.* New York: Alan R. Liss, 1988:595.

227. Papadopoulos EB, Caron P, Castro-Malaspina H, et al. Results of allogeneic bone marrow transplant following 131-I-M195/busulfan/cyclophosphamide (Bu/Cy) in patients with advanced/refractory myeloid malignancies. *Blood* 1993;82[Suppl 1]:80a.

228. Czuczman MS, Straus DJ, Finn R, et al. A phase I trial of 131-I-OKB7 in advanced B cell lymphoma. *J Clin Oncol* 1993;11:2021.

229. Pai LH, Bookman MA, Ozols RF, et al. Clinical evaluation of intraperitoneal *Pseudomonas* exotoxin immunoconjugates OVB3-PE in patients with ovarian cancer. *J Clin Oncol* 1991;9:2095.

230. Vadhan-Raj S, Cordon-Cardo C, Carswell EA, et al. Phase I trial of a mouse monoclonal antibody against GD3 ganglioside in patients with melanoma: induction of inflammatory responses at tumor sites. *J Clin Oncol* 1988;6:1636.

231. Larson SM, Carrasquillo JA, McGuffin RW, et al. Use of I-131 labeled, murine fab against a high molecular weight antigen of human melanoma: preliminary experience. *Radiology* 1987;155:487.

232. Rosen ST, Zimmer AM, Goldman-Leikin R, et al. Radioimmunodetection and radioimmunotherapy of cutaneous T cell lymphomas using an I-131-labeled monoclonal antibody: an Illinois Cancer Council study. *J Clin Oncol* 1987;5(4):562.

233. Rosenblum MG, Lamki LM, Murray JL, et al. Interferon-induced changes in pharmacokinetics and tumor uptake of In-111-labeled antimelanoma antibody 96.5 in melanoma patients. *J Natl Cancer Inst* 1988;80(3):160.

234. Kalofonos HP, Sackier JM, Hatzistylianou M, et al. Kinetics, quantitative analysis and radioimmunolocalization using indium-111-HMFG1 monoclonal antibody in patients with breast cancer. *Br J Cancer* 1989;59:939.

235. Goldenberg DM, Goldenberg H, Sharkey RM, et al. Clinical studies of cancer radioimmunodetection with carcinoembryonic antigen monoclonal antibody fragments labeled with I-123 or Tc99m. *Cancer Res* 1990;50[Suppl]:909s.

236. Breitz HB, Weiden PL, Vanderheyden JL, et al. Clinical experience with Rhenium-186-labeled monoclonal antibodies for radioimmunotherapy: results of phase I trials. *J Nucl Med* 1992;33(6):1099.

237. Colcher D, Esteban J, Carrasquillo JA, et al. Complementation of intracavitary and intravenous administration of a monoclonal antibody (B72.3) in patients with carcinoma. *Cancer Res* 1987;47:4218.

238. Steward JSW, Hird V, Snook D, et al. Intraperitoneal yttrium-90-labeled monoclonal antibody in ovarian cancer. *J Clin Oncol* 1990;8:1941.

239. Rosenblum MG, Kavanagh JJ, Burke TW, et al. Clinical pharmacology, metabolism, and tissue distribution of Y-90-labeled monoclonal antibody B72.3 after intraperitoneal administration. *J Natl Cancer Inst* 1991;83:1629.

240. Larson SM, Carrasquillo JA, Colcher DC, et al. Estimates of radiation absorbed dose for intraperitoneally administered iodine-131 radiolabeled B72.3 monoclonal antibody in patients with peritoneal carcinomatoses. *J Nucl Med* 1991;32:1661.

241. Lashford LS, Davies G, Richardson RB, et al. A pilot study of I-131 monoclonal antibodies in the therapy of leptomeningeal tumors. *Cancer* 1988;61:857.

242. Moseley RP, Davies AG, Richardson RB, et al. Intrathecal administration of 131 I-radiolabelled monoclonal antibody as a treatment for neoplastic meningitis. *Br J Cancer* 1990;62:637.

243. Folli S, Pelegrin A, Chalandon Y, et al. Tumor-necrosis factor can enhance radio-antibody uptake in human colon carcinoma xenografts by increasing vascular permeability. *Int J Cancer* 1993;53:829.

244. Mittal BB, Zimmer AM, Sathiaseelan V, et al. Effects of hyperthermia and iodine-131-labeled anticarcinoembryonic antigen monoclonal antibody on human tumor xenografts in nude mice. *Cancer* 1992;70:2785.

245. Warhoe KA, DeNardo SJ, Wolkov HB, et al. Evidence for external beam irradiation enhancement of radiolabeled monoclonal antibody uptake in breast cancer. *Antibody Immunocon Radiopharmacol* 1992;5(2):227.

246. DeNardo G, DeNardo S, Kukis D, et al. Strategies for enhancement of radioimmunotherapy. *Nucl Med Biol* 1991; 18(6):633.

247. Langmuir VK, Mendoca HL. The combined use of iodine-131-labeled antibody and the hypoxic cytotoxin SR 4233 *in vitro* and *in vivo*. *Radiat Res* 1992;132:351.

248. Santos O, Pant KD, Bland EW, et al. 5-Iododeoxyuridine increases the efficacy of the radioimmunotherapy of human tumors growing in nude mice. *J Nucl Med* 1992;33:1530.

249. Paganelli G, Magnani P, Zito F, et al. Three-step monoclonal antibody tumor targeting in carcinoembryonic antigen-positive patients. *Cancer Res* 1991;51:5960.

250. Sharkey RM, Blumenthal RD, Hansen HJ, et al. Biological considerations for radioimmunotherapy. *Cancer Res* 1990; 50[Suppl]:964s.

251. Lear JL, Kasliwal RK, Feyerabend AJ, et al. Improved tumor imaging with radiolabeled monoclonal antibodies by plasma clearance of unbound antibody with anti-antibody column. *Radiology* 1991;179:509.

252. Greiner JW, Ullmann CD, Nieroda C, et al. Improved radioimmunotherapeutic efficacy of an anticarcinoma monoclonal antibody (I-131-CC49) when given in combination with gamma-interferon. *Cancer Res* 1993;53:600.

253. Houghton AN, Mintzer D, Cardon-Cardo C, et al. Mouse monoclonal antibody detecting GD3 ganglioside: a phase I trial in patients with malignant melanoma. *Proc Natl Acad Sci U S A* 1985;82:1242.

254. Saleh MN, Khazaeli MB, Wheeler RH, et al. Phase I trial of murine monoclonal anti-GD2 antibody 14G2a in metastatic melanoma. *Cancer Res* 1992;52:4342.

255. Goodman GE, Beaumier P, Hellstrom I, et al. Pilot trial of murine monoclonal antibodies in patients with advanced melanoma. *J Clin Oncol* 1985;3:340.

256. Oldham RK, Foon KA, Morgan AC, et al. Monoclonal antibody therapy of malignant melanoma: *in vivo* localization in cutaneous metastasis after intravenous administration. *J Clin Oncol* 1984;2:1235.

257. Sears HF, Atkinson B, Mattis J, et al. The use of monoclonal antibody in phase I clinical trial of human gastrointestinal tumors. *Lancet* 1982;1:762.

258. Welt S, Divgi CR, Kemeny N, et al. Phase I/II study of iodine-131-labeled monoclonal antibody A33 in patients with advanced colon cancer. *J Clin Oncol* 1994;12:1561.

259. Goodman GE, Hellstrom I, Brodzinsky L, et al. Phase I trial of murine monoclonal antibody L6 in breast, colon, ovarian, and lung cancer. *J Clin Oncol* 1990;8:1083.

260. Steffans MG, Boerman OC, Oosterwijk-Wakka JC, et al. Targeting of renal cell carcinoma with iodine-131 labeled chimeric monoclonal antibody G250. *J Clin Oncol* 1997;15:1529.

261. Liu H, Moy P, Kim S, et al. Monoclonal antibodies to the extracellular domain of prostate specific membrane antigen also react with tumor endothelium. *Cancer Res* 1997;57:3629.

262. Dillman RO, Shawler DL, Dillmann JB, et al. Therapy of chronic lymphocytic leukemia and cutaneous T-cell lymphoma with T101 monoclonal antibody. *J Clin Oncol* 1984;2:881.

263. Brown SL, Miller RA, Horning SS, et al. Treatment of B-cell lymphomas with antiidiotype antibodies alone and in combination with alpha interferon. *Blood* 1989;73:651.

264. Maloney DG, Levy R, Miller RA. Monoclonal anti-idiotype therapy of B cell lymphoma. In: DeVita VT Jr, Hellman S, Rosenberg SA, eds. *Biologic therapy of cancer updates*, vol. 2. Philadelphia: JB Lippincott, 1992:1.

265. Waldmann TA, Pastan I, Gansow OA, et al. The multichain interleukin 2 receptor: a target for immunotherapy. *Ann Intern Med* 1992;116:148.

266. Waldmann TA, Goldman CK, Bongiovanni KF, et al. Therapy of patients with human T-cell lymphotropic virus I-induced adult T-cell leukemia with anti-Tac, a monoclonal antibody to the receptor for interleukin 2. *Blood* 1988;72:1805.

267. Waldmann TA, White JD, Goldman CK, et al. The interleukin 2 receptor: a target for monoclonal antibody treatment of human T-cell lymphotrophic virus I-induced adult T-cell leukemia. *Blood* 1993;82:1701.

268. Bajorin DF, Chapman PB, Dimaggio J, et al. Phase I evaluation of a combination of monoclonal antibody R24 and interleukin 2 in patients with metastatic melanoma. *Cancer Res* 1990;50:7490.

269. Ziegler LD, Palazzolo P, Cunningham J, et al. Phase I trial of murine monoclonal antibody L6 in combination with subcutaneous interleukin-2 in patients with advanced carcinoma of the breast, colorectum, and lung. *J Clin Oncol* 1992;10:1470.

270. Ragnhammar P, Fagerberg J, Frödin, et al. Effects of monoclonal antibody 17-1A and GM-CSF in patients with advanced colorectal carcinoma: long-lasting, complete remissions can be induced. *Int J Cancer* 1993;53:751.

271. Mendelsohn J, Shin DM, Donato N, et al. A phase I study of chimerized anti-epidermal growth factor receptor (RGFr) monoclonal antibody, C225, in combination with cisplatin (CDDP) in patients (PTS) with recurrent head and neck squamous cell carcinoma (SCC). *Proceed Am Soc Clin Oncol* 1999;18:389a.

272. Molema G, Meijer DKF, de Leij LFMH. Tumor vasculature targeted therapies, getting the players organized. *Biochem Pharmacol* 1998;55:1939.

273. Welt S, Divgi CR, Scott AM, et al. Antibody targeting in metastatic colon cancer: a phase I study of monoclonal antibody F19 against a cell-surface protein of reactive tumor stromal fibroblasts. *J Clin Oncol* 1994;12:1193.

274. Hale G, Clark MR, Marcus R, et al. Remission induction in non-Hodgkin's lymphoma with reshaped human monoclonal antibody Campath-1H. *Lancet* 1988;2:1394.

275. Sievers EL, Appelbaum FR, Spielberger RT, et al. Selective ablation of acute myeloid leukemia using antibody-targeted chemotherapy: a phase I study of an anti-CD33 calicheamicin immunoconjugate. *Blood* 1999;93:3678.

276. Baselga J, Tripathy D, Mendelson J, et al. Phase II study of weekly intravenous recombinant humanized anti-p185^{HER2} monoclonal antibody in patients with HER2/neu-overexpressing metastatic breast cancer. *J Clin Oncol* 1996;14:737.

277. Jurcic J, DeBlasio T, Dumont L, et al. Molecular remission induction with retinoic acid and anti-CD33 monoclonal antibody HuM195 in acute promyelocytic leukemia. *Clin Cancer Res* 2000;6(2):372.

278. Shan D, Ledbetter JA, Press OW. Apoptosis of malignant human B cells by ligation of CD20 with monoclonal antibodies. *Blood* 1998;91:1644.

279. McLaughlin P, Grillo-López AJ, Link BK, et al. Rituximab chimeric anti-CD20 monoclonal antibody therapy for relapsed indolent lymphoma: half of patients respond to a four-dose treatment program. *J Clin Oncol* 1998;16:2825.

280. Czuczman MS, Grillo-López AJ, White CA, et al. Treatment of patients with low-grade B-cell lymphoma with the combination of chimeric anti-CD20 monoclonal antibody and CHOP chemotherapy. *J Clin Oncol* 1999;17:268.

281. Muss HB, Thor AD, Berry DA, et al. c-erB-2 expression and response to adjuvant therapy in women with node-positive early breast cancer. *N Engl J Med* 1994;330:1260.

282. Baselga J, Norton L, Albanell J, et al. Recombinant humanized anti-HER2 antibody (Herceptin) enhances the antitumor activity of paclitaxel and doxorubicin against HER2/new overexpressing human breast cancer xenografts. *Cancer Res* 1998;13:2325.

283. Epenetos AA, Munro AJ, Stewart S, et al. Antibody-guided irradiation of advanced ovarian cancer with intraperitoneally administered radiolabeled monoclonal antibodies. *J Clin Oncol* 1987;5:1890.

284. Stewart JSW, Hird V, Snook D, et al. Intraperitoneal radioimmunotherapy for ovarian cancer: pharmacokinetics, toxicity, and efficacy of I-131 labeled monoclonal antibodies. *Int J Radiat Oncol Biol Phys* 1990;3:169.

285. Meredith RF, LoBuglio AF. Recent progress in radioimmunotherapy for cancer. *Oncology (Huntingt)* 1997;11(7):979.

286. Halpern SE, Parker BA, Vassos A, et al. 90 Yttrium (90 Y) anti-idiotype monoclonal antibody therapy of non-Hodgkin's lymphoma. *J Nucl Med* 1989;39:778(abst).

287. Kaminski MS, Fig ML, Zasadny KR, et al. Imaging, dosimetry, and radioimmunotherapy with Iodine 131-labeled anti-CD37 antibody in B-cell lymphoma. *J Clin Oncol* 1992;10:1696.

288. Kaminski MS, Zasadny KR, Francis IR, et al. Iodine-131 anti-B1 radioimmunotherapy for B-cell lymphoma. *J Clin Oncol* 1996;14:1974.

289. DeNardo GL, DeNardo SJ, Goldstein DR, et al. Maximum tolerated dose, toxicity, and efficacy of ^{131}I-Lym-1 antibody for fractionated radioimmunotherapy of non-Hodgkin's lymphoma. *J Clin Oncol* 1998;16:3246.

290. Knox SJ, Goris ML, Trisler K, et al. Yttrium-90-labeled anti-CD20 monoclonal antibody therapy of recurrent B-cell lymphoma. *Clin Cancer Res* 1996;2(3):457.

291. Liu SY, Eary JF, Petersdorf SH, et al. Follow-up of relapsed B-cell lymphoma patients treated with Iodine-131-labeled anti-CD20 antibody and autologous stem-cell rescue. *J Clin Oncol* 1998;16:3270.

292. Matthews DC, Appelbaum FR, Eary JF, et al. Development of a marrow transplant regimen for acute leukemia using targeted hematopoietic irradiation delivered by ^{131}I-labeled anti-CD45 antibody, combined with cyclophosphamide and total body irradiation. *Blood* 1995;85:1122.

293. Appelbaum FR, Mathews DC, Eary JF, et al. The use of radiolabeled anti-CD33 antibody to augment marrow irradiation prior to marrow transplantation for acute myelogenous leukemia. *Transplantation* 1992;54:829.

294. Jurcic JG, Caron PC, Miller WH, et al. Reduction of minimal residual disease using 131 I-labeled anti-CD33 (131-I-M195) in relapsed acute promyelocytic leukemia (APL) after remission induction with all-*trans*retinoic acid (RA). *Blood* 1993;82[Suppl 1]:193a.

295. Grossbard ML, Freedman AS, Ritz J, et al. Serotherapy of B-cell neoplasms with anti-B4-blocked ricin: a phase I trial of daily bolus infusion. *Blood* 1992;79:576.

296. Grossbard ML, Gribben JG, Freedman AS, et al. Adjuvant immunotoxin therapy with anti-B4-blocked ricin after autologous bone marrow transplantation for patients with B-cell non-Hodgkin's lymphoma. *Blood* 1993;81:2263.

297. Multani PS, O'Day S, Nadler LM, et al. Phase II clinical trial of bolus infusion anti-B4 blocked ricin immunoconjugate in patients with relapsed B-cell non-Hodgkin's lymphoma. *Clin Cancer Res* 1998;4(11):2599.

298. Baluna R, Sausville EA, Stone MJ, et al. Decreases in levels of serum fibronectin predict the severity of vascular leak syndrome in patients treated with ricin A chain-containing immunotoxins. *Clin Cancer Res* 1996;2(10):1705.

299. Levy R, Miller RA. Therapy of lymphoma directed at idiotypes. *J Natl Cancer Inst Monogr* 1990;10:61.

300. Nourigat C, Badger CC, Bernstein ID. Treatment of lymphoma with radiolabeled antibody: elimination of tumor cells lacking target antigen. *J Natl Cancer Inst* 1990;82:47.

30

TARGETED THERAPY

JEFFREY W. CLARK

Discoveries in laboratories during the past decade have led to an improved understanding of specific biologic processes important for survival, growth, and metastasis of neoplastic cells. The combination of this with technologic advances that allow sophisticated manipulation and analysis of nucleic acids and proteins has generated increased interest in use of antisense oligonucleotides, expressed genes, monoclonal antibodies (mAbs), peptidomimetics, designed small molecules, and other molecularly targeted therapies in the treatment of cancer (Table 30-1). Several of these have sufficient clinical activity to be approved for use. These include the mAbs trastuzumab (Herceptin) (for breast cancer) and rituximab [for follicular B-cell non-Hodgkin's lymphomas (NHLs)] and the immunotoxin denileukin diftitox [diphtheria toxin-interleukin 2 (IL-2) fusion protein, DAB486IL-2] for the treatment of cutaneous T-cell lymphomas. A number of other agents are in clinical trials, and this list is likely to grow.

Targeting a specific gene or protein is simple in concept. Antitumor agents can be designed based on known sequence data rather than depending on empirically screening a large number of compounds. However, there are still many caveats to successful use of these approaches. Targeting one gene may have limited impact on proliferation of neoplastic cells. In many cases, it is not obvious which gene(s) should be targeted. Genes important in the process of becoming a neoplastic cell may not be important for continued proliferation or survival of the cell and, therefore, may be irrelevant targets for treating established malignancies. Inhibition of many genes (or function of these genes), even if they are important for neoplastic cell growth, may only be cytostatic. It would be more useful to target genes whose inhibition (or stimulation) induces cell death (i.e., by apoptosis) or terminal differentiation.[1] Ultimately, these approaches must be capable of eliminating (or at least leading to prolonged growth suppression of) all tumor cells, either by themselves or in combination with other agents, if they are to be effective in curing patients. Agents with cytostatic effects might need to be used in combination with other therapy. It is important that the targeted protein in the neoplastic cell either be sufficiently different (if mutant) or not be critical for survival of normal cells to prevent toxicity.

These arguments seem daunting for successful development of targeted therapies. However, strategies using each of the above-mentioned approaches have been shown to be effective in animal models and, as outlined above, for several human tumors when targeting proteins on the cell surface. Early evidence for success of the bcr-abl kinase inhibitor STI-571 against chronic myelogenous leukemia (CML) indicates that small molecules designed to inhibit specific targets within malignant cells can also have significant antitumor effects. Clearly, a number of genes could be targeted simultaneously or sequentially, and combinations of approaches inhibiting certain genes (or their protein products) and enhancing expression of others may ultimately be used. The complete sequencing of the human genome and improved understanding of complex interactions among different genes and proteins will provide a large range of potential targets in the coming decades. Determining which of these are most fruitful to pursue in treating cancer remains an important challenge.

THEORETIC BASIS FOR TARGETED THERAPY

Current cancer therapy, for the most part, uses drugs that lack selectivity for tumor cells. They are predominantly cytotoxins, lethal for tumors and normal tissues, with a narrow therapeutic index. These agents were discovered through cytotoxic screens rather than an effort to exploit specific biologic or genetic targets. Although they have measurably improved the treatment of many solid tumors and have cured some hematologic malignancies and selected solid tumors, many cancer scientists believe that the explosive growth of knowledge of cancer biology will allow a more rational approach to therapeutic discovery. This allows the targeting of pathways and proteins essential to the survival of cancer cells, and, either quantitatively or qualitatively, unique to cancer.[1–7]

TABLE 30-1. MOLECULARLY TARGETED THERAPIES

Agent	Potential Target(s)
Antisense oligonucleotides	RNA, DNA, proteins
Gene therapy	Neoplastic cells, immune mediator cells, and normal cells (to produce proteins)
Ribozymes	RNA and DNA in tumor cells
Monoclonal antibodies	Growth factor receptors, cell surface antigens, and other cellular proteins
Peptidomimetics/altered peptides	Growth factor receptors, cell surface antigens, extra- and intracellular proteins (e.g., enzymes and signal transduction molecules)
Small molecules	All of the above targets

Recent studies of cancer biology have revealed a number of such pathways and proteins. Many of these are either overexpressed or in some way altered in cancer cells but are not entirely unique to cancer. These include angiogenic pathways [e.g., vascular endothelial growth factor (VEGF) or platelet-derived growth factor (PDGF)–mediated angiogenesis] that provide a blood supply for the expanding tumor; antiapoptotic mechanisms that antagonize cell death, such as overexpression of Bcl-2 or decreased BAX expression; overexpression of growth factor pathways, such as the epidermal growth factor receptor (EGFR) family, including the *HER-2-neu* tyrosine kinase; and enhanced activity of intracellular signaling pathways that promote growth, impede apoptosis, or both.[1–7] Other mechanisms are unique to cancer cells, such as mutant genes. As an example, mutations of genes in signaling pathways can include dysregulation of growth-promoting components, such as the activation of one of the ras family of proteins. In addition, or alternatively, there can be loss of the important brakes on proliferation, such as p53 function, retinoblastoma (RB) protein function, or the phosphate and tensin homolog (PTEN) that regulates the PI3-kinase pathway.[5–8]

Recognition of a potential target for drug discovery is only the first step. The target requires "validation" if it is to warrant concerted attack. A number of theoretic and practical questions must be answered before the investment is justified. Among the most relevant questions are the following:

1. Is the function of the overexpressed or mutated target essential to the transformed behavior of the tumor? Does inhibition of the gene product change the phenotype of the malignant cell? Because many mutations in cancer cells appear late in their progression and may not be essential to maintaining growth or metastasis, these questions must be answered in the affirmative. Experiments in which the subject gene is mutated, deleted, or neutralized with antisense oligonucleotides can help answer these questions.

2. Are the subject gene and its protein found in human tumors, and is there selective expression in tumors versus normal tissues?

3. If overexpressed in tumors, is the protein also expressed in key proliferating normal tissues, such as intestinal epithelium and bone marrow progenitors, or even nonproliferating tissues, such as heart, kidney, or brain? Does a knockout of the gene have fatal consequences for the host (in animal models)? Patterns of drug toxicity are often difficult to predict, but the profile of gene expression in normal tissue may provide helpful clues about potential selectivity of an agent directed against that target.

4. Are there closely related genes that are essential for normal tissue function and survival of the host that might make a molecularly targeted inhibitor nonselective? These considerations become paramount in determining the choice of target and the probability of success. Obviously, even the most validated target may not be amenable to a drug discovery strategy for any number of reasons, the most important being failure to understand the function of the target and related proteins in humans. Unanticipated toxicities, interactions with previously inapparent receptors or proteins, pharmacologic problems in drug distribution, and pharmacokinetics (PK) may defeat the most rational strategy.

The reader is referred to excellent reviews of high-priority molecular targets for cancer therapy.[1–7] The subjects of angiogenesis inhibitors and mAbs are covered elsewhere in this book. The following is a brief review of several of the more prominent pathways that have yielded substantial new leads for cancer treatment.

MOLECULAR TARGETS

The choice of a molecular target is dictated at present by an important consideration: It is vastly easier to design an inhibitor of an overexpressed function than it is to replace an inactive or deleted function. Thus, although suppressor gene mutations, such as those affecting the *p53* gene, play a prominent role in tumorigenesis, it is difficult to restore *p53* function short of introducing a new functional gene. Thus, the primary choices for targeted discovery are dominant or overexpressed functions.[1]

General Approaches to Identifying and Synthesizing Modulators for Molecular Targets

General approaches to development of inhibitors or modulators for identified targets in cancers are described in the following pages. The diversity of approaches is striking, although it is worth remembering that small molecules and antibodies are the only agents with established clear clinical value at this time.

One approach for developing agents targeting specific genes or proteins is empirically screening a large number of compounds for activity and subsequently designing better ones based on structure of the active compound (the approach by which most anticancer agents have been developed). High-throughput screens allowing rapid evaluation of a large number of compounds have recently enhanced the use of this approach. Alternatively, one can design compounds based on structure of the specific region being targeted, using known sequence and other information available about the gene or protein [e.g., x-ray crystallography, nuclear magnetic resonance (NMR) imaging, computer molecular modeling, and analysis]. Clearly, some combination of these two approaches might be most useful—for example, lead identification by random high-throughput screening, followed by lead optimization through structural studies of the inhibitor and target. In the future, this will allow more rational design of antineoplastic molecules, and, at the same time, efficient screening of potentially therapeutic agents with a wide range of structures.

The complexity of molecular structures makes designing compounds based on actual structure (as opposed to DNA sequence) a significant undertaking that requires sophisticated technology (e.g., x-ray crystallography, extensive computer analysis, and molecular modeling). Certain proteins, such as growth factor receptors (GFRs), which are among the most attractive targets for anticancer therapy because of their accessibility and potential importance in proliferation and survival pathways, are large and therefore still difficult to analyze by current analytic approaches. Designed structural modifications to an agent might impact on development of resistance (which remains a major obstacle to the ultimate effectiveness of any treatment), because mechanisms of resistance to the compound cannot be fully predicted beforehand. On the other hand, knowing the surface critical for ligand interaction with the target may allow design of a series of compounds that could overcome resistance due to mutations in the protein being targeted. These could be given either simultaneously, to prevent selection of resistant cells or, possibly, sequentially, to maintain the response for a longer time. The complexity of the body's handling of compounds makes predicting toxicology and PK difficult. At the present time, these can only be determined from careful preclinical and clinical studies.

As with all forms of systemic cancer therapy, the ultimate usefulness of these treatment approaches depends on the ability to effectively deliver the agent to tumor cells, adequate binding to (in the case of mAbs, or other compounds, used to activate the immune system or deliver radioactive compounds) or uptake by neoplastic cells, presence or expression of the agent within cells for a sufficient time to lead to death or differentiation of those cells, the gradient of concentration for the compound in malignant versus normal cells, rate of elimination of the agent in normal and malignant cells, and toxicity of the agent for normal tissues, acutely and chronically. The heterogeneity of neoplastic cells within tumors limits single-drug therapy and is also a problem for single molecularly targeted therapy. Therefore, approaches that target heterogeneous cell populations, including mechanisms for overcoming resistance, need to be part of the strategic plan in designing therapeutic use of these compounds.

A number of issues are potential negative factors for PK of targeted compounds, such as mAbs, antisense oligonucleotides, and peptidomimetics. These include relatively large size as compared to many drugs; complex structures, contributing to decreased absorption, enhanced hepatic clearance, and decreased permeation from blood into tissues; natural nucleases and proteases that rapidly break down unmodified compounds; specific receptors for these agents on cells that contribute to their uptake by certain cells and, therefore, their tissue distribution; and potential immunogenicity, because these compounds often have features (e.g., proteins or peptides) that make them directly immunogenic or inducers of host cytokine release, a property that can limit their long-term use.

ras Pathways

One of the first oncogenes to be recognized in human tumors was the mutation and constitutive activation of *ras*.[9] ras proteins play central roles in transducing signals important for a variety of critical processes in cells, including proliferation and differentiation.[9] One of the key roles played by ras proteins is in transmitting signals from GFRs to downstream signaling molecules. A scheme for *ras* function is shown in Figure 30-1. The ras protein family (K-ras, N-ras, and H-ras) are activated by upstream signaling from tyrosine kinase receptors, such as the EGFRs. ras proteins are activated by binding guanosine triphosphate (GTP) and, subsequently, activate downstream targets in the signaling cascade, including the Raf kinase. In the process, GTP is hydrolyzed to guanosine diphosphate, and ras is inactivated. Mutations at the 12, 13, or 61 codons of the *ras* genes constitutively activate ras by locking it in the GTP-bound state. This leads to activation of Raf and the signal transduction pathway in the absence of growth factor stimulation. *ras* must be bound to the plasma membrane to activate Raf. In concert with other mutations, *ras* is transforming in normal cells. *ras* mutations occur relatively frequently in a number of malignancies. For example, K-*ras* mutations are found in approximately 40% to 50% of colon cancers, 70% to 90% of pancreatic cancers, and 30% of adenocarcinomas of the lung.[9–12] N-*ras* is mutated in approximately 20% to 30% of acute nonlymphocytic leukemias.[13] H-*ras* is mutated in a minority of bladder and head and neck cancers. Thus, as a molecular target, *ras* has attractive features.

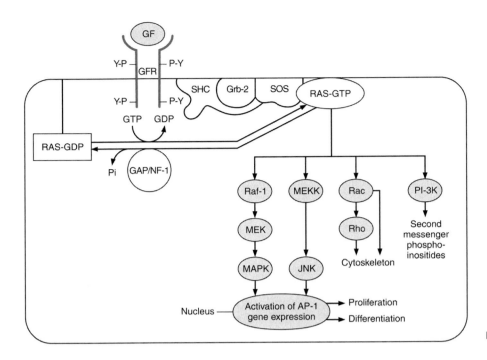

FIGURE 30-1. Ras signaling pathways.

There are several potential methods of inhibiting ras. The unprocessed native protein is inactive and requires sequential posttranslational modification to allow insertion in the plasma membrane, which is required for its active signaling function.[9,14] It must first be farnesylated (attachment of a 15 carbon, lipophilic group) by soluble prenylation enzymes. The carbon terminal (C-terminal) CAAX motif of ras then directs the prenylated protein to the endoplasmic reticulum and Golgi, in which the C-terminal AAX residues are cleaved by a specific protease. The terminal prenylcysteine is then methylated by a prenyl cysteine methyl transferase found in the endomembrane system. The final product is exported to its active site in the plasma membrane. In the case of N- and H-*ras*, this occurs after further lipid attachment (palmitic acid) to another cysteine or cysteines. K-*ras*, which possesses a polybasic region upstream from the C-terminal peptide, does not require palmitylation to localize in the plasma membrane.[14] The sequence of reactions is illustrated in Figure 30-2.

Initial attempts to develop compounds blocking *ras* function have been devoted to the discovery of inhibitors of the farnesylation reaction,[15–18] although there is now considerable interest in exploring inhibition of prenyl cysteine methyl transferase and the *ras* proteases.[14] In addition, targeting of downstream effectors of *ras*, such as the Raf kinase, are also being pursued. Potent and selective farnesyl transferase inhibitors (FTIs) with preference for H-*ras* inhibition have been isolated by selecting lead compounds in high-throughput screening. With subsequent structural refinement, four compounds have entered clinical trial (Table 30-2). Although some evidence of antitumor activity has been seen with several of these compounds, the ultimate clinical use of any of these compounds remains uncertain.

Experience with the FTIs currently in development taught valuable lessons about targeted drug discovery. A number of initial assumptions have proven to be invalid: (a) Contrary to initial knowledge, it is now clear that there is an ever growing number of proteins other than ras proteins that undergo farnesylation. There is evidence arguing that other proteins, such as RhoB, may be the critical target(s) in the inhibition of tumor cell growth by FTIs[19–21]; (b) K-*ras* can be inserted into the cell membrane and, thus, activated through geranyl-geranylation, bypassing FTI inhibition; (c) *ras* plays a role in signaling via a complex set of pathways in cells, and it is not always clear what effects might be produced by inhibition of its function in different cellular circumstances.[14–18] Not surprisingly, given these facts, antitumor activity of FTIs in cell culture does not necessarily correlate with the presence of *ras* mutation. In addition, the FTIs as a class are not selective for tumors but demonstrate a spectrum of toxicities in humans, including diarrhea, hepatotoxicity, neurotoxicity, cardiac conduction abnormalities, and myelosuppression (Table 30-2).

Nonetheless, the FTIs as a class still have a number of features that warrant clinical evaluation and interest. In addition to as yet incompletely defined activity as single agents, they are antiangiogenic, sensitize to irradiation, and display synergy with cytotoxic drugs. Any or all of these properties could result from inhibition of cellular processes, even in cells that lack *ras* mutation, with effects down-

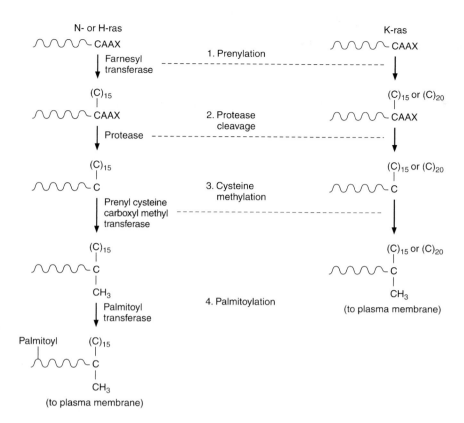

FIGURE 30-2. Posttranslational modification of Ras proteins.

TABLE 30-2. FARNESYL TRANSFERASE INHIBITORS CURRENTLY IN CLINICAL TRIALS

Compound	Route of administration [$t_{1/2}$ (h)]	Best responses	Toxicities
R115777	Oral (~5)	Partial response [breast, non–small cell lung cancer (NSCLC)]	Nausea and vomiting (N/V), diarrhea, headache, fatigue, neurologic (paresthesias, numbness, and confusion), hypotension, skin (rash/hypersensitivity), myelosuppression, increased bilirubin
L-778,123	i.v.	—	Myelosuppression, prolonged blood volume interval corrected for heart rate (QTc), N/V, fatigue
BMS-214662	i.v./oral (~2–4)	Minor response (NSCLC)	N/V, diarrhea, anorexia, fatigue, neurologic (somnolence), myelosuppression, transaminitis
SCH66336	Oral (~4–18)	Partial response (NSCLC)	N/V, diarrhea, anorexia, fatigue, neurologic (confusion), myelosuppression, decreased renal function

Adapted from Hect HI, Cohen DP, et al. Phase I pharmacokinetic trial of the farnesyl transferase inhibitor SCH66366 plus Gemcitabine in advanced cancers. *Proc ASCO* 2000;18; Sharma S, Britten C, et al. A Phase I PK study of farnesyl transferase inhibitor L-778, 123 administered as a seven day continuous infusion in combination with paclitaxel. *Proc ASCO* 2000;18; Lynch TJ, Amrein PC, et al. Phase I clinical trial of the farnesyltransferase (FT) inhibitor BMS-214662 in patients with advanced solid tumors. *Proc ASCO* 2000;18; Howes AJ, Palmer P, et al. A phase II study of the farnesyl transferase inhibitor R115777 in patients with advanced breast cancer. *Proc ASCO* 2000;18; Schellens JH, Klerk GD, et al. Phase I and pharmacologic study with the novel farnesyltransferase inhibitor (FTI) R115777. *Proc ASCO* 2000;18; Ryan DP, Eder JP, et al. Phase 1 clinical trial of the farnesyltransferase (FT) Inhibitor BMS-214662 in patients with advanced solid tumors. *Proc ASCO* 2000;18; Rubin E, Abruzzese JL, et al. Phase I trial of the farnesyl Protein Transferase (FPTase) inhibitor L-778123 on a 14 day or 28 day dosing schedule. *Proc ASCO* 2000;18; Sonnichsen D, Damle B, et al. Pharmacokinetics (PK) and pharmacodynamics (PD) of the farnesyltransferase (FT) inhibitor BMS-214662 in patients with advanced solid tumors. *Proc ASCO* 2000;18; Zujewski J, Horak I, et al. A phase I and Pharmacokinetics study of farnesyltransferase inhibitor, R115777 in advanced cancer. *Proc ASCO* 1999;18:192a; Adjei AA, Erlichman C, et al. A phase I and pharmacologic study of the farnesyl protein transferase (FPT) inhibitor SCH 66366 in patients with locally advanced or metastatic cancer. *Proc ASCO* 1999;19:165a; Hurwitz HI, Colvin OM, et al. Phase I and pharmacokinetic study of SCH66336, a novel FPTI, using a 2 week on, 2 week off schedule. *Proc ASCO* 1999;18:156a, Eskens F, Awada A, et al. Phase I and pharmacologic study of continuous daily oral SCH 66366, a novel farnesyl transferase inhibitor in patients with solid tumors. *Proc ASCO* 1999;18:156a; and Hudes JR, Schol J, et al. Phase I clinical and pharmacokinetic trial of the farnesyltransferase inhibitor R115777 on a 21 day dosing schedule. *Proc ASCO* 1999;18:156a.

stream on the threshold for apoptosis or release of angiogenic factors.

Retinoblastoma Pathway

A second prominent target is the RB pathway (Fig. 30-3).[2,3,6,7] In this pathway, the critical player is the product of the RB gene, a protein that in its underphosphorylated state inhibits E2F, a transcription factor that promotes synthesis of messenger RNAs (mRNAs) for a vast number of proteins involved in DNA synthesis. The function of RB is, in turn, tightly regulated by a complex sequence of protein interactions that regulate its phosphorylation state. The responsible kinases, cdk4, cdk6, or both, are activated by cyclin D and inhibited by p16 and p21. Multiple sites of mutation or alteration in this pathway can lead to malignancy; essentially any mutation or modification that eliminates, inactivates, or phosphorylates RB will activate E2F and promote transformation. These alterations include loss of RB itself in patients with RB, activation of cdk4 in melanoma, overexpression of cyclin D in many human tumors, and a loss of p16 in approximately 50% of human tumors. Virtually all human tumors display an alteration of at least one component of this pathway, most frequently p16 deletion or cyclin D overexpression. Experimental models of RB loss or inactivation have confirmed the tumorigenic effect of mutations in this pathway. Thus, an antitumor therapy targeted at inhibiting RB phosphorylation has compelling logic.

An inhibitor of cdk4, flavopiridol, has entered clinical trial, and its evaluation thus far has disclosed modest antitumor activity in phase I and early phase II.[2,7] It fulfills many of the hypothesized advantages of molecularly targeted therapies. It has limited toxicity for normal proliferating tissues, induces apoptosis in tumor cells, and enhances

cytotoxicity of traditional drugs. However, its mechanism of action, competitive inhibition of the adenosine triphosphate binding site of the kinase, may lead to promiscuous effects on multiple kinases.

It inhibits cdk4 at approximately 100 nmol per L, but lacks specificity for cdk4 in that it has similar affinity for cdk1, cdk2, cdk7, and, at higher (micromolar) concentrations, a number of other kinases. In addition, it suppresses expression of cyclin D1, the important activator of cdk4. Whether its antitumor effects are attributable to cdk4 inhibition remains in question. This can only be answered by detailed studies of the correlation of RB phosphorylation status and antitumor response. The fact that it has antitumor activity, that it potently induces apoptosis in various human tumor cells in a p53-independent manner, and that it has synergy with cytotoxins is reason enough to pursue clinical development of it as well as related compounds.[7]

bcr-abl Kinase

The 9:22 translocation in CML has proven to be a particularly attractive target.[19] The translocation places the Abl tyrosine kinase activity on chromosome 9 in juxtaposition to the breakpoint cluster region of chromosome 22. The resulting protein has a complex variety of functions, including a constitutively active tyrosine kinase. It is capable of transformation in mice. Antisense to the bcr-abl gene reverses the malignant phenotype and induces apoptosis in CML cells *in vitro*. Thus, bcr-abl inhibition should produce significant anti-CML effect. Using high-throughput screening against recombinant bcr-abl protein, Drucker and colleagues identified a peptidomimetic molecule with high affinity for the adenosine triphosphate binding site of the Abl kinase, capable of suppressing proliferation of bcr-abl transfected tumor cells *in vitro* and *in vivo*.[19] It has been strikingly active in initial clinical trials in humans with CML. The compound STI-571 produces clinical hematologic responses in most patients with CML in chronic phase refractory to interferon, at doses that have minimal toxicity (400 mg per m² per day) (and cytogenetic complete remission in 10% of these patients). It also has activity against CML in blast crisis, although the extent of activity in this setting is still being defined. Its maximum tolerated dose has not yet been defined. Exact percentages of responses are not available at this time, and phase I and II trials continue at this writing. Because of its striking activity against CML, it has moved simultaneously into extensive phase II trials in CML and in adult patients with acute lymphoblastic leukemia who have 9:22 translocation. The drug's key features are given in Table 30-3. It also induces remissions in CML in blastic phase, and in transformation, these responses are brief in initial reports.

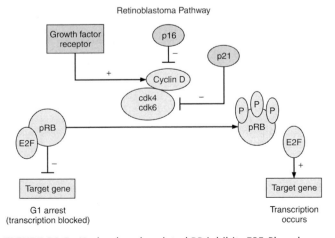

Retinoblastoma Pathway

FIGURE 30-3. Underphosphorylated RB inhibits E2F. Phosphorylation of RB by cdk4/cdk6 kinases releases this inhibition.

TABLE 30-3. KEY FEATURES OF STI-571 bcr-abl TYROSINE KINASE INHIBITOR

2-Phenylaminopyrimidine class of tyrosine kinase inhibitor
Inhibits adenosine triphosphate binding
Selective inhibitor of abl kinase and, to lesser extent, platelet-derived growth factor receptor and c-kit
Daily oral therapy
Half-life between 12 and 14 h
Minimal toxicity at clinically effective doses (maximum tolerated dose not yet defined)
Hematologic responses in almost all chronic phase patients and cytogenetic responses in the majority of patients

This molecule also has inhibitory effects on the PDGF receptor (PDGFR) and the c-kit receptor. It has antitumor activity against tumors overexpressing the PDGFR in animals. Thus, it may have broader activity in humans against PDGFR-expressing tumors, such as gliomas and prostate cancer, and gastrointestinal (GI) stromal tumors (c-kit expressing). STI-571 is clearly the most important drug to arise from molecularly targeted drug discovery to date.

Other Targets

Few mutations associated with human cancer provide such a clear overexpressed target for drug development as the bcr-abl protein. Most epithelial cancers represent the evolution of multiple mutations, and it is unclear whether any single event is critical to the survival of all malignant clones within a given cancer. Candidates that might fit this requirement include apoptosis, telomerase, critical growth factor signaling pathways [e.g., EGFR and HER-2-neu receptor, PTEN gene mutations and deletion in the PI3-kinase pathway, and various angiogenic targets, such as the VEGF and its receptor (see Chapter 35).[20–23] Clinical responses in patients treated with mAbs to HER-2-neu (using trastuzumab), the EGFR (using the IMC-C225 antibody), and an EGFR small molecule inhibitor (ZD 1839, Iressa) offer promise that interruption of growth signals may be a useful strategy for drug design.[21,24–26]

Whether these other targets offer the same degree of specificity, selectivity, and essential role in the proliferation of specific tumors, as is the case for bcr-abl, is still unknown. Of these, the activated and translocated *bcl*-2 gene would seem to be a particularly promising target to fulfill the requirements for validation; an antiapoptotic protein, it is activated and overexpressed in the majority of follicular lymphomas, as well as approximately 50% of high-grade B-cell lymphomas. An antisense to *bcl*-2 induces apoptosis in culture and has antitumor effects in humans when used in patients with NHL (see Antisense Oligonucleotides). In addition, a number of studies suggest enhanced cytotoxicity of various chemotherapeutic agents when *bcl*-2 is inhibited. Thus far, an effective small molecule inhibitor of *bcl*-2 has not been discovered. The reader is referred to an article by Sellers and Fisher for a more complete discussion of the various targets related to apoptosis.[27] There are as yet no effective inhibitors of telomerase ready for clinical testing.

SPECIFIC TARGETING AGENTS

Antisense Oligonucleotides

Antisense oligonucleotides (oligos) are modified single-stranded DNA molecules, usually between 15 and 25 nucleotides in length. They are synthesized to have nucleotide sequences complementary to DNA or mRNA sequences of the specific gene being targeted for inhibition. As drugs, oligos have inherent disadvantages, including large size, significant charge, difficult synthesis, and poor penetration of cells. In part for these reasons, they still have not fulfilled their promise as therapeutic agents. However, development is ongoing with the hope that with greater understanding of their clinical pharmacology, they will prove useful.

Mechanism of Action

When therapy is directed at mRNA, it is based on one of the fundamental features of biology, the specificity of Watson and Crick base pairing. By binding to mRNA, synthesis of the specific protein encoded by that mRNA is ultimately inhibited, and its function blocked. Using mRNA as the target, a number of specific mechanisms can be inhibited or otherwise modified[28–32] (Table 30-4), among these the activation of the RNA degrading enzyme, RNaseH.

Alternatively, specific DNA or protein sequences can be targeted by oligos. The major target in DNA is Hoogsteen and anti-Hoogsteen base pairing in the major groove to produce triple-helical structures leading to inhibition of transcription. Oligos can be coupled to a number of anti-

TABLE 30-4. POTENTIAL MECHANISMS OF MESSENGER RNA (mRNA) FUNCTION OR mRNA MODIFICATION TARGETED BY ANTISENSE OLIGONUCLEOTIDES

Inhibition of mRNA
Translational arrest
Splicing
5' Capping
3' Polyadenylation
Transport
Degradation
Activation of RNaseH, an enzyme present ubiquitously in cells, which degrades RNA complexed to DNA

neoplastic compounds to specifically target them, especially to DNA.

Hybridization to RNA or DNA is a relatively slow process, and, in general, association rates of oligos determine their efficacy.[28-32] The minimum size of oligos required to provide necessary specificity and affinity for these purposes appears to be 15 to 18 bases. A caveat to this specificity is that mismatched oligos can induce degradation of target mRNA, so it is certainly possible that cleavage of nontarget mRNA sequences might occur when specific oligos are used *in vivo*.

Alternatively, the binding of proteins (e.g., transcription factors) to specific DNA or RNA sequences can be targeted. The sequence length required depends on the precise protein-DNA (or RNA) interaction site.[28-32] Normally, non-DNA or RNA binding proteins can also potentially be inhibited by binding to oligos specifically and nonspecifically. An approach to designing specific oligos for this purpose is protein epitope targeting. A large number of partially random oligos are used to screen for binding to a target protein. This allows identification of oligos that bind to specific epitopes. The bound oligos can be amplified by polymerase chain reaction. Identified sequences can then be used to develop improved oligos for targeting the protein therapeutically.

Cellular Pharmacology and Metabolism

Necessary requirements for oligos to be useful therapeutically are outlined in Table 30-5. Oligos appear to bind to the cell surface through receptors, although the exact nature of these remains to be defined.[28-32] This process is saturable. However, it is not clear whether this saturability of uptake will be important for systemic use of oligos. Once bound to the cell surface, oligo uptake into cells appears to occur primarily by pinocytosis, adsorptive endocytosis, or both.[28-32] Although certain studies suggest that a significant proportion of oligos remains in endosomes, the consensus is that retention in endosomes is not a major limitation in their effectiveness. Binding by cellular proteins may modify PK and efficacy of oligos.[28-32]

TABLE 30-5.   REQUIREMENTS FOR OLIGONUCLEO-TIDES TO BE THERAPEUTICALLY USEFUL

Stability *in vivo*
Uptake into and retention in neoplastic cells
Specific and relatively stable interaction with target sequences in RNA, DNA, protein, or a combination of the three, without nonspecific inhibition of other cellular molecules
Absence of significant toxicity to normal cells or organ systems
Limited potential for mutagenicity
Lack of significant immunogenicity
Favorable pharmacokinetics (distribution, metabolism, and excretion) *in vivo* to allow sufficient delivery to tumor cells to inhibit their growth

Uptake of oligos varies among different cell types (studies suggest greater uptake in carcinoma than leukemic cells) and among cells in the same culture. Various factors (e.g., number of oligo receptors, cell-cycle stage, rate of division) can explain differences in oligo uptake. Increased cell density decreases uptake of phosphorothioate oligos.[33] As would be expected, differences in the intracellular degradation of oligos by cells can have a profound effect on their efficacy.[34] Exocytosis also occurs and is a potentially important determinant of the concentration of oligos within cells over time, and, therefore, of their efficacy. Thus, a number of aspects of cellular pharmacology are critical in determining activity of these compounds.

Clinical Pharmacology

Oligos present a special problem as *in vivo* compounds because of the ubiquitous presence of nucleases that rapidly degrade unmodified constructs.[34] Fortunately, the potential clinical use of oligos can be enhanced by medicinal chemical approaches.[28-32] Certain modifications make them potentially better for some purposes, but not as good for others. Modifications can be designed to prevent rapid metabolism, increase cellular uptake, increase targeting to tumor cells, stabilize binding of oligos to the target structure, or increase inhibitory efficacy. Oligos can be conjugated with ribozymes (with catalytic RNase activity; see Ribozymes, Other Nucleases, and Proteases), or other reagents that cleave specific nucleic acid sequences.[35] Peptide nucleic acids can inhibit DNA and RNA function. Attachment of toxic compounds to oligos can target those agents to DNA and enhance cell killing, such as using antisense bcr-abl constructs to deliver compounds specifically to DNA in CML cells.

The most important modifications for *in vivo* use have been chemical alterations of the bases used to construct oligos. This includes using methylphosphonates or phosphorothioates as the phosphodiester backbone, a change that prevents their destruction by nucleases.[28-32] Phosphorothioates appear to be the more advantageous of these analogs, because they have higher affinity than dimethyl phosphonates for nucleic acids, and they are more effective in activating RNaseH. Therefore, phosphorothioates have been the most extensively studied modified oligos. Many other modifications to oligos, including incorporation of methylene, carbonate (or carbamate), sulfonamide, amino acid, peptide, phosphorodithioate, C-5 propyne analogs of cytidine and uridine, and pyrimidines modified at the 5 and 6 positions, also have significant activity *in vitro*.[28-32,36] However, these have not yet been extensively developed for clinical use.

A number of methods have been used to increase specificity of delivery of oligos to tumor cells and uptake by those cells. Molecules such as porphyrin, cholesterol (or cholesteryl), poly-L-lysine, and transferrinpolylysine significantly enhance uptake and retention, although they also reduce the time of the interaction with mRNA or DNA.[28–32] Liposomes (e.g., pH-sensitive liposomes) may provide an effective way of delivering oligos into cells.[37] Complexes of liposomes with compounds (e.g., the Sendai virus protein coat) can significantly enhance their uptake by cells. Coupling of liposomes (with encapsulated oligos) to targeting peptides (i.e., mAbs directed against antigens expressed on the cell surface) offers another means of specific targeting.[38]

Ex vivo use of oligonucleotides does not have many of the problems associated with *in vivo* use. Oligos by themselves, as well as in combination with chemotherapy, are highly effective in inhibiting tumor cell growth *ex vivo*. These strategies may be useful in purging bone marrow of leukemic or other malignant cells.[39]

Alternatives to antisense, with more favorable PK properties, inhibit site-specific interactions between RNA and proteins or nucleotides.[40] For example, the antibiotic neomycin B inhibits the specific interaction between human immunodeficiency virus (HIV) rev protein and the rev-binding site on HIV RNA. In concept, small-molecular-weight inhibitors could be used to block any specific RNA-binding interaction. Although neomycin B itself is too toxic for systemic use, the ability to screen a large number of compounds should provide agents with less toxicity that would still be effective.

Pharmacokinetics

In the excitement over the potential use of antisense therapy for the treatment of cancer, an area that has received less attention and study is the PK of these agents *in vivo*. Until the last 5 years, the paucity of PK data resulted, at least in part, from the high cost of producing sufficient amounts of the compounds for careful PK studies, even in mice. Fortunately, the cost of producing oligos has decreased dramatically with continued improvements in technology. A second problem has been assay methodology for separation of the parent compound and its stepwise oligo cleavage products. These problems have been sufficiently solved for PK studies of oligos to be performed.

Several animal models have been used for evaluating targeting, pharmacology, and effectiveness of these compounds. Most studies suggest that oligos (primarily phosphorothioate analogs, which are resistant to nucleases, water soluble, and readily taken up by cells; to a lesser extent, methylphosphonates have been studied) are fairly rapidly cleared from the circulation.[28–32] Most studies in animals have shown $t_{1/2\alpha}$ ranges from 5 minutes to several hours after bolus administration; human studies to date have been more variable, ranging from 30 minutes to as long as 26 hours after bolus administration and approximately 7 hours after subcutaneous administration.[28,41–58] In any case, overall they have relatively short half-lives, argu-

ing for the need for frequent administration if continued inhibition of the target is to be maintained.

Oligonucleotides are distributed to the majority of tissues, including malignancies. In the absence of central nervous system abnormalities, brain takes up little of systemically delivered phosphorothioate or methylphosphonate oligos.[44–58] Oligo length (at least within the 20 to 50 base range), base sequence, and dose (at least in the range up to 150 mg per kg) do not appear to significantly affect the rate of plasma clearance.[44–50] However, the specific base analog used in constructing the oligos does affect PK.[41–58]

Given the relatively slow uptake of oligos by cells, rapid clearance from the circulation makes delivery of oligos to tumor cells difficult. Mechanisms for enhancing delivery are important considerations if oligos are to be used successfully as systemic agents. In normal tissues, highest concentrations accumulate in the kidney and liver, with up to 40% in the liver at 12 hours.[44–50] This can induce some degree of hepatic inflammation, as indicated by elevations in lactate dehydrogenase and transaminases.[44–58] To a lesser extent, accumulation occurs in other tissues, including intestine, spleen, lungs, heart, and muscle.[45] Route of administration may affect organ distribution, with subcutaneous injection possibly favoring accumulation in spleen and muscle.[45] Oligos are stable in most tissues but are more rapidly metabolized in kidney and liver.[45] Degradation in blood and tissues appears to be primarily due to 3'-exonucleases.[49] Rate of degradation does not appear to be dose dependent as would be expected given the large amount of nucleases present. The $t_{1/2\beta}$ of total-body clearance is approximately 30 to 40 hours.[15,45,49] Clearance of methylphosphonate and unmodified oligos is more rapid than clearance of phosphorothioates.[49] Most of the dose is excreted in urine in 2 to 3 days (with approximately 30% in the first 24 hours) and significantly less via the GI tract.[44–50] Most oligos that are excreted are degraded so that only a small proportion of intact oligos are found in the urine. Modifications to the oligos, including addition of bases, can occur in several tissues, including liver, kidney, and GI tract.[44–50] Interactions with other drugs is poorly understood; there continues to be a need for careful evaluation of PK in the setting of coadministered drugs. However, most studies have not shown significant PK interactions between oligos and chemotherapeutic drugs (see below for further discussion).

Toxicity

Although antisense molecules differ in their sequence and target, they seem to share similar PK and toxicologic properties, independent of effects on the target sequence itself. Although a single dose of 640 mg per kg of anti-HIV phosphorothioate was lethal, single doses of up to 150 mg per kg have been well tolerated in mice.[47,49] Antisense molecules that are cytostatic may require prolonged administration, making potential chronic toxicity an important consideration. Doses up to 100 mg per kg of phosphorothioate oligos for 14 days do not appear to produce serious toxic effects.[44–50] In rhesus monkeys, continuous infusions of oligos at doses up to 1,500 mg for periods as long as 15 days did not produce significant toxicities.[51] Mild elevations in liver functions were seen in the majority of animals, and mild neutropenia was seen in one-third. Many oligos seem to produce complement activation and thrombocytopenia as their dose-limiting toxicities in animals. Oligos can also accumulate in kidneys with potential for nephrotoxicity, although significant nephrotoxicity is primarily seen at higher doses.[44–50]

Most of the clinical trials in humans have indicated that oligonucleotides are generally safe. The most common toxicities have been thrombocytopenia, asthenia, fevers, hypotension, hyperglycemia, and minor changes in renal function (Table 30-6).[52–58] All of these are usually mild and rapidly reverse when the oligonucleotide is discontinued. Local skin reactions are also seen when oligos are delivered subcutaneously. Less common toxicities have included activation of complement and clotting abnormalities.

Clinical Effectiveness

In vivo effectiveness of antisense oligos has been demonstrated in a number of animal model systems.[28–32,41,42] Longer exposure of animals to oligos appears to produce a greater antitumor effect.[41] These results indicate that sufficient quantities of oligos can be delivered over time to a variety of tumors in mice to achieve an antitumor effect at doses that do not produce significant toxicity.

Clinical trials have been completed using antisense constructs alone and in combination with chemotherapy[52–58] (Table 30-6). Antisense constructs to other mutated cancer genes, including *p53* and bcr-abl, as well as to HIV (in patients with HIV-associated malignancies), have been performed. These have shown the following: (a) Target genes can be inhibited in peripheral blood cells and malignant cells in lymph nodes at achievable concentrations of oligonucleotides. (b) Occasional patients have had responses (including a complete response seen in a patient with B-cell NHL treated with Bcl-2 antisense).[53] A proportion of patients have had stable disease. However, overall, most patients have not responded. (c) Combinations of oligonucleotides with chemotherapy can be delivered with acceptable toxicity. In addition, these have not indicated significant PK interactions between oligos and chemotherapeutic agents. Although this remains a potential concern, it does not appear to be a common one. Additional clinical trials are ongoing, and the results will indicate whether sufficient clinical efficacy can be achieved in humans (either of oligonucleotides themselves or combinations with chemotherapy) for this approach to be of value in treating cancer patients. Other routes of administration (*ex*

TABLE 30-6. TOXICITIES OF SOME OF THE OLIGONUCLEOTIDES IN CLINICAL TRIALS FOR CANCER PATIENTS

Compound	Toxicities
Antisense to bcl-2	Fatigue, flulike symptoms (myalgias, arthralgias), transaminitis
Antisense to c-raf-1	Fever, complement activation, prolonged PTT
Antisense to H-ras	Flulike symptoms, fatigue, nausea, self-limiting hemolytic uremic syndrome
Antisense to protein kinase C-alpha	Fever, flulike symptoms, transaminitis, complement activation, prolonged PT, PTT, decreased platelets, hemorrhage

PT, prothrombin time; PTT, partial prothrombin time.
Adapted from Chen H, Ness E, et al. Phase I trial of a second generation oligonucleotide (GEM 123) targeted at type I protein kinase a in patients with refractory solid tumors. *Proc ASCO* 1999;18:159a; Mani S, Shulman K, et al. Phase I trial of protein kinase-C a antisense oligonucleotide (ISIS 3521; ISI 641A) with 5-fluorouracil (5-FU) and leucovorin (LV) in patients with advanced cancer. *Proc ASCO* 1999;18; Advani R, Fisher A, et al. A phase I trial of an antisense oligonucleotide targeted to protein kinase C a (ISIS 3521/ISI641A) delivered as a 24-hour continuous infusion (CI). *Proc ASCO* 1999;18; Dorr A, Bruce J, et al. Phase I and pharmacokinetic trial of ISIS 2503, a 20-Mer antisense oligonucleotide against H-RAS, by 14-day continuous infusion (CIV) in patients with advanced cancer. *Proc ASCO* 1999;18:157a; Gordon MS, Sandler AB, et al. A phase I trial of ISIS 2503, an antisense inhibitor of H-RAS, administered by a 24-hour (hr) weekly infusion to patients (pts) with advanced cancer. *Proc ASCO* 1999;18:157a; Holmlund JT, Rudin CM, et al. Phase I trial of ISIS 5132/ODN 698A, a 20-Mer phosphorothioate antisense oligonucleotide inhibitor of C-RAF kinase, administered by a 24-hour weekly intravenous (IV) infusion to patients with advanced cancer. *Proc ASCO* 1999;18:157a; Daugherty CK, Goh BC, et al. The standard phase II trial design is not acceptable to most patients (pts). *Proc ASCO* 2000;19; Alavi JB, Grossman SA, et al. Efficacy, toxicity and pharmacology of an antisense oligonucleotide directed against protein kinase C-a (ISIS 3521) delivered as a 21 day continuous intravenous infusion in patients with recurrent high grade astrocytomas (HGA). *Proc ASCO* 2000;19; Yuen A, Advani R, et al. A phase I/II trial of ISIS 3521, an antisense inhibitor of protein kinase C Alpha, combined with carboplatin and paclitaxel in patients with with non-small cell lung cancer. *Proc ASCO* 2000; Chi KN, Gleave ME, et al. A phase I trial of an antisense oligonucleotide to BCL-2 (6139) mitoxantrone in patients with metastatic hormone refractory prostate (HRPC). *Proc ASCO* 2000;19; and Scher HI, Morris MJ, et al. A phase I trial of G3139, a bcl2 antisense drug, by continuous infusion (CI) as a single agent and with weekly Taxol. *Proc ASCO* 2000;19:199a.

vivo, intraperitoneal, transcutaneously, intrathecal) are also being explored.

Ribozymes, Other Nucleases, and Proteases

Ribozymes are RNAs that can catalyze a variety of RNA or DNA cleavage reactions (i.e., splicing or site-specific cleavage) via their tertiary structures and therefore function as enzymes, or possibly drugs.[59–65] Their advantage over protein enzymes is that one can, through sequence and structure changes, modify ribozymes to carry out specific functions much more readily than can be done for proteins. As with oligos, they need to be modified to make them nuclease resistant to be useful for *in vivo* purposes. The stability of the RNA being targeted and the turnover rate of ribozyme-substrate interaction are important determinants of the potential usefulness of ribozymes. They need to be targeted to cells by coupling with proteins, genetic vectors, or other compounds to be most useful. Their pharmacology for the most part resembles that of the targeting agent to which they are coupled. Their therapeutic use is currently being pursued primarily as antiviral agents, especially directed against HIV. An ongoing clinical trial is evaluating hairpin ribozymes targeted *ex vivo* for CD8-depleted T cells of HIV-1–infected patients in an attempt to cleave viral RNA.[67] Reinfusion of ribozyme containing T cells has been well tolerated to date, and ribozyme-containing cells can persist for relatively long intervals. No clear-cut evidence of efficacy has yet been seen. Studies are still ongoing for antiviral agents as well as antitumor agents.[64–66]

Gene Therapy

Gene therapy uses the insertion of new genetic information into cells and its expression in those cells to alter their biologic behavior with intended therapeutic benefit. The initial and still a major promise of gene therapy's clinical potential is placement of a normal critical gene into cells that either do not express the gene at all or have a mutated form of the gene. This also could potentially suppress abnormal function of the mutated gene. This strategy is being pursued for inherited genetic disorders and for introducing tumor suppressor genes into neoplastic cells. However, a number of significant hurdles remain to be overcome if we are to be able to treat malignancies with this approach. These include the need to transfect at least the vast majority of malignant cells for this to be clinically useful, inefficiency of gene transfer into cells, difficulties of *in vivo* delivery to neoplastic cells, and the problem of maintaining continued expression of the transduced gene in those cells over time.

Therefore, much of the emphasis in gene therapy as an approach to treating neoplasms has shifted to making cells more immunogenic to activate host-mediated killing of the cells. A number of animal model systems suggest that modification of a subpopulation of tumor cells may lead to an "innocent bystander effect" (by mechanisms that have not been fully elucidated but presumably are, at least in part, immune mediated), whereby nontransfected tumor cells are also eliminated. This approach would not require transfecting every cell to be effective.[67] The fact that the innocent bystander effect is seen with a wide variety of transferred genes suggests that the mechanism(s) involved in mediating this effect may not necessarily all be immunologic, but much more study is required to determine why this occurs and how it might be best used. Alternatively, genes that protect normal cells against toxicity of therapeutic agents used to treat the malignancy could be used to protect the host and allow higher-dose delivery of the toxic agents.

Difficulties remain in ensuring that expression of the transfected gene is appropriately controlled in tumor cells, maintaining expression in these cells during a prolonged period (expression of most genes tends to decrease with time), while preventing deleterious function in normal cells. These need to be adequately addressed for gene therapy to be therapeutically useful.

TABLE 30-7. POTENTIAL APPLICATIONS OF GENE THERAPY

RNA decoys
Transdominant mutant proteins
Intracellular toxins
Intracellular antibodies
Ribozymes
Proteins that make tumor cells more immunogenic
Proteins that make tumor cells susceptible to killing by specific drugs
Proteins that make normal cells resistant to cytotoxic agents
Proteins beneficial to host expressed in immune effector or other host cells

Mechanism of Action

Introduced genetic material can be used to inhibit or augment gene function or produce proteins beneficial to the host by a number of potential mechanisms[68] (Table 30-7): (a) as RNA decoys, in which multiple copies of a sequence can be transcribed and compete with other intracellular sequences for protein binding[69,70]; (b) as transdominant altered proteins that can suppress specific protein function in cells [if these happen to be critical proteins for a signal transduction pathway (e.g., *ras* or *raf*) one could potentially disrupt the entire pathway][71,72]; (c) in production of intracellular toxins leading to cell death[73]; (d) in production of antibodies intracellularly to block function of specific proteins[74]; (e) as ribozymes to catalyze cleavage of specific RNA or DNA sequences[59–64]; (f) in expression of proteins making tumor cells more immunogenic and, therefore, prone to elimination by the host's immune system, as well as generating a systemic immune response against the tumor[75,76]; (g) in expression of genes that make cells susceptible to killing by specific drugs [e.g., the herpesvirus thymidine kinase (TK) gene, which makes cells susceptible to killing by gancyclovir, or the cytosine deaminase gene, which activates 5-fluorocytosine][77,78]; (h) in expression of a gene (i.e., the dihydrofolate reductase or multiple drug resistance type 1) in normal cells that makes them more resistant to killing by cytotoxic agents or radiation therapy[79,80]; or (i) to produce proteins beneficial to the host in an ongoing and controllable manner, either in immune-effector or other host cells, such as fibroblasts.

Cellular Pharmacology and Metabolism

Two major methods for introducing genetic material into cells are (a) physical approaches, such as via liposomal delivery, DNA-ligand complexes, ballistic techniques (in which multiple pellets coated with DNA are rapidly injected into cells), and direct injection of DNA itself, and (b) viral-mediated transfer. Defective retroviral vectors were the initial ones studied for use as a means of getting genes into and expressed in mammalian cells.[81] However, they have a number of limitations for therapeutic use, which has led to development of other viral vectors for this purpose. Limitations of retroviral vectors include the necessity of having active cell division for retroviral vectors to integrate into chromosomes; cells must have the appropriate receptors to take up the vectors; integration of viral DNA into random chromosomal sites raises concerns about potential activation of endogenous genes, which might be transforming, or inactivation of genes important in controlling cell proliferation; and inactivation, such as by complement, when used *in vivo*.

For all these reasons, retroviral vectors have been proposed primarily for *ex vivo* therapy. Construction of other viral vectors that might not carry the same degree of risk for mutagenesis or induction of host genes has been actively pursued. These viral vectors include vaccinia (and other poxviruses), polio, Sindbis (and other RNA viruses), adenovirus, adeno-associated viruses, herpesvirus vectors (e.g., herpes simplex virus 1), and HIV-1, which have all been modified for use in gene therapy.[82–85] As with retroviral vectors, each of these has its potential benefits but also potential problems as delivery systems for gene therapy. There is an ongoing effort to improve each of these vectors that should provide better vector systems for therapeutic use. As an example, a possible method for making these vectors safer is by incorporating the TK gene, rendering the cells they infect susceptible to gancyclovir and, therefore, susceptible to elimination should this be desired. There have also been several clinical trials using vectors containing this gene transfected into CD8 cells.

Physical methods of gene transfer not requiring modified viral vectors also have been used, including liposomal delivery, direct injection of genetic material, *in vivo* lipofection with cationic-lipid-DNA complexes, ballistic techniques to "microinject" large amounts of DNA-coated pellets into cells, and targeted DNA-ligand complexes via cell endocytosis.[82,85–87] Examples of ligands used for this purpose are liver-specific asialoglycoprotein receptors and transferrin receptors. Special efforts have to be made to inhibit lysosomal degradation of introduced DNA. Chloroquine is one of the compounds used for this purpose. Viral particles [e.g., adenovirus (which can disrupt endosomes)] provide another means of preventing DNA degradation.[87,89] These approaches have not been toxic in animal models.[87,90–92] Ultimately, combinations of different delivery systems using the advantages of each may provide the most useful approach to gene therapy.

Clinical Pharmacology

Gene delivery can either be *ex vivo* or *in vivo*. Advantages of *ex vivo* delivery include high efficiency, ability to enrich for

infected cells, and ability to assess for presence of the transduced gene before reinfusing the cells.[93] Cells can be labeled fluorescently for *in vivo* tracking, which allows a means of following the fate of *ex vivo* transfected cells.[94] Targeting vectors to cells via specific receptors is also currently being studied.[95,96] DNA also can be injected directly into tissues to produce desired proteins, such as activators of the immune system.[86,87] Direct injection of the genes for enzymes that activate prodrugs into malignant cells followed by treatment with prodrugs is another approach. Many of the current trials evaluating the efficacy of gene therapy in treating cancer involve *ex vivo* gene [usually an immunomodulatory molecule, such as granulocyte-macrophage colony-stimulating factor (GM-CSF)] introduction into tumor cells (either autologous or allogeneic), with reintroduction of modified inactivated (usually by irradiation) cells into the patient as cancer vaccines.

In vivo, a number of approaches can be used to enhance gene delivery to tumors in specific settings. Liposomal delivery can be used to target cells, such as in the liver or lung. Methods of getting compounds across the blood–brain barrier, such as using the high concentration of transferrin receptors in brain capillary endothelial cells, also might be useful for delivery to lesions in the central nervous system.[97] Cationic liposomes may offer an advantage for targeting delivery to specific tissues. Each of these approaches can be combined with tissue-specific promoter-enhancer elements to limit expression of the gene to tissues of interest (see below).[98–100] A number of factors may be important in the expression of transgenes *in vivo*, including composition of the liposomal lipid, DNA-liposome ratio, and the promoter-enhancer elements that control the expression of the gene.[99] Combinations of viral and physical systems offer yet another approach.

Controlling expression of genes *in vivo* remains an important issue. Expression of genes can be limited to target tissues by using tissue-specific transcriptional regulatory sequences upstream of the gene. An example of this is targeting the active form of a drug by vitally directed enzyme prodrug therapy in which tissue-specific transcriptional regulatory sequences are placed upstream of the drug-activating gene, so its expression is restricted in a tissue-specific manner.[101,102] Expression of most genes has been relatively low and declines with time due to death of transfected cells, as well as loss of gene activity, by mechanisms that are not yet well delineated but may include nucleases.

Although there have been a large number of clinical trials evaluating gene therapy for cancer treatment in humans, a significantly smaller number of these have evaluated PK. Trials in humans that have evaluated the PK of transfected cells have included evaluation of the trafficking of a retrovirally transduced reporter gene (neomycin phosphotransferase) in tumor-infiltrating lymphocyte (TIL) cells reinfused into cancer patients.[103,104] The estimated percentage of cells transduced ranged from 1% to 11%. Circulating cells with the transduced gene were detectable for 3 weeks in all the patients and for as long as 2 months in two patients, indicating that these cells can be relatively long-lived. There was some targeting to tumor sites, as indicated by biopsies of tumor lesions that showed transduced cells present in a proportion of biopsies in three of five patients. However, all five patients also had at least some biopsies that were negative for infiltrating cells. There was no enhanced toxicity from the transduced gene. Another trial evaluated the tumor necrosis factor (TNF) gene transduced into TIL cells.[105] Increased TNF production could be induced in the TILs of the majority of patients, but this production was significantly lower than that seen in the control tumor cell line expressing the gene. Modifications of the vector by insertion of the interferon-γ signal peptide-enhanced TNF production, although it remained significantly below that of the transduced tumor cell line. This indicates that further modifications are necessary before production of specific transduced genes by host cells can be optimized.

Clinical Effectiveness

Transfection of tumor cells with a wide spectrum of cytokines, antisense constructs, foreign major histocompatibility complex genes, or other genes important in mediating various aspects of the immune response, and reintroduction of these cells into animals have been shown to have significant antitumor effects putatively by immune-mediated mechanisms.[75,76,105–108] Most studies suggest that a proportion of tumor cells is killed by an innocent bystander effect (presumably immunologically mediated). However, this effect is seen even with approaches that would not be expected to generate a strong immune response, and the actual mechanisms for the innocent bystander effect remain undetermined.

Gene therapy is undergoing extensive clinical evaluation in humans.[109–112] Approaches demonstrated to be effective in animal studies and currently undergoing clinical trials include (a) inhibition of an oncogene (e.g., K-*ras* or raf); (b) replacement of a functional tumor suppressor gene (e.g., *p53*); (c) transfection of activating enzymes for prodrugs (e.g., *hTK* gene) into tumor cells followed by treatment with the prodrugs (e.g., gancyclovir); (d) transfer of protecting genes (e.g., *MDR1*) into normal (especially hematopoietic) cells, followed by high-dose chemotherapy; (e) transduction of immune effector cells with cytokine genes (e.g., TNF or IL-2) to enhance their effectiveness in killing tumor cells; (f) transduction of tumor cells with immunomodulatory molecules (GM-CSF, IL-2, IL-4, HLA-B7) to make them more susceptible to immunologic destruction, as well as generate a systemic immune response against the tumor; and (g) using vectors expressing antisense messages to inhibit function of critical genes for tumor cell survival or proliferation.[77,103,105–112] There are extensive ongoing efforts to optimize dendritic cell activa-

tion by those approaches using immunomodulatory molecules, such as GM-CSF and IL-4. These approaches have all been successful in treating tumors in animal models, but clearly their potential usefulness in patients is relatively early in development. To date, these approaches for treating cancer patients have had relatively limited toxicity overall and have been shown to be feasible. They have also had limited efficacy, although many of the agents are in early or late phase I testing. Efforts to enhance and prolong the expression of transduced genes *in vivo*, as well as other approaches to enhancing the therapeutic efficacy of these approaches, are being evaluated in ongoing studies.

Monoclonal Antibodies

The ability to generate highly specific antibodies against the antigen of choice makes them excellent candidates for targeting agents. They can be used alone or to deliver radionuclides, toxins, or chemotherapy to malignant cells or specific tissues. mAbs directed against GFRs and other cell surface antigens have undergone extensive testing in treatment of a number of cancers.[113] Two, trastuzumab (for breast cancer) and rituximab (for B-cell NHL), have been approved for treating patients. A number of others (e.g., anti-EGFR and anti-VEGF) are currently undergoing clinical evaluation. Improved targeting of agents, such as radioactive compounds, in an attempt to kill tumor cells continues to be explored. Combinations of antibodies and radiation therapy or chemotherapeutic agents are also being investigated. Radiolabeled antibodies are also useful as imaging agents for cancer. This is also an area of continuing study. See Chapter 28 for a more complete discussion of monoclonal antibodies.

Modified Peptides and Peptidomimetics

Modified peptides or peptidomimetic compounds designed to bind to and inhibit the active sites of proteins are natural candidates for effective inhibitors of protein function. The ubiquitous presence of proteases, the extremely short half-lives of most naturally occurring peptides, and the rapid hepatic and renal clearance make unmodified molecules impractical for clinical use. Therefore, modified compounds, or, more commonly, small organic molecules that mimic peptides functionally, so-called *peptidomimetics*, have been the major focus of study. Modifications include incorporation of altered amino acids (e.g., phosphonates) that are less prone to degradative attack; incorporation of compounds (e.g., benzodiazepine analogs) that structurally mimic amino acids, but are not targets of proteases; and totally synthetic polymers that structurally mimic peptides but are not targets for enzymatic degradation.

For these agents to be effective, a target that is therapeutically relevant must be chosen (Table 30-8). This is an obvious but critical point that can be forgotten in the

TABLE 30-8. PEPTIDOMIMETIC TARGETS

Target	Examples
Cell surface growth factor	Growth factor analogs/receptor antagonists, growth factor–toxin conjugates
Cell surface binding proteins	Laminin peptide antagonists
Enzymes	Farnesyltransferase inhibitors, inhibitors of angiogenesis, metalloproteinase inhibitors, telomerase inhibitors
Protein interaction sites[a]	SH2 and SH3 domains

SH, Src homology.
[a]To date, it has been difficult to synthesize effective specific inhibitors of protein interaction sites, which are readily taken up into cells.

excitement of knowing the sequence or structure of a gene that may not be an ideal candidate from the standpoint of tumor biology. Defining the best genes to target is especially important given the large number of potential targets and the high cost of evaluating each of these. As the human genome project nears completion, the ability to identify optimal targets should be enhanced. Structures of the appropriate active sites of the target protein must be known. Ideally, structures of the specific regions being targeted are known from x-ray crystallography, allowing initial evaluation of potential binding compounds by computer analysis. Those predicted to have the best binding properties can be synthesized. Thus, the process requires production, purification, and crystallization of the known protein, followed by x-ray crystallographic and computer analysis.

An alternative approach is to synthesize short peptidomimetics based on known sequences of active binding sites. These can be used for initial screening and provide the basis for subsequent modifications to improve their efficacy. Clinically, the most extensively studied of the modified peptide compounds to date have been somatostatin analogs.[114,115] Thus, to illustrate pharmacologic features of these compounds, somatostatin analogs are discussed as prototypical examples of synthetic peptide or peptide-like structures. Where appropriate, other peptidomimetics or general features of these types of compounds are discussed. Peptide analogs of luteinizing hormone releasing hormone (LHRH) are also extensively used clinically, but because the antitumor effect is mediated via hormonal manipulation, these are discussed under hormonal therapies.

Mechanisms of Action

Somatostatins are, in general, growth inhibitory for a wide variety of cells, including neoplasms.[114–118] Receptors for somatostatin have been found on a number of tumors, including lung, colon, pancreas, breast, and neuroendocrine tumors.[114–120] Most animal models suggest that biologic effects of these compounds (or analogs) are mediated via binding to receptors, although a few studies have not

shown a direct correlation between receptor numbers and the biologic effect of the compound.[114–120]

Somatostatin itself has too short a half-life (approximately 3 minutes) to be clinically useful. In addition, withdrawal of somatostatin can produce rapid rebound effects. Therefore, a number of analogs have been developed that have greater stability, more selectivity, and possibly induce less of a rebound effect than somatostatin itself.[114,121] Binding of various somatostatin analogs varies between different tissues, suggesting that there are possibly different subtypes of receptors.[114,122] Antiproliferative effects or somatostatin analogs appear to be mediated by a number of mechanisms. One of these is inhibition of centrosomal separation and cell proliferation induced by epidermal growth factor (EGF).[123] This may be due, at least in part, to stimulating a tyrosine phosphatase that inhibits signaling via the EGFR pathway, although additional studies are necessary to further define this.[124] There are also a large number of potential indirect mechanisms of tumor inhibition by somatostatin analogs, including suppression of growth hormone (GH) and prolactin, which can be growth stimulatory for breast cancer; inhibition of GH, with subsequent suppression of a number of growth factors (e.g., insulin-like growth factor I) that are important for tumor cell growth; and suppression of plasma-EGF levels.[114,120] Somatostatin analogs have been shown to inhibit tumor growth *in vitro* and in a number of animal model systems.[114,121] The effect appears to be primarily cytostatic, with return of tumor growth once analogs are removed.

Similar to mAbs directed against GFRs, peptide growth factors can be used to target toxic compounds to cells. Given rapid degradation of growth factors once they are internalized, this is most useful for targeting toxic compounds.[126–134] This approach has been shown to be effective in inhibiting the growth of neoplastic cell lines in culture and tumors in animal models with tolerable toxicity. Human trials also have shown efficacy for this approach using an IL-2–diphtheria hybrid toxin to treat cutaneous T-cell lymphomas and other hematologic malignancies that express the p55 component of the IL-2 receptor.[133]

Given the immunogenicity of toxins, short plasma half-life of most small peptides, and tendency of many growth factors administered *in vivo* to concentrate in organs, such as liver and kidney, these compounds need modification to make them consistently useful therapeutic agents for systemic therapy. A potential means of decreasing systemic side effects and increasing the amount delivered to tumor cells is locally delivered therapy. A recombinant transforming growth factor–alpha *Pseudomonas* exotoxin molecule is undergoing clinical study for intravesical therapy of bladder cancer.[134]

Uncoupled peptide analogs that recognize the binding site of receptors also can be synthesized to bind to and inhibit receptor function directly. These have been shown to be effective *in vitro*, and if these or modified peptides that would be more stable *in vivo* can be effectively delivered to tumors, then they might be clinically useful.[135,136]

Peptides can be modified in a number of ways to enhance their potential as effective therapeutic agents. One of these is coupling them to compounds, such as dextran, that prevent the extremely rapid degradation of peptides that normally occurs in cells and therefore allowing longer retention in these cells.[137] If these constructs are coupled with radioactive or cytotoxic compounds, they can provide a potentially effective delivery system for the toxic compound to tumor targets that express high levels of the GFR or other surface ligands being targeted.

In addition to development of peptidomimetics targeted to cell surface receptors, much of the current interest in these molecules is as inhibitors of specific steps in signal transduction pathways from cell surface to nucleus. The potency of the immunosuppressant drugs cyclosporin A and FK506, which bind to and inhibit intracellular proteins essential in T-cell signaling, has generated a significant impetus to either find or synthesize compounds that might have similar effects in other critical signal transduction pathways.[138] An example of this approach is targeting *ras* genes, as discussed earlier. Clearly, there are a large number of other potential targets for peptidomimetics within cells, including proteins involved in other signaling pathways, enzymes, or sequences important for protein-protein interactions.[139] Many of these are being actively pursued as potential therapeutic targets.

Cellular Pharmacology and Metabolism

Factors important for cellular pharmacologic properties of peptidomimetics targeted to GFRs (or other cell surface antigens) are similar to those for mAbs. Activity, half-life, and metabolism are dependent on whether the ligand-receptor complex is internalized. Internalization is not necessarily essential and might be pharmacologically detrimental for compounds that bind to and inhibit the receptor directly or are ligated to radionuclides. On the other hand, for toxin or chemotherapy conjugates, internalization is essential. Peptidomimetics targeted to intracellular proteins clearly need to be delivered into cells. As discussed above for *ras*, compounds with these properties can be constructed. It is impossible to generalize the pharmacologic properties of different peptidomimetics, because they are affected by the presence, concentration, and properties (e.g., internalization) of proteins to which they bind in plasma as well as on the cell surface.

Clinical Pharmacology

Somatostatin analogs that are significantly more active than the parent compound have been studied extensively. They vary in potency for different somatostatin effects, suggesting some specificity of different analogs. For example, san-

dostatin is 45 times more potent than somatostatin in inhibiting GH release, 11 times more potent in inhibiting glucagon, and 1.3 times more potent in inhibiting insulin.[114] These compounds are rapidly absorbed after subcutaneous injection. Peak plasma concentrations are seen in approximately 25 to 30 minutes. $t_{1/2\alpha}$ values are approximately 10 to 15 minutes, and $t_{1/2\beta}$ values are approximately 100 to 115 minutes when given by subcutaneous injection, and approximately half as long when given by intravenous bolus. Therefore, to have sufficient concentrations for therapeutic effect for any duration, they have to be given by subcutaneous injection three to four times per day, or continuously either intravenously or subcutaneously. Approximately one-third of the dose is excreted unchanged in the urine. There are a number of analogs with different biologic and pharmacologic effects. Somatuline, which has been studied in the treatment of pancreatic cancer, has a plasma half-life of approximately 90 minutes.[114] A long-acting somatostatin analog, an LAR depot form for intramuscular use given once monthly, has been approved for clinical use. Steady-state octreotide serum concentrations are achieved after the third dose. Although effective in treating the carcinoid syndrome and for controlling symptoms related to GH and prolactin-secreting pituitary tumors, it has been only minimally evaluated in other tumor settings.

DAB486IL-2 is rapidly cleared from the serum with a half-life of 7 to 15 minutes and fits a one-compartment model.[133] There was not a significant difference in PK between bolus and 90-minute infusion schedules. Similar to the story with antibodies, there is significant interpatient variability in PK. A significant percentage of patients developed antibodies against the toxin, IL-2, or both.

Given the short half-lives of peptides, a number of approaches to potentially improve their *in vivo* pharmacologic properties have been pursued. For example, polyethylene glycol conjugated to peptides might improve PK by a number of mechanisms, including prolonged plasma half-life, decreased immunogenicity (although occasionally it may actually enhance immunogenicity), increased solubility, resistance to proteolysis, and better coupling to liposomes. Innovative approaches, such as controlled-release polymers, may enhance peptide delivery during a prolonged period.[139] In addition, mathematic models have been developed to define parameters required for *in vivo* use of targeted therapies, and these might be useful in attempting to optimize design of compounds for clinical use.[140,141] Ultimately, clinical trials are necessary to define PK properties and toxicity for any given compound.

Toxicity

Somatostatin analogs are quite nontoxic, with median lethal dose values not being reached in rats. There is no evidence of chronic toxicity in studies conducted up to 2 years in dogs.[114] In addition, they have been given to patients for many years with no discernible long-term side effects. Side effects include pain at the injection site, abdominal pain, cramps, and diarrhea. Chololithiasis can occur.

DAB486IL-2 is well tolerated.[132,133] Flulike symptoms (low-grade fevers and chills) develop in approximately three-fourths of patients but can be treated symptomatically. Hypersensitivity reactions (chest tightness, bronchospasm, and back pain) occur in approximately one-fifth of patients, but again, most of these are controllable or preventable by symptomatic therapy. All patients have some elevations of hepatic enzymes, but this is not accompanied by other liver abnormalities. Renal insufficiency defined the maximum tolerated dose. Anemia, thrombocytopenia, and hemolysis also are seen.

Toxicity profiles of new peptidomimetics will be defined by results of trials using those agents.

Clinical Effectiveness

Unconjugated Peptidomimetics

Clearly, somatostatin analogs have activity in controlling symptoms related to GH and prolactin-secreting pituitary tumors, GI neuroendocrine tumors (especially carcinoid), and diarrhea related to certain chemotherapeutic agents.[114,142] Clinical trials have demonstrated minor activity against prostate cancer, minimal activity in breast and pancreatic cancer, and no activity against small cell lung cancer.[114,143,144] High-dose therapy using somatuline (in the range of 12 mg per day by continuous infusion subcutaneously) has biologic activity as measured by suppression of GH and IGF-I, but evaluation of clinical effectiveness against different tumors is still in progress. As new, potentially more potent, somatostatin analogs are developed, they continue to be evaluated for treating malignancies.[114,144]

Given the relatively low level of antitumor activity of these agents used alone, combinations with other agents have been evaluated in several trials. RC-160 (somatostatin analog) and SB-75 (LH-RH antagonist) inhibit the growth of human pancreatic xenograft in a mouse model, suggesting that this is a potential combination to investigate against this exceedingly difficult to treat tumor.[145] However, no beneficial effects were seen in a large trial using LH-RH (not the antagonist) and somatostatin, alone or in combination, to treat patients with pancreatic cancer, and the LH-RH agonist goserelin plus hydrocortisone produced no responses.[146] Somatostatin analogs appear to enhance the antitumor effects of tamoxifen in preclinical studies.[147] A randomized study suggests that the combination of a somatostatin analog, an antiprolactin agent, and tamoxifen produced a higher response rate and time to disease progression than tamoxifen alone for patients with metastatic breast cancer.[148] However, there was no difference in overall survival. Additional studies are needed to define the true role of somatostatin analogs in this setting.

Evaluation of combinations of somatostatin analogs and other agents or approaches, including chemotherapy and radiation therapy, is ongoing.[149]

Conjugated Peptidomimetics

In addition to combination therapy, a potentially promising approach is using somatostatin analogs to deliver cytotoxic agents to tumors expressing high receptor levels. This approach has produced some responses in early testing of radionuclide-coupled somatostatin analogs, and additional studies are ongoing.[149–153] The only significant toxicities to date have been reversible myelosuppression, especially anemia; decrease in lymphocyte counts; mild thrombocytopenia; and mild increases in creatinine. Other analogs coupled to radionuclides, chemotherapeutic agents, and toxins are also being developed and evaluated as potential therapeutic, as well as imaging, agents.[151–153] Evidence of antitumor activity has been seen using radiolabeled somatostatin analogs to treat neuroendocrine tumors.[152]

DAB389IL-2 has shown effectiveness against a number of hematopoietic malignancies, including Hodgkin's disease and lymphomas [including cutaneous T-cell lymphomas (CTCL)].[133,154,155] The U.S. Food and Drug Administration has approved its use for the treatment of patients with advanced or refractory CTCL. Its use in the other disease settings continues to be evaluated.

CONCLUSION

Sufficient understanding of the biology of cellular processes exists, and tools are now available to manipulate molecular systems for therapeutic benefit to allow rational design and delivery of molecules directed at specific proteins or genes important for survival or growth of malignant cells. Several examples of targeted therapy are in clinical use, including mAbs for treatment of breast cancer and B-cell NHL, as well as an immunotoxin for treatment of CTCL. A number of other agents, especially the small molecule bcr-abl tyrosine kinase inhibitor STI-571, have shown sufficient antitumor activity that they likely will have expanded use in the near future. Thus, this is an exciting time in the development of rationally targeted therapies. However, there is still a significant amount of study necessary to develop additional clinically useful antitumor approaches using targeted agents. Continued improvement in understanding critical processes in cancer development, growth, and metastasis should provide new targets and new agents for attacking these. Technological advances allowing much more sophisticated evaluation of intra- and intercellular processes will play an increasingly important role. As more information is gathered about the immensely complex interaction of proteins in cells, this effort will require the use of mathematic evaluation by powerful computers. However, carefully performed toxicity and pharmacologic studies to determine how to best deliver these therapies to patients remain critical to the process of successful clinical development of any of these agents. Because there is no current method for adequately modeling these by *in vitro* studies, analysis (e.g., by computer models), or both, well-done animal and, most important, human clinical studies remain essential ingredients to development of these compounds as therapeutic agents.

REFERENCES

1. Kaelin Jr WG. Taking aim at novel molecular targets in cancer therapy. *J Clin Invest* 1999;104:1495.
2. Shapiro GI, Harper JW. Anticancer drug targets: cell cycle and checkpoint control. *J Clin Invest* 1999;104:1645–1653.
3. Chabner BA, Boral AL, Multani P. Translational research: walking the bridge between idea and cure—seventeenth Bruce F. Cain Memorial Award lecture. *Cancer Res* 1998;58:4211–4116.
4. Keshet E, Ben-Sasson SA. Anticancer drug targets: approaching angiogenesis. *J Clin Invest* 1999;104:1497–1501.
5. Kaelin Jr WG. Choosing anticancer drug targets in the postgenomic era. *J Clin Invest* 1999;104:1503–1506.
6. Lundberg AS, Weinberg RA. Control of the cell cycle and apoptosis. *Science* 1999; 35:1886–1894.
7. Senderowicz AM, Sausville EA. Preclinical and clinical development of cyclin-dependent kinase modulators. *J Natl Cancer Inst* 2000;92:376–387.
8. Wu X, et al. The PTEN/MMAC1 tumor suppressor phosphatase functions as a negative regulator of the phosphoinositide 3-kinase/AKT pathway. *Proc Natl Acad Sci U S A* 1998;95:15587–15591.
9. Yamamoto T, Taya S, Kaibuchi K. Ras-induced transformation and signaling pathway. *J Biochem* 1999;126:799–803.
10. Gao HG, et al. Distribution of p53 and K-ras mutations in human lung cancer tissues. *Carcinogenesis* 1997;18:473–478.
11. Breivik J, et al. K-ras mutations in colorectal cancer: relations to patient age, sex, and tumor source. *Br J Cancer* 1994;69:367–371.
12. Sakorafas GH, Tsiotou AG, Tsiotos GG. Molecular biology of pancreatic cancer; oncogenes, tumour suppressor genes, growth factors, and their receptor from a clinical perspective. *Cancer Treat Rev* 2000;26:29–52.
13. Baupre DM, Kurzrock R. Ras and leukemia: from basic mechanisms to gene directed therapy. *J Clin Oncol* 1999;17:1071–1079.
14. Choy, E et al. Endomembrane trafficking of ras: the CAAX motif targets proteins to the ER and Golgi. *Cell* 1999;98:69–80.
15. End DW. Farnesyl protein transferase inhibitors and other therapies targeting the Ras signal transduction pathway. *Invest New Drugs* 1999;18:241–258.
16. Waddick KG, Uckum FM. Innovative treatment programs against cancer. I. Ras oncoprotein as a molecular target. *Biochem Pharmacol* 1998;56:1411–1426.
17. Lebowitz PF, Pendergast GC. Non-ras targets of farnesyltransferase inhibitors: focus on Rho. *Oncogene* 1998;17:1439–1445.
18. Gibbs JB. Anticancer drug targets: growth factors and growth factor signaling. *J Clin Invest* 2000;105:9–13.
19. Drucker BJ, Lydon NB. Lessons learned from the development of an Abl tyrosine kinase inhibitor for chronic myelogenous leukemia. *J Clin Invest* 2000;105:3–7.
20. Hahn WC, et al. Inhibition of telomerase limits the growth of human cancer cells. *Nat Med* 1999;5:1164–1170.
21. Rubin, MS, et al. Monoclonal antibody (MoAb) IMC-C225, and anti-epidermal growth factor receptor (EGFr), for patients (pts) with EGFr-positive tumors refractory to or in relapse from previous therapeutic regimens. *Proc ASCO* 2000;19:474a.
22. Leenders WP. Targeting VEGF in anti-angiogenic and anti-tumor therapy: where are we now? *Int J Exp Pathol* 1998;79:339–346.
23. Bridges AJ. The rationale and strategy used to develop a series of highly potent, irreversible, inhibitors of the epidermal growth factor receptor family of kinases. *Curr Med Chem* 1999;6:825–843.
24. Seidman AD, et al. Final report: weekly (w) herceptin (H) and taxol (T) for metastatic breast cancer (MBC): analysis of efficacy by HER2 immunophenotype [Immunohistochemistry (IHC)] and gene amplification [fluorescent in-situ hybridization (FISH)]. *Proc ASCO* 2000;19:83a.
25. Bonner JA, et al. Continued response following treatment with IMC-C225, an EGFr MoAb, combined with RT in advanced head and neck malignancies. *Proc ASCO* 2000;19:4a.
26. Ferry D, et al. Intermittent oral Zd 1839 (Iressa) a novel epidermal growth factor receptor tyrosine kinase inhibitor (Egfr-Tki) shows evidence of good tolerability and activity: final results from a phase I study. *Proc ASCO* 2000;19:3a.
27. Sellers WR, Fisher DE. Apoptosis and cancer drug targeting. *J Clin Invest* 1999;104:1655–1661.
28. Marcusson EG, et al. Preclinical and clinical pharmacology of antisense oligonucleotides. *Mol Biotech* 1999;12:1–11.
29. Curcio LD, Bouffard DY, Scanlon KJ. Oligonucleotides as modulators of cancer gene expression. *Pharmacol Ther* 1997;74:317–332.
30. Dachs GU, et al. Targeting gene therapy to cancer: a review. *Oncol Res* 1997;9:313–325.
31. Alama A, et al. Antisense oligonucleotides as therapeutic agents. *Pharmacol Res* 1997;36:171–178.
32. Calogero A, Hospers GA, Mulders NH. Synthetic oligonucleotides: useful molecules? A review. *Pharm World Sci* 1997;19:264–268.
33. Iwanaga T, Ferriola PC. Cellular uptake of phosphorothioate oligodeoxynucleotides is negatively affected by cell density in a transformed rat tracheal epithelial cell line: implication for antisense approaches. *Biochem Biophys Res Commun* 1993;191:1152–1157.
34. Ryte A, et al. Oligonucleotide degradation contributes to resistance to antisense compounds. *Anticancer Drugs* 1993; 4:197–200.
35. Sarver N, et al. Ribozymes as potential anti-HIV-1 therapeutic agents. *Science* 1990;247:1222–1225.
36. Sanghvi YS, et al. Antisense oligodeoxynucleotides: synthesis, biophysical and biological evaluation of oligodeoxynucleotides containing modified pyrimidines. *Nucleic Acids Res* 1993;21:3197–3203.

37. Pagnan A, et al. Delivery of c-myb antisense oligonucleotides to human neuroblastoma cells via disialoganglioside GD(2)-targeted immunoliposomes: antitumor effects. *J Natl Cancer Inst* 2000;92:253–261.

38. Penichet ML, et al. An antibody-avidin fusion protein specific for the transferrin receptor serves as a vehicle for effective brain targeting: initial applications in anti-HIV antisense therapy in the brain. *J Immunol* 1999;163:4421–4426.

39. Bergan RC. Ex vivo bone marrow purging with oligonucleotides. *Antisense Nucleic Acid Drug Dev* 1997;7:251–255.

40. Zapp ML, Stern S, Green MR. Small molecules that selectively block RNA binding of HIV-1 Rev protein inhibit Rev function and viral production. *Cell* 1993;74:969–978.

41. Ratajczak MZ, et al. In vivo treatment of human leukemia in a scid mouse model with c-myb antisense oligodeoxynucleotides. *Proc Natl Acad Sci U S A* 1992;89:11823–11827.

42. Gray GD, et al. Antisense DNA inhibition of tumor growth induced by c-Ha-ras oncogene in nude mice. *Cancer Res* 1993;53:577–580.

43. Kitajima I, et al. Human T-cell leukemia virus type I tax transformation is associated with increased uptake of oligodeoxynucleotides in vitro and in vivo. *J Biol Chem* 1992;267:25881–25888.

44. Iversen P. In vivo studies with phosphorothioate oligonucleotides: pharmacokinetics prologue. *Anticancer Drug Design* 1991;6:531–538.

45. Agrawal S, Temsamani J, Tang JY. Pharmacokinetics, biodistribution, and stability of oligodeoxynucleotide phosphorothioates in mice. *Proc Natl Acad Sci U S A* 1991;88:7595–7599.

46. Levin AA. A review of the issues in the pharmacokinetics and toxicology of phosphorothioate antisense oligonucleotides. *Biochim Biophys Acta* 1999;1489:69–84.

47. Agrawal S. Temsamani J, Tang JY. Pharmacokinetics, biodistribution, and stability of oligodeoxynucleotide phosphorothioates in mice. *Proc Natl Acad Sci U S A* 1991;88:7595–7599.

48. Karamyshev V, Vlasov V, Zon D. Distribution of oligonucleotide derivatives and their stability in murine tissue. *Biokhimiia* 1993;58:590.

49. Monteith DK, Levin AA. Synthetic oligonucleotides: the development of antisense therapeutics. *Toxicol Pathol* 1999;27:8–13.

50. Vlassov V, Yakubov L. Oligonucleotides in cells and organisms: pharmacological considerations. In: Wickstrom E, ed. *Prospects for antisense nucleic acid therapy of cancer and AIDS.* New York: Wiley, 1991;243.

51. Spinolo J, et al. Toxicity of human p53 antisense oligonucleotide infusions in rhesus macacca. *Proc AACR* 1993;33:3125.

52. Gewirtz AM. Oligonucleotide therapeutics: a step forward. *J Clin Oncol* 2000; 18:1809–1811.

53. Waters JS, et al. Phase I clinical and pharmacokinetic study of Bcl-2 antisense oligonucleotide therapy in patients with non-Hodgkin's lymphoma. *Science* 1992;258:1792–1795.

54. O'Dwyer PJ, et al. c-raf-1 depletion and tumor responses in patients treated with raf-1 antisense oligodeoxynucleotide ISIS 5132 (CGP 69846A*). Clin Cancer Res* 1999;5:647–661.

55. Yuen AR, Sikic BI. Clinical studies of antisense therapy in cancer. *Front Biosci* 2000;5:D588–593.

56. Kronenwett R, Haas R. Antisense strategies for the treatment of hematological malignancies and solid tumors. *Ann Hematol* 1998;77:1–12.

57. Galderisi U, Cascino A, Giordano A. Antisense oligonucleotides as therapeutic agents. *J Cell Physiol* 1999;81:251–257.

58. Agarwal N, Gewirtz AM. Oligonucleotide therapeutics for hematologic disorders. *Biochim Biophys Acta* 1999;1489:85–96.

59. Dropulic B, et al. Ribozymes: use as anti-HIV therapeutic molecules. *Antisense Res Devel* 1993;3:87–94.

60. Cotten M, Birnstiel ML. Ribozyme mediated destruction of RNA in vivo. *EMBO J* 1989;8:3861–3866.

61. Bartel DP, Szostak JW. Isolation of new ribozymes from a large pool of random sequences [see comment]. *Science* 1993;261:1411–1418.

62. Pieken WA, et al. Kinetic characterization of ribonuclease-resistant 2'-modified hammerhead ribozymes. *Science* 1991;253:314–317.

63. Chowrira BM, Burke JM. Extensive phosphorothioate substitution yields highly active and nuclease-resistant hairpin ribozymes. *Nucleic Acids Res* 1992;20:2835–2840.

64. Norris JS, et al. Design and testing of ribozymes for cancer gene therapy. *Adv Exp Med Biol* 2000;465:293–301.

65. Shippy R, et al. The hairpin ribozyme. Discovery, mechanism, and development for gene therapy. *Mol Biotechnol* 1999;12:117–129.

66. Macpherson JL, et al. Ribozymes in gene therapy of HIV-1. *Front Biosci* 1999;4:D497–505.

67. Russell SJ, et al. Decreased tumorigenicity of a transplantable rat sarcoma following transfer and expression of an IL-2 cDNA. *Int J Cancer* 1991;47:244–251.

68. Sarver N, Rossi J. Gene therapy: a bold direction for HIV-treatment. *AIDS Res Hum Retroviruses* 1993;9:483–487.

69. Sullenger BA, et al. Overexpression of TAR sequences renders cells resistant to human immunodeficiency virus replication. *Cell* 1990;63:601–608.

70. Sullenger BA, et al. Analysis of trans-acting response decoy RNA-mediated inhibition of human immunodeficiency virus type 1 transactivation. *J Virol* 1991;65:6811–6816.

71. Malim MH, et al. Stable expression of transdominant Rev protein in human T cells inhibits human immunodeficiency virus replication. *J Exp Med* 1992;176:1197–1201.

72. Yu X, et al. The matrix protein of human immunodeficiency virus type 1 is required for incorporation of viral envelope protein into mature virions. *J Virol* 1992;66:4966–4971.

73. Harrison GS, et al. Inhibition of human immunodeficiency virus-1 production resulting from transduction with a retrovirus containing an HIV-regulated diphtheria toxin A chain gene. *Hum Gene Ther* 1992;3:461–469.

74. Carlson JR. A new use for intracellular antibody expression: inactivation of human immunodeficiency virus type 1 [comment]. *Proc Natl Acad Sci U S A* 1993;90:7427–7428.

75. Tepper R. Cytokines and strategies for anticancer vaccines. *Contemp Oncol* 1993;3:38.

76. Lanzavecchia A. Identifying strategies for immune intervention. *Science* 1993;260:937–944.

77. Borden EC, Schlom J. Williamsburg Conference on Biological and Immunological Treatments for Cancer, 1992. *J Natl Cancer Inst* 1993;85:1288–1293.

78. Culver KW, et al. In vivo gene transfer with retroviral vector-producer cells for treatment of experimental brain tumors [see comments]. *Science* 1992;256:1550–1552.

79. Corey CA, et al. Serial transplantation of methotrexate-resistant bone marrow: protection of murine recipients from drug toxicity by progeny of transduced stem cells. *Blood* 1990;75:337–343.

80. Galski H, et al. Expression of a human multidrug resistance cDNA (MDR1) in the bone marrow of transgenic mice: resistance to daunomycin-induced leukopenia. *Mol Cell Biol* 1989;9:4357–4363.

81. Cornetta K, et al. Amphotropic murine leukemia retrovirus is not an acute pathogen for primates. *Hum Gene Ther* 1990;1:15–30.

82. RC M. Gene therapy protocols. *ASCO Education Book.* 1993;134.

83. Robinson C. Gene therapy—proceeding from laboratory to clinic. *Trends Biotechnol* 1993;11:155.

84. Kotin RM, et al. Site-specific integration by adeno-associated virus. *Proc Natl Acad Sci U S A* 1990;87:2211–2215.

85. Nabel GJ, Felgner PL. Direct gene transfer for immunotherapy and immunization. *Trends Biotechnol* 1993;11:211–215.

86. Cohen J. Naked DNA points way to vaccines [news; comment]. *Science* 1993;259(5102):1691–1692.

87. Ulmer JB, et al. Heterologous protection against influenza by injection of DNA encoding a viral protein [see comments]. *Science* 1993;259:1745–1749.

88. Curiel DT, et al. Adenovirus enhancement of transferrin-polylysine-mediated gene delivery. *Proc Natl Acad Sci U S A* 1991;88:8850–8854.

89. Michael SI, et al. Binding-incompetent adenovirus facilitates molecular conjugate-mediated gene transfer by the receptor-mediated endocytosis pathway. *J Bio Chem* 1993;268:6866–6869.

90. Tomita N, et al. Direct in vivo gene introduction into rat kidney. *Biochem Biophys Res Commun* 1992;186:129–134.

91. Stewart MJ, et al. Gene transfer in vivo with DNA-liposome complexes: safety and acute toxicity in mice. *Hum Gene Ther* 1992;3:267–275.

92. Wagner E, et al. Influenza virus hemagglutinin HA-2 N-terminal fusogenic peptides augment gene transfer by transferrin-polylysine-DNA complexes: toward a synthetic virus-like gene-transfer vehicle. *Proc Natl Acad Sci U S A* 1992; 89:7934–7938.

93. Mitani K, Caskey CT. Delivering therapeutic genes—matching approach and application. *Trends Biotechnol* 1993; 11:162–166.

94. Horan PK, et al. Fluorescent cell labeling for in vivo and in vitro cell tracking. *Methods Cell Biol* 1990;33:469–490.

95. Watson F. Human gene therapy—progress on all fronts. *Trends Biotechnol* 1993;11(4):114–117.

96. Findeis MA, et al. Targeted delivery of DNA for gene therapy via receptors. *Trends Biotechnol* 1993;11:202–205.

97. Bickel U, et al. Pharmacologic effects in vivo in brain by vector-mediated peptide drug delivery. *Proc Natl Acad Sci U S A* 1993;90:2618–2622.

98. Jerome V, Muller R. Tissue-specific, cell cycle-regulated chimeric transcription factors for the targeting of gene expression to tumor cells. *Hum Gene Ther* 1998;9:2653–2659.

99. Philip R, et al. In vivo gene delivery. Efficient transfection of T lymphocytes in adult mice. *J Bio Chem* 1993;268:16087–16090.

100. Zhu N, et al. Systemic gene expression after intravenous DNA delivery into adult mice. *Science* 1993;261:209–211.

101. Huber BE, Richards CA, Krenitsky TA. Retroviral-mediated gene therapy for the treatment of hepatocellular carcinoma: an innovative approach for cancer therapy. *Proc Natl Acad Sci U S A* 1991;88:8039–8043.

102. Sikora K. Gene therapy for cancer. *Trends Biotechnol* 1993;11:197–201.

103. Rosenberg SA, et al. Gene transfer into humans—immunotherapy of patients with advanced melanoma, using tumor-infiltrating lymphocytes modified by retroviral gene transduction [see comments]. *N Engl J Med* 1990;323:570–578.

104. Rosenberg SA. Gene therapy of cancer. *Important Adv Oncol* 1992:17–38.

105. Dranoff G, et al. Vaccination with irradiated tumor cells engineered to secrete murine granulocyte-macrophage colony-stimulating factor stimulates potent, specific, and long-lasting anti-tumor immunity. *Proc Natl Acad Sci U S A* 1993;90:3539–3543.

106. Plautz GE, et al. Immunotherapy of malignancy by in vivo gene transfer into tumors [see comments]. *Proc Natl Acad Sci U S A* 1993;90:4645–4649.

107. Trojan J, et al. Treatment and prevention of rat glioblastoma by immunogenic C6 cells expressing antisense insulin-like growth factor I RNA [see comments]. *Science* 1993;259:94–97.

108. Townsend SE, Allison JP. Tumor rejection after direct costimulation of CD8+ T cells by B7-transfected melanoma cells [see comments]. *Science* 1993;259:368–370.

109. Roskrow MA, Gansbacher B. Recent developments in gene therapy for oncology/hematology. *Crit Rev Oncol Hematol* 1998;28:139–151.

110. Roth JA, Cristiano RJ. Gene therapy for cancer: what have we done and where are we going? *J Natl Cancer Inst* 1997;89:21–39.

111. Sokol DL, Gewirtz AM. Gene therapy: basic concepts and recent advances. *Crit Rev Euk Gene Exp* 1996;6:29–57.

112. Anderson WF. Human gene therapy. *Nature* 1998;392:25–30.

113. Farah RA, et al. The development of monoclonal antibodies for the therapy of cancer. *Crit Rev Euk Gene Exp* 1998; 8:321–356.

114. Parmar H, Phillips RH, Lightman SL. Somatostatin analogs: mechanisms of action. *Rec Results Cancer Res* 1993; 129:1–24.

115. Pollak MN, Schally AV. Mechanisms of antineoplastic action of somatostatin analogs. *Proc Soc Exp Biol Med* 1998;217:143–152.

116. Gillespie TJ, et al. Novel somatostatin analogs for the treatment of acromegaly and cancer exhibit improved in vivo stability and distribution. *J Pharmacol Exp Ther* 1998;285:95–104.

117. O'Byrne KJ, et al. Phase II study of RC-160 (vapreotide), an octapeptide analog of somatostatin, in the treatment of metastatic breast cancer. *Br J Cancer* 1999;79:1413–1418.

118. Brunton VG, Workman P. Cell-signaling targets for antitumour drug development. *Cancer Chemother Pharmacol* 1993;32:1–19.

119. Mendelsohn J. Antibodies to growth factors and receptors. *Biol Ther Cancer* 1991;601.

120. Prevost G, et al. Molecular heterogeneity of somatostatin analog BIM-23014C receptors in human breast carcinoma cells using the chemical cross-linking assay. *Cancer Res* 1992;52:843–850.

121. Schally AV. Oncological applications of somatostatin analogs [published erratum appears in *Cancer Res* 1989;49:1618]. *Cancer Res* 1988;48:6977–6985.

122. Lewin MJ. Somatostatin receptors. *Scan J Gastroenterol* 1986;119:42–46.

123. Moscardo R, Sherline P. Somatostatin inhibits rapid centrosomal separation and cell proliferation induced by epidermal growth factor. *Endocrinology* 1982;3:1394.

124. Liebow C, et al. Somatostatin analogs inhibit growth of pancreatic cancer by stimulating tyrosine phosphatase. *Proc Natl Acad Sci U S A* 1989;86:2003–2007.

125. Dy DY, Whitehead RH, Morris DL. SMS 201.995 inhibits in vitro and in vivo growth of human colon cancer. *Cancer Res* 1992;52:917–923.

126. Szepeshazi K, et al. Growth inhibition of estrogen-dependent and estrogen-independent MXT mammary cancers in mice by the bombesin and gastrin-releasing peptide antagonist RC-3095. *J Natl Cancer Inst* 1992;84:1915–1922.

127. Schally AV, Nagy A. Cancer chemotherapy based on targeting of cytotoxic peptide conjugates to their receptors on tumors. *Eur J Endocrinol* 1999;141:1–14.

128. Yang D, et al. Recombinant heregulin-*Pseudomonas* exotoxin fusion proteins: interactions with the heregulin receptors and antitumor activity in vivo. *Clin Cancer Res* 1998;4:993–1004.

129. Dachs GU, et al. Targeting gene therapy to cancer: a review. *Oncol Res* 1997;9:313–325.

130. Arora N, et al. Vascular endothelial growth factor chimeric toxin is highly active against endothelial cells. *Cancer Res* 1999;59:183–188.

131. Fang K. A toxin conjugate containing transforming growth factor-alpha and ricin A specifically inhibits growth of A431 human epidermoid cancer cells. *Proc Natl Sci Council* 1998;22:76–82.

132. Schally AV, Nagy A. Cancer chemotherapy based on targeting of cytotoxic peptide conjugates to their receptors on tumors. *Eur J Endocrinol* 1999;141:1–14.

133. Hesketh P, Caguioa P, Bukger K. Clinical response in cutaneous T-cell lymphoma to an IL2-diphtheria hybrid toxin (DAB 486IL2). *Blood* 1990;76:352a.

134. Theuer CP, Fitzgerald DJ, Pastan I. A recombinant form of *Pseudomonas* exotoxin A containing transforming growth factor alpha near its carboxyl terminus for the treatment of bladder cancer. *J Urol* 1993;149:1626–1632.

135. Pietrzkowski Z, et al. Inhibition of cellular proliferation by peptide analogs of insulin-like growth factor 1. *Cancer Res* 1992;52:6447–6451.

136. Pietrzkowski Z, et al. Inhibition of growth of prostatic cancer cell lines by peptide analogs of insulin-like growth factor 1. *Cancer Res* 1993;53:1102–1106.

137. Lindstrom A, Carlsson J. Penetration and binding of epidermal growth factor-dextran conjugates in spheroids of human glioma origin. *Cancer Biother* 1993;8:145–158.

138. Brugge JS. New intracellular targets for therapeutic drug design. *Science* 1993;260:918–919.

139. Langer R. New methods of drug delivery. *Science* 1990;249:1527–1533.

140. Mulshine JL, et al. The correct dose: pharmacologically guided end point for anti-growth factor therapy. *Cancer Res* 1992;52:2743s–2746s.

141. Weinstein JN, van Osdol W. Early intervention in cancer using monoclonal antibodies and other biological ligands: micropharmacology and the "binding site barrier." *Cancer Res* 1992;52:2747s–2751s.

142. Buchanan KD. Effects of sandostatin on neuroendocrine tumours of the gastrointestinal system. *Rec Results Cancer Res* 1993;129:45–55.

143. Prevost G, Israel L. Somatostatin and somatostatin analogs in human breast carcinoma. *Rec Results Cancer Res* 1993;129:63–70.

144. Canobbio L, et al. Treatment of advanced pancreatic carcinoma with the somatostatin analog BIM 23014. Preliminary results of a pilot study. *Cancer* 1992;69:648–650.

145. Radulovic S, et al. Somatostatin analog RC-160 and LH-RH antagonist SB-75 inhibit growth of MIA PaCa-2 human pancreatic cancer xenografts in nude mice. *Pancreas* 1993;8:88–97.

146. Philip PA, et al. Hormonal treatment of pancreatic carcinoma: a phase II study of LHRH agonist goserelin plus hydrocortisone. *Br J Cancer* 1993;67:379–382.

147. Pollak M. Enhancement of the anti-neoplastic effects of tamoxifen by somatostatin analogs. *Digestion* 1996;57:29–33.

148. Bontenbal M, et al. Feasibility, endocrine and anti-tumour effects of a triple endocrine therapy with tamoxifen, a somatostatin analog and an antiprolactin in post-menopausal metastatic breast cancer: a randomized study with long-term follow-up. *Br J Cancer* 1998;77:115–122.

149. Robbins RJ. Somatostatin and cancer. *Metab Clin Exp* 1996;45:98–100.

150. Kwekkeboom DJ, Krenning EP. Radiolabeled somatostatin analog scintigraphy in oncology and immune diseases: an overview. *Eur Radiol* 1997;7:1103–1109.

151. Schally AV, Nagy A. Cancer chemotherapy based on targeting of cytotoxic peptide conjugates to their receptors on tumors. *Eur J Endocrinol* 1999;141:1–14.

152. De Jong M, et al. Therapy of neuroendocrine tumors with radiolabeled somatostatin analogs. *QJ Nucl Med* 1999;43:356–366.

153. Pagamelli G, et al. Receptor-mediated radionuclide therapy with 90Y-DOTA-D-Tyr3-Octreotide: preliminary report in cancer patients. *Cancer Biother Radiopharm* 1999;14:477–483.

154. Saleh MN, et al. Antitumor activity of DAB389IL-2 fusion toxin in mycosis fungoides. *J Am Acad Dermatol* 1998;39:63–73.

155. LeMaistre CF, et al. Phase I trial of a ligand fusion-protein (DAB389IL-2) in lymphomas expressing the receptor for interleukin-2. *Blood* 1998;91:399–405.

31

PHYSICAL BARRIERS TO DRUG DELIVERY

BRENDAN D. CURTI

Our understanding of neoplasia has been transformed in the last decade. An illustration of how much our consciousness about oncology has changed can be found by looking at the topics covered in the educational sessions of the annual American Society of Clinical Oncology meetings in 1990 and 1999. In 1990, most sessions were named after disease processes, such as "Breast Cancer," or "Adult Lymphoma."[1] In 1999, the American Society of Clinical Oncology annual meeting held sessions on angiogenesis, signal transduction, tumor suppressor genes, and the use of genomics to complement the sessions on treatments for specific cancer diagnoses.[2] The organizing framework for oncologic research and practice is now molecular and mechanistic. The tools of molecular biology now allow us to take apart the machinery of cancer cells and reassemble the parts. We find new therapeutic modalities as we examine different parts of the cell cycle, the regulation of genes, and the interaction between cancer cells and the host's immune system and vasculature.

It is exciting that there is a new engine for innovation in oncology and that some of the molecular targets suggested by our understanding of cancer cells are being tested. However, this new molecular knowledge has not yet translated into a major change in outcome for cancer patients. The number of cancer deaths in the United States has not changed dramatically in the last decade.[3] There is some cause for hope in that estimated annual percent changes in cancer mortality for some specific sites have improved in 1991 to 1995 compared to 1973 to 1990.[4] However, much of this progress can be attributed to prevention and improvements in detection. The notably successful chemotherapy regimens for lymphoma, leukemia, and testicular cancer were not developed using a molecular rationale, but on the older pharmacologic notions of non–cross-resistance and dose intensity.[5–7] Although both classic and molecular pharmacology may yield effective cancer treatments, it is also apparent that cancer cells possess numerous mechanisms to resist destruction by chemotherapy agents or the immune system. A sampling of resistance mechanisms discovered thus far includes the P170 glycoprotein (multiple drug resistance gene product),[8] up-regulation of thymidylate synthase leading to 5-fluorouracil resistance,[9] and enhanced DNA repair after cisplatin chemotherapy.[9,10] Tumor cells also may evade immune surveillance by expressing essentially normal tissue antigens,[11] inducing defects in T-cell signaling,[12] and by expressing Fas ligand, which can induce apoptosis of T cells.[13] It appears likely that cancer cells possess many as yet undefined additional molecular mechanisms to defeat chemotherapy and immunotherapy strategies. Thus, designing effective treatment regimens for solid tumors may prove extremely difficult, even with a vastly improved knowledge of the molecular events within the tumor.

Although genetic events and receptor-protein interactions are obviously important, recent insights about the macroscopic aspects of tumor physiology complement this molecular knowledge. The study of the physiology and the interstitial space of tumors, pioneered by Gullino in the 1960s and continued most recently by Jain and his colleagues, suggests a new basis for understanding drug delivery problems in tumors.[14–17] Their work has defined tumor nodules *in vivo* as distinct physiologic entities with unique, biophysical properties compared to normal tissues. These properties cannot be deduced or reproduced by *in vitro* work because of the complex interaction of growing tumor cells with the new blood vessels they induce and the surrounding normal tissues. The microenvironment of tumor nodules can generate a number of physical barriers to a wide range of therapeutic agents. These treatment barriers cannot be ignored when attempting to design new and more effective treatment regimens.

The key to understanding the unique properties of a tumor's physiology requires focus on the tumor vasculature and interstitial space. The characteristics of tumor blood vessels, and their behavior in the aggregate, influence the transport processes used for the delivery of nutrients and therapeutic agents and the disposal of metabolic wastes. These vessels also have a profound secondary effect on the properties of the interstitial space of tumors. The emphasis here will be to provide a general discussion of physiologic spaces, transport variables, and the properties of tumor blood vessels. These basic concepts will be used as a framework for the discussion of intratumoral pharmacokinetics, selected models for the transport of therapeutic agents in tumors, and measurements of the physical barriers to drug delivery.

TRANSPORT COMPARTMENTS AND VARIABLES

Several spaces with different physiologic characteristics must be traversed for a therapeutic molecule to reach a neoplastic cell within a tumor nodule. The vascular space is the first compartment encountered by any intravenous agent. The therapeutic molecule must then cross the vascular endothelium and vessel basement membrane before it can percolate through the tumor interstitium to reach a cancer cell. There are potential impediments to transport in each of these physiologic spaces. To understand these impediments, the general mechanisms for transport of any molecule must be discussed.

Convection, diffusion, and transcytosis are the only ways that solutes (i.e., nutrients, toxins, and therapeutic agents) are propelled through physiologic spaces. The relative contribution of these variables to transport depends on the size and physical properties of the molecule and the physiologic space it is moving through (see below). For the purpose of this discussion, active transport across cell membranes is not considered. Each transport variable is discussed separately; this is followed by an explanation of how these variables interact and which are important in tumors.

Convection

Convection is defined as the movement of solute in the direction of solvent flow. This process can be envisioned as water flowing down a pipe. If a solute (e.g., sodium chloride) is dissolved in the water, the salt molecules will travel in the direction of the flowing water. Convection depends on a series of constants that describe how the solute and solvent move together, multiplied by a pressure gradient.[18]

Convection in tumors has been measured in a number of model systems. A fluorescent photobleaching technique has been developed to address this question, and has been applied to single vessels in granulation tissue and VX2 carcinoma grown in a rabbit ear chamber model.[19] The velocity of fluid moving through the interstitium of this preparation was comparable in both granulation tissue and tumor, suggesting that convective flux was the same in this model. Indirect data, using gravimetric or implanted chamber techniques, have been obtained in some animal tumors. These indicate a convective flux from the tumor interstitium to surrounding normal tissues that is 10 to 1,000 times greater than in normal tissues. These numbers represent bulk flow and do not define the events occurring at the

blood vessel–tumor interface. Data obtained from measurements of arterial and venous hematocrits in tissue-isolated tumors (i.e., tumors isolated on a vascular pedicle with one artery entering the tumor nodule and one vein leaving it) show a marked hemoconcentration from the arterial to venous circulation.[20] In models using Walker 256 and MTW-9 mammary carcinomas, the hematocrit of the tumor efferent veins averaged 1.043 times greater than aortic arterial blood. The authors estimated that 4.5% to 10.2% of the perfusing plasma volume was lost into the tumor interstitium. This implies that plasma left the tumor blood vessels and percolated through the tumor, and was discharged into the surrounding normal tissues and absorbed by peritumoral lymphatic vessels or veins (if the fluid remained in the tumor, the nodule would sequester the entire plasma volume of the animal in a brief time). The data suggest a net convective flux away from the tumor. Direct measurements of convection in human tumor nodules do not exist.

Diffusion

Diffusion is defined as the movement of solute along a concentration gradient. The force that causes a drop of ink to spread through a beaker of water is diffusion (stirring the beaker would move the ink drop by convection). Diffusion is dictated by the concentration gradient and a constant that depends on the transport medium.[18]

Diffusion across individual tumor blood vessels was measured in a rabbit ear chamber model using fluorescein-labeled immunoglobulin (Ig).[21] These experiments show that tumor blood vessels have high effective interstitial diffusion coefficients compared to normal tissues. The high diffusion coefficient implies that transport by diffusion was greater across tumor blood vessels than normal vessels in this model. Diffusion varied greatly among tumor blood vessels. Some tumor vessels have diffusion coefficients that are nearly normal, whereas others are approximately four times higher than normal vessels. Again, no direct measurements of diffusion coefficients have been made in humans for immunotherapy or chemotherapy agents.

Transcytosis

Transcytosis occurs when vascular endothelial cells form vesicles that entrap molecules or particles from the luminal surface. These vesicles are transported to the basal portion of the cell and exocytosed. The distribution of endothelial cells that can conduct transcytosis varies among different tissue types and from the arterial to venous end of capillaries.[22] Vesicles can coalesce to form transcapillary channels. These structures may be short lived or permanent. Given the heterogeneous and chaotic array of tumor blood vessels (see below), transcytosis is thought to be insignificant compared to convection and diffusion for anticancer agents (with the possible exception of liposome-encapsulated drugs)[23] and is not included in any of the transport models discussed.

INTERSTITIAL SPACE

Before discussion of the interactions and relative importance of these transport variables in tumors, the composition of the interstitial space must be reviewed, along with an additional physiologic variable—namely, interstitial pressure (IP).

Composition of the Interstitial Space

The interstitial space of tumors is greatly different from that found in normal tissues. Furthermore, the interstitium also varies between different tumor types, sites of metastasis, and perhaps even between different nodules of the same histology.[24,25] Even though the tumor interstitium is quite variable, some generalizations can be made to illustrate the differences between normal tissues and tumors.

There is a range of values in the literature for different components of the interstitial space measured in different tumor models. The volume of the interstitial space of several animal tumor models has been measured and was found to be 36% to 53% of the total tumor volume.[25] This compares with 14% to 34% in normal tissues.[26] The total protein content of the interstitial fluid can be either higher or lower than normal serum, depending on the model studied. Gullino et al.[14] showed by implantable capsules in a rat model that total protein in the interstitial fluid in a variety of tumor implants was consistently lower than aortic serum by approximately 33%. Sylven and Bois[27] compared tumor interstitial fluid sampled by micropipettes to peritoneal fluid in a variety of carcinomas grown subcutaneously in mice. These researchers found that the protein content of the tumor fluid was 5% higher than that of peritoneal samples. The composition of the protein matrix in tumors is also different from normal tissues. The amount of type IV collagen and glycosaminoglycans is much greater in tumors than in the normal interstitial space.[24,28] The amino acid, phospholipid, and cholesterol levels vary but are generally lower in tumors than in normal serum.

Direct measures of the interstitial space pH and oxygen tension in human tumors have been made. Measurements of pH in a series of melanomas ranged from 6.4 to 7.3.[28,29] Some authors have reported tumor pH values less than 6 in squamous cell carcinomas and astrocytomas.[30] The extremely acidic conditions found in the interstitial space of tumors was thought to occur from lactic acid production during anaerobic and aerobic glycolysis. Studies of glycolysis-deficient ras-transfected lung fibroblasts grown as subcutaneous tumors in nude mice have shown that an acidic microenvironment *in vivo* can be generated by tumor cells that do not make lactic acid.[31] In the murine model, there was no significant difference in interstitial pH between glycolysis-deficient and parental tumor cells. These data suggest that alternative pathways exist for tumors to create and maintain an acidic microenvironment. Despite low pH values in the tumor interstitium, intracellular pH appears to be normal.

Direct oxygen tension measurements in human breast cancers have shown partial pressures of oxygen as low as 0 mm Hg.[32,33] Six out of fifteen nodules tested had oxygen tensions between 0.0 and 2.5 mm Hg. Intertumoral oxygen tension differences were more pronounced than intratumoral measurements. Low oxygen tensions do not necessarily abrogate the ability of tumors to use energy. Nuclear magnetic resonance (NMR) spectroscopy has been used to determine the ratio of nucleoside triphosphate to inorganic phosphorus as a measure of energy status in isolated tumor nodules.[34] In this model, hypoxia had no statistically significant effect on tumor lactate release, pH, or the nucleoside triphosphate to inorganic phosphate ratio. Glucose deprivation was much more effective in changing the energy status of the tumor. Temporal changes in oxygenation are also common in tumors. Dewhirst and colleagues measured oxygen tension in real time using polarographic electrodes in 1-cm R-3230AC tumors in Fischer-344 rats.[35] Hypoxia occurred episodically with four to seven events per hour. The duration of hypoxia ranged from less than 1 minute to greater than 40 minutes. Additional evidence on the heterogeneity of tumor pH and oxygen gradients was described by Helmlinger et al.[36] These investigators performed an elegant study of single vessel pH and oxygen measurements at a resolution exceeding 10 μm in human colon adenocarcinoma (LS-174T) xenografts implanted in SCID mice using fluorescence ratio imaging and phosphorescence-quenching microscopy. There was no correlation locally between pH, oxygen profiles, and blood vessel flow. Perfusion of blood vessels did not assure oxygen delivery to the local tissue. Although local conditions within the tumor implants were variable, there was a correlation between mean pH and oxygen profiles. In a separate study, chemotherapy drugs, such as doxorubicin and mitomycin-C, altered tumor blood flow and oxygenation, but not in a consistent direction. Durand and LePard used laser Doppler and image analysis techniques to assess perfusion in human cervical (SiHa) and colon (WiDr) cancer cell lines in nude or SCID mice.[37] Radiosensitivity was used as a surrogate measure of oxygenation. The investigators found a dose- and time-dependent decrease in tumor blood flow and oxygenation from doxorubicin, whereas mitomycin-C caused increases in flow.

One can conclude from these data that the interstitial space of tumors is profoundly different from normal tissues and that tumors display a remarkable degree of metabolic diversity and resilience. These differences represent a mechanism for potential drug resistance if the therapeutic agent is not stable or functional in an acidic or hypoxic environment. The function of immune cells that infiltrate the tumor microenvironment also may be impaired by the low pH and oxygen tension.[38] Murine T cells cultured under pH, glucose, and oxygen tension conditions similar to those reported in tumors showed marked decreases in interleukin 2–induced T-cell proliferation. These observations suggest that anticancer agents should be engineered to function in hypoxic or acidic conditions. Also, the changing microenvironment of established tumors represents a challenge for effective therapy.

INTERSTITIAL PRESSURE

IP is the result of oncotic pressure in the interstitial space, oncotic and hydrostatic pressures in the microvascular space, the reflection coefficient, and the hydraulic conductivity of the vascular wall and interstitial space (e.g., how well water can move through these tissues) (see below). There are a number of methods to measure IP *in vivo*, including implantable capsules, the wick-in-needle technique, and micropuncture techniques.[39,40] The data for IP in normal subcutaneous tissue and muscle tissues show a range of values in the literature from –2 to 4 mm Hg.[41,42] IP was first noted to be elevated in animal tumors in 1950 by Young and colleagues.[43] In 1990, the first IP studies in humans were published.[44–47] These data indicate that many human tumor nodules have IPs much greater than in normal tissues. Table 31-1 shows a summary of published IP data for human tumors. Increased tumor volume in some studies correlated directly with the IP.[45] In a series of patients with cervical carcinoma, there was a correlation between IP and the oxygenation status of the tumor and an inverse correlation with tumor response to radiation therapy.[48] The authors suggested that the hypoxia in the high IP lesions was a factor in the radioresistance of these

lesions. Other studies have failed to show a correlation between IP and oxygenation.[48,49] Trends in IP profiles and response to treatment in a group of melanoma and lymphoma patients have been reported.[47] In the 14 melanoma nodules examined, 11 progressed on a variety of immunotherapies. Ten of these nodules showed an increase in IP over time. Three of three responding nodules showed a decrease in IP profiles over time. All seven non-Hodgkin's lymphoma nodules had a low IP at the start of treatment. Five of these nodules showed a complete response to chemotherapy or radiation therapy, and one was observed off treatment. The only lymphoma nodule that did not respond to treatment showed a significant increase in IP from 1 to 30 mm Hg at the time of tumor progression.

IP in animal tumor models is in equilibrium with microvascular pressure.[50] These authors studied tissue-isolated R-3230AC mammary carcinomas grown in rats. Pressures in superficial postcapillary venules surrounding the tumor were equal to IP in the center and periphery of the tumor. The coupling between the microvascular and IPs derives from the intrinsic leakiness of the neovasculature. By using intravital microscopy to characterize the vascular status of implanted tumors and micropipette techniques to measure IP, the appearance of vascular loops and sprouts in developing tumors correlated with the appearance of elevated IP.[51] Thus, an angiogenic state causes increased IP. There is also a time dependence between pressure changes in the microvascular and interstitial spaces. Fluctuations in arterial pressure are transmitted to the tumor interstitium within seconds (11 ± 6), whereas cessation of blood flow causes only a gradual decline in IP that takes 1,500 ± 900 seconds.[52] The difference in time scales reflects transcapillary events in the former and percolation of fluid out of the interstitium in the latter. Another characteristic of IP is that it is transmitted uniformly through tumor nodules.[53] IP measured by a micropuncture technique (in mammary carcinomas grown as tissue-isolated tumors in rats) was essentially uniform throughout the tumor nodules studied. It should be noted that there was a sharp pressure gradient in the outermost 0.5 mm of the tumor nodules extending into the surrounding normal tissues.

Elevated IP has other consequences on tumor blood flow. A network model examining pressure, flow, and resistance relationships in the arterial and venous circulations of tumors and the surrounding tissue was developed by Zlotecki et al.[54] They used their model to predict the effect of epinephrine, norepinephrine, hydralazine, nitroglycerin, and angiotensin on the tumor vasculature and sought to validate the model using laboratory observations and published data. The major conclusions from this analysis were that arterial control is minimal in tumors, and the steal phenomenon (serial and parallel paths for blood flow) predominates. Vasoconstrictors increased mean arterial pressures, tumor blood flow, and IP, whereas vasodilators had the opposite effect. The model also suggested that elevated IP

TABLE 31-1. PUBLISHED DATA FOR INTRATUMORAL INTERSTITIAL PRESSURE (IP) IN HUMANS

Histology	n	IP (mm Hg)	Reference
Melanoma	12	14.3 ± 12.5	44
	3	33 ± 14	46
	22	29.8	47
Epidermoid carcinomas of the head and neck	19	13.2 ± 8.8	45
Cervical carcinoma	12	15.7 ± 5.7	48
Breast carcinoma	9	15 ± 9	46
Renal cell carcinoma	1	38	46
Colorectal carcinoma (hepatic metastases)	9	21 ± 12	46
Primary brain tumors	11	2.0 ± 2.5[a]	134
Non-Hodgkin's lymphoma	7	4.7	47

[a]After dexamethasone, furosemide, and mannitol treatment.

did not cause vascular collapse. A recently published model also supports the inverse relationship between IP and tumor blood flow, but not the notion that increased IP causes a collapse of tumor vessels.[55] Lowering blood viscosity resulted in improved perfusion in the model. Although the model has limitations, it suggests that lowering IP is essential to drug delivery in tumors. Hemodilution, which lowers blood viscosity, was studied by Lee et al. in a mouse model.[56] When approximately 12% of the blood volume was removed from the animal, the IP decreased by 40%, red blood cell flux (a measure of tumor blood flow) doubled, and oxygenation remained stable. This finding raises issues about the transfusion threshold in patients receiving chemotherapy and the use of growth factors to increase the erythrocyte or leukocyte mass. IP also affects how pressures are transmitted between the arterial and venous sides of the circulation in tumors. Netti et al. devised single vessel models with varying degrees of deformability and permeability embedded in a medium with uniform pressure.[57] The model showed that changes in venous pressure were not completely transmitted to the arterial side of the circulation, efferent tumor blood flow decreases with increasing venous pressure, and hydrostatic pressure profiles along the length of the vessel are less steep than in normal vessels.

Several strategies have been used in animal models to lower IP. There are no patient trials prospectively testing this hypothesis. Radiation caused a modest lowering of IP and improvement in oxygenation in a human xenograft model.[58] These changes occurred before radiation-induced tumor regression. Dexamethasone was tested in the same tumor model in SCID mice and transiently decreased IP by approximately 5 mm Hg with a peak effect at day 4 that disappeared by day 7.[59] It should be noted that most tumors responding to dexamethasone still had elevated IP compared to normal tissues. The authors proposed that the dexamethasone caused a drug-induced decrease in microvascular permeability. Dexamethasone is frequently used in patients with spinal cord compression or brain metastatic deposits to decrease edema, which is a consequence of microvascular permeability.[60] In immunocompetent humans, dexamethasone may exert its effect by altering mediators of angiogenesis or by down-regulating immune cells, which can release proinflammatory cytokines. Lee et al. showed that nicotinamide was able to acutely decrease IP in C3H mice bearing subcutaneous FSa-II tumors.[61] Angiotensin II in similar animal models increased systemic blood pressure and IP,[62] suggesting that increases in local tumor blood flow or systemic blood pressure changes mediated by nicotinamide or other agents also may influence IP. Tumor water content in this study also correlated with IP and may contribute to its pathogenesis. Tumor necrosis factor α (TNF-α) was tested in three melanoma xenograft models to determine its effect on IP.[63] Decrements in IP (8 to 10 mm Hg) were seen 1 to 5 hours after TNF-α treatment, which resolved in 24 hours. Again,

nadir intratumoral IP values were substantially greater than expected normal tissue IP values after TNF-α. Hyperthermia in an animal model also decreased IP and improved therapeutic response as measured by growth delay of the tumors compared with controls, perhaps through damage to small tumor blood vessels.[64] It is interesting to note that several of the strategies proposed to lower IP use agents that inhibit angiogenesis, such as dexamethasone. This provides an additional rationale for combining antiangiogenic agents with chemotherapy or immunotherapy. The timing of chemotherapy after antiangiogenic agents may be crucial in taking advantage of the physiologic alterations in the tumor.

INTERACTION OF TRANSPORT VARIABLES

We have seen, thus far, that tumor blood vessels can have high effective diffusion coefficients and that diffusion and convection are quite different in tumors compared with normal tissues. The interaction of these variables is examined in this section, and the importance of each to the delivery of anticancer drugs in tumors is discussed.

Experimental models looking at the ratio of diffusion to convection for molecules of different sizes traveling through the interstitial space of a tumor provide an estimate of the relative importance of these transport variables.[65] Larger molecules [i.e., those with molecular weights (MWs) greater than approximately 800 d] move much more readily by convection, whereas smaller molecules move easily by diffusion alone. To illustrate the importance of convection for large molecules, one can ask how long it would take an IgG molecule to travel 1 cm by diffusion alone through an interstitial matrix having the same composition as a tumor. The answer is approximately 7 months.[66] Several *in vitro* models have been developed to quantify the rate of chemotherapy delivery by diffusion through multicellular tumor layers.[67] The rate of diffusion for doxorubicin (MW = 579) and mitoxantrone (MW = 517) was approximately fivefold slower than methotrexate (MW = 454) and 5-fluorouracil (MW = 130), which have substantially lower MWs. The diffusion rate for either class of chemotherapy drug was much slower through tumor tissue than through Teflon control membranes. Convection, therefore, is needed to transport large therapeutic molecules over a time scale that is relevant to cancer treatment. We can now try to answer whether convection or diffusion predominates in the interstitial space of tumors.

To determine which transport force predominates in tumors, we focus on what happens at the interface between blood vessels and the interstitium of tumors. Here, the blood vessels of interest are those that participate in the exchange of nutrients or therapeutic agents. These vessels are thought to be postcapillary venules. Because convection is the rate-limiting process for large molecules, it will be examined first. The relation for convective flux, J_C, across a blood vessel wall is given by Starling's law[68]:

$$J_C = L_p S \left[(p_v - p_i) - \sigma_T (\pi_v - \pi_i) \right]$$

where L_p is the hydraulic conductivity of the blood vessel wall; S is the surface area of the vessels; p_v and p_i are the vascular and IPs, respectively; σ_T is the osmotic reflection coefficient (this relates the movement of solute under conditions of high filtration rate and no concentration difference); and π_v and π_i are the osmotic pressures of the intravascular plasma and the interstitial fluid, respectively.

The osmotic pressure components of Starling's law are dictated by the permeability of blood vessels. Dvorak and Clauss, among others, have shown that tumor vessels are extremely leaky to large protein molecules.[69–71] Specific tumor vessel permeability factors also have been described in animal models and malignant pleural effusions in humans.[72,73] Assays of tumor interstitial fluid have shown directly that there is a high protein content.[27] Given that tumor vessels are leaky, the quantity $(\pi_v - \pi_i)$ will approach 0, because proteins would distribute equally between the vessel lumen and the area just outside the vessel (this statement is not applicable to what is happening at a distance from the vessel; however, this difference is not important for the considerations here).

The terms in Starling's law related to hydrostatic pressures in blood vessels and the interstitial space are examined here. As discussed previously, p_v in peripheral tumor vessels is equal to the IP (p_i) in the animal models studies, thus the quantity $(p_v - p_i)$ is 0. This implies that there is no convection across nutrient exchange vessels in tumors. Diffusion, therefore, becomes the only mode of transport available to therapeutic agents at the level of the vasculature most important to the delivery of any therapeutic agent. As we have seen, diffusion may also be impaired in tumors but is more effective in moving small molecules (MW less than 800 d) through the tumor interstitium, but it is an extremely poor mechanism to move larger molecules through this space over a short period of time.

A significant physiologic impediment to the delivery of therapeutic agents, which is particularly relevant to high-molecular-weight molecules, such as biologic response modifiers and IgGs, is strongly suggested by consideration of these data and models. We examine additional mechanisms that may inhibit the delivery of therapeutic agents that stem from the unique geometry and flow characteristics of tumor blood vessels.

TUMOR BLOOD VESSELS

The process of angiogenesis in normal tissues and tumors has been the subject of intensive research in recent years.[74,75] There also have been a number of studies examining the microscopic characteristics of tumor blood vessels

and their overall organization.[76–79] Much less is known about the aggregate flow characteristics of these vessels and how they interact with surrounding normal vessels. New imaging technologies are providing some insight about human tumors *in vivo*, but these studies are often difficult to interpret because of the extreme variability of tumor vessels. This variation encompasses not only the number of blood vessels (ranging from 0.8% to 25.0% of the total tumor volume in the same animal model),[80] but also their characteristics over different tumor histologies, different nodules of the same histology, and different regions within the same nodule. Despite these difficulties, it is possible to make some valid generalizations about features that may impact the transport of drugs to tumors.

Tumor Vessel Characteristics

Normal blood vessels have a relatively uniform structure, consisting of an endothelial lining, basement membrane, and surrounding pericytes.[81] Certain specialized blood vessels, such as those found in the glomerulus or those that make up the blood–brain barrier, have additional unique anatomic and functional characteristics,[82,83] yet they have the same basic framework outlined previously. Normal vessels dilate and contract in a stereotypic way when subjected to a variety of pharmacologic agents.[84,85]

Despite the fact that tumor blood vessels are thought to be recruited from surrounding normal host vessels, they do not have a consistent structural motif. The endothelial lining of tumor vessels is patchy and may include tumor cells in direct contact with flowing blood. The basement membrane is also irregular in distribution and thickness and has a different composition compared to normal vessels.[86,87] There are no pericytes or myocytes associated with tumor vessels.[70] This may account for the fact that tumor vessels have a much diminished response to a variety of vasoactive drugs.[88] Much of this disturbed behavior may be secondary to the angiogenic state induced by tumors. Normally, concentration gradients and controlled release of angiogenic growth factors facilitate the orderly branching patterns of blood vessels. Tumors induce promiscuous release of vessel growth factors. The concentration gradients important to normal vessel formation become randomized, and so does the vessel branching in tumors.[89]

The branching pattern of normal vessels as they progress from large arteries to arterioles, capillaries, postcapillary venules, and veins is orderly and can be described with remarkable precision using a mathematical tool known as *fractal geometry*.[90] Fractal geometry differs from Euclidian geometry in that it can describe the spatial relations of complicated and irregular objects, not just "classic" forms such as cones and cylinders. Fractal geometry is an appropriate tool to model the branching patterns in tumors. By using a statistical method known as *invasion percolation* and several measures of the heterogeneity of the vessel distribution and path, Baish and colleagues developed a network model for the tumor vessels.[91,92] The model predicted high geometric resistance found in tumor vessels despite increased vessel diameter and was better at describing decreased tissue oxygenation. This network modeling approach is much more powerful than describing vessels as simple cylinders embedded in a matrix.

Tumor Vessel Geometry

There are a number of unique blood vessel configurations present in tumors but not in most normal tissues. An elegant characterization of these geometries was published by Less and colleagues,[76] who systematically described the branching pattern and vessel diameters from vascular casts of mammary carcinomas grown as tissue-isolated tumors in rats. These authors noted the presence of vessel true loops (single vessels taking a 360-degree circular path before branching), self-loops (vessels bifurcating and then rejoining without additional branches), trifurcations, and the direct branching of moderate-sized arterioles into capillary networks. They did not observe arterial-venous shunts; however, other authors have observed these structures.[93,94] Vessel diameters and lengths also were measured in this model, showing that tumor vessel diameters were greater and lengths shorter for a given vessel generation number than published values for normal tissues (the generation number denotes the number of branchings that have occurred from the main arterial vessel entering the tumor).

In addition, the overall organization of tumor blood vessels was unique. Some nodules displayed central vascularization, with large vessels occupying the interior portion of the nodule. Other vascular casts showed a pattern of peripheral organization, with the largest number of vessels covering the surface of the nodule. With either of these vascular schemes, the distance between blood vessels and tumor cells could be quite large (in some areas, approaching 1 cm). In a study of the microvasculature architecture of colon tumors in a rat model, changes were documented over time in the pattern of vascularization.[77] Initially, pre-existing host microvessels provided most of the nutrient supply to the tumor. With tumor growth, chaotically arranged new vessels predominated. This finding is consistent with current views of tumor angiogenesis.

The spatial differences and uniqueness of tumor vessel organization illustrate an important and recurring theme in tumor physiology—namely, that tumor nodules are not alike and change over time. Even if an understanding of the dynamics of drug delivery in the setting of peculiar blood vessel geometries is achieved, the relative contribution of each geographic region of the tumor would have to be assessed individually to arrive at an accurate determination of blood flow in a particular nodule.

Flow Characteristics in Tumor Vasculature

A number of experimental methods have been used to study tumor blood flow, including laser Doppler,[95] radioactive tracer washout,[96] perfusion techniques,[97] magnetic resonance imaging,[34] and color Doppler ultrasonography[98] (Table 31-2). Blood flow in tumors can vary significantly, even among tumors of the same size derived from the same cell line.[99] Despite this variability, a number of researchers have concluded that as tumor size increases, total perfusion decreases.[100] This has been measured directly by xenon 133 (^{133}Xe) clearance and is also manifest indirectly by observing the geometric resistance of tumor blood vessels, which increases with tumor weight. The geometric resistance of

TABLE 31-2. COMPARISON OF MEASUREMENT TECHNIQUES FOR INTRATUMORAL FLOW AND PHARMACOKINETICS

Technique	Variable measured	Tracers and contrast agents	Limitations
Doppler sonography	Bulk flow and tumor vascular resistance	Microbubbles, sonicated albumin, galactose compounds (Levovist)	Pharmacokinetics not possible, not all anatomic areas accessible for imaging.
Radiolabeled tracer washout	Bulk flow, antibodies distribution, certain chemotherapy drugs, and cell trafficking	Technetium 99, inert gases, indium 111, other radiolabeled agents	Individual vessels and regions of tumors poorly resolved.
Vascular windows with fluorescence microscopy	Single vessel resolution of flow, transvascular diffusion, and vascular permeability	Variety of radiolabeled agents	Animal models only.
Tissue isolated tumor (*ex vivo* perfusion)	Bulk flow, vascular resistance, and selected chemotherapy agents	Not available	Practical only in animal models. Individual vessels not resolved.
Magnetic resonance spectroscopy	Bulk flow, microvascular density, and angiogenic activity	Gadolinium	Individual tumor vessels and angiogenic activity variably resolved.
Positron emission tomography	Bulk flow, exchanging water space, cell trafficking, intratumoral pharmacokinetics of certain chemotherapy agents and tumor metabolism	Fluorine 18 (^{18}F)–fluorouracil, oxygen 15–labeled water, ^{18}F-fluorodeoxyglucose, carbon 11–methionine	Individual vessels and regions of tumors poorly resolved.

tumor vessels is one to two orders of magnitude higher than normal vessels. Using positron emission tomography (PET) and inhaled oxygen 15 (^{15}O) as a tracer, Wilson and colleagues[101] made direct measurements of total blood flow in human breast tumors. The ^{15}O is converted by carbonic anhydrase in the lung to $H_2^{15}O$, which distributes into arterial blood. These authors determined that the mean blood flow in normal breast tissue was 5.6 mL per dL per minute, compared with 29.8 mL per dL per minute in breast tumors. The blood flow in tumors was apparently higher than in normal tissues, but when the volume of distribution for the tracer was taken into account, there was no significant difference between normal and neoplastic tissue. It is likely that the investigators were measuring convective flux away from the tumor, as described previously. There was no correlation between tumor size or prognosis and tumor blood flow in these patients. The degree of tumor necrosis or vascularity was not examined in this study. NMR with deuterium oxide contrast material also has been used to image tumor blood flow in a tissue-isolated tumor preparation.[34] Variations in tumor perfusion over time and between regions of tumors were much greater than those observed in normal tissues. Most of the measurement techniques described previously depend on the use of rapidly diffusable tracers and assume that the distribution of the tracer within the tumor is relatively uniform. These assumptions were challenged by Eskey and colleagues, who used tissue-isolated tumors (R-3230AC rat mammary carcinoma) to study tracer residence times in the effluent from the tumor.[102] They found that the tracer exited the tumor more rapidly than expected, which was not predicted by a one-compartment model or explained by vascular shunting or flow heterogeneity. Most NMR and PET studies estimate blood flow using one-compartment models; thus, new models are needed for a complete understanding of tumor blood flow.

Tumor blood flow can be altered by a number of factors. Viscosity of blood in tumors has been measured and was found to be greater than normal vessels. Viscosity also varies directly with hematocrit and increases with decreasing blood pressure.[103] The reason that intratumoral blood viscosity is different from that of normal vessels is thought to stem from two causes. Extravasation of plasma from leaky vessels (see above) causes a relative hemoconcentration. Also, red blood cells normally stream in the center of blood vessels as long as the vessel diameter is greater than one red cell diameter. This creates a cell-free marginal layer at the vessel wall, which results in decreased blood viscosity. This is known as the *Fahraeus-Lindqvist effect*. This phenomenon is decreased in tumors secondary to irregular vessels.[100] This ultimately results in nonlinear flow, increased turbulence, increased rouleaux formation, and elevated blood viscosity. Cytokines also can alter tumor blood flow. This was documented by Kluge et al.,[104] who showed that TNF-α and lymphotoxin lower tumor blood flow and increase tumor

vascular resistance. This resulted in a larger decrement in tumor energy consumption as measured by phosphorus 31 (^{31}P) NMR spectroscopy. Hydralazine and some anesthetic agents were shown by other investigators[105,106] to decrease tumor blood flow in some, but not all, mouse models tested. There is also a variable effect of hydralazine on human tumor xenografts in nude mice.

One of the most difficult physiologic barriers to understand and influence is heterogeneous blood flow in tumors. As described previously, IP can change tumor blood flow, but what accounts for the spatial heterogeneity of blood flow in tumors? Baish and colleagues devised network models for a regular mesh of vessels and for a pair of vessels (artery and vein) of equal diameter embedded in a medium with similar characteristics to tumor interstitium. The model looked at factors coupling vascular, transvascular, and interstitial fluid flow. As the leakiness and compliance of blood vessels were increased in these models, blood was diverted away from the center of the tumor. Elevated IP altered the vascular pressure distribution and contributed to the low-flow state in the center of the tumor. This model provides further insight about the difficulties of delivering therapeutic agents to the central areas of tumors, even when tumor blood vessels are highly permeable. A number of clinical trials were designed to increase vessel leakiness as a way to enhance antibody or biologic response modifier penetration into the tumor.[107,108] These strategies are unlikely to be effective.

INTRATUMORAL PHARMACOKINETICS IN HUMANS

The increasing sophistication of NMR and PET scanning now permits real-time intratumoral analysis of some chemotherapy drugs in humans. One of the first reports used fluorine 19 (^{19}F)–labeled 5-fluorouracil imaged by NMR spectroscopy to estimate the accumulation of drug in metastatic adenocarcinoma deposits in humans.[109] Four out of four patients with 5-fluorouracil "trapping" in tumor deposits (time range, 20 to 78 minutes compared to 5 to 15 minutes in blood) had regression in those sites (pelvis, breast, lung, and liver). The three patients who did not show measurable amounts of 5-fluorouracil trapping did not have tumor regression. ^{18}F-labeled fluorouracil PET scanning was used to study patients with liver metastases from colorectal carcinoma.[110,111] A variety of systemic (bolus and infusional) and regional 5-fluorouracil regimens were used in these patient populations. PET scanning was done 120 minutes after drug injection in each study. ^{18}F-labeled fluorouracil trapping was highly variable from patient to patient and at different metastatic sites within the same patient. Patients who achieved higher drug uptake within the tumor were more likely to achieve stable disease or tumor regression and had a significantly longer mean survival.

Another approach was taken by Müller et al., who used microdialysis probes to measure intratumoral and normal tissue uptake of 5-fluorouracil and methotrexate.[112,113] Patients received either the cyclophosphamide, methotrexate, and 5-fluorouracil or the 5-fluorouracil, epirubicin, and cyclophosphamide regimens. The kinetics of 5-fluorouracil clearance were similar in the tumor and subcutaneous tissues. Patients with high intratumoral 5-fluorouracil were significantly more likely to respond. There was no association of response to plasma or normal tissue uptake to drug. Similarly, in the patients having methotrexate measurements, there was no correlation between plasma and tumor drug levels and a high degree of variability among patients. Methotrexate levels in the tumor did not correlate with response.

In animal models, PET has been used to follow interleukin-2–activated natural killer cells or nonactivated lymphocytes.[114] The investigators used carbon-11 methyl iodide as the positron emitter, injected 1×10^7 cells via tail vein in a murine tumor model, and performed PET imaging 30 to 60 minutes after injection. Tumor uptake of natural killer cells was seen in this model, but not to a greater degree than nonactivated cells. Additional studies will need to be done to determine whether PET scanning for adoptive immunotherapy is more informative than other available techniques, such as indium 111 (^{111}In) labeling or gene marking. The half-life of current positron emitters also limits suitability for cellular immunotherapy, in which serial measurements over days or weeks may be more informative.

TRANSPORT MODELS IN TUMORS

Monoclonal antibody studies for therapy, or their use in imaging human tumors after intravenous administration, have shown that the antibodies will localize to the tumor but will be unevenly distributed.[115–117] Common distribution patterns include finding the antibody in the peritumoral area or focally deposited around intratumoral blood vessels. The amount of antibody measured in the tumor is also much less than predicted by *in vitro* binding experiments. This is illustrated by a study by Shockley et al.,[118] who examined a melanoma xenograft model. They found that melanoma-specific antigen concentrations were 15 to 70 times less than that suggested by a three-compartment kinetic model, which translated into markedly lower antibody concentrations in the tumor 72 hours after injection. Another study compared diphtheria toxin and an immunoconjugate of diphtheria toxin and the human transferrin receptor in a human xenograft tumor model.[119] Although the plasma-to-tissue transport constants were high in the tumors, the amount of immunotoxin that localized *in vivo* was 530 times less than predicted by *in vitro* binding affinities. These findings suggest that lower expression of antigen-binding sites and decreased accessibility of the antibody *in vivo* present significant barriers to antibody treatment. Another study used autoradiography to quantify the spatial distribution of diphtheria toxin and a variety of binding and nonbinding diphtheria toxin immunoconjugates.[120] The nonbinding conjugates and unconjugated toxin showed the most homogeneous distribution in RD2 rhabdomyosarcoma xenografts. The reduced penetration of the binding immunoconjugates was attributed to their greater MW and to antigen binding. The growth rate of the RD2 tumor xenografts *in vivo* was inhibited more effectively by the diphtheria toxin, which penetrated into the tumor, but not by immunoconjugate with lower penetration. *In vitro* growth retardation by the two agents was similar. The authors concluded that tumor response may be correlated with the spatial distribution of the therapeutic agent.

Similarly, adoptively transferred cells, such as lymphokine-activated killer cells, are not generally found in tumor sites.[121] Tumor-infiltrating lymphocytes (TIL), which are predominantly CD8[+] T cells, were initially thought to reproducibly reach their tumor targets.[122] An interesting trafficking study was performed using gene-labeled TIL and peripheral blood leukocytes (PBL).[123] TIL were transduced with the amphotropic retroviral vector LNL6, and PBL with G1Na. These investigators showed that marked TIL or PBL could be detected in the peripheral blood up to 99 days after infusion. Marked TIL or PBL could be detected in six out of nine tumor biopsies studied; however, there was no preference in tumor trafficking of TIL compared to PBL. Biopsies of muscle, fat, or skin showed greater accumulation of TIL than in tumor specimens. This is the most convincing evidence thus far that TIL have no particular affinity for tumors and supports the notion that TIL accumulate nonspecifically. Anti–CD3-stimulated CD4[+]-enriched T-cell populations may preferentially accumulate in some tumor sites.[124] The mixed findings from these studies reflect the heterogeneity of tumor blood flow and immune cell interactions with tumor endothelium. The physical properties of activated immune cells, namely decreased cell deformability, may also make it difficult for them to traverse the vascular network of tumors.[125] The dynamics of cell movement are likely to be more complicated than the forces that govern monoclonal antibody or chemotherapy drug movement, because cells can expend energy to move along chemotactic gradients and have additional interactions with the vasculature mediated by adhesion molecules. As discussed previously, concentration gradients of molecules, such as angiogenic and chemotactic factors, may be washed out by the pressure gradients created by elevated IP. Thus, immune cells may lose the signal they need to enter and remain in the tumor.

There are several models that account for physiologic variables such as diffusion, convection, and concentration gradient effects. In the development of monoclonal antibodies, two of the central issues are the binding affinity of the antibody and the distribution of antigen within the tumor mass. Fujimori and colleagues[126] developed a spherical tumor nodule model that looked at the distribution of antibodies with varying affinities and different tumor antigen concentrations. Their model also took into account the effective interstitial diffusion coefficient, capillary permeation, initial concentration of the antibody in the serum, and valence of the antibody. This modeling scheme showed that as the number of antibody-antigen binding events increased or the affinity of the antibody increased, the percolation of the antibody through the tumor decreased. This reduced the heterogeneity of antibody distribution and produced a binding site barrier. Direct evidence for the binding site barrier hypothesis was obtained using double-label immunohistochemistry and autoradiography.[127] Monoclonal antibody D3 was given to guinea pigs bearing intradermally implanted line 10 carcinomas. A low level of D3 antibody binding to antigen significantly impaired antibody penetration in the tumor. An irrelevant antibody distributed uniformly through the tumor, indicating that other physiologic barriers were not present.

Sung et al.[128] developed a plasma and tissue compartmental model that accounted for interstitial fluid flow and used the Langmuir isotherm to estimate antibody-antigen binding. Using this approach, the model predicted that increasing antibody affinity at low doses of antibody would result in increased tumor uptake. When antigen saturation was approached, binding affinity had a smaller effect. Another implication of this model was that if antigen density could be increased, antibody localization also could be increased. This point was illustrated by an animal model comparing two different melanomas with different antigen concentrations grown subcutaneously. The antibodies used had similar affinities for antigen in the tumor studies. The melanoma with the greater antigen density (SK-MEL-2) had greater antibody uptake. Other researchers also have concluded that antigen density is of salient importance to antibody distribution in model systems that used antibodies to epidermal growth factor receptors, carcinoembryonic antigen, and cell surface ovarian carcinoma antigens.[129–131]

Another modeling approach incorporated IP as a variable to explain heterogeneous antibody distribution in tumors. In the model developed by Jain and Baxter,[132] IP opposed the tendency of fluid and macromolecules to leave tumor blood vessels. It also resulted in net convective forces that are directed radially outward and are of a magnitude sufficient to counteract the tendency of any molecule present in the area surrounding the tumor nodule to diffuse back into the substance of the tumor. A number of assumptions were made, including that the tumor was uniformly perfused, that IP was spatially dependent, and that the macromolecules modeled were free to move in the tumor interstitium (i.e., no binding in the tumor). With these constraints, the model predicted that smaller molecules,

such as Fab fragments, reached higher concentrations for a given radial position in the tumor than IgG after bolus injections. Continuous infusion of the antibody resulted in higher intratumoral concentrations of both IgG and Fab. Furthermore, the distribution of IgG, Fab2, or Fab predicted by the model was heterogeneous. Thus, by modeling a physiologic variable and not the binding characteristics of the therapeutic agent, it was concluded that tumors would have regions with different concentrations of macromolecules delivered intravenously.

Gene therapy requires appropriate vectors for delivery, which are often large constructs measuring 100 to 300 nm in diameter. Particles of this size must traverse transvascular pores in tumor vessels. Hobbs and colleagues studied this problem in human and murine tumors implanted in dorsal skin-fold chambers or cranial windows.[133] They also tested the influence of hormone-induced tumor regression on transvascular pore size. Pore size was measured between 200 nm and 1.2 μm. Subcutaneous tumor vessels had larger pores than intracranial tumors, but hormone-induced tumor regression diminished the size of pores in subcutaneous tumors. Thus, the delivery of gene vector therapy or encapsulated therapeutics may face additional physical barriers to delivery, especially in intracranial tumors.

CONCLUSIONS

The chaotic nature of tumor blood vessels and blood flow, the varied composition of the tumor interstitium, and disturbed convection and diffusion in the interstitial space of tumors all create significant physical barriers to the delivery of therapeutic agents to neoplastic cells *in vivo*. This hostile microenvironment is not duplicated or predicted by any *in vitro* system. Similarly, animal models using small tumor nodules that possess a nascent or absent vascular network do not mimic the physiology discussed here. Although there is heightened awareness of angiogenesis as a therapeutic target, there are few efforts seeking to alter the behavior of these new vessels to enhance drug delivery. If the aggregate physiologic behavior of tumor nodules is not taken into account, then any therapy, no matter how rationally designed or effective *in vitro*, is likely to be diminished in patients with large tumors.

A great deal more needs to be understood about tumor blood vessels and the interstitium of human tumors. Recent advances in imaging technologies, such as NMR and PET scanning, are providing additional insights about how cancer therapies interact with their tumor targets *in vivo*. The main conclusion from these studies is that intratumoral pharmacokinetics are far more predictive of tumor response than plasma levels of drug. As forecast by many of the animal and computer models, blood flow and tumor uptake of therapeutic agents is highly variable; thus, physical barriers to drug delivery are real.

Overcoming these barriers may prove to be just as important as thwarting the molecular mechanisms of tumor resistance. Studies of the tumor vasculature and interstitium will answer at least one very important question in cancer therapeutics—namely, does the drug reach its target and stay there? It is only when this is understood that the full potential of chemotherapy, gene therapy, and immunotherapy can be realized.

REFERENCES

1. Leventhal B. *Program/Proceedings, American Society of Clinical Oncology.* 1990;9.
2. Perry MC. *Program/Proceedings, American Society of Clinical Oncology.* 1999;18.
3. Landis SH, Murray T, Boldin S, et al. Cancer statistics, 1998. *CA Cancer J Clin* 1998;48:6–30.
4. Kramer BS, Klausner RD. Grappling with cancer—defeatism versus the reality of progress. *N Engl J Med* 1997;337:931–934.
5. Larson RA, Dodge RK, Burns CP, et al. A five-drug remission induction regimen with intensive consolidation for adults with acute lymphoblastic leukemia: cancer and leukemia group B study 8811. *Blood* 1995;85:2025–2037.
6. Bosl GJ, Motzer RJ. Testicular germ-cell cancer. *N Engl J Med* 1997;337:242–253.
7. Fisher RI, Gaynor ER, Dahlberg S, et al. Comparison of a standard regimen (CHOP) with three intensive chemotherapy regimens for advanced non-Hodgkin's lymphoma. *N Engl J Med* 1993;328:1002–1006.
8. Salmon SE, Dalton WS, Grogan TM, et al. Multidrug-resistant myeloma: laboratory and clinical effects of verapamil as a chemosensitizer. *Blood* 1991;78:44–50.
9. Zhang ZG, Harstick A, Rustum YM. Mechanisms of resistance to fluoropyrimidines. *Semin Oncol* 1992;19:4–9.
10. Parker RJ, Eastman A, Bostick-Bruton F, et al. Acquired cisplatin resistance in human ovarian cancer cells is associated with enhanced repair of cisplatin-DNA lesions and reduced drug accumulation. *J Clin Invest* 1991;87:772–777.
11. Herlyn M, Menrad A, Koprowski H. Structure, function, and clinical significance of human tumor antigens. *J Natl Cancer Inst* 1990;82:1883–1889.
12. Zea AH, Curti BD, Longo DL, et al. Alterations in T cell receptor and signal transduction molecules in melanoma patients. *Clin Cancer Res* 1995;1:1327–1335.
13. Hahne M, Rimoldi D, Schröter M, et al. Melanoma cell expression of Fas (Apo-1/CD95) ligand: implications for tumor immune response. *Science* 1996;274:1363–1366.
14. Gullino PM, Clark SH, Grantham FH. The interstitial fluid of solid tumors. *Cancer Res* 1964;24:780–797.
15. Gullino PM, Grantham FH. Studies on the exchange of fluids between host and tumor. I. A method for growing "tissue-isolated" tumors in laboratory animals. *J Natl Cancer Inst* 1961;27:679–693.
16. Jain RK. Delivery of novel therapeutic agents in tumors: physiological barriers and strategies. *J Natl Cancer Inst* 1989;81:570–576.
17. Jain RK. The next frontier of molecular medicine: delivery of therapeutics. *Nature Med* 1998;4:655–657.
18. Jain RK. Transport of molecules in the tumor interstitium: a review. *Cancer Res* 1987;47:3039–3051.
19. Chary SR, Jain RK. Direct measurement of interstitial convection and diffusion of albumin in normal and neoplastic tissues by fluorescence photobleaching. *Proc Natl Acad Sci U S A* 1989;86:5385–5389.
20. Butler TP, Grantham FH, Gullino PM. Bulk transfer of fluid in the interstitial compartment of mammary tumors. *Cancer Res* 1975;35:3084–3088.
21. Clauss MA, Jain RK. Interstitial transport of rabbit and sheep antibodies in normal and neoplastic tissues. *Cancer Res* 1990;50:3487–3492.
22. Taylor AE, Granger DN. Exchange of macromolecules across the microcirculation. In: Renkin EM, Michel CC, eds. *Handbook of physiology: the cardiovascular system.* Bethesda, MD: American Physiology Society, 1984:467.
23. Gabizon AA. Selective tumor localization and improved therapeutic index of anthracyclines encapsulated in long-circulating liposomes. *Cancer Res* 1992;52:891–896.
24. Gullino PM, Grantham FH, Clark SH. The collagen content of transplanted tumors. *Cancer Res* 1962;22:1031–1034.
25. Gullino PM, Grantham FH, Smith SH. The interstitial water space of tumors. *Cancer Res* 1965;25:277–281.
26. O'Conner SW, Bale WF. Accessibility of circulating immunoglobulin G to the extravascular compartment of solid rat tumors. *Cancer Res* 1984;44:3719–3723.
27. Sylven B, Bois I. Protein content and enzymatic assays of interstitial fluid from some normal tissues and transplanted mouse tumors. *Cancer Res* 1960;20:831–836.
28. Choi HU, Meyer K, Swarm R. Mucopolysaccharide and protein-polysaccharide of a transplantable rat chondrosarcoma. *Proc Natl Acad Sci U S A* 1971;68:877–879.
29. Thistlewaite AJ, Leeper DB, Moylan DJ, et al. pH distribution in human tumors. *Int J Radiat Oncol Biol Phys* 1985;11:1647–1652.
30. Ashby BS. pH studies in human malignant tumors. *Lancet* 1966;2:312–315.
31. Newell K, Franchi A, Pouyssegur J, et al. Studies with glycolysis-deficient cells suggest that production of lactic acid is not the only cause of tumor acidity. *Proc Natl Acad Sci U S A* 1993;90:1127–1131.
32. Vaupel P, Schlenger K, Knoop C, et al. Oxygenation of human tumors: evaluation of tissue oxygen distribution in breast cancers by computerized O_2 tension measurements. *Cancer Res* 1991;51:3316–3322.
33. Vaupel P, Kallinowski F, Okunieff P. Blood flow, oxygen and nutrient supply, and metabolic microenvironment of human tumors: a review. *Cancer Res* 1989;49:6449–6465.
34. Eskey CJ, Koretsky AP, Domach MM, et al. ^{2}H-nuclear magnetic resonance imaging of tumor blood flow: spatial and temporal heterogeneity in a tissue-isolated mammary adenocarcinoma. *Cancer Res* 1992;52:6010–6019.
35. Dewhirst MW, Braun RD, Lanzen JL. Temporal changes in PO2 of R3230AC tumors in Fischer-344 rats. *Int J Radiat Oncol Biol Phys* 1998;42:723–726.
36. Helmlinger G, Yuan F, Dellian M, et al. Interstitial pH and pO_2 gradients in solid tumors *in vivo*: high-resolution measurements reveal a lack of correlation. *Nat Med* 1997;3:177–182.

37. Durand RE, LePard NE. Modulation of tumor hypoxia by conventional chemotherapeutic agents. *Int J Radiat Oncol Biol Phys* 1994;29:481–486.

38. Loeffler DA, Juneau PL, Masserant S. Influence of tumour physico-chemical conditions on interleukin-2-stimulated lymphocyte proliferation. *Br J Cancer* 1992;66:619–622.

39. Guyton AC. A concept of negative interstitial pressure based on pressures in implanted perforated capsules. *Circ Res* 1963;7:399–414.

40. Wiig H, Reed RK, Aukland K. Measurement of interstitial fluid pressure: comparison of methods. *Ann Biomed Eng* 1986;14:139–151.

41. McMaster PD. The pressure and interstitial resistance prevailing in the normal and edematous skin of animals and man. *J Exp Med* 1946;84:473–494.

42. Hargens AR, Mubarak SJ, Owen CA, et al. Interstitial fluid pressure in muscle and compartment syndromes in man. *Microvasc Res* 1977;14:1–10.

43. Young JS, Lumsden CE, Stalker AL. The significance of the "tissue pressure" of normal testicular and neoplastic (Brown-Pierce carcinoma) tissue in the rabbit. *J Path Bacteriol* 1950;62:313–316.

44. Boucher Y, Kirkwood JM, Opacic D, et al. Interstitial hypertension in superficial metastatic melanomas in humans. *Cancer Res* 1991;51:6691–6694.

45. Gutmann R, Leunig M, Feyh J, et al. Interstitial hypertension in head and neck tumors in patients: correlation with tumor size. *Cancer Res* 1992;52:1993–1995.

46. Less JR, Posner MC, Boucher Y, et al. Interstitial hypertension in human breast and colorectal tumors. *Cancer Res* 1992;52:6371–6374.

47. Curti BD, Urba WJ, Alvord WG, et al. Interstitial pressure of subcutaneous nodules in melanoma and lymphoma patients: changes during treatment. *Cancer Res* 1993;53:2204–2207.

48. Roh HD, Boucher Y, Kalnicki S, et al. Interstitial hypertension in carcinoma of uterine cervix in patients: possible correlation with tumor oxygenation and radiation response. *Cancer Res* 1991;51:6695–6698.

49. Boucher Y, Lee I, Jain RK. Lack of general correlation between interstitial fluid pressure and oxygen partial pressure in solid tumors. *Microvasc Res* 1995;50:175–182.

50. Boucher Y, Jain RK. Microvascular pressure is the principal driving force for interstitial hypertension in solid tumors: implications for vascular collapse. *Cancer Res* 1992;52:5110–5114.

51. Boucher Y, Leunig M, Jain RK. Tumor angiogenesis and interstitial hypertension. *Cancer Res* 1996;56:4264–4266.

52. Netti PA, Baxter LT, Boucher Y, et al. Time-dependent behavior of interstitial fluid pressure in solid tumors: implications for drug delivery. *Cancer Res* 1995;55:5451–5458.

53. Boucher Y, Baxter LT, Jain RK. Interstitial pressure gradients in tissue-isolated and subcutaneous tumors: implications for therapy. *Cancer Res* 1990;50:4478–4484.

54. Zlotecki RA, Baxter LT, Boucher Y, et al. Pharmacologic modification of tumor blood flow and interstitial fluid pressure in a human tumor xenograft: network analysis and mechanistic interpretation. *Microvasc Res* 1995;50:429–443.

55. Milosevic MF, Fyles AW, Hill RP. The relationship between elevated interstitial fluid pressure and blood flow in tumors: a bioengineering analysis. *Int J Radiat Oncol Biol Phys* 1999;43:1111–1123.

56. Lee I, Demhartner TJ, Boucher Y, et al. Effect of hemodilution and resuscitation on tumor interstitial fluid pressure, blood flow, and oxygenation. *Microvasc Res* 1994;48:1–12.

57. Netti PA, Roberge S, Boucher Y, et al. Effect of transvascular fluid exchange on pressure-flow relationship in tumors: a proposed mechanism for tumor blood flow heterogeneity. *Microvasc Res* 1996;52:27–46.

58. Znati CA, Rosenstein M, Boucher Y, et al. Effect of radiation on interstitial fluid pressure and oxygenation in a human tumor xenograft. *Cancer Res* 1996;56:964–968.

59. Kristjansen PE, Boucher Y, Jain RK. Dexamethasone reduces the interstitial fluid pressure in a human colon adenocarcinoma xenograft. *Cancer Res* 1993;53:4764–4766.

60. Byrne TN. Spinal cord compression from epidural metastases. *N Engl J Med* 1992;327:614–619.

61. Lee I, Boucher Y, Jain RK. Nicotinamide can lower tumor interstitial fluid pressure: mechanistic and therapeutic implications. *Cancer Res* 1992;52:3237–3240.

62. Zlotecki RA, Boucher Y, Lee I, et al. Effect of angiotensin II induced hypertension on tumor blood flow and interstitial fluid pressure. *Cancer Res* 1993;53:2466–2468.

63. Kristensen CA, Nozue M, Boucher Y, et al. Reduction of interstitial fluid pressure after TNF-alpha treatment of three human melanoma xenografts. *Br J Cancer* 1996;74:533–536.

64. Endrich B, Hammersen F, Messmer K. Hyperthermia-induced changes in tumor microcirculation. *Cancer Res* 1988;107:44–59.

65. Swabb EA, Wei J, Gullino PM. Diffusion and convection in normal and neoplastic tissues. *Cancer Res* 1974;34:2814–2822.

66. Jain RK, Baxter LT. Mechanisms of heterogeneous distribution of monoclonal antibodies and other macromolecules in tumors: significance of elevated interstitial pressure. *Cancer Res* 1988;48:7022–7032.

67. Tunggal JK, Cowan DS, Shaikh H, et al. Penetration of anticancer drugs through solid tissue: a factor that limits the effectiveness of chemotherapy for solid tumors. *Clin Cancer Res* 1999;5:1583–1586.

68. Kedem O, Katchalsky A. Thermodynamic analysis of the permeability of biological membranes to non-electrolytes. *Biochim Biophys Acta* 1989;1000:413–430.

69. Brock TA, Dvorak HF, Senger DR. Tumor-secreted vascular permeability factor increases cytosolic Ca2+ and von Willebrand factor release in human endothelial cells. *Am J Pathol* 1991;138:213–221.

70. Dvorak HF, Nagy JA, Dvorak JT, et al. Identification and characterization of the blood vessels of solid tumors that are leaky to circulating macromolecules. *Am J Pathol* 1988;133:95–109.

71. Keck PJ, Hauser SD, Krivi G, et al. Vascular permeability factor, an endothelial cell mitogen related to PDGF. *Science* 1989;246:1309–1312.

72. Yeo KT, Wang HH, Nagy JA, et al. Vascular permeability factor (vascular endothelial growth factor) in guinea pig and human tumor and inflammatory effusions. *Cancer Res* 1993;53:2912–2918.

73. Senger DR, Perruzzi CA, Feder J, et al. A highly conserved vascular permeability factor secreted by a variety of human and rodent tumor cell lines. *Cancer Res* 1986;46:5629–5632.

74. Fidler IJ, Ellis LM. The implications of angiogenesis for the biology and therapy of cancer metastasis. *Cell* 1994;79:185–188.

75. Folkman J. Seminars in medicine of the Beth Israel Hospital, Boston. Clinical applications of research on angiogenesis. *N Engl J Med* 1995;333:1757–1763.

76. Less JR, Skalak TC, Sevick EM, et al. Microvascular architecture in a mammary carcinoma: branching patterns and vessel dimensions. *Cancer Res* 1991;51:265–273.

77. Skinner SA, Tutton PJM, O'Brien PE. Microvascular architecture of experimental colon tumors in the rat. *Cancer Res* 1990;50:2411–2417.

78. Adachi Y, Mori M, Enjoji M, et al. Microvascular architecture of early gastric carcinoma. *Cancer* 1993;72:32–36.

79. Leunig M, Yuan F, Menger MD, et al. Angiogenesis, microvascular architecture, microhemodynamics, and interstitial fluid pressure during early growth of human adenocarcinoma LS174T in SCID mice. *Cancer Res* 1992;52:6553–6560.

80. Jain RK. Determinants of tumor blood flow: a review. *Cancer Res* 1988;48:2641–2658.

81. Rodkiewicz CM. *Arteries and arterial blood flow.* New York: Springer-Verlag, 1983:1.

82. Waeber B, Burnier M, Nussberger J, et al. Role of atrial natriuretic peptides and neuropeptide Y in blood pressure regulation. *Horm Res* 1990;34:161–165.

83. Vane JR, Anggard EE, Botting RM. Regulatory functions of the vascular endothelium. *N Engl J Med* 1990;323:27–36.

84. Williams GH. Converting-enzyme inhibitors in the treatment of hypertension. *N Engl J Med* 1988;319:1517–1525.

85. Dean CR, Maling T, Dargie HJ, et al. Effect of propranolol on plasma norepinephrine during sodium nitroprusside-induced hypotension. *Clin Pharmacol Ther* 1980;27:156–164.

86. Kaiser HE. Stroma, generally a non-neoplastic structure of the tumor. *Cancer Growth Prog* 1989;3:1–10.

87. Ingerber DE, Folkman J. Extracellular matrix, endothelial cell shape modulation, and control of angiogenesis: potential targets for antitumor differentiation therapy. *Serono Symp Publ* 1988;45:111–115.

88. Hori K, Zhang QH, Saito S, et al. Microvascular mechanisms of change in tumor blood flow due to angiotensin II, epinephrine, and methoxamine: a functional morphometric study. *Cancer Res* 1993;53:5528–5534.

89. Baish JW, Jain RK. Cancer, angiogenesis and fractals. *Nature Med* 1998;4:984.

90. Mandelbrot BB. *The fractal geometry of nature.* New York: WH Freeman, 1983:1.

91. Baish JW, Gazit Y, Berk DA, et al. Role of tumor vascular architecture in nutrient and drug delivery: an invasion percolation-based network model. *Microvasc Res* 1996;51:327–346.

92. Gazit Y, Baish JW, Safabakhsh N, et al. Fractal characteristics of tumor vascular architecture during tumor growth and regression. *Microcirculation* 1997;4:395–402.

93. Warren BA. The vascular morphology of tumors. In: Peterson HI, ed. *Tumor blood circulation: angiogenesis, vascular morphology and blood flow of experimental and human tumors.* Boca Raton, FL: CRC Press, 1979.

94. Gothlin J. Arteriovenous shunting in carcinomas evaluated by a dye dilution technique. *Scand J Urol Nephrol* 1977;11:159–163.

95. Vaupel P, Kluge M, Ambroz MC. Laser Doppler flowmetry in subepidermal tumours and in normal skin of rats during localized ultrasound hyperthermia. *Int J Hyperthermia* 1988;4:307–321.

96. Mantyla M, Heikkonen J, Perkkio J. Regional blood flow in human tumours measured with argon, krypton and xenon. *Br J Radiol* 1988;61:379–382.

97. Tveit E, Weiss L, Lundstam S, et al. Perfusion characteristics and norepinephrine reactivity of human renal carcinoma. *Cancer Res* 1987;47:4709–4713.

98. Alexander AA, Nazarian LN, Capuzzi DMJ, et al. Color Doppler sonographic detection of tumor flow in superficial melanoma metastases: histologic correlation. *J Ultrasound Med* 1998;17:123–126.

99. Lyng H, Skretting A, Rofstad EK. Blood flow in six human melanoma xenograft lines with different growth characteristics. *Cancer Res* 1992;52:584–592.

100. Sevick EM, Jain RK. Geometric resistance to blood flow in solid tumors perfused *ex vivo*: effects of tumor size and perfusion pressure. *Cancer Res* 1989;49:3506–3512.

101. Wilson CBJH, Lammertsma AA, McKenzie CG, et al. Measurements of blood flow and exchanging water space in breast tumors using positron emission tomography: a rapid and noninvasive dynamic method. *Cancer Res* 1992;52:1592–1597.

102. Eskey CJ, Wolmark N, McDowell CL, et al. Residence time distributions of various tracers in tumors: implications for drug delivery and blood flow measurement. *J Natl Cancer Inst* 1994;86:293–299.

103. Sevick EM, Jain RK. Viscous resistance to blood flow in solid tumors: effect of hematocrit on intratumor blood viscosity. *Cancer Res* 1989;49:3513–3519.

104. Kluge M, Elger B, Engel T, et al. Acute effects of tumor necrosis factor alpha or lymphotoxin on global blood flow, laser Doppler flux, and bioenergetic status of subcutaneous rodent tumors. *Cancer Res* 1992;52:2167–2173.

105. Bremner JCM, Counsell CJR, Adams GE, et al. *In vivo* P nuclear magnetic resonance spectroscopy of experimental murine tumours and human tumour xenografts: effects of blood flow modification. *Br J Cancer* 1991;64:862–866.

106. Thomas C, Counsell C, Wood P, et al. Use of fluorine-19 nuclear magnetic resonance spectroscopy and hydralazine for measuring dynamic changes in blood perfusion volume in tumors in mice. *J Natl Cancer Inst* 1992;84:174–180.

107. LeBerthon B, Khawli LA, Alauddin M, et al. Enhanced tumor uptake of macromolecules induced by a novel vasoactive interleukin 2 immunoconjugate. *Cancer Res* 1991;51:2694–2698.

108. Schultz KR, Badger CC, Dombi GW, et al. Effect of interleukin-2 on biodistribution of monoclonal antibody in tumor and normal tissues in mice bearing SL-2 thymoma. *J Natl Cancer Inst* 1992;84:109–113.

109. Presant CA, Wolf W, Albright MJ, et al. Human tumor fluorouracil trapping: clinical correlations of *in vivo* [19]F nuclear magnetic resonance spectroscopy pharmacokinetics. *J Clin Oncol* 1990;8:1868–1873.

110. Moehler M, Dimitrakopoulou-Strauss A, Gutzler F, et al. 18F-labeled fluorouracil positron emission tomography and the prognoses of colorectal carcinoma patients with metastases to the liver treated with 5-fluorouracil. *Cancer* 1998;83:245–253.

111. Dimitrakopoulou-Strauss A, Strauss LG, Schlag P, et al. Fluorine-18-fluorouracil to predict therapy response in liver metastases from colorectal carcinoma. *J Nucl Med* 1998; 39:1197–1202.

112. Müller M, Mader RM, Steiner B, et al. 5-Fluorouracil kinetics in the interstitial tumor space: clinical response in breast cancer patients. *Cancer Res* 1997;57:2598–2601.

113. Müller M, Brunner M, Schmid R, et al. Interstitial methotrexate kinetics in primary breast cancer lesions. *Cancer Res* 1998;58:2982–2985.

114. Melder RJ, Brownell AL, Shoup TM, et al. Imaging of activated natural killer cells in mice by positron emission tomography: preferential uptake in tumors. *Cancer Res* 1993;53:5867–5871.

115. Larson SM. Radioimmunology. Imaging and therapy. *Cancer* 1991;67:1253–1260.

116. Begent RH, Pedley RB. Antibody targeted therapy in cancer: comparison of murine and clinical studies. *Cancer Treat Rev* 1990;17:373–378.

117. Shockley TR, Lin K, Nagy JA, et al. Spatial distribution of tumor-specific monoclonal antibodies in human melanoma xenografts. *Cancer Res* 1992;52:367–376.

118. Shockley TR, Lin K, Sung C, et al. A quantitative analysis of tumor specific monoclonal antibody uptake by human melanoma xenografts: effects of antibody immunological properties and tumor antigen expression levels. *Cancer Res* 1992;52:357–366.

119. Sung C, Youle RJ, Dedrick RL. Pharmacokinetic analysis of immunotoxin uptake in solid tumors: role of plasma kinetics, capillary permeability, and binding. *Cancer Res* 1990;50:7382–7392.

120. Juweid M, Neumann R, Paik C, et al. Micropharmacology of monoclonal antibodies in solid tumors: direct experimental evidence for a binding site barrier. *Cancer Res* 1992;52: 5144–5153.

121. Clark JW, Smith JW II, Steis RG, et al. Interleukin 2 and lymphokine-activated killer cell therapy: analysis of a bolus interleukin 2 and a continuous infusion interleukin 2 regimen. *Cancer Res* 1990;50:7343–7350.

122. Griffith KD, Read EJ, Carrasquillo JA, et al. *In vivo* distribution of adoptively transferred indium-111-labeled tumor infiltrating lymphocytes and peripheral blood lymphocytes

123. Economou JS, Belldegrun AS, Glaspy J, et al. *In vivo* trafficking of adoptively transferred interleukin-2 expanded tumor-infiltrating lymphocytes and peripheral blood lymphocytes. Results of a double gene marking trial. *J Clin Invest* 1996;97:515–521.

124. Curti BD, Ochoa AC, Powers GC, et al. A phase I trial of anti-CD3-stimulated CD4+ T cells, infusional interleukin-2 and cyclophosphamide in patients with advanced cancer. *J Clin Oncol* 1998;16:2752–2760.

125. Sasaki A, Jain RK, Maghazachi AA, et al. Low deformability of lymphokine-activated killer cells as a possible determinant of *in vivo* distribution. *Cancer Res* 1989;49:3742–3746.

126. Fujimori K, Covell DG, Fletcher JE, et al. A modeling analysis of monoclonal antibody percolation through tumors: a binding-site barrier. *J Nucl Med* 1990;31:1191–1198.

127. Sung C, Dedrick RL, Hall WA, et al. The spatial distribution of immunotoxins in solid tumors: assessment by quantitative autoradiography. *Cancer Res* 1993;53:2092–2099.

128. Sung C, Shockley TR, Morrison PF, et al. Predicted and observed effects of antibody affinity and antigen density on monoclonal antibody uptake in solid tumors. *Cancer Res* 1992;52:377–384.

129. Goldenberg A, Masui H, Divgi C, et al. Imaging of human tumor xenografts with an indium-111-labeled anti-epidermal growth factor receptor monoclonal antibody. *J Natl Cancer Inst* 1989;81:1616–1625.

130. Philben VJ, Jakowatz JG, Beatty BG, et al. The effect of tumor CEA content and tumor size on tissue uptake of indium 111-labeled anti-CEA monoclonal antibody. *Cancer* 1986;57:571–576.

131. Boerman O, Massuger L, Makkink K, et al. Comparative *in vitro* binding characteristics and biodistribution in tumor-bearing athymic mice of anti-ovarian carcinoma monoclonal antibodies. *Anticancer Res* 1990;10:1289–1295.

132. Baxter LT, Zhu H, Mackensen DG, et al. Biodistribution of monoclonal antibodies: scale-up from mouse to human using a physiologically based pharmacokinetic model. *Cancer Res* 1995;55:4611–4622.

133. Hobbs SK, Monsky WL, Yuan F, et al. Regulation of transport pathways in tumor vessels: role of tumor type and microenvironment. *Proc Natl Acad Sci U S A* 1998;95:4607–4612.

134. Boucher Y, Salehi H, Witwer B, et al. Interstitial fluid pressure in intracranial tumours in patients and in rodents. *Br J Cancer* 1997;75:829–836.

32

ADOPTIVE CELLULAR THERAPY

CARL H. JUNE

Immunotherapy of cancer is entering into a new era of progress at the preclinical and clinical level. This is due to the exciting developments in basic immunology and tumor biology that have allowed a tremendous increase in our understanding of mechanisms of interactions between the immune system and tumor cells. Adoptive cellular therapy can be considered as a strategy aimed at tumor elimination through direct antineoplastic effects or through indirect effects, such as immune-mediated antiangiogenic effects. Adoptive cellular therapy may also have a role in replacing, repairing, or enhancing the immune function damaged as a consequence of cytotoxic therapy by means of autologous or allogeneic cell infusions. The analysis of the presently available clinical results suggests that, despite some disappointments, there is room for optimism that adoptive immunotherapy and active immunotherapy (vaccination) may eventually become part of the therapeutic arsenal to prevent or combat cancer in a more efficient way. Although adoptive immunotherapy has, thus far, added little to the routine treatment of most human cancer, it can now be considered front-line therapy for patients with chronic myelogenous leukemia (CML) in relapse after allogeneic stem cell or marrow transplantation and for certain Epstein-Barr virus (EBV)–related tumors. This review describes the background, rationale, and current clinical use and experimental approach of adoptive cellular therapies and *ex vivo* cellular vaccination for the treatment of cancer.

HISTORY

The sentinel observations made by William B. Coley in the 1890s that patients with certain malignancies responded to the intratumoral inoculation of live bacterial organisms or bacterial toxins became the impetus for the development of immunotherapy for cancers.[1] In a series of experiments addressing mechanisms of skin allograft rejection, Bellingham and co-workers first coined the term *adoptive immunity* to describe the transfer of lymphocytes

to mediate an effector function.[2] Based on these studies, immunologists have categorized immunotherapies as either active or passive. Active immunizations require an intact host immune system and are typically delivered as prophylactic or therapeutic vaccines. In contrast, passive or adoptive immunotherapies consist of the transfer of serum, antibodies, or lymphocytes to the host and do not require an intact host immune system to generate the response. One characteristic of an adoptively transferred immune response is that the host has never experienced the primary immune response. This is particularly attractive for patients with late-stage tumors who may not have the time or capability to mount a primary immune response. However, as noted below, with the advent of dendritic cell (DC)–transfer therapies, in a practical sense the distinction between active and passive (adoptive) cellular therapy is blurring.

The concept of adoptive cellular therapy for tumor allografts was first reported for rodents more than 45 years ago by Mitchison.[3] The cloning of T-cell growth factors made possible the first *ex vivo* expansion of tumor-specific T cells for adoptive immunotherapy in mouse syngeneic tumor models.[4] There are several excellent reviews of the rationale and experimental basis for adoptive T-cell therapy of tumors.[5–8] In early clinical trials, patients have been given adoptive transfers of autologous, allogeneic, and xenogeneic lymphocytes for a variety of tumors. The results of these early trials were not promising, and this is not surprising, because they were carried out before the principles of T-cell biology and tumor antigens (Ags) were understood. The first 25 years of adoptive cellular therapy have been reviewed by Rosenberg and Terry.[9]

TUMOR IMMUNOLOGY AND CELL BIOLOGY

Rational use of adoptive cellular therapy is predicated on an understanding of the relevant principles of cellular and molecular immunology and cancer cell biology. The reasons for the shortcomings of many previous forms of adoptive cellular therapy are now clear, based on current advances in the basic sciences.

Immunosurveillance

Sir MacFarlane Burnet proposed a theory of immunologic surveillance.[10] The concept of immunosurveillance remains controversial and states that a function of the immune system is to control the outgrowth of cancer cells by eliminating cells bearing malignant mutations. Thus, immunocompromised humans do have a propensity to develop tumors, and the tumors are often found in immunologically privileged sites, such as the brain. However, there is evidence against this concept. For example, athymic nude mice do not develop tumors with greater frequency than normal mice.[11] This concept may be more important for tumors induced by oncogenic viruses, as illustrated by the frequent occurrence of lymphomas in immunosuppressed individuals. Recent evidence shows that patients with melanoma frequently have tumor-specific T-cell immunity that developed spontaneously.[12] Furthermore, as is discussed below, the occurrence of certain immunologically mediated paraneoplastic syndromes also provides strong support for tumor immunosurveillance in some circumstances. In retrospect, the theory of immunosurveillance appears to have been largely correct; however, sophisticated mechanisms used by tumors in many instances probably thwarts the natural immune response.

Immune Escape Mechanisms

Current immunologic dogma is that tumor cells are antigenic but not immunogenic. The fact that tumors frequently survive and prosper in the face of measurable immune responses underscores the importance of regarding living tumors as complex entities rather than clonal aggregates of transformed cells. There are multiple means that tumors use to escape or prevent immune-mediated elimination.[13] These are broadly classified as (a) mechanisms leading to decreased immunogenicity and (b) mechanisms leading to immunosuppression. The concept of tumor immune suppression and evasion arose, in part, from studies with poorly immunogenic tumors. Experiments with transplantable tumors demonstrated that some tumors induced by low-dose carcinogen lacked tumor-rejection Ags and actually grew better in preimmunized mice. For example, North and colleagues found that progressive growth of a tumor in mice evoked the generation of a T-cell–mediated mechanism of immunosuppression, which inhibited the capacity of adoptively transferred tumor-sensitized T cells from eliminating the tumor.[14] This and other forms of tumor-induced immune suppression were initially thought to be due to the generation of suppressor T cells[15]; however, the inability to clone suppressor T cells and the failure to genetically identify their putative major

histocompatibility complex (MHC) restriction element led to the abandonment of the suppressor T-cell notion for twenty years. However, there is a recent resurgence of interest in this concept, with a return to active investigation of a role for regulatory cells in autoimmunity and cancer.[16] Tumor cells often have low expression of MHC class I molecules, and absent or low density of peptide-MHC complexes may cause lack of recognition, a phenomenon termed *immune ignorance*. Tumor cells themselves are poor antigen Ag-presenting cells (APCs), as the lack of cell surface co-stimulatory molecules, such as B7, may induce anergy. Ineffective presentation of tumor Ags by the tumor itself, as well as by APC, leads to a failure to provide the necessary co-stimulatory signals required to activate Ag-specific T cells and the subsequent functional clonal inactivation of tumor-specific T cells.[17,18]

Multiple tumor immunosuppressive events may also blunt, or eliminate, a tumor-specific immune response. For example, tumor cells often secrete suppressive cytokines, such as tumor growth factor β (TGF-β) or interleukin 10 (IL-10), which can down-regulate T-cell responses. Tumor cells may also express an enzyme termed *indoleamine 2,3-dioxygenase*, leading to the catabolism of tryptophan and the subsequent inhibition of T-cell proliferation.[19] Finally, to sustain an ongoing T-cell response, it requires a continued production of IL-2 and perhaps other cytokines, such as IL-15.[20] In the absence of cytokines, cytotoxic T lymphocytes (CTLs) undergo a few cell divisions and die. CTLs require helper T cells to supply these cytokines, and the tumor microenvironment is generally deficient in helper T cells.

Tumor Antigens

Adoptive cellular therapy is based on the premise that tumor cells possess intracellular or surface Ags that are qualitatively or quantitatively distinct from those present on normal cells. Furthermore, the repertoire of the adoptively transferred T cells must be able to recognize the tumor Ags. The initial successes of adoptive T-cell therapy in the 1950s were discredited when it was realized that the tumors were allogeneic and that tumor rejection was simply a form of allograft rejection. However, Klein and Hellström provided strong evidence for specific tumor immunity by demonstrating that, after resection of a methylcholanthrene-induced tumor, the host could subsequently reject challenge with its own resected tumor.[21] Indeed, tumor immunology was not considered as a respectable field until the last decade, when a clear molecular understanding of the nature of antigenic targets presented by tumors became available.

Tumor Ags can be classified according to the type of immune response they elicit: humoral, cellular, CD4+, or CD8+ CTL responses. Humoral Ags must be expressed on the surface of the tumor cells for it to be a therapeutic target, whereas T-cell Ags may be derived from cytosolic and membrane proteins. A classification of human tumor rejection Ags was recently proposed by Gilboa.[22] Tumor Ags may be one of the following types: (a) Non–self-tumor Ags, such as transforming proteins of viral origin for tumors caused by viruses. For example, approximately 30% of all human cancers are caused by transforming viruses, such as EBV and human papilloma virus. (b) Mutated "self"-Ags occur because tumor cells have genetic instability and may accumulate mutations or chromosomal translocations. (c) Overexpressed mutated oncogene products, of which the best examples are *p53* and *HER-2-neu*. (d) In addition, tumor Ags may be normal self-tumor Ags, such as reexpressed embryonic Ags, which were not expressed during the development of the immune system, differentiation Ags which are transiently expressed in tissue development may be reexpressed in tumor cells, and reexpressed retroviral gene products encoded in the mammalian genome (these have been identified for mouse tumors but not yet for human tumors), and tissue-specific Ags, which may be from immunologically privileged sites, or from so-called "dispensable tissue." (e) Self-Ags modified chemically by carcinogens such as methylcholanthrene in the mouse. (f) "Silent" genes, cellular genes that are not normally expressed but become transcriptionally active in tumor cells, such as the thymic leukemia Ag in mice.

There is currently an explosive growth in the understanding of human tumor Ags and the immune response to tumors. This is based on the development of technologies to identify human tumor rejection Ags. In seminal studies, Boon and colleagues developed a genetic approach using CTLs to screen either genomic or complementary DNA libraries derived from tumors to identify MHC class I restricted Ags.[23] Due to technical hurdles consequent to the differences in MHC class I and class II Ag presentation, it has only recently been possible to identify MHC class II restricted tumor rejection Ags by screening of complementary DNA libraries to identify MHC class II restricted Ags recognized by CD4[+] T cells.[24] Thus, at present, there is much less known about the helper T-cell response than the CTL response.

A second major advance in the understanding of the human tumor immune response has been the development of tetramers and other immunoglobulin-based reagents that display Ag-specific binding to T-cell receptors. These reagents permit for the first time the tracking and quantitation of tumor-specific T cells. Initial studies with tetramers of the MHC class I restricted CD8[+] T-cell response in patients with melanoma indicate that tumor-specific T cells are present in approximately 30% of patients with advanced melanoma. In a subset of patients, the tumor-specific T cells are dysfunctional, and chemotherapy appears to ablate the Ag-specific tumor immune response.[12] These are major concerns for adoptive cellular

therapy if this form of immunosuppression proves to be a frequent occurrence.

Principles of T-Cell Growth

Adoptive cellular therapy depends on the ability to optimally select or genetically produce cells with the desired antigenic specificity and then induce cellular proliferation while preserving the effector function, engraftment, and homing abilities of the lymphocytes. Unfortunately, many previous clinical trials were carried out with adoptively transferred cells that were propagated in what are now understood to be suboptimal conditions, which impairs the essential functions of the adoptively transferred cells. Our understanding of T-cell activation through cell surface receptors and proteins now indicates that this is a complex multistaged process of recognition, adhesion, and stimulation. *In vivo*, the generation of Ag-specific T cells requires the interaction of DCs and naïve T cells in a secondary lymphoid organ, usually a lymph node.[25]

For more than half a century, immunologists have sought to understand how self-tolerance is induced and maintained. Bretscher and Cohn first proposed a two-signal model of B-lymphocyte activation that was later modified by Lafferty and Cunningham for T-cell activation and allograft rejection.[26] The essential features of these models were that activation of lymphocytes requires an Ag-specific *signal 1* as well as a second Ag nonspecific event termed *signal 2*. Moreover, these theories and later modifications proposed that signal 1, in the absence of the co-stimulatory signal 2, led to tolerance or apoptosis. Indeed, in some instances, the binding of tumor Ag presented to the T-cell receptor (TCR) in the absence of co-stimulation not only fails to activate the cell, but also leads to functional inactivation.[27] It is now appreciated that antigenic stimulation of T cells leads to at least three distinct outcomes: (a) activation, clonal expansion, and differentiation to produce cells that secrete distinct subsets of cytokines or to express lytic machinery; (b) induction of an unresponsive state termed *anergy*; and (c) induction of apoptosis.[28,29]

The most appropriate methods of *ex vivo* T-cell activation and propagation mimic the physiologic processes whereby DCs generate a constellation of Ag-specific and co-stimulatory signals in the T cells. Polyclonal T cells' proliferation can be induced by mimicking the Ag signal by anti–T-cell receptor antibodies or anti-CD3 antibodies.[30,31] However, anti-CD3 stimulation without the addition of IL-2 or another co-stimulus is not sufficient for full activation of T cells and long-term growth.[32] Enhanced polyclonal T-cell activation and proliferation results when cells are stimulated via the T-cell receptor as well as the CD28 receptor.[33] This culture system has been adapted for clinical use, and starting with an initial apheresis product, it is possible to generate the number of mature T cells found in adults within 2 weeks of *ex vivo* culture.[34,35] Ag-specific T-cell proliferation can be induced by addition of autologous DCs that have been loaded with the desired Ag or by use of tetramers to activate the T cells with the desired specificity.[36–40] DCs are most efficient for the activation of naïve T cells; however, other forms of APC may suffice for previously primed T cells. Schultze and co-workers have shown that CD40-stimulated B cells are an efficient means to propagate Ag-specific T cells.[41] In addition, cell lines can be transfected with the appropriate MHC molecules to create engineered APC to generate Ag-specific T cells and avoid the need to use autologous APC for patient-specific cultures.[42]

Dispensable Tissues: A New Paradigm for Tumor Immunotherapy?

For decades, the goal of most cancer immunotherapy centered on the induction of immune responses against tumor-specific "neoantigens." However, the coalescence of results from many laboratories now indicates that the generation of tissue-specific autoimmune responses represents an alternate approach to cancer immunotherapy that is gaining momentum.[43,44] This is because it is now clear that, for most tumors, there is no special set of tumor protein targets, but rather that tumor Ags are by and large normal self proteins. Furthermore, for many, and perhaps most, tumor proteins, active immunologic tolerance has not been induced, as they have simply been ignored previously by the immune system because they have not been presented in an immunogenic form.[45]

For common tumors derived from "dispensable tissues," such as prostate, pancreas, breast, ovary, and skin, an acceptable toxicity could include the immune-mediated damage or destruction of normal, as well as neoplastic, tissue. Given that many common cancers, such as melanoma, prostate cancer, pancreatic cancer, and breast cancer, are derived from dispensable tissues, the induction of immune responses against tissue-specific Ags shared by these tumors might represent an immunotherapy approach whose autoimmune side effects would represent acceptable "collateral damage." Thus, a new hypothesis in cancer therapy is that the ability to induce tissue-specific autoimmunity could permit the treatment of many important cancers.

The rationale for the induction of tissue-specific, rather than tumor-specific, responses is derived from several observations. First, in the 1980s, immunologists learned that for many peripheral tissues, T-cell tolerance to self-Ags is not maintained purely by clonal deletion of autoreactive T cells in the thymus, but also by peripheral mechanisms that result in the functional silencing of the T cells or ignorance to the peripheral tissue. Autoimmunity is the disruption of this mechanism and leads to the loss of self-tolerance to tissues. Second, in the 1990s it was discovered that patients who experienced immune-based rejection of tumors often had responses that were directed against normal self-Ags. For example, Brichard and colleagues[46] dis-

covered that the target for a melanoma-specific CD8[+] T-cell clone isolated from a melanoma patient was wild-type tyrosinase, a melanosomal enzyme selectively expressed in melanocytes and responsible for one of the steps in melanin biosynthesis. Additional evidence for the relevance of tissue-specific responses in melanoma immunotherapy came from the finding that patients whose tumors responded to IL-2–based immunotherapy occasionally developed vitiligo, an autoimmune depigmentation of patches of skin, whereas vitiligo was essentially never seen among melanoma patients who failed to respond to immunotherapy.[47] Third, recent studies by Linette and colleagues and others using more potent DC-based vaccine strategies indicate that it is now routinely possible to induce vitiligo, as it is now observed in approximately 50% of melanoma patients that are vaccinated with DCs that express melanocyte-specific Ags. Thus, the ability to induce at least some forms of autoimmunity does not appear to be dependent on the presence of rare MHC backgrounds or other unusual polymorphisms.

The ability of adoptive cellular therapies to "break" tolerance to tissue-specific Ags for cancer therapy will probably depend on the antigenic target, as well as other host-specific genetic elements, such as the patient's MHC background. It is likely that the specific Ag, as well as the form of immunologic adjuvant, will be critical in defining the qualitative and quantitative nature of immune responses generated. Under physiologic circumstances, the level of endogenous immunity against an Ag is below a critical threshold necessary for clinical autoimmunity or antitumor immunity. A successful antitumor response would require the elevation of immunity against a particular Ag above a critical threshold. The stringency of tolerance against a particular Ag will dictate how potent the vaccination strategy will have to be to raise the immune response above the threshold level. For Ags that are difficult to elicit responses against, approaches to interfere with the normal down-regulation of the immune responses, such as blocking CTL–A-4 or PD-1 interactions might be required for the induction of clinically evident antitumor immunity.[48–50]

Paraneoplastic Syndromes

One premise for adoptive immunotherapy, especially when using an autologous source of T cells for infusion, is that T-cell immunity occurs in response to tumors, and that clinically evident tumors have developed the means to escape or overwhelm the cellular response. Unfortunately, it has been extraordinarily difficult to demonstrate naturally occurring T-cell immunity to most human tumors. Other than recent tetramer data, paraneoplastic syndromes provide perhaps the clearest examples of naturally occurring tumor immunity in humans. A recent series of studies in a rare subset of patients with occult carcinomas indicates that spontaneous and potent T-cell immunity in fact occurs in some human tumors. Studies indicate that patients with paraneoplastic neurologic disorders often harbor systemic tumors that express proteins whose normal expression is restricted to the central nervous system (CNS). Thus, the expression of these Ags by tumors outside of the normal immunologically privileged site of expression allows for their recognition by the immune system and, consequently, the fortuitous antitumor response. A Purkinje's neuronal protein termed cdr2 has been identified as a target that is responsible for paraneoplastic cerebellar degeneration (PCD) in patients with ovarian and breast tumors.[51] Cdr2 messenger RNA (mRNA) is expressed in almost all tissues, whereas the protein is expressed only in the brain and testis.[52] Previous studies had shown that although tumor immunity and autoimmune neuronal degeneration in PCD correlates with a specific antibody response to the tumor and brain Ag cdr2, this humoral response has not been shown to be pathogenic. In recent studies, Darnell and coworkers have detected expanded populations of MHC class I–restricted cdr2-specific CTLs in the blood of three of three human lymphocyte Ag (HLA)-A2.1[+] PCD patients.[53] Thus, it is likely that tumor-induced peripheral activation of cdr2-specific CTLs contributes to the subsequent development of the autoimmune neuronal degeneration in the CNS. These studies raise the hope that therapeutically induced immunity to this Ag, and, perhaps, other similar "self"-Ags, might be an effective immune-based therapy for a variety of carcinomas. They also raise the possibility that effective immunotherapy against some carcinomas could be subject to CNS toxicity, as they may share immunodominant Ags with CNS tissue.

Limitations to Adoptive Cellular Therapy

The major rationale for the use of T cells is that the cells have the capacity to specifically kill tumor cells, to proliferate, and to persist after transfer and therefore could completely eliminate all residual tumor cells or newly emerging tumor cells. T-cell survival and replication in the host are essential for efficacy, as irradiation of adoptively transferred T cells before their transfer abrogates therapeutic efficacy in most animal models.[54,55] Factors leading to failure or suboptimal efficacy of adoptive cellular therapies can be classified as those due to intrinsic limitations of the infused cells and as immunosuppressive conditions in the tumor-bearing host (Table 32-1). Large tumor burdens present qualitative and quantitative problems for immunotherapy, and as with all therapies, cell transfer therapy has most promise when conducted in the setting of minimal residual disease. Immunologists have long observed a process termed *tumor sneaking through*, by which it is meant that small tumors grow progressively, medium-sized tumors are rejected, and large ones break through again. De Boer and colleagues developed mathematic models studying tumor kinetics in the setting of adoptively transferred T cells.[56] In de Boer's

TABLE 32-1. POTENTIAL EXPLANATIONS FOR LACK OF EFFICACY OF ADOPTIVE T-CELL THERAPY

Limitations of the infused cells
  Ex vivo–expanded T-cell population approaches or reaches replicative senescence or loss of CD28 expression.
  Tumor antigen-specific T cells have been deleted or tolerized in the donor by previous chemotherapy or by the tumor itself.
  Ex vivo expansion of T-cell population introduces failure to home to tumor or lymph nodes.
  Culture process renders transferred T cells immunogenic, leading to failure of sustained engraftment.
Limitations in the host
  Unrealistic effector to target ratio: Host tumor burden exceeds killing capacity of adoptively transferred cells.
  Poor engraftment of adoptively transferred CTLs: lack of CD4 T-cell help, cytokine "addiction."
  Infertile soil: Previous chemotherapy or radiotherapy has ablated stroma and lymph nodes, leading to impaired survival signals and lack of "niche."
  Regulatory cells in the host kill or inactivate adoptively transferred T cells.
  Tumor cells kill or inactivate adoptively transferred T cells.
  Transferred T cells do not recognize tumor-associated antigens due to loss of tumor antigen expression.
  Lack of tumor co-stimulation induces anergy or apoptosis of adoptively transferred cells.

model, the magnitude of the cytotoxic effector cell response depends on the time at which helper T cells become activated: Early helper activity steeply increases the magnitude of the immune response. Thus, tumor rejection is most favored if the tumor-specific CD4[+] helper T cells are induced early, as this helps to magnify the induction of CTLs. Recent studies have shown de Boer's work to be remarkably prescient, as there is an emerging consensus that one of the primary limitations in the immune response to tumors is the development of Ag-specific CD4[+] helper T cells.[57] Given the accumulating evidence that CD4[+] T cells are critical participants in effective antitumor immune responses, a number of potential roles have been suggested. Although it had long been known that CD4[+] T cells provide help for the development of CTLs via the elaboration of lymphokines, more recent evidence has indicated that a critical cellular signaling pathway for delivery of help for CTLs is dependent on CD4[+] T cells. The recent data support a concept whereby interactions between CD40 ligand on the CD4[+] T cell and CD40 on the DC activate and therefore "license" the DC to present Ags to, and co-stimulate the priming of, CD8[+] CTL precursors.[58,59]

Recent studies indicate that T-cell survival in the periphery is dependent on continuous delivery of environmental signals. The nature of the survival signals that are required appears to differ between naïve and memory T cells, and between CD4[+] and CD8[+] T cells.[60] In some cases, T-cell survival is dependent on MHC class II–expressing DCs; it is likely that chemotherapy and radiation can damage these stromal cells that are required for long-term clonal survival of adoptively transferred T cells.

A large body of literature indicates that chemotherapy enhances the effectiveness of adoptively transferred T cells.[5] Multiple reasons appear to account for this observation. Chemotherapy may ablate cells and create niches for the adoptively transferred cells. However, the "space" argument is likely a minor factor, as other studies indicate that a major effect of chemotherapy is to ablate suppressor or regulatory T cells that inhibit the effects of adoptively transferred T cells.[61] The identity of these regulatory cells remains controversial, and candidate cell populations are subsets of CD4[+] cells that secrete IL-10 and TGF-β[62] or have a phenotype of CD4[+] CD25[+].[16] Finally, chemotherapy may enhance the effectiveness of adoptively transferred T cells by killing tumor, leading to enhanced Ag presentation on bone marrow–derived APC and the subsequent loss of immunologic tolerance or ignorance to tumor.[17,63]

A final host-specific factor that can prevent therapeutic efficacy of adoptively transferred T cells is the inactivation of the T cells in the immunosuppressive environment of the host. The priming of tumor–Ag-specific T cells is critical for the initiation of successful antitumor immune responses, yet the fate of such cells during tumor progression is unknown. In a lymphoma model in mice, when naive CD4[+] T cells specific for an Ag expressed by tumor cells were transferred into tumor-bearing mice, transient clonal expansion occurred early after transfer. The adoptively transferred cells then developed a diminished tumor-specific response, suggesting that tolerance to tumor Ags may impose a significant barrier to therapeutic vaccination, at least in the case of tumors that express MHC class II Ags.[18] T cells from patients with Hodgkin's disease have defects in activation that are reversible *in vitro* by stimulation with anti-CD3 and anti-CD28.[64]

Replicative Senescence

T cells have finite clonal life spans *in vitro*,[65] a phenomenon also manifested with other somatic tissue cells and that is commonly known as the *Hayflick's limit*. *In vitro*, the current limit of polyclonal expansion for adult mature T cells is approximately 30 to 40 population doublings.[32,66,67] Several mechanisms, such as progressive gene demethylation, have been proposed to serve as a biologic clock for the cell to count its replicative history. However, currently, the most widely accepted hypothesis to account for replicative senescence is that progressive telomere shortening in cells can trigger replicative arrest. Telomeres are specific structures found at the ends of eukaryotic autosomal and sex chromosomes. The telomere consists of thousands of copies of the hexameric sequence (TTAGGG)n. The length of telomeres is species specific and in humans, telomeres are approximately 5 to 15 kb long. The function of telomeres is to stabilize chromosomal ends, as chromosomes lacking telomeres are genetically unstable and have a propensity to undergo fusion, rearrangement, and translocation. In T

cells, the rate of telomere loss *in vitro* is approximately 50 to 120 base pairs per cell doubling, a rate comparable to that seen in other somatic cells.[68]

In vivo, clonal exhaustion of T cells has been observed under certain immunologically unfavorable conditions of antigenic load and persistence.[69] The mechanisms of clonal exhaustion and its relation to replicative senescence, if any, remain unknown. Telomerase is a reverse transcriptase riboprotein complex that adds telomeric repeats to the 3' end of existing telomeres, using its RNA component as a template. Mutant mice lacking the RNA component of telomerase demonstrate an essential role for telomerase and, hence, telomeres in the maintenance of genomic integrity and in the long-term viability of high-turnover organ systems, such as bone marrow–derived cells.[70] Recent results suggest that the induced expression of the human telomerase catalytic subunit can facilitate organ regeneration and prevent replicative senescence and maintain a normal karyotype in fibroblasts for at least 20 population doublings past the usual onset of growth arrest.[71,72] These exciting results may have relevance to Ag-specific forms of adoptive transfer and immunotherapy, if telomere exhaustion proves rate limiting for clonal T-cell persistence *in vivo*. Replicative senescence could have important implications for adoptive immunotherapy with T cells, particularly in the case of Ag-specific T cells. For example, to obtain one billion clonal T cells of a desired specificity from a single naïve T cell, 27 population doublings are required. Given that most culture systems contain a significant fraction of apoptotic cells, substantially more than 27 cell divisions are required to obtain one billion T cells. It is likely that many previous clinical adoptive immunotherapy trials have been unsuccessful because the prolonged *ex vivo* culture process resulted in a population of cells that had reached replicative senescence. Consistent with this general notion, allogeneic bone marrow transplantation in adults has been shown to result in host reconstitution with populations of T cells with shortened telomeres, estimated to represent 15 years' worth of "aging."[73,74]

Engraftment

Adoptive immunotherapy with *ex vivo*–expanded Ag-specific CTLs has been shown to clear viral infections and eliminate tumors in murine models. In human clinical trials, there is promising data for the use of adoptive immunotherapy to treat infections with human immunodeficiency virus-1 (HIV-1), and cytomegalovirus (CMV) and EBV infections in bone marrow transplant recipients. For therapy of these viral infections, the need for *ex vivo*–expanded CTLs is often short lived until the donor transplant reconstitutes the host immune system. In contrast, in HIV and cancer therapy, long-term engraftment of adoptively transferred CTLs and generation of memory will be necessary. In fact, one major rationale for adoptive immunotherapy is that it establishes a long-lasting memory to provide an ongoing effector response. In the case of T cells, memory is manifested by the clonal survival of the effector cells. The survival of mature T cells is an active process and depends on either biochemical signals derived from the T-cell receptor or from cytokines. Naïve T cells require T-cell receptor interactions with the self-MHC molecules that are expressed on APC, whereas memory T cells survive independent of MHC interactions, and, at least in the case of mouse CD8+ CTLs, survival is dependent on IL-7 and IL-15.[20,60]

Given the concept of clonal persistence, the definition of life span for T lymphocytes is confusing and can either be taken as the time to cell division (i.e., intermitotic survival time) or as the time to cell death. Clonal persistence can be attributed to two distinct mechanisms: the presence of non-cycling, long-lived cell populations or through continued self-renewal by cycling cells. Studies indicate that T cells use both mechanisms.[75,76] Until recently, it was not possible to safely measure T-cell survival in humans. However, it is now possible to label lymphocytes with deuterated glucose, a nonradioactive stable isotope-enriched precursor, to measure DNA replication.[77] Recent measurements using this technique indicate that the half-lives in normal adults of CD4+ T cells and CD8+ T cells are 87 and 77 days, respectively.[78] Indeed, several studies that use distinct techniques to measure lymphocyte life spans in primates have concluded that CD8+ T-cell turnover is slightly more rapid than CD4+ T-cell turnover. The survival of different functional T-cell subsets also varies, as studies after the disappearance rates of cells with radiation-induced chromatin damage indicate that naïve T cells have a longer intermitotic survival, estimated at division occurring on average every 3.5 years, whereas memory cells divide on average every 22 weeks.[79] In HIV-1–infected adults on antiretroviral therapy, deuterated glucose measurements indicate that the half-lives of naïve-phenotype T cells ranges from 116 to more than 365 days, whereas T cells of the memory and effector phenotype persisted with half-lives from 22 to 79 days.[80]

Several studies have assessed the engraftment of adoptively transferred T cells in patients with immunodeficiency. Gene-modified autologous T cells have been shown to survive for more than 8 years in two patients with adenosine deaminase deficiency.[81] T cells marked with the gene encoding neomycin phosphotransferase have been shown to persist for more than 4 months after adoptive transfer to bone marrow allograft recipients.[82] Surprisingly, neomycin or hygromycin-marked syngeneic or autologous T cells initially engraft but do not persist long term in most patients with HIV infection, owing to immune-mediated rejection of the gene-marked cells.[83,84] Survival of adoptively transferred CD4+ T cells in HIV-infected patients is enhanced if the cells express a gene product that confers resistance to HIV infection.[85]

The engraftment efficiency of adoptively transferred T cells in humans has been assessed in recent clinical studies. In early studies, in which tumor-infiltrating lymphocytes (TILs) were retrovirally transduced with the neomycin gene and given to melanoma patients, the frequency of adoptively transferred cells represented approximately 1% of peripheral blood mononuclear cells (PBMC) 1 hour after infusion; however, the frequency fell to less than 1 in 10,000 PBMC within one week after infusion, and trafficking to tumor sites was inefficient.[86] More recent studies from Greenberg and colleagues at the University of Washington used tetramers to track the persistence of adoptively transferred Ag-specific CTL clones in patients with melanoma. They found that the transferred cells achieved initial frequencies of at least 1 in 800 PBMCs in the peripheral blood, and that the median survival of the transferred T cells was approximately 7 days. If patients were given low-dose IL-2 (500,000 U per m^2 per day), then the median survival of the CTL was enhanced.

Together, the above studies indicate that limited *in vivo* survival of adoptively transferred T cells can occur for multiple reasons (Table 36-1). If clonal populations of CD8 cells are being infused, then treatment of the patient with IL-2 can extend survival of the cells. However, if the cells have been cultured *ex vivo* for prolonged times in high concentrations of IL-2, they have shortened survival *in vivo*, due to apoptosis from growth factor withdrawal. In recent experiments using adoptively transferred polyclonal mixtures of CD4+ and CD8+ T cells in HIV-infected patients, the frequency of retrovirally marked cells 2 weeks after infusion was greater than 1%, and the level remained essentially unchanged for at least 6 months. The reasons for the enhanced efficiency of engraftment in this study were due to technical changes in *ex vivo* culture of the cells, as well as the fact that the CD4+ T cells provide helper effects to increase their own survival.[87] IL-2 infusions do not enhance the survival of adoptively transferred populations of T cells that contain adequate CD4 helper T cells. Thus, data from a number of trials indicate that adoptively transferred T cells can persist for extended times. However, detailed kinetic studies have not yet been performed, and it is not yet known if the intermitotic survival times of the transferred cells are the same as for their normal lymphocyte counterparts. Finally, T cells are different from most other tissues, such as in the case of red blood cells, in which survival is related to life span of the cells, and the oldest cells are removed first. The majority of T cells induced after an antigenic challenge die while still "young" through activation-induced cell death as a consequence of the need to maintain T-cell homeostasis at the total population number as well as at the clonal level.[75]

ADOPTIVE CELLULAR THERAPY FOR HUMAN TUMORS

Natural Killer and Lymphokine-Activated Killer Cell Adoptive Therapy

Unlike T cells or B cells, which recognize Ag using clonally restricted receptors generated by gene rearrangement, natural killer (NK) cells appear to use a variety of different, non-rearranging receptors to initiate cytolytic activity and cytokine production. NKs are cytolytic for targets even in the absence of MHC class I expression, and inhibitory receptors expressing immunoreceptor tyrosine-based inhibition (ITIM) motifs prevent NK cells from harming tissues that express normal levels of MHC class I. This latter characteristic, the ability to cause non–MHC-restricted lysis, is a major distinguishing feature of NK cells from T cells. Many receptors have been implicated in NK cell activation, including CD94-NKG2C, NKR-P1, CD2, and CD16.[88] NK cells, unlike T cells, do not have an extensive replicative potential, perhaps due to the fact that telomerase is expressed at much lower levels in NK cells than in T cells.[89]

Human lymphocytes that mediate non–MHC-restricted cytotoxicity can be divided into multiple subpopulations. The physiologic basis for this is based on the differential expression of multiple killer receptors at the single cell level, and the recent appreciation of this explains the previous controversy between the relationship of NK cells and lymphokine-activated killer (LAK) cells. For example, T cells develop NK-like cytotoxicity after activation with anti-CD3 or cytokines, and the most likely explanation for this phenomenon is the *de novo* expression of one or more NK receptors. The ability of NK and LAK cells to kill a variety of tumor cell targets *in vitro* made them attractive candidates for adoptive cellular therapy. This TCR and CD3-independent form of cellular cytotoxicity was originally reported to spare normal tissues; however, autologous human lymphocytes and cultured normal human kidney cells can be killed by LAK cells.[90,91] Another major drawback of NK and LAK cells is a relative inability of these cells to traffic to the tumor.[92]

The availability of recombinant IL-2 enabled the first clinical trials of adoptively transferred autologous NK cells.[93] An extensive series of trials has demonstrated clinical responses in a minority of patients, particularly those with melanoma and renal cell carcinoma.[94,95] Randomized studies at the National Cancer Institute with LAK cells have failed to show clinical efficacy.[96] Subsequent analysis has shown that the IL-2 that was administered concomitant with the LAK cells accounted for the majority of the clinical responses that were observed. The human MHC-nonrestricted cytotoxic T-cell line TALL-104 has been shown to display antitumor effects in several animal models with spontaneous and induced malignancies. For example, the xenogeneic adoptive transfer of human TALL-104 killer cells into a dog with metastatic mammary adenocarcinoma resulted in 50% reduction of the largest lung metastasis and stabilization of the other lesions for 10 weeks, accompanied by the development of tumor-specific immune responses.[97] A phase I trial with TALL-104 cells in patients with metastatic breast carcinoma has recently been completed.

At present, adoptive therapy with NK cells has been largely abandoned. However, it is likely that variations of this form of therapy will be explored again, given that adoptively transferred T cells can not kill MHC class I negative tumors and T-cell therapy will likely select for tumor cell loss variants of this phenotype. Furthermore, it has only recently been appreciated that NK cells express activating and inhibitory receptors (KIR). In addition, the same NK cell can express KIR and activating receptors. Because of the expression of KIR for certain MHC class I allotypes, a person's NK cells will not recognize, and will therefore kill, cells from individuals lacking their own KIR epitopes. Known ligands for some of the NK receptors include HLA-C for KIR and HLA-E for CD94-NKG2C. Once the complexity of the NK system is better understood, it is likely that clinical trials using combinations of tumor-specific T cells and NK cells will be explored.

Adoptive T-Cell Therapy

The principles of adoptive immunotherapy established in animal models have formed the basis for the testing of therapeutic strategies for human tumors. The primary attraction for the use of T cells for adoptive therapy is their ability to specifically target tumor cells that express small peptides, even if the intact target protein itself is not expressed on the cell surface. A second attraction is the potentially long clonal life span of T cells. Finally, unlike NK and LAK cells, adoptively transferred human T cells have been shown to traffic to tumor.[86]

Autologous T-Cell Therapy

In mice, nearly all successful immunotherapies have required the use of large numbers of T cells derived from multiple immunized syngeneic animals. In humans, it is not possible to use this approach, and therefore, a central issue for the development of clinical adoptive immunotherapy strategies has been the development of culture systems to produce adequate numbers of effector T cells. Two basic approaches are being tested (Fig. 32-1). In one case, polyclonal *ex vivo* activation of the T cells is done. This approach is based on the assumptions that tumor-specific T cells are present in the patient but that they have not been primed in the patient, that the *in vivo* function of the cells in the patient is impaired, or both. The cells are activated polyclonally by various means *in vitro* and are then reinfused to the patient in the hope that they will respond directly to tumor or to tumor Ag presented by APC in the patient. The second approach is to isolate and activate Ag-specific T cells *in vitro* and then to clonally expand Ag-specific cells *in vitro* by various approaches.

As to the first approach, one of the first human trials of activated autologous polyclonal T-cell transfers was done by Mazumder and colleagues at the National Cancer Institute.[98] They and others had shown that the *in vitro* activation of T cells from cancer patients with the lectin

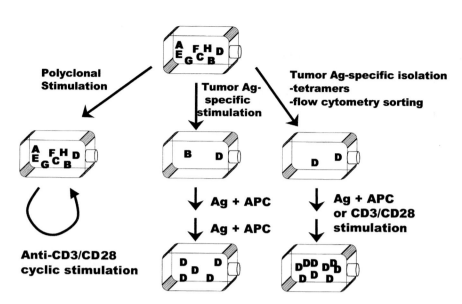

FIGURE 32-1. General approaches for *ex vivo* T-cell expansion. The initial T cells are obtained from peripheral blood, tumor infiltrating lymphocyte, or draining lymph nodes. The starting T-cell repertoire can be expanded by polyclonal stimulation via CD3 and CD28 stimulation or other methods to generate cells with enhanced effector function, or to maintain the T-cell receptor repertoire of the initial population (*left*). Antigen-specific (Ag-specific) cytotoxic T lymphocytes can be generated without prior selection, or enrichment can be done by repeated stimulation with Ag-pulsed Ag-presenting cells (APC) or tumor cells. This process usually requires several rounds of stimulation (*middle*). Selection of cytotoxic T lymphocyte via tetramers can improve the efficiency of Ag-specific T-cell generation, and several methods, such as cyclic anti-CD3 and -CD28 stimulation, can be used for *ex vivo* expansion of these Ag-specific cells (*right*). At least 27 cell divisions are required from a single precursor T cell to generate one billion clonal T cells.

phytohemagglutinin generated cells that were lytic for fresh autologous tumor. In a phase I clinical protocol, ten patients with late-stage cancers were given repeated infusions of up to 10^{11} autologous T cells after *in vitro* culture in phytohemagglutinin for 2 days. Ten patients were treated, and the toxicity encountered included fever and chills in ten of ten patients, headaches in five of ten, and nausea and vomiting in three of ten. No tumor regressions were seen.

Investigators have used mouse tumor models to show that antibodies that bind to the CD3 complex can mimic Ag, and even though all T cells are activated *ex vivo* nonspecifically, it has been demonstrated that subsequent specific antitumor responses can be enhanced. For example, tumor-specific T cells from the spleens of mice immunized with the FBL-3 leukemic cell line could be expanded in number *in vitro* by culture with anti-CD3 and IL-2.[30] In a related approach, Osband and colleagues developed a technique termed *autolymphocyte therapy* for activating human T cells *ex vivo*. PBMCs are activated *ex vivo* for 5 days by low doses of the mitogenic monoclonal antibody OKT3 in conditioned medium, a mixture of previously prepared culture supernatant that contains autologous cytokines in the presence of cimetidine and indomethacin.[99]

In a phase I trial in patients with advanced cancer, Curti and co-workers tested autologous adoptive transfers of T cells activated with anti-CD3 *ex vivo* for 4 days.[100] They showed that the anti-CD3–activated CD4+ T cells could traffic to tumor sites *in vivo* and mediate antitumor effects. Of four lymphoma patients in this study, three had tumor regressions, one of which was a complete response. Patients in this trial were given IL-2 infusions after the T-cell infusion, so that it is not possible to attribute the clinical responses solely to the adoptively transferred T cells.

Repeated *ex vivo* stimulation with anti-CD3 may cause cell death *in vitro* and preferential expansion of CD8+ T cells.[101] Based on a related approach that anti-CD3 and CD28 can more efficiently activate T cells *ex vivo*[32,33] and that tumor-draining lymph node cells cultured with anti-CD3 and anti-CD28 can mediate antitumor effects in mice,[102] we are currently carrying out a phase I trial using the adoptive transfer of anti-CD3– and anti-CD28–activated autologous T cells after high-dose therapy and stem-cell transplantation in patients with refractory lymphoma.

In the second general approach, which is to specifically activate and expand tumor-specific T cells *ex vivo*, infusions of TIL have been tested most extensively. This approach is based on the hypothesis that tumor-specific T cells will be preferentially present in the resected tumor specimens.[103] TIL reactivity to tumor is enhanced compared to deselected peripheral blood T cells, and the antitumor response is generally MHC class I restricted. Furthermore, the TIL are relatively more specific to the tumor of origin. TIL are generated by *in vitro* culture of dissociated tumor cell preparations in the presence of high concentrations of IL-2. In mice, TIL are 50- to 100-fold more potent than NK cells in several tumor models.[104] TIL have proven to be useful for the identification of tumor Ags.[105] The failure to consistently generate TIL from tumor specimens has limited widespread clinical application of the approach.[106] Furthermore, clinical studies with TIL have shown poor engraftment efficiencies in patients.[86] Gene-marked TIL have been infused in patients with melanoma and renal cell carcinoma, and selective trafficking of the TIL to the tumor site could not be demonstrated.[107,108] It is likely that the poor clinical results obtained with TIL to date are in part due to the prolonged 4 to 6 week *in vitro* culture time that leads to replicative senescence and loss of homing abilities in the

TIL. It is also possible that TIL trials have been disappointing because the populations of TIL cells infused also contain regulatory T cells that inhibit the antitumor response.[14,109] Finally, it is possible that the TIL populations that were tested have only contained populations' effector cells, and that the response is limited by a lack of tumor-specific T-helper and memory cells.[110]

Shu and Chang have developed an approach that should circumvent many of the limitations posed by TIL therapy. They and others have shown in mice that tumor-draining lymph nodes harbor T cells that are not capable of mediating tumor rejection in adoptive transfer experiments. In contrast, if the draining lymph node cells are activated *in vitro* with anti-CD3 and IL-2, the cells are now capable of mediating tumor rejection after adoptive transfer.[8] They have shown that for mouse T cells, optimal generation of effector T cells occurs when anti-CD3 is added to the culture for the first 2 days and IL-2 is added subsequently on days 3 to 5 of culture.[111] In further studies, T cells were isolated from vaccine-primed lymph nodes obtained from patients with melanoma, renal cell, and head and neck cancer. In the absence of APCs, activation with anti-CD3 and anti-CD28 greatly enhanced subsequent T-cell expansion in IL-2 (greater than 100-fold), compared to anti-CD3 alone.[112] Thus, these results define conditions whereby tumor-draining lymph node cells could be stimulated in the absence of tumor Ag to develop into specific therapeutic effector cells during an abbreviated period of cell culture. Based on these preclinical studies, Chang and co-workers carried out a phase I trial in patients with late-stage melanoma and renal cell carcinoma.[113] Patients were given intradermal vaccination with irradiated autologous tumor cells and bacillus Calmette-Guérin as an adjuvant. The draining lymph nodes were harvested 7 to 10 days later and the vaccine-primed T cells cultured with anti-CD3 and IL-2. A mean of 8.4×10^{10} cells were administered per patient. The activated lymph node T cells were administered intravenously with the concomitant administration of IL-2. In most cultures, there was a specific release of granulocyte-macrophage colony-stimulating factor (GM-CSF) and interferon-gamma (IFN-γ) after stimulation with autologous, but not allogeneic, tumor. Among the 11 melanoma patients, one had a partial tumor response, and there were two complete and two partial responses among the 12 patients with renal cell carcinoma. Thus, there may be some clinical activity with this approach in patients with metastatic renal cell carcinoma. One potential limitation of this approach is that the infused T cells will be immunogenic with this particular culture process, as they will contain the murine anti-CD3 OKT3 antibody that is bound to the T cells.

Other T-cell culture techniques have been developed to selectively activate or clonally expand, or do both to, tumor-specific T cells with the goal of retaining *in vivo* antitumor reactivity, trafficking, and engraftment potential.

The identification of tumor Ags has permitted the expansion of Ag-specific CTL, which can specifically lyse tumor cells. Theoretically, oligoclonal T-cell lines are preferred to CTL clones for treatment, because a more broadly directed response is likely to minimize the emergence of escape mutants to one epitope. They are also less costly to develop. However, CTL clones are a powerful tool to identify the precise sequence of tumor or viral epitopes, and by virtue of their specificity are the least likely cell preparations to trigger adverse effects, such as autoimmunity. Initial studies have used DCs or other APCs loaded with Ag to activate and expand T-cell clones or lines. The limited general availability of autologous tumor cells to serve as a source of Ag for repeated *in vitro* stimulation of T cells is a practical limitation for clinical therapy. This approach is also not desirable because many tumor cells secrete immunosuppressive cytokines, such as TGF-β or IL-10. When tumor cells themselves are used as APC, only MHC class I–reactive T cells are usually obtained. Obtaining sufficient autologous DC for repeated pulsing of the T cells is also a practical limitation. However, it appears that this limitation will soon be circumvented with the advent of flt3 ligand-mediated DC mobilization protocols. APC should be autologous or MHC-matched for propagation of tumor-specific T cells. The most widely used method for the generation of CTL *in vitro* is to pulse DC with tumor-specific peptides that are presented by the appropriate MHC-restricting allele. It is critical that the correct concentration of peptide be used to pulse the DC. Berzofsky and colleagues showed that if high peptide concentrations are used *in vitro*, only low-avidity T cells are propagated, because the high-avidity T cells die by apoptosis,[114] suggesting that a submaximal concentration of peptides may be required for *in vitro* induction of tumor-reactive CTLs. Furthermore, CTLs generated with peptide-pulsed APCs are often peptide reactive but not reactive with tumors that express the gene of interest, due to low-level expression or impaired Ag processing by the tumor cells. To circumvent this, Greenberg and colleagues have used recombinant vaccinia virus encoding the tyrosinase gene to infect autologous APC and have generated tyrosinase-specific and melanoma-reactive CTL cells from the peripheral blood of five out of eight patients with melanoma.[115] Tyrosinase-specific CD4+ T-cell clones were isolated from six of the eight patients by stimulation with autologous APCs infected with recombinant vaccinia virus, and all of these clones were capable of recognizing autologous tumor cells.

An obstacle to adoptive T-cell therapy with Ag-specific T cells is that each T-cell culture is patient and tumor specific. Thus, if universal tumor Ags could be identified that are presented by most MHC types, a more widely applicable form of cellular therapy could be developed. Recent studies indicate that the catalytic subunit of telomerase (hTERT) may be such a candidate.[116] In cancer patients, CD8+ CTL specific for hTERT peptide could be elicited, and the CTL lysed tumors expressing hTERT in an MHC HLA-A2–restricted manner. More than 85% of human cancers exhibit strong telomerase activity, but normal adult tissues, with few exceptions, do not. They found that endogenous hTERT was naturally processed, presented in the context of HLA-A2, and served as a target for Ag-specific CTL in a variety of primary tumors. These findings suggest that hTERT is a potentially widely applicable target for anticancer immunotherapeutic strategies; however, it remains to be determined whether the approach is safe. For example, given that bone marrow progenitor cells express hTERT, aplastic anemia from autoimmune attack would be a potential toxicity. Furthermore, the feasibility of reproducibly obtaining sufficient numbers of hTERT-reactive CTLs remains to be demonstrated.

Several approaches are being developed to circumvent the need for repeated addition of feeder cells and autologous APC to the cultures. A current obstacle to the routine generation of CTL derives from the inability to simply and rapidly isolate or expand large numbers of highly efficient APCs for repetitive stimulations of Ag-specific T cells *in vitro*, or both. To address the limited replicative potential of DC precursor cells, Schultze has shown that autologous CD40-activated B cells represent a readily available source of APC. They have shown that peripheral blood B cells can be activated and rapidly expanded *in vitro* on feeder cells that are transfected to express CD40. The resulting activated B cells may circumvent the need for DC by providing a source of efficient APCs with which to generate Ag-specific T cells *ex vivo* for autologous adoptive immunotherapy.[41]

Others have made artificial APC, either by coating beads with peptide:MHC "tetramer" complexes, or by transfecting MHC-negative cells with MHC molecules and co-stimulatory molecules. Magnetic beads have been coated with MHC class I molecules loaded with specific peptide, and the beads were used as a substrate for T-cell capture. Low-frequency T cells, as well as T cells that display TCRs with low affinity for the Ag, were captured on the beads. After isolation and expansion, the recovered cells specifically killed target cells *in vitro* and displayed antiviral therapeutic effects *in vivo* in a rodent model.[40] Others have used nonmagnetic microspheres coated with complexes of recombinant MHC molecules to successfully generate CTLs *ex vivo* from naïve precursor cells.[38] Peptide-MHC tetramers specific for the melanoma proteins MART-1 (melanoma Ag recognized by T cell–1) and gp100 have been used to isolate high-avidity tumor-reactive CD8[+] T cells from a heterogeneous population by flow cytometry. The tetramer reactive cells could be cloned, and they retained their functional activity on reexpansion.[117,118] Sadelain and colleagues engineered APC that could be used to stimulate T cells of any patient with a given HLA type.[42] Mouse fibroblasts were retrovirally transduced with a single HLA class I molecular complex, along with the human accessory molecules CD80 (B7.1), CD54 [intercellular

adhesion molecule-1 (ICAM-1)], and CD58 [leukocyte factor Ag-3 (LFA-3)]. These artificial APCs consistently elicited and expanded CTLs specific for the melanoma tumor Ags gp100 and MART-1.

Due to the recent technical advances that permit the generation of tumor-specific CTL, their clinical use has not yet been extensively evaluated. In one study, CTLs were induced *in vitro* by repeated stimulation with inactivated autologous tumor cells and the CTL lines were administered intravenously to 11 patients with advanced cancers once every 2 weeks for 10 weeks. The cell infusions were not toxic, and tumor reduction or decreased tumor markers were observed in four patients.[119] In another recent study, autologous CTLs were generated against primary-cultured malignant gliomas from PBMCs *in vitro* in four patients.[120] The CTLs specifically recognized the corresponding autologous glioma *in vitro*. The CTLs were injected 3 times into the primary tumor–resected cavity via an Ommaya tube, and reduction of the tumor volume was observed in three of the four patients. These results suggest that adoptive immunotherapy with autologous CTL may be a promising approach for malignant gliomas; however, further testing will be required to establish whether there is clinical benefit.

Virally Induced Lymphomas

Virally induced lymphomas that retain some expression of the inciting viral genome are likely to present a good target for adoptive cellular therapy. Unlike most spontaneous tumors, the repertoire of T-cell receptors contains T cells with high-affinity receptors for the viral protein, as a consequence of a lack of deletion of these T cells in the thymus. In patients recovering from allogeneic bone marrow transplantation, a severe defect in the cellular immune system exists, and this often results in the death of the patients from reactivation of systemic CMV or EBV infection. Donor-derived, CMV Ag-specific CD8[+] CTLs have been administered to the patients, and an extremely promising restoration of immune function noted.[121,122] EBV often reactivates after bone marrow or organ transplantation, resulting in aggressive lymphoma. Infusions of allogeneic peripheral blood T cells have proved effective, as well as infusions of EBV-specific T-cell lines. The latter approach has the benefit of reduced risk of inducing or exacerbating graft-versus-host disease (GVHD), because the T cells with allospecificity are eliminated or greatly reduced before infusion. *In vitro* cultured T-cell lines or clones that recognize viral Ags can be effective in suppressing EBV-associated lymphoproliferative disorders. Recent studies indicate that even relatively modest doses of T cells (1×10^6 cells per kg) are an effective treatment or prophylaxis for EBV-associated lymphoma, with complete remissions recorded in most patients.[82,123] Pneumonitis and tumor swelling with respiratory obstruction have been reported as adverse events after CTL infusion for lymphoma.[123]

A single patient with an aggressive EBV-associated lymphoma treated with adoptive immunotherapy using autologous LAK cells was recently reported.[124] The patient had leukapheresis, and autologous PBMCs were cultured in IL-2 for 10 days, and the IL-2–activated LAK cells were returned to the patient in the absence of systemic IL-2 therapy. The patient experienced a complete response.

Donor Lymphocyte Infusions and Allogeneic T-Cell Therapy

The first form of human adoptive T-cell therapy was given "inadvertently" as passenger T cells contained in stem cell infusions from bone marrow harvests. The bone marrow infusions were given to patients receiving allogeneic marrow grafts using myeloablative regimens as therapy for leukemia. At the time, the T cells were regarded as "contaminants" of the stem cell grafts. Weiden and co-workers performed a retrospective analysis of a series of patients treated with total-body irradiation and high-dose cyclophosphamide,[125] and, to their surprise, they discovered that the probability of tumor recurrence was significantly lower in patients receiving allografts than in those who had syngeneic (twin) grafts. Later studies showed that the probability of tumor recurrence was inversely related to the occurrence of GVHD. Resting donor peripheral blood T cells are now given routinely to patients with CML who relapse after a marrow allograft, and this procedure results in the induction of molecular complete remissions in a high proportion of cases.[126–129] This form of therapy is now termed *donor lymphocyte infusion* (DLI).

The mechanisms of DLI-mediated antitumor effects are not yet well understood. It is likely that T cells, DCs, or both, are involved and that the antigenic targets are minor histocompatibility Ags or leukemia-specific Ags. It is noteworthy that the kinetics of the clinical response are delayed, as the time to clinical response after DLI takes weeks to months, and often 6 to 8 months are required for maximal antileukemic effects; these kinetics are typical of an acquired immune response that is mediated by T cells. Recently, Falkenburg and co-workers have used T-cell leukemia-reactive CTL lines generated from a patient's HLA-identical donor to induce a complete remission in a patient with CML.[130] The CTL did not react with normal lymphocytes from the donor or recipient and did not affect donor hematopoietic progenitor cells. The CTL lines were infused at 5-week intervals at a cumulative dose of 3.2×10^9 CTL, and after the third infusion, a complete eradication of the leukemic cells was observed. The interpretation of the clinical benefit in this experiment is difficult because the patient had been given previous DLI, which was terminated due to failure to induce a response and the onset of GVHD. If the observed clinical response that was eventually observed was in fact due to the infused CTL, then it is likely that the CTL engrafted and proliferated *in vitro*. This

is due to the fact that the initial effector to target ratio was only approximately 1 in 1,000 *in vivo* immediately after the CTL infusion, given the patient's estimated leukemic burden of 1 to 3×10^{12} cells.

One critical issue with DLI is that it often results in the induction of chronic GVHD. Under some experimental conditions in transgenic mice, high-avidity T cells reactive for tumor Ags and self-Ags are deleted, and the remaining low-avidity T cells appear to be sufficient to provide protection against subsequent tumor challenge, but do not suffice to provoke autoimmunity.[131] This may explain why clinically evident GVHD doesn't appear necessary for clinically evident antitumor effects. However, clinical trials currently under way are evaluating whether depletion of CD8+ T cells from the adoptively transferred cell population might reduce GVHD while retaining the antileukemic effects.[132,133] Given the early results of these trials, it is likely that CD8+ T lymphocytes are important as effectors of GVHD but may not be essential for the DLI-mediated antitumor effect. Another limitation of DLI is that, although it is effective for CML, it is much less effective for other forms of leukemia, and it is not yet known whether it will have a role for solid tumors. It is possible that CML is especially susceptible to the effects of DLI, because the tumor clone can undergo differentiation to generate MHC class II positive APC *in vivo*, and, consistent with this notion, it is possible to generate DCs from CML cells *in vitro*. Thus, it is possible that the improvement of Ag presentation *in vivo* for other tumors will enhance their susceptibility to DLI, and, similarly, it is possible that the T cells in DLI might be rendered more effective through *in vitro* activation before infusion.

It is possible that the antitumor effects of donor leukocytes can be used for therapeutic benefit outside the setting of allogeneic transplantation. Xenogeneic and allogeneic adoptive T-cell therapy has the obvious advantage that the *in vivo* antitumor effect is not dependent on the condition that all tumor cells express tumor-specific Ags, because alloantigens or minor histocompatibility Ags can serve as targets. Furthermore, the donor repertoire has not been contracted by previous chemotherapy, and therefore it is more likely to contain naïve T cells reactive with tumor Ags. Xenogeneic adoptive lymphocyte transfers have been done in humans by Symes and co-workers.[134] Pigs were immunized with transitional cell carcinoma fragments, and later, the draining porcine lymph node cells were harvested and injected into patients with bladder carcinoma. Two of seven patients had objective responses, and no significant toxicity was observed, in part because of the rapid rejection of the porcine allograft that likely occurred.

Allogeneic MHC mismatched human lymphocytes have also been transferred to patients in a variety of settings without the myeloablative or immunosuppressive conditioning required to permit engraftment. As can be seen in Figure 32-2, the general design of some of these

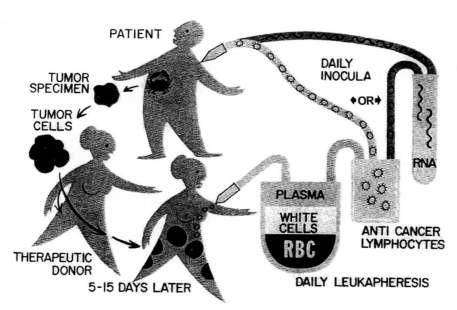

FIGURE 32-2. An approach used by Nadler and Moore in the 1960s. Major histocompatibility complex–unrelated patients with cancer were immunized with viable tumors by subcutaneous injection. The allogeneic donor was then subjected to leukapheresis, and the buffy coat given as a form of donor leukocyte infusion to another cancer-bearing patient. This approach is not endorsed by the author or by the editors, and this experiment is illustrated simply to indicate the general similarity to currently ongoing clinical trials. (RBC, red blood cells.) (Adapted from Nadler SH, Moore GE. Immunotherapy of malignant disease. *Arch Surg* 1969;99:376–381.)

early trials was remarkably similar to current approaches. In spite of the limitations of these early trials due to the failure to obtain engraftment of the adoptively transferred cells, objective tumor regressions were observed when patients were given infusions of allogeneic MHC-mismatched lymphocytes from donors immunized with the recipient's tumor.[135,136] However, in the absence of MHC matching, it is unlikely that allogeneic or xenogeneic T cells can mediate tumor-specific responses, and it is possible that the responses observed in these early trials were due to NK cells.

Terasaki and co-workers performed the first adoptive transfers of HLA-matched allogeneic lymphocytes and observed objective responses in two of six patients with advanced cancers.[137] Haploidentical lymphocytes have been given in conjunction with cyclophosphamide to a small group of patients with various tumors as primary therapy without inducing GVHD.[138] Six patients received infusions of lymphocytes after alloactivation and expansion *in vitro*, and this resulted in a complete response in one patient with lymphoma. More recently, Porter and colleagues gave MHC-matched allogeneic DLI to patients without myeloablative or immunosuppressive conditioning.[139] Donor cells were detected in the blood of 4 of 13 assessable patients 4 weeks after DLI, and 4 of 16 evaluable patients had evidence of GVHD. A history of prior autologous transplantation was associated with late chimerism, as all four patients who had long-term chimerism were treated with primary adoptive immunotherapy for relapsed disease after autologous transplantation. Four of the 18 patients in the trial had objective responses. Slavin and co-workers have obtained similar results in patients with breast cancer given allogeneic lymphocyte infusions after autologous stem cell transplants.[140] The main limitations of these approaches are the generally short-term engraftment, the suboptimal response rate, and the unpredictable onset of GVHD in a subset of patients.

For the full antitumor potential of allogeneic T cells to be realized, it is necessary to achieve long-term donor engraftment. Previously, this was only possible in young patients who could survive the rigorous myeloablative protocols. This fact largely precluded the use of allografting for patients older than 55 years or for younger patients with certain preexisting organ damage. A major step to decrease the rigors of allogeneic stem cell transplants has occurred with the development of nonmyeloablative stem cell transplantation (NMSCT), a procedure in which the preparative regimen is designed only to provide sufficient immunosuppression to achieve engraftment of an allogeneic stem cell graft.[141,142] The nonmyeloablative regimen does not by itself completely eliminate residual host hematopoietic cells, but rather, the allogeneic T cells over the period of weeks to months may either maintain partial hematopoietic chimerism or eliminate all residual host elements and achieve full donor chimerism. Barrett and co-workers have studied the kinetics of engraftment in patients receiving NMSCT, consisting of an allogeneic peripheral blood stem cell transplant from an HLA-matched donor after a preparative regimen of cyclophosphamide and fludarabine.[143] Donor myeloid chimerism gradually supplanted recipient hematopoiesis, and the myeloid compartment became fully donor in all survivors by 200 days after transplantation. In contrast, T-cell engraftment was more rapid, with full chimerism occurring in some patients by day 30 and in other patients by day 200 after cyclosporine withdrawal and DLI. Ten of 14 patients surviving more than 30 days had delayed tumor regression, consistent with a T-cell–mediated tumor rejection.

An unanticipated benefit of NMSCT is that the incidence of acute GVHD is markedly decreased, permitting allogeneic marrow grafts to be done in much older patients. This is likely due to the absence of chemotherapy-induced mucositis that leads to the secretion of cytokines and generation of other danger signals, and the subsequent activation of allogeneic donor T cells. Another attractive feature of NMSCT is that adoptive cell transfers can be given to patients later, as additional immunotherapy months after the graft has been established, creating an ideal platform for adoptive immunotherapy with allogeneic T cells and DCs. Now that older patients can undergo allogeneic adoptive transfers, it will be possible for the first time to determine the efficacy of this approach in patients with the common solid tumors that occur in this age group. For example, it is possible that tumors that are conventionally regarded as poor immunotherapy targets may prove responsive to DLI infusions. Recently, Champlin and co-workers observed the regression of visceral tumor deposits in patients with breast cancer associated with the onset of GVHD, suggesting that that graft-versus-tumor effects may occur against breast cancer.[144] Furthermore, a durable complete response was recently observed in a patient with metastatic renal cell carcinoma after NMSCT.[145] Thus, it is likely that a resurgence of interest in allogeneic cell therapy will occur owing to the advent of NMSCT. NMSCT provides a platform to avoid acute GVHD and to circumvent the difficulties with autologous T-cell therapy in patients who have had previous repertoire contractions due to chemotherapy.

Antigen-Presenting Cells Therapy: Dendritic Cells and Macrophages

Ag-presenting cells initiate the cellular immune response. There are three major classes of bone marrow–derived APC: B cells, macrophages, and DC, and the latter two have been used extensively for various forms of adoptive cellular therapy and vaccine therapy for cancer. The adoptive transfer of autologous activated macrophages, being effector cells and APCs, represents a promising approach for cancer immunotherapy. Studies in many tumor models suggest that macrophages provide an important role in the outcome of tumor immunotherapy.[146] Resting macrophages do not mediate the antitumor effects; rather, activated macrophages are required.[147] Human macrophages can be differentiated from circulating mononuclear precursors present in the blood, and after IFN-γ activation, they acquire antineoplastic properties and adhere to transformed cells. Andreesen and co-workers reported a phase I trial to test the safety of autologous activated macrophages.[148] Autologous macrophages were generated *in vitro* from blood monocytes by culture in autologous serum and recombinant human IFN-γ. The activated macrophages were then harvested from the culture, isolated by elutriation, and reinfused into the patient by intravenous or intra-peritoneal routes. The adoptive transfers were well tolerated, and the disappearance of malignant ascites in two of seven patients was a possible indication of a therapeutic effect. In another phase I study of patients with progressive colorectal cancers, autologous activated macrophages were given after activation with IFN-γ. PBMCs were collected six times by weekly apheresis, cultured for 7 days, and the activated macrophages isolated by elutriation and given as adoptive cellular therapy by intravenous infusion. A mean total of 7.9×10^9 macrophages were given per patient. Clinical tolerance was good; however, no clinical responses were observed in the 14 evaluable patients.[149] Further clinical trials with adoptively transferred macrophages are ongoing[150]; however, most investigators have abandoned this approach in favor of DC-based approaches.

Unlike macrophages, DCs evolved relatively recently, and they probably arose to control T and B cells. DCs are the only APCs capable of efficiently activating a naïve T cell. Once a T cell has undergone initial activation, it has less stringent activation requirements and can be activated by other types of less potent APCs. The existence of several different DC subsets has only been recently appreciated, and it appears that these subsets may have distinct functional roles, such as polarizing the T-cell immune response toward type 1 or type 2 cytokine responses.[151] Subcutaneous injection of only a few million Ag-loaded DCs is sufficient to induce a potent response in humans to the naïve foreign protein Ag keyhole limpet hemocyanin.[152] To date, autologous and allogeneic DC infusions appear safe, but they can break tolerance to self-Ags and have resulted in the induction of vitiligo, leading to a potential concern for induction of other, more serious autoimmune disorders. It is only over the past few years that sufficient DCs have been available for clinical immunotherapy, and this has occurred due to the availability of DC growth factors, such as GM-CSF and flt3 ligand. Furthermore, it has been demonstrated that functional impairments of APC can be observed in cancer patients[153] and that products produced by human tumors can inhibit differentiation of DC.[154] Therefore, adoptive transfer of autologous or allogeneic DCs loaded with tumor Ags may represent a potentially effective method of inducing antitumor immunity in patients with cancer.

Human trials testing adoptive transfers of DC loaded with tumor Ags are ongoing at several institutions. Hsu, Benike, and co-workers conducted the first reported clinical trial of therapeutic vaccination of cancer patients with DC.[155] Patients with malignant B-cell lymphoma for whom conventional chemotherapy had failed were given intravenous infusions of immature autologous DC pulsed *ex vivo* with tumor-specific idiotypic Ag. T-cell–specific immune responses were induced in the patients after several infusions of the Ag-loaded DC, and two of the initial four patients had complete responses, including one molecular remission. In a second promising DC trial, Nestle and co-workers tested the safety and efficacy of autologous DC in patients with metastatic melanoma.[156] Autologous monocyte-derived DCs were pulsed with autologous tumor lysates or peptides, and the Ag-loaded DCs were injected (1×10^6 cells per injection) into uninvolved inguinal lymph nodes. Most patients had induction of tumor-specific immunity, and objective clinical responses were observed in five of 16 evaluable patients, including two durable complete remissions. The mechanism of the effect after the DC infusions remains unknown. It is likely that the DCs work by priming T cells and inducing a cellular immune response, and consistent with this notion is the observation that the patients have not developed humoral responses to the idiotypic protein in the lymphoma trial. Furthermore, given the unexpected clinical benefit to the cancer-bearing patient from the injection of only a few million Ag-loaded DCs, these results suggest the existence of a severe functional defect in endogenous DC surveillance and trafficking in some patients with late-stage cancers.

A major research effort is currently aimed at determining the optimal method to load DCs with Ag. Tumor-specific peptides, protein, mRNA, and apoptotic or necrotic cells have all been used. It is not yet known which methods are the most efficacious or clinically relevant. Approaches aimed at using peptides or cocktails of peptides will probably result in the induction of a potent, but narrowly directed, immune response that may be subject to tumor escape variants. More cumbersome approaches, such as transfecting the DC with whole-cell mRNA derived from the tumor, are promising for their clinical use and potential antigenic breadth of the immune response.[157] Another approach is to fuse tumor cells with DC, and a recent trial reported that injections of irradiated allogeneic DC fused with autologous tumor resulted in objective clinical responses in seven of 17 patients with metastatic renal cell carcinoma.[158] If the promising results with therapeutic vaccination using DC tumor cell heterokaryons are confirmed, it is likely that whole tumor cells or preparations derived from the cells will become the preferred way to load DC with Ag (Fig. 32-3). Approaches in which Ags derived from whole cellular fractions or in the form of mRNA are used to load DC as opposed to peptides carry the potential advantage to encode multiple epitopes for many HLA alleles, thus permitting induction of CTL responses among many cancer patients independent of their HLA repertoire.

The concept of therapeutic vaccination, also referred to as *active immunotherapy*, is based on the notion that the administration of tumor Ags in a highly immunogenic fashion will lead to the development of a therapeutically useful antitumor immunity in cancer patients. For several reasons, the recent ready availability of DC is leading to a blurring between active and passive immunotherapy. In a practical manner, DCs are prepared *ex vivo*, with similar techniques to those that were developed for adoptive T-cell therapy. Furthermore, DCs are not long-lived cells, and

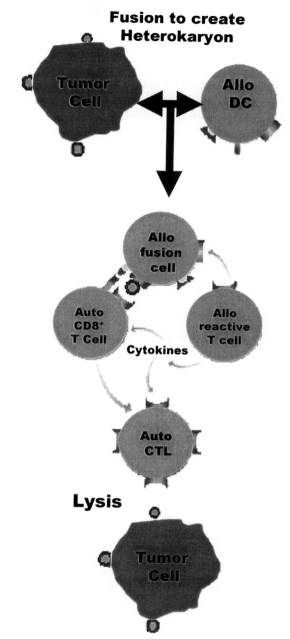

FIGURE 32-3. An approach used by Kugler and colleagues to develop a therapeutic vaccine for metastatic renal cell carcinoma.[158] Heterokaryons were created by electrofusion of autologous tumor cells and allogeneic dendritic cells (DCs) obtained from random blood donors. The DCs were injected intranodally to patients in whom the allo fusion cell may then display tumor antigens, as well as allogeneic major histocompatibility complex antigens. It is possible that the dominant major histocompatibility complex class II restricted allogeneic CD4 T-cell response in the host may function as helper cells to augment the generation of cytotoxic T lymphocytes (CTLs) that are tumor specific. (Adapted from Kufe DW. Smallpox, polio and now a cancer vaccine? *Nat Med* 2000;6:252–253.)

durable tumor memory can only be induced if the DCs elicit long-lived T memory cells. It is likely that the most effective antitumor immunotherapies will consist of combination strategies using passive and active immunity induced by the adoptive transfer of T cells and therapeutic vaccination with Ag-loaded DC.

RANDOMIZED CLINICAL TRIALS

A number of randomized controlled clinical trials testing efficacy of adoptively transferred cells have been reported (Table 32-2). The first tumors in humans treated with adoptive immunotherapy to be subjected to randomized controlled trials were melanoma and renal cell carcinoma. Renal cell carcinoma and melanoma are relatively highly immunogenic tumors that have proven resistant to standard cytotoxic chemotherapy but have shown reproducible responses to immune-based therapy. Infusions of NK cells, LAK cells isolated from peripheral blood, and polyclonal T-cell populations isolated from TILs and nonspecifically expanded *in vitro* with IL-2 suggested the therapeutic potential of tumor-reactive T cells in humans. However, the low response rates and the severe toxicity due to the high doses of IL-2 injected to maintain cell survival dampened the early enthusiasm. Indeed, randomized studies using this approach have not demonstrated efficacy of the adoptively transferred cell populations, as, to date, the responses observed can be attributed to cytokine-mediated antitumor effects alone. Similarly, positive effects in randomized trials

TABLE 32-2. RANDOMIZED CLINICAL TRIALS OF ADOPTIVE IMMUNOTHERAPY

Indication	Description	Reference
Metastatic renal cell cancer and melanoma	Patients were randomized to receive either systemic interleukin 2 (IL-2) alone or IL-2 plus adoptively transferred lymphokine-activated killer cells. Twenty-three patients with renal cell carcinoma and 20 with melanoma were entered into the protocol. There were no objective responses noted.	186
Metastatic renal cell cancer and melanoma	Patients were randomized to receive either systemic IL-2 alone or IL-2 plus adoptively transferred lymphokine-activated killer (LAK) cells. The results suggested a trend toward increased survival when IL-2 was given with LAK cells in patients with melanoma ($p = .09$), but no trend was observed for patients with renal cell cancer.	96
Metastatic renal cell cancer	Adoptive autologous polyclonal T-cell therapy after activation with anti-CD3 and conditioned medium. Ninety patients with metastatic renal cell carcinoma were randomized to receive monthly for 6 mo an infusion of autologous activated peripheral blood lymphocytes plus oral cimetidine or cimetidine alone. Positive results were reported, but later trials did not confirm the initial results.	159, 187
Advanced renal cell cancer	A randomized phase III trial compared continuous intravenous infusion IL-2 alone with IL-2 plus LAK cell adoptive transfers. Seventy-one patients were treated, 36 on the IL-2 arm and 35 on the IL-2 plus LAK arm. Four patients (6%) had major responses (two complete, two partial). The addition of LAK cells did not improve the response rate, as there were no differences between treatment arms with regard to response ($p = .61$) and survival ($p = .67$).	188
Advanced renal cell cancer	A randomized phase I trial was done to determine whether subcutaneous administration of IL-2 in combination with an autologous renal cell vaccine is feasible and can potentiate antitumor immunity. Seventeen patients with metastatic renal cell carcinoma underwent surgical resection with preparation of an autologous tumor cell vaccine. Patients were vaccinated intradermally twice with 10e7 irradiated tumor cells plus bacillus Calmette-Guérin, and once with 10e7 tumor cells alone. Patients were randomized to one of three groups: no adjuvant IL-2, low-dose IL-2, or high-dose IL-2. Four patients developed cellular immunity specific for autologous tumor cells as measured by delayed–type hypersensitivity responses. IL-2 did not have a major effect on the delayed–type hypersensitivity response. Prospective testing of response to recall antigens indicated that only 7 of 12 tested patients were anergic.	160
Metastatic renal cell cancer	A multicenter randomized trial to test the efficacy of tumor-infiltrating lymphocytes (TILs) in combination with low-dose IL-2 compared with IL-2 alone after radical nephrectomy in 178 patients with metastatic renal cell carcinoma was done. Intent-to-treat analysis demonstrated objective response rates of 9.9% vs. 11.4% and 1-year survival rates of 55% vs. 47% in the TIL–recombinant IL-2 (rIL-2) and rIL-2 control groups, respectively. Treatment with TILs did not improve response rate or survival in patients treated with low-dose rIL-2 after nephrectomy.	189
Hepatocellular carcinoma	Patients were treated with spleen-derived LAK cells cultured for 3 to 30 days in rIL-2. These autologous activated spleen cells were administered to patients 2 days after the intraarterial infusion of doxorubicin. Patients randomized to receive splenic LAK cells had a lower recurrence rate that did not reach statistical significance.	164
Non–small cell lung cancer (NSCLC)	A phase II randomized study tested the efficacy of TIL plus IL-2 infusions in 113 patients with stage II, IIIa, or IIIb NSCLC. Three-year survival was significantly better for patients given TIL therapy than for controls.	162
NSCLC	One hundred and seventy-four patients were randomized in a phase III trial to receive either combined immunotherapy consisting of IL-2 and LAK cells or control standard therapy consisting of no adjuvant therapy, radiotherapy, or chemotherapy. There were statistically improved survival rates in the immunotherapy group; however, it is difficult to interpret the results owing to changes in study design that occurred during the trial.	163, 190, 191

of patients with advanced renal cell carcinoma treated with anti-CD3–activated PBMCs cultured in conditioned medium were also reported[159]; however, a larger, multicenter phase III trial failed to confirm the earlier studies. Although further trials are ongoing, thus far, these approaches have not consistently shown benefit in comparison to standard immune-based treatment with biologic response modifiers—most important, high-dose bolus IL-2. In a randomized phase I trial by Fenton and colleagues at the National Cancer Institute,[160] more than half of the patients with advanced renal cell carcinoma entering the trial were found to be anergic to recall Ags, confirming other studies indicating that patients with late-stage tumors can be significantly immunosuppressed and that this may present a significant barrier to overcome if immunotherapy is to be successful. For reasons that remain unclear, some investigators have reported that metastatic ocular melanoma is much less responsive than cutaneous melanoma to adoptive cellular transfers.[161] It is likely that other approaches will be required to establish the usefulness of adoptive immunotherapy in melanoma and renal cell carcinoma, but its promise for these difficult diseases is already evident.

Randomized trials suggest that other tumors may also be responsive to immunotherapy. A single randomized trial of adoptive immunotherapy with TIL and IL-2 infusions indicated a survival advantage for patients with non–small cell lung carcinoma, particularly those with stage IIIB.[162] Similarly, in another randomized trial of patients with non–small cell lung carcinoma, LAK cell infusions and IL-2 therapy in combination with standard therapy were shown to be superior to standard therapy.[163] In both of these trials, it was not possible to discern whether the adoptively transferred cells contributed to the beneficial effects, due to the confounding effects of the concomitant IL-2 infusions. Finally, patients with hepatoma may have immunogenic tumors that are targets for adoptively transferred cells.[164] Together, although there are some intriguing clinical results, there are no published randomized controlled trials that have convincingly demonstrated clinical benefit from adoptively transferred cells. Currently, adoptive immunotherapy does not represent the standard of care for any disease, except for patients with CML, who relapse after an allogeneic marrow grafting procedure.

ADOPTIVE CELLULAR THERAPY: TOXICITY, DOSE, AND SCHEDULING ISSUES

Information on the dose and schedule dependence of adoptively transferred cells is widely scattered in the literature, and from this literature one concludes that there is no standardized dose system. The ideal dose of transferred cells is related to the tumor burden and the homing and persistence (memory) characteristics of the infused cells.[60] Doses of adoptively transferred cells are usually reported as the total number of viable cells administered, or as the total number of viable cells per kg body weight or per square meter body surface area. However, total lymphocyte numbers do not correlate well with body surface area, but rather display a stronger inverse correlation with age. Other variables add to the complexity, particularly the fact that, in the case of T cells or other adoptively transferred cells with high replicative potential, the infused dose may not relate well to the steady-state number of cells. Therefore, dose considerations are more complex than in other areas of transfusion medicine, in which, for example, the maximal level of transfused red cells or platelets occurs immediately after infusion. In our studies of adoptively transferred autologous CD4+ T cells, we often find that the highest number of cells in the host peaks 2 weeks after infusion of the cells. This is because the engraftment potential and the replicative potential of the infused cells depends on complex host variables, such as the number of niches available in the host for engraftment and the antigenic stimulus for clonal expansion or deletion. In most rodent tumor models, T-cell proliferation in the host after transfer is obligatory for therapeutic efficacy.[5]

Cytokines given to the host can also have major impact on the persistence of adoptively transferred T cells. Others have found that the persistence of adoptively transferred CD8+ T cells is enhanced by coadministration of IL-2[165]; however, we have found that when autologous human CD4+ T cells are also given, persistence is not increased by concomitant IL-2 therapy.[87] Finally, recent studies show that IL-2 can induce proliferation and maintain effector CD8+ T cells but may actually delete memory cells, whereas IL-15 and IL-7 appear to select for the persistence of memory CD8+ T cells.[20] Thus, it may be desirable to provide IL-2 at early times in immunotherapy, when tumor cytoreduction is the issue, but to remove IL-2 or provide IL-7 and IL-15 signaling later in therapy to promote antitumor memory.

Immunotherapy has often been advertised as a "non-toxic therapy" when compared to cytotoxic chemotherapy. However, it is instructive to recall that William Coley's first therapeutic vaccines were accompanied by life-threatening toxicity.[1,166] Furthermore, anyone who has experienced the fatigue and malaise accompanied by systemic viral infections, such as infectious mononucleosis, would not be surprised to learn that cellular therapies have many of the same toxicities. Thus, one would expect that, in the setting of therapeutic immunization to treat established malignancy, systemic toxicity will be an expected response, and prophylactic immunization strategies in cases with no or minimal residual disease would be accompanied by less toxicity.

Many types of adverse events have been reported after infusion of human autologous or allogeneic lymphocytes or DCs. The toxicities can be classified as (a) those due to extrinsic factors present in the culture process, (b) those due to accompanying cytokines that may be co-infused with the cells, and (c) those that are intrinsic to the cells themselves.

With regard to the first type of toxicity, with the earlier cell-manufacturing techniques, many cell products were cultured in sources of foreign proteins, such as fetal calf serum. In such cases, patients often developed febrile transfusion reactions that were sometimes severe and could include anaphylaxis. These reactions were usually encountered in cases of multiple cell infusions to the same patient, but instances have occurred in which patients were presensitized to bovine proteins, and the patients have had severe reactions even on the occasion of the first cellular infusion. Hepatitis A has been reported due to the contamination of the culture medium with infectious pooled human serum.[96] With the advent of the widespread use of serum-free culture medium, there has been a substantial reduction in the incidences of immediate-type allergic responses, febrile transfusion reactions, and infectious complications. Similarly, with the development of closed cell culturing and manufacturing processes, there has been a substantially decreased potential for microbial contamination.[167]

With regard to the second type of toxicity, many patients have been given infusions of IL-2 at the time of and after cellular adoptive transfer. IL-2 has a well-known dose- and schedule-dependent toxicity.[168] IL-2 given in high doses and by intravenous bolus injection induces multiorgan dysfunction due to a capillary leak syndrome that is directly mediated by local production of nitric oxide by cells of the monocyte-macrophage lineage. In contrast, low doses and subcutaneous injections of IL-2 induce an influenza-like syndrome, and this can be ameliorated by giving the IL-2 at night. Laboratory abnormalities induced at high and low doses of IL-2 include anemia, lymphopenia with rebound lymphocytosis, and eosinophilia.[169]

The spectrum of the third form of adverse effects intrinsic to the cellular therapy is still being defined and, for the moment, appears to be quite limited. Respiratory obstruction has been reported after CTL infusion for EBV-related lymphomas.[123] This is probably due to a T-cell–induced inflammatory response that results in tumor edema and necrosis. With regard to toxicity of T cells infused under conditions that lead to long-term engraftment, in more than 75 infusions of autologous activated CD4+ and CD8+ T cells given to patients with lymphoma or HIV infection in the absence of concomitant IL-2 infusions, we have observed a dose-dependent induction of fever and headaches in a substantial proportion of patients. These symptoms are self-limited, and they typically resolve within 36 hours after the infusion. The onset of the symptoms is delayed and does not occur immediately on infusion of the cells but several hours after the infusion. The etiology of the symptoms is likely related to secretion of cytokines by the infused cells. These symptoms are not due to allergy to the infused cells, because subsequent infusions of cells do not engender more severe adverse effects. Modest eosinophilia occurs in some patients, and this is likely related to an indirect effect consequent to secretion of IL-2 by the infused T cells. As was mentioned previously, eosinophilia occurs in patients treated with systemic IL-2.

Effector functions of infused T cells can be expected to include tissue damage similar to that encountered in T-cell–mediated autoimmune diseases. In the case of DLI, GVHD and marrow aplasia often occur.[126] Autoimmune thyroiditis with hypothyroidism has been reported to occur after LAK cell infusions and IL-2.[170] Many investigators at the Dana-Farber Cancer Institute have observed vitiligo in a substantial proportion of patients with melanoma after injections of autologous DCs loaded with melanocyte Ags. The passive transfer of antibodies with shared specificities between normal and malignant tissues can also induce autoimmune pathology.[171] Theoretic toxicities associated with T-cell transfer also include leukemia or lymphoma if transformation is induced consequent to the *in vitro* culture process. T-cell lymphomas have developed in nonhuman primates after transplantation with gene-modified stem cells.[172] The etiology of the lymphomas appears to be due to insertional mutagenesis from the presence of replication retrovirus that was generated from recombination from the viral vector that was used to transduce the stem cells. In human trials to date, no cases of malignant transformation of the infused T cells or APC have been reported.

Schedule-dependent efficacy and adverse effects from adoptively transferred cells have been reported. Many studies in rodent tumor models show that the administration of cytotoxic therapy can enhance the effects of adoptively transferred cells. Cyclophosphamide is the preferred drug, and the mechanism is not thought to be through tumor cytoreduction. The mechanism is likely due to multiple effects, including (a) killing of host-regulatory lymphocytes that suppress antitumor immune responses,[7,109] (b) creating "space" in the host so that the adoptively transferred cells can engraft,[60] and perhaps (c) enhanced cross priming of tumor Ags. Cyclophosphamide is generally given 1 or 2 days before the adoptively transferred T cells.[109] Curti and colleagues[100] have examined a related issue concerning the optimal time to harvest autologous CD4+ T cells in relation to the timing of cyclophosphamide administration in patients with advanced cancers. T cells were harvested at steady state, when on the decline or when on the recovery from the cyclophosphamide-induced leukopenia. From that study, they concluded that the best time to harvest autologous T cells was not at steady state, but rather just before the leukopenic nadir that occurred after administration of cyclophosphamide. The best *in vivo* expansion of the infused CD4+ T cells occurred when the cells had been harvested as patients entered the cyclophosphamide-induced nadir. Most of the clinical antitumor responses also occurred in patients treated on this schedule. These results are generally consistent with animal models that predicted a need to ablate immunosuppressive lymphocytes for efficient engraftment and subsequent *in vivo* expansion of adoptively transferred CD4$^+$ T cells. In a recent study of patients with stage III non–small cell lung cancer, investigators tested the sequence of adoptive therapy with autologous TIL and IL-2 followed by standard chemotherapy and radiotherapy and, perhaps not surprisingly, they found that the sequence of immunotherapy followed by chemotherapy is not effective.[173]

In patients with earlier-stage cancers who have not yet had cytotoxic chemotherapy, it is probably best to harvest autologous T cells before initiation of chemotherapy. This is because adults have limited regeneration of T cells from the thymus, and therefore, the repertoire remains contracted for long periods of time and, in many cases, never recovers.[174,175] Naïve T cells are most sensitive to the effects of cytotoxic chemotherapy, and their numbers are severely depleted in heavily pretreated patients. It is not yet known whether the antitumor-specific T cells are derived from primed or naïve T cells in the host, and this likely varies depending on the intrinsic immunogenicity of the tumor. Recent studies with tetramers that can identify tumor Ag–specific T cells show that, in some patients, chemotherapy can ablate the tumor-specific T cells that have an effector phenotype while sparing memory cells.[12] The mechanism for this observation is unknown, but the authors speculated that the effector cells were in the active phases of the cell cycle and were, therefore, rendered relatively susceptible to the cytotoxic effects of the chemotherapy. If these results are confirmed, then they would argue that patients should have their repertoire "archived" by apheresis before undergoing chemotherapy.

Anecdotal evidence suggests that immunotherapy may, in some circumstances, restore tumors to a chemotherapy-sensitive state. I am aware of several patients who had platinum-resistant ovarian cancer who were treated with adoptive cellular therapies or therapeutic vaccines. The patients had responses to the immunotherapy; however, they subsequently experienced disease progression. Interestingly, when chemotherapy was recommenced, they appeared to have tumor that was more sensitive to the drugs than when they had previously been treated. If true, this would suggest a need for further study of this interesting scheduling issue between cytotoxic chemotherapy and immunotherapy.

Finally, there are dose- and schedule-dependent effects that have been observed with DLI *vis à vis* the induction of GVHD. Early studies showed that the infusion of donor T cells soon after a myeloablative transplant conditioning regimen resulted in the marked augmentation of acute GVHD.[176] It has been well established by the work of Kernan and colleagues that the initial dose of infused T cells in the setting of allogeneic marrow transplantation has a major effect on the incidence and severity of acute GVHD.[177] As was discussed earlier, it has only been recently appreciated that donor T cells can be infused with relative freedom from acute GVHD in the setting of NMSCT.[141] Studies by Dazzi and colleagues show that, in

the steady-state setting of relapsed CML, infusions of resting T cells result in a decreased incidence of GVHD by starting with low doses of donor cells and escalating subsequent doses as required.[128] In a nonrandomized trial, they compared a bulk, single-infusion DLI (average, 1.5×10^8 CD3$^+$ cells per kg) to an escalating-dose regimen of DLI, in which increasing numbers of cells (average total 1.9×10^8 CD3$^+$ cells per kg) were given at 20-week average intervals between infusion. They found that antileukemic effects were preserved, but that the incidence of GVHD was much lower using the escalating dose regimen of DLI.

GENETICALLY MODIFIED CELLULAR THERAPY

Genetic modification of T cells and DC *ex vivo* to engineer an improved antitumor effect is an attractive strategy for many settings. Unlike hematopoietic stem cells, currently available vectors provide high-level expression of transgenes in T cells and DCs. The first use of genetically modified T cells was to demonstrate that adoptively transferred cells could persist in the host and traffic to tumor, albeit with low efficiency.[86] A principal limitation of immunotherapy for some tumors is that the tumors are poorly antigenic, in that no T cells are available that have high avidity for tumor-specific Ags, or that no T cells remain in the patient after chemotherapy that have the desired specificity. To address this problem, some clinical trials now in progress attempt to endow T cells with novel receptor constructs by introduction of "T bodies," chimeric receptors that have antibody-based external receptor structures and cytosolic domains that encode signal transduction modules of the TCR.[178] These constructs can function to retarget T cells *in vitro* in an MHC-unrestricted manner. The major issues with the approach currently involve improved receptor design and the immunogenicity of the T-body construct. T cells are also being transduced to express natural TCR alpha beta heterodimers of known specificity and avidity for tumor Ags[179]; however, this approach is of limited general value for humans, because each TCR will be specific for a given MHC allele, such that each vector would be patient specific.

A major limitation to adoptive transfer of CTLs is that they have short-term persistence in the host in the absence of Ag-specific T helper cells. Greenberg and co-workers have transduced human CTLs with chimeric GM-CSF–IL-2 receptors that deliver an IL-2 signal on binding GM-CSF. Stimulation of the CTLs with Ag-caused GM-CSF secretion and resulted in an autocrine growth loop such that the CTL clones proliferated in the absence of exogenous cytokines. This type of genetic modification has potential for increasing the circulating half-life and, by extension, the efficacy of *ex vivo*–expanded CTLs. To date, there is limited clinical experience with engineered T cells; however, in certain instances, they have been shown to persist after adoptive transfer in humans for years.[81,87]

As was noted above, severe and potentially lethal GVHD represents a frequent complication of allogeneic DLI. The promising results with DLI have created increased interest in developing T cells with an inducible suicide phenotype. Expression of herpes simplex virus thymidine kinase in T cells provides a means of ablating transduced T cells *in vivo* by the administration of acyclovir or ganciclovir.[180] Using this strategy, Bonini and colleagues infused donor lymphocytes into 12 patients who, after receiving allogeneic bone marrow transplants, had experienced complications such as cancer relapse or virus-induced lymphomas.[181] The lymphocytes survived for up to 1 year, and complete or partial tumor remissions in five of the eight patients were achieved. Tumor regressions coincided with onset of GVHD, and in most cases, the GVHD was abrogated when gancyclovir was given. Thus, GVHD associated with the therapeutic infusion of donor lymphocytes after allogeneic marrow transplantation could be efficiently controlled by these novel suicide gene strategies in allogeneic lymphocytes. However, subsequent studies that are still unpublished have indicated problems with this approach, in that the herpes simplex virus–thymidine kinase gene confers immunogenicity to the transfused cells, leading to impaired survival and the inability to re-treat a patient with DLI should the tumor recur. Future experiments will be required to develop vectors that are less immunogenic and able to confer even higher gancyclovir sensitivity to transduced human lymphocytes. Recently, investigators at Ariad have developed a suicide system comprised of a fusion protein with a fas signaling domain and a modified FKBP.[182] This system has the advantage that the fas-based suicide switch is expected to be nonimmunogenic. T cells expressing this modified chimeric protein are induced to undergo apoptosis when exposed to a drug that dimerizes the modified FKBP.[183,184] Finally, gene-modified DCs are currently in human clinical trials, and adoptive transfers of gene-modified DC remains promising.[185]

SUMMARY

The basis for tumor immunology is the premise that the immune system is capable of recognizing tumor cells and that the activated immune system can lead to the subsequent rejection of tumors. Although the former premise is now well accepted, the latter remains controversial. As we complete nearly 50 years of research into adoptive immunity for tumors, there are no forms of cellular therapy that have been approved by the U.S. Food and Drug Administration. Allogeneic DLI is being incorporated into the practice of medicine as a valuable and potentially curative indication for selected patients with CML. However, there are several obstacles that investigators must overcome before adoptive immunotherapy can become a more gener-

ally applicable and successful form of prophylaxis or treatment for human tumors. Concerns about the costs of cellular therapy should eventually be overcome if it achieves curative potential or long-lasting tumor immunity for patients with otherwise chemotherapy-refractory indications. Finally, it is likely that adoptive immunotherapy will not be used alone, but rather in combination with other forms of immunotherapy and chemotherapy.

REFERENCES

1. Coley WB. The treatment of malignant tumors by repeated inoculations of erysipelas: with a report of ten original cases. *Am J Med Sci* 1893;105:487–511.
2. Billingham RE, Brent L, Medawar PB. Quantitative studies on tissue transplantation immunity. II. The origin, strength and duration of actively and adoptively acquired immunity. *Proc R Soc* 1954;143:58–80.
3. Mitchison NA. Studies on the immunological response to foreign tumor transplants in the mouse. I. The role of lymph node cells in conferring immunity by adoptive transfer. *J Exp Med* 1955;102:157–177.
4. Cheever MA, Greenberg PD, Fefer A. Specific adoptive therapy of established leukemia with syngeneic lymphocytes sequentially immunized *in vivo* and *in vitro* and nonspecifically expanded by culture with Interleukin 2. *J Immunol* 1981;126:1318–1322.
5. Greenberg PD. Adoptive T cell therapy of tumors: mechanisms operative in the recognition and elimination of tumor cells. *Adv Immunol* 1991;49:281–355.
6. Cheever MA, Chen W. Therapy with cultured T cells: principles revisited. *Immunol Rev* 1997;157:177–194.
7. Melief CJ. Tumor eradication by adoptive transfer of cytotoxic T lymphocytes. *Adv Cancer Res* 1992;58:143–175.
8. Strome SE, Krauss JC, Chang AE, et al. Strategies of lymphocyte activation for the adoptive immunotherapy of metastatic cancer: a review. *J Hematother* 1993;2:63–73.
9. Rosenberg SA, Terry WD. Passive immunotherapy of cancer in animals and man. *Adv Cancer Res* 1997;25:323–388.
10. Burnet FM. The concept of immunological surveillance. *Prog Exp Tumor Res* 1970;13:1–27.
11. Rygaard J, Povlsen CO. The nude mouse vs. the hypothesis of immunological surveillance. *Transplant Rev* 1976;28:43–61.
12. Lee PP, Yee C, Savage PA, et al. Characterization of circulating T cells specific for tumor-associated antigens in melanoma patients. *Nat Med* 1999;5:677–685.
13. Marincola FM, Jaffee EM, Hicklin DJ, et al. Escape of human solid tumors from T-cell recognition: molecular mechanisms and functional significance. *Adv Immunol* 2000;74:181–273.
14. Dye ES, North RJ. T cell-mediated immunosuppression as an obstacle to adoptive immunotherapy of the P815 mastocytoma and its metastases. *J Exp Med* 1981;154:1033–1042.
15. Fisher MS, Kripke ML. Suppressor T lymphocytes control the development of primary skin cancers in ultraviolet-irradiated mice. *Science* 1982;216:1133–1134.

16. Shevach EM. Regulatory T cells in autoimmmunity. *Annu Rev Immunol* 2000;18:423–449.

17. Huang AY, Golumbek P, Ahmadzadeh M, et al. Role of bone marrow-derived cells in presenting MHC class I-restricted tumor antigens. *Science* 1994;264:961–965.

18. Staveley-O'Carroll K, Sotomayor E, Montgomery J, et al. Induction of antigen-specific T cell anergy: an early event in the course of tumor progression. *Proc Natl Acad Sci U S A* 1998;95:1178–1183.

19. Hwu P, Du MX, Lapointe R, et al. Indoleamine 2,3-dioxygenase production by human dendritic cells results in the inhibition of T cell proliferation. *J Immunol* 2000;164:3596–3599.

20. Ku CC, Murakami M, Sakamoto A, et al. Control of homeostasis of CD8+ memory T cells by opposing cytokines. *Science* 2000;288:675–678.

21. Klein G. Tumor antigens. *Annu Rev Microbiol* 1966;20:223–252.

22. Gilboa E. The makings of a tumor rejection antigen. *Immunity* 1999;11:263–270.

23. Lurquin C, Van Pel A, Mariame B, et al. Structure of the gene of tum-transplantation antigen P91A: the mutated exon encodes a peptide recognized with Ld by cytolytic T cells. *Cell* 1989;58:293–303.

24. Wang RF, Wang X, Atwood AC, et al. Cloning genes encoding MHC class II-restricted antigens: mutated CDC27 as a tumor antigen. *Science* 1999;284:1351–1354.

25. Banchereau J, Steinman RM. Dendritic cells and the control of immunity. *Nature* 1998;392:245–252.

26. Bretscher P, Cohn M. A theory of self-nonself discrimination. *Science* 1970;169:1042–1049.

27. Chen L, Ashe S, Brady WA, et al. Costimulation of antitumor immunity by the B7 counterreceptor for the T lymphocyte molecules CD28 and CTLA-4. *Cell* 1992;71:1093–1102.

28. June CH, Bluestone JA, Nadler LM, et al. The B7 and CD28 receptor families. *Immunol Today* 1994;15:321–331.

29. Lenschow DJ, Walunas TL, Bluestone JA. CD28/B7 system of T cell costimulation. *Ann Rev Immunol* 1996;14:233–258.

30. Crossland KD, Lee VK, Chen W, et al. T cells from tumor-immune mice nonspecifically expanded *in vitro* with anti-CD3 plus IL-2 retain specific function *in vitro* and can eradicate disseminated leukemia *in vivo*. *J Immunol* 1991;146:4414–4420.

31. Katsanis E, Xu Z, Anderson PM, et al. Short-term *ex vivo* activation of splenocytes with anti-CD3 plus IL-2 and infusion post-BMT into mice results in *in vivo* expansion of effector cells with potent antilymphoma activity. *Bone Marrow Transplant* 1994;14:563–572.

32. Levine BL, Bernstein W, Craighead N, et al. Effects of CD28 costimulation on long term proliferation of CD4+ T cells in the absence of exogenous feeder cells. *J Immunol* 1997;159:5921–5930.

33. Levine BL, Mosca J, Riley JL, et al. Antiviral effect and *ex vivo* CD4+ T cell proliferation in HIV-positive patients as a result of CD28 costimulation. *Science* 1996;272:1939–1943.

34. Levine BL, Cotte J, Small CC, et al. Large scale production of CD4+ T cells from HIV-infected donors following CD3/CD28 stimulation. *J Hematother* 1998;7:437–448.

35. Garlie NK, LeFever AV, Siebenlist RE, et al. T cells coactivated with immobilized anti-CD3 and anti-CD28 as potential immunotherapy for cancer. *J Immunother* 1998;22:336–345.

36. Rogers J, Mescher MF. Augmentation of *in vivo* cytotoxic T lymphocyte activity and reduction of tumor growth by large multivalent immunogen. *J Immunol* 1992;149:269–276.

37. Altmann DM, Hogg N, Trowsdale J, et al. Cotransfection of ICAM-1 and HLA-DR reconstitutes human antigen-presenting cell function in mouse L cells. *Nature* 1989;338:512–514.

38. Lone YC, Motta I, Mottez E, et al. *In vitro* induction of specific cytotoxic T lymphocytes using recombinant single-chain MHC class I/peptide complexes. *J Immunother* 1998;21:283–294.

39. Valmori D, Pittet MJ, Rimoldi D, et al. An antigen-targeted approach to adoptive transfer therapy of cancer. *Cancer Res* 1999;59:2167–2173.

40. Luxembourg AT, Borrow P, Teyton L, et al. Biomagnetic isolation of antigen-specific CD8+ T cells usable in immunotherapy. *Nat Biotechnol* 1998;16:281–285.

41. Schultze JL, Michalak S, Seamon MJ, et al. CD40-activated human B cells: an alternative source of highly efficient antigen presenting cells to generate autologous antigen-specific T cells for adoptive immunotherapy. *J Clin Invest* 1997;100:2757–2765.

42. Latouche JB, Sadelain M. Induction of human cytotoxic T lymphocytes by artificial antigen-presenting cells. *Nat Biotechnol* 2000;18:405–409.

43. Nanda NK, Sercarz EE. Induction of anti-self-immunity to cure cancer. *Cell* 1995;82:13–17.

44. Pardoll DM. Inducing autoimmune disease to treat cancer. *Proc Natl Acad Sci U S A* 1999;96:5340–5342.

45. Lanzavecchia A. How can cryptic epitopes trigger autoimmunity? *J Exp Med* 1995;181:1945–1948.

46. Brichard V, Van Pel A, Wolfel T, et al. The tyrosinase gene codes for an antigen recognized by autologous cytolytic T lymphocytes on HLA-A2 melanomas. *J Exp Med* 1993;178:489–495.

47. Rosenberg SA, White DE. Vitiligo in patients with melanoma: normal tissue antigens can be targets for cancer immunotherapy. *J Immunother Emphasis Tumor Immunol* 1996;19:81–84.

48. Hurwitz AA, Yu TF, Leach DR, et al. CTLA-4 blockade synergizes with tumor-derived granulocyte-macrophage colony-stimulating factor for treatment of an experimental mammary carcinoma. *Proc Natl Acad Sci U S A* 1998;95:10067–10071.

49. Chappell DB, Restifo NP. T cell-tumor cell: a fatal interaction? *Cancer Immunol Immunother* 1998;47:65–71.

50. Nishimura H, Nose M, Hiai H, et al. Development of lupus-like autoimmune diseases by disruption of the PD-1 gene encoding an ITIM motif-carrying immunoreceptor. *Immunity* 1999;11:141–151.

51. Sakai K, Mitchell DJ, Tsukamoto T, et al. Isolation of a complementary DNA clone encoding an autoantigen recognized by an antineuronal cell antibody from a patient with paraneoplastic cerebellar degeneration. *Ann Neurol* 1990;28:692–698.

52. Corradi JP, Yang C, Darnell JC, et al. A post-transcriptional regulatory mechanism restricts expression of the paraneo-

plastic cerebellar degeneration antigen cdr2 to immune privileged tissues. *J Neurosci* 1997;17:1406–1415.

53. Albert ML, Darnell JC, Bender A, et al. Tumor-specific killer cells in paraneoplastic cerebellar degeneration. *Nat Med* 1998;4:1321–1324.

54. Fefer A. Adoptive chemoimmunotherapy of a Moloney lymphoma. *Int J Cancer* 1971;8:364–373.

55. Wong RA, Alexander RB, Puri RK, et al. *In vivo* proliferation of adoptively transferred tumor-infiltrating lymphocytes in mice. *J Immunother* 1991;10:120–130.

56. de Boer RJ, Hogeweg P, Dullens HF, et al. Macrophage T lymphocyte interactions in the antitumor immune response: a mathematical model. *J Immunol* 1985;134:2748–2758.

57. Pardoll DM, Topalian SL. The role of CD4+ T cell responses in antitumor immunity. *Curr Opin Immunol* 1998;10:588–594.

58. Schoenberger SP, Toes RE, van der Voort EI, et al. T-cell help for cytotoxic T lymphocytes is mediated by CD40-CD40L interactions. *Nature* 1998;393:480–483.

59. Sotomayor EM, Borrello I, Tubb E, et al. Conversion of tumor-specific CD4+ T-cell tolerance to T-cell priming through *in vivo* ligation of CD40. *Nat Med* 1999;5:780–787.

60. Freitas AA, Rocha B. Peripheral T cell survival. *Curr Opin Immunol* 1999;11:152–156.

61. Awwad M, North RJ. Cyclophosphamide (Cy)-facilitated adoptive immunotherapy of a Cy-resistant tumour. Evidence that Cy permits the expression of adoptive T-cell mediated immunity by removing suppressor T cells rather than by reducing tumour burden. *J Immunol* 1988;65:87–92.

62. Groux H, O'Garra A, Bigler M, et al. A CD4+ T-cell subset inhibits antigen-specific T-cell responses and prevents colitis. *Nature* 1997;389:737–742.

63. Matzinger P. Tolerance, danger, and the extended family. *Annu Rev Immunol* 1994;12:991–1045.

64. Renner C, Ohnesorge S, Held G, et al. T cells from patients with Hodgkin's disease have a defective T-cell receptor zeta chain expression that is reversible by T-cell stimulation with CD3 and CD28. *Blood* 1996;88:236–241.

65. Effros RB, Pawelec G. Replicative senescence of T cells: does the Hayflick Limit lead to immune exhaustion? *Immunol Today* 1997;18:450–454.

66. Pawelec G, Rehbein A, Haehnel K, et al. Human T-cell clones in long-term culture as a model of immunosenescence. *Immunol Rev* 1997;160:31–42.

67. Weng N-P, Levine BL, June CH, et al. Human naive and memory T lymphocytes differ in telomeric length and replicative potential. *Proc Natl Acad Sci U S A* 1995;92:11091–11094.

68. Weng N-P, Palmer LD, Levine BL, et al. Tales of tails: regulation of telomere length and telomerase activity during lymphocyte development, differentiation, activation, and aging. *Immunol Rev* 1997;160:43–54.

69. Gallimore A, Glithero A, Godkin A, et al. Induction and exhaustion of lymphocytic choriomeningitis virus-specific cytotoxic T lymphocytes visualized using soluble tetrameric major histocompatibility complex class I-peptide complexes. *J Exp Med* 1998;187:1383–1393.

70. Lee HW, Blasco MA, Gottlieb GJ, et al. Essential role of mouse telomerase in highly proliferative organs. *Nature* 1998;392:569–574.

71. Bodnar AG, Ouellette M, Frolkis M, et al. Extension of life-span by introduction of telomerase into normal human cells. *Science* 1998;279:349–352.

72. Rudolph KL, Chang S, Millard M, et al. Inhibition of experimental liver cirrhosis in mice by telomerase gene delivery. *Science* 2000;287:1253–1258.

73. Wynn RF, Cross MA, Hatton C, et al. Accelerated telomere shortening in young recipients of allogeneic bone-marrow transplants. *Lancet* 1998;351:178–181.

74. Wynn R, Thornley I, Freedman M, et al. Telomere shortening in leucocyte subsets of long-term survivors of allogeneic bone marrow transplantation. *Br J Haematol* 1999;105:997–1001.

75. Freitas AA, Rocha BB. Lymphocyte lifespans: homeostasis, selection and competition. *Immunol Today* 1995;14:25–29.

76. Michie CA, McLean A, Alcock C, et al. Lifespan of human lymphocyte subsets defined by CD45 isoforms. *Nature* 1992;360:264–265.

77. Hellerstein MK. Measurement of T-cell kinetics: recent methodologic advances. *Immunol Today* 1999;20:438–441.

78. Hellerstein M, Hanley MB, Cesar D, et al. Directly measured kinetics of circulating T lymphocytes in normal and HIV-1-infected humans. *Nat Med* 1999;5:83–89.

79. McLean AR, Michie CA. *In vivo* estimates of division and death rates of human T lymphocytes. *Proc Natl Acad Sci U S A* 1995;92:3707–3711.

80. McCune JM, Hanley MB, Cesar D, et al. Factors influencing T-cell turnover in HIV-1-seropositive patients. *J Clin Invest* 2000;105:R1–R8.

81. Blaese RM, Culver KW, Miller AD, et al. T lymphocyte-directed gene therapy for ADA-SCID: initial trial results after 4 years. *Science* 1995;270:475–480.

82. Heslop HE, Ng CY, Li C, et al. Long-term restoration of immunity against Epstein-Barr virus infection by adoptive transfer of gene-modified virus-specific T lymphocytes. *Nat Med* 1996;2:551–555.

83. Walker RE, Carter CS, Muul L, et al. Peripheral expansion of pre-existing mature T cells is an important means of CD4+ T-cell regeneration HIV-infected adults. *Nat Med* 1998;4:852–856.

84. Riddell SR, Elliott M, Lewinsohn DA, et al. T-cell mediated rejection of gene-modified HIV-specific cytotoxic T lymphocytes in HIV-infected patients. *Nat Med* 1996;2:216–223.

85. Ranga U, Woffendin C, Verma S, et al. Retroviral delivery of an antiviral gene in HIV-infected individuals. *Proc Natl Acad Sci U S A* 1998;95:1201–1206.

86. Rosenberg SA, Aebersold P, Cornetta K, et al. Gene transfer into humans—immunotherapy of patients with advanced melanoma, using tumor-infiltrating lymphocytes modified by retroviral gene transduction. *N Engl J Med* 1990;323:570–578.

87. Mitsuyasu RT, Anton P, Deeks SG, et al. Prolonged survival and tissue trafficking following adoptive transfer of CD4ζ gene-modified autologous CD4+ and CD8+ T cells in HIV-infected subjects. *Blood* 2000;96:785–793.

88. Lanier LL. Turning on natural killer cells. *J Exp Med* 2000;191:1259–1262.

89. Franco S, Vyas Y, McKenzie KL, et al. Differential upregulation of telomerase in NK (natural killer) and T lymphocytes *in vitro*. *Blood* 1999;94(Suppl 1):4a.

90. Sondel PM, Hank JA, Kohler PC, et al. Destruction of autologous human lymphocytes by interleukin 2-activated cytotoxic cells. *J Immunol* 1986;137:502–511.

91. Miltenburg AM, Meijer-Paape ME, Daha MR, et al. Lymphokine-activated killer cells lyse human renal cancer cell lines and cultured normal kidney cells. *J Immunol* 1988;63:729–731.

92. Mukherji B, Arnbjarnarson O, Spitznagle LA, et al. Imaging pattern of previously *in vitro* sensitized and interleukin-2 expanded autologous lymphocytes in human cancer. *Int J Rad Appl Instrum B* 1988;15:419–427.

93. Rosenberg SA, Lotze MT, Muul LM, et al. A progress report on the treatment of 157 patients with advanced cancer using lymphokine-activated killer cells and interleukin-2 or high-dose interleukin-2 alone. *N Engl J Med* 1987;316:889–897.

94. Urba WJ, Longo DL. Adoptive cellular therapy. *Cancer Chemother Biol Response Modif* 1990;11:265–280.

95. Chang AE, Geiger JD, Sondak VK, et al. Adoptive cellular therapy of malignancy. *Arch Surg* 1993;128:1281–1290.

96. Rosenberg SA, Lotze MT, Yang JC, et al. Prospective randomized trial of high-dose interleukin-2 alone or in conjunction with lymphokine-activated killer cells for the treatment of patients with advanced cancer. *J Natl Cancer Inst* 1993;85:622–632.

97. Visonneau S, Cesano A, Jeglum KA, et al. Adoptive therapy of canine metastatic mammary carcinoma with the human MHC non-restricted cytotoxic T-cell line TALL-104. *Oncol Rep* 1999;6:1181–1188.

98. Mazumder A, Eberlein TJ, Grimm EA, et al. Phase I study of the adoptive immunotherapy of human cancer with lectin activated autologous mononuclear cells. *Cancer* 1984;53:896–905.

99. Gold JE, Zachary DT, Osband ME. Adoptive transfer of *ex vivo*-activated memory T-cell subsets with cyclophosphamide provides effective tumor-specific chemoimmunotherapy of advanced metastatic murine melanoma and carcinoma. *Int J Cancer* 1955;61:580–586.

100. Curti BD, Ochoa AC, Powers GC, et al. A phase I trial of anti-CD3 stimulated CD4+ T cells, infusional interleukin-2 and cyclophosphamide in patients with advanced cancer. *J Clin Oncol* 1998;16:2752–2760.

101. Curti BD, Ochoa AC, Urba WJ, et al. Influence of interleukin-2 regimens on circulating populations of lymphocytes after adoptive transfer of anti-CD3-stimulated T cells: results from a phase I trial in cancer patients. *J Immunother Emphasis Tumor Immunol* 1996;19:296–308.

102. Harada M, Okamoto T, Omoto K, et al. Specific immunotherapy with tumour-draining lymph node cells cultured with both anti-CD3 and anti-CD28 monoclonal antibodies. *Immunology* 1996;87:447–453.

103. Rosenberg SA, Spiess P, Lafreniere R. A new approach to the adoptive immunotherapy of cancer with tumor-infiltrating lymphocytes. *Science* 1986;233:1318–1321.

104. Spiess PJ, Yang JC, Rosenberg SA. *In vivo* antitumor activity of tumor-infiltrating lymphocytes expanded in recombinant interleukin-2. *J Natl Cancer Inst* 1987;79:1067–1075.

105. van der Bruggen P, Traversari C, Chomez P, et al. A gene encoding an antigen recognized by cytolytic T lymphocytes on a human melanoma. *Science* 1991;254:1643–1647.

106. Hoffman DM, Gitlitz BJ, Belldegrun A, et al. Adoptive cellular therapy. *Semin Oncol* 2000;27:221–233.

107. Merrouche Y, Negrier S, Bain C, et al. Clinical application of retroviral gene transfer in oncology: results of a French study with tumor-infiltrating lymphocytes transduced with the gene of resistance to neomycin. *J Clin Oncol* 1995;13:410–418.

108. Economou JS, Belldegrun AS, Glaspy J, et al. *In vivo* trafficking of adoptively transferred interleukin-2 expanded tumor-infiltrating lymphocytes and peripheral blood lymphocytes. Results of a double gene marking trial. *J Clin Invest* 1996;97:515–521.

109. North RJ. Models of adoptive T-cell-mediated regression of established tumors. *Contemp Top Immunobiol* 1984;13:243–257.

110. Sallusto F, Lenig D, Forster R, et al. Two subsets of memory T lymphocytes with distinct homing potentials and effector functions. *Nature* 1999;401:708–712.

111. Yoshizawa H, Chang AE, Shu S. Specific adoptive immunotherapy mediated by tumor-draining lymph node cells sequentially activated with anti-CD3 and IL-2. *J Immunol* 1991;147:729–737.

112. Li Q, Furman SA, Bradford CR, et al. Expanded tumor-reactive CD4+ T-cell responses to human cancers induced by secondary anti-CD3/anti-CD28 activation. *Clin Cancer Res* 1999;5:461–469.

113. Chang AE, Aruga A, Cameron MJ, et al. Adoptive immunotherapy with vaccine-primed lymph node cells secondarily activated with anti-CD3 and interleukin-2. *J Clin Oncol* 1997;15:796–807.

114. Alexander-Miller MA, Leggatt GR, Berzofsky JA. Selective expansion of high- or low-avidity cytotoxic T lymphocytes and efficacy for adoptive immunotherapy. *Proc Natl Acad Sci U S A* 1996;93:4102–4107.

115. Yee C, Gilbert MJ, Riddell SR, et al. Isolation of tyrosinase-specific CD8+ and CD4+ T cell clones from the peripheral blood of melanoma patients following *in vitro* stimulation with recombinant vaccinia virus. *J Immunol* 1996;157:4079–4086.

116. Vonderheide RH, Hahn WC, Schultze JL, et al. The telomerase catalytic subunit is a widely expressed tumor-associated antigen recognized by cytotoxic T lymphocytes. *Immunity* 1999;10:673–679.

117. Dunbar PR, Chen JL, Chao J, et al. Cutting edge: rapid cloning of tumor-specific CTL suitable for adoptive immunotherapy of melanoma. *J Immunol* 1999;162:6959–6962.

118. Yee C, Savage PA, Lee PP, et al. Isolation of high avidity melanoma-reactive CTL from heterogeneous populations using peptide-MHC tetramers. *J Immunol* 1999;162:2227–2234.

119. Soda H, Koda K, Yasutomi J, et al. Adoptive immunotherapy for advanced cancer patients using *in vitro* activated cytotoxic T lymphocytes. *J Surg Oncol* 1999;72:211–217.

120. Tsurushima H, Liu SQ, Tuboi K, et al. Reduction of end-stage malignant glioma by injection with autologous cytotoxic T lymphocytes. *Jpn J Cancer Res* 1999;90:536–545.

121. Riddell SR, Watanabe KS, Goodrich JM, et al. Restoration of viral immunity in immunodeficient humans by the adoptive transfer of T cell clones. *Science* 1992;257:238–241.

122. Walter EA, Greenberg PD, Gilbert MJ, et al. Reconstitution of cellular immunity against cytomegalovirus in recipients of allogeneic bone marrow by transfer of T-cell clones from the donor. *N Engl J Med* 1995;333:1038–1044.

123. Heslop HE, Rooney CM. Adoptive cellular immunotherapy for EBV lymphoproliferative disease. *Immunol Rev* 1997;157:217–222.

124. Li PK, Tsang K, Szeto CC, et al. Effective treatment of high-grade lymphoproliferative disorder after renal transplantation using autologous lymphocyte activated killer cell therapy. *Am J Kidney Dis* 1998;32:813–819.

125. Weiden PL, Flournoy N, Thomas ED, et al. Antileukemic effect of graft-versus-host disease in human recipients of allogeneic-marrow grafts. *N Engl J Med* 1979;300:1068–1073.

126. Kolb HJ, Mittermuller J, Clemm C, et al. Donor leukocyte transfusions for treatment of recurrent chronic myelogenous leukemia in marrow transplant patients. *Blood* 1990;76:2462–2465.

127. Porter DL, Roth MS, McGarigle C, et al. Induction of graft-versus-host disease as immunotherapy for relapsed chronic myeloid leukemia. *N Engl J Med* 1994;330:100–106.

128. Dazzi F, Szydlo RM, Craddock C, et al. Comparison of single-dose and escalating-dose regimens of donor lymphocyte infusion for relapse after allografting for chronic myeloid leukemia. *Blood* 2000;95:67–71.

129. Collins RH Jr, Shpilberg O, Drobyski WR, et al. Donor leukocyte infusions in 140 patients with relapsed malignancy after allogeneic bone marrow transplantation. *J Clin Oncol* 1997;15:433–444.

130. Falkenburg JH, Wafelman AR, Joosten P, et al. Complete remission of accelerated phase chronic myeloid leukemia by treatment with leukemia-reactive cytotoxic T lymphocytes. *Blood* 1999;94:1201–1208.

131. Morgan DJ, Kreuwel HT, Fleck S, et al. Activation of low avidity CTL specific for a self epitope results in tumor rejection but not autoimmunity. *J Immunol* 1998;160:643–651.

132. Giralt S, Hester J, Huh Y, et al. CD8-depleted donor lymphocyte infusion as treatment for relapsed chronic myelogenous leukemia after allogeneic bone marrow transplantation. *Blood* 1995;86:4337–4343.

133. Alyea EP, Soiffer RJ, Canning C, et al. Toxicity and efficacy of defined doses of CD4(+) donor lymphocytes for treatment of relapse after allogeneic bone marrow transplant. *Blood* 1998;91:3671–3680.

134. Feneley RC, Eckert H, Riddell AG, et al. The treatment of advanced bladder cancer with sensitized pig lymphocytes. *Br J Surg* 1974;61:825–827.

135. Nadler SH, Moore GE. Clinical immunologic study of malignant disease: response to tumor transplants and transfer of leukocytes. *Ann Surg* 1966;164:482–490.

136. Nadler SH, Moore GE. Immunotherapy of malignant disease. *Arch Surg* 1969;99:376–381.

137. Yonemoto RH, Terasaki PI. Cancer immunotherapy with HLA-compatible thoracic duct lymphocyte transplantation. A preliminary report. *Cancer* 1972;30:1438–1443.

138. Kohler PC, Hank JA, Exten R, et al. Clinical response of a patient with diffuse histiocytic lymphoma to adoptive chemoimmunotherapy using cyclophosphamide and alloactivated haploidentical lymphocytes. A case report and phase I trial. *Cancer* 1985;55:552–560.

139. Porter DL, Connors JM, Van Deerlin VM, et al. Graft-versus-tumor induction with donor leukocyte infusions as primary therapy for patients with malignancies. *J Clin Oncol* 1999;17:1234–1243.

140. Or R, Ackerstein A, Nagler A, et al. Allogeneic cell-mediated immunotherapy for breast cancer after autologous stem cell transplantation: a clinical pilot study. *Cytokines Cell Mol Ther* 1998;4:1–6.

141. Giralt S, Estey E, Albitar M, et al. Engraftment of allogeneic hematopoietic progenitor cells with purine analog-containing chemotherapy: harnessing graft-versus-leukemia without myeloablative therapy. *Blood* 1997;89:4531–4536.

142. Slavin S, Nagler A, Naparstek E, et al. Nonmyeloablative stem cell transplantation and cell therapy as an alternative to conventional bone marrow transplantation with lethal cytoreduction for the treatment of malignant and nonmalignant hematologic diseases. *Blood* 1998;91:756–763.

143. Childs R, Clave E, Contentin N, et al. Engraftment kinetics after nonmyeloablative allogeneic peripheral blood stem cell transplantation: full donor T-cell chimerism precedes alloimmune responses. *Blood* 1999;94:3234–3241.

144. Ueno NT, Rondon G, Mirza NQ, et al. Allogeneic peripheral-blood progenitor-cell transplantation for poor-risk patients with metastatic breast cancer. *J Clin Oncol* 1998;16:986–993.

145. Childs RW, Clave E, Tisdale J, et al. Successful treatment of metastatic renal cell carcinoma with a nonmyeloablative allogeneic peripheral-blood progenitor-cell transplant: evidence for a graft-versus-tumor effect. *J Clin Oncol* 1999;17:2044.

146. Evans R, Alexander P. Mechanism of immunologically specific killing of tumour cells by macrophages. *Nature* 1972;236:168–170.

147. Drysdale BE, Agarwal S, Shin HS. Macrophage-mediated tumoricidal activity: mechanisms of activation and cytotoxicity. *Prog Allergy* 1988;40:111–161.

148. Andreesen R, Scheibenbogen C, Brugger W, et al. Adoptive transfer of tumor cytotoxic macrophages generated *in vitro* from circulating blood monocytes: a new approach to cancer immunotherapy. *Cancer Res* 1990;50:7450–7456.

149. Eymard JC, Lopez M, Cattan A, et al. Phase I/II trial of autologous activated macrophages in advanced colorectal cancer. *Eur J Cancer* 1996;32A:1905–1911.

150. Andreesen R, Hennemann B, Krause SW. Adoptive immunotherapy of cancer using monocyte-derived macrophages: rationale, current status, and perspectives. *J Leukoc Biol* 1998;64:419–426.

151. Banchereau J, Briere F, Caux C, et al. Immunobiology of dendritic cells. *Annu Rev Immunol* 2000;18:767–811.

152. Dhodapkar MV, Steinman RM, Sapp M, et al. Rapid generation of broad T-cell immunity in humans after a single injection of mature dendritic cells. *J Clin Invest* 1999;104:173–180.

153. Loercher AE, Nash MA, Kavanagh JJ, et al. Identification of an IL-10-producing HLA-DR-negative monocyte subset in

the malignant ascites of patients with ovarian carcinoma that inhibits cytokine protein expression and proliferation of autologous T cells. *J Immunol* 1999;163:6251–6260.

154. Gabrilovich DI, Chen HL, Girgis KR, et al. Production of vascular endothelial growth factor by human tumors inhibits the functional maturation of dendritic cells. *Nat Med* 1996;2:1096–1103.

155. Hsu FJ, Benike C, Fagnoni F, et al. Vaccination of patients with B-cell lymphoma using autologous antigen-pulsed dendritic cells. *Nat Med* 1996;2:52–58.

156. Nestle FO, Alijagic S, Gilliet M, et al. Vaccination of melanoma patients with peptide- or tumor lysate-pulsed dendritic cells. *Nat Med* 1998;4:328–332.

157. Heiser A, Dahm P, Yancey R, et al. Human dendritic cells transfected with RNA encoding prostate-specific antigen stimulate prostate-specific CTL responses *in vitro*. *J Immunol* 2000;164:5508–5514.

158. Kugler A, Stuhler G, Walden P, et al. Regression of human metastatic renal cell carcinoma after vaccination with tumor cell-dendritic cell hybrids. *Nat Med* 2000;6:332–336.

159. Osband ME, Lavin PT, Babayan PK, et al. Effect of autolymphocyte therapy on survival and quality of life in patients with metastatic renal-cell carcinoma. *Lancet* 1990;335:994–998.

160. Fenton RG, Steis RG, Madara K, et al. A phase I randomized study of subcutaneous adjuvant IL-2 in combination with an autologous tumor vaccine in patients with advanced renal cell carcinoma. *J Immunother Emphasis Tumor Immunol* 1996;19:364–374.

161. Keilholz U, Scheibenbogen C, Brado M, et al. Regional adoptive immunotherapy with interleukin-2 and lymphokine-activated killer (LAK) cells for liver metastases. *Eur J Cancer* 1994;30A:103–105.

162. Ratto GB, Zino P, Mirabelli S, et al. A randomized trial of adoptive immunotherapy with tumor-infiltrating lymphocytes and interleukin-2 versus standard therapy in the postoperative treatment of resected nonsmall cell lung carcinoma. *Cancer* 1996;78:244–251.

163. Kimura H, Yamaguchi Y. A phase III randomized study of interleukin-2 lymphokine-activated killer cell immunotherapy combined with chemotherapy or radiotherapy after curative or noncurative resection of primary lung carcinoma. *Cancer* 1997;80:42–49.

164. Uchino J, Une Y, Kawata A, et al. Postoperative chemoimmunotherapy for the treatment of liver cancer. *Semin Surg Oncol* 1993;9:332–336.

165. Cheever MA, Greenberg PD, Fefer A, et al. Augmentation of the antitumor therapeutic efficacy of long-term cultured T lymphocytes by *in vivo* administration of purified interleukin 2. *J Exp Med* 1982;155:968–980.

166. Old LJ. Tumor immunology: the first century. *Curr Opin Immunol* 1992;4:603–607.

167. Carter CS, Leitman SF, Cullis H, et al. Development of an automated closed system for generation of human lymphokine-activated killer (LAK) cells for use in adoptive immunotherapy. *J Immunol Methods* 1987;101:171–181.

168. Margolin KA. Interleukin-2 in the treatment of renal cancer. *Semin Oncol* 2000;27:194–203.

169. Ettinghausen SE, Moore JG, White DE, et al. Hematologic effects of immunotherapy with lymphokine-activated killer

cells and recombinant interleukin-2 in cancer patients. *Blood* 1987;69:1654–1660.

170. Atkins MB, Mier JW, Parkinson DR, et al. Hypothyroidism after treatment with interleukin-2 and lymphokine-activated killer cells. *N Engl J Med* 1988;318:1557–1563.

171. Livingston PO, Ragupathi G, Musselli C. Autoimmune and antitumor consequences of antibodies against antigens shared by normal and malignant tissues. *J Clin Immunol* 2000;20:85–93.

172. Donahue RE, Kessler SW, Bodine D, et al. Helper virus induced T cell lymphoma in nonhuman primates after retroviral mediated gene transfer. *J Exp Med* 1992;176:1125–1135.

173. Ratto GB, Cafferata MA, Scolaro T, et al. Phase II study of combined immunotherapy, chemotherapy, and radiotherapy in the postoperative treatment of advanced non-small-cell lung cancer. *J Immunother* 2000;23:161–167.

174. Mackall CL, Fleisher TA, Brown MR, et al. Age, thymopoiesis, and CD4+ T-lymphocyte regeneration after intensive chemotherapy. *N Engl J Med* 1995;332:143–149.

175. Mackall CL, Gress RE. Pathways of T-cell regeneration in mice and humans: implications for bone marrow transplantation and immunotherapy. *Immunol Rev* 1997;157:61–72.

176. Sullivan KM, Storb R, Buckner CD, et al. Graft-versus-host disease as adoptive immunotherapy in patients with advanced hematologic neoplasms. *N Engl J Med* 1989;320:828–834.

177. Kernan NA, Collins NH, Juliano L, et al. Clonable T lymphocytes in T cell-depleted bone marrow transplants correlate with development of graft-v-host disease. *Blood* 1986;68:770–773.

178. Eshhar Z, Bach N, Fitzer-Attas CJ, et al. The T-body approach: potential for cancer immunotherapy. *Springer Semin Immunopathol* 1996;18:199–209.

179. Arca MJ, Mule JJ, Chang AE. Genetic approaches to adoptive cellular therapy of malignancy. *Semin Oncol* 1996;23:108–117.

180. Helene M, Lake-Bullock V, Bryson JS, et al. Inhibition of graft-versus-host disease. Use of a T cell-controlled suicide gene. *J Immunol* 1997;158:5079–5082.

181. Bonini C, Ferrari G, Verzeletti S, et al. HSV-TK gene transfer into donor lymphocytes for control of allogeneic graft-versus-leukemia. *Science* 1997;276:1719–1724.

182. Clackson T, Yang W, Rozamus LW, et al. Redesigning an FKBP-ligand interface to generate chemical dimerizers with novel specificity. *Proc Natl Acad Sci U S A* 1998;95:10437–10442.

183. Amara JF, Courage NL, Gilman M. Cell surface tagging and a suicide mechanism in a single chimeric human protein. *Hum Gene Ther* 1999;10:2651–2655.

184. Thomis DC, Marktel S, Bonini C, et al. A Fas-based switch in human T cells for the treatment of graft-versus-disease. *Blood* 2001;97:1249–1257.

185. Kirk CJ, Mule JJ. Gene-modified dendritic cells for use in tumor vaccines. *Hum Gene Ther* 2000;11:797–806.

186. Koretz MJ, Lawson DH, York RM, et al. Randomized study of interleukin 2 (IL-2) alone vs IL-2 plus lymphokine-activated killer cells for treatment of melanoma and renal cell cancer. *Arch Surg* 1991;126:898–903.

187. Graham S, Babayan RM, Lamm DL, et al. The use of *ex vivo*-activated memory T cells (autolymphocyte therapy) in the treatment of metastatic renal cell carcinoma: final results from a randomized, controlled, multisite study. *Semin Urol* 1993;11:27–34.

188. Law TM, Motzer RJ, Mazumdar M, et al. Phase III randomized trial of interleukin-2 with or without lymphokine-activated killer cells in the treatment of patients with advanced renal cell carcinoma. *Cancer* 1995;76:824–832.

189. Figlin RA, Thompson JA, Bukowski RM, et al. Multicenter, randomized, phase III trial of CD8(+) tumor-infiltrating lymphocytes in combination with recombinant interleukin-2 in metastatic renal cell carcinoma. *J Clin Oncol* 1999;17:2521–2529.

190. Kimura H, Yamaguchi Y. Adjuvant immunotherapy with interleukin 2 and lymphokine-activated killer cells after noncurative resection of primary lung cancer. *Lung Cancer* 1995;13:31–44.

191. Kimura H, Yamaguchi Y. Adjuvant chemo-immunotherapy after curative resection of Stage II and IIIA primary lung cancer. *Lung Cancer* 1996;14:301–314.

33

CANCER VACCINES 2001

GLENN DRANOFF

At the dawn of a new millennium, cancer immunology can delight in a renewed beginning. One hundred years ago, William Coley unveiled the first compelling evidence that host defenses could modulate the natural history of cancer. This surgeon induced tumor regressions in some patients harboring advanced sarcoma with the administration of bacterial toxins.[1] Although the mechanisms underlying these striking findings have yet to be elucidated fully, the efforts invested in exploring these phenomena have yielded substantive insights into the host-tumor relationship. As a consequence of this enterprise, cancer immunology today stands on a strong scientific foundation, deeply rooted in molecular genetics, cellular technologies, pathologic analysis, and clinical investigation.

Cancer immunologists today possess the tools to identify immunogenic gene products selectively expressed in cancer cells; the tools to incorporate these gene products into diverse immunotherapy strategies likely to augment antitumor immunity; and the tools to monitor the efficacy and intensity of induced immune responses in tumor-bearing hosts. These impressive capabilities establish a powerful platform through which a deeper understanding of the therapeutic possibilities and limitations of cancer immunotherapy is likely to emerge. Already a large number of cancer vaccination schemes have entered clinical trials, but most of the approaches are in only early stages of testing, with the determination of immunogenicity, toxicity, and feasibility constituting the primary objectives of small phase I and II studies. As these characteristics become more clearly defined, they will serve as key criteria for selecting a few promising strategies for further clinical development, with the undertaking of definitive efficacy testing in the setting of minimal residual disease. The most effective prioritization of cancer immunotherapies will depend on many productive collaborations between basic and clinical investigators.

Toward the realization of this end, this review highlights some of the exciting genetic and cellular advances that frame current laboratory work and some of the provocative human data that inform current clinical investigation in cancer immunology.

CANCER IMMUNOSURVEILLANCE

One way of assessing the immune system's capacity to mediate antitumor effects is to determine whether naturally occurring immune responses are correlated with either the frequency of cancer development or the pace of disease progression. Epidemiologic studies have convincingly demonstrated that multiple congenital and acquired forms of immunodeficiency (both drug- and disease-induced) are associated with a marked increase in specific forms of malignancy, particularly lymphoma, Kaposi's sarcoma, and skin cancer.[2] These malignancies reflect the complex biology of viral infection, however, and their heightened incidence is probably best viewed as a manifestation of compromised antiviral immunity.

The idea that subtle defects in immunity might be linked to cancer development is a more controversial but, perhaps, influential hypothesis. First suggested almost 100 years ago by Paul Ehrlich,[3] the concept of cancer immunosurveillance subsequently was formalized by Lewis Thomas[4] and MacFarlane Burnet,[5] who speculated that T lymphocytes would prove to be critical mediators in such defense. Although the work of Stutman,[6] who failed to detect an increased incidence of spontaneous or chemically induced tumors in nude mice, challenged the notion of immunosurveillance, experiments using gene-targeted mice have provided persuasive evidence in support of a functional defense against carcinogenesis.

Schreiber and colleagues have generated provocative data that reveal that interferon-γ is required for effective tumor surveillance in murine systems.[7] These workers demonstrated that mice rendered interferon-γ resistant (because of deletions in either the cytokine receptor or molecules essential for proper signal transduction) develop tumors after exposure to the mutagen 3-methylcholanthrene at increased frequency and with reduced latency compared with similarly treated wild-type littermates. Moreover, when mice insensitive to interferon-γ were crossed with p53 heterozygous mutant mice, the doubly deficient progeny suffered from a broader spectrum of neoplasms than mice mutant in p53 alone. The host and incipient tumor both seem to participate in the inhibition of disease progression, a process that reflects the complex interplay of innate and specific immunity. The importance of T lymphocytes in tumor defense is also supported by studies in murine systems that reveal a striking inverse correlation between the capacity to mount strong contact hypersensitivity responses to epicutaneously applied polycyclic hydrocarbons (a T-cell–dependent reaction) and susceptibility to carcinogenesis induced by these agents.[8]

To establish whether comparable immunosurveillance systems are functional in humans, investigators first need to identify and characterize specific immune responses that are capable of mediating substantive tumor destruction in patients. One approach to this challenging problem involves, perhaps somewhat paradoxically, the phenotyping of progressive cancers for features indicative of escape from immunologic control. Similar studies of virulence factors devised by successful pathogens have disclosed critical components of the immune response to infection.[9] Within this framework, the fact that defects in the expression of major histocompatibility (MHC) molecules and other proteins involved in antigen presentation are frequently found in clinical cancers[10] is intriguing and suggests that T lymphocytes participate in tumor control. Corroborating this hypothesis is evidence that tumor cells often release soluble factors which inhibit T-lymphocyte priming by professional antigen-presenting cells. One example is vascular endothelial growth factor, which, in addition to exerting well-described angiogenic effects, markedly inhibits dendritic cell development.[11] Tumors also secrete soluble factors, such as transforming growth factor β, which potently inhibit T-cell expansion.[12]

A second approach to understanding the features underlying effective antitumor immunity in humans involves analysis of the immune responses of cancer patients experiencing prolonged survival. Highly compelling data have been marshaled in this regard through the pathologic assessment of the host response to early-stage tumors. The pioneering work of Clark and Mihm demonstrated a striking correlation between the presence of brisk T-lymphocyte infiltrates in the vertical growth phase of primary malignant melanoma and a reduced incidence of recurrent disease and mortality.[13,14] A key insight provided by these studies is that the prognostic value of lymphocytes which circumscribe, but fail to infiltrate and perturb, the neoplasm is equivalent to that associated with the absence of a lymphocyte infiltrate. Remarkably, the development of brisk T-cell infiltrates in melanomas that already have metastasized to regional lymph nodes similarly predicts for better survival than with tumors that fail to evoke this host response.[15]

Investigations aimed at elucidating the differences between T cells that merely circumscribe tumors and those that invade tumors should be a high priority and are likely to yield important insights into cancer-associated T-lymphocyte dysfunction. Interestingly, comparable observations have been made in studies of the pathogenesis of autoimmune diabetes. A peri–islet cell accumulation of T cells is not sufficient to mediate disease in this system; rather, additional events are required before T cells infiltrate and destroy the islets.[16] In this context, genetic mapping studies directed at identifying susceptibility factors underlying autoimmune diabetes in mice and humans[17] may reveal loci that are also relevant to the generation of antitumor immunity.

The prognostic importance of lymphocyte infiltrates in early-stage tumors has been convincingly demonstrated in adenocarcinoma of the colon as well, in which the presence of CD8+ T lymphocytes within nests of primary tumors proves to be as strong a prognostic factor for survival as the widely used Dukes staging system.[18] Moreover, the frequency of lymphocytic infiltrates is inversely correlated with tumor stage, which raises the possibility that advanced cancers develop, at least in part, through escape from immunologic control. Macrophages positioned at the tumor-stromal interface have been shown, in some cases, to express high levels of the B7-1 and B7-2 costimulatory molecules[19]; in these instances, CD4+ and CD8+ T cells are intimately apposed to the activated macrophages, which implies an important functional interaction.

Lymphocyte infiltrates have been reported to a variable degree with many other tumors, including lymphoma, glioblastoma, and carcinomas of the stomach, breast, bladder, testes, and ovary. These observations raise the idea that immunosurveillance may be a general phenomenon and not restricted, as is so often claimed, to malignant melanoma. If this provocative hypothesis can be validated through careful clinicopathologic studies, a deeper understanding of these "spontaneous" host responses may provide the blueprint for devising effective immunotherapy.

CANCER ANTIGENS

One of the critical challenges in understanding the host antitumor response is identifying the cancer antigens provoking immune recognition. Because pathologic analysis has underscored the importance of T lymphocytes in cancer surveillance, antigenic targets of these cells are of particular interest. Basic immunology studies have disclosed that T lymphocytes respond to target antigens as processed peptides, derived from cellular proteins, inserted into the grooves of MHC molecules.[20] This insight provided the foundation for Boon and colleagues to devise the first effective strategy to identify cancer antigens[21]; in this approach, tumor-specific cytolytic T-cell clones were used to screen complementary DNA expression libraries, constructed from tumor samples, which were transfected into recipient cells expressing the appropriate MHC class I molecules. The ability of this innovative scheme to identify antigens mediating tumor destruction was confirmed through the demonstration, in murine systems, that immunization with either P1A or mutated mitogen-activated protein kinase (murine cancer antigens detected through the Boon approach) led to protective immunity against parental tumor challenge.[22] Moreover, initial clinical testing has revealed that vaccination with peptides derived from the MAGE-3 and gp100 gene products (human cancer antigens identified through the Boon approach) induces tumor regressions in some patients with metastatic melanoma.[23,24] A second, closely related strategy, developed by Hunt and collaborators, relies on tumor-specific T cells to screen candidate peptides acid-eluted from tumor-derived MHC molecules[25]; stimulatory peptides are then sequenced using reverse-phase high-performance liquid chromatography or mass spectrometry.

In contrast to using T cells as probes for the screening of complementary DNA expression libraries, Pfreundschuh and colleagues, in a third antigen identification scheme, have used high-titer antitumor immunoglobulin G (IgG) antibodies as a detection system.[26] Underlying this strategy is the hypothesis that, because cancer patients frequently develop coordinated humoral and cellular antitumor responses, at least some of the antigens recognized by high-titer IgG antibodies will be recognized by CD4[+] and CD8[+] T lymphocytes as well (although through different antigen presentation pathways).[27] Indeed, cytokine production by CD4[+] T cells is required for B-cell class switching to IgG isotypes. The predictive value of this hypothesis has been established by the identification of MAGE-1 and tyrosinase through serologic techniques; these antigens previously had been discovered with T-cell cloning methods. Perhaps more impressive, though, is the demonstration that NY-ESO-1, an antigen initially detected by antibody-based cloning, is a target for MHC class I restricted cytotoxic T lymphocytes as well.[28]

These intriguing results suggest that serologically based cloning methods are likely to find broad application, particularly because patient tumors and sera are easy to obtain, and in contrast to the extensive manipulations required to generate T-cell clones, antibodies can be directly used for library screening. That serologically based methods will provide an extensive number of target antigens for most cancers already is clear. An initial report of the application of serologic screening to colorectal carcinoma disclosed a group of antigens recognized only by cancer patients,[29] which raises the possibility that this technology may also yield a panel of new diagnostic tests.

Together, the three cancer antigen discovery schemes have begun to elucidate the rules underlying immune recognition of cancer. Four categories of antigens have been delineated thus far (reviewed in reference 30). The first class, dubbed "cancer-testis" antigens, are oncofetal proteins ectopically expressed in tumors. Although they are widely expressed during fetal development (their function is not yet known), in the adult their expression is restricted to the testis and placenta. Examples of this group are NY-ESO-1 and the MAGE, BAGE, and GAGE gene families. A second class of antigens consists of mutated cellular proteins, some of which contribute to the transformed phenotype, such as cyclin-dependent protein kinase 4, β-catenin, and caspase 8. A third group is composed of short peptides derived from intronic sequences aberrantly expressed in cancer cells; some members are MUM-1, p15, *N*-acetylglucosaminyltransferase V, and a novel form of tyrosinase-related protein-2 (TRP-2).

In contrast to the three preceding groups, in which the basis for their function as cancer antigens can be readily understood, the final class of targets, apparently normal cellular proteins, is more problematic. The mechanism by which the immune system reacts selectively to these antigens in malignant cells and not in normal tissues remains to be clarified fully, but the existence of this group of molecules underscores the delicate balance between autoimmunity and tumor immunity.[31] Indeed, in the case of normal tissues that are not essential for survival such as the prostate, breast, thyroid, and melanocyte, some degree of autoimmunity may be an acceptable toxicity for immunotherapy provided that the antitumor effects are sufficiently potent. The most thoroughly characterized gene products in this group include key components of the melanin biosynthetic pathway, such as tyrosinase, Melan A/MART-1, gp75 (tyrosinase-related protein-1, TRP-1), TRP-2, and gp100/Pmel 17.

OVERCOMING DEFECTIVE ANTITUMOR IMMUNITY

Notwithstanding the elegance of cancer antigen discovery and the provocative association between lymphocyte infiltrates in early-stage cancer and prolonged survival, one may still legitimately question the significance of cancer immune recognition. Are antitumor immune responses the consequences of cancer cell death effectuated by hypoxia, growth factor deficiency, and inefficient protection from apoptosis? Or, conversely, is immune escape a decisive step in the natural history of progressive cancer? The immunotherapist, perhaps somewhat unexpectedly, is likely to play a central role in resolving this fascinating dilemma. If treatment strategies can be devised that consistently augment the generation of antitumor immunity, then randomized clinical trials will conclusively arbitrate whether or not these schemes can modify cancer mortality.

A dominant theme underlying current immunotherapy research is that tumor cells frequently do not stimulate maximal immune responses. This insight derives in large measure from an improved understanding of the mechanisms underlying tumor antigen presentation. A substantial body of evidence now implicates dendritic cells as critical initiators of effective immunity.[32] These cells are specialized to prime antigen-specific T- and B-cell responses because of their abilities to process antigens efficiently into both MHC class I and class II pathways, and their high-level expression of costimulatory molecules. As discussed earlier, however, cancer cells may actively suppress the development and function of dendritic cells in the tumor microenvironment. This stratagem, together with the tumor cell's sparse endowment of antigen-processing ability and costimulatory molecule expression, render it unlikely that T and B lymphocytes are exposed to tumor antigens in an optimal immunologic environment; tumor-specific effectors may instead be driven to abortive or dysfunctional responses.[33]

With this scenario defining a critical defect in antitumor immunity, investigators have devised an array of strategies designed to improve tumor antigen presentation. Perhaps the most direct approach is to force intermingling of tumor cells and dendritic cells. The crafting of *in vitro* methods to propagate large numbers of dendritic cells from hemopoietic progenitors,[34,35] exploiting the activities of granulocyte-macrophage colony-stimulating factor (GM-CSF), has led to several studies which demonstrate that dendritic cells can dramatically enhance antitumor immunity in murine tumor models.[36] Multiple strategies involving the *ex vivo* manipulation of dendritic cells have been shown to stimulate antitumor immunity,[37-40] including pulsing dendritic cells with tumor antigen–derived peptides or whole-tumor-cell lysates and genetically modifying dendritic cells to express tumor antigens. These latter experiments have used replication-defective adenoviral vectors encoding tumor antigens or the electroporation of tumor-derived total RNA.

In contrast to these approaches that involve the *ex vivo* manipulation of dendritic cells, other vaccination schemes attempt to augment dendritic cell function *in vivo*. The systemic infusion of recombinant flt3 ligand induces a marked expansion of dendritic cells in many tissues and mediates impressive antitumor effects in several murine models.[41,42] Vaccination with naked DNA encoding tumor antigens, a potent strategy for generating humoral and cellular responses, involves the *in situ* transfection of dendritic cells.[43] The presence of unmethylated CpG oligonucleotides in plasmid DNA molecules, moreover, has been shown to promote the proliferation and maturation of dendritic cells.[44] Vaccination with heat-shock proteins, which chaperone partially processed cellular proteins, involves uptake by host professional antigen-presenting cells as well.[45]

The generation of antitumor immune responses *in vivo* involves the transition from a nonspecific inflammatory reaction associated with innate immunity to the stimulation of antigen-specific T and B cells by activated dendritic cells. Based on this framework, multiple strategies are being devised to induce an inflammatory focus at the site of tumor antigen deposition. One approach involves the *in vivo* administration of recombinant viral vectors encoding tumor antigens; such vectors have been derived from adenovirus, herpes simplex virus, and vaccinia and fowlpox viruses.[46] Underlying this strategy is the hypothesis that strong, preexisting antiviral immunity creates a favorable mixture of cytokines resulting in the priming of tumor antigen–specific responses. A potential limitation of the approach, however, is that the nascent immune response may remain skewed toward viral targets, with epitope spreading proving to be inefficient.

To obviate this problem, many investigators are exploring the use of a variety of adjuvants admixed with tumor antigen–derived proteins or peptides. QS-21 and DETOX appear to be among the most promising of these agents, which biochemically are complexes of saponins and microbial products. Adjuvant function depends on the abilities of these complexes to serve as depots for sustained antigen delivery and as stimuli for local inflammatory responses.[47] The injection of recombinant cytokines as vaccine adjuvants for defined proteins is also under intensive study, with encouraging results observed with GM-CSF and interleukin 12 (IL-12) in murine systems.[48,49]

The use of recombinant cytokines to enhance immunization efficacy is probably best viewed as derivative to the work of Forni and colleagues.[50] These investigators demonstrated that the peritumoral injection of specific molecules, especially interleukin 2 (IL-2), could modulate the host-cancer relationship and evoke tumor destruction through the recruitment and activation of neutrophils, eosinophils, macrophages, natural killer cells, and lymphocytes. This complex cellular infiltrate, in some cases, engendered the development of protective immunity against wild-type tumor challenge. These provocative findings catalyzed a large number of studies evaluating the antitumor activities of various immunostimulatory molecules. This line of inquiry was considerably advanced with the introduction of gene transfer techniques for the stable modification of tumor cells, as this resulted in gene expression superior to that achieved with inoculation of recombinant proteins (reviewed in reference 51).

Retrovirally mediated gene transfer was the most common system used in these studies because of its versatility in achieving stable, high-level gene expression without the concomitant production of replication-competent virus.[52] Although many molecules were tested for the ability to abrogate tumorigenicity after transduction into tumor cells, IL-12 and IL-2 emerged as the most consistently active gene products across the entire range of studies.[53-55] The mechanisms underlying tumor destruction induced by these cytokines remains incompletely understood, but involves the coordinated activities of CD4+ and CD8+ T lymphocytes, natural killer cells, macrophages, neutrophils, and eosinophils. In addition to direct toxicity to tumor cells, the destruction of the tumor vasculature and inhibition of angiogenesis appear to be critical components.[56]

An intriguing finding in these experiments was that the abrogation of tumorigenicity could sometimes be dissociated from the generation of protective immunity.[57]

Although the basis for this result remains unclear, it motivated a second series of experiments directly comparing the relative abilities of engineered tumor cells to stimulate systemic immunity. Because many gene products failed to abrogate tumorigenicity, these studies required the use of replication-incompetent tumor cells for vaccination. Irradiation served as a suitable method for this purpose, for although it induces a G_2 cell-cycle arrest, it fails to inhibit transgene expression.

Our own group has investigated the vaccination activity of more than 30 different gene products in this manner. We have demonstrated that immunization with irradiated tumor cells engineered to secrete GM-CSF stimulates potent, specific, and long-lasting antitumor immunity in multiple murine tumor models.[58] GM-CSF based vaccinations require both CD4+ and CD8+ T lymphocytes and likely involve the improved uptake and processing of irradiated tumor cells by activated dendritic cells recruited to the immunization site.

CLINICAL INVESTIGATIONS

Armed with a large number of novel vaccination strategies and candidate tumor antigens, clinical investigators have begun the challenging task of assessing the relative immunogenicity, toxicity, and feasibility of these new immunotherapies. Because the initial trials are targeted primarily at establishing safety and toxicity, they predominantly involve patients with advanced disease. At this late stage of illness, however, clonal evolution likely has propagated the most resistant and heterogeneous malignant cells. The immune system probably also has been damaged as a consequence of prior treatments and the suppressive effects of heavy tumor burdens. Given these considerations, achieving substantive antitumor effects consistently may prove difficult in this setting, although discerning preliminary evidence of biologic activity nonetheless should be possible.

The overall vaccination efforts can be broadly divided, based on the choice of immunizing material, into antigen-specific and whole-tumor-cell–based approaches. Encouragingly, early trials of both approaches have disclosed antitumor effects without significant toxicity. With the defined antigens, several different schemes have manifested antitumor activity. Perhaps most surprising is the finding that immunization with free peptides (derived from melanoma antigens) can induce tumor regressions. Seven of 25 melanoma patients injected with three doses of a HLA-A1–presented peptide derived from the MAGE-3 gene product demonstrated objective tumor regressions.[23] Despite these impressive results, no antigen-specific cytotoxic T lymphocytes could be detected in the peripheral blood of these patients, which suggests either that these cells were not involved in the antitumor response (which seems unlikely) or that they localize to tumor sites.

In an effort to enhance the immune response to defined peptides, investigators have begun testing the activity of recombinant cytokines as vaccine adjuvants. The administration of GM-CSF in conjunction with peptides derived from Melan A, tyrosinase, and gp100 has induced tumor regressions in patients with metastatic melanoma; responding patients developed antigen-specific cytotoxic T cells and delayed-type hypersensitivity reactions.[59] The use of GM-CSF as an adjuvant has also shown promising results with idiotype-based vaccinations for multiple myeloma[60] and follicular lymphoma.[61] This intriguing strategy hypothesizes that the immunoglobulin molecule expressed on the surface of malignant B cells can function as a tumor-rejection antigen. When this approach was tested after autologous bone marrow transplantation, a significant proportion of lymphoma patients achieved molecular remissions associated with the induction of CD4+ and CD8+ T-cell and antibody responses. The systemic administration of high-dose IL-2 together with a modified peptide (to increase MHC class I binding affinity) derived from the gp100 protein also induced a significant number of tumor regressions in metastatic melanoma patients,[24] although the relative contributions of IL-2 and peptide remain to be clarified. Lastly, initial clinical testing of bone-marrow–derived dendritic cells pulsed with melanoma antigens or B-cell idiotypes has revealed antitumor effects as well.[62,63]

The development of peptide epitope/MHC molecule tetramers will considerably advance the immunologic monitoring of antigen-specific vaccination strategies. Tetramers are complexes of synthetic peptide epitopes and bacterially produced MHC molecules conjugated to a fluorochrome.[64] Their multimeric nature overcomes the inherent low affinity and fast off-rate of T-cell receptor/MHC-peptide interactions and results in relatively stable T-cell binding. These complexes can thus be effectively used in fluorescence-activated cell sorter analysis of unselected T-cell populations. These reagents can also be used to sort tetramer-binding cells for subsequent functional studies, that is, antigen-specific cytokine production, proliferation, and cytotoxicity.

Not only have tumor-derived peptides and proteins been used for cancer vaccination, but promising results have been obtained using carbohydrate antigens as well. Furthest along in development are those approaches using ganglioside GM_2.[65] Vaccination with admixtures of this molecule in QS-21 after lymph node dissection for stage III malignant melanoma currently has entered phase III testing. Preliminary evidence that immunization with globo H can induce antibody responses and alter the rate of prostate-specific antigen elevation in patients with metastatic prostate carcinoma also has been reported.[66]

Although antigen-specific vaccination strategies clearly augment antitumor immunity, they may ultimately be limited by the development of antigen-loss variants. Indeed, this already has been observed in the context of melanoma peptide vaccination, in which progressive tumors were found to lack the relevant target antigen.[67] In view of this concern, the application of whole-tumor cells might provide a strategy in which such escape would be less likely. The use of allogeneic tumor lines, in this context, presents practical advantages for manufacturing and is readily amenable to testing in large numbers of patients. Immunization with allogeneic melanoma cells in a variety of forms, including intact cells or shed antigens with bacillus Calmette-Guérin (BCG), viral-modified cell lysates, and cell lysates admixed with complex adjuvants has been associated with antitumor effects.[68–71] Some of these approaches have entered phase III testing in settings of minimal residual disease. The clinical use of allogeneic tumor cell lines engineered to express immunostimulatory molecules has been initiated as well. A small study of immunization with IL-2–secreting melanoma cells revealed the development of inflammatory reactions at metastatic sites.[72] Similar studies of GM-CSF and B7-1 transfected cells are under way, but results have not yet been published.

Although allogeneic cell vaccines can be manufactured with relative ease, substantial evidence in murine models suggests that individual tumors harbor distinct antigenic profiles and that vaccination, at least in some cases, may be most effective using autologous tumor cells.[73] In this context, provocative data have been published demonstrating that patients with early-stage colorectal carcinoma experience a 61% reduction in the risk for recurrent disease after vaccination with irradiated, autologous colorectal carcinoma cells admixed with BCG as postoperative therapy.[74] Studies of vaccination with autologous, hapten-modified tumor cells in conjunction with BCG and cyclophosphamide have also shown provocative antitumor effects,[75] although this approach has yet to be evaluated in a randomized study.

Genetically modified autologous tumor cell vaccines have been introduced into clinical trials. Two small studies have evaluated vaccination with lethally irradiated, autologous melanoma cells engineered to secrete interferon-γ.[76,77] A few minor clinical responses have been observed in patients with metastatic disease. These have been associated with the development of immunoglobulin G2a antibodies directed against melanoma cells in enzyme-linked immunosorbent assay and radioimmunoassay analysis. Initial experience with immunization using irradiated, GM-CSF–secreting autologous renal cell carcinoma cells has been presented.[78] Vaccination sites revealed an influx of macrophages, dendritic cells, eosinophils, and lymphocytes. After but not before vaccination, injections of nontransfected tumor cells stimulated reactions composed of lymphocytes, eosinophils, and macrophages. One partial response of almost a year's duration was observed in a group of three patients receiving an active biologic dose of cells.

The results of a phase I trial of 21 metastatic melanoma patients who were vaccinated with irradiated, autologous melanoma cells engineered to secrete GM-CSF have been published.[79] All patients developed impressive admixtures of dendritic cells, macrophages, eosinophils, and T lymphocytes at vaccination sites and, as a consequence of immunization, intense infiltrates of T lymphocytes and eosinophils in response to injections of irradiated, nontransfected melanoma cells. Moreover, although metastatic lesions resected before vaccination were minimally infiltrated with cells of the immune system in all patients, metastatic lesions resected after vaccination were densely infiltrated with T lymphocytes and plasma cells, and showed extensive tumor destruction (at least 80%), fibrosis, and edema in 11 of 16 patients examined. Lymphocytes harvested from the infiltrated metastases displayed potent cytotoxicity and broad cytokine production in response to autologous melanoma cells. High-titer antibodies recognizing melanoma determinants could be demonstrated in immunoblotting and fluorescence-activated cell sorter analysis.

CONCLUSIONS

Cancer immunology has made substantive progress during the 100 years since Coley's pioneering clinical experiments. The introduction of genetic technologies has revolutionized our understanding of cancer antigens and the host-tumor relationship. The recognition that most, if not all, cancer patients develop antitumor immune responses, together with the striking prognostic importance of lymphocyte infiltrates in early-stage tumors, has rejuvenated the concept of cancer immunosurveillance. If this principle can be rigorously established, then it would imply that the development of clinical cancer necessarily involves the subversion of immune defense mechanisms; perhaps, progressive cancer embodies the exception rather than the rule.

The crafting of several novel vaccination strategies provides inviting opportunities to overcome some of the pathways underlying immune escape. Such interventions are likely to find their broadest application in early-stage disease, however, and thus the assessment of immunotherapies in advanced-stage patients must overcome the myopia of focusing on tumor regression as the ultimate arbiter of biologic activity. Indeed, the failure of autologous bone marrow transplantation to prolong survival of high-risk, early-stage breast cancer patients vividly illustrates the inadequacy of relying on tumor regression as the criteria for selecting therapies that may alter cancer's natural history. The critical objective of early vaccination trials must be the determination of immunogenicity, a characteristic that can now be adequately defined using pathologic and laboratory techniques.

ACKNOWLEDGMENT

Supported by the Cancer Research Institute/Partridge Foundation and CA74886.

REFERENCES

1. Nauts H, Fowler G, Bogatko F. A review of the influence of bacterial infection and of bacterial products (Coley's toxins) on malignant tumors in man. *Acta Med Scand* 1953:5–103.

2. Penn I. Depressed immunity and the development of cancer. *Cancer Detect Prev* 1994;18:241–252.

3. Ehrlich P. Über den jetzigen Stand der Karzinomforschung. In: *The Collected Papers of Paul Ehrlich*, vol. 2. London: Pergamon Press, 1957:550.

4. Thomas L. Discussion of Medawar: reactions to homologous tissue antigens in relation to hypersensitivity. In: Lawrence H, ed. *Cellular and humoral aspects of the hypersensitivity state*. New York: Paul Hoeberg, 1959.

5. Burnet F. Immunological surveillance in neoplasia. *Transplant Rev* 1971;7:3–25.

6. Stutman O. Immunodepression and malignancy. *Adv Cancer Res* 1975;22:261–422.

7. Kaplan D, Shankaran V, Dighe A, et al. Demonstration of an interferon γ-dependent tumor surveillance system in immunocompetent mice. *Proc Natl Acad Sci U S A* 1998; 95:7556–7561.

8. Elmets C, Athar M, Tubesing K, et al. Susceptibility to the biological effects of polyaromatic hydrocarbons is influenced by genes of the major histocompatibility complex. *Proc Natl Acad Sci U S A* 1998;95:14915–14919.

9. Hill A. The immunogenetics of human infectious diseases. *Annu Rev Immunol* 1998;16:593–617.

10. Hicklin D, Wang Z, Arienti F, et al. Beta2-microglobulin mutations, HLA class I antigen loss, and tumor progression in melanoma. *J Clin Invest* 1998;101:2720–2729.

11. Gabrilovich D, Chen H, Girgis K, et al. Production of vascular endothelial growth factor by human tumors inhibits the functional maturation of dendritic cells. *Nat Med* 1996;2:1096–1103.

12. De Visser K, Kast W. Effects of TGF-beta on the immune system: implications for cancer immunotherapy. *Leukemia* 1999;13:1188–1199.

13. Clark W, Elder D, Guerry D, et al. Model predicting survival in stage I melanoma based on tumor progression. *J Natl Cancer Inst* 1989;81:1893–1904.

14. Clemente C, Mihm M, Bufalino R, et al. Prognostic value of tumor infiltrating lymphocytes in the vertical growth phase of primary cutaneous melanoma. *Cancer* 1996;77:1303–1310.

15. Mihm M, Clemente C, Cascinelli N. Tumor infiltrating lymphocytes in lymph node melanoma metastases—a histopathologic prognostic indicator and an expression of local immune response. *Lab Invest* 1996;74:43–47.

16. Andre-Schmutz I, Hindelang C, Benoist C, et al. Cellular and molecular changes accompanying the progression from insulitis to diabetes. *Eur J Immunol* 1999;29:245–255.

17. Wicker L, Todd J, Peterson L. Genetic control of autoimmune diabetes in the NOD mouse. *Annu Rev Immunol* 1995;13:179–200.

18. Naito Y, Saito K, Shiiba K, et al. CD8+ T cells infiltrated within cancer cell nests as a prognostic factor in human colorectal cancer. *Cancer Res* 1998;58:3491–3494.

19. Ohtani H, Naito Y, Saito K, et al. Expression of costimulatory molecules B7-1 and B7-2 by macrophages along invasive margin of colon cancer: a possible antitumor immunity. *Lab Invest* 1997;77:231–241.

20. Townsend A, Bodmer H. Antigen recognition by class I-restricted T-lymphocytes. *Annu Rev Immunol* 1989;7:601–624.

21. Boon T, Cerottini J-C, Van den Eynde B, et al. Tumor antigens recognized by T lymphocytes. *Annu Rev Immunol* 1994;12:337–365.

22. Ikeda H, Ohta N, Furukawa K, et al. Mutated mitogen-activated protein kinase: a tumor rejection antigen of mouse sarcoma. *Proc Natl Acad Sci U S A* 1997;94:6375–6379.

23. Marchand M, van Baren N, Weynants P, et al. Tumor regressions observed in patients with metastatic melanoma treated with an antigenic peptide encoded by gene MAGE-3 and presented by HLA-A1. *Int J Cancer* 1999;80:219–230.

24. Rosenberg S, Yang J, Schwartzentruber D, et al. Immunologic and therapeutic evaluation of a synthetic peptide vaccine for the treatment of patients with metastatic melanoma. *Nat Med* 1998;4:321–327.

25. Cox A, Skipper J, Chen Y, et al. Identification of a peptide recognized by five melanoma-specific human cytotoxic T cell lines. *Science* 1994;264:716–719.

26. Sahin U, Tureci O, Schmitt H, et al. Human neoplasms elicit multiple specific immune responses in the autologous host. *Proc Natl Acad Sci U S A* 1995;92:11810–11813.

27. Old L, Chen Y-T. New paths in human cancer serology. *J Exp Med* 1998;187:1163–1167.

28. Jager E, Chen Y-T, Drijfhout J, et al. Simultaneous humoral and cellular immune response against cancer-testis antigen NY-ESO-1: definition of human histocompatibility leukocyte antigen (HLA)-A2-binding peptide epitopes. *J Exp Med* 1998;187:265–270.

29. Scanlan M, Chen Y-T, Williamson B, et al. Characterization of human colon cancer antigens recognized by autologous antibodies. *Int J Cancer* 1998;76:652–658.

30. Gilboa E. The makings of a tumor rejection antigen. *Immunity* 1999;11:263–270.

31. Houghton A. Cancer antigens: immune recognition of self and altered self. *J Exp Med* 1994;180:1–4.

32. Banchereau J, Steinman R. Dendritic cells and the control of immunity. *Nature* 1998;392:245–252.

33. Guinan E, Gribben J, Boussiotis V, et al. Pivotal role of the B7:CD28 pathway in transplantation tolerance and tumor immunity. *Blood* 1994;84:3261–3282.

34. Caux C, Dezutter-Dambuyant C, Schmitt D, et al. GM-CSF and TNF-α cooperate in the generation of dendritic Langerhans cells. *Nature* 1992;360:258–261.

35. Inaba K, Inaba M, Romani N, et al. Generation of large numbers of dendritic cells from mouse bone marrow cultures supplemented with granulocyte/macrophage colony-stimulating factor. *J Exp Med* 1992;176:1693–1702.

36. Young JW, Inaba K. Dendritic cells as adjuvants for class I major histocompatibility complex–restricted antitumor immunity. *J Exp Med* 1996;183:7–11.

37. Mayordomo JT, Zorina T, Storkus WJ, et al. Bone marrow derived dendritic cells pulsed with synthetic tumor peptides elicit protective and therapeutic anti-tumor immunity. *Nat Med* 1995;1:1297–1302.

38. Zitvogel L, Robbins PD, Storkus WJ, et al. Interleukin-12 and B7.1 co-stimulation cooperate in the induction of effec-

tive antitumor immunity and therapy of established tumors. *Eur J Immunol* 1996;26:1335–1341.

39. Paglia P, Chiodoni C, Rodolfo M, et al. Murine dendritic cells loaded in vitro with soluble protein prime cytotoxic T lymphocytes against tumor antigen in vivo. *J Exp Med* 1996;183:317–322.

40. Boczkowski D, Nair SK, Snyder D, et al. Dendritic cells pulsed with RNA are potent antigen-presenting cells in vitro and in vivo. *J Exp Med* 1996;184:465–472.

41. Lynch D, Andreasen A, Maraskovsky E, et al. Flt3 ligand induces tumor regression and antitumor immune responses *in vivo. Nat Med* 1997;3:625–631.

42. Esche C, Subbotin V, Maliszewski C, Lotze M, et al. Flt3 ligand administration inhibits tumor growth in murine melanoma and lymphoma. *Cancer Res* 1998;58:380–383.

43. Akbari O, Panjwani N, Garcia S, et al. DNA vaccination: transfection and activation of dendritic cells as key events for immunity. *J Exp Med* 1999;189:169–177.

44. Hartmann G, Weiner G, Krieg A. CpG DNA: a potent signal for growth, activation, and maturation of human dendritic cells. *Proc Natl Acad Sci U S A* 1999;96:9305–9310.

45. Suto R, Srivastava PK. A mechanism for the specific immunogenicity of heat shock protein-chaperoned peptides. *Science* 1995;269:1585–1588.

46. Restifo N, Rosenberg S. Developing recombinant and synthetic vaccines for the treatment of melanoma. *Curr Opin Oncol* 1999;11:50–57.

47. O'Hagan D. Recent advances in vaccine adjuvants for systemic and mucosal administration. *J Pharm Pharmacol* 1998;50:1–10.

48. Disis ML, Bernhard H, Shiota FM, et al. Granulocyte-macrophage colony-stimulating factor—an effective adjuvant for protein and peptide-based vaccines. *Blood* 1996;88:202–210.

49. Noguchi Y, Richards EC, Chen YT, et al. Influence of interleukin-12 on p53 peptide vaccination against established Meth A sarcoma. *Proc Natl Acad Sci U S A* 1995;92:2219–2223.

50. Forni G, Fujiwara H, Martino F, et al. Helper strategy in tumor immunology: expansion of helper lymphocytes and utilization of helper lymphokines for experimental and clinical immunotherapy. *Cancer Metast Rev* 1988;7:289–309.

51. Dranoff G, Mulligan RC. Gene transfer as cancer therapy. *Adv Immunol* 1995;58:417–454.

52. Mulligan RC. The basic science of gene therapy. *Science* 1993;260:926–932.

53. Fearon ER, Pardoll DM, Itaya T, et al. Interleukin-2 production by tumor cells bypasses T helper function in the generation of an antitumor response. *Cell* 1990;60:397–403.

54. Gansbacher B, Zier K, Daniels B, et al. Interleukin-2 gene transfer into tumor cells abrogates tumorigenicity and induces protective immunity. *J Exp Med* 1990;172:1217–1224.

55. Tahara H, Zeh HJ, Storkus WJ, et al. Fibroblasts genetically engineered to secrete interleukin-12 can suppress tumor growth and induce antitumor immunity to a murine melanoma in vivo. *Cancer Res* 1994;54:182–189.

56. Cavallo F, Di Carlo E, Butera M, et al. Immune events associated with the cure of established tumors and spontaneous metastases by local and systemic interleukin-12. *Cancer Res* 1999;59:414–421.

57. Dranoff G. Cancer gene therapy: connecting basic research with clinical inquiry. *J Clin Oncol* 1998;16:2548–2556.

58. Dranoff G, Jaffee E, Lazenby A, et al. Vaccination with irradiated tumor cells engineered to secrete murine granulocyte-macrophage colony-stimulating factor stimulates potent, specific, and long-lasting anti-tumor immunity. *Proc Natl Acad Sci U S A* 1993;90:3539–3543.

59. Jager E, Ringhoffer M, Dienes HP, et al. Granulocyte-macrophage-colony-stimulating factor enhances immune responses to melanoma-associated peptides in vivo. *Int J Cancer* 1996;67:54–62.

60. Osterborg A, Yi Q, Henriksson L, et al. Idiotype immunization combined with granulocyte-macrophage colony-stimulating factor in myeloma patients induced type I, major histocompatibility complex-restricted, CD8- and CD4-specific T-cell responses. *Blood* 1998;91:2459–2466.

61. Bendandi M, Gocke C, Kobrin C, et al. Complete molecular remissions induced by patient-specific vaccination plus granulocyte-monocyte colony-stimulating factor against lymphoma. *Nat Med* 1999;5:1171–1177.

62. Hsu F, Benike C, Fagnoni F, et al. Vaccination of patients with B-cell lymphoma using autologous antigen-pulsed dendritic cells. *Nat Med* 1996;2:52–58.

63. Nestle F, Alijagic S, Gilliet M, et al. Vaccination of melanoma patients with peptide- or tumor lysate-pulsed dendritic cells. *Nat Med* 1998;4:328–332.

64. Altman J, Moss P, Goulder P, et al. Direct visualization and phenotypic analysis of virus-specific T lymphocytes in HIV-infected individuals. *Science* 1996;274:94–96.

65. Kitamura K, Livingston PO, Fortunato SR, et al. Serological response patterns of melanoma patients immunized with a GM_2 ganglioside conjugate vaccine. *Proc Natl Acad Sci U S A* 1995;92:2805–2809.

66. Slovin S, Ragupathi G, Adluri S, et al. Carbohydrate vaccines in cancer: immunogenicity of a fully synthetic globo H hexasaccharide conjugate in man. *Proc Natl Acad Sci U S A* 1999;96:5710–5715.

67. Jager E, Ringhoffer M, Karbach J, et al. Inverse relationship of melanocyte differentiation antigen expression in melanoma tissues and CD8+ cytotoxic-T-cell responses: evidence for immunoselection of antigen-loss variants in vivo. *Int J Cancer* 1996;66:470–476.

68. Oratz R, Cockerill C, Speyer J, et al. Induction of tumor-infiltrating lymphocytes in human malignant melanoma metastases by immunization to melanoma antigen vaccine. *J Biol Response Mod* 1989;8:355–358.

69. Mitchell MS, Harel W, Kempf RA, et al. Active-specific immunotherapy for melanoma. *J Clin Oncol* 1990;8:856–869.

70. Hersey P, Edwards A, Coates A, et al. Evidence that treatment with vaccinia melanoma cell lysates (VMCL) may improve survival of patients with stage II melanoma. Treatment of stage II melanoma with viral lysates. *Cancer Immunol Immunother* 1987;25:257–265.

71. Morton DL, Foshag LJ, Hoon DSB, et al. Prolongation of survival in metastatic melanoma after active specific immunotherapy with a new polyvalent melanoma vaccine. *Ann Surg* 1992;216:463–482.

72. Belli F, Arienti F, Sule-Suso J, et al. Active immunization of metastatic melanoma patients with interleukin-2-transduced allogeneic melanoma cells: evaluation of efficacy and tolerability. *Cancer Immunol Immunother* 1997;44:197–203.

73. Basombrio MA. Search for common antigenicity among twenty-five sarcomas induced by methylcholanthrene. *Cancer Res* 1970;30:2458–2462.

74. Vermorken J, Claessen A, van Tinteren H, et al. Active specific immunotherapy for stage II and stage III human colon cancer: a randomised trial. *Lancet* 1999;353:345–350.

75. Berd D, Murphy G, Maguire HC, et al. Immunization with haptenized, autologous tumor cells induces inflammation of human melanoma metastases. *Cancer Res* 1991;51:2731–2734.

76. Abdel-Wahab Z, Weltz C, Hester D, et al. A Phase I clinical trial of immunotherapy with interferon-γ gene-modified autologous melanoma cells. *Cancer* 1997;80:401–412.

77. Nemunaitis J, Bohart C, Fing T, et al. Phase I trial of retroviral vector-mediated interferon (IFN)-gamma gene transfer into autologous tumor cells in patients with metastatic melanoma. *Cancer Gene Ther* 1998;5:292–300.

78. Simons JW, Jaffee EM, Weber CE, et al. Bioactivity of autologous irradiated renal cell carcinoma vaccines generated by ex vivo granulocyte-macrophage colony-stimulating factor gene transfer. *Cancer Res* 1997;57:1537–1546.

79. Soiffer R, Lynch T, Mihm M, et al. Vaccination with irradiated, autologous melanoma cells engineered to secrete human granulocyte-macrophage colony stimulating factor generates potent anti-tumor immunity in patients with metastatic melanoma. *Proc Natl Acad Sci U S A* 1998;95:13141–13146.

34

CYTOKINE AND GROWTH FACTOR AND RECEPTOR DATABASE: BIOLOGIC, MOLECULAR, AND PATHOPHYSIOLOGIC PROPERTIES OF LIGAND-RECEPTOR INTERACTIONS

ERIC SCHAFFER
DENNIS D. TAUB

The term *cytokine* is used to describe a diverse group of soluble proteins and peptides that plays a key role in the regulation of humoral and cellular responses to foreign and self-antigens, viruses, parasites, bacteria, and cancer cells. These proteins and peptides operate at nano- to picomolar concentrations, which modulate the functional activities of individual cells, tissues, or entire organ systems. Cytokines typically mediate their interactions between cells via direct and indirect mechanisms, regulating various immune and homeostatic processes. This cytokine-mediated regulation can occur either locally, through cell-cell interactions within a specific tissue microenvironment, or systemically, via circulating cytokines in a fashion similar to that observed in hormone-mediated responses. The majority of cytokines are pleiotropic in their activities, mediating various biologic responses *in vitro* and *in vivo*. In addition, a number of cytokines mediate overlapping effects on individual cell types yielding identical biologic responses. Such overlapping activities may explain the lack of phenotypical changes in a cytokine-deficient host, in that redundant cytokine mediators may compensate for certain deficiencies. Cytokine expression is strictly regulated, in that only cells in response to an inflammatory or activation signal produce many of these factors. Protein and RNA expression is usually transient and can be regulated at various stages of gene expression and translation. The expression of many cytokines also seems to be regulated differentially, depending on cell type, developmental stage, and age.

The biologic activities of cytokines are mediated through specific membrane receptors, which can be expressed on virtually all cell types. Although some receptors are constitutively expressed, cytokine receptor expression is typically under strict regulation and requires specific activation sig-nals to mediate expression. Cytokine receptor proteins have been shown to share a number of similar and distinct features that separate certain cytokine receptors into specific subfamilies. Many receptors are multisubunit structures that bind specific ligands, which typically mediate an immediate intracellular signal due to their intrinsic kinase activity. Many receptors often share common signal transducing receptor components in the same family, which may explain part of the functional redundancy of several cytokines. This functional and signaling cross talk and the ubiquitous distribution of certain cytokine receptors on various cell types have hindered researchers' efforts at defining responsive cell populations and the critical cell-specific functions of cytokines *in vivo*. Thus, as some receptors may bind more than one cytokine with different affinity, avidity, or both, mediating a distinct signal and subsequently biologic effect, a single receptor may mediate distinct biologic responses on a given cell population at different ligand concentrations. In addition to the presence of cell-associated cytokine receptors, several cytokine receptors have also been shown to be active in a soluble form, in which they may play a biologic role in regulating ligand access to the cells.

Many cytokines have been shown to play critical roles in various pathologic and developmental processes, including septic shock, meningitis, asthma, allergy, delayed-type hypersensitivity responses, various acute phase reactions, wound healing, coagulation, embryogenesis and organ development, angiogenesis, and various neuroregulatory processes. Cytokines are also important regulators of cell division, differentiation, chemotaxis, adhesion, cellular trafficking, cell activation, apoptosis, cell survival, and transformation. Neutralization of certain cytokines has been shown to dampen or eliminate ongoing immune and physiologic responses in certain disease models and systems. Thus, the development of antagonists to cytokine mediators is an incredibly hot topic, with many labs and companies studying various forms of inflammation and inflammatory diseases and their control. In addition, given the potent and selective properties of certain cytokines, individual cytokines have been used for therapeutic interventions into various immunodeficient and neoplastic disease states, tissue transplantation, and hematopoietic dysfunction. A greater overall understanding of cytokines and their receptors in normal and pathophysiologic responses may assist us in controlling and manipulating the beneficial and destructive properties of various cytokines.

The current chapter is an updated and extended version of the previous entry by Casciari and colleagues in 1996. Each section of this database describes specific features of a given cytokine and its corresponding receptor(s), including nomenclature listings for each cytokine, structural features (e.g., molecular weight, primary and secondary structures, stability, precursor size), molecular features (e.g., DNA and RNA size, human-rodent homology, chromosomal localization), transgenic and knockout animal models, functional features (e.g., target cells, biologic responses *in vitro* and *in vivo*), and pathophysiologic associations (e.g., disease and symptom associations). We believe that this up-to-date summary provides a powerful and informative reference for researchers studying cytokines as well as individuals who are new to the area of cytokine research.

ABBREVIATIONS USED IN THIS CHAPTER

AcPL	Interleukin 1 receptor accessory protein-like protein
Ag	Antigen
AIDS	Acquired immunodeficiency syndrome
BCGF	B-cell growth factor
BSF	B-cell stimulatory factor
cAMP	Cyclic adenosine monophosphate
CSH	Chorionic somatomammotropin hormone
CXCR	CXC chemokine receptor
ERK	Extracellular signal-regulated kinase
γc	Common gamma chain
gp	Glycoprotein
HBGF	Heparin-binding growth factor
HIV	Human immunodeficiency virus
HVS	Herpesvirus saimiri
Ig	Immunoglobulin
IL-R	Interleukin receptor
JAK	Janus kinase
kb	Kilobase
LAK	Lymphocyte-activated killer
LPS	Lipopolysaccharide
LT	Lymphotoxin
MAPK	Mitogen-activated protein kinase
MCGF	Mast cell growth factor
MHC	Major histocompatibility complex
MIP	Macrophage inflammatory protein
ND	No data
NF-κB	Nuclear factor-κB
NK	Natural killer
PGE2	Prostaglandin E_2
PMA	Phorbol myristate acetate
Rrp	Receptor-related protein
STAT	Signal transduction and transcription-activating factor
TCGF	T-cell growth factor
Th	T helper cell

NOMENCLATURE DATABASE

Cytokine	Full Name	Synonyms
Interleukins		
IL-1α and β	Interleukin 1α and β	Lymphocyte activating factor, leukocyte endogenous mediator, B-cell activating factor, hemopoietin-1, endogenous pyrogen
IL-1ra	Interleukin 1 receptor antagonist	IL-1 receptor antagonist protein
IL-2	Interleukin 2	TCGF, lymphocyte proliferation factor, thymocyte differentiation factor
IL-3	Interleukin 3	Multi-colony stimulating factor, persisting cell-stimulating factor, MCGF-1, hemopoietic-cell growth factor, burst promoting factor
IL-4	Interleukin 4	BSF-1, BCGF-1, TCGF-2, MCGF-2
IL-5	Interleukin 5	T-cell replicating factor-1, BCGF-II, B-cell maturation factor, eosinophil differentiating factor
IL-6	Interleukin 6	Hybridoma-plasmacytoma growth factor, BSF-2, IFN-β-2, hepatocyte stimulating factor
IL-7	Interleukin 7	Lymphopoietin-1
IL-8	Interleukin 8	Monocyte-derived neutrophil chemotactic factor, granulocyte chemotactic peptide, neutrophil attractant protein-1, neutrophil activating factor, leukocyte adhesion inhibitor
IL-9	Interleukin 9	TCGF-3
IL-10	Interleukin 10	B-cell–derived TCGF, cytokine synthesis inhibitory factor
IL-11	Interleukin 11	
IL-12	Interleukin 12	NK cell stimulatory factor, cytotoxic lymphocyte maturation factor
IL-13	Interleukin 13	NC30, P600
IL-14	Interleukin 14	High-molecular-weight BCGF, BCGF-1
IL-15	Interleukin 15	IL-T
IL-16	Interleukin 16	Lymphocyte chemoattractant factor
IL-17	Interleukin 17	Cytotoxic T-cell lymphocyte-associated Ag 8
IL-18	Interleukin 18	IFN-γ inducing factor
Colony-stimulating factors		
EPO	Erythropoietin	Erythrocyte stimulating factor, hemopoietin
M-CSF	Macrophage colony-stimulating factor	CSF-1
G-CSF	Granulocyte colony-stimulating factor	CSF-3, CSF-β
GM-CSF	Granulocyte-macrophage colony-stimulating factor	CSF-2, CSF-α
LIF	Leukemia inhibitory factor	Embryonal stem cell growth factor, differentiation inhibitory activity, differentiation inducing factor, hepatocyte stimulating factor-3
SCF	Stem cell factor	c-kit ligand, steel factor, steel locus factor, MCGF
Tumor necrosis factors		
TNF-α	Tumor necrosis factor α	Cachectin, macrophage toxin
TNF-β	Tumor necrosis factor β	LT, LT-A
Interferons		
IFN-α	Interferon-α 1 and 2	Type I IFN, leukocyte IFN, lymphoblast IFN, B-cell IFN, buffy coat IFN
IFN-β	Interferon-β	Type I IFN, fibroblast IFN
IFN-γ	Interferon-γ	Type II IFN, immune IFN, acid-labile IFN, macrophage activating factor, T-cell replacing factor
Growth factors		
aFGF	Acidic fibroblast growth factor	Prostatropin, HBGF, beta-endothelial cell growth factor, eye-derived growth stimulatory factor, FGF1
bFGF	Basic fibroblast growth factor	Brain cell–derived growth factor, cartilage-derived growth factor, HBGF-2, FGF2
PDGF	Platelet-derived growth factor	
EGF	Epidermal growth factor	β-Urogastrone
TGF-α	Transforming growth factor α	
TGF-β	Transforming growth factor β1, 2, 3	Cartilage-inducing factor-A or B, BSC-1 growth inhibitor
HGF	Hepatic growth factor	Scatter factor, hematopoietin A
NGF	Nerve growth factor	Neurotrophin
PRL	Prolactin	
GH	Growth hormone	Somatotropin
IGF-I	Insulin-like growth factor I	Somatomedin C
IGF-II	Insulin-like growth factor II	Somatomedin A, multiplication stimulating activity

MOLECULAR STRUCTURE DATABASE 1

Cytokine	No. of Amino Acids in Protein	Molecular Size (kd)		Glycosylation (N, O Linked)	Stable Form (If Not Monomer)
		Theoretic	Observed		
IL-1α	159	17.5	17.5	No	
IL-1β	153	17.4	17.5	No	
IL-1ra	152	17.1	18–22	Yes (N, O)	
IL-2	133	15	15–23	Yes (O)	
IL-3	133	15.4	14–17, 22–34	Yes (N)	
IL-4	129	15, 25	15–20	Yes (N)	
IL-5	115	12	18, 45	Yes (N, O)	Homodimer
IL-6	184	21	21, 23–32	Yes (N, O)	
IL-7	148	17	22, 25	Yes (N)	
IL-8	72 (69, 77, 79)	8	8, 16	No	Homodimer
IL-9	126	14	30–40	Yes (N)	
IL-10	160	18.5	17, 19, 21		Homodimer
IL-11	178	23	23	No	
IL-12	p40:306	34.7	40	Yes (N)	
	p35:197	22.5	35, 75 (total)	Yes (N)	Heterodimer
IL-13	131 or 132	14	10, 12		
IL-14	498 (?)	53	50–60		
IL-15	114		14–15	Yes (N)	
IL-16	130	14	14–17	Yes (N)	Homotetramer
IL-17	155	18	15	Yes (N)	Homodimer
IL-18	157	18	18	No	
EPO	166	18	21, 34, 46	Yes (N, O)	
M-CSF	224, 522	24, 58	45, 68–86, 80–100	Yes (N, O)	Homodimer
G-CSF	174, 177	19, 20	19, 20	Yes (O)	
GM-CSF	127	14	18–32, 23, 45	Yes (N, O)	Homodimer
LIF	202	20	32–67	Yes (N)	
SCF	248			Yes (N, O)	
TNF-α	157	17.4	17, 45–50, 51	No	Homotrimer
TNF-β	171		60–70, 251	Yes (N)	Homotrimer (solution), heterodimer (cell)
IFN-α-1	165–166	20	20, 19–26	No	
IFN-α-2	165–166	20	20	No	
IFN-β	166, 165–172	20	20–25	Yes	
IFN-γ	143, 127–134	17	34–50, 45	Yes (N)	Homodimer
aFGF	134, 140, 155		15.5	No	
bFGF	131, 146, 154, 155, 157	18	18, 21, 22.5, 24	No	
PDGF	125 (A), 241 (B)		28–31, 30, 14–18 (A), 16 (B)		AA, AB, BB dimers
EGF	53		6	No	
TGF-α	50		21, 24, 40, 42	Yes	
TGF-β1	112	12.5	25	Yes (N)	Homodimer or heterodimer
TGF-β2	112	12.5	25	Yes (N)	Homodimer or heterodimer
TGF-β3	112	12.5	25	Yes	Homodimer or heterodimer
HGF	674 (α 440, β 234)	75	76–92	Yes (N)	Heterodimer
NGF	118		26		Homodimer
PRL				Yes	
GH	191, 176		20, 22		
IGF-I	70	8			
IGF-II	67	8			

MOLECULAR STRUCTURE DATABASE 2

Cytokine	Disulfide Bonds No.	Disulfide Bonds Biologic Activity Effect	Isoelectric Point (Estimated)	Binding to: Heparin	Binding to: α_2-Macro-globulin	Primary Structure Similar Protein (%)	Primary Structure Human-Murine Homology
IL-1α	0		5.2, 5.4			IL-1β (26), IL-1ra (19)	62
IL-1β	0		6.8–7.0		Yes	IL-ra (26)	67
IL-1ra			6 (5.2)			IL-1α (19) IL-1β (26)	
IL-2	1	Yes	6.8–8.2 (7.23)				65–70
IL-3	1	Yes		Yes			29
IL-4	3	Yes	10.5			IL-5, IL-13 (30)	50
IL-5	1					IL-4	70
IL-6	2	Yes			Yes	IFN-γ, G-CSF (25.7)	42
IL-7	3	Yes	9				85
IL-8	2	Yes	8.5+	Yes		CXC chemokines	
IL-9			6.2–7.3, 10				56
IL-10	2	Yes	8.1			BCRF-1 (70)	73
IL-11	0		11.5				88
IL-12 p40	4	Yes				IL-6Rα	70
p35	3	Yes				IL-6, G-CSF	60
IL-13	2					IL-4 (25)	58
IL-14						Complement Bb	
IL-15	2						73
IL-16			9.1				85
IL-17						HVS-13 (72)	63
IL-18	0					IL-1β (19)	65
EPO	2		4–5, 9.2				78
M-CSF	3	Yes	3–5				70
G-CSF	2	Yes					73
GM-CSF	2		3.4–4.5	Yes			54
LIF			8.5–9.0				78
SCF							82
TNF-α	1	No	5.3 (7.24)	Yes	Yes	TNF-β (30)	80
TNF-β	0		5.8 (8.92)			TNF-α (30)	75
IFN-α-1	2	Yes				IFN-β (30)	
IFN-α-2	2	Yes				IFN-β	62
IFN-β			8.9, 8.6, 7.8			IFN-α (30)	
IFN-γ	0					IL-6	40
aFGF	0		5.4	Yes		bFGF (55)	95
bFGF	0		9.6–9.8	Yes	Yes		94
PDGF	8	Yes	10.2		Yes		
EGF	3						
TGF-α	3					EGF (40)	90
TGF-β1	4				Yes	TGF-β2 (71), β3 (80)	89
TGF-β2	4					TGF-β1 (71), β3 (80)	89
TGF-β3	4					TGF-β1 (80), β2 (80)	97
HGF	1		Basic			Plasminogen (38)	91
NGF	3				Yes		83
PRL							60
GH	2					CSH (85)	66
IGF-I	3					IGF-II (62), proinsulin (43)	89
IGF-II						Insulin (47)	82

MOLECULAR STRUCTURE DATABASE 3

Cytokine	Secondary Structure	3-Dimensional Structural Characteristics
IL-1α	β-Sheet	14 β-strands, capped β-barrel with threefold symmetry
IL-1β	β-Sheet	12 β-strands, tetrahedron core
IL-1ra	β-Sheet	
IL-2	α-Helix	Four antiparallel α-helical bundles
IL-3	α-Helix	Four α-helix bundles
IL-4	α-Helix	Left-handed four α-helix bundles
IL-5	α-Helix	Helical bundles
IL-6	α-Helix	Four α-helix bundles
IL-7	α-Helix	Four α-helix bundles
IL-8	α-Helix and β-sheet	Dimer of three-strand β-sheet and one α-helix
IL-9		
IL-10	α-Helix	Four α-helix bundles
IL-11		
IL-12		
IL-13	α-Helix	Four α-helix bundles
IL-14		
IL-15	α-Helix	Four α-helix bundles
IL-16	β-Sheet	Six β-sheets
IL-17		
IL-18	β-Sheet	12 β-sheets in β-trefoil
EPO	α-Helix (50%), β-sheet (0%), turns (50%)	
M-CSF		
G-CSF	α-Helix and β-sheet	Four α-helix bundles
GM-CSF	α-Helices (47%) and β-sheets (46%)	Two-strand antiparallel β-sheet with four α-helix open bundles
LIF	α-Helix	Four α-helix bundles
SCF		
TNF-α	β-Sheet	Antiparallel β-sandwich
TNF-β	β-Sheet	Antiparallel β-sandwich
IFN-α-1		
IFN-α-2		
IFN-β		
IFN-γ	α-Helix	Six α-helices, antiparallel dimeric
aFGF	β-Sheet (55%), α-helix (10%)	
bFGF	β-Sheet and α-helix	
PDGF		Antiparallel pairs of β-strands, disulfide bond "knots"
EGF	Antiparallel β-sheets	
TGF-α		
TGF-β		Globular dimer with intrachain disulfide bridge
HGF	Kringle domain	Disulfide-linked heterodimer
NGF	β-Sheet	Antiparallel pair of β-strands form complex
PRL		
GH		
IGF-I		
IGF-II		

MOLECULAR STRUCTURE DATABASE 4

Cytokine	Protease Sensitivity	Stability *In Vitro*	Number of Amino Acids in Precursor		
			Total Molecule	**Signal Sequence**	**Prosequence**
IL-1α			271		
IL-1β	Chymotrypsin, trypsin, V8 protease, elastase		269		
IL-1ra			177	25	
IL-2	Trypsin	>12 mo at 4°C	153	20	
IL-3			152	19	
IL-4	Chymotrypsin, trypsin, V8 protease	>3 mo at 4°C	153	24	
IL-5			135	20	
IL-6			212	28	
IL-7	Trypsin		173	25	
IL-8	Trypsin, chymotrypsin		99	27	
IL-9			144	18	
IL-10			178	18	
IL-11			199	21	
IL-12			328 (p40), 197 (p35)	22 (p40)	
IL-13			151, 152	20	
IL-14					
IL-15			162	48	
IL-16			630		
IL-17			155	19	
IL-18			193		36
EPO	Chymotrypsin, trypsin, V8 protease, endoprotease	>24 mo at 4°C	193	27	
M-CSF	Chymotrypsin, subtilisin; not sensitive: trypsin, papain	6 mo at 4°C	256, 554	32	
G-CSF	Subtilisin, pepsin, trypsin, V8 protease		204, 207	30	
GM-CSF	Not sensitive: chymotrypsin, trypsin		144	17	
LIF			202		
SCF			273	25	
TNF-α	Chymotrypsin, trypsin, V8 protease		233	76	
TNF-β	Not sensitive: chymotrypsin, trypsin, V8 protease		205	34	
IFN-α-1	Chymotrypsin, trypsin, V8 protease				
IFN-α-2	Chymotrypsin, trypsin, V8 protease		188		
IFN-β			187		
IFN-γ					
aFGF	Chymotrypsin, trypsin, V8 protease	1 wk at 4°C	155		
bFGF	Chymotrypsin, trypsin, V8 protease	1 wk at 4°C	155, 157		
PDGF			211 (A), 241 (B)	21	66
EGF			1217, 1207, 1168	23, 26, 29	
TGF-α			160	23	17
TGF-β1	Chymotrypsin, trypsin	6 mo at 4°C	390	23	LAP
TGF-β2		6 mo at 4°C	414	20	LAP
TGF-β3		6 mo at 4°C	412	25	LAP
HGF	Acid, heat labile		728	29	25
NGF			285		
PRL			227		
GH			217		
IGF-I			153, 195		
IGF-II			180		

MOLECULAR STRUCTURE DATABASE 5 (GENOMIC DATA)

Cytokine	Chromosomal Location	No. of Exons	DNA Size (kb)	Messenger RNA Size (kb)	Similar DNA (%)	Human-Murine Homology
IL-1α	2q13–21	7	11	2.1–2.2	IL-1β (45)	
IL-1β	2q13–21	7	7.5	1.8	IL-1α (45)	
IL-1ra	2q13–14.1	4	6.4	1.8		
IL-2	4q26–28	4	3.66, 6	1		76
IL-3	5q23–31	5	2.2	1	GM-CSF	
IL-4	5q23–31	4	10	0.9	IL-13 (30)	
IL-5	5q23–31	4	3	0.9		77
IL-6	7p15	5	5	1.3	G-CSF	65
IL-7	8q12–13		>33, 5.3	1.8, 2.4		81
IL-8	4q12–13	4	5.1	1.8	CXC chemokines	
IL-9	5q23–31	5	4	0.8		67
IL-10	1	5	5.1	2	BCRF-1	81
IL-11	19q13	5	7.5	2.5		86
IL-12	p40:5q31, p35:3p1					p40:70
IL-13	5q31	4	4.6	1.3	IL-4 (30)	66
IL-14						
IL-15	4q31		35	1.2, 1.5		
IL-16	15q26		16	2.6		>90
IL-17	2q31			1.2, 1.9	HVS-13 (75%)	72
IL-18	11q22			1.1		65
EPO	7q21	5	2.1	1.6		80
M-CSF	1p21–13	10	21	1.6, 2.3, 2.5, 4.5		
G-CSF	17q11–12	5	2.2	1.6		69
GM-CSF	5q31	4	2.5	0.7		69
LIF	22q12	3	7.6	4.2		80
SCF	12q22					
TNF-α	6p21	4	3		TNF-β (46)	
TNF-β	6p21	4	3	1.4, 1.6	TNF-α (46)	
IFN-α-1	9p22		1–2	1–2	IFN-β (45)	
IFN-α-2	9p22	1	1–2	1–2	IFN-β (45)	
IFN-β	9p21		0.78	0.78	IFN-α (45)	
IFN-γ	12q14	4	6, 4.5	1.2		40
aFGF	5q31	3	19	4.2		
bFGF	4q26–27	3	38	3.7, 4.5, 7		
PDGF	7 (A), 22 (B)			2.0–2.8 (A), 3.5 (B)		
EGF	4q25–27	24	120	4.9		75
TGF-α	2p13	6	70–100	4.5–4.8		
TGF-β1	19q13		>100	2.5		
TGF-β2	1q41		>100	4.1, 5.1, 6.5, 8		
TGF-β3	14q24		>100	3		
HGF	7q21	4, 18	70	1.3, 2.2, 3, 6		
NGF	1p13					
PRL	6p22				GH (16)	
GH	17q22		67		CSH (90)	
IGF-I	12q22	6		0.7, 1.1, 7.6		
IGF-II	11p15	9	30	1.8–5.3, 2.2–6.0		

RECEPTOR DATABASE 1

Cytokine	Receptor	Common Subunit	Molecular Size (kd)	Total Protein	Extra-cellular	Mem-brane	Intra-cellular	Signal
IL-1	IL-1RI (p80)		80	552	319	20	213	17
	IL-RII (p60)		60	398	331	26	29	12
IL-2	IL-2Rα (p55)	γc: IL-4, 7, 9, 13	140, 45	251	219	19	13	21
	IL-2Rβ (p70)		70–75	525	214, 232	25	286, 86	26
IL-3	IL-3Rα	β: IL-5, GM-CSF	110–130	597 (B)				
IL-4	IL-4R	γc: IL-2, 7, 9, 13	130–140					
IL-5	IL-5Rα	β: IL-3, GM-CSF	151	415				
IL-6	IL-6Rα		80	449	339	28	82	19
	gp130		130	597	305	22	270	
IL-7	IL-7Rα	γc: IL-2, 4, 9, 13	65–75, 150–160	439				
IL-8	IL-8RA (CXCR1)			351				
	IL-8RB (CXCR2)			360				
IL-9	IL-9R	γc: IL-2, 4, 7, 13	64	485	233	21	231	37
IL-10	IL-10R		110					
IL-11	IL-11Rα	gp130: IL-6	50	399	342	26	31	23
IL-12	IL-12Rβ1		110	638	516	31	91	
	IL-12Rβ2		130	835	595	24	216	
IL-13	IL-13Rα1	γc: IL-2, 4, 7, 9	65–70	406	322	24	60	21
	IL-13Rα2	IL-4Rα		354	317	20	17	26
IL-14								
IL-15	IL-15Rα	IL-2Rγ		551	214	25	286	26
	IL-15Rβ	IL-2Rγ		231	175	21	37	32
	IL-15RX	IL-2Rγ	60–65					
IL-16	CD4							
IL-17	IL-17R		98	864	291	21	521	31
IL-18	IL-18Rα (IL-1Rrp1)		80	540	310	22	190	19
	IL-18Rβ (AcPL)			600	342	22	222	14
EPO	EPO-R		66	508	226	22	236	
M-CSF	CSF-1R		150	954	493	25	436	19
G-CSF	G-CSF-R (CSF-3R)		130–150		603	26	183	23
GM-CSF	CSF-2Rα	β: IL-3,5	85, 80–135	409				
LIF	LIF-R	gp130		1097				
SCF								
TNF-α	p55		55	426	182	21	221	29
	p75		75	439	235		174	
TNF-β	LT-βR							
IFN-α-1	Type I	IFN-α, β	110–140	530, 557	409	21	100	
IFN-α-2	α, β (p40)	IFN-α, β	102	331	217	21	77	26
IFN-β								
IFN-γ			90	472	228	23	221, 222	
aFGF	FGF-RI		125	822	330	19	425	30
	FGF-RII		145					
bFGF								
PDGF	α, β		180, 185	120–180				23
EGF			170					24
TGF-α			170					
TGF-β1	I		53–65, 53					
	II		73–95, 70–80	565				
	III		250–350, 300					
	IV		60					
	V		400					
TGF-β2								
TGF-β3								
HGF	c-met		170	190				
NGF				75, 140	426			28, 31
PRL								
GH								
IGF-I	α, β		80 (α), 71 (β), 450 (2α, 2β)					
IGF-II			274		207, 150	23	164	40

RECEPTOR DATABASE 2

Cytokine	Receptor	Receptor Family	Binding Data		Receptor Expression Regulated By
			10^3 sites/cell	K_d (pM)	
IL-1	IL-1RI (p80)	Ig	0–30	200 or 2	Up: mitogens, anti-Ig, TGF-β, IL-4, -10, -13
	IL-1RII (p60)	Ig	0–30	100	Down: IL-1, phorbol esters, retinoic acid
IL-2	IL-2Rα (p55)	Hematopoietin	0.2–100.0	5,000–15,000	Up: Ag stimulation, IL-2, IFN-γ
	IL-2Rβ (p70)			500	
	γc			10	
IL-3	IL-3Rα β_c	Hematopoietin	<1	100; 10,000	Up: IL-2;
					Down: IL-3
IL-4	IL-4R	Hematopoietin	0.1–5.0	20–80	Up: LPS, anti-IgM, IL-4
IL-5	IL-5Rα	Hematopoietin	α: 5	α: 300–2,000	
	β_c		α–β: 0.03–0.40	α–β: 0.5	
IL-6	IL-6Rα, gp130	Hematopoietin	3–24	9.8–740.0	
IL-7	IL-7Rα	Hematopoietin	0.2–20.0	0.2–20.0	
IL-8	IL-8RA (CXCR1), IL-8RB (CXCR2)	Rhodopsin	0.3–20.0	0.1–1.2	Down: IL-8
IL-9	IL-9R	Hematopoietin			
IL-10	IL-10R	IFN	0.1–0.3	50–200	
IL-11	IL-11Rα, gp130	Hematopoietin			
IL-12	IL-12Rβ1	Hematopoietin		Alone: 2,000–50,000	
	IL-12Rβ2			Coexpress: 50–5,000	
IL-13	IL-13Rα1	Hematopoietin	200–3,000	4 nmol per L	
	IL-13Rα2			50	
IL-14					
IL-15	IL-15Rα	Hematopoietin		10	α: Up: IL-2, IFN-γ, anti-CD3, PMA
	IL-15Rβ			1 nmol/L	Down: IL-15
	IL-15RX				
IL-16	CD4				
IL-17	IL-17R				
IL-18	IL-18Rα (IL-1Rrp1), IL-18Rβ (AcPL)	Ig			
EPO	EPO-R	Hematopoietin	0.3–3.0	0.1–1.0	Up: Dimethyl sulfoxide
					Down: Tissue plasminogen activator
M-CSF	CSF-1R	CSF-1R, PDGF-R tyrosine kinase	2–120	0.4	Down: M-CSF, phorbol esters, GM-CSF, IL-3, IL-4, IFN-γ, TNF-α
G-CSF		Hematopoietin	0.03–3.00	100	
GM-CSF	CSF-2Rα	Hematopoietin	0.3–10.0	0.9–10.0	Down: phorbol esters, N-formyl-1-methio-nyl-1-leucyl-1-phenylalamine
LIF					
SCF					
TNF-α	p55	TNF, NGF	0.5–5.0	0.1–1.0, 200–500	Up: IFNs, IL-2, lectins
	p75	TNF, NGF	0.5–5.0	0.1–1.0, 30–70	Down: IL-3, phorbol esters
TNF-β	LT-βR				
IFN-α-1	Type I	IFN	0.2–4.0	100	
IFN-α-2	α, β (p40)	IFN			
IFN-β		IFN			
IFN-γ		IFN	0.2–25.0, 23	100–1,000; 135	Up: IL-1, TNF-α
aFGF	I		2–100, 110–160	10–70, 10–100	Down: IFN-γ
	II		1,000–2,000	2,000–10,000	
bFGF					
PDGF	α, β		50–400	0.1–1.0	
EGF			20–50	0.1 or 3–10	Up: EGF, TGF-α, TNF, TGF-β, retinoic acid, phorbol esters
					Down: PDGF, phorbol esters
TGF-α					
TGF-β1	I	Kinase	4	5–50	Up: retinoic acid, phorbol esters
	II		4	5–50	Down: FGF
	III		100	30–300	
	IV				
	V				
TGF-β2					
TGF-β3					
HGF	c-met		0.2–5.0	5–25, 20–30	
NGF		TNF, NGF		23	
PRL					
GH					
IGF-I	α, β			1,500, 100–10,000	
IGF-II				100–10,000, 1,000	

RECEPTOR DATABASE 3

Cytokine	Receptor	Receptor-Mediated Endocytosis	Tyrosine Kinase Activation	Domain	Signal Transduction	Chromosomal Location	Genomic Size (kb Pairs) Gene	Messenger RNA
IL-1	IL-1RI (p80)	Yes	Yes		Diverse; protein kinase C, MAPK, NF-κB	2q12		5
	IL-1RII (p60)		No					
IL-2	IL-2Rα (p55)		Yes		JAK-1, 3; PI-3 kinase; ERK2; STAT5; Lck, Fyn, Syk	10p14–15	25	1.4,
	IL-2Rβ (p70)	Yes	Yes			22q11–12		3.5
	γc		Yes			Xq13		4
IL-3	IL-3Rα		Yes		MAPK, PI-3 kinase, *ras*, STAT5	X/Y autosomal		
	β					22q12–13		
IL-4	IL-4R		Yes		JAK-1, 3; STAT6	16q11–12		
IL-5	IL-5Rα					3p24–26		
	β							
IL-6	IL-6Rα							5.5
	gp130		Yes					
IL-7	IL-7Rα		Yes		JAK-1, 3; STAT1, 5	5p13		
IL-8	IL-8RA (CXCR1)	Yes			PI-3 kinase, MAPK, PLCβ, *ras*	2q35		
	IL-8RB (CXCR2)							
IL-9	IL-9R		Yes		JAK-1, 3; STAT1, 3			
IL-10	IL-10R		Yes		JAK-1; STAT1, 3, 5	11		
IL-11	IL-11Rα		Yes		JAK; STAT1, 3; MAPK; PI-3 kinase			2
	gp130							
IL-12					JAK-2; STAT3, 4			
IL-13	IL-13Rα1,				STAT6			
	IL-13Rα2							
IL-14								
IL-15	IL-15Rα					10p14–p15		
	IL-15Rβ							
	IL-15RX							
IL-16	CD4							
IL-17	IL-17R							
IL-18	IL-18Rα (IL-1Rrp1),							
	IL-18Rβ (AcPL)							
EPO		Yes			JAK-2, STAT5	19p13		2
M-CSF				Yes	SH-2–containing inositol phosphatase	5q33	58	4.3
G-CSF						1p35		3.0–3.7
GM-CSF	α-β	Yes			JAK-1, 2; STAT5	Xp22 or Yp11		
LIF	LIF-R					5p13		
SCF								
TNF-α	p55	Yes						3
	p75							4.5
TNF-β	LT-βR					12p13	9	
IFN-α-1	Type I	Yes	Yes			21q22.1		
IFN-α-2	α/β (p40)		Yes					4.5 (p40)
IFN-β								
IFN-γ			Yes			6q16–22	30	23
aFGF	I		Yes	Yes				
	II							
bFGF								
PDGF	α, β	Yes	Yes	Yes		5q31–32		
EGF				Yes		7		5.5, 9.5
TGF-α				Yes				
TGF-β1	I			Yes				
	II							
	III							
	IV							
	V							
TGF-β2								
TGF-β3								
HGF	c-met			Yes	ERK1, 2; PI-3 kinase	7q21–31		
NGF				Yes	PI-3 kinase	17		
PRL					STAT5a			
GH					STAT5b			
IGF-I	α, β			Yes	AKT1, 2		150	
IGF-II								

FUNCTIONAL DATABASE 1: PROMINENT EFFECTS

Cytokine	Prominent Effects
IL-1α and β	Inflammation mediator; pleiotropic
IL-1ra	Blocks the inflammatory properties of IL-1
IL-2	Stimulates T-cell growth, T-cell action-induced cell death, induces B-cell proliferation and Ig production
IL-3	Growth factor for hemopoietic progenitors and mast cells
IL-4	Stimulates B, T, and mast cell growth and B-cell antibody production
IL-5	Stimulates eosinophil production, B-cell growth and differentiation
IL-6	Stimulates B-cell Ig production, differentiation of T and hematopoietic progenitor cells, acute phase response
IL-7	Promotes B-cell and T-cell development
IL-8	Chemotactic factor for neutrophils; T, B, and LAK cells; basophils; eosinophils
IL-9	Stimulates growth of Th clones, some leukemic cells and mast cells; enhances B-cell Ig production
IL-10	Suppresses T-cell proliferation and cytokine production by Th1, immunosuppression
IL-11	Stimulates hematopoietic progenitors, megakaryocyte maturation, hybridoma growth
IL-12	Activates T and NK cells; induces differentiation of T to Th1 cell phenotype
IL-13	Induces B-cell proliferation and Ig production; suppresses inflammatory cytokine production by monocytes
IL-14	Induces proliferation of activated B cells and inhibition of Ig secretion
IL-15	Stimulates cytotoxic T lymphocytes and LAK; increases cytotoxicity of T and NK cells, chemotactic factor for T cells
IL-16	Chemotactic for T cells, eosinophils, monocytes; suppresses Ag-responsive proliferation
IL-17	Proinflammatory; promotes hematopoietic progenitors; induces stroma to produces inflammatory cytokines
IL-18	Induces IFN-γ and proinflammatory cytokine production by T cells; enhances NK-cell lytic activity
EPO	Induces erythrocyte production
M-CSF	Stimulates proliferation and differentiation of hematopoietic progenitors to macrophages
G-CSF	Stimulates proliferation and differentiation of hematopoietic progenitors to granulocytes
GM-CSF	Stimulates survival, proliferation, differentiation, and function of hematopoietic progenitors
LIF	Induces differentiation of myeloid leukemia cells, acute phase protein response
SCF	Stimulates growth and development of mast cells and hematopoietic stem cells
TNF-α	Major inducer of inflammation, tumor cytolysis, cachexia, fever
TNF-β	Proinflammatory mediator; activates neutrophils, macrophages, fibroblasts; cytotoxic to tumor cells
IFN-α-1,2	Inhibits viral replication
IFN-β	Inhibits viral replication
IFN-γ	Inhibits viral replication; activates macrophages and monocytes; antiproliferative; potentiates IFN-α, β
aFGF	Mitogenic for fibroblasts; promotes angiogenesis; neurotrophic
bFGF	Mitogenic for fibroblasts; promotes angiogenesis; neurotrophic
PDGF	Mitogenic for fibroblasts; stimulates fibronectin production; promotes healing and cytokine release at wounds
EGF	Stimulates cell growth in culture
TGF-α	Stimulates anchorage-independent tumor growth; mitogenic
TGF-β	Stimulates growth of some tumors, cell proliferation; suppresses leukocyte and other cell activation
HGF	Stimulates hepatocyte growth; regulates placental growth and development
NGF	Growth and differentiation factor for neurons
PRL	Growth and differentiation factor; promotes lactation
GH	Promotes cell growth and differentiation, anabolic effects; suppresses insulin; induces IGF-I
IGF-I	Growth and differentiation factor; anabolic effects, inhibits apoptosis, mediates GH actions, neuroprotective
IGF-II	Promotes prenatal growth; promotes cell growth and differentiation

FUNCTIONAL DATABASE 2: POTENTIAL CLINICAL APPLICATIONS

Cytokine	Key *In Vivo* Effects and Potential Clinical Applications
IL-1	Side effects include flulike symptoms, hypotension, acute phase response, capillary leak syndrome; potential antitumor agent, proinflammatory agent, or hematopoiesis stimulator
IL-1ra	Potential antiinflammatory agent
IL-2	Used as antitumor agent to expand tumor-infiltrating lymphocyte and LAK and induce tumor regression; slows CD4$^+$ T-cell loss in AIDS
IL-3	May repopulate bone marrow, expand stem cells; potential antagonists to treat leukemias, allergic diseases
IL-4	Induces Th2 development; may be used as antitumor or antiinflammatory agent
IL-5	Stimulates eosinophil development; potential antitumor agent
IL-6	Causes fever, acute phase reactions, cachexia; potential antagonists to treat rheumatoid arthritis, osteoporosis
IL-7	Stimulates lymphopoiesis; may be immunostimulant
IL-8	Induces neutrophil infiltration; inhibitors may treat inflammation, acute respiratory distress syndrome, psoriasis, rheumatoid arthritis, gout
IL-9	May be used to enhance hematopoiesis
IL-10	Immunosuppressive; potential antiinflammatory agent
IL-11	Promotes hematopoiesis; potentially enhances thrombopoiesis and gastrointestinal tract healing, reduces myelosuppression
IL-12	Potential antitumor or antiinfection agent; delays AIDS immunosuppression
IL-13	Potential antitumor agent; antagonist may be used to block allergy and asthma
IL-14	Potential use as adjuvant in combination with other biologic response modifiers
IL-15	Antitumor and infection activities; antagonist may decrease rheumatoid arthritis and increase engraftment
IL-16	Promotes CD4$^+$ T-cell growth, suppresses HIV; inhibitors may suppress allergic asthma or rheumatoid arthritis
IL-17	Promotes hematopoiesis, some experimental autoimmune disease, graft rejection, and tumorigenicity
IL-18	Antiinfection activity; may be antitumor agent
EPO	Increases erythrocyte production; used to treat certain anemias
M-CSF	Inhibits certain immunity and inflammatory activities; may be used in hematopoiesis and leukemia treatment
G-CSF	Increases neutrophils; may enhance antitumor or antiinfection regimens, treat neutropenia
GM-CSF	Potentiates immune responses; potential treatment for bone marrow transplants, neutropenia, and AIDS
LIF	May be useful in treating certain leukemias, stimulating platelet formation, bone marrow transplants
SCF	Promotes hematopoietic development; may be useful in bone marrow transplants, treating HIV
TNF-α	Activity against virus, tumors, bacteria, malaria; side effects; antagonists may treat arthritis, septicemia
TNF-β	Proinflammatory and antitumor effects; potential antimalarial and antiviral agent; immunosuppression
IFN-α-1, 2	Activity against virus, tumors, bacteria; serious side effects; used to treat hepatitis, herpes, Kaposi's sarcoma
IFN-β	Activity against virus, tumors, bacteria; side effects; used to treat hepatitis, herpes, multiple sclerosis, Kaposi's sarcoma
IFN-γ	Antiviral, antitumor, and antimicrobial effects; potential against tumors, infection, arthritis
aFGF, bFGF	Angiogenic; promotes wound healing; may be used in treating Alzheimer's or Parkinson's disease
PDGF	Promotes wound healing and may promote cell-mediated immunity
EGF	Promotes wound healing, cell growth in gastrointestinal tract, angiogenesis, and liver regeneration
TGF-α	Promotes wound healing and angiogenesis; antagonists may prevent tumor growth and psoriasis
TGF-β1, 2, 3	Promotes wound healing, angiogenesis, stromal growth and development; pro- and antiinflammatory effects
HGF	Involved in liver regeneration, potential target to suppress tumor metastasis and invasion
NGF	May be useful in nerve regeneration and growth
PRL	Promotes lactation, alters endometrial differentiation; potential immune adjuvant
GH	Anabolic effects; may help to decrease catabolism in patients and diabetogenic side effects, and treat dwarfism
IGF-I, II	Anabolic effects; may improve muscle mass in catabolic patients, treat insulin resistance

FUNCTIONAL DATABASE 3: KNOCKOUT EFFECTS

Cytokine	Effects of Disruption of Cytokine or Receptor Genes on Cells or Host
IL-1α	Cytokine: normal growth.
	Receptor (type I): normal response to LPS, reduced IL-6 production.
IL-1β	Cytokine: fever suppression.
IL-1ra	Cytokine: retarded growth, increased fever response, rheumatoid arthritis–like symptoms.
IL-2	Cytokine: ulcerative colitis observed. Possible deficiency in apoptosis in autoimmune T cells. No effects seen on lymphoid development or proliferation.
IL-3	Cytokine: fewer mast cells, nematode resistance.
	Receptor (β$_c$): lung pathology, reduced eosinophil production.
IL-4	Cytokine: deficient in Ig production and Th2 response.
	Receptor: reduced IL-4 and IL-13 response.
IL-5	Cytokine: reduced eosinophil response, loss of acute graft destruction.
IL-6	Cytokine: deficient in acute phase proteins, increased susceptibility to *Listeria*.
IL-7	Cytokine: increased precursor B-cell apoptosis.
	Receptor: deficient lymphopoiesis.
IL-8	Receptor: deficient neutrophil chemotaxis, accumulation of neutrophils and B cells in lymphoid organs.
IL-9	ND.
IL-10	Cytokine: chronic enterocolitis, deficiency in immune suppression, increased Th1 response.
IL-11	Receptor: impaired decidual and fetoplacental development.
IL-12	Cytokine: impaired IFN-γ and CD8$^+$ T-cell responses.
IL-13	Cytokine: decreased IL-5 and IgE production, reduced eosinophil activity, increased IFN-γ, decreased Th2 development, decreased nematode resistance.
IL-14	ND.
IL-15	Cytokine: lymphopenia, reduced NK, NK T cells, intraepithelial lymphocyte, and CD8$^+$ T cells.
	α Receptor: lymphopenia, reduced proliferation and homing, fewer NK, NK T cells, CD8$^+$ T, memory T, and intraepithelial lymphocyte cells.
IL-16	ND.
IL-17	ND.
IL-18	Cytokine: increased susceptibility to *Leishmania* and mycobacterial infection, defective NK and Th1 responses.
EPO	Cytokine: lethal.
M-CSF	ND.
G-CSF	Cytokine: neutropenia, increased susceptibility to *Listeria*.
GM-CSF	Cytokine: accumulation of surfactants in lung, no effect on hematopoiesis.
LIF	Cytokine: reduced nerve stimulation.
SCF	ND.
TNF-α	Receptor: resistant to LPS plus galactosamine, increased susceptibility to *Listeria*.
TNF-β	Cytokine: lack of lymph nodes and Peyer's patches.
IFN-α	Receptor: increased susceptibility to viral infection.
IFN-β	Receptor: increased susceptibility to viral infection.
IFN-γ	Cytokine: increased susceptibility to mycobacteria, but not influenza infection, defects in immune cell function.
	Receptor: increased susceptibility to lymphocytic choriomeningitis virus (but not to vesicular stomatitis virus), mycobacterial infection, and *Listeria*. Altered antibody response, but no deficiency in Th1 response or MHC class-II Ag expression.
aFGF	Cytokine: impaired hematopoiesis.
bFGF	Cytokine: impaired wound healing, brain development, hematopoiesis.
PDGF	Cytokine: impaired placental development.
	Receptor: impaired neural development.
EGF	Cytokine: impaired mammary development, neonatal development.
TGF-α	Cytokine: reduced pulmonary fibrosis in response to lung injury.
TGF-β	Cytokine: multifocal inflammatory disease; increased expression of adhesion molecules and MHC-II.
HGF	Cytokine or receptor: lethal.
NGF	Cytokine: lethal.
PRL	Cytokine or receptor: no apparent pathology.
GH	Cytokine: dwarfism.
	Receptor: reduced IGF-I, fertility, growth.
IGF-I	Cytokine: lethality, impaired growth and development.
IGF-II	Cytokine: lethal.

FUNCTIONAL DATABASE 4: PRODUCER CELLS

Cytokine	Producer Cells
IL-1α, β, ra	Monocytes, macrophages, B cells, T cells, endothelial cells, keratinocytes, astrocytes, kidney mesangial cells
IL-2	Activated CD4+ T; some CD8+ T, NK cells; some B-cell lines
IL-3	T, NK, mast cells, eosinophils
IL-4	Th2, Th0, CD8+ T, CD4+ T, γδ T, mast, stroma cells; basophils
IL-5	Th2 cells, T-cell clones, activated mast cells, Epstein-Barr virus–transformed B cells
IL-6	Macrophages; Th2, T, B, endothelial, gingival mononuclear, tumor, bone marrow stroma cells; keratinocytes; fibroblasts
IL-7	Bone marrow stromal cells, spleen, thymus, liver, gut epithelium
IL-8	Monocytes; fibroblasts; endothelial cells; epithelial cells; neutrophils; T, NK, tumor cells; granulocytes; phagocytes; melanoma; hepatoma; astrocytoma; glioblastoma; keratinocytes; synovial cells; chondrocytes
IL-9	T, Th2 cells; certain lymphomas
IL-10	Th2, activated T, B, mast cells; monocytes; macrophages; Epstein-Barr virus–transformed B cells; melanoma; colon carcinoma
IL-11	Bone marrow–derived stromal cells, fibroblasts, epithelial cells
IL-12	Monocytes, macrophages, dendritic cells, neutrophils, keratinocytes, microglia, B-lymphoblastoid cells
IL-13	Th2, Th0, Th1, CD45RA+ T, CD45RO+ T, CD8+ T, mast cells; basophils; eosinophils; keratinocytes
IL-14	Activated T-, some B-cell lymphomas
IL-15	Monocytes, macrophages, dendritic cells, epithelial cells, bone marrow stroma, fibroblasts, leukemia lines
IL-16	CD8+ T, CD4+ T ; eosinophils; mast cells; fibroblasts; bronchial epithelial cells of asthmatics
IL-17	CD4+ activated memory (CD45RO+) T cells, Th1-Th0
IL-18	Monocytes, macrophages, keratinocytes, pituitary, adrenal, osteoblasts
EPO	Renal cells, hepatocytes, tumor cells
M-CSF	Stoma cells; macrophages; fibroblasts; epithelial cells; T, B, bone marrow stroma cells; endothelial cells; keratinocytes
G-CSF	Fibroblasts, macrophages, endothelial cells, tumor cells, stromal cells
GM-CSF	T cells, macrophages, fibroblasts, endothelial cells, mast cells
LIF	T cells, tumor cells
SCF	Fibroblasts
TNF-α	Macrophages, NK, mast cells, monocytes, T cells, neutrophils, fibroblasts, myocytes, tumor cells, epidermal cells, granulosa cells
TNF-β	NK, T, B cells, myelomas, astrocytes, Hodgkin's and Reed-Sternberg cells
IFN-α	Leukocytes, B, T cells, macrophages, natural interferon-producing cells
IFN-β	Fibroblasts, epithelial cells, sarcomas
IFN-γ	NK, T cells
aFGF	Pituitary gland, cartilage, brain, kidney, adrenal gland, chondrosarcoma, retina
bFGF	Pituitary gland, cartilage, retina, brain, kidney, adrenal gland, chondrosarcoma, macrophages, injured muscle
PDGF	Platelets, macrophages, endothelial cells, muscle, fibroblasts, tumor cells, megakaryocytes, glial cells, astrocytes, myoblasts, mesangial cells, epithelial cells
EGF	Brain, kidney, adrenal medulla, salivary gland
TGF-α	Platelets, placenta, macrophages, embryos, kidney, liver, pituitary cells, brain, keratinocytes, epithelial cells, hepatocytes, gastric mucosal cells, Sertoli's cells, psoriatic epidermis, tumor cells
TGF-β	Platelets, T, B cells, placenta, endothelial cells, muscle, fibroblasts, macrophages, kidney, thymus, bone, keratinocytes, Sertoli's cells, granulosa cells, carcinoma cells, leukemia cells, glioblastoma cells, myocytes, chondrocytes, lung, submaxillary gland, brain
HGF	Fibroblasts, macrophages, platelets, endothelial, mesenchymal and mesodermal cells, placenta
NGF	Neurons, fibroblasts, gliomas
PRL	Pituitary cells, endometrium
GH	Pituitary cells, T cells
IGF-I	Hepatocytes, macrophages, leukocytes, muscle, placenta
IGF-II	Placenta, hepatocytes, macrophages, lymphocytes, muscle, Wilms' tumor cells

FUNCTIONAL DATABASE 5: REGULATION BY CYTOKINES

Cytokine	Cytokine Regulates Production (Up or Down) of
IL-1α, β	Up: IL-1, IL-2, IL-4, IL-5, IL-6, IL-8, IL-11, TNF-α, IFN-β, IFN-γ, M-CSF, G-CSF, GM-CSF, PDGF, NGF, serotonin, prostaglandins, procoagulant, plasminogen activator
IL-1ra	Down: IL-1α, IL-1β, IL-2, IL-8, TNF-α
IL-2	Up: IFN-γ, IL-1, IL-2, IL-4, GM-CSF, TNF-α, TNF-β, PGE2, thromboxane B2
IL-3	Up: IL-1, IL-6, IL-8, TNF-α
IL-4	Up: IL-4
	Down: IFN-γ, IL-1, IL-1ra, IL-6, IL-8, IL-10, IL-12, TNF, GM-CSF, G-CSF
IL-5	
IL-6	Up: NF-IL-6, PDGF
	Down: TNF-α
IL-7	Up: IL-2
IL-8	
IL-9	
IL-10	Down: IFN-γ, TNF-α, IL-1, IL-2, IL-6, IL-8, IL-12, GM-CSF, G-CSF
IL-11	
IL-12	Up: IFN-γ, IL-2, TNF-α, GM-CSF
IL-13	Up: IL-1ra
	Down: IL-1ra, IL-1α, IL-1β, IL-6, IL-8, IL-12, TNF-α, MIP1α, MIP1β, MIP-3
IL-14	
IL-15	Up: IFN-γ, TNF-α, GM-CSF
IL-16	
IL-17	Up: IL-1β, IL-6, IL-8, G-CSF, PGE2, MCP-1, TNF-α
IL-18	Up: IFN-γ, IL-2, GM-CSF, IL-1β, IL-8, TNF-α
	Down: IL-10
EPO	
M-CSF	Up: IL-6
G-CSF	
GM-CSF	Up: IL-1, IL-6, M-CSF, G-CSF, TNF-α
LIF	
SCF	
TNF-α	Up: IL-1, IL-6, IL-8, LIF, TNF-α, M-CSF, G-CSF, GM-CSF, PDGF, NGF, IFN-β, IFN-γ, collagenase, PGE2, oncogene expression, HLA, intercellular adhesion molecule-1
	Down: activated protein C, oncogenes
TNF-β	Up: IL-1, IL-4, IL-8, TNF-α, G-CSF, GM-CSF, PDGF, IFN-β, PGE2, intercellular adhesion molecule-1
	Down: activated protein C
IFN-α-1	Up: IL-1, GM-CSF, TNF-β
	Down: IL-8
IFN-α-2	
IFN-β	Up: IL-1, IL-6, GM-CSF, TNF-α, TNF-β
	Down: IL-8
IFN-γ	Up: IL-1, IL-8, IL-12, M-CSF, GM-CSF, TNF-α, TNF-β, MHC Ag
	Down: IL-1, TNF-α, IL-6, IL-8, IL-4
aFGF	Up: NGF, stromelysin gene expression
	Down: TGF-β
bFGF	Up: NGF, stromelysin gene expression, enhances HGF function
	Down: TGF-β
PDGF	Up: collagen, fibronectin, TGF-β, phospholipase A$_2$, prostaglandins, IFN-γ, monocyte chemotactic and activating factor, growth-related oncogene, IL-6, M-CSF, PDGF
EGF	Up: PDGF, NGF, TGF-β
	Down: TGF-β
TGF-α	
TGF-β	Up: IL-6, IL-1ra, cellular collagen, EGF, TNF, IL-1, IL-8, integrins, collagenase, monokines, NGF, TGF-β
	Down: IL-1, stromelysin gene expression, EGF, TNF-α, IgM, IgG, TGF-β
HGF	Up: collagen, fibronectin, IL-6, TNF-α, chemokines, protease in tumors
NGF	Up: TGF-β
PRL	Up: thymulin
GH	Up: IGF-I
IGF-I	Up: TNF-α, skeletal muscle mitogen, smooth muscle aortic elastin, cardiac β-myosin heavy chain
IGF-II	Up: skeletal muscle mitogen, smooth muscle aortic elastin, cardiac β-myosin heavy chain

FUNCTIONAL DATABASE 6: REGULATION OF CYTOKINES

Cytokine	Secretion or Function of Cytokine Regulated (Up or Down) by
IL-1α, β	Up: IL-1, IL-2, IL-3, IFN-α, IFN-β, IFN-γ, TNF-α, TNF-β, TGF-β, PMA, GM-CSF, Calcium ionophore, indomethacin Down: IL-2, -3, -4, -10, -13, IFN-γ, TGF-β, corticosteroids, prostaglandins, dexamethasone, prednisolone, cAMP
IL-1ra	Up: IL-4, IL-10, TGF-β, immune complexes, Ig-coated surfaces Down: IL-13
IL-2	Up: mitogens, phorbol esters, calcium ionophores, IL-1, IL-2, IL-7, cimetidine, indomethacin Down: AIDS, 1,26-D3, FK-506, cAMP, anti-CD2, hydrocortisone, prostaglandins, cyclosporin-A
IL-3	Up: Ags, mitogens, Fc receptor binding Down: cyclosporin-A, glucocorticoids
IL-4	Up: IL-1, IL-2, IL-4, PAF, mitogens, antigenic peptides, anti-CD3, anti–T-cell receptor, calcium ionophores + TPA Down: IFN-γ, TGF-β, cyclosporin-A
IL-5	Up: IL-1, IL-4, phorbol ester, immune complexes, calcium ionophores, concanavalin A, anti–T-cell receptor
IL-6	Up: IL-1, IL-3, PDGF, TNF-α, TGF-β, mitogen, viruses, cAMP, cycloheximide, TPA, IFN-β, forskolin, phytohemagglutinin + TPA, LPS Down: IL-3, IL-4, IL-10, IFN-γ, dexamethasone
IL-7	Up: LPS
IL-8	Up: IL-1, TNF, LPS, IL-3, PMA + IL-2, IFN-γ, PHA, uric acid, phorbol esters, viruses, poly(rI):rC, concanavalin A Down: TGF-β, IL-4, IL-10, glucocorticoids, IFN-α, IFN-β, IFN-γ, FK506
IL-9	Up: PHA, anti-CD3, phorbol esters, calcium ionophores, viruses
IL-10	Up: concanavalin A, LPS Down: IL-4
IL-11	Up: IL-1, TGF-β, prostaglandins, calcium ionophore Down: IL-4, dexamethasone
IL-12	Up: LPS, viruses, IFN-γ, phorbol ester, calcium ionophore, GM-CSF Down: IL-10, IL-4, IL-13, TGF-β, PGE2
IL-13	Up: anti-CD3, FceRI cross-linking of mast cells and basophils
IL-14	
IL-15	Up: IFN-γ, IL-1β, TNF-α, LPS, ultraviolet B radiation, virus, bacteria
IL-16	Up: histamine, serotonin, anti-CD3, Ag, mitogen
IL-17	Down: PGE2, cAMP
IL-18	
EPO	Up: hypoxia, anemia, salts, cAMP, 3-isobutyryl-1-methylxanthine Down: hyperoxia, polycythemia
M-CSF	Up: LPS, TNF-α, IL-1, phorbol esters, GM-CSF, IFN-γ, PDGF, bacteria, viruses, parasites
G-CSF	Up: IL-1, TNF-α, TNF-β, GM-CSF, endotoxin Down: PGF2, IL-4, IL-10
GM-CSF	Up: IL-1, TNF-α, TNF-β, bacterial endotoxin, PMA, IFN, TNF, IL-2, retroviruses, concanavalin A, calcium ionophore, anti-CD3 Down: cycloheximide, IL-4, IL-10
LIF	Up: IL-1α, TGF-β, LPS, EGF, PMA, TNF-α, retinoic acid
SCF	
TNF-α	Up: TNF-α, TNF-β, IL-1,-3, IFN-α, IFN-β, IFN-γ, GM-CSF, TGF-β, IGF-I, phorbol esters, endotoxin, viruses, bacteria, indomethacin, PAF Down: IL-3, -4, -10, -6, TGF-β, cyclosporin, dexamethasone, prostaglandins
TNF-β	Up: IL-1, IL-2, phorbol esters, mitogens, viruses, thymosin-1, anti-CD3, IFN-α, IFN-β, IFN-γ, TNF-α, TNF-β, Ags Down: IL-4, cyclosporin-A
IFN-α	Up: bacterial products, viruses, mitogens Down: HIV infection
IFN-β	Up: bacteria, viruses, IL-1, TNF-α, TNF-β Down: HIV infection
IFN-γ	Up: IL-2, IL-12, PDGF, Ags, mitogens, PHA, anti-CD16, activated macrophages, TNF-α Down: HIV, 1,25-D3, dexamethasone, cyclosporin-A, IL-4, IL-10
aFGF	
bFGF	Up: TNF-α, TNF-β, IL-1
PDGF	Up: HBGF-1, TPA, IL-1, IL-6, TNF-α, TNF-β, TGF-β, PDGF, EGF, LPS, endotoxin, TPA Down: forskolin, 8-bromo-cAMP, cholera toxin, PGE1
EGF	Up: TGF-β, testosterone Down: TGF-β, estrogen
TGF-α	Up: estrogen, TGF-α, phorbol esters, *ras* oncogene, viruses, LPS
TGF-β	Up: steroids, retinoids, TGF-β, phorbol esters, EGF, NGF, TNF-α, TNF-β, oncogenes, concanavalin A, sac B, 1,26-D3, IL-1 Down: dexamethasone, EGF, TGF-β, retinoids, FGF, follicle-hormone
HGF	Up: PGE2 Down: cortisol, HGF-variant
NGF	Up: steroids, catechols, IL-1, aFGF, bFGF, TNF-α, EGF, TGF-β, prostaglandins
PRL	Up: IL-1, IL-2, IL-6, cortisol Down: IFN-γ, endothelin-3
GH	Down: IGF-I, GH
IGF	Up: growth hormone, acute phase reaction

FUNCTIONAL DATABASE 7: EFFECTS ON VARIOUS CELL TYPES

A or A–	Activates, stimulates, or inhibits cell	M	Affects cell morphology or adhesiveness
C or C–	Affects cell mobility or chemotaxis	P or P–	Promotes or inhibits cell growth or proliferation
D or D–	Promotes or inhibits cell differentiation	S or S–	Induces or inhibits cell secretions
I or I–	Promotes or inhibits antibody production or switching		

Cytokine	T cells	B cells	NK cells	LAK cells	Phagocytes	Granulocytes	Hematologic/ Stem
IL-1	P, P–	I, P	A		A, S		
IL-1ra					A–, M, S–		
IL-2	A, C, P, S	A, D, I, P, S	A, P, S	A	A	P, S	D
IL-3					A	A, P, S	D, P
IL-4	A, D, P	A, I, I–, P, P–	P, S–	A	A, A–, D, M	A–, S–	
IL-5		A, D, I				C, D, P	D, P
IL-6	D, P	I			D		D
IL-7	P	P				A	D
IL-8	C	C, C–		C		A, C, M, P, S	D–
IL-9	P	I					D, P
IL-10	C, M, P, S–	A, D, M, P	S, S–		M, S–		P
IL-11		P				S–	D, P
IL-12	A, D, P, S	I	A, P, S	A	A, S		D, P
IL-13	S–	A, I, P, S			C, D, M, S, S–	M, P	D, D–, P
IL-14		I–, P					
IL-15	A, C, P	P	A, C, P, S	A, P		P	
IL-16	A, C, M, P, P–				C, M	C, M	
IL-17							
IL-18	A, S	A, I–	A				
EPO							D, P
M-CSF					P, S	P	P
G-CSF						M, P	P
GM-CSF					A, C, P	A, C, M, P, S	P
LIF					S		D
SCF	P		P		P	A, C, D, M, P	D, M, P
TNF-α	P, S	D, I, P			A, D, C, S	A, C, M	D, P–
TNF-β	P, S	A, P			D, S	A, C, M	P–
IFN-α	P–	I–, P–	A, A–	A, A–	A, P–, S		D, P–
IFN-β	P–	P–	A		A, S		
IFN-γ	A, C	A, D, I, P	A		A	C	
aFGF							
bFGF						P	
PDGF	S	S			C, P, S	A, C, P–	
EGF							
TGF-α							
TGF-β	C, P–, S	C, I–, P–, S	A–, P–	A–, P–	C, P–, S	C, M, P–	D–, P, P–
HGF							
NGF							
PRL	A, P				A		P, D
GH	D	D, P			A		P, D
IGF	D, P	D, P	A		A, S		P, D

FUNCTIONAL DATABASE 8: EFFECTS ON VARIOUS CELL TYPES

A or A–	Activates, stimulates, or inhibits cell	M	Affects cell morphology or adhesiveness
C or C–	Affects cell mobility or chemotaxis	P or P–	Promotes or inhibits cell growth or proliferation
D or D–	Promotes or inhibits cell differentiation	S or S–	Induces or inhibits cell secretions
I or I–	Promotes or inhibits antibody production or switching		

Cytokine	Endothelial	Hepatocytes	Epithelial	Fibroblasts	Keratinocytes	Muscle	Tumor
IL-1	M, S	S		P, S	P, S	P, S	P
IL-1ra							
IL-2							
IL-3							
IL-4							
IL-5							
IL-6		A, S			P		P
IL-7							
IL-8	M			S–	P		C
IL-9							P
IL-10							
IL-11					P		
IL-12							P–
IL-13	M, S–		S		S		
IL-14							
IL-15						P	
IL-16							
IL-17	S		S	S			
IL-18							
EPO					M, P		
M-CSF							P–
G-CSF	C, P						P
GM-CSF							
LIF	M	A, S					D, P, P–
SCF							
TNF-α	M, P–, S, S–	S–		P, S			P–
TNF-β	M, P–, S			P, S	P–		P–
IFN-α				P–			P–
IFN-β							P–
IFN-γ							P–
aFGF	C, D, P			C, P, S	P	P	C, M
bFGF	C, D, P			C, P, S	P	C, P	P
PDGF	P			C, M, P, S		C, P	C, P
EGF			P	P			C, P
TGF-α	P		P	S			
TGF-β	P, P–	P–	C–, P–	C, P, S	P–	C, P–	C, P
HGF	C, M, P	P, S	C, D, M, P				C, M, P–, S
NGF							P
PRL							P
GH				P		P	P
IGF				P		P, S	

SUGGESTED READING

General Review References

Casciari JJ, et al. Tabular lexicon of cytokine structure and function. In: Chabner BA, Longo DL, eds. *Cancer chemotherapy and biotherapy*, 2nd ed. Philadelphia: Lippincott–Raven Publishers, 1996.

Delves PJ, Roitt IM, ed. *Encyclopedia of immunology*. San Diego: Academic Press, 1998.

Paul WE, ed. *Fundamental immunology*. San Diego: Lippincott, Williams & Wilkins, 1998.

Thomson A, ed. *The cytokine handbook*. San Diego: Academic Press, 1998.

Interleukin 1α and β

Borth W, Luger TA. Identification of alpha 2-macroglobulin as a cytokine binding plasma protein. Binding of interleukin-1 beta to "F" alpha 2-macroglobulin. *J Biol Chem* 1989;264:5818.

Dinarello CA. Interleukin-1. *Cytokine Growth Factor Rev* 1997; 8:253.

Dower SK, et al. Detection and characterization of high affinity plasma membrane receptors for human interleukin 1. *J Exp Med* 1985;162:501.

Glaccum MB, et al. Phenotypic and functional characterization of mice that lack the type I receptor for IL-1. *J Immunol* 1997;159:3364.

Horai R, et al. Production of mice deficient in genes for interleukin (IL)-1alpha, IL-1beta, IL-1alpha/beta, and IL-1 receptor antagonist shows that IL-1beta is crucial in turpentine-induced fever development and glucocorticoid secretion. *J Exp Med* 1998;187:1463.

Kronheim SR, et al. Human interleukin 1. Purification to homogeneity. *J Exp Med* 1985;161:490.

March CJ, et al. Cloning, sequence and expression of two distinct human interleukin-1 complementary DNAs. *Nature* 1985; 315:641.

Martin MU, Falk W. The interleukin-1 receptor complex and interleukin-1 signal transduction. *Eur Cytokine Netw* 1997;8:5.

McMahan CJ, et al. A novel IL-1 receptor, cloned from B cells by mammalian expression, is expressed in many cell types. *EMBO J* 1991;10:2821.

Priestle JP, et al. Crystal structure of the cytokine interleukin-1 beta. *EMBO J* 1988;7:339.

Sims JE, et al. Cloning the interleukin 1 receptor from human T cells. *Proc Natl Acad Sci U S A* 1989;86:8946.

Smith DE, et al. Four new members expand the interleukin-1 superfamily. *J Biol Chem* 2000;275:1169.

Interleukin 1ra

Arend WP. Interleukin-1 receptor antagonist. *Adv Immunol* 1993; 54:167.

Dinarello CA. Induction of interleukin-1 and interleukin-1 receptor antagonist. *Semin Oncol* 1997;24:S9.

Eisenberg SP, et al. Primary structure and functional expression from complementary DNA of a human interleukin-1 receptor antagonist. *Nature* 1990;343:341.

Horai R, et al. Development of chronic inflammatory arthropathy resembling rheumatoid arthritis in interleukin 1 receptor antagonist-deficient mice. *J Exp Med* 2000;191:313.

Horai R, et al. Production of mice deficient in genes for interleukin (IL)-1alpha, IL-1beta, IL-1alpha/beta, and IL-1 receptor antagonist shows that IL-1beta is crucial in turpentine-induced fever development and glucocorticoid secretion. *J Exp Med* 1998;187:1463.

Seckinger P, et al. A urine inhibitor of interleukin 1 activity that blocks ligand binding. *J Immunol* 1987;139:1546.

Interleukin 2

Brandhuber BJ, et al. Three-dimensional structure of interleukin-2. *Science* 1987;238:1707.

Fujita T, et al. Structure of the human interleukin 2 gene. *Proc Natl Acad Sci U S A* 1983;80:7437.

Gillis S, et al. Molecular characterization of interleukin 2. *Immunol Rev* 1982;63:167.

Hatakeyama M, et al. Interleukin-2 receptor beta chain gene: generation of three receptor forms by cloned human alpha and beta chain cDNAs. *Science* 1989;244:551.

Johnston JA, et al. Phosphorylation and activation of the Jak-3 Janus kinase in response to interleukin-2. *Nature* 1994;370:151.

Knight CR, et al. Interleukin-2-activated human effector lymphocytes mediate cytotoxicity by inducing apoptosis in human leukemia and solid tumour target cells. *Immunology* 1993;79:535.

Lee IH, et al. Inhibition of interleukin 2 signaling and signal transducer and activator of transcription (STAT)5 activation during T cell receptor-mediated feedback inhibition of T cell expansion. *J Exp Med* 1999;190:1263.

Lenardo MJ. Interleukin-2 programs mouse alpha beta T lymphocytes for apoptosis. *Nature* 1991;353:858.

Rosenberg SA. Interleukin-2 and the development of immunotherapy for the treatment of patients with cancer. *Cancer J Sci Am* 2000;1:S2.

Russell SM, et al. Interleukin-2 receptor gamma chain: a functional component of the interleukin-4 receptor. *Science* 1993;262:1880.

Sadlack B, et al. Generalized autoimmune disease in interleukin-2-deficient mice is triggered by an uncontrolled activation and proliferation of CD4+ T cells. *Eur J Immunol* 1995;25:3053.

Sadlack B, et al. Ulcerative colitis-like disease in mice with a disrupted interleukin-2 gene. *Cell* 1993;75:253.

Saltzman EM, et al. Stimulation of the antigen and interleukin-2 receptors on T lymphocytes activates distinct tyrosine protein kinases. *J Biol Chem* 1990;265:10138.

Schorle H, et al. Development and function of T cells in mice rendered interleukin-2 deficient by gene targeting. *Nature* 1991;352:621.

Smith KA, Cantrell DA. Interleukin 2 regulates its own receptors. *Proc Natl Acad Sci U S A* 1985;82:864.

Taniguchi T, et al. Structure and expression of a cloned cDNA for human interleukin-2. *Nature* 1983;302:305.

Zhang J, et al. Interleukin 2 receptor signaling regulates the perforin gene through signal transducer and activator of transcription (Stat)5 activation of two enhancers. *J Exp Med* 1999;190:1297.

Interleukin 3

Ahmad F, et al. IL-3 and IL-4 activate cyclic nucleotide phosphodiesterases 3 (PDE3) and 4 (PDE4) by different mechanisms in FDCP2 myeloid cells. *J Immunol* 1999;162:4864.

Bone H, Welham MJ. Shc associates with the IL-3 receptor beta subunit, SHIP and Gab2 following IL-3 stimulation. Contribution of Shc PTB and SH2 domains. *Cell Signal* 2000;12:183.

Frendl G. Interleukin 3: from colony-stimulating factor to pluripotent immunoregulatory cytokine. *Int J Immunopharmacol* 1992;14:421.

Ihle JN, et al. Biologic properties of homogeneous interleukin 3. I. Demonstration of WEHI-3 growth factor activity, mast cell growth factor activity, p cell-stimulating factor activity, colony-stimulating factor activity, and histamine-producing cell-stimulating factor activity. *J Immunol* 1983;131:282.

Lantz CS, et al. Role for interleukin-3 in mast-cell and basophil development and in immunity to parasites. *Nature* 1998;392:90.

Roberts R, et al. Heparan sulphate bound growth factors: a mechanism for stromal cell mediated hemopoiesis. *Nature* 1988;332:376.

Yang YC, et al. Human IL-3 (multi-CSF): identification by expression cloning of a novel hematopoietic growth factor related to murine IL-3. *Cell* 1986;47:3.

Interleukin 4

Arai N, et al. Complete nucleotide sequence of the chromosomal gene for human IL-4 and its expression. *J Immunol* 1989;142:274.

Holter W. Regulation of interleukin 4 production and of interleukin 4-producing cells. *Int Arch Allergy Immunol* 1992;98:273.

Kaplan MH, et al. Stat6-dependent and -independent pathways for IL-4 production. *J Immunol* 1999;163:6536.

Kopf M, et al. IL-4-deficient Balb/c mice resist infection with Leishmania major. *J Exp Med* 1996;184:1127.

Kopf M, et al. Immune responses of IL-4, IL-5, IL-6 deficient mice. *Immunol Rev* 1995;148:45.

Kuhn R, et al. Generation and analysis of interleukin-4 deficient mice. *Science* 1991;254:707.

Mohrs M, et al. Differences between IL-4- and IL-4 receptor alpha-deficient mice in chronic leishmaniasis reveal a protective role for IL-13 receptor signaling. *J Immunol* 1999;162:7302.

Nelms K, et al. The IL-4 receptor: signaling mechanisms and biologic functions. *Annu Rev Immunol* 1999;17:701.

Pritchard MA, et al. The interleukin-4 receptor gene (IL4R) maps to 16p11.2-16p12.1 in human and to the distal region of mouse chromosome 7. *Genomics* 1991;10:801.

Renz H. Soluble interleukin-4 receptor (sIL-4R) in allergic diseases. *Inflamm Res* 1999;48:425.

Russell SM, et al. Interleukin-2 receptor gamma chain: a functional component of the interleukin-4 receptor. *Science* 1993;262:1880.

Yokota T, et al. Isolation and characterization of a human interleukin cDNA clone, homologous to mouse B-cell stimulatory factor 1, that expresses B-cell- and T-cell-stimulating activities. *Proc Natl Acad Sci U S A* 1986;83:5894.

Zurawski SM, et al. Receptors for interleukin-13 and interleukin-4 are complex and share a novel component that functions in signal transduction. *EMBO J* 1993;12:2663.

Interleukin 5

Azuma C, et al. Cloning of cDNA for human T-cell replacing factor (interleukin-5) and comparison with the murine homologue. *Nucleic Acids Res* 1986;14:9149.

Mori A, et al. Transcriptional control of the IL-5 gene by human helper T cells: IL-5 synthesis is regulated independently from IL-2 or IL-4 synthesis. *J Allergy Clin Immunol* 1999;103:S429.

Stock W, et al. Characterization of yeast artificial chromosomes containing interleukin genes on human chromosome 5. *Cytogenet Cell Genet* 1992;61:263.

Sutherland GR, et al. Interleukin-5 is at 5q31 and is deleted in the 5q-syndrome. *Blood* 1988;71:1150.

Takahashi M, et al. Chromosomal mapping of the mouse IL-4 and human IL-5 genes. *Genomics* 1989;4:47.

Takatsu K. Interleukin 5 and B cell differentiation. *Cytokine Growth Factor Rev* 1998;9:25.

Tanabe T, et al. Molecular cloning and structure of the human interleukin-5 gene. *J Biol Chem* 1987;262:16580.

Tavernier J, et al. Interleukin 5 regulates the isoform expression of its own receptor alpha-subunit. *Blood* 2000;95:1600.

Interleukin 6

Akira S, et al. Interleukin-6 in biology and medicine. *Adv Immunol* 1993;54:1.

Gaillard J, et al. Interleukin-6 receptor signaling. II. Bio-availability of interleukin-6 in serum. *Eur Cytokine Netw* 1999;10:337.

Hirano T, et al. Purification to homogeneity and characterization of human B-cell differentiation factor (BCDF or BSFp-2). *Proc Natl Acad Sci U S A* 1985;82:5490.

Hirano T. Interleukin 6 and its receptor: ten years later. *Int Rev Immunol* 1998;16:249.

Kishimoto T, et al. Interleukin-6 family of cytokines and gp130. *Blood* 1995;86:1243.

Kopf M, et al. Impaired immune and acute-phase responses in interleukin-6-deficient mice. *Nature* 1994;368:339.

Matsuda T, et al. Identification of alpha 2-macroglobulin as a carrier protein for IL-6. *J Immunol* 1989;142:148.

Morton CJ, et al. Solution structure of synthetic peptides corresponding to the C-terminal helix of interleukin-6. *Eur J Biochem* 1994;219:97.

Schumann G, et al. Interleukin-6 activates signal transducer and activator of transcription and mitogen-activated protein kinase signal transduction pathways and induces de novo protein synthesis in human neuronal cells. *J Neurochem* 1999;73:2009.

Yuan J, et al. The signaling pathways of interleukin-6 and gamma interferon converge by the activation of different transcription factors which bind to common responsive DNA elements. *Mol Cell Biol* 1994;14:1657.

Interleukin 7

Benbernou N, et al. Interleukin (IL)-7 induces rapid activation of Pyk2, which is bound to Janus kinase 1 and IL-7Ralpha. *J Biol Chem* 2000;275:7060.

Costello R, et al. Interleukin-7, a major T-lymphocyte cytokine. *Eur Cytokine Netw* 1993;4:253.

Goodwin RG, et al. Human interleukin 7: molecular cloning and growth factor activity on human and murine B-lineage cells. *Proc Natl Acad Sci U S A* 1989;86:302.

Hofmeister R, et al. Interleukin-7: physiological roles and mechanisms of action. *Cytokine Growth Factor Rev* 1999;10:41.

Komschlies KL, et al. Administration of recombinant human IL-7 to mice alters the composition of B-lineage cells and T cell subsets, enhances T cell function, and induces regression of established metastases. *J Immunol* 1994;152:5776.

Lu L, et al. Regulation of cell survival during B lymphopoiesis: apoptosis and Bcl-2/Bax content of precursor B cells in bone marrow of mice with altered expression of IL-7 and recombinase-activating gene-2. *J Immunol* 1999;162:1931.

Peschon JJ, et al. Early lymphocyte expansion is severely impaired in interleukin 7 receptor-deficient mice. *J Exp Med* 1994;180:1955.

Russell SM, et al. Interleukin-2 receptor gamma chain: a functional component of the interleukin-4 receptor. *Science* 1993;262:1880.

Interleukin 8

Baggiolini M, et al. Human chemokines: an update. *Annu Rev Immunol* 1997;15:675.

Besemer J, et al. Specific binding, internalization, and degradation of human neutrophil activating factor by human polymorphonuclear leukocytes. *J Biol Chem* 1989;264:17409.

Cacalano G, et al. Neutrophil and B cell expansion in mice that lack the murine IL-8 receptor homolog. *Science* 1994;265:682.

Furutani Y, et al. Cloning and sequencing of the cDNA for human monocyte chemotactic and activating factor (MCAF). *Biochem Biophys Res Commun* 1989;159:249.

Gayle RB 3rd, et al. Importance of the amino terminus of the interleukin-8 receptor in ligand interactions. *J Biol Chem* 1993;268:7283.

Mukaida N, et al. Genomic structure of the human monocyte-derived neutrophil chemotactic factor IL-8. *J Immunol* 1989;143:1366.

Roebuck KA. Regulation of interleukin-8 gene expression. *J Interferon Cytokine Res* 1999;19:429.

Samanta AK, et al. Interleukin 8 (monocyte-derived neutrophil chemotactic factor) dynamically regulates its own receptor expression on human neutrophils. *J Biol Chem* 1990; 265:183.

Strieter RM, et al. Monokine-induced neutrophil chemotactic factor gene expression in human fibroblasts. *J Biol Chem* 1989;264:10621.

Interleukin 9

Demoulin JB, Renauld JC. Interleukin 9 and its receptor: an overview of structure and function. *Int Rev Immunol* 1998;16:345.

Kaushansky K, et al. Genomic cloning, characterization, and multilineage growth-promoting activity of human granulocyte-macrophage colony-stimulating factor. *Proc Natl Acad Sci U S A* 1986;83:3101.

Kelleher K, et al. Human interleukin-9: genomic sequence, chromosomal location, and sequences essential for its expression

in human T-cell leukemia virus (HTLV)-I-transformed human T cells. *Blood* 1991;77:1436.

Nicolaides NC, et al. Interleukin 9: a candidate gene for asthma. *Proc Natl Acad Sci U S A* 1997;94:13175.

Quesniaux VF. Interleukins 9, 10, 11 and 12 and kit ligand: a brief overview. *Res Immunol* 1992;143:385.

Renauld JC, et al. Human P40/IL-9. Expression in activated CD4+ T cells, genomic organization, and comparison with the mouse gene. *J Immunol* 1990;144:4235.

Russell SM, et al. Interleukin-2 receptor gamma chain: a functional component of the interleukin-4 receptor. *Science* 1993;262:1880.

Vermeesch JR, et al. The IL-9 receptor gene, located in the Xq/Yq pseudoautosomal region, has an autosomal origin, escapes X inactivation and is expressed from the Y. *Hum Mol Genet* 1997;6:1.

Yang YC, et al. Expression cloning of cDNA encoding a novel human hematopoietic growth factor: human homologue of murine T-cell growth factor P40. *Blood* 1989;74:1880.

Interleukin 10

Asseman C, et al. An essential role for interleukin 10 in the function of regulatory T cells that inhibit intestinal inflammation. *J Exp Med* 1999;190:995.

Benjamin D. Interleukin-10 (IL-10). *Cancer Treat Res* 1995; 80:305.

Donnelly RP, et al. The interleukin-10 signal transduction pathway and regulation of gene expression in mononuclear phagocytes. *J Interferon Cytokine Res* 1999;19:563.

Kuhn R, et al. Interleukin-10-deficient mice develop chronic enterocolitis. *Cell* 1993;75:263.

Quesniaux VF. Interleukins 9, 10, 11 and 12 and kit ligand: a brief overview. *Res Immunol* 1992;143:385.

Tan JC, et al. Characterization of interleukin-10 receptors on human and mouse cells. *J Biol Chem* 19933;268:21053.

Vieira P, et al. Isolation and expression of human cytokine synthesis inhibitory factor cDNA clones: homology to Epstein-Barr virus open reading frame BCRFI. *Proc Natl Acad Sci U S A* 1991;88:1172.

Wynn TA, et al. IL-10 regulates liver pathology in acute murine Schistosomiasis mansoni but is not required for immune down-modulation of chronic disease. *J Immunol* 1998; 160:4473.

Interleukin 11

Bilinski P, et al. Maternal IL-11Ralpha function is required for normal decidua and fetoplacental development in mice. *Genes Dev* 1998;12:2234.

Paul SR, et al. Molecular cloning of a cDNA encoding interleukin 11, a stromal cell-derived lymphopoietic and hematopoietic cytokine. *Proc Natl Acad Sci U S A* 1990;87:7512.

Quesniaux VF. Interleukins 9, 10, 11 and 12 and kit ligand: a brief overview. *Res Immunol* 1992;143:385.

Schwertschlag US, et al. Hematopoietic, immunomodulatory and epithelial effects of interleukin-11. *Leukemia* 1999;13:1307.

Trepicchio WL, Dorner AJ. Interleukin-11. A gp130 cytokine. *Ann N Y Acad Sci* 1998;856:12.

Interleukin 12

Adorini L. Interleukin-12, a key cytokine in Th1-mediated autoimmune diseases. *Cell Mol Life Sci* 1999;55:1610.

Brunda MJ. Interleukin-12. *J Leukoc Biol* 1994;55:280.

Ely KH, et al. Augmentation of the CD8+ T cell response by IFN-gamma in IL-12-deficient mice during Toxoplasma gondii infection. *J Immunol* 1999;162:5449.

Gately MK, et al. The interleukin-12/interleukin-12-receptor system: role in normal and pathologic immune responses. *Annu Rev Immunol* 1998;16:495.

Gately MK. Interleukin-12: a recently discovered cytokine with potential for enhancing cell-mediated immune responses to tumors. *Cancer Invest* 1993;11:500.

Scott P. IL-12: initiation cytokine for cell-mediated immunity. *Science* 1993;260:496.

Trinchieri G. Immunobiology of interleukin-12. *Immunol Res* 1998;17:269.

Interleukin 13

de Vries JE. The role of IL-13 and its receptor in allergy and inflammatory responses. *J Allergy Clin Immunol* 1998;102:165.

McKenzie AN, et al. Structural comparison and chromosomal localization of the human and mouse IL-13 genes. *J Immunol* 1993;150:5436.

McKenzie GJ, et al. Simultaneous disruption of interleukin (IL)-4 and IL-13 defines individual roles in T helper cell type 2-mediated responses. *J Exp Med* 1999;189:1565.

Minty A, et al. Interleukin-13 is a new human lymphokine regulating inflammatory and immune responses. *Nature* 1993;362:248.

Orchansky PL, et al. Characterization of the cytoplasmic domain of interleukin-13 receptor-alpha. *J Biol Chem* 1999;274:20818.

Russell SM, et al. Interleukin-2 receptor gamma chain: a functional component of the interleukin-4 receptor [see comments]. *Science* 1993;262:1880.

Zurawski SM, et al. Receptors for interleukin-13 and interleukin-4 are complex and share a novel component that functions in signal transduction. *EMBO J* 1993;12:2663.

Interleukin 14

Ambrus JL Jr, et al. Identification of a cDNA for a human high molecular-weight B-cell growth factor. *Proc Natl Acad Sci U S A* 1996;93:8154.

Ambrus JL Jr, et al. Induction of proliferation by high molecular weight B cell growth factor or low molecular weight B cell growth factor is associated with increases in intracellular calcium in different subpopulations of human B lymphocytes. *Cell Immunol* 1991;134:314.

Ambrus JL Jr, et al. Purification to homogeneity of a high molecular weight human B cell growth factor; demonstration of specific binding to activated B cells; and development of a monoclonal antibody to the factor. *J Exp Med* 1985;162:1319.

Ford R, et al. Identification of B-cell growth factors (interleukin-14; high molecular weight-B-cell growth factors) in effusion fluids from patients with aggressive B-cell lymphomas. *Blood* 1995;86:283.

Nakagawa T, et al. Differential effects of interleukin 2 vs B cell growth factor on human B cells. *J Immunol* 1988;140:465.

Interleukin 15

Anderson DM, et al. Chromosomal assignment and genomic structure of IL-15. *Genomics* 1995;25:701.

Grabstein KH, et al. Cloning of a T cell growth factor that interacts with the beta chain of the interleukin-2 receptor. *Science* 1994;264:965.

Lodolce JP, et al. IL-15 receptor maintains lymphoid homeostasis by supporting lymphocyte homing and proliferation. *Immunity* 1998;9:669.

Ma A, et al. The pleiotropic functions of interleukin 15. Not so interleukin 2-like after all. *J Exp Med* 2000;191:753.

Waldmann TA, Tagaya Y. The multifaceted regulation of interleukin-15 expression and the role of this cytokine in NK cell differentiation and host response to intracellular pathogens. *Annu Rev Immunol* 1999;17:19.

Interleukin 16

Baier M, et al. Molecular cloning, sequence, expression, and processing of the interleukin 16 precursor. *Proc Natl Acad Sci U S A* 1997;94:5273.

Cruikshank W, Center DM. Modulation of lymphocyte migration by human lymphokines. II. Purification of a lymphotactic factor (LCF). *J Immunol* 1982;128:2569.

Cruikshank WW, et al. Signaling and functional properties of interleukin-16. *Int Rev Immunol* 1998;16:523.

Krautwald S. IL-16 activates the SAPK signaling pathway in CD4+ macrophages. *J Immunol* 1998;160:5874.

Nicoll J, et al. Identification of domains in IL-16 critical for biological activity. *J Immunol* 1999;163:1827.

Interleukin 17

Fossiez F, et al. Interleukin-17. *Int Rev Immunol* 1998;16:541.

Spriggs MK. Interleukin-17 and its receptor. *J Clin Immunol* 1997;17:366.

Subramaniam SV, et al. Evidence for the involvement of JAK/STAT pathway in the signaling mechanism of interleukin-17. *Biochem Biophys Res Commun* 1999;262:14.

Tartour E, et al. Interleukin 17, a T-cell-derived cytokine, promotes tumorigenicity of human cervical tumors in nude mice. *Cancer Res* 1999;59:3698.

Yao Z, et al. Human IL-17: a novel cytokine derived from T cells. *J Immunol* 1995;155:5483.

Yao Z, et al. Molecular characterization of the human interleukin (IL)-17 receptor. *Cytokine* 1997;9:794.

Interleukin 18

Lebel-Binay S, et al. Interleukin-18: biological properties and clinical implications. *Eur Cytokine Netw* 2000;11:15.

Okamura H, et al. Cloning of a new cytokine that induces IFN-gamma production by T cells. *Nature* 1995;378:88.

Takeda K, et al. Defective NK cell activity and Th1 response in IL-18-deficient mice. *Immunity* 1998;8:383.

Torigoe K, et al. Purification and characterization of the human interleukin-18 receptor. *J Biol Chem* 1997;272:25737.

Ushio S, et al. Cloning of the cDNA for human IFN-gamma-inducing factor, expression in Escherichia coli, and studies on the biologic activities of the protein. *J Immunol* 1996;156:4274.

Erythropoietin

Ghaffari S, et al. BCR-ABL and v-SRC tyrosine kinase oncoproteins support normal erythroid development in erythropoietin receptor-deficient progenitor cells. *Proc Natl Acad Sci U S A* 1999;96:13186.

Koury MJ, Bondurant MC. The molecular mechanism of erythropoietin action. *Eur J Biochem* 1992;210:649.

Lai PH, et al. Structural characterization of human erythropoietin. *J Biol Chem* 1986;261:3116.

Law ML, et al. Chromosomal assignment of the human erythropoietin gene and its DNA polymorphism. *Proc Natl Acad Sci U S A* 1986;83:6920.

Lin FK, et al. Cloning and expression of the human erythropoietin gene. *Proc Natl Acad Sci U S A* 1985;82:7580.

Tilbrook PA, Klinken SP. Erythropoietin and erythropoietin receptor. *Growth Factors* 1999;17:25.

Wang FF, et al. Some chemical properties of human erythropoietin. *Endocrinology* 1985;116:2286.

Watkins PC, et al. Regional assignment of the erythropoietin gene to human chromosome region 7pter—q22. *Cytogenet Cell Genet* 1986;42:214.

Wojchowski DM, et al. Signal transduction in the erythropoietin receptor system. *Exp Cell Res* 1999;253:143.

Youssoufian H, et al. Structure, function, and activation of the erythropoietin receptor. *Blood* 1993;81:2223.

Macrophage Colony-Stimulating Factor

Cerretti DP, et al. Human macrophage-colony stimulating factor: alternative RNA and protein processing from a single gene. *Mol Immunol* 1988;25:761.

Das SK, Stanley ER. Structure-function studies of a colony stimulating factor (CSF-1). *J Biol Chem* 1982;257:13679.

Kawasaki ES, et al. Molecular cloning of a complementary DNA encoding human macrophage-specific colony-stimulating factor (CSF-1). *Science* 1985;230:291.

Ladner MB, et al. Human CSF-1: gene structure and alternative splicing of mRNA precursors. *EMBO J* 1987;6:2693.

Lieschke GJ, et al. Mice lacking both macrophage- and granulocyte-macrophage colony-stimulating factor have macrophages and coexistent osteopetrosis and severe lung disease. *Blood* 1994;84:27.

Ohno R. Granulocyte colony-stimulating factor, granulocyte-macrophage colony-stimulating factor and macrophage colony-stimulating factor in the treatment of acute myeloid leukemia and acute lymphoblastic leukemia. *Leuk Res* 1998;22:1143.

Pettenati MJ, et al. Assignment of CSF-1 to 5q33.1: evidence for clustering of genes regulating hematopoiesis and for their involvement in the deletion of the long arm of chromosome 5 in myeloid disorders. *Proc Natl Acad Sci U S A* 1987;84:2970.

Granulocyte Colony-Stimulating Factor

Avalos BR. The granulocyte colony-stimulating factor receptor and its role in disorders of granulopoiesis. *Leuk Lymphoma* 1998;28:265.

Devlin JJ, et al. Expression of granulocyte colony-stimulating factor by human cell lines. *J Leukoc Biol* 1987;41:302.

Lieschke GJ, et al. Mice lacking granulocyte colony-stimulating factor have chronic neutropenia, granulocyte and macrophage progenitor cell deficiency, and impaired neutrophil mobilization. *Blood* 1994;84:1737.

Nagata S, et al. The chromosomal gene structure and two mRNAs for human granulocyte colony-stimulating factor. *EMBO J* 1986;5:575.

Nomura H, et al. Purification and characterization of human granulocyte colony-stimulating factor (G-CSF). *EMBO J* 1986;5:871.

Ohno R. Granulocyte colony-stimulating factor, granulocyte-macrophage colony-stimulating factor and macrophage colony-stimulating factor in the treatment of acute myeloid leukemia and acute lymphoblastic leukemia. *Leuk Res* 1998;22:1143.

Simmers RN, et al. Localization of the G-CSF gene on chromosome 17 proximal to the breakpoint in the t(15;17) in acute promyelocytic leukemia. *Blood* 1987;70:330.

Tsuchiya M, et al. Isolation and characterization of the cDNA for murine granulocyte colony-stimulating factor. *Proc Natl Acad Sci U S A* 1986;83:7633.

Tweardy DJ, et al. Molecular cloning and characterization of a cDNA for human granulocyte colony-stimulating factor (G-CSF) from a glioblastoma multiforme cell line and localization of the G-CSF gene to chromosome band 17q21. *Oncogene Res* 1987;1:209.

Granulocyte-Macrophage Colony-Stimulating Factor

Burdach S, et al. The physiologic role of interleukin-3, interleukin-5, granulocyte-macrophage colony-stimulating factor, and the beta c receptor system. *Curr Opin Hematol* 1998;5:177.

Dranoff G, et al. Involvement of granulocyte-macrophage colony-stimulating factor in pulmonary homeostasis. *Science* 1994;264:713.

Gasson JC, et al. Purified human granulocyte-macrophage colony-stimulating factor: direct action on neutrophils. *Science* 1984;226:1339.

Hogge GS, et al. Preclinical development of human granulocyte-macrophage colony-stimulating factor-transfected melanoma cell vaccine using established canine cell lines and normal dogs. *Cancer Gene Ther* 1999;6:26.

Huebner K, et al. The human gene encoding GM-CSF is at 5q21-q32, the chromosome region deleted in the 5q-anomaly. *Science* 1985;230:1282.

Kaushansky K, et al. Genomic cloning, characterization, and multilineage growth-promoting activity of human granulocyte-macrophage colony-stimulating factor. *Proc Natl Acad Sci U S A* 1986;83:3101.

Lieschke GJ, et al. Mice lacking both macrophage- and granulocyte-macrophage colony-stimulating factor have macrophages and coexistent osteopetrosis and severe lung disease. *Blood* 1994;84:27.

Roberts R, et al. Heparan sulphate bound growth factors: a mechanism for stromal cell mediated hemopoiesis. *Nature* 1988;332:376.

Stanley E, et al. Granulocyte/macrophage colony-stimulating factor-deficient mice show no major perturbation of hematopoiesis but develop a characteristic pulmonary pathology. *Proc Natl Acad Sci U S A* 1994;91:5592.

Wong GG, et al. Human GM-CSF: molecular cloning of the complementary DNA and purification of the natural and recombinant proteins. *Science* 1985;228:810.

Leukemia Inhibitory Factor

Ekstrom PA, et al. Leukemia inhibitory factor null mice: unhampered in vitro outgrowth of sensory axons but reduced stimulatory potential by nerve segments. *Neurosci Lett* 2000;281:107.

Gadient RA, Patterson PH. Leukemia inhibitory factor, interleukin 6, and other cytokines using the GP130 transducing receptor: roles in inflammation and injury. *Stem Cells* 1999;17:127.

Gough NM, et al. Molecular cloning and expression of the human homologue of the murine gene encoding myeloid leukemia-inhibitory factor. *Proc Natl Acad Sci U S A* 1988;85:2623.

Stahl J, et al. Structural organization of the genes for murine and human leukemia inhibitory factor. Evolutionary conservation of coding and non-coding regions. *J Biol Chem* 1990;265:8833.

Taupin JL, et al. Leukemia inhibitory factor: part of a large ingathering family. *Int Rev Immunol* 1998;16:397.

Turnley AM, Bartlett PF. Cytokines that signal through the leukemia inhibitory factor receptor-beta complex in the nervous system. *J Neurochem* 2000;74:889.

Stem Cell Factor

Ashman LK. The biology of stem cell factor and its receptor C-kit. *Int J Biochem Cell Biol* 1999;31:1037.

Geissler EN, et al. Stem cell factor (SCF), a novel hematopoietic growth factor and ligand for c-kit tyrosine kinase receptor, maps on human chromosome 12 between 12q14.3 and 12qter. *Somat Cell Mol Genet* 1991;17:207.

Lyman SD, Jacobsen SE. c-kit ligand and Flt3 ligand: stem/progenitor cell factors with overlapping yet distinct activities. *Blood* 1998;91:1101.

Martin FH, et al. Primary structure and functional expression of rat and human stem cell factor DNAs. *Cell* 1990;63:203.

Tumor Necrosis Factor α

Aggarwal BB, et al. Human tumor necrosis factor. Production, purification, and characterization. *J Biol Chem* 1985;260:2345.

Bemelmans MH, et al. Tumor necrosis factor: function, release and clearance. *Crit Rev Immunol* 1996;16:1.

Ding AH, Porteu F. Regulation of tumor necrosis factor receptors on phagocytes. *Proc Soc Exp Biol Med* 1992;200:458.

Lantz M, et al. Characterization in vitro of a human tumor necrosis factor-binding protein. A soluble form of a tumor necrosis factor receptor. *J Clin Invest* 1990;86:1396.

Nedwin GE, et al. Human lymphotoxin and tumor necrosis factor genes: structure, homology and chromosomal localization. *Nucleic Acids Res* 1985;13:6361.

Pennica D, et al. Human tumour necrosis factor: precursor structure, expression and homology to lymphotoxin. *Nature* 1984;312:724.

Rothe J, et al. Mice lacking the tumour necrosis factor receptor 1 are resistant to TNF-mediated toxicity but highly susceptible to infection by *Listeria* monocytogenes. *Nature* 1997;364:798.

Smith RA, Baglioni C. The active form of tumor necrosis factor is a trimer. *J Biol Chem* 1987;262:6951.

Tartaglia LA, et al. The two different receptors for tumor necrosis factor mediate distinct cellular responses. *Proc Natl Acad Sci U S A* 1991;88:9292.

Zurawski SM, et al. Receptors for interleukin-13 and interleukin-4 are complex and share a novel component that functions in signal transduction. *EMBO J* 1993;12:2663.

Tumor Necrosis Factor β

Aggarwal BB, et al. Human lymphotoxin. Production by a lymphoblastoid cell line, purification, and initial characterization. *J Biol Chem* 1984;259:686.

Bemelmans MH, et al. Tumor necrosis factor: function, release and clearance. *Crit Rev Immunol* 1996;16:1.

Crowe PD, et al. A lymphotoxin-beta-specific receptor. *Science* 1994;264:707.

De Togni P, et al. Abnormal development of peripheral lymphoid organs in mice deficient in lymphotoxin. *Science* 1994;264:703.

Eck MJ, et al. The structure of human lymphotoxin (tumor necrosis factor-beta) at 1.9-A resolution. *J Biol Chem* 1992;267:2119.

Gray PW, et al. Cloning and expression of cDNA for human lymphotoxin, a lymphokine with tumour necrosis activity. *Nature* 1984;312:721.

Li CB, et al. Cloning and expression of murine lymphotoxin cDNA. *J Immunol* 1987;138:4496.

Nedwin GE, et al. Human lymphotoxin and tumor necrosis factor genes: structure, homology and chromosomal localization. *Nucleic Acids Res* 1985;13:6361.

Pennica D, et al. Human tumour necrosis factor: precursor structure, expression and homology to lymphotoxin. *Nature* 1984;312:724.

Interferon-α

Fitzgerald-Bocarsly P. Human natural interferon-alpha producing cells. *Pharmacol Ther* 1993;60:39.

Haque SJ, Williams BR. Signal transduction in the interferon system. *Semin Oncol* 1998;25:14.

Lutfalla G, et al. Assignment of the human interferon-alpha receptor gene to chromosome 21q22.1 by in situ hybridization. *J Interferon Res* 1990;10:515.

Muller U, et al. Functional role of type I and type II interferons in antiviral defense. *Science* 1994;264:1918.

Novick D, et al. The human interferon alpha/beta receptor: characterization and molecular cloning. *Cell* 1994;77:391.

Pestka S. The interferon receptors. *Semin Oncol* 1997;24:S9.

Interferon-β

Haque SJ, Williams BR. Signal transduction in the interferon system. *Semin Oncol* 1998;25:14.

Lutfalla G, et al. Assignment of the human interferon-alpha receptor gene to chromosome 21q22.1 by in situ hybridization. *J Interferon Res* 1990;10:515.

Muller U, et al. Functional role of type I and type II interferons in antiviral defense. *Science* 1994;264:1918.

Novick D, et al. The human interferon alpha/beta receptor: characterization and molecular cloning. *Cell* 1994;77:391.

Owerbach D, et al. Leukocyte and fibroblast interferon genes are located on human chromosome 9. *Proc Natl Acad Sci U S A* 1981;78:3123.

Pestka S. The interferon receptors. *Semin Oncol* 1997;24:S9.

Interferon-γ

Farrar MA, Schreiber RD. The molecular cell biology of interferon-gamma and its receptor. *Annu Rev Immunol* 1993;11:571.

Flynn JL, et al. An essential role for interferon gamma in resistance to Mycobacterium tuberculosis infection. *J Exp Med* 1993;178:2249.

Gray PW, Goeddel DV. Structure of the human immune interferon gene. *Nature* 1982;298:859.

Igarashi K, et al. Interferon-gamma induces tyrosine phosphorylation of interferon-gamma receptor and regulated association of protein tyrosine kinases, Jak1 and Jak2, with its receptor. *J Biol Chem* 1994;269:14333.

Krakauer T, Oppenheim JJ. IL-1 and tumor necrosis factor-alpha each up-regulate both the expression of IFN-gamma receptors and enhance IFN-gamma-induced HLA-DR expression on human monocytes and a human monocytic cell line (THP-1). *J Immunol* 1993;150:1205.

Novelli F, et al. Environmental signals influencing expression of the IFN-gamma receptor on human T cells control whether IFN-gamma promotes proliferation or apoptosis. *J Immunol* 1994;152:496.

Pestka S, et al. The interferon gamma (IFN-gamma) receptor: a paradigm for the multichain cytokine receptor. *Cytokine Growth Factor Rev* 1997;8:189.

Pfizenmaier K, et al. High affinity human IFN-gamma-binding capacity is encoded by a single receptor gene located in proximity to c-ros on human chromosome region 6q16 to 6q22. *J Immunol* 1988;141:856.

Yuan J, et al. The signaling pathways of interleukin-6 and gamma interferon converge by the activation of different transcription factors which bind to common responsive DNA elements. *Mol Cell Biol* 1994;14:1657.

Acidic Fibroblast Growth Factor

Basilico C, Moscatelli D. The FGF family of growth factors and oncogenes. *Adv Cancer Res* 1992;59:115.

Copeland RA, et al. The structure of human acidic fibroblast growth factor and its interaction with heparin. *Arch Biochem Biophys* 1991;289:53.

Jaye M, et al. Human endothelial cell growth factor: cloning, nucleotide sequence, and chromosome localization. *Science* 1986;233:541.

Johnson DE, Williams LT. Structural and functional diversity in the FGF receptor multigene family. *Adv Cancer Res* 1993;60:1.

Miller DL, et al. Compensation by fibroblast growth factor 1 (FGF1) does not account for the mild phenotypic defects observed in FGF2 null mice. *Mol Cell Biol* 2000;20:2260.

Basic Fibroblast Growth Factor

Abraham JA, et al. Human basic fibroblast growth factor: nucleotide sequence and genomic organization. *EMBO J* 1986;5:2523.

Allouche M, Bikfalvi A. The role of fibroblast growth factor-2 (FGF-2) in hematopoiesis. *Prog Growth Factor Res* 1995;6:35.

Basilico C, Moscatelli D. The FGF family of growth factors and oncogenes. *Adv Cancer Res* 1992;59:115.

Dennis PA, et al. Alpha 2-macroglobulin is a binding protein for basic fibroblast growth factor. *J Biol Chem* 1989;264:7210.

Johnson DE, Williams LT. Structural and functional diversity in the FGF receptor multigene family. *Adv Cancer Res* 1993;60:1.

Miller DL, et al. Compensation by fibroblast growth factor 1 (FGF1) does not account for the mild phenotypic defects observed in FGF2 null mice. *Mol Cell Biol* 2000;20:2260.

Sommer A, et al. A form of human basic fibroblast growth factor with an extended amino terminus. *Biochem Biophys Res Commun* 1987;144:543.

Wright JA, Huang A. Growth factors in mechanisms of malignancy: roles for TGF-beta and FGF. *Histol Histopathol* 1996;11:521.

Platelet-Derived Growth Factor

Benito M, Lorenzo M. Platelet derived growth factor/tyrosine kinase receptor mediated proliferation. *Growth Regul* 1993;3:172.

Betsholtz C, et al. cDNA sequence and chromosomal localization of human platelet-derived growth factor A-chain and its expression in tumour cell lines. *Nature* 1986;320:695.

Claesson-Welsh L, et al. cDNA cloning and expression of the human A-type platelet-derived growth factor (PDGF) receptor establishes structural similarity to the B-type PDGF receptor. *Proc Natl Acad Sci U S A* 1989;86:4917.

Collins T, et al. Cultured human endothelial cells express platelet-derived growth factor B chain: cDNA cloning and structural analysis. *Nature* 1985;316:748.

Heldin CH, et al. Structure of platelet-derived growth factor: implications for functional properties. *Growth Factors* 1993;8:245.

Heldin CH. Structural and functional studies on platelet-derived growth factor. *EMBO J* 1992;11:4251.

Huang JS, et al. Specific covalent binding of platelet-derived growth factor to human plasma alpha 2-macroglobulin. *Proc Natl Acad Sci U S A* 1984;81:342.

Josephs SF, et al. Transforming potential of human c-sis nucleotide sequences encoding platelet-derived growth factor. *Science* 1984;225:636.

Ohlsson R, et al. PDGFB regulates the development of the labyrinthine layer of the mouse fetal placenta. *Dev Biol* 1999;212:124.

Soriano P. The PDGF alpha receptor is required for neural crest cell development and for normal patterning of the somites. *Development* 1997;124:2691.

Epidermal Growth Factor

Gray A, et al. Nucleotide sequence of epidermal growth factor cDNA predicts a 128,000-molecular weight protein precursor. *Nature* 1983;303:722.

Luetteke NC, et al. Targeted inactivation of the EGF and amphiregulin genes reveals distinct roles for EGF receptor ligands in mouse mammary gland development. *Development* 1999;126:2739.

Zabel BU, et al. Chromosomal locations of the human and mouse genes for precursors of epidermal growth factor and the beta subunit of nerve growth factor. *Proc Natl Acad Sci U S A* 1985;82:469.

Tumor Growth Factor α

Derynck R, et al. Human transforming growth factor-beta complementary DNA sequence and expression in normal and transformed cells. *Nature* 1985;316:701.

Madtes DK, et al. Transforming growth factor-alpha deficiency reduces pulmonary fibrosis in transgenic mice. *Am J Respir Cell Mol Biol* 1999;20:924.

Tumor Growth Factor β

Derynck R, et al. A new type of transforming growth factor-beta, TGF-beta 3. *EMBO J* 1988;7:3737.

Derynck R, et al. Human transforming growth factor-beta complementary DNA sequence and expression in normal and transformed cells. *Nature* 1985;316:701.

Engel ME, et al. Signal transduction by transforming growth factor-beta: a cooperative paradigm with extensive negative regulation. *J Cell Biochem Suppl* 1998;31:111.

Kulkarni AB, et al. Transforming growth factor beta 1 null mutation in mice causes excessive inflammatory response and early death. *Proc Natl Acad Sci U S A* 1993;90:770.

LaMarre J, et al. Reaction of alpha 2-macroglobulin with plasmin increases binding of transforming growth factors-beta 1 and beta 2. *Biochim Biophys Acta* 1991;1091:197.

Lawrence DA. Transforming growth factor-beta: a general review. *Eur Cytokine Netw* 1996;7:363.

Madisen L, et al. Transforming growth factor-beta 2: cDNA cloning and sequence analysis. *DNA* 1988;7:1.

Miyazono K, et al. Transforming growth factor-beta: latent forms, binding proteins and receptors. *Growth Factors* 1993;8:11.

Shull MM, et al. Targeted disruption of the mouse transforming growth factor-beta 1 gene results in multifocal inflammatory disease. *Nature* 1992;359:693.

ten Dijke P, et al. Identification of another member of the transforming growth factor type beta gene family. *Proc Natl Acad Sci U S A* 1988;85:4715.

Hepatic Growth Factor

Bottaro DP, et al. Identification of the hepatocyte growth factor receptor as the c-met proto-oncogene product. *Science* 1991;251:802.

Galimi F, et al. The hepatocyte growth factor and its receptor. *Stem Cells 11 Suppl* 1993;2:22.

Jiang WG, et al. Hepatocyte growth factor/scatter factor, liver regeneration and cancer metastasis. *Br J Surg* 1993;80:1368.

Mizuno K, Nakamura T. Molecular characteristics of HGF and the gene, and its biochemical aspects. *EXS* 1993;65:1.

Nakamura T, et al. Molecular cloning and expression of human hepatocyte growth factor. *Nature* 1989;342:440.

Nakamura T, et al. Purification and characterization of a growth factor from rat platelets for mature parenchymal hepatocytes in primary cultures. *Proc Natl Acad Sci U S A* 1986;83:6489.

Rubin JS, et al. Hepatocyte growth factor/scatter factor and its receptor, the c-met proto-oncogene product. *Biochim Biophys Acta* 1993;1155:357.

Somerset DA, et al. Ontogeny of hepatocyte growth factor (HGF) and its receptor (c-met) in human placenta: reduced HGF expression in intrauterine growth restriction. *Am J Pathol* 1998;153:1139.

Nerve Growth Factor

Borsani G, et al. cDNA sequence of human beta-NGF. *Nucleic Acids Res* 1990;18:4020.

Guroff G. Nerve growth factor as a neurotrophic agent. *Ann N Y Acad Sci* 1993;692:51.

Maness LM, et al. The neurotrophins and their receptors: structure, function, and neuropathology. *Neurosci Biobehav Rev* 1994;18:143.

McDonald NQ, et al. New protein fold revealed by a 2.3-A resolution crystal structure of nerve growth factor. *Nature* 1991;354:411.

Ronne H, et al. Nerve growth factor binds to serum alpha-2-macroglobulin. *Biochem Biophys Res Commun* 1979;87:330.

Ullrich A, et al. Human beta-nerve growth factor gene sequence highly homologous to that of mouse. *Nature* 1983;303:821.

Zabel BU, et al. Chromosomal locations of the human and mouse genes for precursors of epidermal growth factor and the beta subunit of nerve growth factor. *Proc Natl Acad Sci U S A* 1985;82:469.

Prolactin

Chikanza IC. Prolactin and neuroimmunomodulation: in vitro and in vivo observations. *Ann N Y Acad Sci* 1999;876:119.

Clevenger CV, et al. Prolactin receptor signal transduction in cells of the immune system. *J Endocrinol* 1998;157:187.

Goffin V, et al. From the molecular biology of prolactin and its receptor to the lessons learned from knockout mice models. *Genet Anal* 1999;15:189.

Woody MA, et al. Prolactin exerts hematopoietic growth-promoting effects in vivo and partially counteracts myelosuppression by azidothymidine. *Exp Hematol* 1999;27:811.

Growth Hormone

Bartke A, et al. Effects of growth hormone overexpression and growth hormone resistance on neuroendocrine and reproductive functions in transgenic and knock-out mice. *Proc Soc Exp Biol Med* 1999;222:113.

Butler AA, et al. Growth hormone (GH) status regulates GH receptor and GH binding protein mRNA in a tissue- and transcript-specific manner but has no effect on insulin-like growth factor-I receptor mRNA in the rat. *Mol Cell Endocrinol* 1996;116:181.

Heemskerk VH, et al. Insulin-like growth factor-1 (IGF-1) and growth hormone (GH) in immunity and inflammation. *Cytokine Growth Factor Rev* 1999;10:5.

Kelley KW, et al. Growth hormone, prolactin, and insulin-like growth factors: new jobs for old players. *Brain Behav Immun* 1992;6:317.

Insulin-Like Growth Factor I

Brissenden JE, et al. Human chromosomal mapping of genes for insulin-like growth factors I and II and epidermal growth factor. *Nature* 1984;310:781.

Butler AA, et al. Insulin-like growth factor-I receptor signal transduction: at the interface between physiology and cell biology. *Comp Biochem Physiol B Biochem Mol Biol* 1998; 121:19.

Heemskerk VH, et al. Insulin-like growth factor-1 (IGF-1) and growth hormone (GH) in immunity and inflammation. *Cytokine Growth Factor Rev* 1999;10:5.

Jansen M, et al. Sequence of cDNA encoding human insulin-like growth factor I precursor. *Nature* 1983;306:609.

Lackey BR, et al. The insulin-like growth factor (IGF) system and gonadotropin regulation: actions and interactions. *Cytokine Growth Factor Rev* 1999;10:201.

LeRoith D, Roberts CT Jr. Insulin-like growth factors. *Ann N Y Acad Sci* 1993;692:1.

LeRoith D. Insulin-like growth factor I receptor signaling—overlapping or redundant pathways? *Endocrinology* 2000;141:1287.

Liu JL, et al. Conditional knockout of mouse insulin-like growth factor-1 gene using the Cre/loxP system. *Proc Soc Exp Biol Med* 2000;223:344.

Nielsen FC. The molecular and cellular biology of insulin-like growth factor II. *Prog Growth Factor Res* 1992;4:257.

Sussenbach JS, et al. Structure and expression of the human insulin-like growth factor genes. *Growth Regul* 1992;2:1.

Insulin-Like Growth Factor II

Brissenden JE, et al. Human chromosomal mapping of genes for insulin-like growth factors I and II and epidermal growth factor. *Nature* 1984;310:781.

Kelley KW, et al. Growth hormone, prolactin, and insulin-like growth factors: new jobs for old players. *Brain Behav Immun* 1992;6:317.

Lackey BR, et al. The insulin-like growth factor (IGF) system and gonadotropin regulation: actions and interactions. *Cytokine Growth Factor Rev* 1999;10:201.

LeRoith D, Roberts CT Jr. Insulin-like growth factors. *Ann N Y Acad Sci* 1993;692:1.

Nielsen FC. The molecular and cellular biology of insulin-like growth factor II. *Prog Growth Factor Res* 1992;4:257.

35

INHIBITORS OF TUMOR ANGIOGENESIS

ANN L. MELLOTT
WILLIAM J. GRADISHAR

Some thirty years ago, Judah Folkman proposed the theory that tumors would be unable to grow beyond a size of 2 to 3 mm in the absence of a new vascular supply.[1] The view is now accepted that primary tumor growth and the development of metastases are dependent on a series of carefully coordinated steps.[2] A necessary step for growth of the primary tumor and metastases is the development of a vascular supply, referred to as *angiogenesis*.[3,4] For every increase in the diameter of a tumor, an increment in angiogenesis must occur.[1] Due to imbalance between oncogene products that signal cellular proliferation and abnormalities of tumor suppressor genes that suppress unregulated growth, tumor cells can proliferate.[5] As a corollary to these observations, Folkman believed that strategies to interfere with tumor angiogenesis might afford a novel way of treating cancer.[1,3]

Several positive and negative endogenous regulators control angiogenesis.[2,6] Whether angiogenesis develops depends on a balance between promoters of angiogenesis [i.e., acidic and basic fibroblast growth factor (aFGF, bFGF), vascular endothelial growth factor (VEGF), etc.],[7] and inhibitors of angiogenesis (i.e., angiostatin,[8,9] endostatin,[9,10] thrombospondin,[11,12] etc.), as well as other factors involved in tumor cell–stromal interactions.[13]

The characterization of natural inhibitors and promoters of angiogenesis has provided an obvious strategy for the development of compounds that potentially interfere with the various steps necessary for tumor angiogenesis. More than three dozen agents that may potentially interfere with tumor angiogenesis are now in various stages of clinical development. This chapter focuses on the early results of select trials evaluating several of these agents. Finally some of the issues unique to the clinical evaluation of agents potentially capable of inhibiting angiogenesis are discussed.

MATRIX METALLOPROTEINASE INHIBITORS

Matrix metalloproteinases (MMPs) are a family of structurally related zinc-containing endopeptidases that are involved in the degradation of extracellular matrix components (ECM).[14,15] MMP gene expression and enzymatic activity is an important physiologic process that plays an important role in embryogenesis, wound healing, and the female reproductive cycle.[14,15] On the other hand, excessive proteolysis by these enzymes plays an important role in several pathologic processes, including arthritis, autoimmune blistering disorders of the skin, periodontitis, and tumor progression. Because MMPs facilitate the breakdown of the basement membrane and the underlying stroma, they have been implicated in tumor invasion and metastasis formation.

At least 17 members of the MMP family have been identified, and all are characterized by the presence of the metal-binding domain responsible for binding of the zinc ion.[16] The MMPs are produced by a variety of different cells, including fibroblasts, epithelial cells, inflammatory cells, and endothelial cells.[17] Several studies have demonstrated high levels of MMPs in the vicinity of a tumor, but whether tumor cells actually produce the MMPs remains unclear.[16,18] MMPs exist as inactive zymogens that are activated by proteolytic cleavage of the amino-terminal domain. The exception is membrane type 1 (MT-1) MMP, which is cell surface bound and is processed before cell surface localization.[19] Physiologic inhibitors known as tissue inhibitors of metalloproteinases (TIMPs) control MMP activity. The TIMP family currently consists of four members: TIMP-1, TIMP-2, TIMP-3, and TIMP-4.[15]

For a primary tumor to progress locally through adjacent normal tissue, the ECM must be digested.[20] Similarly, for metastases to expand at a site distant from the primary tumor, the ECM must be digested and remodeled. MMPs are also directly involved in the angiogenic response, mediating the remodeling and invasion of the ECM by new capillaries.[21,22] MMPs also promote angiogenesis by regulating endothelial cell attachment, proliferation, and migration.[21,22] These observations have led to the possibility that matrix metalloproteinase inhibitors (MMPIs) could be developed that would inhibit tumor progression at both the primary tumor site and sites of metastases. One would speculate that administration of an MMPI would have little or no direct tumor cell cytotoxicity. As a result, use of such agents may be

TABLE 35-1. MATRIX METALLOPROTEINASE INHIBITORS CURRENTLY UNDER INVESTIGATION IN CLINICAL TRIALS

Compound	Company
Marimastat, BB-2516	British Biotech
Ag3340	Agouron Pharmaceuticals, Inc.
CGS-27023A	Novartis Pharma AG
BAY 12-9566 (discontinued)	Bayer Corp
D2163	Chiroscience Group PLC
Ilomastat, GM6001	Glycomed, Inc.
COL-3, Metastat	CollaGenex Pharmaceuticals

most useful in combination with conventional cytotoxic agents.[23] A concern with the long-term administration of MMPIs is the effect they may have on normal physiologic processes that require MMP activity, such as wound repair or reproduction.[24–26] Several MMPIs are now being developed for potential therapeutic application in cancer therapy, periodontal disease, and ophthalmology (Table 35-1).

Clinical Trials with Matrix Metalloproteinase Inhibitors

Marimastat

Marimastat is an orally administered MMPI that has undergone the most extensive testing in humans, with over 4,000 patients participating in clinical trials.[27] The compound was developed as a successor to Batimastat (BB-94), a low-molecular-weight, nonselective MMPI that demonstrated inhibitory activity against MMP-2, MMP-3, and MMP-9.[28] Batimastat did not appear to have a direct cytotoxic effect against tumor cell lines or fibroblasts.[27] The drug had poor bioavailability and was evaluated in humans by administering it intraperitoneally and intrapleurally.[29,30] Preclinical data suggested that a combination of Batimastat and chemotherapy potentiated the antitumor effect when compared with chemotherapy alone.[31] The presumed requirement to administer MMPIs over the long term resulted in an effort to develop oral MMPIs.

Marimastat is classified as a hydroxamate, with a broad spectrum of MMP-inhibitory activity but with better pharmacokinetic properties than Batimastat.[32] Early phase I trials involving patients with various malignancies showed that musculoskeletal complaints were very common (60% of patients) at dosages greater than 50 mg twice daily.[33–39] Joint pain, stiffness, edema, and skin discoloration characterize the syndrome. When the dosage of Marimastat was reduced to 10 mg twice daily, the incidence of musculoskeletal complaints was markedly reduced (30% after 3 to 5 months of therapy).[33–39] The lower daily dose of Marimastat corresponded to a plasma level that resulted in 90% enzyme inhibition. Data from four placebo-controlled trials involving over 1,000 patients showed no increase in adverse events in patients receiving Marimastat other than the musculoskeletal complaints.

Marimastat has been evaluated in treatment of patients with pancreatic, ovarian, colorectal, breast, gastric, and pros-

tatic cancer. Most patients had metastatic disease that had already progressed after treatment with conventional therapy. In the pancreatic, ovarian, colorectal, and prostate cancer studies, tumor markers (cancer antigen 19-9, cancer antigen 125, carcinoembryonic antigen, and prostate-specific antigen, respectively) were used as surrogate markers of the biologic activity of Marimastat.[34] Only patients who had demonstrated a greater than 25% increase in the level of the tumor marker in the 4 weeks before study entry were eligible. The rate of rise of the tumor marker was then evaluated in patients while receiving Marimastat for 4 weeks to determine if the study drug was having a biologic effect. An analysis of individual studies and a meta-analysis of data from all studies showed that Marimastat significantly reduced the rate of rise of the tumor markers in a dose-dependent fashion.[34,40] The effect was identified for dosages of Marimastat greater than 10 mg twice daily, but no significant difference was found in the rate of rise of tumor markers for higher dosages (25 or 50 mg twice daily). The effect on the rate of rise of tumor markers also appeared to be greater with twice-daily dosing than with once-daily dosing.[40]

Randomized study of Marimastat therapy for gastric cancer has been conducted.[41] A total of 369 patients participated, and the analysis was performed when 85% mortality was observed in one arm. At the predefined analysis point, 22.7% of the patients receiving Marimastat were alive compared with 14.1% of the patients receiving placebo. Progression-free survival was significantly higher among those treated with Marimastat. Although a trend was seen toward a survival benefit in Marimastat-treated patients, it did not reach statistical significance. No treatment-related toxicities were observed other than the previously reported musculoskeletal side effects.[41] Similar trials in metastatic breast cancer and non–small cell lung cancer are ongoing.

BAY 12-9566

BAY 12-9566 is an MMPI classified as a carboxylate inhibitor that shows selectivity for MMP-2 and MMP-9 over other MMPs. In clinical trials with BAY 12-9566, dosages of 1.6 g per day were administered.[42] Thrombocytopenia was the most common side effect associated with this dosage.[42] Feasibility studies demonstrated that BAY 12-9566 could be administered alone or in conjunction with chemotherapy. A comparison of gemcitabine with BAY 12-9566 treatment in patients with advanced pancreatic cancer showed superiority in outcome for patients receiving chemotherapy.[43,44] Unfortunately, due to disappointing interim results from a phase III study in small cell lung cancer patients, development of BAY 12-9566 has been discontinued.

Ag3340

Ag3340 is an oral selective MMPI. Ag3340 appears to selectively inhibit MMP-2, MMP-3, MMP-9, and MMP-14.[28,45] Because MMP-1 is not affected by Ag3340, the joint-related toxicities observed with other MMPIs should be less common. Phase I trials of Ag3340 have been completed in patients with advanced tumors and prostate cancer. Feasibility trials have been completed demonstrating that Ag3340 can be administered in conjunction with paclitaxel and carboplatin,[46,47] and mitoxantrone hydrochloride and prednisone.[48] Based on these results, phase III trials are currently under way to evaluate Ag3340 in patients with non–small cell lung cancer receiving treatment with carboplatin/paclitaxel and in patients with hormone-refractory prostate cancer receiving treatment with mitoxantrone/prednisone.

COL-3

Tetracycline and structurally related compounds have been shown to inhibit collagenase and other MMPs in laboratory experiments.[49–52] A chemically altered tetracycline, 6-demethyl-6-deoxy-4-dedimethylaminotetracycline or COL-3, has been developed that retains the ability to inhibit MMPs but lacks an antimicrobial effect.[53,54] Murohara et al. showed that endothelial cell nitric oxide may mediate angiogenesis by promoting endothelial cell migration through an integrin-dependent mechanism.[55] In cell culture, COL-3 concentrations between 2.5 and 10 μg per mL inhibited inducible nitric oxide synthase and nitric acid production.[56] In addition, COL-3 has been shown to inhibit several MMPs (MT-1-MMP, MMP-2, and pro-MMP-2).[57] Evidence also suggests that COL-3 induces apoptosis in certain cell lines.[58]

In animal experiments COL-3 has been shown to decrease the number and size of lung metastases after SCID mice have been inoculated with C8161 cells.[59] The half-life of COL-3 is quite long, 22 hours. In rodent and monkey studies, steady-state plasma concentrations of 10 and 20 μmol per L were associated with mild and severe toxicity, respectively.[53,56,59] A phase I trial of protracted daily treatment with COL-3 in patients with advanced malignancies was reported.[60] The starting dosage was 36 mg per m^2 per day. Although accrual to the trial is not complete, reported toxicities include fatigue, anemia, skin hyperpigmentation, and rare skin reactions secondary to photosensitization. Treatment with COL-3 is also being correlated with plasma levels of MMP-9, VEGF, tumor necrosis factor, E-selectin, and Fas ligand receptors.[60]

The other compounds listed in Table 35-1 are in early-phase clinical trials in patients with advanced cancer.

THALIDOMIDE

Thalidomide or α-phthalimodoglutarimide, was synthesized in the 1950s and marketed as a sedative hypnotic with minimal side effects.[61] Thalidomide was withdrawn from the market after limb defects and deformities of internal organs were described in infants born to mothers who consumed thalidomide during pregnancy.[62]

Thalidomide has pleiotropic effects, including sedation, inhibition of tumor necrosis factor α, and inhibition of angiogenesis in the xenograft model and the Matrigel assay. Thalidomide may interfere with tumor angiogenesis by inhibiting VEGF and bFGF-2.[63–69] The mechanism responsible for the teratogenicity of thalidomide has been postulated to be inhibition or down-regulation of integrin subunits, which inhibits or slows endothelial migration and, as a result, angiogenesis.[70] Thalidomide has been approved by the Food and Drug Administration for treatment of erythema nodosum leprosum, an inflammatory manifestation of leprosy,[71] and is now in clinical trials to assess its efficacy in patients with a variety of malignancies.

In a phase I-II clinical trial of thalidomide involving patients with recurrent glioma, a maximum tolerated dose (MTD) of 300 mg per m^2 was established.[72] Five patients of 46 (11%) had partial tumor responses, and an additional 28 patients maintained a stable disease state. Treatment with thalidomide was associated with sedation and constipation. Thalidomide has also been combined with carboplatin in the same patient population.

Baidas et al. reported the results of a phase II clinical trial of thalidomide in patients with metastatic breast cancer who received either 200 mg or 800 mg per day.[73] Antitumor activity was not observed at either dose level of thalidomide; however, peripheral neuropathy and somnolence were more common at the higher dose level.

Singhal et al. reported on the use of thalidomide as a single agent in the treatment of refractory myeloma.[74] The overall rate of response was 32%, where response was defined as a reduction of at least 25% in the level of the myeloma protein in serum or Bence Jones protein in the urine. A response was associated with a decrease in the percentage of plasma cells in the bone marrow and a prolongation in time to disease progression. Although the mechanism of action of thalidomide in myeloma is not known, inhibition of blood vessel formation in the bone marrow may contribute.

ANTIVASCULAR ENDOTHELIAL GROWTH FACTOR MONOCLONAL ANTIBODY

VEGF is one of the most potent endothelial cell–specific mitogens and a potent promoter of both physiologic and pathologic angiogenesis.[75,76] Recombinant VEGF is under evaluation in clinical trials in patients with a history of myocardial ischemia. The rationale for these investigations is that VEGF induces neovascularization and reduces symptoms of myocardial ischemia. Neutralizing antibodies to VEGF have been shown to inhibit tumor growth and the development of metastases in experimental models.[77–80] A recombinant humanized monoclonal antibody to VEGF (rhuMAb VEGF) is under evaluation as an inhibitor of tumor angiogenesis. A phase I trial of rhuMAb VEGF involving patients with refractory metastatic cancer demonstrated that rhuMAb VEGF was well tolerated without any grade 3 or 4 drug-related toxicities or acute infusion-related toxicities.[81] Although objective responses were not observed, 50% of patients maintained stable disease for longer than 10 weeks. In addition, circulating VEGF levels decreased during treatment with rhuMAb VEGF. Three tumor-related episodes of bleeding were reported, including a hemorrhage into unrecognized brain metastases in a patient with a hepatoma.[81] Phase I trials have also demonstrated that rhuMAb VEGF can be safely combined with chemotherapy without any novel acute toxicities or long-term sequela.[82]

Preliminary results of a phase II trial of rhuMAb VEGF involving patients with metastatic breast cancer have been reported.[83] Patients were treated with an infusion of either 3 mg per kg or 10 mg per kg of rhuMAb VEFG every 2 weeks. Three patients experienced an objective response to single-agent rhuMAb VEGF, including one patient in the higher dose group with a supraclavicular mass who experienced a complete response. The other responses were observed in soft tissue disease. Therapy with rhuMAb VEFG was well tolerated.[83] Ongoing trials include a randomized phase II design comparing rhuMAb VEGF alone or in combination with carboplatin and paclitaxel in patients with stage IIIB or IV non–small cell lung cancer.

SU5416

Flk-1 is a KDR tyrosine kinase receptor for VEGF.[2,84] SU5416 is a synthetic, specific VEGF receptor antagonist that decreases VEGF-stimulated Flk-1 phosphorylation.[85] In xenograft models, SU5416 shows antitumor activity against a broad spectrum of malignancies, including glioblastoma, ovarian cancer, and non–small cell lung cancer.[85] SU5416 appears to be more effective in slower growing tumors.[85] In a phase I trial of SU5416 in patients with advanced, refractory cancer, many patients maintained a stable disease status for longer than 6 months.[86] SU5416 was administered in a twice-weekly dosing schedule and the MTD was established at 245 mg per m². Results of pharmacokinetic evaluation in this trial supported dose-dependent clearance and extensive tissue penetration.[86]

Another phase I trial of SU5416 involving patients with advanced malignancies was reported in which a 5-day loading dose of the drug was followed by five weekly maintenance infusions.[87] Subsequent cycles consisted of six weekly infusions of SU5416. Dose escalations of SU5416 occurred at 33% increments until a final dose of 65 mg per m² (loading dose) and 190 mg per m² (weekly infusion) was reached. One patient with squamous cell lung cancer and lung metastases had a partial response, and three patients were stable at the 12-week evaluation. Toxicity was minimal with the dose and schedule used in this trial.[87]

A dose-escalating (twice-weekly intravenous) schedule of SU5416 involving 20 patients with acquired immunodeficiency syndrome (AIDS)–related Kaposi's sarcoma was reported.[88] Tumor response was defined as resolution or flattening of lesions. Five patients had an objective response, including one patient who had a complete response at the highest dose level (145 mg per m²). Treatment with SU5416 had no detectable effect on viral load or T-cell subsets. Toxicity was generally mild or moderate.[88] Phase II trials of SU5416 involving patients with AIDS-related Kaposi's sarcoma are now under way.

TNP-470

TNP-470 is a synthetic analog of fumagillin, a compound secreted by the fungus *Aspergillus fumigatus fresenius*.[89,90] Fumagillin was isolated as a contaminant from an endothelial cell culture in which growth inhibition was observed. The compound was demonstrated to inhibit tumor growth and angiogenesis *in vivo* and endothelial cell proliferation *in vitro*.[89] Clinical development of fumagillin was not pursued after experiments in animals revealed prohibitive weight loss.[89] TNP-470 was developed to mimic the effects of fumagillin without its side effects. The mechanism whereby TNP-470 affects angiogenesis is presumed to be multifactorial.[91–97] TNP-470 blocks mitogen-induced endothelial cell proliferation by inhibiting or attenuating cyclins, cyclin kinases, and phosphorylation of the retinoblastoma protein.[92] In addition, TNP-470 inhibits the activity of urokinase-type plasminogen activator in endothelial cells.[97] Reports have also been published that TNP-470 is directly cytotoxic to tumor cells.[93]

Phase I trials have been conducted in patients with refractory solid tumors, prostate cancer, cervical cancer, AIDS-associated Kaposi's sarcoma, and pediatric malignancies.[98–101] Either a 1- or 4-hour infusion of TNP-470 was administered in these trials. Treatment schedules included drug administration every other day; Monday, Wednesday, and Friday; or once a week.[98–101] Some schedules also included a rest period without treatment. The most common toxicities reported from the phase I trials included asthenia (42% of patients), nausea (32%), anorexia (18%), and dizziness (16%). Significant weight loss was uncommon. The most common reason for discontinuing therapy was disease progression (71%).[98–101]

MTDs were determined in each of the phase I trials. The two trials evaluating a 1-hour infusion given every other day for 28 days followed by a 14-day rest identified the MTD as 47 and 60 mg per m², respectively. When TNP-470 was administered as a 1-hour infusion (Monday, Wednesday, and Friday) without a rest period, the MTD was 57.4 mg per m². Increasing the infusion of

TNP-470 to 4 hours once a week resulted in an MTD of 177 mg per m². Rare objective tumor responses and disease stabilization were identified in patients participating in the phase I trials.[98–101]

Reports provide preliminary results of phase I studies of the use of TNP-470 in combination with paclitaxel to treat patients with solid tumors.[102,103] In one study, TNP-470 was administered over 1 hour on Monday, Wednesday, and Friday. Paclitaxel was administered every 3 weeks.[102] Dose escalation in each arm proceeded without limiting toxicity. Initial toxicity analysis suggests that myelosuppression and peripheral neuropathy is no greater with combination therapy than with paclitaxel alone. Assessment of neurocognitive function revealed subclinical declines in memory, frontal lobe function, and motor coordination after two courses of combination therapy in a small percentage of patients; these effects resolved after cessation of treatment with TNP-470.[102] In the second study, both paclitaxel and TNP-470 were administered weekly for 3 weeks followed by a 1-week break. Preliminary results suggest that the combination of weekly paclitaxel and TNP-470 is active and can be administered with minimal toxicity.[103]

SQUALAMINE

Squalamine is a noncytotoxic aminosterol, originally derived from the liver of the dogfish shark.[104] Squalamine inhibits mitogen-induced proliferation and the migration of endothelial cells, thereby preventing tumor neovascularization.[104,105] A phase I dose-escalation trial of squalamine involving patients with advanced malignancies has been reported.[106] Patients were treated with a continuous infusion of squalamine for 5 days every 3 weeks. Dose levels of squalamine varied between 6 and 500 mg per m² per day. Squalamine was well tolerated up to 357 mg per m² per day, after which hyperbilirubinemia and transaminase elevations were more common. The antitumor effect has not been reported, although pharmacokinetic analysis suggests that plasma concentrations of squalamine approach those required for an antiangiogenic effect *in vitro*. Preliminary results from a second phase I study have been reported in which 12 patients with advanced malignancies were treated with doses of squalamine ranging from 6 to 255 mg per m². The plasma concentrations achieved over this dose range were in accordance with those achieving an antiangiogenic effect in laboratory experiments.[107]

ANGIOSTATIN

In a series of elegant experiments by O'Reilly and colleagues, an animal model was developed that demonstrated the suppression of remote metastases by the primary tumor mass.[8] Mice were inoculated with Lewis lung carcinoma (LLC, low metastatic phenotype), which resulted in the development of pulmonary metastases. Once the primary tumor mass was removed, the previously dormant metastases grew and exhibited neovascularization.[8] Additional experiments involved fractionation of the biologic fluids of animals bearing LLC tumors to determine if they contained factors that inhibited the proliferation of bovine endothelial cells. This series of experiments resulted in the isolation and characterization of a protein now called *angiostatin*.[8,108]

Angiostatin has been identified as a fragment of plasminogen.[8,108] The exact mechanism by which angiostatin is produced *in vivo* remains unclear. In mice bearing LLC tumors, if the primary tumor was resected and intraperitoneal angiostatin was then given, lung metastases remained small and avascular. In comparison, resected animals that received plasminogen developed grossly visible, bloody lung metastases. These experiments confirm the activity of angiostatin and, interestingly, show that the parent compound plasminogen has no antiangiogenesis activity.[8,108] A great deal of interest exists in evaluating the activity of angiostatin in patients, but because the methods for producing the compound are unreliable, clinical trials in patients have not been initiated.

ENDOSTATIN

Endostatin is a 20-kd carboxy-terminal fragment of collagen XVIII discovered by O'Reilly et al.[10] Recombinant mouse endostatin suppressed the growth of metastases when administered systemically to mice, and the effect is specific to endothelial cells. No significant toxicity has been associated with endostatin administration in animal studies. The other intriguing observation regarding treatment with endostatin is that long-term, intermittent dosing did not lead to acquired resistance.[109] Subcutaneous administration of endostatin to mice with LLC tumors, T241 fibrosarcomas, and B16-F10 melanomas resulted in tumor regression.[109] All tumors became dormant after two to six cycles of therapy, and once endostatin was discontinued, the tumors failed to regrow. Three phase I trials have been initiated to evaluate endostatin in patients with advanced solid tumor malignancies. No results are available at this time.

CARBOXYAMIDO-TRIAZOLE

Carboxyamido-triazole (CAI) is a novel cytostatic agent with antiproliferative, antimetastatic, and antiangiogenic properties.[110,111] It was the first anticancer agent developed as a signal transduction inhibitor to enter clinical trials. The antiproliferative activity of CAI is presumed to be due to inhibition of calcium influx through voltage-sensitive and voltage-insensitive receptor–mediated calcium channels.[110,111] CAI is also able to inhibit several steps in the angiogenesis cascade, including bFGF-induced tyrosine phosphorylation and human umbilical vein endothelial cell proliferation, adhesion, and motility.[111] Evidence also suggests that CAI reduces the expression of MMP-2 by inhibiting fibroblast growth factor–stimulated MMP-2 synthesis.[112] *In vitro* data suggested that a plasma concentration of CAI of between 1 and 10 mg per mL was necessary to inhibit calcium influx and calcium-mediated signal transduction, malignant invasion, and progression.[113–115] The first phase I clinical trial of CAI, in which the drug was administered orally, confirmed that the ideal plasma concentration could be achieved in patients with daily or every-other-day dosing without severe toxicity.[116]

Subsequent phase I clinical trials using either a gelatin capsule or micronized powder formulation of CAI have been completed.[117,118] When the micronized powder formulation was administered daily, the dose-limiting toxicity, consisting of reversible grade 2 or 3 cerebellar ataxia and confusion, was observed at 350 mg per m² per day. Grade 1 or 2 gastrointestinal toxicity was observed in 50% of patients. One minor response was observed, and an additional nine patients showed disease stabilization.[118] In a separate phase I trial in which the gelatin capsule formulation of CAI was administered daily, the MTD was 75 mg per m² per day with dose-limiting cerebellar toxicity observed at 100 mg per m² per day.[117] Gastrointestinal symptoms were common (79% of patients) but mild. Mild to moderate fatigue was also experienced by 66% of patients. One patient with transitional cell cancer of the bladder showed a partial response to CAI therapy.

A phase II trial of CAI in patients with androgen-independent prostate cancer was reported by the National Cancer Institute.[119] The dose of CAI used in the study was calculated so that the plasma steady-state maximum concentrations would be maintained between 2 and 5 mg per mL. Although no responses were detected in 15 patients, 27.7% of patients were noted to have a decrease in serum VEGF concentrations.

TRIAL DESIGN

One of the challenges facing clinical researchers interested in agents that may inhibit angiogenesis is determining the optimal way to assess the clinical efficacy of the agent.[120] The traditional approach for evaluating a new cytotoxic agent is to perform a phase I dose-escalation trial that identifies the MTD of drug. With conventional cytotoxic agents, the MTD frequently correlates with maximal antitumor activity. With agents that inhibit angiogenesis, however, tumor regression may or may not be observed. As a result, the MTD may not accurately reflect the optimal biologic effect of the drug. Although identifying both acute and long-term toxicities associated with any new agent is important, an angiogenesis inhibitor may have a defined optimal biologic dose that is very different from the MTD.[120]

Identifying plasma concentrations of the angiogenesis inhibitor in animals that are optimal for the desired biologic effect is important. Because angiogenesis inhibitors may not cause tumor shrinkage when administered alone, the clinical development of the agent may be abandoned if surrogate end points that reflect the activity of the agent are not considered in trial design. As an example, several clinical trials have attempted to correlate the effect of drug administration on circulating concentrations of certain angiogenesis mitogens (i.e., bFGF, VEGF, etc.), levels of these mitogens in the urine, or levels of tumor markers (i.e., carcinoembryonic antigen, cancer antigen 15-3, etc.). Whether these effects of a new agent legitimately reflect the antiangiogenesis or antitumor activity remains unclear.

Because good surrogate markers are still lacking, clinical trial design continues to rely on traditional end points. In studies of metastatic disease, response rates may be considered, but time to disease progression and overall survival are the more important primary end points. To evaluate the true effect of the new agent, randomized trials with and without the antiangiogenesis inhibitor are crucial. In adjuvant therapy trials, in which patients have no clinical evidence of disease, judging the effect of the new agent is even more challenging. To evaluate the effect of an adjuvant therapy, randomized trials are necessary and frequently involve thousands of patients. The number of patients required for such a trial depends on the risk profile (i.e., risk of death, risk of recurrence) of the patient population being studied. The clinical end points of interest are time to disease recurrence and overall survival. If a low-risk patient population is being evaluated, a long follow-up period and thousands of patients may be required to judge the difference between standard therapy and treatment with the angiogenesis inhibitor. In a high-risk patient population, recurrences may be expected earlier and in greater numbers. As a result, a smaller sample size is required to assess the new agent.

REFERENCES

1. Folkman J. Tumor angiogenesis: therapeutic implications. *N Engl J Med* 1971;285:1182–1186.
2. Jones A, Harris AL. New developments in angiogenesis: a major mechanism for tumor growth and target for therapy. *Cancer J Sci Am* 1998;4:209–217.
3. Folkman J. Seminars in medicine of the Beth Israel Hospital, Boston. Clinical applications of research on angiogenesis. *N Engl J Med* 1995;333:1757–1763.
4. Folkman J. Angiogenesis in cancer, vascular, rheumatoid and other disease. *Nat Med* 1995;1:27–31.
5. Rastinejad F, Polverini PJ, Bouck NP. Regulation of the activity of a new inhibitor of angiogenesis by a cancer suppressor gene. *Cell* 1989;56:345–355.

6. Folkman J, Klagsbrun M. Angiogenic factors. *Science* 1987;235:442–447.

7. Beckner ME. Factors promoting tumor angiogenesis. *Cancer Invest* 1999;17:594–623.

8. O'Reilly MS, Holmgren L, Shing Y, et al. Angiostatin: a novel angiogenesis inhibitor that mediates the suppression of metastases by a Lewis lung carcinoma. *Cell* 1994;79:315–328.

9. Sim BKL. Angiostatin and endostatin endothelial cell-specific endogenous inhibitors of angiogenesis and tumor growth. *Angiogenesis* 1998;2:37–48.

10. O'Reilly MS, Boehm T, Shing Y, et al. Endostatin: an endogenous inhibitor of angiogenesis and tumor growth. *Cell* 1997;88:277–285.

11. Volpert OV, Tolsma SS, Pellerin S, et al. Inhibition of angiogenesis by thrombospondin-2. *Biochem Biophys Res Commun* 1995;217:326–332.

12. Dameron KM, Volpert OV, Tainsky MA, et al. Control of angiogenesis in fibroblasts by p53 regulation of thrombospondin-1. *Science* 1994;265:1582–1584.

13. Liotta LA, Steeg PS, Stetler-Stevenson WG. Cancer metastasis and angiogenesis: an imbalance of positive and negative regulation. *Cell* 1991;64:327–336.

14. Kleiner DE, Stetler-Stevenson WG. Matrix metalloproteinases and metastasis. *Cancer Chemother Pharmacol* 1999;43:S42–51.

15. Stetler-Stevenson WG. Matrix metalloproteinases in angiogenesis: a moving target for therapeutic intervention. *J Clin Invest* 1999;103:1237–1241.

16. Chambers AF, Matrisian LM. Changing views of the role of matrix metalloproteinases in metastasis. *J Natl Cancer Inst* 1997;89:1260–1270.

17. Werb Z. ECM and cell surface proteolysis: regulating cellular ecology. *Cell* 1997;91:439–442.

18. Stetler-Stevenson WG. Dynamics of matrix turnover during pathologic remodeling of the extracellular matrix. *Am J Pathol* 1996;148:1345–1350.

19. Hiraoka N, Allen E, Apel IJ, et al. Matrix metalloproteinases regulate neovascularization by acting as pericellular fibrinolysins. *Cell* 1998;95:365–377.

20. Liotta LA, Tryggvason K, Garbisa S, et al. Metastatic potential correlates with enzymatic degradation of basement membrane collagen. *Nature* 1980;284:67–68.

21. Mignatti P, Rifkin DB. Biology and biochemistry of proteinases in tumor invasion. *Physiol Rev* 1993;73:161–195.

22. Stetler-Stevenson WG, Hewitt R, Corcoran M. Matrix metalloproteinases and tumor invasion: from correlation and causality to the clinic. *Semin Cancer Biol* 1996;7:147–154.

23. Teicher BA. Potentiation of cytotoxic cancer therapies by antiangiogenic agents. In: Teicher BA, ed. *Antiangiogenic agents in cancer therapy.* Totowa, NJ: Humana Press, 1999:277–316.

24. Brenner CA, Adler RR, Rappolee DA, et al. Genes for extracellular-matrix-degrading metalloproteinases and their inhibitor, TIMP, are expressed during early mammalian development. *Genes Dev* 1989;3:848–859.

25. Wolf C, Chenard MP, Durand de Grossouvre P, et al. Breast-cancer-associated stromelysin-3 gene is expressed in basal cell carcinoma and during cutaneous wound healing. *J Invest Dermatol* 1992;99:870–872.

26. Vaes G, Delaisse JM, Eeckhout Y. Relative roles of collagenase and lysosomal cysteine-proteinases in bone resorption. *Matrix Suppl* 1992;1:383–388.

27. Teicher BA. Batimastat and Marimastat in cancer: summary of early clinical data. In: Teicher BA, ed. *Antiangiogenic agents in cancer therapy.* Totowa, NJ: Humana Press, 1999:399–406.

28. Brown PD, Giavazzi R. Matrix metalloproteinase inhibition: a review of anti-tumour activity. *Ann Oncol* 1995;6:967–974.

29. Macaulay VM, O'Byrne KJ, Saunders MP, et al. Phase I study of intrapleural batimastat (BB-94), a matrix metalloproteinase inhibitor, in the treatment of malignant pleural effusions. *Clin Cancer Res* 1999;5:513–520.

30. Beattie GJ, Smyth JF. Phase I study of intraperitoneal metalloproteinase inhibitor BB94 in patients with malignant ascites. *Clin Cancer Res* 1998;4:1899–1902.

31. Giavazzi R, Garofalo A, Ferri C, et al. Batimastat, a synthetic inhibitor of matrix metalloproteinases, potentiates the antitumor activity of cisplatin in ovarian carcinoma xenografts. *Clin Cancer Res* 1998;4:985–992.

32. Rasmussen HS, McCann PP. Matrix metalloproteinase inhibition as a novel anticancer strategy: a review with special focus on batimastat and marimastat. *Pharmacol Ther* 1997;75:69–75.

33. Millar AW, Brown PD, Moore J, et al. Results of single and repeat dose studies of the oral matrix metalloproteinase inhibitor marimastat in healthy male volunteers. *Br J Clin Pharmacol* 1998;45:21–26.

34. Nemunaitis J, Poole C, Primrose J, et al. Combined analysis of studies of the effects of the matrix metalloproteinase inhibitor marimastat on serum tumor markers in advanced cancer: selection of a biologically active and tolerable dose for longer-term studies. *Clin Cancer Res* 1998;4:1101–1109.

35. Wojtowicz-Praga S, Torri J, Johnson M, et al. Phase I trial of Marimastat, a novel matrix metalloproteinase inhibitor, administered orally to patients with advanced lung cancer. *J Clin Oncol* 1998;16:2150–2156.

36. Primrose JN, Bleiberg H, Daniel F, et al. Marimastat in recurrent colorectal cancer: exploratory evaluation of biological activity by measurement of carcinoembryonic antigen. *Br J Cancer* 1999;79:509–514.

37. Steward WP. Marimastat (BB2516): current status of development. *Cancer Chemother Pharmacol* 1999;43:S56–60.

38. Rosemurgy A, Harris J, Langleben A, et al. Marimastat in patients with advanced pancreatic cancer: a dose-finding study. *Am J Clin Oncol* 1999;22:247–252.

39. Tierney GM, Griffin NR, Stuart RC, et al. A pilot study of the safety and effects of the matrix metalloproteinase inhibitor marimastat in gastric cancer. *Eur J Cancer* 1999;35:563–568.

40. Rasmussen HS. Batimastat and Marimastat in cancer: summary of early clinical data. In: Teicher BA, ed. *Antiangiogenic agents in cancer therapy.* Totowa, NJ: Humana Press, 1999:399–406.

41. Fielding J, Scholefield J, Stuart R, et al. A randomized double-blind placebo-controlled study of Marimastat in patients with inoperable gastric adenocarcinoma. *Proc Annu Meet Am Soc Clin Oncol* 2000;19.

42. Goel R, Hirte H, Major P, et al. Clinical pharmacology of the metalloproteinase and angiogenesis inhibitor Bayer 12-9566 in cancer patients. *Proc Annu Meet Am Soc Clin Oncol* 1999;18:615(abst).

43. Moore M, Hamm J, Eisenberg P, et al. A comparison between gemcitabine and matrix metalloproteinase inhibitor BAY12-9566 in patients with advanced pancreatic cancer. *Proc Annu Meet Am Soc Clin Oncol* 2000;19(abst).

44. Goel R, Chouinard E, Steward D, et al. Phase I pharmacokinetic study of the metalloproteinase and angiogenesis inhibitor Bayer 12-9566 in conjunction with 5-fluorouracil/folinic acid. *Proc Annu Meet Am Soc Clin Oncol* 2000;19(abst).

45. Shalinsky DR, Brekken J, Zou H, et al. Broad antitumor and antiangiogenic activities of AG3340, a potent and selective MMP inhibitor undergoing advanced oncology clinical trials. *Ann N Y Acad Sci* 1999;878:236–270.

46. D'Olimpio J, Hande K, Collier M, et al. Phase I study of the matrix metalloproteinase inhibitor AG3340 in combination with paclitaxel and carboplatin for the treatment of patients with advanced solid tumors. *Proc Annu Meet Am Soc Clin Oncol* 1999;18:615(abst).

47. Tolcher A, Rowinsky E, Rizzo J, et al. A phase I pharmacokinetic study of the oral matrix metalloproteinase inhibitor Bay 12-9566 in combination with paclitaxel and carboplatin. *Proc Annu Meet Am Soc Clin Oncol* 1999;18:617(abst).

48. Collier M, Sheperd F, Ahmann F, et al. Novel approach to studying the efficacy of AG3340, a selective inhibitor of matrix metalloproteinases. *Proc Annu Meet Am Soc Clin Oncol* 1999;18:1861(abst).

49. Golub LM, Wolff M, Lee HM, et al. Further evidence that tetracyclines inhibit collagenase activity in human crevicular fluid and from other mammalian sources. *J Periodontal Res* 1985;20:12–23.

50. Golub LM, Goodson JM, Lee HM, et al. Tetracyclines inhibit tissue collagenases. Effects of ingested low-dose and local delivery systems. *J Periodontol* 1985;56:93–97.

51. Golub LM, Ramamurthy N, McNamara TF, et al. Tetracyclines inhibit tissue collagenase activity. A new mechanism in the treatment of periodontal disease. *J Periodontal Res* 1984;19:651–655.

52. Golub LM, Lee HM, Lehrer G, et al. Minocycline reduces gingival collagenolytic activity during diabetes. Preliminary observations and a proposed new mechanism of action. *J Periodontal Res* 1983;18:516–526.

53. Trachtman H, Futterweit S, Greenwald R, et al. Chemically modified tetracyclines inhibit inducible nitric oxide synthase expression and nitric oxide production in cultured rat mesangial cells. *Biochem Biophys Res Commun* 1996;229:243–248.

54. Golub LM, Ramamurthy NS, McNamara TF, et al. Tetracyclines inhibit connective tissue breakdown: new therapeutic implications for an old family of drugs. *Crit Rev Oral Biol Med* 1991;2:297–321.

55. Murohara T, Witzenbichler B, Spyridopoulos I, et al. Role of endothelial nitric oxide synthase in endothelial cell migration. *Arterioscler Thromb Vasc Biol* 1999;19:1156–1161.

56. Amin AR, Patel RN, Thakker GD, et al. Post-transcriptional regulation of inducible nitric oxide synthase mRNA in murine macrophages by doxycycline and chemically modified tetracyclines. *FEBS Lett* 1997;410:259–264.

57. Golub LM, Ramamurthy NS, Llavaneras A, et al. A chemically modified nonantimicrobial tetracycline (CMT-8) inhibits gingival matrix metalloproteinases, periodontal breakdown, and extra-oral bone loss in ovariectomized rats. *Ann N Y Acad Sci* 1999;878:290–310.

58. Lokeshwar BL, Houston-Clark HL, Selzer MG, et al. Potential application of a chemically modified non-antimicrobial tetracycline (CMT-3) against metastatic prostate cancer. *Adv Dent Res* 1998;12:97–102.

59. Seftor RE, Seftor EA, De Larco JE, et al. Chemically modified tetracyclines inhibit human melanoma cell invasion and metastasis. *Clin Exp Metastasis* 1998;16:217–225.

60. Rowinsky E, Eckhardt S, Rizzo J, et al. Protracted daily treatment with COL-3, an oral tetracycline analog, matrix metalloproteinase inhibitor, is feasible: a phase I, pharmacokinetic, and biologic study. *Proc Annu Meet Am Soc Clin Oncol* 2000;19(abst).

61. Tseng S, Pak G, Washenik K, et al. Rediscovering thalidomide: a review of its mechanism of action, side effects, and potential uses. *J Am Acad Dermatol* 1996;35:969–979.

62. Mellin GW, Katzenstein M. The saga of thalidomide. *N Engl J Med* 1962;24:1238–1244.

63. Haslett PA, Corral LG, Albert M, et al. Thalidomide costimulates primary human T lymphocytes, preferentially inducing proliferation, cytokine production, and cytotoxic responses in the CD8+ subset. *J Exp Med* 1998;187:1885–1892.

64. Corral LG, Haslett PA, Muller GW, et al. Differential cytokine modulation and T cell activation by two distinct classes of thalidomide analogues that are potent inhibitors of TNF-alpha. *J Immunol* 1999;163:380–386.

65. Bellamy WT, Richter L, Frutiger Y, et al. Expression of vascular endothelial growth factor and its receptors in hematopoietic malignancies. *Cancer Res* 1999;59:728–733.

66. Geitz H, Handt S, Zwingenberger K. Thalidomide selectively modulates the density of cell surface molecules involved in the adhesion cascade. *Immunopharmacology* 1996;31:213–221.

67. Damiano JS, Cress AE, Hazlehurst LA, et al. Cell adhesion mediated drug resistance (CAM-DR): role of integrins and resistance to apoptosis in human myeloma cell lines. *Blood* 1999;93:1658–1667.

68. Hallek M, Leif Bergsagel P, Anderson KC. Multiple myeloma: increasing evidence for a multistep transformation process. *Blood* 1998;91:3–21.

69. Parman T, Wiley MJ, Wells PG. Free radical-mediated oxidative DNA damage in the mechanism of thalidomide teratogenicity. *Nat Med* 1999;5:582–585.

70. D'Amato RJ, Loughnan MS, Flynn E, et al. Thalidomide is an inhibitor of angiogenesis. *Proc Natl Acad Sci U S A* 1994;91:4082–4085.

71. Sampaio EP, Kaplan G, Miranda A, et al. The influence of thalidomide on the clinical and immunologic manifestation of erythema nodosum leprosum. *J Infect Dis* 1993;168:408–414.

72. Glass J, Gruber ML, Nirenberg A. Phase I/II study of carboplatin and thalidomide in recurrent glioblastoma multiforme. *Proc Annu Meet Am Soc Clin Oncol* 1999;18:551(abst).

73. Baidas SM, Isaacs C, Crawford J, et al. A phase II evaluation of thalidomide in patients with metastatic breast cancer. *Proc Annu Meet Am Soc Clin Oncol* 1999;18:475(abst).

74. Singhal S, Mehta J, Desikan R, et al. Antitumor activity of thalidomide in refractory multiple myeloma. *N Engl J Med* 1999;341:1565–1571.

75. Neufeld G, Cohen T, Gengrinovitch S, et al. Vascular endothelial growth factor (VEGF) and its receptors. *FASEB J* 1999;13:9–22.

76. Ferrara N. Role of vascular endothelial growth factor in the regulation of angiogenesis. *Kidney Int* 1999;56:794–814.

77. Okuda Y, Tsurumaru K, Suzuki S, et al. Hypoxia and endothelin-1 induce VEGF production in human vascular smooth muscle cells. *Life Sci* 1998;63:477–484.

78. Asano M, Yukita A, Matsumoto T, et al. An anti-human VEGF monoclonal antibody, MV833, that exhibits potent anti-tumor activity in vivo. *Hybridoma* 1998;17:185–190.

79. Melnyk O, Zimmerman M, Kim KJ, et al. Neutralizing anti-vascular endothelial growth factor antibody inhibits further growth of established prostate cancer and metastases in a pre-clinical model. *J Urol* 1999;161:960–963.

80. Wang G, Dong Z, Xu G, et al. The effect of antibody against vascular endothelial growth factor on tumor growth and metastasis. *J Cancer Res Clin Oncol* 1998;124:615–620.

81. Gordon MS, Talpaz M, Margolin K, et al. Phase I trial of recombinant humanized monoclonal anti-vascular endothelial growth factor in patients with metastatic cancer. *Proc Annu Meet Am Soc Clin Oncol* 1998;17:809(abst).

82. Margolin K, Gordon M, Talpaz M, et al. Phase Ib trial of intravenous recombinant humanized monoclonal antibody to vascular endothelial growth factor in combination with chemotherapy in patients with advanced cancer: pharmacologic and long-term safety data. *Proc Annu Meet Am Soc Clin Oncol* 1999;18:1678(abst).

83. Sledge G, Miller K, Novotny W, et al. A phase II trial of single-agent rhuMAb VEGF in patients with relapsed metastatic breast cancer. *Proc Annu Meet Am Soc Clin Oncol* 2000;19(abst).

84. Veikkola T, Karkkainen M, Claesson-Welsh L, et al. Regulation of angiogenesis via vascular endothelial growth factor receptors. *Cancer Res* 2000;60:203–212.

85. Fong TA, Shawver LK, Sun L, et al. SU5416 is a potent and selective inhibitor of the vascular endothelial growth factor receptor (Flk-1/KDR) that inhibits tyrosine kinase catalysis, tumor vascularization, and growth of multiple tumor types. *Cancer Res* 1999;59:99–106.

86. Rosen L, Mulay M, Mayers A, et al. Phase I dose escalating trial of SU5416, a novel angiogenesis inhibitor in patients with advanced malignancies. *Proc Annu Meet Am Soc Clin Oncol* 1999;18:618(abst).

87. Stopeck A. Results of a phase I dose-escalation study of the antiangiogenic agent, SU5416, in patients with advanced malignancies. *Proc Annu Meet Am Soc Clin Oncol* 2000;19(abst).

88. Miles S, Aratesh K, Gill P, et al. A multicenter dose-escalating study of SU5416 in AIDS-related Kaposi's sarcoma. *Proc Annu Meet Am Soc Clin Oncol* 2000;19(abst).

89. Ingber D, Fujita T, Kishimoto S, et al. Synthetic analogues of fumagillin that inhibit angiogenesis and suppress tumour growth. *Nature* 1990;348:555–557.

90. Figg WD, Pluda JM, Lush RM, et al. The pharmacokinetics of TNP-470, a new angiogenesis inhibitor. *Pharmacotherapy* 1997;17:91–97.

91. Turk BE, Su Z, Liu JO. Synthetic analogues of TNP-470 and ovalicin reveal a common molecular basis for inhibition of angiogenesis and immunosuppression. *Bioorg Med Chem* 1998;6:1163–1169.

92. Tudan C, Jackson JK, Pelech SL, et al. Selective inhibition of protein kinase C, mitogen-activated protein kinase, and neutrophil activation in response to calcium pyrophosphate dihydrate crystals, formyl-methionyl-leucyl-phenylalanine, and phorbol ester by O-(chloroacetyl-carbamoyl) fumagillol (AGM-1470; TNP-470). *Biochem Pharmacol* 1999;58:1869–1880.

93. Sedlakova O, Sedlak J, Hunakova L, et al. Angiogenesis inhibitor TNP-470: cytotoxic effects on human neoplastic cell lines. *Neoplasma* 1999;46:283–289.

94. Locigno R, Antoine N, Bours V, et al. TNP-470, a potent angiogenesis inhibitor, amplifies human T lymphocyte activation through an induction of nuclear factor-kappaB, nuclear factor-AT, and activation protein-1 transcription factors. *Lab Invest* 2000;80:13–21.

95. Kria L, Ohira A, Amemiya T. TNP-470 (a fungus-derived inhibitor of angiogenesis) reduces proliferation of cultured fibroblasts isolated from primary pterygia: a possible drug therapy for pterygia. *Curr Eye Res* 1998;17:986–993.

96. Castronovo V, Belotti D. TNP-470 (AGM-1470): mechanisms of action and early clinical development. *Eur J Cancer* 1996;32A:2520–2527.

97. Ishikawa H, Satoh H, Kamma H, et al. The effect of TNP-470 on cell proliferation and urokinase-type plasminogen activator and its inhibitor in human lung cancer cell lines. *J Exp Ther Oncol* 1996;1:390–396.

98. Stadler WM, Kuzel T, Shapiro C, et al. Multi-institutional study of the angiogenesis inhibitor TNP-470 in metastatic renal carcinoma. *J Clin Oncol* 1999;17:2541–2545.

99. Kudelka AP, Levy T, Verschraegen CF, et al. A phase I study of TNP-470 administered to patients with advanced squamous cell cancer of the cervix. *Clin Cancer Res* 1997;3:1501–1505.

100. Milkowski DM, Weiss RA. TNP-470. In: Teicher BA, ed. *Antiangiogenic agents in cancer therapy.* Totowa, NJ: Humana Press, 1999:385–398.

101. Bhargava P, Marshall JL, Rizvi N, et al. A phase I and pharmacokinetic study of TNP-470 administered weekly to patients with advanced cancer. *Clin Cancer Res* 1999;5:1989–1995.

102. Herbst R, Tran H, Madden T, et al. Phase I study of the angiogenesis inhibitor TNP-470 in combination with paclitaxel in patients with solid tumors. *Proc Annu Meet Am Soc Clin Oncol* 2000;19(abst).

103. Baidas S, Bhargava P, Isaacs C, et al. Phase I study of the combination of TNP-470 and paclitaxel in patients with advanced cancer. *Proc Annu Meet Am Soc Clin Oncol* 2000;19(abst).

104. Sills AK Jr, Williams JI, Tyler BM, et al. Squalamine inhibits angiogenesis and solid tumor growth in vivo and perturbs embryonic vasculature. *Cancer Res* 1998;58:2784–2792.

105. Schiller JH, Bittner G. Potentiation of platinum antitumor effects in human lung tumor xenografts by the angiogenesis

inhibitor squalamine: effects on tumor neovascularization. *Clin Cancer Res* 1999;5:4287–4294.

106. Bhargava P, Trocky N, Marshall J, et al. A phase I safety, tolerance and pharmacokinetic study of rising dose, rising duration continuous infusion of MSI-1256F (squalamine lactate) in patients with advanced cancer. *Proc Annu Meet Am Soc Clin Oncol* 1999;18:623(abst).

107. Patnaik A, Rowinsky E, Hammond L, et al. A phase I and pharmacokinetic study of the unique angiogenesis inhibitor, squalamine lactate (MSI-1256F). *Proc Annu Meet Am Soc Clin Oncol* 1999;18:622(abst).

108. O'Reilly MS, Holmgren L, Chen C, et al. Angiostatin induces and sustains dormancy of human primary tumors in mice. *Nat Med* 1996;2:689–692.

109. Boehm T, Folkman J, Browder T, et al. Antiangiogenic therapy of experimental cancer does not induce acquired drug resistance. *Nature* 1997;390:404–407.

110. Kohn EC, Sandeen MA, Liotta LA. In vivo efficacy of a novel inhibitor of selected signal transduction pathways including calcium, arachidonate, and inositol phosphates. *Cancer Res* 1992;52:3208–3212.

111. Kohn EC, Alessandro R, Spoonster J, et al. Angiogenesis: role of calcium-mediated signal transduction. *Proc Natl Acad Sci U S A* 1995;92:1307–1311.

112. Kohn EC, Jacobs W, Kim YS, et al. Calcium influx modulates expression of matrix metalloproteinase-2 (72-kDa type IV collagenase, gelatinase A). *J Biol Chem* 1994;269:21505–21511.

113. Gusovsky F, Lueders JE, Kohn EC, et al. Muscarinic receptor-mediated tyrosine phosphorylation of phospholipase C-gamma. An alternative mechanism for cholinergic-induced phosphoinositide breakdown. *J Biol Chem* 1993;268:7768–7772.

114. Felder CC, Ma AL, Liotta LA, et al. The antiproliferative and antimetastatic compound L651582 inhibits muscarinic acetylcholine receptor-stimulated calcium influx and arachidonic acid release. *J Pharmacol Exp Ther* 1991;257:967–971.

115. Kohn EC, Felder CC, Jacobs W, et al. Structure-function analysis of signal and growth inhibition by carboxyamidotriazole, CAI. *Cancer Res* 1994;54:935–942.

116. Figg WD, Cole KA, Reed E, et al. Pharmacokinetics of orally administered carboxyamido-triazole, an inhibitor of calcium-mediated signal transduction. *Clin Cancer Res* 1995;1:797–803.

117. Berlin J, Tutsch KD, Hutson P, et al. Phase I clinical and pharmacokinetic study of oral carboxyamidotriazole, a signal transduction inhibitor. *J Clin Oncol* 1997;15:781–789.

118. Kohn EC, Figg WD, Sarosy GA, et al. Phase I trial of micronized formulation carboxyamidotriazole in patients with refractory solid tumors: pharmacokinetics, clinical outcome, and comparison of formulations. *J Clin Oncol* 1997;15:1985–1993.

119. Bauer KS, Figg WD, Hamilton JM, et al. A pharmacokinetically guided phase II study of carboxyamido-triazole in androgen-independent prostate cancer. *Clin Cancer Res* 1999;5:2324–2329.

120. Gradishar WJ. Endpoints for determination of efficacy of antiangiogenic agents in clinical trials. In: Teicher BA, ed. *Antiangiogenic agents in cancer therapy.* Totowa, NJ: Humana Press, 1999:341–353.

36

PHARMACOGENETICS

ROBERT B. DIASIO

Cancer chemotherapy drugs, like drugs from other therapeutic classes, are associated with significant interpatient variability in response and toxicity. The causes of this variability may include differences in age (particularly age extremes), gender, nutritional state, and general medical condition (cardiovascular, renal, and hepatic function). By far the most important factor responsible for the differences in drug response, however, is now recognized to be genetic variability. The discipline of pharmacogenetics evolved over the past several decades as a result of the realization that differences in drug response and toxicity could be due to an inherited trait, in which changes in the gene coding for a specific protein (e.g., a drug metabolizing enzyme) could lead to major changes in the qualitative or quantitative function of that protein.[1]

More recently, with completion of sequencing of the human genome and assignment of function to the various genes, there has been an appreciation of the considerable variability or polymorphisms that may exist even at the level of a single nucleotide. Increasingly, it should be possible to associate drug response information with these single nucleotide polymorphisms (SNPs) through screening methods.[2] This has given rise to the relatively new discipline of pharmacogenomics,[3] an area that is of major interest to the pharmaceutical industry and those interested in drug development.

In this chapter, we review the basic principles of pharmacogenetics, followed by several specific examples of how genetic polymorphisms can alter the pharmacology of cancer chemotherapy agents. In addition, we highlight the potential role of pharmacogenomics for the future of chemotherapy.

IMPACT OF GENETIC POLYMORPHISMS ON CANCER CHEMOTHERAPY

Although virtually all drugs are susceptible to the consequences of genetic variability, it should be emphasized that cancer chemotherapy drugs in particular are susceptible, because these drugs typically have a relatively narrow therapeutic index, in which the effective dose and the toxic dose

are not very different. Thus, a small change in the metabolism of a cancer chemotherapy drug due to a genetic change, resulting in either decreased protein (enzyme) production or altered protein (enzyme) function, can lead to major changes in drug effect (efficacy or toxicity). Although theoretically there are many different types of genes that can be affected, the genes affecting drug metabolism have been those most often identified with pharmacogenetic syndromes associated with cancer chemotherapy agents.

METHODS

The methods used to evaluate pharmacogenetic syndromes have evolved over the past several decades. Previously, the focus was almost entirely at the phenotypic level, where the investigation was limited to assessment of an individual patient's clinical response or toxicity to a drug compared to other individuals in the same population. Increasingly, there is a genotypic focus, in which as a result of the completion of the human genome sequence, the emphasis has now shifted to associating changes at the level of the DNA sequence, even SNPs, with altered drug response and toxicity.

For the clinical oncologist caring for patients or investigating new drugs in the clinical setting, it is most useful to have a combined (phenotypic and genotypic) approach when evaluating the possibility of a pharmacogenetic syndrome.[4] Listed below are several of the current approaches that can be used.

Clinical Presentation

The clinical presentation has typically been the event that leads the physician to question the possibility of a pharmacogenetic syndrome. For most cancer chemotherapy agents, it has been the appearance of unexpected toxicity (noted in the history, seen in the physical examination, or observed in the routine initial laboratory tests) that is out of proportion to the drug dose given that leads to initial suspicion of a pharmacogenetic syndrome. As noted, the pharmacogenetic syndromes associated with cancer chemotherapy drugs have typically been secondary to changes in genes coding for drug-metabolizing enzymes. This results in a disturbance in the levels of drug or metabolites typically observed for the dose given. The excess drug or metabolites may produce a clinical presentation with symptoms, signs, or laboratory tests suggestive of an overdose, due to a relatively greater amount of drugs (or metabolites) being present.[5] The excess drug or metabolite produces this effect in particular because cancer chemotherapy drugs are often characterized by a relatively low therapeutic index.

Pharmacokinetics

To provide further support for the presence of a pharmacogenetic syndrome, it is often useful to determine whether the levels of drug or key metabolite(s) are elevated. This can be attempted initially by quantitating the levels of drug or key metabolite in plasma (serum), urine, or tissue. However, one may not detect the presence of elevated drug or metabolite levels if the plasma (serum), urine, or tissue samples are not appropriately timed in relation to when the drug was administered. A more useful approach is to administer a known dose of drug under controlled testing conditions, such that plasma (serum), urine, tissue samples, or a combination of the three are collected and assessed over time for drug and potentially metabolite levels. With cancer chemotherapy agents, in which there is a risk of potentially serious toxicity, a test dose of drug may be used to lessen the safety risk. A particularly useful approach has been to administer a radioactive tracer dose of drug to permit not only accurate quantitation of drug, but also the various metabolites, resulting in a further increase in sensitivity. This approach has been successfully used in characterizing pharmacogenetic syndromes associated with cancer chemotherapy drugs.[6]

Identification of Affected Biochemical Pathway

Using the above approaches with supporting drug, metabolite, or possibly, pharmacokinetic data, one may surmise from knowledge of the drug's metabolism where a potential alteration in its biochemical pathway may exist. Preclinical studies may provide guidance regarding not only the metabolic pathway, but also the tissue that may be accessed for detection of the pharmacogenetic syndrome. Subsequent clinical studies using the appropriate institutionally approved protocols may then be undertaken. Although many drug-metabolizing enzymes are localized mainly in the liver, biopsy of this site is an invasive procedure that is best avoided if possible. Other potentially accessible tissues, like peripheral blood mononuclear (PBM) cells or fibroblasts, can sometimes be useful in identifying which enzyme in the metabolism of the drug is altered. Until

recently, studies of drug-metabolizing enzymes responsible for pharmacogenetic syndromes have been limited by the lack of biochemical and molecular knowledge of these enzymes. Enzyme kinetic analysis may also provide insight into the biochemical basis of enzyme deficiency—for example, lower substrate affinity [increased binding affinity (K_m)] or decreased maximal velocity[7] may suggest a possible pharmacogenetic syndrome.

Identification of the specific defect is not only useful in confirming the biochemical mechanism responsible for the pharmacogenetic syndrome, but also may provide insight into developing a useful biochemical test for screening family members and others in population studies (see below).

Family Studies (Pattern of Inheritance)

With cancer chemotherapy drugs, one cannot use the approach to test family members that has been suggested with drugs from other therapeutic classes, in which the response to a test dose of a drug was evaluated.[5] Obviously, such studies with cytotoxic cancer chemotherapy agents cannot be ethically conducted in healthy individuals. Other phenotypic tests, such as assessment of the activity of a drug-metabolizing enzyme or determination of substrate levels, for such an enzyme in family members can prove useful in helping to clarify the pattern of inheritance.

After the identification and confirmation of the metabolic defect in the affected patient described previously, studies can be undertaken in the family of the individual to determine the pattern of inheritance. This can provide insight as to whether the defect is an autosomal or sexual chromosomal inherited trait and as to whether there is a dominant, codominant, or recessive pattern of inheritance.

With availability of data from the human genome project and the functional assignment of enzyme activity to a particular gene, it is becoming possible at a relatively early point in pharmacogenetic investigations to conduct molecular studies to unequivocally delineate the inheritance of a specific gene. Techniques that can unequivocally identify a specific sequence or SNP, such as allele-specific polymerase chain reaction–based (PCR-based) methods, should make this relatively easy to evaluate in the near future.[8]

Population Studies

The next step is to assess the frequency of the pharmacogenetic syndrome within the general population. As with the family studies discussed previously, this can use either phenotypic or genotypic tests. The frequency of individuals identified with phenotypic characteristics can be used with the Hardy-Weinberg equation to estimate the likely number of homozygous and heterozygous individuals in the general population.[4] With the availability of sequence data on the human genome and, more important, the assignment of function to the particular gene (i.e., the specific protein, or, in this case, the drug-metabolizing enzyme, associated with the particular sequence), it may become possible in the near future to use genotypic tests at an early point in the evaluation of a new pharmacogenetic syndrome, providing more accurate data on not only the frequency of homozygotes and heterozygotes of a particular allele, but also the identification of multiple alleles. The existence of multiple alleles associated with a pharmacogenetic syndrome is now recognized to be common (see below). Thus, it is also useful in these early population studies to understand the relative frequency of the various alleles associated with the specific pharmacogenetic syndrome.

After an assessment of phenotypic and genotypic markers in the general population, it may be useful to undertake surveys in other populations. These may include patients affected with specific types of cancer. Of particular relevance are studies in patient populations being treated with the particular chemotherapy agent. This provides information in determining the risk of the pharmacogenetic syndrome in the cancer patient population at risk. It is often useful to examine other demographic factors in these population studies, such as race, age, and gender, to determine risks for specific groups.

Screening Tests

After the identification and characterization of a pharmacogenetic syndrome using the previously described methods, it is often desirable to develop tests that can be used to screen individuals who are to be treated with the specific drug associated with the pharmacogenetic syndrome, particularly with cancer chemotherapy, in which affected individuals may experience life-threatening toxic consequences. The availability of such screening tests should permit the physician to potentially modify the drug dose before administration to avoid the risk of toxicity. In developing the methods described [see sections Identification of Affected Biochemical Pathway, Family Studies (Pattern of Inheritance), and Population Studies], it should be possible to identify potentially useful screening tests that could be used for routine testing. Ideally, these tests should be user friendly, easy to perform, sensitive, specific, and, at the same time, ideally rapid and inexpensive. Also important is the ability to perform these tests in easily accessible tissues, for example, red blood cells (RBCs), plasma, or urine, as opposed to the need for an invasive procedure (e.g., tissue biopsy) that would be impractical for widespread use and pose an unnecessary risk to the individual being tested. As noted, phenotypic and genotypic tests may be used for this purpose. With certain phenotypic tests, such as determination of substrate concentration (for a drug-metabolizing enzyme) or quantitation of enzymatic activity, in which the factor that is being measured is also present normally, it is necessary to determine the "normal" distribution of these markers in a study using a large number of subjects, after

which the discrimination point (separating normal and abnormal individuals) can be determined.[4] Also, it should be noted that although genotypic tests are being used more frequently today, if the specific allele responsible for the pharmacogenetic syndrome is not tested, the diagnosis will be missed. This has led to phenotypic and genotypic tests, often being used together in screening for pharmacogenetic syndromes.

PHARMACOGENETIC SYNDROMES IMPORTANT IN CANCER

There are now several pharmacogenetic syndromes recognized to be associated with certain cancer chemotherapy agents.[4,9–12] Table 36-1 lists the most common and most characterized pharmacogenetic syndromes in oncology, as well as the specific chemotherapy drugs affected. Thiopurine methyl transferase (TPMT) deficiency affecting 6-mercaptopurine (6-MP) and azathioprine is perhaps the best studied, having been the first to be described at the clinical, pharmacokinetic, population, and genetic levels. Because the use of 6-MP has been restricted essentially to leukemias, there has been, until recently, a relatively limited appreciation by the general oncology community of this pharmacogenetic syndrome, as well as of the potential importance of pharmacogenetics in general. Dihydropyrimidine dehydrogenase (DPD) deficiency affecting metabolism of the widely used chemotherapy drug 5-fluorouracil (5-FU) has been more recently identified as a pharmacogenetic syndrome relevant to medical oncology. Because 5-FU is widely used in oncology, including several of the more common malignancies (colorectal, breast, and skin), the potential impact of this pharmacogenetic syndrome to oncologists has been much greater. Knowledge of this syndrome has, in turn, resulted in an increased awareness of other possible pharmacogenetic syndromes in oncology. Most recently, there has been interest in a new pharmacogenetic syndrome associated with uridine diphosphate glucuronosyltransferase (UGT). UGT has an important role in the metabolism of the relatively new chemotherapy agent irinotecan. The expected increased use of this drug, not only as a first-line agent in the treatment of advanced col-

TABLE 36-1. PHARMACOGENETIC SYNDROMES ASSOCIATED WITH CANCER CHEMOTHERAPY RESULTING FROM POLYMORPHISMS IN DRUG METABOLIZING ENZYMES

Polymorphic Enzyme	Chemotherapy Agent
Thiopurine methyltransferase	6-Mercaptopurine Azathioprine
Dihydropyrimidine dehydrogenase	5-Fluorouracil
Uridine diphosphate glucuronosyltransferase	Irinotecan

orectal cancer, but potentially in the treatment of several other malignancies as well, suggests that this pharmacogenetic syndrome will likely be quantitatively more important in oncology. Details on these common polymorphisms, as well as some of the other potentially important polymorphisms, are presented below.

Thiopurine Methyl Transferase Deficiency

Methylation is an important phase II metabolic reaction of many drugs and xenobiotics, including cancer chemotherapeutic drugs.[13] There are several methyltransferases responsible for methylation, all of which use *S*-adenosyl-L-methionine (Ado-Met) as the methyl group donor for methylation. Most of these enzymes have been shown to have genetic polymorphisms.

Importance of Thiopurine Methyl Transferase in Thiopurine Metabolism

Thiopurine *S*-methyltransferase (TPMT, E.C. 2.1.1.67) is a catabolic enzyme important in the metabolism of 6-MP and of the 6-MP prodrug azathioprine, which has been used as an immunosuppressant, particularly in transplantation.[4,9–14] Figure 36-1 shows the reaction catalyzed by this enzyme, as well as its central position in 6-MP metabolism. Although TPMT was one of the first enzymes associated with a pharmacogenetic presentation shown to be relevant to cancer chemotherapy, knowledge of the polymorphic nature of the enzyme did not come from an initial investigation of an unusual clinical presentation, but from an investigation of the methylation reaction.[13] Although obviously important in metabolism of thiopurine drugs, its primary role in metabolism of endogenous compounds remains unclear.

Clinical Presentation

The clinical presentation associated with TPMT deficiency is now well recognized.[15–17] Patients who are completely deficient in TPMT activity typically present with evidence of severe hematologic toxicity manifest as leukopenia, thrombocytopenia, and anemia after exposure to any of the drugs metabolized by this enzyme. Leukopenia has occasionally been life threatening, with death at times occurring when patients who were completely deficient in TPMT activity received a standard dose of thiopurine drug.[18] Patients who are heterozygotes for the mutant TPMT alleles may have activity between normal and completely deficient individuals.

It should be noted that those individuals with high or high-normal TPMT may also be relatively resistant to the action of 6-MP or 6-TG due to the greater proportion of the drug that is catabolized. These patients may not achieve a remission after antileukemia therapy with 6-MP or 6-TG.[18] After demonstrating elevated TPMT activity in such patients, a decision may be made to give these patients an increased dosage of 6-MP or 6-TG.[19]

Effect of Thiopurine Methyl Transferase Deficiency on 6-Mercaptopurine Metabolism and Pharmacokinetics

As implied, studies have demonstrated that an alteration in TPMT activity can have profound effects in patients given 6-MP. If the TPMT activity is relatively low, more 6-MP is theoretically available. However, pharmacokinetic studies have demonstrated that this may not be reflected in the plasma concentrations of 6-MP.[20] A much better assessment can be made by quantitating the RBC–6-TG nucleotide concentrations, which, when relatively elevated, are predictive of toxicity. At the same time, it has been suggested that if the 6-TG nucleotide concentrations were relatively low, this might predict failure to respond and could provide the rationale for increasing the dose of 6-MP to individualize therapy.[21]

Pattern of Inheritance and Population Studies

Family studies performed early in the course of investigation of TPMT deficiency demonstrated that TPMT activ-

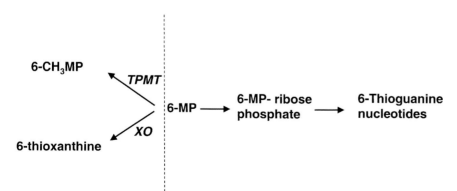

FIGURE 36-1. The metabolism of 6-mercaptopurine (6-MP) in humans showing critical position of thiopurine methyl transferase (TPMT). Anabolic pathway is shown to right of hatched line, whereas catabolic pathways via xanthine oxidase (XO) or TPMT are shown to left of hatched line.

ity is inherited as an autosomal codominant trait.[22] Individuals who had normal activity were hypothesized initially to be homozygous for a wild-type allele, whereas those that were completely deficient were thought to be homozygous for a mutant allele, and finally those with intermediate activity were thought to be heterozygotes with one allele having altered TPMT activity and one allele being wild type. Following identification of the multiple alleles with an appreciation of the degree of TPMT deficiency associated with each allele, the observed variation in TPMT activity has become even clearer, as not all of the abnormal alleles result in the same level of TPMT activity.

Using the RBC assay to assess TPMT activity, studies demonstrated that a trimodal pattern existed in several populations tested, including healthy, otherwise "normal" individuals as well as patients with leukemia (Fig. 36-2). The largest of the three peaks included individuals who were homozygous for the wild-type allele. The middle peak included those who were heterozygous for the wild-type and a mutant allele. The smallest peak represented those individuals who were homozygous for the mutant allele. One can use the Hardy-Weinberg equation to estimate the frequency of individuals who are heterozygotes and homozygotes for the TPMT allele. In the United States, it is estimated that 10% of whites and 10% of African-Americans are likely to have intermediate TPMT activity (i.e., heterozygotes), with approximately 1 in 300 of these individuals having profound TPMT deficiency (i.e., homozygotes for a mutant allele).[23] Complicating the interpretation of TPMT activity in population studies is the fact that TPMT activity can be influenced by many factors, including the patient's age, renal function, and assessment in relation to administration of thiopurine drug and tissue source.[18,24]

Thiopurine Methyl Transferase Gene and Known Mutations

Since the complementary DNA (cDNA) sequence and, subsequently, the structure of the TPMT gene were reported, there have been efforts to determine the mutations responsible for TPMT deficiency.[25,26] The TPMT gene is known to be located on chromosome 6. It is made up of ten exons. Currently, there are at least nine known mutations associated with decreased TPMT activity (Table 36-2).[26] The alleles include (a) point mutations, which result in amino acid substitutions (TPMT*2, TPMT*3A, TPMT*3B, TPMT*3C, TPMT*3D, TPMT*5, and TPMT*6); (b) premature stop codon (TPMT*3D); and (c) destruction of a splice site (TPMT*4).

The mechanism by which the various point mutations result in TPMT deficiency has been extensively studied, demonstrating that for most mutations neither the level of messenger RNA nor the syntheses of TPMT protein are affected.[26] A recent study has demonstrated that in the presence of certain mutations, there is lower TPMT protein and catalytic activity due to rapid proteolysis of the TPMT protein formed via an adenosine triphosphate–dependent proteosomal process.[27] This decreases the half-life of the TPMT protein to 30 minutes compared to 18 hours for the wild-type protein.

Of interest is the fact that at least one allele has been identified with increased TPMT activity. This allele, designated *TPMT*1A*, has a single point mutation with a C to T at nucleotide −178 in exon 1.[28]

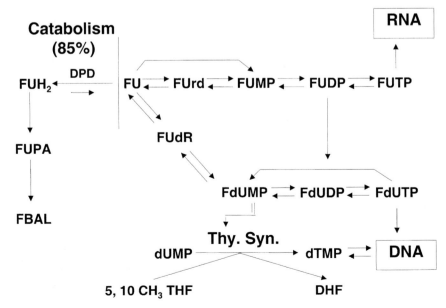

FIGURE 36-2. The metabolism of 5-fluorouracil (5-FU) in humans, showing critical position of dihydropyrimidine dehydrogenase (DPD). Catabolic and anabolic pathways separated by hatched line. DPD is essentially unidirectional step, accounting for approximately 85% of 5-FU metabolism. (DHF, dihydrofolate; dUMP, deoxyuridine monophosphate; dTMP, thymidylate; FBAL, α fluoro-β-alanine; FdUMP, fluorodeoxyuridylate; FdUDP, fluorodeoxyuridine diphosphate; FdUTP, fluorodeoxyuridine triphosphate; FUDP, fluorouridine diphosphate; FUdR, fluorodeoxyuridine; FUH$_2$, dihydrofluorouracil; FUMP, fluorouridine monophosphate; FUPA, fluoroureidopropionic acid; FUrd, fluorouridine; FUTP, fluorouridine triphosphate; 5,10 CH$_3$ THF, 5,10-methylenetetrahydrofolate; Thy. Syn., thymidylate synthase.)

TABLE 36-2. ALLELES OF THIOPURINE METHYL TRANSFERASE (TPMT) ASSOCIATED WITH CHANGE IN ENZYME ACTIVITY

Allele	Type	Enzyme Activity
TPMT*1	Wild type	Normal
TPMT*1A	C-178T in exon 1	Increased
TPMT*2,	G238C (Ala80Pro)	Decreased
TPMT*3A,	G460A (Ala154Thr) and A719G (Tyr240Cys)	Decreased
TPMT*3B,	G460A (Ala154Thr)	Decreased
TPMT*3C,	A719G (Tyr240Cys)	Decreased
TPMT*3D,	G292T (Glu98Stop), G460A (Ala154Thr) and A719G (Tyr240Cys)	Decreased
TPMT*4,	G → A at intron 9/exon 10 splice junction	Decreased
TPMT*5	T146C (Leu49Ser)	Decreased
TPMT*6	A539T (Tyr180Phe)	Decreased
TPMT*8	G644A (Arg215His)	Decreased

Ala, alanine; Arg, arginine; Cys, cysteine; Glu, glutamic acid; His, histidine; Leu, leucine; Phe, phenylalanine; Pro, proline; Ser, serine; Thr, threonine; Tyr, tyrosine.
Adapted from Iyer L. Inherited variations in drug-metabolizing enzymes: significance in clinical oncology. *Mol Diag* 1999;4:327–333; and Krynetski EY, Evans WE. Genetic polymorphism of thiopurine *S*-methyltransferase: molecular mechanisms and clinical importance. *Pharmacol* 2000;61:136–146.

Screening for Thiopurine Methyl Transferase Deficiency

Screening for TPMT deficiency is relatively easy, because TPMT activity can be easily assessed in RBCs.[29] The enzyme activity present in this readily accessible cell source has been shown to correlate well with TPMT activity present in a number of other tissues.[30] This assay has been shown to be capable of distinguishing individuals who are homozygous wild type from individuals who are homozygous deficient and heterozygous for a wild-type and mutant allele. Although it is a relatively unusual situation, it should be noted that spurious results can be obtained in patients who have had RBC transfusions before the screening test.[31]

With isolation of the cDNA, the structure of the TPMT gene, and, subsequently, identification of a number of mutants in large population studies, it has been possible to develop a number of specific genotype tests. This has made possible the development of allele-specific PCR tests to detect several of the more common defects.[32] Although these tests identify the majority of individuals at risk, it should be noted, as with all genotypic tests, that they are not completely predictive, because rare mutants could be completely missed. This has led some investigators[32] to emphasize the continued use of phenotyping methods at the same time genotyping assays are being used. A newer, more potentially powerful, technique is to use automated DNA microarrays to completely genotype a large number of TPMT alleles.[33] This method may become increasingly useful in the future as the sequence database on genes, such as TPMT, from large

population studies increases with clarification and identification of polymorphisms with functional consequences and those that have no functional consequence.

Dihydropyrimidine Dehydrogenase Deficiency

DPD (also known as *dihydrouracil dehydrogenase, dihydrothymine dehydrogenase, uracil reductase, E.C. 1.3.1.2*) is the initial rate-limiting enzymatic step in the catabolism of not only the naturally occurring pyrimidines uracil and thymine, but also the widely used cancer chemotherapy drug 5-FU[34] (Fig. 36-3). DPD has a critical position in the overall metabolism of 5-FU, converting more than 85% of clinically administered 5-FU to 5-FUH$_2$ (an inactive metabolite) in an essentially irreversible enzymatic step.[35] Although anabolism is clearly important in the conversion of 5-FU to the "active" nucleotides fluorodeoxyuridylate, fluorouridine triphosphate, and fluorodeoxyuridine triphosphate, which are responsible for blocking cell replication through inhibition of thymidylate synthase (TS), or through incorporation into RNA or DNA, respectively, catabolism at the level of DPD controls the amount of 5-FU available for anabolism and, thus, occupies a critical position in the overall metabolism of 5-FU.[36]

Importance of Dihydropyrimidine Dehydrogenase in Fluoropyrimidine Pharmacology

The importance of DPD to the clinical pharmacology of 5-FU is summarized in Table 36-3. It is clear that DPD accounts for much of the variability observed with thera-

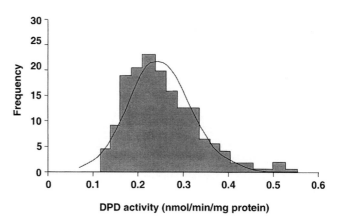

FIGURE 36-3. Distribution of dihydropyrimidine dehydrogenase (DPD) activity in population. DPD activity determined in peripheral blood mononuclear cells of 523 breast cancer patients. Statistical analysis demonstrated that DPD activity followed a normal (gaussian) distribution as is shown by solid line. (Data includes patients from Lu Z, Zhang R, Carpenter JT, et al. Decreased dihydropyrimidine dehydrogenase activity in population of patients with breast cancer: implications for 5-FU-based chemotherapy. *Clin Cancer Res* 1998;4:325–329, as well as more recent patients.)

TABLE 36-3. IMPORTANCE OF DIHYDROPYRIMIDINE DEHYDROGENASE (DPD) IN 5-FLUOROURACIL (5-FU) METABOLISM

Circadian variation of 5-FU related to circadian variation of DPD; implication for time-modified therapy

Variability of 5-FU clinical pharmacokinetics (half-life and clearance) related to variability in DPD

Variability in 5-FU bioavailability related to variability in DPD

Genetic deficiency (pharmacogenetic implication)

Variability in 5-FU antitumor activity (i.e., resistance) may be related to variability in DPD

DPD as therapeutic target for improving 5-FU therapy

peutic use of 5-FU.[36] This includes variable 5-FU levels over 24 hours during a continuous infusion, the widely reported variability in 5-FU pharmacokinetics, the observed variable bioavailability that has led to the recommendation that 5-FU not be administered as an oral agent, and, last, the observed variability in toxicity and drug response (resistance) after the same 5-FU dose. Knowledge of the DPD level as well as the levels of other potentially important molecular markers (e.g., TS) may permit adjustments or modulation of the 5-FU dose that can result in an increase in the therapeutic efficacy of the 5-FU drug.

Clinical Presentation

5-FU has been used as a chemotherapy agent in the clinic, since it was introduced into the clinic in the late 1950s.[37] Over this time, it has ranked as one of the most frequently used cancer chemotherapy drugs in particular, because it has been used to treat several of the more commonly occurring malignancies, such as carcinoma of the breast, colon, and skin. The general impression, with extensive use over the past 40 years, is that 5-FU is reasonably well tolerated as a cancer chemotherapy drug, without the severe toxicity observed with many other cytotoxic agents. Differences in efficacy from patient to patient have been noted, but these variations have been thought to be secondary to both innate and acquired resistance, without much consideration until recently that this could be due to genetic differences.[38]

The first suggestion of a pharmacogenetic syndrome associated with 5-FU was reported in the late 1980s.[39] The affected patient presented with a clinical picture suggestive of a 5-FU overdose. She was hypothesized to have an abnormality in pyrimidine catabolism. The patient had demonstrated increased toxicity (decreased white blood cells, total neutrophils, and platelets) after receiving an initial course of chemotherapy consisting of cyclophosphamide, methotrexate, and 5-FU for treatment of breast cancer. Despite reductions in the dose of each of the drugs, the patient continued to experience similar toxicity on the subsequent two courses, eventually succumbing to sepsis. Although direct confirmation of deficient DPD activity was never obtained, elevated levels of uracil and thymine (substrates for DPD) were dem-

onstrated in the plasma and urine of the patient. Interestingly, elevated levels were also demonstrated in the plasma and urine of the patient's brother, providing a suggestion of an inherited deficiency in DPD.

A second patient was described with a similar clinical presentation of severe fluorouracil-associated toxicity.[40] This patient also had elevated pyrimidine levels in the plasma and urine. Further studies demonstrated deficiency of DPD activity in PBM cells from this patient. Family studies examining DPD activity suggested an autosomal-recessive pattern of inheritance.

Since that time, there have been numerous published reports.[41–47] There are many additional cases that have been detected, but not published, with a current estimate of more than 250 cases of DPD deficiency associated with severe 5-FU toxicity.

Effect of Dihydropyrimidine Dehydrogenase Deficiency on 5-Fluorouracil Metabolism and Pharmacokinetics

The presence of DPD deficiency was hypothesized to produce toxicity by increasing exposure (drug concentration over time) to 5-FU (or a 5-FU derivative or prodrug) through interference with 5-FU catabolism at the level of the DPD enzyme. This enzyme had previously been shown to be a rate-limiting step in pyrimidine catabolism.[34]

To prove that the biochemical step responsible for this syndrome was DPD and that the clinical effect was indeed due to an increased exposure to 5-FU, a clinical pharmacokinetic study was designed using a "test" dose of 5-FU, including radiolabeled drug.[40] Briefly, the patient was given a test dose of 5-FU [25 mg per m², 600 µCi (^{3}H-6)-5-FU] as an IV bolus, after which plasma, urine, and cerebrospinal fluid were sampled at specified times. This patient was observed to have a markedly altered pharmacokinetic pattern, with 5-FU detected in the plasma at unusually high levels for at least 8 hours and 97% of the drug being excreted unchanged in the urine over 24 hours.

This patient, who was shown to be deficient in DPD, had an apparent 5-FU elimination half-life of 159 minutes with a systemic clearance of 71 mL per minute per m². This is in contrast to previous studies[35] in ten patients with excellent performance status and normal liver function, who were given a standard bolus dose of 5-FU (450 mg per m²) with the same radioactive tracer dose [600 µCi (^{3}H-6)-5-FU]. None of these patients experienced toxicity after 5-FU. These patients had an apparent elimination half-life of 13 ± 7 minutes, with a systemic clearance of 594 ± 198 mL per minute per m². The findings in these pharmacokinetic studies were consistent with normal DPD activity. Also of interest is the suggestion of an inverse relationship between DPD activity and 5-FU plasma levels that had been previously demonstrated in cancer patients receiving continuous 5-FU infusion.[48] The PBM-DPD activity appears to reflect the DPD activity in the liver, which is believed to be the major site of 5-FU catabolism.[42]

Pattern of Inheritance

Initial family studies conducted in one of the initial patients with DPD deficiency suggested an autosomal-recessive pattern of inheritance.[40] This was supported by the presence of consanguinity in the family, with evidence of the affected individual's having absent DPD activity with elevated uracil, whereas the parents and children had partial DPD activity with normal uracil levels. Subsequent studies demonstrated that patients with partial deficiency of DPD activity (intermediate between normal and completely deficient individuals), who were thought to be heterozygotes for this disorder, also could develop toxicity. This led to the suspicion that the pattern of inheritance was actually consistent with an autosomal-codominant pattern of inheritance. With the availability of genotyping tests, it has now been confirmed that DPD is inherited as an autosomal codominant.

Population Studies

Initial studies examined the population distribution of DPD activity in PBM cells from 124 healthy individuals (45% men and 55% women). DPD activity was shown to have a normal distribution,[42] with a sixfold range in DPD activity in healthy individuals. No significant difference was observed by gender. Examination of the affect of age in this healthy adult population made up of men and women from 20 to 70 years of age revealed no obvious age-related variation in DPD activity. A comparison of DPD activity in whites and African-Americans suggested no racial difference. Other races have not been examined with sufficient numbers to make any definitive conclusions at this time. These initial studies in healthy individuals permitted establishment of a functional baseline for DPD screening (see below). Fresh and frozen PBM cell samples were used in this study in healthy individuals demonstrating a strong correlation between both fresh and frozen cells, with a similar normal distribution of DPD activity. This has permitted the use of frozen samples from more distant locations for further DPD screening in cancer patients. A similar normal distribution has been observed in human livers from cadaver donors.[49]

A subsequent study examined DPD activity in PBM cells from 151 female breast cancer patients.[50] Figure 36-3 shows an updated population study of DPD activity in breast cancer patients. The distribution pattern of DPD was similar (normal distribution) to the pattern of DPD activity in PBM cells from a healthy population.[42] Of interest, however, the mean DPD activity in the PBM cells from the breast cancer population was shifted to the left and was statistically significantly lower than that observed in the

healthy population. The difference was also shown after cross analysis by age and race. Menopausal status, use of hormonal therapy or chemotherapy, or disease status did not appear related to this finding. The frequency of DPD deficiency in the population of breast cancer patients is similar (approximately 5%) to that of other reported pharmacogenetic syndromes.[1,5]

Dihydropyrimidine Dehydrogenase Gene

At the time DPD deficiency was first described, there was essentially no information on the cDNA or the gene. Indeed, the human DPD enzyme had only recently been isolated to homogeneity.[34] With the availability of the homogeneous protein, it was possible to obtain peptide sequence and antibody necessary for subsequent cloning. Isolation of the human cDNA for DPD soon followed.[51,52] The complete cDNA sequence permitted the complete amino acid sequence to be deduced, which, in turn, revealed several functional domains (reduced form of nicotinamide adenine dinucleotide phosphate, flavin, and two iron-sulfur regions, as well as the uracil binding region), potentially providing insight into critical regions of the molecule that might result in DPD deficiency if mutations affected these regions. The availability of the cDNA also permitted the use of fluorescence *in situ* hybridization, with the assignment of the DPD gene to the region of chromosome 1p22.[53] Although availability of the cDNA permitted initial molecular studies of patients with DPD deficiency, this proved insufficient for characterizing most patients with DPD deficiency at a mechanistic level. This, in turn, motivated an investigation of the DPD gene. The human gene was isolated with detailed analysis of the structure of the DPD gene, demonstrating that the gene consisted of 23 exons with exon length from 50 to more than 1,550 base pairs.[54,55] Several long introns (some larger than 10 kb) have also been shown to be present. These studies also provided valuable information on the intron-exon junctions for subsequent genotyping tests described below. More recently, the DPD promoter was cloned and characterized,[56] permitting this area regulating gene expression to be examined.

Known Mutations of the Dihydropyrimidine Dehydrogenase Gene

There are at least 13 alleles (Table 36-4) that have been reported in the human DPD gene (DPYD).[57,58] Although all of these represent genetic polymorphisms, it is not clear what their relative importance is in terms of frequency in the population and as a cause of DPD deficiency. As can be seen in Table 36-4, many of these suggested alleles have not been fully clarified as to their effect on DPD activity. The mutation that thus far appears to be the most common is DPYD*2A, a G to A mutation in the 5' splicing recogni-

TABLE 36-4. ALLELES OF DIHYDROPYRIMIDINE DEHYDROGENASE GENE (DPYD) POTENTIALLY ASSOCIATED WITH CHANGE IN ENZYME ACTIVITY

Allele	Type	Enzyme activity
DPYD*1	Wild type	Normal
DPYD*2A	G → A at a 5'-splicing donor consensus sequence leading to skipping of exon 14 resulting in truncated protein	Decreased
DPYD*2B	(Same as DPYD*2A) and A1627G (Ile543Val)	Decreased
DPYD*3	ΔC1897 in exon 14 results in truncated protein (frameshift terminates at AA 633)	Decreased *in vivo*
DPYD*4	G1601A (Ser534Asn)	Normal
DPYD*5	A1627G (Ile543Val)	Normal
DPYD*6	G2194A (Val732Ile)	Normal
DPYD*7	ΔTCAT 295-298 in exon 4 results in truncated protein (at AA 633)	ND
DPYD*8	C703T (Arg253Trp)	Decreased *in vivo*
DPYD*9A	T85C (Cys29Arg)	Decreased *in vivo*
DPYD*9B	T85C (Cys29Arg) and G2657A (Arg886His)	Decreased *in vivo*
DPYD*10	G2983T (Val995Phe)	Decreased *in vivo*
DPYD*11	G1003T (Val335Leu)	Decreased *in vivo*
DPYD*12	G62A (Arg21Gln) and G1156T (Glu386Ter)	Decreased *in vivo*

Arg, arginine; Asn, asparagine; Cys, cysteine; Gln, glutamine; Glu, glutamic acid; His, histidine; Ile, isoleucine; Leu, leucine; ND, not determined; Phe, phenylalanine; Ser, serine; Trp, tryptophan; Val, valine.
Adapted from McLeod HL, Collie-Duguild ES, Vreken P, et al. Nomenclature for human DPYD alleles. *Pharmacogenetics* 1998;8:455–459; and Collie-Duguild ES, Etienne MC, Milano G, et al. Known variant DPYD alleles do not explain DPD deficiency in cancer patients. *Pharmacogenetics* 2000;10:217–223.

tion sequence of intron 14, resulting in a 165–base-pair deletion corresponding to exon 14. Several cases of severe life-threatening DPD deficiency have been described with this mutation.[47,59]

Screening for Dihydropyrimidine Dehydrogenase Deficiency

Since DPD deficiency was first described, a number of screening tests have been proposed, including, at first, phenotypic tests, such as measurements of the pyrimidine uracil or thymine (substrates for the enzyme DPD).[39] Although these proved useful for detection of individuals with severe DPD deficiency (e.g., homozygotes for a defective allele), they were less useful in detecting individuals that were partially deficient (e.g., heterozygotes for a defective allele), because even the presence of 50% (or less) of normal DPD activity was sufficient to catabolize uracil and thymine, maintaining normal levels in plasma or urine. Subsequently, direct measurement of DPD activity was used.[40] This technique permitted detection of individuals

with complete or partial deficiency and established the boundaries of normal in the population.[42] The method is most easily used as a radioassay with quantitation of the substrate and the products of the enzyme reaction, using a high-pressure liquid chromatography with an online radiodetector.[60] Another method that has been used quantitates the amount of DPD protein, using an antibody together with a separation method, such as Western blotting, to measure DPD protein. This is a useful screening method for DPD protein in tissues, such as PBM cells[43,44]; liver[49]; and fibroblasts.[61]

Based on the isolation and characterization of the structure of the human DPD gene[54,55] and the demonstration of at least several mutations that may be responsible for DPD deficiency,[57, 58] it should be possible to design specific primers for PCR to detect the presence of specific mutations associated with DPD deficiency. Techniques such as allele-specific PCR should prove to be particularly useful for such common defects as exon skipping of exon 14, which results from a splice defect.[59]

Uridine Diphosphate Glucuronosyltransferase

Glucuronidation is a phase II conjugation reaction in which uridine diphosphate glucuronic acid is used to eliminate xenobiotics or poorly soluble endogenous substrates.[62] The enzymes that catalyze this reaction are known as UGT enzymes. There are two discrete gene families (UGT1 and UGT2), each of which has specific isoforms.[63] The most important and best studied of these isoforms is UGT1A1, the isoform that is known to have an important role in bilirubin disposition.[64] Polymorphism of this specific gene results in the well-characterized hyperbilirubin syndromes of the rare (1 of 1,000,000) Crigler-Najjar syndromes (type I and II) and the relatively common (estimated in up to 15% of the general population) Gilbert syndrome.[65]

The biochemical evaluation of TPMT and DPD and molecular studies of each (cDNA, gene, and mutations) followed as a direct result of the identification of pharmacogenetic syndromes associated with altered drug clearance. In contrast, biochemical studies of UGT1A1 and molecular evaluation (cDNA, gene, and mutations) were completed during an evaluation of hyperbilirubin syndromes before recognition of a pharmacogenetic syndrome associated with a decrease in UGT1A1.

Importance of Uridine Diphosphate Glucuronosyltransferase 1A1 in Irinotecan Pharmacology

As noted elsewhere in this text, irinotecan (CPT-11) is a relatively new cancer chemotherapy drug used primarily in the first-line treatment of advanced colorectal cancer, but

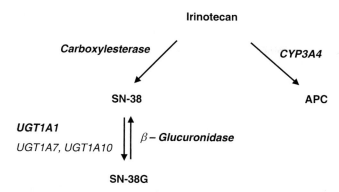

FIGURE 36-4. The metabolism of irinotecan in humans, showing critical position of uridine diphosphate glucuronosyltransferase. SN-38 is the active metabolite of irinotecan. Irinotecan can also be converted to 7-ethyl-10-[4-N-(5-aminopentanoic acid)-1-piperidino] carbonyloxycamptothecin (APC). SN-38 can be glucuronidated to form SN-38G and excreted into the bile, where it can enter the enterohepatic circulation. Glucuronidation is primarily via uridine diphosphate glucuronosyltransferase (UGT)1A1, but may be via UGT1A7 and UGT1A10. SN-38G may be metabolized back to SN-38. (Adapted from Ando Y, Saka H, Asai G, et al. UGT1A1 genotypes and glucuronidation of SN-38, the active metabolite of irinotecan. *Ann Oncol* 1998;9:845–847.)

likely to find indications in several other tumor types in the future.[66] UGT1A1 occupies an important position in irinotecan metabolism (Fig. 36-4), because it has the major role in the disposition and, hence, detoxification, of the active metabolite 7-ethyl-10-hydroxycamptothecin (SN-38).[67] If UGT1A1 is decreased, there should be an excess SN-38 present, which could result in unexpected and severe toxicity. It was hypothesized that the presence of mutations in the UGT1A1 gene could produce a decrease in function or relative amount of UGT1A1, and, in turn, result in delayed clearance of SN-38.

Clinical Presentation

Patients with abnormal UGT1A1 who receive irinotecan often present with severe diarrhea and neutropenia, symptoms suggestive of a irinotecan overdose.[67] The mechanism responsible for toxicity is thought to be due principally to the toxic effect of increasing concentration of SN-38 on the gastrointestinal tract and bone marrow.[68] Although the diarrhea can be severe and potentially life threatening, to date there have been no reported fatalities, in contrast to what has occasionally been seen with TPMT and DPD deficiencies in the presence of thiopurines or 5-FU drugs, respectively.

Effect of Uridine Diphosphate Glucuronosyltransferase 1A1 Deficiency on Irinotecan Metabolism and Pharmacokinetics

Studies have now confirmed that mutations in the UGT1A1 gene can result in decreased UGT1A1 enzyme activity, and this, in turn, could produce the hypothesized

changes in SN-38 levels.[69,70] These mutations affect not only UGT1A1 enzyme activity, but also clearance and profile of irinotecan metabolites,[69-71] and contribute to the marked interpatient variability in pharmacokinetics and toxicity of irinotecan.[69,71] Patients who presented with a clinical picture of Gilbert syndrome and an elevated serum biliary index, and who were subsequently found to be homozygous for the mutant gene, were the patients who had abnormal pharmacokinetics with increased ratios of SN-38 to SN-38 glucuronide (SN-38G).

Pattern of Inheritance

The pattern of inheritance for individuals who are likely to be affected with this pharmacogenetic syndrome is essentially the same as with Gilbert syndrome.[72] Although previous studies of the various hyperbilirubinemic syndromes, including Crigler-Najjar type I and II and Gilbert syndrome, were confusing as to the pattern of inheritance, it is now clear that an autosomal-recessive pattern of inheritance is responsible for both Gilbert and the pharmacogenetic syndrome.

Uridine Diphosphate Glucuronosyltransferase 1A1 Gene and Known Mutations

As noted, the gene for UGT1A1 had earlier been elucidated in the evaluation of the hyperbilirubin syndromes, and, in particular, Gilbert syndrome.[63,64] The gene in humans is located on chromosome 2q37.[73] A number of UGT1A1 mutations have been identified (Table 36-5). Some of these are associated with low or absent enzyme activity, as with the Crigler-Najjar syndromes. Gilbert syndrome, a more common abnormality, is associated with mutations in the promoter region rich in repeated TA sequences, normally

TABLE 36-5. POLYMORPHISMS OF URIDINE DIPHOSPHATE GLUCURONOSYLTRANSFERASE (UGT)1A1 AFFECTING IRINOTECAN METABOLISM

Allele	Type	Enzyme activity
UGT1A1	Wild-type–promoter has (TA)₆TAA	Normal
UGT1A1 28	Extra TA in promoter (TA)₇TAA (Gilbert syndrome)	Decreased
	Two extra TAs in promoter (TA)₈TAA	Decreased
	Missing TA in promoter (TA)₅TAA	Increased
	Several coding region mutations (Crigler-Najjar syndrome)	Decreased or absent
	G295A in coding region resulting in Gly71Arg	Decreased

Arg, arginine; Gly, glycine.
Adapted from Iyer L. Inherited variations in drug-metabolizing enzymes: significance in clinical oncology. *Mol Diag* 1999;4:327–333.

designated as $(TA)_6TAA$. The most common mutation in this region results in an extra TA and is designated as $(TA)_7TAA$. Individuals who are homozygous for the $(TA)_7TAA$ allele [$(TA)_7TAA/(TA)_7TAA$] have enzyme activity approximately 25% of normal, whereas individuals who are heterozygous [$(TA)_7TAA/(TA)_6TAA$] have approximately 50% of the homozygous wild-type [$(TA)_6TAA/(TA)_6TAA$] activity. Additional variant alleles in which there are further alterations of the number of tandem TA repeats have been described, including $(TA)_5TAA$ and $(TA)_8TAA$ variant alleles. An additional mutation has recently been described in the coding region of the UGT1A1 gene, in which there is a substitution of a glycine for an arginine at position 71.

Population Studies

The population studies for the pharmacogenetic syndrome associated with UGT1A1 have made use of data from prior investigations and characterization of the mutations associated with hyperbilirubin syndromes described above.[74] The $(TA)_7TAA$ allele has been shown to vary in different populations. Within the white population, but not Africans or Asians, there is a strong correlation between promoter TA repeat number and bilirubin level.[12] Certain populations, such as the Canadian Inuits, have relatively high frequency (19%) of the [$(TA)_7TAA/(TA)_7TAA$] genotype and thus would be at risk if treated with irinotecan.[75]

Screening for Uridine Diphosphate Glucuronosyltransferase 1A1 Deficiency

The suspicion of UGT1A1 deficiency should be increased in the presence of unexplained hyperbilirubinemia that may be due to Gilbert syndrome.[76] In contrast to TPMT and DPD deficiency, in which a combination of phenotyping and genotyping is usually advised to confirm the existence of a pharmacogenetic syndrome, evaluation of UGT1A1 deficiency usually relies on genotype tests for routine screening. This is particularly true because the liver is the major site of enzyme activity and is not easily accessible for assessment of enzyme activity. Furthermore, extensive genotyping of UGT, particularly in evaluation of the hyperbilirubinemic syndromes, has demonstrated that the most important UGT affected is the UGT1A1 isoform, with several common mutations in the promoter region (Table 36-5) having been shown to be associated with deficiency of UGT1A1 activity.[69,70,74,77] This permits the use of allele-specific PCR methods for screening purposes.

Other Enzymes of Potential Pharmacogenetic Importance to Cancer Chemotherapy Agents

Over the years, a number of other enzymes, including several known to be polymorphic and having potential impor-

tance to the metabolism of cancer chemotherapy drugs, have been examined, with the expectation that relative deficiency might have consequences to cancer patients, either due to the occurrence of increased toxicity or decreased response. Among the enzymes that have been considered are the various cytochrome P-450 enzymes (CYP2D6, CYP2C9, CYP2C19, CYP3A4, CYP3A5, CYP3A7), N-acetyltransferases, aldehyde dehydrogenase, glutathione S-transferases, O^6-alkyl-guanine alkyl transferase, and DT diaphorase (NADP)H-quinone oxidoreductase.[9,10] Despite the known importance of many of these enzymes for pharmacogenetic syndromes associated with drugs from other classes (1,5,7), there is little evidence at this point that polymorphisms of the relevant genes have a significant clinical impact on currently used cancer chemotherapy drugs. However, it must be emphasized that more comprehensive studies are needed to critically evaluate this possibility for other chemotherapy agents. In particular, as noted earlier, one must have a high degree of suspicion for the possibility of a genetic polymorphism, which, in turn, could be the basis for a pharmacogenetic syndrome whenever variability is noted in efficacy or toxicity to a chemotherapeutic agent.

CONCLUSION

In summary, genetic polymorphisms that affect enzymes that have a critical role in drug metabolism are important and likely will become more important in the future in understanding the variability in response and toxicity to cancer chemotherapy agents. Over the past several years, there has been an increasing appreciation of several pharmacogenetic syndromes associated with cancer chemotherapy drugs including polymorphisms affecting TPMT, DPD, and, more recently, UGT. These polymorphisms have been shown to result in an abnormal pattern of metabolism of these drugs, which, in turn, can lead to altered pharmacokinetics and, subsequently, severe, often life-threatening toxicity.

More recently, there has been an additional focus on the role of gene expression in tumors in determining the response to cancer chemotherapy agents. Genes coding for expression of critical enzymes, which are involved in metabolism (both anabolism and catabolism) or are targets for drug action, have been of particular interest. This is illustrated by recent studies (Fig. 36-5) examining the effectiveness of the cancer chemotherapy drug 5-FU, in which response was shown to be related to the expression of the target enzyme TS, and the catabolic enzyme DPD, and the anabolic enzyme thymidylate phosphorylase.[78]

With the completion of sequencing of the human genome and the potential to rapidly screen individuals in the future, together with an increasing understanding of the role of proteins (proteomics) that newly identified genes may code for, there is likely to be a new era in cancer

DPD, TS and TP Gene Expression
vs Response to FU/LV in Colon Cancer

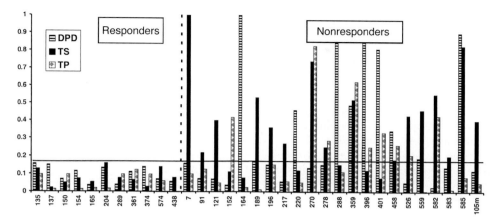

FIGURE 36-5. Pharmacogenomic study in tumor specimens of colorectal cancer patients treated with 5-FU. Quantitative polymerase chain reaction used to measure messenger RNA expression of thymidylate synthase (TS), thymidine phosphorylase (TP), and dihydropyrimidine dehydrogenase (DPD) in tumors. Patients who responded (*left*) had relatively low messenger RNA expression of all three markers (all below *solid horizontal line*, used to divide specimens with low vs. high expression). Patients who were unresponsive (*right*) had elevated expression of one or more markers. (FU, fluorouracil; LV, leucovorin.) (Adapted from Diasio RB, Johnson MR. The importance of pharmacogenetics/pharmacogenomics for the cancer chemotherapy drug 5-fluorouracil, *Pharmacology* 2000;61:299–203; and Salonga D, Danenberg KD, Johnson M, et al. Colorectal tumors responding to 5-fluorouracil have low gene expression levels of dihydropyrimidine dehydrogenase, thymidylate synthase, and thymidine phosphorylase. *Clin Cancer Res* 2000;6:1322–1327.)

chemotherapy. Although pharmacogenetics will remain important, there will be an increasing emphasis on pharmacogenomics, in which the alteration in sequence or a difference in expression of a critical gene will provide the stimulus to investigate the pharmacologic consequences.[3,79] This will include an increasing focus on the importance of SNPs and the role that these subtle nucleotide changes may have in drug response.[2]

REFERENCES

1. Kalow W. Pharmacogenetics: its biological roots and the medical challenge. *Clin Pharmacol Ther* 1993;54:235–241.
2. McCarthy JJ, Hilfiker R. The use of single-nucleotide polymorphism maps in pharmacogenomics. *Nat Biotechnol* 2000;18:505–508.
3. Evans WE, Relling MV. Pharmacogenomics: translating functional genomics into rational therapeutics. *Science* 1999;286:487–491.
4. Lu Z, Diasio RB. Polymorphic drug-metabolizing enzymes. In: Schilsky RL, Milano GA, Ratain MJ, eds. *Principles of antineoplastic drug development and pharmacology.* New York: Marcel Dekker Inc, 1996:281–385.
5. Kalow W. Pharmacoanthropology and the genetics of drug metabolism. In: Kalow W, ed. *Pharmacogenetics of drug metabolism.* New York: Pergamon Press, 1992.
6. Heggie GD, Sommadossi JP, Cross DS, et al. Clinical phar-macokinetics of 5-fluorouracil and its metabolites in plasma, urine, and bile. *Cancer Res* 1987;47:2203–2206.
7. Meyers U, Skoda RC, Zanger UM, et al. The genetic polymorphism of debrisoquine/sparteine metabolism—molecular mechanisms. In: Kalow W, ed. *Pharmacogenetics of drug metabolism.* New York: Pergamon Press, 1992.
8. Sasvari-Szekely M, Gerstner A, Ronai Z, et al. Rapid genotyping of factor V Leiden Mutation using single-tube bi-directional allele-specific amplification and automated ultrathin-layer agarose gel electrophoresis. *Electrophoresis* 2000;21:816–821.
9. Boddy AV, Ratain MJ. Pharmacogenetics in cancer etiology and chemotherapy. *Clin Cancer Res* 1997;3:1025–1030.
10. Iyer L, Ratain MJ. Pharmacogenetics and cancer chemotherapy. *Eur J Cancer* 1998;34:1493–1499.
11. Krynetski EY, Evans WE. Pharmacogenetics of cancer therapy: getting personal. *Am J Hum Genet* 1998;63:11–16.
12. Iyer L. Inherited variations in drug-metabolizing enzymes: significance in clinical oncology. *Mol Diag* 1999;4:327–333.
13. Weinshilboum R. Methyltransferase pharmacogenetics. *Pharmacol Ther* 1989;43:77–90.
14. Diasio RB, LoBuglio AF. Immunomodulators: immunosuppressive agents and immunostimulants. In: Hardman JG, Limbird LE, eds. *The pharmacological basis of therapeutics.* New York: McGraw-Hill, 1996.
15. Evans WE, Horner M, Chu YQ. Altered mercaptopurine metabolism, toxic effects and dosage requirement in a thiopurine methyltransferase-deficient child with acute lymphocytic leukemia. *J Pediatr* 1991;119: 985–989.

16. Lennard L, Gibson BE, Nicole T, et al. Congenital thiopurine methyltransferase deficiency and 6-mercaptopurine toxicity during treatment for acute lymphocytic leukemia. *Arch Dis Child* 1993;69:577–579.

17. Lennard L, Van Loon JA, Weinshilboum RM. Pharmacogenetics of acute azathioprine toxicity; relationship to thiopurine methyltransferase genetic polymorphism. *Clin Pharmacol Ther* 1989;46:149–154.

18. Schutz E, Gummert J, Mohr F, et al. Azathioprine-induced myelosuppression in thiopurine methyltransferase deficient heart transplant recipient. *Lancet* 1993;341:436.

19. Lennard L, Lilleyman JS, Van Loon J, et al. Genetic variation in response to 6-mercaptopurine for childhood acute lymphoblastic leukaemia. *Lancet* 1990;336:225–229.

20. Lennard L, Lilleyman JS. Individualizing therapy with 6-mercaptopurine and 6-thioguanine related to the thiopurine methyltransferase genetic polymorphism. *Ther Drug Monitor* 1996;18:328–334.

21. Lennard L, Keen D, Lilleyman JS. Oral 6-mercaptopurine in childhood leukemia: parent drug pharmacokinetics and active metabolite concentrations. *Clin Pharmacol Ther* 1986;40:287–292.

22. Lilleyman JS, Lennard L. Mercaptopurine metabolism and risk of relapse in childhood lymphoblastic leukaemia. *Lancet* 1994;343:1188–1190.

23. Weinshilboum RM, Sladek SL. Mercaptopurine pharmacogenetics: monogenic inheritance of erythrocyte thiopurine methyltransferase activity. *Am J Hum Genet* 1980;32:651–662.

24. McLeod HL, Lin JS, Scott EP, et al. Thiopurine methyltransferase activity in American white subjects and black subjects. *Clin Pharmacol Ther* 1994;55:15–20.

25. Lee D, Szumlanski C, Houtman J, et al. Thiopurine methyltransferase pharmacogenetics: cloning of human liver cDNA and a processed pseudogene on human chromosome 18Q21.1. *Drug Metab Disp* 1995;23:398–405.

26. Szumlanski C, Otterness D, Her C, et al. Thiopurine methyltransferase pharmacogenetics: human gene cloning and characterization of a common polymorphism. *DNA Cell Biol* 1996;15:17–30.

27. Tai HL, Krynetski EY, Schuetz EG, et al. Enhanced proteolysis of thiopurine S-methyltransferase (TPMT) encoded by mutant alleles in humans (TPMT*3A, TPMT*2): mechanisms for the genetic polymorphism of TPMT activity. *Proc Natl Acad Sci U S A* 1997;94:6444–6449.

28. Spire-Vayrone de la Moureyre C, Debuysere H, Sabbagh N, et al. Detection of known and new mutations in the thiopurine S-methyltransferase gene by single-strand conformation polymorphism analysis. *Hum Mutat* 1998;12:177–185.

29. Weinshilboum RM, Sladek S, Klumpp S. Human erythrocyte thiol methyltransferase: radiochemical microassay and biochemical properties. *Clinica Chimica Acta* 1979;97:59–71.

30. Woodson LC, Dunnette JC, Weinshilboum R. Pharmacogenetics of human thiopurine methyltransferase: kidney-erythrocyte correlation and immunotitration studies. *J Pharmacol Exp Ther* 1982;222:174–181.

31. Yates CR, Krynetski EY, Loennechen T, et al. Molecular diagnosis of thiopurine S-methyltransferase deficiency: genetic basis for azathioprine and mercaptopurine intolerance. *Ann Int Med* 1987;126:608–614.

32. Weinshilboum R. Pharmacogenetics of anticancer drug metabolism. In: Grochow LB, Ames MM, eds. *A clinician's guide to chemotherapy pharmacokinetics and pharmacodynamics.* Baltimore: Williams & Wilkins, 1998.

33. Krynetski EY, Evans WE. Genetic polymorphism of thiopurine S-methyltransferase: molecular mechanisms and clinical importance. *Pharmacology* 2000;61:136–146.

34. Lu Z, Zhang R, Diasio RB. Purification and characterization of dihydropyrimidine dehydrogenase from human liver. *J Biol Chem* 1992;267:17102–17109.

35. Heggie GD, Sommadossi JP, Cross DS, et al. Clinical pharmacokinetics of 5-fluorouracil and its metabolites in plasma, urine, and bile. *Cancer Res* 1987;47:2203–2206.

36. Diasio RB. The role of dihydropyrimidine dehydrogenase (DPD) modulation in 5-FU pharmacology. *Oncology* 1998;12:23–27.

37. Diasio RB, Harris BE. Clinical pharmacology of 5-fluorouracil. *Clin Pharmacokinet* 1989;16:215–237.

38. Diasio RB, Johnson MR. Dihydropyrimidine dehydrogenase (DPD): its role in 5-FU clinical toxicity and tumor resistance. *Clin Cancer Res* 1999;5:2672–2673.

39. Tuchman M, Stoeckeler JS, Kiang DT, et al. Familial pyrimidinemia and pyrimidinuria associated with severe fluorouracil toxicity. *N Engl J Med* 1985;313:245–249.

40. Diasio RB, Beavers TL, Carpenter JT. Familial deficiency of dihydropyrimidine dehydrogenase: biochemical basis for familial pyrimidinemia and severe 5-fluorouracil-induced toxicity. *J Clin Invest* 1988;81:47–51.

41. Harris BE, Carpenter JT, Diasio RB. Severe 5-fluorouracil toxicity secondary to dihydropyrimidine dehydrogenase deficiency: a potentially more common pharmacogenetic syndrome. *Cancer* 1991;68:499–501.

42. Lu Z, Zhang R, Diasio RB. Dihydropyrimidine dehydrogenase activity in human peripheral blood mononuclear cells and liver: population characteristics, newly identified patients, and clinical implication in 5-fluorouracil chemotherapy. *Cancer Res* 1993;53:5433–5438.

43. Takimoto CH, Lu Z-H, Zhang R, et al. Severe neurotoxicity following 5-fluorouracil-based chemotherapy in a patient with dihydropyrimidine dehydrogenase deficiency. *Clin Cancer Res* 1996;2:477–481.

44. Johnson MJ, Hageboutros A, Wang K, et al. Life-threatening toxicity in a dihydropyrimidine dehydrogenase deficient patient following treatment with topical 5-fluorouracil. *Clin Cancer Res* 1999;5:2006–2011.

45. Milano G, Etienne MC, Pierrefite V, et al. Dihydropyrimidine dehydrogenase deficiency and fluorouracil-related toxicity. *Br J Cancer* 1999;79:627–630.

46. Shehata N, Pater A, Tang SC. Prolonged severe 5-fluorouracil-associated neurotoxicity in a patient with dihydropyrimidine dehydrogenase deficiency. *Cancer Invest* 1999;17:201–205.

47. Wei X, McLeod HL, McMurrough J, et al. Molecular basis of the human dihydropyrimidine dehydrogenase deficiency and 5-fluorouracil toxicity. *J Clin Invest* 1996;98:610–615.

48. Harris BE, Song R, Soong SJ, et al. Relationship of dihydropyrimidine dehydrogenase activity and plasma 5-fluorouracil levels: evidence for circadian variation of 5-FU levels in cancer patients receiving protracted continuous infusion. *Cancer Res* 1990;50:197–201.

49. Lu Z, Zhang R, Diasio RB. Dihydropyrimidine dehydrogenase activity in human liver: population characteristics and clinical implication in 5-FU chemotherapy. *Clin Pharmacol Ther* 1995;8:512–522.

50. Lu Z, Zhang R, Carpenter JT, et al. Decreased dihydropyrimidine dehydrogenase activity in population of patients with breast cancer: implications for 5-FU-based chemotherapy. *Clin Cancer Res* 1998;4:325–329.

51. Yokota H, Fernandez-Salguero P, Furuya H, et al. cDNA cloning and chromosome mapping of human dihydropyrimidine dehydrogenase, an enzyme associated with 5-fluorouracil toxicity and congenital thymine uraciluria. *J Biol Chem* 1994;269:23192–23196.

52. Albin N, Johnson MR, Diasio RB. cDNA cloning of bovine liver dihydropyrimidine dehydrogenase. *DNA Sequence* 1996;6:231–238.

53. Takai S, Fernandez-Salguero P, Kimura S, et al. Assignment of the human dihydropyrimidine dehydrogenase gene (DPYD) to chromosome region 1p22 by fluorescence in situ hybridization. *Genomics* 1994;24:613–614.

54. Johnson MJ, Wang K, Tillmanns S, et al. Structural organization of the human dihydropyrimidine dehydrogenase gene. *Cancer Res* 1997;57:1660–1663.

55. Wei X, Elizondo G, Sapone A, et al. Characterization of the human dihydropyrimidine dehydrogenase gene. *Genomics* 1998;51:391–400.

56. Shestopol SA, Johnson MR, Diasio RB. Molecular cloning and characterization of the human dihydropyrimidine dehydrogenase promoter. *Biochim Biophys Acta* 2000;1494:162–169.

57. McLeod HL, Collie-Duguid ES, Vreken P, et al. Nomenclature for human DPYD alleles. *Pharmacogenetics* 1998;8:455–459.

58. Collie-Duguild ESR, Etienne MC, Milano G, et al. Known variant DPYD alleles do not explain DPD deficiency in cancer patients. *Pharmacogenetics* 2000;10:217–223.

59. Johnson MJ, Hageboutros A, Wang K, et al. Life-threatening toxicity in a dihydropyrimidine dehydrogenase deficient patient following treatment with topical 5-fluorouracil. *Clin Cancer Res* 1999;5:2006–2011.

60. Johnson MJ, Yan J, Albin N, et al. Rapid screening for dihydropyrimidine dehydrogenase (dpd) deficiency, a condition associated with 5-fluorouracil toxicity. *J Chromatogr B Biomed Appl* 1997;696:183–191.

61. Diasio RB, Van Kuilenburg ABP, Lu Z, et al. Dihydropyrimidine dehydrogenase (DPD) in fibroblasts of a DPD deficient patient and family members. In: Sahota A, Taylor M, eds. *Purine and pyrimidine metabolism in man.* New York: Plenum Publishing, 1995:7–10.

62. Parkinson A. Biotransformation of xenobiotics. In: Klaasen CD, ed. *Casarett and Doulls toxicology, the basic science of poisons.* New York: McGraw Hill, 1996.

63. Clarke DJ, Burchell B. The uridine diphosphate glucurosyltransferase multigene family: function and regulation. In: Kaufman FC, ed. *Handbook of experimental pharmacology.* Berlin: Springer-Verlag, 1994.

64. Bosma PJ, Seppen J, Goldhoorn B, et al. Bilirubin UDP-glucuronosyltransferase 1 is the only relevant bilirubin glucuronidating isoform in man. *J Biol Chem* 1994;269:17960–17964.

65. Bosma PJ, Chowdhury JR, Bakker C, et al. The genetic basis of the reduced expression of bilirubin UDP-glucuronosyltransferase 1 in Gilbert's syndrome. *N Engl J Med* 1995;333:1171–1175.

66. Iyer L, Ratain MJ. Clinical pharmacology of camptothecins. *Cancer Chemother Pharmacol* 1998;42:S31–43.

67. Gupta E, Lestingi TM, Mick R, et al. Metabolic fate of irinotecan in humans: correlation of glucuronidation with diarrhea. *Cancer Res* 1994;54:3723–3725.

68. Araki E, Ishikawa M, Iigo M, et al. Relationship between development of diarrhea and the concentration of SN-38, an active metabolite of CPT-11, in the intestine and the blood plasma of athymic mice following intraperitoneal administration of CPT-11. *Jpn J Cancer Res* 1993;84:697–702.

69. Ando Y, Saka H, Asai G, et al. UGT1A1 genotypes and glucuronidation of SN-38, the active metabolite of irinotecan. *Ann Oncol* 1998;9:845–847.

70. Iyer L, King CD, Whitington PF, et al. Genetic predisposition to the metabolism of irinotecan (CPT-11). Role of uridine diphosphate glucuronosyltransferase isoform 1A1 in the glucuronidation of its active metabolite (SN-38) in human liver microsomes. *J Clin Invest* 1998;101:847–854.

71. Gupta E, Mick R, Ramirez J, et al. Pharmacokinetic and pharmacodynamic evaluation of the topoisomerase inhibitor irinotecan in cancer patients. *J Clin Oncol* 1997;15:1502–1510.

72. Bosma P, Chowdhury JR, Jansen PH. Genetic inheritance of Gilbert's syndrome. *Lancet* 1995;346:314–315.

73. Tukey RH, Strassburg CP. Human UDP-glucuronosyltransferases: metabolism, expression, and disease. *Annu Rev Pharmacol Toxicol* 2000;40:581–616.

74. Iyer L, Hall D, Das S, et al. Phenotype-genotype correlation of in vitro SN-38 (active metabolite of irinotecan) and bilirubin glucuronidation in human liver tissue with UGT1A1 promoter polymorphism. *Clin Pharmacol Ther* 1999;65:576–582.

75. Monaghan G, Foster B, Jurima-Romet M, et al. UGT1*1 genotyping in a Canadian Inuit population. *Pharmacogenetics* 1997;7:153–156.

76. Wasserman E, Myara A, Lokiec F, et al. Severe CPT-11 toxicity in patients with Gilbert's syndrome: two case reports. *Ann Oncol* 1997;8:1049–1051.

77. Hall D, Ybazeta G, Destro-Bisol G, et al. Variability at the uridine diphosphate glucuronosyltransferase 1A1 promoter in human populations and primates. *Pharmacogenetics* 1999;9:591–599.

78. Salonga D, Danenberg KD, Johnson M, et al. Colorectal tumors responding to 5-fluorouracil have low gene expression levels of dihydropyrimidine dehydrogenase, thymidylate synthase, and thymidine phosphorylase. *Clin Cancer Res* 2000;6:1322–1327.

79. Diasio RB, Johnson MR. The importance of pharmacogenetics/pharmacogenomics for the cancer chemotherapy drug 5-fluorouracil. *Pharmacology* 2000;61:199–203.

37

CHEMOKINE–CHEMOKINE RECEPTOR DATABASE 2001: BIOLOGIC, MOLECULAR, AND PATHOPHYSIOLOGIC PROPERTIES OF CHEMOKINE-RECEPTOR INTERACTIONS

HARRY D. DAWSON
DENNIS D. TAUB

Chemotaxis is the process by which leukocytes are directed to sites of inflammation under the influence of a concentration gradient of soluble chemotactic molecules. On encountering a chemotactic molecule, a responding leukocyte begins to migrate directionally from regions of low ligand concentrations toward the sites of chemoattractant production. Various endogenous compounds have been shown to mediate leukocyte migration, including activated serum components, arachidonic acid metabolites, various lipid mediators, acute-phase proteins, inflammatory cytokines, opioid peptides, and various hormones. Although many of these factors are believed to play some role in inflammation, their relevance to leukocyte locomotion in various pathologic disease states and in normal homing processes has been brought into question. Over the past 15 years, more than 50 unique human and rodent cytokines have been identified as members of a superfamily of chemoattractants called *chemokines*. Chemokines have been shown to induce the directional migration of selected leukocytic cell types, including neutrophils, basophils, eosinophils, monocytes, macrophages, dendritic cells, and lymphocytes. Members of this family were originally characterized as low-molecular-weight peptides with similarities in their primary sequences as well as in the presence of a conserved motif containing either two or four cysteine residues that form disulfide bonds in the tertiary structures of the proteins. Today, four classes of chemokines have been defined by the arrangement of the conserved cysteine residues of the mature secreted protein: the CXC (or α) chemokines, which have one amino acid separating the first two conserved cysteine residues; the CC (or β) chemokines, in which the first two conserved cysteine residues are adjacent; the C (or λ) chemokines, which lack two (the first

and the third) of the four conserved cysteine residues; and the CX_3C (or δ) chemokines, which have three amino acids separating the first two conserved cysteine residues. Besides being highly basic in nature and having the ability to bind heparin and heparan proteoglycans through heparin-binding domains, many chemokines exhibit a significant level of cross-homology at the amino acid (24% to 80%) and nucleotide (25% to 75%) level. As the chemokines are secreted molecules, their complementary DNAs code for a precursor protein that presumably enables the chemokines to be produced, cleaved, and secreted by a wide variety of cell types to yield a mature form at the cell membrane. In addition, all chemokine subfamily members have been shown to mediate their biologic effects through high-affinity G protein–coupled seven-transmembrane cell surface receptors. Because many of these chemokines are active in their monomeric forms (approximately 7 to 14 kd), the biologically active concentration range for these ligands is typically 10^{-8} to 10^{-10} mol per L, a range that strongly correlates with many of the known receptor-ligand affinities. Not only do many chemokines show similarities in protein sequences and secondary structures, but in addition the gene organization of many chemokine subfamily members is highly conserved, with similar numbers of introns and exons. Furthermore, many of the chemokine ligand and receptor subfamilies co-cluster on the same chromosomes, which suggests an evolutionary divergence from a common ancestral gene.

Historically, the chemokine subfamilies were biologically distinguished from one another by their apparent leukocyte specificity in mediating cell migration. The early rule was that CXC chemokines induce neutrophil but not monocyte migration, whereas CC chemokines predomi-

TABLE 37-1. CC CHEMOKINE NOMENCLATURE

Systematic Name	Human Ligand	Mouse Ligand	Rat Ligand	Receptor(s)
CCL1	I-309	TCA-3, P500	I-309, TCA-3	CCR8
CCL2	MCP-1, MCAF	MCP-1, JE	MCP-1, JE	CCR2, CCR10
CCL3	LD78A, LD78B, MIP-1α	MIP-1α	MIP-1α	CCR1, CCR5, CCR10
CCL4	MIP-1β	Act-2, MIP-1β	MIP-1β	CCR5, CCR8
CCL5	RANTES	RANTES	RANTES, SIS-δ	CCR1, CCR3, CCR4, CCR5, US28
CCL6	Unknown	C10, MRP-1	Unknown	Unknown
CCL7	MCP-3	FIC, MARC, NC28	MCP-3	CCR1, CCR2, CCR3, CCR10
CCL8	MCP-2, HC14	MCP-2	Unknown	CCR2, CCR3, CCR5
CCL9/CCL10	Unknown	MRP-2, MIP-1γ	Unknown	Unknown
CCL11	EOT-1	EOT-1	EOT-1	CCR3
CCL12	Unknown	MCP-5	MCP-5	CCR2
CCL13	CKβ-10, MCP-4, NCC-1	Unknown	Unknown	CCR2, CCR3
CCL14	HCC-1, HCC-3, NCC-2	Unknown	Unknown	CCR1
CCL15	HCC-2, LKN-1, MIP-1δ, MIP-5	Unknown	Unknown	CCR1, CCR3
CCL16	HCC-4, LEC, LMC	LEC (pseudogene)	Unknown	CCR1
CCL17	TARC	TARC	Unknown	CCR4
CCL18	DC-CK-1, MIP-4, PARC	AMAC-1	Unknown	Unknown
CCL19	MIP-3β, ELC, exodus-3	MIP-3β	Unknown	CCR7
CCL20	Exodus-1, MIP-3α, LARC	MIP-3α	ST38	CCR6
CCL21	6Ckine, exodus-2, SLC	TCA-4, 6Ckine	Unknown	CCR7
CCL22	DCtactin-β, MDC, STCP-1	ABCD-1	MDC	CCR4
CCL23	MPIF-1, MIP-3, CKβ-8	Unknown	Unknown	CCR1
CCL24	Eotaxin-2, MPIF-2	Unknown	Unknown	CCR3
CCL25	TECK	TECK	Unknown	CCR9
CCL26	EOT-3	Unknown	Unknown	CCR3
CCL27	ALP, CTACK, Eskine	ALP, CTACK	Unknown	Unknown

Adapted from Homey B, Zlotnik A. Chemokines in allergy. *Curr Opin Immunol* 1999;11(6):626–634.

nantly act on monocytes and macrophages with no activity on neutrophils. With the examination of additional leukocyte subsets and the discovery of additional chemokine subfamily members, however, distinguishing chemokine subfamilies based on leukocyte motility and specificity has become invalid. Today, we know that, besides acting on neutrophils and monocytes, both CXC and CC family members are active on a number of cell types, including basophils, eosinophils, lymphocytes, mast cells, endothelial cells, epithelial cells, melanocytes, smooth muscle cells, keratinocytes, and hepatocytes. The CXC chemokine subfamily can be further subdivided into two groups based on the presence of the amino acid motif ELR (glutamic acid–leucine–arginine), that precedes the first cysteine residue near the amino terminus. These ELR-bearing chemokines (e.g., IL-8, GRO-α, GRO-β, GRO-γ, ENA-78, GCP-2, and NAP-2) have been shown to be potent chemoattractants for neutrophils, whereas non–ELR bearing CXC chemokines (e.g., PF-4, IP-10, Mig, and SDF-1α/β) have been shown to be potent chemoattractants for lymphocytes but exhibit little to no activity on neutrophils. Many of the CC, C, and CX$_3$C chemokine family members as well as several CXC chemokines have been shown to induce human lymphocyte migration both *in vitro* and *in vivo*. A detailed summary of all of the chemokine subfamily members, including alternative names and receptor-ligand pairs, can be found in Tables 37-1 through 37-3. Besides chemo-

taxis, chemokines have also been shown to mediate other biologic effects on leukocytes, including respiratory burst, enzyme release, degranulation, intracellular free Ca^{2+} mobilization, cell activation through several kinase signaling pathways, cellular polarization, shape changes, actin polymerization and intracellular structural changes, proliferation, cell surface CD and integrin molecule expression, increased integrin activity, and alterations in cell adherence between cells and adhesion proteins. Additional chemokine activities have been observed on nonleukocytic populations within various tissue- and organ-specific systems (e.g., neuronal cell depolarization and apoptosis), which suggests that these molecules are much more than simple chemoattractants and inflammatory mediators. Studies have demonstrated that several microorganisms possess genes that encode biologically active chemokine- and chemokine receptor–like molecules, which are believed to play a role in microbial binding-entry into various cell types and in many facets of disease pathogenesis.

Critical to an overall understanding of chemokine biology is an understanding of the specific receptors on various cell types that mediate their effects. The chemokine receptor field has exploded over the past several years. Over 50 human and rodent chemokine receptors have been isolated, characterized, and cloned. All of these receptors are members of the rhodopsin or serpentine receptor superfamily and have the characteristic G protein–coupled seven hydro-

TABLE 37-2. CXC CHEMOKINE NOMENCLATURE

Systematic Name	Human Ligand	Mouse Ligand	Rat Ligand	Receptor(s)
CXCL1	GRO-1, GRO-α, MGSA-α	GRO, KC	CINC-1, GRO, KC	CXCR2
CXCL2	GRO-2, GRO-β, MGSA-β, MIP-2α	GRO, KC	CINC-3, CINC-2α	CXCR2
CXCL3	GRO-3, GRO-γ, MIP-2β	GRO, KC	CINC-2β	CXCR2
CXCL4	PF-4, PF-4var1	PF-4alt	PF-4	Unknown
CXCL5	ENA-78	LIX?	LIX?	CXCR2
CXCL6	GCP-2, CKα-3	LIX?	LIX?	CXCR1, CXCR2
CXCL7	NAP-2	Unknown	Unknown	CXCR2
CXCL8	IL-8, MDNCF, NAP-1	Unknown	Unknown	CXCR1, CXCR2
CXCL9	Mig, Humig	Mig	Mig	CXCR3
CXCL10	IP-10	crg-2	mob-1	CXCR3
CXCL11	I-TAC, H174, β-R1	Unknown	Unknown	CXCR3
CXCL12	SDF-1α/β, PBSF	SDF-1α/β, PBSF	SDF-1α/β	CXCR4
CXCL13	BLC, BCA-1	BLC, BCA-1	Unknown	CXCR5
CXCL14	BRAK/bolekine	BRAK	Unknown	Unknown
CXCL15	Unknown	Lungkine	Unknown	Unknown

Adapted from Homey B, Zlotnik A. Chemokines in allergy. *Curr Opin Immunol* 1999;11(6):626–634.

phobic spanning transmembrane regions. A great deal of similarity is found between the tertiary structure of chemokine receptors and that of other G protein–coupled receptors (e.g., C5a receptor, fMLP receptor), yet chemokine receptors initiate unique and specific cellular activities only in response to their specific chemokines. As with other G protein–linked receptors, chemokine receptors are also known to exhibit overlapping ligand specificities (Tables 37-1, 37-2, and 37-3). Chemokine ligand-receptor interactions initiate a characteristic pattern of responses, including shape change, integrin activation, chemotaxis, degranulation, enzyme secretion, and respiratory burst. Depending on the chemokine and leukocyte subtype, receptor ligation has been shown to activate signaling pathways including phosphoinositol hydrolysis (inositol 1,4,5-triphosphate), phospholipase activation, arachidonic acid metabolism, cyclic adenosine monophosphate and cyclic guanosine monophosphate activation and turnover, the activation of a tyrosine and serine/threonine kinases, the activation of PI3K, and the rapid elevation of diacylglycerol and cytosolic Ca^{2+} levels. In addition, chemokine-mediated leukocyte migration and certain other biologic responses have been shown to be desensitized in response to high concentrations of chemokines, which yields the typical bell-shaped dose-response curves. The desensitization process is believed to play an important physiologic role by preventing the remobilization and departure of leukocytes on entering sites of inflammation where the chemokine concentrations are believed to be maximal. Based on the characteristics of shared ligands and shared signaling pathways, the likelihood is that interaction of chemokine ligands with a specific receptor results in a series of signals and responses that are distinct from those that result when the same chemokines interact with a shared receptor.

Given the broad cellular distribution of chemokine receptors and ligand responsiveness, one would predict that chemokines would play a significant role in inflammatory and noninflammatory disease states. To date, a role for chemokines have been demonstrated in a variety of pathophysiologic processes and diseases, including acute and chronic inflammation, asthma, atherosclerosis, rheumatoid arthritis and osteoarthritis, various microbe-mediated inflammatory diseases, tumor growth and metastasis, ischemia-reperfusion injury, hematopoietic progenitor proliferation, apoptosis, wound healing, blood coagulation, extracellular matrix deposition, vasopermeability, and erythema. Several chemokine subfamily members also exert potent proangiogenic effects (e.g., ELR-bearing CXC ligands) and antiangiogenic effects (e.g., non–ELR-bearing CXC ligands) *in vivo*, which may differentially promote and regulate wound repair, inflammation, and tumor cell growth. In addition, chemokine receptors serve as coreceptors for the binding, fusion, and entry of viruses, including cytomegalovirus, human herpesviruses, and human immunodeficiency viruses 1 and 2. This interaction is highly receptor-, cell-, and viral strain–specific. Moreover, muta-

TABLE 37-3. C AND CX$_3$C CHEMOKINE NOMENCLATURE

Systematic Name	Human Ligand	Mouse Ligand	Rat Ligand	Receptor(s)
XCL1	LTN, SCM-1α, ATAC	LTN	Unknown	XCR-1
XCL2	SCM-1β	Unknown	Unknown	XCR-1
CX$_3$CL1	FKN, neurotactin	FKN	FKN	CX$_3$CR-1

Adapted from Homey B, Zlotnik A. Chemokines in allergy. *Curr Opin Immunol* 1999;11(6):626–634.

tions in these receptors can result in host resistance to human and simian immunodeficiency virus infections and affect the progression of the disease course. The future challenge in the study of chemokines is to further the understanding of their roles in the pathogenesis of disease and their potential as targets for therapy. The reviews in references 1 through 9 have been used in preparing this summary of the biologic and molecular properties of chemokines and their receptors.

This chapter presents a highly detailed and comprehensive database of all of the known molecular, biochemical, and biologic properties of human, rodent, and viral chemokines and their receptors. A detailed listing of alternative names, similar proteins, tissue and cellular distribution, regulators of expression, pathologic associations, genomic resources and descriptions, mutations, and knockout/transgenic phenotypes is also provided for each ligand and receptor. Many of the chemokines (L) and their receptors (R) have recently been reassigned a new designation based on their association with each of the ligand subfamilies. The new CXCL, CCL, XCL, and CX3CL designations along with an assigned numerical suffix are currently used to standardize chemokines, given the many alternative names associated with each chemokine ligand. Similarly, new CXCR, CCR, XCR, and CX_3CR designations, along with assigned numerical suffixes, are now used for all chemokine receptor subfamily members. All CXCR, CCR, XCR, and CX_3CR database entries follow the order in which they appear in Tables 37-1 through 37-3. These entries are followed by entries for the Duffy receptor, orphan chemokine receptors, viral chemokines, and viral chemokine receptors. The database provides complete and comprehensive information on this relatively new cytokine subfamily and should be a valuable resource to researchers in many different areas of study, including oncology and hematology.

ABBREVIATIONS USED IN THIS CHAPTER

3D	Three-dimensional		LDL	Low-density lipoprotein
ABCD	Activated B and dendritic cell–derived protein		LEC	Liver-expressed chemokine
Act	Activation gene		LIX	Lipopolysaccharide-induced CXC chemokine
AIDS	Acquired immunodeficiency syndrome		LKN	Leukotactin
AMAC	Alternative macrophage activation-associated chemokine		LMC	Lymphocyte and monocyte chemoattractant
ATAC	Activation-induced, T-cell–derived, and chemokine-related		LN	Lymph node
BCA	B-cell–attracting chemokine		LPL	Lamina propria lymphocyte
BLC	B-lymphocyte chemoattractant		LPS	Lipopolysaccharide
BM	Bone marrow		LTC4	Leukotriene C4
BRAK	Breast and kidney cell chemokine		LTN	Lymphotactin
CCL	CC chemokine		m	Mouse
CCR	CC chemokine receptor		Mφ	Macrophage
CCRL	Chemokine (CC motif) receptor–like		MALP	Mycoplasma macrophage-activating lipopeptide
CINC	Cytokine-induced neutrophil chemotactic factor		MAPK	Mitogen-activated protein kinase
CK	Chemokine		MCAF	Monocyte chemotactic and activating factor
CKR	Chemokine receptor		MCP	Monocyte chemotactic protein
CLA	Cutaneous lymphocyte antigen		MDC	Macrophage-derived chemokine
CMKBR	Chemokine β receptor–like		MDNCF	Monocyte-derived neutrophil chemotactic factor
CMV	Cytomegalovirus		MGSA	Melanoma growth-stimulatory activity
conA	Concanavalin A		Mig	Monokine induced by interferon-γ
CREB	Cyclic AMP responsive element-binding protein		MIP	Macrophage inflammatory protein
crg	Cytokine-responsive gene		MPIF	Myeloid progenitor inhibitory factor
CTACK	Cutaneous T-cell–attracting chemokine		MRP	Macrophage inflammatory protein–related protein
CTL	Cytotoxic C lymphocyte		MS	Multiple sclerosis
CXC	CXC chemokine		N/A	Not applicable
CXCR	CXC chemokine receptor		NAP	Neutrophil-activating peptide
CX$_3$CL	CX$_3$C chemokine		NCC	New CC chemokine
CX$_3$CR	CX$_3$C chemokine receptor		NF-κB	Nuclear factor-κB
DARC	Duffy antigen receptor for chemokines		NK	Natural killer
DC	Dendritic cell		ORF	Open reading frame
DC-CK	Dendritic cell chemokine		PARC	Pulmonary and activation-regulated chemokine
dsRNA	Double-stranded RNA		PBMC	Peripheral blood mononuclear cell
DTH	Delayed-type hypersensitivity		PBP	Platelet basic protein
EAE	Experimental allergic encephalomyelitis		PBSF	Pre–B-cell growth–stimulating factor
EC	Endothelial cell		PF	Platelet factor
ELC	Epstein-Barr virus–induced gene-1 ligand chemokine		PGE$_2$	Prostaglandin E$_2$
ELR	Glutamic acid-leucine-arginine		PHA	Phytohemagglutinin
ENA	Epithelial neutrophil-activating peptide		PI3K	Phosphoinositide 3 kinase
EOT	Eotaxin		PKB	Protein kinase B
FIC	Fibroblast-induced cytokine		PMA	Phorbol myristate acetate
FKN	Fractalkine		PPBP	Pro-platelet basic protein
fMLP	N-formyl-methionyl-leucyl-phenylalanine		r	Rat
GCP	Granulocyte chemotactic protein		RANTES	Regulated on activation, normal T expressed and secreted
GM-CSF	Granulocyte-macrophage colony-stimulating factor		SCM	Single cysteine motif
GPCR	G protein–coupled receptor		SCY	Small inducible cytokine subfamily
GRK	G protein receptor kinase		SDF	Stromal cell–derived factor
GRO	Growth-related oncogene		SEB	Staphylococcal enterotoxin B
h	Human		SLC	Secondary lymphoid-tissue chemokine
HCC	Hemofiltrate CC chemokine		SNP	Single nucleotide polymorphism
HEV	High endothelial venule		STAT	Signal transduction- and transcription-activating factor
HHV	Human herpesvirus		STCP	Stimulated T-cell chemotactic protein-1
HIV	Human immunodeficiency virus		TARC	Thymus and activation-regulated chemokine
HUVEC	Human umbilical vein endothelial cells		TCA	T-cell activation
ICAM-1	Intracellular adhesion molecule-1		TECK	Thymus-expressed chemokine
IEL	Intraepithelial lymphocyte		TG	Thromboglobulin
IFN	Interferon		TGF	Transforming growth factor
Ig	Immunoglobulin		TIL	Tumor infiltrating lymphocyte
IL	Interleukin		TNF	Tumor necrosis factor
IP	Interferon-γ inducible protein		TSST-1	Toxic shock syndrome toxin-1
I-TAC	Human interferon–inducible T-cell α chemoattractant		TYMSTR	T-lymphocyte–expressed seven-transmembrane domain receptor
Jak	Janus kinase		v	Virus
K_d	Dissociation constant		VCAM-1	Vascular cell adhesion molecule-1
kbp	Thousand base pairs		VEGF	Vascular endothelial growth factor
KC	Keratinocyte-derived chemokine		XCL	C chemokine
KSHV	Kaposi's sarcoma–associated herpesvirus		XCR	XC chemokine receptor
LARC	Liver and activation-regulated chemokine			

CC CHEMOKINES

I-309

Systematic name	CCL1.
Other names	CCR8 ligand, P500 (m), SIS-ε, SCYA1, TCA-3 (m).
Similar proteins	m I-309 (42%), hMIP-1δ (33%).[10]
Genbank source	NP_002972 (h), NP_035459 (m).
Amino acids in precursor protein	96 (h), 92 (m).
Size of mature protein (Kd)	8.5 (h).
Amino acids in mature protein	73 (h),[11] 69 (m).[12]
Stable form(s)	Monomer (h).[13]
Glycosylation sites	1 N (h, m).
Disulfide bonds	2 (h, m).
3D structure	Not reported.
Mature protein variants	Two variants, TCA-3 and P500/SIS-ε, are produced by alternate splicing (m).[14]
Tissue and cellular expression	Specific cell types include activated mast cells,[15] activated monocytes,[16] NK cells, and activated T cells.[11,12]
Regulation of expression	
Up	Anti-Fc receptor I (mast cells[15]), conA (T cells[12]), IgG (monocytes[16]), IL-1α (monocytes[16]), IL-1β (monocytes[16]), LPS (monocytes[16]).
Down	Not reported.
Biologic activities	
In vitro	Binds CCR8 (K_d = 0.5–1.2 nmol/L); chemoattractant for monocytes,[17] neutrophils (m),[18] CCR8–transfected cells,[19] mesangial cells,[20] and smooth muscle cells[21]; inhibits cellular infectivity by T-cell–trophic, M-trophic, dual-trophic strains of HIV[22]; induces intracellular Ca^{2+} mobilization in CCR8–transfected cells[22,23]; prevents glucocorticoid-induced apoptosis in thymic lymphoma cells[24]; stimulates the production of nitric oxide from neutrophils and Mφs, stimulates exocytosis of lysozyme and elastase, stimulates production of superoxide and hydrogen peroxide from neutrophils and Mφs.[25]
In vivo	Chemoattractant for neutrophils and monocytes (m).[18]
Pathologic association(s)	DTH,[26] EAE/MS,[27] acute tubulointerstitial nephritis.[28]
Genbank source (gene)	M57506 (h), X52401 (m).
Gene coding region (kbp)	3.7 (h), 4.2 (m).
Chromosomal location	17q11.2[29] (h), 11:47.32 cM (m).
Exons	3 (h, m).[12]
Introns	2 (h, m).[12]
Natural mutations/polymorphisms	EAE.[30]
Genbank source (RNA)	NM_002981 (h), NM_011329 (m).
Size of RNA (kbp)	0.5 (h, m).
RNA splice variants	2 (m).

CC CHEMOKINES

Monocyte Chemotactic Protein-1 (MCP-1)

Systematic name	CCL2.
Other names	D1Kyo2, HC11, glioma-derived chemotactic factor-2, JE, lymphocyte-derived chemotactic factor, MCAF, monocyte secretory protein JE (m), mouse competence gene JE, platelet-derived growth factor-inducible gene, SCYA2, small inducible gene JE,[31] smooth muscle cell–derived chemotactic factor, SP6, TSG8, tumor-derived chemotactic factor.
Similar proteins	mJE (55%), hMCP-2 (62%), hMCP-3 (71%), hMCP-4 (61%), hEOT-1 (66%), hMIP-1α (37%), hMIP-1β (37%), hDC-CK-1 (33%),[32] hMIP-1δ (32%), hHCC-1 (32%), hI-309 (32%).
Genbank source	NP_002973 (h), NP_035463 (m), P14844 (r).
Amino acids in precursor protein	99 (h), 148 (m, r).[31,33]
Size of mature protein (Kd)	8.7–13.0 (h), 20–25 (m, r).[34,35]
Amino acids in mature protein	76 (h), 125 (m, r).
Stable form(s)	Monomer/dimer[13,36] (h).
Glycosylation sites	3 N (h, m).[37]
Disulfide bonds	2 (h, m, r).
3D structure	Three antiparallel β sheets, COOH terminal α helix.[38]
Mature protein variants	Several different forms differing in glycosylation state.[37] Other forms generated by amino-terminal processing by CD26/dipeptidyl-peptidase IV.[39]
Tissue and cellular expression	Expressed at a low level in normal tissues. Relatively high levels are found in breast milk.[40] Specific cell types include B cells, articular chondrocytes, ECs, pulmonary type-2–like epithelial cells, eosinophils,[41] fibroblasts, glioblastoma cells, mast cells, Mφs, monocytes, mesangial cells, osteoblastic cells, ovarian carcinoma cells, smooth muscle cells.
Regulation of expression	
Up	C5a (eosinophils[41]); conA (PBMCs[42]); fMLP (eosinophils[41]); dsRNA (PBMCs[42]); HIV/Tat (astrocytes[43]); IFN-β (PBMCs[42]); IL-1β (astrocytes,[44] glial cells,[44] HUVECs,[45] keratinocytes,[46] PBMCs[42]); IL-4 (ECs[47]); IL-9 (lung ECs[48]); LPS (astrocytes,[44] DCs,[49] glial cells[44]); lysophosphatidylcholine (ECs[50]); macrophage colony-stimulating factor (ECs[51]); MALP-2 (Mφs[52]); oxidized LDL (ECs,[53] HUVECs[45]); LPS (PBMCs[42]); platelet-derived growth factor (fibroblasts[54]); SEB (PBMCs[55]); shear stress (ECs[56]); TNF-α (astrocytes,[57] glial cells[44]), ECs[58]); TSST-1 (PBMCs[55]).
Down	Glucocorticoids (ECs[59]), nitric oxide (ECs[60]).
Biologic activities	
In vitro	Binds to CCR2B (K_d = 1–2 nmol/L)[61] and CCR10 (K_d = 0.4–16 nmol/L)[62]; chemoattractant for basophils,[63] B cells,[1] DCs,[34] monocytes,[64] NK cells,[65] and activated T cells[66,67]; induces basophil and mast cell release of histamine and LTC4[63,68,69]; induces synthesis of IL-4 by basophils[63]; induces recruitment of β-arrestin, GRK2, and GRK3 to CCR2B and subsequent phosphorylation and desensitization of CCR2B[70,71]; stimulates the release of arachidonic acid from monocytes[72]; stimulates release of *N*-acetyl-β-D-glucosaminidase from monocytes[64]; induces adhesion of monocytes to ECs under flow conditions[73]; induces tissue factor production in EC cells[74]; acts as costimulator during T-cell activation[75]; up-regulates CD11b/CD18 and CD11c/CD18 on monocytes; induces intracellular Ca^{2+} mobilization in monocytes[76]; induces respiratory burst in monocytes[76]; augments tumoricidal activity of monocytes[77]; induces T cells to adopt a T_H2-like phenotype[78]; blocks entry of M-tropic strains of HIV-1 into DCs[79]; enhances CTL-mediated cytolysis of target cells.[1]
In vivo	Chemoattractant for monocytes[80] and T cells[67]; anorexic[81]; angiogenic[82]; augments monocyte antitumor activity; MCP-1–overexpressing transgenic mice were more susceptible to infection with several pathogens[83]; MCP-1 (–/–) mice exhibit impaired monocytes recruitment to thioglycollate[84] and DTH lesions, reduced formation of lung granulomas in response to *Schistosoma mansoni* egg antigen,[84] impaired production of IL-4, IL-5, and IFN-γ.[84] MCP-1 (–/–) mice were resistant to atherosclerosis in two models, (LDL) receptor-deficient mice fed a high cholesterol diet[85] and transgenic mice overexpressing human apolipoprotein B.[86]

(continued)

CC CHEMOKINES

Monocyte Chemotactic Protein-1 (MCP-1) (*Continued*)

Pathologic association(s)	Acute tubulointerstitial nephritis,[28] adult respiratory distress syndrome, alcohol-induced hepatitis,[87] aging,[88] asthma, atherosclerosis,[89] breast cancer,[90] cervical cancer,[91,92] contact dermatitis, cystic fibrosis, endometriosis,[93] glomerulonephritis,[94] Guillain-Barré syndrome/autoimmune neuritis,[95] HIV/AIDS,[96] leishmaniasis,[97,98] lichen planus,[99] myocardial infarction,[100] ovarian cancer,[101,102] pulmonary fibrosis,[103] pulmonary granulomatosis, psoriasis, renal ischemia, reperfusion injury, rheumatoid arthritis, sepsis,[104] sarcoidosis, spinal cord injury,[105] systemic sclerosis,[103] transplant rejection, ulcerative colitis,[106] uveoretinitis, wound healing.[107]
Genbank source (gene)	D26087 (h), M19681 (m), AF079313 (r).
Gene coding region (kbp)	3.2 (h), 2.4 (m), 3.6 (r).
Chromosomal location	17q11.2-q12 (h), 11:46.5 cM[31] (m), 10 (r).
Exons	3 (h, m).[37]
Introns	2 (h, m).[37]
Natural mutations/polymorphisms	Two SNPs in human MCP-1 promoter region, MCP-1-2518 G/A and -2076 A/T.[108] Cells from individuals with MCP-1 -2518 G secrete more MCP-1 than those with MCP-1-2518. In the mouse a polymorphism in the MCP-1 gene was predictive of susceptibility to EAE/MS.[30] Numerous SNPs in mouse gene[31] but no linkage with pathology has been established.
Genbank source (RNA)	NM_002982 (h), NM_011333 (m), M57441 (r).
Size of RNA (kbp)	0.7 (h), 0.5 (m), 0.6 (r).
RNA splice variants	Not reported.

CC CHEMOKINES

Macrophage Inflammatory Protein-1α (MIP-1α)

Systematic name	CCL3.
Other names	BB-10010, CCL3L1, heparin-binding chemotaxis protein, G_0 switch19 (G0S19-1), G0S19-2, L2G25B,[109] LD78α,[110] LD78β,[110] MIP-1αP, MIP-1αS, pAT464.1, pAT464.2, SCYA3, SCYA3L1, SIS-α, SIS-β, stem cell inhibitor,[111] T-cell–secreted protein, TCA-A, TY-5 (m).
Similar proteins	hMIP-1δ (75%), hDC-CK-1 (61%),[32] hMIP-1β (60%), hMPIF (51%),[112] hHCC-1 (46%), hEOT-1 (33%), hMDC (31%).
Genbank source	NP_002974 (h), NP_035467 (m), AAA80608 (r).
Amino acids in precursor protein	92 (h, m, r).[113]
Size of mature protein (Kd)	7.5 (h, m, r).
Amino acids in mature protein	66 (h), 69 (m, r).
Stable form(s)	Monomer/dimer/tetramer.[114]
Glycosylation sites	0 N (h, m, r).
Disulfide bonds	2 (h, m, r).
3D structure	Three antiparallel β sheets, COOH terminal α helix.[114]
Mature protein variants	Two forms, LD78α and LD78β (h),[110,115] arise from transcription from two different loci. In addition, BB-10010 is a genetically engineered version (Asp26Ala) of MIP-1α that has been developed for clinical trials.
Tissue and cellular expression	Highly expressed in lung, pancreas, and spleen. Expressed at low level in breast milk.[116] Specific cell types include chondrocytes,[117] Mϕs, monocytes, neutrophils,[110] and T cells.[118]
Regulation of expression	
Up	β-amyloid (monocytes[119]), IL-1β (astrocytes,[120] microglia[44]), isopentenyl pyrophosphate (γ/δ T cells[121]), LPS (astrocytes,[44] microglia,[44] neutrophils[118]), MALP-2 (Mϕs[52]), PHA (PBMCs, T cells[118]), TNF-α (astrocytes,[44] microglia[44]), TSST-1 (PBMCs[55]), SEB (PBMCs[55]).
Down	IFN-γ (activated neutrophils[122]), IL-10 (neutrophils[118]), IL-13 (Mϕs,[123] monocytes[123]).
Biologic activities	
In vitro	Binds CCR1 (K_d = 3.2–4.0 nmol/L) CCR5 (K_d = 0.4 nmol/L), CCR10 (K_d = 0.1–64 nmol/L),[124,125] and heparin sulfate[126]; chemoattractant for astrocytes,[127] basophils,[128] B cells,[129] blood-derived DCs,[130] eosinophils,[131] monocytes,[132] neutrophils (r),[133] NK cells,[65] activated T cells (CD8+ > CD4+)[134]; induces intracellular Ca^{2+} mobilization in blood-derived DCs,[130] eosinophils, monocytes, neutrophils, vascular smooth muscle cells,[89] and T cells; stimulates release of N-acetyl-β-D-glucosaminidase from monocytes[64]; activates STAT1 and STAT3 in T cells[135]; acts as costimulator during T-cell activation[75]; induces basophil and mast cell release of histamine[68,69]; inhibits hemopoietic progenitor proliferation and colony formation[136]; stimulates[137] or inhibits[138] adenyl cyclase; enhances osteoclast differentiation[139]; stimulates the release of arachidonic acid from monocytes[72]; LD78β form inhibits the cellular entry of HIV strains through CCR5[115,140]; inhibits erythroid progenitor cell proliferation[141]; enhances CTL-mediated cytolysis of target cells.[1]
In vivo	Chemoattractant for neutrophils,[133,142] monocytes, and T cells[143]; inhibits hemopoietic progenitor proliferation[136]; pyrogenic[144]; decreases neutropenia in patients with advanced breast cancer when administered concomitantly with 5-fluorouracil, doxorubicin hydrochloride (Adriamycin), and cyclophosphamide chemotherapy[145]; MIP-1α (–/–) mice exhibit decreased resistance to coxsackievirus–induced cardiopulmonary inflammation[146]; decreases influenza-induced lung inflammation[146]; decreases development of herpes virus–induced corneal stromal keratitis[147]; decreases leukocyte recruitment and cryptococcal clearance from the brain.
Pathologic association(s)	Alcohol-induced hepatitis,[87] atherosclerosis,[89,148] atopic dermatitis,[149] EAE/MS,[27,150] glomerulonephritis,[94] Guillain-Barré syndrome/autoimmune neuritis,[95] hemophagocytic syndrome,[151] hepatocellular carcinoma,[152] HIV/AIDS dementia,[153] leishmaniasis,[97] lichen planus,[99] osteoarthritis,[117] ovarian carcinoma,[101] psoriasis, pulmonary fibrosis,[103] respiratory distress syndrome, rheumatoid arthritis,[117,154] sarcoidosis,[155] systemic sclerosis,[103] upper respiratory tract infection.[156]

(continued)

CC CHEMOKINES

Macrophage Inflammatory Protein-1α (MIP-1α) (*Continued*)

Genbank source (gene)	D90144 (h), M73061 (m).
Gene coding region (kbp)	3.2 (h), 3.6 (m).
Chromosomal location	17q21.1-q21.3 (h),[157] 11:47.59 cM (m).[158]
Exons	3 (h, m).[157,159]
Introns	2 (h, m).[157,159]
Natural mutations/polymorphisms	One SNP in promoter region of LD78A.[160] A human pseudogene, LD78γ, has also been described.[110]
Genbank source (RNA)	NM_002983 (h), NM_011337 (m), U22414 (r).
Size of RNA (kbp)	0.8 (h, m, r).
RNA splice variants	Not reported.

CC CHEMOKINES

Macrophage Inflammatory Protein-1β (MIP-1β)

Systematic name	CCL4.
Other names	AT744.1, AT744.2, Act-2, pAT744 gene product, G-26, H400, HC21, lymphocyte activation gene-1, MAD-5, SCYA4, SIS-γ.
Similar proteins	mMIP-1β (76%), rMIP-1β (77%), hMIP-1α (60%), hMPIF (41%),[161] hHCC-1 (46%), hDC-CK-1 (42%),[32] hEOT-1 (37%),[162] hMDC (34%).
Genbank source	NP_002984 (h), P14097 (m), P50230 (r).
Amino acids in precursor protein	92 (h, m, r).
Size of mature protein (Kd)	7.8 (h).
Amino acids in mature protein	69 (h, m, r).
Stable form(s)	Monomer/dimer/tetramer.[114]
Glycosylation sites	0 N (h, m, r).
Disulfide bonds	2 (h, m, r).
3D structure	Three antiparallel β sheets, COOH terminal α helix.[163]
Mature protein variants	Not reported.
Tissue and cellular expression	Specific cell types include activated astrocytes, chondrocytes,[117] activated microglia, neutrophils, activated T cells, and thymocytes.
Regulation of expression	
Up	EOT-1 (thymocytes[164]), IL-1β (astrocytes,[120] microglia[44]), isopentenyl pyrophosphate (γ/δ T cells[121]), LPS (astrocytes,[44] microglia,[44] LPS (microglia[118]), PHA (T cells), SEB (PBMCs[55]), TNF-α (astrocytes,[44] microglia[44]), TSST-1 (PBMCs[55]).
Down	IL-10 (neutrophils[118]).
Biologic activities	
In vitro	Binds CCR5 (K_d = 0.2–0.4 nmol/L), CCR8, and heparin sulfate[126]; induces phosphorylation/activation of RAFTK/pyk2 in T cells[165]; chemoattractant for DCs,[166] NK cells,[167] activated T cells (CD4+ > CD8+),[134] and CCR5–transfected cells[168]; stimulates release of N-acetyl-β-D-glucosaminidase from monocytes[64]; acts as costimulator during T-cell activation[75]; induces basophil release of histamine[68]; induces intracellular Ca^{2+} mobilization in DCs,[166] monocytes, and T cells; blocks entry of M-tropic strains of HIV-1 into DCs[79]; enhances CTL-mediated cytolysis of target cells.[1]
In vivo	Chemoattractant for monocytes, neutrophils, and T cells[143]; pyrogenic.[144]
Pathologic association(s)	EAE/MS,[27] hepatocellular carcinoma,[152] HIV/AIDS dementia,[153] Kawasaki's disease,[169] osteoarthritis,[117] rheumatoid arthritis,[117] systemic sclerosis.[103]
Genbank source (gene)	X62502 (m).
Gene coding region (kbp)	3.0 (m).
Chromosomal location	17q21.1 (h), 11:47.59 cM (m).
Exons	3 (h).
Introns	2 (h).
Natural mutations/polymorphisms	Not reported.
Genbank source (RNA)	NM_002984 (h), M23503 (m), U06434 (r).
Size of RNA (kbp)	0.7 (h), 0.3 (r).
RNA splice variants	Not reported.

CC CHEMOKINES

Regulated on Activation, Normal T Expressed and Secreted (RANTES)

Systematic name	CCL5.
Other names	D17S136E, SCYA5, SIS-δ (r), T-cell–specific protein p288.
Similar proteins	mRANTES (80%), rRANTES (80%), hDC-CK-1 (32%),[32] hLEC (37%), hEOT-1 (34%),[162] hEOT-2 (32%),[170] hMDC (31%), hMPIF-1 (31%), hMIP-3β (30%).
Genbank source	NP_002976 (h), A46539 (m), P50231 (r).
Amino acids in precursor protein	91 (h, m), 92 (r).
Size of mature protein (Kd)	8.0 (h).[171]
Amino acids in mature protein	68 (h, m, r).
Stable form(s)	Monomer/dimer/tetramer.[114]
Glycosylation sites	0 N (h, m, r).
Disulfide bonds	2 (h, m, r).
3D structure	Three antiparallel β sheets, COOH terminal α helix.[172]
Mature protein variants	Other forms generated by amino-terminal processing by CD26/dipeptidyl-peptidase IV.[173]
Tissue and cellular expression	Relatively high levels are found in breast milk.[40] Specific cell types include astrocytes,[174] activated ECs,[171] activated epithelial cells,[171] activated fibroblasts,[171] megakaryocytes,[175] mesangial cells, activated monocytes,[171] platelets,[176] activated T cells.[171]
Regulation of expression	
Up	EOT-1 (thymocytes[164]), IFN-γ (ECs[177]), IL-1β (astrocytes[174]), LPS (DCs[49]), IFN-γ + TNF-α (astrocytes,[174] ECs,[171] fibroblasts,[171,174] renal epithelial cells,[171] mesangial cells,[171] smooth muscle cells[178]).
Down	Glucocorticoids (activated ECs[179,180]), IL-4 (IFN-γ– and TNF-α–stimulated EC cells,[171] IL-1β–stimulated fibroblasts,[171] TNF-α–stimulated fibroblasts[171]), IL-13 (IFN-γ– and TNF-α–stimulated EC cells[171]).
Biologic activities	
In vitro	Binds to CCR1 (K_d = 7–8 nmol/L), CCR3 (K_d = 3 nmol/L), CCR4, CCR5, US28,[181] and heparin sulfate[126]; chemoattractant for basophils,[128] B cells,[1] DCs,[166] eosinophils,[131] mast cells,[182] monocytes,[64,183] NK cells[65]; induces intracellular Ca^{2+} mobilization in DCs[166]; activates Akt/PKB in monocytes[184]; stimulates release of *N*-acetyl-β-D-glucosaminidase from monocytes[64]; induces basophil release of histamine[68]; recruits pleckstrin and PI3Kγ to the cell membrane in NK cells[185]; induces phosphorylation/activation of RAFTK/pyk2 in T cells[165,186]; induces activation and assembly of focal adhesion complexes[186]; stimulates phosphorylation/activation of ZAP-70[186]; recruits GRK2 and GRK3 to CCR5[187]; induces phosphorylation and desensitization of CCR5[187]; activates STAT1 and STAT3 in T cells[135]; acts as costimulator during T-cell activation[75]; blocks entry of M-tropic strains of HIV-1 into DCs[79]; enhances CTL-mediated cytolysis of target cells.[1]
In vivo	Chemoattractant for eosinophils,[188] mast cells,[189] monocytes,[188] and T cells[143]; anorexic[81]; augments T_H1 immune responses[190]; inhibits IL-4 production.[189]
Pathologic association(s)	Asthma,[8,191] arthritis,[192] atherosclerosis,[89,148,193] atopic dermatitis,[194] autoimmune diabetes,[195] endometriosis,[196] glomerular nephritis,[197] Kawasaki's disease,[169] lichen planus,[99] EAE/MS,[27,198] sarcoidosis,[155] T_H1-mediated immune responses,[190] transplant rejection,[199] upper respiratory tract infection.[156]
Genbank source (gene)	AB23654 (h), U02298 (m).
Gene coding region (kbp)	7.3 (h),[200] 4.5 (m).[201]
Chromosomal location	17q1.2-q12,[202] 11:47 cM (m).
Exons	3 (h, m).[200,201]
Introns	2 (h, m).[200,201]
Natural mutations/polymorphisms	Three SNPs identified in promoter region. RANTES-28G promoter SNP is associated with higher rate of RANTES transcription and a reduced HIV progression rate[203]; RANTES-401A promoter SNP is associated with higher rate of atopic dermatitis.[204]
Genbank source (RNA)	NM_002985 (h), M77747 (m), U06436 (r).
Size of RNA (kbp)	1.2 (h) 0.6 (m, r).[171]
RNA splice variants	Not reported.

CC CHEMOKINES

C10

Systematic name	CCL6.
Other names	MRP-1,[205] SCYA6.
Similar proteins	hMIP-1δ.
Genbank source	AAA37329 (m).
Amino acids in precursor protein	116 (m).
Size of mature protein (Kd)	10.7 (m).
Amino acids in mature protein	95 (m).
Stable form(s)	Not reported.
Glycosylation sites	0 N (m).
Disulfide bonds	3 (m).
3D structure	Not reported.
Mature protein variants	Not reported.
Tissue and cellular expression	Highly expressed in uterus.[206] Specific cell types include eosinophils,[207] activated Mφs,[207] and activated neutrophils.
Regulation of expression	
Up	IL-3 (Mφs,[208] microglia,[208] neutrophils[208]), IL-4 (Mφs,[208] neutrophils[208]), GM-CSF (Mφs,[208] neutrophils[208]).
Down	Not reported.
Biologic activities	
In vitro	Binds to unknown receptor; chemoattractant for B cells, monocytes, NK cells, and T cells[208,209]; inhibits megakaryocyte colony formation.[210]
In vivo	Chemoattractant for monocytes[209] and T cells (CD4$^+$ > CD8$^+$).[209]
Pathologic association(s)	Chronic inflammation,[207] EAE/MS,[209] experimental allergic airway inflammation.[211]
Genbank source (gene)	L11237 (m).
Gene coding region (kbp)	5.1 (m).
Chromosomal location	11:47.51 cM (m).[212]
Exons	4 (m).[212]
Introns	3 (m).[212]
Natural mutations/polymorphisms	Several SNPs,[30] currently no reported links to known pathologies.
Genbank source (RNA)	M58004 (m).
Size of RNA (kbp)	1.3 (m).
RNA splice variants	Not reported.

CC CHEMOKINES

Monocyte Chemotactic Protein-3 (MCP-3)

Systematic name	CCL7.
Other names	Chemotactic protein-3 (r), FIC (m), MARC (m), NC28 (m),[213] SCYA7.
Similar proteins	mMCP-3 (59%), hMCP-1 (71%), hMCP-4 (59%), hMCP-2 (58%), hEOT-1 (65%), hEOT-2 (40%), hMPIF-1 (37%), hDC-CK-1 (34%), hEOT-3 (34%), hMDC (31%), hSLC (30%).
Genbank source	CAB59723 (h), AAB30997 (m), AAF24172 (r).
Amino acids in precursor protein	109 (h),[214] 97 (m, r).
Size of mature protein (Kd)	11/13/17/18 (h),[37] 8.5 (m).[37]
Amino acids in mature protein	76 (h), 74 (m, r).
Stable form(s)	Monomer/dimer (h).[36,215]
Glycosylation sites	3 N (h, m).[37]
Disulfide bonds	2 (h, m, r).
3D structure	Three antiparallel β sheets, COOH terminal α helix, α/β sandwich.[215]
Mature protein variants	Several forms differing in glycosylation state have been isolated.[37]
Tissue and cellular expression	Specific cell types include monocytes,[213] platelets,[176] and tumor cells.[216]
Regulation of expression	
Up	IFN-γ (ECs,[217] fibroblasts,[218] monocytes[217]), IL-1β (ECs,[217] monocytes[217]), IL-4 (fibroblasts[218]), IL-9 (ECs[48]), LPS (ECs[217]), PHA (PBMCs[213]), TNF-α (ECs,[217] fibroblasts,[218] monocytes[217]).
Down	IL-13 (PBMCs[213]).
Biologic activities	
In vitro	Binds CCR1 (K_d = 0.7–8 nmol/L),[219] CCR2B (K_d = 7 nmol/L),[219] CCR3 (K_d = 3 nmol/L), CCR10 (K_d = 1 nmol/L),[125,220] and US28[181]; chemoattractant for basophils,[221] B cells,[1] DCs,[166] activated eosinophils,[222] monocytes,[64,216] activated NK cells,[223] and activated T cells[67]; stimulates release of *N*-acetyl-β-D-glucosaminidase from monocytes[64]; induces unprimed and IL-3 treated basophil release of histamine[221]; induces intracellular Ca^{2+} mobilization in DCs[166]; enhances CTL-mediated cytolysis of target cells.[1]
In vivo	Chemoattractant for monocytes[216] and T cells[67]; antitumor.[224]
Pathologic association(s)	Acute tubulointerstitial nephritis,[28] allergy,[225] atherosclerosis,[226] autoimmune diabetes,[195] chronic sinusitis,[227] EAE/MS,[27,228] restenosis,[226] stroke,[229] ulcerative colitis.[106]
Genbank source (gene)	X72309 (h), AF154245 (r).
Gene coding region (kbp)	2.9 (h), 2.4 (r).
Chromosomal location	17q11.2-q12 (h).[214]
Exons	3 (h).[37]
Introns	2 (h).[37]
Natural mutations/polymorphisms	Five SNPs, designated MCP-3*A1 through MCP-3*A5[214,230] (h).
Genbank source (RNA)	X72308 (h), S71251 (m).
Size of RNA (kbp)	1.1 (h), 0.8 (m).
RNA splice variants	Not reported.

CC CHEMOKINES

Monocyte Chemotactic Protein-2 (MCP-2)

Systematic name	CCL8
Other names	HC14 (m),[231] SCYA8.
Similar proteins	mMCP-5 (55%), hMCP-1 (62%), hMCP-3 (58%), hMCP-4 (56%), hEOT-1 (66%).
Genbank source	NP_005614 (h).
Amino acids in precursor protein	109 (h).
Size of mature protein (Kd)	9.0 (h).
Amino acids in mature protein	76 (h).
Stable form(s)	Monomer/homodimer (h).[36]
Glycosylation sites	1 N/0 O (h).[37]
Disulfide bonds	2 (h).
3D structure	Not reported.
Mature protein variants	At least two isoforms and other forms generated by processing by CD26/dipeptidyl-peptidase IV.[232]
Tissue and cellular expression	Highly expressed in colon, heart, lung, ovary, pancreas, peripheral blood, placenta, small intestine, skeletal muscle, spinal cord, and thymus.[233] Specific cell types include activated fibroblasts and tumor cells.[216]
Regulation of expression	
Up	IFN-γ (epithelial cells, fibroblasts,[234] osteosarcoma cells), IFN-γ + IL-1β (epithelial cells,[234] fibroblasts[234]), IL-1β (epithelial cells, fibroblasts,[235] osteosarcoma cells), dsRNA (fibroblasts[235]).
Down	Not reported.
Biologic activities	
In vitro	Binds CCR1 (K_d = 5 nmol/L),[236] CCR2B (K_d = 3 nmol/L),[236] CCR3, and CCR5 (K_d = 5 nmol/L)[168]; chemoattractant for basophils, DCs,[34] activated eosinophils, mast cells, monocytes,[64,216] activated NK cells,[223] activated T cells,[67] and CCR5–transfected cells[168]; stimulates release of *N*-acetyl-β-D-glucosaminidase from monocytes,[64] blocks entry of HIV into CCR5–transfected cells[168]; induces CCR5 internalization in CCR5–transfected cells.[168]
In vivo	Chemoattractant for monocytes[216] and T cells.[67]
Pathologic association(s)	EAE/MS,[228] sepsis.[104]
Genbank source (gene)	X99886 (h).
Gene coding region (kbp)	3.0 (h).
Chromosomal location	17q11.2 (h).[233]
Exons	3 (h).[37]
Introns	2 (h).[37]
Natural mutations/polymorphisms	Two SNPs in coding region designated MCP-246 Lys MCP-246 Glu.[232]
Genbank source (RNA)	NM_005623 (h).
Size of RNA (kbp)	1.0/1.5/2.4 (h).[233]
RNA splice variants	Not reported.

CC CHEMOKINES

Macrophage Inflammatory Protein-1γ (MIP-1γ)

Systematic name	CCL9/CCL10.
Other names	C10-like chemokine, CCF-18, MRP-2, MMRP2, SCYA9.
Similar proteins	mC10 (45%).
Genbank source	NP_035468 (m).
Amino acids in precursor protein	122 (m).
Size of mature protein (Kd)	11.6 (m).[205]
Amino acids in mature protein	101 (m).
Stable form(s)	Not reported.
Glycosylation sites	0 N (m).
Disulfide bonds	3 (m).
3D structure	Not reported.
Mature protein variants	Not reported.
Tissue and cellular expression	Expressed in most normal tissues. Found as a normal constituent in serum of healthy mice.[237] Specific cell types include DCs, Mφs, and myeloid cell lines.
Regulation of expression	
Up	Not reported.
Down	Not reported.
Biologic activities	
In vitro	Receptor unknown; chemoattractant for CD4+ and CD8+ T cells; induces intracellular Ca^{2+} mobilization in CD4+ and CD8+ T cells; inhibits hematopoietic progenitor cells proliferation.[205]
In vivo	Pyrogenic.[237]
Pathologic association(s)	Not reported.
Genbank source (gene)	Not reported.
Gene coding region (kbp)	Not reported.
Chromosomal location	11:47.0 cM (m).
Exons	Not reported.
Introns	Not reported.
Natural mutations/polymorphisms	Not reported.
Genbank source (RNA)	NM_011338 (m).
Size of RNA (kbp)	1.3 (m).
RNA splice variants	Not reported.

CC CHEMOKINES

Eotaxin-1 (EOT-1)

Systematic name	CCL11.
Other names	Eosinophil chemotactic protein, SCYA11.
Similar proteins	mEOT-1 (63%),[162] rEOT-1 (62%),[238] hMCP-1 (66%), hMCP-2 (66%), hMCP-3 (65%), hMCP-4 (63%), hEOT-2 (39%), hEOT-3 (37%), hSLC (32%), hMIP-1β (37%),[162] hRANTES (34%),[162] hMIP-1α (33%), hDC-CK-1 (33%).[32]
Genbank source	NP_002977 (h), NP_035460 (m), P97545 (r).
Amino acids in precursor protein	97 (h, m, r).[238,239]
Size of mature protein (Kd)	8.4 (h, m, r).
Amino acids in mature protein	72 (h), 74 (m, r).[238]
Stable form(s)	Monomer.[240]
Glycosylation sites	0 N/1 O (h, m, r).[241]
Disulfide bonds	2 (h, m, r).
3D structure	Three antiparallel β sheets, COOH terminal α helix.[240]
Mature protein variants	Three variants (h).[218]
Tissue and cellular expression	Highly expressed in colon and small intestine.[162,242] Specific cell types include ECs,[239] fibroblasts,[243] Mφs,[238] smooth muscle cells.[244]
Regulation of expression	
Up	C5a (eosinophils[245]), IFN-γ (ECs[239]), IL-1α (fibroblasts[243]), IL-1β (ECs,[246] smooth muscle cells[244]), IL-4 (ECs,[48] fibroblasts[218,247]), IL-9 (lung ECs[48]), IL-5 (eosinophils[248]), IL-18 (bronchial epithelial cells,[249] Mφs[249]), PMA (U937 cells[250]), TNF-α (ECs,[246] eosinophils,[248] fibroblasts,[243] Mφs,[246] smooth muscle cells,[244] U937 cells[250]).
Down	Glucocorticoids (ECs,[246] eosinophils[248]), IL-10 (activated smooth muscle cells[251]).
Biologic activities	
In vitro	Binds to CCR3 (K_d = 0.15–0.20 nmol/L); chemoattractant for basophils,[221,252] eosinophils,[253] T cells, and thymocytes[164]; activates MAPK p42/p44 through CCR3; blocks entry of M-tropic strains of HIV-1 into DCs[79]; induces IL-3–treated basophil release of histamine[221]; induces oxygen radical production from eosinophils[254]; induces intracellular Ca^{2+} mobilization in basophils,[252] eosinophils,[254] and thymocytes[164]; induces actin polymerization in eosinophils[254]; induces CD11b expression in eosinophils[254]; up-regulates the expression of ICAM-1 and VCAM-1 on ECs[255]; induces secretion of IL-8, MIP-1β, and RANTES from thymocytes.[164]
In vivo	Chemoattractant for eosinophils[256]; EOT-1 (–/–) mice exhibit a reduction in the basal and allergen-induced eosinophils.[257,258]
Pathologic association(s)	Asthma,[8,259–261] atopic dermatitis,[8,262] graft vasculopathy,[263] nephrotic syndrome,[264] chronic sinusitis.[265]
Genbank source (gene)	U46572 (h), U77462 (m).
Gene coding region (kbp)	2.7 (h).
Chromosomal location	17q2.1.1-q2.1.2 (h),[253] 11:47.0 cM (m).[239]
Exons	3 (h).[37]
Introns	2 (h).[37]
Natural mutations/polymorphisms	Numerous SNPs in 3' UTR.[266]
Genbank source (RNA)	NM_002986 (h), NM_011330 (m), Y08358 (r).
Size of RNA (kbp)	0.8/1.1 (h),[162,242] 1.0 (m), 1.0 (r).
RNA splice variants	Not reported.

CC CHEMOKINES

Monocyte Chemotactic Protein-5 (MCP-5)

Systematic name	CCL12.
Other names	MCP-1–related chemokine, SCYA12.
Similar proteins	hMCP-1 (66%).[267]
Genbank source	AAB50053 (m).
Amino acids in precursor protein	104 (m).
Size of mature protein (Kd)	9.3 (m).
Amino acids in mature protein	82 (m).
Stable form(s)	Monomer.
Glycosylation sites	0 N (m).[37]
Disulfide bonds	2 (m).
3D structure	Not reported.
Mature protein variants	Not reported.
Tissue and cellular expression	Highly expressed in lung, LNs, and thymus.[267] Specific cell types include activated Mϕs.[267]
Regulation of expression	
Up	IFN-γ (Mϕs[267]), LPS (Mϕs[267,268]).
Down	Not reported.
Biologic activities	
In vitro	Binds to CCR2B; chemoattractant for monocytes[267] and CCR2B–transfected cells[267]; induces intracellular Ca^{2+} mobilization in CCR2B–transfected cells.[267]
In vivo	Not reported.
Pathologic association(s)	Allergic inflammation,[269] autoimmune diabetes,[195] spinal cord injury.[105]
Genbank source (gene)	Not reported.
Gene coding region (kbp)	Not reported.
Chromosomal location	11:47.0 cM (m).[267]
Exons	Not reported.
Introns	Not reported.
Natural mutations/polymorphisms	Several SNPs that may be linked to EAE/MS.[30]
Genbank source (RNA)	U50712 (m).
Size of RNA (kbp)	0.5 (m).
RNA splice variants	Not reported.

CC CHEMOKINES

Monocyte Chemotactic Protein-4 (MCP-4)

Systematic name	CCL13.
Other names	CKβ-10, NCC-1, SCYA13, SCYL1.
Similar proteins	hEOT-1 (63%), hMCP-1 (61%), hMCP-3 (59%), hMCP-2 (56%), hEOT-3 (41%), hDC-CK-1 (32%).[32]
Genbank source	NP_005399 (h).
Amino acids in precursor protein	98 (h).
Size of mature protein (Kd)	8.6 (h).[37]
Amino acids in mature protein	75 (h).
Stable form(s)	Not reported.
Glycosylation sites	0 N/0 O (h).[37]
Disulfide bonds	2 (h).
3D structure	Not reported.
Mature protein variants	Not reported.
Tissue and cellular expression	Highly expressed in colon,[270] heart,[271] lung,[271] small intestine,[270,272] and thymus.[272] Specific cell types include monocyte-derived DCs,[273] activated fibroblasts, bronchial ECs, Mφs,[272] and smooth muscle cells.[272]
Regulation of expression	
Up	IFN-γ (fibroblasts[274]), IL-1α (fibroblasts[274]), IL-4 (fibroblasts[274]), serum (smooth muscle cells[272]), TNF-α (ECs,[275] epithelial cells,[275] fibroblasts[274]).
Down	Glucocorticoids (ECs[271]).
Biologic activities	
In vitro	Binds to CCR2B (K_d = 7 nmol/L),[272] and CCR3; chemoattractant for basophils,[221] DCs,[166] eosinophils,[271] monocytes,[276] CD4+ and CD8+ T cells[276]; stimulates the release of histamine and LTC4 from basophils[271]; induces intracellular Ca2+ mobilization in DCs,[166] monocytes,[272] and CCR2B–transfected cell lines[272,275]; blocks entry of M-tropic strains of HIV-1 into DCs.[79]
In vivo	Not reported.
Pathologic association(s)	Allergic sinusitis,[275] asthma,[260,277] atherosclerosis,[148,272] chronic sinusitis.[227]
Genbank source (gene)	AJ000979 (h).
Gene coding region (kbp)	3.2 (h).
Chromosomal location	17q11.2 (h).[29]
Exons	3 (h).[274]
Introns	2 (h).[274]
Natural mutations/polymorphisms	Not reported.
Genbank source (RNA)	NM_005408 (h).
Size of RNA (kbp)	0.9 (h).
RNA splice variants	Not reported.

CC CHEMOKINES

Hemofiltrate CC Chemokine-1 (HCC-1)

Systematic name	CCL14.
Other names	CC chemokine-2, CKβ-1, HCC-3, macrophage colony inhibition factor, NCC-2, SCYA14, SCYL2.
Similar proteins	hMIP-1α (46%), hMIP-1β (46%), hDC-CK-1 (40%), hMIP-1δ (39%),[10] hLEC (38%), hEOT-3 (38%), hMCP-1 (32%), MIP-1δ (32%).
Genbank source	NP_004157 (h).
Amino acids in precursor protein	93 (h).
Size of mature protein (Kd)	8.7 (h).[278]
Amino acids in mature protein	74 (h).
Stable form(s)	Not reported.
Glycosylation sites	0 N/0 O (h).
Disulfide bonds	2 (h).
3D structure	Not reported.
Mature protein variants	Not reported.
Tissue and cellular expression	Highly expressed in BM, gut, liver, heart muscle, skeletal muscle, and spleen.[278] Found in normal plasma (1–80 nmol/L).[278]
Regulation of expression	
Up	Not reported.
Down	Not reported.
Biologic activities	
In vitro	Binds CCR1 (K_d = 100 nmol/L)[138]; chemoattractant for DCs,[166] monocytes,[138] and CCR1-transfected cells[138]; induces the proliferation of CD34+ myeloid progenitor cells[278]; induces intracellular Ca^{2+} mobilization in DCs,[166] monocytes,[138] and CCR1-transfected cells[138]; inhibits adenyl cyclase in CCR1-transfected cells.[138]
In vivo	Not reported.
Pathologic association(s)	Not reported.
Genbank source (gene)	Z49269 (h).
Gene coding region (kbp)	4.0 (h).
Chromosomal location	17q11.2 (h).[279]
Exons	3 (h).[10]
Introns	2 (h).[10]
Natural mutations/polymorphisms	Not reported.
Genbank source (RNA)	NM_004166 (h).
Size of RNA (kbp)	0.9 (h).
RNA splice variants	Not reported.

CC CHEMOKINES

Macrophage Inflammatory Protein-1δ (MIP-1δ)

Systematic name	CCL15.
Other names	HCC-2,[10] HMRB-2β, MIP-5, LKN-1,[280] NCC-3,[29] SCYA15, SCYL3.
Similar proteins	hMPIF (73%), hHCC-1 (39%), hMIP-3α (77%), hMIP-1α (75%), hSLC (68%).[10]
Genbank source	NP_004158 (h).
Amino acids in precursor protein	113 (h).
Size of mature protein (Kd)	8.0/12.2 (h).[10]
Amino acids in mature protein	92 (h).
Stable form(s)	Monomer (h).[281]
Glycosylation sites	0 N/0 O (h).
Disulfide bonds	3 (h).[10]
3D structure	Three antiparallel β sheets, COOH terminal α helix.[281]
Mature protein variants	Not reported.
Tissue and cellular expression	Highly expressed in intestine, liver, and lung.[282] Specific cell types include B cells, monocyte-derived DCs, NK cells, monocytes, and T cells.[283]
Regulation of expression	
Up	Not reported.
Down	Not reported.
Biologic activities	
In vitro	Binds CCR1 (K_d = 3–4 nmol/L)[284] and CCR3 (K_d = 2.5 nmol/L)[282]; chemoattractant for immature DCs,[49,285] eosinophils,[10] monocytes,[282] neutrophils[10,282–284] and T cells[10,283]; stimulates the release of *N*-acetyl-β-D-glucosaminidase from monocytes[10]; induces intracellular Ca^{2+} mobilization in CCR1– and CCR3–transfected cells[283,286]; inhibits hemopoietic progenitor colony formation.[280]
In vivo	Not reported.
Pathologic association(s)	Not reported.
Genbank source (gene)	AF088219 (h).
Gene coding region (kbp)	4.0 (h).
Chromosomal location	17q11.2 (h).[29]
Exons	4 (h).[279]
Introns	3 (h).[279]
Natural mutations/polymorphisms	Not reported.
Genbank source (RNA)	NM_004167 (h).
Size of RNA (kbp)	1.0 (h).
RNA splice variants	2 (h).

CC CHEMOKINES

Liver-Expressed Chemokine (LEC)

Systematic name	CCL16.
Other names	HCC-4, IL-10–inducible chemokine, LCC-1 (m), LMC, NCC-4,[287] monotactin-1, SCYA16, SCYL4.
Similar proteins	hHCC-1 (38%), hRANTES (36%), hMIP-1β (35%), hMIP-1α [hLD78α (32%), hLD78β (33%)], hDC-CK-1 (31%), hEOT-1 (31%).
Genbank source	NP_004581 (h).
Amino acids in precursor protein	120 (h).
Size of mature protein (Kd)	11.0 (h).[286]
Amino acids in mature protein	100 (h).
Stable form(s)	Not reported.
Glycosylation sites	1 N (h).
Disulfide bonds	2 (h).
3D structure	Not reported.
Mature protein variants	Not reported.
Tissue and cellular expression	Highly expressed in adult and fetal liver.[287,288] Specific cell types include activated monocytes.[289]
Regulation of expression	
Up	IFN-γ (monocytes), IL-10 (monocytes[289]), LPS (monocytes).
Down	Not reported.
Biologic activities	
In vitro	Binds CCR1; chemoattractant for monocytes and lymphocytes[286]; inhibits proliferation of myeloid progenitors in colony-formation assays.[286]
In vivo	Not reported.
Pathologic association(s)	Not reported.
Genbank source (gene)	AF088219 (h).
Gene coding region (kbp)	5.0 (h).[290]
Chromosomal location	17q11.2 (h),[29] 11:47.0 cM (m).[290]
Exons	3 (h).[290]
Introns	2 (h).[290]
Natural mutations/polymorphisms	Not reported.
Genbank source (RNA)	NM_004590 (h); pseudogene is present in mouse.[290]
Size of RNA (kbp)	0.6 (h), 1.5 (h).[288]
RNA splice variants	2 (h).[287]

CC CHEMOKINES

Thymus- and Activation-Regulated Chemokine (TARC)

Systematic name	CCL17.
Other names	A-152E5.3, ABCD-2 (m),[291] dendrokine, SCYA17, T-cell–directed CC chemokine.
Similar proteins	mTARC (66%),[291] hMDC (32%), hDC-CK-1 (32%).[32]
Genbank source	NP_002978 (h), CAB45256 (m).
Amino acids in precursor protein	94 (h), 93 (m).
Size of mature protein (Kd)	8.0 (h), 7.9 (m).
Amino acids in mature protein	71 (h), 70 (m).[291]
Stable form(s)	Not reported.
Glycosylation sites	0 N (h, m).
Disulfide bonds	2 (h, m).
3D structure	Not reported.
Mature protein variants	Not reported.
Tissue and cellular expression	Constitutively expressed in thymus, and at lower levels in lung, colon, and small intestine. Specific cell types include activated B cells,[291] monocyte-derived DCs,[273,292] thymic DCs,[292] LN DCs,[292] ECs,[293] activated keratinocytes,[294] and Reed-Sternberg cells.[295]
Regulation of expression	
Up	Anti-CD40 (DCs[291]), anti-IgM (B cells[291]),GM-CSF (DCs[291]), LPS (DCs[292]), PHA (PBMCs), TNF-α (DCs[291]).
Down	Not reported.
Biologic activities	
In vitro	Binds CCR4 (K_d = 0.6 nmol/L)[296]; chemoattractant for subsets of activated CD4+/CD4- T cells (T_H2)[291,292] and CCR4–transfected cells[296]; induces activated T-cell adhesion to ICAM-1 under flow conditions[293]; induces intracellular Ca^{2+} mobilization in CCR4–transfected cells.[296]
In vivo	Not reported.
Pathologic association(s)	Atopic dermatitis,[294] bacteria-induced hepatic failure,[297] Hodgkin's lymphoma,[295] lichen planus,[293] psoriasis.[293]
Genbank source (gene)	D43767 (h), AF192527 (m).
Gene coding region (kbp)	Not reported.
Chromosomal location	16q13[298] (h).
Exons	3 (m).[291]
Introns	2 (m).[291]
Natural mutations/polymorphisms	Not reported.
Genbank source (RNA)	NM_002987 (h), AJ242587 (m).
Size of RNA (kbp)	0.6 (h), 0.5 (m).
RNA splice variants	3 (m).[291]

CC CHEMOKINES

Dendritic Cell Chemokine-1 (DC-CK-1)

Systematic name	CCL18.
Other names	AMAC-1,[299] CC chemokine-1, CKβ-7, DCtactin, MIP-4, PARC,[32] SCYA18
Similar proteins	hMIP-1α [LD78α (61%), LD78β, (60%)], hMIP-1β (42%), hHCC-1 (40%), hRANTES (37%), hMCP-3 (34%), hMCP-1 (33%), hMCP-4 (32%), hEOT-1 (33%), TARC (30%).
Genbank source	NP_002979 (h).
Amino acids in precursor protein	89 (h).[300]
Size of mature protein (Kd)	7.8 (h).[299]
Amino acids in mature protein	69 (h).
Stable form(s)	Not reported.
Glycosylation sites	0 N/0 O (h).
Disulfide bonds	2 (h).
3D structure	Not reported.
Mature protein variants	Not reported.
Tissue and cellular expression	Highly expressed in lung.[32] Specific cell types include immature and mature activated DCs[301] and activated Mφs.[299,301]
Regulation of expression	
Up	CD40 ligand (Mφs,[301] DCs[301]), IL-4 (Mφs,[299] DCs[302]), IL-4 + glucocorticoids (Mφs[299]), IL-4 + GM-CSF (DCs[302]), IL-10 (Mφs[299]), IL-13 (Mφs[299]), LPS (Mφs, DCs[301]), TNF-α (Mφs, DCs[301]).
Down	Not reported.
Biologic activities	
In vitro	Binds to unknown receptor (K_d = 1.9 nmol/L)[32]; chemoattractant for naïve CD4+ T cells[302] and naïve CD8+ T cells[302]; induces Ca^{2+} mobilization in naïve and activated T cells.[303]
In vivo	Chemoattractant for CD4+ and CD8+ T cells.[303]
Pathologic association(s)	Atherosclerosis,[304] Hodgkin's lymphoma.[295]
Genbank source (gene)	AB012113 (h).
Gene coding region (kbp)	13.2 (h).[300]
Chromosomal location	17q11.2 (h).[305]
Exons	3 (h).[303]
Introns	2 (h).[303]
Natural mutations/polymorphisms	Not reported.
Genbank source (RNA)	NM_002988 (h).
Size of RNA (kbp)	0.8, 1.1 (h).[303]
RNA splice variants	Not reported.

CC CHEMOKINES

Macrophage Inflammatory Protein-3β (MIP-3β)

Systematic name	CCL19.
Other names	CKβ-11, Epstein-Barr virus–induced gene-1 ligand chemokine, exodus-3, SCYA19.
Similar proteins	mMIP-3β (78%),[306] hSLC (32%), hMIP-1β (31%), hMIP-3α (30%), hRANTES (30%).
Genbank source	NP_006265 (h), NP_036018 (m).
Amino acids in precursor protein	98 (h), 108 (m).
Size of mature protein (Kd)	8.8/12.0 (h),[307] 9.4 (m).[306]
Amino acids in mature protein	77 (h),[307] 83 (m).
Stable form(s)	Not reported.
Glycosylation sites	0 N (h),[307] 1 N[306] (m).
Disulfide bonds	2 (h, m).
3D structure	Not reported.
Mature protein variants	Not reported.
Tissue and cellular expression	Highly expressed in appendix,[307,308] LNs,[308] tonsil,[307,308] and thymus.[307,308] Specific cell types include B cells,[309] DCs,[306] activated monocytes,[308] CD4+ T cells,[309] CD8+ T cells,[309] memory T cells.
Regulation of expression	
Up	LPS (monocytes[304,308]), IFN-γ (monocytes,[308] smooth muscle cells[304]), PHA (T cells[309]), and TNF-α (bone marrow stromal cells,[310] smooth muscle cells[304]).
Down	IL-10 (LPS-activated monocytes[308]).
Biologic activities	
In vitro	Binds to CCR7 (K_d = 0.1–10 nmol/L)[311,312]; chemoattractant for immature B cells,[313] mature B cells,[309] activated B cells,[306,314] BM-derived DCs,[315,316] Mφ progenitors,[310] NK cells,[313,317] naïve T cells,[306,314] activated T cells,[309,318] CD4+ and CD8+ thymocytes[313,319]; induces intracellular Ca2+ mobilization in activated NK cells[317] and activated T cells[309]; inhibits synthesis of TNF-α and IL-12 in activated monocytes and IFN-γ by T cells[320]; induces synthesis of IL-10 in activated monocytes and T cells[320]; induces T-cell adhesion to ICAM-1 under flow conditions.[321]
In vivo	Mice with the *paucity of LN T cells (plt)* mutation lack expression of MIP-3β (and SLC) and exhibit major defects in T-cell organization in secondary lymphoid tissue as well as reduced entry of cells into HEVs.[322]
Pathologic association(s)	Atherosclerosis.[304]
Genbank source (gene)	Not reported.
Gene coding region (kbp)	Not reported.
Chromosomal location	9p13 (h).[307]
Exons	Not reported.
Introns	Not reported.
Natural mutations/polymorphisms	Not reported.
Genbank source (RNA)	NM_006274 (h), NM_011888 (m).
Size of RNA (kbp)	0.7 (h, m).[308]
RNA splice variants	Not reported.

CC CHEMOKINES

Macrophage Inflammatory Protein-3α (MIP-3α)

Systematic name	CCL20.
Other names	Exodus-1, LARC,[323] mexikine, ST38 (r),[324] SCYA20, SCYA201.[324]
Similar proteins	mMIP-3α (64%),[324] rMIP-3α (61%),[324] hSLC (31%).[325]
Genbank source	NP_004582 (h), CAA07714 (m), AAB61459 (r).
Amino acids in precursor protein	96 (h, r), 97 (m).
Size of mature protein (Kd)	8.0 (h), 8.0 (m), 8.2 (r).[324]
Amino acids in mature protein	73 (h, r),[324] 75 (m).[326]
Stable form(s)	Not reported.
Glycosylation sites	0 N (h, m, r).
Disulfide bonds	2 (h, m, r).
3D structure	Not reported.
Mature protein variants	Not reported.
Tissue and cellular expression	Constitutively expressed in appendix, colon,[326] liver, LNs, fetal lung, and small intestine.[326] Specific cell types include activated astrocytes, DCs,[327] activated ECs,[326,328] eosinophils,[327] activated fibroblasts,[328] activated Mφs,[327] and activated T cells.[328]
Regulation of expression	
Up	LPS (microglia,[324] Mφs,[324] monocytes[326]), IL-1β (astrocytes[324]), TNF-α (astrocytes,[324] Mφs,[324] microglia[324]).
Down	IL-10 (LPS-activated monocytes[308]).
Biologic activities	
In vitro	Binds to CCR6 (K_d = 0.9–1.3 nmol/L)[327,329,330]; chemoattractant for naïve B cells,[326] immature[331] and mature DCs,[327] eosinophils,[332] NK cells,[317] T cells,[327,333] and γ/δ T cells[326]; induces intracellular Ca^{2+} mobilization in eosinophils,[332] activated NK cells,[317] memory T cells,[333] and TILs[328]; induces phosphorylation/activation of MAPK (p42/44) and stimulation of PI3K activity[332]; inhibits proliferation of myeloid progenitors in colony-formation assays[334]; induces memory CD4+ T-cell adhesion to ICAM-1 under flow conditions.[321]
In vivo	Not reported.
Pathologic association(s)	EAE/MS,[324] pancreatic cancer,[335] spinal cord injury.[105]
Genbank source (gene)	AJ007862 (m).
Gene coding region (kbp)	4.0 (h).
Chromosomal location	2q33-q37 (h),[323] 1 (m).[324]
Exons	4 (m).[326]
Introns	4 (m).[326]
Natural mutations/polymorphisms	Not reported.
Genbank source (RNA)	NM_004591 (h), AB015136 (m), U90447 (r).
Size of RNA (kbp)	0.9/1.0/1.3 (h),[323] 0.8 (m, r).[324]
RNA splice variants	2 (m).[326]

CC CHEMOKINES

Secondary Lymphoid-Tissue Chemokine (SLC)

Systematic name	CCL21.
Other names	6Ckine, CKβ-9, exodus-2, SCYA21, Scya21a (m), Scya21b (m), secondary lymphoid organ chemokine, thymus-derived chemotactic agent-4.
Similar proteins	mSLC (72%), hMIP-1δ (68%),[10] hMIP-3β (32%), hMIP-1α (31%), hMCP-1 (31%), hMCP-2 (32%), hMCP-3 (30%), hEOT-1 (32%).
Genbank source	NP_002980 (h), AAB61440 (m).
Amino acids in precursor protein	134 (h), 133 (m).
Size of mature protein (Kd)	12.2 (h, m).[325]
Amino acids in mature protein	111 (h),[325] 110 (m).
Stable form(s)	Monomer.
Glycosylation sites	0 N (h, m).[325]
Disulfide bonds	3 (h, m).
3D structure	Not reported.
Mature protein variants	Two forms, 6Ckine-leu and 6Ckine-ser, are transcribed from two different loci (m).[336]
Tissue and cellular expression	Highly expressed in appendix,[325] HEVs,[337] lung, LNs,[325] spleen,[325] and thymus.[325] Specific cell types include lymphatic ECs.[337]
Regulation of expression	
Up	Not reported.
Down	Not reported.
Biologic activities	
In vitro	Binds to CCR7 (K_d = 0.1–10 nmol/L)[312] and possibly CXCR3 (m)[338,339]; chemoattractant for mature DCs,[316] CD34+ Mϕ progenitor cells,[340] NK cells,[313] resting and activated T cells,[318,325] CLA-T cells,[341] CD4+ thymocytes,[319] CD8+ thymocytes,[319] and CCR7–transfected cell lines[311]; inhibits hemopoietic progenitor proliferation and colony formation[340]; induces actin polymerization in CD34+ hematopoietic progenitor cells[340]; induces CD4+ T-cell adhesion to ICAM-1 under flow conditions[321]; induces intracellular Ca2+ mobilization in T cells[311,325] and in CCR7–transfected cells[311]; enhances the growth of M- and T-tropic strains of HIV.[342]
In vivo	Angiostatic,[338] expression pattern correlates with CTL trafficking during an antiviral response.[318] Mice with the *paucity of LN T cells (plt)* mutation have severely reduced expression of SLC (and MIP-3β)[322,336] and exhibit defects in T-cell organization in secondary lymphoid tissue as well as reduced entry of cells into HEVs. The mutation has been described as a deletion of the 6Ckine-ser gene.[336]
Pathologic association(s)	HIV.[342]
Genbank source (gene)	AJ005654 (h), AF171085/AF171086 (m).
Gene coding region (kbp)	7.3/7.7 (m).
Chromosomal location	9p13 (h),[325] 4 (m).
Exons	4 (h, m).
Introns	3 (h, m).
Natural mutations/polymorphisms	Not reported.
Genbank source (RNA)	NM_002989 (h), AF006637 (m).
Size of RNA (kbp)	0.9 (h),[325] 0.6 (m).
RNA splice variants	Not reported.

CC CHEMOKINES

Macrophage-Derived Chemokine (MDC)

Systematic name	CCL22.
Other names	ABCD-1(m), DCtactin-β, DC/β-CK, STCP-1, SCYA22.
Similar proteins	mMDC (65%), rMDC (65%), hMIP-1β (34%), hTARC (32%), hRANTES (31%), hMIP-1α (31%), hMCP-3 (31%), hMCP-1 (30%).[343]
Genbank source	NP_002981 (h), NP_033163 (m), AAD55764 (r).
Amino acids in precursor protein	93 (h), 92 (m), 81 (r).
Size of mature protein (Kd)	8.0 (h).
Amino acids in mature protein	69 (h), 68 (m).
Stable form(s)	Monomer.
Glycosylation sites	0 N (h, m, r).
Disulfide bonds	2 (h, m, r).
3D structure	Not reported.
Mature protein variants	At least two forms are generated by amino-terminal processing by CD26/dipeptidyl-peptidase IV.[344]
Tissue and cellular expression	Expressed at high levels in appendix, LNs, lung, spleen, and thymus.[345] Specific cell types include B cells, BM-derived DCs,[273] thymic medullary epithelial cells, Mφs,[273] and T cells.[346]
Regulation of expression	
Up	Anti-CD3/anti-CD28 (T cells, CD45RO+ > CD45RA,+ T_H2 > T_H1[346]), anti-CD40 + IL-4 (B cells[347]), IL-1β (Mφs,[348]), IL-4 (monocytes[349]), IL-13 (monocytes[349]), TNF-α (Mφs[348]), LPS (Mφs[348]).
Down	IFN-γ (DCs,[349] monocytes[349]).
Biologic activities	
In vitro	Binds to CCR4 (K_d = 0.2–0.7 nmol/L)[296]; chemoattractant for DCs,[343] eosinophils,[350] IL-2 activated NK cells,[343] monocytes,[343] activated T cells (T_H2),[347,351] thymocytes,[352] and CCR4–transfected cells[296]; induces intracellular Ca^{2+} mobilization in activated T cells[345] and CCR4–transfected cells[296]; suppresses infection of CD8+ T-cell–depleted PBMCs by T-cell–tropic and M-tropic strains of HIV[353]; desensitizes intracellular Ca^{2+} mobilization and chemotaxis in response to TARC in CCR4–transfected cells[296]; stimulates activation/phosphorylation of MAPK (p42/44)[354]; activates CREB.[354]
In vivo	Not reported.
Pathologic association(s)	Atopic dermatitis,[346] mycosis fungoides.[346]
Genbank source (gene)	Not reported.
Gene coding region (kbp)	Not reported.
Chromosomal location	16q13.[296]
Exons	3 (h, m).[345,347]
Introns	2 (h, m).[345,347]
Natural mutations/polymorphisms	Not reported.
Genbank source (RNA)	NM_002990 (h), NM_009137 (m), AF163477 (r).
Size of RNA (kbp)	2.9 (h), 2.2 (m), 1.7 (r).
RNA splice variants	Not reported.

CC CHEMOKINES

Myeloid Progenitor Inhibitory Factor-1 (MPIF-1)

Systematic name	CCL23.
Other names	C6 β-chemokine, CKβ-8,[161] HMRP-2α, MIP-3, SCYA23.
Similar proteins	hMIP-1δ (68%), hMIP-1α (51%),[112] hMIP-1β (41%),[161] hMCP-3 (37%), hMCP-1 (33%), hI-309 (32%), hRANTES (31%).
Genbank source	NP_005055 (h).
Amino acids in precursor protein	137 (h).
Size of mature protein (Kd)	8.8/11.5 (h).[112,355]
Amino acids in mature protein	99 (h).
Stable form(s)	Not reported.
Glycosylation sites	0 N/0 N (h).[112]
Disulfide bonds	3 (h).[161,355]
3D structure	Not reported.
Mature protein variants	Two variants produced by alternative splicing.[356,357]
Tissue and cellular expression	Highly expressed in BM, liver, and lung.[112] Specific cell types include activated DCs[358] and activated monocytes.[161]
Regulation of expression	
Up	IFN-γ (monocytes[161]), IL-1β (monocytes[161]).
Down	Anti-CD40 (DCs[358]), IFN-γ (DCs[358]).
Biologic activities	
In vitro	Binds to CCR1 (K_d = 5 nmol/L)[359] and heparin; chemoattractant for monocytes[112,161] and resting T cells; induces intracellular Ca^{2+} mobilization in DCs,[359] monocytes,[112] and CCR1–transfected cells[359]; inhibits generation of colony-forming unit granulocyte-macrophage from mouse and human BM-derived precursors[112]; stimulates the release of arachidonic acid from monocytes.[358]
In vivo	Not reported.
Pathologic association(s)	Not reported.
Genbank source (gene)	AF088219 (h).
Gene coding region (kbp)	4.9 (h).
Chromosomal location	17q11.2 (h).[279]
Exons	4 (h).[279]
Introns	3 (h).[279]
Natural mutations/polymorphisms	Not reported.
Genbank source (RNA)	NM_005064 (h).
Size of RNA (kbp)	0.8 (h).[112]
RNA splice variants	2 (h).[356,357]

CC CHEMOKINES

Eotaxin-2 (EOT-2)

Systematic name	CCL24.
Other names	CKβ-6, MPIF-2, SCYA24.
Similar proteins	hMCP-4 (43%), hMIP-1α (42%), hMCP-3 (40%),[170] hEOT-1 (39%), hRANTES (32%).[170]
Genbank source	NP_002982 (h).
Amino acids in precursor protein	119 (h).
Size of mature protein (Kd)	8.7/10.6 (h).[112]
Amino acids in mature protein	93 (h).
Stable form(s)	Not reported.
Glycosylation sites	1 N (h).
Disulfide bonds	2 (h).
3D structure	Not reported.
Mature protein variants	Five variants (h).[170]
Tissue and cellular expression	Not found in normal tissue. Specific cell types include activated monocytes[112] and activated T cells.[112]
Regulation of expression	
Up	Anti-CD3 (T cells[112]), GM-CSF (monocytes[112]).
Down	Not reported.
Biologic activities	
In vitro	Binds to CCR3 (K_d = 0.20 nmol/L)[360]; chemoattractant for basophils,[170] eosinophils,[170] and resting T cells; stimulates the release of histamine and LTC4 from basophils[170]; suppresses colony formation by multipotential hematopoietic progenitors[112]; induces actin polymerization in eosinophils[361]; stimulates the release of reactive oxygen species from eosinophils[361]; induces intracellular Ca^{2+} mobilization in eosinophils[112,361] and CCR3–transfected cells.[360]
In vivo	Chemoattractant for eosinophils.[170]
Pathologic association(s)	Asthma.[277]
Genbank source (gene)	Not reported.
Gene coding region (kbp)	Not reported.
Chromosomal location	7q11.23.[362]
Exons	3 (h).[37]
Introns	2 (h).[37]
Natural mutations/polymorphisms	Not reported.
Genbank source (RNA)	NM_002991 (h).
Size of RNA (kbp)	0.4 (h).
RNA splice variants	Not reported.

CC CHEMOKINES

Thymus-Expressed Chemokine (TECK)

Systematic name	CCL25.
Other names	CKβ-15, SCYA25.
Similar proteins	mTECK (49%).[363]
Genbank source	NP_005615 (h), NP_033164 (m).
Amino acids in precursor protein	151 (h), 144 (m).
Size of mature protein (Kd)	14.3 (h), 14.0 (m).
Amino acids in mature protein	127 (h), 121 (m).
Stable form(s)	Not reported.
Glycosylation sites	0 N (h, m).
Disulfide bonds	2 (h, m).
3D structure	Not reported.
Mature protein variants	Not reported.
Tissue and cellular expression	Highly expressed in brain, liver, small intestine, and thymus.[363] Specific cell types include thymus-derived DCs,[363] intestinal and thymic epithelial cells.[364,365]
Regulation of expression	
Up	LPS (small intestine,[363] spleen,[363] thymus,[363]).
Down	Not reported.
Biologic activities	
In vitro	Binds to CCR9[366,367]; chemoattractant for activated DCs, Mφs, immature thymocytes, and mature thymocytes[363,366,368]; induces intracellular Ca^{2+} mobilization in CCR9–expressing cells[366,369]; inhibits proliferation of myeloid progenitor cells.[370]
In vivo	Not reported.
Pathologic association(s)	Not reported.
Genbank source (gene)	U86358 (h), AJ249480 (m).
Gene coding region (kbp)	1.0 (h, m).[363]
Chromosomal location	19p13.2 (h),[371] 8 (m).[363]
Exons	Not reported.
Introns	Not reported.
Natural mutations/polymorphisms	Not reported.
Genbank source (RNA)	NM_005624 (h), NM_009138 (m).
Size of RNA (kbp)	0.8/1.0 (h), 1.0 (m).
RNA splice variants	Not reported.

CC CHEMOKINES

Eotaxin-3 (EOT-3)

Systematic name	CCL26.
Other names	IMAC, MIP-4α, TSC-1, SCYA26.[372]
Similar proteins	hMIP-1β (42%), hMCP-4 (41%), hMIP-1α (38%), hMCP-3 (38%), hDK-CK-1 (38%), hHCC-1 (38%), hEOT-1 (37%), hRANTES (37%), hMCP-2 (35%), hEOT-2 (34%), hMPIF-1 (32%), hMCP-1 (31%), hMIP-3β (31%).
Genbank source	NP_006063 (h).
Amino acids in precursor protein	94 (h).[372]
Size of mature protein (Kd)	8.4/10.6/12.8 (h).[373]
Amino acids in mature protein	71 (h).
Stable form(s)	Not reported.
Glycosylation sites	0 N (h).
Disulfide bonds	2 (h).
3D structure	Not reported.
Mature protein variants	Not reported.
Tissue and cellular expression	Highly expressed in heart,[372,373] liver,[372] and ovary.[373] Specific cell types include vascular ECs.[374]
Regulation of expression	
Up	IL-4 (vascular ECs[374]), IL-13 (vascular ECs[374]).
Down	Not reported.
Biologic activities	
In vitro	Binds to CCR3 (K_d = 3–10 nmol/L)[373,374]; chemoattractant for basophils (weak),[373] eosinophils (weak),[373] monocytes,[372] and T cells[372]; induces intracellular Ca^{2+} mobilization in eosinophils[374] and CCR3–transfected cells.[373]
In vivo	Chemoattractant for eosinophils.[374]
Pathologic association(s)	Not reported.
Genbank source (gene)	Not reported.
Gene coding region (kbp)	Not reported.
Chromosomal location	7q11.2 (h).[372]
Exons	3 (h).[373]
Introns	2 (h).[372]
Natural mutations/polymorphisms	Not reported.
Genbank source (RNA)	NM_006072 (h).
Size of RNA (kbp)	0.3/0.5/0.6/1.8 (h).
RNA splice variants	Not reported.

CC CHEMOKINES

ALP

Systematic name	CCL27.
Other names	ESkine, CTACK,[341] IL-11Rα-locus chemokine,[375] SCYA27, skinkine.
Similar proteins	mSCYA27 (62%), hTECK, hMIP-3α, hSLC, hMIP-3β, hRANTES, vMC148.
Genbank source	NP_006655 (h), NP_035466 (m).
Amino acids in precursor protein	112 (h), 120 (m).
Size of mature protein (Kd)	10.1 (h), 10.9 (m).
Amino acids in mature protein	87 (h), 95 (m).
Stable form(s)	Not reported.
Glycosylation sites	1 N (h, m, r).
Disulfide bonds	2 (h).
3D structure	Not reported.
Mature protein variants	An alternatively spliced version, PESKY, is highly expressed in brain and testes but is not secreted.
Tissue and cellular expression	Highly expressed in heart, liver, placenta, skin,[375] and testes. PESKY is highly expressed in brain, testes, kidney, and liver. Specific cell types include keratinocytes.[341]
Regulation of expression	
Up	IL-1β (keratinocytes[341]), TNF-α (keratinocytes[341]).
Down	Not reported.
Biologic activities	
In vitro	Binds to unknown receptor; chemoattractant for subsets of activated CD4+ T cells preferentially expressing the CLA antigen.[341]
In vivo	Not reported.
Pathologic association(s)	Not reported.
Genbank source (gene)	Not reported.
Gene coding region (kbp)	Not reported.
Chromosomal location	9p13 (h),[375] 4 (m).
Exons	3 (m).
Introns	2 (m).
Natural mutations/polymorphisms	Not reported.
Genbank source (RNA)	NM_006664 (h), NM_011336 (m), AI058901 (r).
Size of RNA (kbp)	0.4 (h, m, r).
RNA splice variants	PESKY.

CC CHEMOKINE RECEPTORS

Chemokine (CC) Receptor-1 (CCR1)

Other names	CC CKR-1,[376] CMKBR1,[377] CKR-1, HM145,[378] HM145, LD78 receptor,[378] MIP-1α receptor,[379] RANTES receptor.[379]
Similar proteins	mCCR1 (79%),[377] rCCR1 (99%),[380] hCCR3 (54%), hCCR8 (40%),[381] hCCR9 (33%), hCXCR1 (32%), hCXCR2 (32%).
Genbank source	NP_001286 (h), NP_034042 (m), 741970 (r).
Size of mature protein (Kd)	41.1 (h), 40.9 (m).
Amino acids in mature protein	355 (h, m, r).
Stable form(s)	Monomer.
Glycosylation sites	1 N (h), 0 N (m).
Disulfide bonds	1 (h, m, r).
3D structure	Seven transmembrane regions.
Mature protein variants	Not reported.
Tissue and cellular expression	Highly expressed in brain.[382] Specific cell types include astrocytes,[127] basophils,[63] B cells,[379] immature DCs,[166] eosinophils,[382] CD34+ hematopoietic progenitor cells,[383] monocytes,[382] neurons,[384] neutrophils,[382] NK cells, vascular smooth muscle cells,[89] T cells ($T_H1 > T_H2$), and γ/δ T cells.[121]
Regulation of expression	
Up	INF-α (monocytes[385]), IFN-γ (neutrophils,[386] mesangial cells,[387] U937 cells[388]), IL-2 (T cells[389]), IL-5 (eosinophils[390]), IL-12 (T cells[391]), LPS (DCs[49]).
Down	Anti-CD3 (T cells,[389] memory T cells,[392] γ/δ T cells[121]), LPS (monocytes[393]).
Biologic activities	
In vitro	Binds HCC-1 (K_d = 100 nmol/L),[138] LKN-1, MCP-2 (K_d = 2–135 nmol/L),[124,236] MCP-3 (K_d = 1.5 nmol/L), MIP-1α (K_d = 2–4 nmol/L),[124,284] MIP-1δ (K_d = 1 nmol/L),[284] MPIF-1,[359] and RANTES; binds MIP-1β (K_d = 33 nmol/L)[124] and MCP-1 (K_d = 150 nmol/L)[124] with lower affinity; engagement of CCR1 by MIP-1α leads to activation of G_{ao}, G_{as}, and G_{a2} G proteins in NK cells[394]; engagement of CCR1 by RANTES leads to activation of G_{ai}, G_{ao}, G_{as}, and G_{a2} G proteins in NK cells[394]; coreceptor for some strains of HIV-2.[395]
In vivo	CCR1 (–/–) mice exhibit decreased numbers of colony-forming unit granulocyte-macrophage and colony-forming unit granulocyte erythroid megakaryocyte macrophage in the spleen and circulating blood[396]; increases mortality from *Aspergillus fumigatus;* reduces formation of lung granulomas in response to *S. mansoni* egg antigen[397]; increases IFN-γ and decreases IL-4 production in response to *S. mansoni* egg antigen[397]; reduces pancreatitis-induced pulmonary inflammation[398]; enhances T_H1 responses and increases pathology in a model of nephritis.[399] Neutrophils from CCR1 (–/–) mice fail to mobilize Ca²⁺ in response to MIP-1α or MIP-1δ.[284]
Pathologic association(s)	Adult respiratory distress syndrome,[398] bleomycin-induced lung fibrosis,[400] nephritis,[399] pancreatitis.[398]
Genbank source (gene)	D10925 (h), U28404 (m).
Gene coding region (kbp)	1.7 (m).
Chromosomal location	3p21 (h),[382] 9:72.00 cM (m).
Exons	2 (h).[379]
Introns	1 (h).[379]
Natural mutations/polymorphisms	Not reported.
Genbank source (RNA)	NM_001295 (h), NM_009912 (m).
Size of RNA (kbp)	3.0 (h),[376] 1.1 (m).
RNA splice variants	Not reported.

CC CHEMOKINE RECEPTORS

Chemokine (CC) Receptor-2 (CCR2)

Other names	CMKBR2, CKR-2, fibroblast-induced cytokine receptor, JE receptor (m), MCP-1 receptor, CCR2A, CC-CKR-2A, CKR2A, MCP-1RA, CCR2B, CC-CKR-2B, CKR2B, MCP-1RB.
Similar proteins	mCCR2 (80%),[61] rCCR2 (79%), hCCR3 (51%), hCCR4 (47%), hCCR8 (39%).
Genbank source	NP_000638 (h), NP_034045 (m), AAC03242 (r).
Size of mature protein (Kd)	41.9 (h), 42.8 (m).
Amino acids in mature protein	CCR2B; 360 (h).
Stable form(s)	Monomer.
Glycosylation sites	1 N (h), 0 N (m).
Disulfide bonds	1 (h, m, r).
3D structure	Seven transmembrane regions.
Mature protein variants	CCR2A and CCR2B (h).[401]
Tissue and cellular expression	Highly expressed in kidney, lung, spleen, and thymus.[61] CCR2A is expressed only in cytoplasm, whereas CCR2B is expressed on cell surface. Specific cell types include basophils,[63] immature DCs,[166] monocytes,[401] activated NK cells, vascular smooth muscle cells,[89] activated T cells.[389]
Regulation of expression	
Up	IL-2 (monocytes,[393] NK cells,[402] T cells[389]), oxidized LDL (monocytes[403]).
Down	Anti-CD3 (T cells,[389] memory T cells[392]), IFN-γ (monocytes[404]), TNF-α (monocytes[393,404]), IL-1β (monocytes[393,404]), LPS (monocytes[393,405]), oxidized LDL (monocytes[406]).
Biologic activities	
In vitro	CCR2A: binds MCP-1 (K_d = 0.3 nmol/L)[401]; CCR2B: binds MCP-1 (K_d = 1.2 nmol/L),[61] MCP-2 (K_d = 3 nmol/L),[236] MCP-3 (K_d = 7 nmol/L),[61,219] MCP-4 (K_d = 7 nmol/L),[272] MCP-5, and vMIP-II; coreceptor for syncytia-inducing strains of HIV-1, dual-tropic strains of HIV-1, and T-cell tropic strains of HIV-2.[395] Engagement of CCR2B by MCP-1 leads to activation of G_{ai}, G_{ao}, G_{as}, and G_{a2} G proteins in NK cells[394]; engagement of CCR2B by MCP-1 leads to recruitment of GRK3 and phosphorylation of CCR2B[70]; engagement of CCR2B by MCP-1 and MCP-3 induces intracellular Ca^{2+} mobilization in monocytes and CCR2B–transfected cells[70,401]; engagement of CCR2B by MCP-1 leads to inhibition of adenyl cyclase in CCR2B–transfected cells.[401]
In vivo	Mice lacking CCR2 (–/–) exhibit failure to clear *Listeria monocytogenes* infection[407]; impairs ability to recruit Mϕs due to thioglycollate[407,408] or to *S. mansoni* egg antigen[409]; reduces T_H1 cytokine production in response to purified protein derivative or conA[410]; reduces lung granuloma size to PPD challenge[410] or schistosomal antigen[409]; reduces liver granuloma formation due to yeast β-glucan challenge[408]; reduces allergen-induced airway hyperreactivity[411]; reduces MCP-1–induced adhesion to ECs[408]; increases myeloid progenitor cell cycling and apoptosis.[412] Mice lacking CCR2 (–/–) and apolipoprotein E (–/–) exhibit decreased atherosclerotic lesion formation compared with mice expressing CCR2 (+/+) and lacking apolipoprotein E (–/–).[413,414]
Pathologic association(s)	Atherosclerosis,[406,413] HIV,[395] nephritis,[399] ovarian carcinoma.[415]
Genbank source (gene)	U80924 (h), U77349 (r).
Gene coding region (kbp)	5.4 (h), 1.4 (r).
Chromosomal location	3p21 (h),[416] 9:72.00 cM (m).
Exons	3 (h).[401]
Introns	2 (h).[401]
Natural mutations/polymorphisms	Individuals with the CCR2-Val64Ile (+/–) mutation have a reduced HIV progression rate,[4,417] higher risk of developing insulin-dependent diabetes mellitus,[418] and lower risk of developing sarcoidosis.[419]
Genbank source (RNA)	NM_000647 (h), NM_009915 (m).
Size of RNA (kbp)	1.4/2.2 (h),[401,420] 3.8 (m).[61]
RNA splice variants	2 (h).[401]

CC CHEMOKINE RECEPTORS

Chemokine (CC) Receptor-3 (CCR3)

Other names	CMKBR3, CC CKR3,[421] EOT-1 receptor, MIP-1α receptor–like-2,[377] CCR1–like-2 (Cmkbr112, m), Scya3r-rs2.[377]
Similar proteins	mCCR3 (70%), rCCR3 (69%), hCCR1 (54%), hCCR2B (51%).
Genbank source	NP_001828 (h), NP_034044 (m), AAC03337 (r).
Size of mature protein (Kd)	40.6 (h), 41.8 (m), 41.6 (r).
Amino acids in mature protein	355 (h), 359 (m), 359 (r).
Stable form(s)	Monomer.
Glycosylation sites	1 N (h), 0 N (m, r).
Disulfide bonds	1 (h, m, r).
3D structure	Seven transmembrane regions.
Mature protein variants	Not reported.
Tissue and cellular expression	Highly expressed in colon,[242] small intestine,[242] and spleen. Specific cell types include basophils,[221] immature DCs,[422] eosinophils, microglia,[423] monocytes,[385] fetal neurons,[424] adult neurons,[425] neutrophils,[386] T cells (T$_H$2),[426] thymocytes (CD8+).[164]
Regulation of expression	
Up	IFN-α (monocytes,[385] U937 cells[385]), IFN-γ (neutrophils,[386] U937 cells[388]), IL-2 + IL-4 (T cells[427]), IL-5 (eosinophils[390]).
Down	EOT-1 (eosinophils[428]), RANTES (eosinophils[428]), activation (memory T cells; anti-CD3[392]).
Biologic activities	
In vitro	Binds EOT-1 (K_d = 0.15–0.20 nmol/L), EOT-2 (K_d = 0.15–0.20 nmol/L),[360] EOT-3 (K_d = 3–10 nmol/L),[373,374] MIP-1α (K_d = 12 nmol/L),[124] MIP-1β (K_d = 85 nm),[124] MIP-1δ, vMCK-1,[429] MCP-2, MCP-3, MCP-4,[275] and RANTES; coreceptor for some dual-tropic strains of HIV-1[430] and HIV-2[395,431]; engagement of CCR3 by EOT-1 leads to activation of MAPKs (p38)[432] and association of Src family kinases (Hck and c-Fgr) with CCR3[433]; engagement of CCR3 by RANTES leads to activation of G$_{ai}$, G$_{ao}$, G$_{as}$, or G$_{a2}$ G proteins in NK cells[394]; engagement of CCR3 by MCP-3, MIP-1α, and RANTES leads to intracellular Ca^{2+} mobilization in CCR2–transfected cells.[421]
In vivo	Not reported.
Pathologic association(s)	Alzheimer's disease,[434] asthma,[259,435] atopic dermatitis,[8] HIV.[430]
Genbank source (gene)	AB023887 (h), U28406 (m), AF003954 (r).
Gene coding region (kbp)	1.1 (h), 1.4 (m),[377] 1.1 (r).[436]
Chromosomal location	3p21.3[416] (h), 9:72.0 (m).
Exons	Not reported.
Introns	Not reported.
Natural mutations/polymorphisms	Four SNPs identified in humans. Arg275Glu and Leu351Pro, T51C.[437,438]
Genbank source (RNA)	NM_001837 (h), NM_009914 (m), CAA73830 (r).
Size of RNA (kbp)	1.6/4.0 (h),[421] 1.1 (m),[439] 1.1 (r).[436]
RNA splice variants	Not reported.

CC CHEMOKINE RECEPTORS

Chemokine (CC) Receptor-4 (CCR4)

Other names	CC-CKR-4,[440] CMKBR4 (m), K5-5.[441]
Similar proteins	mCCR4 (85%),[440] hCCR8 (84%), hCCR1 (49%),[441] hCCR2B (47%),[441] hCCR6 (36%).[330]
Genbank source	NP_005499 (h), NP_034046 (m).
Size of mature protein (Kd)	41.4 (h), 41.5 (m).
Amino acids in mature protein	360 (h, m).
Stable form(s)	Monomer.
Glycosylation sites	2 N (h), 3 N (m).
Disulfide bonds	1 (h, m).
3D structure	Seven transmembrane regions.
Mature protein variants	Not reported.
Tissue and cellular expression	Highly expressed in thymus[440,441] and spleen.[441] Specific cell types include basophils,[441] DCs, CD34+ hematopoietic progenitor cells,[383] megakaryocytes,[441] neurons,[354] NK cells, platelets,[441] activated T cells (T_H2),[442] memory CD4+ T cells.[293]
Regulation of expression	
Up	Anti-CD3 (T cells[442]), IL-5 (basophils[441]).
Down	Not reported.
Biologic activities	
In vitro	Binds MDC (K_d = 0.18 nmol/L),[296] MIP-1α (K_d = 14 nmol/L),[440,443] MCP-1,[443] RANTES (K_d = 9 nmol/L),[440,443] and TARC (K_d = 0.5 nmol/L)[296,443]; coreceptor for some strains of HIV-1[444] and HIV-2[395]; engagement of CCR4 by TARC[443] or MDC[296] leads to intracellular Ca^{2+} mobilization in CCR4–transfected cells; engagement of CCR4 by TARC[443] or MDC[296] leads to chemotaxis of CCR4–transfected cells.
In vivo	Not reported.
Pathologic association(s)	Atopic dermatitis,[294] HIV/AIDS,[444] lichen planus,[293] psoriasis.[293]
Genbank source (gene)	AB023888 (h).
Gene coding region (kbp)	1.3 (h).
Chromosomal location	3p24-p24 (h),[416] 9:61.00 cM (m).
Exons	Not reported.
Introns	Not reported.
Natural mutations/polymorphisms	Five SNPs.[438]
Genbank source (RNA)	NM_005508 (h), NM_009916 (m).
Size of RNA (kbp)	1.7/4.0 (h), 1.5 (m).[440]
RNA splice variants	Not reported.

CC CHEMOKINE RECEPTORS

Chemokine (CC) Receptor-5 (CCR5)

Other names	AM4-7 (m),[445] chemR13,[446] CKR5, CC-CKR-5, CMKBR5 (m), MIP-1α receptor-2, CCR5-2; CCR5 32-BP deletion mutation.
Similar proteins	mCCR5 (82%), rCCR5 (83%), hCCRL-2 (41%),[447] hCCR8 (40%), hCCR9 (35%).
Genbank source	NP_000570 (h), CAA63867 (m), O08556 (r).
Size of mature protein (Kd)	40.5 (h), 40.8 (m), 41.0 (r).
Amino acids in mature protein	352 (h), 351 (m),[445] 354 (r).
Stable form(s)	Monomer/dimer[448] (h).
Glycosylation sites	1 N/1 O (h), 1 N (m, r).
Disulfide bonds	1 (h, m, r).
3D structure	Seven transmembrane regions.
Mature protein variants	CCR5A and CCR5B.[449]
Tissue and cellular expression	Highly expressed in heart,[445] liver,[445] spleen,[445] and thymus.[445] Specific cell types include immature DCs,[166] eosinophils, immature DCs,[166] microglia,[423] Mφs, neurons,[384] NK cells, activated T cells (T$_H$1),[450] naïve T cells,[450] and γ/δ T cells.[121]
Regulation of expression	
Up	Excitotoxic brain injury,[451] HIV-1 Tat (Mφs), IL-10 (Mφs, monocytes[452]), IFN-γ (Mφs[453]), U937 cells,[388] IL-2 (CD4+ T cells[454,455]), IL-12 (CD4+ T cells[454,455]), TNF-α (CD4+ T cells).[454,455]
Down	Anti-CD3 (memory T cells,[392] γ/δ T cells[121]), IL-10 (CD4+ T cells[454]), IL-16 (DCs, Mφs[456]), LPS (monocytes[393]).
Biologic activities	
In vitro	Binds MIP-1α (K_d = 0.2–0.4 nmol/L),[124] MIP-1β (K_d = 0.2–0.4 nmol/L), RANTES, MCP-2 (K_d = 5 nmol/L),[168] MCP-3, and MCP-4. Coreceptor for M-trophic strains of HIV-1 and some HIV-2 strains[395]; engagement of CCR5 by MIP-1β leads to activation/phosphorylation of RAFTK/pyk2, phosphorylation of paxillin, Jun N-terminal kinase/stress-associated protein kinase and MAPK (p38)[457]; engagement of CCR5 by MIP-1α leads to activation of G$_{ao}$, G$_{as}$, and G$_{a2}$ G proteins in NK cells[394]; engagement of CCR5 by RANTES leads to activation of G$_{ai}$, G$_{ao}$, G$_{as}$, and G$_{a2}$ G proteins in NK cells[394]; engagement of CCR5 by RANTES leads to recruitment of GRK2 and GRK3 to CCR5, and subsequent phosphorylation and desensitization of CCR5[187]; engagement of CCR5 by MCP-2 leads to internalization in CCR5–transfected cells[168]; engagement of CCR5 by MCP-2, MIP-1α, MIP-1β, and RANTES leads to intracellular Ca^{2+} mobilization in CCR5–transfected cells.[445]
In vivo	CCR5 (–/–) mice exhibit increased susceptibility to LPS endotoxemia,[458] decreased ability to clear *Listeria* infection,[458] enhanced DTH reaction,[458] increased humoral responses to T-cell–dependent antigenic challenge,[458] and greater susceptibility to death from experimental challenge with *Cryptococcus neoformans*.[459]
Pathologic association(s)	Alzheimer's disease,[434] graft-versus-host disease,[460] EAE/MS,[198] nephritis,[399] rheumatoid arthritis.[154]
Genbank source (gene)	AF031237 (h), AF019772 (m), U77350 (r).
Gene coding region (kbp)	8.0 (h), 1.1 (m), 1.7 (r).
Chromosomal location	3p21 (h), 9:72.00 cM (m).
Exons	4 (h).[449]
Introns	2 (h).[449]

(continued)

CC CHEMOKINE RECEPTORS

Chemokine (CC) Receptor-5 (CCR5) (*Continued*)

Natural mutations/polymorphisms	Individuals who have the CCR5 Δ32 (–/–) deletion have natural resistance to HIV-1 infection,[4] whereas individuals who are heterozygous for the CCR5 Δ32 (+/–) deletion have a reduced HIV progression rate.[4] HIV-infected individuals who have the CCR5 Δ32 (–/–) deletion polymorphism also have a reduced risk of developing asthma[461] and non-Hodgkin's lymphoma.[462] Individuals with the CCR5-m303 (–/–) mutation have a reduced HIV progression rate.[4] Individuals with the CCR5P1 (–/–) promoter allele polymorphism have an increased HIV progression rate, whereas those with the CCR5P1 G59029A (–/–) mutation have a reduced HIV progression rate.[4] Individuals with CCR5 A59356G (+/+) phenotype have an increased mother-to-child HIV transmission rate.[463] Individuals with the CCR5 Δ32 (–/–) phenotype also have reduced morbidity associated with rheumatoid arthritis[464] but are not protected against MS.[465] Many other mutations/polymorphisms have been identified, including T59353C, A59402G, ARG223GLN, CYS303TER, and ALA335VAL. The functional consequences of these phenotypes are unknown.
Genbank source (RNA)	NM_000579 (h), X94151 (m), Y12009 (r).
Size of RNA (kbp)	3.7 (h), 3.1, 4.0 (m),[445] 1.5 (r).
RNA splice variants	CCR5A and CCR5B.[449]

CC CHEMOKINE RECEPTORS

Chemokine (CC) Receptor-6 (CCR6)

Other names	Barney,[330] BN-1,[330] C-C CKR-6, chemokine receptor–like-3,[466] CMKBR6, DC chemokine receptor-2, DRY6, GPCR29, GPCRCY4, GCY-4, IL-8–related receptor, KY411 (m), LARC receptor, seven-transmembrane receptor lymphocyte-22.[328]
Similar proteins	mCCR6 (72%), rCCR6 (?%), hCCR9 (35%), hCCR7 (42%),[327] hCXCR1 (38%),[330] hCXCR2 (38%),[330] hTYMSTR (37%), hCCR4 (36%).[330]
Genbank source	NP_004358 (h), BAA23776 (m).
Size of mature protein (Kd)	42.5 (h).
Amino acids in mature protein	374 (h), 367 (m).
Stable form(s)	Monomer.
Glycosylation sites	3 N (h), 2 N (m).
Disulfide bonds	1 (h, m).
3D structure	Seven transmembrane regions.[467]
Mature protein variants	Not reported.
Tissue and cellular expression	Highly expressed in liver, lung, LNs, spleen, and thymus.[468] Specific cell types include B cells,[329,333,468] CD34+ DCs,[330,333] lung DCs,[327] ECs, eosinophils,[330,332] fibroblasts, NK cells, T cells,[327,329,468] and memory T cells.[333]
Regulation of expression	
Up	TGF-β1 (DCs[469]).
Down	Anti-CD3 (memory T cells[392]), anti-CD40 (CD34+ DCs[331]), IL-4 (CD34+ DCs[470]), PMA + ionomycin (DCs[330]), TNF-α (CD34+ DCs[331]), LPS (CD34+ DCs[331]).
Biologic activities	
In vitro	Binds MIP-3α (K_d = 0.9–1.3 nmol/L)[327,329,330] and β-defensins[471]; engagement of CCR6 by MIP-3α on eosinophils induces intracellular Ca^{2+} mobilization, phosphorylation/activation of MAPK (p42/44), and stimulation of PI3K activity[332]; engagement of CCR6 by MIP-3α leads to activation of G_{ao}, G_{as}, or G_{a2} G proteins in NK cells.[394]
In vivo	Not reported.
Pathologic association(s)	Pancreatic cancer.[335]
Genbank source (gene)	U45984 (h).
Gene coding region (kbp)	3.7 (h).
Chromosomal location	6q27 (h).[467]
Exons	Not reported.
Introns	Not reported.
Natural mutations/polymorphisms	Not reported.
Genbank source (RNA)	NM_004367 (h), AB009369 (m).
Size of RNA (kbp)	3.0 (h), 3.5 (m).
RNA splice variants	2[467] (h).

CC CHEMOKINE RECEPTORS

Chemokine (CC) Receptor-7 (CCR7)

Other names	Burkitt's lymphoma receptor-2, CKR7, CMKBR7, Epstein-Barr virus–induced gene-1, MIP-3β receptor, SLC receptor.
Similar proteins	mCCR7 (86%),[472] rCCR7 (?%), hCCR6 (42%),[327] hCCR9 (39%), hTYMSTR (32%).
Genbank source	NP_001829 (h), NP_031745 (m).
Size of mature protein (Kd)	42.9 (h, m).
Amino acids in mature protein	378 (h), 378 (m).
Stable form(s)	Monomer.
Glycosylation sites	1 N (h, m).
Disulfide bonds	1 (h, m).
3D structure	Seven transmembrane regions.
Mature protein variants	Not reported.
Tissue and cellular expression	Highly expressed in LNs, Peyer's patches, spleen, and thymus.[472,473] Specific cell types include B cells,[311,472,473] mature DCs, NK cells,[313] resting and activated T cells (T_H1 > T_H2).[311,450]
Regulation of expression	
Up	Anti-CD3 (T cells,[474] memory T cells),[392] anti-CD40 (CD34+ DCs[331]), TNF-α (CD34+ DCs[331]), LPS (CD34+ DCs[331]), HHV-6 (CD4+ T cells),[475] HHV-7 (CD4+ T cells[475]).
Down	Anti-CD3 (T cells,[392] antigen-activated CD8+ T cells[318]).
Biologic activities	
In vitro	Binds SLC (K_d = 0.1–10 nmol/L[311,312]) and MIP-3β (K_d = 0.1–10 nmol/L[312]); engagement of CCR7 by SLC or MIP-3β induces intracellular Ca^{2+} mobilization[311,312]; activation/phosphorylation of MAPK (p42/44)[312] and phosphorylation of p125FAK[312]; engagement of CCR7 by MIP-3β leads to activation of G_{ai}, G_{as}, and G_{as} G proteins in NK cells.[394]
In vivo	Expression pattern correlated with CTL trafficking during an antiviral response[318] and with T-cell trafficking during an inflammatory response.[476] CCR7 (–/–) mice exhibit severely impaired antibody responses, complete lack of responses to induced contact sensitivity or DTH reactions, lack of naïve T-cell and DC colonization in secondary lymphoid organs, an expansion of T cells in the blood and BM, and impaired migration of activated DCs to LNs.[477]
Pathologic association(s)	Adult T-cell leukemia,[478] asthma.[479]
Genbank source (gene)	L31584 (h).
Gene coding region (kbp)	2.2 (h).
Chromosomal location	17q12-q21.2 (h).[472]
Exons	3 (h).[472]
Introns	2 (h).[472]
Natural mutations/polymorphisms	Not reported.
Genbank source (RNA)	NM_001838 (h), NM_007719 (m).
Size of RNA (kbp)	2.1 (h, m).
RNA splice variants	Not reported.

CC CHEMOKINE RECEPTORS

Chemokine (CC) Receptor-8 (CCR8)

Other names	ChemR1,[381] CY6, chemokine receptor–like-1, CMKBR8, chemokine β receptor–like-2, CKR8, GPCR-CY6, I-309 receptor, small inducible cytokine 3 receptor-2 (Scya3r2), TCA-3 receptor, TER1.
Similar proteins	mCCR8 (71%),[19] hCCR4 (43%),[381] hCCR5 (40%), hCCR1 (40%),[381] hCCR2B (39%).
Genbank source	NP_005201 (h), NP_031746 (m).
Size of mature protein (Kd)	40.8 (h), 40.0 (m).
Amino acids in mature protein	355 (h), 353 (m).
Stable form(s)	Monomer.
Glycosylation sites	0 N (h), 1 N (m).
Disulfide bonds	1 (h, m).
3D structure	Seven transmembrane regions.
Mature protein variants	Not reported.
Tissue and cellular expression	Highly expressed in colon,[466] spleen,[466] and thymus.[19,480] Specific cell types include B cells, immature DCs, Mφs,[480] monocytes,[22] neurons,[481] activated T cells (T_H2),[23,442,482] γ/δ T cells,[121] and thymocytes.
Regulation of expression	
Up	Anti-CD3 (T cells,[442] memory T cells[392]).
Down	Anti-CD3 (γ/δ T cells[121]).
Biologic activities	
In vitro	Binds I-309 (K_d = 0.1–2 nmol/L[23,483]) and possibly TARC and MIP-1β[484,485]; binds MCP-3 (K_d = 80 nmol/L)[483] with low affinity; binds vMIP-1 (K_d = 15 nmol/L),[483,486] vMIP-II, vMCC-1, and vMC148R[483,487,488] with high affinity; binds vMIP-III (K_d = 250 nmol/L)[483] and vCXC1 with low affinity; coreceptor for T cell-tropic, M-tropic, dual tropic, and brain cell–tropic strains of HIV[481,489]; engagement of CCR8 by I-309 or vMIP-1 induces intracellular Ca^{2+} mobilization in CCR8–transfected cells.[23,486]
In vivo	Not reported.
Pathologic association(s)	Not reported.
Genbank source (gene)	Z79782 (h), AF001277 (m).
Gene coding region (kbp)	2.6 (h),[490] 1.7 (m).[482]
Chromosomal location	3p22 (h),[23] 9 (m).[482]
Exons	1 (m).[491]
Introns	Not reported.
Natural mutations/polymorphisms	Not reported.
Genbank source (RNA)	NM_005201 (h), NM_007720 (m).
Size of RNA (kbp)	1.4/4.0 (h),[23] 1.1 (m).
RNA splice variants	Not reported.

CC CHEMOKINE RECEPTORS

Chemokine (CC) Receptor-9 (CCR9)

Other names	GPCR-9-6, GPCR28, HEK293.
Similar proteins	mCCR9 (86%), hCCR7 (39%), hCCR6 (35%), hCCR5 (35%), hCCR1 (33%), hTYMSTR (32%).
Genbank source	NP_006632 (h), CAB43480 (m).
Size of mature protein (Kd)	40.7 (h).
Amino acids in mature protein	CCR9A 369 (h, m).[367]
Stable form(s)	Monomer.
Glycosylation sites	1 N (h).
Disulfide bonds	1 (h).
3D structure	Seven transmembrane regions.
Mature protein variants	Two splice variants, CCR9A and CCR9B (h).[492]
Tissue and cellular expression	Highly expressed in thymus,[365] lower levels are expressed in LNs, small intestine, and spleen.[369] Specific cell types include B cells, subsets of peripheral blood memory CD4+ T cells and CD8+ T cells associated with mucosal homing, the majority of CD4+/CD8,+ CD4+ and CD8+, and 50% of CD4−/CD8− thymocytes.[368]
Regulation of expression	
Up	Anti-CD3 (thymocytes[369]).
Down	Anti-CD3 (T cells[368]).
Biologic activities	
In vitro	Binds TECK.[366,367]
In vivo	Not reported.
Pathologic association(s)	Not reported.
Genbank source (gene)	U45982 (h).
Gene coding region (kbp)	2.6 (h).
Chromosomal location	3p21.3-p22 (h), 9F1-F4 (m).[365]
Exons	2 (m).[369]
Introns	Not reported.
Natural mutations/polymorphisms	Not reported.
Genbank source (RNA)	NM_006641 (h), AJ123336 (m).
Size of RNA (kbp)	1.2 (h), 1.6/3.1 (m).[365]
RNA splice variants	2 (h).[492]

CC CHEMOKINE RECEPTORS

Chemokine (CC) Receptor-10 (CCR10)

Other names	Chemokine binding protein-2, CMKBR9, D6,[124] the chemokine receptor formerly known as CCR9.
Similar proteins	mCCR10 (71%), rCCR10 (72%),[62] hCCR4.
Genbank source	NP_001287 (h), 4502911 (m), AAB61572 (r).
Size of mature protein (Kd)	Not reported.
Amino acids in mature protein	384 (h, m),[124] 382 (r).
Stable form(s)	Monomer.
Glycosylation sites	1 N (h).[125]
Disulfide bonds	1 (h).
3D structure	Seven transmembrane regions.
Mature protein variants	Not reported.
Tissue and cellular expression	Highly expressed in brain, heart, kidney, liver, muscle, ovary, placenta, spleen,[62] and thymus.[124,125,220] Specific cell types include neurons.[354]
Regulation of expression	
Up	Not reported.
Down	Not reported.
Biologic activities	
In vitro	Binds EOT-1 (K_d = 46 nmol/L),[125] HCC-1 (K_d = 27 nmol/L),[125] MIP-1α (K_d = 0.1–64 nmol/L),[124,125] MIP-1β (K_d = 0.4–1.7 nmol/L),[62,124,125] MCP-1 (K_d = 0.4–16 nmol/L),[62,124,125,220] MCP-2 (K_d = 0.8 nmol/L),[125] MCP-3 (K_d = 1 nmol/L),[125,220] MCP-4 (K_d = 6–8 nmol/L),[125,220] mMCP-5,[124] and RANTES (K_d = 4–5 nmol/L)[62,125,220]; engagement of mCCR10 by mMIP-1α,[124] mMIP-1β (0.8 nmol/L),[124] or mRANTES induces intracellular Ca^{2+} mobilization in mCCR10–transfected cells; engagement of hCCR10 by human chemokines has no effect on intracellular Ca^{2+} mobilization in hCCR10–transfected cells.
In vivo	Not reported.
Pathologic association(s)	Not reported.
Genbank source (gene)	Not reported.
Gene coding region (kbp)	Not reported.
Chromosomal location	3p21.32-p21.31 (h).[220]
Exons	Not reported.
Introns	Not reported.
Natural mutations/polymorphisms	Not reported.
Genbank source (RNA)	NM_001296 (h), Y12879 (m), RNU92803 (r).
Size of RNA (kbp)	4.0/6.0 (h),[125] 3.2 (m),[124] 1.3 (r).[62]
RNA splice variants	Not reported.

CXC CHEMOKINES

Growth-Related Oncogene-α (GRO-α)

Systematic name	CXCL1.
Other names	CINC-1 (r), fibroblast secretory protein (FSP), GRO1 oncogene, KC (m), MGSA-α, N51 (m), NAP-3, SCYB1.
Similar proteins	mKC, rCINC-1, hENA-78 (52%),[493] hGCP-2 (44%), hIL-8 (42%), hGRO-1β (90%).[494]
Genbank source	NP_001502 (h), NP_032202 (m), P14095 (r).
Amino acids in precursor protein	107 (h), 96 (m, r).
Size of mature protein (Kd)	8.0 (h, m), 7.8 (r).
Amino acids in mature protein	73 (h), 72 (m, r).
Stable form(s)	Monomer/dimer (h).
Glycosylation sites	0 N (h, m, r).
Disulfide bonds	2 (h, m, r).
3D structure	Six-stranded β sheet, two COOH terminus α helices, ELR+.[495]
Mature protein variants	Several N-terminal truncated variants (h).[496]
Tissue and cellular expression	Highly expressed in bronchial epithelium.[497] Relatively high levels are found in breast milk[40] and in normal human serum.[498] Specific cell types include chondrocytes,[117] ECs, epithelial cells, fibroblasts, melanoma cells,[499] monocytes, Mφs, and neutrophils.[500]
Regulation of expression	
Up	IL-1β (ECs,[493] HUVECs,[501] retinal pigment epithelial cells[502]), LPS (neutrophils[500]), oxidized LDL (HUVECs[45]), TNF-α (ECs,[58] epithelial cells,[497] neutrophils[500]).
Down	IL-10 (activated neutrophils[500]).
Biologic activities	
In vitro	Binds to CXCR2 (K_d = 0.5 nmol/L),[503] DARC, and vORF-74[504]; chemoattractant for ECs,[505] neutrophils,[506] mast cells[507]; induces intracellular Ca^{2+} mobilization in mast cells,[507] neutrophils, and CXCR2–transfected cells[503,508]; activates Akt/PKB in neutrophils or CXCR1–transfected cells[184]; stimulates the growth of melanoma cells.[499]
In vivo	Angiogenic[509]; chemoattractant for neutrophils[510,511]; stimulates the growth of melanoma cells.[512]
Pathologic association(s)	Colon cancer,[513] contact hypersensitivity,[511] glomerulonephritis,[514] *Helicobacter pylori* infection,[515] melanoma,[499] osteoarthritis,[117] prostate cancer,[516] psoriasis,[517] rheumatoid arthritis,[117] stroke,[518] squamous cell carcinoma, spinal cord injury,[105] ulcerative colitis.[519]
Genbank source (gene)	X54489 (h), U20634 (m), D11445 (r).
Gene coding region (kbp)	1.8 (h), 2.5 (r).
Chromosomal location	4q21[520] (h), 5:51.00 cM (m).[521]
Exons	4 (h, r).[522]
Introns	3 (h, r).[522]
Natural mutations/polymorphisms	One SNP (h). Mouse GRO-α is highly polymorphic.[523]
Genbank source (RNA)	NM_001511 (h), NM_008176 (m), D11444 (r).
Size of RNA (kbp)	1.1 (h), 0.9 (m), 0.9 (r).
RNA splice variants	Not reported.

CXC CHEMOKINES

Growth-Related Oncogene-β (GRO-β)

Systematic name	CXCL2.
Other names	CINC-2α, CINC-3, MGSA-β, GRO-2, MIP-2,[524] MIP-2α,[524] SCYB2.
Similar proteins	mMIP-2 (62%), rGRO-β, hGRO-α (90%),[494] hIL-8 (41%).
Genbank source	NP_002080 (h), CAA37807 (m), P30348 (r).
Amino acids in precursor protein	107 (h), 100 (m, r).
Size of mature protein (Kd)	8.0 (h), 6.0 (m), 7.7 (r).
Amino acids in mature protein	73 (h, m), 69 (r).
Stable form(s)	Monomer/dimer (h).
Glycosylation sites	0 N (h, m, r).
Disulfide bonds	2 (h, m, r).
3D structure	ELR⁺.
Mature protein variants	Not reported.
Tissue and cellular expression	Specific cell types include ECs, fibroblasts, epithelial cells, Mφs, monocytes, neutrophils, tumor cells.
Regulation of expression	
Up	LPS (epithelial cells[525]), IL-1β (epithelial cells,[525] HUVECs[501], retinal pigment epithelial cells[502]); MALP-2 (Mφs[52]), oxidized LDL (HUVECs[45]).
Down	Not reported.
Biologic activities	
In vitro	Binds to CXCR2 (K_d = 0.8 nmol/L)[503] and vORF-74[504]; chemoattractant for ECs[505] and neutrophils; induces intracellular Ca²⁺ mobilization in neutrophils and CXCR2–transfected cells.[503]
In vivo	Angiogenic,[509] antitumor.[509]
Pathologic association(s)	Acetaminophen-induced liver injury,[526] melanoma.[499]
Genbank source (gene)	X54489 (h).
Gene coding region (kbp)	1.8 (h).
Chromosomal location	4q21 (h),[527] 5:51.00 cM (m).
Exons	4 (h).
Introns	3 (h).
Natural mutations/polymorphisms	Two SNPs.
Genbank source (RNA)	NM_002089 (h), X53798 (m), U45965 (r).
Size of RNA (kbp)	1.1 (h), 1.1 (m), 1.1 (r).
RNA splice variants	Not reported.

CXC CHEMOKINES

Growth-Related Oncogene-γ (GRO-γ)

Systematic name	CXCL3.
Other names	CINC-2-β (r), GRO-3, MIP-2β,[524] SCYB3.
Similar proteins	hGRO-α (86%),[494] hIL-8 (40%).
Genbank source	NP_002081 (h), Q10746 (r).
Amino acids in precursor protein	106 (h), 100 (r).
Size of mature protein (Kd)	8.0 (h).
Amino acids in mature protein	68 (h, r).
Stable form(s)	Monomer/dimer (h).
Glycosylation sites	0 N (h, r).
Disulfide bonds	2 (h, r).
3D structure	ELR+.
Mature protein variants	Several N-terminal truncated variants (h).[496]
Tissue and cellular expression	Highly expressed in bronchial epithelium[497] and colon.[513] Specific cell types include ECs, fibroblasts, epithelial cells, monocytes, Mφs, neutrophils, and tumor cells.
Regulation of expression	
Up	IL-1β (keratinocytes,[46] retinal pigment epithelial cells[502]), TNF-α (epithelial cells[497]).
Down	Not reported.
Biologic activities	
In vitro	Binds to CXCR2 (K_d = 0.7 nmol/L)[503] and vORF-74[504]; chemoattractant for ECs[505] and neutrophils; induces intracellular Ca^{2+} mobilization in neutrophils and CXCR2–transfected cells.[503]
In vivo	Angiogenic.[506,528]
Pathologic association(s)	Melanoma.[499]
Genbank source (gene)	X54489 (h).
Gene coding region (kbp)	1.8 (h).
Chromosomal location	4q21 (h),[527] 5:51.00 cM (m).
Exons	4 (h).
Introns	3 (h).
Natural mutations/polymorphisms	Not reported.
Genbank source (RNA)	NM_002081 (h).
Size of RNA (kbp)	1.1 (h).
RNA splice variants	Not reported.

CXC CHEMOKINES

Platelet Factor-4 (PF-4)

Systematic name	CXCL4.
Other names	CXCL4V1, endothelial cell growth inhibitor, heparin-neutralizing protein, megakaryo-cyte-stimulatory-factor, oncostatin A, PF-4alt (m), PF-4var1, SCYB4.
Similar proteins	hIL-8 (84%), hIP-10 (30%).
Genbank source	NP_002695 (h), BAA75660 (m), P06765 (r).
Amino acids in precursor protein	128 (h), 132 (m, r).[529,530]
Size of mature protein (Kd)	PF-4 and PF-4alt (h).
Amino acids in mature protein	70 (h), 76 (r).
Stable form(s)	Monomer/dimer/tetramer (h).
Glycosylation sites	0 N (h).
Disulfide bonds	2 (h).
3D structure	Three antiparallel β sheets, COOH terminal α helix, ELR−.[531]
Mature protein variants	PF-4 and PFalt (h).
Tissue and cellular expression	Formed by processing of PBP. Cell types include megakaryocytes and platelets.
Regulation of expression	
Up	Ets-1 (megakaryocytes[532]), GATA-1 (megakaryocytes[532]), IL-6 (megakaryocytes[533]), thrombin (platelets).
Down	Not reported.
Biologic activities	
In vitro	Binds to cell surface–bound chondroitin sulfate[534] and to heparin sulfate[126]; chemoat-tractant for fibroblasts[535]; weak chemoattractant for IL-5–stimulated eosino-phils,[536,537] monocytes,[538] IgE-stimulated mast cells,[182] and neutrophils[538]; promotes adherence of eosinophils and neutrophils to ECs[539] and increases ICAM-1 expression on ECs[540]; inhibits VEGF and fibroblast growth factor binding to receptors[541] and inhibits the mitogenic activity of VEGF[541]; stimulates fibroblast proliferation and inhibits EC cell, mesangial cell, and myoblast proliferation[542–545]; inhibits human megakaryocyte colony formation[546]; supports the survival of myeloid progenitors and protects them from apoptosis induced by cytotoxic drugs[547,548]; induces the dif-ferentiation of monocytes into Mϕs; induces basophil and mast cell release of histamine[69,549] and TNF-α–primed neutrophil degranulation[550]; enhances primary T- and B-cell immune response in normal and immunosuppressed mice[551]; mediates cell-contact–dependent CD8+ T-cell–mediated B-cell suppression[552]; enhances LPS-induced tissue factor activity in monocytes[553]; up-regulates CD86 expression on Mϕs[554]; induces TNF-α production from monocytes[554]; prevents spontaneous mono-cyte apoptosis.[554]
In vivo	Anorexic[81]; angiostatic[555,556]; antitumor[542,557]; chemoattractant for monocytes and neu-trophils; induces fibrosis; decreases bone resorption; prevents induction of low-dose tolerance to pneumococcal polysaccharides.[558]
Pathologic association(s)	Atopic dermatitis,[529] Crohn's disease,[559] heparin-induced thrombocytopenia,[560] ischemic heart disease, septicemia,[561] wound healing.
Genbank source (gene)	M25897 (h), M15254 (r).
Gene coding region (kbp)	1.0 (h), 1.7 (r).
Chromosomal location	4q12-21 (h),[562] 14 (r).[563]
Exons	3 (h, r).[530,564]
Introns	2 (h, r).[530,564]
Natural mutations/polymorphisms	One SNP (h).[565]
Genbank source (RNA)	NM_002704 (h), AB017491 (m).
Size of RNA (kbp)	0.4 (h), 0.5 (m), 0.8 (r).
RNA splice variants	Not reported.

CXC CHEMOKINES

Epithelial Neutrophil-Activating Peptide-78 (ENA-78)

Systematic name	CXCL5.
Other names	Alveolar macrophage chemotactic factor-2, LIX (m, r; also see CXCL6), SCYB5.
Similar proteins	hGCP-2 (77%), NAP-2 (53%), GRO-α (52%), lungkine (H) (35%), hIL-8 (34%).
Genbank source	NP_002985 (h).
Amino acids in precursor protein	114 (h), (m, r; see GCP-2).
Size of mature protein (Kd)	8.4 (h).[493]
Amino acids in mature protein	78 (h).
Stable form(s)	Monomer/dimer.
Glycosylation sites	0 N (h).
Disulfide bonds	2 (h).
3D structure	ELR+.
Mature protein variants	Several N-terminal truncated variants (h).[496]
Tissue and cellular expression	Specific cell types include ECs,[566] epithelial cells,[566] fibroblasts,[566] Mϕs, mesothelial cells,[566] monocytes,[566] neutrophils,[566] platelets,[176] and tumor cell lines.[567]
Regulation of expression	
Up	fMLP (monocytes), IL-1β (ECs,[493] fibroblasts, monocytes, smooth muscle cells), LPS (monocytes, neutrophils), RelA/NF-κB,[568] TNF-α (ECs,[493] monocytes, smooth muscle cells).
Down	Glucocorticoids (monocytes[493]), IFN-α (monocytes[569]), IFN-γ (monocytes[569]).
Biologic activities	
In vitro	Binds to CXCR2 (K_d = 1 nmol/L)[503] and vORF-74[504]; chemoattractant for ECs[505] and neutrophils; induces intracellular Ca^{2+} mobilization in neutrophil and CXCR2–transfected cells.[508]
In vivo	Prevents injury and mortality in a model of acetaminophen-induced liver injury.[526]
Pathologic association(s)	Adult respiratory distress syndrome,[493] asthma, chronic pancreatitis,[493] Crohn's disease,[493] *Helicobacter pylori* infection,[570] rheumatoid arthritis,[493] spinal cord injury,[105] ulcerative colitis.[493]
Genbank source (gene)	Not reported.
Gene coding region (kbp)	Not reported.
Chromosomal location	4q13-q21 (h),[527] 5:53.0 cM (m).
Exons	4 (h).[493]
Introns	3 (h).[493]
Natural mutations/polymorphisms	Not reported.
Genbank source (RNA)	NM_002994 (h).
Size of RNA (kbp)	1.2 (h).
RNA splice variants	Not reported.

CXC CHEMOKINES

Granulocyte Chemotactic Protein-2 (GCP-2)

Systematic name	CXCL6.
Other names	CKα-3, LIX (m, r; also see CXCL5), SCYB6.
Similar proteins	hENA-78 (77%),[493] hGRO-α (44%), hNAP-2 (44%), hIL-8 (30%).
Genbank source	NP_002984 (h), NP_033167 (m), P97885 (r).
Amino acids in precursor protein	114 (h); LIX, 132 (m), 130 (r).
Size of mature protein (Kd)	6.0/8.1 (h).
Amino acids in mature protein	77 (h); LIX, 92 (m), 93 (r).
Stable form(s)	Monomer.
Glycosylation sites	0 N (h).
Disulfide bonds	2 (h, m, r).
3D structure	ELR+.
Mature protein variants	Four (67–, 70–, 73–, and 75–amino acid forms) (h).[506]
Tissue and cellular expression	Highly expressed in heart, liver, lung, and pancreas.[506] Specific cell types include amnion cells, carcinoma cells, fibroblasts,[567] and osteosarcoma cells.[571]
Regulation of expression	
Up	IL-1β (fibroblasts,[506] osteosarcoma cells[506]), LPS, dsRNA (fibroblasts[506]), PMA (osteosarcoma cells[506]), TNF-α.
Down	Dexamethasone, IFN-γ (fibroblasts[567]).
Biologic activities	
In vitro	Binds to CXCR1[508] and CXCR2[508]; chemoattractant for ECs[505] and neutrophils[506]; induces intracellular Ca^{2+} mobilization in neutrophils[506] and in CXCR1– and CXCR2–transfected cells.[508,572]
In vivo	Angiogenic[506,528]; chemoattractant for neutrophils[572]; induces plasma leakage.[572]
Pathologic association(s)	Lung cancer,[528] spinal cord injury.[105]
Genbank source (gene)	U83303 (h).
Gene coding region (kbp)	3.5 (h).
Chromosomal location	4q12-q21 (h).[527]
Exons	4 (h).
Introns	3 (h).
Natural mutations/polymorphisms	Not reported.
Genbank source (RNA)	NM_002993 (h), NM_009141 (m), U90448 (r).
Size of RNA (kbp)	1.6 (h), 1.5 (m).
RNA splice variants	Not reported.

CXC CHEMOKINES

β-Thromboglobulin (β-TG)

Systematic name	CXCL7.
Other names	SCYB7.
Similar proteins	hIP-10 (30%).
Genbank source	NP_002695 (h).
Amino acids in precursor protein	128 PPBP (h), 94 PBP (h).
Size of mature protein (Kd)	8.8 (h).
Amino acids in mature protein	81 (h).
Stable form(s)	Monomer (h).
Glycosylation sites	0 N (h).
Disulfide bonds	2 (h).[573]
3D structure	Not reported.
Mature protein variants	Not reported.
Tissue and cellular expression	Formed by processing of PBP or connective tissue–activating peptide-III. Specific cell types include platelets (stored in α-granules).
Regulation of expression	
Up	Not reported.
Down	Not reported.
Biologic activities	
In vitro	Chemoattractant for fibroblasts[535]; weak chemoattractant for neutrophils; stimulates mitogenesis of fibroblasts[574]; stimulates extracellular matrix and plasminogen activator synthesis by fibroblasts[574]; inhibits the maturation of human megakaryocytes.[575]
In vivo	Distinct activities from other PBP-derived proteins.[576]
Pathologic association(s)	Ischemic heart disease, schistosomiasis, thromboembolic risk.
Genbank source (gene)	Not reported.
Gene coding region (kbp)	1.1 (h).
Chromosomal location	4q12-q13 (h).[527]
Exons	3 (h).
Introns	2 (h).
Natural mutations/polymorphisms	Described gene duplication of β-TG gene, designated β-TG2.
Genbank source (RNA)	NM_002704 (h).
Size of RNA (kbp)	0.8 (h).
RNA splice variants	Not reported.

CXC CHEMOKINES

Connective Tissue–Activating Peptide-III (CTAP-III)

Systematic name	CXCL7.
Other names	Histamine-releasing factor, low-affinity platelet factor-4, SCYB7.
Similar proteins	PF-4.
Genbank source	NP_002695 (h).
Amino acids in precursor protein	128 PPBP (h), 94 PBP (h).
Size of mature protein (Kd)	8.4 (h).
Amino acids in mature protein	85 (h).
Stable form(s)	Monomer/dimer/tetramer (h).[573]
Glycosylation sites	0 N (h).
Disulfide bonds	2 (h).[573]
3D structure	Not reported.
Mature protein variants	Multiple variants described.[574]
Tissue and cellular expression	Formed by processing of PBP. Found in relatively high amounts in plasma and in synovial fluid. Specific cell types include platelets.[574]
Regulation of expression	
Up	Not reported.
Down	Not reported.
Biologic activities	
In vitro	Chemoattractant for ECs,[505] fibroblasts, and monocytes; weak chemoattractant for neutrophils[577]; induces synthesis and secretion of plasminogen activator from fibroblasts[578]; mitogenic for fibroblasts; induces the synthesis and secretion of hyaluronic acid, glycosaminoglycans, proteoglycan core protein, plasminogen activator, and PGE_2; induces histamine in basophils[579]; stimulates 2-deoxy-glucose uptake in cultures of human synovial cells, chondrocytes, and dermal fibroblasts[580]; inhibits human megakaryocyte colony formation.[546]
In vivo	Chemoattractant for monocytes.[581]
Pathologic association(s)	Rheumatoid arthritis.[574]
Genbank source (gene)	Not reported.
Gene coding region (kbp)	1.1 (h).
Chromosomal location	4q12-q13 (h).[562]
Exons	3 (h).
Introns	2 (h).
Natural mutations/polymorphisms	Not reported.
Genbank source (RNA)	NM_002704 (h).
Size of RNA (kbp)	0.8 (h).
RNA splice variants	Not reported.

CXC CHEMOKINES

Neutrophil-Activating Peptide-2 (NAP-2)

Systematic name	CXCL7.
Other names	SCYB7.
Similar proteins	hENA-78 (53%),[493] hIL-8 (48%), hGCP (44%).
Genbank source	NP_002695 (h).
Amino acids in precursor protein	128 PPBP (h), 94 PBP (h).
Size of mature protein (Kd)	7.8 (h).
Amino acids in mature protein	70 (h).
Stable form(s)	Monomer/dimer/tetramer (h).[582]
Glycosylation sites	0 N (h).
Disulfide bonds	2 (h).[573]
3D structure	Three antiparallel β sheets, COOH terminal α helix, ELR$^+$ (h).[582]
Mature protein variants	Two (h).[583]
Tissue and cellular expression	Formed by processing of PBP or connective tissue–activating peptide-III by neutrophil cathepsin G.[584] Cell types include ECs[585] and platelets.
Regulation of expression	
Up	LPS (ECs[585]), serum (platelets[583]), thrombin (platelets[583]).
Down	Not reported.
Biologic activities	
In vitro	Binds to CXCR2 (K_d = 7 nmol/L)[503] and vORF-74[504]; chemoattractant for ECs[505] and neutrophils[577,586]; stimulates the release of histamine and leukotriene B$_4$ from IL-3–treated basophils; induces intracellular Ca^{2+} mobilization in neutrophils and CXCR2–transfected cells[503]; induces elastase release from neutrophils; supports the survival of myeloid progenitor cells.
In vivo	Angiogenic; inhibits megakaryocytopoiesis; induces neutrophil infiltration.[581]
Pathologic association(s)	Autoantibodies to NAP-2 present in patients with heparin-associated thrombocytopenia.[587]
Genbank source (gene)	Not reported.
Gene coding region (kbp)	1.1 (h).
Chromosomal location	4q12-q13 (h).[562]
Exons	3 (h).
Introns	2 (h).
Natural mutations/polymorphisms	Not reported.
Genbank source (RNA)	NM_002704 (h).
Size of RNA (kbp)	0.8 (h).
RNA splice variants	Not reported.

CXC CHEMOKINES

Interleukin 8 (IL-8)

Systematic name	CXCL8.
Other names	Anionic neutrophil-activating peptide, apoptosis-inducing factor, β-TG-like protein, chemotaxin, fibroblast-derived neutrophil chemotactic factor, GCP-1, lung carcinoma–derived chemotaxin, lymphocyte-derived neutrophil-activating factor, lymphocyte-derived neutrophil-activating peptide, monocyte-derived neutrophil-activating protein, MDNCF, neutrophil-activating factor, NAP-1, neutrophil chemotactic factor, 3-10C, SCYB8.
Similar proteins	hPF-4 (84%), hNAP-2 (48%), hGRO-α (42%), hGRO-β (41%), hGRO-γ (40%), hENA-78 (34%), hGCP-2 (30%), hSDF-1α (30%).
Genbank source	AAA59158 (h), N/A (m, r).
Amino acids in precursor protein	99 (h); N/A (m, r).[588]
Size of mature protein (Kd)	8.0 (h).
Amino acids in mature protein	77, 72, 71, 69 (h).[589]
Stable form(s)	Monomer/dimer.[13]
Glycosylation sites	0 N (h).
Disulfide bonds	2 (h).
3D structure	Three antiparallel β sheets, COOH terminal α helix, ELR+.[590]
Mature protein variants	At least four forms (h).[589]
Tissue and cellular expression	Relatively high levels are found in breast milk.[40] Specific cell types include amnion cells, astrocytes,[591] carcinoma cell lines, chondrocytes,[117] ECs,[592] eosinophils,[593] epithelial cells, fibroblasts, hepatocytes,[594] keratinocytes, Mφs, mast cells, mesangial cells,[595] mesothelial cells, monocytes, NK cells,[596] neutrophils,[597] sarcoma cell lines, smooth muscle cells, stromal cells, synovial cells, T cells.[598,599]
Regulation of expression	
Up	Anti-CD16 + IL-2 (NK cells[596]), cholesterol (ECs[600]), conA (T cells[601]), eosinophil major basic protein (neutrophils[602]), EOT-1 (thymocytes[164]), GM-CSF (neutrophils[603]), hypoxia (ECs,[604] glioblastoma cells,[605,606] ovarian carcinoma cells,[607] pancreatic carcinoma cells[608]), IFN-γ + TNF-α (keratinocytes[609]), IL-1β (astrocytes,[591] fibroblasts,[610] hepatocytes,[594] HUVECs,[501] keratinocytes[46]), IL-7 (monocytes[611]), IL-17 (glial cells[612]), oxidized LDL (HUVECs[45]), leukoregulin (fibroblasts[613]), LPS (fibroblasts,[614] monocytes,[615] neutrophils[118]), PHA (T cells[598,599]), PMA (epithelial cells[616]), dsRNA (fibroblasts[610]), TNF-α (astrocytes,[57,591] hepatocytes[594]).
Down	Glucocorticoids (ECs,[617,618] monocytes[493]), IFN-α (monocytes,[569] PBMCs[603]), IFN-β (fibroblasts[619]), IFN-γ (monocytes[569]), IL-10 (microglia,[620] neutrophils[118]).
Biologic activities	
In vitro	Binds CXCR1 (K_d = 1.3 nmol/L), CXCR2 (K_d = 0.4–2.5 nmol/L),[503] DARC, vECRF-3, vORF-74,[621] and heparin sulfate (K_d = 0.4–2.6 mmol/L)[126]; chemoattractant for basophils, B cells,[622] ECs,[505] activated eosinophils,[623] fibroblasts, keratinocytes, mast cells,[507] smooth muscle cells,[624] neutrophils, activated NK cells,[625] and T cells[626,627]; inhibits hemopoietic progenitor proliferation and colony formation; induces actin polymerization in neutrophils; stimulates the release of elastase, gelatinase B, β-glucuronidase, lactoferrin, myeloperoxidase, and vitamin B_{12}–binding protein from neutrophils; induces intracellular Ca^{2+} mobilization in basophils, eosinophils, mast cells,[507] neutrophils,[628] and CXCR1– and CXCR2–transfected cells[508]; induces respiratory burst in neutrophils via CXCR1; stimulates the release of peroxidase from eosinophils, primes neutrophils for responses to fMLP, PMA, and platelet activating factor; up-regulates expression of CD11b/CD18, CD11c/CD18, CD35, and fMLP receptor on neutrophils; promotes basophil, monocyte, and neutrophil adhesion to cytokine-stimulated EC monolayers; induces adhesion of monocytes to ECs under flow conditions[73]; stimulates the release of histamine and leukotriene B_4 from IL-3–treated basophils; stimulates smooth muscle cells to proliferate and release PGE_2[624]; stimulates proliferation of keratinocytes; activates G_{a14}, G_{a15}, or G_{a16} and G_i proteins[629] and stimulates guanine nucleotide exchange to Rho; activates/induces phosphorylation of Akt/PKB in neutrophils or CXCR1–transfected cells[184]; stimulates the growth of neurons.[630]

(continued)

CXC CHEMOKINES

Interleukin 8 (IL-8) (*Continued*)

In vivo	Anorexic[81]; angiogenic[631]; chemoattractant for neutrophils[632]; eosinophils,[633] and T cells[633]; induces leukopenia and neutrophilia; induces plasma leakage[634]; induces release of hemopoietic progenitor cells from BM.
Pathologic association(s)	Acute glomerulonephritis, adult respiratory distress syndrome, alcohol-induced hepatitis, asthma,[635] atherosclerosis,[600,636] atopic dermatitis,[149] bacteremia, bladder inflammation, bronchial carcinoma, chronic pancreatitis,[493] Crohn's disease,[493] contact dermatitis, cutaneous T-cell lymphoma,[637] cystic fibrosis,[638] emphysema,[635] gastric carcinoma,[639] gastritis, gingivitis, glioblastoma,[606] gouty arthritis, hepatocellular carcinoma,[152] *Helicobacter pylori* infection,[640] Kawasaki's disease,[169] lymphoma, meningococcal infections, mycobacterial infections, nasal polyps, non–small cell lung cancer,[641] ocular inflammation, osteoarthritis,[117] ovarian carcinoma,[642] palmoplantar pustulosis, pancreatitis, parturition, peritonitis, pertussis, pregnancy, prostate cancer,[516] psoriasis,[643] pulmonary reperfusion injury, pulmonary fibrosis, red cell incompatibility, relapsing fever, rheumatoid arthritis,[117] sarcoidosis, β-thalassemia, transplant rejection, ulcerative colitis,[106] uremia, uveoretinitis, wound healing.
Genbank source (gene)	M28130 (h).
Gene coding region (kbp)	5.2 (h).
Chromosomal location	4q12-q13 (h).[527]
Exons	4 (h).[644]
Introns	3 (h).[644]
Natural mutations/polymorphisms	Three SNPs identified.[645] Differential expression in diffuse panbronchitis.[646]
Genbank source (RNA)	M17017 (h).
Size of RNA (kbp)	1.6 (h).
RNA splice variants	Not reported.

CXC CHEMOKINES

Monokine Induced by Interferon-γ (Mig)

Systematic name	CXCL9.
Other names	CMK, Humig, m119 (m),[647] SCYB9.
Similar proteins	mMig (69%), hMig (40%), hIP-10 (37%).
Genbank source	NP_002407 (h), NP_032625 (m).
Amino acids in precursor protein	125 (h), 126 (m).
Size of mature protein (Kd)	8.0–14.3 (h).
Amino acids in mature protein	103 (h), 105 (m).
Stable form(s)	Monomer.
Glycosylation sites	0 N/0 O (h).[648]
Disulfide bonds	2 (h, m).
3D structure	ELR⁻.
Mature protein variants	Several ranging from 78 to 103 amino acids generated by COOH terminus processing.[648]
Tissue and cellular expression	Specific cell types include activated monocytes and Mφs[648] and activated neutrophils.[603]
Regulation of expression	
Up	IFN-γ (ECs,[618] fibroblasts,[649] keratinocytes,[649] Mφs,[650] monocytes,[648] THP-1 cells[648]), IFN-γ + IL-1β (ECs[618]), IFN-γ + TNF-α (ECs[618]).
Down	IL-4 (activated neutrophils[603]), IL-10 (activated neutrophils[603]).
Biologic activities	
In vitro	Binds to CXCR3 (K_d = 0.9–4.9 nmol/L)[651,652]; chemoattractant for NK cells,[167] activated T cells,[648] and TILs[648]; inhibits hemopoietic progenitor proliferation and colony formation[653]; induces intracellular Ca^{2+} mobilization in activated T cells and TILs[648]; stimulates the proliferation of mesangial cells.[654]
In vivo	Angiostatic[655]; antitumor[656–659]; antiviral.[660]
Pathologic association(s)	Atherosclerosis,[661] B-cell lymphoma,[662–664] chronic lymphocytic leukemia,[664] contact dermatitis,[665] cutaneous T-cell lymphoma,[666] Epstein-Barr virus infection,[667,668] graft rejection,[669] hemophagocytic syndrome,[151] hepatocellular carcinoma,[152] lichen planus,[99] EAE/MS,[198] non–small cell lung carcinoma,[659] pancreatitis,[670] experimental protozoan infection,[671] experimental viral infection.[671]
Genbank source (gene)	X72755 (h).
Gene coding region (kbp)	Not reported.
Chromosomal location	4q21 (h).[672]
Exons	Not reported.
Introns	Not reported.
Natural mutations/polymorphisms	Two SNPs.
Genbank source (RNA)	NM_002416 (h), NM_008599 (m).
Size of RNA (kbp)	2.5 (h), 1.6 (m).[647]
RNA splice variants	Several (h).[648]

CXC CHEMOKINES

Interferon-γ Inducible Protein 10 kd (IP-10)

Systematic name	CXCL10.
Other names	crg-2 (m),[673] mob-1 (r),[674] C7 (m),[675] Ifi10, pIFN-γ-31,[676] SCYB10.
Similar proteins	mIP-10 (60%),[677] rIP-10 (70%),[677] hI-TAC (40%), hMig (37%), hPF-4 (30%), hβ-TG (30%)
Genbank source	NP_001556 (h), AAA75249 (m), AAC52811 (r).
Amino acids in precursor protein	98 (h, m, r).[675]
Size of mature protein (Kd)	8.6/10.0 (h),[677] 8.7 (m).
Amino acids in mature protein	77 (h, m, r).[675]
Stable form(s)	Monomer.
Glycosylation sites	0 N (h, m, r).
Disulfide bonds	2 (h, m, r).
3D structure	ELR-.[678]
Mature protein variants	Four variants (h).[571]
Tissue and cellular expression	Highly expressed in kidney, liver, LNs, spleen, and thymus.[677] Specific cell types include amnion cells, astrocytes, carcinomas, bronchial ECs,[618] fibroblasts, hepatocytes, keratinocytes,[679,680] Mφs, monocytes, neutrophils,[603] sarcomas, splenic stromal cells, synovial cells, T cells, thymic stromal cells, and thymocytes.
Regulation of expression	
Up	Anti-CD3 (T cells), activator protein-1,[681] CD40 ligand (IFN-γ–activated ECs[661]), IFN-α (neutrophils,[603] PBMCs[603]), IFN-γ (astrocytes,[682] ECs,[618] fibroblasts,[676] keratinocytes,[679] mesangial cells,[683] neutrophils[684]), IL-1β (ECs,[618] IFN-γ–activated ECs,[661] fibroblasts,[685] synovial cells[685]), LPS (astrocytes,[686] DCs,[49] mesangial cells,[683] microglia,[686] synovial cells[685]), platelet-derived growth factor (Mφs),[687] RelA/NF-κB,[688] dsRNA (fibroblasts[689]), STAT-1,[681] TNF-α (astrocytes,[57] ECs[618] IFN-γ–activated ECs[661]).
Down	IL-4 (Mφs,[690] monocytes,[690] activated neutrophils[603]), IL-10 (activated neutrophils[603]), nitric oxide (IFN-γ–activated ECs[661]).
Biologic activities	
In vitro	Binds to CXCR3 (K_d = 0.04–0.3 nmol/L),[651,652] vORF-74,[504] and heparin sulfate[126]; chemoattractant for monocytes,[167] NK cells,[167,691] smooth muscle cells,[692] and activated T cells[167]; mitogen for smooth muscle cells[692]; inhibits EC proliferation[693]; inhibits hemopoietic progenitor proliferation and colony formation[694]; induces intracellular Ca^{2+} mobilization in NK cells[691]; induces T-cell adhesion to ICAM-1 and VCAM-1[695]; increases NK cell activity[167]; inhibits constitutive signaling of vORF-74 receptor.[696]
In vivo	Chemoattractant for monocytes,[697] neutrophils, and T cells[697]; anorexic[81]; angiostatic[693]; antitumor[657,658,663,698]; antiviral.[660]
Pathologic association(s)	Atherosclerosis,[661] adult respiratory distress syndrome,[699] autoimmune diabetes,[195] DTH,[700] contact dermatitis,[665] psoriasis,[700] EAE/MS,[150,198] colorectal cancer,[701] cutaneous T-cell lymphoma,[666] glomerular nephritis,[702] hemophagocytic syndrome,[151] leprosy,[700] lichen planus,[99] restenosis,[692] sarcoidosis,[703] spinal cord injury,[105] tuberculosis,[618] uveoretinitis, ulcerative colitis,[106] wound healing,[107] viral meningitis.[704]
Genbank source (gene)	L07417 (m).
Gene coding region (kbp)	4.2 (m).
Chromosomal location	4q21 (h).[527]
Exons	4 (h, m).[679,705]
Introns	3 (h),[679] 4 (m).[705]
Natural mutations/polymorphisms	Two SNPs.[677]
Genbank source (RNA)	NM_001565 (h), M33266 (m), U22520 (r).
Size of RNA (kbp)	1.2 (h), 1.1 (m), 1.1 (r).
RNA splice variants	Not reported.

CXC CHEMOKINES

Interferon-Inducible T-Cell α Chemoattractant (I-TAC)

Systematic name	CXCL11.
Other names	IP-9,[706] β-R1,[707] H174,[708] SCYB9B, SCYB11.
Similar proteins	IP-10 (40%), hMig (40%).
Genbank source	NP_005400 (h).
Amino acids in precursor protein	94 (h).[709]
Size of mature protein (Kd)	8.3 (h).
Amino acids in mature protein	72 (h).
Stable form(s)	Monomer.
Glycosylation sites	0 N (h).
Disulfide bonds	2 (h).
3D structure	ELR⁻.[708]
Mature protein variants	Not reported.
Tissue and cellular expression	Highly expressed in lung, pancreas, thymus, and brain.[57] Specific cell types include activated astrocytes, neutrophils,[603] activated monocytes,[661] ECs,[661,709] fibroblasts,[709] keratinocytes.[706]
Regulation of expression	
Up	IFN-α (astrocytoma cell lines,[708] monocytes,[708] PBMCs[603]), IFN-β (astrocytomas,[707,708] monocytes[708]), IFN-γ (astrocytes,[57] astrocytoma cell lines,[708] ECs,[618] monocytes[57,708,709]), IFN-γ + IL-1β (ECs[618]), IFN-γ + TNF-α (ECs[618,710]), IL-1β (astrocytes,[57] monocytes[57]).
Down	IL-4 (activated neutrophils[603]), IL-10 (activated neutrophils[603]).
Biologic activities	
In vitro	Binds to CXCR3 (K_d = 0.3–36 nmol/L)[57]; chemoattractant for activated T cells[57,709] and CXCR3–transfected cells[57]; induces intracellular Ca^{2+} mobilization in activated T cells[57] and in CXCR3–transfected cells.
In vivo	Not reported.
Pathologic association(s)	Atherosclerosis,[661] allergic contact dermatitis,[665,706] lichen planus,[706] mycosis fungoides.[706]
Genbank source (gene)	Y15221 (h).
Gene coding region (kbp)	3.4 (h).
Chromosomal location	4q21.2 (h).[711]
Exons	4 (h).[709]
Introns	3 (h).[709]
Natural mutations/polymorphisms	Not reported.
Genbank source (RNA)	NM_005409 (h).
Size of RNA (kbp)	0.9/1.4 (h).[57,709]
RNA splice variants	Not reported.

CXC CHEMOKINES

Stromal Cell–Derived Factor-1 (SDF-1)

Systematic name	CXCL12.
Other names	Intracrine-α, intercrine reduced in hepatomas,[712] PBSF, SCYB12, thymic lymphoma cell-stimulating factor-α/β, TPA (tumor promoter 12-O-tetradecanoylphorbol 13-acetate)–repressed gene-1.[713]
Similar proteins	mSDF-1 (92%), rSDF-1 (90%), hIL-8 (30%).
Genbank source	P48061 (h), I81182 (m), AAF01066 (r).
Amino acids in precursor protein	SDF-1α/β 89/93 (h, m), 89 (r).
Size of mature protein (Kd)	SDF-1α/β 7.8/8.0 (h, m, r).
Amino acids in mature protein	SDF-1β 72 (h, m), 68 (r).
Stable form(s)	Monomer (h, m, r).
Glycosylation sites	0 N (h, m, r).
Disulfide bonds	2 (h, m, r).
3D structure	Three antiparallel β sheets, COOH terminal α helix,[714,715] ELR$^-$.[678]
Mature protein variants	Two major variants, SDF-1α and SDF-1β.[716] Other forms generated by processing by CD26/dipeptidyl-peptidase IV.[717]
Tissue and cellular expression	Highly expressed in a large number of tissues, including brain, heart, kidney, lung, liver, spleen, thymus.[718] Specific cell types include BM stromal cells,[718] DCs,[719,720] BM ECs,[720] activated fibroblasts,[720,721] mesothelial cells,[722] and capillary pericytes.[720]
Regulation of expression	
Up	LPS (astrocytes[723]).
Down	Not reported.
Biologic activities	
In vitro	Binds to CXCR4 (K_d = 5–10 nmol/L),[724] vORF-74,[504] and heparin sulfate (K_d = 35–40 nmol/L)[725]; chemoattractant for T cells,[726] B cells,[727,728] pre–B cells,[729] pro–B cells,[729] DCs,[166] monocytes,[726] CD34$^+$ hematopoietic progenitor cells,[730,731] megakaryocytes,[732] ECs,[733] activated NK cells[734]; induces intracellular Ca^{2+} mobilization in B cells,[728] DCs,[166] ECs,[735] activated NK cells,[734] T cells,[726] and CXCR4–transfected cells[729,730]; induces dimerization and phosphorylation of CXCR4[736]; stimulates phosphorylation of focal adhesion complex components crk and paxillin[737] and induces actin polymerization[726]; activates p85/p110PI3K,[738] protein kinase B,[739] phospholipase Cb3,[740] RAFTK/pyk2[737] Jak2 and Jak3,[736] SHP-1 phosphatase,[736] MAPK kinase,[737] MAPK (p42/44),[737] CREB,[354] and NF-κB[737]; causes association of G$_{ai}$, Jak2 and Jak3, STAT1, STAT2, STAT3, and STAT5 with CXCR4[736]; activates G$_{ao}$, G$_{as}$, and G$_{aq}$ G proteins in NK cells[394]; induces the synthesis of VEGF in ECs[741]; induces CD4$^+$ T-cell adhesion to ICAM-1[321] and CD34$^+$ hematopoietic progenitor cell adhesion to P-selectin, E-selectin, VCAM-1, and ICAM-1 under flow conditions[742]; down-regulates expression of CXCR4 on B cells[727,728] and T cells[743]; stimulates proliferation and maturation of pre–B cells[744] and CD34$^+$ hematopoietic progenitor cells[745]; inhibits cytokine-induced hematopoietic progenitor cell adhesion to fibronectin[746]; inhibits cellular infection with T-cell tropic forms of HIV-1 (SDF-1β > SDF-1α)[747,748]; inhibits constitutive signaling of vORF-74 receptor.[749]
In vivo	Angiogenic[741]; chemoattractant for CD34$^+$ hematopoietic progenitor cells.[730] The SDF-1 (–/–) phenotype is embryonically or perinatally lethal; SDF-1 (–/–) mice exhibit impaired B lymphopoiesis and BM myelopoiesis,[750] defective formation of the large blood vessels supplying the gastrointestinal tract and other organs, defective cardiogenesis,[750] and defective cerebellar neuron migration.[751]
Pathologic association(s)	Inflammatory skin disease,[720] hepatocellular carcinoma,[712] HIV,[752] non-Hodgkin's lymphoma.[462]
Genbank source (gene)	Not reported.
Gene coding region (kbp)	Not reported.
Chromosomal location	10q11.1 (h),[716] 6:53.0 cM (m),[753] 4q42.1[753] (r).
Exons	SDF-1α/β 4/3 (h).

(continued)

CXC CHEMOKINES

Stromal Cell–Derived Factor-1 (SDF-1) (*Continued*)

Introns	SDF-1α/β 3 (h).
Natural mutations/polymorphisms	Individuals who have the (+/+) SDF1-3'A polymorphism in the SDF-β 3' untranslated region have an accelerated progression to AIDS but prolonged survival after AIDS diagnosis.[754,755] HIV-infected individuals who have the (–/+) or (+/+) SDF1-3'A polymorphism in the SDF-β 3' untranslated region have a two- or fourfold risk of developing non-Hodgkin's lymphoma.[462]
Genbank source (RNA)	U16752 (h), D43805 (m), AF189725 (r).
Size of RNA (kbp)	3.2 (h), 1.7 (m),[744] 0.3 (r).
RNA splice variants	SDF-1α and SDF-1β.[716]

CXC CHEMOKINES

B-Cell–Attracting Chemokine-1 (BCA-1)

Systematic name	CXCL13.
Other names	Angie, angie-2, BLC-1, Burkitt's lymphoma receptor-1 ligand, B-cell homing chemokine.
Similar proteins	mBCA-1 (48%).
Genbank source	NP_006410 (h), AAC14401 (m).
Amino acids in precursor protein	109 (h, m).[756,757]
Size of mature protein (Kd)	Not reported.
Amino acids in mature protein	87 (h).[756]
Stable form(s)	Monomer.
Glycosylation sites	0 N (m).
Disulfide bonds	2 (h, m).
3D structure	ELR⁻.
Mature protein variants	Not reported.
Tissue and cellular expression	Highly expressed in appendix,[756] intestine,[757] liver,[756] LNs,[756] spleen,[756] and stomach.[756] Specific cell types include DCs and stromal cells.
Regulation of expression	
Up	TNF-α (DCs[758]).
Down	Not reported.
Biologic activities	
In vitro	Binds to CXCR5; induces intracellular Ca²⁺ mobilization in B cells[756,757] and CXCR5–transfected cells[756,757]; chemoattractant for B cells[756,757] and activated CD4⁺ T cells.[759]
In vivo	Not reported.
Pathologic association(s)	Gastric lymphoma,[760] *Helicobacter pylori* infection.[760]
Genbank source (gene)	Not reported.
Gene coding region (kbp)	Not reported.
Chromosomal location	4q21 (h).[757]
Exons	Not reported.
Introns	Not reported.
Natural mutations/polymorphisms	One SNP identified (11868).
Genbank source (RNA)	NM_006419 (h), AF044196 (m).
Size of RNA (kbp)	1.4 (h),[756] 1.2 (m).[757]
RNA splice variants	Not reported.

CXC CHEMOKINES

Breast and Kidney Cell Chemokine (BRAK)

Systematic name	CXCL14.
Other names	Bolekine, kidney-expressed chemokine, NJAC, SCYB14.
Similar proteins	mBRAK (97%), hGRO-β (30%), hGRO-γ (30%).
Genbank source	NP_004878 (h), AAD34157 (m).
Amino acids in precursor protein	99 (h), 99 (m).
Size of mature protein (Kd)	8.0 (h, m).
Amino acids in mature protein	75 (h, m).
Stable form(s)	Not reported.
Glycosylation sites	0 N (h, m).
Disulfide bonds	2 (h).
3D structure	Not reported.
Mature protein variants	Not reported.
Tissue and cellular expression	Highly expressed in most normal tissues.[761]
Regulation of expression	
Up	Not reported.
Down	Not reported.
Biologic activities	
In vitro	Not reported.
In vivo	Not reported.
Pathologic association(s)	Not reported.
Genbank source (gene)	Not reported.
Gene coding region (kbp)	6.6 (h).
Chromosomal location	5q31 (h).[761]
Exons	4 (h).
Introns	3 (h).
Natural mutations/polymorphisms	Not reported.
Genbank source (RNA)	NM_004887 (h), AF192557 (m).
Size of RNA (kbp)	0.4/1.5 (h), 1.9 (m).
RNA splice variants	Not reported.

CXC CHEMOKINES

Lungkine (LGK)

Systematic name	CXCL15.
Other names	CINC-2β–like, SCYB15.
Similar proteins	hPBP (35%), hENA-78 (35%), hIL-8 (31%).
Genbank source	NP_035469 (m).
Amino acids in precursor protein	167 (m).
Size of mature protein (Kd)	Not reported.
Amino acids in mature protein	141 (m).[510]
Stable form(s)	Monomer.
Glycosylation sites	0 N (h).
Disulfide bonds	2 (h).
3D structure	Not reported.
Mature protein variants	Not reported.
Tissue and cellular expression	Highly expressed in lung.[510] Specific cell types include lung ECs.[510]
Regulation of expression	
Up	Not reported.
Down	Not reported.
Biologic activities	
In vitro	Chemoattractant for neutrophils.[510]
In vivo	Chemoattractant for neutrophils.[510]
Pathologic association(s)	Asthma.[510]
Genbank source (gene)	Not reported.
Gene coding region (kbp)	Not reported.
Chromosomal location	5 (m).[510]
Exons	Not reported.
Introns	Not reported.
Natural mutations/polymorphisms	Not reported.
Genbank source (RNA)	NM_011339 (m).
Size of RNA (kbp)	2.0, 1.2 (m).[510]
RNA splice variants	2 (m).

CXC CHEMOKINE RECEPTORS

Chemokine (CXC) Receptor-1 (CXCR1)

Other names	CDw128a, CMKAR1, IL-8 receptor-α, IL-8 receptor-type 1.
Similar proteins	rCXCR1 (71%),[762] hCXCR2 (77%),[763] hCCR6 (38%),[330] hCXCR3 (36%), hCXCR4 (36%), hCCR1 (32%).
Genbank source	NP_000625 (h), N/A (m), AAC52962 (r).
Size of mature protein (Kd)	44.0–59.0 (h), 40.0 (r).[762]
Amino acids in mature protein	350 (h),[764] 349 (r).[762]
Stable form(s)	Monomer.
Glycosylation sites	5 N (h), N/A (m), 1 N (r).
Disulfide bonds	1 (h, r), N/A (m).
3D structure	Seven transmembrane regions.
Mature protein variants	T276S (h).
Tissue and cellular expression	Highly expressed in lung.[762] Specific cell types include basophils,[63] DCs, ECs,[735] activated eosinophils,[623] mast cells,[507] alveolar Mϕs, NK cells, neutrophils, T-cell subsets (CD8+/CD56+).[765]
Regulation of expression	
Up	Ets PU.1 transcription factor (neutrophils[766]), GM-CSF (neutrophils[767]).
Down	Anti-CD45 (neutrophils[768]), hypoxia/reoxygenation (neutrophils[769]), IL-8 (neutrophils[770,771]), LPS (neutrophils[767]), TNF-α (neutrophils[772]).
Biologic activities	
In vitro	Binds IL-8 (K_d = 1.3 nmol/L) and GCP-2; engagement of CXCR1 by IL-8 induces intracellular Ca^{2+} mobilization in neutrophils and CXCR1–transfected cell lines,[773] stimulation of PI3K activity,[773] phosphorylation/activation of phospholipase Cβ3,[773] stimulation of guanosine triphosphatase activity[773]; engagement of CXCR1 by IL-8 activates MAPK (p42/44) in neutrophils[774]; engagement of CXCR1 by IL-8 activates phospholipase D[775]; engagement of CXCR1 by IL-8 leads to activation of G$_{ao}$ and G$_{as}$ G proteins in NK cells.[394]
In vivo	Not reported.
Pathologic association(s)	Psoriasis.[776]
Genbank source (gene)	L19592 (h), N/A (m), U71089 (r).
Gene coding region (kbp)	4.0 (h), N/A (m), 1.4 (r).
Chromosomal location	2q34-35 (h),[777] N/A (m).
Exons	2[778] (h), N/A (m).
Introns	1 (h),[778] N/A (m).
Natural mutations/polymorphisms	Not reported.
Genbank source (RNA)	NM_000634 (h), N/A (m).
Size of RNA (kbp)	2.9 (h), N/A (m).
RNA splice variants	Not reported.

CXC CHEMOKINE RECEPTORS

Chemokine (CXC) Receptor-2 (CXCR2)

Other names	CDw128b, GRO receptor, IL-8 receptor-β, IL-8 receptor type 2, MGSA receptor.
Similar proteins	mCXCR2 (71%), rCXCR2 (70%),[762] hCXCR1 (77%), hCXCR3 (38%), hCCR6 (38%),[330] hCCR1 (32%).
Genbank source	NP_001548 (h), NP_034039 (m), CAA54824 (r).
Size of mature protein (Kd)	40.0 (h), 40.4 (m), 40.5 (r).
Amino acids in mature protein	360 (h), 359 (m, r).[762,779]
Stable form(s)	Monomer (h, m, r).
Glycosylation sites	1 N (h, m), 4 N (r).
Disulfide bonds	1 (h, m, r).
3D structure	Seven transmembrane regions.
Mature protein variants	Not reported.
Tissue and cellular expression	Highly expressed in lung and spleen.[762] Specific cell types include basophils,[63] DCs,[166] ECs,[735] keratinocytes, melanocytes, mast cells,[507] neurons,[780,781] neutrophils,[762,779] NK cells, T-cell subsets (CD8+/CD56+).[765]
Regulation of expression	
Up	Not reported.
Down	Anti-CD45 (neutrophils[768]), IL-8 (neutrophils[770,771]), TNF-α (neutrophils[772,782]).
Biologic activities	
In vitro	Binds ENA-78 (K_d = 1 nmol/L),[503] GCP-2, GRO-α (K_d = 0.5 nmol/L),[503] GRO-β (K_d = 0.8 nmol/L),[503] GRO-γ (K_d = 0.7 nmol/L),[503] iIL-8 (K_d = 0.4–2.5 nmol/L),[503] NAP-2 (K_d = 7 nmol/L),[503] and vCXC-1 (K_d = 0.2–3 nmol/L)[783]; engagement of CXCR2 by IL-8 leads to phosphorylation of CXCR2 by PKC[773]; engagement of CXCR2 by IL-8 leads to activation of G_{ao} and G_{as} G proteins in NK cells.[394]
In vivo	CXCR2 (–/–) mice exhibit impaired neutrophil recruitment to thioglycollate, an increase in myelopoiesis and lymphadenopathy secondary to B-cell expansion,[784] less pathology in a model of LPS-induced uveitis,[785] increased susceptibility to systemic candidiasis.[786]
Pathologic association(s)	Acetaminophen-induced liver injury,[526] adenovirus-induced liver injury,[787] Alzheimer's disease,[780,781] melanoma,[499] nephritis,[399] *Nocardia asteroides* infection,[788] psoriasis.[776]
Genbank source (gene)	U11869 (h), U31207 (m), U70988 (r).
Gene coding region (kbp)	3.3 (h), 1.9 (m), 1.4 (r).
Chromosomal location	2q35 (h),[789] 1:40.00 cM (m).[790]
Exons	3 (h).[791]
Introns	2 (h).[791]
Natural mutations/polymorphisms	Not reported.
Genbank source (RNA)	NM_001557 (h), NM_009909 (m), X77797 (r).
Size of RNA (kbp)	2.8 (h), 1.9 (m), 1.3 (r).
RNA splice variants	IL8RB3, IL8RB4, IL8RB7 (h).

CXC CHEMOKINE RECEPTORS

Chemokine (CXC) Receptor-3 (CXCR3)

Other names	CKR-L2, Cmkar3 (m), GPCR9, IP-10 receptor,[792] Mig receptor.
Similar proteins	mCXCR3 (86%),[338] hGPCR-2 (41%), hCXCR2 (38%), hCXCR1 (36%).
Genbank source	NP_001495 (h), NP_034040 (m).
Size of mature protein (Kd)	40.6 (h), 41.0 (m).[338]
Amino acids in mature protein	368 (h), 367 (m).[338]
Stable form(s)	Monomer (h, m).
Glycosylation sites	2 N (h), 3 N (m).[338]
Disulfide bonds	1 (h, m).
3D structure	Seven transmembrane regions.
Mature protein variants	Not reported.
Tissue and cellular expression	Highly expressed in heart,[338] lung,[338] spleen,[338] and thymus.[792] Specific cell types include B cells,[338] eosinophils, ECs,[338] NK cells,[651,793] CD4+ T cells (T$_H$1),[338,794] CD4+ NK1.1+ T cells,[338] CD4−CD8− thymocytes,[338] CD8+ T cells.[338]
Regulation of expression	
Up	Anti-CD3 (naïve T cells,[795] prothymocytes[338]), conA (T cells[792]).
Down	Anti-CD3 [CD4+ T cells (T$_H$1),[338] CD4−CD8− thymocytes, memory T cells[392]].
Biologic activities	
In vitro	Binds IP-10 (K_d = 0.04–0.3 nmol/L[651,652]), Mig (K_d = 0.9–4.9 nmol/L[651,652]), I-TAC (K_d = 0.3–36 nmol/L[57,706]), and SLC (K_d = unknown[338,339,651,652]); engagement of CXCR3 by IP-10, I-TAC, Mig, or SLC (m) leads to intracellular Ca^{2+} mobilization[57,338,652]; engagement of CXCR3 by IP-10 leads to activation of G$_{ai}$, G$_{ao}$, and G$_{aq}$ G proteins in NK cells.[394]
In vivo	Not reported.
Pathologic association(s)	Allergy,[665] atherosclerosis,[661] B-cell lymphoma,[664] chronic lymphocytic leukemia,[664,796] contact dermatitis,[665] EAE/MS,[150,198] extranodal marginal zone lymphoma,[664] hepatocellular carcinoma,[152] proliferative glomerulonephritis,[399,654] rheumatoid arthritis,[793,797] sarcoidosis,[703] splenic marginal zone lymphoma,[664] ulcerative colitis.[793]
Genbank source (gene)	U32674 (h).
Gene coding region (kbp)	1.3 (h).
Chromosomal location	8p12-p11.2 (h),[798] Xq13 (h),[651] X:41.5 (m).[338]
Exons	2 (h).[798]
Introns	1 (h).[798]
Natural mutations/polymorphisms	Not reported.
Genbank source (RNA)	NM_001504 (h), NM_009910 (m).
Size of RNA (kbp)	1.7/3.6 (m).[338]
RNA splice variants	Not reported.

CXC CHEMOKINE RECEPTORS

Chemokine (CXC) Receptor-4 (CXCR4)

Other names	Cmkar4 (mouse gene), D2S201E, FB22, fusin, HM89, human serum transmembrane segment receptor, LCR1 (r), leukocyte-derived seven-transmembrane-domain receptor, neuropeptide Y receptor-Y3 (NPY3R), neuropeptide Y receptor-I, pre–B-cell–derived chemokine receptor, SDF-1α/β receptor, seven-transmembrane segment receptor.
Similar proteins	mCXCR4 (91%), rCXCR4 (91%), hCXCR1 (36%), hAGTR1 (36%).
Genbank source	NP_003458 (h), NP_034041 (m), O08565 (r).
Size of mature protein (Kd)	39.7 (h), 40.4 (m), 39.3 (r).
Amino acids in mature protein	352 (h), 359 (m), 349 (r).
Stable form(s)	Monomer/dimer (h).[736]
Glycosylation sites	1 N/1 O (h, m, r).
Disulfide bonds	1 (h, m, r).
3D structure	Seven transmembrane regions.
Mature protein variants	CXCR4 and CXCR4lo (h),[799] CXCR4A and CXCR4B (m).[800]
Tissue and cellular expression	Highly expressed in brain, colon, heart, and lung.[801] Specific cell types include astrocytes,[802] B cells,[803] CD34+ hematopoietic progenitor cells,[745] DCs, vascular ECs,[733] colon ECs,[804] Langerhans' cells,[805] mast cells, megakaryocytes,[732] microglia,[802] monocytes, Mϕs, NK cells (weak),[806] neurons,[802] neutrophils, platelets,[732] and T cells.[743]
Regulation of expression	
Up	T-cell activation,[807] cyclic adenosine monophosphate (T cells[808]), basic fibroblast growth factor (ECs[741]), 1,25-dihydroxyvitamin D$_3$ (HL-60 cells, U937 cells[809]), HIV TATA transactivator (T cells[810]), glucocorticoids (T cells[811]), IL-2 (NK cells[734]), IL-4 (T cells,[811,812] Langerhans' cells[805]), phosphorylation by phospholipase C β3,[740] TGF-β (Langerhans' cells[805]), VEGF (ECs[741]).
Down	Activation (T cells, PHA, CD3, IL-2, *Staphylococcus* enterotoxin A[807]), HHV-6,[813] HHV-7,[813] HIV gp120 (T cells[814]), IFN-γ (Langerhans' cells,[805] PBMCs,[815] T cells, U937 cells[815]), IFN-α (Langerhans' cells,[805] PBMCs,[815] U937 cells[815]), IFN-β (Langerhans' cells[805]), IFN-γ (ECs,[733] Langerhans' cells,[805] PBMCs,[815] T cells, U937 cells[815]), IL-1β (ECs[733]), IL-12 (T cells[816]), IL-16,[456] LPS (astrocytes,[723] ECs[733]), phosphorylation by protein kinase C,[740] PMA (T cells[743]), SDF-1α (T cells[743,817]), TNF-α (ECs[733]).
Biologic activities	
In vitro	Binds SDF-1α/β (K_d = 5–10 nmol/L)[724] and HIV gp120; coreceptor for T-cell–tropic strains of HIV-1; engagement of CXCR4 by SDF-1α/β induces intracellular Ca^{2+} mobilization in astrocytes,[723] neurons,[723] T cells, and CXCR4–transfected cells; engagement of CXCR4 by SDF-1α/β induces formation of IP-3,[739] activation of MAPK kinase, activation/phosphorylation of MAPK (p42/44), decrease in cyclic adenosine monophosphate formation, activation/phosphorylation of RAFTK/pyk2, activation of NF-κB, phosphorylation of crk and paxillin, stimulation of PI3K activity[737]; engagement of CXCR4 by SDF-1α leads to activation of G$_{ao}$, G$_{as}$, and G$_{aq}$ G proteins in NK cells.[394]
In vivo	Engraftment of BM.[818] The CXCR4 (–/–) phenotype is embryonically or perinatally lethal. CXCR4 (–/–) mice exhibit impaired B lymphopoiesis and BM myelopoiesis, defective formation of the large blood vessels supplying the gastrointestinal tract and other organs, defective cardiogenesis, and defective cerebellar neuron migration.[751,819]
Pathologic association(s)	Allograft rejection,[820] EAE/MS,[436] glioma,[821] hepatocellular carcinoma,[712] HIV.[7]
Genbank source (gene)	AF005058 (h), U65580 (m).
Gene coding region (kbp)	5.1 (h), 3.7 (m).
Chromosomal location	2q21 (h), 1:67.40 cM (m).
Exons	2 (h, m).
Introns	1 (h, m).
Natural mutations/polymorphisms	Two SNPs have been identified in the coding region,[822] A204G and T278C.
Genbank source (RNA)	NM_003467 (h), NM_009911 (m), U90610 (r).
Size of RNA (kbp)	1.7 (h), 1.9 (m), 1.3 (r).
RNA splice variants	CXCR4A and CXCR4B (m).[800]

CXC CHEMOKINE RECEPTORS

Chemokine (CXC) Receptor-5 (CXCR5)

Other names	Burkitt's lymphoma receptor-1, GPCR6 (m),[823] guanosine triphosphate-binding protein, neurolymphatic receptor (m, r).[824]
Similar proteins	mCXCR5 (83%),[825] rCXCR5 (81%).
Genbank source	NP_001707 (h), NP_031577 (m), P34997 (r).
Size of mature protein (Kd)	41.9 (h), 42.1 (m), 42.0 (r).
Amino acids in mature protein	372 (h), 374 (m, r).[824,826]
Stable form(s)	Monomer.
Glycosylation sites	2 N (h, m, r).
Disulfide bonds	1 (h, m, r).
3D structure	Seven transmembrane regions.[827]
Mature protein variants	Monocyte-derived receptor-15 (h).
Tissue and cellular expression	Highly expressed in neuronal tissue[826] and spleen. Specific cell types include mature B cells[825] and activated CD4+ T cells.[825]
Regulation of expression	
Up	Anti-CD3 (T cells,[759] memory T cells[392]), octamer-2 (B cells[828]), RelA/NF-κB (B cells[828]).
Down	Anti-CD3 (memory T cells[825]), anti-CD40 (B cells[825]).
Biologic activities	
In vitro	Binds B-cell–attracting chemokine-1.
In vivo	CXCR5 (–/–) mice exhibit absence of Peyer's patches and splenic B-cell germinal centers and severe defects in B-cell homing.[829]
Pathologic association(s)	B-cell lymphoma,[826] colorectal cancer,[830] gastric lymphoma,[760] *Helicobacter pylori* infection,[760] HIV.[831]
Genbank source (gene)	Not reported.
Gene coding region (kbp)	Not reported.
Chromosomal location	11 (h), 9:25.00 cM (m).
Exons	2 (m).[825]
Introns	1 (m).[825]
Natural mutations/polymorphisms	One SNP identified; however, no pathologic links have been reported.
Genbank source (RNA)	NM_001716 (h), NM_007551 (m), X71463 (r).
Size of RNA (kbp)	2.8 (h), 5.5/2.5 (m), 5.5/1.3 (r).
RNA splice variants	Monocyte-derived receptor–15 (h).[832]

C CHEMOKINES AND RECEPTOR

Protein Lymphotactin-1α (LTN-1α)/Lymphotactin-1β (LTN-1β)

Systematic name	XCL1/XCL2.
Other names	XCL1: ATAC,[833] CD8[+] T-cell–specific protein, CL1, LPTN, lymphotaxin, SCM-1α,[834] SCYC1. XCL2: SCM-1β,[834] SCM-2, SCYC2.
Similar proteins	XCL1: hLTN-1β (97%), mLTN-1α (61%), rLTN-1α (57%).
Genbank source	NP_002986 (h), NP_032536 (m), P51672 (r).
Amino acids in precursor protein	114 (h, m, r).
Size of mature protein (Kd)	10.3/12–18 (h),[835] 15.0 (m).[836]
Amino acids in mature protein	92 (h, m, r).[834,837,838]
Stable form(s)	Monomer.
Glycosylation sites	1 O (h, m).[836,837]
Disulfide bonds	1 (h, m, r).
3D structure	Not reported.
Mature protein variants	Not reported.
Tissue and cellular expression	Specific cell types include TCR α/β[+] CD4[-]/CD8[-] thymocytes,[838] activated CD8[+] T cells,[833,836] IEL γ/δ T cells,[839] NK cells,[840] activated basophils,[841] activated mast cells,[841] activated CD4[+] NK1.1[+] T cells, DCs.
Regulation of expression	
Up	Anti-CD3 (T cells[836]), anti-Fcε receptor I (mast cell[841]), IL-2 (NK cells[840]), IL-4 (activated mast cells[841]), IL-12 (NK cells[840]), isopentenyl pyrophosphate (γ/δ T cells[121]), PHA (T cells[833]), TGF-β (activated mast cells[841]).
Down	CD28 costimulation (T$_H$1 T cells[836]), cyclosporin A (T cells,[833] activated mast cells[841]).
Biologic activities	
In vitro	Binds to XCR-1 (K_d = 10 nmol/L), chemoattractant for NK cells,[842,843] CD4[+] T cells,[837] and CD8[+] T cells[842,843]; moderately inhibits cellular infection with M-tropic and T cell-tropic strains of HIV-1[844]; induces intracellular Ca[2+] mobilization in NK cells[691] and T cells[838,845]; inhibits hemopoietic progenitor colony formation.[370]
In vivo	Chemoattractant for CD8[+] T cells[843] and NK cells[843]; antitumor activity when given with IL-2[846]; systemic and mucosal adjuvant.[847]
Pathologic association(s)	Glomerulonephritis,[848] graft rejection.[849]
Genbank source (gene)	D43768 (h), D63789 (h), U15607 (m).
Gene coding region (kbp)	5.7 (h).[834]
Chromosomal location	1q24.1-24.3 (h),[833] 1:87.00 cM (m).
Exons	3 (m).[836]
Introns	2 (m).[836]
Natural mutations/polymorphisms	Not reported.
Genbank source (RNA)	NM_002995 (h), NM_008510 (m), U23377 (r).
Size of RNA (kbp)	0.3/1.2 (h),[835] 0.5 (m), 0.3 (r).
RNA splice variants	Not reported.

C CHEMOKINES AND RECEPTOR

Chemokine (XC) Receptor-1 (XCR-1)

Other names	GPCR-5,[850] SCM-1 receptor, XCR-1.
Similar proteins	mXCR-1 (71%),[851] hCCR4, hCCR1.
Genbank source	NP_005274 (h), NP_035928 (m).
Size of mature protein (Kd)	Not reported.
Amino acids in mature protein	333 (h),[852] 332 (m).[851]
Stable form(s)	Monomer (h, m).
Glycosylation sites	Not reported.
Disulfide bonds	Not reported.
3D structure	Seven transmembrane regions.
Mature protein variants	Not reported.
Tissue and cellular expression	Highly expressed in placenta.[851] Specific cell types include NK cells[851] and CD8+ T cells.[851]
Regulation of expression	
Up	Not reported.
Down	Not reported.
Biologic activities	
In vitro	Binds LTN-1α (K_d = 10 nmol/L)[851,852] and vMIP-II; engagement of XCR1 by LTN-1α leads to activation of G_{ai}, G_{ao}, and G_{aq} G proteins in NK cells.[394]
In vivo	Not reported.
Pathologic association(s)	Not reported.
Genbank source (gene)	L36149 (h).
Gene coding region (kbp)	1.3 (h).
Chromosomal location	3p21.3-p21.1[850] (h).
Exons	Not reported.
Introns	Not reported.
Natural mutations/polymorphisms	Not reported.
Genbank source (RNA)	NM_005283 (h), NM_011798 (m).
Size of RNA (kbp)	5.0 (h),[852] 2.4 (m).[851]
RNA splice variants	Not reported.

CX$_3$C CHEMOKINE AND RECEPTOR

Fractalkine (FKN)

Systematic name	CX$_3$CL1.
Other names	Activated B and dendritic cell–derived protein-3 (m),[291] C3Xkine, neurotactin, NTT, SCYD1, type 1 membrane protein.
Similar proteins	mFKN, rFKN (66%).[853]
Genbank source	NP_002987 (h), NP_033168 (m), AAC33834 (r).
Amino acids in precursor protein	397 (h), 395 (m), 393 (r).
Size of mature protein (Kd)	Soluble, 8.5 (h, m); membrane, 90 (h).
Amino acids in mature protein	Membrane bound, 373 (h), 373 (m), 369 (r)[854]; soluble, 76 (h).
Stable form(s)	Monomer[855] (h).
Glycosylation sites	1 N (h, m, r).
Disulfide bonds	2 (h, m, r).
3D structure	Three antiparallel β sheets, COOH terminal α helix.[855,856]
Mature protein variants	Membrane bound and secreted forms.[856]
Tissue and cellular expression	Highly expressed in brain, kidney, lung, skeletal muscle, heart, and testis.[857] Specific cell types include activated B cells,[291] DCs,[858,859] pulmonary ECs, thymic ECs,[860] umbilical vein ECs,[861] Langerhans' cells,[859] monocytes, neurons,[854,862] neutrophils, and T cells.
Regulation of expression	
Up	Anti-CD40 (B cells[291,860]), anti-μ (B cells[860]), IL-1β (astrocytes,[863] umbilical vein ECs,[861] DCs,[291] Langerhans' cells[859]), LPS (DCs[291]), TNF-α (astrocytes,[863] DCs,[291] umbilical vein ECs[861]).
Down	Not reported.
Biologic activities	
In vitro	Soluble FKN binds to CX$_3$CR-1 (K_d = 0.9–5.3 nmol/L)[854]; soluble FKN is a chemoattractant for monocytes,[861] NK cells,[317] and T cells[861]; EC cell membrane–bound FKN mediates leukocyte capture and adhesion in a G protein–independent fashion[864,865]; induces intracellular Ca^{2+} mobilization in activated NK cells[317]; stimulates activation/phosphorylation of MAPK (p42/44)[354]; activates CREB.[354]
In vivo	Not reported.
Pathologic association(s)	Glomerulonephritis,[866] HIV-1 encephalitis.[867]
Genbank source (gene)	U84487 (h).
Gene coding region (kbp)	3.3 (h), 3.1 (m).[857]
Chromosomal location	16q13 (h),[868] 8 (m).[857]
Exons	Not reported.
Introns	Not reported.
Natural mutations/polymorphisms	Not reported.
Genbank source (RNA)	NM_002996 (h), NM_009142 (m), AF030358 (r).
Size of RNA (kbp)	1.8/4.0/7.0 (m).[857]
RNA splice variants	At least 2 (h).[861]

CX₃C CHEMOKINE AND RECEPTOR

Chemokine (CX₃C) Receptor-1 (CX₃CR1)

Other names	CMKBR-1,[382] CMKDR1, FKN receptor, GPCR13, G protein–coupled receptor V28, RBS11 (r),[380] V28,[869] VT28.
Similar proteins	mCX3CR-1 (83%), rCX3CR-1 (82%), hCCR1.
Genbank source	NP_001328 (h), AAC72408 (m), P35411 (r).
Size of mature protein (Kd)	40.4 (h), 40.3 (m, r).
Amino acids in mature protein	355 (h), 354 (m, r).
Stable form(s)	Monomer (h, m, r).
Glycosylation sites	0 N (h, r).
Disulfide bonds	1 (h, m, r).
3D structure	Seven transmembrane regions.
Mature protein variants	Not reported.
Tissue and cellular expression	Highly expressed in brain,[380,869] lung,[870] intestine,[380] kidney,[380] spinal cord,[380] spleen,[869] testes,[380] and uterus.[380] Specific cell types include microglia,[871] monocytes,[872] neutrophils,[869] NK cells,[872] T cells (CD45RO⁺ > CD45RA⁺).[860,872]
Regulation of expression	
Up	IL-2 (CD4⁺ T cells,[872] CD8⁺ T cells[872]).
Down	LPS (microglia[871]), PHA (CD4⁺ T cells,[872] CD8⁺ T cells[872]).
Biologic activities	
In vitro	Binds FKN (K_d = 0.9–5.3 nmol/L[854]) and vMIP-II (K_d = 0.2 nmol/L)[873]; coreceptor for syncytia-inducing strains of HIV-1, dual-tropic strains of HIV-1, and T-cell–tropic strains of HIV-2[489]; mediates cell capture and adhesion to FKN-expressing EC cells in a G protein–independent fashion[864,865]; engagement of XCR1 by FKN leads to activation of G_{ai}, G_{a2}, and G_{aq} G proteins in NK cells.[394]
In vivo	Not reported.
Pathologic association(s)	EAE/MS,[436] HIV,[489] HIV-1 encephalitis,[867] glomerulonephritis.[866]
Genbank source (gene)	Not reported.
Gene coding region (kbp)	Not reported.
Chromosomal location	3p21[869] (h).
Exons	1 (h).[869]
Introns	0 (h).[869]
Natural mutations/polymorphisms	Not reported.
Genbank source (RNA)	NM_001337 (h), AF102269 (m), U04808 (r).
Size of RNA (kbp)	3.2 (h), 1.2 (m), 3.0 (r).
RNA splice variants	Not reported.

DUFFY AND ORPHAN CHEMOKINE RECEPTORS

Duffy Antigen Receptor for Chemokines (DARC)

Other names	Chemokine binding protein-1, glycoprotein D, gpFy.
Similar proteins	mDARC (59%).
Genbank source	NP_002027 (h), NP_034175 (m).
Size of mature protein (Kd)	35.7/47.0 (h),[874] 36.7 (m).
Amino acids in mature protein	337 (h, m).
Stable form(s)	Monomer.
Glycosylation sites	2 N (h), 3 N (m).[875]
Disulfide bonds	2 (h, m).
3D structure	Seven transmembrane regions.[876]
Mature protein variants	Several variants (h).[877]
Tissue and cellular expression	Highly expressed in brain[875,878] and liver (m).[875] Specific cell types include ECs,[879] erythrocytes, and neurons.[780]
Regulation of expression	
Up	Not reported.
Down	Not reported.
Biologic activities	
In vitro	Binds GRO-α (K_d = 21 nmol/L),[880] IL-8 (K_d = 5–20 nmol/L),[874,881] MCP-1, RANTES (K_d = 7.0 nmol/L),[880] and TARC. Also binds *Plasmodium vivax*[882] and HIV.[883]
In vivo	Acts as an erythrocyte receptor for *P. vivax*.[882]
Pathologic association(s)	EAE/MS,[884] hemolytic uremic syndrome,[885] malaria.[882]
Genbank source (gene)	X85785 (h), AF016697 (m).
Gene coding region (kbp)	2.5 (h), 1.6 (m).
Chromosomal location	1q21-q22 (h), 1:94 cM (m).
Exons	2 (h, m).[875,886]
Introns	1 (h, m).[875,886]
Natural mutations/polymorphisms	Nine SNPs have been identified. Of these, three major allelic versions have been described, Fy^{a-}, Fy^{b-}.[887] Individuals who have (+/+) -365T to C promoter mutant genotype are resistant to *P. vivax* infection.[888]
Genbank source (RNA)	NM_002036 (h), NM_010045 (m).
Size of RNA (kbp)	1.4 (h), 1.4/1.8/8.5/10.2 (m).[875]
RNA splice variants	Several variants (h).[877]

DUFFY AND ORPHAN CHEMOKINE RECEPTORS

Chemokine (CC Motif) Receptor–Like-2 (CCRL-2)

Other names	CKR-X, CRAM-A, CRAM-B, human chemokine receptor.
Similar proteins	LPS-inducible CC chemokine receptor–related gene (m) (51%), hCCR1 (43%),[447] hCCR2 (42%),[447] hCCR5 (41%).[447]
Genbank source	NP_003956 (h).
Size of mature protein (Kd)	39.5 (h).
Amino acids in mature protein	344 (h).
Stable form(s)	Monomer.
Glycosylation sites	2 (h).
Disulfide bonds	1 (h).
3D structure	Not reported.
Mature protein variants	Not reported.
Tissue and cellular expression	Highly expressed in BM, fetal liver, heart, LNs, lung, and spleen.
Regulation of expression	
Up	Not reported.
Down	Not reported.
Biologic activities	
In vitro	Orphan CC chemokine receptor.
In vivo	Not reported.
Pathologic association(s)	Not reported.
Genbank source (gene)	Not reported.
Gene coding region (kbp)	Not reported.
Chromosomal location	Xq13, 3p21.
Exons	Not reported.
Introns	Not reported.
Natural mutations/polymorphisms	Not reported.
Genbank source (RNA)	NM_003965 (h).
Size of RNA (kbp)	1.6 (h).
RNA splice variants	Not reported.

DUFFY AND ORPHAN CHEMOKINE RECEPTORS

G Protein–Coupled Receptor-1 (GPR1)

Other names	None.
Similar proteins	rGPCR-1 (78%).
Genbank source	NP_005270 (h), P46090 (r).
Size of mature protein (Kd)	41.4 (h).
Amino acids in mature protein	355 (h), 353 (r).
Stable form(s)	Monomer.
Glycosylation sites	1 N (h).
Disulfide bonds	1 (h).
3D structure	Seven transmembrane regions.[889]
Mature protein variants	Not reported.
Tissue and cellular expression	Highly expressed in hippocampus (h).[890] Specific cell types include alveolar Mφs,[889] microglia,[891] and T cells.[891]
Regulation of expression	
Up	Not reported.
Down	Not reported.
Biologic activities	
In vitro	Orphan chemokine receptor ?; coreceptor for strains of HIV-1 and HIV-2.[891,892]
In vivo	Not reported.
Pathologic association(s)	HIV/AIDS.
Genbank source (gene)	U13666 (h), S74702 (r).
Gene coding region (kbp)	1.1 (r).
Chromosomal location	15q21.6 (h).[890]
Exons	1 (h).
Introns	0 (h).
Natural mutations/polymorphisms	Not reported.
Genbank source (RNA)	NM_005279 (h).
Size of RNA (kbp)	1.1 (h).
RNA splice variants	Not reported.

DUFFY AND ORPHAN CHEMOKINE RECEPTORS

G Protein–Coupled Receptor-15 (GPCR15)

Other names	Brother of Bonzo, GPCRF.
Similar proteins	hCCR5.
Genbank source	NP_005281 (h).
Size of mature protein (Kd)	40.8 (h).
Amino acids in mature protein	360 (h).
Stable form(s)	Monomer.
Glycosylation sites	0 N (h).
Disulfide bonds	0 (h).
3D structure	Seven transmembrane regions.[889,893]
Mature protein variants	Not reported.
Tissue and cellular expression	Highly expressed in colon and spleen.[894] Specific cell types include alveolar Mφs and T cells.[889,894]
Regulation of expression	
Up	Not reported.
Down	Not reported.
Biologic activities	
In vitro	Orphan chemokine receptor ?; coreceptor for M-tropic strains of HIV-1 and some strains of HIV-2.[395,894]
In vivo	Not reported.
Pathologic association(s)	HIV/AIDS.
Genbank source (gene)	U34806 (h).
Gene coding region (kbp)	1.2 (h).
Chromosomal location	3q11.2-q13.1.[850]
Exons	Not reported.
Introns	Not reported.
Natural mutations/polymorphisms	Not reported.
Genbank source (RNA)	NM_005290 (h).
Size of RNA (kbp)	1.1 (h).
RNA splice variants	Not reported.

DUFFY AND ORPHAN CHEMOKINE RECEPTORS

LPS-Inducible CC Chemokine Receptor–Related Gene (L-CCR)

Other names	Not reported.
Similar proteins	hCCRL-2 (51%), mCCR5 (36%), mCCR1 (35%).
Genbank source	BAA25879 (m).
Size of mature protein (Kd)	Not reported.
Amino acids in mature protein	360 (m).
Stable form(s)	Monomer.
Glycosylation sites	Not reported.
Disulfide bonds	1 (h).
3D structure	Not reported.
Mature protein variants	Not reported.
Tissue and cellular expression	Specific cell types include activated Mφs.[895]
Regulation of expression	
Up	LPS (Mφs[895]).
Down	Not reported.
Biologic activities	
In vitro	Orphan chemokine receptor.
In vivo	Not reported.
Pathologic association(s)	Not reported.
Genbank source (gene)	Not reported.
Gene coding region (kbp)	Not reported.
Chromosomal location	Not reported.
Exons	Not reported.
Introns	Not reported.
Natural mutations/polymorphisms	Not reported.
Genbank source (RNA)	AB009384 (m).
Size of RNA (kbp)	1.9 (m).
RNA splice variants	Not reported.

DUFFY AND ORPHAN CHEMOKINE RECEPTORS

CXC Chemokine Receptor RDC-1 (RDC-1)

Other names	GPCRN-1, vasoactive intestinal peptide-1 receptor (withdrawn).[896,897]
Similar proteins	mRDC (92%), hCXCR2 (30%).
Genbank source	AAA62370 (h), AAB71343 (m), CAA09370 (r).
Size of mature protein (Kd)	60.0 (h, m, r).
Amino acids in mature protein	362 (h, m, r).
Stable form(s)	Monomer.
Glycosylation sites	3 N (h, m).[790]
Disulfide bonds	1 (h, m).
3D structure	Not reported.
Mature protein variants	Not reported.
Tissue and cellular expression	Highly expressed in heart, kidney, lung, spleen,[790] and testis. Specific cell types include astrocytes, neutrophils,[790] and T cells.[898]
Regulation of expression	
Up	Not reported.
Down	Not reported.
Biologic activities	
In vitro	Orphan CXC chemokine receptor[898]; coreceptor for M- and T-tropic strains of HIV-1 and some strains of HIV-2.[898]
In vivo	Not reported.
Pathologic association(s)	HIV.[898]
Genbank source (gene)	Not reported.
Gene coding region (kbp)	Not reported.
Chromosomal location	1:67.40 cM[790] (m).
Exons	Not reported.
Introns	Not reported.
Natural mutations/polymorphisms	Not reported.
Genbank source (RNA)	U67784 (h), AF000236 (m), AJ010828 (r).
Size of RNA (kbp)	1.7 (h), 1.9 (m), 1.4 (r).
RNA splice variants	Not reported.

DUFFY AND ORPHAN CHEMOKINE RECEPTORS

TYMSTR

Other names	BONZO, seven-transmembrane-domain receptor from lymphocyte clone 33.
Similar proteins	hCCR7 (37%), hCCR6 (37%), CCR9 (32%).
Genbank source	NP_006555 (h).
Size of mature protein (Kd)	39.2 (h).
Amino acids in mature protein	342 (h).
Stable form(s)	Monomer.
Glycosylation sites	1 N (h).
Disulfide bonds	1 (h).
3D structure	Seven transmembrane regions.[893]
Mature protein variants	One variant (h).
Tissue and cellular expression	Highly expressed in appendix, BM, LNs, peripheral blood, placenta, small intestine, spleen, and thymus.[894,899] Specific cell types include astrocytes,[900] monocytes,[894] TILs,[899] and activated T cells.[899,901]
Regulation of expression	
Up	PHA + ionomycin (T cells[899]).
Down	Not reported.
Biologic activities	
In vitro	Orphan CC chemokine receptor; coreceptor for M- and T-tropic strains of HIV-1 and for some strains of HIV-2.[395,899,901]
In vivo	Not reported.
Pathologic association(s)	HIV/AIDS.[395]
Genbank source (gene)	Not reported.
Gene coding region (kbp)	Not reported.
Chromosomal location	3 (h).[901]
Exons	Not reported.
Introns	Not reported.
Natural mutations/polymorphisms	Not reported.
Genbank source (RNA)	NM_006564 (h).
Size of RNA (kbp)	2.0 (h).
RNA splice variants	Not reported.

VIRAL CHEMOKINE AND CHEMOKINE RECEPTOR HOMOLOGS

Mouse Cytomegalovirus Chemokine-1 (vMCK-1)/mCMV-2 (vMCK-2)

Other names	M131, ORF HJ1.
Similar proteins	mMIP-1α, mMIP-1β, mRANTES.[902]
Genbank source	AAD44683 (v).
Amino acids in precursor protein	vMCK-1: 116 (v).
Size of mature protein (Kd)	vMCK-1: 7.8. vMCK-2: 31.4.[903]
Amino acids in mature protein	vMCK-1: 81 (v). vMCK-2: 280.
Stable form(s)	Not reported.
Glycosylation sites	Not reported.
Disulfide bonds	2 (v).
3D structure	Not reported.
Mature protein variants	Not reported.
Tissue and cellular expression	mCMV encoded.[902]
Regulation of expression	
Up	Induces intracellular Ca^{2+} mobilization in Mϕs and CCR3–transfected cells.[429]
Down	Not reported.
Biologic activities	
In vitro	Not reported.
In vivo	Angiogenic.[429] The presence of an intact M131 gene determines the pathogenicity of mCMV.[904]
Pathologic association(s)	Not reported.
Genbank source (gene)	U68299/AF124602 (v).
Gene coding region (kbp)	0.9 (v).
Chromosomal location	N/A.
Exons	N/A.
Introns	N/A.
Natural mutations/polymorphisms	Not reported.
Genbank source (RNA)	Not reported.
Size of RNA (kbp)	0.9 (m).[902]
RNA splice variants	Not reported.

VIRAL CHEMOKINE AND CHEMOKINE RECEPTOR HOMOLOGS

Molluscum Contagiosum Protein 148R (vMC148R)

Other names	Molluscum contagiosum chemokine homolog, viral molluscum contagiosum chemokine-1.
Similar proteins	hMIP-1α.
Genbank source	AAC55276 (v).
Amino acids in precursor protein	104 (v).
Size of mature protein (Kd)	9.0 (v).[905]
Amino acids in mature protein	Not reported.
Stable form(s)	Monomer.
Glycosylation sites	Not reported.
Disulfide bonds	2 (v).
3D structure	Not reported.
Mature protein variants	Not reported.
Tissue and cellular expression	Molluscum contagiosum virus encoded.
Regulation of expression	
Up	Not reported.
Down	Not reported.
Biologic activities	
In vitro	Binds to CCR8 (K_d = 0.3 mol/L)[483,487,488,905]; blocks I-309–stimulated intracellular Ca^{2+} mobilization and chemotaxis in CCR8–transfected cells.[905]
In vivo	Not reported.
Pathologic association(s)	Molluscum contagiosum virus–induced skin tumors.[488]
Genbank source (gene)	U60315 (v).
Gene coding region (kbp)	0.3 (v).
Chromosomal location	N/A.
Exons	Not reported.
Introns	Not reported.
Natural mutations/polymorphisms	Two subtype variants, MC148R1 and MC148R2.
Genbank source (RNA)	Not reported.
Size of RNA (kbp)	0.3 (v).
RNA splice variants	Not reported.

VIRAL CHEMOKINE AND CHEMOKINE RECEPTOR HOMOLOGS

Viral Macrophage Inflammatory Protein-I (vMIP-I)

Other names	Open reading frame K6,[906] vMIP-IA.
Similar proteins	vMIP-II (60%), hMIP-1α (43%).
Genbank source	AAC57095 (v).
Amino acids in precursor protein	95 (v).
Size of mature protein (Kd)	Not reported.
Amino acids in mature protein	Not reported.
Stable form(s)	Monomer.
Glycosylation sites	Not reported.
Disulfide bonds	Not reported.
3D Structure[907]	
Mature protein variants	Not reported.
Tissue and cellular expression	HHV-8 encoded.
Regulation of expression	
Up	Not reported.
Down	Not reported.
Biologic activities	
In vitro	Binds to CCR8[483,486];induces intracellular Ca^{2+} mobilization in T cells[483] and CCR8–transfected cells[486]; vMIP-I partially inhibits CCR5–mediated HIV infection of PBMCs[908]; chemoattractant for T cells ($T_H2 > T_H1$).[486]
In vivo	Angiogenic.[908]
Pathologic association(s)	Kaposi's sarcoma,[909] lymphoma.
Genbank source (gene)	U75698 (v).
Gene coding region (kbp)	0.3 (v).
Chromosomal location	N/A.
Exons	N/A.
Introns	N/A.
Natural mutations/polymorphisms	N/A.
Genbank source (RNA)	Not reported.
Size of RNA (kbp)	Not reported.
RNA splice variants	Not reported.

VIRAL CHEMOKINE AND CHEMOKINE RECEPTOR HOMOLOGS

Viral Macrophage Inflammatory Protein-II (vMIP-II)

Other names	1609-1325, open reading frame K4, vMIP-1B.
Similar proteins	vMIP-I (60%), hMIP-1α (52%).
Genbank source	AAC57093 (v).
Amino acids in precursor protein	94 (v).
Size of mature protein (Kd)	Not reported.
Amino acids in mature protein	Not reported.
Stable form(s)	Not reported.
Glycosylation sites	Not reported.
Disulfide bonds	Not reported.
3D structure	Not reported.
Mature protein variants	Not reported.
Tissue and cellular expression	HHV-8 encoded.
Regulation of expression	
Up	Not reported.
Down	Not reported.
Biologic activities	
In vitro	Binds to CCR3, CCR8 (K_d = 28 nmol/L),[483,905] CX3CR-1 (K_d = 0.2 nmol/L),[873] and XCR-1[910]; chemoattractant for eosinophils,[908] monocytes,[911] T cells (T_H2 > T_H1),[911] and CCR8–transfected Jurkat cells[908]; partially inhibits HIV infection of PBMCs[908] and a CD4+ cell line expressing CCR3[908]; induces intracellular Ca^{2+} mobilization in eosinophils[908]; inhibits MCP-1–, MIP-1α–, RANTES–, and FKN-induced chemotaxis of activated leukocytes[873]; partially or fully inhibits intracellular Ca^{2+} mobilization through CCR1, CCR2B, CCR3, CCR4, CCR5, CCR8, CXCR3, CXCR4, CX_3CR-1, and XCL-1 ligands[905]; inhibits constitutive signaling of vORF-74 receptor.[749]
In vivo	Angiogenic[908]; inhibits MIP-1α–, MIP-1β–, and RANTES-induced inflammation in a rat model of experimental glomerulonephritis.[873]
Pathologic association(s)	Kaposi's sarcoma.[908]
Genbank source (gene)	U75698 (v).
Gene coding region (kbp)	0.3 (v).
Chromosomal location	N/A.
Exons	N/A.
Introns	N/A.
Natural mutations/polymorphisms	Not reported.
Genbank source (RNA)	Not reported.
Size of RNA (kbp)	Not reported.
RNA splice variants	Not reported.

VIRAL CHEMOKINE AND CHEMOKINE RECEPTOR HOMOLOGS

Viral Macrophage Inflammatory Protein-III (vMIP-III)

Other names	BCK, ORF K4.1.
Similar proteins	hEOT-1 (38%), hTARC (35%), hMIP-1β, MCP-1.
Genbank source	AAC56951 (v).
Amino acids in precursor protein	114 (v).[912]
Size of mature protein (Kd)	9.6 (v).[913]
Amino acids in mature protein	88 (v).[913]
Stable form(s)	Not reported.
Glycosylation sites	0 N/0 O (v).[913]
Disulfide bonds	2 (v).[912]
3D structure	Not reported.
Mature protein variants	Not reported.
Tissue and cellular expression	HHV-8 encoded.
Regulation of expression	
Up	Not reported.
Down	Not reported.
Biologic activities	
In vitro	Binds weakly to CCR4 and CCR5[913]; chemoattractant for T cells ($T_H2 > T_H1$).[913]
In vivo	Angiogenic.[913]
Pathologic association(s)	Kaposi's sarcoma.[913]
Genbank source (gene)	U83351 (v).
Gene coding region (kbp)	0.3 (v).
Chromosomal location	N/A.
Exons	N/A.
Introns	N/A.
Natural mutations/polymorphisms	N/A.
Genbank source (RNA)	Not reported.
Size of RNA (kbp)	Not reported.
RNA splice variants	Not reported.

VIRAL CHEMOKINE AND CHEMOKINE RECEPTOR HOMOLOGS

Viral CXC Chemokine-1 (vCXC1)

Other names	ORF UL146.
Similar proteins	hIL-8.
Genbank source	AAA85885 (v).
Amino acids in precursor protein	117 (v).
Size of mature protein (Kd)	14.0–25.0 (v).[783]
Amino acids in mature protein	95 (v), 100 (v).
Stable form(s)	Not reported.
Glycosylation sites	3 (v).
Disulfide bonds	Not reported.
3D structure	Not reported.
Mature protein variants	Several.[783]
Tissue and cellular expression	CMV encoded.
Regulation of expression	
Up	Not reported.
Down	Not reported.
Biologic activities	
In vitro	Binds to CXCR2 (K_d = 0.2–3 nmol/L)[783]; binds to CCR8 with low affinity; chemoattractant for neutrophils[783]; induces intracellular Ca^{2+} mobilization in neutrophils[783]; stimulates degranulation of neutrophils[783]; desensitizes signaling to NAP-2, GRO-α, GRO-β, GRO-γ, and ENA-78.[783]
In vivo	Not reported.
Pathologic association(s)	Not reported.
Genbank source (gene)	U33331 (v).
Gene coding region (kbp)	0.4.
Chromosomal location	N/A.
Exons	N/A.
Introns	N/A.
Natural mutations/polymorphisms	N/A.
Genbank source (RNA)	Not reported.
Size of RNA (kbp)	Not reported.
RNA splice variants	Not reported.

VIRAL CHEMOKINE AND CHEMOKINE RECEPTOR HOMOLOGS

Viral CXC Chemokine-2 (vCXC2)

Other names	ORF UL147.
Similar proteins	hIL-8, hMIG.
Genbank source	AAA85886 (v).
Amino acids in precursor protein	159 (v).
Size of mature protein (Kd)	Not reported.
Amino acids in mature protein	Not reported.
Stable form(s)	Not reported.
Glycosylation sites	Not reported.
Disulfide bonds	Not reported.
3D structure	Not reported.
Mature protein variants	Not reported.
Tissue and cellular expression	CMV encoded.
Regulation of expression	
Up	Not reported.
Down	Not reported.
Biologic activities	
In vitro	Not reported.
In vivo	Not reported.
Pathologic association(s)	Not reported.
Genbank source (gene)	U33331 (v).
Gene coding region (kbp)	0.4 (v).
Chromosomal location	N/A.
Exons	N/A.
Introns	N/A.
Natural mutations/polymorphisms	N/A.
Genbank source (RNA)	Not reported.
Size of RNA (kbp)	Not reported.
RNA splice variants	Not reported.

VIRAL CHEMOKINE AND CHEMOKINE RECEPTOR HOMOLOGS

Human Herpesvirus-6–Encoded Open Reading Frame U38 (vORF U83)

Other names	Not reported.
Similar proteins	Not reported.
Genbank source	BAA78303 (v).
Amino acids in precursor protein	113 (v).[914]
Size of mature protein (Kd)	10.0 (v).[914]
Amino acids in mature protein	93 (v).[914]
Stable form(s)	Not reported.
Glycosylation sites	1 N (v).[914]
Disulfide bonds	2 (v).[914]
3D structure	Not reported.
Mature protein variants	Not reported.
Tissue and cellular expression	HHV-6 encoded.
Regulation of expression	
Up	Not reported.
Down	Not reported.
Biologic activities	
In vitro	Chemoattractant for THP-1 cells[914]; induces intracellular Ca^{2+} mobilization in THP-1 cells.[914]
In vivo	Not reported.
Pathologic association(s)	Lymphoproliferative disorders.[914]
Genbank source (gene)	AB021506 (v).
Gene coding region (kbp)	0.3 (v).
Chromosomal location	N/A.
Exons	N/A.
Introns	N/A.
Natural mutations/polymorphisms	Not reported.
Genbank source (RNA)	Not reported.
Size of RNA (kbp)	Not reported.
RNA splice variants	Not reported.

VIRAL CHEMOKINE AND CHEMOKINE RECEPTOR HOMOLOGS

Open Reading Frame-74 (vORF-74)

Other names	KSHV-GPCR, v-GPCR, VG74.
Similar proteins	hCXCR2, hCXCR1.
Genbank source	AAB51506 (v).
Size of mature protein (Kd)	38.7 (v).
Amino acids in mature protein	342 (v).
Stable form(s)	Monomer.
Glycosylation sites	3 N (v).
Disulfide bonds	0 (v).
3D structure	Not reported.
Mature protein variants	Not reported.
Tissue and cellular expression	HHV-8 or KSHV encoded.
Regulation of expression	
Up	Not reported.
Down	Not reported.
Biologic activities	
In vitro	Binds ENA-78,[504] GRO-α (K_d = 0.1 nmol/L),[504] GRO-β (K_d = 0.2 nmol/L),[504] GRO-γ (K_d = 0.4 nmol/L),[504] IL-8,[504] IP-10,[504] NAP-2,[504] SDF-1α,[504] and vMIP-II[504]; vORF-74 constitutively signals through protein kinase C, Jun N-terminal kinase/stress-associated protein kinase, and p38MAPK[915,916]; engagement of vORF-74 by GRO-α or IL-8 leads to activation of phospholipase C and generation of inositol triphosphate[917]; transformation of EC cells via transfection with vORF-74 leads to cell proliferation and production of VEGF.[915]
In vivo	Oncogene[915,916]; transgenic expression of vORF-74 in mice leads to Kaposi's sarcoma–like lesions.[918]
Pathologic association(s)	Kaposi's sarcoma,[919] primary effusion B-cell lymphoma.[920]
Genbank source (gene)	U82242 (v).
Gene coding region (kbp)	1.0 (v).
Chromosomal location	N/A.
Exons	Not reported.
Introns	Not reported.
Natural mutations/polymorphisms	Not reported.
Genbank source (RNA)	Not reported.
Size of RNA (kbp)	Not reported.
RNA splice variants	Not reported.

VIRAL CHEMOKINE AND CHEMOKINE RECEPTOR HOMOLOGS

Cytomegalovirus US28 Protein (vUS28)

Other names	HHRF3.
Similar proteins	hCCR1.
Genbank source	AAA98741 (v).
Size of mature protein (Kd)	41.0 (v).
Amino acids in mature protein	354 (v).
Stable form(s)	Monomer.
Glycosylation sites	1 N (v).
Disulfide bonds	0 (v).
3D structure	Not reported.
Mature protein variants	Four variants described.[376]
Tissue and cellular expression	CMV encoded.
Regulation of expression	
Up	Not reported.
Down	Not reported.
Biologic activities	
In vitro	Binds FKN (K_d = 0.4 nmol/L), MCP-1 (K_d = 0.6 nmol/L), MCP-3, MIP-1α (K_d = 1.2 nmol/L), MIP-1β (K_d = 7.5 nmol/L), and RANTES (K_d = 0.3 nmol/L)[181,921,922]; engagement of US28 by MCP-3 and RANTES activates G_{ai} and G_{a16} and stimulates intracellular Ca^{2+} mobilization in US28-transfected cells[181]; coreceptor for some strains of HIV[489,923]; engagement of US28 by RANTES or MCP-1 induces smooth muscle cell chemotaxis[924]; acts as a sequestrant for MCP-1, MCP-3, MIP-1α, MIP-1β, and RANTES[925]; coreceptor for CMV.[921]
In vivo	Not reported.
Pathologic association(s)	CMV-induced vascular disease,[924] HIV/AIDS.[489]
Genbank source (gene)	L20501 (v).
Gene coding region (kbp)	1.1 (v).
Chromosomal location	N/A.
Exons	N/A.
Introns	N/A.
Natural mutations/polymorphisms	Not reported.
Genbank source (RNA)	Not reported.
Size of RNA (kbp)	1.3/2.9 (v).[925]
RNA splice variants	Not reported.

REFERENCES

1. Taub DD. Chemokine-leukocyte interactions. The voodoo that they do so well. *Cytokine Growth Factor Rev* 1996;7(4):355–376.

2. Baggiolini M. Chemokines and leukocyte traffic. *Nature* 1998;392(6676):565–568.

3. Luster AD. Chemokines—chemotactic cytokines that mediate inflammation. *N Engl J Med* 1998;338(7):436–445.

4. Locati M, Murphy PM. Chemokines and chemokine receptors: biology and clinical relevance in inflammation and AIDS. *Annu Rev Med* 1999;50:425–440.

5. Reape TJ, Groot PH. Chemokines and atherosclerosis. *Atherosclerosis* 1999;147(2):213–225.

6. Lalani AS, McFadden G. Evasion and exploitation of chemokines by viruses. *Cytokine Growth Factor Rev* 1999;10(3–4):219–233.

7. Berger EA, Murphy PM, Farber JM. Chemokine receptors as HIV-1 coreceptors: roles in viral entry, tropism, and disease. *Annu Rev Immunol* 1999;17:657–700.

8. Homey B, Zlotnik A. Chemokines in allergy. *Curr Opin Immunol* 1999;11(6):626–634.

9. Ransohoff RM. Mechanisms of inflammation in MS tissue: adhesion molecules and chemokines. *J Neuroimmunol* 1999;98(1):57–68.

10. Pardigol A, et al. HCC-2, a human chemokine: gene structure, expression pattern, and biological activity. *Proc Natl Acad Sci U S A* 1998;95(11):6308–6313.

11. Miller MD, et al. A novel polypeptide secreted by activated human T lymphocytes. *J Immunol* 1989;143(9):2907–2916.

12. Burd PR, et al. Cloning and characterization of a novel T cell activation gene. *J Immunol* 1987;139(9):3126–3131.

13. Paolini JF, et al. The chemokines IL-8, monocyte chemoattractant protein-1, and I-309 are monomers at physiologically relevant concentrations [published erratum appears in *J Immunol* 1996;156(8):following 3088]. *J Immunol* 1994;153(6):2704–2717.

14. Miller MD, et al. Sequence and chromosomal location of the I-309 gene. Relationship to genes encoding a family of inflammatory cytokines. *J Immunol* 1990;145(8):2737–2744.

15. Oh CK, et al. Two different negative regulatory elements control the transcription of T-cell activation gene 3 in activated mast cells. *Biochem J* 1997;323(Pt 2):511–519.

16. Selvan RS, Zhou LJ, Krangel MS. Regulation of I-309 gene expression in human monocytes by endogenous interleukin-1. *Eur J Immunol* 1997;27(3):687–694.

17. Miller MD, Krangel MS. The human cytokine I-309 is a monocyte chemoattractant. *Proc Natl Acad Sci U S A* 1992;89(7):2950–2954.

18. Luo Y, et al. Biologic activities of the murine beta-chemokine TCA3. *J Immunol* 1994;153(10):4616–4624.

19. Goya I, et al. Identification of CCR8 as the specific receptor for the human beta-chemokine I-309: cloning and molecular characterization of murine CCR8 as the receptor for TCA-3. *J Immunol* 1998;160(4):1975–1981.

20. Luo Y, Dorf ME. Beta-chemokine TCA3 binds to mesangial cells and induces adhesion, chemotaxis, and proliferation. *J Immunol* 1996;156(2):742–748.

21. Luo Y, D'Amore PA, Dorf ME. Beta-chemokine TCA3 binds to and activates rat vascular smooth muscle cells. *J Immunol* 1996;157(5):2143–2148.

22. Horuk R, et al. The CC chemokine I-309 inhibits CCR8-dependent infection by diverse HIV-1 strains. *J Biol Chem* 1998;273(1):386–391.

23. Roos RS, et al. Identification of CCR8, the receptor for the human CC chemokine I-309. *J Biol Chem* 1997;272(28):17251–17254.

24. Van Snick J, et al. I-309/T cell activation gene-3 chemokine protects murine T cell lymphomas against dexamethasone-induced apoptosis. *J Immunol* 1996;157(6):2570–2576.

25. Devi S, et al. Biologic activities of the beta-chemokine TCA3 on neutrophils and macrophages. *J Immunol* 1995;154(10):5376–5383.

26. Doyle HA, Murphy JW. Role of the C-C chemokine, TCA3, in the protective anticryptococcal cell-mediated immune response. *J Immunol* 1999;162(8):4824–4833.

27. Godiska R, et al. Chemokine expression in murine experimental allergic encephalomyelitis. *J Neuroimmunol* 1995;58(2):167–176.

28. Ou ZL, Natori Y. Gene expression of CC chemokines in experimental acute tubulointerstitial nephritis [see comments]. *J Lab Clin Med* 1999;133(1):41–47.

29. Naruse K, et al. A YAC contig of the human CC chemokine genes clustered on chromosome 17q11.2. *Genomics* 1996;34(2):236–240.

30. Teuscher C, et al. Sequence polymorphisms in the chemokines Scya1 (TCA-3), Scya2 [monocyte chemoattractant protein (MCP)-1], and Scya12 (MCP-5) are candidates for eae7, a locus controlling susceptibility to monophasic remitting/nonrelapsing experimental allergic encephalomyelitis. *J Immunol* 1999;163(4):2262–2266.

31. Smith A, et al. Sigje, a member of the small inducible gene family that includes platelet factor 4 and melanoma growth stimulatory activity, is on mouse chromosome 11. *Cytogenet Cell Genet* 1989;52(3–4):194–196.

32. Hieshima K, et al. A novel human CC chemokine PARC that is most homologous to macrophage-inflammatory protein-1 alpha/LD78 alpha and chemotactic for T lymphocytes, but not for monocytes. *J Immunol* 1997;159(3):1140–1149.

33. Yoshimura T, Takeya M, Takahashi K. Molecular cloning of rat monocyte chemoattractant protein-1 (MCP-1) and its expression in rat spleen cells and tumor cell lines. *Biochem Biophys Res Commun* 1991;174(2):504–509.

34. Xu LL, et al. Human recombinant monocyte chemotactic protein and other C-C chemokines bind and induce directional migration of dendritic cells *in vitro*. *J Leukoc Biol* 1996;60(3):365–371.

35. Jones ML, et al. Potential role of monocyte chemoattractant protein 1/JE in monocyte/macrophage-dependent IgA immune complex alveolitis in the rat. *J Immunol* 1992;149(6):2147–2154.

36. Kim KS, et al. Structural characterization of a monomeric chemokine: monocyte chemoattractant protein-3. *FEBS Lett* 1996;395(2–3):277–282.

37. Van Coillie E, Van Damme J, Opdenakker G. The MCP/eotaxin subfamily of CC chemokines. *Cytokine Growth Factor Rev* 1999;10(1):61–86.

38. Lubkowski J, et al. The structure of MCP-1 in two crystal forms provides a rare example of variable quaternary interactions. *Nat Struct Biol* 1997;4(1):64–69.

39. Proost P, et al. Posttranslational modifications affect the activity of the human monocyte chemotactic proteins MCP-1 and MCP-2: identification of MCP-2(6–76) as a natural chemokine inhibitor. *J Immunol* 1998;160(8):4034–4041.

40. Michie CA, et al. Physiological secretion of chemokines in human breast milk. *Eur Cytokine Netw* 1998;9(2):123–129.

41. Izumi S, et al. Expression and regulation of monocyte chemoattractant protein-1 by human eosinophils. *Eur J Immunol* 1997;27(4):816–824.

42. Van Damme J, et al. Isolation of human monocyte chemotactic proteins and study of their producer and responder cells by immunotests and bioassays. *Methods Enzymol* 1997;287:109–127.

43. Conant K, et al. Induction of monocyte chemoattractant protein-1 in HIV-1 Tat-stimulated astrocytes and elevation in AIDS dementia. *Proc Natl Acad Sci U S A* 1998;95(6):3117–3121.

44. Peterson PK, et al. Differential production of and migratory response to beta chemokines by human microglia and astrocytes. *J Infect Dis* 1997;175(2):478–481.

45. De Waard V, et al. Serial analysis of gene expression to assess the endothelial cell response to an atherogenic stimulus. *Gene* 1999;226(1):1–8.

46. Bickel M, et al. Chemokine expression in human oral keratinocyte cell lines and keratinized mucosa. *J Dent Res* 1996;75(11):1827–1834.

47. Rollins BJ, Pober JS. Interleukin-4 induces the synthesis and secretion of MCP-1/JE by human endothelial cells. *Am J Pathol* 1991;138(6):1315–1319.

48. Dong Q, et al. IL-9 induces chemokine expression in lung epithelial cells and baseline airway eosinophilia in transgenic mice. *Eur J Immunol* 1999;29(7):2130–2139.

49. Foti M, et al. Upon dendritic cell (DC) activation chemokines and chemokine receptor expression are rapidly regulated for recruitment and maintenance of DC at the inflammatory site. *Int Immunol* 1999;11(6):979–986.

50. Takahara N, et al. Lysophosphatidylcholine stimulates the expression and production of MCP-1 by human vascular endothelial cells. *Metabolism* 1996;45(5):559–564.

51. Shyy YJ, et al. Human monocyte colony-stimulating factor stimulates the gene expression of monocyte chemotactic protein-1 and increases the adhesion of monocytes to endothelial monolayers. *J Clin Invest* 1993;92(4):1745–1751.

52. Deiters U, Muhlradt PF. Mycoplasmal lipopeptide MALP-2 induces the chemoattractant proteins macrophage inflammatory protein 1 alpha (MIP-1 alpha), monocyte chemoattractant protein 1, and MIP-2 and promotes leukocyte infiltration in mice. *Infect Immun* 1999;67(7):3390–3398.

53. Cushing SD, et al. Minimally modified low density lipoprotein induces monocyte chemotactic protein 1 in human endothelial cells and smooth muscle cells. *Proc Natl Acad Sci U S A* 1990;87(13):5134–5138.

54. Alberta JA, et al. Platelet-derived growth factor stimulation of monocyte chemoattractant protein-1 gene expression is mediated by transient activation of the phosphoinositide 3-kinase signal transduction pathway. *J Biol Chem* 1999;274(43):31062–31067.

55. Krakauer T. Induction of CC chemokines in human peripheral blood mononuclear cells by staphylococcal exotoxins and its prevention by pentoxifylline. *J Leukoc Biol* 1999;66(1):158–164.

56. Shyy YJ, et al. Fluid shear stress induces a biphasic response of human monocyte chemotactic protein 1 gene expression in vascular endothelium. *Proc Natl Acad Sci U S A* 1994;91(11):4678–4682.

57. Cole KE, et al. Interferon-inducible T cell alpha chemoattractant (I-TAC): a novel non-ELR CXC chemokine with potent activity on activated T cells through selective high affinity binding to CXCR3. *J Exp Med* 1998;187(12):2009–2021.

58. Weber KS, et al. Differential immobilization and hierarchical involvement of chemokines in monocyte arrest and transmigration on inflamed endothelium in shear flow. *Eur J Immunol* 1999;29(2):700–712.

59. Mukaida N, et al. Dexamethasone inhibits the induction of monocyte chemotactic-activating factor production by IL-1 or tumor necrosis factor. *J Immunol* 1991;146(4):1212–1215.

60. Tsao PS, et al. Nitric oxide regulates monocyte chemotactic protein-1. *Circulation* 1997;96(3):934–940.

61. Kurihara T, Bravo R. Cloning and functional expression of mCCR2, a murine receptor for the C-C chemokines JE and FIC. *J Biol Chem* 1996;271(20):11603–11607.

62. Bonini JA, Steiner DF. Molecular cloning and expression of a novel rat CC-chemokine receptor (rCCR10rR) that binds MCP-1 and MIP-1 beta with high affinity. *DNA Cell Biol* 1997;16(9):1023–1030.

63. Ochensberger B, et al. Regulation of cytokine expression and leukotriene formation in human basophils by growth factors, chemokines and chemotactic agonists. *Eur J Immunol* 1999;29(1):11–22.

64. Uguccioni M, et al. Actions of the chemotactic cytokines MCP-1, MCP-2, MCP-3, RANTES, MIP-1 alpha and MIP-1 beta on human monocytes. *Eur J Immunol* 1995;25(1):64–68.

65. Maghazachi AA, al-Aoukaty A, Schall TJ. C-C chemokines induce the chemotaxis of NK and IL-2-activated NK cells. Role for G proteins. *J Immunol* 1994;153(11):4969–4977.

66. Carr MW, et al. Monocyte chemoattractant protein 1 acts as a T-lymphocyte chemoattractant. *Proc Natl Acad Sci U S A* 1994;91(9):3652–3656.

67. Taub DD, et al. Monocyte chemotactic protein-1 (MCP-1), -2, and -3 are chemotactic for human T lymphocytes. *J Clin Invest* 1995;95(3):1370–1376.

68. Kuna P, et al. Characterization of the human basophil response to cytokines, growth factors, and histamine releasing factors of the intercrine/chemokine family. *J Immunol* 1993;150(5):1932–1943.

69. Nitschke M, et al. Effects of basophil-priming and stimulating cytokines on histamine release from isolated human skin mast cells. *Arch Dermatol Res* 1996;288(8):463–468.

70. Franci C, et al. Phosphorylation by a G protein-coupled kinase inhibits signaling and promotes internalization of the monocyte chemoattractant protein-1 receptor. Critical role of carboxyl-tail serines/threonines in receptor function. *J Immunol* 1996;157(12):5606–5612.

71. Aragay AM, et al. Monocyte chemoattractant protein-1-induced CCR2B receptor desensitization mediated by the G protein-coupled receptor kinase 2. *Proc Natl Acad Sci U S A* 1998;95(6):2985–2990.

72. Locati M, et al. Rapid induction of arachidonic acid release by monocyte chemotactic protein-1 and related chemokines. Role of Ca^{2+} influx, synergism with platelet-activating factor and significance for chemotaxis. *J Biol Chem* 1994;269(7):4746–4753.

73. Gerszten RE, et al. MCP-1 and IL-8 trigger firm adhesion of monocytes to vascular endothelium under flow conditions. *Nature* 1999;398(6729):718–723.

74. Schecter AD, et al. Tissue factor is induced by monocyte chemoattractant protein-1 in human aortic smooth muscle and THP-1 cells. *J Biol Chem* 1997;272(45):28568–28573.

75. Taub DD, et al. Chemokines and T lymphocyte activation: I. Beta chemokines costimulate human T lymphocyte activation *in vitro*. *J Immunol* 1996;156(6):2095–2103.

76. Rollins BJ, Walz A, Baggiolini M. Recombinant human MCP-1/JE induces chemotaxis, calcium flux, and the respiratory burst in human monocytes. *Blood* 1991;78(4):1112–1116.

77. Singh RK, Fidler IJ. Synergism between human recombinant monocyte chemotactic and activating factor and lipopolysaccharide for activation of antitumor properties in human blood monocytes. *Lymphokine Cytokine Res* 1993;12(5):285–291.

78. Karpus WJ, Kennedy KJ. MIP-1 alpha and MCP-1 differentially regulate acute and relapsing autoimmune encephalomyelitis as well as Th1/Th2 lymphocyte differentiation. *J Leukoc Biol* 1997;62(5):681–687.

79. Ayehunie S, et al. Human immunodeficiency virus-1 entry into purified blood dendritic cells through CC and CXC chemokine coreceptors. *Blood* 1997;90(4):1379–1386.

80. Ernst CA, et al. Biochemical and biologic characterization of murine monocyte chemoattractant protein-1. Identification of two functional domains. *J Immunol* 1994;152(7):3541–3549.

81. Plata-Salaman CR, Borkoski JP. Chemokines/intercrines and central regulation of feeding. *Am J Physiol* 1994;266(5 Pt 2):R1711–R1715.

82. Goede V, et al. Induction of inflammatory angiogenesis by monocyte chemoattractant protein-1. *Int J Cancer* 1999;82(5):765–770.

83. Gu L, et al. *In vivo* properties of monocyte chemoattractant protein-1. *J Leukoc Biol* 1997;62(5):577–580.

84. Lu B, et al. Abnormalities in monocyte recruitment and cytokine expression in monocyte chemoattractant protein 1-deficient mice. *J Exp Med* 1998;187(4):601–608.

85. Gu L, et al. Absence of monocyte chemoattractant protein-1 reduces atherosclerosis in low density lipoprotein receptor-deficient mice. *Mol Cell* 1998;2(2):275–281.

86. Gosling J, et al. MCP-1 deficiency reduces susceptibility to atherosclerosis in mice that overexpress human apolipoprotein B. *J Clin Invest* 1999;103(6):773–778.

87. Fisher NC, et al. Serum concentrations and peripheral secretion of the beta chemokines monocyte chemoattractant protein 1 and macrophage inflammatory protein 1 alpha in alcoholic liver disease. *Gut* 1999;45(3):416–420.

88. Inadera H, et al. Increase in circulating levels of monocyte chemoattractant protein-1 with aging. *J Interferon Cytokine Res* 1999;19(10):1179–1182.

89. Hayes IM, et al. Human vascular smooth muscle cells express receptors for CC chemokines. *Arterioscler Thromb Vasc Biol* 1998;18(3):397–403.

90. Neumark E, et al. MCP-1 expression as a potential contributor to the high malignancy phenotype of murine mammary adenocarcinoma cells. *Immunol Lett* 1999;68(1):141–146.

91. Riethdorf S, et al. Expression of the MCP-1 gene and the HPV 16 E6/E7 oncogenes in squamous cell carcinomas of the cervix uteri and metastases. *Pathobiology* 1998;66(6):260–267.

92. Kleine-Lowinski K, et al. Monocyte-chemo-attractant-protein-1 (MCP-1)-gene expression in cervical intra-epithelial neoplasias and cervical carcinomas. *Int J Cancer* 1999; 82(1):6–11.

93. Akoum A, et al. Increased monocyte chemotactic protein-1 level and activity in the peripheral blood of women with endometriosis. Le Groupe d'Investigation en Gynecologie. *Am J Obstet Gynecol* 1996;175(6):1620–1625.

94. Wada T, et al. MIP-1 alpha and MCP-1 contribute to crescents and interstitial lesions in human crescentic glomerulonephritis. *Kidney Int* 1999;56(3):995–1003.

95. Zou LP, et al. Dynamics of production of MIP-1 alpha, MCP-1 and MIP-2 and potential role of neutralization of these chemokines in the regulation of immune responses during experimental autoimmune neuritis in Lewis rats. *J Neuroimmunol* 1999;98(2):168–175.

96. Weiss L, et al. Plasma levels of monocyte chemoattractant protein-1 but not those of macrophage inhibitory protein-1 alpha and RANTES correlate with virus load in human immunodeficiency virus infection. *J Infect Dis* 1997;176(6): 1621–1624.

97. Ritter U, et al. Differential expression of chemokines in patients with localized and diffuse cutaneous American leishmaniasis. *J Infect Dis* 1996;173(3):699–709.

98. Hashimoto S, et al. Correlation of plasma monocyte chemoattractant protein-1 (MCP-1) and monocyte inflammatory protein-1 alpha (MIP-1 alpha) levels with disease activity and clinical course of sarcoidosis. *Clin Exp Immunol* 1998;111(3):604–610.

99. Spandau U, et al. MIG is a dominant lymphocyte-attractant chemokine in lichen planus lesions. *J Invest Dermatol* 1998;111(6):1003–1009.

100. Matsumori A, et al. Plasma levels of the monocyte chemotactic and activating factor/monocyte chemoattractant protein-1 are elevated in patients with acute myocardial infarction. *J Mol Cell Cardiol* 1997;29(1):419–423.

101. Negus RP, et al. Quantitative assessment of the leukocyte infiltrate in ovarian cancer and its relationship to the expression of C-C chemokines. *Am J Pathol* 1997;150(5):1723–1734.

102. Hefler L, et al. Monocyte chemoattractant protein-1 serum levels in ovarian cancer patients. *Br J Cancer* 1999;81(5): 855–859.

103. Hasegawa M, Sato S, Takehara K. Augmented production of chemokines [monocyte chemotactic protein-1 (MCP-1), macrophage inflammatory protein-1 alpha (MIP-1 alpha) and MIP-1 beta] in patients with systemic sclerosis: MCP-1 and MIP-1 alpha may be involved in the development of pulmonary fibrosis. *Clin Exp Immunol* 1999;117(1):159–165.

104. Bossink AW, et al. Plasma levels of the chemokines monocyte chemotactic proteins-1 and -2 are elevated in human sepsis. *Blood* 1995;86(10):3841–3847.

105. McTigue DM, et al. Selective chemokine mRNA accumulation in the rat spinal cord after contusion injury. *J Neurosci Res* 1998;53(3):368–376.

106. Uguccioni M, et al. Increased expression of IP-10, IL-8, MCP-1, and MCP-3 in ulcerative colitis. *Am J Pathol* 1999;155(2):331–336.

107. Engelhardt E, et al. Chemokines IL-8, GRO alpha, MCP-1, IP-10, and Mig are sequentially and differentially expressed during phase-specific infiltration of leukocyte subsets in human wound healing. *Am J Pathol* 1998;153(6):1849–1860.

108. Rovin BH, Lu L, Saxena R. A novel polymorphism in the MCP-1 gene regulatory region that influences MCP-1 expression. *Biochem Biophys Res Commun* 1999;259(2):344–348.

109. Kwon BS, Weissman SM. cDNA sequences of two inducible T-cell genes. *Proc Natl Acad Sci U S A* 1989;86(6):1963–1967.

110. Nakao M, Nomiyama H, Shimada K. Structures of human genes coding for cytokine LD78 and their expression. *Mol Cell Biol* 1990;10(7):3646–3658.

111. Grove M, et al. Sequence of the murine haemopoietic stem cell inhibitor/macrophage inflammatory protein 1 alpha gene. *Nucleic Acids Res* 1990;18(18):5561.

112. Patel VP, et al. Molecular and functional characterization of two novel human C-C chemokines as inhibitors of two distinct classes of myeloid progenitors. *J Exp Med* 1997;185(7):1163–1172.

113. Shi MM, Godleski JJ, Paulauskis JD. Molecular cloning and posttranscriptional regulation of macrophage inflammatory protein-1 alpha in alveolar macrophages. *Biochem Biophys Res Commun* 1995;211(1):289–295.

114. Czaplewski LG, et al. Identification of amino acid residues critical for aggregation of human CC chemokines macrophage inflammatory protein (MIP)-1 alpha, MIP-1 beta, and RANTES. Characterization of active disaggregated chemokine variants. *J Biol Chem* 1999;274(23):16077–16084.

115. Nibbs RJ, et al. LD78beta, a non-allelic variant of human MIP-1 alpha (LD78alpha), has enhanced receptor interactions and potent HIV suppressive activity. *J Biol Chem* 1999;274(25):17478–17483.

116. Rudloff S, et al. Inflammation markers and cytokines in breast milk of atopic and nonatopic women. *Allergy* 1999;54(3):206–211.

117. Borzi RM, et al. Flow cytometric analysis of intracellular chemokines in chondrocytes *in vivo*: constitutive expression and enhancement in osteoarthritis and rheumatoid arthritis. *FEBS Lett* 1999;455(3):238–242.

118. Kasama T, et al. Regulation of neutrophil-derived chemokine expression by IL-10. *J Immunol* 1994;152(7):3559–3569.

119. Meda L, et al. Proinflammatory profile of cytokine production by human monocytes and murine microglia stimulated with beta-amyloid[25–35]. *J Neuroimmunol* 1999;93(1–2):45–52.

120. Miyamoto Y, Kim SU. Cytokine-induced production of macrophage inflammatory protein-1 alpha (MIP-1 alpha) in cultured human astrocytes. *J Neurosci Res* 1999;55(2):245–251.

121. Cipriani B, et al. Activation of C-C beta-chemokines in human peripheral blood gammadelta T cells by isopentenyl pyrophosphate and regulation by cytokines. *Blood* 2000;95(1):39–47.

122. Cassatella MA. Interferon-gamma inhibits the lipopolysaccharide-induced macrophage inflammatory protein-1 alpha gene transcription in human neutrophils. *Immunol Lett* 1996;49(1–2):79–82.

123. Berkman N, et al. Interleukin 13 inhibits macrophage inflammatory protein-1 alpha production from human alveolar macrophages and monocytes. *Am J Respir Cell Mol Biol* 1996;15(3):382–389.

124. Nibbs RJB, et al. Cloning and characterization of a novel murine beta chemokine receptor, D6. Comparison to three other related macrophage inflammatory protein-1 alpha receptors, CCR-1, CCR-3, and CCR-5. *J Biol Chem* 1997;272(19):12495–12504.

125. Nibbs RJ, et al. Cloning and characterization of a novel promiscuous human beta-chemokine receptor D6. *J Biol Chem* 1997;272(51):32078–32083.

126. Kuschert GS, et al. Glycosaminoglycans interact selectively with chemokines and modulate receptor binding and cellular responses. *Biochemistry* 1999;38(39):12959–12968.

127. Tanabe S, et al. Murine astrocytes express a functional chemokine receptor. *J Neurosci* 1997;17(17):6522–6528.

128. Bischoff SC, et al. RANTES and related chemokines activate human basophil granulocytes through different G protein-coupled receptors. *Eur J Immunol* 1993;23(3):761–767.

129. Schall TJ, et al. Human macrophage inflammatory protein alpha (MIP-1 alpha) and MIP-1 beta chemokines attract distinct populations of lymphocytes. *J Exp Med* 1993;177(6):1821–1826.

130. Sozzani S, et al. Migration of dendritic cells in response to formyl peptides, C5a, and a distinct set of chemokines. *J Immunol* 1995;155(7):3292–3295.

131. Rot A, et al. RANTES and macrophage inflammatory protein 1 alpha induce the migration and activation of normal human eosinophil granulocytes. *J Exp Med* 1992;176(6):1489–1495.

132. Wang JM, et al. Human recombinant macrophage inflammatory protein-1 alpha and -beta and monocyte chemotactic and activating factor utilize common and unique receptors on human monocytes. *J Immunol* 1993;150(7):3022–3029.

133. Takano K, et al. Rat macrophage inflammatory protein-1 alpha, a CC chemokine, acts as a neutrophil chemoattractant *in vitro* and *in vivo*. *Inflammation* 1999;23(5):411–424.

134. Taub DD, et al. Preferential migration of activated CD4+ and CD8+ T cells in response to MIP-1 alpha and MIP-1 beta. *Science* 1993;260(5106):355–358.

135. Wong M, Fish EN. RANTES and MIP-1 alpha activate stats in T cells. *J Biol Chem* 1998;273(1):309–314.

136. Dunlop DJ, et al. Demonstration of stem cell inhibition and myeloprotective effects of SCI/rhMIP1 alpha *in vivo*. *Blood* 1992;79(9):2221–2225.

137. Mantel C, et al. Macrophage inflammatory protein-1 alpha enhances growth factor-stimulated phosphatidylcholine metabolism and increases cAMP levels in the human growth factor-dependent cell line M07e, events associated with growth suppression. *J Immunol* 1995;154(5):2342–2350.

138. Tsou CL, et al. Identification of C-C chemokine receptor 1 (CCR1) as the monocyte hemofiltrate C-C chemokine (HCC)-1 receptor. *J Exp Med* 1998;188(3):603–608.

139. Kukita T, et al. Macrophage inflammatory protein-1 alpha (LD78) expressed in human bone marrow: its role in regulation of hematopoiesis and osteoclast recruitment. *Lab Invest* 1997;76(3):399–406.

140. Menten P, et al. The LD78beta isoform of MIP-1 alpha is the most potent CCR5 agonist and HIV-1-inhibiting chemokine. *J Clin Invest* 1999;104(4):R1–R5.

141. Su S, et al. Inhibition of immature erythroid progenitor cell proliferation by macrophage inflammatory protein-1 alpha by interacting mainly with a C-C chemokine receptor, CCR1. *Blood* 1997;90(2):605–611.

142. Wolpe SD, Cerami A. Macrophage inflammatory proteins 1 and 2: members of a novel superfamily of cytokines. *FASEB J* 1989;3(14):2565–2573.

143. Taub DD, et al. Chemokine-induced human lymphocyte infiltration and engraftment in huPBL-SCID mice. *Methods Enzymol* 1997;287:265–291.

144. Minano FJ, et al. Hypothalamic interaction between macrophage inflammatory protein-1 alpha (MIP-1 alpha) and MIP-1 beta in rats: a new level for fever control? *J Physiol (Lond)* 1996;491(Pt 1):209–217.

145. Clemons MJ, et al. A randomized phase-II study of BB-10010 (macrophage inflammatory protein-1 alpha) in patients with advanced breast cancer receiving 5-fluorouracil, adriamycin, and cyclophosphamide chemotherapy. *Blood* 1998;92(5):1532–1540.

146. Cook DN, et al. Requirement of MIP-1 alpha for an inflammatory response to viral infection. *Science* 1995;269(5230):1583–1585.

147. Tumpey TM, et al. Absence of macrophage inflammatory protein-1 alpha prevents the development of blinding herpes stromal keratitis. *J Virol* 1998;72(5):3705–3710.

148. Wilcox JN, et al. Local expression of inflammatory cytokines in human atherosclerotic plaques. *J Atheroscler Thromb* 1994;1[Suppl 1]:S10–S13.

149. Hatano Y, et al. Macrophage inflammatory protein 1 alpha expression by synovial fluid neutrophils in rheumatoid arthritis. *Ann Rheum Dis* 1999;58(5):297–302.

150. Balashov KE, et al. CCR5(+) and CXCR3(+) T cells are increased in multiple sclerosis and their ligands MIP-1 alpha and IP-10 are expressed in demyelinating brain lesions. *Proc Natl Acad Sci U S A* 1999;96(12):6873–6878.

151. Teruya-Feldstein J, et al. MIP-1 alpha expression in tissues from patients with hemophagocytic syndrome. *Lab Invest* 1999;79(12):1583–1590.

152. Yoong KF, et al. Expression and function of CXC and CC chemokines in human malignant liver tumors: a role for human monokine induced by gamma-interferon in lymphocyte recruitment to hepatocellular carcinoma. *Hepatology* 1999;30(1):100–111.

153. Nuovo GJ, Alfieri ML. AIDS dementia is associated with massive, activated HIV-1 infection and concomitant expression of several cytokines. *Mol Med* 1996;2(3):358–366.

154. Suzuki N, et al. Selective accumulation of CCR5+ T lymphocytes into inflamed joints of rheumatoid arthritis. *Int Immunol* 1999;11(4):553–559.

155. Oshima M, et al. Expression of C-C chemokines in bronchoalveolar lavage cells from patients with granulomatous lung diseases. *Lung* 1999;177(4):229–240.

156. Bonville CA, Rosenberg HF, Domachowske JB. Macrophage inflammatory protein-1 alpha and RANTES are present in nasal secretions during ongoing upper respiratory tract infection. *Pediatr Allergy Immunol* 1999;10(1):39–44.

157. Hirashima M, et al. Nucleotide sequence of the third cytokine LD78 gene and mapping of all three LD78 gene loci to human chromosome 17. *DNA Seq* 1992;3(4):203–212.

158. Wilson SD, et al. Clustering of cytokine genes on mouse chromosome 11. *J Exp Med* 1990;171(4):1301–1314.

159. Widmer U, et al. Genomic structure of murine macrophage inflammatory protein-1 alpha and conservation of potential regulatory sequences with a human homolog, LD78. *J Immunol* 1991;146(11):4031–4040.

160. Al-Sharif FM, et al. A new microsatellite marker within the promoter region of the MIP-1A gene. *Immunogenetics* 1999;49(7–8):740–741.

161. Forssmann U, et al. CKbeta8, a novel CC chemokine that predominantly acts on monocytes. *FEBS Lett* 1997;408(2):211–216.

162. Ponath PD, et al. Cloning of the human eosinophil chemoattractant, eotaxin. Expression, receptor binding, and functional properties suggest a mechanism for the selective recruitment of eosinophils. *J Clin Invest* 1996;97(3):604–612.

163. Lodi PJ, et al. High-resolution solution structure of the beta chemokine hMIP-1 beta by multidimensional NMR. *Science* 1994;263(5154):1762–1767.

164. Franz-Bacon K, et al. Human thymocytes express CCR-3 and are activated by eotaxin. *Blood* 1999;93(10):3233–3240.

165. Dikic I, Dikic I, Schlessinger J. Identification of a new Pyk2 isoform implicated in chemokine and antigen receptor signaling. *J Biol Chem* 1998;273(23):14301–14308.

166. Sozzani S, et al. Receptor expression and responsiveness of human dendritic cells to a defined set of CC and CXC chemokines. *J Immunol* 1997;159(4):1993–2000.

167. Taub DD, et al. Alpha and beta chemokines induce NK cell migration and enhance NK-mediated cytolysis. *J Immunol* 1995;155(8):3877–3888.

168. Gong W, et al. Monocyte chemotactic protein-2 activates CCR5 and blocks CD4/CCR5-mediated HIV-1 entry/replication. *J Biol Chem* 1998;273(8):4289–4292.

169. Wong M, Silverman ED, Fish EN. Evidence for RANTES, monocyte chemotactic protein-1, and macrophage inflammatory protein-1 beta expression in Kawasaki disease. *J Rheumatol* 1997;24(6):1179–1185.

170. Forssmann U, et al. Eotaxin-2, a novel CC chemokine that is selective for the chemokine receptor CCR3, and acts like eotaxin on human eosinophil and basophil leukocytes. *J Exp Med* 1997;185(12):2171–2176.

171. Nelson PJ, Pattison JM, Krensky AM. Gene expression of RANTES. *Methods Enzymol* 1997;287:148–162.

172. Chung CW, et al. The three-dimensional solution structure of RANTES. *Biochemistry* 1995;34(29):9307–9314.

173. Proost P, et al. Amino-terminal truncation of chemokines by CD26/dipeptidyl-peptidase IV. Conversion of RANTES into a potent inhibitor of monocyte chemotaxis and HIV-1-infection. *J Biol Chem* 1998;273(13):7222–7227.

174. Barnes DA, et al. Induction of RANTES expression by astrocytes and astrocytoma cell lines. *J Neuroimmunol* 1996;71(1–2):207–214.

175. Von Luettichau I, et al. RANTES chemokine expression in diseased and normal human tissues. *Cytokine* 1996;8(1):89–98.

176. Power CA, et al. Chemokine and chemokine receptor mRNA expression in human platelets. *Cytokine* 1995;7(6):479–482.

177. Marfaing-Koka A, et al. Regulation of the production of the RANTES chemokine by endothelial cells. Synergistic induction by IFN-gamma plus TNF-alpha and inhibition by IL-4 and IL-13. *J Immunol* 1995;154(4):1870–1878.

178. John M, et al. Human airway smooth muscle cells express and release RANTES in response to T helper 1 cytokines: regulation by T helper 2 cytokines and corticosteroids. *J Immunol* 1997;158(4):1841–1847.

179. Stellato C, et al. Expression of the chemokine RANTES by a human bronchial epithelial cell line. Modulation by cytokines and glucocorticoids. *J Immunol* 1995;155(1):410–418.

180. Berkman N, et al. Expression of RANTES in human airway epithelial cells: effect of corticosteroids and interleukin-4, -10 and -13. *Immunology* 1996;87(4):599–603.

181. Billstrom MA, et al. Intracellular signaling by the chemokine receptor US28 during human cytomegalovirus infection. *J Virol* 1998;72(7):5535–5544.

182. Taub D, et al. Bone marrow-derived murine mast cells migrate, but do not degranulate, in response to chemokines. *J Immunol* 1995;154(5):2393–2402.

183. Schall TJ, et al. Selective attraction of monocytes and T lymphocytes of the memory phenotype by cytokine RANTES. *Nature* 1990;347(6294):669–671.

184. Tilton B, et al. G-Protein-coupled receptors and Fcgamma-receptors mediate activation of Akt/protein kinase B in human phagocytes. *J Biol Chem* 1997;272(44):28096–28101.

185. Al-Aoukaty A, Rolstad B, Maghazachi AA. Recruitment of pleckstrin and phosphoinositide 3-kinase gamma into the cell membranes, and their association with G beta gamma after activation of NK cells with chemokines. *J Immunol* 1999;162(6):3249–3255.

186. Bacon KB, et al. RANTES induces tyrosine kinase activity of stably complexed p125FAK and ZAP-70 in human T cells. *J Exp Med* 1996;184(3):873–882.

187. Oppermann M, et al. Differential effects of CC chemokines on CC chemokine receptor 5 (CCR5) phosphorylation and identification of phosphorylation sites on the CCR5 carboxyl terminus. *J Biol Chem* 1999;274(13):8875–8885.

188. Meurer R, et al. Formation of eosinophilic and monocytic intradermal inflammatory sites in the dog by injection of human RANTES but not human monocyte chemoattractant protein 1, human macrophage inflammatory protein 1 alpha, or human interleukin 8. *J Exp Med* 1993;178(6):1913–1921.

189. Conti P, et al. Massive infiltration of basophilic cells in inflamed tissue after injection of RANTES. *Immunol Lett* 1997;58(2):101–106.

190. Chensue SW, et al. Differential expression and cross-regulatory function of RANTES during mycobacterial (type 1) and schistosomal (type 2) antigen-elicited granulomatous inflammation. *J Immunol* 1999;163(1):165–173.

191. Berkman N, et al. Expression of RANTES mRNA and protein in airways of patients with mild asthma. *Am J Respir Crit Care Med* 1996;154(6 Pt 1):1804–1811.

192. Barnes DA, et al. Polyclonal antibody directed against human RANTES ameliorates disease in the Lewis rat adjuvant-induced arthritis model. *J Clin Invest* 1998;101(12):2910–2919.

193. Pattison JM, et al. RANTES chemokine expression in transplant-associated accelerated atherosclerosis. *J Heart Lung Transplant* 1996;15(12):1194–1199.

194. Gluck J, Rogala B. Chemokine RANTES in atopic dermatitis. *Arch Immunol Ther Exp (Warsz)* 1999;47(6):367–372.

195. Bradley LM, et al. Islet-specific Th1, but not Th2, cells secrete multiple chemokines and promote rapid induction of autoimmune diabetes. *J Immunol* 1999;162(5):2511–2520.

196. Hornung D, et al. Immunolocalization and regulation of the chemokine RANTES in human endometrial and endometriosis tissues and cells. *J Clin Endocrinol Metab* 1997;82(5):1621–1628.

197. Lloyd CM, et al. RANTES and monocyte chemoattractant protein-1 (MCP-1) play an important role in the inflammatory phase of crescentic nephritis, but only MCP-1 is involved in crescent formation and interstitial fibrosis. *J Exp Med* 1997;185(7):1371–1380.

198. Sorensen TL, et al. Expression of specific chemokines and chemokine receptors in the central nervous system of multiple sclerosis patients. *J Clin Invest* 1999;103(6):807–815.

199. Pattison J, et al. RANTES chemokine expression in cell-mediated transplant rejection of the kidney. *Lancet* 1994;343(8891):209–211.

200. Nelson PJ, et al. Genomic organization and transcriptional regulation of the RANTES chemokine gene. *J Immunol* 1993;151(5):2601–2612.

201. Danoff TM, et al. Cloning, genomic organization, and chromosomal localization of the Scya5 gene encoding the murine chemokine RANTES. *J Immunol* 1994;152(3):1182–1189.

202. Donlon TA, et al. Localization of a human T-cell-specific gene, RANTES (D17S136E), to chromosome 17q11.2-q12. *Genomics* 1990;6(3):548–553.

203. Liu H, et al. Polymorphism in RANTES chemokine promoter affects HIV-1 disease progression. *Proc Natl Acad Sci U S A* 1999;96(8):4581–4585.

204. Nickel RG, et al. Atopic dermatitis is associated with a functional mutation in the promoter of the C-C chemokine RANTES. *J Immunol* 2000;164(3):1612–1616.

205. Youn BS, et al. A novel chemokine, macrophage inflammatory protein-related protein-2, inhibits colony formation of bone marrow myeloid progenitors. *J Immunol* 1995;155(5):2661–2667.

206. Pollard JW, Lin EY, Zhu L. Complexity in uterine macrophage responses to cytokines in mice. *Biol Reprod* 1998;58(6):1469–1475.

207. Wu Y, Prystowsky MB, Orlofsky A. Sustained high-level production of murine chemokine C10 during chronic inflammation. *Cytokine* 1999;11(7):523–530.

208. Orlofsky A, Lin EY, Prystowsky MB. Selective induction of the beta chemokine C10 by IL-4 in mouse macrophages. *J Immunol* 1994;152(10):5084–5091.

209. Asensio VC, et al. C10 is a novel chemokine expressed in experimental inflammatory demyelinating disorders that promotes recruitment of macrophages to the central nervous system. *Am J Pathol* 1999;154(4):1181–1191.

210. Gewirtz AM, et al. Chemokine regulation of human megakaryocytopoiesis. *Blood* 1995;86(7):2559–2567.

211. Hogaboam CM, et al. Immunomodulatory role of C10 chemokine in a murine model of allergic bronchopulmonary aspergillosis. *J Immunol* 1999;162(10):6071–6079.

212. Berger MS, et al. The gene for C10, a member of the beta-chemokine family, is located on mouse chromosome 11 and

contains a novel second exon not found in other chemokines. *DNA Cell Biol* 1993;12(9):839–847.

213. Minty A, et al. Molecular cloning of the MCP-3 chemokine gene and regulation of its expression. *Eur Cytokine Netw* 1993;4(2):99–110.

214. Opdenakker G, et al. The human MCP-3 gene (SCYA7): cloning, sequence analysis, and assignment to the C-C chemokine gene cluster on chromosome 17q11.2-q12. *Genomics* 1994;21(2):403–408.

215. Meunier S, et al. Determination of the three-dimensional structure of CC chemokine monocyte chemoattractant protein 3 by 1H two-dimensional NMR spectroscopy. *Biochemistry* 1997;36(15):4412–4422.

216. Van Damme J, et al. Structural and functional identification of two human, tumor-derived monocyte chemotactic proteins (MCP-2 and MCP-3) belonging to the chemokine family. *J Exp Med* 1992;176(1):59–65.

217. Polentarutti N, et al. Expression of monocyte chemotactic protein-3 in human monocytes and endothelial cells. *Eur Cytokine Netw* 1997;8(3):271–274.

218. Teran LM, et al. Th1- and Th2-type cytokines regulate the expression and production of eotaxin and RANTES by human lung fibroblasts. *Am J Respir Cell Mol Biol* 1999;20(4):777–786.

219. Combadiere C, et al. Monocyte chemoattractant protein-3 is a functional ligand for CC chemokine receptors 1 and 2B. *J Biol Chem* 1995;270(50):29671–29675.

220. Bonini JA, et al. Cloning, expression, and chromosomal mapping of a novel human CC-chemokine receptor (CCR10) that displays high-affinity binding for MCP-1 and MCP-3. *DNA Cell Biol* 1997;16(10):1249–1256.

221. Uguccioni M, et al. High expression of the chemokine receptor CCR3 in human blood basophils. Role in activation by eotaxin, MCP-4, and other chemokines. *J Clin Invest* 1997;100(5):1137–1143.

222. Dahinden CA, et al. Monocyte chemotactic protein 3 is a most effective basophil- and eosinophil-activating chemokine. *J Exp Med* 1994;179(2):751–756.

223. Allavena P, et al. Induction of natural killer cell migration by monocyte chemotactic protein-1, -2 and -3. *Eur J Immunol* 1994;24(12):3233–3236.

224. Fioretti F, et al. Reduced tumorigenicity and augmented leukocyte infiltration after monocyte chemotactic protein-3 (MCP-3) gene transfer: perivascular accumulation of dendritic cells in peritumoral tissue and neutrophil recruitment within the tumor. *J Immunol* 1998;161(1):342–346.

225. Humbert M, et al. Bronchial mucosal expression of the genes encoding chemokines RANTES and MCP-3 in symptomatic atopic and nonatopic asthmatics: relationship to the eosinophil-active cytokines interleukin (IL)-5, granulocyte macrophage-colony-stimulating factor, and IL-3. *Am J Respir Cell Mol Biol* 1997;16(1):1–8.

226. Wang X, et al. Expression of monocyte chemotactic protein-3 mRNA in rat vascular smooth muscle cells and in carotid artery after balloon angioplasty. *Biochim Biophys Acta* 2000;1500(1):41–48.

227. Wright ED, et al. Monocyte chemotactic protein expression in allergy and non-allergy-associated chronic sinusitis. *J Otolaryngol* 1998;27(5):281–287.

228. McManus C, et al. MCP-1, MCP-2 and MCP-3 expression in multiple sclerosis lesions: an immunohistochemical and in situ hybridization study. *J Neuroimmunol* 1998;86(1):20–29.

229. Wang X, et al. Molecular cloning and expression of the rat monocyte chemotactic protein-3 gene: a possible role in stroke. *Brain Res Mol Brain Res* 1999;71(2):304–312.

230. Fiten P, et al. Microsatellite polymorphisms in the gene promoter of monocyte chemotactic protein-3 and analysis of the association between monocyte chemotactic protein-3 alleles and multiple sclerosis development. *J Neuroimmunol* 1999;95(1–2):195–201.

231. Chang HC, et al. Cloning and expression of a gamma-interferon-inducible gene in monocytes: a new member of a cytokine gene family. *Int Immunol* 1989;1(4):388–397.

232. Van Coillie E, et al. Functional comparison of two human monocyte chemotactic protein-2 isoforms, role of the amino-terminal pyroglutamic acid and processing by CD26/dipeptidyl peptidase IV. *Biochemistry* 1998;37(36):12672–12680.

233. Van Coillie E, et al. The human MCP-2 gene (SCYA8): cloning, sequence analysis, tissue expression, and assignment to the CC chemokine gene contig on chromosome 17q11.2. *Genomics* 1997;40(2):323–331.

234. Van Coillie E, et al. Transcriptional control of the human MCP-2 gene promoter by IFN-gamma and IL-1 beta in connective tissue cells. *J Leukoc Biol* 1999;66(3):502–511.

235. Van Coillie E, et al. Human monocyte chemotactic protein-2: cDNA cloning and regulated expression of mRNA in mesenchymal cells. *Biochem Biophys Res Commun* 1997;231(3):726–730.

236. Gong X, et al. Monocyte chemotactic protein-2 (MCP-2) uses CCR1 and CCR2B as its functional receptors. *J Biol Chem* 1997;272(18):11682–11685.

237. Poltorak AN, et al. MIP-1 gamma: molecular cloning, expression, and biological activities of a novel CC chemokine that is constitutively secreted *in vivo*. *J Inflamm* 1995;45(3):207–219.

238. Ishi Y, et al. Cloning of rat eotaxin: ozone inhalation increases mRNA and protein expression in lungs of brown Norway rats. *Am J Physiol* 1998;274(1 Pt 1):L171–L176.

239. Rothenberg ME, Luster AD, Leder P. Murine eotaxin: an eosinophil chemoattractant inducible in endothelial cells and in interleukin 4-induced tumor suppression. *Proc Natl Acad Sci U S A* 1995;92(19):8960–8964.

240. Crump MP, et al. Solution structure of eotaxin, a chemokine that selectively recruits eosinophils in allergic inflammation. *J Biol Chem* 1998;273(35):22471–22479.

241. Noso N, et al. Delayed production of biologically active O-glycosylated forms of human eotaxin by tumor-necrosis-factor-alpha-stimulated dermal fibroblasts. *Eur J Biochem* 1998;253(1):114–122.

242. Kitaura M, et al. Molecular cloning of human eotaxin, an eosinophil-selective CC chemokine, and identification of a specific eosinophil eotaxin receptor, CC chemokine receptor 3. *J Biol Chem* 1996;271(13):7725–7730.

243. Bartels J, et al. Human dermal fibroblasts express eotaxin: molecular cloning, mRNA expression, and identification of eotaxin sequence variants. *Biochem Biophys Res Commun* 1996;225(3):1045–1051.

244. Ghaffar O, et al. Constitutive and cytokine-stimulated expression of eotaxin by human airway smooth muscle cells. *Am J Respir Crit Care Med* 1999;159(6):1933–1942.

245. Nakajima T, et al. Intracellular localization and release of eotaxin from normal eosinophils. *FEBS Lett* 1998;434(3): 226–230.

246. Lilly CM, et al. Expression of eotaxin by human lung epithelial cells: induction by cytokines and inhibition by glucocorticoids. *J Clin Invest* 1997;99(7):1767–1773.

247. Mochizuki M, et al. IL-4 induces eotaxin in human dermal fibroblasts. *Int Arch Allergy Immunol* 1999;120[Suppl 1]:19–23.

248. Han SJ, et al. Interleukin (IL)-5 downregulates tumor necrosis factor (TNF)-induced eotaxin messenger RNA (mRNA) expression in eosinophils. Induction of eotaxin mRNA by TNF and IL-5 in eosinophils. *Am J Respir Cell Mol Biol* 1999;21(3):303–310.

249. Campbell E, et al. Differential roles of IL-18 in allergic airway disease: induction of eotaxin by resident cell populations exacerbates eosinophil accumulation. *J Immunol* 2000;164(2):1096–1102.

250. Nakamura H, et al. Differential regulation of eotaxin expression by TNF-alpha and PMA in human monocytic U-937 cells. *Am J Physiol* 1998;275(3 Pt 1):L601–L610.

251. Chung KF, et al. Induction of eotaxin expression and release from human airway smooth muscle cells by IL-1beta and TNFalpha: effects of IL-10 and corticosteroids. *Br J Pharmacol* 1999;127(5):1145–1150.

252. Yamada H, et al. Eotaxin is a potent chemotaxin for human basophils. *Biochem Biophys Res Commun* 1997;231(2):365–368.

253. Garcia-Zepeda EA, et al. Genomic organization, complete sequence, and chromosomal location of the gene for human eotaxin (SCYA11), an eosinophil-specific CC chemokine. *Genomics* 1997;41(3):471–476.

254. Tenscher K, et al. Recombinant human eotaxin induces oxygen radical production, Ca^{2+}-mobilization, actin reorganization, and CD11b upregulation in human eosinophils via a pertussis toxin-sensitive heterotrimeric guanine nucleotide-binding protein. *Blood* 1996;88(8):3195–3199.

255. Hohki G, et al. The effects of eotaxin on the surface adhesion molecules of endothelial cells and on eosinophil adhesion to microvascular endothelial cells. *Biochem Biophys Res Commun* 1997;241(1):136–141.

256. Rothenberg ME, et al. Eotaxin triggers eosinophil-selective chemotaxis and calcium flux via a distinct receptor and induces pulmonary eosinophilia in the presence of interleukin 5 in mice. *Mol Med* 1996;2(3):334–348.

257. Rothenberg ME, et al. Targeted disruption of the chemokine eotaxin partially reduces antigen-induced tissue eosinophilia. *J Exp Med* 1997;185(4):785–790.

258. Matthews AN, et al. Eotaxin is required for the baseline level of tissue eosinophils. *Proc Natl Acad Sci U S A* 1998;95(11):6273–6278.

259. Ying S, et al. Enhanced expression of eotaxin and CCR3 mRNA and protein in atopic asthma. Association with airway hyperresponsiveness and predominant co-localization of eotaxin mRNA to bronchial epithelial and endothelial cells. *Eur J Immunol* 1997;27(12):3507–3516.

260. Taha RA, et al. Eotaxin and monocyte chemotactic protein-4 mRNA expression in small airways of asthmatic and non-asthmatic individuals. *J Allergy Clin Immunol* 1999;103(3 Pt 1):476–483.

261. Lilly CM, et al. Elevated plasma eotaxin levels in patients with acute asthma. *J Allergy Clin Immunol* 1999;104(4 Pt 1):786–790.

262. Yawalkar N, et al. Enhanced expression of eotaxin and CCR3 in atopic dermatitis. *J Invest Dermatol* 1999;113(1):43–48.

263. Chen J, et al. Eotaxin and capping protein in experimental vasculopathy. *Am J Pathol* 1998;153(1):81–90.

264. Haltia A, et al. mRNA differential display analysis of nephrotic kidney glomeruli. *Exp Nephrol* 1999;7(1):52–58.

265. Minshall EM, et al. Eotaxin mRNA and protein expression in chronic sinusitis and allergen-induced nasal responses in seasonal allergic rhinitis. *Am J Respir Cell Mol Biol* 1997;17(6):683–690.

266. Nickel RG, et al. Positional candidate gene approach and functional genomics strategy in atopy gene discovery. *Int Arch Allergy Immunol* 1999;118(2–4):282–284.

267. Sarafi MN, et al. Murine monocyte chemoattractant protein (MCP)-5: a novel CC chemokine that is a structural and functional homologue of human MCP-1. *J Exp Med* 1997;185(1):99–109.

268. Kopydlowski KM, et al. Regulation of macrophage chemokine expression by lipopolysaccharide *in vitro* and *in vivo*. *J Immunol* 1999;163(3):1537–1544.

269. Jia GQ, et al. Distinct expression and function of the novel mouse chemokine monocyte chemotactic protein-5 in lung allergic inflammation. *J Exp Med* 1996;184(5):1939–1951.

270. Godiska R, et al. Monocyte chemotactic protein-4: tissue-specific expression and signaling through CC chemokine receptor-2. *J Leukoc Biol* 1997;61(3):353–360.

271. Stellato C, et al. Production of the novel C-C chemokine MCP-4 by airway cells and comparison of its biological activity to other C-C chemokines. *J Clin Invest* 1997;99(5):926–936.

272. Berkhout TA, et al. Cloning, *in vitro* expression, and functional characterization of a novel human CC chemokine of the monocyte chemotactic protein (MCP) family (MCP-4) that binds and signals through the CC chemokine receptor 2B. *J Biol Chem* 1997;272(26):16404–16413.

273. Hashimoto S, et al. Serial analysis of gene expression in human monocyte-derived dendritic cells. *Blood* 1999;94(3):845–852.

274. Hein H, et al. Genomic organization, sequence analysis and transcriptional regulation of the human MCP-4 chemokine gene (SCYA13) in dermal fibroblasts: a comparison to other eosinophilic beta-chemokines. *Biochem Biophys Res Commun* 1999;255(2):470–476.

275. Garcia-Zepeda EA, et al. Human monocyte chemoattractant protein (MCP)-4 is a novel CC chemokine with activities on monocytes, eosinophils, and basophils induced in allergic and nonallergic inflammation that signals through the CC chemokine receptors (CCR)-2 and -3. *J Immunol* 1996;157(12):5613–5626.

276. Uguccioni M, et al. Monocyte chemotactic protein 4 (MCP-4), a novel structural and functional analogue of MCP-3 and eotaxin. *J Exp Med* 1996;183(5):2379–2384.

277. Ying S, et al. Eosinophil chemotactic chemokines [eotaxin, eotaxin-2, RANTES, monocyte chemoattractant protein-3 (MCP-3), and MCP-4], and C-C Chemokine Receptor 3 expression in bronchial biopsies from atopic and nonatopic (intrinsic) asthmatics. *J Immunol* 1999;163(11):6321–6329.

278. Schulz-Knappe P, et al. HCC-1, a novel chemokine from human plasma. *J Exp Med* 1996;183(1):295–299.

279. Nomiyama H, et al. Organization of the chemokine gene cluster on human chromosome 17q11.2 containing the genes for CC chemokine MPIF-1, HCC-2, HCC-1, LEC, and RANTES. *J Interferon Cytokine Res* 1999;19(3):227–234.

280. Youn BS, et al. Molecular cloning of leukotactin-1: a novel human beta-chemokine, a chemoattractant for neutrophils, monocytes, and lymphocytes, and a potent agonist at CC chemokine receptors 1 and 3. *J Immunol* 1997;159(11):5201–5215.

281. Sticht H, et al. Solution structure of the human CC chemokine 2: a monomeric representative of the CC chemokine subtype. *Biochemistry* 1999;38(19):5995–6002.

282. Coulin F, et al. Characterisation of macrophage inflammatory protein-5/human CC cytokine-2, a member of the macrophage-inflammatory-protein family of chemokines. *Eur J Biochem* 1997;248(2):507–515.

283. Wang W, et al. Molecular cloning and functional characterization of human MIP-1 delta, a new C-C chemokine related to mouse CCF-18 and C10. *J Clin Immunol* 1998;18(3):214–222.

284. Zhang S, et al. Differential effects of leukotactin-1 and macrophage inflammatory protein-1 alpha on neutrophils mediated by CCR1. *J Immunol* 1999;162(8):4938–4942.

285. Dieu-Nosjean MC, et al. Regulation of dendritic cell trafficking: a process that involves the participation of selective chemokines. *J Leukoc Biol* 1999;66(2):252–262.

286. Youn BS, et al. Isolation and characterization of LMC, a novel lymphocyte and monocyte chemoattractant human CC chemokine, with myelosuppressive activity. *Biochem Biophys Res Commun* 1998;247(2):217–222.

287. Shoudai K, et al. Isolation of cDNA encoding a novel human CC chemokine NCC-4/LEC. *Biochim Biophys Acta* 1998;1396(3):273–277.

288. Yang JY, Spanaus KS, Widmer U. Cloning, characterization and genomic organization of LCC-1 (Scya16), a novel human CC chemokine expressed in liver. *Cytokine* 2000;12(2):101–109.

289. Hedrick JA, et al. Characterization of a novel CC chemokine, HCC-4, whose expression is increased by interleukin-10. *Blood* 1998;91(11):4242–4247.

290. Fukuda S, et al. Genomic organization of the genes for human and mouse CC chemokine LEC. *DNA Cell Biol* 1999;18(4):275–283.

291. Schaniel C, et al. Three chemokines with potential functions in T lymphocyte-independent and -dependent B lymphocyte stimulation. *Eur J Immunol* 1999;29(9):2934–2947.

292. Lieberam I, Forster I. The murine beta-chemokine TARC is expressed by subsets of dendritic cells and attracts primed CD4(+) T cells. *Eur J Immunol* 1999;29(9):2684–2694.

293. Campbell JJ, et al. The chemokine receptor CCR4 in vascular recognition by cutaneous but not intestinal memory T cells. *Nature* 1999;400(6746):776–780.

294. Vestergaard C, et al. Overproduction of Th2-specific chemokines in NC/Nga mice exhibiting atopic dermatitis-like lesions. *J Clin Invest* 1999;104(8):1097–1105.

295. Van den Berg A, Visser L, Poppema S. High expression of the CC chemokine TARC in Reed-Sternberg cells. A possible explanation for the characteristic T-cell infiltrate in Hodgkin's lymphoma. *Am J Pathol* 1999;154(6):1685–1691.

296. Imai T, et al. Macrophage-derived chemokine is a functional ligand for the CC chemokine receptor 4. *J Biol Chem* 1998;273(3):1764–1768.

297. Yoneyama H, et al. Pivotal role of TARC, a CC chemokine, in bacteria-induced fulminant hepatic failure in mice. *J Clin Invest* 1998;102(11):1933–1941.

298. Nomiyama H, et al. Assignment of the human CC chemokine gene TARC (SCYA17) to chromosome 16q13. *Genomics* 1997;40(1):211–213.

299. Kodelja V, et al. Alternative macrophage activation-associated CC-chemokine-1, a novel structural homologue of macrophage inflammatory protein-1 alpha with a Th2-associated expression pattern. *J Immunol* 1998;160(3):1411–1418.

300. Tasaki Y, et al. Chemokine PARC gene (SCYA18) generated by fusion of two MIP-1 alpha/LD78alpha-like genes. *Genomics* 1999;55(3):353–357.

301. Sallusto F, et al. Distinct patterns and kinetics of chemokine production regulate dendritic cell function. *Eur J Immunol* 1999;29(5):1617–1625.

302. Adema GJ, et al. A dendritic-cell-derived C-C chemokine that preferentially attracts naive T cells. *Nature* 1997;387(6634):713–717.

303. Guan P, et al. Genomic organization and biological characterization of the novel human CC chemokine DC-CK-1/PARC/MIP-4/SCYA18. *Genomics* 1999;56(3):296–302.

304. Reape TJ, et al. Expression and cellular localization of the CC chemokines PARC and ELC in human atherosclerotic plaques. *Am J Pathol* 1999;154(2):365–374.

305. Yoshie O, Imai T, Nomiyama H. Novel lymphocyte-specific CC chemokines and their receptors. *J Leukoc Biol* 1997;62(5):634–644.

306. Ngo VN, Tang HL, Cyster JG. Epstein-Barr virus-induced molecule 1 ligand chemokine is expressed by dendritic cells in lymphoid tissues and strongly attracts naive T cells and activated B cells. *J Exp Med* 1998;188(1):181–191.

307. Yoshida R, et al. Molecular cloning of a novel human CC chemokine EBI1-ligand chemokine that is a specific functional ligand for EBI1, CCR7. *J Biol Chem* 1997;272(21):13803–13809.

308. Rossi DL, et al. Identification through bioinformatics of two new macrophage proinflammatory human chemokines: MIP-3 alpha and MIP-3 beta. *J Immunol* 1997;158(3):1033–1036.

309. Yoshida R, et al. EBI1-ligand chemokine (ELC) attracts a broad spectrum of lymphocytes: activated T cells strongly up-regulate CCR7 and efficiently migrate toward ELC. *Int Immunol* 1998;10(7):901–910.

310. Kim CH, et al. Macrophage-inflammatory protein-3 beta/EBI1-ligand chemokine/CK beta-11, a CC chemokine, is a chemoattractant with a specificity for macrophage progenitors among myeloid progenitor cells. *J Immunol* 1998;161(5):2580–2585.

311. Yoshida R, et al. Secondary lymphoid-tissue chemokine is a functional ligand for the CC chemokine receptor CCR7. *J Biol Chem* 1998;273(12):7118–7122.

312. Sullivan SK, et al. Pharmacological and signaling analysis of human chemokine receptor CCR-7 stably expressed in HEK-293 cells: high-affinity binding of recombinant ligands MIP-

3 beta and SLC stimulates multiple signaling cascades. *Biochem Biophys Res Commun* 1999;263(3):685–690.

313. Kim CH, et al. CCR7 ligands, SLC/6Ckine/Exodus2/TCA4 and CKbeta-11/MIP-3 beta/ELC, are chemoattractants for CD56(+)CD16(-) NK cells and late stage lymphoid progenitors. *Cell Immunol* 1999;193(2):226–235.

314. Kim CH, et al. CK beta-11/macrophage inflammatory protein-3 beta/EBI1-ligand chemokine is an efficacious chemoattractant for T and B cells. *J Immunol* 1998;160(5):2418–2424.

315. Vecchi A, et al. Differential responsiveness to constitutive vs. inducible chemokines of immature and mature mouse dendritic cells. *J Leukoc Biol* 1999;66(3):489–494.

316. Kellermann SA, et al. The CC chemokine receptor-7 ligands 6Ckine and macrophage inflammatory protein-3 beta are potent chemoattractants for *in vitro-* and *in vivo-*derived dendritic cells. *J Immunol* 1999;162(7):3859–3864.

317. Al-Aoukaty A, et al. MIP-3 alpha, MIP-3 beta and fractalkine induce the locomotion and the mobilization of intracellular calcium, and activate the heterotrimeric G proteins in human natural killer cells. *Immunology* 1998;95(4):618–624.

318. Potsch C, Vohringer D, Pircher H. Distinct migration patterns of naive and effector CD8 T cells in the spleen: correlation with CCR7 receptor expression and chemokine reactivity. *Eur J Immunol* 1999;29(11):3562–3570.

319. Campbell JJ, Pan J, Butcher EC. Cutting edge: developmental switches in chemokine responses during T cell maturation. *J Immunol* 1999;163(5):2353–2357.

320. Byrnes HD, et al. Macrophage inflammatory protein-3 beta enhances IL-10 production by activated human peripheral blood monocytes and T cells. *J Immunol* 1999;163(9):4715–4720.

321. Campbell JJ, et al. Chemokines and the arrest of lymphocytes rolling under flow conditions. *Science* 1998;279(5349):381–384.

322. Gunn MD, et al. Mice lacking expression of secondary lymphoid organ chemokine have defects in lymphocyte homing and dendritic cell localization [see comments]. *J Exp Med* 1999;189(3):451–460.

323. Hieshima K, et al. Molecular cloning of a novel human CC chemokine liver and activation-regulated chemokine (LARC) expressed in liver. Chemotactic activity for lymphocytes and gene localization on chromosome 2. *J Biol Chem* 1997;272(9):5846–5853.

324. Utans-Schneitz U, et al. A novel rat CC chemokine, identified by targeted differential display, is upregulated in brain inflammation [published erratum appears in *J Neuroimmunol* 1999;94(1–2):222]. *J Neuroimmunol* 1998;92(1–2):179–190.

325. Nagira M, et al. Molecular cloning of a novel human CC chemokine secondary lymphoid-tissue chemokine that is a potent chemoattractant for lymphocytes and mapped to chromosome 9p13. *J Biol Chem* 1997;272(31):19518–19524.

326. Tanaka Y, et al. Selective expression of liver and activation-regulated chemokine (LARC) in intestinal epithelium in mice and humans. *Eur J Immunol* 1999;29(2):633–642.

327. Power CA, et al. Cloning and characterization of a specific receptor for the novel CC chemokine MIP-3 alpha from lung dendritic cells. *J Exp Med* 1997;186(6):825–835.

328. Liao F, et al. STRL22 is a receptor for the CC chemokine MIP-3 alpha. *Biochem Biophys Res Commun* 1997;236(1):212–217.

329. Baba M, et al. Identification of CCR6, the specific receptor for a novel lymphocyte-directed CC chemokine LARC. *J Biol Chem* 1997;272(23):14893–14898.

330. Greaves DR, et al. CCR6, a CC chemokine receptor that interacts with macrophage inflammatory protein 3 alpha and is highly expressed in human dendritic cells. *J Exp Med* 1997;186(6):837–844.

331. Dieu MC, et al. Selective recruitment of immature and mature dendritic cells by distinct chemokines expressed in different anatomic sites. *J Exp Med* 1998;188(2):373–386.

332. Sullivan SK, et al. MIP-3 alpha induces human eosinophil migration and activation of the mitogen-activated protein kinases (p42/p44 MAPK). *J Leukoc Biol* 1999;66(4):674–682.

333. Liao F, et al. CC-chemokine receptor 6 is expressed on diverse memory subsets of T cells and determines responsiveness to macrophage inflammatory protein 3 alpha. *J Immunol* 1999;162(1):186–194.

334. Hromas R, et al. Cloning and characterization of exodus, a novel beta-chemokine. *Blood* 1997;89(9):3315–3322.

335. Kleeff J, et al. Detection and localization of Mip-3 alpha/LARC/Exodus, a macrophage proinflammatory chemokine, and its CCR6 receptor in human pancreatic cancer. *Int J Cancer* 1999;81(4):650–657.

336. Vassileva G, et al. The reduced expression of 6Ckine in the plt mouse results from the deletion of one of two 6Ckine genes. *J Exp Med* 1999;190(8):1183–1188.

337. Campbell JJ, et al. 6-C-kine (SLC), a lymphocyte adhesion-triggering chemokine expressed by high endothelium, is an agonist for the MIP-3 beta receptor CCR7. *J Cell Biol* 1998;141(4):1053–1059.

338. Soto H, et al. The CC chemokine 6Ckine binds the CXC chemokine receptor CXCR3. *Proc Natl Acad Sci U S A* 1998;95(14):8205–8210.

339. Jenh CH, et al. Cutting edge: species specificity of the CC chemokine 6Ckine signaling through the CXC chemokine receptor CXCR3: human 6Ckine is not a ligand for the human or mouse CXCR3 receptors. *J Immunol* 1999;162(7):3765–3769.

340. Kim CH, Broxmeyer HE. SLC/exodus2/6Ckine/TCA4 induces chemotaxis of hematopoietic progenitor cells: differential activity of ligands of CCR7, CXCR3, or CXCR4 in chemotaxis vs. suppression of progenitor proliferation. *J Leukoc Biol* 1999;66(3):455–461.

341. Morales J, et al. CTACK, a skin-associated chemokine that preferentially attracts skin-homing memory T cells. *Proc Natl Acad Sci U S A* 1999;96(25):14470–14475.

342. Nagira M, et al. Enhanced HIV-1 replication by chemokines constitutively expressed in secondary lymphoid tissues. *Virology* 1999;264(2):422–426.

343. Godiska R, et al. Human macrophage-derived chemokine (MDC), a novel chemoattractant for monocytes, monocyte-derived dendritic cells, and natural killer cells. *J Exp Med* 1997;185(9):1595–1604.

344. Proost P, et al. Truncation of macrophage-derived chemokine by CD26/dipeptidylpeptidase IV beyond its predicted cleavage site affects chemotactic activity and CC chemokine receptor 4 interaction. *J Biol Chem* 1999;274(7):3988–3993.

345. Chang M, et al. Molecular cloning and functional characterization of a novel CC chemokine, stimulated T cell chemotactic protein (STCP-1) that specifically acts on activated T lymphocytes. *J Biol Chem* 1997;272(40):25229–25237.
346. Galli G, et al. Macrophage-derived chemokine production by activated human T cells *in vitro* and *in vivo:* preferential association with the production of type 2 cytokines. *Eur J Immunol* 2000;30(1):204–210.
347. Schaniel C, et al. A novel CC chemokine ABCD-1, produced by dendritic cells and activated B cells, exclusively attracts activated T lymphocytes. *Curr Top Microbiol Immunol* 1999;246:95–101.
348. Rodenburg RJ, et al. Expression of macrophage-derived chemokine (MDC) mRNA in macrophages is enhanced by interleukin-1 beta, tumor necrosis factor alpha, and lipopolysaccharide. *J Leukoc Biol* 1998;63(5):606–611.
349. Bonecchi R, et al. Divergent effects of interleukin-4 and interferon-gamma on macrophage-derived chemokine production: an amplification circuit of polarized T helper 2 responses. *Blood* 1998;92(8):2668–2671.
350. Bochner BS, et al. Macrophage-derived chemokine induces human eosinophil chemotaxis in a CC chemokine receptor 3- and CC chemokine receptor 4-independent manner. *J Allergy Clin Immunol* 1999;103(3 Pt 1):527–532.
351. Imai T, et al. Selective recruitment of CCR4-bearing Th2 cells toward antigen-presenting cells by the CC chemokines thymus and activation-regulated chemokine and macrophage-derived chemokine. *Int Immunol* 1999;11(1):81–88.
352. Chantry D, et al. Macrophage-derived chemokine is localized to thymic medullary epithelial cells and is a chemoattractant for CD3(+), CD4(+), CD8(low) thymocytes. *Blood* 1999;94(6):1890–1898.
353. Pal R, et al. Inhibition of HIV-1 infection by the beta-chemokine MDC [see comments]. *Science* 1997;278(5338):695–698.
354. Meucci O, et al. Chemokines regulate hippocampal neuronal signaling and gp120 neurotoxicity. *Proc Natl Acad Sci U S A* 1998;95(24):14500–14505.
355. Navale V, et al. Peptide mapping and disulfide bond analysis of myeloid progenitor inhibitory chemokine and keratinocyte growth factor by matrix-assisted laser desorption ionization mass spectrometry. *Anal Biochem* 1999;267(1):125–134.
356. Youn BS, et al. Characterization of CKbeta8 and CKbeta8-1: two alternatively spliced forms of human beta-chemokine, chemoattractants for neutrophils, monocytes, and lymphocytes, and potent agonists at CC chemokine receptor 1. *Blood* 1998;91(9):3118–3126.
357. Macphee CH, et al. Identification of a truncated form of the CC chemokine CK beta-8 demonstrating greatly enhanced biological activity. *J Immunol* 1998;161(11):6273–6279.
358. Nardelli B, et al. Dendritic cells and MPIF-1: chemotactic activity and inhibition of endogenous chemokine production by IFN-gamma and CD40 ligation. *J Leukoc Biol* 1999;65(6):822–828.
359. Nardelli B, et al. Characterization of the signal transduction pathway activated in human monocytes and dendritic cells by MPIF-1, a specific ligand for CC chemokine receptor 1. *J Immunol* 1999;162(1):435–444.
360. White JR, et al. Cloning and functional characterization of a novel human CC chemokine that binds to the CCR3 receptor and activates human eosinophils. *J Leukoc Biol* 1997;62(5):667–675.
361. Elsner J, et al. Eotaxin-2 activates chemotaxis-related events and release of reactive oxygen species via pertussis toxin-sensitive G proteins in human eosinophils. *Eur J Immunol* 1998;28(7):2152–2158.
362. Nomiyama H, et al. Assignment of the human CC chemokine MPIF-2/eotaxin-2 (SCYA24) to chromosome 7q11.23. *Genomics* 1998;49(2):339–340.
363. Vicari AP, et al. TECK: a novel CC chemokine specifically expressed by thymic dendritic cells and potentially involved in T cell development. *Immunity* 1997;7(2):291–301.
364. Wilkinson B, Owen JJ, Jenkinson EJ. Factors regulating stem cell recruitment to the fetal thymus. *J Immunol* 1999;162(7):3873–3881.
365. Wurbel MA, et al. The chemokine TECK is expressed by thymic and intestinal epithelial cells and attracts double- and single-positive thymocytes expressing the TECK receptor CCR9. *Eur J Immunol* 2000;30(1):262–271.
366. Youn BS, et al. TECK, an efficacious chemoattractant for human thymocytes, uses GPR-9-6/CCR9 as a specific receptor. *Blood* 1999;94(7):2533–2536.
367. Zaballos A, et al. Cutting edge: identification of the orphan chemokine receptor GPR-9-6 as CCR9, the receptor for the chemokine TECK. *J Immunol* 1999;162(10):5671–5675.
368. Zabel BA, et al. Human G Protein-coupled receptor GPR-9-6/CC chemokine receptor 9 is selectively expressed on intestinal homing T lymphocytes, mucosal lymphocytes, and thymocytes and is required for thymus-expressed chemokine-mediated chemotaxis. *J Exp Med* 1999;190(9):1241–1256.
369. Norment AM, et al. Murine CCR9, a chemokine receptor for thymus-expressed chemokine that is up-regulated following pre-TCR signaling. *J Immunol* 2000;164(2):639–648.
370. Broxmeyer HE, et al. Effects of CC, CXC, C, and CX3C chemokines on proliferation of myeloid progenitor cells, and insights into SDF-1-induced chemotaxis of progenitors. *Ann N Y Acad Sci* 1999;872:142–162; discussion 163.
371. Nomiyama H, et al. The human CC chemokine TECK (SCYA25) maps to chromosome 19p13.2. *Genomics* 1998;51(2):311–312.
372. Guo RF, et al. Molecular cloning and characterization of a novel human CC chemokine, SCYA26. *Genomics* 1999;58(3):313–317.
373. Kitaura M, et al. Molecular cloning of a novel human CC chemokine (Eotaxin-3) that is a functional ligand of CC chemokine receptor 3. *J Biol Chem* 1999;274(39):27975–27980.
374. Shinkai A, et al. A novel human CC chemokine, eotaxin-3, which is expressed in IL-4-stimulated vascular endothelial cells, exhibits potent activity toward eosinophils. *J Immunol* 1999;163(3):1602–1610.
375. Ishikawa-Mochizuki I, et al. Molecular cloning of a novel CC chemokine, interleukin-11 receptor alpha-locus chemokine (ILC), which is located on chromosome 9p13 and a potential homologue of a CC chemokine encoded by molluscum contagiosum virus. *FEBS Lett* 1999;460(3):544–548.
376. Neote K, et al. Molecular cloning, functional expression, and signaling characteristics of a C-C chemokine receptor. *Cell* 1993;72(3):415–425.

377. Gao JL, Murphy PM. Cloning and differential tissue-specific expression of three mouse beta chemokine receptor-like genes, including the gene for a functional macrophage inflammatory protein-1 alpha receptor. *J Biol Chem* 1995;270(29):17494–17501.

378. Nomura H, Nielsen BW, Matsushima K. Molecular cloning of cDNAs encoding a LD78 receptor and putative leukocyte chemotactic peptide receptors. *Int Immunol* 1993; 5(10):1239–1249.

379. Gao JL, et al. Structure and functional expression of the human macrophage inflammatory protein 1 alpha/RANTES receptor. *J Exp Med* 1993;177(5):1421–1427.

380. Harrison JK, Barber CM, Lynch KR. cDNA cloning of a G-protein-coupled receptor expressed in rat spinal cord and brain related to chemokine receptors. *Neurosci Lett* 1994;169(1–2):85–89.

381. Samson M, et al. Molecular cloning and chromosomal mapping of a novel human gene, ChemR1, expressed in T lymphocytes and polymorphonuclear cells and encoding a putative chemokine receptor. *Eur J Immunol* 1996;26(12):3021–3028.

382. Combadiere C, Ahuja SK, Murphy PM. Cloning, chromosomal localization, and RNA expression of a human beta chemokine receptor-like gene. *DNA Cell Biol* 1995;14(8):673–680.

383. Durig J, et al. Expression of macrophage inflammatory protein-1 receptors in human CD34(+) hematopoietic cells and their modulation by tumor necrosis factor-alpha and interferon-gamma. *Blood* 1998;92(9):3073–3081.

384. Hesselgesser J, et al. CD4-independent association between HIV-1 gp120 and CXCR4: functional chemokine receptors are expressed in human neurons. *Curr Biol* 1997;7(2):112–121.

385. Zella D, et al. Recombinant IFN-alpha (2b) increases the expression of apoptosis receptor CD95 and chemokine receptors CCR1 and CCR3 in monocytoid cells. *J Immunol* 1999;163(6):3169–3175.

386. Bonecchi R, et al. Up-regulation of CCR1 and CCR3 and induction of chemotaxis to CC chemokines by IFN-gamma in human neutrophils. *J Immunol* 1999;162(1):474–479.

387. Banas B, et al. Chemokine and chemokine receptor expression in a novel human mesangial cell line. *J Am Soc Nephrol* 1999;10(11):2314–2322.

388. Zella D, et al. Interferon-gamma increases expression of chemokine receptors CCR1, CCR3, and CCR5, but not CXCR4 in monocytoid U937 cells. *Blood* 1998;91(12):4444–4450.

389. Loetscher P, et al. Interleukin-2 regulates CC chemokine receptor expression and chemotactic responsiveness in T lymphocytes. *J Exp Med* 1996;184(2):569–577.

390. Zimmermann N, et al. Molecular analysis of CCR-3 events in eosinophilic cells. *J Immunol* 2000;164(2):1055–1064.

391. Colantonio L, et al. Upregulation of integrin alpha6/beta1 and chemokine receptor CCR1 by interleukin-12 promotes the migration of human type 1 helper T cells. *Blood* 1999;94(9):2981–2989.

392. Sallusto F, et al. Switch in chemokine receptor expression upon TCR stimulation reveals novel homing potential for recently activated T cells. *Eur J Immunol* 1999;29(6):2037–2045.

393. Sica A, et al. Bacterial lipopolysaccharide rapidly inhibits expression of C-C chemokine receptors in human monocytes. *J Exp Med* 1997;185(5):969–974.

394. Maghazachi AA. Intracellular signalling pathways induced by chemokines in natural killer cells. *Cell Signal* 1999;11(6):385–390.

395. Owen SM, et al. Genetically divergent strains of human immunodeficiency virus type 2 use multiple coreceptors for viral entry. *J Virol* 1998;72(7):5425–5432.

396. Broxmeyer HE, et al. Dominant myelopoietic effector functions mediated by chemokine receptor CCR1. *J Exp Med* 1999;189(12):1987–1992.

397. Gao JL, et al. Impaired host defense, hematopoiesis, granulomatous inflammation and type 1-type 2 cytokine balance in mice lacking CC chemokine receptor 1. *J Exp Med* 1997;185(11):1959–1968.

398. Gerard C, et al. Targeted disruption of the beta-chemokine receptor CCR1 protects against pancreatitis-associated lung injury. *J Clin Invest* 1997;100(8):2022–2207.

399. Topham PS, et al. Lack of chemokine receptor CCR1 enhances Th1 responses and glomerular injury during nephrotoxic nephritis. *J Clin Invest* 1999;104(11):1549–1557.

400. Tokuda A, et al. Pivotal role of CCR1-positive leukocytes in bleomycin-induced lung fibrosis in mice. *J Immunol* 2000;164(5):2745–2751.

401. Wong LM, et al. Organization and differential expression of the human monocyte chemoattractant protein 1 receptor gene. Evidence for the role of the carboxyl-terminal tail in receptor trafficking. *J Biol Chem* 1997;272(2):1038–1045.

402. Polentarutti N, et al. IL-2-regulated expression of the monocyte chemotactic protein-1 receptor (CCR2) in human NK cells: characterization of a predominant 3.4-kilobase transcript containing CCR2B and CCR2A sequences. *J Immunol* 1997;158(6):2689–2694.

403. Weber KS, et al. Expression of CCR2 by endothelial cells: implications for MCP-1 mediated wound injury repair and *in vivo* inflammatory activation of endothelium. *Arterioscler Thromb Vasc Biol* 1999;19(9):2085–2093.

404. Tangirala RK, Murao K, Quehenberger O. Regulation of expression of the human monocyte chemotactic protein-1 receptor (hCCR2) by cytokines. *J Biol Chem* 1997;272(12):8050–8056.

405. Xu L, et al. Identification of a novel mechanism for endotoxin-mediated down-modulation of CC chemokine receptor expression. *Eur J Immunol* 2000;30(1):227–235.

406. Han KH, et al. Chemokine receptor CCR2 expression and monocyte chemoattractant protein-1-mediated chemotaxis in human monocytes. A regulatory role for plasma LDL. *Arterioscler Thromb Vasc Biol* 1998;18(12):1983–1991.

407. Kurihara T, et al. Defects in macrophage recruitment and host defense in mice lacking the CCR2 chemokine receptor. *J Exp Med* 1997;186(10):1757–1762.

408. Kuziel WA, et al. Severe reduction in leukocyte adhesion and monocyte extravasation in mice deficient in CC chemokine receptor 2. *Proc Natl Acad Sci U S A* 1997;94(22):12053–12058.

409. Warmington KS, et al. Effect of C-C chemokine receptor 2 (CCR2) knockout on type-2 (schistosomal antigen-elicited) pulmonary granuloma formation: analysis of cellular recruitment and cytokine responses. *Am J Pathol* 1999;154(5):1407–1416.

410. Boring L, et al. Impaired monocyte migration and reduced type 1 (Th1) cytokine responses in C-C chemokine receptor 2 knockout mice. *J Clin Invest* 1997;100(10):2552–2561.

411. Campbell EM, et al. Monocyte chemoattractant protein-1 mediates cockroach allergen-induced bronchial hyperreactivity in normal but not CCR2-/- mice: the role of mast cells. *J Immunol* 1999;163(4):2160–2167.

412. Reid S, et al. Enhanced myeloid progenitor cell cycling and apoptosis in mice lacking the chemokine receptor, CCR2. *Blood* 1999;93(5):1524–1533.

413. Boring L, et al. Decreased lesion formation in CCR2-/-mice reveals a role for chemokines in the initiation of atherosclerosis. *Nature* 1998;394(6696):894–897.

414. Dawson TC, et al. Absence of CC chemokine receptor-2 reduces atherosclerosis in apolipoprotein E-deficient mice. *Atherosclerosis* 1999;143(1):205–211.

415. Sica A, et al. Defective expression of the monocyte chemotactic protein-1 receptor CCR2 in macrophages associated with human ovarian carcinoma. *J Immunol* 2000;164(2): 733–738.

416. Samson M, et al. The genes encoding the human CC-chemokine receptors CC-CKR1 to CC-CKR5 (CMKBR1-CMKBR5) are clustered in the p21.3-p24 region of chromosome 3. *Genomics* 1996;36(3):522–526.

417. Smith MW, et al. Contrasting genetic influence of CCR2 and CCR5 variants on HIV-1 infection and disease progression. Hemophilia Growth and Development Study (HGDS), Multicenter AIDS Cohort Study (MACS), Multicenter Hemophilia Cohort Study (MHCS), San Francisco City Cohort (SFCC), ALIVE Study. *Science* 1997;277(5328):959–965.

418. Szalai C, et al. Chemokine receptor CCR2 and CCR5 polymorphisms in children with insulin-dependent diabetes mellitus. *Pediatr Res* 1999;46(1):82–84.

419. Hizawa N, et al. The role of the C-C chemokine receptor 2 gene polymorphism V64I (CCR2-64I) in sarcoidosis in a Japanese population. *Am J Respir Crit Care Med* 1999;159(6):2021–2023.

420. Charo IF, et al. Molecular cloning and functional expression of two monocyte chemoattractant protein 1 receptors reveals alternative splicing of the carboxyl-terminal tails. *Proc Natl Acad Sci U S A* 1994;91(7):2752–2756.

421. Combadiere C, Ahuja SK, Murphy PM. Cloning and functional expression of a human eosinophil CC chemokine receptor [published erratum appears in *J Biol Chem* 1995;270(50):30235]. *J Biol Chem* 1995;270(28):16491–16494.

422. Rubbert A, et al. Dendritic cells express multiple chemokine receptors used as coreceptors for HIV entry. *J Immunol* 1998;160(8):3933–3941.

423. Albright AV, et al. Microglia express CCR5, CXCR4, and CCR3, but of these, CCR5 is the principal coreceptor for human immunodeficiency virus type 1 dementia isolates. *J Virol* 1999;73(1):205–213.

424. Klein RS, et al. Chemokine receptor expression and signaling in macaque and human fetal neurons and astrocytes: implications for the neuropathogenesis of AIDS. *J Immunol* 1999;163(3):1636–1646.

425. Zhang L, et al. *In vivo* distribution of the human immunodeficiency virus/simian immunodeficiency virus coreceptors: CXCR4, CCR3, and CCR5. *J Virol* 1998;72(6):5035–5045.

426. Sallusto F, Mackay CR, Lanzavecchia A. Selective expression of the eotaxin receptor CCR3 by human T helper 2 cells. *Science* 1997;277(5334):2005–2007.

427. Jinquan T, et al. Eotaxin activates T cells to chemotaxis and adhesion only if induced to express CCR3 by IL-2 together with IL-4. *J Immunol* 1999;162(7):4285–4292.

428. Zimmermann N, Conkright JJ, Rothenberg ME. CC chemokine receptor-3 undergoes prolonged ligand-induced internalization. *J Biol Chem* 1999;274(18):12611–12618.

429. Saederup N, et al. Cytomegalovirus-encoded beta chemokine promotes monocyte-associated viremia in the host. *Proc Natl Acad Sci U S A* 1999;96(19):10881–10886.

430. Choe H, et al. The beta-chemokine receptors CCR3 and CCR5 facilitate infection by primary HIV-1 isolates. *Cell* 1996;85(7):1135–1148.

431. Sol N, et al. Usage of the coreceptors CCR-5, CCR-3, and CXCR-4 by primary and cell line-adapted human immunodeficiency virus type 2. *J Virol* 1997;71(11):8237–8244.

432. Boehme SA, et al. Activation of mitogen-activated protein kinase regulates eotaxin-induced eosinophil migration. *J Immunol* 1999;163(3):1611–1618.

433. El-Shazly A, et al. Novel association of the src family kinases, hck and c-fgr, with CCR3 receptor stimulation: a possible mechanism for eotaxin-induced human eosinophil chemotaxis. *Biochem Biophys Res Commun* 1999;264(1):163–170.

434. Xia MQ, et al. Immunohistochemical study of the beta-chemokine receptors CCR3 and CCR5 and their ligands in normal and Alzheimer's disease brains. *Am J Pathol* 1998;153(1):31–37.

435. Zeibecoglou K, et al. Increased mature and immature CCR3 messenger RNA+ eosinophils in bone marrow from patients with atopic asthma compared with atopic and nonatopic control subjects. *J Allergy Clin Immunol* 1999;103(1 Pt 1):99–106.

436. Jiang Y, et al. Chemokine receptor expression in cultured glia and rat experimental allergic encephalomyelitis. *J Neuroimmunol* 1998;86(1):1–12.

437. Zimmermann N, Bernstein JA, Rothenberg ME. Polymorphisms in the human CC chemokine receptor-3 gene. *Biochim Biophys Acta* 1998;1442(2–3):170–176.

438. Kato H, et al. New variations of human CC-chemokine receptors CCR3 and CCR4. *Genes Immun* 1999;1:97–104.

439. Post TW, et al. Molecular characterization of two murine eosinophil beta chemokine receptors. *J Immunol* 1995; 155(11):5299–5305.

440. Hoogewerf A, et al. Molecular cloning of murine CC CKR-4 and high affinity binding of chemokines to murine and human CC CKR-4. *Biochem Biophys Res Commun* 1996;218(1):337–343.

441. Power CA, et al. Molecular cloning and functional expression of a novel CC chemokine receptor cDNA from a human basophilic cell line. *J Biol Chem* 1995;270(33):19495–19500.

442. D'Ambrosio D, et al. Selective up-regulation of chemokine receptors CCR4 and CCR8 upon activation of polarized human type 2 Th cells. *J Immunol* 1998;161(10):5111–5115.

443. Imai T, et al. The T cell-directed CC chemokine TARC is a highly specific biological ligand for CC chemokine receptor 4. *J Biol Chem* 1997;272(23):15036–15042.

444. Xiao L, et al. Adaptation to promiscuous usage of CC and CXC-chemokine coreceptors *in vivo* correlates with HIV-1 disease progression. *AIDS* 1998;12(13):F137–F143.

445. Meyer A, et al. Cloning and characterization of a novel murine macrophage inflammatory protein-1 alpha receptor [published erratum appears in *J Biol Chem* 1996;271(38):23601]. *J Biol Chem* 1996;271(24):14445–14451.

446. Samson M, et al. Molecular cloning and functional expression of a new human CC-chemokine receptor gene. *Biochemistry* 1996;35(11):3362–3367.

447. Fan P, et al. Cloning and characterization of a novel human chemokine receptor. *Biochem Biophys Res Commun* 1998;243(1):264–268.

448. Benkirane M, et al. Mechanism of transdominant inhibition of CCR5-mediated HIV-1 infection by ccr5delta32. *J Biol Chem* 1997;272(49):30603–30606.

449. Mummidi S, et al. The human CC chemokine receptor 5 (CCR5) gene. Multiple transcripts with 5'-end heterogeneity, dual promoter usage, and evidence for polymorphisms within the regulatory regions and noncoding exons. *J Biol Chem* 1997;272(49):30662–30671.

450. Randolph DA, et al. The role of CCR7 in T(H)1 and T(H)2 cell localization and delivery of B cell help *in vivo*. *Science* 1999;286(5447):2159–2162.

451. Galasso JM, Harrison JK, Silverstein FS. Excitotoxic brain injury stimulates expression of the chemokine receptor CCR5 in neonatal rats. *Am J Pathol* 1998;153(5):1631–1640.

452. Houle M, et al. IL-10 up-regulates CCR5 gene expression in human monocytes. *Inflammation* 1999;23(3):241–251.

453. Hariharan D, et al. Interferon-gamma upregulates CCR5 expression in cord and adult blood mononuclear phagocytes. *Blood* 1999;93(4):1137–1144.

454. Patterson BK, et al. Regulation of CCR5 and CXCR4 expression by type 1 and type 2 cytokines: CCR5 expression is downregulated by IL-10 in CD4-positive lymphocytes. *Clin Immunol* 1999;91(3):254–262.

455. Zou W, et al. Acute upregulation of CCR-5 expression by CD4+ T lymphocytes in HIV-infected patients treated with interleukin-2. ANRS 048 IL-2 Study Group. *AIDS* 1999;13(4):455–463.

456. Hermann E, et al. Recombinant interleukin-16 selectively modulates surface receptor expression and cytokine release in macrophages and dendritic cells. *Immunology* 1999;97(2):241–248.

457. Ganju RK, et al. Beta-chemokine receptor CCR5 signals via the novel tyrosine kinase RAFTK. *Blood* 1998;91(3):791–797.

458. Zhou Y, et al. Impaired macrophage function and enhanced T cell-dependent immune response in mice lacking CCR5, the mouse homologue of the major HIV-1 coreceptor. *J Immunol* 1998;160(8):4018–4025.

459. Huffnagle GB, et al. Cutting edge: role of C-C chemokine receptor 5 in organ-specific and innate immunity to *Cryptococcus neoformans*. *J Immunol* 1999;163(9):4642–4646.

460. Murai M, et al. Active participation of CCR5(+)CD8(+) T lymphocytes in the pathogenesis of liver injury in graft-versus-host disease. *J Clin Invest* 1999;104(1):49–57.

461. Hall IP, et al. Association of CCR5 delta32 with reduced risk of asthma [Letter]. *Lancet* 1999;354(9186):1264–1265.

462. Rabkin CS, et al. Chemokine and chemokine receptor gene variants and risk of non-Hodgkin's lymphoma in human immunodeficiency virus-1-infected individuals. *Blood* 1999;93(6):1838–1842.

463. Kostrikis LG, et al. A polymorphism in the regulatory region of the CC-chemokine receptor 5 gene influences perinatal transmission of human immunodeficiency virus type 1 to African-American infants. *J Virol* 1999;73(12):10264–10271.

464. Garred P, et al. CC chemokine receptor 5 polymorphism in rheumatoid arthritis. *J Rheumatol* 1998;25(8):1462–1465.

465. Bennetts BH, et al. The CCR5 deletion mutation fails to protect against multiple sclerosis. *Hum Immunol* 1997;58(1):52–59.

466. Zaballos A, et al. Molecular cloning and RNA expression of two new human chemokine receptor-like genes. *Biochem Biophys Res Commun* 1996;227(3):846–853.

467. Liao F, Lee HH, Farber JM. Cloning of STRL22, a new human gene encoding a G-protein-coupled receptor related to chemokine receptors and located on chromosome 6q27. *Genomics* 1997;40(1):175–180.

468. Varona R, et al. Molecular cloning, functional characterization and mRNA expression analysis of the murine chemokine receptor CCR6 and its specific ligand MIP-3 alpha. *FEBS Lett* 1998;440(1–2):188–194.

469. Yang D, et al. Cutting edge: immature dendritic cells generated from monocytes in the presence of TGF-beta1 express functional C-C chemokine receptor 6. *J Immunol* 1999;163(4):1737–1741.

470. Carramolino L, et al. Down-regulation of the beta-chemokine receptor CCR6 in dendritic cells mediated by TNF-alpha and IL-4. *J Leukoc Biol* 1999;66(5):837–844.

471. Yang D, et al. Beta-defensins: linking innate and adaptive immunity through dendritic and T cell CCR6. *Science* 1999;286(5439):525–528.

472. Schweickart VL, et al. Cloning of human and mouse EBI1, a lymphoid-specific G-protein-coupled receptor encoded on human chromosome 17q12-q21.2. *Genomics* 1994;23(3):643–650.

473. Birkenbach M, et al. Epstein-Barr virus-induced genes: first lymphocyte-specific G protein-coupled peptide receptors. *J Virol* 1993;67(4):2209–2220.

474. Burgstahler R, et al. Expression of the chemokine receptor BLR2/EBI1 is specifically transactivated by Epstein-Barr virus nuclear antigen 2. *Biochem Biophys Res Commun* 1995;215(2):737–743.

475. Hasegawa H, et al. Induction of G protein-coupled peptide receptor EBI 1 by human herpesvirus 6 and 7 infection in CD4+ T cells. *J Virol* 1994;68(8):5326–5329.

476. Sallusto F, et al. Two subsets of memory T lymphocytes with distinct homing potentials and effector functions. *Nature* 1999;401(6754):708–712.

477. Forster R, et al. CCR7 coordinates the primary immune response by establishing functional microenvironments in secondary lymphoid organs. *Cell* 1999;99(1):23–33.

478. Hasegawa H, et al. Increased chemokine receptor CCR7/EBI1 expression enhances the infiltration of lymphoid organs by adult T-cell leukemia cells. *Blood* 2000;95(1):30–38.

479. Syed F, et al. CCR7 (EBI1) receptor down-regulation in asthma: differential gene expression in human CD4+ T lymphocytes. *QJM* 1999;92(8):463–471.

480. Tiffany HL, et al. Identification of CCR8: a human monocyte and thymus receptor for the CC chemokine I-309. *J Exp Med* 1997;186(1):165–170.

481. Jinno A, et al. Identification of the chemokine receptor TER1/CCR8 expressed in brain-derived cells and T cells as a new coreceptor for HIV-1 infection. *Biochem Biophys Res Commun* 1998;243(2):497–502.

482. Zingoni A, et al. The chemokine receptor CCR8 is preferentially expressed in Th2 but not Th1 cells. *J Immunol* 1998;161(2):547–551.

483. Dairaghi DJ, et al. HHV8-encoded vMIP-I selectively engages chemokine receptor CCR8. Agonist and antagonist profiles of viral chemokines. *J Biol Chem* 1999;274(31): 21569–21574.

484. Bernardini G, et al. Identification of the CC chemokines TARC and macrophage inflammatory protein-1 beta as novel functional ligands for the CCR8 receptor. *Eur J Immunol* 1998;28(2):582–588.

485. Garlisi CG, et al. The assignment of chemokine-chemokine receptor pairs: TARC and MIP-1 beta are not ligands for human CC-chemokine receptor 8. *Eur J Immunol* 1999;29(10):3210–3215.

486. Endres MJ, et al. The Kaposi's sarcoma-related herpesvirus (KSHV)-encoded chemokine vMIP-I is a specific agonist for the CC chemokine receptor (CCR)8. *J Exp Med* 1999;189(12):1993–1998.

487. Krathwohl MD, et al. Functional characterization of the C—C chemokine-like molecules encoded by molluscum contagiosum virus types 1 and 2. *Proc Natl Acad Sci U S A* 1997;94(18):9875–9880.

488. Damon I, Murphy PM, Moss B. Broad spectrum chemokine antagonistic activity of a human poxvirus chemokine homolog. *Proc Natl Acad Sci U S A* 1998;95(11):6403–6407.

489. Rucker J, et al. Utilization of chemokine receptors, orphan receptors, and herpesvirus-encoded receptors by diverse human and simian immunodeficiency viruses. *J Virol* 1997;71(12):8999–9007.

490. Napolitano M, et al. Molecular cloning of TER1, a chemokine receptor-like gene expressed by lymphoid tissues. *J Immunol* 1996;157(7):2759–2763.

491. Youn BS, et al. Molecular cloning and characterization of a cDNA, CHEMR1, encoding a chemokine receptor with a homology to the human C-C chemokine receptor, CCR-4. *Blood* 1997;89(12):4448–4460.

492. Yu CR, et al. CCR9A and CCR9B: two receptors for the chemokine CCL25/TECK/Ckbeta-15 that differ in their sensitivities to ligand. *J Immunol* 2000;164(3):1293–1305.

493. Walz A, et al. Regulation and function of the CXC chemokine ENA-78 in monocytes and its role in disease. *J Leukoc Biol* 1997;62(5):604–611.

494. Haskill S, et al. Identification of three related human GRO genes encoding cytokine functions. *Proc Natl Acad Sci U S A* 1990;87(19):7732–7736.

495. Hanzawa H, et al. Solution structure of CINC/Gro investigated by heteronuclear NMR. *J Biochem (Tokyo)* 1998; 123(1):62–70.

496. Wuyts A, et al. Isolation of the CXC chemokines ENA-78, GRO alpha and GRO gamma from tumor cells and leukocytes reveals NH$_2$-terminal heterogeneity. Functional comparison of different natural isoforms. *Eur J Biochem* 1999;260(2):421–429.

497. Becker S, et al. Constitutive and stimulated MCP-1, GRO alpha, beta, and gamma expression in human airway epithe-

lium and bronchoalveolar macrophages. *Am J Physiol* 1994;266(3 Pt 1):L278–L286.

498. Kanda Y, et al. GRO-alpha in human serum: differences related to age and sex. *Am J Reprod Immunol* 1997;38(1):33–38.

499. Luan J, et al. Mechanism and biological significance of constitutive expression of MGSA/GRO chemokines in malignant melanoma tumor progression. *J Leukoc Biol* 1997; 62(5):588–597.

500. Gasperini S, et al. Regulation of GRO alpha production in human granulocytes. *J Inflamm* 1995;45(3):143–151.

501. Introna M, et al. IL-1 inducible genes in human umbilical vein endothelial cells. *Eur Heart J* 1993;14[Suppl K]:78–81.

502. Jaffe GJ, et al. Expression of three forms of melanoma growth stimulating activity (MGSA)/gro in human retinal pigment epithelial cells. *Invest Ophthalmol Vis Sci* 1993;34(9):2776–2785.

503. Ahuja SK, Murphy PM. The CXC chemokines growth-regulated oncogene (GRO) alpha, GRO beta, GRO gamma, neutrophil-activating peptide-2, and epithelial cell-derived neutrophil-activating peptide-78 are potent agonists for the type B, but not the type A, human interleukin-8 receptor. *J Biol Chem* 1996;271(34):20545–20550.

504. Rosenkilde MM, et al. Agonists and inverse agonists for the herpesvirus 8-encoded constitutively active seven-transmembrane oncogene product, ORF-74. *J Biol Chem* 1999;274(2):956–961.

505. Strieter RM, et al. The functional role of the ELR motif in CXC chemokine-mediated angiogenesis. *J Biol Chem* 1995;270(45):27348–27357.

506. Van Damme J, et al. Granulocyte chemotactic protein-2 and related CXC chemokines: from gene regulation to receptor usage. *J Leukoc Biol* 1997;62(5):563–569.

507. Lippert U, et al. Expression and functional activity of the IL-8 receptor type CXCR1 and CXCR2 on human mast cells. *J Immunol* 1998;161(5):2600–2608.

508. Wolf M, et al. Granulocyte chemotactic protein 2 acts via both IL-8 receptors, CXCR1 and CXCR2. *Eur J Immunol* 1998;28(1):164–170.

509. Cao Y, et al. gro-beta, a -C-X-C- chemokine, is an angiogenesis inhibitor that suppresses the growth of Lewis lung carcinoma in mice. *J Exp Med* 1995;182(6):2069–2077.

510. Rossi DL, et al. Lungkine, a novel CXC chemokine, specifically expressed by lung bronchoepithelial cells. *J Immunol* 1999;162(9):5490–5497.

511. Dilulio NA, et al. Groalpha-mediated recruitment of neutrophils is required for elicitation of contact hypersensitivity. *Eur J Immunol* 1999;29(11):3485–3495.

512. Haghnegahdar H, et al. The tumorigenic and angiogenic effects of MGSA/GRO proteins in melanoma. *J Leukoc Biol* 2000;67(1):53–62.

513. Cuenca RE, Azizkhan RG, Haskill S. Characterization of GRO alpha, beta and gamma expression in human colonic tumours: potential significance of cytokine involvement. *Surg Oncol* 1992;1(4):323–329.

514. Wu X, et al. Cytokine-induced neutrophil chemoattractant mediates neutrophil influx in immune complex glomerulonephritis in rat. *J Clin Invest* 1994;94(1):337–344.

515. Suzuki H, et al. Enhanced levels of C-X-C chemokine, human GRO alpha, in *Helicobacter pylori*-associated gastric disease. *J Gastroenterol Hepatol* 1998;13(5):516–520.

516. Moore BB, et al. Distinct CXC chemokines mediate tumor-igenicity of prostate cancer cells. *Am J Pathol* 1999;154(5): 1503–1512.

517. Kulke R, et al. Co-localized overexpression of GRO-alpha and IL-8 mRNA is restricted to the suprapapillary layers of psoriatic lesions. *J Invest Dermatol* 1996;106(3):526–530.

518. Liu T, et al. Cytokine-induced neutrophil chemoattractant mRNA expressed in cerebral ischemia. *Neurosci Lett* 1993;164(1–2):125–128.

519. Isaacs KL, Sartor RB, Haskill S. Cytokine messenger RNA profiles in inflammatory bowel disease mucosa detected by polymerase chain reaction amplification. *Gastroenterology* 1992;103(5):1587–1595.

520. Richmond A, et al. Molecular characterization and chromosomal mapping of melanoma growth stimulatory activity, a growth factor structurally related to beta-thromboglobulin. *EMBO J* 1988;7(7):2025–2033.

521. Modi WS, et al. Assignment of the mouse and cow CXC chemokine genes. *Cytogenet Cell Genet* 1998;81(3–4):213–216.

522. Konishi K, et al. Structure of the gene encoding rat neutrophil chemo-attractant Gro. *Gene* 1993;126(2):285–286.

523. Sakaguchi AY, et al. Mouse melanoma growth stimulatory activity gene (Mgsa) is polymorphic and syntenic with the W, patch, rumpwhite, and recessive spotting loci on chromosome 5. *Genomics* 1989;5(3):629–632.

524. Tekamp-Olson P, et al. Cloning and characterization of cDNAs for murine macrophage inflammatory protein 2 and its human homologues. *J Exp Med* 1990;172(3):911–919.

525. Ohno Y, et al. Macrophage inflammatory protein-2: chromosomal regulation in rat small intestinal epithelial cells. *Proc Natl Acad Sci U S A* 1997;94(19):10279–10284.

526. Hogaboam CM, et al. Novel CXCR2-dependent liver regenerative qualities of ELR-containing CXC chemokines. *FASEB J* 1999;13(12):1565–1574.

527. O'Donovan N, Galvin M, Morgan JG. Physical mapping of the CXC chemokine locus on human chromosome 4. *Cytogenet Cell Genet* 1999;84(1–2):39–42.

528. Strieter RM, et al. Role of C-X-C chemokines as regulators of angiogenesis in lung cancer. *J Leukoc Biol* 1995;57(5): 752–762.

529. Watanabe O, et al. Significantly elevated expression of PF4 (platelet factor 4) and eotaxin in the NOA mouse, a model for atopic dermatitis. *J Hum Genet* 1999;44(3):173–176.

530. Doi T, Greenberg SM, Rosenberg RD. Structure of the rat platelet factor 4 gene: a marker for megakaryocyte differentiation. *Mol Cell Biol* 1987;7(2):898–904.

531. Zhang X, et al. Crystal structure of recombinant human platelet factor 4. *Biochemistry* 1994;33(27):8361–8366.

532. Minami T, et al. Both Ets-1 and GATA-1 are essential for positive regulation of platelet factor 4 gene expression. *Eur J Biochem* 1998;258(2):879–889.

533. Ravid K, Kuter DJ, Rosenberg RD. rmIL-6 stimulates the transcriptional activity of the rat PF4 gene. *Exp Hematol* 1995;23(5):397–401.

534. Petersen F, et al. A chondroitin sulfate proteoglycan on human neutrophils specifically binds platelet factor 4 and is involved in cell activation. *J Immunol* 1998;161(8):4347–4355.

535. Senior RM, et al. Chemotactic activity of platelet alpha granule proteins for fibroblasts. *J Cell Biol* 1983;96(2):382–385.

536. Warringa RA, et al. Modulation of eosinophil chemotaxis by interleukin-5. *Am J Respir Cell Mol Biol* 1992;7(6):631–636.

537. Burgers JA, et al. Human platelets secrete chemotactic activity for eosinophils. *Blood* 1993;81(1):49–55.

538. Deuel TF, et al. Platelet factor 4 is chemotactic for neutrophils and monocytes. *Proc Natl Acad Sci U S A* 1981; 78(7):4584–4587.

539. Hayashi N, et al. Effect of platelet-activating factor and platelet factor 4 on eosinophil adhesion. *Int Arch Allergy Immunol* 1994;104[Suppl 1(1)]:57–59.

540. Griffioen AW, et al. Angiogenesis inhibitors overcome tumor induced endothelial cell anergy. *Int J Cancer* 1999;80(2):315–319.

541. Gengrinovitch S, et al. Platelet factor-4 inhibits the mitogenic activity of VEGF121 and VEGF165 using several concurrent mechanisms. *J Biol Chem* 1995;270(25):15059–15065.

542. Tanaka T, et al. Viral vector-mediated transduction of a modified platelet factor 4 cDNA inhibits angiogenesis and tumor growth. *Nat Med* 1997;3(4):437–442.

543. Gupta SK, Hassel T, Singh JP. A potent inhibitor of endothelial cell proliferation is generated by proteolytic cleavage of the chemokine platelet factor 4. *Proc Natl Acad Sci U S A* 1995;92(17):7799–7803.

544. Peng H, et al. Suppression by platelet factor 4 of the myogenic activity of basic fibroblast growth factor. *Arch Histol Cytol* 1997;60(2):163–174.

545. Gentilini G, et al. Inhibition of human umbilical vein endothelial cell proliferation by the CXC chemokine, platelet factor 4 (PF4), is associated with impaired downregulation of p21(Cip1/WAF1). *Blood* 1999;93(1):25–33.

546. Han ZC, et al. Negative regulation of human megakaryocytopoiesis by human platelet factor 4 (PF4) and connective tissue-activating peptide (CTAP-III). *Int J Cell Cloning* 1990;8(4):253–259.

547. Aidoudi S, et al. *In vivo* effect of platelet factor 4 (PF4) and tetrapeptide AcSDKP on haemopoiesis of mice treated with 5-fluorouracil. *Br J Haematol* 1996;94(3):443–448.

548. Han ZC, et al. Platelet factor 4 and other CXC chemokines support the survival of normal hematopoietic cells and reduce the chemosensitivity of cells to cytotoxic agents. *Blood* 1997;89(7):2328–2335.

549. Brindley LL, Sweet JM, Goetzl EJ. Stimulation of histamine release from human basophils by human platelet factor 4. *J Clin Invest* 1983;72(4):1218–1223.

550. Petersen F, et al. TNF-alpha renders human neutrophils responsive to platelet factor 4. Comparison of PF-4 and IL-8 reveals different activity profiles of the two chemokines. *J Immunol* 1996;156(5):1954–1962.

551. Barone AD, et al. The expression in *Escherichia coli* of recombinant human platelet factor 4, a protein with immunoregulatory activity. *J Biol Chem* 1988;263(18):8710–8715.

552. Crisi GM, et al. Induction of inhibitory activity for B cell differentiation in human CD8 T cells with pokeweed mitogen, dimaprit, and cAMP upregulating agents: countersup-

pressive effect of platelet factor 4. *Cell Immunol* 1996;172(2):205–216.

553. Engstad CS, et al. A novel biological effect of platelet factor 4 (PF4): enhancement of LPS-induced tissue factor activity in monocytes. *J Leukoc Biol* 1995;58(5):575–581.

554. Scheuerer B, et al. The CXC-chemokine platelet factor 4 promotes monocyte survival and induces monocyte differentiation into macrophages. *Blood* 2000;95(4):1158–1166.

555. Maione TE, et al. Inhibition of angiogenesis by recombinant human platelet factor-4 and related peptides. *Science* 1990;247(4938):77–79.

556. Jouan V, et al. Inhibition of *in vitro* angiogenesis by platelet factor-4-derived peptides and mechanism of action. *Blood* 1999;94(3):984–993.

557. Sharpe RJ, et al. Induction of local inflammation by recombinant human platelet factor 4 in the mouse. *Cell Immunol* 1991;137(1):72–80.

558. Yin JZ, et al. Prevention by a platelet-derived factor (platelet factor 4) of induction of low dose tolerance to pneumococcal polysaccharides. *Cell Immunol* 1988;115(2):221–227.

559. Simi M, et al. Raised plasma concentrations of platelet factor 4 (PF4) in Crohn's disease. *Gut* 1987;28(3):336–338.

560. Pouplard C, et al. Antibodies to platelet factor 4-heparin after cardiopulmonary bypass in patients anticoagulated with unfractionated heparin or a low-molecular-weight heparin: clinical implications for heparin-induced thrombocytopenia. *Circulation* 1999;99(19):2530–2536.

561. Lorenz R, Brauer M. Platelet factor 4 (PF4) in septicaemia. *Infection* 1988;16(5):273–276.

562. Wenger RH, Hameister H, Clemetson KJ. Human platelet basic protein/connective tissue activating peptide-III maps in a gene cluster on chromosome 4q12-q13 along with other genes of the beta-thromboglobulin superfamily. *Hum Genet* 1991;87(3):367–368.

563. Remmers EF, et al. Map of seven polymorphic markers on rat chromosome 14: linkage conservation with human chromosome 4. *Mamm Genome* 1993;4(2):90–94.

564. Eisman R, et al. Structural and functional comparison of the genes for human platelet factor 4 and PF4alt. *Blood* 1990;76(2):336–344.

565. Guzzo C, et al. An Eco R1 polymorphism of a human platelet factor 4 (PF4) gene. *Nucleic Acids Res* 1987;15(1):380.

566. Strieter RM, et al. The detection of a novel neutrophil-activating peptide (ENA-78) using a sensitive ELISA. *Immunol Invest* 1992;21(6):589–596.

567. Froyen G, et al. Cloning, bacterial expression and biological characterization of recombinant human granulocyte chemotactic protein-2 and differential expression of granulocyte chemotactic protein-2 and epithelial cell-derived neutrophil activating peptide-78 mRNAs. *Eur J Biochem* 1997;243(3):762–769.

568. Chang MS, et al. Cloning and characterization of the human neutrophil-activating peptide (ENA-78) gene. *J Biol Chem* 1994;269(41):25277–25282.

569. Schnyder-Candrian S, et al. Interferon-alpha and interferon-gamma down-regulate the production of interleukin-8 and ENA-78 in human monocytes. *J Leukoc Biol* 1995;57(6):929–935.

570. Shimoyama T, et al. Chemokine mRNA expression in gastric mucosa is associated with *Helicobacter pylori* cagA positivity and severity of gastritis. *J Clin Pathol* 1998;51(10):765–770.

571. Proost P, et al. Identification of a novel granulocyte chemotactic protein (GCP-2) from human tumor cells. *In vitro* and *in vivo* comparison with natural forms of GRO, IP-10, and IL-8. *J Immunol* 1993;150(3):1000–1010.

572. Wuyts A, et al. Characterization of synthetic human granulocyte chemotactic protein 2: usage of chemokine receptors CXCR1 and CXCR2 and *in vivo* inflammatory properties. *Biochemistry* 1997;36(9):2716–2723.

573. Proudfoot AE, et al. Structure and bioactivity of recombinant human CTAP-III and NAP-2. *J Protein Chem* 1997;16(1):37–49.

574. Castor CW, et al. Connective tissue activation. XXXVI. The origin, variety, distribution, and biologic fate of connective tissue activating peptide-III isoforms: characteristics in patients with rheumatic, renal, and arterial disease. *Arthritis Rheum* 1993;36(8):1142–1153.

575. Abgrall JF, et al. Inhibitory effect of highly purified human platelet beta-thromboglobulin on *in vitro* human megakaryocyte colony formation. *Exp Hematol* 1991;19(3):202–205.

576. Van Damme J, et al. The neutrophil-activating proteins interleukin 8 and beta-thromboglobulin: *in vitro* and *in vivo* comparison of NH2-terminally processed forms. *Eur J Immunol* 1990;20(9):2113–2118.

577. Walz A, et al. Effects of the neutrophil-activating peptide NAP-2, platelet basic protein, connective tissue-activating peptide III and platelet factor 4 on human neutrophils. *J Exp Med* 1989;170(5):1745–1750.

578. Ragsdale CG, et al. Connective tissue activating peptide III. Induction of synthesis and secretion of plasminogen activator by synovial fibroblasts. *Arthritis Rheum* 1984;27(6):663–667.

579. Kuna P, et al. IL-8 inhibits histamine release from human basophils induced by histamine-releasing factors, connective tissue activating peptide III, and IL-3. *J Immunol* 1991;147(6):1920–1924.

580. Tai PK, et al. Regulation of glucose transporters by connective tissue activating peptide-III isoforms. *J Biol Chem* 1992;267(27):19579–19586.

581. Van Osselaer N, et al. Increased microvascular permeability *in vivo* in response to intradermal injection of neutrophil-activating protein (NAP-2) in rabbit skin. *Am J Pathol* 1991;138(1):23–37.

582. Young H, et al. NMR structure and dynamics of monomeric neutrophil-activating peptide 2. *Biochem J* 1999;338(Pt 3):591–598.

583. Piccardoni P, et al. Thrombin-activated human platelets release two NAP-2 variants that stimulate polymorphonuclear leukocytes. *Thromb Haemost* 1996;76(5):780–785.

584. Car BD, Baggiolini M, Walz A. Formation of neutrophil-activating peptide 2 from platelet-derived connective-tissue-activating peptide III by different tissue proteinases. *Biochem J* 1991;275(Pt 3):581–584.

585. Beck GC, et al. Release of CXC-chemokines by human lung microvascular endothelial cells (LMVEC) compared with macrovascular umbilical vein endothelial cells. *Clin Exp Immunol* 1999;118(2):298–303.

586. Ludwig A, et al. The CXC-chemokine neutrophil-activating peptide-2 induces two distinct optima of neutrophil chemo-

taxis by differential interaction with interleukin-8 receptors CXCR-1 and CXCR-2. *Blood* 1997;90(11):4588–4597.

587. Kaplan KL, Francis CW. Heparin-induced thrombocytopenia. *Blood Rev* 1999;13(1):1–7.

588. Yoshimura T, Johnson DG. cDNA cloning and expression of guinea pig neutrophil attractant protein-1 (NAP-1). NAP-1 is highly conserved in guinea pig. *J Immunol* 1993;151(11):6225–6236.

589. Schmid J, Weissmann C. Induction of mRNA for a serine protease and a beta-thromboglobulin-like protein in mitogen-stimulated human leukocytes. *J Immunol* 1987;139(1):250–256.

590. Clore GM, Gronenborn AM. NMR and X-ray analysis of the three-dimensional structure of interleukin-8. *Cytokines* 1992;4:18–40.

591. Aloisi F, et al. Production of hemolymphopoietic cytokines (IL-6, IL-8, colony-stimulating factors) by normal human astrocytes in response to IL-1 beta and tumor necrosis factor-alpha. *J Immunol* 1992;149(7):2358–2366.

592. Brown Z, et al. Chemokine gene expression and secretion by cytokine-activated human microvascular endothelial cells. Differential regulation of monocyte chemoattractant protein-1 and interleukin-8 in response to interferon-gamma. *Am J Pathol* 1994;145(4):913–921.

593. Braun RK, et al. Human peripheral blood eosinophils produce and release interleukin-8 on stimulation with calcium ionophore. *Eur J Immunol* 1993;23(4):956–960.

594. Thornton AJ, Ham J, Kunkel SL. Kupffer cell-derived cytokines induce the synthesis of a leukocyte chemotactic peptide, interleukin-8, in human hepatoma and primary hepatocyte cultures. *Hepatology* 1991;14(6):1112–1122.

595. Brown Z, et al. Cytokine-activated human mesangial cells generate the neutrophil chemoattractant, interleukin 8. *Kidney Int* 1991;40(1):86–90.

596. Smyth MJ, et al. IL-8 gene expression and production in human peripheral blood lymphocyte subsets. *J Immunol* 1991;146(11):3815–3823.

597. Bazzoni F, et al. Phagocytosing neutrophils produce and release high amounts of the neutrophil-activating peptide 1/interleukin 8. *J Exp Med* 1991;173(3):771–774.

598. Zipfel PF, et al. Mitogenic activation of human T cells induces two closely related genes which share structural similarities with a new family of secreted factors. *J Immunol* 1989;142(5):1582–1590.

599. Zipfel PF, Bialonski A, Skerka C. Induction of members of the IL-8/NAP-1 gene family in human T lymphocytes is suppressed by cyclosporin A. *Biochem Biophys Res Commun* 1991;181(1):179–183.

600. Wang N, et al. Interleukin 8 is induced by cholesterol loading of macrophages and expressed by macrophage foam cells in human atheroma. *J Biol Chem* 1996;271(15):8837–8842.

601. Gregory H, et al. Structure determination of a human lymphocyte derived neutrophil activating peptide (LYNAP). *Biochem Biophys Res Commun* 1988;151(2):883–890.

602. Page SM, et al. Stimulation of neutrophil interleukin-8 production by eosinophil granule major basic protein. *Am J Respir Cell Mol Biol* 1999;21(2):230–237.

603. Gasperini S, et al. Gene expression and production of the monokine induced by IFN-gamma (MIG), IFN-inducible T cell alpha chemoattractant (I-TAC), and IFN-gamma-inducible protein-10 (IP-10) chemokines by human neutrophils. *J Immunol* 1999;162(8):4928–4937.

604. Karakurum M, et al. Hypoxic induction of interleukin-8 gene expression in human endothelial cells. *J Clin Invest* 1994;93(4):1564–1570.

605. Desbaillets I, et al. Upregulation of interleukin 8 by oxygen-deprived cells in glioblastoma suggests a role in leukocyte activation, chemotaxis, and angiogenesis. *J Exp Med* 1997;186(8):1201–1212.

606. Desbaillets I, et al. Regulation of interleukin-8 expression by reduced oxygen pressure in human glioblastoma. *Oncogene* 1999;18(7):1447–1456.

607. Xu L, et al. Hypoxia-induced elevation in interleukin-8 expression by human ovarian carcinoma cells. *Cancer Res* 1999;59(22):5822–5829.

608. Shi Q, et al. Constitutive and inducible interleukin 8 expression by hypoxia and acidosis renders human pancreatic cancer cells more tumorigenic and metastatic. *Clin Cancer Res* 1999;5(11):3711–3721.

609. Barker JN, et al. Modulation of keratinocyte-derived interleukin-8 which is chemotactic for neutrophils and T lymphocytes. *Am J Pathol* 1991;139(4):869–876.

610. Wuyts A, Proost P, Van Damme J. Interleukin-8 and other CXC chemokines. In: Thomson AW, ed. *The cytokine handbook*. San Diego: Academic Press, 1998:271–311.

611. Standiford TJ, et al. IL-7 up-regulates the expression of IL-8 from resting and stimulated human blood monocytes. *J Immunol* 1992;149(6):2035–2039.

612. Kehlen A, et al. Interleukin-17 stimulates the expression of IkappaB alpha mRNA and the secretion of IL-6 and IL-8 in glioblastoma cell lines. *J Neuroimmunol* 1999;101(1):1–6.

613. Mauviel A, et al. Leukoregulin, a T cell-derived cytokine, induces IL-8 gene expression and secretion in human skin fibroblasts. Demonstration and secretion in human skin fibroblasts. Demonstration of enhanced NF-kappa B binding and NF-kappa B-driven promoter activity. *J Immunol* 1992;149(9):2969–2976.

614. Xing Z, et al. Lipopolysaccharide induces expression of granulocyte/macrophage colony-stimulating factor, interleukin-8, and interleukin-6 in human nasal, but not lung, fibroblasts: evidence for heterogeneity within the respiratory tract. *Am J Respir Cell Mol Biol* 1993;9(3):255–263.

615. Yoshimura T, et al. Purification of a human monocyte-derived neutrophil chemotactic factor that has peptide sequence similarity to other host defense cytokines. *Proc Natl Acad Sci U S A* 1987;84(24):9233–9237.

616. Roebuck KA, et al. Stimulus-specific regulation of chemokine expression involves differential activation of the redox-responsive transcription factors AP-1 and NF-kappaB. *J Leukoc Biol* 1999;65(3):291–298.

617. Kwon OJ, et al. Inhibition of interleukin-8 expression by dexamethasone in human cultured airway epithelial cells. *Immunology* 1994;81(3):389–394.

618. Sauty A, et al. The T cell-specific CXC chemokines IP-10, Mig, and I-TAC are expressed by activated human bronchial epithelial cells. *J Immunol* 1999;162(6):3549–3558.

619. Oliveira IC, et al. Downregulation of interleukin 8 gene expression in human fibroblasts: unique mechanism of transcriptional inhibition by interferon. *Proc Natl Acad Sci U S A* 1992;89(19):9049–9053.

620. Ehrlich LC, et al. IL-10 down-regulates human microglial IL-8 by inhibition of NF-kappaB activation. *Neuroreport* 1998;9(8):1723–1726.

621. Yang W, Wang D, Richmond A. Role of clathrin-mediated endocytosis in CXCR2 sequestration, resensitization, and signal transduction. *J Biol Chem* 1999;274(16):11328–11333.

622. Schratzberger P, et al. Interleukin-8-induced human peripheral blood B-lymphocyte chemotaxis *in vitro*. *Immunol Lett* 1997;58(3):167–170.

623. Petering H, et al. The biologic role of interleukin-8: functional analysis and expression of CXCR1 and CXCR2 on human eosinophils. *Blood* 1999;93(2):694–702.

624. Yue TL, et al. Interleukin-8. A mitogen and chemoattractant for vascular smooth muscle cells. *Circ Res* 1994;75(1):1–7.

625. Sebok K, et al. IL-8 induces the locomotion of human IL-2-activated natural killer cells. Involvement of a guanine nucleotide binding (Go) protein. *J Immunol* 1993;150(4):1524–1534.

626. Tanaka J, et al. T-cell chemotactic activity of cytokine LD78: a comparative study with interleukin-8, a chemotactic factor for the T-cell CD45RA+ phenotype. *Int Arch Allergy Immunol* 1993;100(3):201–208.

627. Xu L, et al. Modulation of IL-8 receptor expression on purified human T lymphocytes is associated with changed chemotactic responses to IL-8. *J Leukoc Biol* 1995;57(2):335–342.

628. Schorr W, Swandulla D, Zeilhofer HU. Mechanisms of IL-8-induced Ca^{2+} signaling in human neutrophil granulocytes. *Eur J Immunol* 1999;29(3):897–904.

629. Wu D, LaRosa GJ, Simon MI. G protein-coupled signal transduction pathways for interleukin-8. *Science* 1993;261(5117):101–113.

630. Araujo DM, Cotman CW. Trophic effects of interleukin-4, -7 and -8 on hippocampal neuronal cultures: potential involvement of glial-derived factors. *Brain Res* 1993;600(1):49–55.

631. Koch AE, et al. Interleukin-8 as a macrophage-derived mediator of angiogenesis. *Science* 1992;258(5089):1798–1801.

632. Foster SJ, et al. Acute inflammatory effects of a monocyte-derived neutrophil-activating peptide in rabbit skin. *Immunology* 1989;67(2):181–183.

633. Burrows LJ, et al. Intraperitoneal injection of human recombinant neutrophil-activating factor/interleukin 8 (hrNAF/IL-8) produces a T cell and eosinophil infiltrate in the guinea pig lung. Effect of PAF antagonist WEB2086. *Ann N Y Acad Sci* 1991;629:422–424.

634. Beaubien BC, et al. A novel neutrophil chemoattractant generated during an inflammatory reaction in the rabbit peritoneal cavity *in vivo*. Purification, partial amino acid sequence and structural relationship to interleukin 8. *Biochem J* 1990;271(3):797–801.

635. Kanazawa H, et al. Clinical significance of serum concentration of interleukin 8 in patients with bronchial asthma or chronic pulmonary emphysema. *Respiration* 1996;63(4):236–240.

636. Apostolopoulos J, Davenport P, Tipping PG. Interleukin-8 production by macrophages from atheromatous plaques. *Arterioscler Thromb Vasc Biol* 1996;16(8):1007–1012.

637. Lawlor F, Camp R, Greaves M. Epidermal interleukin 1 alpha functional activity and interleukin 8 immunoreactivity are increased in patients with cutaneous T-cell lymphoma [Letter; comment]. *J Invest Dermatol* 1992;99(4):514–515.

638. Dean TP, et al. Interleukin-8 concentrations are elevated in bronchoalveolar lavage, sputum, and sera of children with cystic fibrosis. *Pediatr Res* 1993;34(2):159–161.

639. Kitadai Y, et al. Expression of interleukin-8 correlates with vascularity in human gastric carcinomas. *Am J Pathol* 1998;152(1):93–100.

640. Crabtree JE. Role of cytokines in pathogenesis of *Helicobacter pylori*-induced mucosal damage. *Dig Dis Sci* 1998;43[9 Suppl]:46S–55S.

641. Arenberg DA, et al. Inhibition of interleukin-8 reduces tumorigenesis of human non-small cell lung cancer in SCID mice. *J Clin Invest* 1996;97(12):2792–2802.

642. Yoneda J, et al. Expression of angiogenesis-related genes and progression of human ovarian carcinomas in nude mice. *J Natl Cancer Inst* 1998;90(6):447–454.

643. Schroder JM. Biochemical and biological characterization of NAP-1/IL-8-related cytokines in lesional psoriatic scale. *Adv Exp Med Biol* 1991;305:97–107.

644. Mukaida N, Shiroo M, Matsushima K. Genomic structure of the human monocyte-derived neutrophil chemotactic factor IL-8. *J Immunol* 1989;143(4):1366–1371.

645. Fey MF, Tobler A. An interleukin-8 (IL-8) cDNA clone identifies a frequent HindIII polymorphism. *Hum Genet* 1993;91(3):298.

646. Emi M, et al. Association of diffuse panbronchiolitis with microsatellite polymorphism of the human interleukin 8 (IL-8) gene. *J Hum Genet* 1999;44(3):169–172.

647. Farber JM. A macrophage mRNA selectively induced by gamma-interferon encodes a member of the platelet factor 4 family of cytokines. *Proc Natl Acad Sci U S A* 1990;87(14):5238–5242.

648. Liao F, et al. Human Mig chemokine: biochemical and functional characterization. *J Exp Med* 1995;182(5):1301–1314.

649. Farber JM. Mig and IP-10: CXC chemokines that target lymphocytes. *J Leukoc Biol* 1997;61(3):246–257.

650. Farber JM. HuMig: a new human member of the chemokine family of cytokines. *Biochem Biophys Res Commun* 1993;192(1):223–230.

651. Loetscher M, et al. Lymphocyte-specific chemokine receptor CXCR3: regulation, chemokine binding and gene localization. *Eur J Immunol* 1998;28(11):3696–3705.

652. Weng Y, et al. Binding and functional properties of recombinant and endogenous CXCR3 chemokine receptors. *J Biol Chem* 1998;273(29):18288–18291.

653. Schwartz GN, et al. Suppressive effects of recombinant human monokine induced by IFN-gamma (rHuMig) chemokine on the committed and primitive hemopoietic progenitors in liquid cultures of CD34+ human bone marrow cells. *J Immunol* 1997;159(2):895–904.

654. Romagnani P, et al. Role for interactions between IP-10/Mig and CXCR3 in proliferative glomerulonephritis. *J Am Soc Nephrol* 1999;10(12):2518–2526.

655. Strieter RM, et al. The role of CXC chemokines as regulators of angiogenesis. *Shock* 1995;4(3):155–160.

656. Sgadari C, et al. Mig, the monokine induced by interferon-gamma, promotes tumor necrosis *in vivo*. *Blood* 1997;89(8):2635–2643.

657. Kanegane C, et al. Contribution of the CXC chemokines IP-10 and Mig to the antitumor effects of IL-12. *J Leukoc Biol* 1998;64(3):384–392.

658. Tannenbaum CS, et al. The CXC chemokines IP-10 and Mig are necessary for IL-12-mediated regression of the mouse RENCA tumor. *J Immunol* 1998;161(2):927–932.

659. Addison CL, et al. The CXC chemokine, monokine induced by interferon-gamma, inhibits non-small cell lung carcinoma tumor growth and metastasis. *Hum Gene Ther* 2000;11(2):247–261.

660. Mahalingam S, Farber JM, Karupiah G. The interferon-inducible chemokines MuMig and Crg-2 exhibit antiviral activity *in vivo*. *J Virol* 1999;73(2):1479–1491.

661. Mach F, et al. Differential expression of three T lymphocyte-activating CXC chemokines by human atheroma-associated cells. *J Clin Invest* 1999;104(8):1041–1050.

662. Tosato G, et al. Regression of experimental Burkitt's lymphoma induced by Epstein-Barr virus-immortalized human B cells. *Blood* 1994;83(3):776–784.

663. Sgadari C, et al. Interferon-inducible protein-10 identified as a mediator of tumor necrosis *in vivo*. *Proc Natl Acad Sci U S A* 1996;93(24):13791–13796.

664. Jones D, et al. The chemokine receptor CXCR3 is expressed in a subset of B-cell lymphomas and is a marker of B-cell chronic lymphocytic leukemia. *Blood* 2000;95(2):627–632.

665. Flier J, et al. The CXCR3 activating chemokines IP-10, Mig, and IP-9 are expressed in allergic but not in irritant patch test reactions. *J Invest Dermatol* 1999;113(4):574–578.

666. Tensen CP, et al. Epidermal interferon-gamma inducible protein-10 (IP-10) and monokine induced by gamma-interferon (Mig) but not IL-8 mRNA expression is associated with epidermotropism in cutaneous T cell lymphomas. *J Invest Dermatol* 1998;111(2):222–226.

667. Teruya-Feldstein J, et al. The role of Mig, the monokine induced by interferon-gamma, and IP-10, the interferon-gamma-inducible protein-10, in tissue necrosis and vascular damage associated with Epstein-Barr virus-positive lymphoproliferative disease. *Blood* 1997;90(10):4099–4105.

668. Setsuda J, et al. Interleukin-18, interferon-gamma, IP-10, and Mig expression in Epstein-Barr virus-induced infectious mononucleosis and posttransplant lymphoproliferative disease. *Am J Pathol* 1999;155(1):257–265.

669. Koga S, et al. T cell infiltration into class II MHC-disparate allografts and acute rejection is dependent on the IFN-gamma-induced chemokine Mig. *J Immunol* 1999;163(9):4878–4885.

670. Saurer L, et al. Differential expression of chemokines in normal pancreas and in chronic pancreatitis. *Gastroenterology* 2000;118(2):356–367.

671. Amichay D, et al. Genes for chemokines MuMig and Crg-2 are induced in protozoan and viral infections in response to IFN-gamma with patterns of tissue expression that suggest nonredundant roles *in vivo*. *J Immunol* 1996;157(10):4511–4520.

672. Lee HH, Farber JM. Localization of the gene for the human MIG cytokine on chromosome 4q21 adjacent to INP10 reveals a chemokine "mini-cluster." *Cytogenet Cell Genet* 1996;74(4):255–258.

673. Vanguri P, Farber JM. Identification of CRG-2. An interferon-inducible mRNA predicted to encode a murine monokine. *J Biol Chem* 1990;265(25):15049–15057.

674. Liang P, et al. Ras activation of genes: Mob-1 as a model. *Proc Natl Acad Sci U S A* 1994;91(26):12515–12519.

675. Ohmori Y, Hamilton TA. A macrophage LPS-inducible early gene encodes the murine homologue of IP-10. *Biochem Biophys Res Commun* 1990;168(3):1261–1267.

676. Luster AD, Unkeless JC, Ravetch JV. Gamma-interferon transcriptionally regulates an early-response gene containing homology to platelet proteins. *Nature* 1985;315(6021):672–676.

677. Neville LF, Mathiak G, Bagasra O. The immunobiology of interferon-gamma inducible protein 10 kD (IP-10): a novel, pleiotropic member of the C-X-C chemokine superfamily. *Cytokine Growth Factor Rev* 1997;8(3):207–219.

678. Clark-Lewis I, et al. Structure-activity relationships of chemokines. *J Leukoc Biol* 1995;57(5):703–711.

679. Luster AD, Ravetch JV. Biochemical characterization of a gamma interferon-inducible cytokine (IP-10). *J Exp Med* 1987;166(4):1084–1097.

680. Boorsma DM, et al. Chemokine IP-10 expression in cultured human keratinocytes. *Arch Dermatol Res* 1998;290(6):335–341.

681. Ohmori Y, Hamilton TA. The interferon-stimulated response element and a kappa B site mediate synergistic induction of murine IP-10 gene transcription by IFN-gamma and TNF-alpha. *J Immunol* 1995;154(10):5235–5244.

682. Ransohoff RM, et al. Astrocyte expression of mRNA encoding cytokines IP-10 and JE/MCP-1 in experimental autoimmune encephalomyelitis. *FASEB J* 1993;7(6):592–600.

683. Gomez-Chiarri M, et al. Expression of IP-10, a lipopolysaccharide- and interferon-gamma-inducible protein, in murine mesangial cells in culture. *Am J Pathol* 1993;142(2):433–439.

684. Cassatella MA, et al. Regulated production of the interferon-gamma-inducible protein-10 (IP-10) chemokine by human neutrophils. *Eur J Immunol* 1997;27(1):111–115.

685. Bedard PA, Golds EE. Cytokine-induced expression of mRNAs for chemotactic factors in human synovial cells and fibroblasts. *J Cell Physiol* 1993;154(2):433–441.

686. Ren LQ, et al. Lipopolysaccharide-induced expression of IP-10 mRNA in rat brain and in cultured rat astrocytes and microglia. *Brain Res Mol Brain Res* 1998;59(2):256–263.

687. Tannenbaum CS, et al. Lipopolysaccharide-inducible macrophage early genes are induced in Balb/c 3T3 cells by platelet-derived growth factor. *J Biol Chem* 1989;264(7):4052–4057.

688. Ohmori Y, et al. Kappa B binding activity in a murine macrophage-like cell line. Sequence-specific differences in kappa B binding and transcriptional activation functions. *J Biol Chem* 1994;269(26):17684–17690.

689. Memet S, et al. Direct induction of interferon-gamma- and interferon-alpha/beta-inducible genes by double-stranded RNA. *J Interferon Res* 1991;11(3):131–141.

690. Larner AC, et al. IL-4 attenuates the transcriptional activation of both IFN-alpha and IFN-gamma-induced cellular gene expression in monocytes and monocytic cell lines. *J Immunol* 1993;150(5):1944–1950.

691. Maghazachi AA, et al. Interferon-inducible protein-10 and lymphotactin induce the chemotaxis and mobilization of intracellular calcium in natural killer cells through pertussis

toxin-sensitive and -insensitive heterotrimeric G-proteins. *FASEB J* 1997;11(10):765–774.

692. Wang X, et al. Interferon-inducible protein-10 involves vascular smooth muscle cell migration, proliferation, and inflammatory response. *J Biol Chem* 1996;271(39):24286–24293.

693. Luster AD, Greenberg SM, Leder P. The IP-10 chemokine binds to a specific cell surface heparan sulfate site shared with platelet factor 4 and inhibits endothelial cell proliferation. *J Exp Med* 1995;182(1):219–231.

694. Sarris AH, et al. Human interferon-inducible protein 10: expression and purification of recombinant protein demonstrate inhibition of early human hematopoietic progenitors. *J Exp Med* 1993;178(3):1127–1132.

695. Lloyd AR, et al. Chemokines regulate T cell adherence to recombinant adhesion molecules and extracellular matrix proteins. *J Immunol* 1996;156(3):932–938.

696. Geras-Raaka E, et al. Human interferon-gamma-inducible protein 10 (IP-10) inhibits constitutive signaling of Kaposi's sarcoma-associated herpesvirus G protein-coupled receptor. *J Exp Med* 1998;188(2):405–408.

697. Taub DD, Longo DL, Murphy WJ. Human interferon-inducible protein-10 induces mononuclear cell infiltration in mice and promotes the migration of human T lymphocytes into the peripheral tissues and human peripheral blood lymphocytes-SCID mice. *Blood* 1996;87(4):1423–1431.

698. Luster AD, Leder P. IP-10, a -C-X-C- chemokine, elicits a potent thymus-dependent antitumor response *in vivo. J Exp Med* 1993;178(3):1057–1065.

699. Abdullah F, et al. The novel chemokine mob-1: involvement in adult respiratory distress syndrome. *Surgery* 1997;122(2):303–312.

700. Kaplan G, et al. The expression of a gamma interferon-induced protein (IP-10) in delayed immune responses in human skin. *J Exp Med* 1987;166(4):1098–1108.

701. Zhang R, et al. Mob-1, a Ras target gene, is overexpressed in colorectal cancer. *Oncogene* 1997;14(13):1607–1610.

702. Gomez-Chiarri M, et al. Interferon-inducible protein-10 is highly expressed in rats with experimental nephrosis. *Am J Pathol* 1996;148(1):301–311.

703. Agostini C, et al. Involvement of the IP-10 chemokine in sarcoid granulomatous reactions. *J Immunol* 1998;161(11):6413–6420.

704. Lahrtz F, et al. Chemotactic activity on mononuclear cells in the cerebrospinal fluid of patients with viral meningitis is mediated by interferon-gamma inducible protein-10 and monocyte chemotactic protein-1. *Eur J Immunol* 1997;27(10):2484–2489.

705. Ohmori Y, Hamilton TA. Cooperative interaction between interferon (IFN) stimulus response element and kappa B sequence motifs controls IFN gamma- and lipopolysaccharide-stimulated transcription from the murine IP-10 promoter. *J Biol Chem* 1993;268(9):6677–6688.

706. Tensen CP, et al. Human IP-9: a keratinocyte-derived high affinity CXC-chemokine ligand for the IP-10/Mig receptor (CXCR3). *J Invest Dermatol* 1999;112(5):716–722.

707. Rani MRS, et al. Characterization of beta-R1, a gene that is selectively induced by interferon beta (IFN-beta) compared with IFN-alpha. *J Biol Chem* 1996;271(37):22878–22884.

708. Luo Y, et al. The CXC-chemokine, H174: expression in the central nervous system. *J Neurovirol* 1998;4(6):575–585.

709. Laich A, et al. Structure and expression of the human small cytokine B subfamily member 11 (SCYB11/formerly SCYB9B, alias I-TAC) gene cloned from IFN-gamma-treated human monocytes (THP-1). *J Interferon Cytokine Res* 1999;19(5):505–513.

710. Tensen CP, et al. Genomic organization, sequence and transcriptional regulation of the human CXCL 11(1) gene. *Biochim Biophys Acta* 1999;1446(1–2):167–172.

711. Erdel M, et al. The human gene encoding SCYB9B, a putative novel CXC chemokine, maps to human chromosome 4q21 like the closely related genes for MIG (SCYB9) and INP10 (SCYB10). *Cytogenet Cell Genet* 1998;81(3–4):271–272.

712. Begum NA, et al. Loss of hIRH mRNA expression from premalignant adenomas and malignant cell lines. *Biochem Biophys Res Commun* 1996;229(3):864–868.

713. Jiang W, et al. Molecular cloning of TPAR1, a gene whose expression is repressed by the tumor promoter 12-O-tetradecanoylphorbol 13-acetate (TPA). *Exp Cell Res* 1994;215(2):284–293.

714. Crump MP, et al. Solution structure and basis for functional activity of stromal cell-derived factor-1; dissociation of CXCR4 activation from binding and inhibition of HIV-1. *EMBO J* 1997;16(23):6996–7007.

715. Dealwis C, et al. Crystal structure of chemically synthesized [N33A] stromal cell-derived factor 1 alpha, a potent ligand for the HIV-1 "fusin" coreceptor. *Proc Natl Acad Sci U S A* 1998;95(12):6941–6946.

716. Shirozu M, et al. Structure and chromosomal localization of the human stromal cell-derived factor 1 (SDF1) gene. *Genomics* 1995;28(3):495–500.

717. Proost P, et al. Processing by CD26/dipeptidyl-peptidase IV reduces the chemotactic and anti-HIV-1 activity of stromal-cell-derived factor-1 alpha. *FEBS Lett* 1998;432(1–2):73–76.

718. Tashiro K, et al. Signal sequence trap: a cloning strategy for secreted proteins and type I membrane proteins. *Science* 1993;261(5121):600–603.

719. Aiuti A, et al. Human CD34(+) cells express CXCR4 and its ligand stromal cell-derived factor-1. Implications for infection by T-cell tropic human immunodeficiency virus. *Blood* 1999;94(1):62–73.

720. Pablos JL, et al. Stromal-cell derived factor is expressed by dendritic cells and endothelium in human skin. *Am J Pathol* 1999;155(5):1577–1586.

721. Iyer VR, et al. The transcriptional program in the response of human fibroblasts to serum [see comments]. *Science* 1999;283(5398):83–87.

722. Coulomb-L'Hermin A, et al. Stromal cell-derived factor 1 (SDF-1) and antenatal human B cell lymphopoiesis: expression of SDF-1 by mesothelial cells and biliary ductal plate epithelial cells. *Proc Natl Acad Sci U S A* 1999;96(15):8585–8590.

723. Bajetto A, et al. Expression of chemokine receptors in the rat brain. *Ann N Y Acad Sci* 1999;876:201–209.

724. Hesselgesser J, et al. Identification and characterization of the CXCR4 chemokine receptor in human T cell lines: ligand binding, biological activity, and HIV-1 infectivity. *J Immunol* 1998;160(2):877–883.

725. Amara A, et al. Stromal cell-derived factor-1 alpha associates with heparan sulfates through the first beta-strand of the chemokine. *J Biol Chem* 1999;274(34):23916–23925.

726. Bleul CC, et al. A highly efficacious lymphocyte chemoattractant, stromal cell-derived factor 1 (SDF-1) [see comments]. *J Exp Med* 1996;184(3):1101–1109.

727. Bleul CC, Schultze JL, Springer TA. B lymphocyte chemotaxis regulated in association with microanatomic localization, differentiation state, and B cell receptor engagement. *J Exp Med* 1998;187(5):753–762.

728. Vicente-Manzanares M, et al. The chemokine SDF-1 alpha triggers a chemotactic response and induces cell polarization in human B lymphocytes. *Eur J Immunol* 1998;28(7):2197–2207.

729. D'Apuzzo M, et al. The chemokine SDF-1, stromal cell-derived factor 1, attracts early stage B cell precursors via the chemokine receptor CXCR4. *Eur J Immunol* 1997;27(7):1788–1793.

730. Aiuti A, et al. The chemokine SDF-1 is a chemoattractant for human CD34+ hematopoietic progenitor cells and provides a new mechanism to explain the mobilization of CD34+ progenitors to peripheral blood. *J Exp Med* 1997;185(1):111–120.

731. Mohle R, et al. The chemokine receptor CXCR-4 is expressed on CD34+ hematopoietic progenitors and leukemic cells and mediates transendothelial migration induced by stromal cell-derived factor-1. *Blood* 1998;91(12):4523–4530.

732. Wang JF, Liu ZY, Groopman JE. The alpha-chemokine receptor CXCR4 is expressed on the megakaryocytic lineage from progenitor to platelets and modulates migration and adhesion. *Blood* 1998;92(3):756–764.

733. Gupta SK, et al. Chemokine receptors in human endothelial cells. Functional expression of CXCR4 and its transcriptional regulation by inflammatory cytokines. *J Biol Chem* 1998;273(7):4282–4287.

734. Maghazachi AA. Role of the heterotrimeric G proteins in stromal-derived factor-1 alpha-induced natural killer cell chemotaxis and calcium mobilization [published erratum appears in *Biochem Biophys Res Commun* 1997;237(3):759]. *Biochem Biophys Res Commun* 1997;236(2):270–274.

735. Murdoch C, Monk PN, Finn A. CXC chemokine receptor expression on human endothelial cells. *Cytokine* 1999;11(9):704–712.

736. Vila-Coro AJ, et al. The chemokine SDF-1 alpha triggers CXCR4 receptor dimerization and activates the JAK/STAT pathway. *FASEB J* 1999;13(13):1699–1710.

737. Ganju RK, et al. The alpha-chemokine, stromal cell-derived factor-1 alpha, binds to the transmembrane G-protein-coupled CXCR-4 receptor and activates multiple signal transduction pathways. *J Biol Chem* 1998;273(36):23169–23175.

738. Vicente-Manzanares M, et al. Involvement of phosphatidylinositol 3-kinase in stromal cell-derived factor-1 alpha-induced lymphocyte polarization and chemotaxis. *J Immunol* 1999;163(7):4001–4012.

739. Sotsios Y, et al. The CXC chemokine stromal cell-derived factor activates a Gi-coupled phosphoinositide 3-kinase in T lymphocytes. *J Immunol* 1999;163(11):5954–5963.

740. Haribabu B, et al. Regulation of human chemokine receptors CXCR4. Role of phosphorylation in desensitization and internalization. *J Biol Chem* 1997;272(45):28726–28731.

741. Salcedo R, et al. Vascular endothelial growth factor and basic fibroblast growth factor induce expression of CXCR4 on human endothelial cells: *in vivo* neovascularization induced by stromal-derived factor-1 alpha. *Am J Pathol* 1999;154(4):1125–1135.

742. Peled A, et al. The chemokine SDF-1 stimulates integrin-mediated arrest of CD34(+) cells on vascular endothelium under shear flow. *J Clin Invest* 1999;104(9):1199–1211.

743. Signoret N, et al. Phorbol esters and SDF-1 induce rapid endocytosis and down modulation of the chemokine receptor CXCR4. *J Cell Biol* 1997;139(3):651–664.

744. Nagasawa T, Kikutani H, Kishimoto T. Molecular cloning and structure of a pre-B-cell growth-stimulating factor. *Proc Natl Acad Sci U S A* 1994;91(6):2305–2309.

745. Lataillade JJ, et al. Chemokine SDF-1 enhances circulating CD34(+) cell proliferation in synergy with cytokines: possible role in progenitor survival. *Blood* 2000;95(3):756–768.

746. Gotoh A, et al. SDF-1 suppresses cytokine-induced adhesion of human haemopoietic progenitor cells to immobilized fibronectin. *Br J Haematol* 1999;106(1):171–174.

747. Bleul CC, et al. The lymphocyte chemoattractant SDF-1 is a ligand for LESTR/fusin and blocks HIV-1 entry. *Nature* 1996;382(6594):829–833.

748. Oberlin E, et al. The CXC chemokine SDF-1 is the ligand for LESTR/fusin and prevents infection by T-cell-line-adapted HIV-1 [published erratum appears in *Nature* 1996;384(6606):288]. *Nature* 1996;382(6594):833–835.

749. Geras-Raaka E, et al. Kaposi's sarcoma-associated herpesvirus (KSHV) chemokine vMIP-II and human SDF-1 alpha inhibit signaling by KSHV G protein-coupled receptor. *Biochem Biophys Res Commun* 1998;253(3):725–727.

750. Nagasawa T, et al. Defects of B-cell lymphopoiesis and bone-marrow myelopoiesis in mice lacking the CXC chemokine PBSF/SDF-1. *Nature* 1996;382(6592):635–638.

751. Ma Q, et al. Impaired B-lymphopoiesis, myelopoiesis, and derailed cerebellar neuron migration in CXCR4- and SDF-1-deficient mice. *Proc Natl Acad Sci U S A* 1998;95(16):9448–9453.

752. Derdeyn CA, et al. Correlation between circulating stromal cell-derived factor 1 levels and CD4+ cell count in human immunodeficiency virus type 1-infected individuals. *AIDS Res Hum Retroviruses* 1999;15(12):1063–1071.

753. Nomura M, et al. Genetic mapping of the mouse stromal cell-derived factor gene (Sdf1) to mouse and rat chromosomes. *Cytogenet Cell Genet* 1996;73(4):286–289.

754. Van Rij RP, et al. The role of a stromal cell-derived factor-1 chemokine gene variant in the clinical course of HIV-1 infection. *AIDS* 1998;12(9):F85–F90.

755. Winkler C, et al. Genetic restriction of AIDS pathogenesis by an SDF-1 chemokine gene variant. ALIVE Study, Hemophilia Growth and Development Study (HGDS), Multicenter AIDS Cohort Study (MACS), Multicenter Hemophilia Cohort Study (MHCS), San Francisco City Cohort (SFCC). *Science* 1998;279(5349):389–393.

756. Legler DF, et al. B cell-attracting chemokine 1, a human CXC chemokine expressed in lymphoid tissues, selectively attracts B lymphocytes via BLR1/CXCR5. *J Exp Med* 1998;187(4):655–660.

757. Gunn MD, et al. A B-cell-homing chemokine made in lym-

phoid follicles activates Burkitt's lymphoma receptor-1. *Nature* 1998;391(6669):799–803.

758. Ngo VN, et al. Lymphotoxin alpha/beta and tumor necrosis factor are required for stromal cell expression of homing chemokines in B and T cell areas of the spleen. *J Exp Med* 1999;189(2):403–412.

759. Ansel KM, et al. *In vivo*-activated CD4 T cells upregulate CXC chemokine receptor 5 and reprogram their response to lymphoid chemokines. *J Exp Med* 1999;190(8):1123–1134.

760. Mazzucchelli L, et al. BCA-1 is highly expressed in *Helicobacter pylori*-induced mucosa-associated lymphoid tissue and gastric lymphoma. *J Clin Invest* 1999;104(10):R49–R54.

761. Hromas R, et al. Cloning of BRAK, a novel divergent CXC chemokine preferentially expressed in normal versus malignant cells. *Biochem Biophys Res Commun* 1999;255(3):703–706.

762. Dunstan CAN, et al. Identification of two rat genes orthologous to the human interleukin-8 receptors. *J Biol Chem* 1996;271(51):32770–32776.

763. Murphy PM, Tiffany HL. Cloning of complementary DNA encoding a functional human interleukin-8 receptor. *Science* 1991;253(5025):1280–1283.

764. Holmes WE, et al. Structure and functional expression of a human interleukin-8 receptor. *Science* 1991;253(5025):1278–1280.

765. Oin S, et al. Expression of monocyte chemoattractant protein-1 and interleukin-8 receptors on subsets of T cells: correlation with transendothelial chemotactic potential. *Eur J Immunol* 1996;26(3):640–647.

766. Wilkinson NC, Navarro J. PU.1 regulates the CXCR1 promoter. *J Biol Chem* 1999;274(1):438–443.

767. Lloyd AR, et al. Granulocyte-colony stimulating factor and lipopolysaccharide regulate the expression of interleukin 8 receptors on polymorphonuclear leukocytes. *J Biol Chem* 1995;270(47):28188–28192.

768. Mitchell GB, et al. CD45 modulation of CXCR1 and CXCR2 in human polymorphonuclear leukocytes. *Eur J Immunol* 1999;29(5):1467–1476.

769. Grutkoski PS, et al. Regulation of IL-8RA (CXCR1) expression in polymorphonuclear leukocytes by hypoxia/reoxygenation. *J Leukoc Biol* 1999;65(2):171–178.

770. Samanta AK, Oppenheim JJ, Matsushima K. Interleukin 8 (monocyte-derived neutrophil chemotactic factor) dynamically regulates its own receptor expression on human neutrophils. *J Biol Chem* 1990;265(1):183–189.

771. Chuntharapai A, Kim KJ. Regulation of the expression of IL-8 receptor A/B by IL-8: possible functions of each receptor. *J Immunol* 1995;155(5):2587–2594.

772. Jawa RS, et al. Tumor necrosis factor alpha regulates CXC chemokine receptor expression and function. *Shock* 1999;11(6):385–390.

773. Richardson RM, et al. Differential cross-regulation of the human chemokine receptors CXCR1 and CXCR2. Evidence for time-dependent signal generation. *J Biol Chem* 1998;273(37):23830–23836.

774. Jones SA, Moser B, Thelen M. A comparison of post-receptor signal transduction events in Jurkat cells transfected with either IL-8R1 or IL-8R2. Chemokine mediated activation of p42/p44 MAP-kinase (ERK-2). *FEBS Lett* 1995;364(2):211–214.

775. Schumacher C, et al. High- and low-affinity binding of GRO alpha and neutrophil-activating peptide 2 to interleukin 8 receptors on human neutrophils. *Proc Natl Acad Sci U S A* 1992;89(21):10542–10546.

776. Kulke R, et al. The CXC receptor 2 is overexpressed in psoriatic epidermis. *J Invest Dermatol* 1998;110(1):90–94.

777. Mollereau C, et al. The high-affinity interleukin 8 receptor gene (IL8RA) maps to the 2q33-q36 region of the human genome: cloning of a pseudogene (IL8RBP) for the low-affinity receptor. *Genomics* 1993;16(1):248–251.

778. Ahuja SK, et al. Comparison of the genomic organization and promoter function for human interleukin-8 receptors A and B. *J Biol Chem* 1994;269(42):26381–26389.

779. Harada A, et al. Cloning of a cDNA encoding a mouse homolog of the interleukin-8 receptor. *Gene* 1994;142(2):297–300.

780. Horuk R, et al. Expression of chemokine receptors by subsets of neurons in the central nervous system. *J Immunol* 1997;158(6):2882–2890.

781. Xia M, et al. Interleukin-8 receptor B immunoreactivity in brain and neuritic plaques of Alzheimer's disease. *Am J Pathol* 1997;150(4):1267–1274.

782. Asagoe K, et al. Down-regulation of CXCR2 expression on human polymorphonuclear leukocytes by TNF-alpha. *J Immunol* 1998;160(9):4518–4525.

783. Penfold ME, et al. Cytomegalovirus encodes a potent alpha chemokine. *Proc Natl Acad Sci U S A* 1999;96(17):9839–9844.

784. Cacalano G, et al. Neutrophil and B cell expansion in mice that lack the murine IL-8 receptor homolog [see comments] [published erratum appears in *Science* 1995;270(5235):365]. *Science* 1994;265(5172):682–684.

785. Brito BE, et al. Murine endotoxin-induced uveitis, but not immune complex-induced uveitis, is dependent on the IL-8 receptor homolog. *Curr Eye Res* 1999;19(1):76–85.

786. Balish E, et al. Mucosal and systemic candidiasis in IL-8Rh-/-BALB/c mice. *J Leukoc Biol* 1999;66(1):144–150.

787. Hogaboam CM, et al. Macrophage inflammatory protein-2 gene therapy attenuates adenovirus- and acetaminophen-mediated hepatic injury. *Gene Ther* 1999;6(4):573–584.

788. Moore TA, et al. Bacterial clearance and survival are dependent on CXC chemokine receptor-2 ligands in a murine model of pulmonary nocardia asteroides infection. *J Immunol* 2000;164(2):908–915.

789. Lloyd A, et al. Assignment of genes for interleukin-8 receptors (IL8R) A and B to human chromosome band 2q35. *Cytogenet Cell Genet* 1993;63(4):238–240.

790. Heesen M, et al. Cloning and chromosomal mapping of an orphan chemokine receptor: mouse RDC1. *Immunogenetics* 1998;47(5):364–370.

791. Sprenger H, et al. Structure, genomic organization, and expression of the human interleukin-8 receptor B gene. *J Biol Chem* 1994;269(15):11065–11072.

792. Tamaru M, et al. Cloning of the murine interferon-inducible protein 10 (IP-10) receptor and its specific expression in lymphoid organs. *Biochem Biophys Res Commun* 1998;251(1):41–48.

793. Qin S, et al. The chemokine receptors CXCR3 and CCR5 mark subsets of T cells associated with certain inflammatory reactions. *J Clin Invest* 1998;101(4):746–754.

794. Bonecchi R, et al. Differential expression of chemokine receptors and chemotactic responsiveness of type 1 T helper cells (Th1s) and Th2s. *J Exp Med* 1998;187(1):129–134.

795. Loetscher M, et al. Chemokine receptor specific for IP10 and mig: structure, function, and expression in activated T-lymphocytes [see comments]. *J Exp Med* 1996;184(3):963–969.

796. Trentin L, et al. The chemokine receptor CXCR3 is expressed on malignant B cells and mediates chemotaxis. *J Clin Invest* 1999;104(1):115–121.

797. Loetscher P, et al. CCR5 is characteristic of Th1 lymphocytes. *Nature* 1998;391(6665):344–345.

798. Marchese A, et al. Cloning and chromosomal mapping of three novel genes, GPR9, GPR10, and GPR14, encoding receptors related to interleukin 8, neuropeptide Y, and somatostatin receptors. *Genomics* 1995;29(2):335–344.

799. Gupta SK, Pillarisetti K. Cutting edge: CXCR4-Lo: molecular cloning and functional expression of a novel human CXCR4 splice variant. *J Immunol* 1999;163(5):2368–2372.

800. Heesen M, et al. Alternate splicing of mouse fusin/CXC chemokine receptor-4: stromal cell-derived factor-1 alpha is a ligand for both CXC chemokine receptor-4 isoforms. *J Immunol* 1997;158(8):3561–3564.

801. Federsppiel B, et al. Molecular cloning of the cDNA and chromosomal localization of the gene for a putative seven-transmembrane segment (7-TMS) receptor isolated from human spleen. *Genomics* 1993;16(3):707–712.

802. Lavi E, et al. CXCR-4 (Fusin), a co-receptor for the type 1 human immunodeficiency virus (HIV-1), is expressed in the human brain in a variety of cell types, including microglia and neurons. *Am J Pathol* 1997;151(4):1035–1042.

803. Bleul CC, et al. The HIV coreceptors CXCR4 and CCR5 are differentially expressed and regulated on human T lymphocytes [see comments]. *Proc Natl Acad Sci U S A* 1997; 94(5):1925–1930.

804. Dwinell MB, et al. Chemokine receptor expression by human intestinal epithelial cells. *Gastroenterology* 1999; 117(2):359–367.

805. Zoeteweij JP, et al. Cytokines regulate expression and function of the HIV coreceptor CXCR4 on human mature dendritic cells. *J Immunol* 1998;161(7):3219–3223.

806. Hori T, et al. Detection and delineation of CXCR-4 (fusin) as an entry and fusion cofactor for T cell-tropic HIV-1 by three different monoclonal antibodies. *J Immunol* 1998;160(1):180–188.

807. Carroll RG, et al. Differential regulation of HIV-1 fusion cofactor expression by CD28 costimulation of CD4+ T cells. *Science* 1997;276(5310):273–276.

808. Cole SW, Jamieson BD, Zack JA. cAMP up-regulates cell surface expression of lymphocyte CXCR4: implications for chemotaxis and HIV-1 infection. *J Immunol* 1999; 162(3):1392–1400.

809. Gupta SK, Pillarisetti K, Lysko PG. Modulation of CXCR4 expression and SDF-1 alpha functional activity during differentiation of human monocytes and macrophages. *J Leukoc Biol* 1999;66(1):135–143.

810. Secchiero P, et al. Extracellular HIV-1 tat protein up-regulates the expression of surface CXC-chemokine receptor 4 in resting CD4+ T cells. *J Immunol* 1999;162(4):2427–2431.

811. Wang J, et al. IL-4 and a glucocorticoid up-regulate CXCR4 expression on human CD4+ T lymphocytes and enhance HIV-1 replication. *J Leukoc Biol* 1998;64(5):642–649.

812. Abbal C, et al. TCR-mediated activation of allergen-specific CD45RO(+) memory T lymphocytes results in down-regulation of cell-surface CXCR4 expression and a strongly reduced capacity to migrate in response to stromal cell-derived factor-1. *Int Immunol* 1999;11(9):1451–1462.

813. Yasukawa M, et al. Down-regulation of CXCR4 by human herpesvirus 6 (HHV-6) and HHV-7. *J Immunol* 1999; 162(9):5417–5422.

814. Deng X, et al. A synthetic peptide derived from human immunodeficiency virus type 1 gp120 downregulates the expression and function of chemokine receptors CCR5 and CXCR4 in monocytes by activating the 7-transmembrane G-protein-coupled receptor FPRL1/LXA4R. *Blood* 1999; 94(4):1165–1173.

815. Shirazi Y, Pitha PM. Interferon downregulates CXCR4 (fusin) gene expression in peripheral blood mononuclear cells. *J Hum Virol* 1998;1(2):69–76.

816. Galli G, et al. Enhanced HIV expression during Th2-oriented responses explained by the opposite regulatory effect of IL-4 and IFN-gamma of fusin/CXCR4. *Eur J Immunol* 1998;28(10):3280–3290.

817. Amara A, et al. HIV coreceptor downregulation as antiviral principle: SDF-1 alpha-dependent internalization of the chemokine receptor CXCR4 contributes to inhibition of HIV replication. *J Exp Med* 1997;186(1):139–146.

818. Peled A, et al. Dependence of human stem cell engraftment and repopulation of NOD/SCID mice on CXCR4. *Science* 1999;283(5403):845–848.

819. Zou YR, et al. Function of the chemokine receptor CXCR4 in haematopoiesis and in cerebellar development [see comments]. *Nature* 1998;393(6685):595–599.

820. Eitner F, et al. Chemokine receptor (CXCR4) mRNA-expressing leukocytes are increased in human renal allograft rejection. *Transplantation* 1998;66(11):1551–1557.

821. Sehgal A, et al. CXCR-4, a chemokine receptor, is overexpressed in and required for proliferation of glioblastoma tumor cells. *J Surg Oncol* 1998;69(2):99–104.

822. Cohen OJ, et al. CXCR4 and CCR5 genetic polymorphisms in long-term nonprogressive human immunodeficiency virus infection: lack of association with mutations other than CCR5-Delta32. *J Virol* 1998;72(7):6215–6217.

823. Wilkie TM, et al. Identification, chromosomal location, and genome organization of mammalian G-protein-coupled receptors. *Genomics* 1993;18(2):175–184.

824. Kouba M, et al. Cloning of a novel putative G-protein-coupled receptor (NLR) which is expressed in neuronal and lymphatic tissue. *FEBS Lett* 1993;321(2–3):173–178.

825. Forster R, et al. Selective expression of the murine homologue of the G-protein-coupled receptor BLR1 in B cell differentiation, B cell neoplasia and defined areas of the cerebellum. *Cell Mol Biol (Noisy-le-grand)* 1994;40(3):381–387.

826. Kaiser E, et al. The G protein-coupled receptor BLR1 is involved in murine B cell differentiation and is also expressed in neuronal tissues. *Eur J Immunol* 1993;23(10):2532–2539.

827. Emrich T, Forster R, Lipp M. Topological characterization of the lymphoid-specific seven transmembrane receptor BLR1 by epitope-tagging and high level expression. *Biochem Biophys Res Commun* 1993;197(1):214–220.

828. Wolf I, et al. Downstream activation of a TATA-less promoter by Oct-2, Bob1, and NF-kappaB directs expression of the homing receptor BLR1 to mature B cells. *J Biol Chem* 1998;273(44):28831–28836.

829. Forster R, et al. A putative chemokine receptor, BLR1, directs B cell migration to defined lymphoid organs and specific anatomic compartments of the spleen. *Cell* 1996;87(6):1037–1047.

830. Cao J, et al. Characterization of colorectal-cancer-related cDNA clones obtained by subtractive hybridization screening. *J Cancer Res Clin Oncol* 1997;123(8):447–451.

831. Forster R, et al. Abnormal expression of the B-cell homing chemokine receptor BLR1 during the progression of acquired immunodeficiency syndrome. *Blood* 1997;90(2):520–525.

832. Barella L, et al. Sequence variation of a novel heptahelical leucocyte receptor through alternative transcript formation. *Biochem J* 1995;309(Pt 3):773–779.

833. Muller S, et al. Cloning of ATAC, an activation-induced, chemokine-related molecule exclusively expressed in CD8+ T lymphocytes. *Eur J Immunol* 1995;25(6):1744–1748.

834. Yoshida T, et al. Molecular cloning of a novel C or gamma type chemokine, SCM-1. *FEBS Lett* 1995;360(2):155–159.

835. Yoshida T, et al. Structure and expression of two highly related genes encoding SCM-1/human lymphotactin. *FEBS Lett* 1996;395(1):82–88.

836. Hautamaa D, et al. Murine lymphotactin: gene structure, post-translational modification and inhibition of expression by CD28 costimulation. *Cytokine* 1997;9(6):375–382.

837. Dorner B, et al. Purification, structural analysis, and function of natural ATAC, a cytokine secreted by CD8(+) T cells. *J Biol Chem* 1997;272(13):8817–8823.

838. Kelner GS, et al. Lymphotactin: a cytokine that represents a new class of chemokine. *Science* 1994;266(5189):1395–1399.

839. Boismenu R, et al. Chemokine expression by intraepithelial gamma delta T cells. Implications for the recruitment of inflammatory cells to damaged epithelia. *J Immunol* 1996;157(3):985–992.

840. Hennemann B, et al. Expression of SCM-1 alpha/lymphotactin and SCM-1 beta in natural killer cells is upregulated by IL-2 and IL-12. *DNA Cell Biol* 1999;18(7):565–571.

841. Rumsaeng V, et al. Lymphotactin gene expression in mast cells following Fc(epsilon) receptor I aggregation: modulation by TGF-beta, IL-4, dexamethasone, and cyclosporin A. *J Immunol* 1997;158(3):1353–1360.

842. Giancarlo B, et al. Migratory response of human natural killer cells to lymphotactin. *Eur J Immunol* 1996;26(12):3238–3241.

843. Hedrick JA, et al. Lymphotactin is produced by NK cells and attracts both NK cells and T cells *in vivo*. *J Immunol* 1997;158(4):1533–1540.

844. Greco G, Mackewicz C, Levy JA. Sensitivity of human immunodeficiency virus infection to various alpha, beta and gamma chemokines. *J Gen Virol* 1999;80(Pt 9):2369–2373.

845. Kennedy J, et al. Molecular cloning and functional characterization of human lymphotactin. *J Immunol* 1995;155(1):203–209.

846. Dilloo D, et al. Combined chemokine and cytokine gene transfer enhances antitumor immunity. *Nat Med* 1996;2(10):1090–1095.

847. Lillard JW Jr, et al. Lymphotactin acts as an innate mucosal adjuvant. *J Immunol* 1999;162(4):1959–1965.

848. Natori Y, Ou ZL, and Yamamoto-Shuda Y. Expression of lymphotactin mRNA in experimental crescentic glomerulo-nephritis. *Clin Exp Immunol* 1998;113(2):265–268.

849. Wang JD, et al. Lymphotactin: a key regulator of lymphocyte trafficking during acute graft rejection. *Immunology* 1998;95(1):56–61.

850. Heiber M, et al. Isolation of three novel human genes encoding G protein-coupled receptors. *DNA Cell Biol* 1995;14(1):25–35.

851. Yoshida T, et al. Molecular cloning of mXCR1, the murine SCM-1/lymphotactin receptor. *FEBS Lett* 1999;458(1):37–40.

852. Yoshida T, et al. Identification of single C motif-1/lymphotactin receptor XCR1. *J Biol Chem* 1998;273(26):16551–16554.

853. Nishiyori A, et al. Localization of fractalkine and CX3CR1 mRNAs in rat brain: does fractalkine play a role in signaling from neuron to microglia? *FEBS Lett* 1998;429(2):167–172.

854. Harrison JK, et al. Role for neuronally derived fractalkine in mediating interactions between neurons and CX3CR1-expressing microglia. *Proc Natl Acad Sci U S A* 1998;95(18):10896–10901.

855. Mizoue LS, et al. Solution structure and dynamics of the CX3C chemokine domain of fractalkine and its interaction with an N-terminal fragment of CX3CR1. *Biochemistry* 1999;38(5):1402–1414.

856. Fong AM, et al. Ultrastructure and function of the fractalkine mucin domain in CX(3)C chemokine domain presentation. *J Biol Chem* 2000;275(6):3781–3786.

857. Rossi DL, et al. Cloning and characterization of a new type of mouse chemokine. *Genomics* 1998;47(2):163–170.

858. Kanazawa N, et al. Fractalkine and macrophage-derived chemokine: T cell-attracting chemokines expressed in T cell area dendritic cells. *Eur J Immunol* 1999;29(6):1925–1932.

859. Papadopoulos EJ, et al. Fractalkine, a CX3C chemokine, is expressed by dendritic cells and is up-regulated upon dendritic cell maturation. *Eur J Immunol* 1999;29(8):2551–2559.

860. Foussat A, et al. Fractalkine receptor expression by T lymphocyte subpopulations and *in vivo* production of fractalkine in human. *Eur J Immunol* 2000;30(1):87–97.

861. Bazan JF, et al. A new class of membrane-bound chemokine with a CX3C motif. *Nature* 1997;385(6617):640–644.

862. Schwaeble WJ, et al. Neuronal expression of fractalkine in the presence and absence of inflammation. *FEBS Lett* 1998;439(3):203–207.

863. Maciejewski-Lenoir D, et al. Characterization of fractalkine in rat brain cells: migratory and activation signals for CX3CR-1-expressing microglia. *J Immunol* 1999;163(3):1628–1635.

864. Fong AM, et al. Fractalkine and CX3CR1 mediate a novel mechanism of leukocyte capture, firm adhesion, and activation under physiologic flow. *J Exp Med* 1998;188(8):1413–1419.

865. Haskell CA, Cleary MD, Charo IF. Molecular uncoupling of fractalkine-mediated cell adhesion and signal transduc-

tion. Rapid flow arrest of CX3CR1-expressing cells is independent of G-protein activation. *J Biol Chem* 1999; 274(15):10053–10058.

866. Feng L, et al. Prevention of crescentic glomerulonephritis by immunoneutralization of the fractalkine receptor CX3CR1 rapid communication. *Kidney Int* 1999;56(2):612–620.

867. Tong N, et al. Neuronal fractalkine expression in HIV-1 encephalitis: roles for macrophage recruitment and neuroprotection in the central nervous system. *J Immunol* 2000;164(3):1333–1339.

868. Nomiyama H, et al. Human chemokines fractalkine (SCYD1), MDC (SCYA22) and TARC (SCYA17) are clustered on chromosome 16q13. *Cytogenet Cell Genet* 1998; 81(1):10–11.

869. Raport CJ, et al. The orphan G-protein-coupled receptor-encoding gene V28 is closely related to genes for chemokine receptors and is expressed in lymphoid and neural tissues. *Gene* 1995;163(2):295–299.

870. Combadiere C, et al. Gene cloning, RNA distribution, and functional expression of mCX3CR1, a mouse chemotactic receptor for the CX3C chemokine fractalkine. *Biochem Biophys Res Commun* 1998;253(3):728–732.

871. Boddeke EW, et al. Functional expression of the fractalkine (CX3C) receptor and its regulation by lipopolysaccharide in rat microglia. *Eur J Pharmacol* 1999;374(2):309–313.

872. Imai T, et al. Identification and molecular characterization of fractalkine receptor CX3CR1, which mediates both leukocyte migration and adhesion. *Cell* 1997;91(4):521–530.

873. Chen S, et al. *In vivo* inhibition of CC and CX3C chemokine-induced leukocyte infiltration and attenuation of glomerulonephritis in Wistar-Kyoto (WKY) rats by vMIP-II. *J Exp Med* 1998;188(1):193–198.

874. Horuk R, et al. A receptor for the malarial parasite *Plasmodium vivax*: the erythrocyte chemokine receptor. *Science* 1993;261(5125):1182–1184.

875. Luo H, et al. Cloning, characterization, and mapping of a murine promiscuous chemokine receptor gene: homolog of the human Duffy gene [Letter]. *Genome Res* 1997;7(9):932–941.

876. Lomize AL, Pogozheva ID, Mosberg HI. Structural organization of G-protein-coupled receptors. *J Comput Aided Mol Des* 1999;13(4):325–353.

877. Hadley TJ, Peiper SC. From malaria to chemokine receptor: the emerging physiologic role of the Duffy blood group antigen. *Blood* 1997;89(9):3077–3091.

878. Horuk R, et al. The Duffy antigen receptor for chemokines: structural analysis and expression in the brain. *J Leukoc Biol* 1996;59(1):29–38.

879. Peiper SC, et al. The Duffy antigen/receptor for chemokines (DARC) is expressed in endothelial cells of Duffy negative individuals who lack the erythrocyte receptor. *J Exp Med* 1995;181(4):1311–1317.

880. Lu ZH, et al. The promiscuous chemokine binding profile of the Duffy antigen/receptor for chemokines is primarily localized to sequences in the amino-terminal domain. *J Biol Chem* 1995;270(44):26239–26245.

881. Darbonne WC, et al. Red blood cells are a sink for interleukin 8, a leukocyte chemotaxin. *J Clin Invest* 1991;88(4): 1362–1369.

882. Miller LH, et al. Erythrocyte receptors for (*Plasmodium knowlesi*) malaria: Duffy blood group determinants. *Science* 1975;189(4202):561–563.

883. Lachgar A, et al. Binding of HIV-1 to RBCs involves the Duffy antigen receptors for chemokines (DARC). *Biomed Pharmacother* 1998;52(10):436–439.

884. Whitney LW, et al. Analysis of gene expression in multiple sclerosis lesions using cDNA microarrays. *Ann Neurol* 1999;46(3):425–428.

885. Liu XH, et al. Up-regulation of Duffy antigen receptor expression in children with renal disease. *Kidney Int* 1999;55(4):1491–1500.

886. Iwamoto S, et al. Genomic organization of the glycoprotein D gene: Duffy blood group Fya/Fyb alloantigen system is associated with a polymorphism at the 44-amino acid residue. *Blood* 1995;85(3):622–626.

887. Olsson ML, et al. A clinically applicable method for determining the three major alleles at the Duffy (FY) blood group locus using polymerase chain reaction with allele-specific primers. *Transfusion* 1998;38(2):168–173.

888. Tournamille C, et al. Disruption of a GATA motif in the Duffy gene promoter abolishes erythroid gene expression in Duffy-negative individuals. *Nat Genet* 1995;10(2):224–228.

889. Farzan M, et al. Two orphan seven-transmembrane segment receptors which are expressed in CD4-positive cells support simian immunodeficiency virus infection. *J Exp Med* 1997;186(3):405–411.

890. Marchese A, et al. Cloning of human genes encoding novel G protein-coupled receptors. *Genomics* 1994;23(3):609–618.

891. Shimizu N, et al. An orphan G protein-coupled receptor, GPR1, acts as a coreceptor to allow replication of human immunodeficiency virus types 1 and 2 in brain-derived cells. *J Virol* 1999;73(6):5231–5239.

892. Edinger AL, et al. Use of GPR1, GPR15, and STRL33 as coreceptors by diverse human immunodeficiency virus type 1 and simian immunodeficiency virus envelope proteins. *Virology* 1998;249(2):367–378.

893. Brussel A, et al. Sequences and predicted structures of chimpanzee STRL33 (Bonzo) and gpr15 (BOB). *AIDS Res Hum Retroviruses* 1999;15(14):1315–1319.

894. Deng HK, et al. Expression cloning of new receptors used by simian and human immunodeficiency viruses. *Nature* 1997;388(6639):296–300.

895. Shimada T, et al. A novel lipopolysaccharide inducible C-C chemokine receptor related gene in murine macrophages. *FEBS Lett* 1998;425(3):490–494.

896. Sreedharan SP, et al. Cloning and expression of the human vasoactive intestinal peptide receptor. *Proc Natl Acad Sci U S A* 1991;88(11):4986–4990.

897. Sreedharan SP, et al. Cloning and functional expression of a human neuroendocrine vasoactive intestinal peptide receptor. *Biochem Biophys Res Commun* 1993;193(2):546–553.

898. Shimizu N, et al. A putative G protein-coupled receptor, RDC1, is a novel coreceptor for human and simian immunodeficiency viruses. *J Virol* 2000;74(2):619–626.

899. Liao F, et al. STRL33, a novel chemokine receptor-like protein, functions as a fusion cofactor for both macrophage-

tropic and T cell line-tropic HIV-1. *J Exp Med* 1997;185(11):2015–2023.

900. Sabri F, et al. Nonproductive human immunodeficiency virus type 1 infection of human fetal astrocytes: independence from CD4 and major chemokine receptors. *Virology* 1999;264(2):370–384.

901. Loetscher M, et al. TYMSTR, a putative chemokine receptor selectively expressed in activated T cells, exhibits HIV-1 coreceptor function. *Curr Biol* 1997;7(9):652–660.

902. MacDonald MR, Li XY, Virgin HW 4th. Late expression of a beta chemokine homolog by murine cytomegalovirus. *J Virol* 1997;71(2):1671–1678.

903. MacDonald MR, et al. Spliced mRNA encoding the murine cytomegalovirus chemokine homolog predicts a beta chemokine of novel structure. *J Virol* 1999;73(5):3682–3691.

904. Fleming P, et al. The murine cytomegalovirus chemokine homolog, m131/129, is a determinant of viral pathogenicity. *J Virol* 1999;73(8):6800–6809.

905. Luttichau BH, et al. A highly selective CC chemokine receptor (CCR)8 antagonist encoded by the poxvirus molluscum contagiosum. *J Exp Med* 2000;191(1):171–180.

906. Russo JJ, et al. Nucleotide sequence of the Kaposi sarcoma-associated herpesvirus (HHV8). *Proc Natl Acad Sci U S A* 1996;93(25):14862–14867.

907. Shao W, et al. Accessibility of selenomethionine proteins by total chemical synthesis: structural studies of human herpesvirus-8 MIP-II. *FEBS Lett* 1998;441(1):77–82.

908. Boshoff C, et al. Angiogenic and HIV-inhibitory functions of KSHV-encoded chemokines. *Science* 1997;278(5336):290–294.

909. Sturzl M, et al. Expression of the human herpesvirus 8-encoded viral macrophage inflammatory protein-1 gene in Kaposi's sarcoma lesions [Letter]. *AIDS* 1998;12(9):1105–1106.

910. Shan L, et al. Identification of viral macrophage inflammatory protein (vMIP)-II as a ligand for GPR5/XCR1. *Biochem Biophys Res Commun* 2000;268(3):938–941.

911. Sozzani S, et al. The viral chemokine macrophage inflammatory protein-II is a selective Th2 chemoattractant. *Blood* 1998;92(11):4036–4039.

912. Nicholas J, et al. A single 13-kilobase divergent locus in the Kaposi sarcoma-associated herpesvirus (human herpesvirus 8) genome contains nine open reading frames that are homologous to or related to cellular proteins. *J Virol* 1997;71(3):1963–1974.

913. Stine JT, et al. KSHV-encoded CC chemokine vMIP-III is a CCR4 agonist, stimulates angiogenesis, and selectively chemoattracts TH2 cells. *Blood* 2000;95(4):1151–1157.

914. Zou P, et al. Human herpesvirus 6 open reading frame U83 encodes a functional chemokine. *J Virol* 1999;73(7):5926–5933.

915. Bais C, et al. G-protein-coupled receptor of Kaposi's sarcoma-associated herpesvirus is a viral oncogene and angiogenesis activator. *Nature* 1998;391(6662):86–89.

916. Geras-Raaka E, et al. Inhibition of constitutive signaling of Kaposi's sarcoma-associated herpesvirus G protein-coupled receptor by protein kinases in mammalian cells in culture. *J Exp Med* 1998;187(5):801–806.

917. Gershengorn MC, et al. Chemokines activate Kaposi's sarcoma-associated herpesvirus G protein-coupled receptor in mammalian cells in culture [see comments]. *J Clin Invest* 1998;102(8):1469–1472.

918. Yang BT, et al. Transgenic expression of the chemokine receptor encoded by human herpesvirus 8 induces an angioproliferative disease resembling Kaposi's sarcoma. *J Exp Med* 2000;191(3):445–454.

919. Kirshner JR, et al. Expression of the open reading frame 74 (G-protein-coupled receptor) gene of Kaposi's sarcoma (KS)-associated herpesvirus: implications for KS pathogenesis. *J Virol* 1999;73(7):6006–6014.

920. Cobo F, et al. Expression of potentially oncogenic HHV-8 genes in an EBV-negative primary effusion lymphoma occurring in an HIV-seronegative patient. *J Pathol* 1999;189(2):288–293.

921. Kledal TN, Rosenkilde MM, Schwartz TW. Selective recognition of the membrane-bound CX3C chemokine, fractalkine, by the human cytomegalovirus-encoded broad-spectrum receptor US28. *FEBS Lett* 1998;441(2):209–214.

922. Kuhn DE, Beall CJ, Kolattukudy PE. The cytomegalovirus US28 protein binds multiple CC chemokines with high affinity. *Biochem Biophys Res Commun* 1995;211(1):325–330.

923. Pleskoff O, et al. Identification of a chemokine receptor encoded by human cytomegalovirus as a cofactor for HIV-1 entry. *Science* 1997;276(5320):1874–1878.

924. Streblow DN, et al. The human cytomegalovirus chemokine receptor US28 mediates vascular smooth muscle cell migration. *Cell* 1999;99(5):511–520.

925. Bodaghi B, et al. Chemokine sequestration by viral chemoreceptors as a novel viral escape strategy: withdrawal of chemokines from the environment of cytomegalovirus-infected cells. *J Exp Med* 1998;188(5):855–866.

INDEX

Note: Page numbers followed by *f* indicate figures; page numbers followed by *t* indicate tables.

Anthracyclines—*continued*
 dosage and administration of, 514
 drug interactions of, 513–514
 features of, 501t
 leukemogenic potential of, 76
 mechanism of action of, 500–511
 mechanisms of resistance to, 511–513
 pharmacokinetics of, 514–515
 structures of, 501f
 topoisomerase inhibition by, 503–504, 513
 toxicity of, 501t, 515–520
Anthraquinones, 509f, 730
Antiandrogens, 97–99
 bicalutamide, 98
 flutamide, 97–98
 synthetic, 97f
 withdrawal of, 98–99
Antibody-dependent cellular cytotoxicity,
  859–861, 865
Antibody-dependent enzyme-prodrug
  therapy, 866, 867f
Antibody-directed enzyme therapy
  (ADEPT), 169
Antiestrogens, 103–113, 112f. *See also*
  Tamoxifen
 pure, 112–113
Antifolates. *See also* Methotrexate; *specific drugs*
 cellular pharmacology of, 140–154, 142f
  intracellular transformation of, 144–146
  transmembrane transport of, 142–144
 CNS effects of, 165–167
 dosage of, 167
 mechanism of action of, 139
 mechanisms of resistance to, 140–154
  binding to dihydrofolate reductase,
   146–150
 pharmacokinetics of, 156–160
 sites of action of, 140f
 structure of, 139–140, 141f
 toxicity of, 161–165
Antigen-presenting cells therapy, 938–940
Antimicrotubule agents, 329
 dolastatins, 355–356
 estramustine, 356–358
 taxanes, 343–355
 vinca alkaloids, 330–343
Antiprogestins, 115–116, 116f
Antisense oligonucleotides, 897–900
 cellular pharmacology of, 898
 clinical effectiveness of, 900
 clinical pharmacology, 898–899
 mechanism of action of, 897–898, 897t
 metabolism of, 898, 898t
 pharmacokinetics of, 899
 toxicity of, 899–900, 900t
Antitumor activity, initial detection of, 24
Antivascular endothelial growth factor monoclonal antibody, 990. *See also*
   Vascular endothelial growth
   factor (VEGF)
Apoptosis, drug resistance and, 8–9, 9f
Arabinosylcytosine. *See* Ara-C
Ara-C, 265–277
 alternate schedules of administration of, 274
 alternatives to, 278t
 carcinogenicity of, 71
 cellular pharmacology of, 267f, 268–272

clinical pharmacology of, 272
 combination therapy using, 8
  with mitoxantrone, 521
 cytotoxicity of, 271t, 272, 272f
 dosage and administration of, 661, 663
 dose randomization of, 266t
 drug interactions of, 275–277, 276f
 features of, 267t
 interaction with fludarabine, 302
 mechanism of action of, 265–268
 mechanisms of resistance to, 270–272, 270f
 metabolism of, 268–272, 268f
 pharmacokinetics of, 45, 45f, 271f,
   272–274, 273f
 pharmacology of, 268f, 269t
 structure of, 266f
 toxicity of, 274–275
Arachnoiditis, due to treatment with methotrexate, 166
ARCON regimen, 731
Aromatase, 100, 101f, 117
 nonsteroidal inhibitors of, 120–122
 regulation of, 117–118
 steroidal inhibitors of, 118–120
Arzoxifene, 113
L-Asparaginase, 647–653
 allergic reactions to, 650–651
 cellular pharmacology of, 648–649
 chemical modification of, 649
 clinical pharmacology of, 649–653
 combination therapy with methotrexate,
   652t
 dosage and administration of, 649–650,
   650f
 drug interactions of, 652–653
 features of, 648t
 hydrolysis of, 648
 mechanism of action of, 647–648
 mechanism of resistance to, 648–649
 properties of, 647–648
 sources of, 648f
 structure of, 647
 toxicity of, 650–653, 651t, 652t
L-Aspartate analogs, 653t
Autologous bone marrow transplantation. *See*
   Bone marrow transplantation,
   autologous
5-Azacytidine, 278–281, 281f
 assay methods for, 280
 cellular pharmacology of, 280
 clinical pharmacology of, 280–281
 features of, 279t
 mechanism of action of, 279–280
 pharmacokinetics of, 280–281
 structure of, 279, 279f
 toxicity of, 281
5-Azacytosine, structure of, 266f
5-Aza-cytosine arabinoside, structure of, 266f
Azathioprine
 carcinogenicity of, 80
 clinical pharmacology of, 298
 drug interactions of, 299
 features of, 296t
 mechanism of action of, 295, 297f
 structure of, 296f
Azidothymidine (AZT)
 bioavailability of, 37

combination therapy with 5-FU,
   226–227
Aziridines, 375–376, 376f
Azoospermia
 caused by amsacrine, 52
 caused by combination therapy, 53
AZT. *See* Azidothymidine (AZT)

B
Bacillus Calmette-Guérin, 934
 adjuvant activity of, 956
Basic fibroblast growth factor (bFGF), 28
BAY 12-9566, 989
B-cell stimulating factor 2, 833
BCNU, 373
 alkylation by, 378f
 brain tumor therapy with, 657
 decomposition of, 389f
 dosage and administration of, 660, 663
bcr-abl kinase
 features of, 897t
 molecular targeting of, 896–897
Benzotriazine dioxide. *See* Tirapazamine
Bicalutamide, 98
Bifunctional antibodies, 865–866, 866f
Bioavailability, drug administration route
   and, 37
Biologic agents, interactions with chemotherapy of, 13–14
Biotoxin-conjugated antibodies, 867, 868f
1,3-bis-(2-chloroethyl)-L-nitrosourea. *See*
   BCNU
Bischloroethylamines, 373
 structure of, 374f
Bischloroethylnitrosourea. *See* BCNU
Bischloroethylsulfide. *See* Nitrogen mustard
Bisdioxopiperazines, 559–560
Bisphosphonates, 700–704
 for breast cancer, 703–704, 703t
 for hypercalcemia, 701
 mechanism of action of, 700–701
 for multiple myeloma, 702–703, 702t
 pharmacology of, 700
 properties of, 701t
 for prostate cancer, 704
 structure of, 701f
Bispiperazinedione, structure of, 539f
Bleomycin, 466–477
 carcinogenicity of, 71
 cellular pharmacokinetics of, 472–473
 cellular pharmacology of, 470–472
 clinical pharmacokinetics of, 473f
 DNA cleavage by, 468–470, 468f, 469f,
   470f
 dosage and administration of, 476–477
 drug interactions of, 477
 features of, 467t
 interaction with radiotherapy of, 13
 interactions with topisomerase II inhibitors, 560
 mechanism of action of, 466–468, 468f
 radiation and, 477
 resistance to, 472
 structure of, 466–468, 467f
 toxicity of, 473–476
  cutaneous, 476
  pulmonary, 473–476, 475f